	insulin (regular)	isoproterenol	lactated Ringer's	lidocaine	methylprednisolone sodium succinate	mezlocillin	midazolam	morphine sulfate	nafcillin	norepinephrine	normal saline solution	ondansetron	oxacillin	penicillin G potassium	phenylephrine	phenytoin	phytonadione	piperacillin	potassium chloride	procainamide	ranitidine	sodium bicarbonate	ticarcillin	tobramycin	vancomycin	verapamil
acyclovir			4		4		4	4					4	4				4	4		4	4	4	4		
albumin																										
amikacin		24			24	4	24	24	4		8		8		24		4		24	24				24	24	
aminophylline		24	24	?		24		24											4	24						
amiodarone	24	24		24			24	24		24	24					4	24		24	24				4	4	24
ampicillin	2						4		8							3	4	?	?			?				
calcium gluconate		24	24			24					24								4				1		48	
cefazolin	2		24			24		24	4							?					?	24			24	
cefoxitin	24		24			4		24	4								24		24		24					
ceftazidime						4		24	4							?	6									
cimetidine	24	24			24	24			48	4		24		24		24		24				24	24			24
ciprofloxacin		48	24			24									24	24		24		24				24		24
clindamycin		24		24		4		24	4		24		48	24		?	24		48	24				24		24
dexamethasone sodium phosphate						4			4							4	24	4								24
dextrose 5% in water (D5W)		24		24	?	24		24	24		48	6	6	24		24	24	24	48	24	24	24	24	24	24	24
D5W in lactated Ringer's	24		24					24		24	24				24		24									24
D5W in normal saline solution	24		24	?			24		48	?		24		24	24		24		48					24		24
diazepam																			?							24
diphenhydramine					4	¼		4			24					4	1									
dobutamine	24	24	24		4	4		24	24			24				?	24	48								24
dopamine		48	24	18	4	4		48		24						24	48									24
epinephrine		24			4	4		4	24		3		4				24									24
erythromycin lactobionate		18			24	4		22									24	24								24
esmolol		24			24	8	24	24	24			24		24	24		24							24	24	24
gentamicin	2		24		24	1		24	4		1						24									24
heparin sodium	2	24		24	?	24	1			4	4	4	?	4	6	24	4	24	24	6						24
hydrocortisone sodium succinate	4	4	24		?	4		24	4	4		4	24	4		24		24								24
insulin (regular)			24		24	1					2					4		24	3	2	2	2				48
isoproterenol		24						24										24								24
lactated Ringer's		24		24	?	72		24			24		24		24		24	24		24				24	24	24
lidocaine	24		24			4	48				24								24	24	24					48
methylprednisolone sodium succinate		?			24	4			?					24				?		48	2					24
mezlocillin		72						48																		
midazolam	24				24		24		24		24							24	24					24	24	
morphine sulfate	1		4	4	24		4	4	4		4	4	1	4		4		4	4		1	3	4	1	4	24
nafcillin		24	48			4		24			24								24			24				
norepinephrine		24		24		4		24											4		24			24		24
normal saline solution		24		24	?	48		24	48	24		24		24	24	24	48	24	24	24	48	24	24	48	24	24
ondansetron					24	4						48					4	4		4		4	4		4	
oxacillin		24				4		24											4		24					
oxytocin	2					1												4		24						24
penicillin G potassium					24											24			24							24
phenylephrine																			24			24				
phenytoin																						24				48
phytonadione																			4			24				
piperacillin		24				24		24								24			24							24
potassium chloride	4		24	?	24	4	24		24	4		4			24		4	24	4	48	24					24
procainamide			24						24									4							48	
ranitidine	24	24		24	48		1		4	48	4		24	4		24		4	48	24			24	24	24	24
sodium bicarbonate	3		24	2			3	24		24			24			24	24	24	24	24				24	24	24
ticarcillin	2	24					24					24							24							24
tobramycin	2	24			24	1			48										24							24
vancomycin	2	24			24	4			24	4									24							24
verapamil	48	24	24	48	24			24			24		24	24		48		24	24	48			24	24	24	

Kalpana Roy

Springhouse
Nurse's
Drug Guide
2005

SIXTH EDITION

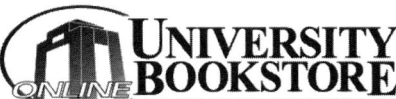

UNIVERSITY BOOKSTORE

ONLINE

340 Carroll Avenue • Dekalb Illinois, 60115-2869

- Office: (815) 753-1081
- Fax: (815) 753-1099
- UPS Orders (800) 999-6488

STORE HOURS:
FALL & SPRING

Monday-Thursday	8:00-6:00
Friday	8:00-4:30
Saturday SUMMER	12:00-4:30
Monday-Friday	8:00-4:30

E-mail: universitybookstore@niu.edu
Web site: www.niubookstore.niu.edu

Springhouse
Nurse's
Drug Guide
2005

SIXTH EDITION

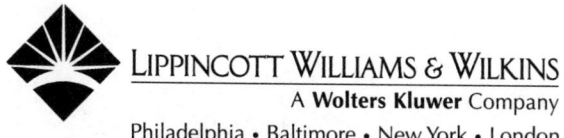

LIPPINCOTT WILLIAMS & WILKINS
A **Wolters Kluwer** Company
Philadelphia • Baltimore • New York • London
Buenos Aires • Hong Kong • Sydney • Tokyo

Staff

Executive Publisher
Judith A. Schilling McCann, RN, MSN

Editorial Director
William J. Kelly

Clinical Director
Joan M. Robinson, RN, MSN

Senior Art Director
Arlene Putterman

Art Director
Elaine Kasmer

Clinical Manager
Eileen Cassin Gallen, RN, BSN

Drug Information Editor
Melissa M. Devlin, PharmD

Editorial Project Manager
Christiane L. Brownell

Clinical Project Manager
Minh N. Luu, RN, BSN, JD

Editor
Lynne Christensen

Clinical Editors
Lisa M. Bonsall, RN, MSN, CRNP;
Christine M. Damico, RN, MSN, CPNP;
Shari A. Regina-Cammon, RN, MSN, CCRN;
Kimberly Zalewski, RN, MSN

Copy Editors
Leslie Dworkin, Tom Groff, Patricia Turkington,
Jenifer F. Walker

Digital Composition Services
Diane Paluba (manager), Joyce Rossi Biletz,
Donald G. Knauss

Manufacturing
Patricia K. Dorshaw (director), Beth Welsh

Editorial Assistants
Carol Caputo, Tara Carter-Bell

Indexer
Deb Tourtlotte

The clinical procedures described and recommended in this publication are based on research and consultation with nursing, medical, pharmaceutical, and legal authorities. To the best of our knowledge, these procedures reflect currently accepted practice; nevertheless, they can't be considered absolute and universal recommendations. For individual application, all recommendations must be considered in light of the patient's clinical condition and, before the administration of new or infrequently used drugs, in light of the latest package-insert information. The authors and publisher disclaim responsibility for adverse effects resulting directly or indirectly from the suggested procedures, from undetected errors, or from the reader's misunderstanding of the text.

©2005 by Lippincott Williams & Wilkins. All rights reserved. This book is protected by copyright. No part of it may be reproduced, stored in a retrieval system, or transmitted, in any form or by any means—electronic, mechanical, photocopy, recording, or otherwise—without prior written permission of the publisher, except for brief quotations embodied in critical articles and reviews and testing and evaluation materials provided by publisher to instructors whose schools have adopted its accompanying textbook. Printed in the United States of America. For information, write Lippincott Williams & Wilkins, 323 Norristown Road, Suite 200, Ambler, PA 19002-2758.

Visit our Web site at eDrugInfo.com

SNDG6–D   N O S A J J
06 05 04 10 9 8 7 6 5 4 3 2 1
ISBN 1-58255-321-1
ISSN 1088-8063

Contents

PharmDisk 6.0   Inside back cover

Drug updates on the Internet   eDrugInfo.com

Contributors and consultants

At the time of publication, the contributors and consultants held the following positions.

Tricia M. Berry, PharmD
Assistant Professor of Pharmacy Practice
St. Louis College of Pharmacy

Jane Bliss-Holtz, DNSc, RC
Nurse Researcher
Ann May Center for Nursing
Jersey Shore Medical Center
Neptune, N.J.

Cheryl Brady, RN, MSN
Adjunct Faculty
Kent State University
East Liverpool, Ohio

Rosanne Burke, RN, MSN, CCRC
Research Coordinator
National Institutes of Health
Bethesda, Md.

Michael J. Burman, RPh
Product Information Specialist III
Wyeth Pharmaceuticals
Collegeville, Pa.

Lawrence P. Carey, PharmD
Assistant Professor, Physician Assistant Studies
Philadelphia University

Susan M. Carver, RN, BSN, DNC
Dermatology Nurse
Minneapolis VA Medical Center

Wendy Tagan Conroy, MSN, APRN, FNP, BC
St. Francis Hospital and Medical Center
Hartford, Conn.

Jason C. Cooper, PharmD
Clinical Pharmacist
St. Francis Hospital
Charleston, S.C.

Michele A. Danish, RPh, PharmD
Pharmacy Clinical Manager
St. Joseph Health Services
N. Providence, R.I.

Linda Dean, MSN, CRNP, ACRN
Director, Clinical Education, HIV/AIDS
Medicine Division
MCP Hahnemann University
Philadelphia

Teresa S. Dunsworth, PharmD, BCPS
Associate Professor of Clinical Pharmacy
West Virginia University
Morgantown

Patricia L. Eells, RN, MS, CPNP
The Children's Hospital
Denver

Jennifer L. Faulkner, PharmD
Clinical Psychiatric Specialist
Central Texas Veteran's Health Care System
Temple

Amy S. Flusche, RPh, BS, PharmD
Assistant Professor
St. Louis College of Pharmacy

S. Kim Genovese, RNC, MSN, MSA, CARN
Associate Professor of Nursing
Purdue University, North Central
Westville, Ind.

Mary Jo Gerlach, RN, MSNEd
Assistant Professor, Adult Nursing (Retired)
Medical College of Georgia
School of Nursing
Athens, Ga.

Jennifer J. Gorrell, PharmD
Clinical Coordinator
Boone Memorial Hospital
Madison, W.Va.

Tanya Gurvich, PharmD
Clinical Pharmacologist
Glendale (Calif.) Adventist FPRP

Connie S. Heflin, RN, MSN
Professor
Paducah (Ky.) Community College

AnhThu Hoang, PharmD
North York, Ontario, Canada

Erin P. Jaynes, RN, MSN
Administrative Nurse Specialist
Medical College of Ohio
Toledo

Julia Kleckner, PharmD
Pharmacy Manager
Option Care
Upper Darby, Pa.

Michelle Kosich, PharmD
Pharmacy Clinical Coordinator
Mercy-Fitzgerald Hospital
Darby, Pa,

Nancy L. Kranzley, RN, MS
Pulmonary Clinical Nurse Specialist
Cincinnati Therapy Centers

Lisa M. Kutney, RPh, PharmD
Freelance Medical Writer
Ivyland, Pa.

Kristi L. Lenz, PharmD
Oncology Clinical Pharmacy Specialist
Medical University of South Carolina
Charleston

Thomas P. Lodise, PharmD
Assistant Professor
Albany (N.Y.) College of Pharmacy

Yun Lu, RPh, PharmD, MS, BCPS,
Clinical Pharmacy Specialist
Hennepin County Medical Center
Minneapolis

Randall A. Lynch, RPh, PharmD
Assistant Director, Pharmacy
Presbyterian Medical Center, University of
    Pennsylvania Health System
Philadelphia

Nicole M. Maisch, PharmD
Assistant Clinical Professor
St. John's University College of Pharmacy and
    Allied Health Professions
Jamaica, N.Y.

Marie Maloney, PharmD
Clinical Pharmacist
University Medical Center
Tucson, Ariz.

Luana Martindale, RN, MSN
Associate Professor
University of Arkansas at Little Rock

George Melko, RPh, PharmD
Manager, Regulatory Affairs
AstraZeneca Pharmaceuticals
Wayne, Pa.

William O'Hara, PharmD
Clinical Team Leader
Thomas Jefferson University Hospital
Philadelphia

Christine K. O'Neil, PharmD, BCPS
Associate Professor
Duquesne University
Pittsburgh

Nicole T. Passerrello, PharmD
Clinical Pharmacy Specialist, Neonatal and
    Pediatrics
Charleston (W. Va.) Area Medical Center,
    Women & Children's Hospital

Christine Price, PharmD
Clinical Coordinator
Department of Pharmaceutical Services,
    Morton Plant Mease Health Care
Dunedin, Fla.

Barbara Reville, MS, CRNP, AOCN, BC
Clinical Instructor
University of Pennsylvania School of Nursing
Philadelphia

Mary Clare A. Schafer, RN, BSN, MS, ONC
Orthopaedic Specialist, Infection Control
    Coordinator, Osteoporosis Program
    Coordinator
Rehabilitation Hospital of South Jersey
Vineland, N.J.

Michele F. Shepherd, PharmD, MS, BCPS,
    FASHP
Clinical Specialist
Abbott Northwestern Hospital
Minneapolis, Minn.

Wendy J. Smith, RN, MSN, ACNP, AOCN
The West Clinic
Memphis, Tenn.

Janis Smith-Love, MSN, ARNP-C, CCRN, CEN
Advanced Registered Nurse Practitioner
Broward General Medical Center
Ft. Lauderdale, Fla.

Joseph F. Steiner, PharmD
Dean & Professor of Pharmacy Practice
College of Pharmacy, Idaho State University
Pocatello, Idaho

Charles S. Sweet, PhD
Adjunct Faculty, Temple University, Nursing
    Department
Gwynedd-Mercy College, Natural Science
    Department
Gwynedd Valley, Pa.

Catherine Ultrino, RN, MS, OCN
Staff Nurse
Kindred Care Hospital
Tampa, Fla.

Connie J. Webb, BS Pharm
Pharmacist
Hospital of the Florida Suncoast
Largo

Barbara S. Wiggins, PharmD
Pharmacy Clinical Specialist
University of Virginia Health System
Charlottesville, Va.

Diana Wong, PharmD
Pharmacy Practice Management Resident
University of California, San Francisco

Foreword

During my thirty years of teaching pharmacology to nursing students, I have had the opportunity to review many drug reference guides for content as well as accuracy. As an educator and a licensed pharmacist, I judge a drug reference not only on its applicability to the student but also to the practicing health professional. I can think of no other nursing drug guide that fulfills these criteria better than *Springhouse Nurse's Drug Guide 2005*. The new 6th edition of this well-received drug guide has all of the unique and popular features of previous editions that have set it apart from other drug guides while adding several new features that only increase its usefulness.

The early chapters are devoted to important aspects of drug usage, such as calculating dosages, administering drugs by different routes, and avoiding medication errors. A section outlining appropriate drug classifications precedes the individual drug monographs and assists the reader in grouping drugs sharing similar actions, an important learning tool especially for the student user.

The drug monographs themselves make up the bulk of the book and contain a wealth of useful, pertinent information. A listing of common American brand names and those available in Canada and Australia follow phonetic pronunciation of the generic drug name. Among the other distinct features of the *Springhouse Nurse's Drug Guide 2005* monographs are the designation of indications as either approved or off-label and the classification of adverse reactions as either common, uncommon, life-threatening, or common and life-threatening. This latter feature is of enormous value in properly responding to an adverse drug reaction depending on its potential for serious harm. Every monograph containing an I.V. drug provides information about properly preparing, administering, monitoring, and storing I.V. drugs. The I.V. compatibility table on the inside front cover complements these I.V. administration sections. A new feature in the Interactions section of each monograph is the highlighting of rapid-onset interactions that must be given immediate attention. The breakdown of drug-herb, drug-food, and drug-lifestyle interactions in addition to drug-drug interactions provides important information for monitoring drug therapy in the outpatient setting, where OTC drug use and patient behavior often can result in problematic interactions. Following the detailed presentation of the pharmacology of each drug, a section devoted to the nursing process provides additional information to help the reader make proper decisions to guarantee safe and effective drug use.

An extensive section on herbal medications provides further data on these widely used products, with additional interactions between herbs and foods prominently noted. Color photographs of commonly used drugs are displayed mid-guide and cross-referenced to the appropriate monograph page, aiding the user in visually identifying many common oral drugs. Users can test their drug knowledge using the enclosed free CD-ROM, which contains a pharmacology review and self-test, a drug-class match game, and a link to eDrugInfo.com, a Web site with drug news and updates.

As in previous editions, the appendices offer a wealth of relevant information for students as well as practitioners, including a critical section on look-alike and sound-alike drug names. Increasingly, these similarities are contributing to serious medication errors, and several manufactures have initiated labeling changes to avoid just such errors. Nurses need to be especially vigilant in this regard, and *Springhouse Nurse's Drug Guide 2005* provides valuable information to help avoid these errors.

Endorsed by the National Student Nurses' Association (NSNA), the *Guide* remains an invaluable addition to the labcoat and library of every nurse, whether prospective or practicing. This nearly 1,500-page guide provides one of the most comprehensive, topical, and accurate drug references currently available. Students will find it to be a useful reference during their academic careers and beyond, while practitioners will appreciate the instant retrieval of essential drug information. The often-overwhelming volume of new drug information has been made exceedingly manageable within the pages of *Springhouse Nurses' Drug Guide 2005.* I will continue to use and recommend the *Guide* enthusiastically.

Roger T. Malseed, PhD
Adjunct Associate Professor
University of Pennsylvania School of Nursing
Philadelphia

How to use *Springhouse Nurse's Drug Guide 2005*

Springhouse Nurse's Drug Guide 2005 is the premier drug reference for all nursing students—beginning to advanced. Tightly organized entries offer consistent, practical drug information for more than 750 common generic drugs, presented in a clear writing style that be ginning students can understand. The book is a must-have for advanced students as well; it includes comprehensive pharmacokinetic and pharmacodynamic information and route-onset-peak-duration tables that give readers a clear understanding of drug actions. Because each entry also follows a nursing process organization, the book even helps students formulate accurate patient care plans. Students of all levels will find that *Springhouse Nurse's Drug Guide 2005* offers a comprehensive, convenient resource for all aspects of drug information.

The book begins with introductory material crucial to safe, accurate drug administration. Chapter 1 discusses drug therapy as it relates to the nursing process. Chapter 2 explains how to calculate dosages and provides examples for each step in the calculations. Chapter 3 discusses how to administer drugs by commonly used routes and includes illustrations to guide students through the steps of each procedure. Chapter 4 focuses on common medication errors and explains how to avoid them.

Drug classifications

Springhouse Nurse's Drug Guide 2005 provides complete overviews of 40 pharmacologic and therapeutic drug classifications, from alkylating drugs to xanthine derivatives. Following the class name is an alphabetical list of examples of drugs in that class; the drug highlighted in color represents the prototype drug for the class. The text then provides class-specific information on indications, actions, adverse reactions, contraindications, and precautions. Look for the special Lifespan logo (⚇) for contraindications and precautions for specific populations including children, pregnant and breast-feeding women, and elderly patients.

Alphabetical listing of drugs

Drug entries in this text appear alphabetically by generic name for quick reference. The generic name is followed by a pronunciation guide and an alphabetical list of brand (trade) names. Brands that don't need a prescription are designated with a dagger (†); those available only in Canada with a closed diamond (♦); those available only in Australia with an open diamond (◇); and those that contain alcohol with a single asterisk (*). The mention of a brand name in no way implies endorsement of that product or guarantees its legality.

Each entry then identifies the drug's pharmacologic and therapeutic classifications; that is, its chemical category and its major clinical use. Listing both classifications helps you grasp the multiple, varying, and sometimes overlapping uses of drugs within a single pharmacologic class and among different classes. Each entry then lists the drug's pregnancy risk category and, if appropriate, its controlled substance schedule.

Indications and dosages

The next section lists the drug's indications and provides dosage information for adults, children, and elderly patients, as applicable. Off-label indications (uses that are clinically accepted but not approved by the FDA) are designated with a double dagger (‡). Dosage instructions reflect current clinical trends in therapeutics and can't be considered as absolute or universal recommendations. For individual application, dosage instructions must be considered in light of the patient's clinical condition.

When giving a drug to an impaired patient or another patient who requires an adjusted dose, look for the Adjust-a-Dose label and logo (◨) at the end of the indication.

I.V. administration

This new section, only found in monographs for drugs that can be given I.V., addresses preparation, administration, and storage information, as well as cautions and other information about the safe use of I.V. drugs.

Contraindications and precautions

This section specifies conditions in which the drug should not be used and details recommendations for cautious use. The Lifespan logo (⚖) draws your attention to contraindications and precautions for special populations, such as children, pregnant and breast-feeding women, and elderly patients.

Adverse reactions

This section lists adverse reactions to each drug by body system. The most common adverse reactions (those experienced by at least 10% of people taking the drug in clinical trials) are in *italic* type; less common reactions are in roman type; life-threatening reactions are in ***bold italic*** type; and reactions that are common *and* life-threatening are in **BOLD CAPITAL** letters.

Interactions

This section lists each drug's confirmed, clinically significant interactions with other drugs (additive effects, potentiated effects, and antagonistic effects), herbs, foods, and lifestyle (such as alcohol use or smoking).

Drug interactions are listed under the drug that is adversely affected. For example, antacids that contain magnesium may decrease absorption of tetracycline. Therefore, this interaction is listed under tetracycline. To determine the possible effects of using two or more drugs simultaneously, check the interactions section for each of the drugs in question.

A new feature to this edition shows in color the drugs that cause interactions that arise quickly and require immediate attention, called rapid-onset interactions.

Effects on lab test results

This section lists increased and decreased levels, counts, and other laboratory test results that may be caused by the drug.

Pharmacokinetics

This section describes absorption, distribution, metabolism, and excretion, along with the drug's half-life. It also provides a quick reference table highlighting onset, peak, and duration for each route of administration. Values for half-life, onset, peak, and duration are for patients with normal renal function, unless specified otherwise.

Action

This section explains the drug's chemical and therapeutic actions. For example, although all antihypertensives lower blood pressure, they don't all do so by the same pharmacologic process.

Available forms

This section lists all available preparations for each drug (for example, tablets, capsules, solutions for injection) and all available dosage forms and strengths. As with the brand names discussed above, over-the-counter dosage forms and strengths are marked with a dagger (†); those available only in Canada with a closed diamond (♦); those available only in Australia with an open diamond (◇); and those that contain alcohol with an asterisk (*).

Nursing Process

This section uses the nursing process as its organizational framework. It also contains an Alert logo (⚡) to call your attention to vital, need-to-know information or serve as a warning about a common drug error.

• Assessment focuses on observation and monitoring of key patient data, such as vital signs, weight, intake and output, and laboratory values.

• Nursing diagnoses represent those most commonly applied to drug therapy. In actual use, nursing diagnoses must be relevant to an individual patient; therefore, they may not include the listed examples and may include others not listed.

• Planning and implementation offers detailed recommendations for drug administration, including full coverage of P.O., I.M., S.C., and other routes.

• Patient teaching focuses on explaining the drug's purpose, promoting compliance, and ensuring proper use and storage of the drug. It also includes instructions for preventing or minimizing adverse reactions.

• Evaluation identifies the expected patient outcomes for the listed nursing diagnoses.

Because nursing considerations in this text emphasize drug-specific recommendations, they don't include standard recommendations that apply to all drugs, such as "assess the six rights of drug therapy before administration" or "teach the patient the name, dose, frequency, route, and strength of the prescribed drug."

Photoguide to tablets and capsules

To make drug identification easier and to enhance patient safety, *Springhouse Nurse's Drug Guide 2005* offers a full-color photoguide to the most commonly prescribed tablets and capsules. Shown in their actual sizes, the drugs are arranged alphabetically by generic names. Trade names and most common dosage strengths are included. Page references appear under each drug name so you can turn quickly to information about the drug.

Herbal medicines

Herbal medicine entries appear alphabetically by name, followed by a phonetic spelling.

Reported uses

This section lists reported uses of herbal medicines. Some of these uses are based on anecdotal claims; other uses have been studied. However, a listing in this section should not be considered a recommendation; herbal medicines aren't regulated by the FDA.

Dosages

This section lists the routes and general dosage information for each form of the herb and, where available, in accordance with its reported use. This information has been gathered from the herbal literature, anecdotal reports, and available clinical data. However, not all uses have specific dosage information; often, no consensus exists. Dosage notations reflect current clinical trends and should not be considered as recommendations by the publisher.

Cautions

This section lists any condition, especially a disease, in which use of the herbal remedy is undesirable. It also provides recommendations for cautious use, as appropriate.

Adverse reactions

This section lists undesirable effects that may follow use of an herbal supplement. Some of these effects have not been reported but are theoretically possible, given the chemical composition or action of the herb.

Interactions

This section lists each herb's clinically significant interactions, actual or potential, with other herbs, drugs, foods, or lifestyle choices. Each statement describes the effect of the interaction and then offers a specific suggestion for avoiding the interaction. As with adverse reactions, some interactions have not been proven but are theoretically possible.

Action

This section describes the herb's chemical and therapeutic actions.

Common forms

This section lists the available preparations for each herbal medicine as well as dosage forms and strengths.

Nursing considerations

This section offers helpful information, such as monitoring techniques and methods for the prevention and treatment of adverse reactions. Patient teaching tips that focus on educating the patient about the herb's purpose, preparation, administration, and storage are also included, as are suggestions for promoting patient compliance with the therapeutic regimen and steps the patient can take to prevent or minimize the risk or severity of adverse reactions.

Appendices and index

The appendices include a list of look-alike and sound-alike drug names for use in preventing drug errors, a listing of opioid analgesic combination products detailing the components of each product, a list of dialyzable drugs, a glossary explaining unfamiliar medical words and phrases, a list of drugs that shouldn't be crushed, a table of equivalents, a new English-to-Spanish translator of common drug-related phrases, and a list of normal laboratory test values.

The comprehensive index lists drug classifications, generic drugs, brand names, indications, and herbal medicines included in this book.

PharmDisk 6.0

The CD-ROM included with this book (inside the back cover) offers two exciting Windows-based software programs. "Pharmacology Self-test" tests your knowledge with 300 multiple-choice questions. And a challenging interactive game helps you learn drug classifications. *PharmDisk 6.0* also provides a link to eDrugInfo.com.

eDrugInfo.com

This Web site keeps *Springhouse Nurse's Drug Guide 2005* current by providing the following features:
• updates on new drugs, new indications, and new warnings
• patient teaching aids on new drugs
• news summaries of pertinent drug information.

The Web site also gives you:
• information on herbs
• links to pharmaceutical companies, government agencies, and other drug information sites
• a bookstore full of nursing books, software, and more.

Plus, registering with eDrugInfo.com entitles you to e-mail notifications when new drug updates are posted.

Guide to abbreviations

ACE	angiotensin-converting enzyme	EEG	electroencephalogram
ACT	activated clotting time	EENT	eyes, ears, nose, throat
ADH	antidiuretic hormone	FDA	Food and Drug Administration
AIDS	acquired immunodeficiency syndrome	g	gram
		G	gauge
ALT	alanine transaminase	GABA	gamma-aminobutyric acid
APTT	activated partial thromboplastin time	GFR	glomerular filtration rate
		GGT	gamma-glutamyltransferase
AST	aspartate transaminase	GI	gastrointestinal
AV	atrioventricular	gtt	drops
b.i.d.	twice daily	GU	genitourinary
BPH	benign prostatic hyperplasia	G6PD	glucose-6-phosphate dehydrogenase
BUN	blood urea nitrogen		
cAMP	cyclic adenosine monophosphate	H	histamine
		HDL	high-density lipoprotein
CBC	complete blood count	HIV	human immunodeficiency virus
CK	creatine kinase	HMG-CoA	beta-hydroxy-beta-methylglutaryl coenzyme A
CMV	cytomegalovirus		
CNS	central nervous system	hr	hour
COMT	catechol-O-methyltransferase	h.s.	at bedtime
COPD	chronic obstructive pulmonary disease	ICU	intensive care unit
		I.D.	intradermal
CPK	creatine phosphokinase	I.M.	intramuscular
CSF	cerebrospinal fluid	INR	international normalized ratio
CV	cardiovascular	IPPB	intermittent positive-pressure breathing
CVA	cerebrovascular accident		
CYP	cytochrome P450	IU	international unit
DIC	disseminated intravascular coagulation	I.V.	intravenous
		kg	kilogram
D_5W	dextrose 5% in water	L	liter
dl	deciliter	lb	pound
DNA	deoxyribonucleic acid	LDH	lactate dehydrogenase
ECG	electrocardiogram		

LDL	low-density lipoprotein		S.C.	subcutaneous
M	molar		SIADH	syndrome of inappropriate antidiuretic hormone
m^2	square meter			
MAO	monoamine oxidase		S.L.	sublingual
mcg	microgram		SSRI	selective serotonin reuptake inhibitor
mEq	milliequivalent			
mg	milligram		T_3	triiodothyronine
MI	myocardial infarction		T_4	thyroxine
min	minute		tbs	tablespoon
ml	milliliter		t.i.d.	three times daily
mm^3	cubic millimeter		tsp	teaspoon
Na	sodium		USP	United States Pharmacopeia
NG	nasogastric		UTI	urinary tract infection
NSAID	nonsteroidal anti-inflammatory drug		WBC	white blood cell
OTC	over-the-counter			
oz	ounce			
PABA	para-aminobenzoic acid			
$Paco_2$	carbon dioxide partial pressure			
Pao_2	oxygen partial pressure			
PCA	patient-controlled analgesia			
P.O.	by mouth			
P.R.	by rectum			
p.r.n.	as needed			
PT	prothrombin time			
PTT	partial thromboplastin time			
PVC	premature ventricular contraction			
q	every			
q.i.d.	four times daily			
RBC	red blood cell			
RDA	recommended daily allowance			
REM	rapid eye movement			
RNA	ribonucleic acid			
RSV	respiratory syncytial virus			
SA	sinoatrial			

1

Drug therapy and the nursing process

Springhouse Nurse's Drug Guide uses the nursing process in its organizational outline for good reason. The nursing process guides nursing decisions about the proper way to give drugs to ensure the patient's safety and to meet medical and legal standards. This process provides thorough assessment, appropriate nursing diagnoses, effective planning and implementation, and consistent evaluation.

Assessment

Data collection begins with the patient history. After taking the patient's history, perform a thorough physical examination. Also, evaluate the patient's knowledge and understanding of the drug therapy he's about to receive.

History

When taking a history, investigate the patient's allergies, use of drugs and herbs, medical history, lifestyle and beliefs, and socioeconomic status.

Allergies

Specify the drug or food to which the patient is allergic. Describe the reaction he has; its situation, time, and setting; and any contributing factors, such as a significant change in eating habits or the simultaneous use of stimulants, tobacco, alcohol, or illegal drugs. Don't forget to place an allergy label conspicuously on the front of the patient's chart and place an allergy band on the patient.

Drugs and herbs

Take a complete drug history that includes both prescription and over-the-counter drugs. Also, find out which herbs, if any, the patient takes. Investigate the patient's reasons for using a drug or herb and his knowledge of its use. Explore the patient's thoughts and attitudes about drug use to find out if he may encounter problems with drug therapy. Note any special

procedures he'll need to perform, such as monitoring his glucose level or checking his heart rate, and make sure he can perform them correctly.

After the patient starts taking the drug, discuss the effects of therapy to determine whether new symptoms or adverse drug reactions have developed. Also, talk about measures the patient has taken to recognize, minimize, or avoid adverse drug reactions or accidental overdose. Ask the patient where he stores his medication and what system he uses to help himself remember to take it as prescribed.

Medical history

Note any chronic disorders the patient has, and record the date of diagnosis, the prescribed treatment, and the name of the prescriber. Careful attention during this part of the history can uncover one of the most important problems with drug therapy: incompatible drug regimens.

Lifestyle and beliefs

Ask about the patient's support systems, marital status, childbearing status, attitudes toward health and health care, and daily patterns of activity. These elements all affect patient compliance and, therefore, the patient's care plan.

Also, ask about the patient's diet. Certain foods can influence the effectiveness of many drugs. Don't forget to inquire about the patient's use of alcohol, tobacco, caffeine, and illegal drugs, such as marijuana, cocaine, and heroin. Note the substance used and the amount and frequency of use.

Socioeconomic status

Note the patient's age, educational level, occupation, and insurance coverage. These characteristics help determine the plan of care, the likelihood of compliance, and the possible need for financial assistance, counseling, or other social services.

Physical examination

Examine the patient closely for expected drug effects and for adverse reactions. Every drug has a desired effect on one body system, but it also may have one or more undesired effects on that or another body system. For example, chemotherapeutic drugs destroy cancer cells, but they also affect normal cells and typically cause hair loss, diarrhea, and nausea. Besides looking for adverse drug effects, investigate whether the patient has any sensory impairments or changes in mental state.

Sensory impairment

Assess the patient for sensory impairments that could influence his care plan. For example, impaired vision or paralysis can hinder the patient's ability to give himself a subcutaneous injection, break a scored tablet, or open a drug vial. Hearing impairment can prevent a patient from finding out from you all that he needs to know about the drug he's taking.

Mental state

Note whether the patient is alert, oriented, and able to interact appropriately. Assess whether he can think clearly and converse properly. Check his short-term and long-term memory; he needs both to follow the prescribed regimen correctly. Also, determine whether the patient can read and at what level.

Understanding drug therapy

A patient is more likely to comply if he understands the reason for drug therapy. During your assessment, evaluate your patient's understanding of his therapy and the reason for it. Pay particular attention to his emotional acceptance of the need for drug therapy. For instance, a young patient being prescribed an antihypertensive may need more education than an older patient to ensure compliance.

Nursing diagnosis

Using the information you gathered during assessment, define drug-related problems by formulating each problem into a relevant nursing diagnosis. The most common problem statements related to drug therapy are "Deficient knowledge," "Ineffective health maintenance," and "Noncompliance." Nursing diagnoses provide the framework for planning interventions and outcome criteria, also known as patient goals.

Planning and implementation

Make sure that your outcome criteria state the desired patient behaviors or responses that should result from nursing care. Such criteria should be:
- measurable
- objective
- concise
- realistic for the patient
- attainable by nursing management.

Express patient behavior in terms of expectations, and specify a time frame. An example of a good outcome statement is "Before discharge, the patient verbalizes major adverse effects related to his chemotherapy."

After developing outcome criteria, determine the interventions needed to help the patient reach the desired goals. Appropriate interventions may include administration procedures and techniques, legal and ethical concerns, patient teaching, and special actions for pregnant, breast-feeding, pediatric, and geriatric patients. Interventions also may be independent nursing actions, such as turning a bedridden patient every 2 hours.

Evaluation

The final piece of the nursing process is a formal and systematic process for determining the effectiveness of nursing care. This evaluation process lets you determine whether outcome criteria were met, so you can make informed decisions about subsequent interventions. If you stated the outcome criteria in measurable terms, then you can evaluate easily whether the criteria were met.

For example, if a patient experiences relief from headache pain within 1 hour after receiving an analgesic, the outcome criterion was met. If the headache was the same or worse, the outcome criterion wasn't met. In that case, you'll need to reassess the patient, which may produce a new plan, new data that might invalidate the original nursing diagnosis, or new nursing interventions that are more specific or more appropriate for the patient. For instance, this reassessment could lead to a higher dosage, a different analgesic, or the discovery of the underlying cause of the headache pain.

Evaluation enables you to design and implement a revised plan of care, to continuously reevaluate the effectiveness of your interventions for each outcome, and to provide the highest quality of care to your patient.

2

Essentials of dosage calculations

Because nurses frequently perform drug and intravenous (I.V.) fluid calculations, it's important to understand how drugs are weighed and measured, how to convert between systems and measures, how to compute drug dosages, and how to make adjustments for children.

Systems of drug weights and measures

Prescribers use several systems of measurement when ordering drugs, including the metric, household, and apothecaries' systems. The metric and household systems are so widely used that most brands of medication cups for liquid measurements are standardized in both systems. The apothecaries' system isn't widely used but may still be encountered in practice. A fourth system, the avoirdupois system, is rarely used. This system uses solid units of measure, such as the ounce and the pound. Additionally, some special systems of measurement—such as units, international units, and milliequivalents—have been developed by drug manufacturers and only pertain to particular drugs or biological agents.

Metric system

The metric system is the international system of measurement, the most widely used system, and the system used by the U.S. Pharmacopoeia. It has units for both liquid and solid measures. Among its many advantages, the metric system enables accuracy in calculating small drug dosages. It uses Arabic numerals, which are commonly used by health care professionals worldwide. And most manufacturers standardize newly developed drugs in the metric system.

Liquid measures

In the metric system, one liter (L) is equal to about 1 quart in the apothecaries' system. Liters are often used when ordering and administering I.V. solutions. Milliliters are frequently used to give parenteral and some oral drugs. One milliliter (ml) equals $\frac{1}{1,000}$ of a liter.

Solid measures

The gram (g) is the basis for solid measures or units of weight in the metric system. One milligram (mg) equals $\frac{1}{1,000}$ of a gram. Drugs are frequently ordered in grams, milligrams, or an even smaller unit, the microgram (mcg), depending on the drug. One microgram equals $\frac{1}{1,000}$ of a milligram. Body weight is usually recorded in kilograms (kg). One kilogram equals 1,000 g.

The following are examples of drug orders using the metric system:
• 30 ml milk of magnesia P.O. at bedtime
• Ancef 1 g I.V. q 6 hours
• Lanoxin 0.125 mg P.O. daily.

Household system

Most foods, recipes, over-the-counter drugs, and home remedies use the household system. Health care professionals seldom use this system for drug administration; however, knowledge of household measures may be useful in some clinical situations.

Liquid measures

Liquid measurements in the household system include teaspoons (tsp) and tablespoons (tbs). For medical purposes, these measurements have been standardized to 5 milliliters and 15 milliliters, respectively. Using these standardized amounts, 3 teaspoons equal 1 tablespoon, 6 teaspoons equal 1 ounce, and so forth. Patients who need to measure doses by teaspoon or tablespoon should do so using standardized medical devices to make sure they receive exactly the prescribed amount. Advise patients not to use an ordinary spoon to measure a teaspoonful of a drug because the amount will most likely be inaccurate. Teaspoon sizes vary from 4 to 6 milliliters or more.

The following are examples of drug orders using the household system:
• 2 tsp Bactrim P.O. twice daily

• Riopan 2 tbs P.O. 1 hour before meals and at bedtime.

Apothecaries' system

Two unique features distinguish the apothecaries' system from other systems: the use of Roman numerals and the placement of the unit of measurement before the Roman numeral. For example, a measurement of 5 grains would be written as *grains V*.

In the apothecaries' system, equivalents among the various units of measure are close approximations of one another. By contrast, equivalents in the metric system are exact. When using apothecaries' equivalents for calculations and conversions, the calculations, although not precise, must fall within acceptable standards.

The apothecaries' system is the only system of measurement that uses both symbols and abbreviations to represent units of measure. Although the use of the apothecaries' system is becoming less common in healthcare, you must still be able to read dosages that have been written in the apothecaries' system and convert them to the metric system.

Liquid measures

The smallest unit of liquid measurement in the apothecaries' system is the minim (♏), which is about the size of a drop of water. Fifteen to sixteen minims equal about one ml.

Solid measures

The grain (gr) is the smallest solid measure or unit of weight in the apothecaries' system. It equals about 60 milligrams. One dram equals about 60 grains.

The following are examples of drug orders using the apothecaries' system:
• Robitussin f℥ (fluidrams) IV P.O. every 6 hours
• Mylanta f℥ (fluidounce) I P.O. 1 hour after meals
• Tylenol gr X P.O. every 4 hours as needed for headache.

Units, international units, and milliequivalents

For some drugs, you'll need to use a measuring system developed by drug manufacturers. Three of the most common special systems of measurement are units, international units, and milliequivalents.

Units

Insulin is one of several drugs measured in units. Although many types of insulin exist, all are measured in units. The international standard of U-100 insulin means that 1 ml of insulin solution contains 100 units of insulin, regardless of type. Heparin, an anticoagulant, is also measured in units, as are several antibiotics, available in liquid, solid, and powder forms for oral or parenteral use. Each manufacturer of drugs made available in units provides specific information about the measurement of each drug.

The following are examples of drug orders using units:
• Inject 14 units NPH insulin S.C. this a.m.
• Heparin 5,000 units S.C. q 12 hours
• Nystatin 200,000 units P.O. q 12 hours.
The unit is not a standard measure. Thus, different drugs, although each measured in units, may have no relationship to one another in quality or activity.

Units should never be abbreviated as "U" because of the potential for confusing this with a "0."

International units

International units (IU) are used to measure biologicals, such as vitamins, enzymes, and hormones. For instance, the activity of calcitonin, a synthetic hormone used in calcium regulation, is expressed in international units.

The following are examples of drug orders using international units:
• 100 IU calcitonin (salmon) S.C. daily
• 8 IU somatropin S.C. three times a week.

Milliequivalents

Electrolytes may be measured in milliequivalents (mEq). Drug manufacturers provide information about the number of metric units needed to provide a prescribed number of milliequivalents. Potassium chloride (KCl), for example, is usually ordered in milliequivalents.

The following are examples of drug orders using milliequivalents:
• 30 mEq KCl P.O. b.i.d.
• 1 L dextrose 5% in normal saline solution with 40 mEq KCl to be run at 125 ml/hour.

Conversions between measurement systems

Sometimes you may need to convert from one measurement system to another, particularly when a drug is ordered in one system but available only in another system. To perform conversion calculations, you need to know the equivalent measurements for the different systems of measurement. One of the most commonly used methods for converting drug measurements is the fraction method.

Fraction method

The fraction method for converting between measurement systems involves an equation consisting of two fractions. Set up the first fraction by placing the ordered dosage over an unknown number of units of the available dosage.

For example, say a prescriber orders 7.5 ml of acetaminophen elixir to be given by mouth. To find the equivalent in teaspoons, first set up a fraction in which the top of the fraction (numerator) represents the ordered dosage in milliliters and the bottom of the fraction (denominator) represents the unknown (x) number of teaspoons:

$$\frac{7.5 \text{ ml}}{x \text{ tsp}}$$

Then, set up the second fraction, which appears on the right side of the equation. This fraction consists of the standard equivalents between the ordered and the available measures. Because milliliters must be converted to teaspoons, the right side of the equation appears as:

$$\frac{5 \text{ ml}}{1 \text{ tsp}}$$

The same unit of measure should appear in the numerator of both fractions. Likewise, the same unit of measure should appear in both denominators. The entire equation should appear as:

$$\frac{7.5 \text{ ml}}{x \text{ tsp}} = \frac{5 \text{ ml}}{1 \text{ tsp}}$$

To solve for x, cross multiply.

$$x \text{ tsp} \times 5 \text{ ml} = 7.5 \text{ ml} \times 1 \text{ tsp}$$

$$x \text{ tsp} = \frac{7.5 \text{ ml} \times 1 \text{ tsp}}{5 \text{ ml}}$$

$$x \text{ tsp} = \frac{7.5 \times 1 \text{ tsp}}{5}$$

$$x \text{ tsp} = 1.5 \text{ tsp}$$

The patient should receive 1.5 teaspoons of acetaminophen elixir.

Computing drug dosages

Computing a drug dosage is a two-step process that you complete after verifying the drug order. Determine whether the ordered drug is available in units in the same system of measurement. If not, convert the measurement for the ordered drug to the system used for the available drug.

If the ordered units of measurement are available, calculate how much of the available dosage form should be given. For example, if the prescribed dose is 250 mg, determine the quantity of tablets, powder, or liquid that would equal 250 mg. To determine that quantity, use one of the methods described below.

Fraction method

When using the fraction method to compute a drug dosage, write an equation consisting of two fractions. First, set up a fraction showing the number of units to be given over x, which represents the quantity of the dosage form you are trying to find. In this case, the dosage form is tablets (tab).

On the other side of the equation, set up a fraction showing the number of units of the drug in its dosage form over the quantity of dosage forms that supply that number of units. The number of units and the quantity of dosage forms are specific for each drug. In most cases, the stated quantity equals 1. Information provided on the drug label should supply the details needed to form the second fraction.

For example, if the number of units to be administered equals 250 mg, the first fraction in the equation would appear as:

$$\frac{250 \text{ mg}}{x \text{ tab}}$$

The drug label states that each tablet contains 125 mg, so the second fraction would appear as:

$$\frac{125 \text{ mg}}{1 \text{ tab}}$$

Note that the same units of measure appear in the numerators and the same units appear in the denominators. Note also that the units of measure in the denominators differ from the units in the numerators.

The entire equation would appear as:

$$\frac{250 \text{ mg}}{x \text{ tab}} = \frac{125 \text{ mg}}{1 \text{ tab}}$$

Solving for x determines the quantity of the dosage form—2 tablets, in this example.

Ratio method

To use the ratio method, write the amount of the drug to be given and the x quantity of the dosage form as a ratio. Using the example shown above, you'd write:

$$250 \text{ mg} : x \text{ tab}$$

Next, complete the equation by forming a second ratio from the number of units in each tablet (or whatever the drug form is). The manufacturer's label provides this information. Again using the example from above, the entire equation is:

$$250 \text{ mg} : x \text{ tab} :: 125 \text{ mg} : 1 \text{ tab}$$

Solve for x by multiplying the inner portions (means) and outer portions (extremes) of the equation. The patient should receive 2 tablets.

Desired-available method

You can also use the desired-available method, also known as the dose-over-on hand (D/H) method. This method converts ordered units into available units and computes the drug dosage all in one step. The desired-available equation appears as:

$$\frac{x}{\text{quantity}} = \frac{\text{ordered}}{\text{units}} \times \frac{\text{conversion}}{\text{fraction}} \times \frac{\text{quantity of dosage form}}{\text{stated quantity of drug within each dosage form}}$$

For example, say you receive an order for grains (gr) X of a drug. The drug is available only in 300-mg tablets. To determine what number of tablets to give the patient, substitute gr X (the ordered number of units) for the first element of the equation. Then use the conver-

sion fraction as the second portion of the formula. The conversion factor is:

$$\frac{60 \text{ mg}}{\text{gr I}}$$

The measure in the denominator must be the same as the measure in the ordered units. In this case, the order specified gr X. As a result, grains appears in the denominator of the conversion fraction.

The third element of the equation shows the dosage form over the stated drug quantity for that dosage form. Because the drug is available in 300-mg tablets, the fraction appears as:

$$\frac{1 \text{ tab}}{300 \text{ mg}}$$

The dosage form should always appear in the numerator, and the quantity of drug in each dosage form should always appear in the denominator. The completed equation is:

$$x \text{ tab} = \text{gr X} \times \frac{60 \text{ mg}}{\text{gr I}} \times \frac{1 \text{ tab}}{300 \text{ mg}}$$

Solving for x shows that the patient should receive 2 tablets.

The desired-available method has the advantage of using only one equation. However, you need to memorize an equation more elaborate than the one used in the fraction method or the ratio method. Relying on your memorization of a more complicated equation may increase the chance of error.

Dimensional analysis

A variation of the ratio method, dimensional analysis (also known as factor analysis or factor labeling) eliminates the need to memorize formulas and requires only one equation to determine the answer. To compare the two methods at a glance, read the following problem and solutions, then read the paragraphs that follow for a detailed explanation.

Say the prescriber orders 0.25 g of streptomycin sulfate I.M. The vial reads 2 ml = 1 g. How many milliliters should you give?

Dimensional analysis

$$\frac{0.25 \text{ g}}{1} \times \frac{2 \text{ ml}}{1 \text{ g}} = 0.5 \text{ ml}$$

Ratio method

$$1 \text{ g} : 2 \text{ ml} :: 0.25 \text{ g} : x \text{ ml}$$

$$x = 2 \times 0.25$$

$$x = 0.5 \text{ ml}$$

When using dimensional analysis, you arrange a series of ratios, called factors, in a single (although sometimes lengthy) fractional equation. Each factor, written as a fraction, consists of two quantities and their related units of measurement. For instance, if 1,000 ml of a drug should be given over 8 hours, the relationship between the dose and time is expressed by the fraction

$$\frac{1{,}000 \text{ ml}}{8 \text{ hr}}$$

When a problem includes a quantity or a unit of measurement that doesn't have an equivalent in the problem, these numbers appear in the numerator of the fraction, and 1 becomes the denominator. In the problem and solutions above, 0.25 g is such a number.

Some mathematical problems contain all of the information needed to identify the factors, set up the equation, and find the solution. Other problems require the use of a conversion factor. Conversion factors are equivalents (for example, 1 g = 1,000 mg) that you can memorize or get from a conversion chart. Because the two quantities and units of measurement are equivalent, they can serve as the numerator or the denominator; thus, the conversion factor 1 g = 1,000 mg can be written in fraction form as

$$\frac{1{,}000 \text{ mg}}{1 \text{ g}} \text{ or } \frac{1 \text{ g}}{1{,}000 \text{ mg}}$$

The factors given in the problem plus any conversion factors needed to solve the problem are called *knowns*. The quantity of the answer, of course, is the *unknown*. When setting up an equation in dimensional analysis, work backward, beginning with the unit of measurement of the answer. After plotting all the knowns, find the solution by following this sequence:
• Cancel similar quantities and units of measurement.
• Multiply the numerators.
• Multiply the denominators.
• Divide the numerator by the denominator.

Mastering dimensional analysis can take practice, but you may find your efforts well rewarded. To understand more fully how dimensional analysis works, review the following problem and the steps taken to solve it.

A prescriber orders grains X of a drug. The pharmacy supplies the drug in 300-mg tablets (tab). How many tablets should you administer?
• Write down the unit of measurement of the answer, followed by an "equal to" symbol.

$$\text{tab} =$$

• Search the problem for the quantity with the same unit of measurement (if one doesn't exist, use a conversion factor); place this in the numerator and its related quantity and unit of measurement in the denominator.

$$\text{tab} = \frac{1 \text{ tab}}{300 \text{ mg}}$$

• Separate the first factor from the next with a multiplication symbol.

$$\text{tab} = \frac{1 \text{ tab}}{300 \text{ mg}} \times$$

• Place the unit of measurement of the denominator of the first factor in the numerator of the second factor; search the problem for the quantity with the same unit of measurement (if one doesn't exist, as in this example, use a conversion factor); place this in the numerator and its related quantity and unit of measurement in the denominator, and follow with a multiplication symbol. Repeat this step until all known factors are included in the equation.

$$\text{tab} = \frac{1 \text{ tab}}{300 \text{ mg}} \times \frac{60 \text{ mg}}{\text{gr I}} \times \frac{\text{gr X}}{1}$$

• Treat the equation as a large fraction. First, cancel similar units of measurement in the numerator and the denominator. What remains should be what you began with: the unit of measurement of the answer. If not, recheck your equation to find and correct the error. Next, multiply the numerators and then the denominators. Finally, divide the numerator by the denominator.

$$\text{tab} = \frac{1 \text{ tab}}{300 \text{ mg}} \times \frac{60 \text{ mg}}{\text{gr I}} \times \frac{\text{gr X}}{1}$$

$$= \frac{60 \times 10 \text{ tab}}{300}$$

$$= \frac{600 \text{ tab}}{300}$$

$$= 2 \text{ tab}$$

For more practice, study the following examples, which use dimensional analysis to solve various mathematical problems common to dosage calculations and drug administration.

1. A patient weighs 140 lb. What is his weight in kilograms (kg)?

1st factor (conversion factor): $\dfrac{1 \text{ kg}}{2.2 \text{ lb}}$

2nd factor: $\dfrac{140 \text{ lb}}{1}$

$$kg = \frac{1 \text{ kg}}{2.2 \text{ lb}} \times 140 \text{ lb}$$

$$= \frac{140}{2.2}$$

$$= 63.6 \text{ kg}$$

2. A physician prescribes 75 mg of a drug. The pharmacy stocks a multidose vial containing 100 mg/ml. How many milliliters should you give?

1st factor: $\dfrac{1 \text{ ml}}{100 \text{ mg}}$

2nd factor: $\dfrac{75 \text{ mg}}{1}$

$$ml = \frac{1 \text{ ml}}{100 \text{ mg}} \times \frac{75 \text{ mg}}{1}$$

$$= 0.75 \text{ ml}$$

3. A nurse practitioner prescribes 1 tsp of a cough elixir. The pharmacist sends up a bottle whose label reads 1 ml = 50 mg. How many milligrams should you give?

1st factor: $\dfrac{50 \text{ mg}}{1 \text{ ml}}$

2nd factor (conversion factor): $\dfrac{5 \text{ ml}}{1 \text{ tsp}}$

3rd factor: $\dfrac{1 \text{ tsp}}{1}$

$$mg = \frac{50 \text{ mg}}{1 \text{ ml}} \times \frac{5 \text{ ml}}{1 \text{ tsp}} \times \frac{1 \text{ tsp}}{1}$$

$$= 50 \text{ mg} \times 5$$

$$= 250 \text{ mg}$$

4. A physician prescribes 1,000 ml of an I.V. solution to be given over 8 hours. The I.V. tubing delivers 15 gtt/ml/minute. What is the infusion rate in gtt/minute?

1st factor: $\dfrac{15 \text{ gtt}}{1 \text{ ml}}$

2nd factor: $\dfrac{1,000 \text{ ml}}{8 \text{ hr}}$

3rd factor (conversion factor): $\dfrac{1 \text{ hr}}{60 \text{ min}}$

$$gtt/minute = \frac{15 \text{ gtt}}{1 \text{ ml}} \times \frac{1,000 \text{ ml}}{8 \text{ hr}} \times \frac{1 \text{ hr}}{60 \text{ min}}$$

$$= \frac{15 \text{ gtt} \times 1,000 \times 1}{8 \times 60 \text{ min}}$$

$$= \frac{15,000 \text{ gtt}}{480 \text{ min}}$$

$$= 31.3 \text{ or } 31 \text{ gtt/min}$$

5. A physician prescribes 10,000 units of heparin added to 500 ml of 5% dextrose and water at 1,200 units/hour. How many drops per minute should you give if the I.V. tubing delivers 10 gtt/ml?

1st factor: $\dfrac{10 \text{ gtt}}{1 \text{ ml}}$

2nd factor: $\dfrac{500 \text{ ml}}{10,000 \text{ units}}$

3rd factor: $\dfrac{1,200 \text{ units}}{1 \text{ hr}}$

4th factor (conversion factor): $\dfrac{1 \text{ hr}}{60 \text{ min}}$

$$\frac{gtt}{minute} = \frac{10 \text{ gtt}}{1 \text{ ml}} \times \frac{500 \text{ ml}}{10,000 \text{ units}} \times \frac{1,200 \text{ units}}{1 \text{ hr}} \times \frac{1 \text{ hr}}{60 \text{ min}}$$

$$= \frac{10 \times 500 \times 1,200 \text{ gtt}}{10,000 \times 60 \text{ min}}$$

$$= \frac{6,000,000 \text{ gtt}}{600,000 \text{ min}}$$

$$= 10 \text{ gtt/min}$$

Special computations

The fraction, ratio, and desired-available methods and dimensional analysis can be used to compute drug dosages when the ordered drug and the available form of the drug occur in the same units of measure. These methods can also be used when the quantity of a particular dosage form differs from the units in which the dosage form is given.

For example, if a patient is to receive 1,000 mg of a drug available in liquid form and measured in milligrams, with 100 mg contained in 6 ml, how many milliliters should the patient receive? Because the ordered and the available dosages are in milligrams, no initial conversions are needed. The fraction method would be used to determine the number of milliliters the patient should receive, in this case, 60 ml.

Because the drug will be given in ounces (oz), the number of ounces should be determined using a conversion method. For the fraction method of conversion, the equation would appear as:

$$\frac{60 \text{ ml}}{x \text{ oz}} = \frac{30 \text{ ml}}{1 \text{ oz}}$$

Solving for x shows that the patient should receive 2 oz of the drug.

To use the desired-available method, change the order of the elements in the equation to correspond with the situation. The revised equation should appear as:

$$\begin{array}{c} x \\ \text{quantity} \\ \text{to give} \end{array} = \frac{\begin{array}{c} \text{ordered} \\ \text{units} \end{array}}{1} \times \frac{\begin{array}{c} \text{quantity} \\ \text{of dosage} \\ \text{form} \\ \hline \text{stated} \\ \text{quantity of} \\ \text{drug within} \\ \text{each dosage} \\ \text{form} \end{array}}{} \times \begin{array}{c} \text{conversion} \\ \text{fraction} \end{array}$$

Placing the given information into the equation results in:

$$x \text{ oz} = \frac{1,000 \text{ mg}}{1} \times \frac{6 \text{ ml}}{100 \text{ mg}} \times \frac{1 \text{ oz}}{30 \text{ ml}}$$

Solving for x shows that the patient should receive 2 oz of the drug.

Inexact nature of dosage computations

Converting drug measurements from one system to another and then determining the amount of a dosage form to give can easily produce inexact dosages. A rounding error made during computation or discrepancies in the dosage may occur, depending on the conversion standard used in calculation. Or, you may determine a precise amount to be given, only to find that giving that amount is impossible. For example, precise computations may indicate that a patient should receive 0.97 tablet. Giving such an amount is impossible.

The following rule helps avoid calculation errors and discrepancies between theoretical and real dosages: No more than a 10% variation should exist between the dosage ordered and the dosage to be given. For example, if you determine that a patient should receive 0.97 tablet, you can safely give 1 tablet.

Computing parenteral dosages

The methods for computing drug dosages can be used not just for oral but also for parenteral routes. The following example shows how to determine a parenteral drug dosage. Say a prescriber orders 75 mg of Demerol. The package label reads: meperidine (Demerol), 100 mg/ml. By using the fraction method to determine the number of milliliters the patient should receive, your equation should look like this:

$$\frac{75 \text{ mg}}{x \text{ ml}} = \frac{100 \text{ mg}}{1 \text{ ml}}$$

To solve for x, cross multiply:

$$x \text{ ml} \times 100 \text{ mg} = 75 \text{ mg} \times 1 \text{ ml}$$

$$x \text{ ml} = \frac{75 \text{ mg} \times 1 \text{ ml}}{100 \text{ mg}}$$

$$x \text{ ml} = \frac{75 \text{ ml}}{100}$$

$$x \text{ ml} = 0.75 \text{ ml}$$

The patient should receive 0.75 ml.

Reconstituting powders for injection

Although a pharmacist usually reconstitutes powders for parenteral use, nurses sometimes perform this function by following the directions on the drug label. The label gives the total quantity of drug in the vial or ampule, the amount and type of diluent to be added to the powder, and the strength and expiration date of the resulting solution.

When you add diluent to a powder, the powder increases the fluid volume. That's why the label calls for less diluent than the total volume of the prepared solution. For example, a label may tell you to add 1.7 ml of diluent to a vial of powdered drug to obtain a 2-ml total volume of prepared solution.

To determine the amount of solution to give, use the manufacturer's information about the concentration of the solution. For example, if you want to give 500 mg of a drug and the concentration of the prepared solution is 1 g (1,000 mg)/10 ml, use the following equation:

$$\frac{500 \text{ mg}}{x \text{ ml}} = \frac{1,000 \text{ mg}}{10 \text{ ml}}$$

The patient would receive 5 ml of the prepared solution.

Intravenous drip rates and flow rates

Make sure you know the difference between I.V. drip and flow rates and also how to calculate each rate. I.V. drip rate refers to the number of drops of solution to be infused per minute. Flow rate refers to the number of milliliters of fluid to be infused over 1 hour.

To calculate an I.V. drip rate, first set up a fraction showing the volume of solution to be delivered over the number of minutes in which that volume should be infused. For example, if a patient should receive 100 ml of solution in 1 hour, the fraction would be written as:

$$\frac{100 \text{ ml}}{60 \text{ min}}$$

Multiply the fraction by the drip factor (the number of drops [gtt] contained in 1 ml) to determine the number of drops per minute to be infused, or the drip rate. The drip factor varies among different I.V. sets and should appear on the package that contains the I.V. tubing administration set.

Following the manufacturer's directions for drip factor is a crucial step. Standard administration sets have drip factors of 10, 15, or 20 gtt/ml. A microdrip, or minidrip, set has a drip factor of 60 gtt/ml.

Use the following equation to determine the drip rate of an I.V. solution:

$$\text{gtt/min} = \frac{\text{total no. of ml}}{\text{total no. of min}} \times \frac{\text{drip}}{\text{factor}}$$

The equation applies to I.V. solutions that infuse over many hours or to small-volume infusions such as those used for antibiotics, usually given in less than 1 hour. For example, if an order requires 1,000 ml of 5% dextrose in normal saline solution to infuse over 12 hours and the administration set delivers 15 gtt per ml, what should the drip rate be?

$$x \text{ gtt/min} = \frac{1,000 \text{ ml}}{720 \text{ min}} \times 15 \text{ gtt/ml}$$

$$x \text{ gtt/min} = 20.83 \text{ gtt/min}$$

The drip rate would be rounded to 21 gtt per minute.

You'll use flow-rate calculations when working with I.V. infusion pumps to set the number of milliliters to be delivered in 1 hour. To perform this calculation, you should know the total volume in milliliters to be infused and the amount of time for the infusion. Use the following equation:

$$\text{flow rate} = \frac{\text{total volume ordered}}{\text{number of hours}}$$

Quick methods for calculating drip rates

Keep in mind that quicker methods exist for computing I.V. solution administration rates. To give an I.V. solution through a microdrip set, adjust the flow rate (number of milliliters per hour) to equal the drip rate (gtt per minute).

Using this method, the flow rate would be divided by 60 minutes and then multiplied by the drip factor, which also equals 60. Because the flow rate and the drip factor are equal, the two arithmetic operations cancel each other out. For example, if 125 ml/hour represented the ordered flow rate, the equation would be:

$$\text{drip rate (125)} = \frac{125 \text{ ml}}{60 \text{ min}} \times 60$$

Rather than spending time calculating the equation, you can use the number assigned to the flow rate as the drip rate.

For I.V. administration sets that deliver 15 gtt/ml, the flow rate divided by 4 equals the drip rate. For sets with a drip factor of 10, the flow rate divided by 6 equals the drip rate.

Critical care calculations

Many drugs given on the critical care unit are used to treat life-threatening disorders; you must be able to perform calculations swiftly and accurately, prepare the drug for infusion, give the drug, and then observe the patient closely to evaluate the drug's effectiveness. Three calculations must be performed before giving critical care drugs:
• Calculate the concentration of the drug in the I.V. solution.
• Figure the flow rate needed to deliver the desired dose.
• Determine the needed dosage.

Calculating concentration

To calculate the drug's concentration, use the following formula:

concentration in mg/ml = mg of drug/ml of fluid

To express the concentration in mcg/ml, multiply the answer by 1,000.

Figuring flow rate

To determine the I.V. flow rate per minute, use the following formula:

$$\frac{dose/min}{x \text{ ml/min}} = \frac{concentration \text{ of solution}}{1 \text{ ml of fluid}}$$

To calculate the hourly flow rate, first multiply the ordered dose, given in milligrams or micrograms per minute, by 60 minutes to determine the hourly dose. Then use the following equation to compute the hourly flow rate:

$$\frac{hourly \text{ dose}}{x \text{ ml/hr}} = \frac{concentration \text{ of solution}}{1 \text{ ml of fluid}}$$

Determining dosage

To determine the dosage in milligrams per kilogram of body weight per minute, first determine the concentration of the solution in milligrams per milliliter. (If a drug is ordered in micrograms, convert milligrams to micrograms by multiplying by 1,000.) To determine the dose in milligrams per hour, multiply the

hourly flow rate by the concentration using the formula:

$$\frac{dose \text{ in}}{mg/hr} = \frac{hourly}{flow \text{ rate}} \times concentration$$

Then calculate the dose in milligrams per minute. Divide the hourly dose by 60 minutes:

$$dose \text{ in mg/min} = \frac{dose \text{ in mg/hr}}{60 \text{ min}}$$

Divide the dose per minute by the patient's weight, using the following formula:

$$mg/kg/min = \frac{mg/min}{patient's \text{ weight in kg}}$$

Finally, make sure that the drug is being given within a safe and therapeutic range. Compare the amount in milligrams per kilogram per minute to the safe range shown in a drug reference book.

The following examples show how to calculate an I.V. flow rate using the different formulas.

Example 1

A patient has frequent runs of ventricular tachycardia that subside after 10 to 12 beats. The prescriber orders 2 g (2,000 mg) of lidocaine in 500 ml of D_5W to infuse at 2 mg/minute. What's the flow rate in milliliters per minute? Milliliters per hour?

First, find the concentration of the solution by setting up a proportion with the unknown concentration in one fraction and the ordered dose in the other fraction:

$$\frac{x \text{ mg}}{1 \text{ ml}} = \frac{2,000 \text{ mg}}{500 \text{ ml}}$$

Cross multiply the fractions:

$$x \text{ mg} \times 500 \text{ ml} = 2,000 \text{ mg} \times 1 \text{ ml}$$

Solve for x by dividing each side of the equation by 500 ml and canceling units that appear in both the numerator and denominator:

$$\frac{x \text{ mg} \times 500 \text{ ml}}{500 \text{ ml}} = \frac{2,000 \text{ mg} \times 1 \text{ ml}}{500 \text{ ml}}$$

$$x = \frac{2,000 \text{ mg}}{500}$$

$$x = 4 \text{ mg}$$

The concentration of the solution is 4 mg/ml. Next, calculate the flow rate per minute needed to deliver the ordered dose of 2 mg/minute. To do this, set up a proportion with the unknown flow rate per minute in one fraction and the concentration of the solution in the other fraction:

$$\frac{2 \text{ mg}}{x \text{ ml}} = \frac{4 \text{ mg}}{1 \text{ ml}}$$

Cross multiply the fractions:

$$x \text{ ml} \times 4 \text{ mg} = 1 \text{ ml} \times 2 \text{ mg}$$

Solve for x by dividing each side of the equation by 4 mg and canceling units that appear in both the numerator and denominator:

$$\frac{x \text{ ml} \times 4 \text{ mg}}{4 \text{ mg}} = \frac{1 \text{ ml} \times 2 \text{ mg}}{4 \text{ mg}}$$

$$x = \frac{2 \text{ ml}}{4}$$

$$x = 0.5 \text{ ml}$$

The patient should receive 0.5 ml/minute of lidocaine. Because lidocaine must be given with an infusion pump, compute the hourly flow rate. Set up a proportion with the unknown flow rate per hour in one fraction and the flow rate per minute in the other fraction:

$$\frac{x \text{ ml}}{60 \text{ min}} = \frac{0.5 \text{ ml}}{1 \text{ min}}$$

Cross multiply the fractions:

$$x \text{ ml} \times 1 \text{ min} = 0.5 \text{ ml} \times 60 \text{ min}$$

Solve for x by dividing each side of the equation by 1 minute and canceling units that appear in both the numerator and denominator:

$$\frac{x \text{ ml} \times 1 \text{ min}}{1 \text{ min}} = \frac{0.5 \text{ ml} \times 60 \text{ min}}{1 \text{ min}}$$

$$x = 30 \text{ ml}$$

Set the infusion pump to deliver 30 ml/hour.

Example 2

A 200-lb patient is scheduled to receive an I.V. infusion of dobutamine at 10 mcg/kg/minute. The package insert says to dilute 250 mg of the drug in 50 ml of D_5W. Because the drug vial contains 20 ml of solution, the total to be infused is 70 ml (50 ml of D_5W plus 20 ml of solution). How many micrograms of the drug should the patient receive each minute? Each hour?

First, compute the patient's weight in kilograms. To do this, set up a proportion with the weight in pounds and the unknown weight in kilograms in one fraction and the number of pounds per kilogram in the other fraction:

$$\frac{200 \text{ lb}}{x \text{ kg}} = \frac{2.2 \text{ lb}}{1 \text{ kg}}$$

Cross multiply the fractions:

$$x \text{ kg} \times 2.2 \text{ lb} = 1 \text{ kg} \times 200 \text{ lb}$$

Solve for x by dividing each side of the equation by 2.2 lb and canceling units that appear in both the numerator and denominator.

$$\frac{x \text{ kg} \times 2.2 \text{ lb}}{2.2 \text{ lb}} = \frac{1 \text{ kg} \times 200 \text{ lb}}{2.2 \text{ lb}}$$

$$x = \frac{200 \text{ kg}}{2.2}$$

$$x = 90.9 \text{ kg}$$

The patient weighs 90.9 kg. Next, determine the dose in micrograms per minute by setting up a proportion with the patient's weight in kilograms and the unknown dose in micrograms per minute in one fraction and the known dose in micrograms per kilogram per minute in the other fraction:

$$\frac{90.9 \text{ kg}}{x \text{ mcg/min}} = \frac{1 \text{ kg}}{10 \text{ mcg/min}}$$

Cross multiply the fractions:

$$x \text{ mcg/min} \times 1 \text{ kg} = 10 \text{ mcg/min} \times 90.9 \text{ kg}$$

Solve for x by dividing each side of the equation by 1 kg and canceling units that appear in both the numerator and denominator:

$$\frac{x \text{ mcg/min} \times 1 \text{ kg}}{1 \text{ kg}} = \frac{10 \text{ mcg/min} \times 90.9 \text{ kg}}{1 \text{ kg}}$$

$$x = 909 \text{ mcg/min}$$

The patient should receive 909 mcg of dobutamine every minute. Finally, determine the hourly dose by multiplying the dose per minute by 60:

$$909 \text{ mcg/min} \times 60 \text{ min/hr} = 54,540 \text{ mcg/hr}$$

The patient should receive 54,540 mcg of dobutamine every hour.

Pediatric dosage considerations

To determine the correct pediatric dosage of a drug, prescribers, pharmacists, and nurses usually use two computation methods. One is based on weight in kilograms; the other uses the child's body surface area. Other methods are less accurate and not recommended.

Dosage range per kilogram of body weight

Currently, many pharmaceutical companies provide information on the safe dosage ranges for drugs given to children. The companies usually provide the dosage ranges in milligrams per kilogram of body weight and, in many cases, give similar information for adult dosage ranges. The following example and explanation show how to calculate the safe pediatric dosage range for a drug, using the company's suggested safe dosage range provided in milligrams per kilogram.

For a child, a prescriber orders a drug with a suggested dosage range of 10 to 12 mg/kg of body weight/day. The child weighs 12 kg. What is the safe daily dosage range for the child?

You must calculate the lower and upper limits of the dosage range provided by the manufacturer. First, calculate the dosage based on 10 mg/kg of body weight. Then, calculate the dosage based on 12 mg/kg of body weight. The answers represent the lower and upper limits of the daily dosage range, expressed in mg/kg of the child's weight.

Body surface area

A second method for calculating safe pediatric dosages uses the child's body surface area. This method may provide a more accurate calculation because the child's body surface area is thought to parallel the child's organ growth and maturation and metabolic rate.

You can determine the body surface area of a child by using a three-column chart called a nomogram. Mark the child's height in the first column and weight in the third column. Then draw a line between the two marks. The point at which the line intersects the vertical scale in the second column is the child's estimated body surface area in square meters. To calculate the

child's approximate dose, use the body surface area measurement in the following equation:

$$\frac{\text{body surface area of child}}{\text{average adult body surface area } (1.73 m^2)} \times \frac{\text{average}}{\text{adult dose}} = \frac{\text{child's}}{\text{dose}}$$

The following example illustrates the use of the equation. The nomogram shows that a 25-lb (11.3-kg) child who is 33 inches (84 cm) tall has a body surface area of 0.52 m². To determine the child's dose of a drug with an average adult dose of 100 mg, the equation would appear as:

$$\frac{0.52 \text{ m}^2}{1.73 \text{ m}^2} \times 100 \text{ mg} = \frac{30.06 \text{ mg}}{\text{(child's dose)}}$$

The child should receive 30 mg of the drug. Keep in mind that many facilities have guidelines that determine acceptable calculation methods for pediatric dosages. If you work in a pediatric setting, make sure to familiarize yourself with your facility's policies about pediatric dosages.

3

Drug administration

You will give drugs by many routes, including oral (P.O.), intravenous (I.V.), intramuscular (I.M.), subcutaneous (S.C.), topical, ophthalmic, rectal (P.R.), buccal and sublingual (S.L.), inhalation, nasogastric (NG), otic, and vaginal. No matter which route you use, you'll need to follow established procedures to make sure you give the right drug in the right dose to the right patient at the right time and by the right route, and, immediately after giving the drug, you'll need to provide the right documentation. These procedures include checking the order, medication record, and label; confirming the patient's identity; following standard safety procedures; addressing all of the patient's questions; and correctly documenting the administration of the drug in the patient's medical record.

Check the order

Make sure that you have a written order for every drug given. Verbal orders should be used only in emergencies and should be signed by the prescriber within the time period specified by your facility. If your facility has a computerized order system, it may allow prescribers to order drugs electronically from the pharmacy. The computer may indicate whether the pharmacy has the drug and trigger the pharmacy staff to fill the prescription. A computerized order also may generate a patient record on which you can document medication administration. In fact, you may be able to document administration right on the computer.

Computer systems offer several advantages over paper systems. For instance, drugs may arrive on the unit or floor more quickly. Documentation is quicker and easier. Prescribers can see at a glance which drugs have been given. Errors won't result from poor handwriting (although typing mistakes may occur). Finally, computerized records are easier to store than paper records.

Check the medication record

Check the order on the patient's medication record against the prescriber's order.

Check the label

Before giving a drug, check its label three times to make sure you're giving the prescribed drug and the prescribed dose. First, check the label when you take the container from the shelf or drawer. Next, check the label right before pouring the drug into the medication cup or drawing it into the syringe. Finally, check the label again before returning the container to the shelf or drawer. If you're giving a unit-dose drug, you'll be opening the container at the patient's bedside. Check the label for the third time immediately after pouring the drug and again before discarding the wrapper.

Don't give a drug from a poorly labeled or unlabeled container. Also, don't attempt to label a drug or to reinforce a label that is falling off or improperly placed. Instead, return the drug to the pharmacist for verification and proper labeling.

Confirm the patient's identity

Before giving the drug, ask the patient his full name, and confirm his identity by checking his name and medical record number on his patient identification wristband against the medication administration record. Don't rely on information that can vary during a hospital stay, such as a room or bed number. Check again that you have the correct drug, and make sure the patient isn't allergic to it.

If the patient has any drug allergies, check to make sure the chart and medication administration record are labeled accordingly and that the patient is wearing an allergy wristband identifying the allergen.

Follow safety procedures

Whenever you give a drug, follow these safety procedures:
• Never give a drug poured or prepared by someone else.
• Never allow the medication cart or tray out of your sight once you've prepared a dose.
• Never leave a drug at a patient's bedside.

• Always observe the patient during drug administration; make sure that the patient swallows oral drugs or appropriately and effectively uses an inhaler. If the patient is giving the drug to himself, observe the patient to make sure his technique is correct.

• Never return unwrapped or prepared drugs to stock containers; instead, dispose of them, and notify the pharmacy.

• Keep the medication cart locked at all times.

• Follow standard precautions, as appropriate.

Respond to questions

If the patient questions you about his drug or dosage, check his medication record again. If the drug you're giving is correct, reassure the patient and explain the reason for the drug. Explain any changes to his medication regimen or drug dosage. Instruct him, as appropriate, about possible adverse reactions, and ask him to report anything that he feels may be an adverse reaction.

Oral administration

Because oral drug administration is usually the safest, most convenient, and least expensive, most drugs are given by this method. Drugs for oral administration are available in many forms: tablets, enteric-coated tablets, capsules, syrups, elixirs, oils, liquids, suspensions, powders, and granules. Some require special preparation before administration, such as mixing with juice to make them more palatable.

Oral drugs are sometimes prescribed in higher dosages than their parenteral equivalents because, after the drugs are absorbed through the gastrointestinal (GI) system, the liver breaks them down before they reach the systemic circulation.

Equipment and preparation

• Check the chart and the medication administration record.

• Gather the prescribed drug and medication cup.

• If necessary, gather a mortar and pestle for crushing pills and an appropriate buffer, such as jelly and applesauce for crushed pills or juice, water, and milk for liquid drugs. These variations commonly are used for children or elderly patients.

Implementation

• Wash your hands.

• Confirm the patient's identity by asking his full name and checking the name and medical record number on his wristband.

• Make sure that the patient is not allergic to the drug or any of its components.

• Assess the patient's condition, including level of consciousness and vital signs, as needed. Changes in the patient's condition may warrant withholding the drug.

• Give the patient the drug. If appropriate, crush the drug to facilitate swallowing or mix it with an appropriate vehicle or liquid to aid swallowing, minimize adverse effects, or promote absorption.

• Stay with the patient until he has swallowed the drug. If he seems confused or disoriented, check his mouth to make sure he has swallowed it. Return and reassess the patient's response within 1 hour after giving the drug.

Nursing considerations

• To avoid damaging or staining the patient's teeth, give acid or iron preparations through a straw. An unpleasant-tasting liquid usually can be made more palatable if taken through a straw because the liquid contacts fewer taste buds.

• If the patient can't swallow a whole tablet or capsule, ask the pharmacist if the drug is available in liquid form or if it can be given by another route. If not, ask the pharmacist if the tablet can be crushed or if capsules can be opened and mixed with food.

• Don't crush sustained-action, buccal, S.L., and enteric-coated drugs because these drugs may become ineffective if crushed.

Intravenous bolus administration

In this method, rapid I.V. administration allows drug levels to quickly peak in the bloodstream. This method also may be used for drugs that can't be given I.M. because they're toxic or because the patient has a reduced ability to absorb them. It may also be used to deliver drugs that can't be diluted. Bolus doses may be injected directly into a vein or through an existing I.V. line.

Equipment and preparation

• Check the chart and the medication administration record. Gather the prescribed drug, 20G needle and syringe, diluent (if needed), tourniquet, alcohol sponge, sterile 2″ × 2″ gauze pad, gloves, adhesive bandage, and tape. Other materials may include a winged device primed with normal saline solution and a second syringe (and needle) filled with normal saline solution.

• Draw the drug into the syringe and dilute if needed.

Implementation

• Confirm the patient's identity by asking his full name and checking the name and medical record number on his wristband.

• Wash your hands and put on gloves.

To give a direct injection

• Select the largest vein suitable to dilute the drug and minimize irritation.

• Apply a tourniquet above the site to distend the vein, and clean the site with an alcohol sponge working outward in a circle.

• If you're using the needle of the drug syringe, insert it at a 30-degree angle with the bevel up. The bevel should reach ¼″ (0.6 cm) into the vein. Insert a winged device bevel-up at a 10- to 25-degree angle. Lower the angle once you enter the vein. Advance the needle into the vein. Tape the wings in place when you see blood return, and attach the syringe containing the drug.

• Check for blood backflow.

• Remove the tourniquet, and inject the drug at the ordered rate.

• Check for blood backflow to ensure that the needle remained in place and the entire amount of injected drug entered the vein.

• For a winged device, flush the line with normal saline solution from the second syringe to ensure complete delivery.

• Withdraw the needle and apply pressure to the site with the sterile gauze pad for at least 3 minutes to prevent hematoma.

• Apply an adhesive bandage when the bleeding stops.

• Remove and discard your gloves. Wash your hands.

To inject through an existing line

• Wash your hands, and put on gloves.

• Check the compatibility of the drug.

• If the drug isn't compatible with the I.V. solution, flush the line with normal saline solution before and after the injection.

• Close the flow clamp, wipe the injection port with an alcohol sponge, and inject the drug as you would a direct injection.

• Open the flow clamp and readjust the flow rate.

• Remove and discard your gloves. Wash your hands.

Nursing considerations

• If the existing I.V. line is capped, making it an intermittent infusion device, verify patency and placement of the device before injecting the drug. Then flush the device with normal saline solution, give the drug, and follow with the appropriate flush.

• Immediately report signs of acute allergic reaction or anaphylaxis. If extravasation occurs, stop the injection, estimate the amount of infiltration, and notify the prescriber.

• When giving diazepam or chlordiazepoxide hydrochloride through a steel needle winged device or an I.V. line, flush with bacteriostatic water to prevent precipitation.

Intravenous administration through a secondary line

A secondary I.V. line is a complete I.V. set connected to the lower Y-port (secondary port) of a primary line instead of to the I.V. catheter or needle. It features an I.V. container, long tubing, and either a microdrip or a macrodrip system, and it can be used for continuous or intermittent drug infusion. When used continuously, it permits drug infusion and titration while the primary line maintains a constant total infusion rate.

A secondary I.V. line used only for intermittent drug administration is called a piggyback set. In this case, the primary line maintains venous access between drug doses. A piggyback set includes a small I.V. container, short tubing, and usually a macrodrip system, and it connects to the primary line's upper Y-port (piggyback port).

Equipment and preparation

• Check the chart and the medication administration record.

• Gather the prescribed I.V. drug, diluent (if needed), prescribed I.V. solution, administration set with secondary injection port, 22G 1″ needle or a needleless system, alcohol sponges, 1″ (2.5 cm) adhesive tape, time tape, labels, infusion pump, extension hook, and solution for intermittent piggyback infusion.
• Wash your hands.
• Inspect the I.V. container for cracks, leaks, or contamination.
• Check the expiration date.
• Check compatibility with the primary solution.
• Determine whether the primary line has a secondary injection port.
• If necessary, add the drug to the secondary I.V. solution (usually 50- to 100-ml "minibags" of normal saline solution or D_5W). To do so, remove any seals from the secondary container and wipe the main port with an alcohol sponge.
• Inject the prescribed drug and agitate the solution to mix the drug.
• Label the I.V. mixture.
• Insert the administration set spike, and attach the needle or needleless system.
• Open the flow clamp and prime the line. Then close the flow clamp.
• Some drugs come in vials that can hang directly on an I.V. pole. In this case, inject diluent directly into the drug vial. Then spike the vial, prime the tubing, and hang the set.

Implementation
• If the drug is incompatible with the primary I.V. solution, replace the primary solution with a fluid that's compatible with both solutions, and flush the line before starting the drug infusion.
• Hang the container of the secondary set and wipe the injection port of the primary line with an alcohol sponge.
• Insert the needle or needleless system from the secondary line into the injection port, and tape it securely to the primary line.
• To run the container of the secondary set by itself, lower the primary set's container with an extension hook. To run both containers simultaneously, place them at the same height.
• Open the clamp and adjust the drip rate.
• For continuous infusion, set the secondary solution to the desired drip rate; then adjust the

primary solution to the desired total infusion rate.
• For intermittent infusion, wait until the secondary solution has completely infused; then adjust the primary drip rate, as needed.
• If the secondary solution tubing is being reused, close the clamp on the tubing and follow your facility's policy: Either remove the needle or needleless system and replace it with a new one, or leave it taped to the injection port and label it with the time it was first used.
• Leave the empty container in place until you replace it with a new dose of drug at the prescribed time. If the tubing won't be reused, discard it appropriately with the I.V. container.

Nursing considerations
• If institutional policy allows, use a pump for drug infusion. Place a time tape on the secondary container to help prevent an inaccurate administration rate.
• When reusing secondary tubing, change it when your facility's policy requires, usually every 2 or 3 days. Inspect the injection port for leakage with each use; change it more often, if needed.
• Except for lipids, don't piggyback a secondary I.V. line to a total parenteral nutrition line because it risks contamination.

Intramuscular administration
You'll use I.M. injections to deposit up to 5 ml of drug deep into well-vascularized muscle for rapid systemic action and absorption.

Equipment and preparation
• Check the chart and the medication administration record.
• Gather the prescribed drug, diluent or filter needle (if needed), 3- to 5-ml syringe, 20G to 25G 1″ to 3″ needle, gloves, and alcohol sponges.
• The prescribed drug must be sterile. The needle may be packaged separately or already attached to the syringe. Needles used for I.M. injections are longer than those used for S.C. injections because they must reach deep into the muscle. Needle length also depends on the injection site, the patient's size, and the amount of S.C. fat covering the muscle. A larger needle

gauge can accommodate viscous solutions and suspensions.

• Check the drug for abnormal changes in color and clarity. If in doubt, ask the pharmacist.

• Use alcohol to wipe the stopper that tops the drug vial, and draw up the prescribed amount of drug.

• Provide privacy and explain the procedure to the patient.

• Position and drape him appropriately, making sure that the site is well lit and exposed.

Implementation

• Wash your hands.

• Confirm the patient's identity by asking his full name and checking the name and medical record number on his wristband.

• Select an appropriate injection site. Avoid any site that looks inflamed, edematous, or irritated. Also, avoid using injection sites that contain moles, birthmarks, scar tissue, or other lesions. The dorsogluteal and ventrogluteal muscles are used most commonly for I.M. injections.

Dorsogluteal muscle

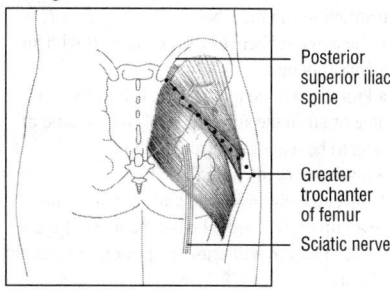

Posterior superior iliac spine

Greater trochanter of femur

Sciatic nerve

Ventrogluteal muscle

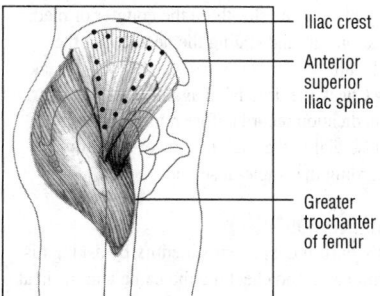

Iliac crest

Anterior superior iliac spine

Greater trochanter of femur

• The deltoid muscle may be used for injections of 2 ml or less.

Deltoid muscle

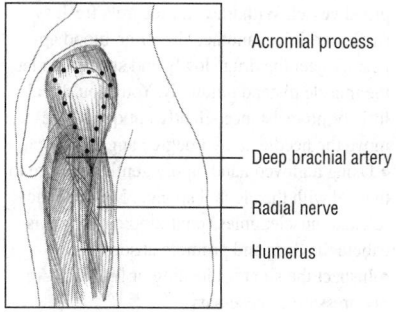

Acromial process

Deep brachial artery

Radial nerve

Humerus

• The vastus lateralis muscle is used most often in children; the rectus femoris may be used in infants.

Vastus lateralis and rectus femoris muscles

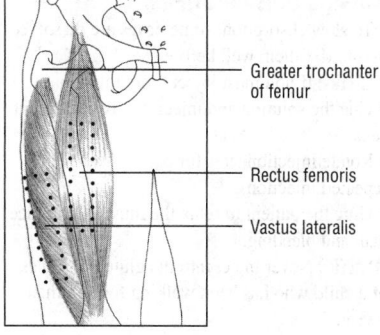

Greater trochanter of femur

Rectus femoris

Vastus lateralis

• Loosen, but don't remove, the needle sheath.

• Gently tap the site to stimulate nerve endings and minimize pain.

• Clean the site with an alcohol sponge, starting at the site and moving outward in expanding circles to about 2″ (5 cm). Allow the skin to dry because wet alcohol stings in the puncture.

• Put on gloves.

• With the thumb and index finger of your nondominant hand, gently stretch the skin.

• With the syringe in your dominant hand, remove the needle sheath with the free fingers of the other hand.

• Position the syringe perpendicular to the skin surface and a couple of inches from the skin. Tell the patient that he will feel a prick. Then quickly and firmly thrust the needle into the muscle.

• Pull back slightly on the plunger to aspirate for blood. If blood appears, the needle is in a blood vessel. Withdraw it, prepare a fresh syringe, and inject another site. If no blood appears, inject the drug slowly and steadily to let the muscle distend gradually. You should feel little or no resistance. Gently but quickly remove the needle at a 90-degree angle.

• Using a gloved hand, apply gentle pressure to the site with the alcohol sponge. Massage the relaxed muscle, unless contraindicated, to distribute the drug and promote absorption.

• Inspect the site for bleeding or bruising. Apply pressure as necessary.

• Discard all equipment properly. Don't recap needles; put them in an appropriate biohazard container to avoid needle-stick injuries.

• Remove and discard your gloves. Wash your hands.

Nursing considerations

• To slow absorption, some drugs are dissolved in oil. Mix them well before use.

(§) **ALERT:** If you must inject more than 5 ml, divide the solution and inject it at two different sites.

• Rotate injection sites for patients who need repeated injections.

• Urge the patient to relax the muscle to reduce pain and bleeding.

(§) **ALERT:** Never inject into the gluteal muscles of a child who has been walking for less than 1 year.

• Keep in mind that I.M. injections can damage local muscle cells and elevate CK levels, which can be confused with elevated levels caused by MI. Diagnostic tests can be used to differentiate between them.

Subcutaneous administration

Injection of drug S.C. allows slower, more sustained administration than I.M. injection. Drugs and solutions delivered S.C. are injected through a relatively short needle using sterile technique.

Equipment and preparation

• Check the chart and the medication administration record.

• Gather gloves, drug, needle of appropriate gauge and length, 1- to 3-ml syringe, and alcohol sponges. Other materials may include antiseptic cleanser, filter needle, insulin syringe, and insulin pump.

• Inspect the drug to make sure it's not cloudy and is free of precipitates.

For single-dose ampules

• Wrap the neck of the ampule in an alcohol sponge and snap off the top, directing it away from you.

• If desired, attach a filter needle to the needle, slightly tip the ampule, and withdraw the desired amount of the drug.

• Tap the syringe to disperse air bubbles.

• Cover the needle with the needle sheath by placing the sheath on the counter or medication cart and sliding the needle into the sheath.

• Before discarding the ampule, check the label against the patient's medication record.

• Discard the filter needle and the ampule.

• Attach the appropriate-sized needle to the syringe.

For single-dose and multidose vials

• Reconstitute powdered drugs according to the instructions on the label.

• Clean the rubber stopper on the vial with an alcohol sponge.

• Pull the syringe plunger back until the volume of air in the syringe equals the volume of drug to be withdrawn from the vial.

• Insert the needle into the vial.

• Inject the air, invert the vial, and keep the bevel tip of the needle below the level of the solution as you withdraw the prescribed amount of drug.

• Tap the syringe to disperse air bubbles.

• Cover the needle with the needle sheath by placing the sheath on the counter or medication cart and sliding the needle into the sheath.

• Check the drug label against the patient's medication record before returning the multidose vial to the shelf or drawer or before discarding the single-dose vial.

Implementation

• Confirm the patient's identity by asking his full name and checking the name and medical record number on his wristband.

• Select the injection site from those shown, and tell the patient where you'll be giving the injection.

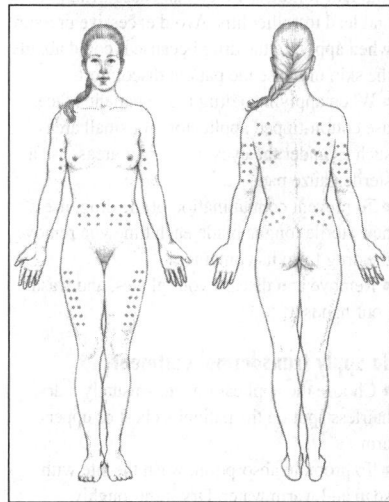

• Wash your hands and put on gloves. Position and drape the patient if necessary.
• Clean the injection site with an alcohol sponge. Loosen the protective needle sheath.
• With your nondominant hand, pinch the skin around the injection site firmly to elevate the S.C. tissue, forming a 1″ (2.5 cm) fat fold, as shown.

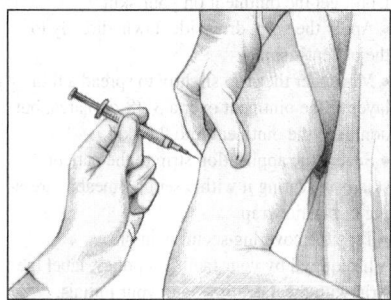

• Holding the syringe in your dominant hand, grip the needle sheath between the fourth and fifth fingers of your nondominant hand while continuing to pinch the skin around the injection site with the index finger and thumb of your nondominant hand. Pull the sheath back to uncover the needle. Don't touch the needle.
• Position the needle with its bevel up.

• Tell the patient he'll feel a prick as you insert the needle. Do so quickly, in one motion, at a 45-degree or 90-degree angle, as shown below. The needle length and the angle you use depend on the amount of S.C. tissue at the site. Some drugs, such as heparin, should always be injected at a 90-degree angle.

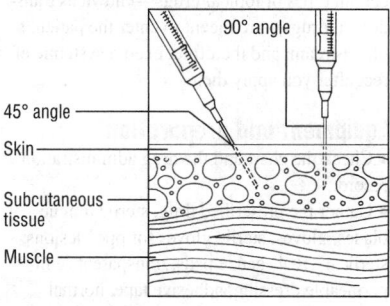

• Release the skin to avoid injecting the drug into compressed tissue and irritating the nerves. Except for insulin and heparin, pull the plunger back slightly to check for blood return. If blood appears, withdraw the needle, prepare another syringe, and repeat the procedure. If no blood appears, slowly inject the drug.
• After injection, remove the needle at the same angle you used to insert it. Cover the site with an alcohol sponge, and massage the site gently.
• Remove the alcohol sponge, and check the injection site for bleeding or bruising.
• Don't recap the needle. Follow your facility's policy to dispose of the injection equipment.
• Remove and discard your gloves. Wash your hands.

Nursing considerations
⑤ **ALERT:** Don't aspirate for blood return when giving insulin or heparin. It isn't necessary with insulin and may cause a hematoma with heparin.
• Don't massage the site after giving heparin.
⑤ **ALERT:** Repeated injections in the same site can cause lipodystrophy, a natural immune response. Rotating injection sites can minimize this complication.

Topical administration

Topical drugs, such as patches, lotions, and ointments, are applied directly to the skin. They're commonly used for local, rather than systemic, effects. Keep in mind, however, that certain types of topical drugs—known as transdermal drugs—are meant to enter the patient's bloodstream, and therefore, exert a systemic effect after you apply them.

Equipment and preparation
- Check the chart and the drug administration record.
- Gather the prescribed drug, sterile tongue blades, gloves, sterile gloves for open lesions, sterile 4″ × 4″ gauze pads, transparent semipermeable dressing, adhesive tape, normal saline solution, cotton-tipped applicators, gloves, and linen savers, if necessary.

Implementation
- Confirm the patient's identity by asking his full name and checking the name and medical record number on his wristband.
- Explain the procedure to the patient because, after discharge, he may have to apply the drug by himself.
- Premedicate the patient with an analgesic if the procedure is uncomfortable. Give the drug time to take effect.
- Wash your hands to reduce the risk of cross-contamination, and glove your dominant hand.
- Help the patient to a comfortable position, and expose the area to be treated. Make sure the skin or mucous membrane is intact (unless the drug has been ordered to treat a skin lesion). Application of drug to broken or abraded skin may cause unwanted systemic absorption and further irritation.
- If necessary, clean debris from the skin. You may have to change your gloves if they become soiled.

To apply paste, cream, or ointment
- Open the container. Place the cap upside down to avoid contaminating its inner surface.
- Remove a tongue blade from its sterile wrapper, and cover one end of it with drug from the tube or jar. Then transfer the drug from the tongue blade to your gloved hand.

- Apply the drug to the affected area with long, smooth strokes that follow the direction of hair growth. This technique avoids forcing the drug into hair follicles, which can cause irritation and lead to folliculitis. Avoid excessive pressure when applying the drug because it could abrade the skin or cause the patient discomfort.
- When applying a drug to the patient's face, use cotton-tipped applicators for small areas, such as under the eyes. For larger areas, use a sterile gauze pad.
- To prevent contamination of the drug, use a new sterile tongue blade each time you remove the drug from its container.
- Remove and discard your gloves, and wash your hands.

To apply transdermal ointment
- Choose the application site—usually a dry, hairless spot on the patient's chest or upper arm.
- To promote absorption, wash the site with soap and warm water. Dry it thoroughly.
- Put on gloves.
- If the patient has a previously applied medication strip at another site, remove it and wash this area to clear away any drug residue.
- If the area you choose is hairy, clip excess hair rather than shaving it; shaving causes irritation, which the drug may worsen.
- Squeeze the prescribed amount of ointment onto the application strip or measuring paper. Don't get the ointment on your skin.
- Apply the strip, drug side down, directly to the patient's skin.
- Maneuver the strip slightly to spread a thin layer of the ointment over a 3″ (8-cm) area, but don't rub the ointment into the skin.
- Secure the application strip to the patient's skin by covering it with a semipermeable dressing or plastic wrap.
- Tape the covering securely in place.
- If required by your facility's policy, label the strip with the date, time, and your initials.
- Remove your gloves and wash your hands.

To apply a transdermal patch
- Remove the old patch.
- Choose a dry, hairless application site.
- As with the transdermal ointment, clip (don't shave) hair from the chosen site. Wash the area with warm water and soap, and dry it thoroughly.

- Open the drug package and remove the patch.
- Without touching the adhesive surface, remove the clear plastic backing.
- Apply the patch to the site without touching the adhesive.
- If required by your facility's policy, label the patch with the date, time, and your initials.

To remove ointment
- Wash your hands and put on gloves.
- Gently swab ointment from the patient's skin using a sterile 4″ × 4″ gauze pad saturated with normal saline solution.
- Don't wipe too hard because you could irritate the skin.
- Remove and discard your gloves, and wash your hands.

Nursing considerations
- To prevent skin irritation from drug accumulation, never apply a drug without first removing previous applications.
- Always wear gloves to prevent absorption by your skin.
- Never apply ointment to the eyelids or ear canal unless ordered. The ointment may congeal and occlude the tear duct or ear canal.
- Inspect the treated area frequently for allergic or other adverse reactions.
- Don't apply a topical drug to scarred or callused skin because this may impair absorption.
- Don't place a defibrillator paddle on a transdermal patch. The aluminum on the patch can cause electrical arcing during defibrillation, resulting in smoke and thermal burns. If a patient has a patch on a standard paddle site, remove the patch before applying the paddle.

Ophthalmic administration

Ophthalmic drugs—drops or ointments—serve both diagnostic and therapeutic purposes. During an ophthalmic examination, drugs can be used to anesthetize the eye, dilate the pupil, and stain the cornea to identify anomalies. Therapeutic uses include eye lubrication and treatment of glaucoma and infections.

Equipment and preparation
- Check the chart and the medication administration record.
- Gather the prescribed ophthalmic medication, sterile cotton balls, gloves, warm water or normal saline solution, sterile gauze pads, and facial tissue. An ocular dressing also may be used.
- Make sure the drug is labeled for ophthalmic use. Then check the expiration date. Remember to date the container after first use.
- Inspect ocular solutions for cloudiness, discoloration, and precipitation, keeping in mind that some medications are suspensions and normally appear cloudy. Don't use solutions that appear abnormal.

Implementation
- Make sure you know which eye you are treating because different drugs or doses may be ordered for each eye.
- Confirm the patient's identity by asking his full name and checking the name and medical record number on his wristband.
- Wash your hands and put on gloves.
- If the patient has an eye dressing, remove it by pulling it down and away from his forehead. Avoid contaminating your hands. Don't apply pressure to the area around the eyes.
- To remove exudates or meibomian gland secretions, clean around the eye with sterile cotton balls or sterile gauze pads moistened with warm water or normal saline solution. Have the patient close his eye; then gently wipe the eyelids from the inner to the outer canthus. Use a fresh cotton ball or gauze pad for each stroke, and use a different cotton ball or pad for each eye.
- Have the patient sit or lie on his back. Instruct him to tilt his head back and toward his affected eye so that any excess drug can flow away from the tear duct, minimizing systemic absorption through the nasal mucosa.
- Remove the dropper cap from the drug container, and draw the drug into the dropper. Or, if the bottle has a dropper tip, remove the cap and hold or place it upside down to prevent contamination.
- Before instilling eyedrops, instruct the patient to look up and away. This moves the cornea away from the lower lid and minimizes the risk of touching it with the dropper.

To instill eyedrops
- Steady the hand that's holding the dropper by resting it against the patient's forehead. With your other hand, gently pull down the lower lid of the affected eye, and instill the drops in the

conjunctival sac. Never instill eyedrops directly onto the eyeball.

• After instilling the eyedrops, instruct the patient to close his eyes gently, without squeezing the lids shut. Then tell the patient to blink.

•When teaching elderly patients how to instill eyedrops, keep in mind that they may have difficulty sensing drops in the eye. Suggest chilling the drug slightly because the cold drops will be easier to feel when they come in contact with the eye.

To apply eye ointment

• Squeeze a small ribbon of drug on the edge of the conjunctival sac from the inner to the outer canthus. Cut off the ribbon by turning the tube. Don't touch the eye with the tip of the tube.

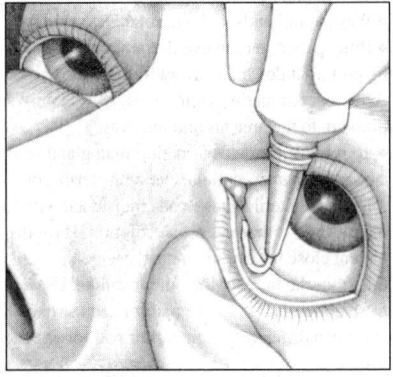

• After applying ointment, instruct the patient to close his eyes gently, without squeezing the lids shut. If you applied ointment, tell him to roll his eyes behind closed lids to help distribute the drug over the eyeball.

• Use a clean tissue to remove any excess drug that leaks from the eye. Use a fresh tissue for each eye to prevent cross-contamination.

• Apply a new eye dressing, if necessary.

• Remove and discard your gloves. Wash your hands.

Nursing considerations

• When administering an eye medication that may be absorbed systemically, gently press your thumb on the inner canthus for 1 to 2 minutes after instillation while the patient closes his eyes. Avoid applying pressure around the eye.

• Urge the patient not to rub his eyes.

• To maintain the drug container's sterility, don't put the cap down after opening the container, and never touch the tip of the dropper or bottle to the eye area. Discard any solution remaining in the dropper before returning it to the bottle. If the dropper or bottle tip has become contaminated, discard it and use another sterile dropper. Never share eyedrops between patients.

Rectal administration

A rectal suppository is a small, solid, medicated mass, usually cone shaped, with a cocoa butter or glycerin base. It may be inserted to stimulate peristalsis and defecation or to relieve pain, vomiting, and local irritation. An ointment is a semisolid drug used to produce local effects. It may be applied externally to the anus or internally to the rectum.

Equipment and preparation

• Check the chart and the medication administration record.

• Gather the rectal suppository or tube of ointment and applicator, 4″ × 4″ gauze pads, gloves, and a water-soluble lubricant. A bedpan also may be needed.

• To prevent softening of the drug and possible decreased effectiveness, store rectal suppositories in the refrigerator until needed. A soft suppository is also harder to handle and insert than a hard one. To harden a softened suppository, hold it (in its wrapper) under cold running water.

Implementation

• Confirm the patient's identity by asking his full name and checking the name and medical record number on his wristband.

• Wash your hands.

To insert a rectal suppository

• Place the patient on his left side in Sims' position. Drape him with the bedcovers, exposing only his buttocks.

• Put on gloves. Unwrap the suppository, and lubricate it with water-soluble lubricant.

• Lift the patient's upper buttock with your nondominant hand to expose the anus.

• Instruct the patient to take several deep breaths through his mouth to relax the anal sphincter and reduce anxiety and discomfort during drug insertion.
• Using the index finger of your dominant hand, insert the suppository—tapered end first—about 3″ (8 cm) until you feel it pass the internal anal sphincter, as shown.

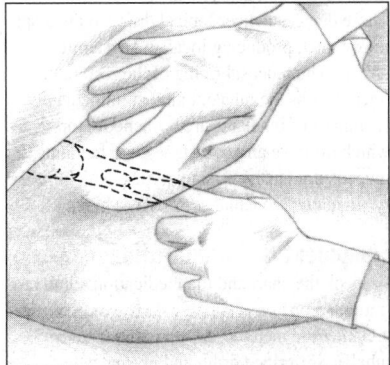

• Direct the tapered end of the suppository toward the side of the rectum so it contacts the membranes.
• Encourage the patient to lie quietly and, if possible, to contract his anal sphincter and buttocks together to retain the suppository for the correct length of time. Press on the patient's anus with a gauze pad, if necessary, until the urge to defecate passes.
• Discard the used equipment and gloves. Wash your hands thoroughly.

To apply an ointment
• For external application, put on gloves and use a gauze pad to spread the drug over the anal area. For internal application, attach the end of the applicator to the tube of ointment, and coat the applicator with water-soluble lubricant.
• Expect to use about 1″ (2.5 cm) of ointment. To gauge how much pressure to use during application, try squeezing a small amount from the tube before you attach the applicator.
• Lift the patient's upper buttock with your nondominant hand to expose the anus.
• Tell the patient to take several deep breaths through his mouth to relax the anal sphincter and reduce anxiety and discomfort during inser-

tion. Then gently insert the applicator, directing it toward the umbilicus.
• Squeeze the tube to eject drug.
• Remove the applicator, and place a folded 4″ × 4″ gauze pad between the patient's buttocks to absorb excess ointment.
• Disassemble the tube and applicator, and recap the tube. Clean the applicator with soap and warm water and store or discard it. Remove and discard your gloves. Then wash your hands thoroughly.

Nursing considerations
• Because eating and drinking stimulates peristalsis, a suppository for relieving constipation should be inserted about 30 minutes before mealtime to help soften the stool and facilitate defecation. A medicated retention suppository should be inserted between meals.
• Tell the patient not to expel the suppository. If retaining it is difficult, place the patient on a bedpan.
• Make sure that the patient's call button is handy, and watch for his signal because he may be unable to suppress the urge to defecate.
• Inform the patient that the suppository may discolor his next bowel movement.

Buccal and sublingual administration
Certain drugs are given buccally (between the cheek and teeth) or S.L. (under the tongue) to bypass the digestive tract and facilitate absorption into the bloodstream. When using either administration method, observe the patient carefully to make sure he doesn't swallow the drug or develop mucosal irritation.

Equipment and preparation
• Check the chart and the medication administration record.
• Gather the prescribed drug, medication cup, and gloves.

Implementation
• Wash your hands. Put on gloves if you'll be placing the drug into the patient's mouth.
• Confirm the patient's identity by asking his full name and checking the name and medical record number on his wristband.

• For buccal administration, place the tablet in the patient's buccal pouch, between the cheek and teeth, as shown below.

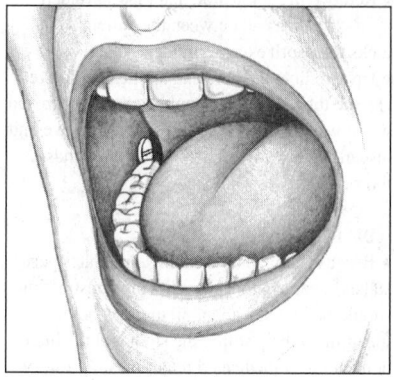

• For S.L. administration, place the tablet under the patient's tongue, as shown below.

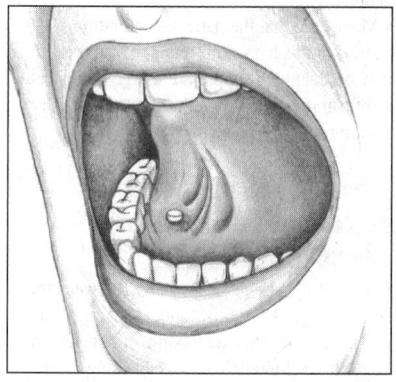

• Remove and discard your gloves, and wash your hands.
• Instruct the patient to keep the drug in place until it dissolves completely to ensure absorption. Caution the patient against chewing the tablet or touching it with his tongue to prevent accidental swallowing.
• Tell the patient not to smoke before the drug has dissolved because because nicotine constricts blood vessels and slows drug absorption.

Nursing considerations
• Don't give liquids until a buccal tablet is absorbed, in some cases up to 1 hour.
• If the patient has angina, tell him to wet the nitroglycerin tablet with saliva and keep it under his tongue until it's fully absorbed.

• Make sure a patient with angina knows how to take the medication, how many doses to take, and when to call for emergency help.

Inhalation administration
Hand-held oropharyngeal inhalers include the metered-dose inhaler and the turbo-inhaler. These devices deliver topical drugs to the respiratory tract, producing local and systemic effects. The mucosal lining of the respiratory tract absorbs the inhalant almost immediately. Examples of inhalants are bronchodilators, which improve airway patency and facilitate mucous drainage, and mucolytics, which liquefy tenacious bronchial secretions.

Equipment and preparation
• Check the chart and the medication administration record.
• Gather the metered-dose inhaler or turbo-inhaler, prescribed drug, and normal saline solution.

Implementation
• Confirm the patient's identity by asking his full name and checking the name and medical record number on his wristband.
• Wash your hands.

To use a metered-dose inhaler
• Shake the inhaler bottle. Remove the cap and insert the stem into the small hole on the flattened portion of the mouthpiece, as shown.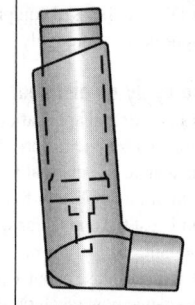
• Place the inhaler about 1″ (2.5 cm) in front of the patient's open mouth.
• Tell the patient to exhale.
• If you're using a spacer, which can make the inhaler more effective, tell the patient to place the mouthpiece of the spacer in his mouth and to press his lips firmly around the mouthpiece.
• As you push the bottle down against the mouthpiece, instruct the patient to inhale slowly through his mouth and to continue inhaling until his lungs feel full. Compress the bottle against the mouthpiece only once.

• Remove the inhaler and tell the patient to hold his breath for several seconds. Then instruct him to exhale slowly through pursed lips to keep distal bronchioles open and allow increased absorption and diffusion of the drug.

• Have the patient gargle with normal saline solution or water to remove the drug from his mouth and the back of his throat. This step helps prevent oral fungal infections. Warn the patient not to swallow after gargling, but rather to spit out the liquid.

To use a turbo-inhaler

• Hold the mouthpiece in one hand. With the other hand, slide the sleeve away from the mouthpiece as far as possible, as shown.

• Unscrew the tip of the mouthpiece by turning it counterclockwise.

• Press the colored portion of the drug capsule into the propeller stem of the mouthpiece.

• Screw the inhaler together again.

• Holding the inhaler with the mouthpiece at the bottom, slide the sleeve all the way down and then up again to puncture the capsule and release the drug. Do this only once.

• Have the patient exhale completely and tilt his head back. Instruct him to place the mouthpiece in his mouth, close his lips around it, and inhale once. Tell him to hold his breath for several seconds.

• Remove the inhaler from the patient's mouth, and tell him to exhale as much air as possible.

• Repeat the procedure until the entire amount of drug in the device is inhaled.

• Have the patient gargle and spit with normal saline solution or water, if desired, to remove the drug from his mouth and the back of his throat.

Nursing considerations

• Teach the patient how to use the inhaler so he can continue treatments after discharge, if needed. Explain that overdose can cause the drug to lose its effectiveness. Tell him to record the date and time of each inhalation and his response.

• Be aware that some inhalants may cause restlessness, palpitations, nervousness, and other

systemic effects. They also can cause hypersensitivity reactions, such as a rash, urticaria, or bronchospasms.

• Give inhalants cautiously to patients with heart disease because these drugs may potentiate coronary insufficiency, cardiac arrhythmias, or hypertension. If paradoxical bronchospasm occurs, stop the drug and use a different drug.

• If the patient is prescribed a bronchodilator and a corticosteroid, give the bronchodilator first so the air passages can open fully before the patient uses the corticosteroid.

• Instruct the patient to keep an extra inhaler handy.

• Instruct the patient to discard the inhaler after taking the prescribed number of doses and to then start a new inhaler.

• Urge the patient to notify his prescriber if he notices an increased use of or need for an inhaler or his symptoms are not relieved with the prescribed regimen.

Nasogastric administration

Besides providing an alternative means of nourishment for patients who can't eat normally, an NG tube allows for the instillation of drugs directly into the GI system.

Equipment and preparation

• Check the chart and the medication administration record.

• Gather equipment for use at the bedside, including prescribed drug, towel or linen-saver pad, 50- or 60-ml piston-type catheter-tip syringe, feeding tubing, two 4″ × 4″ gauze pads, stethoscope, gloves, diluent (juice, water, or a nutritional supplement), cup for mixing drug and fluid, spoon, 50-ml cup of water, and rubber band. You may also need pill-crushing equipment and a clamp, if it's not already attached to the tube.

• Make sure that liquids are at room temperature to avoid abdominal cramping and that the cup, syringe, spoon, and gauze are clean.

Implementation

• Wash your hands and put on gloves.

• Confirm the patient's identity by asking his full name and checking the name and medical record number on his wristband.

• Unpin the tube from the patient's gown. To avoid soiling the sheets during the procedure, fold back the bed linens and drape the patient's chest with a towel or linen-saver pad.

• Help the patient into Fowler's position, if his condition allows.

• After unclamping the tube, auscultate the patient's abdomen about 3″ (8 cm) below the sternum as you gently insert 10 ml of air into the tube with the 50- or 60-ml syringe. You should hear the air bubble entering the stomach. Gently draw back on the piston of the syringe. The appearance of gastric contents indicates that the tube is patent and is properly placed in the stomach.

• If no gastric contents appear or if you meet resistance, the tube may be lying against the gastric mucosa. Withdraw the tube slightly or turn the patient to free it.

• Clamp the tube, detach the syringe, and lay the end of the tube on the 4″ × 4″ gauze pad.

• If the drug is in tablet form, crush it before mixing it with the diluent. Make sure the particles are small enough to pass through the eyes at the distal end of the tube. Keep in mind that some drugs (extended release, enteric-coated, or S.L. drugs, for example) shouldn't be crushed. Ask a pharmacist if you aren't sure. Also, check to see if the drug comes in liquid form or if a capsule form may be opened and the contents poured into a diluent. Pour liquid drugs into the diluent and stir well.

• Reattach the syringe, without the piston, to the end of the tube. Holding the tube upright at a level slightly above the patient's nose, open the clamp and pour the drug in slowly and steadily, as shown below.

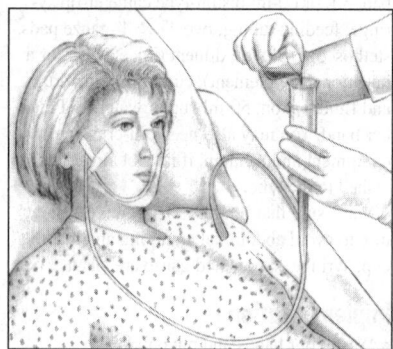

• To keep air from entering the patient's stomach, hold the tube at a slight angle and add more drug before the syringe empties. If the drug flows smoothly, slowly give the entire

dose. If it doesn't flow, it may be too thick. If so, dilute it with water. If you suspect that tube placement is inhibiting flow, stop the procedure and reevaluate the placement.

• Watch the patient's reaction. Stop immediately if you see signs of discomfort.

• As the last of the drug flows out of the syringe, start to irrigate the tube by adding 30 to 50 ml of water (15 to 30 ml for a child). Irrigating clears drug from the tube and reduces the risk of clogging.

• When the water stops flowing, clamp the tube. Detach the syringe, and discard it properly.

• Fasten the tube to the patient's gown, and make the patient comfortable.

• Leave the patient in Fowler's position or on his right side with his head partially elevated for at least 30 minutes to facilitate flow and prevent esophageal reflux.

• Remove and discard your gloves, and wash your hands.

Nursing considerations

• If you must give a tube feeding as well as instill a drug, give the drug first to make sure the patient receives the entire drug.

• Certain drugs—such as phenytoin (Dilantin)—bind with tube feedings, decreasing the availability of the drug. Stop the tube feeding for 2 hours before and after the dose, according to your facility's policy.

• If residual stomach contents exceed 150 ml, withhold the drug and feeding, and notify the prescriber. Excessive stomach contents may indicate intestinal obstruction or paralytic ileus.

• Never crush enteric-coated, buccal, S.L., or sustained-release drugs.

• If the NG tube is on suction, turn it off for 20 to 30 minutes after giving a drug.

Otic administration

Eardrops may be instilled to treat infection and inflammation, to soften cerumen for later removal, to produce local anesthesia, or to facilitate removal of an insect trapped in the ear.

Equipment and preparation

• Check the chart and the medication administration record.

• Gather the eardrops, some gloves, a light, and facial tissue or cotton-tipped applicators. Cotton balls and a bowl of warm water may be needed, as well.

• First, warm the drug to body temperature in the bowl of warm water, or carry the drug in your pocket for 30 minutes before giving. If necessary, test the temperature of the drug by placing a drop on your wrist because if the drug is too hot, it may burn the patient's eardrum.

• To avoid injuring the ear canal, check the dropper before use to make sure it's not chipped or cracked.

Implementation

• Wash your hands and put on gloves.

• Confirm the patient's identity by asking his full name and checking the name and medical record number on his wristband.

• Have the patient lie on the side opposite from the affected ear.

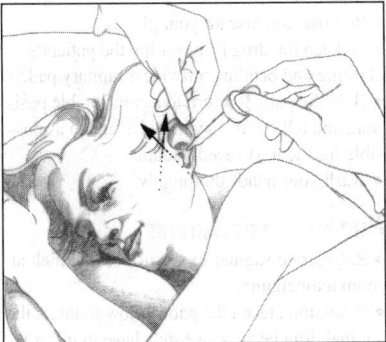

• Straighten the patient's ear canal. For an adult, pull the auricle up and back. For a child under age 3, gently pull the auricle down and back because the ear canal is straighter at this age.

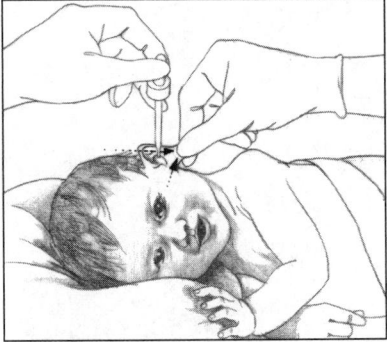

• Using a light, examine the ear canal for drainage. If you see drainage, gently clean the canal with the tissue or cotton-tipped applicators because drainage can reduce the effectiveness of the drug. Never insert an applicator past the point where you can see it.

• Compare the label on the eardrops to the order on the patient's medication record. Check the label again while drawing the drug into the dropper. Check the label for the final time before giving the eardrops.

• Straighten the patient's ear canal once again, and instill the proper number of drops. To avoid patient discomfort, aim the dropper so that the drops fall against the sides of the ear canal, not on the eardrum. Hold the ear canal in position until you see the drug disappear down the canal. Then release the ear.

• To avoid damaging the ear canal with the dropper, especially with a struggling child, it may be necessary to gently rest the hand that is holding the dropper against the patient's head to secure a safe position before giving the drug.

• Instruct the patient to remain on his side for 5 to 10 minutes to allow the drug to run down into the ear canal.

• Tuck a cotton ball with a small amount of petroleum jelly on it loosely into the opening of the ear canal to prevent the drug from leaking out. Be careful not to insert it too deeply into the canal because doing so may prevent secretions from draining and increase pressure on the eardrum.

• Clean and dry the outer ear.

• If needed, repeat the procedure in the other ear after 5 to 10 minutes.

• Help the patient into a comfortable position.

• Remove your gloves and wash your hands.

Nursing considerations

• Some conditions make the normally tender ear canal even more sensitive, so be especially gentle.

• To prevent injury to the eardrum, never insert a cotton-tipped applicator into the ear canal past the point where you can see the tip.

• After instilling eardrops to soften cerumen, irrigate the ear to facilitate its removal. If the patient has vertigo, keep the side rails of his bed up and assist him as needed during the procedure. Also, move slowly to avoid worsening his vertigo.

• If necessary, teach the patient to instill the eardrops himself so that he can continue treatment at home. Review the procedure, and let the patient try it himself while you observe.

Vaginal administration

Vaginal drugs can be inserted as topical treatment for infection, particularly *Trichomonas vaginalis* and vaginal candidiasis or inflammation. Suppositories melt when they contact the vaginal mucosa, and the drug diffuses topically.

Vaginal drugs usually come with a disposable applicator that enables placement of drug in the anterior and posterior fornices. Vaginal administration is most effective when the patient can remain lying down afterward to retain the drug.

Equipment and preparation

• Check the chart and the medication administration record.
• Gather the prescribed drug and applicator (if needed), gloves, water-soluble lubricant, and a small sanitary pad.

Implementation

• If possible, give vaginal drugs h.s. when the patient is lying down.
• Confirm the patient's identity by asking her full name and checking the name and medical record number on her wristband.
• Wash your hands, explain the procedure to the patient, and provide privacy.
• Ask the patient to void.
• Ask the patient if she would rather insert the drug herself. If so, provide appropriate instructions. If not, proceed with the following steps.
• Help her into the lithotomy position. Drape the patient, exposing only the perineum.
• Remove the suppository from the wrapper and lubricate it with water-soluble lubricant.
• Put on gloves, and expose the vagina by spreading the labia. If you see discharge, wash the area with several cotton balls soaked in warm, soapy water. Clean each side of the perineum and then the center, using a fresh cotton ball for each stroke. While the labia are still separated, insert the suppository or vaginal applicator about 3″ to 4″ (7.6 to 10 cm) into the vagina.

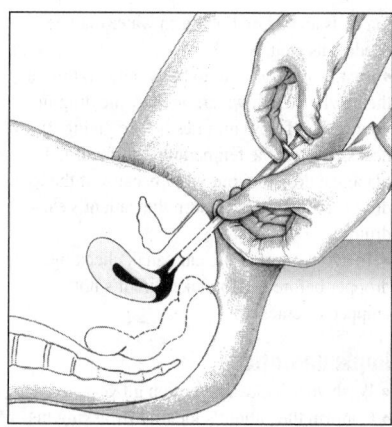

• After insertion, wash the applicator with soap and warm water, and store or discard it, as appropriate. Label it so it will be used only for one patient.
• Remove and discard your gloves.
• To keep the drug from soiling the patient's clothing and bedding, provide a sanitary pad.
• Help the patient return to a comfortable position, and tell her to stay in bed as much as possible for the next several hours.
• Wash your hands thoroughly.

Nursing considerations

• Refrigerate vaginal suppositories that melt at room temperature.
• If possible, teach the patient how to insert the vaginal drug because she may have to insert it herself after she is discharged. Give her instructions in writing, if possible.
• Instruct the patient not to insert a tampon after inserting a vaginal drug because the tampon will absorb the drug and decrease its effectiveness.

4

Avoiding medication errors

In the state where you practice nursing, a number of different health care professionals may be legally permitted to prescribe, dispense, and give medications—such as doctors, nurse practitioners, dentists, podiatrists, and optometrists. Most often, however, doctors prescribe medications, pharmacists dispense them, and nurses give them to patients.

That means you're almost always on the front line when it comes to patients and their drugs. It also means that you bear a major share of the responsibility for avoiding medication errors. Besides faithfully following your facility's drug administration policies, you can help prevent medication errors by studying and avoiding the common slip-ups that allow them to happen. This chapter outlines some common causes of medication errors.

Name game
Drugs with similar-sounding names can be easy to confuse. Even different-sounding names can look similar when written out rapidly by hand on a medication order: For example, Soriatane and Loxitane, which are both capsules. If the patient's drug order doesn't seem right for his diagnosis, call the prescriber to clarify the order.

⊛ ALERT: Many nurses have confused an order for morphine with one for hydromorphone (Dilaudid). Both drugs come in 4-mg prefilled syringes. If you give morphine when the prescriber really ordered hydromorphone, the patient could develop respiratory depression or even arrest. Consider posting a prominent notice in the place where opioids are kept that warns the staff about this common mix-up. Or, try attaching a fluorescent sticker printed with NOT MORPHINE to each hydromorphone syringe.

Drug names aren't the only words you can confuse. Patient names can cause trouble as well if you fail to verify each person's identity. This problem can be especially troublesome if two patients have the same first name.

Consider this clinical scenario. Robert Brewer, age 5, was hospitalized for measles. Robert Brinson, also age 5, was admitted after a severe asthma attack. The boys were assigned to adjacent rooms on a small pediatric unit. Each had a nonproductive cough. When Robert Brewer's nurse came to give him an expectorant, the child's mother told her that Robert had already inhaled a medication through a mask.

The nurse quickly figured out that another nurse, new to the unit, had given Robert Brinson's medication (acetylcysteine, a mucolytic) to Robert Brewer in error. Fortunately, no harmful adverse effects arose. Had the nurse checked her patient's identity more carefully, however, the error wouldn't have occurred.

Always check each patient's full name. Also, teach each patient (or parent) to offer an identification bracelet for inspection and to state his full name when anyone enters the room with the intention of giving a medication. (See *Reducing medication errors through patient teaching, page 32.*) Also, urge patients to tell you if an identification bracelet falls off, is removed, or gets lost. Replace it right away.

Allergy alert
Once you've verified your patient's full name, check to see if he is wearing an allergy bracelet. If the patient is wearing an allergy bracelet, the allergy bracelet should have the name of the allergen conspicuously written on it. The allergy information also should be labeled on the front of the patient's chart and on his medication record. Whether the patient is wearing an allergy bracelet or not, take the time to double check and ask the patient whether he has any drug allergies—even if he's in distress. Consider this real-life example.

A doctor issued a stat order for chlorpromazine (Thorazine) for a distressed patient. By the time the nurse arrived with the drug, the patient had grown more distressed and was demanding relief. Unnerved by the patient's demeanor, the nurse gave the drug without checking the patient's medication administration record or documenting the order—and the patient had an allergic reaction to it.

Any time you're in a tense situation with a patient who needs or wants medication fast, re-

Reducing medication errors through patient teaching

You aren't the only one who's at risk for making medication errors. Patients are at an even higher risk because they know so much less about drugs than you do. Although inpatient deaths from medication errors rose more than twofold from 1983 to 1993, outpatient deaths rose more than eightfold. Clearly, patient teaching is a crucial aspect of your nursing responsibility in minimizing medication errors and their consequences—especially with more patients receiving outpatient instead of inpatient care.

To help minimize medication errors, teach your patient about his diagnosis and the purpose of his drug therapy. Make sure he knows the name of each drug in his regimen, what each drug is for, how much of each drug he's supposed to take, and when and how he's supposed to take it. Use an interpreter if he doesn't speak English. Ideally, the patient should go home with his drug information in clear and legible writing. Explaining the drug therapy regimen to the patient's family and others closely involved with his care also helps to reduce drug errors.

Remember that some types of drug therapy can be quite confusing for patients. One patient who went home with a warfarin prescription took the 2.5 and 5 mg tablets at the same time rather than 2.5 and 5 mg on alternating days. He eventually was hospitalized with GI bleeding—a problem that might have been avoided had he better understood his dosage regimen. Likewise, any regimen that requires a patient to take more than one drug greatly increases the complexity of the therapy and the chance of confusion and drug errors. The patient may need special help to establish a practical, workable dosing schedule.

Also, ask if your patient takes over-the-counter drugs at home in addition to his prescribed drugs. Make a special point of asking about herbal remedies and other nutritional supplements. Some herbal remedies have drug-like effects and can cause or contribute to a drug-related problem. What's more, because these preparations aren't regulated like drugs are, government assurance standards don't apply to their labeling or manufacturing, and their ingredients can be misrepresented, substituted, or contaminated.

Finally, tell your patient which kinds of drug-related problems warrant a call to his prescriber. Encourage him to report anything about his drug therapy that concerns or worries him.

---

sist the temptation to act first and document later. Skipping that crucial assessment step could easily lead to a medication error.

⊛ **ALERT:** A patient who is severely allergic to peanuts could have an anaphylactic reaction to ipratropium bromide (Atrovent) aerosol given by metered-dose inhaler. Ask your patient or his parents whether he's allergic to peanuts before you give this drug. If you find that he has such an allergy, you'll need to use the nasal spray and inhalation solution form of the drug. Because it doesn't contain soy lecithin, it's safe for patients allergic to peanuts.

Compound errors

Many medication errors stem from compound problems—a mistake that could have been caught at any of several steps along the way. For a drug to be given correctly, each member of the health care team must fulfill the appropriate role. The prescriber must write the order correctly and legibly. The pharmacist must evaluate whether the order is appropriate and then fill it correctly. And the nurse must evaluate whether the order is appropriate and then give it correctly.

A breakdown anywhere along this chain of events easily can lead to a medication error. That's why it's so important for members of the health care team to act as a real team, so they can check each other and catch any problems that might arise before those problems affect the patient's health. Do your best to foster an environment in which professionals can double-check each other.

For instance, the pharmacist can help clarify the number of times a drug should be given each day. He can help you label drugs in the most appropriate way. He can remind you to always return unused or discontinued medications to the pharmacy.

You can—indeed, you must—clarify any prescriber's order that doesn't seem clear or correct. You also must correctly handle and store any multidose vials obtained from the pharmacist. Only give drugs that you've prepared personally. And never give a drug that has an ambiguous label or no label at all. Here's an actual example of what could happen if you do.

A nurse placed an unlabeled cup of phenol (used in neurolytic procedures) next to a cup of guanethidine (a postganglionic-blocking drug). The doctor accidentally injected the phenol instead of the guanethidine, causing severe tissue damage to a patient's arm. The patient needed emergency surgery and later developed neurologic complications as a result of receiving the wrong and unlabeled injection.

Obviously, this was a compound problem. The nurse should have labeled each cup clearly, and the doctor shouldn't have given an unlabeled drug to a patient.

Here's another example of a compound problem: In the neonatal intensive care unit, a nurse prepared and gave a dose of aminophylline to an infant. He didn't have anyone else check his work. After receiving the drug, the infant developed tachycardia and other signs of theophylline toxicity. She later died. The nurse thought the order read 7.4 ml of aminophylline; instead, it read 7.4 mg.

This tragedy might have been avoided if the doctor had written a clearer order, if the nurse had clarified the order, if a pharmacist had prepared and dispensed the drug, or if another nurse had checked the dose calculation. To help prevent such problems, many facilities require that a pharmacist prepare and dispense non-emergency parenteral doses whenever commercial unit doses aren't available.

Here's another example: A container of 5% acetic acid, used to clean tracheostomy tubing, was left near nebulization equipment in the room of a 10-month-old infant. A respiratory therapist mistook the liquid for normal saline solution and used it to dilute albuterol for the child's nebulizer treatment. During treatment, the child experienced bronchospasm, hypercapnic dyspnea, tachypnea, and tachycardia.

Leaving dangerous chemicals near patients is extremely risky, especially when the container labels don't warn of toxicity. To prevent such problems, read the label on every drug you prepare, and never give any drug that isn't labeled or is labeled poorly.

Route trouble

Many drug errors stem at least in part from problems related to the route of administration. The risk of error increases when a patient has several lines running for different purposes. Consider this example:

A nurse prepared a dose of digoxin elixir for a patient who had both a central intravenous (I.V.) line and a jejunostomy tube. She mistakenly gave the drug into the central I.V. line. Fortunately, the patient had no adverse reaction. To help prevent such mix-ups in route of administration, prepare all oral medications in a syringe that has a tip small enough to fit an abdominal tube but too big to fit a central line.

Here's another error that could have been avoided: To clear air bubbles from a 9-year-old patient's insulin infusion, a nurse disconnected the tubing and raised the pump rate to 200 ml/hour to flush the bubbles through quickly. She then reconnected the tubing and restarted the infusion, but she forgot to reset the drip rate back to 2 units/hour. The child received 50 units of insulin before the error was detected. To prevent this kind of error, never increase a drip rate to clear bubbles from a line. Instead, remove the tubing from the pump, disconnect it from the patient, and use the flow-control clamp to establish gravity flow.

Risky abbreviations

Abbreviating drug names is risky, as in this example. Cancer patients with anemia may receive epoetin alfa, commonly abbreviated EPO, to stimulate red blood cell production. In one case, when a cancer patient was admitted to a hospital, the doctor wrote, "May take own supply of EPO." However, the patient wasn't anemic. Sensing that something was wrong, the pharmacist interviewed the patient, who confirmed that he was taking "EPO," or evening primrose oil, to lower his cholesterol level. Ask all prescribers to spell out drug names.

Unclear orders

A patient was supposed to receive one dose of the antineoplastic lomustine to treat brain cancer. (Lomustine typically is given as a single oral dose once every 6 weeks.) The doctor's order read, "Administer h.s." Because a nurse misinterpreted the order to mean every night, the patient received nine daily doses, developed severe thrombocytopenia and leukopenia, and died.

If you're unfamiliar with a drug, check a drug book before giving it. If a prescriber uses "h.s." but doesn't specify the frequency of administration, ask him to clarify the order.

When documenting orders, note "h.s. nightly" or "h.s. one dose today."

Color changes

In two reports, alert nurses noticed that antineoplastics prepared in the pharmacy didn't look the way they should. The first error involved a 6-year-old child who was to receive 12 mg of methotrexate intrathecally. In the pharmacy, a 1-g vial was mistakenly selected instead of a 20-mg vial, and the drug was reconstituted with 10 ml of normal saline. The vial containing 100 mg/ml was incorrectly labeled as containing 2 mg/ml, and 6 ml of the solution was drawn into a syringe. Although the syringe label indicated 12 mg of drug, the syringe actually contained 600 mg of drug.

When the nurse received the syringe and noted that the drug's color didn't appear right, she returned it to the pharmacy for verification. The pharmacist retrieved the vial used to prepare the dose and drew the remaining solution into another syringe. The solutions in both syringes matched, and no one noticed the vial's 1-g label. The pharmacist concluded that a manufacturing change caused the color difference.

The child received the 600-mg dose and experienced seizures 45 minutes later. A pharmacist responding to the emergency detected the error. The child received an antidote and recovered.

A similar case involved a 20-year-old patient with leukemia who received mitomycin instead of mitoxantrone. The nurse had questioned the drug's unusual bluish tint, but the pharmacist assured her that the color difference was due to a change in manufacturer. Fortunately, the patient didn't suffer any harm.

If a familiar drug seems to have an unfamiliar appearance, investigate the cause. If the pharmacist cites a manufacturing change, ask him to double-check whether he has received verification from the manufacturer. Always document the appearance discrepancy, your actions, and the pharmacist's response in the patient record.

Stress levels

A nurse-anesthetist gave the sedative midazolam (Versed) to the wrong patient. When she discovered the error, she reached for what she thought was a vial of the antidote flumazenil (Romazicon), withdrew 2.5 ml of the drug, and gave it. When the patient didn't respond, she realized she'd reached for a vial of ondansetron (Zofran), an antiemetic, instead. Another practitioner assisted with proper I.V. administration of flumazenil, and the patient recovered without harm.

Committing a serious error can cause enormous stress and cloud your judgment. If you're involved in a drug error, ask another professional to give the antidote.

Clearly, you carry a great deal of responsibility for making sure that the right patient gets the right drug in the right concentration at the right time by the right route. By staying aware of potential trouble spots, you can minimize your risk of making medication errors and maximize the therapeutic effects of your patients' drug regimens.

Drug
Classifications

Alkylating drugs

altretamine
busulfan
carboplatin
carmustine
chlorambucil
cisplatin
cyclophosphamide
dacarbazine
ifosfamide
lomustine
mechlorethamine hydrochloride
melphalan
thiotepa

Indications

▶ Various tumors, especially those having large volume and slow cell-turnover rate.

Contraindications and precautions

• Contraindicated in patients hypersensitive to these drugs.
• Use cautiously in patients receiving other cell-destroying drugs or radiation therapy.
≋ Lifespan: Alkylating drugs appear in breast milk. Instruct women to stop breast-feeding during therapy to avoid possible adverse effects in their infants. In children, safety and effectiveness of many alkylating drugs haven't been established. Geriatric patients have an increased risk of adverse reactions; monitor them closely.

Adverse reactions

The most common adverse reactions are bone marrow depression, leukopenia, thrombocytopenia, fever, chills, sore throat, nausea, vomiting, diarrhea, flank or joint pain, anxiety, swelling of feet or lower legs, hair loss, and redness or pain at injection site.

Action

Alkylating drugs appear to act independently of a specific cell-cycle phase. They are polyfunctional compounds that can be divided chemically into five groups: nitrogen mustards, ethylenimines, alkyl sulfonates, triazines, and nitrosoureas. Highly reactive, these drugs primarily target nucleic acids and form links with the nuclei of different molecules. This allows the drugs to cross-link double-stranded DNA

and to prevent strands from separating for replication, which may contribute to these drugs' ability to destroy cells.

NURSING PROCESS

✏ Assessment
• Perform a complete assessment before therapy begins.
• Monitor patient for adverse reactions throughout therapy.
• Monitor hematocrit, platelet and total and differential leukocyte counts, and BUN, ALT, AST, LDH, bilirubin, creatinine, uric acid, and other levels as needed.
• Monitor vital signs and patency of catheter or I.V. line throughout administration.

⊕ Key nursing diagnoses
• Ineffective protection related to thrombocytopenia
• Risk for infection related to immunosuppression
• Risk for deficient fluid volume related to adverse GI effects

▷ Planning and implementation
• Follow established procedures for safe and proper handling, administration, and disposal of chemotherapeutic drugs.
• Treat extravasation promptly.
• While giving carboplatin or cisplatin, keep epinephrine, corticosteroids, and antihistamines available. Anaphylactoid reactions may occur.
• Give ifosfamide with mesna to prevent hemorrhagic cystitis.
• Give lomustine 2 to 4 hours after meals. Nausea and vomiting usually last less than 24 hours, although loss of appetite may last for several days.
• Maintain adequate hydration before and for 24 hours after cisplatin treatment.
• Be aware that allopurinol may be prescribed to prevent drug-induced hyperuricemia.
Patient teaching
• Tell patient to avoid people with bacterial or viral infections because chemotherapy can increase susceptibility. Urge him to report signs of infection promptly.
• Review proper oral hygiene, including cautious use of toothbrush, dental floss, and toothpicks.

• Advise patient to complete dental work before therapy begins or to delay it until blood counts are normal.
• Warn patient that he may bruise easily because of drug's effect on blood count.

☑ Evaluation
• Patient develops no serious bleeding complications.
• Patient remains free from infection.
• Patient maintains adequate hydration.

Alpha-adrenergic blockers (peripherally-acting)

doxazosin mesylate (non-selective)
prazosin hydrochloride (non-selective)
tamsulosin hydrochloride (selective)
terazosin hydrochloride (non-selective)

Indications

▶ Mild to moderate urinary obstruction in men with BPH, hypertension.

Contraindications and precautions

• Contraindicated in patients with MI, coronary insufficiency, or angina or with hypersensitivity to these drugs or any of their components.
⚖ **Lifespan:** In pregnant or breast-feeding women, use cautiously. In children, safety and effectiveness of many alpha-adrenergic blockers haven't been established; use cautiously. In elderly patients, hypotensive effects may be more pronounced.

Adverse reactions

Alpha-adrenergic blockers may cause severe orthostatic hypotension and syncope, especially with the first few doses—often called the "first-dose effect." The most common adverse effects of alpha$_1$ blockade are dizziness, headache, drowsiness, somnolence, and malaise. These drugs also may cause orthostatic hypotension, tachycardia, palpitations, fluid retention (from excess renin secretion), nasal and ocular congestion, and aggravation of respiratory tract infection.

Action

Selective alpha-adrenergic blockers have readily observable effects. They decrease vascular resistance and increase vein capacity, thereby lowering blood pressure and causing nasal and scleroconjunctival congestion, ptosis, orthostatic and exercise hypotension, mild to moderate miosis, interference with ejaculation, and pink, warm skin. They also relax nonvascular smooth muscle, especially in the prostate capsule, which reduces urinary problems in men with BPH. Because alpha$_1$ blockers don't block alpha$_2$ receptors, they don't cause transmitter overflow.

Nonselective alpha-adrenergic blockers antagonize both alpha$_1$ and alpha$_2$ receptors. Generally, alpha-adrenergic blockade results in tachycardia, palpitations, and increased renin secretion because of abnormally large amounts of norepinephrine (because of transmitter overflow) released from adrenergic nerve endings as a result of the blockade of alpha$_1$ and alpha$_2$ receptors. Norepinephrine's effects are counterproductive to the major uses of nonselective alpha-adrenergic blockers.

NURSING PROCESS

☑ Assessment
• Monitor vital signs, especially blood pressure.
• Monitor patient closely for adverse reactions.

☑ Key nursing diagnoses
• Decreased cardiac output related to hypotension
• Acute pain related to headache
• Excessive fluid volume related to fluid retention

☑ Planning and implementation
• Give at bedtime to minimize dizziness or light-headedness.
• Begin therapy with small dose to avoid first-dose syncope.
Patient teaching
• Warn patient not to rise suddenly from a lying or sitting position.
• Urge patient to avoid hazardous tasks that require mental alertness until the full effects of drug are known.
• Advise patient that alcohol, excessive exercise, prolonged standing, and heat exposure will intensify adverse effects.

• Tell patient to promptly report dizziness or irregular heartbeat.

☑ Evaluation
• Patient maintains adequate cardiac output.
• Patient's headache is relieved.
• Patient has no edema.

Aminoglycosides
amikacin sulfate
gentamicin sulfate
neomycin sulfate
streptomycin sulfate
tobramycin sulfate

Indications

▶ Septicemia; postoperative, pulmonary, intra-abdominal, and urinary tract infections; skin, soft tissue, bone, and joint infections; aerobic gram-negative bacillary meningitis that is not susceptible to other antibiotics; serious staphylococcal, *Pseudomonas aeruginosa,* and *Klebsiella* infections; enterococcal infections; nosocomial pneumonia; anaerobic infections involving *Bacteroides fragilis;* tuberculosis; initial empiric therapy in febrile, leukopenic patient.

Contraindications and precautions

• Contraindicated in patients hypersensitive to these drugs.
• Use cautiously in patients with a neuromuscular disorder and in those taking neuromuscular blockades.
• Use at reduced dosages in patients with renal impairment.
⚖ Lifespan: In pregnant women, use cautiously. In breast-feeding women, safety hasn't been established. In neonates and premature infants, the half-life of aminoglycosides is prolonged because of their immature renal systems. In infants and children, dosage adjustment may be needed. Geriatric patients have an increased risk of nephrotoxicity and commonly need reduced dosages and longer dosing intervals; they're also susceptible to ototoxicity and superinfection.

Adverse reactions
Ototoxicity and nephrotoxicity are the most serious complications. Neuromuscular blockade also may occur. Oral forms most commonly cause nausea, vomiting, and diarrhea. Parenteral drugs may cause vein irritation, phlebitis, and sterile abscess.

Action
Aminoglycosides are bactericidal. They bind directly and irreversibly to 30S ribosomal subunits, inhibiting bacterial protein synthesis. They're active against many aerobic gram-negative and some aerobic gram-positive organisms.

NURSING PROCESS

⚐ Assessment
• Obtain patient's history of allergies.
• Monitor patient for adverse reactions.
• Obtain results of culture and sensitivity tests before first dose, and check tests periodically to assess drug effectiveness.
• Monitor vital signs, electrolyte levels, hearing ability, and renal function studies before and during therapy.
• Draw blood for peak level 1 hour after I.M. injection and 30 minutes to 1 hour after I.V. infusion; for trough level, draw sample just before next dose. Time and date all blood samples. Don't use heparinized tube to collect blood samples because it interferes with results.

⊕ Key nursing diagnoses
• Risk for injury related to nephrotoxicity and ototoxicity
• Risk for infection related to drug-induced superinfection
• Risk for deficient fluid volume related to adverse GI reactions

▶ Planning and implementation
• Keep patient hydrated to minimize chemical irritation of renal tubules.
• Don't add or mix other drugs with I.V. infusions, particularly penicillins, which inactivate aminoglycosides. If other drugs must be given I.V., temporarily stop infusion of primary drug.
• Follow manufacturer's instructions for reconstitution, dilution, and storage of drugs; check expiration dates.
• Shake oral suspensions well before giving.

• Give I.M. dose deep into the gluteal muscles mass or midlateral thigh; rotate injection sites to minimize tissue injury. Apply ice to injection site to relieve pain.

• Giving I.V. dose too rapidly may cause neuromuscular blockade. Infuse I.V. dose continuously or intermittently over 30 to 60 minutes for adults, 1 to 2 hours for infants; dilution volume for children is determined individually.

Patient teaching

• Teach signs and symptoms of hypersensitivity and other adverse reactions. Urge patient to report unusual effects promptly.

• Emphasize importance of adequate fluid intake.

☑ Evaluation

• Patient maintains pretreatment renal and hearing functions.

• Patient is free from infection.

• Patient maintains adequate hydration.

Angiotensin-converting enzyme inhibitors

benazepril hydrochloride
captopril
enalapril maleate
fosinopril sodium
lisinopril
moexipril hydrochloride
perindopril erbumine
quinapril hydrochloride
ramipril
trandolapril

Indications

▶ Hypertension, heart failure, left ventricular dysfunction (LVD), MI (with ramipril and lisinopril), and diabetic nephropathy (with captopril).

Contraindications and precautions

• Contraindicated in patients hypersensitive to these drugs.

• Use cautiously in patients with impaired renal function or serious autoimmune disease and in those taking other drugs known to decrease WBC count or immune response.

☀ **Lifespan:** Women of childbearing age taking ACE inhibitors should report suspected pregnancy immediately to prescriber. High risks of fetal morbidity and mortality are linked to ACE inhibitors, especially in the second and third trimesters. Some ACE inhibitors appear in breast milk. To avoid adverse effects in infants, instruct patient to stop breast-feeding during therapy. In children, safety and effectiveness haven't been established; give drug only if potential benefit outweighs risk. Geriatric patients may need lower doses because of impaired drug clearance.

Adverse reactions

The most common adverse effects of therapeutic doses are headache, fatigue, hypotension, tachycardia, dysgeusia, proteinuria, hyperkalemia, rash, cough, and angioedema of face and limbs. Severe hypotension may occur at toxic drug levels.

Action

ACE inhibitors prevent conversion of angiotensin I to angiotensin II, a potent vasoconstrictor. Besides decreasing vasoconstriction and thus reducing peripheral arterial resistance, inhibiting angiotensin II decreases adrenocortical secretion of aldosterone. This reduces sodium and water retention and extracellular fluid volume. ACE inhibition also causes increased levels of bradykinin, which results in vasodilation. This decreases heart rate and systemic vascular resistance.

NURSING PROCESS

⚕ Assessment

• Observe patient for adverse reactions.

• Monitor vital signs regularly and WBC count and electrolyte level periodically.

⊕ Key nursing diagnoses

• Risk for trauma related to orthostatic hypotension

• Ineffective protection related to hyperkalemia

• Acute pain related to headache

▶ Planning and implementation

• Stop diuretic 2 to 3 days before beginning ACE inhibitor to reduce risk of hypotension. If drug doesn't adequately control blood pressure, diuretics may be restarted.

• Give a reduced dosage if the patient has impaired renal function.

• Give potassium supplements, and potassium-sparing diuretics cautiously because ACE inhibitors may cause potassium retention.

• Stop ACE inhibitors if patient becomes pregnant. These drugs can cause birth defects or fetal death in the second and third trimesters.

• Give captopril and moexipril 1 hour before meals.

Patient teaching

• Tell patient that drugs may cause a dry, persistent, tickling cough that stops when therapy stops.

• Urge patient to report light-headedness, especially in the first few days of therapy, so the dosage can be adjusted. Also, tell him to report signs of infection (such as sore throat and fever) because these drugs may decrease WBC count; facial swelling or difficulty breathing because these drugs may cause angioedema; and loss of taste, for which therapy may stop.

• Advise patient to avoid sudden position changes to minimize orthostatic hypotension.

• Warn patient to seek medical approval before taking self-prescribed cold preparations.

• Tell women to report pregnancy at once.

• Warn patient to use salt substitutes containing potassium cautiously because ACE inhibitors may cause potassium retention.

☑ Evaluation

• Patient sustains no injury from orthostatic hypotension.

• Patient's WBC count remains normal throughout therapy.

• Patient's headache is relieved by mild analgesic.

Antacids

aluminum hydroxide
calcium carbonate
magaldrate
magnesium hydroxide
magnesium oxide
sodium bicarbonate

Indications

▶ Hyperacidity.

Contraindications and precautions

• Calcium carbonate, magaldrate, and magnesium oxide are contraindicated in patients with severe renal disease. Sodium bicarbonate is contraindicated in patients with hypertension, renal disease, or edema; patients who are vomiting; patients receiving diuretics or continuous GI suction; and patients on sodium-restricted diets.

• In patients with mild renal impairment, give magnesium oxide cautiously.

• Give aluminum preparations, calcium carbonate, and magaldrate cautiously in elderly patients; in those receiving antidiarrheals, antispasmodics, or anticholinergics; and in those with dehydration, fluid restriction, chronic renal disease, or suspected intestinal absorption.

⚖ Lifespan: Breast-feeding women may take antacids. In infants, serious adverse effects are more likely from changes in fluid and electrolyte balance; monitor them closely. Geriatric patients have an increased risk of adverse reactions; monitor them closely; also, give these patients aluminum preparations, calcium carbonate, magaldrate, and magnesium oxide cautiously.

Adverse reactions

Antacids containing aluminum may cause aluminum intoxication, constipation, hypophosphatemia, intestinal obstruction, and osteomalacia. Antacids containing magnesium may cause diarrhea or hypermagnesemia (in renal failure). Calcium carbonate, magaldrate, magnesium oxide, and sodium bicarbonate may cause milk-alkali syndrome or rebound hyperacidity.

Action

Antacids reduce the total acid load in the GI tract and elevate gastric pH to reduce pepsin activity. They also strengthen the gastric mucosal barrier and increase esophageal sphincter tone.

NURSING PROCESS

☑ Assessment

• Assess patient's condition before therapy and regularly thereafter.

• Record number and consistency of stools.

• Observe patient for adverse reactions.

• Monitor patient receiving long-term, high-dose aluminum carbonate and hydroxide for fluid and electrolyte imbalance, especially if patient is on a sodium-restricted diet.
• Monitor phosphate level in a patient taking aluminum carbonate or hydroxide.
• Watch for signs of hypercalcemia in a patient taking calcium carbonate.
• Monitor magnesium level in a patient with mild renal impairment who takes magaldrate.

▣ Key nursing diagnoses
• Constipation related to adverse effects of aluminum-containing antacid
• Diarrhea related to adverse effects of magnesium-containing antacid
• Ineffective protection related to drug-induced electrolyte imbalance

▶ Planning and implementation
• Manage constipation with laxatives or stool softeners, or switch patient to a magnesium preparation.
• If patient suffers from diarrhea, give an anti-diarrheal, and switch patient to an antacid containing aluminum.
• Shake container well, and give with small amount of water or juice to facilitate passage. When giving through an NG tube, make sure the tube is patent and placed correctly. After instilling the drug, flush the tube with water to ensure passage to the stomach and to clear the tube.
Patient teaching
• Warn patient not to take antacids randomly or to switch antacids without prescriber's consent.
• Tell patient not to take calcium carbonate with milk or other foods high in vitamin D.
• Warn patient not to take sodium bicarbonate with milk because doing so could cause hypercalcemia.

☑ Evaluation
• Patient regains normal bowel pattern.
• Patient states that diarrhea is relieved.
• Patient maintains normal electrolyte balance.

Antianginals
Beta blockers
atenolol
metoprolol
nadolol
propranolol hydrochloride
Calcium channel blockers
amlodipine besylate
diltiazem hydrochloride
nicardipine hydrochloride
nifedipine
verapamil hydrochloride
Nitrates
isosorbide dinitrate
isosorbide mononitrate
nitroglycerin

Indications

▶ Moderate to severe angina (beta blockers); classic, effort-induced angina and Prinzmetal's angina (calcium channel blockers); recurrent angina (long-acting nitrates and topical, transdermal, transmucosal, and oral extended-release nitroglycerin); acute angina (S.L. nitroglycerin and S.L. or chewable isosorbide dinitrate); unstable angina (I.V. nitroglycerin).

Contraindications and precautions

• Beta blockers are contraindicated in patients hypersensitive to them and in patients with cardiogenic shock, sinus bradycardia, heart block greater than first degree, bronchial asthma, or heart failure unless failure results from tachyarrhythmia that is treatable with propranolol. Calcium channel blockers are contraindicated in patients with severe hypotension or heart block greater than first degree (except with functioning pacemaker). Nitrates are contraindicated in patients with severe anemia, cerebral hemorrhage, head trauma, glaucoma, or hyperthyroidism.
• Use beta blockers cautiously in patients with nonallergic bronchospastic disorders, diabetes mellitus, or impaired hepatic or renal function. Use calcium channel blockers cautiously in patients with hepatic or renal impairment, bradycardia, heart failure, or cardiogenic shock. Use nitrates cautiously in patients with hypotension or recent MI.

⚖ **Lifespan:** In pregnant women, use beta blockers cautiously. Recommendations for breast-feeding vary by drug; use beta blockers and calcium channel blockers cautiously. In children, safety and effectiveness haven't been established. Check with prescriber before giving these drugs to children. Geriatric patients have an increased risk of adverse reactions; use cautiously.

Adverse reactions

Beta blockers may cause bradycardia, heart failure, cough, diarrhea, disturbing dreams, dizziness, dyspnea, fatigue, fever, hypotension, lethargy, nausea, peripheral edema, and wheezing. Calcium channel blockers may cause bradycardia, confusion, constipation, depression, diarrhea, dizziness, edema, elevated liver enzyme levels (transient), fatigue, flushing, headache, hypotension, insomnia, nervousness, and rash. Nitrates may cause alcohol intoxication (from I.V. preparations containing alcohol), flushing, headache, orthostatic hypotension, reflex tachycardia, rash, syncope, and vomiting.

Action

Beta blockers decrease catecholamine-induced increases in heart rate, blood pressure, and myocardial contraction. Calcium channel blockers inhibit the flow of calcium through muscle cells, which dilates coronary arteries and decreases systemic vascular resistance, known as afterload. Nitrates decrease afterload and left ventricular end-diastolic pressure, or preload, and increase blood flow through collateral coronary vessels.

NURSING PROCESS

⚕ **Assessment**
● Monitor vital signs. With I.V. nitroglycerin, monitor blood pressure and pulse rate every 5 to 15 minutes while adjusting dosage and every hour thereafter.
● Monitor the effectiveness of the drug.
● Observe patient for adverse reactions.

⊕ **Key nursing diagnoses**
● Risk for injury related to adverse reactions
● Excessive fluid volume related to adverse CV effects of beta blockers or calcium channel blockers
● Acute pain related to headache

▷ **Planning and implementation**
● Have patient sit or lie down when receiving the first nitrate dose; take his pulse and blood pressure before giving dose and when drug action starts.
● Don't give a beta blocker or calcium channel blocker to relieve acute angina.
● Withhold the dose and notify prescriber if patient's heart rate is slower than 60 beats/ minute or systolic blood pressure is lower than 90 mm Hg.
Patient teaching
● Warn patient not to stop drug abruptly without prescriber's approval.
● Teach patient to take his pulse before taking a beta blocker or calcium channel blocker. Tell him to withhold the dose and alert the prescriber if his pulse rate is slower than 60 beats/ minute.
● Instruct patient taking nitroglycerin S.L. to go to the emergency department if three tablets taken 5 minutes apart don't relieve angina.
● Tell patient to report serious or persistent adverse reactions.

☑ **Evaluation**
● Patient sustains no injury from adverse reactions.
● Patient maintains normal fluid balance.
● Patient's headache is relieved with mild analgesic.

Antiarrhythmics
Class Ia
disopyramide
moricizine hydrochloride
procainamide hydrochloride
quinidine bisulfate
quinidine gluconate
quinidine sulfate
Class Ib
lidocaine hydrochloride
mexiletine hydrochloride
phenytoin sodium
tocainide hydrochloride
Class Ic
flecainide acetate
propafenone hydrochloride

Class II (beta blockers)
acebutolol
esmolol hydrochloride
propranolol hydrochloride
Class III
amiodarone hydrochloride
bretylium tosylate
dofetilide
ibutilide fumarate
sotalol hydrochloride
Class IV (calcium channel blocker)
verapamil hydrochloride

Indications

▶ Atrial and ventricular arrhythmias.

Contraindications and precautions

• Contraindicated in patients hypersensitive to these drugs.
• Many antiarrhythmics are contraindicated or require cautious use in patients with cardiogenic shock, digitalis toxicity, and second- or third-degree heart block (unless patient has a pacemaker).
⚖ Lifespan: In pregnant women, use only if the potential benefits to the mother outweigh the risks to the fetus. Many antiarrhythmics appear in breast milk. In breast-feeding women, use cautiously. In children, monitor them closely because they have an increased risk of adverse reactions. In elderly patients, use these drugs cautiously because these patients may exhibit physiologic alterations in CV system.

Adverse reactions

Most antiarrhythmics can aggravate existing arrhythmias or cause new ones. They also may produce hypersensitivity reactions; hypotension; GI problems, such as nausea, vomiting, or altered bowel elimination; and CNS disturbances, such as dizziness or fatigue. Some antiarrhythmics may worsen heart failure. Class II drugs may cause bronchoconstriction.

Action

Class I drugs reduce the inward current carried by sodium ions, which stabilizes neuronal cardiac membranes. Class Ia drugs deprss phase 0, prolong the action potential, and stabilize cardiac membranes. Class Ib drugs depress phase 0, shorten the action potential, and stabilize cardiac membranes. Class Ic drugs block the transport of sodium ions, which decreases conduction velocity but not repolarization rate. Class II drugs decrease the heart rate, myocardial contractility, blood pressure, and AV node conduction. Class III drugs prolong the action potential and refractory period. Class IV drugs decrease myocardial contractility and oxygen demand by inhibiting calcium ion influx; they also dilate coronary arteries and arterioles.

NURSING PROCESS

⚗ Assessment
• Monitor ECG continuously when therapy starts and dosage is adjusted.
• Monitor patient's vital signs frequently and assess for signs of toxicity and adverse reactions.
• Measure apical pulse rate before giving drug.
• Monitor drug level as indicated.

⊞ Key nursing diagnoses
• Decreased cardiac output related to arrhythmias or myocardial depression
• Ineffective protection related to adverse reactions
• Noncompliance related to long-term therapy

▷ Planning and implementation
• Don't crush sustained-release tablets.
• Take safety precautions if adverse CNS reactions occur.
• Notify prescriber about adverse reactions.
Patient teaching
• Stress the importance of taking drug exactly as prescribed.
• Teach patient to take his pulse before each dose. Tell him to notify prescriber if his pulse is irregular or slower than 60 beats/minute.
• Instruct patient to avoid hazardous activities that require mental alertness if adverse CNS reactions occur.
• Tell patient to limit fluid and salt intake if his prescribed drug causes fluid retention.

☑ Evaluation
• Patient maintains adequate cardiac output, as evidenced by normal vital signs and adequate tissue perfusion.
• Patient has no serious adverse reactions.
• Patient states importance of compliance with therapy.

Antibiotic antineoplastics

bleomycin sulfate
daunorubicin hydrochloride
doxorubicin hydrochloride
epirubicin hydrochloride
idarubicin hydrochloride
mitomycin
mitoxantrone hydrochloride
procarbazine hydrochloride
valrubicin

Indications

▶ Various tumors.

Contraindications and precautions

• Contraindicated in patients hypersensitive to these drugs.
☀ Lifespan: In pregnant women, avoid antineoplastics. Breast-feeding during therapy isn't recommended. In children, safety and effectiveness of some drugs haven't been established. In geriatric patients, use cautiously because they have an increased risk of adverse reactions.

Adverse reactions

The most common adverse reactions include nausea, vomiting, diarrhea, fever, chills, sore throat, anxiety, confusion, flank or joint pain, swelling of the feet or lower legs, hair loss, redness or pain at the injection site, bone marrow depression, and leukopenia.

Action

Although classified as antibiotics, these drugs destroy cells, thus ruling out their use as antimicrobials alone. They interfere with proliferation of malignant cells in several ways. Their action may be cell-cycle-phase nonspecific, cell-cycle-phase specific, or both. Some of these drugs act like alkylating drugs or antimetabolites. By binding to or complexing with DNA, antibiotic antineoplastics directly or indirectly inhibit DNA, RNA, and protein synthesis.

NURSING PROCESS

Assessment

• Perform a complete assessment before therapy begins.

• Monitor patient for adverse reactions.
• Monitor vital signs and patency of catheter or I.V. line.
• Monitor hemoglobin, hematocrit, platelet and total and differential leukocyte counts, ALT, AST, LDH, bilirubin, creatinine, uric acid, and BUN levels.
• Monitor pulmonary function tests in a patient receiving bleomycin. Assess lung function regularly.
• Monitor ECG before and during treatment with daunorubicin and doxorubicin.

Key nursing diagnoses

• Ineffective protection related to thrombocytopenia
• Risk for infection related to immunosuppression
• Risk for deficient fluid volume related to adverse GI effects

Planning and implementation

• Follow established procedures for safe and proper handling, administration, and disposal of chemotherapeutic drugs.
• Try to ease anxiety in patient and his family before treatment.
• Keep epinephrine, corticosteroids, and antihistamines available during bleomycin therapy. Anaphylactoid reactions may occur.
• Treat extravasation promptly.
• Ensure adequate hydration during idarubicin therapy.
• Stop procarbazine and notify prescriber if patient becomes confused or neuropathies develop.

Patient teaching
• Warn patient to avoid close contact with persons who have received the oral poliovirus vaccine.
• Advise patient to avoid exposure to persons with bacterial or viral infections because chemotherapy increases susceptibility. Urge him to report signs of infection immediately.
• Review proper oral hygiene, including cautious use of toothbrush, dental floss, and toothpicks. Chemotherapy can increase the risk of microbial infection, delayed healing, and bleeding gums.
• Urge patient to complete dental work before therapy begins or to delay it until blood counts are normal.
• Warn patient that he may bruise easily.

• Tell patient to report redness, pain, or swelling at injection site immediately. Local tissue injury and scarring may result if I.V. infiltration occurs.
• Warn patient taking procarbazine to avoid hazardous activities that require alertness until drug's CNS effects are known. Also advise him to take procarbazine at bedtime and in divided doses to reduce nausea and vomiting.
• Advise patient taking daunorubicin, doxorubicin, or idarubicin that his urine may turn orange or red for 1 to 2 days after therapy begins.

Evaluation
• No serious bleeding complications develop.
• Patient remains free from infection.
• Patient maintains adequate hydration.

Anticholinergics

atropine sulfate
benztropine mesylate
dicyclomine hydrochloride
scopolamine
scopolamine butylbromide
scopolamine hydrobromide

Indications

▶ Prevention of motion sickness, preoperative reduction of secretions and blockage of cardiac reflexes, adjunct treatment of peptic ulcers and other GI disorders, blockage of cholinomimetic effects of cholinesterase inhibitors or other drugs, and (for benztropine) various spastic conditions, including acute dystonic reactions, muscle rigidity, parkinsonism, and extrapyramidal disorders.

Contraindications and precautions

• Contraindicated in patients hypersensitive to these drugs and in those with angle-closure glaucoma, renal or GI obstructive disease, reflux esophagitis, or myasthenia gravis.
• Use cautiously in patients with heart disease, GI infection, open-angle glaucoma, prostatic hypertrophy, hypertension, hyperthyroidism, ulcerative colitis, autonomic neuropathy, or hiatal hernia with reflux esophagitis.

Lifespan: In breast-feeding women, avoid anticholinergics because these drugs may decrease milk production, and some may appear in breast milk and may cause infant toxicity. In children, safety and effectiveness haven't been established. Patients older than age 40 may be more sensitive to these drugs. In geriatric patients, use cautiously and give a reduced dosage as indicated.

Adverse reactions

Therapeutic doses commonly cause dry mouth, decreased sweating or anhidrosis, headache, mydriasis, blurred vision, cycloplegia, urinary hesitancy and retention, constipation, palpitations, and tachycardia. These reactions usually disappear when therapy stops. Toxicity can cause signs and symptoms resembling psychosis (disorientation, confusion, hallucinations, delusions, anxiety, agitation, and restlessness); dilated, nonreactive pupils; blurred vision; hot, dry, flushed skin; dry mucous membranes; dysphagia; decreased or absent bowel sounds; urine retention; hyperthermia; tachycardia; hypertension; and increased respirations.

Action

Anticholinergics competitively antagonize the actions of acetylcholine and other cholinergic agonists at muscarinic receptors.

NURSING PROCESS

Assessment
• Monitor patient regularly for adverse reactions.
• Check vital signs at least every 4 hours.
• Measure urine output; check for urine retention.
• Assess patient for changes in vision and for signs of impending toxicity.

Key nursing diagnoses
• Urine retention related to adverse effect on bladder
• Constipation related to adverse effect on GI tract
• Acute pain related to headache

Planning and implementation
• Provide ice chips, cool drinks, or hard candy to relieve dry mouth.
• Relieve constipation with stool softeners or bulk laxatives.

• Give a mild analgesic for headache.
• Notify prescriber of urine retention, and be prepared for catheterization.

Patient teaching
• Teach patient how and when to take the drug; caution him not to take other drugs unless prescribed.
• Warn patient to avoid hazardous tasks if he experiences dizziness, drowsiness, or blurred vision. Inform him that the drug may increase his sensitivity to or intolerance of high temperatures, resulting in dizziness.
• Advise patient to avoid alcohol because it may cause additive CNS effects.
• Urge patient to drink plenty of fluids and to eat a high-fiber diet to prevent constipation.
• Tell patient to notify prescriber promptly if he experiences confusion, rapid or pounding heartbeat, dry mouth, blurred vision, rash, eye pain, significant change in urine volume, or pain or difficulty on urination.
• Advise women to report planned or known pregnancy.

☑ Evaluation
• Patient maintains normal voiding pattern.
• Patient regains normal bowel patterns.
• Patient is free from pain.

Anticoagulants

Coumarin derivative
warfarin sodium
Heparin derivative
heparin sodium
Low–molecular-weight heparins (LMWHs)
dalteparin sodium
enoxaparin sodium
tinzaparin sodium
Selective factor Xa inhibitor
fondaparinux sodium
Thrombin inhibitors
argatroban
bivalirudin

Indications

▶ Pulmonary emboli, deep vein thrombosis, thrombus, blood clotting, DIC, unstable angina, MI, atrial fibrillation.

Contraindications and precautions

• Contraindicated in patients hypersensitive to these drugs or any of their components; in patients with aneurysm, active bleeding, CV hemorrhage, hemorrhagic blood dyscrasias, hemophilia, severe hypertension, pericardial effusions, or pericarditis; and in patients undergoing major surgery, neurosurgery, or ophthalmic surgery.
• Use cautiously in patients with severe diabetes, renal impairment, severe trauma, ulcerations, or vasculitis.
⚖ **Lifespan:** Heparin may be used in pregnancy only if clearly necessary. In pregnant women and in women who have just had a threatened or complete spontaneous abortion, warfarin is contraindicated. Women should avoid breastfeeding during therapy. Infants, especially neonates, may be more susceptible to anticoagulants because of vitamin K deficiency. Geriatric patients are at greater risk for hemorrhage because of altered hemostatic mechanisms or age-related deterioration of hepatic and renal functions.

Adverse reactions

Anticoagulants commonly cause bleeding and may cause hypersensitivity reactions. Warfarin may cause agranulocytosis, alopecia (long-term use), anorexia, dermatitis, fever, nausea, tissue necrosis or gangrene, urticaria, and vomiting. Heparin derivatives may cause thrombocytopenia and may increase liver enzyme levels.

Action

Heparin derivatives accelerate formation of an antithrombin III-thrombin complex. It inactivates thrombin and prevents conversion of fibrinogen to fibrin. The coumarin derivative, warfarin, inhibits vitamin-K–dependent activation of clotting factors II, VII, IX, and X, which are formed in the liver. Thrombin inhibitors directly bind to thrombin and inhibit its action. Selective factor Xa inhibitors bind to antithrombin III, which in turn initiates the neutralization of factor Xa.

NURSING PROCESS

☜ Assessment
• Monitor patient closely for bleeding and other adverse reactions.
• Check PT, INR, PTT, or APTT.

• Monitor vital signs, hemoglobin, and hematocrit.
• Assess patient's urine, stools, and emesis for blood.

⊞ **Key nursing diagnoses**
• Ineffective protection related to drug's effects on body's normal clotting and bleeding mechanisms
• Risk for deficient fluid volume related to bleeding
• Noncompliance related to long-term warfarin therapy

▷ **Planning and implementation**
• Don't give heparin I.M., and avoid I.M. injections of any anticoagulant, if possible.
• Keep protamine sulfate available to treat severe bleeding caused by heparin. Keep vitamin K available to treat frank bleeding caused by warfarin.
• Notify prescriber about serious or persistent adverse reactions.
• Maintain bleeding precautions throughout therapy.
Patient teaching
• Urge patient to take drug exactly as prescribed. If he's taking warfarin, tell him to take it at night and to have blood drawn for PT or INR in the morning for accurate results.
• Advise patient to consult his prescriber before taking any other drug, including OTC medications or herbal remedies.
• Review bleeding-prevention precautions to take in everyday living. Urge patient to make repairs and to remove safety hazards from home to reduce risk of injury.
• Advise patient not to increase his intake of green, leafy vegetables because vitamin K may antagonize anticoagulant effects.
• Instruct patient to report bleeding or other adverse reactions promptly.
• Encourage patient to keep appointments for blood tests and follow-up examinations.
• Advise women to report planned or known pregnancy.

☑ **Evaluation**
• Patient has no adverse change in health status.
• Patient has no evidence of bleeding or hemorrhaging.

• Patient demonstrates compliance with therapy, as evidenced by normal bleeding and clotting values.

Anticonvulsants

acetazolamide sodium
carbamazepine
clonazepam
clorazepate dipotassium
diazepam
divalproex sodium
fosphenytoin sodium
gabapentin
lamotrigine
levetiracetam
magnesium sulfate
oxcarbazepine
phenobarbital
phenobarbital sodium
phenytoin sodium
phenytoin sodium (extended)
primidone
tiagabine hydrochloride
topiramate
valproate sodium
valproic acid

Indications

▶ Seizure disorders; acute, isolated seizures not caused by seizure disorders; status epilepticus; prevention of seizures after trauma or craniotomy.

Contraindications and precautions

• Contraindicated in patients hypersensitive to these drugs.
• Carbamazepine is contraindicated within 14 days of MAO inhibitor use.
⚘ **Lifespan:** In breast-feeding women, the safety of many anticonvulsants hasn't been established. Children, especially young ones, are sensitive to the CNS depression of some anticonvulsants; use cautiously. Geriatric patients are sensitive to CNS effects and may require lower doses. Also, some anticonvulsants may take longer to be eliminated because of decreased renal function, and parenteral use is more likely to cause apnea, hypotension, bradycardia, and cardiac arrest.

Adverse reactions

Anticonvulsants can cause adverse CNS effects, such as confusion, somnolence, tremor, and ataxia. Many anticonvulsants also cause GI effects, such as vomiting; CV disorders, such as arrhythmias and hypotension; and hematologic disorders, such as leukopenia, bone marrow depression, thrombocytopenia, and agranulocytosis. Stevens-Johnson syndrome and other severe rashes and abnormal liver function tests may occur with certain anticonvulsants.

Action

Anticonvulsants include six classes of drugs: selected hydantoin derivatives, barbiturates, benzodiazepines, succinimides, iminostilbene derivatives (carbamazepine), and carboxylic acid derivatives. Two miscellaneous anticonvulsants are acetazolamide and magnesium sulfate. Some hydantoin derivatives and carbamazepine inhibit the spread of seizure activity in the motor cortex. Some barbiturates and succinimides limit seizure activity by increasing the threshold for motor cortex stimuli. Selected benzodiazepines and carboxylic acid derivatives may increase inhibition of GABA in brain neurons. Acetazolamide inhibits carbonic anhydrase. Magnesium sulfate interferes with the release of acetylcholine at the myoneural junction.

NURSING PROCESS

⚗ Assessment
• Monitor drug level and patient's response as indicated.
• Monitor patient for adverse reactions.
• Assess patient's compliance with therapy at each follow-up visit.

🔲 Key nursing diagnoses
• Risk for trauma related to adverse reactions
• Impaired physical mobility related to sedation
• Noncompliance related to long-term therapy

⟫ Planning and implementation
• Give oral forms with food to reduce GI irritation.
• Phenytoin binds with tube feedings, thus decreasing absorption of drug. Turn off tube feedings for 2 hours before and after giving phenytoin, according to your facility's policy.

• Adjust dosage according to patient's response.
• Take safety precautions if patient has adverse CNS reactions.
Patient teaching
• Instruct patient to take drug exactly as prescribed and not to stop drug without medical supervision.
• Urge patient to avoid hazardous activities that require mental alertness if adverse CNS reactions occur.
• Advise patient to wear or carry medical identification at all times.

🔳 Evaluation
• Patient sustains no trauma from adverse reactions.
• Patient maintains physical mobility.
• Patient complies with therapy and has no seizures.

Antidepressants, tricyclic

amitriptyline hydrochloride
amitriptyline pamoate
amoxapine
clomipramine hydrochloride
desipramine hydrochloride
doxepin hydrochloride
imipramine hydrochloride
imipramine pamoate
nortriptyline hydrochloride

Indications

▶ Depression, anxiety (doxepin hydrochloride), obsessive-compulsive disorder (clomipramine), enuresis in children older than age 6 (imipramine).

Contraindications and precautions

• Contraindicated in patients hypersensitive to these drugs and in patients with urine retention or angle-closure glaucoma.
• Tricyclic antidepressants (TCAs) are contraindicated within 2 weeks of MAO inhibitor therapy.
• Use cautiously in patients with suicidal tendencies, schizophrenia, paranoia, seizure disorders, CV disease, or impaired hepatic function.

⚘ Lifespan: In breast-feeding women, safety hasn't been established; use cautiously. In children younger than age 12, TCAs aren't recommended. Geriatric patients are more sensitive to therapeutic and adverse effects; they need lower dosages.

Adverse reactions

Adverse reactions include sedation, anticholinergic effects, and orthostatic hypotension. The tertiary amines (amitriptyline, doxepin, and imipramine) exert the strongest sedative effects; tolerance usually develops in a few weeks. Amoxapine is most likely to cause seizures, especially with overdose.

Action

TCAs may inhibit reuptake of norepinephrine and serotonin in CNS nerve terminals (presynaptic neurons), thus enhancing the concentration and activity of neurotransmitters in the synaptic cleft. TCAs also exert antihistaminic, sedative, anticholinergic, vasodilatory, and quinidine-like effects.

NURSING PROCESS

🗓 Assessment

• Observe patient for mood changes to monitor drug effectiveness; benefits may not appear for 3 to 6 weeks.
• Check vital signs regularly for tachycardia or decreased blood pressure; observe patient carefully for other adverse reactions and report changes. Check ECG in patients older than age 40 before starting therapy.
• Monitor patient for anticholinergic adverse reactions, such as urine retention or constipation, which may require dosage reduction.

🗷 Key nursing diagnoses

• Disturbed thought processes related to adverse effects
• Risk for injury related to sedation and orthostatic hypotension
• Noncompliance related to long-term therapy

⯈ Planning and implementation

• Make sure patient swallows each dose; depressed patient may hoard pills for suicide attempt, especially when symptoms begin to improve.

• Don't withdraw drug abruptly; instead, gradually reduce dosage over several weeks to avoid rebound effect or other adverse reactions.
Patient teaching
• Explain to patient the rationale for therapy and its anticipated risks and benefits. Inform patient that full therapeutic effect may not occur for several weeks.
• Teach patient how and when to take the drug. Warn him not to increase dosage, stop taking the drug, or take any other drug, including OTC medicines and herbal remedies, without medical approval.
• Because overdose with TCAs commonly is fatal, entrust a reliable family member with the drug, and warn him to store drug safely away from children.
• Advise patient not to take drug with milk or food to minimize GI distress. Suggest taking full dose at bedtime if daytime sedation is a problem.
• Tell patient to avoid alcohol.
• Advise patient to avoid hazardous tasks that require mental alertness until full effects of drug are known.
• Warn patient that excessive exposure to sunlight, heat lamps, or tanning beds may cause burns and abnormal hyperpigmentation.
• Urge diabetic patient to monitor his glucose level carefully because drug may alter it.
• Recommend sugarless gum or hard candy, artificial saliva, or ice chips to relieve dry mouth.
• Advise patient to report adverse reactions promptly.

🗹 Evaluation

• Patient regains normal thought processes.
• Patient sustains no injury from adverse reactions.
• Patient complies with therapy, and his depression is alleviated.

Antidiarrheals

bismuth subgallate
bismuth subsalicylate
calcium polycarbophil
diphenoxylate hydrochloride and atropine sulfate
kaolin and pectin mixtures
loperamide

octreotide acetate
opium tincture
opium tincture, camphorated

Indications

▶ Mild, acute, or chronic diarrhea. Octreotide acetate is only indicated for diarrhea caused by tumors.

Contraindications and precautions

• Contraindicated in patients hypersensitive to these drugs.

⚖ **Lifespan:** Some antidiarrheals may appear in breast milk; check individual drugs for specific recommendations. For infants younger than age 2, don't give kaolin and pectin mixtures. For children or teenagers recovering from flu or chickenpox, consult prescriber before giving bismuth subsalicylate. For geriatric patients, use caution when giving antidiarrheal drugs, especially opium preparations.

Adverse reactions

Bismuth preparations may cause salicylism (with high doses) or temporary darkening of tongue and stools. Kaolin and pectin mixtures may cause constipation and fecal impaction or ulceration. Opium preparations may cause dizziness, light-headedness, nausea, physical dependence (with long-term use), and vomiting.

Action

Bismuth preparations may have a mild water-binding capacity, may absorb toxins, and provide a protective coating for the intestinal mucosa. Kaolin and pectin mixtures decrease fluid in the stool by absorbing bacteria and toxins that cause diarrhea. Opium preparations increase smooth muscle tone in the GI tract, inhibit motility and propulsion, and decrease digestive secretions.

NURSING PROCESS

🔾 Assessment

• Assess patient's condition before therapy and regularly thereafter.
• Monitor fluid and electrolyte balance.
• Observe patient for adverse reactions.

📵 Key nursing diagnoses

• Constipation related to adverse effect of bismuth preparations on GI tract
• Risk for injury related to adverse CNS reactions
• Risk for deficient fluid volume related to GI upset

▶ Planning and implementation

• Take safety precautions if patient experiences adverse CNS reactions.
• Don't substitute opium tincture for paregoric.
• Notify prescriber about serious or persistent adverse reactions.

Patient teaching
• Instruct patient to take drug exactly as prescribed; warn him that excessive use of opium preparations can lead to dependence.
• Instruct patient to notify prescriber if diarrhea lasts for more than 2 days and to report adverse reactions.
• Warn patient to avoid hazardous activities that require alertness if CNS depression occurs.

✔ Evaluation

• Patient doesn't develop constipation.
• Patient isn't injured during therapy.
• Patient maintains adequate hydration.

Antihistamines

azelastine hydrochloride
brompheniramine maleate
cyproheptadine hydrochloride
desloratadine
diphenhydramine hydrochloride
fexofenadine hydrochloride
hydroxyzine embonate
hydroxyzine hydrochloride
hydroxyzine pamoate
loratadine
meclizine hydrochloride
promethazine hydrochloride
promethazine theoclate
triprolidine hydrochloride

Indications

▶ Allergic rhinitis, urticaria, pruritus, vertigo, motion sickness, nausea and vomiting, sedation, dyskinesia, parkinsonism.

Contraindications and precautions

• Contraindicated in patients hypersensitive to these drugs and in those with angle-closure glaucoma, stenosing peptic ulcer, pyloroduodenal obstruction, or bladder neck obstruction. Also contraindicated in those taking MAO inhibitors.

⚥ Lifespan: During breast-feeding, antihistamines shouldn't be used; many of these drugs appear in breast milk and may cause unusual excitability in the infant. Neonates, especially premature infants, may experience seizures. Children, especially those younger than age 6, may experience paradoxical hyperexcitability with restlessness, insomnia, nervousness, euphoria, tremors, and seizures; administer cautiously. Geriatric patients usually are more sensitive to the adverse effects of antihistamines, especially dizziness, sedation, hypotension, and urine retention; use cautiously and monitor these patients closely.

Adverse reactions

Most antihistamines cause drowsiness and impaired motor function early in therapy. They also can cause dry mouth and throat, blurred vision, and constipation. Some antihistamines, such as promethazine, may cause cholestatic jaundice, which may be a hypersensitivity reaction, and may predispose patients to photosensitivity.

Action

Antihistamines are structurally related chemicals that compete with histamine for histamine H_1-receptor sites on smooth muscle of bronchi, GI tract, and large blood vessels, binding to cellular receptors and preventing access to and subsequent activity of histamine. They don't directly alter histamine or prevent its release.

NURSING PROCESS

▨ Assessment

• Monitor patient for adverse reactions.
• Monitor blood counts during long-term therapy; watch for signs of blood dyscrasia.

⊕ Key nursing diagnoses

• Risk for injury related to sedation
• Impaired oral mucous membrane related to dry mouth
• Constipation related to anticholinergic effect of antihistamines

▷ Planning and implementation

• Reduce GI distress by giving antihistamines with food.
• Provide sugarless gum, hard candy, or ice chips to relieve dry mouth.
• Increase fluid intake or humidify air to decrease adverse effect of thickened secretions.

Patient teaching

• Advise patient to take drug with meals or snacks to prevent GI upset.
• Suggest that patient use warm water rinses, artificial saliva, ice chips, or sugarless gum or candy to relieve dry mouth. Tell him to avoid overusing mouthwash, which may worsen dryness and destroy normal flora.
• Warn patient to avoid hazardous activities until full CNS effects of drug are known.
• Tell patient to seek medical approval before using alcohol, tranquilizers, sedatives, pain relievers, or sleeping medications.
• For accurate diagnostic skin test results, advise patient to stop taking antihistamines 4 days before test.

▧ Evaluation

• Patient sustains no injury from sedation.
• Patient maintains normal mucous membranes by using preventive measures throughout therapy.
• Patient maintains normal bowel function.

Antihypertensives

ACE inhibitors
benazepril hydrochloride
captopril
enalaprilat
enalapril maleate
fosinopril sodium
lisinopril
moexipril hydrochloride
perindopril erbumine
quinapril hydrochloride
ramipril
trandolapril

Angiotensin II receptor blockers
candesartan cilexetil
eprosartan mesylate
irbesartan
losartan potassium

telmisartan
valsartan
Beta blockers
acebutolol
atenolol
bisoprolol fumarate
carvedilol
labetalol hydrochloride
metoprolol tartrate
nadolol
pindolol
propranolol hydrochloride
timolol maleate
Calcium channel blockers
amlodipine besylate
diltiazem hydrochloride
felodipine
nicardipine hydrochloride
nifedipine
nisoldipine
verapamil hydrochloride
Centrally acting alpha-adrenergic blockers (sympatholytics)
clonidine hydrochloride
guanfacine hydrochloride
methyldopa
Peripherally acting alpha-adrenergic blockers
doxazosin mesylate
prazosin hydrochloride
tamsulosin hydrochloride
terazosin hydrochloride
Rauwolfia alkaloid
reserpine
Vasodilators
diazoxide
hydralazine hydrochloride
minoxidil
nitroprusside sodium

Indications

▶ Essential and secondary hypertension.

Contraindications and precautions

• Contraindicated in patients hypersensitive to these drugs and in those with hypotension.
• Use cautiously in patients with hepatic or renal dysfunction.
⚖ Lifespan: In breast-feeding women, use cautiously; some antihypertensives appear in breast milk. In children, safety and effective-ness of many antihypertensives haven't been established; give these drugs cautiously and monitor patients closely. Geriatric patients are more susceptible to adverse reactions and may need lower maintenance doses; monitor them closely.

Adverse reactions

Most antihypertensives commonly cause ortho-static hypotension, changes in heart rate, head-ache, nausea, and vomiting. Other reactions vary greatly among different drug types. Cen-trally acting sympatholytics may cause consti-pation, depression, dizziness, drowsiness, dry mouth, headache, palpitations, severe rebound hypertension, and sexual dysfunction; methyl-dopa also may cause aplastic anemia and thrombocytopenia. Rauwolfia alkaloids may cause anxiety, depression, drowsiness, dry mouth, hyperacidity, impotence, nasal stuffi-ness, and weight gain. Vasodilators may cause heart failure, ECG changes, diarrhea, dizziness, palpitations, pruritus, and rash.

Action

Antihypertensives reduce blood pressure through various mechanisms. For information on the action of ACE inhibitors, alpha-adrenergic blockers, angiotensin II receptor blockers, beta blockers, calcium channel blockers, and diuret-ics, see their individual drug class entries. Cen-trally acting sympatholytics stimulate central alpha-adrenergic receptors, reducing cerebral sympathetic outflow, thereby decreasing periph-eral vascular resistance and blood pressure. Rauwolfia alkaloids bind to and gradually de-stroy the norepinephrine-containing storage vesicles in central and peripheral adrenergic neurons. Vasodilators act directly on smooth muscle to reduce blood pressure.

NURSING PROCESS

⚖ Assessment
• Obtain baseline blood pressure and pulse rate and rhythm; recheck regularly.
• Monitor patient for adverse reactions.
• Monitor patient's weight and fluid and elec-trolyte status.
• Monitor patient's compliance with treatment.

⊞ Key nursing diagnoses
● Risk for trauma related to orthostatic hypotension
● Risk for deficient fluid volume related to GI upset
● Noncompliance related to long-term therapy or adverse reactions

▷▷ Planning and implementation
● Give drug with food or h.s., as indicated.
● Follow manufacturer's guidelines when mixing and administering parenteral drugs.
● Take steps to prevent or minimize orthostatic hypotension.
● Maintain patient's nonpharmacologic therapy, such as sodium restriction, calorie reduction, stress management, and exercise program.
Patient teaching
● Instruct patient to take drug exactly as prescribed. Warn him not to stop taking drug abruptly.
● Review adverse reactions caused by drug, and urge patient to notify prescriber of serious or persistent reactions.
● Advise patient to avoid sudden changes in position to prevent dizziness, light-headedness, or fainting.
● Warn patient to avoid hazardous activities until full effects of drug are known. Also, warn patient to avoid physical exertion, especially in hot weather.
● Advise patient to consult prescriber before taking any OTC medications or herbal remedies; serious drug interactions can occur.
● Encourage patient to comply with therapy.

☑ Evaluation
● Patient isn't caused trauma by orthostatic hypotension.
● Patient maintains adequate hydration.
● Patient complies with therapy, as evidenced by normal blood pressure.

Antilipemics

atorvastatin calcium
cholestyramine
colesevelam hydrochloride
ezetimibe
fenofibrate
fluvastatin sodium

gemfibrozil
lovastatin
pravastatin sodium
rosuvastatin calcium
simvastatin

Indications

▶ Hyperlipidemia, hypercholesterolemia.

Contraindications and precautions

● Contraindicated in patients hypersensitive to these drugs. Also, bile-sequestering drugs are contraindicated in patients with complete biliary obstruction. Fibric acid derivatives are contraindicated in patients with primary biliary cirrhosis or significant hepatic or renal dysfunction. HMG-CoA reductase inhibitors are contraindicated in patients with active liver disease or persistently elevated transaminase levels.
● Use bile-sequestering drugs cautiously in constipated patients. Use fibric acid derivatives cautiously in patients with peptic ulcer. Use cholesterol synthesis inhibitors cautiously in patients who consume large amounts of alcohol or who have a history of liver or renal disease.
⚱ **Lifespan:** In pregnant women, use bile-sequestering drugs and fibric acid derivatives cautiously and avoid using cholesterol synthesis inhibitors. In breast-feeding women, avoid using fibric acid derivatives and cholesterol synthesis inhibitors; give bile-sequestering drugs cautiously. In children ages 10 to 17, certain antilipemics have been approved to treat heterozygous familial hypercholesterolemia. Geriatric patients have an increased risk of severe constipation; use bile-sequestering drugs cautiously and monitor patients closely.

Adverse reactions

Antilipemics commonly cause GI upset. Bile-sequestering drugs may cause cholelithiasis, constipation, bloating, and steatorrhea. Fibric acid derivatives may cause cholelithiasis and GI or CNS effects. Use of gemfibrozil with lovastatin may cause myopathy. HMG-CoA reductase inhibitors may affect liver function or cause rash, pruritus, increased CK levels, rhabdomyolysis, and myopathy.

Action

Antilipemics lower elevated lipid levels. Bile-sequestering drugs (cholestyramine and cole-sevelam) lower LDL level by forming insoluble complexes with bile salts, thus triggering cholesterol to leave the bloodstream and other storage areas to make new bile acids. Fibric acid derivatives (gemfibrozil) reduce cholesterol formation, increase sterol excretion, and decrease lipoprotein and triglyceride synthesis. HMG-CoA reductase inhibitors (atorvastatin, fluvastatin, lovastatin, pravastatin, rosuvastatin, simvastatin) interfere with the activity of enzymes that generate cholesterol in the liver.

NURSING PROCESS

Assessment
• Monitor cholesterol and lipid levels before and periodically during therapy.
• Monitor CK level when therapy begins and every 6 months thereafter. Also, check CK level if a patient who takes a cholesterol synthesis inhibitor complains of muscle pain.
• Monitor patient for adverse reactions.

Key nursing diagnoses
• Risk for deficient fluid volume related to adverse GI reactions
• Constipation related to adverse effect on bowel
• Noncompliance related to long-term therapy

Planning and implementation
• Mix powder form of bile-sequestering drugs with 120 to 180 ml of liquid. Never give dry powder alone because patient may inhale it accidentally.
• Give lovastatin with evening meal, simvastatin in the evening, and fluvastatin and pravastatin at bedtime.
Patient teaching
• Instruct patient to take drug exactly as prescribed. If he takes a bile-sequestering drug, warn him never to take the dry form.
• Stress importance of diet in controlling lipid levels.
• Advise patient to drink 2 to 3 L of fluid daily and to report persistent or severe constipation.

Evaluation
• Patient maintains adequate fluid volume.

• Patient doesn't experience severe or persistent constipation.
• Patient complies with therapy, as evidenced by normal lipid and cholesterol levels.

Antimetabolite antineoplastics
capecitabine
cytarabine
cytarabine liposomal
fludarabine phosphate
fluorouracil
hydroxyurea
mercaptopurine
methotrexate
pentostatin
thioguanine

Indications
▶ Various tumors.

Contraindications and precautions
• Contraindicated in patients hypersensitive to these drugs.
⚘ **Lifespan:** Pregnant women should be informed of the risks to the fetus. Breast-feeding isn't recommended for women taking these drugs. In children, safety and effectiveness of some drugs haven't been established. Geriatric patients have an increased risk of adverse reactions; monitor them closely.

Adverse reactions
The most common adverse effects include nausea, vomiting, diarrhea, fever, chills, hair loss, flank or joint pain, redness or pain at injection site, anxiety, bone marrow depression, leukopenia, thrombocytopenia, anemia, and swelling of the feet or lower legs.

Action
Antimetabolites are structurally similar to naturally occurring metabolites and can be divided into three subcategories: purine, pyrimidine, and folinic acid analogues. Most of these drugs interrupt cell reproduction at a specific phase of the cell cycle. Purine analogues are incorporated into DNA and RNA, interfering with nucleic acid synthesis (by miscoding) and replication. They also may inhibit synthesis of purine bases

through pseudofeedback mechanisms. Pyrimidine analogues inhibit enzymes in metabolic pathways that interfere with biosynthesis of uridine and thymine. Folic acid antagonists prevent conversion of folic acid to tetrahydrofolate by inhibiting the enzyme dihydrofolic acid reductase.

NURSING PROCESS

⚗ Assessment
• Perform a complete assessment before therapy begins.
• Monitor patient for adverse reactions.
• Monitor vital signs and patency of catheter or I.V. line throughout administration.
• Monitor hematocrit, platelet and total and differential leukocyte counts, ALT, AST, LDH, bilirubin, creatinine, uric acid, and BUN levels.

⊞ Key nursing diagnoses
• Ineffective protection related to thrombocytopenia
• Risk for infection related to immunosuppression
• Risk for deficient fluid volume related to adverse GI effects

▷ Planning and implementation
• Follow established procedures for safe and proper handling, administration, and disposal of drugs.
• Try to ease anxiety in patient and his family before treatment.
• Give an antiemetic before giving drug to lessen nausea.
• Give cytarabine with allopurinol to decrease the risk of hyperuricemia. Encourage patient to drink a lot of fluids.
• Provide diligent mouth care to prevent stomatitis with cytarabine, fluorouracil, or methotrexate therapy.
• Anticipate the need for leucovorin rescue with high-dose methotrexate therapy.
• Treat extravasation promptly.
• Anticipate diarrhea, possibly severe, with prolonged fluorouracil therapy.
Patient teaching
• Teach patient proper oral hygiene, including cautious use of toothbrush, dental floss, and toothpicks. Chemotherapy can increase the risk of microbial infection, delayed healing, and bleeding gums.

• Advise patient to complete dental work before therapy begins or to delay it until blood counts are normal.
• Tell patient to defer immunizations if possible until hematologic stability is confirmed.
• Warn patient that he may bruise easily because of drug's effect on platelets.
• Advise patient to avoid close contact with persons who have taken oral poliovirus vaccine and who have been exposed to persons with bacterial or viral infection because chemotherapy may increase susceptibility. Urge patient to notify prescriber promptly if he develops signs or symptoms of infection.
• Instruct patient to report redness, pain, or swelling at injection site. Local tissue injury and scarring may result from tissue infiltration at infusion site.

☑ Evaluation
• Patient doesn't have serious bleeding complications.
• Patient doesn't have an infection.
• Patient maintains adequate hydration.

Antiparkinsonians
amantadine hydrochloride
benztropine mesylate
bromocriptine mesylate
diphenhydramine hydrochloride
entacapone
levodopa
levodopa and carbidopa
pergolide mesylate
pramipexole dihydrochloride
ropinirole hydrochloride
selegiline hydrochloride
tolcapone
trihexyphenidyl hydrochloride

Indications

▶ Signs and symptoms of Parkinson's and drug-induced extrapyramidal reactions.

Contraindications and precautions

• Contraindicated in patients hypersensitive to these drugs.

• Use cautiously in patients with prostatic hyperplasia or tardive dyskinesia and in debilitated patients.

• Neuroleptic malignantlike syndrome involving muscle rigidity, increased body temperature, and mental status changes may occur with abrupt withdrawal of antiparkinsonians.

⚄ Lifespan: Antiparkinsonians may appear in breast milk; a decision should be made to stop the drug or stop breast-feeding, taking into account the importance of the drug to the mother. In children, safety and effectiveness haven't been established. Geriatric patients have an increased risk for adverse reactions; monitor them closely.

Adverse reactions

Anticholinergics may cause decreased sweating or anhidrosis, dry mouth, headache, mydriasis, blurred vision, cycloplegia, urinary hesitancy and urine retention, constipation, palpitations, and tachycardia. Dopaminergics may cause nausea, vomiting, muscle cramps, dystonias, headache, orthostatic hypotension, confusion, arrhythmias, hallucinations, and disturbing dreams. Amantadine also causes irritability, insomnia, and livedo reticularis (with prolonged use).

Action

Antiparkinsonians include synthetic anticholinergics, dopaminergics, and the antiviral amantadine. Anticholinergics probably prolong the action of dopamine by blocking its reuptake into presynaptic neurons and by suppressing central cholinergic activity. Dopaminergics act in the brain by increasing dopamine availability, thus improving motor function. Entacapone is a reversible inhibitor of peripheral COMT, which is responsible for elimination of various catecholamines, including dopamine. Blocking this pathway when giving levodopa and carbidopa should result in higher levels of levodopa, thereby allowing greater dopaminergic stimulation in the CNS and leading to a greater effect in treating parkinsonian symptoms. Amantadine is thought to increase dopamine release in the substantia nigra.

NURSING PROCESS

⚖ Assessment
• Obtain baseline assessment of patient's impairment, and reassess regularly to monitor drug effectiveness.
• Monitor patient for adverse reactions.
• Monitor vital signs, especially during dosage adjustments.

⚄ Key nursing diagnoses
• Risk for injury related to adverse CNS effects
• Urine retention related to anticholinergic effect on bladder
• Disturbed sleep pattern related to amantadine-induced insomnia

▷ Planning and implementation
• Give drug with food to prevent GI irritation.
• Adjust dosage according to patient's response and tolerance.
• Never withdraw drug abruptly.
• Institute safety precautions.
• Provide ice chips, drinks, or sugarless hard candy or gum to relieve dry mouth. Increase fluid and fiber intake to prevent constipation, as appropriate.
• Notify prescriber about urine retention, and be prepared to catheterize patient, if necessary.
Patient teaching
• Instruct patient to take drug exactly as prescribed, and warn him not to stop drug suddenly.
• Advise patient to take drug with food to prevent GI upset.
• Teach patient how to manage anticholinergic effects, if needed.
• Instruct patient to avoid hazardous tasks if adverse CNS effects occur. Tell him to avoid alcohol during therapy.
• Encourage patient to report severe or persistent adverse reactions.

☑ Evaluation
• Patient remains free from injury.
• Patient's voiding pattern doesn't change.
• Patient's sleep pattern isn't altered by amantadine.

Antivirals

abacavir sulfate
acyclovir sodium
amantadine hydrochloride
amprenavir
atazanavir sulfate
cidofovir
delavirdine mesylate
didanosine
efavirenz
emtricitabine
enfuvirtide
famciclovir
fosamprenavir calcium
foscarnet sodium
ganciclovir
indinavir sulfate
lamivudine
lamivudine and zidovudine
lopinavir and ritonavir
nelfinavir mesylate
nevirapine
oseltamivir phosphate
ribavirin
rimantadine hydrochloride
ritonavir
saquinavir mesylate
stavudine
valacyclovir hydrochloride
valganciclovir
zalcitabine
zanamivir
zidovudine

Indications

▶ Viral infections.

Contraindications and precautions

● Contraindicated in patients hypersensitive to these drugs.

≋ Lifespan: In breast-feeding women, some antivirals are contraindicated, while others require cautious use. For infants and children, recommendations vary with the antiviral prescribed. Geriatric patients have an increased risk of adverse reactions; monitor them closely.

Adverse reactions

Antivirals may cause anorexia, chills, confusion, depression, diarrhea, dry mouth, edema, fatigue, hallucinations, headache, nausea, and vomiting.

Action

Acyclovir, cidofovir, didanosine, famciclovir, ganciclovir, valacyclovir, valganciclovir, and zalcitabine interfere with DNA synthesis and replication. Amantadine prevents the release of infectious viral nucleic acid into the host cell and possibly prevents viruses from penetrating cells. Foscarnet blocks the pyrophosphate-binding site. Rimantadine prevents viral uncoating. Abacavir, amprenavir, indinavir, ritonavir, saquinavir, and stavudine inhibit the activity of HIV protease. Delavirdine, efavirenz, lamivudine, nevirapine, and zidovudine inhibit reverse transcriptase.

NURSING PROCESS

℞ Assessment
● Obtain baseline assessment of patient's viral infection, and reassess regularly to monitor drug's effectiveness.
● Monitor renal and hepatic function, CBC, and platelet count regularly. Monitor electrolytes, such as calcium, phosphate, magnesium, potassium, in patients receiving foscarnet.
● Inspect patient's I.V. site regularly for signs of irritation, phlebitis, inflammation, or extravasation.
● If patient has a history of heart failure, watch closely for worsening or recurrence during amantadine therapy.
● Monitor patient's cardiac status during ribavirin therapy.

⊕ Key nursing diagnoses
● Ineffective protection related to adverse hematologic reactions
● Risk for deficient fluid volume related to GI upset
● Noncompliance related to long-term therapy

▶ Planning and implementation
● Adjust dosage of selected antiviral for patient with decreased renal function, especially during parenteral therapy.

• Follow manufacturer's guidelines for reconstituting and giving an antiviral.

• Obtain an order for an antiemetic or antidiarrheal, if needed.

• Take safety precautions if patient has adverse CNS reactions. For example, place bed in low position, raise bed rails, and supervise ambulation and other activities.

• Notify prescriber about serious or persistent adverse reactions.

Patient teaching

• Instruct patient to take drug exactly as prescribed, even if he feels better.

• Urge patient to notify prescriber promptly about severe or persistent adverse reactions.

• Encourage patient to keep appointments for follow-up care.

☑ Evaluation

• Patient doesn't have any serious adverse hematologic effects.

• Patient maintains adequate hydration.

• Patient complies with therapy, and viral infection is eradicated.

Barbiturates

amobarbital
amobarbital sodium
pentobarbital sodium
phenobarbital
phenobarbital sodium
primidone
secobarbital sodium

Indications

▶ Sedation, preanesthetic, short-term treatment of insomnia, seizure disorders.

Contraindications and precautions

• Contraindicated in patients hypersensitive to these drugs and in those with bronchopneumonia, other severe pulmonary insufficiency, or liver dysfunction.

• Use cautiously in patients with blood pressure alterations, pulmonary disease, and CV dysfunction.

⚠ **Lifespan:** During pregnancy, use of barbiturates can cause fetal abnormalities; avoid use. Barbiturates appear in breast milk and may re-

sult in infant CNS depression; use cautiously. Premature infants are more susceptible to depressant effects of barbiturates because of their immature hepatic metabolism. Children may experience hyperactivity, excitement, or hyperalgesia. Use cautiously and monitor children carefully. Geriatric patients may experience hyperactivity, excitement, or hyperalgesia; use cautiously.

Adverse reactions

Drowsiness, lethargy, vertigo, headache, and CNS depression are common with barbiturates. After hypnotic doses, a hangover effect, subtle distortion of mood, and impaired judgment and motor skills may continue for many hours. After dosage reduction or discontinuation, rebound insomnia or increased dreaming or nightmares may occur. Barbiturates cause hyperalgesia in subhypnotic doses. They also can cause paradoxical excitement at low doses, confusion in elderly patients, and hyperactivity in children. High fever, severe headache, stomatitis, conjunctivitis, or rhinitis may precede potentially fatal skin eruptions. Withdrawal symptoms may occur after as little as 2 weeks of uninterrupted therapy.

Action

Barbiturates act throughout the CNS, especially in the mesencephalic reticular activating system, which controls the CNS arousal mechanism. The main anticonvulsant actions are reduced nerve transmission and decreased excitability of the nerve cell. Barbiturates decrease presynaptic and postsynaptic membrane excitability by promoting the actions of GABA. They also depress respiration and GI motility and raise the seizure threshold.

NURSING PROCESS

☑ Assessment

• Assess patient's level of consciousness and sleeping patterns before and during therapy to evaluate drug effectiveness. Monitor neurologic status for alteration or deterioration.

• Assess vital signs frequently, especially during I.V. administration.

• Monitor seizure character, frequency, and duration for changes.

• Observe patient to prevent hoarding or self-dosing, especially if patient is depressed, suicidal, or drug-dependent.

⊞ Key nursing diagnoses
• Risk for injury related to sedation
• Disturbed thought processes related to confusion
• Impaired adjustment related to drug dependence

▶ Planning and implementation
• When giving parenteral drug, avoid extravasation, which may cause local tissue damage and tissue necrosis; inject I.V. or deep I.M. only. Don't exceed 5 ml for any I.M. injection site to avoid tissue damage.
• Keep resuscitative measures available. Too-rapid I.V. administration may cause respiratory depression, apnea, laryngospasm, or hypotension.
• Take seizure precautions, as needed.
• Institute safety measures to prevent falls and injury. Raise side rails, assist patient out of bed, and keep call light within easy reach.
• Stop drug slowly. Abrupt discontinuation may cause withdrawal symptoms.
Patient teaching
• Explain that barbiturates can cause physical or psychological dependence.
• Instruct patient to take drug exactly as prescribed. Warn him not to change the dosage or take other drugs, including OTC medications or herbal remedies, without prescriber's approval.
• Reassure patient that a morning hangover is common after therapeutic use of barbiturates.
• Advise patient to avoid hazardous tasks, driving a motor vehicle, or operating machinery while taking drug and to review other safety measures to prevent injury.
• Instruct patient to report skin eruption or other significant adverse effects.

☑ Evaluation
• Patient sustains no injury from sedation.
• Patient maintains normal thought processes.
• Patient doesn't develop physical or psychological dependence.

Beta blockers
Beta₁ blockers
acebutolol
atenolol
bisoprolol fumarate
esmolol hydrochloride
metoprolol tartrate
Beta₁ and beta₂ blockers
carvedilol
labetalol hydrochloride
nadolol
pindolol
propranolol hydrochloride
sotalol hydrochloride
timolol maleate

Indications

▶ Hypertension (most drugs), angina pectoris (atenolol, metoprolol, nadolol, and propranolol), arrhythmias (acebutolol, esmolol, propranolol, and sotalol), glaucoma (betaxolol and timolol), prevention of MI (atenolol, metoprolol, propranolol, and timolol), prevention of recurrent migraine and other vascular headaches (propranolol and timolol), pheochromocytomas or essential tremors (selected drugs), heart failure (atenolol, bisoprolol, carvedilol, metoprolol).

Contraindications and precautions

• Contraindicated in patients hypersensitive to these drugs and in patients with cardiogenic shock, sinus bradycardia, heart block greater than first degree, bronchial asthma, and heart failure unless failure is caused by tachyarrhythmia treatable with propranolol.
• Use cautiously in patients with nonallergic bronchospastic disorders, diabetes mellitus, or impaired hepatic or renal function.
⚛ Lifespan: In pregnant women, use cautiously. Drugs appear in breast milk. In children, safety and effectiveness of drug haven't been established; use only if the potential benefits outweigh the potential risks. Geriatric patients may need reduced maintenance doses because of increased bioavailability or delayed metabolism and may also have increased adverse effects; use cautiously.

Adverse reactions

Therapeutic doses may cause bradycardia, fatigue, and dizziness; some may cause other CNS disturbances, such as nightmares, depression, memory loss, and hallucinations. Toxic doses can produce severe hypotension, bradycardia, heart failure, or bronchospasm.

Action

Beta blockers compete with beta agonists for available beta-receptors; individual drugs differ in their ability to affect beta receptors. Some drugs are considered nonselective: they block beta$_1$ receptors in cardiac muscle and beta$_2$ receptors in bronchial and vascular smooth muscle. Several drugs are cardioselective and, in lower doses, primarily inhibit beta$_1$ receptors. Some beta blockers have intrinsic sympathomimetic activity and stimulate and block beta receptors, thereby decreasing cardiac output. Others stabilize cardiac membranes, which affects cardiac-action potential.

NURSING PROCESS

⚚ Assessment
• Check apical pulse rate daily; alert prescriber about extremes, such as a pulse rate lower than 60 beats/minute.
• Monitor blood pressure, ECG, and heart rate and rhythm frequently; be alert for progression of AV block or bradycardia.
• If patient has heart failure, weigh him regularly; watch for weight gain of more than 2.25 kg (5 lb) per week.
• Observe diabetic patients for sweating, fatigue, and hunger. Signs of hypoglycemic shock may be masked.

⊕ Key nursing diagnoses
• Risk for injury related to adverse CNS effects
• Excessive fluid volume related to edema
• Decreased cardiac output related to bradycardia or hypotension

⧁ Planning and implementation
• Discontinue a beta blocker before surgery for pheochromocytoma. Before any surgical procedure, notify anesthesiologist that patient is taking a beta blocker.
• Keep glucagon nearby to reverse beta blocker overdose.

Patient teaching
• Teach patient to take drug exactly as prescribed, even when he feels better.
• Warn patient not to stop drug suddenly. Stopping suddenly can worsen angina or precipitate MI.
• Tell patient not to take OTC medications or herbal remedies without prescriber's approval.
• Explain potential adverse reactions, and stress importance of reporting unusual effects.

☑ Evaluation
• Patient remains free from injury.
• Patient has no signs of edema.
• Patient maintains normal blood pressure and heart rate.

Calcium channel blockers
amlodipine besylate
diltiazem hydrochloride
felodipine
nicardipine hydrochloride
nifedipine
nisoldipine
verapamil hydrochloride

Indications
▶ Prinzmetal's variant angina, chronic stable angina, unstable angina, mild-to-moderate hypertension, arrhythmias.

Contraindications and precautions
• Contraindicated in patients hypersensitive to these drugs and in those with second- or third-degree heart block (except those with a pacemaker) and cardiogenic shock.
⚖ Lifespan: In pregnant women, use cautiously. Calcium channel blockers may appear in breast milk; instruct patient to stop breastfeeding during therapy. In neonates and infants, adverse hemodynamic effects of parenteral verapamil are possible, but safety and effectiveness of other calcium channel blockers haven't been established; avoid use, if possible. In geriatric patients, the half-life of calcium channel blockers may be increased as a result of decreased clearance; use cautiously.

Adverse reactions

Adverse reactions vary among the drugs. Verapamil may cause bradycardia, various degrees of heart block, worsening of heart failure, and hypotension after rapid I.V. administration. Prolonged oral verapamil therapy may cause constipation. Nifedipine may cause hypotension, peripheral edema, flushing, light-headedness, and headache. The most common adverse reactions with diltiazem are anorexia and nausea, and the drug may also induce various degrees of heart block, bradycardia, heart failure, and peripheral edema.

Action

The main physiologic action of calcium channel blockers is to inhibit calcium influx across the slow channels of myocardial and vascular smooth muscle cells. By inhibiting calcium flow into these cells, calcium channel blockers reduce intracellular calcium concentrations. This, in turn, dilates coronary arteries, peripheral arteries, and arterioles and slows cardiac conduction.

When used to treat Prinzmetal's variant angina, calcium channel blockers inhibit coronary spasm, which then increases oxygen delivery to the heart. Peripheral artery dilation decreases total peripheral resistance, which reduces afterload. This, in turn, decreases the amount of oxygen used by the myocardium. Inhibiting calcium flow into the specialized cardiac conduction cells (specifically, those in the SA and AV nodes) slows conduction through the heart. Of the calcium channel blockers, verapamil and diltiazem have the greatest effect on the AV node, which slows the ventricular rate in atrial fibrillation or flutter and converts supraventricular tachycardia to a normal sinus rhythm.

NURSING PROCESS

Assessment

• Monitor cardiac rate and rhythm and blood pressure carefully when therapy starts or dosage increases.
• Monitor fluids and electrolytes.
• Monitor patient for adverse reactions.

Key nursing diagnoses

• Decreased cardiac output related to adverse CV reactions

• Constipation related to oral verapamil therapy
• Noncompliance related to long-term therapy

Planning and implementation

• Don't give calcium supplements while patient takes a calcium channel blocker; they may decrease the drug's effectiveness.
• Expect to decrease dosage gradually; don't stop calcium channel blockers abruptly.

Patient teaching
• Teach patient to take drug exactly as prescribed, even if he feels better.
• Instruct patient to take a missed dose as soon as possible, unless it's almost time for his next dose. Warn him never to take a double dose.
• Warn patient not to stop drug suddenly; abrupt discontinuation can produce serious adverse effects.
• Urge patient to report irregular heartbeat, shortness of breath, swelling of hands and feet, pronounced dizziness, constipation, nausea, or hypotension.

Evaluation

• Patient maintains adequate cardiac output throughout therapy, as evidenced by normal blood pressure and pulse rate.
• Patient regains normal bowel pattern.
• Patient complies with therapy, as evidenced by absence of symptoms related to disorder.

Cephalosporins

First generation
cefadroxil monohydrate
cefazolin sodium
cephalexin monohydrate
Second generation
cefaclor
cefotetan disodium
cefoxitin sodium
cefprozil
cefuroxime axetil
cefuroxime sodium
loracarbef
Third generation
cefdinir
cefditoren pivoxil
cefoperazone sodium
cefotaxime sodium

cefpodoxime proxetil
ceftazidime
ceftibuten
ceftizoxime sodium
ceftriaxone sodium

Indications

▶ Infections of the lungs, skin, soft tissue, bones, joints, urinary and respiratory tracts, blood, abdomen, and heart; CNS infections caused by susceptible strains of *Neisseria meningitidis, Haemophilus influenzae,* and *Streptococcus pneumoniae;* meningitis caused by *Escherichia coli* or *Klebsiella;* infections that develop after surgical procedures classified as contaminated or potentially contaminated; penicillinase-producing *N. gonorrhoeae;* otitis media and ampicillin-resistant middle ear infection caused by *H. influenzae.*

Contraindications and precautions

• Contraindicated in patients hypersensitive to these drugs.
• Use cautiously in patients with renal or hepatic impairment, history of GI disease, or allergy to penicillins.
⚜ **Lifespan:** In breast-feeding women, use cautiously because drugs appear in breast milk. In neonates and infants, half-life is prolonged; use cautiously. Geriatric patients are susceptible to superinfection and coagulopathies, commonly have renal impairment, and may need a lower dosage; use cautiously.

Adverse reactions

Many cephalosporins have similar adverse effects. Hypersensitivity reactions range from mild rashes, fever, and eosinophilia to fatal anaphylaxis and are more common in patients with penicillin allergy. Adverse GI reactions include nausea, vomiting, diarrhea, abdominal pain, glossitis, dyspepsia, and tenesmus. Hematologic reactions include positive direct and indirect antiglobulin in Coombs' test, thrombocytopenia or thrombocythemia, transient neutropenia, and reversible leukopenia. Minimal elevation of liver function test results occurs occasionally. Adverse renal effects may occur with any cephalosporin; they are most common in older patients, those with decreased renal function, and those taking other nephrotoxic drugs.

Local venous pain and irritation are common after I.M. injection; these reactions occur more often with higher doses and long-term therapy. Disulfiram-type reactions occur when cefoperazone or cefotetan are given within 3 days of alcohol use. Bacterial and fungal superinfections may result from suppression of normal flora.

Action

Cephalosporins are chemically and pharmacologically similar to penicillin; they act by inhibiting bacterial cell wall synthesis, causing rapid cell destruction. Their sites of action are enzymes known as penicillin-binding proteins. The affinity of certain cephalosporins for these proteins in various microorganisms helps explain the differing actions of these drugs. They are bactericidal; they act against many aerobic gram-positive and gram-negative bacteria and some anaerobic bacteria but don't kill fungi or viruses.

First-generation cephalosporins act against many gram-positive cocci, including penicillinase-producing *Staphylococcus aureus* and *Staphylococcus epidermidis; Streptococcus pneumoniae,* group B streptococci, and group A beta-hemolytic streptococci; susceptible gram-negative organisms include *Klebsiella pneumoniae, E. coli, Proteus mirabilis,* and *Shigella.*

Second-generation cephalosporins are effective against all organisms attacked by first-generation drugs and have additional activity against *Moraxella catarrhalis, H. influenzae, Enterobacter, Citrobacter, Providencia, Acinetobacter, Serratia,* and *Neisseria.* Bacteroides fragilis is susceptible to cefotetan and cefoxitin.

Third-generation cephalosporins are less active than first- and second-generation drugs against gram-positive bacteria, but are more active against gram-negative organisms, including those resistant to first- and second-generation drugs. They have the greatest stability against beta-lactamases produced by gram-negative bacteria. Susceptible gram-negative organisms include *E. coli, Klebsiella, Enterobacter, Providencia, Acinetobacter, Serratia, Proteus, Morganella,* and *Neisseria.* Some third-generation drugs are active against *B. fragilis* and *Pseudomonas.*

NURSING PROCESS

⚙ Assessment

• Review patient's history of allergies. Try to determine whether previous reactions were true hypersensitivity reactions or adverse effects (such as GI distress) that patient interpreted as allergy.

• Monitor patient continuously for possible hypersensitivity reactions or other adverse effects.

• Obtain culture and sensitivity specimen before giving first dose; check test results periodically to assess drug's effectiveness.

• Monitor renal function study; dosage of certain cephalosporins must be lowered in a patient with severe renal impairment. In patient with decreased renal function, monitor BUN and creatinine levels and urine output for significant changes.

• Monitor PT and platelet count, and assess patient for signs of hypoprothrombinemia, which may occur, with or without bleeding, during therapy with cefoperazone, cefonicid, cefotetan, or ceftriaxone. It usually occurs in elderly, debilitated, malnourished, and immunocompromised patients and in patients with renal impairment or impaired vitamin K synthesis.

• Monitor patient receiving long-term therapy for possible bacterial and fungal superinfection, especially elderly and debilitated patients and those receiving immunosuppressants or radiation therapy.

• Monitor at-risk patients for fluid retention while they are taking sodium salts of cephalosporins.

⊕ Key nursing diagnoses

• Ineffective protection related to hypersensitivity

• Risk for infection related to superinfection

• Risk for deficient fluid volume related to adverse GI reactions

▶ Planning and implementation

• Give these drugs at least 1 hour before bacteriostatic antibiotics, such as tetracyclines, erythromycins, and chloramphenicol; the antibiotics keep bacteria from growing by decreasing cephalosporin uptake by bacterial cell walls.

• Refrigerate oral suspensions, which are stable for 14 days; shake well before giving to ensure correct dosage.

• Follow manufacturer's directions for reconstitution, dilution, and storage of drugs; check expiration dates.

• Give I.M. dose deep into gluteal muscle mass or midlateral thigh; rotate injection sites to minimize tissue injury.

• Don't add or mix other drugs with I.V. infusions, particularly aminoglycosides, which will be inactivated if mixed with cephalosporins. If other drugs must be given I.V., temporarily stop infusion of primary drug.

• Ensure adequate dilution of I.V. infusion and rotate site every 48 hours to help minimize local vein irritation; using a small-gauge needle in a larger available vein may be helpful.

Patient teaching

• Make sure patient understands how and when to take drug. Urge him to comply with instructions for around-the-clock dosage and to complete the prescribed regimen.

• Advise patient to take oral drug with food if GI irritation occurs.

• Review proper storage and disposal of drug, and remind him to check expiration date.

• Teach signs and symptoms of hypersensitivity and other adverse reactions, and emphasize importance of reporting unusual effects.

• Teach signs and symptoms of bacterial and fungal superinfection, especially if patient is elderly or debilitated or has low resistance from immunosuppressants or irradiation. Emphasize importance of reporting signs and symptoms promptly.

• Warn patient not to ingest alcohol in any form within 3 days of treatment with cefoperazone or cefotetan.

• Advise patient to add yogurt or buttermilk to diet to prevent intestinal superinfection resulting from suppression of normal intestinal flora.

• Advise diabetic patient to monitor glucose level with Diastix, not Clinitest.

• Urge patient to keep follow-up appointments.

☑ Evaluation

• Patient has no evidence of hypersensitivity.

• Patient is free from infection.

• Patient maintains adequate hydration.

Corticosteroids

betamethasone
betamethasone sodium phosphate
cortisone acetate
dexamethasone
dexamethasone acetate
dexamethasone sodium phosphate
fludrocortisone acetate
hydrocortisone
hydrocortisone acetate
hydrocortisone cypionate
hydrocortisone sodium phosphate
hydrocortisone sodium succinate
methylprednisolone
methylprednisolone acetate
methylprednisolone sodium succinate
prednisolone
prednisolone acetate
prednisolone sodium phosphate
prednisolone steaglate
prednisolone tebutate
prednisone
triamcinolone
triamcinolone diacetate
triamcinolone hexacetonide

Indications

▶ Hypersensitivity; inflammation, particularly of eye, nose, and respiratory tract; to initiate immunosuppression; replacement therapy in adrenocortical insufficiency, dermatological diseases, respiratory disorders, rheumatic disorders.

Contraindications and precautions

• Contraindicated in patients hypersensitive to these drugs or their components and in those with systemic fungal infection.
• Use cautiously in patients with GI ulceration, renal disease, hypertension, osteoporosis, varicella, vaccinia, exanthema, diabetes mellitus, hypothyroidism, thromboembolic disorder, seizures, myasthenia gravis, heart failure, tuberculosis, ocular herpes simplex, hypoalbuminemia, emotional instability, or psychosis.
⚘ **Lifespan:** In pregnant women, avoid use, if possible, because of risk to fetus. Women should stop breast-feeding because these drugs appear in breast milk and could cause serious

adverse effects in infants. In children, long-term use should be avoided, if possible, because stunted growth may result. Geriatric patients may have an increased risk of adverse reactions; monitor them closely.

Adverse reactions

Systemic corticosteroid therapy may suppress the hypothalamic-pituitary-adrenal (HPA) axis. Excessive use may cause cushingoid symptoms and various systemic disorders, such as diabetes and osteoporosis. Other effects may include euphoria, psychosis, insomnia, edema, hypertension, peptic ulcer, increased appetite, weight gain, fluid and electrolyte imbalances, dermatologic disorders, and immunosuppression.

Action

Corticosteroids suppress cell-mediated and humoral immunity in three ways: by reducing levels of leukocytes, monocytes, and eosinophils; by decreasing immunoglobulin binding to cell-surface receptors; and by inhibiting interleukin synthesis. They reduce inflammation by preventing hydrolytic enzyme release into the cells, preventing plasma exudation, suppressing polymorphonuclear leukocyte migration, and disrupting other inflammatory processes.

NURSING PROCESS

Assessment
• Establish baseline blood pressure, fluid and electrolyte status, and weight; reassess regularly.
• Monitor patient closely for adverse reactions.
• Evaluate drug effectiveness at regular intervals.

Key nursing diagnoses
• Ineffective protection related to suppression of HPA axis with long-term therapy
• Risk for injury related to severe adverse reactions
• Risk for infection related to immunosuppression

Planning and implementation
• Give drug early in the day to mimic circadian rhythm.
• Give drug with food to prevent GI irritation.
• Take precautions to avoid exposing patient to infection.

- Don't stop drug abruptly.
- Notify prescriber of severe or persistent adverse reactions.
- Avoid prolonged use of corticosteroids, especially in children.

Patient teaching
- Teach patient to take drug exactly as prescribed, and warn him never to stop the drug suddenly.
- Tell patient to notify prescriber if stress level increases; dosage may need to be temporarily increased.
- Instruct patient to take oral drug with food.
- Urge patient to report black tarry stools, bleeding, bruising, blurred vision, emotional changes, or other unusual effects.
- Encourage patient to wear or carry medical identification at all times.

☑ Evaluation
- Patient doesn't have evidence of adrenal insufficiency.
- Patient remains free from injury.
- Patient is free from infection.

Diuretics, loop
bumetanide
ethacrynate sodium
ethacrynic acid
furosemide
torsemide

Indications

▶ Edema from heart failure, hepatic cirrhosis, or nephrotic syndrome; mild-to-moderate hypertension; adjunct treatment in acute pulmonary edema or hypertensive crisis.

Contraindications and precautions

- Contraindicated in patients hypersensitive to these drugs and in patients with anuria, hepatic coma, or severe electrolyte depletion.
- Use cautiously in patients with severe renal disease.
- Use cautiously in patients with severe hypersensitivity to sulfonamides because allergic reaction may occur.
- ☀ **Lifespan:** In pregnant women, use cautiously. In breast-feeding women, don't use. In

neonates, use cautiously; the usual pediatric dose can be used, but dosage intervals should be extended. Geriatric patients are more susceptible to drug-induced diuresis, and reduced dosages may be indicated; monitor these patients closely.

Adverse reactions

Therapeutic doses commonly cause metabolic and electrolyte disturbances, particularly potassium depletion. They also may cause hypochloremic alkalosis, hyperglycemia, hyperuricemia, and hypomagnesemia. Rapid parenteral administration may cause hearing loss (including deafness) and tinnitus. High doses can produce profound diuresis, leading to hypovolemia and CV collapse. Photosensitivity also may occur.

Action

Loop diuretics inhibit sodium and chloride reabsorption in the ascending loop of Henle, thus increasing excretion of sodium, chloride, and water. Like thiazide diuretics, loop diuretics increase excretion of potassium. Loop diuretics produce more diuresis and electrolyte loss than thiazide diuretics.

NURSING PROCESS

☑ Assessment
- Monitor blood pressure and pulse rate, especially during rapid diuresis. Establish baseline values before therapy begins, and watch for significant changes.
- Establish baseline CBC (including WBC count), liver function test results, and electrolytes, carbon dioxide, magnesium, BUN, and creatinine levels. Review periodically.
- Assess patient for evidence of excessive diuresis: hypotension, tachycardia, poor skin turgor, excessive thirst, or dry and cracked mucous membranes.
- Monitor patient for edema and ascites. Observe the legs of ambulatory patients and the sacral area of patients on bed rest.
- Weigh patient each morning immediately after voiding and before breakfast, in the same type of clothing, and on the same scale. Weight provides a reliable indicator of patient's response to diuretic therapy.
- Monitor and record patient's intake and output daily.

⊕ Key nursing diagnoses
- Risk for deficient fluid volume related to excessive diuresis
- Impaired urine elimination related to change in diuresis pattern
- Ineffective protection related to electrolyte imbalance

▶ Planning and implementation
- Give diuretics in morning to ensure that major diuresis occurs before bedtime. To prevent nocturia, give diuretics before 6 p.m.
- Reduce dosage for patient with hepatic dysfunction, and increase dosage for patient with renal impairment, oliguria, or decreased diuresis. Inadequate urine output may result in circulatory overload, which causes water intoxication, pulmonary edema, and heart failure. Increase dosage of insulin or oral hypoglycemic in diabetic patient, and reduce dosage of other antihypertensives.
- Take safety measures for all ambulatory patients until response to diuretic is known.
- Consult dietitian about need for potassium supplements.
- Keep urinal or commode readily available to patient.

Patient teaching
- Explain rationale for therapy and importance of following prescribed regimen.
- Review adverse effects, and urge patient to report symptoms promptly, especially chest, back, or leg pain; shortness of breath; dyspnea; increased edema or weight; and excess diuresis evidenced by weight loss of more than 0.9 kg (2 lb) daily.
- Advise patient to eat potassium-rich foods and to avoid high-sodium foods, such as lunch meat, smoked meats, and processed cheeses. Instruct him not to add table salt to foods.
- Encourage patient to keep follow-up appointments to monitor effectiveness of therapy.

☑ Evaluation
- Patient maintains adequate hydration.
- Patient states importance of taking diuretic early in the day to prevent nocturia.
- Patient complies with therapy, as evidenced by improvement in underlying condition.

Diuretics, thiazide and thiazide-like

Thiazide
chlorothiazide
hydrochlorothiazide
Thiazide-like
indapamide
metolazone

Indications

▶ Edema from right-sided heart failure, mild-to-moderate left-sided heart failure, or nephrotic syndrome; edema and ascites caused by hepatic cirrhosis; hypertension; diabetes insipidus, particularly nephrogenic diabetes insipidus.

Contraindications and precautions

- Contraindicated in patients hypersensitive to these drugs and in those with anuria.
- Use cautiously in patients with severe renal disease, impaired hepatic function, or progressive liver disease.
- ⚞ **Lifespan:** In pregnant women, use cautiously. In breast-feeding women, thiazides are contraindicated because they appear in breast milk. In children, safety and effectiveness haven't been established. Geriatric patients are more susceptible to drug-induced diuresis, and reduced dosages may be needed; monitor patient closely.

Adverse reactions

Therapeutic doses cause electrolyte and metabolic disturbances, most commonly potassium depletion. Other abnormalities include hypochloremic alkalosis, hypomagnesemia, hyponatremia, hypercalcemia, hyperuricemia, hyperglycemia, and elevated cholesterol levels. Photosensitivity also may occur.

Action

Thiazide and thiazide-like diuretics interfere with sodium transport across the tubules of the cortical diluting segment in the nephron, thereby increasing renal excretion of sodium, chloride, water, potassium, and calcium.

Thiazide diuretics also exert an antihypertensive effect. Although the exact mechanism is unknown, direct arteriolar dilation may be partially responsible. In diabetes insipidus, thiazides cause a paradoxical decrease in urine volume and an increase in renal concentration of urine, possibly because of sodium depletion and decreased plasma volume. This increases water and sodium reabsorption in the kidneys.

NURSING PROCESS

⚚ Assessment

• Monitor patient's intake, output, and electrolyte level regularly.
• Weigh patient each morning immediately after voiding and before breakfast, in the same type of clothing, and on the same scale. Weight provides a reliable indicator of patient's response to diuretic therapy.
• Monitor diabetic patient's glucose level. Diuretics may cause hyperglycemia.
• Monitor creatinine and BUN levels regularly. Drug isn't as effective if these levels are more than twice normal. Also, monitor uric acid level.

⬢ Key nursing diagnoses

• Risk for deficient fluid volume related to excessive diuresis
• Impaired urine elimination related to change in diuresis pattern
• Ineffective protection related to electrolyte imbalance

⯈ Planning and implementation

• Give drug in the morning to prevent nocturia.
• Provide a high-potassium diet.
• Give potassium supplements to maintain acceptable potassium level.
• Keep urinal or commode readily available to patient.
Patient teaching
• Explain the rationale for therapy and the importance of following the prescribed regimen.
• Tell patient to take drug at the same time each day to prevent nocturia. Suggest taking drug with food to minimize GI irritation.
• Urge patient to seek prescriber's approval before taking any other drug, including OTC medications and herbal remedies.
• Advise patient to record his weight each morning after voiding and before breakfast, in the same type of clothing, and on the same scale.

• Review adverse effects, and urge the patient to report symptoms promptly, especially chest, back, or leg pain; shortness of breath; dyspnea; increased edema or weight; or excess diuresis evidenced by weight loss of more than 0.9 kg [2 lb] daily. Warn him about photosensitivity reactions that usually occur 10 to 14 days after initial sun exposure.
• Advise patient to eat potassium-rich foods and to avoid high-sodium foods, such as lunch meat, smoked meats, processed cheeses. Instruct him not to add table salt to foods.
• Encourage patient to keep follow-up appointments to monitor effectiveness of therapy.

☑ Evaluation

• Patient maintains adequate hydration.
• Patient states importance of taking diuretic early in the day to prevent nocturia.
• Patient complies with therapy, as evidenced by improvement in underlying condition.

Estrogens

esterified estrogens
estradiol
estradiol cypionate
estradiol valerate
estrogenic substances, conjugated
estrone
estropipate

Indications

▶ Prevention of moderate to severe vasomotor symptoms linked to menopause, such as hot flushes and dizziness; stimulation of vaginal tissue development, cornification, and secretory activity; inhibition of hormone-sensitive cancer growth; female hypogonadism; female castration; primary ovulation failure; ovulation control; prevention of conception.

Contraindications and precautions

• Contraindicated in women with thrombophlebitis or thromboembolic disorders, unexplained abnormal genital bleeding, or estrogen-dependent neoplasia.
• Use cautiously in patients with hypertension; metabolic bone disease; migraines; seizures; asthma; cardiac, renal, or hepatic impairment;

blood dyscrasia; diabetes; family history of breast cancer; or fibrocystic disease.

≛ **Lifespan:** In pregnant or breast-feeding women, use is contraindicated. In adolescents whose bone growth isn't complete, use cautiously because of effects on epiphyseal closure. Postmenopausal women with long-term estrogen use have an increased risk of endometrial cancer. Postmenopausal women also have increased risk for breast cancer, heart attack, stroke, and blood clots when taking estrogen plus progestin long-term.

Adverse reactions

Acute adverse reactions include abdominal cramps, swollen feet or ankles, bloating caused by fluid and electrolyte retention, breast swelling and tenderness, weight gain, nausea, loss of appetite, headache, photosensitivity, loss of libido, and changes in menstrual bleeding patterns, such as spotting and prolongation or absence of bleeding.

Long-term effects include elevated blood pressure (sometimes into the hypertensive range), cholestatic jaundice, benign hepatomas, endometrial carcinoma (rare), and thromboembolic disease (risk increases markedly with cigarette smoking, especially in women older than age 35).

Action

Estrogens promote the development and maintenance of the female reproductive system and secondary sexual characteristics. They inhibit the release of pituitary gonadotropins and have various metabolic effects, including retention of fluid and electrolytes, retention and deposition in bone of calcium and phosphorus, and mild anabolic activity. Of the six naturally occurring estrogens in humans, estradiol, estrone, and estriol are present in significant quantities.

Estrogens and estrogenic substances given as drugs have effects related to endogenous estrogen's mechanism of action. They can mimic the action of endogenous estrogen when used as replacement therapy and can inhibit ovulation or the growth of certain hormone-sensitive cancers. Conjugated estrogens and estrogenic substances are normally obtained from the urine of pregnant mares. Other estrogens are manufactured synthetically.

NURSING PROCESS

⊠ Assessment
● Monitor patient regularly to detect improvement or worsening of symptoms; observe patient for adverse reactions.
● If patient has diabetes mellitus, watch closely for loss of diabetes control.
● Monitor PT of patient receiving warfarin-type anticoagulant. Adjust anticoagulant dosage.

⊞ Key nursing diagnoses
● Excessive fluid volume related to drug-induced fluid retention
● Risk of injury related to adverse effects
● Noncompliance related to long-term therapy

▷ Planning and implementation
● Notify pathologist of patient's estrogen therapy when sending specimens for evaluation.
● Give drug once daily for 3 weeks, followed by 1 week without drugs; repeat as needed.

Patient teaching
● Urge patient to read the package insert describing adverse reactions. Follow this with a verbal explanation. Tell patient to keep the package insert for later reference.
● Advise patient to take drug with meals or at bedtime to relieve nausea. Reassure patient that nausea usually disappears with continued therapy.
● Teach patient how to apply estrogen ointments or transdermal estrogen. Review symptoms that accompany a systemic reaction to ointments.
● Teach patient how to insert intravaginal estrogen suppository. Advise her to use sanitary pads instead of tampons when using suppository.
● Teach patient how to perform routine monthly breast self-examination.
● Tell patient to stop taking drug immediately if she becomes pregnant because estrogens can harm fetus.
● Remind patient not to breast-feed during estrogen therapy.
● If patient is receiving cyclic therapy for postmenopausal symptoms, explain that withdrawal bleeding may occur during the week off, but that fertility hasn't been restored and ovulation won't occur.
● Explain that medical supervision is essential during prolonged therapy.

• Tell man on long-term therapy about possible temporary gynecomastia and impotence, which will disappear when therapy ends.

• Instruct patient to notify prescriber immediately if patient experiences abdominal pain; pain, numbness, or stiffness in legs or buttocks; pressure or pain in chest; shortness of breath; severe headaches; visual disturbances, such as blind spots, flashing lights, or blurriness; vaginal bleeding or discharge; breast lumps; swelling of hands or feet; yellow skin and sclera; dark urine; or light-colored stools.

• Urge diabetic patient to report symptoms of hyperglycemia or glycosuria.

☑ Evaluation

• Patient experiences only minimal fluid retention.

• Patient doesn't develop serious complications of estrogen therapy.

• Patient complies with therapy, as evidenced by improvement in condition or absence of pregnancy.

Hematinics, oral

ferrous fumarate
ferrous gluconate
ferrous sulfate

Indications

▶ Prevention and treatment of iron-deficiency anemia.

Contraindications and precautions

• Contraindicated in patients with hemochromatosis, hemolytic anemia, or hemosiderosis.

• Use cautiously in patients with peptic ulcer disease, regional enteritis, ulcerative colitis, or sensitivity to sulfites or tartrazine.

☀ Lifespan: In breast-feeding women, iron supplements are commonly recommended; no adverse effects are known. With children, caution parents about possible lethal effects of iron overdose. In elderly patients, iron-induced constipation is common; stress proper diet high in fiber to minimize this effect. Elderly patients also may need higher doses because reduced gastric secretions and achlorhydria may lower their capacity for iron absorption.

Adverse reactions

Because iron is corrosive, GI intolerance occurs in 5% to 20% of patients; symptoms include nausea, vomiting, anorexia, constipation, and dark stools. Liquid forms may stain teeth.

Action

Iron is an essential component of hemoglobin. It's needed in adequate amounts for erythropoiesis and for efficient oxygen transport in the blood. After absorption into the blood, iron is immediately bound to transferrin, a plasma protein that transports iron to bone marrow, where it's used during hemoglobin synthesis. Some iron is also used during synthesis of myoglobin and other nonhemoglobin heme units.

NURSING PROCESS

☲ Assessment

• Monitor patient for adverse reactions, especially those related to bowel function.

• Monitor hemoglobin and reticulocyte count during therapy.

⊕ Key nursing diagnoses

• Risk for deficient fluid volume related to GI upset

• Constipation related to adverse effect on bowel function

• Noncompliance related to adverse effects or long-term use

▷ Planning and implementation

• Dilute liquid forms in juice (preferably orange juice, which promotes iron absorption) or water, but not in milk or antacids. To avoid staining teeth, give liquid preparations through a straw. Don't give antacids within 1 hour before or 2 hours after an iron product, if possible, to prevent interference with absorption.

• Don't crush tablets or capsules; if patient has trouble swallowing, use a liquid form.

Patient teaching

• Explain rationale for therapy, and urge patient to follow the prescribed regimen.

• Tell patient to continue his regular dosage schedule if he misses a dose, and warn him not to take double doses.

• Advise patient to dilute liquid form in juice (preferably orange juice) or water. Suggest that he use a straw to avoid staining his teeth.

• Review possible adverse effects. Tell patient that oral iron may turn stools black, and reassure him that this is harmless. Teach dietary measures to help prevent constipation.

• Explain the toxicity of iron, and emphasize importance of keeping iron away from children to prevent poisoning. As few as three or four tablets can cause serious iron poisoning.

• Urge patient to report diarrhea or constipation because prescriber may want to adjust dosage, modify diet, or order further tests.

• Explain that iron therapy may be required for 4 to 6 months after anemia resolves. Encourage compliance.

☑ Evaluation

• Patient maintains adequate hydration.

• Patient regains normal bowel pattern.

• Patient complies with therapy, as evidenced by return of normal hemoglobin and resolution of iron deficiency anemia.

Histamine$_2$-receptor antagonists
cimetidine
famotidine
nizatidine
ranitidine hydrochloride

Indications

▶ Acute duodenal or gastric ulcer, Zollinger-Ellison syndrome, gastroesophageal reflux.

Contraindications and precautions

• Contraindicated in patients hypersensitive to these drugs.

• Use cautiously in patients with impaired renal or hepatic function.

⚖ Lifespan: In pregnant women, use cautiously. In breast-feeding women, H$_2$-receptor antagonists are contraindicated because they may appear in breast milk. In children, safety and effectiveness haven't been established. Geriatric patients have increased risk of adverse reactions, particularly those affecting the CNS; use cautiously.

Adverse reactions

H$_2$-receptor antagonists rarely cause adverse reactions. Mild and transient diarrhea, thrombo-

cytopenia, dizziness, fatigue, headache, cardiac arrhythmias, and gynecomastia are possible.

Action

All H$_2$-receptor antagonists inhibit the action of H$_2$-receptors in gastric parietal cells, reducing gastric acid output and concentration, regardless of stimulants, such as histamine, food, insulin, and caffeine, or basal conditions.

NURSING PROCESS

🔍 Assessment

• Monitor patient for adverse reactions, especially hypotension and arrhythmias.

• Periodically monitor laboratory tests, such as CBC and renal and hepatic studies.

🔑 Key nursing diagnoses

• Risk for infection related to drug-induced neutropenia

• Decreased cardiac output related to adverse CV effects (cimetidine)

• Fatigue related to drug's CNS effects

▷ Planning and implementation

• Give once-daily dose h.s., twice-daily doses in morning and evening, and multiple doses with meals and h.s. A once-daily dose h.s. promotes compliance.

• Don't exceed recommended infusion rates when giving drugs I.V.; doing so increases risk of adverse CV effects. Continuous I.V. infusion may suppress acid secretion more effectively.

• Give antacids at least 1 hour before or after H$_2$-receptor antagonists. Antacids can decrease drug absorption.

• Adjust dosage for patient with renal disease.

• Don't stop drug abruptly.

Patient teaching

• Teach patient how and when to take drug, and warn him not to stop drug suddenly.

• Review possible adverse reactions, and urge him to report unusual effects.

• Caution patient to avoid smoking during therapy; smoking stimulates gastric acid secretion and worsens the disease.

☑ Evaluation

• Patient is free from infection.

• Patient maintains a normal heart rhythm.

• Patient states appropriate management plan for combating fatigue.

Hypoglycemics, oral

acarbose
glimepiride
glipizide
glyburide
metformin hydrochloride
miglitol
nateglinide
pioglitazone hydrochloride
repaglinide
rosiglitazone maleate

Indications

▶ Mild to moderately severe, stable, nonketotic, non–insulin-dependent diabetes mellitus that can't be controlled by diet alone.

Contraindications and precautions

● Contraindicated in patients hypersensitive to these drugs and in patients with diabetic ketoacidosis with or without coma. Metformin is also contraindicated in patients with renal disease or metabolic acidosis and generally should be avoided in patients with hepatic disease.
● Use sulfonylureas cautiously in patients with renal or hepatic disease. Use metformin cautiously in patients with adrenal or pituitary insufficiency and in debilitated and malnourished patients. Alpha-glucosidase inhibitors should be used cautiously in patients with mild to moderate renal insufficiency. Use thiazolidinediones cautiously in patients with edema or heart failure.
⚖ Lifespan: In pregnant or breast-feeding women, use is contraindicated; oral hypoglycemics appear in small amounts in breast milk and may cause hypoglycemia in the infant. In children, oral hypoglycemics aren't effective in type 1 diabetes mellitus. Geriatric patients may be more sensitive to these drugs, usually need lower dosages, and are more likely to develop neurologic symptoms of hypoglycemia; monitor these patients closely. In geriatric patients, avoid chlorpropamide use because of its long duration of action.

Adverse reactions

Sulfonylureas cause dose-related reactions that usually respond to decreased dosage: headache, nausea, vomiting, anorexia, heartburn, weakness, and paresthesia. Hypoglycemia may follow excessive dosage, increased exercise, decreased food intake, or alcohol use.

The most serious adverse reaction linked to metformin is lactic acidosis. It's rare and most likely to occur in patients with renal dysfunction. Other reactions to metformin include GI upset, megaloblastic anemia, rash, dermatitis, and unpleasant or metallic taste.

Action

Oral hypoglycemics come in several types. Sulfonylureas are sulfonamide derivatives that aren't antibacterial. They lower glucose levels by stimulating insulin release from the pancreas. These drugs work only in the presence of functioning beta cells in the islet tissue of the pancreas. After prolonged administration, they produce hypoglycemia by acting outside of the pancreas, including reduced glucose production by the liver and enhanced peripheral sensitivity to insulin. The latter may result from an increased number of insulin receptors or from changes after insulin binding. Sulfonylureas are divided into first-generation drugs, such as chlorpropamide, and second-generation drugs, such as glyburide, glimepiride, and glipizide. Although their mechanisms of action are similar, the second-generation drugs carry a more lipophilic side chain, are more potent, and cause fewer adverse reactions. Their most important difference is their duration of action.

Meglitinides, such as nateglinide and repaglinide, are non-sulfonylurea hypoglycemics that stimulate the release of insulin from the pancreas.

Metformin decreases hepatic glucose production, reduces intestinal glucose absorption, and improves insulin sensitivity by increasing peripheral glucose uptake and utilization. With metformin therapy, insulin secretion remains unchanged, and fasting insulin levels and all-day insulin response may decrease.

Alpha-glucosidase inhibitors, such as acarbose and miglitol, delay digestion of carbohydrates, resulting in a smaller rise in glucose levels.

Rosiglitazone and pioglitazone are thiazolidinediones, which lower glucose levels by improving insulin sensitivity. These drugs are potent and highly selective agonists for receptors found in insulin-sensitive tissues, such as adipose, skeletal muscle, and liver.

NURSING PROCESS

✍ Assessment
● Monitor patient's glucose level regularly. Increase monitoring during periods of increased stress, such as infection, fever, surgery, or trauma.
● Monitor patient for adverse reactions.
● Assess patient's compliance with drug therapy and other aspects of diabetic treatment.

🖉 Key nursing diagnoses
● Risk for injury related to hypoglycemia
● Risk for deficient fluid volume related to adverse GI effects
● Noncompliance related to long-term therapy

▶ Planning and implementation
● Give sulfonylurea 30 minutes before morning meal for once-daily dosing or 30 minutes before morning and evening meals for twice-daily dosing. Give metformin with morning and evening meals. Alpha-glucosidase inhibitors should be taken with the first bite of each main meal three times daily.
● Patients who take a thiazolidinedione should have liver enzyme levels measured at the start of therapy, every 2 months for the first year of therapy, and periodically thereafter.
● Keep in mind that a patient transferring from one oral hypoglycemic to another (except chlorpropamide) usually needs no transition period.
● Anticipate patient's need for insulin during periods of increased stress.
Patient teaching
● Emphasize importance of following the prescribed regimen. Urge patient to adhere to diet, weight reduction, exercise, and personal hygiene recommendations.
● Explain that therapy relieves symptoms but doesn't cure the disease.
● Teach patient how to recognize and treat hypoglycemia.

☑ Evaluation
● Patient sustains no injury.
● Patient maintains adequate hydration.
● Patient complies with therapy, as evidenced by normal or near-normal glucose level.

Laxatives
Bulk-forming
calcium polycarbophil
methylcellulose
psyllium
Emollient
docusate calcium
docusate potassium
docusate sodium
Hyperosmolar
glycerin
lactulose
magnesium citrate
magnesium hydroxide
magnesium sulfate
sodium phosphates
Stimulant
bisacodyl
senna

Indications

▶ Constipation, irritable bowel syndrome, diverticulosis.

Contraindications and precautions

● Contraindicated in patients with GI obstruction or perforation, toxic colitis, megacolon, nausea and vomiting, or acute surgical abdomen.
● Use cautiously in patients with rectal or anal conditions, such as rectal bleeding or large hemorrhoids.
⚖ Lifespan: For breast-feeding women, recommendations vary for individual drugs. Infants and children have an increased risk of fluid and electrolyte disturbances; use cautiously. In elderly patients, dependence is more likely to develop because of age-related changes in GI function; monitor these patients closely.

Adverse reactions

All laxatives may cause flatulence, diarrhea, abdominal discomfort, weakness, and dependence. Bulk-forming laxatives may cause intestinal obstruction, impaction, or (rarely) esophageal obstruction. Emollient laxatives may cause a bitter taste or throat irritation. Hyperosmolar laxatives may cause fluid and electrolyte imbalances. Stimulant laxatives may cause urine discoloration, malabsorption, and weight loss.

Action

Laxatives promote movement of intestinal contents through the colon and rectum in several ways: bulk-forming, emollient, hyperosmolar, and stimulant.

NURSING PROCESS

⚕ Assessment
• Obtain baseline assessment of patient's bowel patterns and GI history before giving.
• Monitor patient for adverse reactions.
• Monitor bowel pattern throughout therapy. Assess bowel sounds and color and consistency of stools.
• Monitor patient's fluid and electrolyte status during administration.

⚙ Key nursing diagnoses
• Diarrhea related to adverse GI effects
• Acute pain related to abdominal discomfort
• Impaired health maintenance related to laxative dependence

⯈ Planning and implementation
• Don't crush enteric-coated tablets.
• Time administration so that bowel evacuation doesn't interfere with sleep.
• Make sure patient has easy access to bedpan or bathroom.
• Institute measures to prevent constipation.
Patient teaching
• Advise patient that therapy should be short-term. Point out that abuse or prolonged use can cause nutritional imbalances.
• Tell patient that stool softeners and bulk-forming laxatives may take several days to achieve results.
• Encourage patient to remain active and to drink plenty of fluids if he's taking a bulk-forming laxative.
• Explain that stimulant laxatives may cause harmless urine discoloration.
• Teach patient about including foods high in fiber into diet.

☑ Evaluation
• Patient regains normal bowel pattern.
• Patient states that pain is relieved with stool evacuation.

• Patient discusses dangers of laxative abuse and importance of limiting laxative use.

Nonsteroidal anti-inflammatory drugs
celecoxib
diclofenac potassium
diclofenac sodium
diflunisal
etodolac
ibuprofen
indomethacin
indomethacin sodium trihydrate
ketoprofen
ketorolac tromethamine
mefenamic acid
meloxicam
nabumetone
naproxen
naproxen sodium
oxaprozin
piroxicam
rofecoxib
sulindac
valdecoxib

Indications

▶ Mild to moderate pain, inflammation, stiffness, swelling, or tenderness caused by headache, arthralgia, myalgia, neuralgia, dysmenorrhea, rheumatoid arthritis, juvenile arthritis, osteoarthritis, or dental or surgical procedures.

Contraindications and precautions

• Contraindicated in patients with GI lesions or GI bleeding and in patients hypersensitive to these drugs.
• Use cautiously in patients with cardiac decompensation, hypertension, fluid retention, or coagulation defects.
⚖ Lifespan: In pregnant women, use cautiously in the first and second trimesters; don't use in the third trimester. For breast-feeding women, NSAIDs aren't recommended. In children younger than age 14, safety of long-term therapy hasn't been established. Patients older than age 60 may be more susceptible to toxic effects

of NSAIDs because of decreased renal function.

Adverse reactions

Adverse reactions chiefly involve the GI tract, particularly erosion of the gastric mucosa. The most common symptoms are dyspepsia, heartburn, epigastric distress, nausea, and abdominal pain. CNS reactions also may occur. Flank pain with other evidence of nephrotoxicity occurs occasionally. Fluid retention may aggravate hypertension or heart failure.

Action

The analgesic effect of NSAIDs may result from interference with the prostaglandins involved in pain. Prostaglandins appear to sensitize pain receptors to mechanical stimulation or to other chemical mediators. NSAIDs inhibit synthesis of prostaglandins peripherally and possibly centrally.

Like salicylates, NSAIDs exert an antiinflammatory effect that may result in part from inhibition of prostaglandin synthesis and release during inflammation. The exact mechanism isn't clear.

NURSING PROCESS

☞ Assessment
• Assess patient's level of pain and inflammation before therapy begins, and evaluate drug effectiveness after administration.
• Monitor patient for signs and symptoms of bleeding. Assess bleeding time if patient needs surgery.
• Monitor ophthalmic and auditory function before and periodically during therapy to detect toxicity.
• Monitor CBC, platelet count, PT, and hepatic and renal function studies periodically to detect abnormalities.
• Watch for bronchospasm in patients with aspirin hypersensitivity, rhinitis or nasal polyps, and asthma.

⊞ Key nursing diagnoses
• Risk for injury related to adverse reactions
• Excessive fluid volume related to fluid retention
• Disturbed sensory perception (visual and auditory) related to toxicity

⊠ Planning and implementation
• Administer oral NSAIDs with 8 oz (240 ml) of water to ensure adequate passage into the stomach. Have patient sit up for 15 to 30 minutes after taking drug to prevent lodging in esophagus.
• Crush tablets or mix with food or fluid to aid swallowing. Give with antacids to minimize GI upset.

Patient teaching
• Encourage patient to take drug as directed to achieve desired effect. Explain that he may not notice benefits of drug for 2 to 4 weeks.
• Review methods to prevent or minimize GI upset.
• Work with patient on long-term therapy to arrange for monitoring of laboratory values, especially BUN and creatinine levels, liver function test results, and CBC.
• Instruct patient to notify prescriber about severe or persistent adverse reactions.

☑ Evaluation
• Patient remains free from injury.
• Patient shows no signs of edema.
• Patient maintains normal visual and auditory function.

Opioids
alfentanil hydrochloride
codeine phosphate
codeine sulfate
difenoxin
diphenoxylate
fentanyl citrate
hydromorphone hydrochloride
meperidine hydrochloride
methadone hydrochloride
morphine sulfate
oxycodone hydrochloride
oxymorphone hydrochloride
propoxyphene hydrochloride
propoxyphene napsylate
sufentanil citrate

Indications

▶ Moderate to severe pain from acute and some chronic disorders; diarrhea; dry, nonproductive cough; management of opiate dependence; anesthesia support; sedation.

Contraindications and precautions

• Contraindicated in patients hypersensitive to these drugs and in those who have recently taken an MAO inhibitor. Also contraindicated in those with acute or severe bronchial asthma or respiratory depression.
• Use cautiously in patients with head injury, increased intracranial or intraocular pressure, and hepatic or renal dysfunction.
• Use cautiously in patients with mental illnesses and emotional disturbances, and in patients exhibiting drug-seeking behaviors.
⚞ **Lifespan:** In pregnant or breast-feeding women, use cautiously; codeine, meperidine, methadone, morphine, and propoxyphene appear in breast milk. Breast-feeding infants of women taking methadone may develop physical dependence. In children, safety and effectiveness haven't been established. Geriatric patients may be more sensitive to opioids; lower doses are usually indicated.

Adverse reactions

Respiratory and circulatory depression (including orthostatic hypotension) are the major hazards of opioids. Other adverse CNS effects include dizziness, visual disturbances, mental clouding, depression, sedation, coma, euphoria, dysphoria, weakness, faintness, agitation, restlessness, nervousness, and seizures. Adverse GI effects include nausea, vomiting, constipation, and biliary colic. Urine retention or hypersensitivity also may occur. Tolerance to the drug and psychological or physical dependence may follow prolonged therapy.

Action

Opioids act as agonists at specific opiate-receptor binding sites in the CNS and other tissues, altering the patient's perception of and emotional response to pain.

NURSING PROCESS

⚗ **Assessment**
• Obtain baseline assessment of patient's pain, and reassess frequently to determine drug effectiveness.
• Evaluate patient's respiratory status before each dose; watch for respiratory rate below patient's baseline level and for restlessness, which may be compensatory signs of hypoxia. Respiratory depression may last longer than the analgesic effect.
• Monitor patient for other adverse reactions.
• Monitor patient for tolerance and dependence. The first sign of tolerance to opioids is usually a shortened duration of effect.

⚎ **Key nursing diagnoses**
• Ineffective breathing pattern related to respiratory depression
• Risk for injury related to orthostatic hypotension
• Ineffective individual coping related to drug dependence

⚎ **Planning and implementation**
• Keep resuscitative equipment and an opioid antagonist, such as naloxone, available.
• Give I.V. drug by slow injection, preferably in diluted solution. Rapid I.V. injection increases the risk of adverse effects.
• Give drug I.M. or S.C. cautiously to a patient with decreased platelet count and to a patient who is chilled, hypovolemic, or in shock; decreased perfusion may lead to drug accumulation and toxicity. Rotate injection sites to avoid induration.
• Carefully note the strength of solution when measuring a dose. Oral solutions of varying concentrations are available.
• For maximum effectiveness, give on a regular dosage schedule rather than p.r.n.
• Institute safety precautions.
• Encourage postoperative patient to turn, cough, and breathe deeply every 2 hours to avoid atelectasis.
• Give oral forms with food if GI irritation occurs.
• Withdrawal symptoms—including tremors, agitation, nausea, and vomiting—may occur if drug is stopped abruptly. Monitor patient with these symptoms carefully and provide supportive therapy.

Patient teaching
• Teach patient to take drug exactly as prescribed. Urge him to call prescriber if he isn't experiencing desired effect or is experiencing significant adverse reactions.
• Warn patient to avoid hazardous activities until drug's effects are known.

• Advise patient to avoid alcohol while taking opioid; alcohol will cause additive CNS depression.

• Suggest measures to prevent constipation, such as increasing fiber in diet and using a stool softener.

• Instruct patient to breathe deeply, cough, and change position every 2 hours to avoid respiratory complications.

☑ **Evaluation**

• Patient maintains adequate ventilation, as evidenced by normal respiratory rate and rhythm and pink color.

• Patient remains free from injury.

• Patient doesn't become tolerant to drug.

Penicillins

Natural penicillins
penicillin G benzathine
penicillin G potassium
penicillin G procaine
penicillin G sodium
penicillin V potassium

Aminopenicillins
amoxicillin and clavulanate potassium
amoxicillin trihydrate
ampicillin
ampicillin sodium and sulbactam sodium
ampicillin trihydrate

Penicillinase-resistant penicillins
dicloxacillin sodium
nafcillin sodium
oxacillin sodium

Extended-spectrum penicillins
carbenicillin indanyl sodium
piperacillin sodium and tazobactam sodium
ticarcillin disodium
ticarcillin disodium and clavulanate potassium

Indications

▶ Streptococcal pneumonia; enterococcal and nonenterococcal Group D endocarditis; diphtheria; anthrax; meningitis; tetanus; botulism; actinomycosis; syphilis; relapsing fever; Lyme disease; pneumococcal infections; rheumatic fever; bacterial endocarditis; neonatal Group B streptococcal disease; septicemia; gynecologic infections; infections of urinary, respiratory, and GI tracts; infections of skin, soft tissue, bones, and joints.

Contraindications and precautions

• Contraindicated in patients hypersensitive to these drugs.

• Use cautiously in patients with history of asthma or drug allergy, mononucleosis, renal impairment, CV diseases, hemorrhagic condition, or electrolyte imbalance.

⚖ Lifespan: In pregnant women, use cautiously. For breast-feeding patients, recommendations vary depending on the drug. For children, dosage recommendations have been established for most penicillins. Geriatric patients are susceptible to superinfection and renal impairment, which decreases excretion of penicillins; use cautiously and at a lower dosage.

Adverse reactions

With all penicillins, hypersensitivity reactions range from mild rash, fever, and eosinophilia to fatal anaphylaxis. Hematologic reactions include hemolytic anemia, transient neutropenia, leukopenia, and thrombocytopenia.

Certain adverse reactions are more common with specific classes: For example, bleeding episodes are usually seen with high doses of extended-spectrum penicillins, whereas GI adverse effects are most common with ampicillin. In patients with renal disease, high doses, especially of penicillin G, irritate the CNS by causing confusion, twitching, lethargy, dysphagia, seizures, and coma. Hepatotoxicity may occur with penicillinase-resistant penicillins; hyperkalemia and hypernatremia have been reported with extended-spectrum penicillins.

Local irritation from parenteral therapy may be severe enough to warrant administration by subclavian or centrally placed catheter or discontinuation of therapy.

Action

Penicillins are generally bactericidal. They inhibit synthesis of the bacterial cell wall, causing rapid cell destruction. They're most effective against fast-growing susceptible bacteria. Their sites of action are enzymes known as penicillin-binding proteins (PBPs). The affinity of certain penicillins for PBPs in various microorganisms helps explain the different activities of these drugs.

Susceptible aerobic gram-positive cocci include *Staphylococcus aureus;* nonenterococcal Group D streptococci; Groups A, B, D, G, H, K, L, and M streptococci; *Streptococcus viridans;* and enterococcus (usually with an aminoglycoside). Susceptible aerobic gram-negative cocci include *Neisseria meningitidis* and non–penicillinase-producing *N. gonorrhoeae.*

Susceptible aerobic gram-positive bacilli include *Corynebacterium, Listeria,* and *Bacillus anthracis.* Susceptible anaerobes include *Peptococcus, Peptostreptococcus, Actinomyces, Clostridium, Fusobacterium, Veillonella,* and non–beta-lactamase–producing strains of *Streptococcus pneumoniae.* Susceptible spirochetes include *Treponema pallidum, T. pertenue, Leptospira, Borrelia recurrentis,* and, possibly, *B. burgdorferi.*

Aminopenicillins have uses against more organisms, including many gram-negative organisms. Like natural penicillins, aminopenicillins are vulnerable to inactivation by penicillinase. Susceptible organisms include *Escherichia coli, Proteus mirabilis, Shigella, Salmonella, Streptococcus pneumoniae, N. gonorrhoeae, Haemophilus influenzae, Staphylococcus aureus, Staphylococcus epidermidis* (non–penicillinase-producing *Staphylococcus*), and *Listeria monocytogenes.*

Penicillinase-resistant penicillins are semisynthetic penicillins designed to remain stable against hydrolysis by most staphylococcal penicillinases and thus are the drugs of choice against susceptible penicillinase-producing staphylococci. They also act against most organisms susceptible to natural penicillins.

Extended-spectrum penicillins offer a wider range of bactericidal action than the other three classes and usually are given in combination with aminoglycosides. Susceptible strains include *Enterobacter, Klebsiella, Citrobacter, Serratia, Bacteroides fragilis, Pseudomonas aeruginosa, Proteus vulgaris, Providencia rettgeri,* and *Morganella morganii.* These penicillins are also vulnerable to beta-lactamase and penicillinases.

NURSING PROCESS

Assessment

- Assess patient's history of allergies. Try to find out whether previous reactions were true hypersensitivity reactions or adverse reactions (such as GI distress) that patient interpreted as allergy.
- Keep in mind that a patient who has never had a penicillin hypersensitivity reaction may still have future allergic reactions; monitor patient continuously for possible allergic reactions or other adverse effects.
- Obtain culture and sensitivity tests before giving first dose; repeat tests periodically to assess drug's effectiveness.
- Monitor vital signs, electrolytes, and renal function studies.
- Assess patient's consciousness and neurologic status when giving high doses; CNS toxicity can occur.
- Coagulation abnormalities, even frank bleeding, can follow high doses, especially of extended-spectrum penicillins. Monitor PT, INR, and platelet counts. Assess patient for signs of occult or frank bleeding.
- Monitor patients, especially elderly patients, debilitated patients, and patients receiving immunosuppressants or radiation, receiving long-term therapy for possible superinfection.

Key nursing diagnoses

- Ineffective protection related to hypersensitivity
- Risk for infection related to superinfection
- Risk for deficient fluid volume related to adverse GI reactions

Planning and implementation

- Give penicillin at least 1 hour before bacteriostatic antibiotics, such as tetracyclines, erythromycins, and chloramphenicol; these drugs inhibit bacterial cell growth and decrease rate of penicillin uptake by bacterial cell walls.
- Follow manufacturer's directions for reconstituting, diluting, and storing drugs; check expiration dates.
- Give oral penicillin at least 1 hour before or 2 hours after meals to enhance GI absorption.
- Refrigerate oral suspensions, which will be stable for 14 days; shake well before giving to ensure correct dosage.

• Give I.M. dose deep into gluteal muscle mass or midlateral thigh, rotate injection sites to minimize tissue injury, and apply ice to injection site to relieve pain. Don't inject more than 2 g of drug per injection site.

• With I.V. infusions, don't add or mix another drug, especially an aminoglycoside, which will become inactive if mixed with a penicillin. If other drugs must be given I.V., temporarily stop infusion of primary drug.

• Infuse I.V. drug continuously or intermittently over 30 minutes. Rotate infusion site every 48 hours. Intermittent I.V. infusion may be diluted in 50 to 100 ml sterile water, normal saline solution, D_5W, D_5W and half-normal saline solution, or lactated Ringer's solution.

Patient teaching

• Make sure patient understands how and when to take drug. Urge him to complete the prescribed regimen, comply with instructions for around-the-clock scheduling, and keep follow-up appointments.

• Teach patient signs and symptoms of hypersensitivity and other adverse reactions. Urge him to report unusual reactions.

• Tell patient to check drug's expiration date and to discard unused drug. Warn him not to share drug with family or friends.

☑ Evaluation

• Patient shows no signs of hypersensitivity.
• Patient is free from infection.
• Patient maintains adequate hydration.

Phenothiazines

chlorpromazine hydrochloride
fluphenazine
mesoridazine besylate
perphenazine
prochlorperazine
promazine hydrochloride
promethazine
thioridazine hydrochloride
thiothixene
trifluoperazine hydrochloride

Indications

▶ Agitated psychotic states, hallucinations, manic-depressive illness, excessive motor and

autonomic activity, nausea and vomiting, moderate anxiety, behavioral problems caused by chronic organic mental syndrome, tetanus, acute intermittent porphyria, intractable hiccups, itching, symptomatic rhinitis.

Contraindications and precautions

• Contraindicated in patients with CNS depression, bone marrow suppression, heart failure, circulatory collapse, coronary artery or cerebrovascular disorders, subcortical damage, or coma. Also contraindicated in patients receiving spinal and epidural anesthetics and adrenergic blockers.

• Use cautiously in debilitated patients and in those with hepatic, renal, or CV disease; respiratory disorders; hypocalcemia; seizure disorders; suspected brain tumor or intestinal obstruction; glaucoma; and prostatic hyperplasia.

⚞ Lifespan: In pregnant women, use only if clearly necessary; safety hasn't been established. Women shouldn't breast-feed during therapy because most phenothiazines appear in breast milk and directly affect prolactin levels. For children younger than age 12, phenothiazines aren't recommended unless otherwise specified; use cautiously for nausea and vomiting. Acutely ill children, such as those with chickenpox, measles, CNS infections, or dehydration have a greatly increased risk of dystonic reactions. Geriatric patients are more sensitive to therapeutic and adverse effects, especially cardiac toxicity, tardive dyskinesia, and other extrapyramidal effects; use cautiously and give reduced doses, adjusting dosage to patient response.

Adverse reactions

Phenothiazines may produce extrapyramidal symptoms, such as dystonic movements, torticollis, oculogyric crises, parkinsonian symptoms, ranging from akathisia during early treatment to tardive dyskinesia after long-term use. A neuroleptic malignant syndrome resembling severe parkinsonism may occur, most often in young men taking fluphenazine. The progression of elevated liver enzyme levels to obstructive jaundice usually indicates an allergic reaction. Other adverse reactions include orthostatic hypotension with reflex tachycardia, fainting, dizziness, confusion, agitation, hallucinations, arrhythmias, anorexia, dry mouth, urine retention, nausea, vomiting, abdominal pain, constipation, local gastric irritation, seizures, endocrine effects, hematologic disorders, visual disturbances, skin eruptions, and photosensitivity.

Action

Phenothiazines are believed to function as dopamine antagonists by blocking postsynaptic dopamine receptors in various parts of the CNS. Their antiemetic effects result from blockage of the chemoreceptor trigger zone. They also produce varying degrees of anticholinergic effects and alpha-adrenergic–receptor blocking.

NURSING PROCESS

⚗ Assessment

• Check vital signs regularly for decreased blood pressure, especially before and after parenteral therapy, or tachycardia; observe patient carefully for other adverse reactions.
• Check intake and output for urine retention or constipation, which may require dosage reduction.
• Monitor bilirubin level weekly for the first 4 weeks. Establish baseline CBC, ECG (for quinidine-like effects), liver and renal function test results, electrolyte level (especially potassium), and eye examination findings. Monitor these findings periodically thereafter, especially in patients receiving long-term therapy.
• Observe patient for mood changes and monitor progress.
• Monitor patient for involuntary movements. Check patient receiving prolonged treatment at least once every 6 months.

🔲 Key nursing diagnoses

• Risk for injury related to adverse reactions
• Impaired mobility related to extrapyramidal symptoms
• Noncompliance related to long-term therapy

▶ Planning and implementation

• Don't stop drug abruptly. Although physical dependence doesn't occur with antipsychotic drugs, rebound worsening of psychotic symptoms may occur, and many drug effects may persist.
• Follow manufacturer's guidelines for reconstitution, dilution, administration, and storage of drugs; slightly discolored liquids may or

may not be acceptable for use. Check with pharmacist.

Patient teaching

• Teach patient how and when to take drug. Tell him not to increase the dosage or stop taking the drug without prescriber's approval. Suggest taking the full dose at bedtime if daytime sedation occurs.
• Explain that full therapeutic effect may not occur for several weeks.
• Teach signs and symptoms of adverse reactions, and urge patient to report unusual effects, especially involuntary movements.
• Instruct patient to avoid beverages and drugs containing alcohol, and warn him not to take other drugs, including OTC or herbal products, without prescriber's approval.
• Advise patient to avoid hazardous tasks until full effects of drug are established. Explain that sedative effects will lessen after several weeks.
• Inform patient that excessive exposure to sunlight, heat lamps, or tanning beds may cause photosensitivity reactions. Advise him to avoid exposure to extreme heat or cold.
• Explain that phenothiazines may cause pink or brown discoloration of urine.

☑ Evaluation

• Patient remains free from injury.
• Patient doesn't develop extrapyramidal symptoms.
• Patient complies with therapy, as evidenced by improved thought processes.

Skeletal muscle relaxants

baclofen
carisoprodol
chlorzoxazone
cyclobenzaprine hydrochloride
methocarbamol

Indications

▶ Painful musculoskeletal disorders, spasticity caused by multiple sclerosis.

Contraindications and precautions

• Contraindicated in patients hypersensitive to these drugs.

• Use cautiously in patients with impaired renal or hepatic function.

❉ **Lifespan:** In breast-feeding women and in children, recommendations vary for use. Geriatric patients have an increased risk of adverse reactions; monitor them carefully.

Adverse reactions

Skeletal muscle relaxants may cause ataxia, confusion, depressed mood, dizziness, drowsiness, dry mouth, hallucinations, headache, hypotension, nervousness, tachycardia, tremor, and vertigo. Baclofen also may cause seizures.

Action

All skeletal muscle relaxants, except baclofen, reduce impulse transmission from the spinal cord to skeletal muscle. Baclofen's mechanism of action is unclear.

NURSING PROCESS

𝔸 Assessment
• Monitor patient for hypersensitivity reactions.
• Assess degree of relief obtained to determine when dosage can be reduced.
• Watch for increased seizures in epileptic patient receiving baclofen.
• Monitor CBC results closely.
• In patient receiving cyclobenzaprine, monitor platelet counts.
• In patient receiving methocarbamol, watch for orthostatic hypotension.
• In patient receiving long-term baclofen or chlorzoxazone therapy, monitor hepatic function and urinalysis results.
• In patient receiving long-term therapy, assess compliance.

⊕ Key nursing diagnoses
• Risk for trauma related to baclofen-induced seizures
• Disturbed thought processes related to confusion
• Noncompliance related to long-term therapy

▷ Planning and implementation
• After long-term therapy and unless patient has severe adverse reactions, don't stop baclofen or carisoprodol abruptly to avoid withdrawal symptoms, such as insomnia, headache, nausea, and abdominal pain.
• Institute safety precautions as needed.

• To prevent GI distress, give oral forms of drug with meals or milk.
• Obtain an order for a mild analgesic to relieve drug-induced headache.

Patient teaching
• Tell patient to take drug exactly as prescribed. Tell him not to stop baclofen or carisoprodol suddenly after long-term therapy to avoid withdrawal symptoms.
• Instruct patient to avoid hazardous activities that require mental alertness until CNS effects of drug are known.
• Advise patient to avoid alcohol use during therapy.
• Advise patient to follow prescriber's advice regarding rest and physical therapy.
• Instruct patient receiving cyclobenzaprine or baclofen to report urinary hesitancy.
• Inform patient taking methocarbamol or chlorzoxazone that urine may be discolored.

☑ Evaluation
• Patient remains free from seizures.
• Patient exhibits normal thought processes.
• Patient complies with therapy, as evidenced by pain relief or improvement of spasticity.

Sulfonamides

co-trimoxazole (trimethoprim and sulfamethoxazole)
sulfasalazine

Indications

▶ Bacterial infections, nocardiosis, toxoplasmosis, chloroquine-resistant *Plasmodium falciparum* malaria.

Contraindications and precautions

• Contraindicated in patients hypersensitive to these drugs.
• Use cautiously in patients with renal or hepatic impairment, bronchial asthma, severe allergy, or G6PD deficiency.

❉ **Lifespan:** In pregnant women at term and in breast-feeding women, use is contraindicated; sulfonamides appear in breast milk. In infants younger than age 2 months, sulfonamides are contraindicated unless there is no therapeutic alternative. In children with fragile

X chromosome and mental retardation, use cautiously. Geriatric patients are susceptible to bacterial and fungal superinfection and have an increased risk of folate deficiency anemia and adverse renal and hematologic effects.

Adverse reactions

Many adverse reactions stem from hypersensitivity, including rash, fever, pruritus, erythema multiforme, erythema nodosum, Stevens-Johnson syndrome, toxic epidermal necrolysis, Lyell's syndrome, exfoliative dermatitis, photosensitivity, joint pain, conjunctivitis, leukopenia, and bronchospasm. GI reactions include nausea, vomiting, anorexia, stomatitis, pancreatitis, diarrhea, and folic acid malabsorption. Hematologic reactions include granulocytopenia, thrombocytopenia, agranulocytosis, hypoprothrombinemia and, in G6PD deficiency, hemolytic anemia. Renal effects usually result from crystalluria caused by precipitation of sulfonamide in renal system.

Action

Sulfonamides are bacteriostatic. They inhibit biosynthesis of tetrahydrofolic acid, which is needed for bacterial cell growth. They're active against some strains of staphylococci, streptococci, *Nocardia asteroides* and *brasiliensis, Clostridium tetani* and *perfringens, Bacillus anthracis, Escherichia coli,* and *Neisseria gonorrhoeae* and *meningitidis.* Sulfonamides are also active against organisms that cause UTIs, such as *E. coli, Proteus mirabilis* and *vulgaris, Klebsiella, Enterobacter,* and *Staphylococcus aureus,* and genital lesions caused by *Haemophilus ducreyi* (chancroid).

NURSING PROCESS

Assessment
- Assess patient's history of allergies, especially to sulfonamides or to any drug containing sulfur, such as thiazides, furosemide, and oral sulfonylureas.
- Monitor patient for adverse reactions; patients with AIDS have a much higher risk of adverse reactions.
- Obtain culture and sensitivity tests before first dose; check test results periodically to assess drug effectiveness.
- Monitor urine cultures, CBC, and urinalysis before and during therapy.

- During long-term therapy, monitor patient for possible superinfection.

Key nursing diagnoses
- Ineffective protection related to hypersensitivity
- Risk for infection related to superinfection
- Risk for deficient fluid volume related to adverse GI reactions

Planning and implementation
- Give oral dose with 8 oz (240 ml) of water. Give 3 to 4 L of fluids daily, depending on drug; patient's urine output should be at least 1,500 ml daily.
- Follow manufacturer's directions for reconstituting, diluting, and storing drugs; check expiration dates.
- Shake oral suspensions well before giving to ensure correct dosage.

Patient teaching
- Urge patient to take drug exactly as prescribed, to complete the prescribed regimen, and to keep follow-up appointments.
- Advise patient to take oral drug with full glass of water and to drink plenty of fluids; explain that tablet may be crushed and swallowed with water to ensure maximal absorption.
- Teach signs and symptoms of hypersensitivity and other adverse reactions. Urge patient to report bloody urine, difficulty breathing, rash, fever, chills, or severe fatigue.
- Advise patient to avoid direct sun exposure and to use a sunscreen to help prevent photosensitivity reactions.
- Tell diabetic patient that sulfonamides may increase effects of oral hypoglycemics. Tell him not to use Clinitest to monitor glucose level.
- Inform patient taking sulfasalazine that it may cause an orange-yellow discoloration of urine or skin and may permanently stain soft contact lenses yellow.

Evaluation
- Patient exhibits no signs of hypersensitivity.
- Patient is free from infection.
- Patient maintains adequate hydration.

Tetracyclines

doxycycline
doxycycline hyclate
doxycycline hydrochloride
minocycline hydrochloride
oxytetracycline hydrochloride
tetracycline hydrochloride

Indications

▶ Bacterial, protozoal, rickettsial, and fungal infections.

Contraindications and precautions

• Contraindicated in patients hypersensitive to these drugs.
• Use cautiously in patients with renal or hepatic impairment.
⚠ Lifespan: In pregnant or breast-feeding women, use is contraindicated; tetracyclines appear in breast milk. Children younger than age 8 shouldn't take tetracyclines; these drugs can cause permanent tooth discoloration, enamel hypoplasia, and a reversible decrease in bone calcification. Elderly patients may have decreased esophageal motility; use these drugs cautiously and monitor patients for local irritation from slow passage of oral forms. Elderly patients are also more susceptible to superinfection.

Adverse reactions

The most common adverse effects involve the GI tract and are dose-related; they include anorexia; flatulence; nausea; vomiting; bulky, loose stools; epigastric burning; and abdominal discomfort. Superinfections also are common. Photosensitivity reactions may be severe. Renal failure may be caused by Fanconi's syndrome after use of outdated tetracycline. Permanent discoloration of teeth occurs if drug is given during tooth formation in children younger than age 8.

Action

Tetracyclines are bacteriostatic but may be bactericidal against certain organisms. They bind reversibly to 30S and 50S ribosomal subunits, which inhibits bacterial protein synthesis.

Susceptible gram-positive organisms include *Bacillus anthracis, Actinomyces israelii,*

Clostridium perfringens, C. tetani, Listeria monocytogenes, and *Nocardia.*

Susceptible gram-negative organisms include *Neisseria meningitidis, Pasteurella multocida, Legionella pneumophila, Brucella, Vibrio cholerae, Yersinia enterocolitica, Y. pestis, Bordetella pertussis, Haemophilus influenzae, H. ducreyi, Campylobacter fetus, Shigella,* and many other common pathogens.

Other susceptible organisms include *Rickettsia akari, R. typhi, R. prowazekii, R. tsutsugamushi, Coxiella burnetii, Chlamydia trachomatis, C. psittaci, Mycoplasma pneumoniae, M. hominis, Leptospira, Treponema pallidum, T. pertenue,* and *Borrelia recurrentis.*

NURSING PROCESS

☑ Assessment
• Assess patient's allergic history.
• Monitor patient for adverse reactions.
• Obtain culture and sensitivity tests before first dose; check cultures periodically to assess drug effectiveness.
• Check expiration dates before giving. Outdated tetracyclines may cause nephrotoxicity.
• Monitor patient for bacterial and fungal superinfection, especially if patient is elderly, debilitated, or receiving immunosuppressants or radiation therapy; watch especially for oral candidiasis.

⊞ Key nursing diagnoses
• Ineffective protection related to hypersensitivity
• Risk for infection related to superinfection
• Risk for deficient fluid volume related to adverse GI reactions

▶ Planning and implementation
• Give all oral tetracyclines except doxycycline and minocycline 1 hour before or 2 hours after meals for maximum absorption; don't give drug with food, milk or other dairy products, sodium bicarbonate, iron compounds, or antacids, which may impair absorption.
• Give water with and after oral drug to help it pass to the stomach because incomplete swallowing can cause severe esophageal irritation. Don't give drug within 1 hour of bedtime to prevent esophageal reflux.

• Follow manufacturer's directions for reconstituting and storing; keep drug refrigerated and away from light.

• Monitor I.V. injection sites and rotate routinely to minimize local irritation. I.V. administration may cause severe phlebitis.

Patient teaching

• Urge patient to take drug exactly as prescribed, to complete the prescribed regimen, and to keep follow-up appointments.

• Warn patient not to take drug with food, milk or other dairy products, sodium bicarbonate, or iron compounds because they may interfere with absorption. Advise him to wait 3 hours after taking tetracycline before taking an antacid.

• Instruct patient to check expiration dates and to discard any expired drug.

• Teach signs and symptoms of adverse reactions, and urge patient to report them promptly.

• Advise patient to avoid direct exposure to sunlight and to use a sunscreen to help prevent photosensitivity reactions.

☑ **Evaluation**

• Patient shows no signs of hypersensitivity.

• Patient is free from infection.

• Patient maintains adequate hydration.

Thyroid hormones

levothyroxine sodium
liothyronine sodium
thyroid, desiccated

Indications

▶ Hypothyroidism, simple goiter, goitrogenesis.

Contraindications and precautions

• Contraindicated in patients with MI, thyrotoxicosis, or uncorrected adrenal insufficiency.

• Use cautiously in patients with angina pectoris, hypertension, other CV disorders, renal insufficiency, endocrine disorders, ischemia, or myxedema.

⚖ **Lifespan:** During pregnancy, women may continue thyroid replacement. Minimal amounts of exogenous thyroid hormones appear in breast milk. However, problems haven't been

reported in breast-feeding infants. Children may have partial hair loss during first few months of therapy; reassure child and parents that this is temporary. In patients older than age 60, initial hormone replacement dosage should be 25% less than the usual recommended starting dosage.

Adverse reactions

Adverse reactions include nervousness, insomnia, tremor, tachycardia, palpitations, nausea, headache, fever, and sweating.

Action

Thyroid hormones have catabolic and anabolic effects and influence normal metabolism, growth, and development. Affecting every organ system, these hormones are vital to normal CNS function. Thyroid-stimulating hormone increases iodine uptake by the thyroid, increases formation and release of thyroid hormone, and is produced from bovine anterior pituitary glands.

NURSING PROCESS

⬥ **Assessment**

• Assess patient's thyroid function test results regularly.

• Monitor pulse rate and blood pressure.

• Monitor patient for signs of thyrotoxicosis or inadequate dosage, including diarrhea, fever, irritability, listlessness, rapid heartbeat, vomiting, and weakness.

• Monitor PT and INR in patients taking anticoagulants.

⬥ **Key nursing diagnoses**

• Risk for injury related to adverse CV reactions

• Disturbed sleep pattern related to insomnia

• Noncompliance related to long-term therapy

▶ **Planning and implementation**

• Thyroid hormone dosage varies widely. Begin treatment at lowest level, adjusting to higher doses according to patient's symptoms and laboratory data, until euthyroid state is reached.

• Give thyroid hormones at same time each day, preferably in the morning to prevent insomnia.

• Thyroid medications may be supplied either in micrograms (mcg) or in milligrams (mg). Don't confuse these dose measurements.

Patient teaching

• Instruct patient to take drug exactly as prescribed. Suggest taking dose in morning to prevent insomnia.

• Advise patient to report signs and symptoms of overdose (chest pain, palpitations, sweating, nervousness) or aggravated CV disease (chest pain, dyspnea, tachycardia).

• Tell patient who has achieved a stable response not to change brands.

• Inform parents that child may lose hair during first months of therapy, but reassure them that this is temporary.

• Urge patient to keep follow-up appointments and have regular laboratory testing of thyroid levels.

☑ Evaluation

• Patient sustains no injury from adverse reactions.

• Patient gets adequate sleep during the night.

• Patient complies with therapy, as evidenced by normal thyroid hormone levels and resolution of underlying disorder.

Xanthine derivatives

aminophylline
theophylline

Indications

▶ Asthma and bronchospasm from emphysema and chronic bronchitis.

Contraindications and precautions

• Contraindicated in patients hypersensitive to these drugs.

• Use cautiously in patients with arrhythmias, cardiac or circulatory impairment, cor pulmonale, hepatic or renal disease, active peptic ulcers, hyperthyroidism, or diabetes mellitus.

⚖ Lifespan: In pregnant women, use cautiously. In breast-feeding women, avoid these drugs because they appear in breast milk, and infants may have serious adverse reactions. Small children may have excessive CNS stimulation;

monitor them closely. In elderly patients, use cautiously.

Adverse reactions

Adverse effects are dose-related, except for hypersensitivity, and can be controlled by dosage adjustment. Common reactions include hypotension, palpitations, arrhythmias, restlessness, irritability, nausea, vomiting, urine retention, and headache.

Action

Xanthine derivatives are structurally related; they directly relax smooth muscle, stimulate the CNS, induce diuresis, increase gastric acid secretion, inhibit uterine contractions, and exert weak inotropic and chronotropic effects on the heart. Of these drugs, theophylline exerts the greatest effect on smooth muscle.

The action of xanthine derivatives isn't completely caused by inhibition of phosphodiesterase. Current data suggest that inhibition of adenosine receptors or unidentified mechanisms may be responsible for therapeutic effects. By relaxing smooth muscle of the respiratory tract, they increase airflow and vital capacity. They also slow onset of diaphragmatic fatigue and stimulate the respiratory center in the CNS.

NURSING PROCESS

Assessment

• Monitor theophylline level closely; therapeutic level ranges from 10 to 20 mcg/ml.

• Monitor patient closely for adverse reactions, especially toxicity.

• Monitor vital signs.

⊞ Key nursing diagnoses

• Disturbed sleep pattern related to CNS effects

• Urine retention related to adverse effects on bladder

• Noncompliance related to long-term therapy

▷ Planning and implementation

• Don't crush or allow patient to chew timed-release preparations.

• Calculate dosage from lean body weight because theophylline doesn't distribute into fatty tissue.

• Adjust daily dosage in elderly patients and in those with heart failure or hepatic disease.

• Provide patient with nondrug sleep aids, such as a back rub or milk-based beverage.

Patient teaching

• Tell patient to take drug exactly as prescribed.

• Advise patient to check with prescriber before using any other drug, including OTC medications or herbal remedies, or before switching brands.

• If patient smokes, tell him that doing so may decrease theophylline level. Urge him to notify prescriber if he quits smoking because the dosage will need adjustment to avoid toxicity.

☑ **Evaluation**

• Patient sleeps usual number of hours without interruption.

• Patient's voiding pattern doesn't change.

• Patient complies with therapy, as evidenced by maintenance of therapeutic level.

Alphabetical
Listing of Drugs

A

abacavir sulfate
(uh-BACK-ah-veer SUL-fayt)
Ziagen

Pharmacologic class: nucleoside analogue
reverse transcriptase inhibitor
Therapeutic class: antiretroviral
Pregnancy risk category: C

Indications and dosages

▶ **HIV-1 infection.** *Adults:* 300 mg P.O. b.i.d.
with other antiretrovirals.
Children ages 3 months to 16 years: 8 mg/kg
P.O. b.i.d. (maximum, 300 mg P.O. b.i.d.) with
other antiretrovirals.

Contraindications and precautions

• Contraindicated in patients hypersensitive to
drug or its components.
• Use cautiously in patients at high-risk of liver
disease. Lactic acidosis and severe hepatomegaly with steatosis may occur in patients (more
women than men) taking nucleoside analogues,
such as abacavir and other antiretrovirals. Obesity and prolonged nucleoside exposure may be
risk factors.
❧ **Lifespan:** In pregnant women, use only if
potential benefits outweigh risk. In elderly patients, use cautiously as they may have decreased renal or hepatic function.

Adverse reactions

CNS: insomnia, sleep disorders, headache,
fever.
GI: *nausea, vomiting,* diarrhea, loss of appetite,
anorexia.
Hepatic: *hepatotoxicity.*
Metabolic: *lactic acidosis.*
Skin: rash.
Other: *fatal hypersensitivity reaction.*

Interactions

Drug-lifestyle. *Alcohol use:* Decreases elimination of abacavir, increasing overall exposure to
drug. Discourage using together.

Effects on lab test results

• May increase GGT, glucose, and triglyceride
levels.

Pharmacokinetics

Absorption: Rapid and extensive; the mean absolute bioavailability of the tablet is 83%. Systemic exposure is comparable for oral solution
and tablets; they may be used interchangeably.
Distribution: Distributed into extravascular
space; about 50% binds to plasma proteins.
Metabolism: In the liver, alcohol dehydrogenase and glucuronyl transferase metabolize the
drug to form two inactive metabolites. CYP enzymes don't significantly metabolize the drug.
Excretion: Mainly in urine, with about 1% unchanged. About 16% of a dose is eliminated in
feces. *Half-life:* 1 to 2 hours.

Route	Onset	Peak	Duration
P.O.	Unknown	Unknown	Unknown

Action

Chemical effect: Inhibits the activity of HIV-1
reverse transcriptase after metabolism, thereby
stopping viral DNA growth.
Therapeutic effect: Reduces the symptoms of
HIV-1 infection.

Available forms

Oral solution: 20 mg/ml
Tablets: 300 mg

NURSING PROCESS

⚖ Assessment

• Assess patient's condition before therapy and
regularly thereafter.
• Watch for hypersensitivity reaction.
• Monitor glucose level during therapy.
• Assess patient for risk factors of liver disease.
Lactic acidosis and severe hepatomegaly with
steatosis may occur, especially in woman or patient who is obese or has prolonged exposure to
nucleosides. Stop treatment if patient has symptoms of lactic acidosis or pronounced hepatotoxicity, which may include hepatomegaly and
steatosis, even without elevated transaminase
levels.
• Evaluate patient's and family's knowledge of
drug therapy.

⊞ Nursing diagnoses

• Risk for infection secondary to presence of HIV
• Ineffective individual coping related to HIV infection
• Deficient knowledge related to drug therapy

⊠ Planning and implementation

• Drug should always be given with other antiretrovirals, never alone.
• Register pregnant woman taking abacavir with the Antiretroviral Pregnancy Registry at 1-800-258-4263.
• Don't restart drug after a hypersensitivity reaction because more severe signs and symptoms will recur within hours and may include life-threatening hypotension. To aid in reporting of hypersensitivity reactions, register patient with the Abacavir Hypersensitivity Registry at 1-800-270-0425.
⊛ ALERT: Drug may cause fatal hypersensitivity reactions. If a patient develops evidence of hypersensitivity—such as fever, rash, fatigue, nausea, vomiting, diarrhea, or abdominal pain—stop the drug and notify the prescriber immediately.
⊛ ALERT: Don't use triple antiretroviral therapy with abacavir, lamivudine, and tenofovir as a new treatment because of a high rate of early virologic resistance. Monitor patients currently taking this combination and consider changing therapies.
Patient teaching
• Inform patient that abacavir can cause a life-threatening hypersensitivity reaction. Tell patient to stop drug and seek medical attention immediately if evidence of hypersensitivity develops—such as fever, rash, severe fatigue, achiness, a generally ill feeling, or GI signs or symptoms, such as nausea, vomiting, diarrhea, or stomach pain.
• Give written information about drug with each new prescription and refill. Patient also should receive—and be instructed to carry—a warning card summarizing abacavir hypersensitivity reaction.
• Explain that the drug neither cures HIV nor reduces the risk of transmitting HIV to others. Its long-term effects are unknown.
• Tell patient to take drug exactly as prescribed.
• Inform patient that drug can be taken with or without food.

☑ Evaluation

• Patient has reduced signs and symptoms of infection.
• Patient demonstrates adequate coping mechanisms.
• Patient and family state understanding of drug therapy.

abciximab
(ab-SIKS-ih-mahb)
ReoPro

Pharmacologic class: fab fragment of chimeric human-murine monoclonal antibody 7E3
Therapeutic class: platelet-aggregation inhibitor
Pregnancy risk category: C

Indications and dosages

▶ **Adjunct for percutaneous coronary intervention (PCI) to prevent acute cardiac ischemic complications in patients at high risk for abrupt closure of treated coronary vessel.** *Adults:* 0.25 mg/kg as I.V. bolus 10 to 60 minutes before PCI, followed by continuous I.V. infusion of 0.125 mcg/kg/minute (maximum, 10 mcg/minute) for 12 hours.
▶ **Patients with unstable angina not responding to conventional medical therapy who are to undergo PCI within 24 hours.** *Adults:* 0.25 mg/kg as I.V. bolus; then an 18- to 24-hour infusion of 10 mcg/minute, concluding 1 hour after PCI.

▽ I.V. administration

• Inspect solution for particulate matter before injecting it. If you see opaque particles, discard solution and obtain new vial. Withdraw drug for I.V. bolus injection through sterile, non-pyrogenic, low–protein-binding 0.2- or 0.22-micron filter into syringe.
• Give I.V. bolus 10 to 60 minutes before procedure.
• Withdraw 4.5 ml of drug for continuous I.V. infusion through sterile, nonpyrogenic, low–protein-binding 0.2- or 0.22-micron filter into syringe. Inject into 250 ml of sterile normal saline solution or D_5W, and infuse at 17 ml/hour for 12 hours via continuous infusion pump equipped with in-line filter.

Reactions may be *common,* uncommon, *life-threatening,* or COMMON AND LIFE-THREATENING.

- Give drug in separate I.V. line; don't add another drug to infusion solution.
- Discard unused portion.

Contraindications and precautions

- Contraindicated in patients hypersensitive to a drug component or to murine proteins and in patients with active internal bleeding, bleeding diathesis, platelet count less than 100,000/mm³, intracranial neoplasm, intracranial arteriovenous malformation, intracranial aneurysm, severe uncontrolled hypertension, a history of CVA within 2 years or with significant residual neurologic deficit, or a history of vasculitis. Also contraindicated within 6 weeks of major surgery, trauma, or GI or GU bleeding; when oral anticoagulants have been given within 7 days unless PT is less than or equal to 1.2 times control; and when I.V. dextran is used before or during PCI.
- Use cautiously in patients who weigh less than 75 kg (165 lb), have history of GI disease, or are receiving thrombolytic drugs because these patients are at increased risk for bleeding. Conditions that increase risk of bleeding include PCI within 12 hours of onset of symptoms for acute MI, PCI lasting longer than 70 minutes, failed PCI, and use of heparin.
- ⚜ Lifespan: In pregnant or breast-feeding women, use cautiously. In children, safety and effectiveness of drug haven't been established. In patients older than age 65, use cautiously.

Adverse reactions

CNS: hypoesthesia, confusion, headache, pain.
CV: hypotension, chest pain, *bradycardia*, peripheral edema.
EENT: abnormal vision.
GI: nausea, vomiting, abdominal pain.
Hematologic: *bleeding, thrombocytopenia,* anemia, leukocytosis.
Musculoskeletal: *back pain.*
Respiratory: pleural effusion, pleurisy, pneumonia.

Interactions

Drug-drug. *Antiplatelets, heparin, NSAIDs, other anticoagulants, thrombolytics:* May increase risk of bleeding. Monitor patient closely.

Effects on lab test results

- May increase WBC count. May decrease hemoglobin, hematocrit, and platelet count.

Pharmacokinetics

Absorption: Administered I.V.
Distribution: Rapidly binds to platelet receptors.
Metabolism: Unknown.
Excretion: Unknown. *Half-life:* Initially, less than 10 minutes; second phase, about 30 minutes.

Route	Onset	Peak	Duration
I.V.	Almost immediate	Almost immediate	24 hr

Action

Chemical effect: Prevents binding of fibrinogen, von Willebrand factor, and other adhesive molecules to receptor sites on activated platelets.
Therapeutic effect: Inhibits platelet aggregation.

Available forms

Injection: 2 mg/ml

NURSING PROCESS

🔖 Assessment

- Note patient's history. Patients at risk for abrupt closure include those undergoing PCI with at least one of the following: unstable angina, non-Q wave MI, acute Q wave MI within 12 hours of onset of symptoms, two type B lesions in artery to be dilated, one type B lesion in artery to be dilated in a woman older than age 65 or a patient with diabetes, one type C lesion in artery to be dilated, and angioplasty of infarct-related lesion within 7 days of MI.
- Assess vital signs and evaluate bleeding studies before therapy.
- Monitor patient closely for bleeding. Bleeding caused by therapy falls into two categories: that observed at arterial access site used for cardiac catheterization, and internal bleeding involving GI or GU tract or retroperitoneal sites.
- Be alert for adverse reactions and drug interactions.
- Evaluate patient's and family's knowledge of drug therapy.

🔖 Nursing diagnoses

- Ineffective cerebral or cardiopulmonary tissue perfusion related to patient's underlying condition

- Risk for deficient fluid volume related to drug-induced bleeding
- Deficient knowledge related to drug therapy

⟩ Planning and implementation

- Institute bleeding precautions. Keep patient on bed rest for 6 to 8 hours after removing sheath or stopping infusion, whichever is later.
- Drug is intended for use with aspirin and heparin.

⊛ **ALERT:** Keep epinephrine, dopamine, theophylline, antihistamines, and corticosteroids available in case of anaphylaxis.

Patient teaching

- Teach patient about his disease and therapy.
- Stress the importance of reporting adverse reactions.

☑ Evaluation

- Patient maintains adequate tissue perfusion.
- Patient maintains adequate hydration.
- Patient and family state understanding of drug therapy.

---

acarbose

(ay-KAR-bohs)
Precose

Pharmacologic class: alpha-glucosidase inhibitor
Therapeutic class: antidiabetic
Pregnancy risk category: B

Indications and dosages

▶ **Adjunct to diet to lower glucose level in patients with type 2 (non-insulin–dependent) diabetes mellitus whose hyperglycemia can't be managed by diet alone or by diet and a sulfonylurea.** *Adults:* Initially, 25 mg P.O. t.i.d. with the first bite of each main meal. Subsequent dosage adjustment made q 4 to 8 weeks, based on glucose level and tolerance 1 hour after a meal. Maintenance dosage is 50 to 100 mg P.O. t.i.d.

▶ **Adjunct to insulin or metformin in patients with type 2 (non-insulin–dependent) diabetes mellitus whose hyperglycemia can't be managed by diet, exercise, and insulin or metformin alone.** *Adults:* Initially, 25 mg P.O. t.i.d. with first bite of each main meal. Subsequent dosage adjustment made q 4 to 8 weeks,

based on glucose level and tolerance 1 hour after a meal. Maintenance dosage is 50 to 100 mg P.O. t.i.d. Maximum dosage for patients weighing 60 kg (132 lb) or less is 50 mg P.O. t.i.d.; for patients weighing more than 60 kg, maximum dosage is 100 mg P.O. t.i.d.

Contraindications and precautions

- Contraindicated in patients hypersensitive to drug and in patients with diabetic ketoacidosis, cirrhosis, inflammatory bowel disease, colonic ulceration, partial intestinal obstruction, predisposition to intestinal obstruction, chronic intestinal disease with disorder of digestion or absorption, and conditions that may deteriorate because of increased intestinal gas formation.
- Drug isn't recommended in patients with severe renal impairment.
- Use cautiously in patients receiving sulfonylurea or insulin. Drug may increase the hypoglycemic potential of sulfonylurea.

⚖ **Lifespan:** In pregnant or breast-feeding women, drug isn't recommended. In children, safety and efficacy haven't been established.

Adverse reactions

GI: abdominal pain, diarrhea, flatulence.

Interactions

Drug-drug. *Calcium channel blockers, corticosteroids, estrogens, hormonal contraceptives, isoniazid, nicotinic acid, phenothiazines, phenytoin, sympathomimetics, thiazides and other diuretics, thyroid products:* May cause hyperglycemia and loss of glucose control during use or hypoglycemia when withdrawn. Monitor glucose level.
Digestive enzyme preparations containing carbohydrate-splitting enzymes (such as amylase, pancreatin), intestinal adsorbents (such as activated charcoal): May reduce effect of acarbose. Don't give together.
Digoxin: May decrease digoxin level. Monitor digoxin level.
Drug-herb. *Aloe, bilberry leaf, bitter melon, burdock, dandelion, fenugreek, garlic, ginseng:* May improve glucose control and allow reduced antidiabetic dosage. Urge patient to discuss herbal products with prescriber before use.

Effects on lab test results

- May increase ALT and AST levels. May decrease calcium and vitamin B_6 levels.

Reactions may be *common,* uncommon, *life-threatening,* or COMMON AND LIFE-THREATENING.

• May decrease hemoglobin and hematocrit.

Pharmacokinetics

Absorption: Minimal.
Distribution: Acts locally within GI tract.
Metabolism: Exclusively in the GI tract, primarily by intestinal bacteria and—to a lesser extent—by digestive enzymes.
Excretion: Almost completely excreted by the kidneys. *Half-life:* 2 hours.

Route	Onset	Peak	Duration
P.O.	Unknown	1 hr	2-4 hr

Action

Chemical effect: Delays carbohydrate digestion and glucose absorption.
Therapeutic effect: Lessens postprandial hyperglycemia.

Available forms

Tablets: 25 mg, 50 mg, 100 mg

NURSING PROCESS

⚘ Assessment

• Monitor glucose level 1 hour after a meal to determine effectiveness and to identify appropriate dose. Report hypoglycemia or hyperglycemia to prescriber.
• Monitor glycosylated hemoglobin every 3 months.
• Monitor transaminase level every 3 months in first year of therapy and periodically thereafter in patient receiving doses in excess of 50 mg t.i.d. Report abnormalities to prescriber.
• Obtain baseline creatinine level; drug isn't recommended in patient with a creatinine level greater than 2 mg/dl.
• Evaluate patient's and family's knowledge of drug therapy.

⊕ Nursing diagnoses

• Risk for imbalanced fluid volume related to adverse GI effect
• Imbalanced nutrition: less than body requirements related to patient's underlying condition
• Deficient knowledge related to drug therapy

▷ Planning and implementation

• With doses exceeding 50 mg t.i.d., watch for high transaminase and bilirubin levels and low calcium and vitamin B_6 levels.

• Drug may increase hypoglycemic potential of sulfonylureas. Closely monitor patient receiving both drugs. If hypoglycemia occurs, treat with dextrose, I.V. glucose infusion, or glucagon. Report hypoglycemia to prescriber.
• Insulin therapy may be needed during increased stress, such as infection, fever, surgery, or trauma.

Patient teaching

• Tell patient to take drug daily with first bite of each of three main meals.
• Explain that therapy relieves symptoms but doesn't cure the disease.
• Stress importance of adhering to specific diet, weight reduction, exercise, and hygiene programs. Show patient how to monitor glucose level and to recognize and treat hyperglycemia.
• Teach patient to recognize hypoglycemia and to treat symptoms with a form of dextrose rather than with a product containing table sugar.
• Urge patient to carry medical identification at all times.

☑ Evaluation

• Patient maintains adequate fluid volume balance.
• Patient doesn't experience hypoglycemia.
• Patient and family state understanding of drug therapy.

acebutolol
(as-ih-BYOO-tuh-lol)
Sectral

Pharmacologic class: beta blocker
Therapeutic class: antihypertensive, antiarrhythmic
Pregnancy risk category: B

Indications and dosages

▶ **Hypertension.** *Adults:* 400 mg P.O. as single daily dose or in divided doses b.i.d. Maximum, 1,200 mg daily.
▶ **Suppression of PVCs.** *Adults:* 400 mg P.O. in divided doses b.i.d. Increase dosage to provide adequate clinical response. Usual dosage is 600 to 1,200 mg daily.
▶ **Stable angina‡.** *Adults:* Initially, 200 mg P.O. b.i.d. Increase dose up to 800 mg daily until angina is controlled. Patients with severe stable angina may require higher doses.

⧉ **Adjust-a-dose:** For patients with renal impairment, decrease dose by 50% if creatinine clearance is less than 50 ml/minute; decrease dose by 75% if creatinine clearance is less than 25 ml/minute. In geriatric patients, don't exceed 800 mg daily.

Contraindications and precautions

• Contraindicated in patients with persistently severe bradycardia, second- or third-degree heart block, overt heart failure, or cardiogenic shock.
• Use cautiously in patients with heart failure, peripheral vascular disease, bronchospastic disease, diabetes, or hepatic impairment.
⚘ **Lifespan:** In pregnant women, use cautiously. In breast-feeding women, use is contraindicated. In children, safety of drug hasn't been established. In elderly patients, use cautiously and at a reduced dose.

Adverse reactions

CNS: *fatigue,* headache, dizziness, fever, insomnia.
CV: chest pain, edema, *bradycardia, heart failure,* hypotension.
GI: nausea, constipation, diarrhea, dyspepsia, flatulence, vomiting, *mesenteric arterial thrombosis.*
GU: impotence.
Metabolic: *hypoglycemia,* increased risk of developing type 2 diabetes mellitus.
Musculoskeletal: arthralgia, myalgia.
Respiratory: dyspnea, cough, *bronchospasm.*
Skin: rash.

Interactions

Drug-drug. *Alpha-adrenergic stimulants:* Increases hypertensive response. Use together cautiously.
Digoxin, diltiazem: May cause excessive bradycardia and increase depression of the myocardium. Use together cautiously.
Insulin, oral antidiabetics: May alter dosage requirements in previously stabilized patient with diabetes. Observe patient carefully.
NSAIDs: Decreases antihypertensive effect. Monitor blood pressure and adjust dosage.
Reserpine: Additive effect. Monitor patient closely.
Verapamil: May increase the effects of both drugs. Monitor cardiac function closely and decrease dosages as necessary.

Prazosin: May increase the risk of orthostatic hypotension in the early phases of use together. Assist patient to stand slowly until effects are known.

Effects on lab test results

• May increase AST and ALT levels.
• May cause positive antinuclear antibody test result.
• May cause false results with glucose or insulin tolerance tests.

Pharmacokinetics

Absorption: Well absorbed after oral administration.
Distribution: About 25% protein-bound; minimal quantities detected in CSF.
Metabolism: Undergoes extensive first-pass metabolism in liver.
Excretion: 30% to 40% of dose is excreted in urine; the remainder, in feces and bile. *Half-life:* 3 to 4 hours.

Route	Onset	Peak	Duration
P.O.	1-1½ hr	2½ hr	Up to 24 hr

Action

Chemical effect: Antihypertensive action unknown. May reduce cardiac output, decrease sympathetic outflow to peripheral vasculature, and inhibit renin release. Antiarrhythmic action decreases myocardial contractility and heart rate and has mild intrinsic sympathomimetic activity.
Therapeutic effect: Lowers blood pressure and heart rate and restores normal sinus rhythm.

Available forms

Capsules: 200 mg, 400 mg

NURSING PROCESS

⧉ **Assessment**
• Assess patient's blood pressure and heart rate and rhythm before and during therapy.
• Monitor patient's energy level.
• Be alert for adverse reactions and drug interactions.
• Evaluate patient's and family's knowledge of drug therapy.

🔷 Nursing diagnoses
- Risk for injury related to patient's underlying condition
- Fatigue related to drug-induced CNS adverse reactions
- Deficient knowledge related to drug therapy

▶ Planning and implementation
- Drug may be removed by hemodialysis.
- Check apical pulse before giving drug; if slower than 60 beats/minute, withhold drug and call prescriber.
- 🔷 **ALERT:** Don't stop drug abruptly; doing so may worsen angina and MI, or cause rebound hypertension.
- Before surgery, notify anesthesiologist about patient's drug therapy.
- 🔷 **ALERT:** Don't confuse Sectral with Factrel or Septra.

Patient teaching
- Teach patient how to take his pulse, and instruct him to withhold dose and notify prescriber if pulse rate is slower than 60 beats/minute.
- Warn patient that drug may cause dizziness. Instruct him to avoid sudden position changes and to sit down immediately if he feels dizzy.
- Explain the importance of taking drug as prescribed, even when feeling well.
- Tell diabetic patient to monitor glucose level closely because this drug may mask the symptoms of hypoglycemia.

☑ Evaluation
- Patient's blood pressure and heart rate and rhythm are normal.
- Patient effectively combats fatigue.
- Patient and family state understanding of drug therapy.

acetaminophen
(APAP, paracetamol)
(as-ee-tuh-MlH-nuh-fin)

Abenol; Aceta Elixir*†; Acetaminophen Uniserts†; Aceta Tablets†; Actamin†; Actimol†; Aminofen†; Anacin-3†; Anacin-3 Children's Elixir*†; Anacin-3 Children's Tablets†; Anacin-3 Extra Strength†; Anacin-3, Infants'†; Apacet Capsules†; Apacet Elixir*†; Apacet Extra Strength Caplets†;

Apacet, Infants'†; Apo-Acetaminophen ♦ †; Arthritis Pain Formula Aspirin Free†; Atasol Caplets ♦ †; Atasol Drops ♦ †; Atasol Elixir*†; Atasol Tablets ♦ †; Banesin†; Dapa†; Dapa X-S†; Datril Extra-Strength; Dorcol Children's Fever and Pain Reducer†; Dymadon ◇ †; Exdol†; Feverall Junior Strength ◇ ; Feverall Children's Sprinkle Caps ◇ ; Genapap Children's Elixir†; Genapap Children's Tablets†; Genapap Extra Strength Caplets†; Genapap, Infants'†; Genapap Regular Strength Tablets†; Genebs Extra Strength Caplets†; Genebs Regular Strength Tablets†; Genebs X-Tra†; Halenol Elixir*†; Liquiprin Infants' Drops†; Meda Cap†; Neopap†; Oraphen-PD†; Panadol†; Panadol, Children's†; Panadol Extra Strength†; Panadol, Infants'†; Panadol Maximum Strength Caplets†; Redutemp†; Ridenol Caplets†; Robigesic†; Rounox†; Snaplets-FR†; St. Joseph Aspirin-Free Fever Reducer for Children†; Suppap-120†; Suppap-325†; Suppap-650†; Tapanol Extra Strength Caplets†; Tapanol Extra Strength Tablets†; Tempra†; Tempra D.S.†; Tempra, Infants'†; Tempra Syrup†; Tylenol Arthritis Strength; Tylenol Children's Elixir†; Tylenol Children's Chewable Tablets†; Tylenol Extended Relief†; Tylenol Extra Strength Caplets†; Tylenol Infants' Drops†; Tylenol Junior Strength Caplets†; Valorin†; Valorin Extra†

Pharmacologic class: para-aminophenol derivative
Therapeutic class: nonopioid analgesic, antipyretic
Pregnancy risk category: B

Indications and dosages

▶ **Mild pain or fever.** *Adults and children older than age 12:* 325 to 650 mg P.O. or P.R. q 4 hours, p.r.n.; or 1 g P.O. t.i.d. or q.i.d., p.r.n. Alternatively, 2 extended-release caplets P.O. q 8 hours. Maximum, 4 g daily. Dosage for long-term therapy shouldn't exceed 2.6 g daily unless monitored by prescriber.
Children ages 11 to 12: 480 mg P.O. or P.R. q 4 to 6 hours p.r.n.
Children ages 9 to 10: 400 mg P.O. or P.R. q 4 to 6 hours p.r.n.

Children ages 6 to 8: 320 mg P.O. or P.R. q 4 to 6 hours p.r.n.
Children ages 4 to 5: 240 mg P.O. or P.R. q 4 to 6 hours p.r.n.
Children ages 2 to 3: 160 mg P.O. or P.R. q 4 to 6 hours p.r.n.
Children ages 12 to 23 months: 120 mg P.O. q 4 to 6 hours p.r.n.
Infants ages 4 to 11 months: 80 mg P.O. q 4 to 6 hours p.r.n.
Infants age 3 months or younger: 40 mg P.O. q 4 to 6 hours p.r.n.

▶ **Osteoarthritis.** *Adults:* Up to 1 g P.O. q.i.d.

Contraindications and precautions

• Contraindicated in patients hypersensitive to drug.
• Use cautiously in patients with history of chronic alcohol abuse; hepatotoxicity may occur after therapeutic doses.
⚖ Lifespan: In pregnant or breast-feeding women, use cautiously.

Adverse reactions

Hematologic: hemolytic anemia, *neutropenia, leukopenia, pancytopenia, thrombocytopenia.*
Hepatic: *liver damage* (with toxic doses), jaundice.
Metabolic: *hypoglycemia.*
Skin: rash, urticaria.

Interactions

Drug-drug. *Barbiturates, carbamazepine, hydantoins, isoniazid, rifampin, sulfinpyrazone:* High doses or long-term use of these drugs may reduce therapeutic effects and enhance hepatotoxic effects of acetaminophen. Avoid use together.
Warfarin: May increase hypoprothrombinemic effects with long-term use with high doses of acetaminophen. Monitor PT and INR closely.
Zidovudine: May increase risk of bone marrow suppression because of impaired zidovudine metabolism. Monitor patient closely.
Drug-food. *Caffeine:* May enhance analgesic effects of acetaminophen. Monitor patient for effect.
Drug-lifestyle. *Alcohol use:* May increase risk of liver damage. Discourage using together.

Effects on lab test results

• May decrease hemoglobin, hematocrit, and neutrophil, WBC, RBC, and platelet counts.

• May produce false-positive decrease in glucose level. May alter laboratory tests for urinary 5-hydroxyindoleacetic acid.

Pharmacokinetics

Absorption: Rapid and complete.
Distribution: 25% protein-bound. Plasma levels don't correlate well with analgesic effect but do correlate with toxicity.
Metabolism: 90% to 95% metabolized in liver.
Excretion: In urine. *Half-life:* 1 to 4 hours.

Route	Onset	Peak	Duration
P.O., P.R.	Unknown	1-3 hr	1-3 hr

Action

Chemical effect: May produce analgesic effect by blocking pain impulses, probably by inhibiting prostaglandin or other substances that sensitize pain receptors. May relieve fever by action in hypothalamic heat-regulating center.
Therapeutic effect: Relieves pain and reduces fever.

Available forms

Caplets (extended-release): 650 mg
Capsules: 500 mg†
Elixir: 120 mg/5 ml, 130 mg/5 ml*†, 160 mg/ 5 ml*†, 325 mg/5 ml*†
Granules: 80 mg/packet†, 325 mg/capful†
Infant drops: 100 mg/ml†
Oral liquid: 160 mg/5 ml†, 500 mg/15 ml†
Oral solution: 48 mg/ml†, 100 mg/ml†
Oral suspension: 100 mg/ml†, 120 mg/5 ml ◊, 160 mg/ml†
Powder for solution: 1 g/packet
Sprinkles: 80 mg/capsule, 160 mg/capsule
Suppositories: 120 mg†, 125 mg†, 300 mg†, 325 mg†, 650 mg†
Tablets: 160 mg†, 325 mg†, 500 mg†, 650 mg†
Tablets (chewable): 80 mg†, 160 mg†
Tablets for solution: 325 mg
Wafers: 120 mg†

NURSING PROCESS

📈 **Assessment**

• Assess patient's pain or temperature before and during therapy.
• Assess patient's medication history. Many OTC products and combination prescription pain products contain acetaminophen; calculate total daily dosage accordingly.

Reactions may be *common*, uncommon, *life-threatening*, or COMMON AND LIFE-THREATENING.

- Be alert for adverse reactions and drug interactions.
- Evaluate patient's and family's knowledge of drug therapy.

Nursing diagnoses
- Acute pain related to patient's underlying condition
- Risk for injury related to drug-induced liver damage with toxic doses
- Deficient knowledge related to drug therapy

Planning and implementation
- Give liquid form to children and other patients who have trouble swallowing.
- **ALERT:** When giving oral preparation, calculate dosage based on level of drug because drops and elixir have different concentrations.
- Use P.R. in young children or other patient for whom oral forms aren't practical.

Patient teaching
- **ALERT:** Tell patient that drug is for short-term use only. Prescriber should be consulted if child takes drug for longer than 5 days or, for adults, longer than 10 days.
- **ALERT:** Tell patient not to use drug for temperature above 103.1° F (39.5° C), fever persisting longer than 3 days, or recurrent fever unless directed by prescriber.
- Warn patient that high doses or unsupervised long-term use can cause liver damage. Excessive alcohol use may increase risk of hepatotoxicity.
- Tell patient to keep track of daily acetaminophen intake, including OTC and prescription medications. Warn patient not to exceed total recommended dose of acetaminophen per day because of risk of hepatotoxicity.
- Tell breast-feeding woman that drug appears in breast milk in levels less than 1% of dose. She may use drug safely for short-term therapy that doesn't exceed recommended doses.

Evaluation
- Patient reports pain relief with drug.
- Patient's liver function test results remain normal.
- Patient and family state understanding of drug therapy.

acetazolamide
(ah-see-tuh-ZOH-luh-mighd)
Acetazolam, Apo-Acetazolamide, Diamox, Diamox Sequels

acetazolamide sodium
Diamox

Pharmacologic class: carbonic anhydrase inhibitor
Therapeutic class: adjunct therapy for open-angle glaucoma, agent for perioperative treatment of acute angle-closure glaucoma, anticonvulsant, agent for management of edema and for prevention and treatment of acute mountain sickness
Pregnancy risk category: C

Indications and dosages

▶ **Secondary glaucoma and preoperative management of acute angle-closure glaucoma.** *Adults:* 250 mg P.O. q 4 hours, or 250 mg P.O. or I.V. b.i.d. for short-term therapy. For some acute glaucomas, 500 mg P.O., then 125 mg to 250 mg P.O. q 4 hours. Give at 100 to 500 mg/minute.
▶ **Edema in heart failure.** *Adults:* 250 to 375 mg (5 mg/kg) P.O. daily in a.m.
▶ **Chronic open-angle glaucoma.** *Adults:* 250 mg to 1 g P.O. daily in divided doses q.i.d., or 500 mg extended-release P.O. b.i.d.
▶ **Prevention or amelioration of acute mountain sickness.** *Adults:* 500 mg to 1 g P.O. daily in divided doses q 8 to 12 hours, or 500 mg extended-release P.O. b.i.d. Therapy should start 24 to 48 hours before ascent and continue for 48 hours while at high altitude.
▶ **Adjunct treatment of myoclonic, refractory generalized tonic-clonic, absence, or mixed seizures.** *Adults and children:* 8 to 30 mg/kg P.O. daily in divided doses. Optimum dosage, 375 mg to 1 g daily. When given with other anticonvulsants, the initial dose is 250 mg daily.
▶ **Drug-induced edema.** *Adults:* 250 to 375 mg (5 mg/kg) P.O. as a single dose for 1 to 2 days with one drug-free day.
▶ **Periodic paralysis.** *Adults:* 250 mg P.O. b.i.d. or t.i.d., not to exceed 1.5 g daily.

▼ I.V. administration

• Reconstitute 500-mg vial with at least 5 ml of sterile water for injection.
• Inject 100 to 500 mg/minute into large vein, using 21G or 23G needle; intermittent or continuous infusion isn't recommended.
• Use within 24 hours.

Contraindications and precautions

• Contraindicated in patients hypersensitive to drug and in those undergoing long-term therapy for chronic noncongestive angle-closure glaucoma. Also contraindicated in patients with hyponatremia, hypokalemia, renal or hepatic impairment, adrenal gland failure, and hyperchloremic acidosis.
• Use cautiously in patients with respiratory acidosis, emphysema, or COPD, and in patients receiving other diuretics.
⚠ Lifespan: In pregnant women, use cautiously. In breast-feeding women, drug is contraindicated. In children, safety and efficacy of drug haven't been established.

Adverse reactions

CNS: drowsiness, paresthesia, confusion.
EENT: transient myopia.
GI: nausea, vomiting, anorexia, altered taste.
GU: crystalluria, renal calculi, hematuria.
Hematologic: *aplastic anemia,* hemolytic anemia, *leukopenia.*
Metabolic: *hyperchloremic acidosis,* asymptomatic hyperuricemia, hypokalemia.
Skin: rash.
Other: *pain at injection site,* sterile abscesses.

Interactions

Drug-drug. *Amphetamines, anticholinergics, mecamylamine, procainamide, quinidine, tricyclic antidepressants:* May decrease renal clearance of these drugs, increasing toxicity. Monitor patient closely.
Lithium: May increase lithium secretion. Monitor patient.
Methenamine: May reduce effectiveness of acetazolamide. Avoid using together.
Salicylates: May cause accumulation and toxicity of acetazolamide, including CNS depression and metabolic acidosis. Monitor patient closely.

Effects on lab test results

• May increase uric acid level. May decrease potassium level.

• May decrease hemoglobin, hematocrit, thyroid iodine uptake, and WBC count.
• May cause false-positive urine protein test results.

Pharmacokinetics

Absorption: Well absorbed from GI tract.
Distribution: Distributed throughout body tissues.
Metabolism: None.
Excretion: Primarily in urine. *Half-life:* 10 to 15 hours.

Route	Onset	Peak	Duration
P.O.			
tablets	1-1½ hr	2-4 hr	8-12 hr
capsules	2 hr	8-12 hr	18-24 hr
I.V.	2 min	15 min	4-5 hr

Action

Chemical effect: Blocks action of carbonic anhydrase, promoting renal excretion of sodium, potassium, bicarbonate, and water, and decreases secretion of aqueous humor in eye. As anticonvulsant, may inhibit carbonic anhydrase in CNS and decrease abnormal paroxysmal or excessive neuronal discharge. In acute mountain sickness, carbonic anhydrase inhibitors produce respiratory and metabolic acidosis that may stimulate ventilation, increase cerebral blood flow, and promote release of oxygen from hemoglobin.
Therapeutic effect: Lowers intraocular pressure, controls seizure activity, and may improve respiratory function.

Available forms

Capsules (extended-release): 500 mg
Injection: 500 mg/vial
Tablets: 125 mg, 250 mg

NURSING PROCESS

🔲 Assessment

• Assess patient's underlying condition before and during therapy, including eye discomfort and intraocular pressure in those with glaucoma, edema in those with heart failure, and neurologic status in those with seizures.
• Closely monitor intake and output.
• Be alert for adverse reactions and drug interactions.

Reactions may be *common,* uncommon, *life-threatening,* or COMMON AND LIFE-THREATENING.

• Evaluate patient's and family's knowledge of drug therapy.

🔷 **Nursing diagnoses**
• Excessive fluid volume related to patient's underlying condition
• Impaired urine elimination related to diuretic action of drug
• Deficient knowledge related to drug therapy

▶ **Planning and implementation**
• Give oral preparation early in the morning to avoid nocturia. Give second dose early in the afternoon.
• If patient can't swallow oral forms, ask pharmacist if he can make a suspension using crushed tablets in flavored syrup. Although concentrations up to 500 mg/5 ml are possible, concentrations of 250 mg/5 ml are more palatable. Refrigeration improves palatability but doesn't improve stability. Suspensions are stable for 1 week.
• Diuretic effect decreases with acidosis but is reestablished by stopping drug for several days and then restarting it or by using intermittent administration.
⚠ **ALERT:** Don't confuse acetazolamide with acetohexamide. Also don't confuse acetazolamide sodium (Diamox) with acyclovir sodium (Zovirax); these vials may appear similar.
• Withhold drug and notify prescriber if hypersensitivity or adverse reactions occur.
Patient teaching
• Advise patient to take drug early in the day to avoid sleep interruption caused by nocturia.
• Teach patient to monitor fluid volume by measuring weight, intake, and output daily.
• Encourage patient to avoid high-sodium foods and to choose high-potassium foods.
• Teach patient to recognize and report signs and symptoms of fluid and electrolyte imbalance.

☑ **Evaluation**
• Patient is free from edema.
• Patient adjusts lifestyle to accommodate altered patterns of urine elimination.
• Patient and family state understanding of drug therapy.

acetylcysteine
(as-ee-til-SIS-teen)
Mucomyst, Mucomyst-10, Mucosil-10, Mucosil-20, Parvolex◊

Pharmacologic class: amino acid (L-cysteine) derivative
Therapeutic class: mucolytic, antidote for acetaminophen overdose
Pregnancy risk category: B

Indications and dosages

▶ **Pneumonia, bronchitis, tuberculosis, cystic fibrosis, emphysema, atelectasis (adjunct), complications of thoracic and CV surgery.**
Adults and children: 1 to 2 ml of 10% or 20% solution by direct instillation into trachea as often as hourly; or 3 to 5 ml of 20% solution or 6 to 10 ml of 10% solution by nebulization q 2 to 3 hours p.r.n.
▶ **Acetaminophen toxicity.** *Adults and children:* Initially, 140 mg/kg P.O., followed by 70 mg/kg P.O. q 4 hours for 17 doses; or, where available ◊, 300 mg/kg by I.V. infusion.
▶ **Prevention of acute renal failure related to radiographic contrast media‡.** *Adults:* 600 mg P.O. b.i.d. given the day before and on the day of contrast media administration for a total of four doses. Or, if for hydration, give with ½ normal saline solution injection for I.V. infusion at 1 ml/kg/hr for 12 hours before and 12 hours after contrast media administration.

▼ I.V. administration ◊
• Dilute calculated dose in D₅W. Dilute initial dose of 150 mg/kg in 200 ml of D₅W and infuse over 15 minutes.
• Dilute second dose of 50 mg/kg in 500 ml of D₅W and infuse over 4 hours.
• Dilute final dose of 100 mg/kg in 1,000 ml of D₅W and infuse over 16 hours.

Contraindications and precautions
• Contraindicated in patients hypersensitive to drug.
• Use cautiously in debilitated patients with severe respiratory insufficiency.
⚠ **Lifespan:** In pregnant and breast-feeding women and in elderly patients with severe respiratory insufficiency, use cautiously.

Adverse reactions

EENT: rhinorrhea, hemoptysis.
GI: stomatitis, nausea, vomiting.
Respiratory: BRONCHOSPASM.

Interactions

Drug-drug. *Activated charcoal:* Limits acetylcysteine's effectiveness. Avoid using together in treating drug toxicity.

Effects on lab test results

None reported.

Pharmacokinetics

Absorption: Most inhaled acetylcysteine acts directly on mucus in lungs; remainder is absorbed by pulmonary epithelium. After oral administration, drug is absorbed from GI tract.
Distribution: Unknown.
Metabolism: Metabolized in liver.
Excretion: Unknown. *Half-life:* 6¼ hours.

Route	Onset	Peak	Duration
P.O., I.V., inhalation	Unknown	Unknown	Unknown

Action

Chemical effect: Increases production of respiratory tract fluids to help liquefy and reduce viscosity of tenacious secretions. Also, restores glutathione in liver to treat acetaminophen toxicity.
Therapeutic effect: Thins respiratory secretions and reverses toxic effects of acetaminophen.

Available forms

Injection: 200 mg/ml ◊
Solution: 10%, 20%

NURSING PROCESS

🔖 Assessment

• Assess patient's respiratory secretions before and frequently during therapy.
• Be alert for adverse reactions and drug interactions.
• Evaluate patient's and family's knowledge of drug therapy.

🔲 Nursing diagnoses

• Ineffective airway clearance related to patient's underlying condition

• Impaired oral mucous membrane related to drug-induced stomatitis
• Deficient knowledge related to drug therapy

⟩ Planning and implementation

• Dilute oral doses with cola, fruit juice, or water before giving to treat acetaminophen overdose. Dilute 20% solution to a concentration of 5% by adding 3 ml of diluent to each ml of acetylcysteine. If patient vomits within 1 hour of initial or maintenance dose, repeat dose.
• Use plastic, glass, stainless steel, or another nonreactive metal when giving by nebulization.
• Hand-bulb nebulizers aren't recommended because output is too small and particle size is too large.
• Before aerosol administration, have patient clear airway by coughing.
• After opening, store in refrigerator, and use within 4 days.
⚕ **ALERT:** Drug is physically or chemically incompatible with tetracyclines, erythromycin lactobionate, amphotericin B, and ampicillin sodium. If given by aerosol inhalation, these drugs should be nebulized separately. Iodized oil, trypsin, and hydrogen peroxide are physically incompatible with acetylcysteine; don't add these drugs to nebulizer.
• Have suction equipment available in case patient can't effectively clear his air passages.
• Alert prescriber if patient's respiratory secretions thicken or become purulent or if bronchospasm occurs.
⚕ **ALERT:** Acetylcysteine is given to treat acetaminophen overdose within 24 hours after ingestion. Start treatment immediately; don't wait for drug level determinations.
⚕ **ALERT:** Don't confuse acetylcysteine with acetylcholine.
Patient teaching
• Instruct patient to follow directions on drug label exactly. Explain importance of using drug as directed.
• If patient's condition doesn't improve within 10 days, tell him to notify prescriber. Drug shouldn't be used for prolonged period without direct medical supervision.
• Teach patient how to use and clean nebulizer.
• Inform patient that drug may have foul taste or smell.
• Instruct patient to clear his airway by coughing before aerosol administration to achieve maximum effect.

Reactions may be *common,* uncommon, *life-threatening,* or COMMON AND LIFE-THREATENING.

• Instruct patient to rinse mouth with water after nebulizer treatment because it may leave sticky coating on oral cavity.

✔ Evaluation
• Patient has clear lung sounds, decreased respiratory secretions, and reduced frequency and severity of cough.
• Patient's oral mucous membranes remain unchanged.
• Patient and family state understanding of drug therapy.

activated charcoal
(AK-tih-vay-ted CHAR-kohl)
Actidose†, Actidose-Aqua†, CharcoAid†, CharcoCaps†, Insta-Char Pediatric†, Liqui-Char†, SuperChar†

Pharmacologic class: adsorbent
Therapeutic class: antidote
Pregnancy risk category: C

Indications and dosages
▶ **Flatulence, dyspepsia.** *Adults:* 600 mg to 5 g P.O. t.i.d. after meals.
▶ **Poisoning.** *Adults:* Initially, 1 g/kg (30 to 100 g) P.O. or five to ten times amount of poison ingested as suspension in 180 to 240 ml of water.
Children: Five to ten times estimated weight of poison ingested, with minimum dose being 30 g P.O. in 240 ml of water to make a slurry, preferably within 30 minutes of poisoning. Larger dose is necessary if food is in stomach.
▶ **To relieve GI disturbances (such as halitosis, anorexia, nausea, and vomiting) in uremic patients‡.** *Adults:* 20 to 50 g P.O. daily.

Contraindications and precautions
None reported.

Adverse reactions
GI: black stools, nausea, constipation.

Interactions
Drug-drug. *Acetylcysteine, ipecac:* Render charcoal ineffective. Don't give together, and don't perform gastric lavage until all charcoal is removed.

Effects on lab test results
None reported.

Pharmacokinetics
Absorption: None.
Distribution: None.
Metabolism: None.
Excretion: In feces.

Route	Onset	Peak	Duration
P.O.	Immediate	Unknown	Unknown

Action
Chemical effect: Adheres to many drugs and chemicals, inhibiting their absorption from GI tract.
Therapeutic effect: Used as antidote for selected poisons and overdoses.

Available forms
Capsules: 260 mg†
Oral suspension: 0.625 g/5 ml†, 0.83 g/5 ml†, 1 g/5 ml†, 1.25 g/5 ml†
Powder: 30 g†, 50 g†
Tablets: 200 mg ◊ †, 300 mg ◊ †, 325 mg†, 650 mg†

NURSING PROCESS

⚕ Assessment
• Obtain history of substance reportedly ingested, including time of ingestion, if possible. Drug isn't effective for all drugs and toxic substances.
• Be alert for adverse reactions and drug interactions.
• Evaluate patient's and family's knowledge of drug therapy.

⚕ Nursing diagnoses
• Risk for injury related to ingestion of toxic substance or overdose
• Risk for deficient fluid volume related to drug-induced vomiting
• Deficient knowledge related to drug therapy

▶ Planning and implementation
• Commonly used for treating poisoning or overdose with acetaminophen, aspirin, atropine, barbiturates, cardiac glycosides, poisonous mushrooms, oxalic acid, parathion, phenol, phenytoin, propantheline, propoxyphene, strychnine, or tricyclic antidepressants. Check

with poison control center for use in other types of poisonings or overdoses.

• Give after emesis is complete because drug absorbs and inactivates syrup of ipecac.

⊛ **ALERT:** Don't give to semiconscious or unconscious persons unless airway is protected and NG tube is in place for instillation.

• Mix powder form (most effective) with tap water to form consistency of thick syrup. Add small amount of fruit juice or flavoring to make mix more palatable.

• Give by NG tube after lavage, if needed.

• Don't give in ice cream, milk, or sherbet, which may reduce absorption.

• Repeat dose if patient vomits shortly after administration.

• Keep airway, oxygen, and suction equipment nearby.

• Follow treatment with stool softener or laxative to prevent constipation.

⊛ **ALERT:** Don't confuse Actidose with Actos.

Patient teaching

• Warn patient that feces will be black.

• Instruct patient to report respiratory difficulty immediately.

☑ Evaluation

• Patient doesn't experience injury from ingesting toxic substance or from overdose.

• Patient exhibits no signs of deficient fluid volume.

• Patient and family state understanding of drug therapy.

acyclovir sodium
(ay-SIGH-kloh-veer SOH-dee-um)
Aciclovir ◇, **Acihexal** ◇, **Avirax** ♦, **Zovirax**†

Pharmacologic class: synthetic purine nucleoside
Therapeutic class: antiviral
Pregnancy risk category: B

Indications and dosages

▶ **Initial and recurrent episodes of mucocutaneous herpes simplex virus (HSV-1 and HSV-2) infections in immunocompromised patients; severe initial episodes of herpes genitalis in immunocompetent patients.** *Adults and children age 12 and older:* 5 mg/kg I.V. at

constant rate over 1 hour q 8 hours for 7 days (5 days for herpes genitalis).
Children younger than age 12: 250 mg/m² I.V. at constant rate over 1 hour q 8 hours for 7 days (5 days for herpes genitalis).

▶ **Initial genital herpes.** *Adults:* 200 mg P.O. q 4 hours during waking hours (total of 5 capsules daily) for 10 days.

▶ **Genital herpes in immunocompromised patients‡.** *Adults:* 400 mg P.O. three to five times daily.

▶ **Intermittent therapy for recurrent genital herpes.** *Adults:* 200 mg P.O. q 4 hours during waking hours (total of 5 capsules daily) for 5 days. Start therapy at first sign of recurrence.

▶ **Long-term suppressive therapy for recurrent genital herpes.** *Adults:* 400 mg P.O. b.i.d. for up to 12 months.

▶ **Long-term suppressive or maintenance therapy for recurrent HSV infections in patients with HIV‡.** *Adults and children older than age 12:* 200 mg P.O. t.i.d. or 400 mg P.O. b.i.d.
Children age 12 and younger: 600 to 1,000 mg P.O. daily in three to five divided doses.

▶ **Chickenpox.** *Adults and children age 2 and older weighing more than 40 kg (88 lb):* 800 mg P.O. q.i.d. for 5 days.

▶ **Acute herpes zoster.** *Adults:* 800 mg P.O. q 4 hours, five times daily for 7 to 10 days. Give within 48 hours of rash onset.

▶ **Disseminated herpes zoster‡.** *Adults:* 5 to 10 mg/kg I.V. q 8 hours for 7 to 10 days. Infuse over at least 1 hour.

▶ **Herpes simplex encephalitis.** *Adults:* 10 mg/kg infused at a constant rate over 1 hour, q 8 hours for 10 days.
Children ages 6 months to 12 years: 500 mg/m² at a constant rate over at least 1 hour, q 8 hours for 10 days.

▶ **Varicella zoster in immunocompromised patients.** *Adults and children age 12 and older:* 10 mg/kg I.V. infused at a constant rate over 1 hour, q 8 hours for 7 days. Obese patients should be given 10 mg/kg (ideal body weight). Don't exceed maximum dose equivalent to 500 mg/m² q 8 hours.
Children younger than age 12: 20 mg/kg I.V. q 8 hours for 7 days, or 500 mg/m² at a constant rate over at least 1 hour, q 8 hours for 7 days.

▶ **Acute herpes zoster ophthalmicus‡.** *Adults:* 600 mg P.O. q 4 hours five times daily for 10 days, preferably within 3 days of rash on-set, but no longer than 7 days.

▶ **Rectal herpes infection‡.** *Adults:* 400 mg P.O. five times daily for 10 days or until re-solved; Or, give 800 mg P.O. q 8 hours for 7 to 10 days.

🔲 **Adjust-a-dose:** For patients with renal impair-ment, if creatinine clearance is less than 10 ml/minute, decrease the normal oral dose (200 to 400 mg) to 200 mg q 12 hours. For normal oral doses more than 400 mg, consult package insert. In patients with renal failure, give 100% of the I.V. dose q 8 hours if creatinine clearance ex-ceeds 50 ml/minute; 100% of the dose q 12 hours if creatinine clearance is between 25 and 50 ml/minute; 100% of the dose q 24 hours if the creatinine clearance is between 10 to 25 ml/minute; and 50% of the dose q 24 hours if it falls below 10 ml/minute.

▶ **Recurrent herpes labialis (cold sores).** *Adults and children age 12 and older:* Apply cream five times daily for four days. Start ther-apy as early as possible following onset of signs and symptoms.

▼ I.V. administration

• Dissolve the contents of the 500-mg vial in 10 ml of sterile water for injection, or the 1,000-mg vial in 20 ml sterile water for injec-tion, to yield 50 mg/ml. Don't use bacteriostatic water containing benzyl alcohol or parabens.
• Add the calculated dose to the selected type and volume of I.V. solution for administration. The infusion concentration should be 7 mg/ml or less. Concentrated solutions (10 mg/ml or more) increase the risk of phlebitis.
• Give I.V. infusion over at least 1 hour to pre-vent renal tubular damage. Don't give by bolus injection.
• Ensure I.V. infusion is accompanied by ade-quate hydration. Monitor intake and output closely during administration.

Contraindications and precautions

• Contraindicated in patients hypersensitive to drug.
• Use cautiously in patients with underlying neurologic problems, renal disease, or dehydra-tion and in those receiving other nephrotoxic drugs.
⚕ **Lifespan:** In pregnant or breast-feeding women, use cautiously. In children younger than age 2, safety and efficacy of drug haven't been established.

Adverse reactions

CNS: *encephalopathic changes* (including lethargy, obtundation, tremor, confusion, hallu-cinations, agitation, *seizures, coma,* headache [with I.V. dosage]).
CV: hypotension.
GI: nausea, vomiting, diarrhea.
GU: hematuria.
Skin: rash, itching, *vesicular eruptions.*
Other: inflammation, phlebitis at injection site.

Interactions

Drug-drug. *Phenytoin:* May decrease pheny-toin level. Monitor patient closely.
Probenecid: Increases acyclovir level. Monitor patient for possible toxicity.
Valproic acid: Decreases valproic acid level. Monitor patient closely.
Zidovudine: May cause drowsiness or lethargy. Use together cautiously.

Effects on lab test results

• May increase BUN, creatinine, and liver en-zyme levels.
• May decrease hemoglobin and hematocrit. May increase or decrease platelet, neutrophil, and WBC counts.

Pharmacokinetics

Absorption: Slow and only 15% to 30% is ab-sorbed. Not affected by food.
Distribution: Widely distributed to organ tis-sues and body fluids. CSF levels equal about 50% of serum levels. 9% to 33% binds to plas-ma proteins.
Metabolism: Primarily inside viral cell to its active form. About 10% of dose is metabolized extracellularly.
Excretion: Up to 92% of systemically absorbed acyclovir is excreted unchanged by kidneys via glomerular filtration and tubular secretion. *Half-life:* 2 to 3½ hours with normal renal function; up to 19 hours with renal impairment.

Route	Onset	Peak	Duration
P.O.	Unknown	Unknown	Unknown
I.V.	Immediate	Immediate	Unknown

Action

Chemical effect: Becomes incorporated into viral DNA and inhibits viral multiplication.
Therapeutic effect: Kills susceptible viruses.

Available forms

Capsules: 200 mg
Cream: 5%, in 2-g tubes†
Injection: 500 mg/vial, 1 g/vial
Suspension: 200 mg/5 ml
Tablets: 400 mg, 800 mg

NURSING PROCESS

☲ Assessment

• Assess infection before and regularly during therapy.
• Monitor patient for renal toxicity. Bolus injection, dehydration, renal disease, and use of other nephrotoxic drugs increase risk.
• Monitor patient's mental status when giving drug I.V. Encephalopathic changes are more likely in patients with neurologic disorders or in those who have had neurologic reactions to cytotoxic drugs.
• If adverse GI reactions occur with oral administration, monitor patient's hydration.
• Evaluate patient's and family's knowledge of drug therapy.

⊕ Nursing diagnoses

• Infection related to presence of virus
• Risk for deficient fluid volume related to adverse GI reactions to oral drug
• Deficient knowledge related to drug therapy

⬗ Planning and implementation

⊛ **ALERT:** Don't give I.M., S.C., or by bolus injection.
⊛ **ALERT:** Don't confuse Zovirax with Zyvox. They both come in a 400-mg tablet strength.
⊛ **ALERT:** Don't confuse acyclovir sodium (Zovirax) with acetazolamide sodium (Diamox). The vials may look alike.
Patient teaching
• Tell patient that drug effectively manages herpes infection but doesn't eliminate or cure it.
• Warn patient that drug won't prevent spread of infection to others.
• Help patient to recognize early symptoms of herpes infection (tingling, itching, pain) so he can take drug before infection fully develops.

• Tell patient to alert nurse if he has pain or discomfort at I.V. injection site.

☑ Evaluation

• Patient's infection is eradicated.
• Patient maintains adequate hydration.
• Patient and family state understanding of drug therapy.

adalimumab

(ay-da-LIM-yoo-mab)
Humira

Pharmacologic class: tumor necrosis factor (TNF)–alpha blocker
Therapeutic class: antirheumatic
Pregnancy risk category: B

Indications and dosages

▶ **Moderately to severely active rheumatoid arthritis that hasn't responded well to disease-modifying antirheumatics.** *Adults:* 40 mg S.C. q other week. May increase to 40 mg q week if patient isn't taking methotrexate.

Contraindications and precautions

• Contraindicated in patients hypersensitive to drug or its components. Don't start drug if patient is immunosuppressed or has a chronic or localized active infection.
• Use cautiously in patients with a history of recurrent infection, those with underlying conditions that predispose them to infections, and those who have lived in areas where tuberculosis and histoplasmosis are common. Use cautiously in patients with CNS-demyelinating disorders.
⚐ **Lifespan:** In pregnant women, give only if clearly needed and benefits outweigh risks since no well-controlled studies exist. Breast-feeding women should stop nursing or stop using the drug because of the risk for serious adverse reactions; it's unknown whether drug appears in breast milk or would be absorbed systemically by a breast-feeding infant. In children, safety and efficacy of drug haven't been established. In elderly patients, use cautiously because serious infections and malignancies are more common in these patients.

Reactions may be *common,* uncommon, *life-threatening,* or COMMON AND LIFE-THREATENING.

Adverse reactions

CNS: headache.
CV: hypertension.
EENT: sinusitis.
GI: nausea, abdominal pain.
GU: UTI, hematuria.
Metabolic: hypercholesterolemia, hyperlipidemia.
Musculoskeletal: back pain.
Respiratory: upper respiratory tract infection, bronchitis.
Skin: rash.
Other: *malignancy,* flu syndrome, *accidental injury,* allergic reactions, injection site reactions (erythema, itching, hemorrhage, pain, swelling).

Interactions

Drug-drug. *Live-virus vaccines:* May cause immunosuppression and susceptibility to disease. Avoid using together.

Effects on lab test results

• May increase cholesterol level.

Pharmacokinetics

Absorption: Average absolute bioavailability is 64%.
Distribution: Levels in synovial fluid are 31% to 96% of those in serum.
Metabolism: Clearance may be higher if anti-adalimumab antibodies are present and lower in patients age 40 and older.
Excretion: Unknown. *Half-life:* Ranges from 10 to 20 days.

Route	Onset	Peak	Duration
S.C.	Variable	Variable	Unknown

Action

Chemical effect: A recombinant human IgG$_1$ monoclonal antibody that blocks human TNF-alpha. TNF-alpha takes part in normal inflammatory and immune responses and also in the inflammation and joint destruction of rheumatoid arthritis.
Therapeutic effect: Reduces signs and symptoms of rheumatoid arthritis.

Available forms

Injection: 40 mg/0.8 ml

NURSING PROCESS

Assessment
• Assess patient for immunosupression or active infection before therapy and regularly thereafter.
• Monitor patient for hypersensitivity reaction.

Nursing diagnoses
• Alteration in mobility status related to rheumatoid arthritis
• Deficient knowledge related to signs and symptoms of immunosupression and/or infection
• Deficient knowledge related to drug therapy.

Planning and implementation
• Drug can be given alone or with methotrexate or other disease-modifying antirheumatics.
• Give first dose under supervision of experienced health care provider.
• Evaluate patient for latent tuberculosis and, if present, start treatment before giving drug.
• Serious infections and sepsis, including tuberculosis and invasive opportunistic fungal infections, may occur. If patient develops new infection during treatment, monitor patient closely.
• **ALERT:** The needle cover contains latex and shouldn't be handled by those with latex sensitivity.
• Stop drug if patient develops a severe infection, anaphylaxis, other serious allergic reaction, or evidence of a lupuslike syndrome.
Patient teaching
• Tell patient to report evidence of tuberculosis or infection.
• If appropriate, teach patient or caregiver how to give drug.
• Tell patient to rotate injection sites and to avoid tender, bruised, red, or hard skin.
• Teach patient to dispose of used vials, needles, and syringes safely.
• Tell patient to refrigerate drug in its original container before use.

Evaluation
• Patient experiences reduced signs and symptoms of rheumatoid arthritis.
• Patient remains free from infection during therapy.
• Patient and family state understanding of drug therapy.

adefovir dipivoxil
(uh-DEPH-uh-veer dih-pih-VOCKS-ul)
Hepsera

Pharmacologic class: acyclic nucleotide analogue
Therapeutic class: antiviral
Pregnancy risk category: C

Indications and dosages

▶ **Chronic hepatitis B infection.** *Adults:* 10 mg P.O. daily.
Adjust-a-dose: For patients with renal impairment, if creatinine clearance is 20 to 49 ml/minute, give 10 mg P.O. q 2 days. If creatinine clearance is 10 to 19 ml/minute, give 10 mg P.O. q 3 days. In patients receiving hemodialysis, give 10 mg P.O. q 7 days, after dialysis session.

Contraindications and precautions

• Contraindicated in patients hypersensitive to any component of the drug.
• Use cautiously and at a reduced dose in patients with renal impairment and in those receiving nephrotoxic drugs.
Lifespan: In pregnant women, use drug only if benefits outweigh risks. Women should avoid breast-feeding; it's unknown if drug appears in breast milk. In children, safety and efficacy of drug haven't been established. In elderly patients, use cautiously because of increased risk of renal or CV dysfunction.

Adverse reactions

CNS: *asthenia,* headache, fever.
EENT: pharyngitis, sinusitis.
GI: abdominal pain, diarrhea, dyspepsia, flatulence, nausea, vomiting.
GU: ***renal failure,*** renal insufficiency, hematuria, glycosuria.
Hepatic: ***hepatomegaly with steatosis, hepatic failure.***
Metabolic: ***lactic acidosis.***
Respiratory: cough.
Skin: pruritus, rash.

Interactions

Drug-drug. *Ibuprofen:* May increase adefovir bioavailability. Monitor patient closely.
Nephrotoxic drugs, such as aminoglycosides, cyclosporine, NSAIDs, tacrolimus, vancomycin: Increases risk of nephrotoxicity. Use together cautiously.

Effects on lab test results

• May increase ALT, amylase, AST, CK, creatinine, and lactic acid levels.

Pharmacokinetics

Absorption: Readily absorbed from the GI tract with a bioavailability of 59%.
Distribution: Up to 4% bound to plasma and serum proteins.
Metabolism: Rapidly converted to adefovir diphosphate, an active metabolite.
Excretion: Undergoes renal elimination. *Half-life:* Unknown.

Route	Onset	Peak	Duration
P.O.	Unknown	1-4 hr	Unknown

Action

Chemical effect: Inhibits hepatitis B virus reverse transcriptase, which breaks the viral DNA chain.
Therapeutic effect: Reduces symptoms of hepatitis B.

Available forms

Tablets: 10 mg

NURSING PROCESS

Assessment

• Assess patient's condition before therapy and regularly thereafter.
• Watch for hypersensitivity reaction.
• Monitor renal function, especially in patients with renal dysfunction and in those taking nephrotoxic drugs.
• Monitor hepatic function.

Nursing diagnoses

• Risk for lactic acidosis, hepatomegaly, and steatosis secondary to liver disease.
• Deficient knowledge related to drug therapy.

Planning and implementation

• The ideal length of treatment hasn't been established.
• Patients receiving drug should be offered HIV antibody testing. Drug may promote resistance

to antiretrovirals in patients with unrecognized or untreated HIV infection.
• Monitor hepatic function. Notify prescriber if patient develops signs or symptoms of lactic acidosis and severe hepatomegaly with steatosis. Drug may have to be stopped.
• Severe exacerbations of hepatitis may result from stopping drug. Monitor hepatic function closely in patients who stop taking drug.
⊛ **ALERT:** Patients may develop lactic acidosis and severe hepatomegaly with steatosis during treatment. Risk is higher in women, obese patients, and those taking other antiretrovirals.
• Overdose causes GI adverse effects. Treating overdose includes monitoring for evidence of toxicity and giving supportive therapy. Dialysis may also be helpful.
• Pregnant women exposed to drug may call the Antiretroviral Pregnancy Registry at 1-800-258-4263, to monitor fetal outcome.
Patient teaching
• Inform patient that drug may be taken without regard to meals.
• Tell patient to immediately report weakness, muscle pain, trouble breathing, stomach pain with nausea and vomiting, dizziness, light-headedness, fast or irregular heartbeat, and feeling cold, especially in arms and legs.
• Warn patient not to stop taking drug unless directed because it could cause hepatitis to become worse.
• Instruct women to tell their prescriber if they become pregnant or are breast-feeding. Advise breast-feeding women to stop either breast-feeding or taking the drug.

☑ **Evaluation**
• Patient remains free from lactic acidosis, hepatomegaly, and steatosis during therapy.
• Patient and family state understanding of drug therapy.

adenosine
(uh-DEN-oh-seen)
Adenocard

Pharmacologic class: nucleoside
Therapeutic class: antiarrhythmic
Pregnancy risk category: C

Indications and dosages
▶ **Conversion of paroxysmal supraventricular tachycardia (PSVT) to sinus rhythm.**
Adults: 6 mg I.V. by rapid bolus injection over 1 to 2 seconds. If PSVT isn't eliminated in 1 to 2 minutes, give 12 mg by rapid I.V. bolus and repeat, if needed.

▽ I.V. administration
• Check solution for crystals that may form if solution is cold. If crystals are visible, gently warm solution to room temperature. Don't use cloudy solutions.
• Give by rapid I.V. injection over 1 to 2 seconds. Give directly into vein if possible; if I.V. line is used, inject drug into most proximal port.
• Drug has a very short half-life; follow with rapid saline flush to ensure that drug reaches systemic circulation quickly.
• Don't give single dose that exceeds 12 mg.
• Discard unused drug; it doesn't contain preservatives.

Contraindications and precautions
• Contraindicated in patients hypersensitive to drug and in those with second- or third-degree heart block or sick-sinus syndrome unless artificial pacemaker is present. Drug decreases conduction through AV node and may produce transient first-, second-, or third-degree heart block. Patients for whom significant heart block develops shouldn't receive additional doses.
• Use cautiously in patients with asthma because bronchoconstriction may occur.
⚶ **Lifespan:** In pregnant and breast-feeding women and in children, safety of drug hasn't been established.

Adverse reactions
CNS: apprehension, burning sensation, dizziness, heaviness in arms, light-headedness, numbness, tingling in arms.
CV: chest pressure, chest pain, *facial flushing,* headache, hypotension, palpitations.
EENT: metallic taste, blurred vision, tightness in throat.
GI: nausea.
Musculoskeletal: back pain, neck pain.
Respiratory: dyspnea, shortness of breath, hyperventilation.
Skin: diaphoresis.
Other: groin pressure.

Interactions

Drug-drug. *Carbamazepine:* Higher degree of heart block may occur. Monitor patient.

Digoxin, verapamil: In rare cases, combined use causes ventricular fibrillation. Use together cautiously.

Dipyridamole: May potentiate adenosine's effects. A smaller dose may be needed.

Methylxanthines: May antagonize adenosine's effects. A patient receiving theophylline or caffeine may require a higher dose or may not respond to therapy.

Drug-herb. *Guarana:* May decrease therapeutic response. Discourage using together.

Drug-food. *Caffeine:* May antagonize adenosine's effects. May require higher dose.

Effects on lab test results

None reported.

Pharmacokinetics

Absorption: Administered I.V.
Distribution: Rapidly taken up by erythrocytes and vascular endothelial cells.
Metabolism: Metabolized within tissues to inosine and adenosine monophosphate.
Excretion: Unknown. *Half-life:* Less than 10 seconds.

Route	Onset	Peak	Duration
I.V.	Immediate	Immediate	Extremely short

Action

Chemical effect: Acts on AV node to slow conduction and inhibit reentry pathways. Drug also is useful in treating PSVT with accessory bypass tracts (Wolff-Parkinson-White syndrome).
Therapeutic effect: Restores normal sinus rhythm.

Available forms

Injection: 3 mg/ml in 2-ml vials, 2-ml and 5-ml syringes

NURSING PROCESS

🔧 Assessment
• Monitor patient's heart rate and rhythm before and during therapy.
• Be alert for adverse reactions and drug interactions.

• Evaluate patient's and family's knowledge of drug therapy.

🔛 Nursing diagnoses
• Decreased cardiac output related to arrhythmias
• Ineffective protection related to drug-induced proarrhythmias
• Deficient knowledge related to drug therapy

▶ Planning and implementation
• If ECG disturbances occur, withhold drug, obtain rhythm strip, and notify prescriber immediately.
⊕ ALERT: Have emergency equipment and drugs on hand to treat new arrhythmias.
Patient teaching
• Teach patient and family about his disease and therapy.
• Stress importance of alerting health care provider if chest pain or dyspnea occurs.
• Advise patient to avoid caffeine.

✅ Evaluation
• Patient's arrhythmias are corrected and his heart maintains normal sinus rhythm.
• Patient doesn't experience proarrhythmias.
• Patient and family state understanding of drug therapy.

albumin 5%
(al-BYOO-min)
Albuminar-5, Albutein 5%, Buminate 5%, Plasbumin-5

albumin 25%
Albuminar-25, Albutein 25%, Buminate 25%, Plasbumin-25

Pharmacologic class: blood derivative
Therapeutic class: plasma volume expander
Pregnancy risk category: C

Indications and dosages

▶ **Hypovolemic shock.** *Adults:* Initially, 500 ml 5% solution by I.V. infusion; repeat, p.r.n. Dosage varies with patient's condition and response. Maximum, 250 g in 48 hours.
Children: 10 to 20 ml/kg 5% solution by I.V. infusion, repeated in 15 to 30 minutes if response

isn't adequate. Or, 2.5 to 5 ml/kg 25% solution
I.V.; repeat after 10 to 30 minutes, if needed.
▶ **Hypoproteinemia.** *Adults:* 1,000 to 1,500 ml
5% solution by I.V. infusion daily, with maximum rate of 5 to 10 ml/minute; or 200 to 300 ml
25% solution by I.V. infusion daily, with maximum rate of 3 ml/minute. Dosage varies with
patient's condition and response.
▶ **Hyperbilirubinemia.** *Infants:* 1 g albumin
(4 ml 25%)/kg I.V. 1 to 2 hours before transfusion.

▼ I.V. administration

• Dilute with normal saline solution or D$_5$W.
Use solution promptly and discard any unused
solution because it doesn't contain preservatives.
Don't use cloudy solutions or those containing
sediment. Solution should be clear amber.
• Minimize waste when preparing and giving
drug. This product is expensive, and random
shortages are common.
• Avoid infusing 10 ml/minute or faster. Infusion rate is individualized according to patient's
age, condition, and diagnosis. Albumin 5% is
infused undiluted; albumin 25% may be undiluted or diluted with normal saline or D$_5$W injection.
• Follow storage instructions on bottle. Freezing
may cause bottle to break.
⚠ **ALERT:** Don't give more than 250 g in 48
hours.

Contraindications and precautions

• Contraindicated in patients hypersensitive to
drug.
• Use cautiously in patients with hypertension,
cardiac disease, severe pulmonary infection, severe chronic anemia, or hypoalbuminemia with
peripheral edema.
⚕ **Lifespan:** In pregnant women, use cautiously.

Adverse reactions

CNS: fever.
CV: *vascular overload,* hypotension, altered
pulse rate.
GI: increased salivation, nausea, vomiting.
Respiratory: altered respiration.
Skin: urticaria, rash.
Other: chills.

Interactions

None significant.

Effects on lab test results

• May increase albumin level.

Pharmacokinetics

Absorption: Administered I.V.
Distribution: Albumin accounts for about 50%
of plasma proteins; it is distributed into intravascular space and extravascular sites, including
skin, muscle, and lungs.
Metabolism: Unknown.
Excretion: Unknown, although liver, kidneys,
or intestines may provide elimination mechanisms for albumin. *Half-life:* 15 to 20 days.

Route	Onset	Peak	Duration
I.V.	15 min for hydrated patient	15 min for hydrated patient	Up to several hr with reduced blood volume

Action

Chemical effect: Albumin 5% supplies colloid
to blood and expands plasma volume. Albumin
25% provides intravascular oncotic pressure in
5:1 ratio, causing fluid shift from interstitial
spaces to circulation and slightly increasing protein level.
Therapeutic effect: Relieves shock by increasing plasma volume and corrects plasma protein
deficiency.

Available forms

albumin 5% injection: 50-ml, 250-ml, 500-ml,
1,000-ml vials
albumin 25% injection: 10-ml, 20-ml, 50-ml,
100-ml vials

NURSING PROCESS

⚗ Assessment
• Assess patient's underlying condition.
• Be alert for adverse reactions.
• Monitor fluid intake and output, hemoglobin,
hematocrit, and protein and electrolyte levels.
• Monitor blood pressure frequently during
therapy.
• Evaluate patient's and family's knowledge of
drug therapy.

🔖 Nursing diagnoses
• Deficient fluid volume related to patient's underlying condition

● Excessive fluid volume related to adverse effects of drug
● Deficient knowledge related to drug therapy

▶ **Planning and implementation**
● One volume of albumin 25% is equivalent to five volumes of albumin 5% in producing hemodilution and relative anemia.
● Withhold fluids in patient with cerebral edema for 8 hours after infusion to avoid fluid overload.
● If hypotension occurs, slow, or stop infusion. Use vasopressor, if needed.
Patient teaching
● Explain how and why albumin is given.
● Tell patient to report chills, fever, dyspnea, nausea, or rash immediately.

☑ **Evaluation**
● Patient's deficient fluid volume is resolved.
● Patient doesn't experience fluid overload.
● Patient and family state understanding of drug therapy.

albuterol sulfate (salbutamol sulfate)

(al-BYOO-ter-ohl SUHL-fayt)
AccuNeb, Airomir◇, Asmol CFC-free◇, Proventil, Proventil HFA, Proventil Repetabs, Ventolin, Ventolin CFC-free◇, Ventolin HFA, Ventolin Obstetric injection◇, Ventolin Rotacaps◇, Volmax

Pharmacologic class: adrenergic
Therapeutic class: bronchodilator
Pregnancy risk category: C

Indications and dosages

▶ **Prevention of exercise-induced bronchospasm.** *Adults and children age 4 and older:* Two aerosol inhalations 15 to 30 minutes before exercise.
▶ **To prevent or treat bronchospasm in patients with reversible obstructive airway disease.** *Aerosol inhalation. Adults and children age 4 and older:* One or two inhalations q 4 to 6 hours. More frequent administration and more inhalations aren't recommended. Proventil isn't indicated for use in children younger than age 12.

Solution for inhalation. Adults and children age 12 and older: 2.5 mg t.i.d. or q.i.d. by nebulizer. To prepare solution, use 0.5 ml of 0.5% solution diluted with 2.5 ml normal saline solution. Or, use 3 ml of 0.083% solution.
Children ages 2 to 11: Initially, 0.1 to 0.15 mg/kg by nebulizer, with subsequent dosing adjusted to response. Don't exceed 2.5 mg t.i.d. or q.i.d. by nebulization.
Syrup. Adults and children age 15 and older: 2 to 4 mg (1 to 2 tsp) P.O. t.i.d. or q.i.d. Maximum, 8 mg P.O. q.i.d.
Children ages 6 to 14: 2 mg (1 tsp) P.O. t.i.d. or q.i.d. Maximum, 24 mg daily in divided doses.
Children ages 2 to 5: Initially, 0.1 mg/kg P.O. t.i.d. Starting dose shouldn't exceed 2 mg (1 tsp) t.i.d. Maximum, 4 mg (2 tsp) t.i.d.
Tablets. Adults and children older than age 12: 2 to 4 mg P.O. t.i.d. or q.i.d. Maximum, 8 mg q.i.d.
Children ages 6 to 12: 2 mg P.O. t.i.d. or q.i.d. Maximum, 6 mg q.i.d.
Elderly patients and patients sensitive to beta stimulators: 2 mg P.O. t.i.d. or q.i.d. tablets or syrup. Maximum, 8 mg t.i.d. or q.i.d.
Extended-release tablets. Adults and children older than age 12: 4 to 8 mg P.O. q 12 hours. Maximum, 16 mg b.i.d.
Children ages 6 to 12: 4 mg P.O. q 12 hours. Maximum, 12 mg b.i.d.

Contraindications and precautions

● Contraindicated in patients hypersensitive to drug or its components.
● Use cautiously in patients with CV disorders (including coronary insufficiency and hypertension), hyperthyroidism, or diabetes mellitus and in those unusually responsive to adrenergics.
● Use extended-release tablets cautiously in patients with GI narrowing.
⚞ **Lifespan:** With pregnant women, use cautiously. Breast-feeding women shouldn't take drug. In children, safety of drug hasn't been established in those younger than age 6 for tablets and Repetabs, younger than age 4 for aerosol and capsules for inhalation, and younger than age 2 for inhalation solution and syrup. In elderly patients, use cautiously.

Adverse reactions

CNS: *tremor, nervousness,* dizziness, insomnia, headache.

Reactions may be *common,* uncommon, *life-threatening,* or COMMON AND LIFE-THREATENING.

CV: tachycardia, palpitations, hypertension.
EENT: drying and irritation of nose and throat.
GI: heartburn, nausea, vomiting.
Metabolic: hypokalemia, weight loss.
Musculoskeletal: muscle cramps.
Respiratory: *bronchospasm.*

Interactions

Drug-drug. *CNS stimulants:* Increases CNS stimulation. Avoid using together.
Levodopa: Increases risk of arrhythmias. Monitor patient closely.
MAO inhibitors, tricyclic antidepressants: Increases adverse CV effects. Monitor patient closely.
Propranolol, other beta blockers: Mutual antagonism. Monitor patient carefully.
Drug-herb. *Herbs containing caffeine:* Additive adverse effects. Discourage using together.
Drug-food. *Caffeine:* Increases CNS stimulation. Discourage using together.

Effects on lab test results

• May decrease potassium level.

Pharmacokinetics

Absorption: After inhalation, drug appears to be absorbed over several hours from respiratory tract; however, most of dose is swallowed and absorbed through GI tract. After oral administration, drug is well absorbed through GI tract.
Distribution: Doesn't cross blood-brain barrier.
Metabolism: Extensively metabolized in liver to inactive compounds.
Excretion: Rapidly excreted in urine and feces.
Half-life: About 4 hours.

Route	Onset	Peak	Duration
P.O.	15-30 min	2-3 hr	6-12 hr
Inhalation	5-15 min	1-1½ hr	3-6 hr

Action

Chemical effect: Relaxes bronchial and uterine smooth muscle by acting on $beta_2$-adrenergic receptors.
Therapeutic effect: Improves ventilation.

Available forms

Aerosol inhaler: 90 mcg/metered spray, 100 mcg/metered spray
Capsules: 200 mcg ◊
Solution for inhalation: 0.083%, 0.5%
Syrup: 2 mg/5 ml

Tablets: 2 mg, 4 mg
Tablets (extended-release): 4 mg, 8 mg

NURSING PROCESS

Assessment
• Obtain baseline assessment of patient's respiratory status, and assess frequently throughout therapy.
• Be alert for adverse reactions and drug interactions.
• Evaluate patient's and family's knowledge of drug therapy.

Nursing diagnoses
• Impaired gas exchange related to underlying respiratory condition
• Risk for injury related to drug-induced adverse reactions
• Deficient knowledge related to drug therapy

Planning and implementation
• Pleasant-tasting syrup may be taken by children as young as age 2. Syrup contains no alcohol or sugar.
• Wait at least 2 minutes between nebulized doses if more than one dose is ordered. If corticosteroid inhaler also is used, first have patient use bronchodilator, wait 5 minutes, and then have patient use corticosteroid inhaler. This permits bronchodilator to open air passages for maximum corticosteroid effectiveness.
• Aerosol form may be prescribed for use 15 minutes before exercise to prevent exercise-induced bronchospasm.
• Patients may use tablets and aerosol together.
⑤ ALERT: Don't confuse albuterol with atenolol or Albutein.

Patient teaching
• Warn patient to stop drug immediately if paradoxical bronchospasm occurs.
• Give patient clear instructions for using metered-dose inhaler: Clear nasal passages and throat. Breathe out, expelling as much air from lungs as possible. Place mouthpiece well into mouth and inhale deeply as dose is released. Hold breath for several seconds, remove mouthpiece, and exhale slowly.
• Advise patient to wait at least 2 minutes before repeating procedure if more than one inhalation is ordered.

• Warn patient to avoid accidentally spraying inhalant form into eyes, which may blur vision temporarily.

• Tell patient to reduce intake of foods and herbs containing caffeine, such as coffee, cola, and chocolate, when using a bronchodilator.

• Show patient how to check his pulse rate. Instruct him to check pulse before and after using bronchodilator and to call prescriber if pulse rate increases more than 20 to 30 beats/minute.

☑ Evaluation

• Patient's respiratory signs and symptoms improve.

• Patient has no injury from adverse drug reactions.

• Patient and family state understanding of drug therapy.

alefacept
(ALE-fuh-sept)
Amevive

Pharmacologic class: immunosuppressive
Therapeutic class: antipsoriatic
Pregnancy risk category: B

Indications and dosages

▶ **Moderate to severe chronic plaque psoriasis in candidates for systemic therapy or phototherapy.** *Adults:* 15 mg I.M. once weekly for 12 weeks. Another 12-week course may be given if CD4+ T lymphocyte count is normal and at least 12 weeks have passed since the previous treatment.

▧ **Adjust-a-dose:** If CD4+ T lymphocyte count is below 250 cells/mm³, withhold dose. Stop drug if CD4+ count remains below 250 cells/mm³ for 1 month.

Contraindications and precautions

• Contraindicated in patients hypersensitive to drug or its components and in patients with a history of systemic malignancy or clinically important infection.

• Use cautiously in patients at high risk for malignancy and in those with chronic or recurrent infections.

☀ **Lifespan:** In pregnant women, use only if clearly needed; effects on fetus aren't known. Breast-feeding women should stop nursing or

stop using the drug; it's not known whether drug appears in breast milk. In children, safety and efficacy of drug haven't been established. In elderly patients, give drug cautiously because of their increased rate of infection and malignancies.

Adverse reactions

CNS: dizziness.
CV: *coronary artery disorder, MI.*
EENT: pharyngitis.
GI: nausea.
Hematologic: *lymphopenia.*
Musculoskeletal: myalgia.
Respiratory: cough.
Skin: pruritus.
Other: infection; chills; *malignancy;* hypersensitivity reaction; antibody formation; *injection site pain, inflammation,* bleeding, edema, or mass.

Interactions

Drug-drug. *Immunosuppressants, phototherapy:* Increases risk of excessive immunosuppression. Avoid using together.

Effects on lab test results

• Decreases CD4+ and CD8+ T lymphocyte counts.

Pharmacokinetics

Absorption: Unknown.
Distribution: 63% bioavailable after I.M. injection. I.V. distribution unknown.
Metabolism: Unknown.
Excretion: Unknown. *Half-life:* 11 days for I.V. use.

Route	Onset	Peak	Duration
I.V., I.M.	Unknown	Unknown	Unknown

Action

Chemical effect: An immunosuppressive protein that interferes with lymphocyte activation and reduces subsets of CD2+ T lymphocytes, which reduces circulating total CD4+ and CD8+ T lymphocyte counts.
Therapeutic effect: Reduces symptoms of psoriasis.

Available forms

Powder for injection: 15-mg single-dose vial

NURSING PROCESS

🔁 Assessment
• Monitor CD4+ T lymphocyte count weekly for the 12-week course. Ensure that patient has normal CD4+ T lymphocyte count before starting therapy.
• Monitor patient carefully for evidence of infection or malignancy, and stop drug if it appears.

⊕ Nursing diagnoses
• Impaired skin integrity related to psoriasis
• Risk for infection related to immunosuppressive drug therapy
• Deficient knowledge related to drug therapy

⟩ Planning and implementation
Ⓢ ALERT: Rotate I.M. injection sites so that the new injection is given at least 1 inch away from the old site and not in an area that is bruised, tender, or hard.
• Overdose may cause chills, headache, arthralgia, and sinusitis. Provide supportive care, and closely monitor total lymphocyte and CD4+ T lymphocyte counts.
• Enroll pregnant women receiving drug into the Biogen Pregnancy Registry by phoning 1-866-263-8483 so that drug effects can be studied.

Patient teaching
• Warn patient about potential adverse reactions.
• Urge patient to report evidence of infection immediately.
• Inform patient that blood tests will be done regularly to monitor WBC count.
• Tell patient to notify prescriber if she is or could be pregnant within 8 weeks of receiving drug.

✓ Evaluation
• Patient's psoriasis improves.
• Patient remains free from infection.
• Patient and family state understanding of drug therapy.

alemtuzumab
(ah-lem-TOO-zeh-mab)
Campath

Pharmacologic classification: monoclonal antibody
Therapeutic classification: antineoplastic
Pregnancy risk category: C

Indications and dosages

▶ **B-cell chronic lymphocytic leukemia in patients treated with alkylating drugs, and for whom fludarabine therapy has failed.** *Adults:* Initially, 3 mg I.V. infusion over 2 hours daily; if tolerated, increase dose to 10 mg daily; then increase to 30 mg daily. Escalation to 30 mg usually can be accomplished in 3 to 7 days. As maintenance, give 30 mg I.V. three times weekly on nonconsecutive days (such as Monday, Wednesday, Friday) for up to 12 weeks. Don't give a single dose greater than 30 mg or a weekly dose greater than 90 mg.
Ⓢ **Adjust-a-dose:** At the first occurrence of absolute neutrophil count (ANC) of 250/mm³ or less or platelet count of 25,000/mm³ or less, stop therapy; resume at same dose when ANC of 500/mm³ or more or platelet count of 50,000/mm³ or more. If delay between doses is 7 days or longer, start therapy at 3 mg; increase to 10 mg, then 30 mg as tolerated. At the second occurrence of ANC of 250/mm³ or less or platelet count of 25,000/mm³ or less, stop therapy; when ANC returns to 500/mm³ or more or platelet count to 50,000/mm³ or more, resume at 10 mg; if delay between doses is 7 days or longer, start therapy at 3 mg; increase to 10 mg only. At the third occurrence of ANC of 250/mm³ or less or platelet count of 25,000/mm³ or less, stop therapy. For a decrease of ANC or platelet count ≤ 50% of the baseline value in patients starting therapy with a baseline ANC of 500/mm³ or less or a baseline platelet count 25,000/mm³ or less, stop therapy; when ANC or platelet count returns to baseline, resume therapy. If the delay between dosing is 7 days or longer, start therapy at 3 mg and increase to 10 mg, then 30 mg, as tolerated.

▽ I.V. administration
• Don't use solution if discolored or contains precipitate. Don't shake ampule before use. Fil-

ter with a sterile, low–protein-binding, 5-micron filter before dilution. Add to 100 ml normal saline solution or D_5W. Gently invert bag to mix solution.

• Premedicate with 50 mg diphenhydramine and 650 mg acetaminophen 30 minutes before initial infusion and before each dose increase. May give 200 mg hydrocortisone to decrease severe infusion-related adverse events. Give antiinfective prophylaxis while patient is receiving therapy, such as TMP-sulfa DS b.i.d. three times weekly and 250 mg famciclovir (or equivalent) b.i.d. Prophylaxis should continue for 2 months, or until CD4+ count is 200 cells/mm³ or more, whichever occurs later.

• Don't give as I.V. push or bolus.
• Infuse over 2 hours.
• Protect solution from light.
• Use within 8 hours of dilution.

Contraindications and precautions

• Contraindicated in patients with active systemic infections, underlying immunodeficiency (such as HIV), or type I hypersensitivity or anaphylactic reactions to drug or any of its components.

⚠ **Lifespan:** In pregnant women, benefits of drug should be weighed against risks to the fetus because immunoglobolin G crosses the placenta and causes fetal B and T lymphocyte depletion. Breast-feeding women should stop breast-feeding during treatment and for at least 3 months after taking last dose of drug. In children, safety and efficacy of drug haven't been established.

Adverse reactions

CNS: fever, insomnia, depression, somnolence, asthenia, headache, dysthenias, dizziness, fatigue, malaise, tremor.
CV: edema, peripheral edema, hypotension, hypertension, tachycardia, SUPRAVENTRICULAR TACHYCARDIA.
EENT: epistaxis, rhinitis, *pharyngitis.*
GI: anorexia, nausea, vomiting, diarrhea, stomatitis, ulcerative stomatitis, mucositis, abdominal pain, dyspepsia, constipation.
Hematologic: NEUTROPENIA, *anemia, pancytopenia,* THROMBOCYTOPENIA, purpura.
Musculoskeletal: pain, skeletal pain, back pain, myalgias.
Respiratory: dyspnea, cough, bronchitis, pneumonitis, *bronchospasm.*

Skin: rash, urticaria, pruritus, increased sweating.
Other: SEPSIS, infection, herpes simplex, rigors, chills, candidiasis.

Interactions

None reported.

Effects on lab test results

• May decrease hemoglobin, hematocrit, and CD4+, lymphocyte, neutrophil, WBC, RBC, and platelet counts.
• May interfere with diagnostic tests that use antibodies.

Pharmacokinetics

Absorption: Administered I.V.
Distribution: Binds to various tissues.
Metabolism: Unknown.
Excretion: Unknown. *Half-life:* 12 days.

Route	Onset	Peak	Duration
I.V.	Unknown	Unknown	Unknown

Action

Chemical effect: Binds to CD_{52} and causes antibody-dependent destruction of leukemic cells following cell-surface binding.
Therapeutic effect: Destroys leukemic cells.

Available forms

Ampules: 10 mg/ml, in 3-ml ampules

NURSING PROCESS

📋 **Assessment**

• Assess patient's underlying condition before therapy for signs or symptoms of active infection or compromised immune function.
• Obtain baseline CBC and platelet count before starting therapy.
• Monitor blood pressure and be alert for hypotensive symptoms during drug administration.
⊛ **ALERT:** Monitor hematologic studies carefully during therapy. Even with normal dosages, patients may experience signs and symptoms of hematologic toxicity, including myelosuppression, bone marrow dysplasia, and thrombocytopenia. Initial doses of greater than 3 mg aren't well tolerated. Extremely high doses can cause acute bronchospasm, cough, shortness of breath, anuria, and death. If these occur, stop drug and provide supportive treatment.

Reactions may be *common,* uncommon, *life-threatening,* or COMMON AND LIFE-THREATENING.

• Monitor CBC and platelet counts weekly during therapy and more frequently if anemia, neutropenia, or thrombocytopenia worsens.

• After treatment, monitor CD4+ count until it reaches 200 cells/mm³ or more.

🖰 Nursing diagnoses

• Risk for infection related to immunocompromised state.

• Fatigue due to drug therapy.

• Deficient knowledge related to alemtuzumab therapy.

▶ Planning and implementation

• Irradiate blood if transfusions are needed to protect against graft versus host disease.

• Don't immunize with live viral vaccines.

• If therapy is stopped for longer than 7 days, restart with gradual dose increase.

(!) ALERT: Don't confuse alemtuzumab with trastuzumab.

Patient teaching

• Tell patient to report immediately infusion reactions, such as rigors, chills, fever, nausea, or vomiting.

• Advise patient to report immediately signs or symptoms of infection.

• Inform patient that blood tests will be done frequently during therapy to observe for adverse effects.

• Tell women of childbearing age and men to use effective contraceptive methods during therapy and for at least 6 months following completion of therapy.

🗹 Evaluation

• Patient remains free from infection.

• Patient doesn't suffer any harmful drug-induced adverse reactions.

• Patient and family state understanding of drug therapy.

---

alendronate sodium
(ah-LEN-droh-nayt SOH-dee-um)
Fosamax

Pharmacologic class: inhibitor of osteoclast-mediated bone resorption
Therapeutic class: antiosteoporotic
Pregnancy risk category: C

Indications and dosages

▶ **Osteoporosis in postmenopausal women; to increase bone mass in men with osteoporosis.** *Adults:* 10 mg P.O. daily or 70-mg tablet P.O. once weekly with water at least 30 minutes before first food, beverage, or medication of the day.

▶ **Prevention of osteoporosis in postmenopausal women.** *Women:* 5 mg P.O. daily or 35-mg tablet P.O. once weekly taken with water at least 30 minutes before first food, beverage, or medication of the day.

▶ **Corticosteroid-induced osteoporosis, given with calcium and vitamin D supplements.** *Adults:* 5 mg P.O. daily.
Postmenopausal women not receiving estrogen replacement therapy: 10 mg P.O. daily.

▶ **Paget's disease of bone.** *Adults:* 40 mg P.O. daily for 6 months taken with water at least 30 minutes before first food, beverage, or drug of the day.

Contraindications and precautions

• Contraindicated in patients with hypocalcemia, severe renal insufficiency, or hypersensitivity to drug or its components.

• Use cautiously in patients with dysphagia, esophageal diseases, gastritis, duodenitis, ulcers, or mild to moderate renal insufficiency.

⚖ **Lifespan:** In pregnant women, use only if benefits outweigh the risks to fetus. In breastfeeding women and in children, safety of drug hasn't been established.

Adverse reactions

CNS: headache.
GI: abdominal pain, nausea, dyspepsia, constipation, diarrhea, flatulence, acid regurgitation, esophageal ulcer, vomiting, dysphagia, abdominal distention, gastritis, taste perversion.
Musculoskeletal: musculoskeletal pain.

Interactions

Drug-drug. *Antacids, calcium supplements, and many other oral medications:* Interferes with alendronate absorption. Give 30 minutes after alendronate dose.
Aspirin, NSAIDs: May increase risk of upper GI reactions with alendronate doses greater than 10 mg daily. Monitor patient closely.
Drug-food. *Any food:* May decrease absorption of drug. Don't give drug with food.

Effects on lab test results

None reported.

Pharmacokinetics

Absorption: Absorbed from GI tract; food or beverages can significantly decrease bioavailability.
Distribution: Distributed to soft tissues but rapidly redistributed to bone or excreted in urine; about 78% protein-bound.
Metabolism: Doesn't appear to be metabolized.
Excretion: Excreted in urine. *Terminal half-life:* More than 10 years.

Route	Onset	Peak	Duration
P.O.	1 mo	3-6 mo	3 wk after therapy

Action

Chemical effect: Suppresses osteoclast activity on newly formed resorption surfaces, reducing bone turnover.
Therapeutic effect: Increases bone mass.

Available forms

Tablets: 5 mg, 10 mg, 35 mg, 40 mg, 70 mg

NURSING PROCESS

☜ Assessment
• Obtain history of patient's underlying disorder before therapy.
• Monitor calcium and phosphate levels throughout therapy.
• Be alert for adverse reactions and drug interactions.
• Evaluate patient's and family's knowledge of drug therapy.

⊕ Nursing diagnoses
• Risk for injury related to decreased bone mass
• Risk for deficient fluid volume related to drug-induced GI upset
• Deficient knowledge related to drug therapy

▶ Planning and implementation
• Hypocalcemia and other disturbances of mineral metabolism (such as vitamin D deficiency) should be corrected before therapy begins.
• Give drug in the morning at least 30 minutes before first meal, fluid, or other oral drug administration.
⊛ **ALERT:** Don't confuse Fosamax with Flomax.

Patient teaching
• Advise patient to take drug with 6 to 8 ounces of water upon rising. Drug is absorbed better when taken on an empty stomach.
⊛ **ALERT:** Warn patient not to lie down for at least 30 minutes after taking drug to aid passage to stomach and reduce potential for esophageal irritation.
• Tell patient to take calcium and vitamin D supplements if daily dietary intake is inadequate.
• Show patient how to perform weight-bearing exercises, which help increase bone mass.
• Urge patient to limit or restrict smoking and alcohol use, if appropriate.

☑ Evaluation
• Patient remains free from bone fracture.
• Patient maintains adequate hydration.
• Patient and family state understanding of drug therapy.

alfentanil hydrochloride
(al-FEN-tah-nil high-droh-KLOR-ighd)
Alfenta

Pharmacologic class: opioid
Therapeutic class: analgesic, adjunct to anesthetic, primary anesthetic
Pregnancy risk category: C
Controlled substance schedule: II

Indications and dosages

▶ **Adjunct to general anesthetic.** *Adults:* Initially, 8 to 50 mcg/kg I.V.; then increments of 3 to 15 mcg/kg I.V. q 5 to 20 minutes.
▶ **Monitored analgesic care.** *Adults:* Initially, 3 to 8 mcg/kg I.V., then 3 to 5 mcg/kg q 5 to 20 minutes.
▶ **Primary anesthetic.** *Adults:* Initially, 130 to 245 mcg/kg I.V.; then maintain on 0.5 to 1.5 mcg/kg/minute I.V.
◿ **Adjust-a-dose:** Reduce dosage in elderly and debilitated patients.

▽ I.V. administration

• Drug is compatible with D_5W, D_5W in lactated Ringer's solution, and normal saline solution. Infusions containing 25 to 80 mcg/ml are used most often.

Reactions may be *common*, uncommon, *life-threatening*, or COMMON AND LIFE-THREATENING.

• Drug should be given only by those specifically trained in use of I.V. anesthetics.
• Stop infusion no less than 10 to 15 minutes before surgery ends.
• Use tuberculin syringe to give small volumes of drug accurately.
• Keep narcotic antagonist (naloxone) and resuscitation equipment available.

Contraindications and precautions

• Contraindicated in patients hypersensitive to drug.
• Use cautiously in patients with head injury, pulmonary disease, decreased respiratory reserve, or hepatic or renal impairment.
⚘ Lifespan: In pregnant or breast-feeding women, use cautiously. In children younger than age 12, use isn't recommended. In elderly patients, use cautiously and at a reduced dose.

Adverse reactions

CNS: blurred vision, agitation, anxiety, headache, confusion.
CV: hypotension, hypertension, *bradycardia,* tachycardia, palpitations, orthostatic hypotension.
GI: nausea, vomiting.
Musculoskeletal: intraoperative muscle movement.
Respiratory: chest wall rigidity, *bronchospasm, respiratory depression, hypercapnia.*
Skin: itching.

Interactions

Drug-drug. *Cimetidine:* May cause CNS toxicity. Monitor patient.
CNS depressants: May have additive effects. Use together cautiously.
Diazepam: With high doses of alfentanil, may cause CV depression and decrease blood pressure. Use together cautiously.

Effects on lab test results

• May increase amylase and lipase levels.

Pharmacokinetics

Absorption: Administered I.V.
Distribution: More than 90% is protein-bound.
Metabolism: In liver.
Excretion: In urine. *Half-life:* About 1½ hours.

Action

Chemical effect: Binds with opiate receptors in CNS, altering perception of and emotional response to pain through unknown mechanism.
Therapeutic effect: Enhances anesthesia and relieves pain.

Available forms

Injection: 500 mcg/ml

NURSING PROCESS

⚕ Assessment

• Assess patient's CV and respiratory status before and during therapy.
• Drug decreases rate and depth of respirations. Monitor arterial oxygen saturation to assess effects of respiratory depression.
• Be alert for adverse reactions and drug interactions.
• Evaluate patient's and family's knowledge of drug therapy.

🔁 Nursing diagnoses

• Ineffective health maintenance related to need for surgery
• Ineffective breathing pattern related to drug-induced respiratory depression
• Deficient knowledge related to drug therapy

▷ Planning and implementation

• Notify prescriber immediately if assessment findings are different than expected. Patient who has developed tolerance to other opioids may become tolerant to alfentanil as well.
⚠ ALERT: Don't confuse alfentanil with Anafranil, fentanyl, or sufentanil; or Alfenta with Sufenta.
Patient teaching
• Explain anesthetic effect of drug.
• Inform patient that another analgesic will be available after effects of drug have worn off.

☑ Evaluation

• Patient regains previous health after alfentanil administration and recovers from surgery.
• Patient's respiratory status returns to normal after effects of drug wear off.
• Patient and family state understanding of drug therapy.

Route	Onset	Peak	Duration
I.V.	1 min	1½-2 min	5-10 min

alfuzosin hydrochloride
(al-FYOO-zoe-sin)
UroXatral

Pharmacologic class: Selective post-synaptic alpha$_1$-adrenergic antagonist
Therapeutic class: BPH drug
Pregnancy risk category: B

Indications and dosages

▶ **BPH.** *Men:* 10 mg P.O. after the same meal daily.

Contraindications and precautions

• Contraindicated in patients hypersensitive to drug or any of its components and in those with moderate or severe hepatic insufficiency (Child-Pugh categories B and C). Also contraindicated for hypertension.
• Use cautiously in patients with severe renal insufficiency, congenital or acquired prolonged QT interval, or symptomatic hypotension and in those who have had a hypotensive response to other medications.
⚠ **Lifespan:** In women and children, drug is contraindicated.

Adverse reactions

CNS: dizziness, headache, fatigue, pain.
CV: angina, orthostatic hypotension.
EENT: sinusitis, pharyngitis.
GI: abdominal pain, dyspepsia, constipation, nausea.
GU: impotence.
Respiratory: upper respiratory tract infection, bronchitis.

Interactions

Drug-drug. *Alpha blockers:* Although not adequately studied, interaction may occur. Don't use together.
Antihypertensives: May cause hypotension. Monitor blood pressure and use together cautiously.
Atenolol: May cause reductions in blood pressure and heart rate. Monitor blood pressure and heart rate.
Cimetidine: Increases azulfosin levels. Use together cautiously.

CYP 3A4 inhibitors (itraconazole, ketoconazole, and ritonavir): Increases alfuzosin level. Don't use together.
Drug-food. *Any food:* Absorption is 50% lower while fasting. Give with food.

Effects on lab test results

None significant.

Pharmacokinetics

Absorption: When taken with food, bioavailability is 49% and peak levels are achieved in 8 hours. Absorption is 50% lower while fasting; therefore drug should be taken immediately following a meal.
Distribution: 82% to 90% bound to plasma proteins.
Metabolism: Extensively metabolized, via three pathways: oxidation, O-demethylation, and N-dealkylation, by the liver to inactive metabolites. CYP 3A4 is the principal enzyme involved in metabolism.
Excretion: 11% of dose is excreted unchanged in the urine. *Elimination half-life:* 10 hours.

Route	Onset	Peak	Duration
P.O.	Unknown	8 hr	Unknown

Action

Chemical effect: Drug exhibits selectivity for alpha$_1$-adrenergic receptors in the lower urinary tract. Blockade of these adrenoreceptors can cause smooth muscle in the bladder, neck, and prostate to relax.
Therapeutic effect: Improves urine flow and reduces symptoms of BPH.

Available forms

Tablets (extended-release): 10 mg

NURSING PROCESS

▨ Assessment
• Assess patient's condition before therapy and regularly thereafter.
• Monitor patient for adverse reactions.
• Evaluate patient's and family's knowledge of drug therapy.

▣ Nursing diagnoses
• Risk of injury related to adverse reactions from drug therapy
• Deficient knowledge related to drug therapy

Planning and implementation
• Prostate cancer and BPH may cause similar symptoms. Make sure prostate cancer is ruled out before starting drug therapy.
• Orthostatic hypotension may occur within a few hours following drug therapy. Provide safety precautions.
• Stop drug if angina appears or worsens.
⑤ **ALERT:** If overdose leads to hypotension, provide CV support by restoring blood pressure and heart rate. Have patient lie down and give I.V. fluids and vasopressors, if needed.
Patient teaching
• Tell patient to take drug with food and with the same meal each day.
• Advise patient to rise slowly to prevent orthostatic hypotension.
• Warn patient that the symptoms related to hypotension, such as dizziness, may occur and caution him to avoid driving, operating machinery, or performing other hazardous tasks until the effects of the drug are known.
• Advise patient not to crush or chew tablets.

✓ Evaluation
• Patient remains free from any adverse effects.
• Patient and family state understanding of drug therapy.

allopurinol
(al-oh-PYOOR-ih-nol)
Allorin ◇, Apo-Allopurinol ♦, Capurate, Zyloprim

allopurinol sodium
Aloprim

Pharmacologic class: xanthine oxidase inhibitor
Therapeutic class: antigout drug
Pregnancy risk category: C

Indications and dosages
▶ **Gout, primary or secondary to hyperuricemia.** *Adults:* Mild gout, 200 to 300 mg P.O. daily; severe gout with large tophi, 400 to 600 mg P.O. daily. Dosage varies with severity of disease; can be given as single dose or in divided doses; doses larger than 300 mg should be divided. Maximum dosage, 800 mg daily.

▶ **Hyperuricemia secondary to malignancies.** *Adults:* 200 to 400 mg/m²/day I.V. as a single infusion or in equally divided doses q 6, 8, or 12 hours.
Children: Initially, 200 mg/m²/day I.V. as a single infusion or in equally divided doses q 6, 8, or 12 hours. Then, titrate according to uric acid level. For children ages 6 to 10, 300 mg P.O. daily or divided t.i.d. For children younger than age 6, 50 mg P.O. t.i.d.
▶ **Prevention of acute gouty attacks.** *Adults:* 100 mg P.O. daily; increase at weekly intervals by 100 mg without exceeding maximum dose (800 mg), until uric acid level falls to 6 mg/100 ml or less.
▶ **Prevention of uric acid nephropathy during cancer chemotherapy.** *Adults:* 600 to 800 mg P.O. daily for 2 to 3 days, with high fluid intake.
▶ **Recurrent calcium oxalate calculi.** *Adults:* 200 to 300 mg P.O. daily in single or divided doses.
⑤ **Adjust-a-dose:** For patients with renal impairment, if creatinine clearance is 10 to 20 ml/minute, give 200 mg P.O. or I.V. daily; if less than 10 ml/minute, give 100 mg P.O. or I.V. daily; if less than 3 ml/minute, give 100 mg P.O. or I.V. at extended intervals.

▼ I.V. administration
• Dissolve contents of vial in 25 ml sterile water for injection. Dilute solution to desired concentration (no greater than 6 mg/ml) with normal saline solution for injection or D₅W. Don't use solution that contains sodium bicarbonate.
• Drug is incompatible with many other drugs. Check with pharmacist before mixing drug with other drugs.
• Store solution at 68° to 77° F (20° to 25° C) and use within 10 hours. Don't use if solution has particulates or is discolored.

Contraindications and precautions
• Contraindicated in patients hypersensitive to drug and in those with idiopathic hemochromatosis.
⚠ **Lifespan:** In pregnant or breast-feeding women, use cautiously.

Adverse reactions
CNS: drowsiness, headache.
EENT: cataracts, retinopathy, severe furunculosis of nose.

GI: nausea, vomiting, diarrhea, abdominal pain.
GU: *renal failure,* uremia.
Hematologic: *agranulocytosis,* anemia, *aplastic anemia, thrombocytopenia.*
Hepatic: *hepatitis.*
Skin: rash, usually maculopapular; *exfoliative lesions;* urticarial and purpuric lesions; *erythema multiforme;* ichthyosis; *toxic epidermal necrolysis.*

Interactions

Drug-drug. *ACE inhibitors:* Higher risk of hypersensitivity reaction. Monitor patient closely.
Amoxicillin, ampicillin, bacampicillin: Increases risk of rash. Avoid using together.
Anticoagulants, dicumarol: Potentiates anticoagulant effect. Adjust dosage, if needed.
Antineoplastics: May increase potential for bone marrow suppression. Monitor patient carefully.
Azathioprine, mercaptopurine (purinethol): May increase levels of these drugs. Adjust dosage, if needed.
Chlorpropamide: May increase hypoglycemic effect. Avoid using together.
Diazoxide, diuretics, mecamylamine, pyrazinamide: May increase uric acid level. Adjust allopurinol dosage, if needed.
Ethacrynic acid, thiazide diuretics: May increase risk of allopurinol toxicity. Reduce allopurinol dosage and closely monitor renal function.
Uricosurics: Additive effect. May be used to therapeutic advantage.
Urine-acidifying drugs: May increase possibility of kidney stone formation. Monitor patient carefully.
Xanthines: May increase theophylline level. Adjust theophylline dosage.
Drug-lifestyle. *Alcohol use:* May increase uric acid level. Discourage using together.

Effects on lab test results

• May increase alkaline phosphatase, AST, ALT, BUN, and creatinine levels.
• May decrease hemoglobin, hematocrit, and granulocyte and platelet counts.

Pharmacokinetics

Absorption: 80% to 90%.
Distribution: Distributed widely throughout body except brain, where levels are 50% of those found elsewhere.
Metabolism: To oxypurinol by xanthine oxidase.

Excretion: Primarily in urine; minute amount excreted in feces. *Half-life:* Allopurinol, 1 to 2 hours; oxypurinol, about 15 hours.

Route	Onset	Peak	Duration
P.O.	2-3 days	½-2 hr	1-2 wk
I.V.	Unknown	½ hr	Unknown

Action

Chemical effect: Reduces uric acid production by inhibiting the necessary biochemical reactions.
Therapeutic effect: Alleviates gout symptoms.

Available forms

Capsules ◊ : 100 mg, 300 mg
Injection: 500 mg/30 ml vial
Tablets (scored): 100 mg, 200 mg ◊ , 300 mg

NURSING PROCESS

⚒ Assessment

• Assess patient's history. Gout may be secondary to such diseases as acute or chronic leukemia, polycythemia vera, multiple myeloma, and psoriasis.
• Assess patient's uric acid level, joint stiffness, and pain before and during therapy. Optimal benefits may require 2 to 6 weeks of therapy.
• Monitor fluid intake and output. Daily urine output of at least 2 L and maintenance of neutral or slightly alkaline urine are desirable.
• Monitor CBC and hepatic and renal function at start of therapy and periodically during therapy.
• Be alert for adverse reactions and drug interactions.
• Evaluate patient's and family's knowledge of drug therapy.

⊞ Nursing diagnoses

• Acute pain (joint) related to patient's underlying condition
• Risk for infection related to drug-induced agranulocytosis
• Deficient knowledge related to drug therapy

▷ Planning and implementation

• Give drug with or immediately after meals to minimize adverse GI reactions.
• Have patient drink plenty of fluids while taking drug, unless contraindicated.

• Notify prescriber if renal insufficiency occurs during treatment; this usually warrants dosage reduction.

⑤ **ALERT:** Don't confuse Zyloprim with ZORprin.

• Give colchicine with allopurinol. This combination prophylactically treats acute gout attacks that may occur in first 6 weeks of therapy.

Patient teaching

• Advise patient to refrain from driving or performing hazardous tasks requiring mental alertness until CNS effects of drug are known.

• Advise patient taking allopurinol for recurrent calcium oxalate stones to reduce intake of animal protein, sodium, refined sugars, oxalate-rich foods, and calcium.

• Tell patient to stop drug at first sign of rash, which may precede severe hypersensitivity or other adverse reaction. Rash is more common in patients taking diuretics and in those with renal disorders. Tell patient to report all adverse reactions immediately.

• Advise patient to avoid alcohol use during drug therapy.

☑ **Evaluation**

• Patient expresses relief from joint pain.

• Patient is free from infection.

• Patient and family state understanding of drug therapy.

almotriptan malate
(AL-moh-trip-tan MAH-layt)
Axert

Pharmacologic class: serotonin 5-HT₁ receptor agonist
Therapeutic class: antimigraine drug
Pregnancy risk category: C

Indications and dosages

▶ **Acute migraine with or without aura.**
Adults: 6.25-mg or 12.5-mg tablet P.O., with one additional dose after 2 hours if headache is unresolved or recurs. Maximum, two doses within 24 hours.

◼ **Adjust-a-dose:** For patients with hepatic or renal impairment, initially, 6.25 mg P.O. daily, with a maximum daily dose of 12.5 mg.

Contraindications and precautions

• Contraindicated in patients hypersensitive to drug or its components. Also contraindicated in those with angina pectoris, history of MI, silent ischemia, uncontrolled hypertension, other CV disease, hemiplegic and basilar migraine, and coronary artery vasospasm, such as with Prinzmetal's variant angina.

• Don't give within 24 hours after other serotonin agonists or ergotamine drugs.

• Use cautiously in patients with renal or hepatic impairment and in those with cataracts because of the potential for corneal opacities.

• Also use cautiously in patients with risk factors for coronary artery disease (CAD), such as obesity, diabetes, and family history of CAD.

⚹ **Lifespan:** In breast-feeding women, use cautiously because it isn't known whether drug appears in breast milk. In children, safety and efficacy of drug haven't been established.

Adverse reactions

CNS: paresthesia, headache, dizziness, somnolence.
CV: *coronary artery vasospasm, transient myocardial ischemia, MI, ventricular tachycardia, ventricular fibrillation.*
GI: nausea, dry mouth.

Interactions

Drug-drug. *MAO inhibitors, verapamil:* May increase almotriptan level. No dosage adjustment is necessary.
CYP 3A4 inhibitors, such as ketoconazole: May increase almotriptan level. Monitor patient for adverse reactions. Reduce dosage, if needed.
Ergot-containing drugs, serotonin₁B/1D agonists: May cause additive effects. Avoid using within 24 hours of almotriptan.
SSRIs: May cause additive serotonin effects, resulting in weakness, hyperreflexia, or incoordination. Monitor patient closely if given together.

Effects on lab test results

None reported.

Pharmacokinetics

Absorption: Rapid and extensive; reaches peak level in 1 to 3 hours. Food doesn't affect absorption.
Distribution: High with minimal protein-binding.

Metabolism: No active metabolites. Monoamine oxidase-A and CYP 3A4 and 2D6 are responsible for the majority of metabolism.
Excretion: 75% is eliminated through renal excretion. *Half-life:* 3 to 4 hours.

Route	Onset	Peak	Duration
P.O.	1-3 hr	1-3 hr	3-4 hr

Action

Chemical effect: Binds selectively to various serotonin receptors, primarily serotonin$_{1B/1D}$ receptors, resulting in cranial vessel constriction, which inhibits migraine headache.
Therapeutic effect: Blocks neuropeptide release to the pain pathways to prevent migraine headaches.

Available forms

Tablets: 6.25 mg, 12.5 mg

NURSING PROCESS

⚖ Assessment
• Assess patient's condition before and during drug therapy.
• Obtain list of patient's medication intake within 24 hours to prevent drug interactions. Use caution when giving drug to patient who is taking an MAO inhibitor or a CYP 3A4 or 2D6 inhibitor. Don't give drug with other serotonin agonist or ergotamine derivatives.
• Be alert for any adverse reactions.
• Monitor ECG in patients with risk factors for CAD or with symptoms similar to those of CAD, such as chest or throat tightness, pain, and heaviness.
• Evaluate patient's and family's knowledge of drug therapy.

⊕ Nursing diagnoses
• Acute pain related to presence of acute migraine attack
• Risk for injury related to drug-induced interactions
• Deficient knowledge related to almotriptan therapy

▷ Planning and implementation
• Give dose as soon as patient complains of migraine symptoms.
• Repeat dose after 2 hours if needed.

• Don't give more than two doses within 24 hours.
ⓈALERT: Don't confuse Axert with Antivert.
Patient teaching
• Advise patient to take drug only when he is having a migraine.
• Teach patient to avoid possible migraine triggers, such as cheese, chocolate, citrus fruits, caffeine, and alcohol.
• Tell patient to repeat dose only once within 24 hours and no sooner than 2 hours after initial dose.
• Inform patient that other commonly prescribed migraine medications may interact with this drug.
• Tell patient to report chest, throat, jaw, or neck tightness, pain, or heaviness immediately and to stop drug until further notice from prescriber.
• Advise patient to use caution while driving or operating machinery.

☑ Evaluation
• Patient's symptoms are alleviated and patient is free from pain.
• Serious complications from drug interactions don't develop.
• Patient and family state understanding of drug therapy.

alosetron hydrochloride
(a-LOE-se-tron high-droh-KLOR-ighd)
Lotronex

Pharmacologic class: selective 5-HT$_3$ receptor antagonist
Therapeutic class: GI drug
Pregnancy risk category: B

Indications and dosages

▶ **Irritable bowel syndrome (IBS) in women with severe diarrhea.** *Women:* Initially, 1 mg P.O. daily for 4 weeks. If response is inadequate, the dose may be increased to 1 mg P.O. b.i.d. May be taken with or without food. If adequate relief is not achieved at 1 mg b.i.d. after 4 weeks, stop drug.

Contraindications and precautions

• Only physicians enrolled in the prescribing program are allowed to prescribe this drug.

• Contraindicated in men, women hypersensitive to drug or its components, and in those with a history of chronic or severe constipation, sequelae from constipation, intestinal obstruction, stricture, toxic megacolon, GI perforation, GI adhesions, ischemic colitis, impaired intestinal circulation, thrombophlebitis, or hypercoagulable state. Also contraindicated in women with current or history of Crohn's disease, ulcerative colitis, or diverticulitis. Women shouldn't take drug if they are constipated or if their chief bowel symptom is constipation.

⚥ Lifespan: In breast-feeding women, use cautiously because it's unknown whether drug or its metabolites appear in breast milk. In children, use hasn't been studied and, therefore, isn't recommended. In elderly women, use cautiously because they may be at greater risk for complications of constipation.

Adverse reactions

CNS: headache, sedation, abnormal dreams, anxiety, sleep and depressive disorders.
CV: *arrhythmias, hypertension.*
EENT: *photophobia, allergic rhinitis, throat and tonsil discomfort and pain, bacterial ear, nose, and throat infections.*
GI: *constipation,* nausea, GI discomfort and pain, abdominal discomfort and pain, abdominal distention, gaseous symptoms, viral GI infections, proctitis, hemorrhoids, dyspeptic symptoms, *ileus, perforation, ischemic colitis, small bowel mesenteric ischemia.*
GU: UTI, polyuria, diuresis.
Respiratory: *cough.*
Skin: rash, acne, folliculitis.

Interactions

Drug-drug. *Hydralazine, isoniazid, procainamide:* May slow metabolism and increase level of these drugs because of inhibition of N-acetyltransferase. Monitor patient for toxicity.

Effects on lab test results

• May increase ALT, AST, alkaline phosphatase, and bilirubin levels.

Pharmacokinetics

Absorption: Rapid. Mean absolute bioavailability is 50% to 60%. Food decreases rate of absorption by 25%.
Distribution: 82% bound to plasma proteins.

Metabolism: Extensively metabolized in the liver by CYP enzymes (2C9, 3A4, 1A2). 11% metabolized by other hepatic mechanisms.
Excretion: 7% unchanged in urine. Radiolabeled dose 73% in urine and 24% in feces. *Half-life:* 1½ hours.

Route	Onset	Peak	Duration
P.O.	Unknown	1 hr	Variable

Action

Chemical effect: Selectively inhibits 5-HT$_3$ receptors on enteric neurons in the GI tract. Inactive cation channels block neuronal depolarization, which results in decreased visceral pain, colonic transit, and GI secretions, which usually contribute to the symptoms of IBS.
Therapeutic effect: Relieves pain and decreases frequency of loose stools caused by IBS.

Available forms

Tablets: 1 mg

NURSING PROCESS

✎ Assessment
⚠ **ALERT:** Contraindicated in men.
• Don't use in patient whose main symptom is constipation.
• Assess patient before and during drug therapy.

⊕ Nursing diagnoses
• Diarrhea related to underlying IBS condition
• Acute pain related to underlying IBS condition
• Deficient knowledge related to drug therapy

▷ Planning and implementation
• If patient develops constipation, therapy should be suspended and the usual care of laxatives and fiber should be prescribed until the constipation resolves.
⚠ **ALERT:** Fatalities have occurred among patients who developed ischemic colitis and serious complications of constipation. If patient complains of rectal bleeding or sudden worsening of abdominal pain, therapy should be discontinued and acute ischemic colitis should be ruled out.
• Acute symptoms of toxicity include labored respiration, ataxia, subdued behavior, tremors, and seizures. No antidote exists for overdose.

Treatment for overdose includes supportive care.

Patient teaching

⊛ **ALERT:** Explain to patient that she must be enrolled in the Prescribing Program. Counsel patient about the risks and benefits of the drug, give instruction, answer questions, and provide information about the drug. The patient must review and sign a patient-physician agreement. A special program sticker must be affixed to all written prescriptions; no telephone, facsimile, or computerized prescriptions are permitted.

• Instruct patient not to start drug if she is constipated.

⊛ **ALERT:** Urge patient to be alert for constipation or signs and symptoms of ischemic colitis, such as rectal bleeding, bloody diarrhea, or worsened abdominal pain or cramping. Tell her to stop drug and consult prescriber immediately if symptoms occur.

• Explain that this drug isn't a cure but may alleviate some of the symptoms of IBS. If the drug doesn't adequately control symptoms after twice-daily therapy, advise patient to stop taking drug and contact prescriber.

• Inform patient that most women notice their symptoms improving after about 1 week of therapy, but some may take up to 4 weeks to experience relief from abdominal pain, discomfort, and diarrhea. Symptoms usually return within 1 week of stopping therapy.

☑ Evaluation

• Patient's symptoms, including pain and frequency of loose stools, related to IBS are relieved.

• Patient and family state understanding of drug therapy.

---

alprazolam
(al-PRAH-zoh-lam)
Apo-Alpraz ◆ , Novo-Alprazol ◆ ,
Nu-Alpraz ◆ , Xanax, Xanax XR

Pharmacologic class: benzodiazepine
Therapeutic class: anxiolytic
Pregnancy risk category: D
Controlled substance schedule: IV

Indications and dosages

▶ **Anxiety.** *Adults:* Usual initial dose, 0.25 to 0.5 mg P.O. t.i.d. Maximum, 4 mg daily in divided doses.

◪ **Adjust-a-dose:** For elderly or debilitated patients or those with advanced liver disease, usual initial dose is 0.25 mg P.O. b.i.d. or t.i.d. Maximum, 4 mg daily in divided doses.

▶ **Panic disorders.** *Adults:* 0.5 mg P.O. t.i.d., increased q 3 to 4 days in increments of no more than 1 mg. Maximum, 10 mg daily in divided doses. Or, initially 0.5 to 1 mg extended-release P.O. daily. Increase dose by no more than 1 mg daily at intervals of 3 to 4 days. Usual dosage is 3 to 6 mg P.O. once daily, preferably in the morning. Individualize dosage as necessary. Maximum dosage is 10 mg daily. If dosage reduction is necessary, decrease by no more than 0.5 mg every 3 days.

▶ **Social phobias‡.** *Adults:* 2 to 8 mg P.O. daily.

Contraindications and precautions

• Contraindicated in patients hypersensitive to drug or other benzodiazepines and in those with acute angle-closure glaucoma. Also, contraindicated with azole antifungals.

• Use cautiously in patients with hepatic, renal, or pulmonary disease. Also use cautiously in patients with cardiac disease; hypotension may occur.

⚵ **Lifespan:** In pregnant women, use cautiously because infants can be at risk for withdrawal symptoms. In breast-feeding women, drug isn't recommended. In children, safety of drug hasn't been established. In elderly patients, use cautiously because they may be more sensitive to sedation and ataxia.

Adverse reactions

CNS: *drowsiness, light-headedness, sedation, somnolence, difficulty speaking, impaired coordination, memory impairment, fatigue, depression,* mental impairment, ataxia, paresthesia, dyskinesia, emergence of anxiety between doses, hypoesthesia, lethargy, *confusion, anxiety,* vertigo, malaise, *headache, dizziness,* tremor, *irritability, insomnia,* nervousness, restlessness, agitation, nightmare, syncope, akathisia, mania, *suicidal thoughts.*

CV: palpitation, chest pain, hypotension.
EENT: sore throat, allergic rhinitis, blurred vision, nasal congestion.

Reactions may be *common,* uncommon, *life-threatening*, or COMMON AND LIFE-THREATENING.

GI: *dry mouth, constipation,* nausea, increased or decreased appetite, anorexia, *diarrhea,* vomiting, dyspepsia, abdominal pain.
GU: dysmenorrhea, premenstrual syndrome, difficulty urinating.
Metabolic: increased or decreased weight.
Musculoskeletal: arthralgia, myalgia, limb and back pain; muscle rigidity, cramps, or twitch.
Respiratory: upper respiratory tract infection, dyspnea, hyperventilation.
Skin: pruritus, increased sweating, dermatitis.
Other: hot flushes, influenza, injury, decreased or increased libido, sexual dysfunction, dependence.

Interactions

Drug-drug. *Anticonvulsants, antidepressants, antihistamines, barbiturates, benzodiazepines, general anesthetics, opioids, phenothiazines:* May increase CNS depressant effects. Avoid using together.
Carbamazepine, propoxyphene: May decrease alprazolam concentrations. Use together cautiously.
Cimetidine, fluoxetine, fluvoxamine, hormonal contraceptives, nefazodone: Increased alprazolam concentrations. Use together cautiously and consider alprazolam dosage reduction.
Fluconazole, ketoconazole, itraconazole, miconazole: May increase and prolong levels, CNS depression, and psychomotor impairment. Don't use together.
Tricyclic antidepressants: Increased levels of these drugs. Monitor patient closely.
Drug-herb. *Calendula, hops, lemon balm, skullcap, valerian:* May enhance sedative effects. Discourage using together.
Kava: May enhance CNS sedation. Discourage using together.
Drug-lifestyle. *Alcohol use:* May cause additive CNS effects. Strongly discourage use together.
Smoking: May decrease effectiveness of drug. Help patient to quit smoking.

Effects on lab test results

• May increase ALT and AST levels.

Pharmacokinetics

Absorption: Well absorbed.
Distribution: Wide; 80% of dose is bound to plasma protein.

Metabolism: In liver by CYP 3A4 pathway equally to alpha-hydroxyalprazolam and inactive metabolites.
Excretion: Alpha-hydroxyalprazolam and other metabolites are excreted in urine. *Half-life:* Immediate-release is 12 to 15 hours; extended-release is 11 to 16 hours.

Route	Onset	Peak	Duration
P.O.	Unknown	1-2 hr	Unknown
P.O. extended	Unknown	Unknown	Unknown

Action

Chemical effect: Unknown. Probably potentiates effects of GABA, an inhibitory neurotransmitter, and depresses CNS at limbic and subcortical levels of brain.
Therapeutic effect: Decreases anxiety.

Available forms

Oral solution: 0.5 mg/5 ml, 1 mg/ml (concentrate)
Tablets: 0.25 mg, 0.5 mg, 1 mg, 2 mg
Tablets (extended-release): 0.5 mg, 1 mg, 2 mg, 3 mg

NURSING PROCESS

Assessment
• Assess patient's anxiety before and frequently after therapy.
• In patient receiving repeated or prolonged therapy, monitor liver, renal, and hematopoietic function test results periodically.
• Be alert for adverse reactions and drug interactions.
• Evaluate patient's and family's knowledge of drug therapy.

Nursing diagnoses
• Anxiety related to patient's underlying condition
• Risk for injury related to drug-induced CNS reactions
• Deficient knowledge related to drug therapy

Planning and implementation
• Drug shouldn't be given for everyday stress or for use longer than 4 months.
• When giving drug, check to see that patient has swallowed tablets before leaving.

⊕ ALERT: Paradoxic excitation has occurred. Episodes of hostility, mania, hypomania, and insomnia have been reported.

⊕ ALERT: Don't stop drug abruptly after long-term use; withdrawal symptoms may occur. Abuse or addiction is possible.

⊕ ALERT: Don't confuse alprazolam with alprostadil; also don't confuse Xanax with Zantac or Tenex.

• To switch patient from immediate-release to extended-release tablets, calculate the total daily dose of immediate-release tablets and give the same dose of extended-release tablets once daily.

• Withdrawal symptoms include seizures, status epilepticus, impaired concentration, muscle cramps or twitch, diarrhea, blurred vision, decreased appetite or weight loss.

Patient teaching

• Warn patient to avoid hazardous activities that require alertness and psychomotor coordination until CNS effects of drug are known.

• Tell patient to avoid alcohol use and smoking while taking drug.

• Advise patient to take drug as prescribed and not to stop without prescriber's approval. Inform him of potential for dependence if taken longer than directed.

• Instruct patient to swallow extended-release tablets whole; don't chew or crush them.

• Teach patient how to manage or avoid adverse reactions, such as constipation and drowsiness.

☑ Evaluation

• Patient is less anxious.

• Patient doesn't experience injury from adverse CNS reactions.

• Patient and family state understanding of drug therapy.

---

alprostadil
(al-PROS-tuh-dil)
Prostin VR Pediatric

Pharmacologic class: prostaglandin
Therapeutic class: ductus arteriosus patency adjunct
Pregnancy risk category: NR

Indications and dosages

▶ **Temporary maintenance of patent ductus arteriosus until surgery can be performed.**
Infants: 0.05 to 0.1 mcg/kg per minute by I.V. infusion. When therapeutic response is achieved, reduce infusion rate to lowest effective dosage. Maximum dosage is 0.4 mcg/kg/minute. Alternatively, drug can be given through umbilical artery catheter placed at ductal opening.

▼ I.V. administration

• Before giving, dilute 500 mcg of drug with sodium chloride or dextrose injection. Dilute to appropriate volume for pump delivery system.

⊕ ALERT: Don't use diluents that contain benzyl alcohol. Fatal toxic syndrome may occur.

• Drug isn't recommended for direct injection or intermittent infusion. Give by continuous infusion using constant-rate pump. Infuse through large peripheral or central vein or through umbilical artery catheter placed at level of ductus arteriosus. If flushing occurs as a result of peripheral vasodilation, reposition catheter.

• Reduce infusion rate if fever or significant hypotension develops in infant.

• If apnea and bradycardia develop, stop infusion immediately. This may be a sign of drug overdose.

• Keep respiratory and emergency equipment available.

• In prolonged infusions, infant may develop gastric outlet obstruction, morphologic changes in pulmonary arteries, and proliferation of long bones.

• Discard solution after 24 hours.

Contraindications and precautions

⚖ **Lifespan:** In neonates with bleeding tendencies, use cautiously because drug inhibits platelet aggregation. In neonates with respiratory distress syndrome or in premature infants with a patent ductus arteriosus, drug is contraindicated. Infants on long-term infusions may experience cortical growth of long bones.

Adverse reactions

CNS: fever, *seizures.*
CV: flushing, *bradycardia, cardiac arrest,* hypotension, tachycardia.
GI: diarrhea.
Hematologic: *DIC.*

Respiratory: APNEA.
Other: *sepsis.*

Interactions

None significant.

Effects on lab test results

• May decrease potassium level.

Pharmacokinetics

Absorption: Administered I.V.
Distribution: Rapid.
Metabolism: About 68% of dose is metabolized in one pass through lung, primarily by oxidation; 100% is metabolized within 24 hours.
Excretion: All metabolites are excreted in urine within 24 hours. *Half-life:* About 5 to 10 minutes.

Route	Onset	Peak	Duration
I.V.	5-10 min	20 min	1-3 hr

Action

Chemical effect: Relaxes smooth muscle of ductus arteriosus.
Therapeutic effect: Improves cardiac circulation.

Available forms

Injection: 500 mcg/ml

NURSING PROCESS

🔬 Assessment

• Obtain baseline assessment of infant's cardiopulmonary status before therapy.
• Measure drug's effectiveness by monitoring blood oxygenation of infants with restricted pulmonary blood flow and by systemic blood pressure and blood pH of infants with restricted systemic blood flow.
• Be alert for adverse reactions throughout therapy.
• Evaluate parent's knowledge of drug therapy.

🔲 Nursing diagnoses

• Ineffective cardiopulmonary tissue perfusion related to underlying condition
• Risk for injury related to drug-induced adverse reactions
• Deficient knowledge related to drug therapy

➢ Planning and implementation

• A differential diagnosis should be made between respiratory distress syndrome and cyanotic heart disease before drug is given. Don't use drug in neonates with respiratory distress syndrome.
⊛ **ALERT:** Don't confuse alprostadil with alprazolam.
Patient teaching
• Keep parents informed of infant's status.
• Explain that parents will be allowed as much time and physical contact with infant as possible.

☑ Evaluation

• Patient demonstrates stable and effective cardiopulmonary status as indicated by adequate cardiac and pulmonary parameters and peripheral systemic perfusion.
• Patient isn't injured by adverse drug reactions.
• Parents state understanding of drug therapy.

alteplase (tissue plasminogen activator, recombinant; t-PA)
(AL-teh-plays)
Actilyse ◇ , Activase, Cathflo Activase

Pharmacologic class: enzyme
Therapeutic class: thrombolytic enzyme
Pregnancy risk category: C

Indications and dosages

▶ **Lysis of thrombi obstructing coronary arteries in acute MI.** *Adults:* 100 mg I.V. infusion over 3 hours as follows: 60 mg in first hour, with 6 to 10 mg given as bolus over first 1 to 2 minutes. Then, 20 mg/hour infusion for 2 hours. Adults weighing less than 65 kg (143 lb) should receive 1.25 mg/kg using the same method (60% in first hour with 10% as bolus, then 20% of total dose per hour for 2 hours). Don't exceed 100-mg dose. Higher doses may increase risk of intracranial bleeding.
▶ **Management of acute massive pulmonary embolism.** *Adults:* 100 mg I.V. infusion over 2 hours. Heparin begun at end of infusion when APTT or PT returns to twice normal or less. Don't exceed 100-mg dose. Higher doses may increase risk of intracranial bleeding. Also,‡ may infuse 30 or 50 mg via intrapulmonary ar-

tery over 1½ or 2 hours, respectively, with heparin therapy.

▶ **Management of acute ischemic CVA.**
Adults: 0.9 mg/kg (maximum 90 mg) I.V. over 60 minutes with 10% of the total dose given as initial bolus over 1 minute.

▶ **Restoration of function to central venous access devices as assessed by the ability to withdraw blood.** *Adults and children older than age 2:* For patients weighing 30 kg (66 lb) or more, instill 2 mg Cathflo Activase in 2 ml sterile water into catheter. For patients weighing 10 kg (22 lb) to 30 kg (66 lb), instill 110% of the internal lumen volume of the catheter, not to exceed 2 mg. After 30 minutes of dwell time, assess catheter function by aspirating blood. If function is restored, aspirate 4 to 5 ml of blood to remove Cathflo Activase and residual clot, and gently irrigate the catheter with normal saline solution. If catheter function isn't restored after 120 minutes, instill a second dose.

▶ **Prevention of reocclusion after thrombolysis for acute MI‡.** *Adults:* 3.3 mcg/kg/minute by I.V. infusion for 4 hours with heparin therapy immediately following initial thrombolytic infusion.

▶ **Lysis of arterial occlusion in a peripheral vessel or bypass graft.** *Adults:* 0.05 to 0.1 mg/kg/hour infused via the intrapulmonary artery for 1 to 8 hours.

▼ I.V. administration

● Reconstitute drug with sterile water (without preservatives) for injection only. Check manufacturer's label for specific information. Don't use vial if vacuum seal isn't present. Reconstitute with large-bore (18G) needle, directing stream of sterile water at lyophilized cake. Don't shake, but make sure that drug is dissolved completely. Slight foaming is common, and solution should be clear or pale yellow.

● Drug may be given as reconstituted (1 mg/ml) or diluted with equal volume of normal saline solution or D₅W to make 0.5 mg/ml solution. Adding other drugs to infusion isn't recommended.

● Reconstitute alteplase solution immediately before use, and give within 8 hours because it contains no preservatives. Drug may be stored temporarily at 35° to 86° F (2° to 30° C), but it's stable for only 8 hours at room temperature. Discard unused solution.

Restoration of function to central venous catheter

● Reconstitute Cathflo Activase with 2.2 ml sterile water, dissolve completely into a colorless to pale yellow solution that yields a concentration of 1 mg/ml. Solutions are stable for up to 8 hours at room temperature.

● Assess the cause of catheter dysfunction before using Cathflo Activase. Some conditions that may occlude a catheter include: incorrect catheter position, mechanical failure, constriction by a suture, and lipid deposits or drug precipitates within the catheter lumen. Don't attempt to suction because of the risk of damage to the vascular wall or collapse of soft-walled catheters.

● Don't use excessive pressure while instilling Cathflo Activase into the catheter, which could cause catheter rupture or expulsion of the clot into the circulation.

Contraindications and precautions

● Contraindicated in patients with active internal bleeding, intracranial neoplasm, arteriovenous malformation, aneurysm, severe uncontrolled hypertension, history of CVA, known bleeding diathesis, or intraspinal or intracranial trauma or surgery within past 2 months.

● Use cautiously in patients who had major surgery within past 10 days; in those receiving anticoagulants; and in those with organ biopsy; trauma (including cardiopulmonary resuscitation); GI or GU bleeding; cerebrovascular disease; hypertension; acute pericarditis or subacute bacterial endocarditis; septic thrombophlebitis; diabetic hemorrhagic retinopathy; or mitral stenosis, atrial fibrillation, or other conditions that may lead to left-sided heart thrombus.

⚖ **Lifespan:** During pregnancy, the first 10 days postpartum, and lactation, use cautiously. In children, safety of drug hasn't been established. In patients age 75 and older, use cautiously.

Adverse reactions

CNS: *cerebral hemorrhage,* fever.
CV: hypotension, *arrhythmias,* edema.
GI: nausea, vomiting.
Hematologic: *severe, spontaneous bleeding.*
Musculoskeletal: arthralgia.
Skin: urticaria.
Other: bleeding at puncture sites, hypersensitivity reactions, *anaphylaxis.*

Reactions may be *common,* uncommon, *life-threatening,* or COMMON AND LIFE-THREATENING.

Interactions

Drug-drug. *Aspirin, coumarin anticoagulants, dipyridamole, heparin:* May increase risk of bleeding. Monitor patient carefully.
Nitroglycerin: May decrease tPA antigen concentrations. Avoid using together. If use together is unavoidable, use the lowest effective dose of nitroglycerin.
Drug-herb. *Dong quai, garlic, ginkgo:* May increase risk of bleeding. Discourage using together.

Effects on lab test results

None reported.

Pharmacokinetics

Absorption: Administered I.V.
Distribution: Rapidly cleared from plasma by liver (about 80% cleared within 10 minutes after infusion stops).
Metabolism: Primarily hepatic.
Excretion: Over 85% excreted in urine, 5% in feces. *Half-life:* Less than 10 minutes.

Route	Onset	Peak	Duration
I.V.	Immediate	45 min	4 hr

Action

Chemical effect: Binds to fibrin in thrombus and locally converts plasminogen to plasmin, which initiates local fibrinolysis.
Therapeutic effect: Dissolves blood clots in coronary arteries and lungs.

Available forms

Injection: 50-mg (29 million IU), 100-mg (58 million IU) vials
Lyophilized powder for intracatheter instillation: 2 mg single-patient vials
Solution for intracatheter clearance: 2-mg single-use vials

NURSING PROCESS

🗝 Assessment

• Assess patient's cardiopulmonary status (including ECG, vital signs, and coagulation studies) before and during therapy.
• Be alert for adverse reactions and drug interactions.
• Monitor patient for internal bleeding, and check puncture site frequently.

• Evaluate patient's and family's knowledge of drug therapy.

🔷 Nursing diagnoses

• Ineffective cardiopulmonary tissue perfusion related to patient's underlying condition
• Risk for injury related to adverse effects of drug therapy
• Deficient knowledge related to drug therapy

⟩ Planning and implementation

• Recanalization of occluded coronary arteries and improvement of heart function require starting drug as soon as possible after onset of symptoms.
• Heparin is frequently started after treatment with alteplase to reduce risk of rethrombosis.
• For arterial puncture, select site on arm and apply pressure for 30 minutes afterward. Also use pressure dressings, sand bags, or ice packs on recent puncture sites to prevent bleeding.
• Notify prescriber if severe bleeding occurs and doesn't stop with intervention; alteplase and heparin infusions will need to be discontinued.
⑤ **ALERT:** Have antiarrhythmics available. Coronary thrombolysis is linked to arrhythmias induced by reperfusion of ischemic myocardium.
• Avoid invasive procedures during thrombolytic therapy.
Patient teaching
• Tell patient to report immediately chest pain, dyspnea, changes in heart rate or rhythm, nausea, and bleeding.

✓ Evaluation

• Patient's cardiopulmonary assessment findings demonstrate improved perfusion.
• Patient has no serious adverse drug reactions.
• Patient and family state understanding of drug therapy.

aluminum hydroxide

(uh-LOO-mih-num high-DROKS-ighd)
AlternaGEL†, Alu-Cap†, Alu-Tab†, Amphojel†, Dialume†

Pharmacologic class: aluminum salt
Therapeutic class: antacid
Pregnancy risk category: C

Indications and dosages

▶ **Antacid; relief from peptic ulcer or gastric symptoms; hyperphosphatemia.** *Adults:* 500 to 1,500 mg tablet or capsule P.O. 1 hour after meals and h.s.; or 5 to 30 ml suspension, p.r.n. 1 hour after meals and h.s.

Contraindications and precautions

• Use cautiously in patients with chronic renal disease.

⚕ **Lifespan:** In pregnant women, consult prescriber before giving.

Adverse reactions

GI: anorexia, constipation, intestinal obstruction.
Metabolic: hypophosphatemia.

Interactions

Drug-drug. *Allopurinol, antibiotics (including tetracyclines), corticosteroids, diflunisal, digoxin, ethambutol, H_2-receptor antagonists, iron, isoniazid, penicillamine, phenothiazines, thyroid hormones:* May decrease pharmacologic effect because of possible impaired absorption. Give aluminum hydroxide separately.
Ciprofloxacin, gatifloxacin, levofloxacin, lomefloxacin, moxifloxacin, norfloxacin, ofloxacin: May decrease effects of quinolone. Give antacid at least 6 hours before or 2 hours after the quinolone.
Enteric-coated drugs: May release prematurely in stomach. Separate doses by at least 1 hour.

Effects on lab test results

• May increase gastrin level. May decrease phosphate level.

Pharmacokinetics

Absorption: Small amounts absorbed.
Distribution: None.
Metabolism: None.
Excretion: Excreted in feces. *Half-life:* Unknown.

Route	Onset	Peak	Duration
P.O.	Varies: liquids more rapid than tablets or capsules	Unknown	20-60 min if fasting; 3 hr if taken 1 hr after meal

Action

Chemical effect: Reduces total acid load in GI tract, elevates gastric pH to reduce pepsin activity, strengthens gastric mucosal barrier, and increases esophageal sphincter tone.
Therapeutic effect: Relieves GI discomfort.

Available forms

Capsules: 400 mg†, 500 mg†
Liquid: 600 mg/5 ml†
Suspension: 450 mg/5 ml†, 675 mg/5 ml†
Tablets: 300 mg†, 500 mg†, 600 mg†

NURSING PROCESS

☞ Assessment
• Assess patient's discomfort before therapy and regularly thereafter.
• In patient with restricted sodium intake, monitor long-term, high-dose use. Each tablet, capsule, or 5 ml of suspension contains 2 to 3 mg of sodium.
• Be alert for adverse reactions and drug interactions.
• Evaluate patient's and family's knowledge of drug therapy.

☷ Nursing diagnoses
• Acute pain related to gastric hyperacidity
• Constipation related to drug's adverse effects
• Deficient knowledge related to drug therapy

▶ Planning and implementation
• Shake suspension well; give with small amount of milk or water to ease passage.
• When giving through NG tube, make sure tube is patent and placed correctly; after instilling, flush tube with water to ensure passage to stomach and to clear tube.
• Don't give other oral medications within 2 hours of antacid administration. This may cause premature release of enteric-coated drugs in stomach.

Patient teaching
• Advise patient not to take aluminum hydroxide indiscriminately or to switch antacids without prescriber's advice.
• Instruct patient to shake suspension well and to follow with sips of water or juice.
• Warn patient that drug may color stool white or cause white streaks.
• Teach patient how to prevent constipation.

☑ **Evaluation**
● Patient's pain is relieved.
● Patient maintains normal bowel function.
● Patient and family state understanding of drug therapy.

amantadine hydrochloride
(uh-MAN-tah-deen high-droh-KLOR-ighd)
Symadine, Symmetrel

Pharmacologic class: synthetic cyclic primary amine
Therapeutic class: antiviral, antiparkinsonian
Pregnancy risk category: C

Indications and dosages

▶ **Prophylactic or symptomatic treatment of influenza type A virus; respiratory tract illnesses in geriatric or debilitated patients.**
Adults older than age 64: 100 mg P.O. once daily. Treatment should continue for 24 to 48 hours after symptoms disappear. Prophylaxis should start as soon as possible after initial exposure and continue for at least 10 days. When inactivated influenza A vaccine is unavailable, may continue prophylactic treatment for the duration of known influenza A in the community because of repeated or suspected exposures. If used with influenza vaccine, dose is continued for 2 to 4 weeks until protection develops from vaccine.
Adults age 64 and younger and children age 10 and older: 200 mg P.O. daily in single dose or divided b.i.d.
Children ages 1 to 9: 4.4 to 8.8 mg/kg P.O. daily in single dose or divided b.i.d. Maximum, 150 mg daily.
▶ **Drug-induced extrapyramidal reactions.**
Adults: 100 mg P.O. b.i.d. Occasionally, patients whose responses aren't optimal may benefit from an increase to 300 mg P.O. daily in divided doses.
▶ **Idiopathic parkinsonism, parkinsonian syndrome.** *Adults:* 100 mg P.O. b.i.d.; in patients who are seriously ill or receiving other antiparkinsonians, 100 mg daily for at least 1 week, then 100 mg b.i.d., p.r.n.

Contraindications and precautions

● Contraindicated in patients hypersensitive to drug.

● Use cautiously in patients with seizure disorders, heart failure, peripheral edema, hepatic disease, mental illness, eczematoid rash, renal impairment, orthostatic hypotension, or CV disease. Adjust dosage in patients with renal impairment.
⚖ **Lifespan:** In pregnant and breast-feeding women, use cautiously. In children younger than age 1, safety of drug hasn't been established. In elderly patients, use cautiously.

Adverse reactions

CNS: depression, fatigue, confusion, dizziness, psychosis, hallucinations, anxiety, irritability, ataxia, insomnia, weakness, headache, lightheadedness, difficulty concentrating.
CV: peripheral edema, orthostatic hypotension, *heart failure.*
GI: anorexia, nausea, constipation, vomiting, dry mouth.
GU: urine retention.
Skin: livedo reticularis.

Interactions

Drug-drug. *Anticholinergics:* May increase adverse anticholinergic effects. Use together cautiously.
CNS stimulants: May cause additive CNS stimulation. Use together cautiously.
Hydrochlorothiazide, sulfamethoxazole, triamterene, trimethoprim: May increase amantadine levels. Use together cautiously.
Quinidine, quinine: May reduce renal clearance of amantadine. Use together cautiously.
Thioridazine: May worsen tremor in elderly patients. Monitor these patients closely.
Drug-herb. *Jimsonweed:* May adversely affect CV function. Discourage using together.

Effects on lab test results

None reported.

Pharmacokinetics

Absorption: Well absorbed from GI tract.
Distribution: Distributed widely throughout body; crosses blood-brain barrier.
Metabolism: About 10% of drug is metabolized.
Excretion: About 90% is excreted unchanged in urine, primarily by tubular secretion. Portion of drug may be excreted in breast milk. Excretion rate depends on urine pH. *Half-life:* About

24 hours; with renal dysfunction, may be prolonged to 10 days.

Route	Onset	Peak	Duration
P.O.			
antiparkinsonian	48 hr	2-4 hr	Unknown
antiviral	Unknown	Unknown	Unknown

Action

Chemical effect: May interfere with influenza A virus penetration into susceptible cells. In parkinsonism, action is unknown.
Therapeutic effect: Protects against and reduces symptoms of influenza A viral infection and extrapyramidal symptoms.

Available forms

Capsules: 100 mg
Syrup: 50 mg/5 ml

NURSING PROCESS

⚕ Assessment
• Obtain baseline assessment of patient's exposure to influenza A virus or history of Parkinson's disease.
• Watch for adverse reactions and drug interactions.
• Monitor patient's hydration status if adverse GI reactions occur.
• Evaluate patient's and family's knowledge of drug therapy.

⊕ Nursing diagnoses
• Ineffective health maintenance related to patient's underlying condition
• Risk for deficient fluid volume related to adverse GI reactions
• Deficient knowledge related to drug therapy

⊠ Planning and implementation
• Elderly patients are more susceptible to neurologic adverse effects. Giving drug in two daily doses rather than as single dose may reduce these effects.
• Give drug after meals for best absorption.
• **ALERT:** Don't confuse amantadine with rimantadine.
Patient teaching
• Advise patient to take drug several hours before bedtime to prevent insomnia.

• Advise patient not to stand or change positions too quickly to prevent orthostatic hypotension.
• Instruct patient to report adverse reactions, especially dizziness, depression, anxiety, nausea, and urine retention.
• Warn patient with parkinsonism not to stop drug abruptly because doing so could cause a parkinsonian crisis.

☑ Evaluation
• Patient exhibits improved health.
• Patient maintains adequate hydration.
• Patient and family state understanding of drug therapy.

amifostine
(am-eh-FOS-teen)
Ethyol

Pharmacologic class: organic thiophosphate cytoprotective drug
Therapeutic class: antimetabolite
Pregnancy risk category: C

Indications and dosages

▶ **To reduce cumulative renal toxicity from repeated administration of cisplatin in patients with advanced ovarian cancer or non–small-cell lung cancer.** *Adults:* 910 mg/m² daily as a 15-minute I.V. infusion, starting 30 minutes before chemotherapy. If hypotension occurs and blood pressure doesn't return to normal within 5 minutes after stopping treatment, subsequent cycles should use 740 mg/m².
▶ **To reduce moderate to severe xerostomia in patients undergoing postoperative radiation treatment for head or neck cancer.** *Adults:* 200 mg/m² daily as a 3-minute I.V. infusion, starting 15 to 30 minutes before standard fraction radiation therapy.

▼ I.V. administration

• Inspect vial for particulate matter and discoloration before use. Don't use if cloudy or if precipitate has formed.
• Reconstitute each single-dose vial with 9.5 ml of sterile normal saline solution. Don't use other solutions to reconstitute drug. Reconstituted solution (500 mg amifostine/10 ml) is chemically

stable for up to 5 hours at room temperature (about 77° F [25° C]) or up to 24 hours under refrigeration (35° to 46° F [2° to 8° C]).

• Drug can be prepared in polyvinyl chloride bags in concentrations of 5 to 40 mg/ml and has the same stability as when it is reconstituted in single-use vial.

⊛ **ALERT:** Don't infuse for longer than 15 minutes; longer infusion raises the risk of adverse reactions.

• Hydrate patient adequately before infusion. Give antiemetic before and with amifostine infusion. Monitor patient's blood pressure before and immediately after infusion, and periodically thereafter.

Contraindications and precautions

• Contraindicated in patients hypersensitive to aminothiol compounds or mannitol. Don't use drug in patients receiving chemotherapy for potentially curable malignancies (including certain malignancies of germ cell origin), except for patients involved in clinical studies. Also contraindicated in hypotensive or dehydrated patients and in those receiving antihypertensives that can't be stopped during the 24 hours preceding amifostine administration.

• Use cautiously in patients with ischemic heart disease, arrhythmias, heart failure, or history of CVA or transient ischemic attacks.

• Common adverse effects, such as nausea, vomiting, and hypotension, are likely to have serious consequences; use cautiously.

⚖ **Lifespan:** In breast-feeding women, drug isn't recommended because it's unknown whether drug or its metabolites appear in breast milk. In children and in elderly patients, use cautiously because safety of drug hasn't been established.

Adverse reactions

CNS: dizziness, somnolence.
CV: hypotension, flushing or feeling of warmth, chills or feeling of coldness.
EENT: sneezing.
GI: nausea, vomiting.
Metabolic: hypocalcemia.
Respiratory: hiccups.
Other: allergic reactions ranging from rash to rigors.

Interactions

Drug-drug. *Antihypertensives, other drugs that could potentiate hypotension:* May potentiate hypotension. Monitor patient closely.

Effects on lab test results

• May decrease calcium level.

Pharmacokinetics

Absorption: Administered I.V.
Distribution: Less than 10% remains in plasma 6 minutes after administration.
Metabolism: Metabolized to an active free thiol metabolite.
Excretion: Renally excreted. *Elimination half-life:* 8 minutes.

Route	Onset	Peak	Duration
I.V.	5-8 min	Unknown	Unknown

Action

Chemical effect: Dephosphorylated by alkaline phosphatase to pharmacologically active free thiol metabolite. Free thiol in normal tissues is available to bind to and detoxify reactive metabolites of cisplatin.
Therapeutic effect: Reduces toxic effects of cisplatin on renal tissue.

Available forms

Injection: 500 mg anhydrous base and 500 mg mannitol in 10-ml vial

NURSING PROCESS

℞ **Assessment**

• Patients should be adequately hydrated before receiving drug. Keep patient supine during infusion.

• Monitor blood pressure every 5 minutes during infusion. If hypotension occurs and requires interrupting therapy, notify prescriber and place patient in Trendelenburg's position. Then give an infusion of normal saline solution, using a separate I.V. line. If blood pressure returns to normal within 5 minutes and patient is asymptomatic, restart infusion so full dose of drug can be given. If full dose can't be given, subsequent doses should be limited to 740 mg/m².

• Antiemetics, including 20 mg I.V. dexamethasone and a serotonin 5-HT₃ receptor antagonist, should be given before and with drug. Addition-

al antiemetics may be needed based on the chemotherapeutics given.
- Monitor patient's fluid balance when drug is given with highly emetogenic chemotherapy.
- Monitor calcium level in patients at risk for hypocalcemia, such as those with nephrotic syndrome. Give calcium supplements if needed.
- Evaluate patient's and family's knowledge of drug therapy.

Nursing diagnoses
- Ineffective health maintenance related to neoplastic disease
- Deficient knowledge related to drug therapy

Planning and implementation
- If possible, stop antihypertensive therapy 24 hours before giving drug. If antihypertensive therapy can't be stopped, don't use amifostine because severe hypotension may occur.
Patient teaching
- Instruct patient to remain supine throughout infusion.

Evaluation
- Patient shows positive response to drug.
- Patient and family state understanding of drug therapy.

amikacin sulfate
(am-eh-KAY-sin SUL-fayt)
Amikin

Pharmacologic class: aminoglycoside
Therapeutic class: antibiotic
Pregnancy risk category: D

Indications and dosages

▶ **Serious infections caused by sensitive strains of *Pseudomonas aeruginosa, Escherichia coli, Proteus, Klebsiella, Serratia, Enterobacter, Acinetobacter, Providencia, Citrobacter, Staphylococcus;* meningitis.** *Adults and children:* 15 mg/kg daily divided q 8 to 12 hours I.M. or I.V. infusion.
Neonates: Initially, loading dose of 10 mg/kg I.V., followed by 7.5 mg/kg q 12 hours.
Adjust-a-dose: For patients with renal impairment, initially, 7.5 mg/kg I.M. or I.V. Subsequent doses and frequency determined by drug level and renal function test results.

▶ **Uncomplicated UTI.** *Adults:* 250 mg I.M. or I.V. b.i.d.
▶ ***Mycobacterium avium* complex, with other drugs‡.** *Adults:* 15 mg/kg I.V. daily, in divided doses q 8 to 12 hours.
Adjust-a-dose: For patients with renal impairment, initially, 7.5 mg/kg I.M or I.V. Subsequent doses and frequency determined by drug level. Keep peak level between 15 and 35 mcg/ml; trough level shouldn't exceed 10 mcg/ml.

I.V. administration
- For adults, dilute in 100 to 200 ml of D_5W or normal saline solution. Volume for children depends on dose.
- Infants should receive a 1- to 2-hour infusion. For adults, infuse over 30 to 60 minutes.
- After I.V. infusion, flush line with normal saline solution or D_5W.

Contraindications and precautions
- Contraindicated in patients hypersensitive to drug or other aminoglycosides.
- Use cautiously in patients with impaired renal function or neuromuscular disorders.
Lifespan: In pregnant women, use cautiously and only if benefit outweighs risk to fetus. In breast-feeding women, don't give drug. In neonates and infants, use cautiously. In elderly patients, use cautiously because they are more likely to have ototoxicity.

Adverse reactions
CNS: headache, lethargy, *neuromuscular blockade.*
EENT: ototoxicity.
GU: *nephrotoxicity.*
Hepatic: *hepatic necrosis.*
Other: hypersensitivity reactions, *anaphylaxis.*

Interactions
Drug-drug. *Acyclovir, amphotericin B, cephalothin, cisplatin, methoxyflurane, other aminoglycosides, vancomycin:* May increase nephrotoxicity. Use together cautiously.
Atracurium, doxacurium, mivacurium, pancuronium, rocuronium, tubocurarine, vecuronium: May increase the effects of nondepolarizing neuromuscular blockade, including prolonged respiratory depression. Use together only when necessary. Dose of nondepolarizing muscle relaxant may need to be reduced.

Dimenhydrinate: May mask symptoms of ototoxicity. Use cautiously.

Indomethacin: May increase trough and peak levels of amikacin. Monitor amikacin level closely.

I.V. loop diuretics (such as furosemide): May increase ototoxicity. Use together cautiously.

Parenteral penicillins (such as ticarcillin): May cause amikacin inactivation in vitro. Don't mix.

Effects on lab test results

• May increase BUN, creatinine, nonprotein nitrogen, and urine urea levels.

Pharmacokinetics

Absorption: Rapidly absorbed after I.M. administration.

Distribution: Distributed widely; protein-binding is minimal; drug crosses placenta.

Metabolism: None.

Excretion: Primarily in urine by glomerular filtration. *Half-life:* 2 to 3 hours (adults); 30 to 86 hours (patients with severe renal damage).

Route	Onset	Peak	Duration
I.V.	Immediate	Immediate	8-12 hr
I.M.	Unknown	1 hr	8-12 hr

Action

Chemical effect: Inhibits protein synthesis by binding directly to 30S ribosomal subunit. Generally bactericidal.

Therapeutic effect: Kills susceptible bacteria and many aerobic gram-negative organisms (including most strains of *Pseudomonas aeruginosa*) and some aerobic gram-positive organisms. Ineffective against anaerobes.

Available forms

Injection: 50 mg/ml, 250 mg/ml

NURSING PROCESS

🩺 Assessment

• Assess patient's infection, hearing, weight, and renal function test values before therapy and regularly thereafter.

• Watch for signs of ototoxicity, including tinnitus, vertigo, and hearing loss.

• Monitor amikacin level. Obtain blood for peak amikacin level 1 hour after I.M. injection and 30 minutes to 1 hour after infusion ends; for trough level, draw blood just before next dose.

Don't collect blood in heparinized tube because heparin is incompatible with aminoglycosides. Peak level above 35 mcg/ml and trough level above 10 mcg/ml may raise the risk of toxicity.

• Be alert for signs of nephrotoxicity, including cells or casts in urine, oliguria, proteinuria, decreased creatinine clearance, and increased BUN and creatinine levels.

• Evaluate patient's and family's knowledge of drug therapy.

🩺 Nursing diagnoses

• Risk for infection related to bacteria

• Impaired urine elimination related to amikacin-induced nephrotoxicity

• Deficient knowledge related to drug therapy

⟩ Planning and implementation

• Obtain specimen for culture and sensitivity tests before first dose. Therapy may begin before receiving results.

• Therapy usually lasts 7 to 10 days.

• Drug potency isn't affected if solution turns light yellow.

• Patient should be well hydrated while taking drug to minimize renal tubule irritation.

• If no response occurs after 5 days, therapy may be stopped and new specimens obtained for culture and sensitivity testing.

⑤ ALERT: Don't confuse Amikin with Amicar or amikacin with anakinra.

Patient teaching

• Tell patient to immediately report changes in hearing or in appearance or elimination pattern of urine. Teach patient how to measure intake and output.

• Emphasize importance of drinking 2 L of fluid daily, unless contraindicated.

• Teach patient to watch for and promptly report signs of superinfection, such as continued fever and other signs of new infections, especially of upper respiratory tract.

✓ Evaluation

• Patient's infection is eradicated.

• Patient's renal function test values remain unchanged.

• Patient and family state understanding of drug therapy.

amiloride hydrochloride
(uh-MIL-uh-righd high-droh-KLOR-ighd)
Kaluril, Midamor

Pharmacologic class: potassium-sparing diuretic
Therapeutic class: diuretic, antihypertensive
Pregnancy risk category: B

Indications and dosages

▶ **Hypertension; edema caused by heart failure, usually in patients also taking thiazide or other potassium-wasting diuretics.** *Adults:* 5 mg P.O. daily. Increase to 10 mg daily, if necessary. Maximum, 20 mg daily.
▶ **Lithium-induced polyuria‡.** *Adults:* 5 to 10 mg P.O. b.i.d.

Contraindications and precautions

• Contraindicated in patients with potassium level higher than 5.5 mEq/L; in those receiving other potassium-sparing diuretics, such as spironolactone; in those with anuria, acute or chronic renal insufficiency, diabetic nephropathy, or hypersensitivity to drug.
• Use cautiously, if at all, in patients with diabetes mellitus.
• Also use cautiously in patients with severe hepatic insufficiency and in debilitated patients.
⚠ Lifespan: In pregnant women, use cautiously. In breast-feeding women, drug is contraindicated. In neonates and infants, use cautiously. In children, safety of drug hasn't been established. In elderly patients, use cautiously.

Adverse reactions

CNS: headache, weakness, dizziness.
CV: orthostatic hypotension.
GI: nausea, anorexia, diarrhea, vomiting, abdominal pain, constipation.
GU: impotence.
Hematologic: *aplastic anemia.*
Metabolic: *hyperkalemia.*

Interactions

Drug-drug. *ACE inhibitors, salt substitutes containing potassium, potassium-sparing diuretics, potassium supplements:* May cause hyperkalemia. Monitor potassium level closely.

Lithium: May decrease lithium clearance, increasing risk of lithium toxicity. Monitor lithium level.
NSAIDs: May decrease diuretic's effectiveness. Monitor patient for lack of therapeutic effect.
Drug-food. *Foods high in potassium, salt substitutes containing potassium:* May cause hyperkalemia. Monitor potassium level closely.

Effects on lab test results

• May increase BUN and potassium levels. May decrease sodium level.
• May decrease hemoglobin, hematocrit, and neutrophil count. May cause abnormal liver function test values.

Pharmacokinetics

Absorption: About 50% of dose is absorbed from GI tract; food decreases absorption to 30%.
Distribution: Wide extravascular distribution.
Metabolism: Insignificant.
Excretion: Primarily in urine. *Half-life:* 6 to 9 hours.

Route	Onset	Peak	Duration
P.O.	2 hr	6-10 hr	24 hr

Action

Chemical effect: Inhibits sodium reabsorption and potassium excretion in distal tubule.
Therapeutic effect: Reduces blood pressure; promotes sodium and water excretion while blocking potassium excretion.

Available forms

Tablets: 5 mg

NURSING PROCESS

🔲 **Assessment**
• Assess patient's blood pressure, urine output, weight, electrolyte levels, and degree of edema before therapy and regularly thereafter.
• Be alert for adverse reactions and drug interactions.
• Evaluate patient's and family's knowledge of drug therapy.

🔲 **Nursing diagnoses**
• Excessive fluid volume related to fluid retention

- Risk for injury related to potential for drug-induced hyperkalemia
- Deficient knowledge related to drug therapy

⟫ Planning and implementation
- Give with meals to prevent nausea.
- Give early in the day to prevent nocturia.
- If potassium level exceeds 6.5 mEq/L, alert prescriber immediately and stop drug.
- Have patient follow a low-potassium diet.
- **⟳ ALERT:** Don't confuse amiloride with amiodarone.

Patient teaching
- Advise patient to avoid sudden posture changes and to rise slowly to avoid orthostatic hypotension.
- Warn patient to limit potassium-rich foods (such as oranges and bananas), salt substitutes containing potassium, and potassium supplements to prevent serious hyperkalemia.
- Teach patient and family to identify and report signs of hyperkalemia.
- Teach patient and family to monitor patient's fluid volume by recording daily weight and intake and output.

☑ Evaluation
- Patient's fluid retention is relieved.
- Patient's potassium level remains normal.
- Patient and family state understanding of drug therapy.

amino acid infusions, crystalline
(uh-MEEN-oh AS-id in-FYOO-zhuns)
Aminosyn, Aminosyn II, Aminosyn-PF, FreAmine III, Novamine, Travasol, Trophamine

amino acid infusions in dextrose
Aminosyn II with Dextrose

amino acid infusions with electrolytes
Aminosyn with Electrolytes, Aminosyn II with Electrolytes, FreAmine III with Electrolytes, ProcalAmine with Electrolytes, Travasol with Electrolytes

amino acid infusions with electrolytes in dextrose
Aminosyn II with Electrolytes in Dextrose

amino acid infusions for hepatic failure
HepatAmine

amino acid infusions for high metabolic stress
Aminosyn-HBC, BranchAmin, FreAmine HBC

amino acid infusions for renal failure
Aminess, Aminosyn-RF, NephrAmine, RenAmin

Pharmacologic class: protein substrate
Therapeutic class: parenteral nutritional therapy and caloric
Pregnancy risk category: C

Indications and dosages
▶ **Total parenteral nutrition in patients who can't or won't eat.** *Adults:* 1 to 1.7 g/kg I.V. daily.
Children: 2 to 3 g/kg I.V. daily.
▶ **Nutritional support in patients with cirrhosis, hepatitis, or hepatic encephalopathy.** *Adults:* 80 to 120 g of amino acids (12 to 18 g of nitrogen) I.V. daily using formulation for hepatic failure.
▶ **Nutritional support in patients with high metabolic stress.** *Adults:* 1.7 g/kg I.V. daily using formulation for high metabolic stress.

▼ I.V. administration
- Control infusion rate carefully with infusion pump. If infusion rate falls behind, notify prescriber; don't increase rate to catch up.
- Peripheral infusions should be limited to 2.5% amino acids and 10% dextrose.
- Prescriber will individualize dosage according to patient's metabolic and clinical response as determined by nitrogen balance and body weight corrected for fluid balance.
- If patient has chills, fever, or other signs of sepsis, replace I.V. tubing and bottle and send them to laboratory so a culture can be taken.

Contraindications and precautions

• Contraindicated in patients with anuria; inborn errors of amino acid metabolism, such as maple syrup urine disease and isovaleric acidemia; severe uncorrected electrolyte or acid-base imbalances; hyperammonemia; or decreased circulating blood volume.

• Use cautiously in patients with renal insufficiency or impairment, cardiac disease, or hepatic impairment.

• Also use cautiously in diabetic patients; insulin may be needed to prevent hyperglycemia. Give cautiously to patients with cardiac insufficiency because it may cause circulatory overload. Patients with fluid restriction may tolerate only 1 to 2 L.

⚠ **Lifespan:** In children and neonates, especially those of low birth weight, use cautiously.

Adverse reactions

CNS: confusion, unconsciousness, headache, dizziness.

CV: flushing, hypervolemia, *heart failure* (in susceptible patients), worsening of hypertension (in predisposed patients), thrombophlebitis, *thrombosis.*

GI: nausea, vomiting.

GU: glycosuria, osmotic diuresis.

Hepatic: fatty liver.

Metabolic: *rebound hypoglycemia,* hyperglycemia, *metabolic acidosis,* alkalosis, hypophosphatemia, *hyperosmolar hyperglycemic nonketotic syndrome,* hyperammonemia, electrolyte imbalances, dehydration (if hyperosmolar solutions are used).

Respiratory: *pulmonary edema.*

Skin: feeling of warmth.

Other: chills, hypersensitivity reactions, tissue sloughing at infusion site caused by extravasation, catheter sepsis.

Interactions

Drug-drug. *Tetracyclines:* May reduce protein-sparing effects of infused amino acids because of its antianabolic activity. Monitor patient.

Effects on lab test results

• May increase ammonia and liver enzyme levels. May decrease phosphate, magnesium, and potassium levels. May increase or decrease glucose level.

Pharmacokinetics

Absorption: Administered I.V.
Distribution: Unknown.
Metabolism: Unknown.
Excretion: Unknown. *Half-life:* Unknown.

Route	Onset	Peak	Duration
I.V.	Immediate	Immediate	Unknown

Action

Chemical effect: Provides substrate for protein synthesis or helps to conserve existing body protein. Formulations for hepatic failure and high metabolic stress contain essential and nonessential amino acids, with high levels of branched chain amino acids isoleucine, leucine, and valine. Formulations for renal impairment contain histidine and minimal amounts of essential amino acids; nonessential amino acids are synthesized from excess ammonia in blood of uremic patient, thus lowering azotemia.

Therapeutic effect: Provides body with needed calories and protein.

Available forms

Injection: 250 ml, 500 ml, 1,000 ml, 2,000 ml containing amino acids in varying concentrations.

Crystalline: Aminosyn, 3.5%, 5%, 7%, 8.5%, 10%. Aminosyn II, 3.5%, 5%, 7%, 8.5%, 10%. Aminosyn-PF, 7%, 10%. FreAmine III, 8.5%, 10%. Novamine, 11.4%, 15%. Travasol, 5.5%, 8.5%, 10%. TrophAmine, 6%, 10%.

In dextrose: Aminosyn II, 3.5% in 5% dextrose, 3.5% in 25% dextrose, 4.25% in 10% dextrose, 4.25% in 20% dextrose, 4.25% in 25% dextrose, 5% in 25% dextrose.

With electrolytes: Aminosyn, 3.5%, 7%, 8.5%. Aminosyn II, 3.5%, 7%, 8.5%, 10%. FreAmine III, 3%, 8.5%. ProcalAmine, 3%. Travasol, 3.5%, 5.5%, 8.5%.

With electrolytes in dextrose: Aminosyn II, 3.5% with electrolytes in 5% dextrose, 4.25% with electrolytes in 10% dextrose.

For hepatic failure: HepatAmine, 8%.

For high metabolic stress: Aminosyn-HBC, 7%. BranchAmin, 4%. FreAmine HBC, 6.9%.

For renal failure: Aminess, 5.2%. Aminosyn-RF, 5.2%. NephrAmine, 5.4%. RenAmin, 6.5%.

NURSING PROCESS

⚕ Assessment
● Assess electrolyte, glucose, BUN, calcium, and phosphate levels before therapy and regularly thereafter.
● Be alert for adverse reactions and drug interactions.
● Check infusion site frequently for erythema, inflammation, irritation, tissue sloughing, necrosis, and phlebitis.
● Evaluate patient's and family's knowledge of drug therapy.

🔹 Nursing diagnoses
● Altered nutrition (less than body requirements) related to patient's underlying condition
● Risk for deficient fluid volume related to adverse drug reactions
● Deficient knowledge related to drug therapy

❯ Planning and implementation
🟡 **ALERT:** Don't confuse Aminosyn with Amikacin.
Patient teaching
● Tell patient to report discomfort at injection site or unusual symptoms.

✅ Evaluation
● Patient's nutritional status improves.
● Patient maintains adequate hydration.
● Patient and family state understanding of drug therapy.

aminophylline (theophylline and ethylenediamine)
(uh-mih-NOF-il-in)
Aminophyllin, Phyllocontin, Phyllocontin-350, Somophyllin, Somophyllin-DF, Truphylline

Pharmacologic class: xanthine derivative
Therapeutic class: bronchodilator
Pregnancy risk category: C

Indications and dosages
❯ **Symptomatic relief of bronchospasm.** *Patients currently receiving theophylline products who require rapid relief of symptoms:* Loading dose is 6 mg/kg (equivalent to 4.7 mg/kg anhy-

drous theophylline) I.V. infusion at a rate of 25 mg/minute or less, then maintenance infusion.
Adults (nonsmokers): 0.7 mg/kg/hour I.V. for 12 hours; then 0.5 mg/kg/hour.
Otherwise healthy adult smokers: 1 mg/kg/hour I.V. for 12 hours; then 0.8 mg/kg/hour.
Older patients and adults with cor pulmonale: 0.6 mg/kg/hour I.V. for 12 hours; then 0.3 mg/kg/hour.
Adults with heart failure or liver disease: 0.5 mg/kg/hour I.V. for 12 hours; then 0.1 to 0.2 mg/kg/hour.
Children ages 9 to 16: 1 mg/kg/hour I.V. for 12 hours; then 0.8 mg/kg/hour.
Children ages 6 months to 8 years: 1.2 mg/kg/hour for 12 hours; then 1 mg/kg/hour.
Patients currently receiving theophylline products: Aminophylline infusion of 0.63 mg/kg (0.5 mg/kg anhydrous theophylline) increases level of theophylline by 1 mcg/ml. Some clinicians recommend a dose of 3.1 mg/kg (2.5 mg/kg anhydrous theophylline) with no obvious signs of theophylline toxicity.
❯ **Chronic bronchial asthma.** Dosage is highly individualized. Rectal dosage is same as oral dosage.
Adults: 600 to 1,600 mg P.O. daily in divided doses t.i.d. or q.i.d.
Children: 12 mg/kg P.O. daily in divided doses t.i.d. or q.i.d.
❯ **Periodic apnea related to Cheyne-Stokes respirations, promote diuresis, paroxysmal nocturnal dyspnea‡.** *Adults:* 200 to 400 mg I.V. bolus.
❯ **To reduce severe bronchospasm in infants with cystic fibrosis‡.** *Infants:* 10 to 12 mg/kg I.V. daily.

▼ I.V. administration
● Because I.V. drug can burn, dilute with compatible I.V. solution and inject at no more than 25 mg/minute.
● Exceeding recommended I.V. infusion rates increases the risk of adverse reactions. Drug is compatible with most I.V. solutions except invert sugar, fructose, and fat emulsions.
● Theophylline concentration should range from 10 to 20 mcg/ml; toxicity may occur with level above 20 mcg/ml.
● Aminophylline is a soluble salt of theophylline. Dosage is adjusted by monitoring re-

sponse, tolerance, pulmonary function, and theophylline level.

Contraindications and precautions

• Contraindicated in patients with active peptic ulcer disease, seizure disorders (unless anticonvulsants are given), and hypersensitivity to xanthine compounds (caffeine, theobromine) or ethylenediamine.

• Use cautiously in patients with heart failure or other cardiac or circulatory impairment, COPD, cor pulmonale, renal or hepatic disease, hyperthyroidism, diabetes mellitus, peptic ulcer, severe hypoxemia, or hypertension.

⚠ Lifespan: In pregnant or breast-feeding women, young children, and elderly patients, use cautiously.

Adverse reactions

CNS: nervousness, restlessness, dizziness, headache, insomnia, light-headedness, *seizures,* muscle twitching.
CV: palpitations, tachycardia, extrasystole, flushing, hypotension, *arrhythmias.*
GI: nausea, vomiting, anorexia, dyspepsia, heavy feeling in stomach, diarrhea, bitter aftertaste.
Respiratory: increased respiratory rate, *respiratory arrest.*
Skin: urticaria, local irritation with rectal suppositories.

Interactions

Drug-drug. *Adenosine:* May decrease antiarrhythmic effectiveness. Higher doses of adenosine may be needed.
Alkali-sensitive drugs: May reduce drug's activity. Don't add to I.V. fluids containing aminophylline.
Allopurinol (high doses), cimetidine, influenza virus vaccine, macrolide antibiotics (such as erythromycin), hormonal contraceptives, quinolone antibiotics (such as ciprofloxacin): May decrease hepatic clearance of theophylline and increase theophylline level. Monitor patient for toxicity.
Amiodarone, ticlopidine, verapamil: May increase theophylline level. Use together cautiously.
Barbiturates, carbamazepine, nicotine, phenytoin, rifampin: May enhance metabolism and decrease theophylline level. Monitor patient for decreased aminophylline effect.

Carteolol, pindolol, propranolol, timolol: May act antagonistically reducing the effects of one or both drugs. Monitor patient closely.
Ephedrine, other sympathomimetics: Theophylline may exhibit synergistic toxicity with these drugs, predisposing patient to arrhythmias. Monitor patient closely.
Isoniazid, ketoconazole: May decrease theophylline absorption.
Lithium: Theophylline may increase lithium level. Monitor patient closely.
Drug-herb. *Caffeine-containing herbs (such as guarana):* May increase adverse effects. Discourage using together.
St. John's wort: May decrease level and effectiveness of drug. Monitor patient for lack of therapeutic effect. Discourage using together.
Drug-food. *Caffeinated foods, colas:* May increase CNS adverse effects. Advise patient to monitor caffeine intake.
Drug-lifestyle. *Smoking:* May increase clearance and decrease half-life of theophylline. Higher doses may be needed to achieve desired effect.

Effects on lab test results

• May increase glucose and free fatty acid levels.

Pharmacokinetics

Absorption: Well absorbed except for suppository form, which is unreliable and slow. Food may alter rate but not extent of absorption of oral doses.
Distribution: In all tissues and extracellular fluids except fatty tissue.
Metabolism: Converted to theophylline, then metabolized to inactive compounds.
Excretion: 10% in urine as theophylline. *Half-life:* Depends on many variables, including smoking status, illness, age, and formulation used.

Route	Onset	Peak	Duration
P.O.			
tablets	15-60 min	2 hr	Varies
extended-release	Unknown	4-7 hr	Varies
solution	15-60 min	1 hr	Varies
I.V.	15 min	Immediate	Varies
P.R.	Varies	Varies	Varies

Reactions may be *common,* uncommon, *life-threatening,* or **COMMON AND LIFE-THREATENING.**

Action

Chemical effect: Inhibits phosphodiesterase, the enzyme that degrades cAMP, thereby relaxing smooth muscle of bronchial airways and pulmonary blood vessels.
Therapeutic effect: Eases breathing.

Available forms

Injection: 250 mg/10 ml, 500 mg/20 ml, 500 mg/2 ml, 100 mg/100 ml in half-normal saline solution, 200 mg/100 ml in half-normal saline solution
Oral liquid: 105 mg/5 ml
Rectal suppositories: 250 mg, 500 mg
Tablets: 100 mg, 200 mg
Tablets (extended-release): 350 mg ◆

NURSING PROCESS

🗲 Assessment

• Monitor drug effectiveness by regularly auscultating lungs and noting respiratory rate and results of laboratory studies, such as arterial blood gas analysis.
• Monitor patient's hydration status if adverse GI reactions occur.
• Be alert for adverse reactions and drug interactions.
• Evaluate patient's and family's knowledge of drug therapy.

🔛 Nursing diagnoses

• Impaired gas exchange related to bronchospasm
• Risk for deficient fluid volume related to drug-induced adverse GI reactions
• Deficient knowledge related to drug therapy

⊠ Planning and implementation

• Make sure that patient hasn't had recent theophylline therapy before giving loading dose.
• Give drug with full glass of water at meals. Food in stomach delays absorption. Enteric-coated tablets may delay and impair absorption.
• Give suppository only if patient can't take drug orally. Schedule after bowel evacuation, if possible; may be retained better if given before meal. Have patient remain recumbent for 15 to 20 minutes after insertion.
• **ALERT:** Don't confuse aminophylline with amitriptyline or ampicillin.

Patient teaching

• Supply instructions for home care and dosage schedule. Some patients may need an around-the-clock schedule.
• Warn elderly patients that dizziness is common at start of therapy.
• Warn patient to check with prescriber or pharmacist before combining aminophylline with other drugs; OTC products and herbal remedies may contain ephedrine. Excessive CNS stimulation may result.
• Advise patient to avoid switching brands without consulting prescriber.
• Tell patient to notify prescriber if he quits smoking. Dosage may need to be reduced.
• Advise patient to notify prescriber if he experiences anxiety, insomnia, irritability, or diarrhea, as these are signs of toxicity.

☑ Evaluation

• Patient's appearance, vital signs, and laboratory test results demonstrate improved gas exchange.
• Patient remains hydrated throughout therapy.
• Patient and family state understanding of drug therapy.

amiodarone hydrochloride

(am-ee-OH-dah-rohn high-droh-KLOR-ighd)
Cordarone, Cordarone X ◆, Pacerone

Pharmacologic class: benzofuran derivative
Therapeutic class: ventricular antiarrhythmic
Pregnancy risk category: D

Indications and dosages

▶ **Recurrent ventricular fibrillation, unstable ventricular tachycardia, atrial fibrillation‡, angina‡, and hypertrophic cardiomyopathy‡.**
Adults: Loading dose of 800 to 1,600 mg P.O. daily for 1 to 3 weeks until initial therapeutic response occurs, then 650 to 800 mg P.O. daily for 1 month, then 200 to 600 mg P.O. daily as maintenance dosage. Or, for first 24 hours, 150 mg I.V. over 10 minutes (mix in 100 ml D_5W); then 360 mg I.V. over 6 hours (mix 900 mg in 500 ml D_5W); then maintenance dose of 540 mg I.V. over 18 hours at 0.5 mg/minute. After first 24 hours, continue a maintenance infusion of 0.5 mg/minute in a concentration of 1 to 6 mg/ml. For infusions longer than 1 hour, concentra-

tions shouldn't exceed 2 mg/ml unless you use a central venous catheter. Don't use for longer than 3 weeks.

▶ **Conversion from I.V. to P.O.** *Adults:* After daily dose of 720 mg I.V. (assuming rate of 0.5 mg/minute) for less than 1 week, start 800 to 1,600 mg P.O. daily; for 1 to 3 weeks, give 600 to 800 mg P.O. daily; and for longer than 3 weeks, give 400 mg P.O. daily.

▶ **Supraventricular arrhythmias‡.** *Adults:* 600 to 800 mg P.O. for 1 to 4 weeks or until supraventricular tachycardia is controlled. Maintenance dose is 100 to 400 mg P.O. daily.

▼ I.V. administration

• Drug may be given I.V. where facilities for close monitoring of cardiac function and resuscitation are available. Initial dosage of 5 mg/kg should be mixed in 250 ml of D_5W.

• Repeat doses should be given through central venous catheter. Patient should receive maximum of 1.2 g in up to 500 ml D_5W daily.

• Maintain ECG monitoring during start and alteration of dosage. Notify prescriber of significant change.

Contraindications and precautions

• Contraindicated in patients hypersensitive to drug, and in those with severe sinus node disease, bradycardia, second- or third-degree AV block (unless artificial pacemaker is present), and bradycardia-induced syncope.

• Use cautiously in patients receiving other antiarrhythmics and in patients with pulmonary or thyroid disease, as use may result in fatal toxicity.

⑤ **ALERT:** I.V. Cordarone contains benzyl alcohol, which has caused "gasping syndrome" in neonates younger than age 1 month. Monitor patient for symptoms of sudden onset of gasping respiration, hypotension, bradycardia, and CV collapse.

⚘ **Lifespan:** In pregnant women, use cautiously. In breast-feeding women, drug is contraindicated. In children, safety of drug hasn't been established. In fetuses, infants, and toddlers, I.V. Cordarone may leach out plasticizers such as DEHP, which can adversely affect male reproductive tract development.

Adverse reactions

CNS: peripheral neuropathy, extrapyramidal symptoms, headache, malaise, fatigue.

CV: *bradycardia,* hypotension, *arrhythmias, heart failure, heart block, sinus arrest.*
EENT: corneal microdeposits, vision disturbances.
GI: nausea, vomiting, constipation.
Hepatic: hepatic dysfunction.
Metabolic: hypothyroidism, hyperthyroidism.
Musculoskeletal: muscle weakness.
Respiratory: SEVERE PULMONARY TOXICITY (PNEUMONITIS, ALVEOLITIS).
Skin: photosensitivity, blue-gray skin.
Other: gynecomastia.

Interactions

Drug-drug. *Antiarrhythmics:* Amiodarone may reduce hepatic or renal clearance of certain antiarrhythmics (especially flecainide and procainamide); use of amiodarone with other antiarrhythmics (especially disopyramide, mexiletine, procainamide, and propafenone) may induce torsades de pointes. Monitor ECG closely.
Antihypertensives: May increase hypotensive effect. Use together cautiously.
Beta blockers, calcium channel blockers: May increase cardiac depressant effects and potentiate slowing of sinus node and AV conduction. Use together cautiously.
Digoxin: May increase digoxin level by an average of 70% to 100%. Monitor digoxin level closely.
Cholestyramine: May decrease amiodarone level and half-life. Avoid using together.
Cimetidine: May increase amiodarone level. Avoid using together.
Cyclosporine: May increase cyclosporine level. Monitor patient for cyclosporine toxicity.
Phenytoin: May decrease phenytoin metabolism. Monitor phenytoin level.
Quinidine: May increase quinidine concentrations producing potentially fatal cardiac arrhythmias. Monitor quinidine concentrations closely if combination cannot be avoided. Adjust quinidine as needed.
Theophylline: May increase theophylline level and lead to toxicity. Monitor theophylline level.
Warfarin: May increase INR by an average of 100% within 1 to 4 weeks of therapy. Warfarin dosage should be decreased 33% to 50% when amiodarone is started. Monitor patient closely.
Drug-herb. *Pennyroyal:* May change the rate at which toxic metabolites of pennyroyal form. Discourage using together.

Drug-lifestyle. *Sun exposure:* May cause photosensitivity reaction. Advise against prolonged or unprotected sun exposure.

Effects on lab test results

- May increase ALT, AST, alkaline phosphatase, and GGT levels.
- May increase PT and INR. May alter thyroid function test results.

Pharmacokinetics

Absorption: Slow and variable.
Distribution: Wide, accumulating in adipose tissue and in organs with marked perfusion, such as lungs, liver, and spleen. Drug is 96% protein-bound.
Metabolism: Extensive in liver to active metabolite, desethyl amiodarone.
Excretion: Mainly hepatic through biliary tree. *Half-life:* 25 to 110 days (usually 40 to 50 days).

Route	Onset	Peak	Duration
P.O.	2-21 days	3-7 hr	Varies
I.V.	Unknown	Unknown	Unknown

Action

Chemical effect: Unknown; thought to prolong refractory period and duration of action potential and decrease repolarization.
Therapeutic effect: Abolishes ventricular arrhythmia.

Available forms

Injection: 50 mg/ml
Tablets: 100 mg, 200 mg, 400 mg

NURSING PROCESS

◢ Assessment

- Assess CV status before therapy.
- Review pulmonary, liver, and thyroid function test results before and regularly during therapy.
- Continuously monitor cardiac status of patient receiving I.V. amiodarone to evaluate its effectiveness.
- Watch for adverse reactions and drug interactions.
- Monitor patient carefully for pulmonary toxicity, which can be fatal. Risk increases in patients receiving more than 400 mg daily.
- Monitor electrolytes, particularly potassium and magnesium levels.

- Evaluate patient's and family's knowledge of drug therapy.

⊞ Nursing diagnoses

- Decreased cardiac output related to ventricular arrhythmia
- Risk for injury related to drug-induced adverse reactions
- Deficient knowledge related to drug therapy

⟩ Planning and implementation

- Adverse reactions commonly limit drug's use.
- **⑤ ALERT:** Drug may pose life-threatening risks for patients already at risk for sudden death. Drug may cause fatal toxicities, including hepatic and pulmonary toxicity. Drug should be used only in patients with life-threatening, recurrent ventricular arrhythmias unresponsive to other antiarrhythmics or when alternative drugs can't be tolerated. Drug may also be used to treat atrial fibrillation, atrial flutter, paroxysmal supraventricular tachycardia, and, at low doses, heart failure.
- Divide oral loading dose into three equal doses and give with meals to decrease GI intolerance. Maintenance dosage may be given once daily or divided into two doses taken with meals if GI intolerance occurs.
- Instillation of methylcellulose ophthalmic solution during amiodarone therapy is recommended to minimize corneal microdeposits.
- **⑤ ALERT:** Don't confuse amiodarone with amiloride.

Patient teaching

- Stress importance of taking drug exactly as prescribed.
- Emphasize importance of close follow-up and regular diagnostic studies to monitor drug action and assess for adverse reactions.
- Warn patient that drug may cause blue-gray skin pigmentation.
- Advise patient to use sunscreen to prevent photosensitivity reaction (burning or tingling skin followed by erythema and possible blistering).
- Inform patient that adverse effects are more prevalent at high doses but are generally reversible when therapy stops. Resolution of adverse reactions may take up to 4 months.

☑ Evaluation

- Patient's arrhythmia is corrected.
- Patient has no injury from adverse reactions.

- Patient and family state understanding of drug therapy.

amitriptyline hydrochloride
(am-ih-TRIP-tuh-leen high-droh-KLOR-ighd)
Apo-Amitriptyline ♦, Endep ◇, Tryptanol ◇

Pharmacologic class: tricyclic antidepressant
Therapeutic class: antidepressant
Pregnancy risk category: C

Indications and dosages

▶ **Depression.** *Adults:* 50 to 100 mg P.O. h.s., gradually increasing to 150 mg daily; maximum dosage is 300 mg daily, if needed.
Elderly patients and adolescents: 10 mg P.O. t.i.d. and 20 mg h.s. daily.
▶ **Anorexia or bulimia related to depression or as adjunctive therapy for neurogenic pain‡.** *Adults:* If outpatient, initially 75 to 100 mg P.O. in divided doses daily. If inpatient, 100 to 300 mg P.O. in divided doses daily. After maximum effect is achieved, gradually lower dose to maintenance dose of 50 to 100 mg or less P.O. daily for a minimum of 3 months.

Contraindications and precautions

- Contraindicated during acute recovery phase of MI, in patients hypersensitive to drug, and within 14 days of MAO inhibitor therapy.
- Use cautiously in patients with history of seizures, urine retention, prostatic hypertrophy, angle-closure glaucoma, or increased intraocular pressure; in those with hyperthyroidism, CV disease, diabetes, or impaired liver function; and in those receiving thyroid medications.
⚠ **Lifespan:** In pregnant women, use cautiously. In breast-feeding women, drug is contraindicated. In children younger than age 12, don't use drug. In elderly patients, who may experience increased falls and increased anticholinergic effects while taking this drug, use cautiously.

Adverse reactions

CNS: *drowsiness,* dizziness, excitation, tremors, weakness, confusion, headache, *CVA,* nervousness, EEG alterations, *seizures,* extrapyramidal reactions.
CV: *orthostatic hypotension,* tachycardia, ECG changes, hypertension, *MI, arrhythmias.*

EENT: blurred vision, tinnitus, mydriasis.
GI: *dry mouth, constipation,* nausea, vomiting, anorexia, paralytic ileus.
GU: *urine retention.*
Hematologic: *agranulocytosis, thrombocytopenia.*
Skin: diaphoresis, rash, urticaria, photosensitivity reaction.
Other: hypersensitivity reactions.

Interactions

Drug-drug. *Barbiturates, CNS depressants:* May enhance CNS depression. Avoid using together.
Cimetidine, methylphenidate: May increase tricyclic antidepressant level. Monitor patient for enhanced antidepressant effect.
Clonidine: May cause loss of blood pressure control with potentially life threatening elevations in blood pressure. Don't use together.
Epinephrine, norepinephrine: May increase hypertensive effect. Use cautiously.
Guanethidine: May antagonize antihypertensive action of guanethidine. Monitor patient.
MAO inhibitors: Especially at high dosage, may cause severe excitation, hyperpyrexia, or seizures. Avoid using within 14 days of each other.
Drug-herb. *St. John's wort, SAMe, yohimbe:* May cause serotonin level to become too high. Discourage using together.
Drug-lifestyle. *Alcohol use:* May enhance CNS depression. Discourage using together.
Smoking: May lower drug level. Monitor patient for lack of effect.
Sun exposure: May increase risk of photosensitivity reactions. Advise against prolonged or unprotected sun exposure.

Effects on lab test results

- May increase or decrease glucose level.
- May increase liver function test values and eosinophil count. May decrease granulocyte, platelet, and WBC counts.

Pharmacokinetics

Absorption: Rapid.
Distribution: Distributed widely into body, including CNS and breast milk. Drug is 96% protein-bound.
Metabolism: By liver to active metabolite nortriptyline; significant first-pass effect may ac-

count for variable levels in different patients taking same dosage.
Excretion: Primarily in urine.

Route	Onset	Peak	Duration
P.O., I.M.	Unknown	2-12 hr	Unknown

Action

Chemical effect: Unknown, but tricyclic antidepressant increases norepinephrine, serotonin, or both in CNS by blocking their reuptake by presynaptic neurons.
Therapeutic effect: Relieves depression.

Available forms

Syrup: 10 mg/5 ml
Tablets: 10 mg, 25 mg, 50 mg, 75 mg, 100 mg, 150 mg

NURSING PROCESS

🔬 Assessment
• Assess patient's depression before therapy.
• Be alert for adverse reactions and drug interactions.
• Evaluate patient's and family's knowledge of drug therapy.

💬 Nursing diagnoses
• Ineffective individual coping related to depression
• Risk for injury related to adverse CNS reactions
• Deficient knowledge related to drug therapy

▶ Planning and implementation
• Oral therapy should replace injection as soon as possible.
• Give full dose h.s. when possible.
• Don't withdraw drug abruptly.
• If signs of psychosis occur or increase, reduce dosage. Allow patient only minimum supply of drug.
• Because hypertensive episodes may occur during surgery in patients receiving tricyclic antidepressants, drug should be gradually stopped several days before surgery.
⚠ **ALERT:** Don't confuse amitriptyline with nortriptyline or aminophylline, Elavil with Equanil or Mellaril, or Endep with Depen.
Patient teaching
• Advise patient to take full dose h.s., but warn him of possible morning orthostatic hypotension.

• Tell patient to avoid using alcohol and smoking while taking drug.
• Warn patient to avoid hazardous activities until full CNS effects of drug are known. Drowsiness and dizziness usually subside after a few weeks.
• Advise patient to consult prescriber before taking other prescription drugs, OTC medications, or herbal remedies.
• Teach patient to relieve dry mouth with sugarless hard candy or gum. Saliva substitutes may be needed.
• Advise patient to use sunblock, wear protective clothing, and avoid prolonged exposure to strong sunlight.
• Warn patient not to stop drug therapy abruptly. After abrupt withdrawal of long-term therapy, patient may experience nausea, headache, and malaise. These symptoms don't indicate addiction.
• Tell patient to watch for urine retention and constipation. Instruct him to increase fluids and suggest stool softener or high-fiber diet, p.r.n.
• Advise patient that effects of drug may be apparent for 2 to 3 weeks.

✅ Evaluation
• Patient's behavior and communication indicate improvement of depression.
• Patient doesn't experience injury from CNS adverse reactions.
• Patient and family state understanding of drug therapy.

amlodipine besylate
(am-LOH-dih-peen BES-eh-layt)
Norvasc

Pharmacologic class: dihydropyridine calcium channel blocker
Therapeutic class: antianginal, antihypertensive
Pregnancy risk category: C

Indications and dosages

▶ **Chronic stable angina; vasospastic angina (Prinzmetal's [variant] angina).** *Adults:* Initially, 10 mg P.O. daily.
◻ **Adjust-a-dose:** For small, frail, or elderly patients or patients with hepatic insufficiency, begin therapy at 5 mg daily. Most patients need 10 mg daily for adequate results.

▶ **Hypertension.** *Adults:* Initially, 5 mg P.O. daily.

◈ **Adjust-a-dose:** For small, frail, or elderly patients, patients currently receiving other antihypertensives, and patients with hepatic insufficiency, begin therapy at 2.5 mg daily. Dosage adjusted based on patient response and tolerance. Maximum, 10 mg daily.

Contraindications and precautions

• Contraindicated in patients hypersensitive to drug.
• Use cautiously in patients receiving other peripheral vasodilators (especially those with severe aortic stenosis) and in those with heart failure.
• In patients with severe hepatic disease, use cautiously and in reduced dosage because drug is metabolized by liver.
※ **Lifespan:** In pregnant women, use cautiously. In breast-feeding women, drug is contraindicated. In children, safety of drug hasn't been established.

Adverse reactions

CNS: headache, fatigue, somnolence.
CV: edema, dizziness, flushing, palpitations.
GI: nausea, abdominal pain, dyspepsia.

Interactions

Drug-food. *Grapefruit juice:* May increase drug level and adverse effects. Tell patient not to take drug with grapefruit juice. However, if he has been stabilized on the drug while routinely drinking grapefruit juice, caution him not to abruptly stop doing so.

Effects on lab test results

None reported.

Pharmacokinetics

Absorption: Absolute bioavailability from 64% to 90%.
Distribution: About 93% of circulating drug is bound to plasma proteins.
Metabolism: About 90% of drug is converted to inactive metabolites in liver.
Excretion: Primarily in urine. *Half-life:* 30 to 50 hours.

Route	Onset	Peak	Duration
P.O.	Unknown	6-9 hr	24 hr

Action

Chemical effect: Inhibits calcium ion influx across cardiac and smooth-muscle cells, thus decreasing myocardial contractility and oxygen demand. Also dilates coronary arteries and arterioles.
Therapeutic effect: Reduces blood pressure and prevents angina.

Available forms

Tablets: 2.5 mg, 5 mg, 10 mg

NURSING PROCESS

⬛ **Assessment**
• Assess patient's blood pressure or angina before therapy and regularly thereafter.
• Monitor patient carefully for pain. In some patients, especially those with severe obstructive coronary artery disease, increased frequency, duration, or severity of angina or even acute MI has developed after start of calcium channel blocker therapy or at time of dosage increase.
• Be alert for adverse reactions.
• Evaluate patient's and family's knowledge of drug therapy.

⬛ **Nursing diagnoses**
• Acute pain related to increased oxygen demand in cardiac tissue
• Risk for injury related to hypertension
• Deficient knowledge related to drug therapy

⬛ **Planning and implementation**
• Adjust dosage based on patient response and tolerance.
• Give S.L. nitroglycerin as needed for acute angina.
⬤ **ALERT:** Don't confuse amlodipine with amiloride.
Patient teaching
• Tell patient that S.L. nitroglycerin may be taken as needed for acute angina. If patient continues nitrate therapy during adjustment of amlodipine dosage, urge continued compliance.
• Advise patient to continue taking drug even when feeling better.

⬛ **Evaluation**
• Patient's blood pressure is normal.
• Patient states anginal pain occurs with less frequency and severity.

• Patient and family state understanding of drug therapy.

amoxicillin and clavulanate potassium

(uh-moks-uh-SIL-in and KLAV-yoo-lan-ayt poh-TAH-see-um)
Augmentin, Augmentin ES-600, Augmentin XR, Clavulin ◆

Pharmacologic class: aminopenicillin, beta-lactamase inhibitor
Therapeutic class: antibiotic
Pregnancy risk category: B

Indications and dosages

▶ **Lower respiratory tract infections, otitis media, sinusitis, skin and skin-structure infections, and UTI caused by susceptible strains of gram-positive and gram-negative organisms.** *Adults:* 250 mg (based on amoxicillin component) P.O. q 8 hours. For more severe infections, 500 mg q 8 hours, or 875 mg P.O. q 12 hours.
Children: 20 to 40 mg/kg (based on amoxicillin component) P.O. daily in divided doses q 8 hours.
Neonates and infants younger than age 12 weeks: 30 mg/kg (based on amoxicillin component) P.O. daily in divided doses q 12 hours.
▶ **Recurrent or persistent acute otitis media caused by Streptococcus pneumoniae, Haemophilus influenzae, or Moraxella catarrhalis, in children with antibiotic exposure within the previous 3 months and who either are age 2 or younger or attend daycare.** *Infants and children ages 3 months to 12 years:* 90 mg/kg daily Augmentin ES-600 (based on amoxicillin component) P.O. q 12 hours for 10 days. Experience with this drug in patients weighing 40 kg (88 lb) or more is unavailable.
▶ **Community-acquired pneumonia or acute bacterial sinusitis due to confirmed, or suspected beta-lactamase producing pathogens (H. influenzae, M. catarrhalis, H. parainfluenzae, K. pneumoniae, or methicillin-susceptible S. aureus) and S. pneumoniae with reduced susceptibility to penicillin.** *Adults and children age 16 and older:* 2,000 mg/125 mg Augmentin XR q 12 hours for 7 to 10 days for pneumonia, or 10 days for sinusitis. Take with meals.

Contraindications and precautions

• Contraindicated in patients hypersensitive to drug or other penicillins and in those with a history of amoxicillin-related cholestatic jaundice or hepatic dysfunction.
• Augmentin XR is contraindicated in patients with renal impairment and a creatinine clearance less than 30 ml/minute and in hemodialysis patients. Augmentin XR is also contraindicated for the treatment of infections due to *S. pneumoniae* with penicillin MICs 4 mcg/ml or more.
• Use cautiously in patients with other drug allergies, especially to cephalosporins (possible cross-sensitivity), and in those with mononucleosis (high risk of maculopapular rash) or hepatic impairment.
⚹ **Lifespan:** In pregnant and breast-feeding women, use cautiously. In children younger than age 16, safety and efficacy of Augmentin XR haven't been established.

Adverse reactions

CNS: agitation, anxiety, insomnia, confusion, behavioral changes, dizziness.
GI: nausea, vomiting, *diarrhea*, indigestion, gastritis, stomatitis, glossitis, mucocutaneous candidiasis, abdominal pain, black "hairy" tongue, enterocolitis, *pseudomembranous colitis.*
GU: vaginitis, vaginal candidiasis.
Hematologic: anemia, *thrombocytopenia, thrombocytopenic purpura,* eosinophilia, *leukopenia, agranulocytosis.*
Other: hypersensitivity reactions (*rash,* urticaria, pruritus, *angioedema, anaphylaxis*), overgrowth of nonsusceptible organisms, serum sickness-like reactions (urticaria or skin rash accompanied by arthritis, arthralgia, myalgia and frequently fever).

Interactions

Drug-drug. *Allopurinol:* May cause rash. Monitor patient.
Probenecid: May increase level of amoxicillin and other penicillins. Probenecid may be used for this purpose.

Effects on lab test results

• May increase eosinophil count. May decrease hemoglobin, hematocrit, and granulocyte, platelet, and WBC counts.

• May cause false-positive urine glucose determinations with copper sulfate tests, such as Benedict's solution and Clinitest.

Pharmacokinetics

Absorption: Well absorbed.

Distribution: Both drugs are distributed into pleural fluid, lungs, and peritoneal fluid, with high urine levels. Amoxicillin also is distributed into synovial fluid, liver, prostate, muscle, and gallbladder and penetrates into middle ear effusions, maxillary sinus secretions, tonsils, sputum, and bronchial secretions. Both drugs have minimal protein-binding.

Metabolism: Amoxicillin is metabolized only partially; clavulanate potassium, extensively.

Excretion: Amoxicillin is excreted principally in urine; clavulanate potassium is excreted by glomerular filtration. *Half-life:* Amoxicillin, 1 to 1½ hours (7½ hours in severe renal impairment); clavulanate, about 1 to 1½ hours (4½ hours in severe renal impairment).

Route	Onset	Peak	Duration
P.O.	Unknown	1-2½ hr	6-8 hr
P.O. Augmentin ES-600	Unknown	1-4 hr	Unknown
Augmentin XR	Unknown	1-6 hr	Unknown

Action

Chemical effect: Prevents bacterial cell-wall synthesis during replication. Clavulanic acid increases amoxicillin's effectiveness by inactivating beta lactamases, which destroy amoxicillin.

Therapeutic effect: Kills susceptible bacteria.

Available forms

Oral suspension: 125 mg amoxicillin trihydrate and 31.25 mg clavulanic acid/5 ml (after reconstitution); 200 mg amoxicillin trihydrate and 28.5 mg clavulanic acid/5 ml (after reconstitution); 250 mg amoxicillin trihydrate and 62.5 mg clavulanic acid/5 ml (after reconstitution); 400 mg amoxicillin trihydrate and 57 mg clavulanic acid/5 ml (after reconstitution); 600 mg amoxicillin trihydrate and 42.9 mg clavulanic acid/5 ml (after reconstitution)

Tablets: 875 mg amoxicillin trihydrate, 125 mg clavulanic acid

Tablets (chewable): 125 mg amoxicillin trihydrate, 31.25 mg clavulanic acid; 200 mg amoxicillin trihydrate, 28.5 mg clavulanic acid; 250 mg amoxicillin trihydrate, 62.5 mg clavulanic acid; 400 mg amoxicillin trihydrate, 57 mg clavulanic acid

Tablets (extended-release): 1,000 mg amoxicillin trihydrate, 62.5 mg clavulanic acid

Tablets (film-coated): 250 mg amoxicillin trihydrate, 125 mg clavulanic acid; 500 mg amoxicillin trihydrate, 125 mg clavulanic acid

NURSING PROCESS

☒ Assessment

• Before therapy begins, assess patient's infection, ask him about past allergic reactions to penicillin (although negative history is no guarantee against allergic reaction), and obtain specimen for culture and sensitivity tests. Therapy may begin pending results.

• Be alert for adverse reactions and drug interactions.

• Monitor hydration status if adverse GI reactions occur.

• Evaluate patient's and family's knowledge of drug therapy.

⊞ Nursing diagnoses

• Infection related to susceptible bacteria
• Risk for deficient fluid volume related to drug-induced adverse GI reactions
• Deficient knowledge related to drug therapy

▶ Planning and implementation

• Give drug with food to prevent GI distress. Adverse effects, especially diarrhea, are more common than with amoxicillin alone.

• Give drug at least 1 hour before bacteriostatic antibiotics.

⊕ **ALERT:** Both 250-mg and 500-mg film-coated tablets contain 125 mg of clavulanic acid. Therefore, two 250-mg film-coated tablets don't equal one 500-mg film-coated tablet. Also, don't interchange the oral suspensions because of clavulanic acid content.

⊕ **ALERT:** Augmentin ES-600 is intended for children only.

• This drug combination is particularly useful with amoxicillin-resistant organisms.

• After reconstitution, refrigerate oral suspension and discard after 10 days.

⊕ **ALERT:** Don't confuse amoxicillin with amoxapine.

⊛ **ALERT:** Augmentin (250 mg or 500 mg amoxicillin) and Augmentin XR extended-release tablets aren't interchangeable because of the different amounts of clavulanic acid in each and the fact that Augmentin XR is an extended-release formulation. Don't give 2 Augmentin 500 mg tablets to replace 1 Augmentin XR 1,000 mg tablet.

Patient teaching
• Tell patient to take entire quantity of drug exactly as prescribed, even after he feels better.
• Tell patient to call prescriber if rash develops (sign of allergic reaction).
• Instruct patient to take drug with food to prevent GI distress.

☑ **Evaluation**
• Patient is free from infection.
• Patient maintains adequate hydration.
• Patient and family state understanding of drug therapy.

---

amoxicillin trihydrate (amoxycillin trihydrate)

(uh-moks-uh-SIL-in trigh-HIGH-drayt)
Alphamox ◇ **, Amoxil, Apo-Amoxi** ◆ **, Cilamox** ◇ **, DisperMox, Moxacin** ◇ **, Novamoxin** ◆ **, Nu-Amoxi** ◆ **, Trimox**

Pharmacologic class: aminopenicillin
Therapeutic class: antibiotic
Pregnancy risk category: B

Indications and dosages

▶ **Systemic infections, acute and chronic UTI caused by susceptible strains of gram-positive and gram-negative organisms.**
Adults: 250 mg P.O. q 8 hours.
Children: 20 to 40 mg/kg P.O. daily, divided into doses given q 8 hours.
Adults and children weighing more than 20 kg (44 lb) who have severe infections or infections caused by susceptible organisms: 500 mg P.O. q 8 hours or 875 mg P.O. q 12 hours may be needed.
▶ **Uncomplicated gonorrhea.** *Adults:* 3 g P.O. as a single dose.
Children older than age 2: 50 mg/kg given with 25 mg/kg probenecid as a single dose.

▶ **Endocarditis prophylaxis for dental procedures.** *Adults:* Initially, 3 g P.O. 1 hour before procedure; then 1.5 g 6 hours later.
Children: Initially, 50 mg/kg P.O. 1 hour before procedure; then half of initial dose 6 hours later.
▶ ***Helicobacter pylori* eradication to reduce the risk of duodenal ulcer with clarithromycin or lansoprazole.** *Adults:* For dual therapy, amoxicillin 1 g P.O. and lansoprazole 30 mg P.O., each q 8 hours for 14 days. For triple therapy, amoxicillin 1 g P.O., clarithromycin 500 mg P.O., lansoprazole 30 mg P.O.; each q 12 hours for 14 days.
▶ **Postexposure prophylaxis to penicillin-susceptible anthrax.** *Adults and children age 9 and older:* 500 mg P.O. t.i.d. for 60 days.
Children younger than age 9: 80 mg/kg daily P.O., divided t.i.d. for 60 days.
▶ **Lyme disease‡.** *Adults:* 250 to 500 mg P.O. t.i.d. or q.i.d. for 10 to 30 days.
Children: 25 to 50 mg/kg daily (maximum, 1 to 2 g daily) P.O. in three divided doses for 10 to 30 days.
▶ **Acute complicated UTI in nonpregnant women‡.** *Adults:* 3 g P.O. as a single dose.

Contraindications and precautions

• Contraindicated in patients hypersensitive to drug or other penicillins.
• Use cautiously in patients with other drug allergies, especially to cephalosporins (possible cross-sensitivity), and in those with mononucleosis (high risk of maculopapular rash).
⚘ **Lifespan:** In pregnant or breast-feeding women, use cautiously.

Adverse reactions

CNS: *seizures.*
GI: nausea, vomiting, diarrhea.
Hematologic: anemia, *thrombocytopenia, thrombocytopenic purpura,* eosinophilia, *leukopenia, agranulocytosis.*
Other: hypersensitivity reactions (erythematous maculopapular rash, urticaria, *anaphylaxis*), overgrowth of nonsusceptible organisms.

Interactions

Drug-drug. *Allopurinol:* May increase risk of rash. Monitor patient.
Probenecid: May increase level of amoxicillin and other penicillins. Probenecid may be used for this purpose.

Effects on lab test results
• May increase eosinophil count. May decrease hemoglobin, hematocrit, and granulocyte, platelet, and WBC counts.
• May cause false-positive urine glucose determinations with copper sulfate tests (such as Benedict's solution and Clinitest).

Pharmacokinetics
Absorption: About 80%.
Distribution: Distributed into pleural, peritoneal, and synovial fluids; lungs; prostate; muscle; liver; and gallbladder. Also penetrates middle ear, maxillary sinus and bronchial secretions, tonsils, and sputum. Amoxicillin readily crosses placenta and is 17% to 20% protein-bound.
Metabolism: Only partially metabolized.
Excretion: Principally in urine by renal tubular secretion and glomerular filtration; also excreted in breast milk. *Half-life:* 1 to 1½ hours (7½ hours in severe renal impairment).

Route	Onset	Peak	Duration
P.O.	Unknown	1-2 hr	6-8 hr

Action
Chemical effect: Inhibits cell-wall synthesis during bacterial multiplication.
Therapeutic effect: Kills susceptible bacteria.

Available forms
Capsules: 250 mg, 500 mg
Pediatric drops: 50 mg/ml (after reconstitution)
Suspension: 125 mg/5 ml, 200 mg/5 ml, 250 mg/5 ml, 400 mg/5 ml
Tablets (chewable): 200 mg, 400 mg
Tablets (film-coated): 500 mg, 875 mg
Tablets (for oral suspension): 200 mg, 400 mg, 600 mg

NURSING PROCESS

⚏ Assessment
• Before therapy, assess patient's infection, ask him about allergic reactions to drug or other forms of penicillin (although negative history doesn't guarantee against future reaction), and obtain specimen for culture and sensitivity tests. Therapy may begin pending test results.
• Be alert for adverse reactions and drug interactions.

• Monitor patient's hydration status if adverse GI reactions occur.
• Evaluate patient's and family's knowledge of drug therapy.

⚏ Nursing diagnoses
• Infection related to susceptible bacteria
• Risk for deficient fluid volume related to drug-induced adverse GI reactions
• Deficient knowledge related to drug therapy

⚏ Planning and implementation
• Give amoxicillin at least 1 hour before bacteriostatic antibiotics.
• May be taken with or without food.
• Trimox oral suspension may be stored at room temperature for up to 2 weeks. Check individual product labels for storage information.
• For DisperMox, mix 1 tablet in 10 ml of water and have patient drink mixture. Rinse container with a small amount of water to make sure the entire table is taken. Don't let the patient chew, swallow, or allow tablet to dissolve in mouth.
⚏ **ALERT:** Don't confuse amoxicillin with amoxapine.
Patient teaching
• If drug allergy develops, advise patient to wear or carry medical identification stating penicillin allergy.
• Tell patient to take entire quantity of drug exactly as prescribed, even after he feels better.
• Tell patient to call prescriber if rash (most common), fever, or chills develop.
• Inform patient drug may be taken with or without food.
• Warn patient never to use leftover amoxicillin for a new illness or to share it with others.

⚏ Evaluation
• Patient is free from infection.
• Patient maintains adequate hydration.
• Patient and family state understanding of drug therapy.

amphotericin B
(am-foh-TER-ah-sin bee)
Fungilin Oral ◆ , Fungizone Intravenous

Pharmacologic class: polyene macrolide
Therapeutic class: antifungal
Pregnancy risk category: B

Indications and dosages

▶ **Systemic fungal infections (histoplasmosis, coccidioidomycosis, blastomycosis, cryptococcosis, disseminated candidiasis, aspergillosis, mucormycosis).** *Adults:* Test dose of 1 mg I.V. in 20 ml of D₅W infused over 20 to 30 minutes is recommended. If tolerated, start daily dosage at 0.25 to 0.3 mg/kg by slow I.V. infusion (0.1 mg/ml) over 2 to 6 hours. Increase dose gradually, as patient develops tolerance, to maximum of 1 mg/kg daily. Don't exceed 1.5 mg/kg daily. Alternate-day dosing is recommended for total daily doses of 1.5 mg/kg. If drug is stopped for 1 week or longer, resume with initial dose and increase gradually.

▶ **Fungal endocarditis, fungal septicemia‡.** *Adults and children:* Test dose of 1 mg I.V. in 20 ml of D₅W infused over 20 minutes. If patient tolerates initial test dose, then give daily dose of 0.25 to 0.3 mg/kg, gradually increasing by 5 to 10 mg daily until daily dose is 1 mg/kg or 1.5 mg/kg q alternate day. Duration of therapy depends on severity and nature of infection.

▶ **Infections of GI tract caused by *Candida albicans.*** *Adults:* 100 mg P.O. q.i.d. for 2 weeks.

▶ **Oral and perioral candidal infections.** *Adults:* 1 lozenge q.i.d. for 7 to 14 days. Tell patient to allow lozenge to dissolve slowly.

▶ **Candidal cystitis‡.** *Adults:* Bladder irrigation in levels of 5 to 50 mcg/ml instilled periodically or continuously for 5 to 7 days.

▶ **Prophylaxis of fungal infection in bone marrow transplant recipients‡.** *Adults:* 0.1 mg/kg/day as I.V. infusion.

▼ I.V. administration

• Reconstitute with 10 ml sterile water only. To avoid precipitation, don't mix with solutions containing sodium chloride, other electrolytes, or bacteriostatic drugs (such as benzyl alcohol). Don't use if solution contains precipitate or foreign matter.

• Give drug parenterally only in hospitalized patients, under close supervision, after diagnosis of potentially fatal fungal infection is confirmed. Be prepared to give an initial test dose; 1 mg is added to 20 ml of D₅W and infused over 20 to 30 minutes.

• Use an infusion pump and in-line filter with a mean pore diameter larger than 1 micron. Infuse over 2 to 6 hours; rapid infusion may cause CV collapse.

• Use I.V. sites in distal veins. If thrombosis occurs, alternate sites.

• Reconstituted solution is stable for 1 week in refrigerator, 24 hours at room temperature, and 8 hours in room light.

• Give antibiotics separately; don't mix or piggyback with amphotericin B.

• Amphotericin B appears to be compatible with limited amounts of heparin sodium, hydrocortisone sodium succinate, and methylprednisolone sodium succinate.

• Store dry form at 36° to 46° F (2° to 8° C). Protect from light.

Ⓢ**ALERT:** If patient has severe adverse infusion reactions to initial dose, stop infusion and notify prescriber and give antipyretics, antihistamines, antiemetics, or small doses of corticosteroids. To prevent reactions during subsequent infusions, premedicate with these drugs or give amphotericin B on an alternate-day schedule.

Contraindications and precautions

• Contraindicated in patients hypersensitive to drug.

• Use cautiously in patients with impaired renal function.

⚖ **Lifespan:** In pregnant women, use cautiously. In breast-feeding women, drug is contraindicated. In children, safety of drug hasn't been fully established, but therapy has been successful.

Adverse reactions

CNS: fever, malaise, headache, peripheral neuropathy, *seizures,* peripheral nerve pain, paresthesia (with I.V. use).
CV: hypotension, *arrhythmias, asystole,* phlebitis, thrombophlebitis.
GI: anorexia, weight loss, nausea, vomiting, dyspepsia, diarrhea, epigastric cramps, *hemorrhagic gastroenteritis.*
GU: abnormal renal function with hypokalemia, azotemia, hyposthenuria, hypomagnesemia, renal tubular acidosis, nephrocalcinosis, *permanent renal impairment,* anuria, oliguria.
Hematologic: normochromic normocytic anemia, *thrombocytopenia, agranulocytosis.*
Hepatic: *acute liver failure.*
Metabolic: hypokalemia.
Musculoskeletal: arthralgia, myalgia.
Skin: burning, stinging, irritation, tissue damage with extravasation, pain at injection site.

Other: chills, generalized pain; *anaphylactoid reactions.*

Interactions

Drug-drug. *Corticosteroids:* May cause potassium depletion. Monitor potassium level.
Digoxin: May increase risk of digitalis toxicity in potassium-depleted patients. Monitor patient closely.
Flucytosine: May increase flucytosine toxicity. Monitor patient closely.
Other nephrotoxic drugs (such as antibiotics, antineoplastics): May increase risk of nephrotoxicity. Give cautiously.
Skeletal muscle relaxants: May increase effects of muscle relaxants. Monitor patient for increased effects.
Thiazide diuretics: May increase potassium loss. Monitor patient for signs of hypokalemia; monitor potassium level.

Effects on lab test results

● May increase urine urea, uric acid, BUN, creatinine, alkaline phosphatase, ALT, AST, GGT, LDH, and bilirubin levels. May decrease potassium and magnesium levels. May increase or decrease glucose level.
● May decrease platelet and granulocyte counts, hemoglobin, and hematocrit. May increase or decrease WBC and eosinophil counts.

Pharmacokinetics

Absorption: Poor.
Distribution: Distributed well into pleural cavities and joints; less so into aqueous humor, bronchial secretions, pancreas, bone, muscle, and parotid gland. Drug is 90% to 95% bound to plasma proteins.
Metabolism: Not well defined.
Excretion: Up to 5% excreted unchanged in urine. *Half-life:* Initially, 24 hours; second phase, about 15 days.

Route	Onset	Peak	Duration
P.O.	Unknown	Unknown	Unknown
I.V.	Immediate	Immediate	Unknown

Action

Chemical effect: May bind to sterol in fungal cell membrane and alter cell permeability, allowing leakage of intracellular components.
Therapeutic effect: Decreases activity of or kills susceptible fungi.

Available forms

Lozenges: 10 mg ◇
Oral suspension: 100 mg/ml ◇
Powder for injection: 50-mg lyophilized cake

NURSING PROCESS

⚕ Assessment

● Obtain history of fungal infection and samples for culture and sensitivity tests before first dose. Reevaluate condition during therapy.
● Be alert for adverse reactions and drug interactions.
● Monitor patient's pulse, respiratory rate, temperature, and blood pressure every 30 minutes for at least 4 hours after giving drug I.V.; fever, shaking chills, anorexia, nausea, vomiting, headache, tachypnea, and hypotension may appear 1 to 3 hours after start of I.V. infusion. Symptoms are usually more severe with initial doses.
● Monitor BUN, creatinine or creatinine clearance, and electrolyte levels; CBC; and liver function test results at least weekly.
● Drug is linked to rhinocerebral phycomycosis, especially in patients with uncontrolled diabetes. Leukoencephalopathy also may occur. Monitor pulmonary function. Acute reactions are characterized by dyspnea, hypoxemia, and infiltrates.
● Evaluate patient's and family's knowledge of drug therapy.

⚕ Nursing diagnoses

● Infection related to presence of susceptible fungal infection
● Risk for injury related to drug-induced adverse reactions
● Deficient knowledge related to drug therapy

▶ Planning and implementation

● Lozenge form of drug should be dissolved slowly.
● **ALERT:** Different amphotericin B preparations aren't interchangeable, and dosages vary.
● If BUN level exceeds 40 mg/dl, or if creatinine level exceeds 3 mg/dl, prescriber may reduce or stop drug until renal function improves. Drug may be stopped if alkaline phosphatase or bilirubin level increases.

Patient teaching
• Teach patient signs and symptoms of hypersensitivity, and stress importance of reporting them immediately.
• Warn patient that therapy may take several months; teach personal hygiene and other measures to prevent spread and recurrence of lesions.
• Urge patient to comply with prescribed regimen and recommended follow-up.
• With oral form, instruct patient to let lozenges dissolve slowly.
• With I.V. therapy, warn patient that discomfort at injection site and adverse reactions may occur during therapy, which may last several months.

☑ **Evaluation**
• Patient is free from fungal infection.
• Patient doesn't experience injury as a result of drug-induced adverse reactions.
• Patient and family state understanding of drug therapy.

amphotericin B lipid complex
(am-foe-TER-ah-sin bee LIP-id KOM-pleks)
Abelcet

Pharmacologic class: polyene antibiotic
Therapeutic class: antifungal
Pregnancy risk category: B

Indications and dosages
▶ **Treatment of invasive fungal infections** including *Aspergillus fumigatus, Candida albicans, C. guillermondii, C. stellatoideae,* and *C. tropicalis, Coccidioidomyces sp., Cryptococcus sp., Histoplasma sp.,* and *Blastomyces sp.* **in patients refractory to or intolerant of conventional amphotericin B therapy.**
Adults and children: 5 mg/kg daily as a single I.V. infusion. Give by continuous I.V. infusion at 2.5 mg/kg/hour.

▼ I.V. administration
• To prepare, shake the vial gently until you see no yellow sediment. Using aseptic technique, draw the calculated dose into one or more 20-ml syringes, using an 18G needle. You'll need more than one vial. Attach a 5-micron filter needle to the syringe and inject the dose into an I.V. bag of D₅W. One filter needle can be used for up to four vials of drug. The volume of D₅W should

be sufficient to yield a final concentration of 1 mg/ml.
• For children and patients with CV disease, the recommended final concentration is 2 mg/ml.
• Shake the bag and check the contents for foreign matter.
• Don't mix with saline solution or infuse in the same I.V. line as other drugs. Don't use an in-line filter.
• If infusing through an existing I.V. line, flush first with D₅W.
• Infusions are stable for up to 48 hours when refrigerated at 36° to 46° F (2° to 8° C) and for up to 6 hours at room temperature.
• Refrigerate and protect from light. Don't freeze.
• Discard unused drug; it contains no preservatives.
• Slowing the infusion rate also may decrease the risk of infusion-related reactions.
• For infusions lasting longer than 2 hours, shake the I.V. bag every 2 hours to ensure an even suspension.

Contraindications and precautions
• Contraindicated in patients hypersensitive to amphotericin B or its components.
• Use cautiously in patients with renal impairment.
⚖ **Lifespan:** In pregnant women, safety hasn't been established; use only if benefits outweigh risks to the fetus. In breast-feeding women, a decision must be made to stop breast-feeding or stop drug.

Adverse reactions
CNS: fever, headache, pain.
CV: chest pain, *cardiac arrest*, hypertension, hypotension.
GI: abdominal pain, diarrhea, nausea, vomiting, *GI hemorrhage.*
GU: *renal failure.*
Hematologic: anemia, *leukopenia, thrombocytopenia.*
Hepatic: bilirubinemia.
Metabolic: hypokalemia.
Respiratory: dyspnea, respiratory disorder, *respiratory failure.*
Skin: rash.
Other: chills, infection, MULTIPLE ORGAN FAILURE, *sepsis.*

Interactions

Drug-drug. *Antineoplastics:* May increase risk of renal toxicity, bronchospasm, and hypotension. Use cautiously.

Digoxin: May increase risk of digoxin toxicity and induced hypokalemia. Monitor potassium level closely.

Corticosteroids, corticotropin: May enhance hypokalemia, which may lead to cardiac dysfunction. Monitor electrolytes and cardiac function.

Cyclosporin A: May increase renal toxicity. Monitor patient closely.

Flucytosine: May increase risk of flucytosine toxicity due to increased cellular uptake or impaired renal excretion. Use cautiously.

Imidazoles (clotrimazole, fluconazole, itraconazole, ketoconazole, miconazole): May decrease efficacy of amphotericin B because of inhibition of ergosterol synthesis. Clinical significance is unknown.

Leukocyte transfusions: May cause acute pulmonary toxicity. Avoid using together.

Nephrotoxic drugs (aminoglycosides, pentamidine): May increase risk of renal toxicity. Use cautiously. Monitor renal function closely.

Skeletal muscle relaxants: May enhance effects of skeletal muscle relaxants because of drug-induced hypokalemia. Monitor potassium level closely.

Zidovudine: May increase myelotoxicity and nephrotoxicity. Monitor renal and hematologic function.

Effects on lab test results

- May increase BUN, creatinine, alkaline phosphatase, ALT, AST, bilirubin, GGT, and LDH levels. May decrease potassium level.
- May decrease hemoglobin, hematocrit, and WBC and platelet counts.

Pharmacokinetics

Absorption: Administered I.V.
Distribution: Well distributed. Volume increases with dose. Amphotericin B lipid complex yields measurable amphotericin B levels in spleen, lung, liver, lymph nodes, kidney, heart, and brain.
Metabolism: Unknown.
Excretion: Although rapidly cleared from blood, amphotericin B lipid complex has a terminal half-life of about a week, probably because of slow elimination from tissues.

Route	Onset	Peak	Duration
I.V.	Unknown	Unknown	Unknown

Action

Chemical effect: Amphotericin B binds to sterols in fungal cell membranes, resulting in enhanced cellular permeability and cell damage. It has fungistatic or fungicidal effects, depending on fungal susceptibility.
Therapeutic effect: Decreases activity of or kills susceptible fungi.

Available forms

Suspension for injection: 50 mg/10-ml vial; 100 mg/20-ml vial

NURSING PROCESS

⚷ Assessment

- Obtain history of fungal infection and samples for culture and sensitivity tests before therapy. Reevaluate condition during therapy.
- Be alert for adverse reactions and drug interactions.
- Assess renal function before therapy starts.
- Monitor liver function, creatinine, and electrolyte levels (especially magnesium and potassium), and CBC during therapy.
- Evaluate patient's and family's knowledge of drug therapy.

⟐ Nursing diagnoses

- Risk for infection related to presence of susceptible fungal infection
- Risk for injury related to drug-induced adverse reactions
- Deficient knowledge related to drug therapy

⟩ Planning and implementation

- If severe respiratory distress develops, stop the infusion, provide supportive therapy for anaphylaxis, and notify prescriber. Don't resume the infusion.
- ⊛ **ALERT:** Different amphotericin B preparations aren't interchangeable, and dosages vary.
- Premedicate patient with acetaminophen, antihistamines, and corticosteroids to prevent or lessen the severity of infusion-related reactions, such as fever, chills, nausea, and vomiting, which occur 1 to 2 hours after the start of infusion.

Patient teaching
- Inform patient that fever, chills, nausea, and vomiting may occur during the infusion and that

---

these reactions usually subside with subsequent doses.

• Instruct patient to report any redness or pain at the infusion site.

• Teach patient to recognize and report any symptoms of acute hypersensitivity, such as respiratory distress.

• Tell patient to expect frequent laboratory testing to monitor kidney and liver function.

☑ **Evaluation**

• Patient is free from fungal infection.

• Patient has no injury from adverse drug reactions.

• Patient and family state understanding of drug therapy.

amphotericin B liposomal
(am-foh-TER-ah-sin bee lye-po-SO-mal)
AmBisome

Pharmacologic class: polyene antibiotic
Therapeutic class: antifungal
Pregnancy risk category: B

Indications and dosages

▶ **Empirical therapy for presumed fungal infection in febrile, neutropenic patients.** *Adults and children:* 3 mg/kg I.V. infusion daily.

▶ **Systemic fungal infections caused by** *Aspergillus sp., Candida sp.,* **or** *Cryptococcus sp.* **refractory to amphotericin B deoxycholate or in patients with renal impairment or unacceptable toxicity that precludes the use of amphotericin B deoxycholate.** *Adults and children:* 3 to 5 mg/kg I.V. infusion daily.

▶ **Visceral leishmaniasis in immunocompetent patients.** *Adults and children:* 3 mg/kg I.V. infusion daily on days 1 to 5, 14, and 21. A repeat course of therapy may be beneficial if initial treatment fails to achieve parasitic clearance.

▶ **Visceral leishmaniasis in immunocompromised patients.** *Adults and children:* 4 mg/kg I.V. infusion daily on days 1 to 5, 10, 17, 24, 31, and 38. Expert advice regarding further treatment is recommended if initial therapy fails or relapse occurs.

▶ **Cryptococcal meningitis in HIV-infected patients.** *Adults and children:* 6 mg/kg daily I.V. infusion over 2 hours. Infusion time may be reduced to 1 hour if well tolerated or increased if discomfort occurs.

▽ **I.V. administration**

• Reconstitute each 50-mg vial of amphotericin B liposomal with 12 ml of sterile water for injection to yield a solution of 4 mg amphotericin B per ml. Don't reconstitute with bacteriostatic water for injection, and don't allow bacteriostatic drug into the solution. Don't reconstitute with saline solution; instead, add saline solution to the reconstituted concentration, or mix with other drugs.

• After reconstitution, shake vial vigorously for 30 seconds or until particulate matter disappears. Withdraw calculated amount of reconstituted solution into a sterile syringe and inject through a 5-micron filter into the appropriate amount of D_5W to a final concentration of 1 to 2 mg/ml. Lower concentrations (0.2 to 0.5 mg/ml) may be appropriate for children to provide sufficient volume for infusion.

• Flush existing I.V. line with D_5W before infusing drug. If this isn't feasible, give drug through a separate line.

• Use a controlled infusion device and an in-line filter with a mean pore diameter larger than 1 micron. Initially, infuse drug over at least 2 hours. Infusion time may be reduced to 1 hour if the treatment is well tolerated. If the patient has discomfort during infusion, the duration of infusion may be increased.

• Observe patient closely for adverse reactions during infusion. If anaphylaxis occurs, stop the infusion immediately, provide supportive therapy, and notify the prescriber.

• Refrigerate unopened drug at 36° to 46° F (2° to 8° C). Once reconstituted, the product may be stored for up to 24 hours at 36° to 46° F (2° to 8° C). Don't freeze.

Contraindications and precautions

• Contraindicated in patients hypersensitive to drug or its components.

• Use cautiously in patients with renal impairment.

⚖ **Lifespan:** In pregnant women and elderly patients, use cautiously.

Adverse reactions

CNS: anxiety, confusion, fever, headache, insomnia, asthenia, pain.

CV: chest pain, hypotension, tachycardia, hypertension, edema, vasodilation.
EENT: *epistaxis,* rhinitis.
GI: *GI hemorrhage,* nausea, vomiting, abdominal pain, diarrhea.
GU: hematuria.
Hepatic: hepatomegaly.
Metabolic: hyperglycemia, hypernatremia, hypocalcemia, hypokalemia, hypomagnesemia.
Musculoskeletal: back pain.
Respiratory: cough, dyspnea, hypoxia, pleural effusion, lung disorder, hyperventilation.
Skin: *pruritus, rash,* sweating.
Other: chills, infection, *anaphylaxis, sepsis, blood product infusion reaction.*

Interactions

Drug-drug. *Antineoplastics:* May enhance potential for renal toxicity, bronchospasm, and hypotension. Use cautiously.
Corticosteroids, corticotropin: May potentiate hypokalemia, which could result in cardiac dysfunction. Monitor potassium level and cardiac function.
Digoxin: May increase risk of digoxin toxicity in potassium-depleted patients. Monitor potassium level closely.
Flucytosine: May increase flucytosine toxicity by increasing cellular uptake or impairing renal excretion of flucytosine. Monitor renal function closely.
Imidazole antifungals (clotrimazole, ketoconazole, miconazole): May induce fungal resistance to amphotericin B. Use combination therapy with caution.
Leukocyte transfusions: May increase risk of acute pulmonary toxicity. Avoid using together.
Other nephrotoxic drugs (antibiotics, antineoplastics): May increase risk of nephrotoxicity. Give cautiously. Monitor renal function closely.
Skeletal muscle relaxants: May enhance effects of skeletal muscle relaxants because of amphotericin-induced hypokalemia. Monitor potassium level.

Effects on lab test results

• May increase BUN, creatinine, glucose, sodium, alkaline phosphatase, ALT, AST, bilirubin, GGT, and LDH levels. May decrease potassium, calcium, and magnesium levels.

Pharmacokinetics

Absorption: Administered I.V.

Distribution: Unknown.
Metabolism: Unknown.
Excretion: Unknown. *Initial half-life:* 7 to 10 hours with 24 hour dosing; *terminal elimination half-life:* about 4 to 6 days.

Route	Onset	Peak	Duration
I.V.	Unknown	Unknown	Unknown

Action

Chemical effect: Binds to the sterol component of a fungal cell membrane, leading to alterations in cell permeability and to cell death.
Therapeutic effect: Decreases activity of or kills susceptible fungi. Treats visceral protozoal infections.

Available forms

Injection: 50-mg vial

NURSING PROCESS

⚕ Assessment

• Obtain history of fungal infection and samples for culture and sensitivity tests before therapy. Reevaluate condition during therapy.
• Carefully assess patients who are also receiving chemotherapy or bone marrow transplantation because they are at greater risk for additional adverse reactions, including seizures, arrhythmias, thrombocytopenia, and respiratory failure.
• Monitor CBC, liver function test results, and creatinine, BUN, and CBC and electrolyte levels, particularly magnesium and potassium.
• Monitor patient for signs of hypokalemia, such as ECG changes, muscle weakness, cramping, and drowsiness.
• Watch for adverse reactions. Patients who receive drug may have fewer chills, decreased BUN level, a lower risk of hypokalemia, and less vomiting than patients who receive regular amphotericin B.
• Evaluate patient's and family's knowledge of drug therapy.

⚕ Nursing diagnoses

• Risk for infection related to presence of susceptible fungal or parasite infections
• Risk for injury related to drug-induced adverse reactions
• Deficient knowledge related to drug therapy

⟩ Planning and implementation

⊛ **ALERT:** Different amphotericin B preparations aren't interchangeable, and dosages vary.

• To lessen the risk or severity of adverse reactions, premedicate patient with antipyretics, antihistamines, antiemetics, or corticosteroids.

• Therapy may take several weeks to months.

Patient teaching

• Teach patient signs and symptoms of hypersensitivity, and stress importance of reporting them immediately.

• Warn patient that therapy may take several months; teach personal hygiene and other measures to prevent spread and recurrence of lesions.

• Instruct patient to report adverse reactions.

• Instruct patient to watch for and report signs of hypokalemia, such as muscle weakness, cramping, and drowsiness.

• Advise patient that frequent laboratory testing will be performed.

✓ Evaluation

• Patient is free from fungal or parasite infection.

• Patient doesn't experience injury as a result of drug-induced adverse reactions.

• Patient and family state understanding of drug therapy.

---

ampicillin
(am-pih-SIL-in)
**Apo-Ampi ♦ , Novo-Ampicillin ♦ ,
Nu-Ampi ♦ , Omnipen, Principen**

ampicillin sodium
**Ampicin ♦ , Ampicyn Injection ◇ ,
Omnipen-N, Penbritin ♦ , Polycillin-N,
Totacillin-N**

ampicillin trihydrate
**Ampicyn Oral ◇ , D-Amp, Omnipen,
Penbritin ◇ , Polycillin, Principen 250,
Principen 500, Totacillin**

Pharmacologic class: aminopenicillin
Therapeutic class: antibiotic
Pregnancy risk category: B

Indications and dosages

▶ **Prophylaxis of neonatal group B streptococcus infections‡.** *Adults:* 2 g I.V. given to the mother 4 hours before delivery, then 1 to 2 g I.V. q 4 to 6 hours until delivery.

▶ **Meningitis.** *Adults:* 8 to 14 g (or 150 mg to 200 mg/kg) I.V. daily in divided doses q 3 to 4 hours.

Children ages 2 months to 12 years: Up to 400 mg/kg I.V. daily for 3 days; then up to 300 mg/kg I.M. divided q 4 hours.

▶ **Uncomplicated gonorrhea.** *Adults and children weighing more than 45 kg (99 lb):* 3.5 g P.O. with 1 g probenecid in a single dose.

▶ **Endocarditis prophylaxis for dental procedures.** *Adults:* 2 g I.V. or I.M. 30 minutes before procedure.

Children: 50 mg/kg I.V. or I.M. 30 minutes before procedure.

▶ **Enterococcal endocarditis.** *Adults:* 12 g daily by continuous I.V. infusion or in six equally divided doses with gentamicin for 4 to 6 weeks.

⊠ **Adjust-a-dose:** For patient with severe renal impairment, if creatinine clearance is 10 ml/minute or less, increase dose interval to 12 to 16 hours.

▽ I.V. administration

• Reconstitute with bacteriostatic water for injection. Use 5 ml for 125-mg, 250-mg, or 500-mg vials; 7.4 ml for 1-g vials; and 14.8 ml for 2-g vials.

• Give direct I.V. injections over 3 to 5 minutes for doses of 500 mg or less; over 10 to 15 minutes for larger doses. Don't exceed 100 mg/minute.

• Alternatively, dilute in 50 to 100 ml of normal saline solution and give by intermittent infusion over 15 to 30 minutes. Don't mix with solutions containing dextrose or fructose because these solutions promote rapid breakdown of ampicillin.

• Use initial dilution within 1 hour. Follow manufacturer's directions for stability data when ampicillin is further diluted for I.V. infusion.

• Give intermittently to prevent vein irritation. Change site every 48 hours.

• Don't give I.V. unless prescribed and infection is severe or patient can't take oral dose.

Contraindications and precautions

• Contraindicated in patients hypersensitive to drug or other penicillins.

• Use cautiously in patients with other drug allergies, especially to cephalosporins (possible

---

cross-sensitivity), and in those with mononucleosis (high risk of maculopapular rash).
☆ **Lifespan:** In pregnant or breast-feeding women, use cautiously.

Adverse reactions

CNS: *seizures.*
CV: vein irritation, thrombophlebitis.
GI: nausea, vomiting, diarrhea, glossitis, stomatitis.
Hematologic: anemia, *thrombocytopenia,* thrombocytopenic purpura, eosinophilia, *leukopenia, agranulocytosis.*
Other: hypersensitivity reactions (maculopapular rash, urticaria, *anaphylaxis*), overgrowth of nonsusceptible organisms, pain at injection site.

Interactions

Drug-drug. *Allopurinol:* May increase risk of rash. Monitor patient.
Probenecid: May increase level of ampicillin and other penicillins. Probenecid may be used for this purpose.

Effects on lab test results

• May increase eosinophil count. May decrease hemoglobin, hematocrit, and platelet, WBC, and granulocyte counts.
• May cause false-positive urine glucose determinations with copper sulfate tests (Clinitest).

Pharmacokinetics

Absorption: About 42% is absorbed after an oral dose; unknown after I.M. administration.
Distribution: Distributed into pleural, peritoneal, and synovial fluids; lungs; prostate; liver; and gallbladder. Also penetrates middle ear effusions, maxillary sinus and bronchial secretions, tonsils, and sputum. Ampicillin is minimally protein-bound at 15% to 25%.
Metabolism: Only partially.
Excretion: Excreted in urine by renal tubular secretion and glomerular filtration. *Half-life:* About 1 to 1½ hours (10 to 24 hours in severe renal impairment).

Route	Onset	Peak	Duration
P.O.	Unknown	2 hr	6-8 hr
I.V.	Immediate	Immediate	Unknown
I.M.	Unknown	1 hr	Unknown

Action

Chemical effect: Inhibits cell-wall synthesis during microorganism multiplication.
Therapeutic effect: Kills susceptible bacteria, including non-penicillinase–producing gram-positive bacteria and many gram-negative organisms.

Available forms

Capsules: 250 mg, 500 mg
Infusion: 500 mg, 1 g, 2 g
Injection: 125 mg, 250 mg, 500 mg, 1 g, 2 g, 10-g bulk package
Oral suspension: 125 mg/5 ml, 250 mg/5 ml (after reconstitution)

NURSING PROCESS

🔍 Assessment
• Obtain history of patient's infection before therapy, and reassess for improvement regularly thereafter.
• Ask patient about previous allergic reaction to penicillin. A negative history of penicillin allergy doesn't rule out future reaction.
• Obtain specimen for culture and sensitivity tests before giving first dose.
• Be alert for adverse reactions and drug interactions.
• Monitor patient's hydration status if adverse GI reactions occur.
• Evaluate patient's and family's knowledge of drug therapy.

🔷 Nursing diagnoses
• Risk for infection related to presence of susceptible bacterial infection
• Risk for deficient fluid volume related to drug-induced adverse GI reactions
• Deficient knowledge related to drug therapy

▶ Planning and implementation
• Give 1 hour before or 2 hours after meals. When given orally, drug may cause adverse GI reactions. Food may interfere with absorption.
• Don't give I.M. unless infection is severe or patient can't take oral dose.
• Give ampicillin at least 1 hour before bacteriostatic antibiotics.
• In children with meningitis, give with parenteral chloramphenicol for 24 hours pending culture results.

Reactions may be *common,* uncommon, *life-threatening,* or **COMMON AND LIFE-THREATENING.**

• Stop drug immediately if anaphylaxis occurs. Notify prescriber and prepare to give immediate treatment, such as epinephrine, corticosteroids, antihistamines, and other resuscitative measures.

Patient teaching
• Tell patient to take entire quantity of drug exactly as prescribed, even after he feels better.
• Tell patient to call prescriber if a rash (most common), fever, or chills develop.
• Warn patient never to use leftover ampicillin for a new illness or to share it with others.
• Advise patient to take oral ampicillin 1 hour before or 2 hours after meals for best absorption.

☑ Evaluation
• Patient is free from infection.
• Patient maintains adequate hydration.
• Patient and family state understanding of drug therapy.

ampicillin sodium and sulbactam sodium
(am-pih-SIL-in SOH-dee-um and sul-BAC-tam SOH-dee-um)
Unasyn

Pharmacologic class: aminopenicillin and beta-lactamase inhibitor
Therapeutic class: antibiotic
Pregnancy risk category: B

Indications and dosages

▶ **Intra-abdominal, gynecologic, and skin and skin-structure infections caused by susceptible gram-positive, gram-negative, and beta-lactamase-producing strains.** *Adults:* Dosage expressed as total drug (each 1.5-g vial contains 1 g ampicillin sodium and 0.5 g sulbactam sodium). 1.5 to 3 g I.M. or I.V. q 6 hours. Maximum daily dosage is 4 g sulbactam (12 g of combined drugs).

▶ **Skin and skin-structure infections caused by susceptible organisms.** *Children older than age 1:* 300 mg/kg I.V. daily in equally divided doses q 6 hours. Children should receive a maximum of 14 days of therapy. Children weighing 40 kg (88 lb) or more may receive the usual adult dosage.

▶ **Pelvic inflammatory disease.** *Adults and children:* 3 g (2 g ampicillin and 1 g sulbactam) I.V. or I.M. q 6 hours, given with doxycycline 100 mg P.O. q 12 hours. Continue parenteral therapy for 24 hours after clinical improvement. Continue with oral doxycycline 100 mg P.O. b.i.d. to complete the 14-day cycle.

▼ I.V. administration

• When preparing injection, reconstitute powder with any of the following diluents: normal saline solution, D_5W, lactated Ringer's solution, 1/6 M sodium lactate, dextrose 5% in half-normal saline solution for injection, or 10% inert sugar. Stability varies with diluent, temperature, and concentration of solution.
• After reconstitution, allow vials to stand for a few minutes to allow foam to dissipate to permit visual inspection of contents for particles.
• Give dose by injection over 10 to 15 minutes, or dilute in 50 to 100 ml of a compatible diluent and infuse over 15 to 30 minutes. If permitted, give intermittently to prevent vein irritation. Change site every 48 hours.
• Don't add or mix with other drugs because they might be physically or chemically incompatible.

Contraindications and precautions

• Contraindicated in patients hypersensitive to drug or other penicillins.
• Use cautiously in patients with other drug allergies, especially to cephalosporins (possible cross-sensitivity), and in those with mononucleosis (high risk of maculopapular rash).
⚠ Lifespan: In pregnant and breast-feeding women, use cautiously. In children younger than age 1, safety of drug hasn't been established. In children age 1 and older, drug can be used I.V. for skin and skin-structure infections. Children shouldn't receive the drug I.M.

Adverse reactions

CV: vein irritation, thrombophlebitis.
GI: nausea, vomiting, *diarrhea,* glossitis, stomatitis.
Hematologic: anemia, *thrombocytopenia,* thrombocytopenic purpura, eosinophilia, *leukopenia, agranulocytosis.*
Other: hypersensitivity reactions (erythematous maculopapular rash, urticaria, *anaphylaxis*), overgrowth of nonsusceptible organisms, pain at injection site.

Interactions

Drug-drug. *Allopurinol:* May increase risk of rash. Monitor patient.

Hormonal contraceptives: May decrease efficacy of hormonal contraceptives. Advise patient to use barrier contraception until course of therapy is complete.

Probenecid: May increase ampicillin level. Probenecid may be used for this purpose.

Effects on lab test results

- May increase BUN, creatinine, ALT, AST, alkaline phosphatase, bilirubin, LDH, CK, and GGT levels.
- May increase eosinophil count. May decrease hemoglobin, hematocrit, and platelet, WBC, and granulocyte counts.
- May cause false-positive urine glucose determinations with copper sulfate tests (Clinitest).

Pharmacokinetics

Absorption: Unknown.

Distribution: Both drugs are distributed into pleural, peritoneal, and synovial fluids; lungs; prostate; liver; and gallbladder. They also penetrate middle ear effusions, maxillary sinus and bronchial secretions, tonsils, and sputum. Ampicillin is minimally protein-bound at 15% to 25%; sulbactam is about 38% protein-bound.

Metabolism: Both drugs are metabolized only partially.

Excretion: Both drugs are excreted in urine by renal tubular secretion and glomerular filtration. *Half-life:* 1 to 1½ hours (10 to 24 hours in severe renal impairment).

Route	Onset	Peak	Duration
I.V.	Immediate	Immediate	Unknown
I.M.	Unknown	Unknown	Unknown

Action

Chemical effect: Ampicillin inhibits cell-wall synthesis during microorganism multiplication; sulbactam inactivates bacterial beta-lactamase, the enzyme that inactivates ampicillin and provides bacterial resistance to it.

Therapeutic effect: Kills susceptible bacteria.

Available forms

Injection: Vials and piggyback vials containing 1.5 g (1 g ampicillin sodium with 0.5 g sulbactam sodium); 3 g (2 g ampicillin sodium with 1 g sulbactam sodium)

NURSING PROCESS

◤ Assessment

- Obtain history of patient's infection before therapy and observe for improvement in condition throughout therapy.
- Ask patient about previous allergic reaction to penicillin. A negative history of penicillin allergy doesn't rule out future reaction.
- Obtain specimen for culture and sensitivity tests before administering first dose.
- Be alert for adverse reactions and drug interactions.
- Monitor patient's hydration status if adverse GI reactions occur.
- Evaluate patient's and family's knowledge of drug therapy.

◤ Nursing diagnoses

- Risk for infection related to presence of susceptible bacterial infection
- Risk for deficient fluid volume related to drug-induced adverse GI reactions
- Deficient knowledge related to drug therapy

◤ Planning and implementation

- When giving drug I.M., reconstitute with sterile water for injection or with 0.5% or 2% lidocaine hydrochloride. Add 3.2 ml to a 1.5-g vial (or 6.4 ml to a 3-g vial) to yield a concentration of 375 mg/ml. Give deeply into muscle.
- Dosage should be altered in patients with renal impairment.
- Give drug at least 1 hour before bacteriostatic antibiotics.
- Stop drug immediately if anaphylaxis occurs. Notify prescriber and prepare to give immediate treatment, such as epinephrine, corticosteroids, antihistamines; and other resuscitative measures.

Patient teaching
- Tell patient to call prescriber if rash (most common), fever, or chills develop.
- Advise women taking hormonal contraceptives to use an additional form of contraception during drug therapy.

◤ Evaluation

- Patient is free from infection.
- Patient maintains adequate hydration.
- Patient and family state understanding of drug therapy.

Reactions may be *common,* uncommon, *life-threatening,* or COMMON AND LIFE-THREATENING.

amprenavir
(am-PREH-nah-veer)
Agenerase

Pharmacologic class: HIV protease inhibitor
Therapeutic class: antiviral
Pregnancy risk category: C

Indications and dosages

▶ **HIV-1 infection, with other antiretrovirals.**
Adults and children ages 13 to 16 weighing 50 kg (110 lb) or more: 1,200 mg (eight 150-mg capsules) P.O. b.i.d. with other antiretrovirals.
Children ages 4 to 12 or 13 to 16 weighing less than 50 kg (110 lb): Give 20 mg/kg P.O. capsules b.i.d. or 15 mg/kg P.O. t.i.d. (maximum, 2,400 mg daily) with other antiretrovirals. Or, give 22.5 mg/kg (1.5 ml/kg) oral solution P.O. b.i.d. or 17 mg/kg (1.1 ml/kg) P.O. t.i.d. (maximum, 2,800 mg daily) with other antiretrovirals.
☒ Adjust-a-dose: For patients with hepatic impairment and a Child-Pugh score of 5 to 8, reduce dosage to 450 mg capsules P.O. b.i.d. For patients with hepatic impairment and a Child-Pugh score of 9 to 12, reduce dosage to 300 mg capsules P.O. b.i.d.

Contraindications and precautions

• Contraindicated in patients hypersensitive to drug or its components. Coadministration with drugs dependent on the CYP 3A4 enzyme pathway is contraindicated.
• Use cautiously in patients with moderate or severe hepatic impairment, diabetes mellitus, sulfonamide allergy, or hemophilia A or B.
• Drug can cause severe or life-threatening rash, including Stevens-Johnson syndrome. Therapy should be stopped if patient develops a severe or life-threatening rash or a moderate rash with systemic signs and symptoms.
⚘ Lifespan: In pregnant women, use only if potential benefits outweigh risks; no adequate studies exist. In children age 4 and younger, drug is contraindicated because of risk of toxicity.

Adverse reactions

CNS: *paresthesia,* depressive or mood disorders.
GI: nausea, vomiting, diarrhea or loose stools, taste disorders.

Hepatic: hypertriglyceridemia, hypercholesterolemia.
Metabolic: hyperglycemia.
Skin: *rash, Stevens-Johnson syndrome.*

Interactions

Drug-drug. *Antacids:* Interferes with absorption. Separate administration by at least 1 hour.
Antiarrhythmics, such as amiodarone; lidocaine (systemic); quinidine; anticoagulants, such as warfarin; tricyclic antidepressants: Levels of these drugs may be affected. Monitor patient closely.
Calcium channel blockers, dihydroergotamine, midazolam, rifampin, triazolam: May cause serious and life-threatening interactions. Avoid using together.
Cimetidine, indinavir, nelfinavir, ritonavir: May increase amprenavir level. Monitor patient closely for increased adverse effects.
Efavirenz: May decrease exposure of amprenavir to the body. Increase dose accordingly.
Ethinyl estradiol and norethindrone: Loss of virologic response and possible resistance to amprenavir. Tell patient to use alternative method of birth control.
HMG-CoA reductase inhibitors, such as atorvastatin, lovastatin, and simvastatin: May increase levels of these drugs; therefore, may increase risk of myopathy, including rhabdomyolysis. Avoid using together.
Indinavir, nelfinavir, ritonavir: Increased plasma levels of amprenavir. Monitor patient closely.
Ketoconazole: May increase levels of both drugs. Monitor patient closely for adverse reactions.
Macrolides: May increase amprenavir level. No adjustment necessary.
Methadone: May decrease amprenavir level. Alternative antiretroviral or pain therapy should be considered. Dosage of methadone may need to be increased.
Psychotherapeutic agents: May increase CNS effects. Monitor patient closely.
Rifabutin: May decrease exposure of amprenavir to the body and increase rifabutin level by 200%. Decrease rifabutin dose to 150 mg daily or 300 mg two to three times weekly.
Saquinavir: May decrease exposure of amprenavir to the body. Monitor patient closely.
Sildenafil: May substantially increase sildenafil levels, causing an increase in sildenafil-associated effects, including hypotension, and

---

Rapid onset   *Liquid form contains alcohol.   ◆Canada   ◇Australia   †OTC   ‡Off-label use

priapism. Don't exceed 25 mg of sildenafil in a 48-hour period.

Drug-herb. *St. John's wort:* May decrease amprenavir level. Avoid using together.

Drug-food. *Grapefruit juice:* May affect blood levels of amprenavir. Monitor patient closely. *High-fat meals:* May reduce drug absorption. Discourage taking drug with a high-fat meal.

Effects on lab test results

• May increase glucose, triglyceride, and cholesterol levels.

Pharmacokinetics

Absorption: Rapid.
Distribution: Apparent volume of distribution is about 430 L. In vitro, about 90% of drug binds to plasma proteins.
Metabolism: By CYP 3A4 enzymes in the liver.
Excretion: Minimal, in urine and feces. *Elimination half-life:* 7 to 10½ hours.

Route	Onset	Peak	Duration
P.O.	Unknown	1-2 hr	Unknown

Action

Chemical effect: Inhibits HIV-1 protease by binding to the active site of HIV-1 protease, which causes immature noninfectious viral particles to form.
Therapeutic effect: Reduces symptoms of HIV-1 infection.

Available forms

Capsules: 50 mg, 150 mg
Oral solution: 15 mg/ml

NURSING PROCESS

⬛ Assessment

• Assess patient for appropriateness of drug therapy.
• Because drug may interact with other drugs, obtain patient's complete drug history.
• Patients with moderate or severe hepatic impairment, diabetes mellitus, known sulfonamide allergy, or hemophilia A or B must be monitored very closely while taking this drug.
• Determine whether patient is pregnant or plans to become pregnant.
• Evaluate patient's and family's knowledge about drug therapy.

⬛ Nursing diagnoses

• Risk for infection secondary to presence of HIV
• Ineffective individual coping related to HIV infection
• Deficient knowledge related to drug therapy

⬛ Planning and implementation

• Don't give patient high-fat foods because they may decrease absorption of oral drug.
⬛ **ALERT:** Amprenavir capsules aren't interchangeable with amprenavir oral solution on a milligram-per-milligram basis.
• Monitor coagulation studies. Drug provides high daily doses of vitamin E.
• Protease inhibitors cause spontaneous bleeding in some patients with hemophilia A or B. In some patients, additional factor VIII may be required. Often, treatment with protease inhibitors is continued or restarted.

Patient teaching
• Inform patient that drug doesn't cure HIV infection and that opportunistic infections and other complications may develop. Also, explain that drug doesn't reduce the risk of transmitting HIV to others.
• Tell patient that drug can be taken with or without food, but that he shouldn't take it with a high-fat meal because doing so may decrease drug absorption.
• Urge patient to report adverse reactions, especially rash.
• Warn patient that he may experience a redistribution of body fat, including central obesity, dorsocervical fat enlargement (buffalo hump), peripheral wasting, breast enlargement, and cushingoid appearance.
• Advise patient to take drug every day as prescribed, always with other antiretrovirals. Warn against changing the dosage or stopping the drug without prescriber's approval.
• If patient takes an antacid or didanosine, tell him to do so 1 hour before or after amprenavir to avoid interfering with amprenavir absorption.
• If patient misses a dose by more than 4 hours, tell him to wait and take the next dose at the regularly scheduled time. If he misses a dose by less than 4 hours, tell him to take the dose as soon as possible and then take the next dose at the regularly scheduled time. Caution against doubling the dose.
• Advise patient not to take supplemental vitamin E because high levels of this vitamin may

worsen the blood coagulation defect of vitamin K deficiency caused by anticoagulant therapy or malabsorption.

• If patient uses a hormonal contraceptive, warn her to use another contraceptive during amprenavir therapy.

• Urge patient to notify prescriber about planned, suspected, or known pregnancy during therapy.

• Advise patients taking sildenafil of the increased risk of adverse affects, including hypotension, visual changes, and priapism. These patients should promptly report symptoms to their prescribers and shouldn't exceed 25 mg of sildenafil in a 48-hour period.

☑ Evaluation

• Patient exhibits reduced signs and symptoms of infection.

• Patient demonstrates adequate coping mechanisms.

• Patient and family state understanding of drug therapy.

anakinra
(ann-u-KIN-ruh)
Kineret

Pharmacologic classification: lymphokine
Therapeutic classification: immuno-regulatory drug; antirheumatic
Pregnancy risk category: B

Indications and dosages

▶ **Moderate-to-severe active rheumatoid arthritis (RA) after one failure with disease-modifying antirheumatics.** *Adults:* 100 mg S.C. daily.

Contraindications and precautions

• Contraindicated in patients hypersensitive to *Escherichia coli*–derived proteins or components of the product. Don't use in immunosuppressed patients or in patients with chronic or active infection.

• Use caution with other tumor necrosis factor (TNF) blockers because of the increased risk of neutropenia.

⚕ **Lifespan:** In pregnant women, use only if necessary; no adequate, well-controlled studies exist. In breast-feeding women, use cautiously

because it's unknown whether drug appears in breast milk. In patients with juvenile RA, safety and efficacy of drug haven't been established. In elderly patients, use drug cautiously because they have a greater risk of infection and are more likely to have renal impairment.

Adverse reactions

CNS: headache.
EENT: sinusitis.
GI: abdominal pain, diarrhea, nausea.
Hematologic: *neutropenia.*
Respiratory: upper respiratory tract infection.
Other: infection (cellulitis, pneumonia, bone and joint), flulike symptoms, injection site reactions (erythema, ecchymosis, inflammation, pain).

Interactions

Drug-drug. *Etanercept, other TNF blockers:* May increase risk of severe infection. Use together cautiously.
Vaccines: May decrease effectiveness of vaccines or increase risk of secondary transmission of infection with live vaccines. Avoid using together.

Effects on lab test results

• May increase differential percentage of eosinophils. May decrease neutrophil, WBC, and platelet counts.

Pharmacokinetics

Absorption: Unknown.
Distribution: Absolute bioavailability is 95%.
Metabolism: Unknown.
Excretion: Renal. Clearance increases with increasing creatinine clearance and body weight. Mean plasma clearance decreases 70% to 75% in patients with creatinine clearance less than 30 ml/minute. *Half-life:* 4 to 6 hours.

Route	Onset	Peak	Duration
S.C.	Unknown	3-7 hr	Unknown

Action

Chemical effect: A recombinant, non-glycosylated form of the human interleukin-1 receptor antagonist (IL-1Ra). The level of naturally occurring IL-1Ra in synovium and synovial fluid from patients with RA isn't enough to compete with the elevated level of locally produced IL-1. Drug blocks the activity of IL-1

by competitively inhibiting IL-1 from binding to the interleukin-1–type receptors.
Therapeutic effect: Decreases inflammation and cartilage degradation.

Available forms

Injection: 100 mg/ml in prefilled glass syringe

NURSING PROCESS

Assessment
• Before therapy, assess patient for signs and symptoms of chronic or active infection. Don't start treatment if patient has active infection.
• Obtain neutrophil count before treatment, monthly for the first 3 months of treatment, and then quarterly for up to 1 year.
• Monitor patient for infections and injection site reactions.

Nursing diagnoses
• Risk of infection related to anakinra therapy
• Risk of pain due to underlying rheumatoid arthritis
• Risk of impaired skin integrity due to injection site reaction

Planning and implementation
• Inject the entire contents of the prefilled syringe S.C.
• Stop drug if patient develops a serious infection.
• **ALERT:** Don't confuse anakinra with amikacin.
Patient teaching
• Tell patient to store drug in refrigerator and not to freeze or expose to excessive heat. Tell patient to allow drug to come to room temperature before injecting.
• Teach patient proper technique for administration and disposal of syringes in a puncture-resistant container. Also, warn patient not to reuse needles.
• Urge patient to rotate injection sites.
• Review with patient the signs and symptoms of allergic and other adverse reactions and the symptoms of infection. Urge patient to contact prescriber immediately if they arise. Inform patient that injection site reactions are common, are usually mild, and typically last 14 to 28 days.
• Tell patient to avoid live-virus vaccines while taking anakinra.

Evaluation
• Patient is free from infection or adverse reactions during drug therapy.
• Patient's symptoms of RA are relieved.
• Patient and family state understanding of drug therapy and give drug properly.

anastrozole
(uh-NAS-truh-zohl)
Arimidex

Pharmacologic class: nonsteroidal aromatase inhibitor
Therapeutic class: antineoplastic
Pregnancy risk category: D

Indications and dosages

▶ **First-line treatment of postmenopausal women with hormone–receptor-positive or hormone–receptor-unknown locally advanced or metastatic breast cancer; advanced breast cancer in postmenopausal women with disease progression following tamoxifen therapy; adjuvant treatment of postmenopausal women with hormone–receptor-positive early breast cancer.** *Adults:* 1 mg P.O. daily.

Contraindications and precautions

⚖ **Lifespan:** In pregnant women, drug isn't recommended. In breast-feeding women, use cautiously. In children, safety of drug hasn't been established.

Adverse reactions

CNS: pain, asthenia, headache, dizziness, depression, paresthesia.
CV: chest pain, edema, *thromboembolic disease,* peripheral edema, *vasodilation.*
EENT: pharyngitis.
GI: nausea, vomiting, diarrhea, constipation, dry mouth, abdominal pain, anorexia.
GU: pelvic pain, *vaginal hemorrhage,* vaginal dryness.
Metabolic: weight gain, increased appetite.
Musculoskeletal: back pain, bone pain.
Respiratory: dyspnea, increased cough.
Skin: rash, sweating.
Other: *hot flushes.*

Interactions

None reported.

Effects on lab test results
• May increase liver enzyme levels.

Pharmacokinetics
Absorption: Food affects extent of absorption.
Distribution: 40% bound to plasma proteins.
Metabolism: Metabolized in liver.
Excretion: Excreted in urine. *Half-life:* About 50 hours.

Route	Onset	Peak	Duration
P.O.	Unknown	Unknown	Unknown

Action
Chemical effect: Significantly lowers estradiol level.
Therapeutic effect: Hinders cancer cell growth.

Available forms
Tablets: 1 mg

NURSING PROCESS

Assessment
• Obtain history of patient's neoplastic disease before therapy.
• Be alert for adverse reactions.
• Evaluate patient's and family's knowledge of drug therapy.

Nursing diagnoses
• Ineffective health maintenance related to neoplastic disease
• Risk for deficient fluid volume related to drug-induced adverse GI reactions
• Deficient knowledge related to drug therapy

Planning and implementation
• Rule out pregnancy before treatment begins.
• Give drug under supervision of a prescriber experienced in using antineoplastics.
• Patients with hormone–receptor–negative disease and patients who didn't respond to previous tamoxifen therapy rarely respond to anastrozole.
• Patients with advanced breast cancer should continue therapy until tumor progression is evident.
Patient teaching
• Instruct patient to report adverse reactions.
• Stress importance of follow-up care.

Evaluation
• Patient has positive response to therapy.
• Patient maintains adequate hydration.
• Patient and family state understanding of drug therapy.

antihemophilic factor (AHF, Factor VIII)
(an-tigh-hee-moh-FIL-ik FAK-tor)
Helixate FS, Hemofil M, Hyate:C, Koate-DVI, Kogenate, Kogenate FS, Monoclate-P, Recombinate, Refacto

Pharmacologic class: blood derivative
Therapeutic class: antihemophilic
Pregnancy risk category: C

Indications and dosages
Drug provides hemostasis in factor VIII deficiency and hemophilia A. Dosage depends on the patient's weight, severity of hemorrhage, and presence of inhibitors.

The dose can be calculated by multiplying the desired level (as a percent of normal) with the body weight divided by 2. For example, if you want a peak level of 40% in a 40 kg child, multiply 40% by 40 and divide by 2 to get 800 international units.

$$\text{AHF/international unit required (dose)} = \frac{\text{desired factor VIII increase (\% normal)} \times \text{body weight (kg)}}{2}$$

▶ **Mild bleeding.** *Adults and children:* 10 to 20 international units/kg daily. A level of 20% to 40% of normal is desired.
▶ **Moderate bleeding and minor surgery.** *Adults and children:* Initially, 15 to 30 international units/kg, then repeat one dose at 12 to 24 hours, if needed. A level of 30% to 60% of normal is desired.
▶ **Severe bleeding and bleeding near vital organs.** *Adults and children:* Initially, 40 to 50 international units/kg, then 20 to 25 international unit/kg q 8 to 12 hours, p.r.n. A level of 80% to 100% of normal is desired.
▶ **Major surgery.** *Adults and children:* 50 international units/kg 1 hour before surgery, then

repeat p.r.n. 6 to 12 hours after first dose. A level of 80% to 100% of normal is desired pre- and post-operatively.

▼ I.V. administration

• Refrigerate concentrate until ready to use. Warm concentrate and diluent bottles to room temperature before reconstituting. To mix drug, gently roll vial between your hands.
• Use reconstituted solution within 3 hours.
⊛ **ALERT:** One AHF unit equals the activity present in 1 ml normal pooled plasma less than 1 hour old. Don't confuse commercial product with blood-bank–produced cryoprecipitated factor VIII from individual donors. Drug is for I.V. use only; use plastic syringe because solution adheres to glass surfaces.
• Store away from heat, and don't refrigerate. Refrigeration after reconstitution may cause active ingredient to precipitate.
• Don't shake or mix with other I.V. solutions.
⊛ **ALERT:** Kogenate FS and Helixate FS should be refrigerated at all times at temperatures of 36° to 46° F (2° to 8° C) to ensure potency through the expiration date. Previously, Kogenate FS and Helixate FS could be stored at room temperature for up to 2 months.

Contraindications and precautions

• Contraindicated in patients hypersensitive to drug or to murine (mouse) protein.
• Use cautiously in patients with hepatic disease because of susceptibility to hepatitis, which may be transmitted in AHF.
⚘ **Lifespan:** In pregnant women, use cautiously. In breast-feeding women, safety of drug hasn't been established. In neonates and infants, use cautiously.

Adverse reactions

CNS: *fever,* headache, paresthesia, clouding or loss of consciousness, somnolence, lethargy.
CV: flushing, tachycardia, hypotension, tightness in chest.
EENT: visual disturbances.
GI: nausea, vomiting.
Hematologic: hemolysis (in patients with blood type A, B, or AB).
Hepatic: *hepatitis B.*
Musculoskeletal: backache.
Respiratory: wheezing.
Skin: *erythema,* urticaria.

Other: *chills,* hypersensitivity reactions, rigor, stinging at injection site, *HIV.*

Interactions

None significant.

Effects on lab test results

• May increase fibrinogen level.
• May decrease hemoglobin and hematocrit.

Pharmacokinetics

Absorption: Administered I.V.
Distribution: Unknown.
Metabolism: Rapid.
Excretion: Consumed during blood clotting.
Half-life: 4 to 24 hours (average, 12 hours).

Route	Onset	Peak	Duration
I.V.	Immediate	1-2 hr	Unknown

Action

Chemical effect: Directly replaces deficient clotting factor that converts prothrombin to thrombin.
Therapeutic effect: Causes blood clotting.

Available forms

Injection: Vials, with diluent. Units specified on label.

NURSING PROCESS

⚗ Assessment

• Obtain thorough history of patient's underlying condition (including hematocrit, results of coagulation studies, and vital signs) before therapy begins and regularly throughout therapy.
• Inhibitors to factor VIII develop in some patients, leading to decreased response to drug.
• Assess patient for adverse reactions to drug.
• Evaluate patient's and family's knowledge of drug therapy.

⊞ Nursing diagnoses

• Ineffective health maintenance related to bleeding caused by underlying condition
• Risk for injury related to drug-induced adverse reactions
• Deficient knowledge related to drug therapy

▷ Planning and implementation

• Give hepatitis B vaccine before giving drug.

Reactions may be *common,* uncommon, *life-threatening,* or COMMON AND LIFE-THREATENING.

• Take baseline pulse before giving drug. If pulse rate increases significantly, flow rate should be reduced or administration stopped.

• A porcine product is available for patients with congenital hemophilia A who have antibodies to human factor VIII:C.

Patient teaching

• Educate patient about drug therapy.

• Inform patient about risks of drug therapy, such as contracting hepatitis or HIV.

• Instruct patient to call prescriber if adverse reactions develop.

☑ **Evaluation**

• Patient's vital signs and blood studies are within normal parameters with no bleeding.

• Patient doesn't experience injury as a result of drug therapy.

• Patient and family state understanding of drug therapy.

anti-inhibitor coagulant complex
(an-tigh-in-HIB-eh-tor koh-AG-yoo-lant KOM-pleks)
Autoplex T, Feiba VH Immuno

Pharmacologic class: blood derivative
Therapeutic class: antihemophilic
Pregnancy risk category: C

Indications and dosages

▶ **Prevention and control of hemorrhagic episodes in patients with hemophilia A for whom inhibitor antibodies to antihemophilic factor have developed; management of bleeding in patients with acquired hemophilia who have spontaneously acquired inhibitors to factor VIII.** Drug controls hemorrhage in hemophilia A patients who have a factor VIII inhibitor level above 10 Bethesda units. Patients with a level of 2 to 10 Bethesda units may receive the drug if they have severe hemorrhage or respond poorly to factor VIII infusion. Dosage is highly individualized and varies among manufacturers.

For Autoplex T, give 25 to 100 units/kg I.V. depending on the severity of hemorrhage. If no hemostatic improvement occurs within 6 hours after initial administration, repeat dosage.

For Feiba VH Immuno, give 50 to 100 units/ kg I.V. q 6 or 12 hours until patient shows signs of improvement. Maximum daily dose is 200 units/kg.

▶ **Joint hemorrhage.** *Adults and children:* 50 to 100 units/kg Feiba VH Immuno q 12 hours until patient's condition improves.

▶ **Mucous membrane hemorrhage.** *Adults and children:* 50 units/kg Feiba VH Immuno q 6 hours, increasing to 100 units/kg q 6 hours if hemorrhage continues. Maximum daily dose, 200 units/kg.

▶ **Soft-tissue hemorrhage.** *Adults and children:* 100 units/kg Feiba VH Immuno q 12 hours. Maximum daily dose, 200 units/kg.

▶ **Other severe hemorrhages.** *Adults and children:* 100 units/kg Feiba VH Immuno q 12 hours (occasionally, q 6 hours).

▽ I.V. administration

• Warm drug and diluent to room temperature before reconstitution. Use filter needle provided by manufacturer to withdraw reconstituted solution from vial into syringe; filter needle should then be replaced with a sterile injection needle for infusion. Infuse as soon as possible. Complete Autoplex T infusions within 1 hour after reconstitution; Feiba VH Immuno infusions, within 3 hours.

• Base the rate of infusion on patient's response. Begin Autoplex T infusions at 1 ml/ minute; if well tolerated, increase infusion rate gradually to 10 ml/minute. Don't exceed 2 units/kg with Feiba VH Immuno.

• Keep epinephrine readily available to treat anaphylaxis.

• If flushing, lethargy, headache, transient chest discomfort, or changes in blood pressure or pulse rate develop because of rapid infusion, stop drug and notify prescriber. Symptoms usually disappear when infusion stops. Infusion then may be resumed at a slower rate.

Contraindications and precautions

• Contraindicated in patients with signs of fibrinolysis, in those with DIC, and in those with a normal coagulation mechanism.

• Use cautiously in patients with liver disease.

⚠ **Lifespan:** In pregnant women, use cautiously. In breast-feeding women, safety of drug hasn't been established.

Adverse reactions

CNS: fever, dizziness, headache, lethargy, drowsiness.

CV: flushing, hypotension, transient chest discomfort, changes in pulse rate, *acute MI, thromboembolic events.*
GI: nausea.
Hematologic: *DIC.*
Hepatic: *risk of hepatitis B.*
Respiratory: dyspnea.
Skin: rash, urticaria.
Other: chills, hypersensitivity reactions, *risk of HIV.*

Interactions

Drug-drug. *Antifibrinolytic drugs:* May alter effects of anti-inhibitor coagulant complex. Don't use together.

Effects on lab test results

None reported.

Pharmacokinetics

Absorption: Administered I.V.
Distribution: Unknown.
Metabolism: Unknown.
Excretion: Unknown. *Half-life:* Unknown.

Route	Onset	Peak	Duration
I.V.	10-30 min	Unknown	Unknown

Action

Chemical effect: Unknown. May be related to presence of activated factors, which leads to more complete activation of factor X in conjunction with tissue factor, phospholipid, and ionic calcium, and allows coagulation to proceed beyond those stages that require factor VIII.
Therapeutic effect: Causes blood clotting.

Available forms

Injection: Number of units of factor VIII correctional activity indicated on label of vial

NURSING PROCESS

⚗ Assessment

• Obtain history of patient's underlying condition (including hematocrit, results of coagulation studies, and vital signs) before therapy and regularly throughout therapy.
• Be alert for adverse reactions and drug interactions.
• Evaluate patient's and family's knowledge of drug therapy.

⊕ Nursing diagnoses

• Ineffective health maintenance related to bleeding caused by underlying condition
• Risk for injury related to drug-induced adverse reactions
• Deficient knowledge related to drug therapy

⟩ Planning and implementation

• Give hepatitis B vaccine before giving drug.
Patient teaching
• Teach patient about anti-inhibitor coagulant complex therapy.
• Reassure patient that because of the manufacturing process used, risk of HIV transmission is extremely low.

☑ Evaluation

• Patient's vital signs and blood studies are within normal parameters with no bleeding.
• Patient doesn't experience injury as a result of anti-inhibitor coagulant complex therapy.
• Patient and family state understanding of drug therapy.

antithrombin III, human (ATIII, heparin cofactor I)
(an-tigh-THROM-bin three, HYOO-mun)
ATnativ, Thrombate III

Pharmacologic class: glycoprotein
Therapeutic class: anticoagulant, antithrombotic
Pregnancy risk category: C

Indications and dosages

▶ **Thromboembolism from hereditary ATIII deficiency.** *Adults and children:* Initial dose is quantity needed to increase ATIII activity to 120% of normal activity 30 minutes after administration. Usual dose is 50 to 100 IU/minute I.V. Don't exceed 100 IU/minute. Dose based on anticipated 1% increase in ATIII activity produced by 1 IU/kg of body weight using the formula: Dose (IU) is equal to desired activity (%) minus baseline activity (%) times weight (kg) divided by 1.4 (IU/kg). Maintenance dosage is quantity required to increase ATIII activity to 80% of normal activity and is given at 24-hour intervals. To calculate dosage, multiply desired ATIII activity (as % of normal) minus baseline

ATIII activity (as % of normal) by body weight (kg). Divide by actual increase in ATIII activity (%) produced by 1 IU/kg as determined 30 minutes after administration of initial dose. Treatment usually continues for 2 to 8 days but may be prolonged in pregnancy or during surgery or immobilization.

▽ I.V. administration

• Reconstitute drug using provided 10 ml of sterile water, normal saline solution, or D_5W. Don't shake vial. Filter through the sterile needle supplied in the package before use. Dilute further in same diluent solution, if desired.
• Give within 3 hours of reconstitution. Infuse I.V. over 10 to 20 minutes.
• Store drug at 36° to 46° F (2° to 8° C).

Contraindications and precautions

❅ **Lifespan:** In children and neonates, safety and efficacy of drug haven't been established; use cautiously.

Adverse reactions

CV: vasodilation, lowered blood pressure.
GU: diuresis.

Interactions

Drug-drug. *Heparin:* May increase anticoagulant effect of both drugs. Reduced heparin dose may be needed.

Effects on lab test results

None reported.

Pharmacokinetics

Absorption: Administered I.V.
Distribution: Binding to epithelium and redistribution into extravascular compartment removes ATIII from blood. Special receptors on hepatocytes bind ATIII clotting factor complexes, rapidly removing them from circulation.
Metabolism: Unknown.
Excretion: Unknown. *Half-life:* 2 to 3 days.

Route	Onset	Peak	Duration
I.V.	Immediate	Unknown	4 days

Action

Chemical effect: Replaces ATIII in patients with hereditary ATIII deficiency, normalizing coagulation inhibition and inhibiting throm-

boembolism. Also deactivates plasmin but to a lesser extent than clotting factor.
Therapeutic effect: Prevents or decreases blood clotting.

Available forms

Injection: 500 IU/vial, 1,000 IU/vial

NURSING PROCESS

✎ Assessment

• Obtain history of patient's underlying condition before therapy, and reassess regularly throughout therapy.
• Because of risk of fatality from neonatal thromboembolism in children of parents with hereditary ATIII deficiency, be ready to determine neonate's ATIII levels immediately after birth.
• Obtain ATIII activity levels twice daily until dosage requirement stabilizes, then daily immediately before dose. Functional assays are preferred because quantitative immunologic test results may be normal despite decreased ATIII activity.
• Be alert for adverse reactions and drug interactions.
• Watch for dyspnea and increased blood pressure, which may occur if given too rapidly.
• Evaluate patient's and family's knowledge of drug therapy.

⊕ Nursing diagnoses

• Ineffective tissue perfusion related to underlying condition
• Deficient knowledge related to drug therapy

▷ Planning and implementation

• Drug isn't recommended for long-term prophylaxis of thrombotic episodes.
Patient teaching
• Tell patient to report difficulty breathing and any other sudden symptoms immediately while drug is being given; rate adjustment may be needed.
• Inform patient that risk of contracting hepatitis or HIV is minimal.

☑ Evaluation

• Patient has adequate tissue perfusion.
• Patient and family state understanding of drug therapy.

aprepitant

(uh-pre-Pl-tant)
Emend

Pharmacologic class: substance P and neurokinin-1 receptor antagonist
Therapeutic classification: centrally-acting antiemetic
Pregnancy risk category: B

Indications and dosages

▶ **Adjunct to corticosteroids and 5-HT$_3$– receptor antagonist for the prevention of both acute and delayed nausea and vomiting caused by highly emetogenic chemotherapy, including cisplatin.** *Adults:* 125 mg P.O. on day 1 of treatment (1 hour before chemotherapy), then 80 mg P.O. q a.m. on days 2 and 3. Single doses up to 600 mg of aprepitant have been well tolerated.

Contraindications and precautions

• Contraindicated in patients hypersensitive to drug or any of its components, and in those also receiving pimozide because drug may increase pimozide level, causing life-threatening reactions such as ventricular arrhythmias.
• Administration beyond 3 days per cycle of chemotherapy isn't recommended because of the potential for CYP 3A4- and 2C9-related drug interactions.
⚠ **Lifespan:** In pregnant women, use with caution; drug hasn't been well studied in pregnant women. In breast-feeding women, use cautiously; it's unknown whether drug appears in breast milk.

Adverse reactions

CNS: dizziness, *fatigue,* headache, insomnia.
EENT: tinnitus.
GI: abdominal pain, *anorexia, constipation, diarrhea,* gastritis, *nausea,* vomiting.
GU: proteinuria.
Hematologic: *neutropenia, febrile neutropenia.*
Respiratory: *hiccups.*
Skin: drug-induced rash with uritcaria, *Stevens-Johnson syndrome.*
Other: *angioedema.*

Interactions

Drug-drug. *Benzodiazepines, such as alprazolam and midazolam:* May increase levels of these drugs. Monitor patient for increased sedation and other CNS effects. Decrease the dose of benzodiazepines by 50% if use together is necessary.
Chemotherapy metabolized by CYP 3A4, such as etoposide, ifosfamide, irinotecan, taxanes, and vinca alkaloids: May increase levels of these drugs, leading to increased toxicity. Avoid using together whenever possible.
Corticosteroids: May increase levels of these drugs, leading to increased toxicity. Decrease the dose of corticosteroids by 50% if use together is necessary.
CYP 3A4 inducers (carbamazepine, phenytoin, rifampin): May decrease aprepitant level and decrease antiemetic effect. Avoid using together whenever possible.
CYP 3A4 inhibitors (azole antifungals, diltiazem, erythromycin, nelfinavir, ritonavir): May increase aprepitant level, leading to increased toxicity. Avoid using together whenever possible.
Diltiazem: May increase diltiazem level. Monitor heart rate and blood pressure. Avoid using together whenever possible.
Hormonal contraceptives: May decrease the effectiveness of these drugs. Women should be advised to use an additional form of birth control if use together is necessary.
Phenytoin: May decrease phenytoin level. Monitor phenytoin levels carefully. An increased dose may be needed when used together. Avoid using together whenever possible.
SSRIs: May decrease the effectiveness of these drugs. Avoid using together whenever possible.
Tolbutamide: May decrease the effectiveness of tolbutamide. Monitor glucose level carefully if use together is necessary.
Warfarin: May decrease the effectiveness of warfarin. Monitor INR levels carefully in the 2 weeks after each treatment, especially days 7 to 10. Avoid using together whenever possible.
Drug-herb. *St. John's wort:* May decrease the drug's antiemetic effects. Discourage use together.
Drug-food. *Grapefruit juice:* May increase drug level, leading to increased toxicity. Discourage use together.

Reactions may be *common,* uncommon, *life-threatening,* or COMMON AND LIFE-THREATENING.

Effects on lab test results

• May increase creatinine, AST, and ALT levels.
• May decrease neutrophil counts.

Pharmacokinetics

Absorption: Well absorbed, with an average bioavailability of 60% to 65%. Food doesn't appear to have an effect. Peak level occurs approximately 4 hours after each dose.
Distribution: 95% protein-bound. May cross the placenta and blood-brain barrier.
Metabolism: Extensively metabolized in the liver by CYP 3A4 and to a lesser degree by CYP 1A2 and 2C19.
Excretion: In the urine and in the feces. *Half-life:* 9 to 13 hours.

Route	Onset	Peak	Duration
P.O.	Unknown	4 hr	9-13 hr

Action

Chemical effect: Selectively antagonizes substance P and neurokinin-1 receptors in the brain.
Therapeutic effect: Inhibits emesis caused by cytotoxic chemotherapy.

Available forms

Capsules: 80 mg, 125 mg

NURSING PROCESS

⚡ Assessment

• Monitor patients for potential drug and herbal interactions thoroughly before giving.
• Assess patient's condition before administration and regularly thereafter.
• Watch for hypersensitivity reactions.
• Monitor therapy with other drugs for potential interactions, particularly drugs metabolized by the liver.

✣ Nursing diagnoses

• Imbalanced nutrition: less than body requires related to chemotherapy-induced nausea and vomiting
• Ineffective individual coping related to effects of chemotherapy
• Deficient knowledge related to drug therapy

▶ Planning and implementation

• Give the first dose of drug 1 hour before chemotherapy.

• Give drug with other antiemetics, usually a 5HT$_3$ antagonist and a corticosteroid.
• Don't give for longer than 3 days per chemotherapy cycle.
• Don't give to treat established nausea and vomiting. Make sure patient has other antiemetics to treat breakthrough emesis.
• Higher doses may lead to drowsiness and headache. Provide supportive treatment for overdose; because of the drug's mechanism of action, antiemetics may not be effective. Don't attempt to remove by hemodialysis because removal doesn't occur.
• Monitor CBC, liver function tests, and creatinine periodically during drug therapy.

Patient teaching

• Advise patient that drug is given with other antiemetics and shouldn't be taken alone to prevent chemotherapy-induced nausea and vomiting.
• Tell patient that you will give the first dose 1 hour before each cycle of chemotherapy, and that he should take the second and third doses of the drug in the morning on days 2 and 3 of treatment, with or without food.
• Instruct patient to treat breakthrough emesis with other antiemetics.
• Advise patient to tell his oncologist if he starts or stops any other drugs or herbal supplements during therapy because of the drug's many drug and herb interactions.
• Advise women of childbearing age who are taking hormonal contraceptives to use an additional form of birth control during therapy.

✓ Evaluation

• Patient doesn't experience chemotherapy-induced nausea or vomiting.
• Patient maintains adequate nutrition and hydration during chemotherapy treatments.
• Patient and family state understanding of drug therapy.

aprotinin
(uh-proh-TIN-in)
Trasylol

Pharmacologic class: naturally occurring protease inhibitor
Therapeutic class: systemic hemostatic drug
Pregnancy risk category: B

Indications and dosages

▶ **To reduce blood loss or need for transfusion in patients undergoing coronary artery bypass grafts.** *Adults:* Start with 10,000 kallikrein inactivator units (KIU) test dose at least 10 minutes before loading dose. If no allergic reaction occurs, anesthesia may be induced while loading dose of 2 million KIU is given slowly over 20 to 30 minutes. When loading dose is complete, sternotomy may be performed. Before bypass, cardiopulmonary bypass circuit is primed with 2 million KIU of drug by replacing an aliquot of priming fluid with drug. A continuous infusion at 500,000 KIU/hour is then given until patient leaves operating room. This is known as regimen A. A second regimen, called regimen B, may be given, which is half the dosage of regimen A (except for test dose).

▽ I.V. administration

• Give a test dose. In patients who have previously received drug, pretreat with an antihistamine.
• Drug is incompatible with amino acids, corticosteroids, fat emulsions, heparin, and tetracyclines. Don't add any drugs to I.V. container, and use a separate I.V. line.
• Give all doses through a central line.
• To avoid hypotension, make sure patient is lying down during loading dose.
• If symptoms of hypersensitivity (such as skin eruptions, itching, dyspnea, nausea, or tachycardia) occur, stop infusion immediately, call prescriber, and provide supportive treatment.
• Store drug between 36° and 77° F (2° and 25° C). Protect from freezing.

Contraindications and precautions

• Contraindicated in patients hypersensitive to beef because drug is prepared from bovine lung.
⚜ Lifespan: In pregnant women, use cautiously. In breast-feeding women and in children, safety of drug hasn't been established.

Adverse reactions

CNS: fever, *cerebral embolism, CVA.*
CV: *cardiac arrest, heart failure, MI, ventricular tachycardia,* atrial fibrillation, atrial flutter, hypotension, *supraventricular tachycardia.*
GU: *nephrotoxicity, renal failure.*

Respiratory: pneumonia, respiratory disorder, *bronchospasm, pulmonary edema.*
Other: hypersensitivity reactions, *anaphylaxis.*

Interactions

Drug-drug. *Captopril:* May decrease hypotensive effects of captopril. Monitor blood pressure.
Fibrinolytics: May inhibit fibrinolytics. Monitor patient for clinical effects.
Heparin: May prolong ACT when determined by the celite surface activation method. Kaolin-based ACTs should be used while patient is taking both drugs.

Effects on lab test results

• May increase AST, ALT, creatinine, and glucose levels. May decrease potassium level.
• May prolong ACT and APTT.
• May falsely prolong whole blood clotting times when determined by surface activation methods.

Pharmacokinetics

Absorption: Administered I.V.
Distribution: Rapid.
Metabolism: Unknown.
Excretion: 25% to 40% in urine over 48 hours.
Half-life: About 10 hours.

Route	Onset	Peak	Duration
I.V.	Unknown	Unknown	Unknown

Action

Chemical effect: Inhibits fibrinolysis by affecting kallikrein and plasmin, prevents triggering of contact phase of coagulation pathway, and increases resistance of platelets to damage from mechanical injury and high plasmin levels that occur during cardiopulmonary bypass.
Therapeutic effect: Decreases bleeding and turnover of coagulation factors.

Available forms

Injection: 10,000 KIU/ml (1.4 mg/ml) in 100-ml and 200-ml vials

NURSING PROCESS

℞ Assessment

• Obtain history of allergies. Patients with a history of allergic reactions to drugs or other sub-

stances may be at higher risk for developing an allergic reaction to aprotinin.
- Obtain history of patient's bleeding status before therapy and reassess regularly thereafter.
- Be alert for adverse reactions.
- Monitor laboratory studies.
- Evaluate patient's and family's knowledge of drug therapy.

🔲 **Nursing diagnoses**
- Risk for deficient fluid volume related to potential bleeding during surgery
- Risk for injury related to drug-induced adverse reactions
- Deficient knowledge related to drug therapy

▶ **Planning and implementation**
- Patients who have previously received drug have a higher risk of anaphylaxis. In these patients, pretreat with an antihistamine, and give a test dose.

Patient teaching
- Inform patient and family about aprotinin's use with cardiopulmonary bypass surgery and its adverse reactions.

✔ **Evaluation**
- Patient's bleeding during surgery is minimal.
- Patient doesn't experience injury as a result of aprotinin therapy.
- Patient and family state understanding of drug therapy.

---

argatroban
(are-GA-troe-ban)
Argatroban

Pharmacologic class: direct thrombin inhibitor
Therapeutic class: anticoagulant
Pregnancy risk category: B

Indications and dosages

▶ **Prevention or treatment of thrombosis in patients with heparin-induced thrombocytopenia.** *Adults:* 2 mcg/kg/minute, given as a continuous I.V. infusion; adjust dose until steady state APTT is one and a half to three times the initial baseline value, not to exceed 100 seconds; maximum dose is 10 mcg/kg/minute.

The standard infusion rates for 2 mcg/kg/minute are shown below.

Body weight (kg)	Infusion rate (ml/hr)
50	6
60	7
70	8
80	10
90	11
100	12
110	13
120	14
130	16
140	17

⊠ **Adjust-a-dose:** For patients with moderate hepatic impairment, initial dose should be reduced to 0.5 mcg/kg/minute, given as a continuous infusion. Monitor APTT closely and adjust dosage as needed.
▶ **Anticoagulation in patients with or at risk for heparin-induced thrombocytopenia (HIT) during percutaneous coronary interventions (PCI).** *Adults:* 350 mcg/kg I.V. bolus over 3 to 5 minutes. Start a continuous I.V. infusion at 25 mcg/kg/minute. Activated clotting time (ACT) should be checked 5 to 10 minutes after the bolus dose is completed.
⊠ **Adjust-a-dose:** See table below.

ACT	Additional I.V. bolus	Continuous I.V. infusion
< 300 sec	150 mcg/kg	30 mcg/kg/min***
300-450 sec	None needed	25 mcg/kg/min
> 450 sec	None needed	15 mcg/kg/min***

***Check ACT again after 5 to 10 minutes

In case of dissection, impending abrupt closure, thrombus formation during the procedure, or inability to achieve or maintain an ACT longer than 300 seconds, give an additional bolus of 150 mcg/kg and increase infusion rate to 40 mcg/kg/minute. Check ACT again after 5 to 10 minutes.
⑤ **ALERT:** ACT should be checked every 20 to 30 minutes during a prolonged PCI.

▽ **I.V. administration**
- Dilute in normal saline solution, D₅W, or lactated Ringer's injection to a final concentration of 1 mg/ml.

- Each 2.5-ml vial should be diluted 1:100 by mixing it with 250 ml of diluent.
- Mix the constituted solution by repeatedly turning over the diluent bag for 1 minute.
- Don't mix other drugs with argatroban infusion.
- Prepared solutions are stable for up to 24 hours at 77° F (25° C).

Contraindications and precautions

- Contraindicated in patients hypersensitive to drug or its components and in patients with active bleeding.
- Use cautiously in patients with hepatic disease; disease states that create an increased risk of hemorrhage, such as severe hypertension; very recent lumbar puncture, spinal anesthesia, or major surgery, especially involving the brain, spinal cord, or eye; and hematologic conditions linked to increased bleeding tendencies, such as congenital or acquired bleeding disorders and GI lesions and ulcerations.
- ⚖ Lifespan: In breast-feeding women, a decision should be made to stop breast-feeding or drug because it's unknown whether drug appears in breast milk. In children, safety and efficacy haven't been established.

Interactions

Drug-drug. *Oral anticoagulants, antiplatelet drugs:* May prolong PT and INR and increase risk of bleeding. Avoid using together.
Thrombolytics: May increase risk of intracranial bleeding. Avoid using together.

Adverse reactions

CNS: fever, pain.
CV: atrial fibrillation, *cardiac arrest, cerebrovascular disorder, hemorrhage,* hypotension, *ventricular tachycardia,* vasodilation.
GI: abdominal pain, diarrhea, *GI bleeding,* hemoptysis, nausea, vomiting.
GU: abnormal renal function, groin bleeding, *hematuria,* UTI.
Hematologic: anemia.
Respiratory: cough, dyspnea, pneumonia.
Skin: rash, bullous eruptions.
Other: brachial bleeding, infection, *sepsis, allergic reactions (in patients also receiving thrombolytic therapy for acute MI).*

Effects on lab test results

- May increase WBC and platelet counts, APTT, ACT, and INR. May decrease hemoglobin and hematocrit.

Pharmacokinetics

Absorption: Administered I.V.
Distribution: Mainly in the extracellular fluid. Drug is 54% protein-bound, of which 34% is bound to a_1-acid glycoprotein and 20% to albumin.
Metabolism: Mainly in the liver by hydroxylation. The formation of four metabolites is catalyzed in the liver by CYP 3A4 and 5. The primary metabolite is 20% weaker than that of the parent drug. The other metabolites are detected in low levels in urine.
Excretion: Primarily in the feces, presumably through the biliary tract. *Half-life:* 39 to 51 minutes.

Route	Onset	Peak	Duration
I.V.	Rapid	1-3 hr	Until infusion stops

Action

Chemical effect: Reversibly binds to the thrombin active site and inhibits reactions catalyzed or induced by thrombin, including fibrin formation, activation of coagulation factors V, VIII, and XIII and protein C, and platelet aggregation. Inhibits the action of both free and clot-related thrombin.
Therapeutic effect: Prevents clot formation.

Available forms

Injection: 100 mg/ml

NURSING PROCESS

✐ Assessment
- Assess patient for increased risk of bleeding or overt bleeding before starting drug therapy.
- Obtain baseline coagulation tests, platelet counts, hemoglobin, and hematocrit before therapy. Check APTT and ACT. Note abnormalities and notify prescriber.
- Stop all parenteral anticoagulants before giving drug.
- Evaluate patient's and family's knowledge of drug therapy.

Reactions may be *common,* uncommon, *life-threatening*, or **COMMON AND LIFE-THREATENING.**

⚕ Nursing diagnoses
- Ineffective tissue perfusion due to blood clots
- Increased risk for injury related to increased APTT and increased risk of bleeding from drug therapy.
- Deficient knowledge related to argatroban therapy and anticoagulant safety precautions.

▷ Planning and implementation
- If an unexplained drop in hematocrit or blood pressure or another unexplained symptom occurs, suspect a hemorrhage and notify prescriber.
- ⊛ **ALERT:** Excessive anticoagulation, with or without bleeding, may occur in overdose. Symptoms of acute toxicity include loss of reflex, tremors, clonic seizures, limb paralysis, and coma. No specific antidote is available. Discontinue immediately and monitor APTT and other coagulation tests. Provide symptomatic and supportive therapy.
- To convert to oral anticoagulant therapy, give warfarin with argatroban at doses of up to 2 mcg/kg/minute until the INR is above 4. After stopping argatroban, repeat the INR in 4 to 6 hours. If the repeat INR is below the desired therapeutic range, resume argatroban. Repeat the procedure daily until the desired therapeutic range is reached on warfarin alone.
- ⊛ **ALERT:** Don't confuse Aggrastat (tirofiban) with argatroban.

Patient teaching
- Advise patient that drug can cause bleeding, and urge him to report immediately any unusual bruising, bleeding (nosebleeds, bleeding gums, ecchymosis, or hematuria), or tarry or bloody stools.
- Advise patient to avoid activities that carry a risk of injury or cuts, and instruct him to use a soft toothbrush and electric razor while taking argatroban.
- Tell patient to notify prescriber if she is pregnant, breast-feeding, or recently had a baby.
- Tell patient to notify prescriber if he has stomach ulcers or liver disease; if he's had recent surgery, radiation treatments, falls, or other injury; or if wheezing, difficulty breathing, or rash occurs.

☑ Evaluation
- Patient doesn't have any unnecessary bruising or bleeding.

- Patient doesn't develop blood clots while on drug.
- Patient and family state understanding of drug therapy.

---

aripiprazole
(air-uh-PIP-rah-zol)
Abilify

Pharmacological class: psychotropic
Therapeutic class: atypical antipsychotic
Pregnancy risk category: C

Indications and dosages

▶ **Schizophrenia.** *Adults:* Initially, 10 to 15 mg P.O. daily, increasing to a maximum daily dose of 30 mg if needed, after at least 2 weeks. Maintenance doses of 15 mg P.O. daily may be effective.
⊠ Adjust-a-dose: Give half the dose when given with CYP 3A4 or CYP 2D6 inhibitors, particularly ketoconazole, quinidine, fluoxetine, or paroxetine. Double the dose when given with CYP 3A4 inducers, such as carbamazepine. Give original dose once other drugs are stopped.

Contraindications and precautions

- Contraindicated in patients hypersensitive to drug.
- Use cautiously in patients with CV disease, cerebrovascular disease, or conditions that could predispose the patient to hypotension, such as dehydration or hypovolemia. Also use cautiously in patients with history of seizures or with conditions that lower the seizure threshold and in those at risk for aspiration pneumonia, such as those with Alzheimer's disease. Use caution in patients who engage in strenuous exercise, are exposed to extreme heat, take anticholinergic medications, or are susceptible to dehydration.
- ☙ **Lifespan:** In pregnant women, use only if the benefits outweigh the risks. Breast-feeding women shouldn't breast feed during drug therapy; it's unknown whether drug appears in breast milk. In children, safety and efficacy of drug haven't been established. In elderly patients, use cautiously because they may experience greater sensitivity to drug.

Adverse reactions

CNS: *headache, anxiety, insomnia, lightheadedness, somnolence, akathisia,* tremor, asthenia, depression, nervousness, hostility, *suicidal thoughts,* manic behavior, confusion, abnormal gait, cogwheel rigidity, *seizures,* fever, tardive dyskinesia, cognitive and motor impairment, *neuroleptic malignant syndrome.*
CV: peripheral edema, chest pain, hypertension, tachycardia, orthostatic hypotension, *bradycardia.*
EENT: rhinitis, blurred vision, increased salivation, conjunctivitis, ear pain.
GI: *nausea, vomiting, constipation,* anorexia, diarrhea, abdominal pain, esophageal dysmotility.
GU: urinary incontinence.
Hematologic: anemia.
Metabolic: weight gain, weight loss, hyperglycemia.
Musculoskeletal: neck pain, neck stiffness, muscle cramps.
Respiratory: dyspnea, pneumonia, cough.
Skin: rash, dry skin, ecchymosis, pruritus, sweating, ulcer.
Other: flulike syndrome, inability to regulate body temperature.

Interactions

Drug-drug. *Antihypertensives:* Enhances antihypertensive and orthostatic hypotensive effects. Monitor blood pressure.
Carbamazepine and other CYP 3A4 inducers: Decreases level and effectiveness of aripiprazole. Double the usual dose of aripiprazole and monitor the patient closely.
Ketoconazole and other CYP 3A4 inhibitors; quinidine, fluoxetine, paroxetine, and other CYP 2D6 inhibitors: May increase level and toxicity of aripiprazole. Halve the usual dose of aripiprazole and monitor patient closely.
Drug-food. *Grapefruit juice:* May increase drug level. Advise patient to avoid grapefruit juice during treatment.
Drug-lifestyle. *Alcohol use:* May increase CNS effects. Discourage using together.

Effects on lab test results

• May increase CPK level.

Pharmacokinetics

Absorption: Good. Absolute bioavailability is 87% and isn't affected by food.

Distribution: Extensive. Protein-binding, primarily to albumin, is 99% for drug and major metabolites.
Metabolism: Extensively metabolized through the CYP 3A4 and CYP 2D6 systems, with one active metabolite.
Excretion: In urine and feces. *Elimination half-life:* About 75 hours in patients with normal metabolism and about 146 hours in those unable to metabolize the drug through CYP 2D6.

Route	Onset	Peak	Duration
P.O.	Unknown	3-5 hr	Unknown

Action

Chemical effect: May exhibit its antipsychotic effects through partial agonist activity at D2 and serotonin $5-HT_{1A}$ receptors and antagonist activity at serotonin $5-HT_{2A}$ receptors.
Therapeutic effect: Decreases psychotic behaviors.

Available forms

Tablets: 5 mg, 10 mg, 15 mg, 20 mg, 30 mg

NURSING PROCESS

Assessment
• Assess patient's condition before and after therapy.
• Assess for potential compliance issues with drug regimen.
• Be alert for adverse reactions and drug interactions.
• Evaluate patient and family's knowledge of drug therapy.

Nursing diagnoses
• Risk for recurrence of signs and symptoms of schizophrenia if not compliant with medication regimen
• Potential noncompliance with medication regimen related to underlying mental illness
• Deficient knowledge related to drug therapy

Planning and implementation
ALERT: Neuroleptic malignant syndrome may occur. Monitor patient for hyperpyrexia, muscle rigidity, altered mental status, irregular pulse or blood pressure, tachycardia, diaphoresis, and cardiac arrhythmias. If signs and symptoms of

---

neuroleptic malignant syndrome occur, stop drug immediately.

- Monitor patient for signs and symptoms of tardive dyskinesia. Elderly patients, especially elderly women, are at higher risk of developing this adverse effect. If it occurs, stop drug.

⚠ **ALERT:** Drug may cause hyperglycemia. Monitor diabetic patient's glucose level regularly.

- Give the smallest dose for the shortest time. Periodically reassess need for treatment.
- To reduce risk of overdose, make sure only a small quantity of tablets has been prescribed.
- Overdose may cause somnolence and vomiting. Give activated charcoal within the first hours of overdose; 50% of a 15-mg dose is absorbed within the first hour. Dialysis isn't helpful because drug is highly protein-bound.

Patient teaching

- Tell patient to use caution when driving or operating hazardous machinery because psychoactive drugs may impair judgment, thinking, or motor skills.
- Tell patient that drug may be taken without regard to meals.
- Advise patient to avoid taking drug with grapefruit juice.
- Inform patient that gradual improvement in symptoms should occur over several weeks rather than immediately.
- Tell patient to avoid alcohol use while taking drug.
- Advise patient to limit strenuous activity while taking drug to avoid dehydration and becoming overheated.

☑ **Evaluation**

- Patient demonstrates reduced signs and symptoms of schizophrenia.
- Patient is compliant with drug regimen.
- Patient and family state understanding of drug therapy.

arsenic trioxide
(AR-sen-ik try-OX-ide)
Trisenox

Pharmacologic class: antineoplastic
Therapeutic class: antileukemia drug
Pregnancy risk category: D

Indications and dosages

▶ **Acute promyelocytic leukemia (APL) in patients who have relapsed from or are refractory to retinoid and anthracycline chemotherapy.** *Adults and children age 5 and older:* During induction phase, 0.15 mg/kg I.V. daily until bone marrow remission. Maximum 60 doses. During consolidation phase, 0.15 mg/kg I.V. daily for 25 doses over a period of up to 5 weeks, beginning 3 to 6 weeks after completion of induction therapy.

▼ I.V. administration

- Follow facility policy for preparation and handling of antineoplastics; the active ingredient is a carcinogen.
- Dilute with 100 to 250 ml of D_5W or normal saline solution. After dilution, drug is stable for 24 hours at room temperature and for 48 hours if refrigerated.
- Give I.V. over 1 to 2 hours. If vasomotor reactions occur, extend to 4 hours.

Contraindications and precautions

- Contraindicated in patients hypersensitive to arsenic.
- Use cautiously in patients with heart failure or a history of torsades de pointes, prolonged QT interval, or conditions that result in hypokalemia or hypomagnesemia.

⚘ **Lifespan:** Women of childbearing age should avoid becoming pregnant during therapy. In breast-feeding women, avoid use; arsenic appears in breast milk and may cause fetal harm. In children younger than age 5, safety and efficacy haven't been established.

Adverse reactions

CNS: *fever;* headache, insomnia, paresthesia, dizziness, *pain,* tremor, *seizures,* somnolence, *coma,* anxiety, depression, agitation, confusion, fatigue, weakness.
CV: *hemorrhage,* tachycardia, PROLONGED QT INTERVAL, COMPLETE AV BLOCK, *palpitations, edema, chest pain,* ECG abnormalities, *hypotension, flushing, facial edema, hypertension.*
EENT: *eye irritation, epistaxis, blurred vision,* dry eye, earache, tinnitus, *sore throat, postnasal drip,* facial and eyelid edema, *sinusitis,* nasopharyngitis, painful red eye.
GI: *nausea, vomiting, diarrhea, anorexia, abdominal pain, constipation, loose stools, dyspepsia,* oral blistering, fecal incontinence, *GI*

hemorrhage, dry mouth, abdominal tenderness or distension, bloody diarrhea, oral candidiasis.
GU: *renal failure,* renal impairment, oliguria, incontinence, *vaginal hemorrhage,* intermenstrual bleeding.
Hematologic: *leukocytosis, anemia,* THROMBOCYTOPENIA, NEUTROPENIA, DIC, lymphadenopathy.
Metabolic: hypokalemia, hypomagnesemia, hyperglycemia, hypocalcemia, *hypoglycemia,* acidosis, weight gain, weight loss, HYPERKALEMIA.
Musculoskeletal: arthralgia, myalgia, bone pain, back pain, neck pain, limb pain.
Respiratory: cough, dyspnea, hypoxia, pleural effusion, wheezing, decreased breath sounds, crepitations, rales, hemoptysis, tachypnea, rhonchi, upper respiratory tract infection.
Skin: *dermatitis, pruritus, dry skin, erythema, increased sweating,* night sweats, petechiae, hyperpigmentation, urticaria, skin lesions, local exfoliation, *pallor,* ecchymosis.
Other: drug hypersensitivity; *erythema, or edema at injection site; rigors; herpes simplex infection;* bacterial infection; herpes zoster; *sepsis.*

Interactions

Drug-drug. *Drugs that can lead to electrolyte abnormalities (diuretics or amphotericin B):* May increase risk of electrolyte abnormalities. Use cautiously.
Drugs that can prolong QT interval (antiarrhythmics or thioridazine): May further prolong QT interval. Use cautiously and monitor ECG closely.

Effects on lab test results

• May increase AST, ALT, BUN, magnesium, calcium, and creatinine levels. May decrease sodium level. May increase or decrease glucose and potassium levels.
• May decrease hemoglobin, hematocrit, and RBC, WBC, neutrophil, and platelet counts.

Pharmacokinetics

Absorption: Administered I.V.
Distribution: Stored mainly in the liver, kidneys, heart, lungs, hair, and nails.
Metabolism: Metabolized in the liver.
Excretion: Excreted in urine in the methylated form.

Route	Onset	Peak	Duration
I.V.	Unknown	Unknown	Unknown

Action

Chemical effect: Causes morphologic changes and DNA fragmentation resulting in death of promyelocytic leukemic cells.
Therapeutic effect: Destroys promyelocytic leukemic cells.

Available forms

Injection: 1 mg/ml

NURSING PROCESS

Assessment

⚠ **ALERT:** May cause fatal arrhythmias and complete AV block.
• Monitor patient closely for altered blood pressure.
• Perform ECG; obtain potassium, calcium, magnesium, and creatinine levels; and correct electrolyte abnormalities before starting therapy.
• Monitor electrolyte levels and hematologic and coagulation profiles at least twice weekly during treatment. Keep potassium levels above 4 mEq/dL and magnesium levels above 1.8 mg/dL.
• Monitor patient for syncope and rapid or irregular heart rate. If these occur, stop drug, hospitalize patient, and monitor electrolyte levels and QT interval. Drug may be restarted when electrolyte abnormalities are corrected and QTc interval falls below 460 msec.
• Monitor ECG at least weekly during therapy. QT interval commonly is prolonged between 1 and 5 weeks after infusion and returns to baseline about 8 weeks after infusion. If QTc interval is longer than 500 msec at any time during therapy, assess patient carefully and stop drug.
• Evaluate patient's and family's knowledge of drug therapy.

Nursing diagnoses

• Risk of decreased cardiac output due to drug-induced toxicity
• Risk for infection related to drug-induced thrombocytopenia or neutropenia
• Deficient knowledge related to arsenic trioxide therapy

ⓑ Planning and implementation

• Monitor patient carefully for adverse reactions or drug toxicity. Symptoms of acute arsenic toxicity include confusion, muscle weakness, and seizures. If overdose occurs, stop drug immediately. Give 3 mg/kg dimercaprol I.M. q 4 hours until life-threatening toxicity subsides; then give 250 mg penicillamine P.O. up to q.i.d.

ⓢ **ALERT:** May cause fatal APL differentiation syndrome, characterized by fever, dyspnea, weight gain, pulmonary infiltrates, and pleural or pericardial effusions with or without leukocytosis. If it occurs, give high-dose steroids.

Patient teaching

• Tell patient to report immediately fever, shortness of breath, bloody stools, or weight gain.

• Instruct patient to tell prescriber about all drugs currently being taken and to check with prescriber before starting any new drug.

• Inform patient with diabetes that drug may cause hyperglycemia or hypoglycemia, and instruct him to monitor glucose level closely.

• Caution women of childbearing age to avoid becoming pregnant during therapy.

☑ Evaluation

• Patient tolerates therapy and responds positively to drug therapy.

• Patient doesn't have infection or life-threatening adverse events.

• Patient and family state understanding of drug therapy.

asparaginase (L-asparaginase)

(as-PAR-ah-jin-ays)
Elspar, Kidrolase ◆

Pharmacologic class: enzyme (L-asparagine amidohydrolase), cell-cycle–phase specific, G1 phase
Therapeutic class: antineoplastic
Pregnancy risk category: C

Indications and dosages

▶ **Acute lymphocytic leukemia (ALL) (with other drugs).** *Adults and children:* For ALL Regimen I treatment period, on day 22 of treatment, give 1,000 IU/kg I.V. daily for 10 days, injected over 30 minutes or by slow I.V. push; or for ALL Regimen II treatment protocol, give

6,000 IU/m^2 I.M. at intervals specified in protocol.

▶ **Sole induction drug for remission of ALL.** *Adults and children:* 200 IU/kg I.V. daily for 28 days.

▼ I.V. administration

• Follow facility policy to reduce risks. Preparing and giving parenteral form may carry carcinogenic, mutagenic, and teratogenic risks.

• Reconstitute with 5 ml of either sterile water or normal saline solution for injection. Don't shake vial. Don't use cloudy solutions.

• Give injection over 30 minutes through a running infusion of normal saline solution for injection or D$_5$W injection.

• If drug contacts skin or mucous membranes, wash with copious amounts of water for at least 15 minutes.

• Filtration through a 5-micron filter during administration will remove particles without decreasing potency.

• Keep epinephrine, diphenhydramine, and I.V. corticosteroids available to treat anaphylaxis.

• Refrigerate unopened dry powder. Reconstituted solution is stable for 8 hours if refrigerated.

Contraindications and precautions

• Contraindicated in patients with pancreatitis or history of pancreatitis and previous hypersensitivity unless desensitized.

• Use cautiously in patients with hepatic dysfunction.

⚖ Lifespan: In pregnant women, use cautiously. In breast-feeding women, drug shouldn't be used.

Adverse reactions

CNS: fever, chills, confusion, drowsiness, depression, hallucinations, nervousness, lethargy, somnolence.

GI: *vomiting, anorexia, nausea,* cramps, weight loss, **HEMORRHAGIC PANCREATITIS.**

GU: azotemia, *renal impairment,* uric acid nephropathy, glycosuria, polyuria, *increased blood ammonia level.*

Hematologic: anemia, *hypofibrinogenemia, thrombocytopenia, leukopenia.*

Hepatic: *hepatotoxicity.*

Metabolic: *hyperuricemia, hyperglycemia.*

Skin: rash, urticaria.
Other: ANAPHYLAXIS, *fatal hyperthermia.*

Interactions

Drug-drug. *Methotrexate:* May decrease methotrexate's effectiveness when given immediately before or with methotrexate. Monitor levels of methotrexate. Watch patient for signs of decreased effect.
Prednisone, vincristine: May increase toxicity. Monitor patient closely.

Effects on lab test results

• May increase BUN, AST, ALT, bilirubin, glucose, uric acid, and ammonia levels. May decrease calcium, fibrinogen, and albumin levels, and levels of other clotting factors. May increase or decrease total lipid level.
• May decrease hemoglobin, hematocrit, thyroid function test values, and WBC and platelet counts.

Pharmacokinetics

Absorption: Unknown.
Distribution: Primarily within intravascular space, with detectable levels in thoracic and cervical lymph. Minimal amount crosses blood-brain barrier.
Metabolism: Hepatic sequestration by reticuloendothelial system may occur.
Excretion: Unknown. *Half-life:* 8 to 30 hours.

Route	Onset	Peak	Duration
I.V.	Almost immediate	Almost immediate	23-33 days after stopping drug
I.M.	Almost immediate	4-24 hr after stopping drug	23-33 days

Action

Chemical effect: Destroys amino acid asparagine, which is needed for protein synthesis in acute lymphocytic leukemia. This leads to death of leukemic cell.
Therapeutic effect: Kills leukemia cells.

Available forms

Injection: 10,000 IU vial

NURSING PROCESS

🧠 Assessment
• Obtain history of patient's leukemia.

• Monitor effectiveness by evaluating CBC and bone marrow function test results. Bone marrow regeneration may take 5 to 6 weeks.
• Be alert for adverse reactions and drug interactions.
• Evaluate patient's and family's knowledge of drug therapy.

💠 Nursing diagnoses
• Ineffective health maintenance related to leukemic condition
• Ineffective protection related to drug-induced adverse reactions
• Deficient knowledge related to drug therapy

▶ Planning and implementation
• Give drug in a hospital under close supervision.
• Drug shouldn't be used alone to induce remission unless combination therapy is inappropriate. Not recommended for maintenance therapy.
• Increase patient's fluid intake to prevent tumor lysis, which can result in uric acid nephropathy. Start allopurinol before therapy begins.
⊛ **ALERT:** Repeated doses increase the risk of hypersensitivity reactions. Perform an I.D. skin test before initial dose and repeat after an interval of a week or more, between doses. To perform skin test, give 2 IU of drug I.D. Observe site for at least 1 hour for erythema or a wheal, which indicates a positive response. An allergic reaction to the drug may still develop in a patient with a negative skin test.
• Give a desensitization dose of 1 IU I.V. Dose is doubled q 10 minutes if no reaction occurs, until total amount given equals patient's total dose for that day.
• Limit I.M. dose at single injection site to 2 ml.
• Because patient may vomit, give parenteral fluids for 24 hours or until patient can tolerate oral fluids.

Patient teaching
• Tell patient to watch for signs of infection (fever, sore throat, fatigue) and bleeding (easy bruising, nosebleeds, bleeding gums, tarry or bloody stools). Instruct patient to take temperature daily.
• Encourage patient to maintain an adequate fluid intake to increase urine output and facilitate excretion of uric acid.
• Tell patient that drowsiness may occur during therapy or for several weeks after treatment

---

ends. Warn patient to avoid hazardous activities requiring mental alertness.

☑ Evaluation
• Patient is free from leukemia.
• Patient doesn't experience injury as a result of drug-induced adverse reactions.
• Patient and family state understanding of drug therapy.

aspirin (acetylsalicylic acid)
(AS-prin)
Ancasal ◆ †, Arthrinol ◆ †, Artria S.R. †, ASA†, ASA Enseals†, Aspergum†, Aspro Preparations ◇, Astrin ◆ †, Bayer Aspirin†, Bex Powders ◇, Coryphen ◆ †, Easprin†, Ecotrin†, Empirin†, Entrophen ◆ †, Halfprin, Measurin ◆ †, Norwich Extra Strength†, Novasen ◆ †, Riphen-10 ◆ †, Sal-Adult ◆ †, Sal-Infant ◆ †, Sloprin ◇, Supasa ◆ †, Triaphen-10 ◆ †, Vincent's Powders ◇, ZORprin†

Pharmacologic class: salicylate
Therapeutic class: nonopioid analgesic, antipyretic, anti-inflammatory, antiplatelet drug
Pregnancy risk category: C (D in third trimester)

Indications and dosages
▶ **Arthritis.** *Adults:* Initially, 2.4 to 3.6 g P.O. daily in divided doses. Maintenance dosage is 3.6 to 5.4 g P.O. daily in divided doses. *Children:* 60 to 130 mg/kg P.O. daily in divided doses.
▶ **Mild pain or fever.** *Adults:* 325 to 650 mg P.O. or P.R. q 4 hours, p.r.n. *Children:* For mild pain only, 65 mg/kg P.O. or P.R. daily in four to six divided doses.
▶ **Prevention of thrombosis.** *Adults:* 1.3 g P.O. daily in two to four divided doses.
▶ **Reduction of risk of MI in patients with previous MI or unstable angina.** *Adults:* 160 to 325 mg P.O. daily.
▶ **Kawasaki syndrome (mucocutaneous lymph node syndrome).** *Adults:* 80 to 100 mg/kg P.O. daily in four divided doses during febrile phase. Some patients may need up to 120 mg/kg. When fever subsides, decrease dosage to 3 to 8 mg/kg once daily, adjusted according to salicylate level.

▶ **Prophylaxis for transient ischemic attack (TIA).** *Adults:* 50 to 325 mg P.O. daily.
▶ **TIA.** *Adults:* 160 to 325 mg P.O. immediately within 48 hours of onset of CVA.
▶ **Prevention of reocclusion in coronary revascularization procedures.** *Adults:* 325 mg P.O. q 6 hours after surgery and for 1 year.
▶ **Rheumatic fever‡.** *Adults:* 4.9 to 7.8 g P.O. daily in divided doses q 4 to 6 hours for 1 to 2 weeks. Decrease to 60 to 70 mg/kg daily for 1 to 6 weeks, then gradually withdraw over 1 to 2 weeks. *Children:* 90 to 130 mg/kg P.O. daily in divided doses q 4 to 6 hours.
▶ **Pericarditis after acute MI‡.** *Adults:* 160 to 325 mg P.O. daily.
▶ **Stent implantation‡.** *Adults:* 160 to 325 mg P.O. q 2 hours before stent placement and continued indefinitely.

Contraindications and precautions
• Contraindicated in patients hypersensitive to drug and those with G6PD deficiency; bleeding disorders such as hemophilia, von Willebrand's disease, and telangiectasia; and NSAID-induced sensitivity reactions.
• Use cautiously in patients with GI lesions, impaired renal function, hypoprothrombinemia, vitamin K deficiency, thrombocytopenia, thrombotic thrombocytopenic purpura, or severe hepatic impairment.
⚕ Lifespan: In pregnant women, use cautiously. In breast-feeding women, safety hasn't been established.
⚠ ALERT: Because of the link with Reye's syndrome, the Centers for Disease Control and Prevention recommends not giving salicylates to children or teenagers who have or are recovering from chickenpox or flulike illness. In elderly patients, use cautiously because GI and renal adverse effects may be exacerbated.

Adverse reactions
EENT: *tinnitus, hearing loss.*
GI: *nausea, vomiting, GI distress, occult bleeding, dyspepsia, **GI bleeding.***
GU: *transient renal insufficiency.*
Hematologic: *prolonged bleeding time, **thrombocytopenia.***
Hepatic: *hepatitis.*
Skin: *rash,* bruising, urticaria.
Other: *angioedema,* hypersensitivity reactions, (*anaphylaxis,* asthma), *Reye's syndrome.*

Interactions

Drug-drug. *Ammonium chloride, other urine acidifiers:* May increase levels of aspirin products. Watch for aspirin toxicity.
Antacids in high doses (and other urine alkalinizers): May decrease levels of aspirin products. Watch for decreased aspirin effect.
Beta blockers: May decrease antihypertensive effect. Avoid long-term aspirin use if patient is taking antihypertensives.
Corticosteroids: May enhance salicylate elimination. Watch for decreased salicylate effect.
Heparin: Increases risk of bleeding. Monitor coagulation studies and patient closely if used together.
Methotrexate: May increase risk of methotrexate toxicity. Monitor patient closely.
NSAIDs: May alter pharmacokinetics of these drugs, leading to lower levels and decreased effectiveness. Avoid using together. May also increase risk of GI bleeding. Monitor patient closely.
Oral anticoagulants: May increase risk of bleeding. Monitor patient for signs of bleeding.
Oral antidiabetics: May increase hypoglycemic effect. Monitor patient closely.
Probenecid, sulfinpyrazone: May decrease uricosuric effect. Avoid aspirin during therapy with these drugs.
Steroids: May increase risk of GI bleeding. Monitor patient closely.
Drug-herb. *Dong quai, feverfew, garlic, ginger, horse chestnut, red clover:* May increase risk of bleeding. Monitor patient for increased effects, and discourage using together.
Drug-food. *Caffeine:* May increase the absorption of aspirin. Monitor patient for increased effects.
Drug-lifestyle. *Alcohol use:* May increase risk of GI bleeding. Discourage using together.

Effects on lab test results

• May increase liver function test values. May decrease WBC and platelet counts.

Pharmacokinetics

Absorption: Absorbed rapidly and completely from GI tract.
Distribution: Distributed widely into most body tissues and fluids. Protein-binding to albumin is concentration-dependent; it ranges from 75% to 90%, and decreases as level increases.

Metabolism: Hydrolyzed partially in GI tract to salicylic acid, with almost complete metabolism in liver.
Excretion: Excreted in urine as salicylate and its metabolites. *Half-life:* 15 to 20 minutes.

Route	Onset	Peak	Duration
P.O.			
buffered	5-30 min	1-2 hr	1-4 hr
enteric-coated	5-30 min	4-8 hr	1-4 hr
extended-release	5-30 min	1-2 hr	1-4 hr
regular	5-30 min	25-40 min	1-4 hr
solution	5-30 min	15-60 min	1-4 hr
P.R.	5-30 min	3-4 hr	1-4 hr

Action

Chemical effect: Produces analgesia by blocking prostaglandin synthesis (peripheral action). Drug and other salicylates may prevent lowering of pain threshold that occurs when prostaglandins sensitize pain receptors to stimulation. Exerts its anti-inflammatory effect by inhibiting prostaglandin synthesis; also may inhibit synthesis or action of other mediators of inflammatory response. Relieves fever by acting on hypothalamic heat-regulating center to cause peripheral vasodilation, which increases peripheral blood supply and promotes sweating, which leads to heat loss and to cooling by evaporation. In low doses, aspirin also appears to impede clotting by blocking prostaglandin synthesis, which prevents formation of platelet-aggregating substance thromboxane A_2.
Therapeutic effect: Relieves pain, reduces fever and inflammation, and decreases risk of transient ischemic attacks and MI.

Available forms

Capsules: 325 mg†, 500 mg†
Chewing gum: 227.5 mg†
Suppositories: 60 mg†, 65 mg†, 120 mg†, 125 mg†, 130 mg†, 195 mg†, 200 mg†, 300 mg†, 325 mg†, 600 mg†, 650 mg†
Tablets†: 325 mg, 500 mg, 600 mg, 650 mg
Tablets (chewable): 81 mg†
Tablets (enteric-coated): 165 mg, 325 mg†, 500 mg†, 650 mg†, 975 mg
Tablets (extended-release): 800 mg
Tablets (timed-release): 650 mg†

⚗ Assessment

- Obtain history of patient's pain or fever before therapy, and monitor patient throughout therapy.
- Be alert for adverse reactions and drug interactions.
- During long-term therapy, monitor salicylate level. Therapeutic level in arthritis is 10 to 30 mg/dl. With long-term therapy, mild toxicity may occur at levels of 20 mg/dl. Tinnitus may occur at levels of 30 mg/dl and above but doesn't reliably indicate toxicity, especially in very young patients and those older than age 60.
- Evaluate patient's and family's knowledge of drug therapy.

🔲 Nursing diagnoses

- Acute pain related to underlying condition
- Risk for injury related to drug-induced adverse GI reactions
- Deficient knowledge related to drug therapy

▶ Planning and implementation

- Give aspirin with food, milk, antacid, or large glass of water to reduce adverse GI reactions.
- If patient has trouble swallowing, crush aspirin, combine it with soft food, or dissolve it in liquid. Give immediately after mixing with liquid because drug doesn't stay in solution. Don't crush enteric-coated aspirin.
- Enteric-coated products are slowly absorbed and not suitable for acute effects. These products cause less GI bleeding and may be more suited for long-term therapy, such as for arthritis.
- Give P.R. after a bowel movement or at night to maximize absorption.
- Hold dose and notify prescriber if bleeding, salicylism (tinnitus, hearing loss), or adverse GI reactions develop.
- Stop aspirin 5 to 7 days before elective surgery.
- ⚠ **ALERT:** Don't confuse aspirin with Asendin or Afrin.

Patient teaching

- Encourage patient to retain suppository for as long as possible, preferably at least 10 hours to maximize absorption.
- Advise patient receiving high-dose prolonged treatment to watch for petechiae, bleeding gums, and signs of GI bleeding and to maintain adequate fluid intake. Encourage use of a soft toothbrush.
- Because of many possible drug interactions involving aspirin, warn patient who takes prescription form to check with prescriber or pharmacist before taking OTC combinations containing aspirin or herbal preparations.
- Explain that various OTC preparations contain aspirin. Warn patient to read labels carefully to avoid overdose.
- Advise patient to avoid alcohol use during drug therapy.
- Advise patient to restrict intake of caffeine during drug therapy.
- Instruct patient to take aspirin with food or milk.
- Instruct patient not to chew enteric-coated products.
- Emphasize safe storage of medications in the home. Teach patient to keep aspirin and other drugs out of children's reach. Aspirin is a leading cause of poisoning in children. Encourage use of child-resistant containers in households with children, even if only as occasional visitors.

✔ Evaluation

- Patient states that aspirin has relieved pain.
- Patient remains free from adverse GI effects throughout drug therapy.
- Patient and family state understanding of drug therapy.

atazanavir sulfate

(att-uh-za-NUH-veer sul-FAYT)
Reyataz

Pharmacologic class: azapeptide HIV-1 protease inhibitor
Therapeutic class: antiretroviral
Pregnancy risk category: B

Indications and dosages

▶ **HIV-1 infection.** *Adults:* 400 mg P.O. once daily with food. When giving with efavirenz, give 300 mg atazanavir and 100 mg ritonavir with 600 mg efavirenz, all as a single daily dose with food.
▷ **Adjust-a-dose:** For patients with Child-Pugh Class B, reduce dosage to 300 mg P.O. once daily.

Contraindications and precautions

• Contraindicated in patients hypersensitive to drug or its components. Also contraindicated with drugs, such as midazolam, triazolam, dihydroergotamine, ergotamine, ergonovine, methylergonovine, cisapride, pimozide, that are highly dependent on CYP 3A4 for clearance and for which elevated levels are linked to life-threatening effects.

• Use cautiously in patients with preexisting conduction system disease or hepatic impairment.

⚖ Lifespan: In pregnant women, drug should be used only if potential benefits outweigh risk; no adequate, well-controlled studies exist. To help monitor maternal-fetal outcomes of pregnant women, register pregnant women in the Antiretroviral Pregnancy Registry (1-800-258-4263). Women shouldn't breast-feed; it's unknown whether drug appears in breast milk. In children, an optimal dosing regimen hasn't been established. In children younger than age 3, the drug shouldn't be used because of a risk for kernicterus. In elderly patients, use cautiously because they are more likely to have hepatic, renal, or cardiac impairment and other diseases and to be taking other drugs.

Adverse reactions

CNS: *headache,* fever, pain, fatigue, depression, insomnia, dizziness, peripheral neurology symptoms.
GI: *nausea, abdominal pain,* vomiting, diarrhea.
Hepatic: hepatitis, jaundice or scleral icterus.
Metabolic: lipidystrophy, lactic acidosis, lipohypertrophy.
Musculoskeletal: back pain, arthralgia.
Respiratory: increased cough.
Skin: *rash.*

Interactions

Drug-drug. *Antacids and buffered medications:* May decrease atazanavir levels. Give atazanvir 2 hours before or 1 hour after these medications.
Amiodarone, lidocaine (systemic), quinidine: May increase levels of these drugs. Monitor levels.
Atorvastatin: May increase atorvastatin level and the risk of myopathy and rhabdomyolysis. Use together cautiously.
Pimozide: May cause life-threatening reactions, such as cardiac arrhythmias. Don't use together.

Clarithromycin: May increase clarithromycin and atazanavir levels and decrease 14-OH clarithromycin levels. Reduce clarithromycin dose by 50% when giving with atazanavir. Because levels of the active metabolite 14-OH clarithromycin are significantly reduced, consider alternative therapy for indications other than infections caused by *Mycobacterium avium* complex.
Cyclosporine, sirolimus, tacrolimus: May increase immunosuppressant levels. Monitor immunosuppressant levels.
Didanosine buffered formulations: May decrease atazanavir level. Give atazanavir 2 hours before or 1 hour after didanosine buffered formulations.
Dihydroergotamine, ergonovine, ergotamine, methylergonovine: May cause life-threatening reactions, such as acute ergot toxicity characterized by peripheral vasospasm and ischemia of the limbs and other tissues. Don't use together.
Diltiazem: May increase diltiazem and desacetyl-diltiazem. Use cautiously. Reduce dose of dilitazem by 50%. Monitor ECG.
Efavirenz: May decrease atazanavir levels. If used together, give 300 mg atazanavir with 100 mg ritonavir with 600 mg efavirenz all as a single daily dose with food, because this combination results in atazanavir exposure that approximates the exposure to 400 mg of atazanavir alone. Atazanavir shouldn't be given with efavirenz without ritonavir.
Ethinyl estradiol and norethindrone: May increase ethinyl estradiol and norethindrone. Use cautiously. The lowest effective dose of each hormonal contraceptive component should be used.
Felodipine, nicardpine, nifedipine, verapamil: May increase calcium channel blocker levels. Use cautiously. Adjust dose of the calcium channel blocker. Monitor ECG.
H_2-receptor antagonists: May decrease atazanavir levels. Give 12 hours apart.
Irinotecan: May interfere with the metabolism of irinotecan resulting in increased irinotecan toxicities. Don't use together.
Lovastatin, simvastatin: May cause serious reactions, such as myopathy and rhabdomyolysis. Don't use together.
Midazolam, triazolam: May cause life-threatening reactions, such as prolonged or increased sedation or respiratory depression. Don't use together.

Proton pump inhibitors: May substantially decrease atazanavir levels and reduce its therapeutic effect. Use together isn't recommended.

Rifabutin: May increase rifabutin levels. Reduce rifabutin dose by up to 75.

Rifampin: May decrease level of most protease inhibitors resulting in loss of therapeutic effect and development or resistance. Don't use together.

Ritonavir: May increase atazanavir levels. Give 300 mg atazanavir once daily with 100 mg ritonavir once daily, with food.

Saquinavir (soft gelatin capsules): May increase saquinavir level. Appropriate dose for this combination hasn't been established.

Sildenafil: May increase sildenafil level. Use together may result in increased sildenafil-associated adverse events, including hypotension, visual changes, and priapism. Use sildenafil with caution at a reduced dose of 25 mg every 48 hours and monitor patient for adverse events.

Tenofovir: May decrease atazanavir level, causing resistence. Give both drugs with ritonavir.

Tricyclic antidepressants: May increase levels of tricyclic antidepressants. Monitor levels.

Warfarin: May increase warfarin levels. Monitor INR.

Drug-herb. *St. John's wort:* May reduce atazanavir level, resulting in loss of therapeutic effect and development of resistance. Discourage use together.

Effects on lab test results

● May increase AST, ALT, total bilirubin, amylase, and lipase levels.

● My decrease hemoglobin and neutrophil count.

Pharmacokinetics

Absorption: Rapid. Peak level occurs in approximately 2½ hours. Food enhances bioavailability.

Distribution: 86% protein-bound and binds to alpha-1-acid glycoprotein and albumin to a similar extent.

Metabolism: Extensively metabolized, primarily by the liver.

Excretion: In urine and feces. About 7% excreted unchanged in urine. *Elimination half-life:* About 7 hours.

Route	Onset	Peak	Duration
P.O.	Unknown	2½ hr	Unknown

Action

Chemical effect: Selectively inhibits the virus-specific process of viral Gag and Gag-Pol polyproteins in HIV-1 infected cells, thus preventing formation of mature virions.

Therapeutic effect: Treats symptoms of HIV infection.

Available forms

Capsules: 100 mg, 150 mg, 200 mg

NURSING PROCESS

◪ Assessment

● Monitor cardiac status during therapy.

● Test women for pregnancy before starting therapy.

● Monitor liver function tests periodically during therapy.

● Evaluate patient's and family's knowledge of drug therapy.

◫ Nursing diagnoses

● Infection related to underlying HIV infection

● Risk of injury related to adverse reactions

● Deficient knowledge related to drug therapy

▶ Planning and implementation

● Drug may prolong PR interval.

● Most patients experience asymptomatic elevations in indirect bilirubin which may be accompanied by yellowing of the skin or whites of the eyes. Hyperbilirubinemia is reversible when drug is stopped.

● Various degrees of cross-resistance among protease inhibitors may occur. Resistance to this drug doesn't preclude the subsequent use of other protease inhibitors. Give drug with other antiretrovirals.

● Patients should remain under the care of a physician while taking drug.

● At high doses, jaundice caused by indirect (unconjugated) hyperbilirubinemia (without associated liver function test changes) or prolonged PR interval may occur.

● Treat overdose with general supportive measures, including monitoring of vital signs and ECG, and observations of the patient's clinical status. Induce vomiting or use gastric lavage to eliminate unabsorbed drug. Also give activated

charcoal to aid removal of unabsorbed drug.
Since drug is highly metabolized by the liver
and is highly protein-bound, dialysis is unlikely
to be beneficial.

Patient teaching
• Tell patient that sustained decreases in HIV
RNA have been linked to a reduced risk of progression to AIDS and death.
• Tell patient he should remain under the care of
a physician while taking drug.
• Advise patient to take drug with food every
day, and to take other antiretrovirals, as prescribed.
• Inform patient that drug isn't a cure for HIV
and that he may develop opportunistic infections and other complications of HIV disease.
Also explain that the drug doesn't reduce the
risk of transmitting HIV to others.
• Tell patient not to alter dose or stop therapy
without consulting his prescriber.
• If a dose is missed, advise patient to take the
dose as soon as possible and then return to his
normal schedule. However, if he skips a dose,
tell him not to double the next dose.
• Tell patient to consult prescriber if he experiences dizziness or lightheadedness.
• Tell patient that elevations in indirect bilirubin
may occur and to report yellowing of the skin or
the whites of the eyes.
• Inform patient that redistribution or accumulation of body fat may occur.
• Recommend that HIV-infected mothers avoid
breast-feeding to prevent postnatal transmission
of HIV.

☑ **Evaluation**
• Patient remains free from infection.
• Patient doesn't suffer injury from adverse
reactions.
• Patient and family state understanding of drug
therapy.

atenolol
(uh-TEN-uh-lol)
Apo-Atenol ♦ , Noten ◇ , Nu-Atenol ♦ ,
Tenormin

Pharmacologic class: beta blocker
Therapeutic class: antihypertensive, anti-
anginal
Pregnancy risk category: D

Indications and dosages

▶ **Hypertension.** *Adults:* Initially, 50 mg P.O.
daily as a single dose. Increase dosage to
100 mg once daily after 7 to 14 days. Doses
over 100 mg are unlikely to produce further
benefit.
◙ **Adjust-a-dose:** Adjust dosage in patients with
creatinine clearance less than 35 ml/minute.
In elderly patients, initially, 25 mg P.O. daily
and increase slowly until desired response.
▶ **Angina pectoris.** *Adults:* 50 mg P.O. once
daily. Increase p.r.n. to 100 mg daily after
7 days for optimal effect. Maximum dosage is
200 mg daily.
▶ **To reduce CV mortality rate and risk of
reinfarction in patients with acute MI.** *Adults:*
5 mg I.V. over 5 minutes, followed by another
5 mg 10 minutes later. After another 10 minutes,
50 mg P.O., followed by 50 mg P.O. in 12 hours.
Thereafter, 100 mg P.O. daily (as a single dose
or 50 mg b.i.d.) for at least 7 days.
▶ **To slow rapid ventricular response to atrial tachyarrhythmias after acute MI without
left ventricular dysfunction and AV block‡.**
Adults: 2.5 to 5 mg I.V. over 2 to 5 minutes,
p.r.n. to control rate. Maximum, 10 mg over a
10- to 15-minute period.

▽ I.V. administration

• Mix doses with D_5W, normal saline solution,
or dextrose and sodium chloride solutions.
• Give by slow injection, not to exceed 1 mg/
minute.
• Solution is stable for 48 hours after mixing.

Contraindications and precautions

• Contraindicated in patients with sinus bradycardia, greater than first-degree heart block,
overt cardiac failure, or cardiogenic shock.
• Use cautiously in patients at risk for heart failure and in those with bronchospastic disease, diabetes, and hyperthyroidism.
⚖ **Lifespan:** In pregnant women, don't use unless absolutely necessary because fetal harm can
occur. In breast-feeding women, use cautiously.
In children, safety of drug hasn't been established.

Adverse reactions

CNS: fever, fatigue, lethargy.
CV: BRADYCARDIA, PROFOUND HYPOTENSION,
intermittent claudication, *second- or third-
degree AV block.*

Reactions may be *common,* uncommon, *life-threatening,* or COMMON AND LIFE-THREATENING.

GI: nausea, vomiting, diarrhea, dry mouth.
Metabolic: increased risk of type 2 diabetes.
Respiratory: dyspnea, *bronchospasm.*
Skin: rash.

Interactions

Drug-drug. *Antihypertensives:* May enhance hypotensive effect. Use together cautiously.
Digoxin, diltiazem: May cause excessive bradycardia and may increase depressant effect on myocardium. Use together cautiously.
Insulin, oral antidiabetics: May alter dosage requirements in previously stabilized patient with diabetes. Observe patient carefully.
I.V. lidocaine: May reduce hepatic metabolism of lidocaine, increasing the risk of toxicity. Give bolus doses of lidocaine at a slower rate and monitor lidocaine levels closely.
Prazosin: May increase the risk of orthostatic hypotension in the early phases of use together. Assist patient to stand slowly until effects are known.
Reserpine: May cause hypotension. Use with caution.
Verapamil: May increase the effects of both drugs. Monitor cardiac function closely and decrease dosages as necessary.

Effects on lab test results

• May increase BUN, creatinine, potassium, uric acid, glucose, transaminase, alkaline phosphatase, triglyceride, and LDH levels. May decrease glucose level.
• May increase platelet count.

Pharmacokinetics

Absorption: About 50% to 60%.
Distribution: Distributed into most tissues and fluids except brain and CSF. About 5% to 15% protein-bound.
Metabolism: Minimal.
Excretion: From 40% to 50% of dose is excreted unchanged in urine; remainder is excreted as unchanged drug and metabolites in feces. *Half-life:* 6 to 7 hours (increases as renal function decreases).

Route	Onset	Peak	Duration
P.O.	1 hr	2-4 hr	24 hr
I.V.	5 min	5 min	12 hr

Action

Chemical effect: Selectively blocks beta$_1$ receptors; decreases cardiac output, peripheral resistance, and cardiac oxygen consumption; and depresses renin secretion.
Therapeutic effect: Decreases blood pressure, relieves angina, and reduces CV mortality rate and risk of reinfarction after acute MI.

Available forms

Injection: 5 mg/10 ml
Tablets: 25 mg, 50 mg, 100 mg

NURSING PROCESS

Assessment
• Obtain history of patient's underlying condition.
• If prescribed for hypertension, monitor drug's effectiveness by frequently checking patient's blood pressure. Full antihypertensive effect may not occur for 1 to 2 weeks after therapy starts. For angina pectoris, monitor frequency and severity of anginal pain, and for reducing CV mortality rate and risk of reinfarction after acute MI, monitor signs of reinfarction.
• Be alert for adverse reactions and drug interactions.
• Evaluate patient's and family's knowledge of drug therapy.

Nursing diagnoses
• Risk for injury related to underlying condition
• Decreased cardiac output related to drug-induced adverse CV reactions
• Deficient knowledge related to drug therapy

Planning and implementation
• Adjust dosage in patients with renal insufficiency and those receiving hemodialysis.
• Check patient's apical pulse before giving drug; if slower than 60 beats/minute, withhold drug and call prescriber.
• Give as a single daily dose.
• Be prepared to treat shock or hypoglycemia because this drug masks common signs of these conditions.
• Notify prescriber immediately if patient shows signs of decreased cardiac output.
⑤ **ALERT:** Withdraw drug gradually over 1 to 2 weeks to avoid serious adverse reactions.
⑤ **ALERT:** Don't confuse atenolol with timolol or albuterol.

Patient teaching
• Warn patient that stopping drug abruptly can worsen angina and MI. Drug should be withdrawn gradually over a 2-week period.
• Counsel patient to take drug at same time every day.
• Tell woman to notify prescriber if she becomes pregnant. Drug will need to be discontinued.
• Teach patient how to take his pulse. Tell patient to withhold drug and call prescriber if pulse rate is slower than 60 beats/minute.

☑ **Evaluation**
• Patient's underlying condition improves with drug therapy.
• Patient's cardiac output remains unchanged throughout drug therapy.
• Patient and family state understanding of drug therapy.

atomoxetine hydrochloride
(ATT-oh-mocks-uh-teen high-droh-KLOR-ighd)
Strattera

Pharmacological class: selective norepinephrine reuptake inhibitor
Therapeutic class: attention deficit hyperactivity disorder (ADHD)
Pregnancy risk category: C

Indications and dosages

▶ **Adjunct therapy for ADHD.** *Children weighing more than 70 kg (154 lb):* Initially, 40 mg P.O. daily; increase after a minimum of 3 days to a target total daily dose of 80 mg P.O. as a single dose in the morning or two evenly divided doses in the morning and late afternoon or early evening. After 2 to 4 weeks, increase total dosage to a maximum of 100 mg, if needed. *Children weighing 70 kg or less:* Initially, 0.5 mg/kg P.O. daily; increase after a minimum of 3 days to a target total daily dose of 1.2 mg/kg P.O. as a single dose in the morning or two evenly divided doses in the morning and late afternoon or early evening. Don't exceed 1.4 mg/kg or 100 mg daily, whichever is less.
◨ **Adjust-a-dose:** For patients with moderate hepatic impairment, reduce to 50% of the normal dose; in those with severe hepatic impairment, reduce to 25% of the normal dose.

Contraindications and precautions

• Contraindicated in patients hypersensitive to drug or its components, in those who have used an MAO inhibitor within the past 14 days, and in those with narrow-angle glaucoma.
• Use cautiously in patients with hypertension, tachycardia, or CV or cerebrovascular disease.
⚖ **Lifespan:** In pregnant and breast-feeding women, use cautiously. In children younger than age 6, safety and efficacy of drug haven't been established.

Adverse reactions

CNS: dizziness, *headache,* somnolence, crying, irritability, mood swings, pyrexia, fatigue, *insomnia,* sedation, depression, tremor, early morning awakening, paresthesia, abnormal dreams, sleep disorder.
CV: orthostatic hypotension, tachycardia, hypertension, palpitations.
EENT: ear infection, rhinorrhea, sore throat, nasal congestion, nasopharyngitis, sinus congestion, mydriasis, sinusitis.
GI: abdominal pain, constipation, dyspepsia, nausea, vomiting, decreased appetite, gastroenteritis, dry mouth, flatulence.
GU: urinary retention, urinary hesitation, ejaculatory problems, difficulty in micturition, dysmenorrhea, erectile disturbance, impotence, delayed menses, menstrual disorder, prostatitis.
Metabolic: weight loss.
Musculoskeletal: arthralgia, myalgia.
Respiratory: *cough,* upper respiratory tract infection.
Skin: dermatitis, pruritus, increased sweating.
Other: decreased libido, influenza, rigors, hot flashes.

Interactions

Drug-drug. *Albuterol:* Increases CV effects. Use together cautiously.
MAO inhibitors: May cause hyperthermia, rigidity, myoclonus, autonomic instability with possible rapid fluctuations of vital signs, and mental status changes. Don't combine with an MAO inhibitor, and separate atomoxetine and MAO inhibitor doses by 14 days.
Pressor agents: Increases blood pressure. Use together cautiously.
Strong CYP 2D6 inhibitors (fluoxetine, paroxetine, quinidine): May increase atomoxetine level. In children weighing less than 70 kg, adjust dosage to 0.5 mg/kg daily and increase only to

1.2 mg/kg daily if symptoms don't improve after 4 weeks. In children and adults weighing more than 70 kg, start at 40 mg daily and increase only to 80 mg daily if symptoms don't improve after 4 weeks.

Effects on lab test results

None reported.

Pharmacokinetics

Absorption: Rapid.
Distribution: Distributes primarily into total body water. It's 98% bound to plasma proteins, primarily albumin.
Metabolism: Metabolized primarily through CYP 2D6. The major oxidative metabolite formed is 4-hydroxyatomoxetine. Absolute bioavailability is about 63% in patients with extensive metabolism and 94% in those with poor metabolism.
Excretion: More than 80% of the dose in urine, and less than 17% of the dose via feces. Less than 3% of the dose is excreted unchanged. *Half-life:* 21½ hours.

Route	Onset	Peak	Duration
P.O.	Rapid	1-2 hr	Unknown

Action

Chemical effect: Unknown. May relate to selective inhibition of the presynaptic norepinephrine transporter.
Therapeutic effect: Decreases symptoms of ADHD.

Available forms

Capsules: 10 mg, 18 mg, 25 mg, 40 mg, 60 mg

NURSING PROCESS

⚡ Assessment
• Assess patient's condition before therapy and regularly thereafter.
• Watch for hypersensitivity reaction.
• Evaluate patient's and family's knowledge related to disease and drug therapy.

⊕ Nursing diagnoses
• Alteration in patient's comprehension and concentration related to underlying disease
• Risk for imbalanced nutrition: less than the body requires, related to side effect of medication

• Deficient knowledge related to disease process
• Deficient knowledge related to drug therapy

▶ Planning and implementation
• Use drug as part of a total treatment program for ADHD, with psychological, educational, and social intervention.
• Effectiveness for longer than 10 weeks hasn't been evaluated. Periodically reevaluate patients taking drug for extended periods to determine drug's usefulness.
• Monitor growth during treatment. If growth or weight gain is unsatisfactory, consider stopping therapy.
• Monitor blood pressure and pulse at baseline, after each dose increase, and periodically during treatment.
• Monitor patient for urinary hesitancy or retention and sexual dysfunction.
• Stop drug without tapering.
• In case of overdose, monitor patient closely and provide supportive care. Perform gastric lavage and give activated charcoal to prevent absorption.

Patient teaching
• Tell pregnant women, women planning to become pregnant, and breast-feeding women to consult prescriber before taking drug.
• Tell patient to use caution when operating a vehicle or machinery until the effects of drug are known.

☑ Evaluation
• Patient has reduced signs and symptoms of underlying disease.
• Patient maintains adequate nutritional status.
• Patient and family state understanding of disease and drug therapy.

atorvastatin calcium
(uh-TOR-vah-stah-tin KAL-see-um)
Lipitor

Pharmacologic class: HMG-CoA reductase inhibitor
Therapeutic class: antilipemic
Pregnancy risk category: X

Indications and dosages

▶ **Adjunct to diet to reduce elevated LDL, total cholesterol, apo B, and triglyceride levels and to increase HDL level in patients with primary hypercholesterolemia (heterozygous familial and nonfamilial) and mixed dyslipidemia (Fredrickson Types IIa and IIb.** *Adults:* Initially, 10 or 20 mg P.O. once daily. Start dosage at 40 mg once daily for patients who require a reduction in LDL cholesterol level more than 45%. Increase dose, p.r.n., to maximum of 80 mg daily as single dose. Base dosage on lipid levels drawn within 2 to 4 weeks after starting therapy.

▶ **Alone or as an adjunct to lipid-lowering treatments such as LDL apheresis to reduce total cholesterol and LDL cholesterol levels in patients with homozygous familial hypercholesterolemia.** *Adults:* 10 to 80 mg P.O. daily.

▶ **Heterozygous familial hypercholesterolemia.** *Children ages 10 to 17:* 10 mg P.O. once daily. Adjust dosage after 4 weeks to 20 mg daily.

Contraindications and precautions

• Contraindicated in patients hypersensitive to drug and in those with active liver disease or conditions linked with unexplained persistent increases in transaminase levels. Also contraindicated in patients with serious, acute conditions that suggest myopathy and in those at risk for renal failure caused by rhabdomyolysis from trauma; major surgery; severe metabolic, endocrine, and electrolyte disorders; severe acute infection; hypotension; or uncontrolled seizures.
• Adolescent girls must be at least 1 year postmenarche.
⚞ Lifespan: In pregnant or breast-feeding women and in women who may become pregnant, drug is contraindicated.

Adverse reactions

CNS: *headache,* asthenia, fever, malaise.
EENT: sinusitis, pharyngitis.
GI: abdominal pain, constipation, diarrhea, dyspepsia, flatulence.
Musculoskeletal: back pain, arthralgia, myalgia.
Skin: rash.
Other: infection, accidental injury, flulike syndrome, hypersensitivity reaction.

Interactions

Drug-drug. *Antacids:* May decrease bioavailability. Give separately.
Azole antifungals, cyclosporine, erythromycin, fibric acid derivatives, niacin: May increase risk of myopathy. Avoid using together.
Colestipol and other bile-acid sequestrants: May decrease atorvastatin level; however, these drugs may be used together for therapeutic effect. Monitor patient.
Digoxin: May increase digoxin level. Monitor digoxin level.
Erythromycin: May increase drug level. Monitor patient.
Fluconazole, itraconazole, ketoconazole: May increase level and adverse effects of atorvastatin. Avoid this combination. If they must be given together, reduce dose of atorvastatin.
Hormonal contraceptives: May increase hormone levels. Consider when selecting a hormonal contraceptive.
Warfarin: May increase anticoagulant effect. Monitor INR and patient for bleeding.

Effects on lab test results

• May increase ALT and AST levels.

Pharmacokinetics

Absorption: Rapid.
Distribution: 98% bound to plasma proteins.
Metabolism: By liver.
Excretion: In bile.

Route	Onset	Peak	Duration
P.O.	Unknown	1-2 hr	Unknown

Action

Chemical effect: Selectively inhibits HMG-CoA reductase, which converts HMG-CoA to mevalonate, a precursor of sterols.
Therapeutic effect: Lowers cholesterol and lipoprotein levels.

Available forms

Tablets: 10 mg, 20 mg, 40 mg, 80 mg

NURSING PROCESS

▨ **Assessment**
• Monitor patient's lipid and cholesterol levels at baseline and periodically thereafter.
• Evaluate patient's and family's knowledge of drug therapy.

⊞ Nursing diagnoses
- Risk for injury related to elevated cholesterol levels
- Deficient knowledge related to drug therapy

▷ Planning and implementation
- Use drug only after diet and other nonpharmacologic treatments prove ineffective. Patient should follow a standard low-cholesterol diet before and during therapy.
- Drug can be given as a single dose at any time of the day, with or without food.
- After starting drug and upon adjustment, monitor lipid levels within 2 to 4 weeks and adjust dosage accordingly.
- Before starting treatment, perform a baseline lipid profile to exclude secondary causes of hypercholesterolemia. Liver function test results and lipid levels should be obtained before therapy, after 6 and 12 weeks, or following a dosage increase and periodically thereafter.

⚠ ALERT: Don't confuse Lipitor with Levatol.

Patient teaching
- Teach patient about proper dietary management, weight control, and exercise and explain their role in controlling elevated lipid levels.
- Warn patient to avoid alcohol.
- Tell patient to inform prescriber of adverse reactions such as muscle pain, tenderness, or weakness, especially if accompanied by fever or malaise.
- Urge woman to notify prescriber immediately if pregnancy is suspected.

☑ Evaluation
- Patient's cholesterol level is within normal limits.
- Patient and family state understanding of drug therapy.

atovaquone
(uh-TOH-vuh-kwohn)
Mepron

Pharmacologic class: ubiquinone analogue
Therapeutic class: antiprotozoal
Pregnancy risk category: C

Indications and dosages

▶ **Prevention of _Pneumocystis carinii_ pneumonia in patients who are intolerant to co-trimoxazole, including HIV-infected individuals.** _Adults and children age 13 and older:_ 1,500 mg (10 ml) P.O. daily with food.
Infants ages 1 to 3 months and children older than 24 months‡: 30 mg/kg P.O. once daily.
Infants ages 4 to 24 months: 45 mg/kg P.O. daily‡.

▶ **Mild to moderate _P. carinii_ pneumonia in patients who can't tolerate co-trimoxazole.** _Adults and children age 13 and older:_ 750 mg P.O. b.i.d. for 21 days.

▶ **Prevention of toxoplasmosis in HIV-infected patients‡.** _Adults and children age 13 and older:_ 1,500 mg P.O. daily.

Contraindications and precautions
- Contraindicated in patients hypersensitive to drug.
- Use cautiously with other highly protein-bound drugs because drug is more than 99.9% protein-bound. Also use cautiously in those with liver disease.

⚕ **Lifespan:** In pregnant and breast-feeding women, use cautiously. In children, safety of drug hasn't been established. In elderly patients, use cautiously.

Adverse reactions

CNS: asthenia, dizziness, _headache,_ dreams, insomnia.
EENT: visual difficulties.
GI: _abdominal pain,_ diarrhea, anorexia, _nausea, vomiting,_ dyspepsia, gastritis, oral ulcers.
Respiratory: cough.
Skin: pruritus.

Interactions

Drug-drug. _Highly protein-bound drugs:_ May compete for receptor sites affecting drug levels. Use cautiously.
Rifabutin, rifampin: May decrease atovaquone's steady-state levels. Avoid using together.

Effects on lab test results
- May increase alkaline phosphatase, ALT, and AST levels.
- May decrease hemoglobin, hematocrit, and WBC count.

Pharmacokinetics

Absorption: Limited. Bioavailability is increased twofold when given with meals. Fat enhances absorption significantly.

Distribution: 99.9% bound to plasma proteins.
Metabolism: Not metabolized.
Excretion: Undergoes enterohepatic cycling and is primarily excreted in feces. Less than 0.6% is excreted in urine. *Half-life:* 2 to 3 days.

Route	Onset	Peak	Duration
P.O.	Unknown	1-8 hr (1st peak); 1-4 days (2nd peak)	Unknown

Action

Chemical effect: Unknown; may interfere with electron transport in protozoal mitochondria, inhibiting enzymes needed for synthesis of nucleic acids and adenosine triphosphate.
Therapeutic effect: Kills *Pneumocystis carinii* protozoa.

Available forms

Suspension: 750 mg/5 ml

NURSING PROCESS

Assessment
- Obtain history of patient's protozoal respiratory infection and reassess regularly.
- Be alert for adverse reactions.
- Monitor patient's hydration if adverse GI reactions occur.
- Evaluate patient's and family's knowledge of drug therapy.

Nursing diagnoses
- Infection related to presence of susceptible protozoal organisms
- Risk for deficient fluid volume related to drug-induced adverse GI reactions
- Deficient knowledge related to drug therapy

Planning and implementation
- Give drug with food to improve bioavailability.
Patient teaching
- Instruct patient to take drug with meals because food enhances absorption significantly.
- Warn patient not to perform hazardous activities if dizziness occurs.
- Emphasize importance of taking drug as prescribed, even if patient is feeling better.
- Tell patient to notify prescriber if serious adverse reactions occur.

Evaluation
- Patient's infection is eradicated.
- Patient remains adequately hydrated throughout therapy.
- Patient and family state understanding of drug therapy.

atovaquone and proguanil hydrochloride
(uh-TOH-vuh-kwohn and pro-GWAN-ill high-droh-KLOR-ighd)
Malarone, Malarone Pediatric

Pharmacologic class: hydroxynapthalenedione and biguanide hydrochloride
Therapeutic class: antimalarial
Pregnancy risk category: C

Indications and dosages

▶ **Prevention of** *Plasmodium falciparum* **malaria in areas where chloroquine resistance has been reported.** *Adults and children weighing more than 40 kg (88 lb):* One adult-strength tablet (250 mg atovaquone and 100 mg proguanil) P.O. once daily with food or milk. Begin 1 or 2 days before entering a malaria-endemic area. Continue prophylactic treatment during stay and for 7 days after return.
Children weighing 31 to 40 kg (68 to 88 lb): Three pediatric-strength tablets P.O. once daily with food or milk, beginning 1 or 2 days before entering endemic area. Total daily dose is 187.5 mg atovaquone and 75 mg proguanil. Treatment should continue during stay and for 7 days after return.
Children weighing 21 to 30 kg (46 to 66 lb): Two pediatric-strength tablets P.O. once daily with food or milk, beginning 1 or 2 days before entering endemic area. Total daily dose is 125 mg atovaquone and 50 mg proguanil. Treatment should continue during stay and for 7 days after return.
Children weighing 11 to 20 kg (24 to 44 lb): One pediatric-strength tablet P.O. daily with food or milk, beginning 1 or 2 days before entering endemic area. Continue treatment during stay and for 7 days after return.
▶ **Acute, uncomplicated** *P. falciparum* **malaria.** *Adults and children weighing more than 40 kg:* Four adult-strength tablets, with food or

milk, P.O. once daily for 3 consecutive days. Total daily dose is 1 g atovaquone and 400 mg
proguanil.
Children weighing 31 to 40 kg: Three adult-
strength tablets P.O. once daily, with food or
milk, for 3 consecutive days. Total daily dose is
750 mg atovaquone and 300 mg proguanil.
Children weighing 21 to 30 kg: Two adult-
strength tablets P.O. once daily, with food or
milk, for 3 consecutive days. Total daily dose is
500 mg atovaquone and 200 mg proguanil.
Children weighing 11 to 20 kg: One adult-
strength tablet P.O. once daily, with food or
milk, for 3 consecutive days.
Children weighing 9 to 10 kg: Three pediatric-
strength tablets P.O. daily, with food or milk, for
3 consecutive days.
Children weighing 5 to 8 kg: Two pediatric-
strength tablets P.O. daily, with food or milk, for
3 consecutive days.

Contraindications and precautions

• Contraindicated in patients hypersensitive to
atovaquone, proguanil, or any component of the
formulation. Not intended for patients with severe malaria or for those with a fresh breakout
of *P. falciparum* infection after treatment with
Malarone or failure of preventative treatment
with Malarone.
• Use cautiously in patients with severe renal
impairment because proguanil is renally eliminated. Use cautiously in vomiting patients.
⚘ **Lifespan:** In breast-feeding women, use
cautiously because drug appears in breast milk
in small amounts. In children weighing less than
5 kg, safety and efficacy of drug haven't been
established. In elderly patients, use cautiously
because they may respond differently than
younger patients and are more likely to have decreased renal function.

Adverse reactions

CNS: asthenia, dizziness, dreams, hallucina-
tions, *headache.*
EENT: visual difficulties.
GI: *abdominal pain,* diarrhea, anorexia, dyspep-
sia, oral ulcers, gastritis, *nausea, vomiting.*
Respiratory: cough.
Skin: pruritus.
Other: *anaphylaxis,* flulike syndrome.

Interactions

Drug-drug. *Metoclopramide:* May decrease
atovaquone bioavailability. Consider alternative
antiemetics.
Drugs containing proguanil: Proguanil is eliminated renally and a high level may cause renal
impaiment. Avoid using together.
Rifampin: May reduce atovaquone level by
about 50%. Avoid using together.
Tetracycline: May reduce atovaquone level by
about 40%. Monitor patient closely for signs
and symptoms of parasitemia.

Effects on lab test results

• May increase alkaline phosphatase, ALT, AST,
and creatinine levels.
• May decrease hemoglobin, hematocrit, and
WBC count.

Pharmacokinetics

Absorption: Bioavailability of atovaquone is
23% when tablets are taken with food. Atovaquone bioavailability varies considerably. Dietary fat increases the rate and extent of atovaquone absorption compared with fasting.
Proguanil is well absorbed without regard to
food. Absorption of both drugs is decreased in
patients with diarrhea and vomiting.
Distribution: Atovaquone is more than 99%
protein-bound; proguanil, 75%.
Metabolism: Atovaquone undergoes virtually
no metabolism. Proguanil is metabolized in the
liver to cycloguanil (primarily by CYP 2C19)
and 4-chlorophenylbiguanide.
Excretion: More than 94% of atovaquone is
eliminated unchanged in the feces over 21 days.
The kidneys eliminate 40% to 60% of proguanil
and its metabolites. Half-life in children is decreased. *Atovaquone half-life:* 2 to 3 days in
adults. *Proguanil half-life:* 12 to 21 hours in
adults and children.

Route	Onset	Peak	Duration
P.O.	Unknown	Unknown	Unknown

Action

Chemical effect: May interfere with nucleic
acid replication in the malarial parasite by inhibiting biosynthesis of pyrimidine compounds
in two different pathways. Atovaquone selectively inhibits parasitic mitochondrial electron
transport. Proguanil disrupts deoxythymidilate

synthesis through inhibition of dihydrofolate reductase.
Therapeutic effect: Prevents and treats symptoms of malaria.

Available forms

Tablets: 250 mg atovaquone and 100 mg proguanil (adult-strength); 62.5 mg atovaquone and 25 mg proguanil (pediatric-strength)

NURSING PROCESS

☘ Assessment
• Assess patient for signs and symptoms of malaria.
• Assess patient and travel plans for need for antimalarial prophylaxis.
• Be alert for adverse reactions.
• Monitor patient's liver and renal function during drug therapy.

⊞ Nursing diagnoses
• Risk of infection related to exposure to *P. falciparum* in malaria-endemic areas
• Deficient knowledge related to drug therapy

▷ Planning and implementation
• Atovaquone absorption may be decreased by persistent diarrhea or vomiting. Consider another antimalarial for a patient with persistent diarrhea or vomiting and give antiemetics.
• If treatment or prophylaxis fails, give another antimalarial.
• Give drug at the same time each day with food or milk.
• Store tablets at controlled room temperature 59° to 86° F (15° to 30° C).
Patient teaching
• Tell patient to take dose at the same time each day with food or milk.
• If patient vomits within 1 hour after taking a dose, tell him to take a repeat dose.
• Advise patient to contact prescriber if he can't complete the course of therapy as prescribed.
• Instruct patient that, in addition to drug therapy, malaria prophylaxis should include the use of protective clothing, bed nets, and insect repellents.

☑ Evaluation
• Patient doesn't have malaria.
• Patient and family state understanding of antimalarial drug therapy.

atracurium besylate
(uh-trah-KYOO-ree-um BES-eh-layt)
Tracrium

Pharmacologic class: nondepolarizing neuromuscular blocker
Therapeutic class: skeletal muscle relaxant
Pregnancy risk category: C

Indications and dosages

▶ **Adjunct to general anesthesia, to facilitate endotracheal intubation and cause skeletal muscle relaxation during surgery or mechanical ventilation.** *Adults and children older than age 2:* 0.4 to 0.5 mg/kg by I.V. bolus. Maintenance dosage of 0.08 to 0.1 mg/kg within 20 to 45 minutes of initial dose should be given during prolonged surgical procedures. Maintenance dosages may be given q 15 to 25 minutes in patients receiving balanced anesthesia. For prolonged surgical procedures, a constant infusion of 5 to 9 mcg/kg/minute may be used after initial bolus.
Children ages 1 month to 2 years: Initial dose, 0.3 to 0.4 mg/kg. Frequent maintenance doses may be needed.

▽ I.V. administration

• Don't use lactated Ringer's solution. In lactated Ringer's solution for injection, atracurium is stable for 8 hours at a concentration of 0.5 mg/ml. Because of increased drug degradation in this solution, it isn't recommended.
• Don't mix with acidic or alkaline solution; precipitate may form.
• Drug usually is given by rapid I.V. bolus injection but may be given by intermittent or continuous infusion. At 0.2 to 0.5 mg/ml, drug is compatible for 24 hours in D_5W, normal saline solution injection, or dextrose 5% in normal saline solution injection.

Contraindications and precautions

• Contraindicated in patients hypersensitive to drug.
• Use cautiously in patients with CV disease; severe electrolyte disorders; bronchogenic carcinoma; hepatic, renal, or pulmonary impairment; neuromuscular diseases; myasthenia gravis; and in debilitated patients.

✿ **Lifespan:** In pregnant women, breast-feeding women, and elderly patients, use cautiously.

Adverse reactions

CV: *flushing,* increased heart rate, *bradycardia,* hypotension.
Respiratory: *prolonged dose-related apnea,* wheezing, increased bronchial secretions.
Skin: erythema, pruritus, urticaria.
Other: *anaphylaxis.*

Interactions

Drug-drug. *Amikacin, gentamicin, neomycin, streptomycin, tobramycin:* May increase the effects of nondepolarizing muscle relaxant, including prolonged respiratory depression. Use together only when necessary and reduce dose of nondepolarizing muscle relaxant.
Carbamazepine, phenytoin: May decrease the effects of atracurium causing it to be less effective. Increase dose of atracurium.
Kanamycin; polymyxin antibiotics (colistin, polymyxin B sulfate); clindamycin; general anesthetics (such as enflurane, halothane, isoflurane); quinidine: May potentiate neuromuscular blockade, leading to increased skeletal muscle relaxation and prolongation of effect. Use cautiously during surgical and postoperative periods.
Lithium, magnesium salts, opioid analgesics: May potentiate neuromuscular blockade, which may lead to increased skeletal muscle relaxation and, possibly, respiratory paralysis. Reduce dose of atracurium.

Effects on lab test results

None reported.

Pharmacokinetics

Absorption: Administered I.V.
Distribution: Distributed into extracellular space. About 82% protein-bound.
Metabolism: Rapidly metabolized by Hofmann elimination and by nonspecific enzymatic ester hydrolysis. The liver doesn't appear to play a major role.
Excretion: Drug and its metabolites are excreted in urine and feces. *Half-life:* 20 minutes.

Route	Onset	Peak	Duration
I.V.	2 min	3-5 min	35-70 min

Action

Chemical effect: Prevents acetylcholine from binding to receptors on muscle end plate, thus blocking depolarization and resulting in skeletal muscle paralysis.
Therapeutic effect: Relaxes skeletal muscles.

Available forms

Injection: 10 mg/ml

NURSING PROCESS

⚗ Assessment

● Obtain history of patient's neuromuscular status before therapy and reassess regularly.
● Be alert for adverse reactions and interactions.
● Monitor respirations closely until patient fully recovers from neuromuscular blockade, as evidenced by tests of muscle strength (hand grip, head lift, and ability to cough).
● A nerve stimulator and train-of-four monitoring are recommended to confirm antagonism of neuromuscular blockade and recovery of muscle strength. Before attempting pharmacologic reversal with neostigmine, some evidence of spontaneous recovery should be seen.
● Evaluate patient's and family's knowledge of drug therapy.

⊞ Nursing diagnoses

● Risk for injury related to underlying condition
● Impaired spontaneous ventilation related to drug-induced respiratory paralysis
● Deficient knowledge related to drug therapy

❯ Planning and implementation

● Give sedatives or general anesthetics before neuromuscular blockers. Neuromuscular blockers don't decrease consciousness or alter pain threshold.
● **ALERT:** Use this drug only under direct medical supervision by personnel skilled in use of neuromuscular blockers and techniques for maintaining a patent airway. Don't use unless facilities and equipment for mechanical ventilation, oxygen therapy, and intubation as well as an antagonist are immediately available.
● Don't give by I.M. injection.
● Prior use of succinylcholine doesn't prolong duration of action but quickens onset and may deepen neuromuscular blockade.
● Explain all events to patient because he can still hear.

• Give analgesics for pain. Patient may have pain but be unable to express it.
• Keep airway clear. Have emergency equipment and drugs immediately available.
• After spontaneous recovery starts, reverse atracurium-induced neuromuscular blockade with an anticholinesterase (such as neostigmine or edrophonium). These drugs usually are given with an anticholinergic (such as atropine).

Patient teaching
• Instruct patient and family about drug therapy.
• Reassure patient and family that patient will be monitored at all times and that respiratory life support will be used during paralysis.
• Reassure patient that pain medication will be given as needed.

☑ Evaluation
• Patient's underlying condition is resolved without causing injury.
• Patient sustains spontaneous ventilation after effects of atracurium besylate wear off.
• Patient and family state understanding of drug therapy.

atropine sulfate
(AH-troh-peen SUL-fayt)
AtroPen Auto-Injector, Sal-Tropine

Pharmacologic class: anticholinergic, belladonna alkaloid
Therapeutic class: antiarrhythmic, vagolytic
Pregnancy risk category: C

Indications and dosages

▶ **Symptomatic bradycardia, bradyarrhythmia (junctional or escape rhythm).** *Adults:* Usually 0.5 to 1 mg I.V. push; repeat q 3 to 5 minutes to maximum of 2 mg, p.r.n. Lower doses (less than 0.5 mg) can cause bradycardia. *Children:* 0.02 mg/kg I.V. to a maximum of 1 mg; or 0.3 mg/m² ; may repeat q 5 minutes.
▶ **Anticholinesterase insecticide poisoning.** *Adults and children:* 1 to 2 mg I.M. or I.V. repeated q 20 to 30 minutes until muscarinic symptoms disappear or signs of atropine toxicity appear. Patient with severe poisoning may require up to 6 mg q hour.
▶ **Preoperatively for decreasing secretions and blocking cardiac vagal reflexes.** *Adults and children weighing 20 kg (44 lb) or more:*

0.4 mg I.M. or S.C. 30 to 60 minutes before anesthesia.
Children weighing less than 20 kg: 0.1 mg I.M. for 3 kg, 0.2 mg I.M. for 4 to 9 kg, 0.3 mg I.M. for 10 to 20 kg 30 to 60 minutes before anesthesia.
▶ **Adjunct in peptic ulcer disease; functional GI disorders such as irritable bowel syndrome.** *Adults:* 0.4 to 0.6 mg P.O. q 4 to 6 hours.
Children: 0.01 mg/kg or 0.3 mg/m² (not to exceed 0.4 mg) q 4 to 6 hours.

▼ I.V. administration
• Give by direct I.V. into a large vein or I.V. tubing over 1 to 2 minutes.

Contraindications and precautions
• Contraindicated in patients hypersensitive to drug and those with acute angle-closure glaucoma, obstructive uropathy, obstructive disease of GI tract, paralytic ileus, toxic megacolon, intestinal atony, unstable CV status in acute hemorrhage, asthma, or myasthenia gravis.
• Use cautiously in patients with Down syndrome.
⚜ **Lifespan:** In pregnant women, use cautiously. Use in breast-feeding women isn't recommended. In children and elderly patients, use cautiously because they may have increased adverse effects.

Adverse reactions
CNS: *headache, restlessness,* ataxia, disorientation, hallucinations, delirium, ***coma,*** *insomnia, dizziness,* excitement, agitation, confusion.
CV: *tachycardia, palpitations, angina,* ***arrhythmias,*** flushing.
EENT: photophobia, *blurred vision, mydriasis.*
GI: *dry mouth,* thirst, *constipation,* nausea, vomiting.
GU: urine retention.
Hematologic: leukocytosis.
Other: *anaphylaxis.*

Interactions
Drug-drug. *Antacids:* May decrease absorption of anticholinergics. Give at least 1 hour apart.
Anticholinergics, drugs with anticholinergic effects (such as amantadine, antiarrhythmics, antiparkinsonians, glutethimide, meperidine, phenothiazines, tricyclic antidepressants): May

cause additive anticholinergic effects. Use together cautiously.

Ketoconazole, levodopa: May decrease absorption. Avoid using together.

Methotrimeprazine: May produce extrapyramidal symptoms. Monitor patient carefully.

Potassium chloride wax matrix tablets: May increase risk of mucosal lesions. Use cautiously.

Effects on lab test results
• May increase WBC count.

Pharmacokinetics
Absorption: Well absorbed after P.O. and I.M. administration; unknown for S.C. administration.

Distribution: Throughout the body, including CNS. Only 18% binds with plasma protein.

Metabolism: In liver to several metabolites.

Excretion: Primarily through kidneys; small amount may be excreted in feces and expired air. *Half-life:* Initial, 2 hours; second phase, 12½ hours.

Route	Onset	Peak	Duration
P.O.	½-1 hr	2 hr	4 hr
I.V.	Immediate	2-4 min	4 hr
I.M.	30 min	1-1½ hr	4 hr
S.C.	Unknown	Unknown	4 hr

Action
Chemical effect: Inhibits acetylcholine at parasympathetic neuroeffector junction, blocking vagal effects on SA node. This enhances conduction through AV node and speeds heart rate.

Therapeutic effect: Increases heart rate, decreases secretions preoperatively, and slows GI motility. Antidote for anticholinesterase insecticide poisoning.

Available forms
Injection: 0.05 mg/ml, 0.1 mg/ml, 0.3 mg/ml, 0.4 mg/ml, 0.5 mg/ml, 0.6 mg/ml, 0.8 mg/ml, 1 mg/ml, 1.2 mg/ml

Tablets: 0.4 mg, 0.6 mg

NURSING PROCESS

🜛 Assessment
• Obtain history of patient's underlying condition and reassess regularly.

• Be alert for adverse reactions and drug interactions.

• Monitor patients, especially those receiving doses of 0.4 to 0.6 mg, for paradoxical initial bradycardia, which is caused by a drug effect in CNS and usually disappears within 2 minutes.

⚠ **ALERT:** Watch for tachycardia in cardiac patients because it may cause ventricular fibrillation.

• Evaluate patient's and family's knowledge of drug therapy.

🜛 Nursing diagnoses
• Ineffective health maintenance related to underlying condition
• Risk for injury related to drug-induced adverse reactions
• Deficient knowledge related to drug therapy

▷ Planning and implementation
• Give with or without food.
• If ECG disturbances occur, withhold drug, obtain a rhythm strip, and notify prescriber immediately.
• Have emergency equipment and drugs on hand to treat new arrhythmias. Other anticholinergic drugs may increase vagal blockage.
• Use physostigmine salicylate as antidote for atropine overdose.

Patient teaching
• Teach patient about atropine sulfate therapy.
• Instruct patient to ask for assistance with activities if adverse CNS reactions occur.
• Teach patient how to handle distressing anticholinergic effects.

☑ Evaluation
• Patient's underlying condition improves.
• Patient has no injury as a result of therapy.
• Patient and family state understanding of drug therapy.

---

auranofin
(or-AN-uh-fin)
Ridaura

Pharmacologic class: gold salt
Therapeutic class: antiarthritic
Pregnancy risk category: C

Indications and dosages

▶ **Psoriatic arthritis‡, active systemic lupus erythematosus‡, Felty's syndrome‡, rheumatoid arthritis.** *Adults:* 6 mg P.O. daily, either as 3 mg b.i.d. or 6 mg once daily. After 4 to 6 months, increase dosage to 9 mg daily. Stop drug if no response at 9 mg daily for 3 months.

Contraindications and precautions

• Contraindicated in patients with history of severe gold toxicity, necrotizing enterocolitis, pulmonary fibrosis, exfoliative dermatitis, bone marrow aplasia, severe hematologic disorders, or history of severe toxicity resulting from previous exposure to other heavy metals. Also contraindicated in patients with urticaria, eczema, colitis, severe debilitation, hemorrhagic conditions, or systemic lupus erythematosus and in patients who recently received radiation therapy.
• Use cautiously with other drugs that cause blood dyscrasia. Also use cautiously in patients who have renal, hepatic, or inflammatory bowel disease; rash; or a history of bone marrow depression.
🜲 **Lifespan:** In breast-feeding women, drug isn't recommended. In children, safety of drug hasn't been established.

Adverse reactions

CNS: confusion, *seizures.*
EENT: metallic taste.
GI: *diarrhea, abdominal pain, nausea, vomiting,* stomatitis, enterocolitis, anorexia, dyspepsia, flatulence.
GU: proteinuria, hematuria, glomerulonephritis, *acute renal failure,* nephrotic syndrome.
Hematologic: *thrombocytopenia, aplastic anemia, agranulocytosis, leukopenia,* eosinophilia.
Hepatic: jaundice.
Respiratory: interstitial pneumonitis.
Skin: *rash, pruritus, dermatitis,* exfoliative dermatitis.

Interactions

Drug-drug. *Phenytoin:* May raise phenytoin level. Watch for toxicity.

Effects on lab test results

• May increase BUN, creatinine, ALT, AST, and alkaline phosphatase levels.

• May increase eosinophil count. May decrease hemoglobin, hematocrit, and platelet, granulocyte, and WBC counts.

Pharmacokinetics

Absorption: 25% absorbed through GI tract.
Distribution: Distributed widely in body tissues. Synovial fluid levels are about 50% of blood levels. Drug is 60% protein-bound.
Metabolism: Unknown.
Excretion: 60% of absorbed drug is excreted in urine and remainder in feces. *Half-life:* 26 days.

Route	Onset	Peak	Duration
P.O.	1-3 mo	2 hr	Unknown

Action

Chemical effect: Unknown. May inhibit sulfhydryl systems, which alters cellular metabolism and reduces inflammation. Also may alter enzyme function and immune response and suppress phagocytic activity.
Therapeutic effect: Relieves symptoms of rheumatoid arthritis.

Available forms

Capsules: 3 mg

NURSING PROCESS

🜚 **Assessment**
• Obtain history of patient's joint pain and stiffness before therapy and reassess regularly.
• Be alert for adverse reactions and drug interactions.
• Monitor patient's hydration status if adverse GI reactions occur.
• Monitor patient's platelet count and CBC regularly.
• Evaluate patient's and family's knowledge of drug therapy.

⊕ **Nursing diagnoses**
• Acute pain related to presence of rheumatoid arthritis
• Risk for deficient fluid volume related to drug-induced adverse GI reactions
• Deficient knowledge related to drug therapy

▶ **Planning and implementation**
• Store at controlled room temperature and in a light-resistant container.

• Continue to give other drugs, such as NSAIDs.

• Notify prescriber and stop drug if patient's platelet count falls below 100,000/mm³, if hemoglobin drops suddenly, if granulocyte count is less than 1,500/mm³, if WBC count is less than 4,000/mm³, or eosinophil count is greater than 75%.

• If urinalysis shows proteinuria or hematuria, notify prescriber and stop drug because nephrotic syndrome or glomerulonephritis may occur.

Patient teaching

• Encourage patient to take drug as prescribed and not to alter dosage schedule.

• Tell patient to continue taking other drugs, such as NSAIDs, as prescribed.

• Remind patient to see prescriber monthly to monitor platelet counts.

• Advise patient to have regular urinalysis.

• Tell patient to continue taking drug if he experiences mild diarrhea (the most common adverse reaction) and to contact prescriber immediately if he notices blood in stool.

• Advise patient to report rashes or other skin problems immediately. Pruritus often precedes dermatitis; any pruritic skin eruption that occurs while patient is receiving auranofin should be considered a reaction to the drug until proven otherwise. Advise patient to stop therapy until reaction subsides and to notify prescriber.

• Advise patient that stomatitis is often preceded by a metallic taste, which should be reported to prescriber immediately. Promote careful oral hygiene during therapy.

• Reassure patient that he may not experience drug's beneficial effect for up to 3 months. If response is inadequate and maximum dosage has been reached, expect prescriber to stop drug.

• Warn patient not to give drug to others.

☑ Evaluation

• Patient expresses that arthritic pain has been relieved.

• Patient maintains fluid volume balance throughout therapy.

• Patient and family state understanding of drug therapy.

aurothioglucose
(or-oh-thigh-oh-GLOO-kohs)
Gold-50 ◊ , Solganal

gold sodium thiomalate
(gohld SOH-dee-um thee-oh-MAH-layt)
Myochrysine

Pharmacologic class: gold salt
Therapeutic class: antiarthritic
Pregnancy risk category: C

Indications and dosages

▶ **Rheumatoid arthritis.** *aurothioglucose.*
Adults: Initially, 10 mg I.M., followed by 25 mg for second and third doses at weekly intervals. Then, 50 mg weekly until 0.8 to 1 g has been given. If improvement occurs without toxicity, continue 50 mg at 3- to 4-week intervals indefinitely as maintenance therapy.
Children ages 6 to 12: One-fourth usual adult dosage of aurothioglucose, not to exceed 25 mg per dose.
gold sodium thiomalate. Adults: Initially, 10 mg gold sodium thiomalate I.M., followed by 25 mg in 1 week. Then, 25 to 50 mg weekly until 14 to 20 doses have been given. If improvement occurs without toxicity, continue 25 to 50 mg q 2 weeks for four doses; then 25 to 50 mg q 3 weeks for four doses; then 25 to 50 mg every month indefinitely as maintenance therapy. If relapse occurs during maintenance therapy, resume injections at weekly intervals.
Children: 1 mg/kg gold sodium thiomalate I.M. weekly for 20 weeks. The maximum single dose for children younger than age 12 is 50 mg. If response is good, may be given q 3 to 4 weeks indefinitely.

▶ **Palindromic rheumatism‡.** *Adults:* 10 to 50 mg gold sodium thiomalate I.M. weekly dose until a total of 1 g.

▶ **Pemphigus‡.** *Adults:* Initial dose of 10 mg gold sodium thiomalate I.M. for the first week, 25 mg I.M. for the second week, then 50 mg I.M. weekly until corticosteroids are eliminated from the drug regimen. Maintenance dosage of 25 to 50 mg I.M. q 2 weeks.

Contraindications and precautions

• Contraindicated in patients hypersensitive to drug or with a history of severe toxicity from exposure to gold or other heavy metals, hepatitis, or exfoliative dermatitis; severe, uncontrollable diabetes; renal disease; hepatic dysfunction; uncontrolled heart failure; systemic lupus erythematosus; colitis; Sjögren's syndrome; urticaria; eczema; hemorrhagic conditions; severe hematologic disorders; or recent radiation therapy.

• Use cautiously, if at all, in patients with rash, marked hypertension, compromised cerebral or CV circulation, or history of renal or hepatic disease, drug allergies, or blood dyscrasia.

⚠ Lifespan: In pregnant women, use cautiously. In breast-feeding women, drug isn't recommended. In children younger than age 6, safety of drug hasn't been established.

Adverse reactions

CNS: *dizziness,* syncope, *seizures.*
CV: *bradycardia,* hypotension.
EENT: corneal gold deposition, corneal ulcers.
GI: stomatitis, difficulty swallowing, nausea, vomiting, metallic taste.
GU: albuminuria, proteinuria, nephrotic syndrome, nephritis, *acute tubular necrosis, acute renal failure.*
Hematologic: *thrombocytopenia, aplastic anemia, agranulocytosis, leukopenia,* eosinophilia.
Hepatic: *hepatitis,* jaundice.
Skin: diaphoresis, photosensitivity reaction, *rash, dermatitis.*
Other: *anaphylaxis, angioedema.*

Interactions

None significant.

Effects on lab test results

• May increase BUN, creatinine, ALT, AST, and alkaline phosphatase levels.
• May increase eosinophil count. May decrease hemoglobin, hematocrit, and platelet, granulocyte, and WBC counts.

Pharmacokinetics

Absorption: Slow and erratic because drug is in oil suspension.
Distribution: Distributed widely throughout body in lymph nodes, bone marrow, kidneys, liver, spleen, and tissues. About 85% to 90% is protein-bound.
Metabolism: Not broken down into elemental form.

Excretion: About 70% in urine; 30% in feces.
Half-life: 14 to 40 days.

Route	Onset	Peak	Duration
I.M.	Unknown	3-6 hr	Unknown

Action

Chemical effect: Unknown. May inhibit sulfhydryl systems, which alters cellular metabolism and reduces inflammation. Also may alter enzyme function and immune response and suppress phagocytic activity.
Therapeutic effect: Relieves signs and symptoms of rheumatoid arthritis.

Available forms

aurothioglucose
Injection (suspension): 50 mg/ml in sesame oil with aluminum monostearate 2% and propylparaben 0.1% in 10-ml container
gold sodium thiomalate
Injection: 50 mg/ml with benzyl alcohol

NURSING PROCESS

📝 Assessment
• Obtain history of patient's rheumatoid arthritis before therapy and reassess regularly.
• Be alert for adverse reactions.
• Analyze urine for protein and sediment changes before each injection.
• Monitor CBC, including platelet count, before every second injection.
• Evaluate patient's and family's knowledge of drug therapy.

🔲 Nursing diagnoses
• Acute joint pain related to presence of rheumatoid arthritis
• Risk for injury related to drug-induced adverse reactions
• Deficient knowledge related to drug therapy

▶ Planning and implementation
• Give only under constant supervision of prescriber who is thoroughly familiar with drug's toxicities and benefits.
ⓢ **ALERT:** Rash and dermatitis occur in 20% of patients and may lead to fatal exfoliative dermatitis if drug isn't stopped.
• Drugs are typically used only in active rheumatoid arthritis that hasn't responded ade-

---

quately to salicylates, rest, and physical therapy. May use earlier before disease progresses.

● Give all gold salts I.M., preferably intra-gluteally. Drug is pale yellow; don't use if it darkens.

● Immerse vial of aurothioglucose suspension in warm water, and shake vigorously before injecting.

● When giving gold sodium thiomalate, have patient lie down and remain recumbent for 10 to 20 minutes after injection to minimize hypotension.

● Observe patient for 30 minutes after administration because of possible anaphylactoid reaction.

● If adverse reactions develop and are mild, some rheumatologists resume gold therapy after 2 to 3 weeks' rest.

● Monitor platelet count if patient develops purpura or ecchymoses.

● Keep dimercaprol on hand to treat acute toxicity.

Patient teaching

● Inform patient that benefits of therapy may not appear for 3 to 4 months or longer.

● Advise patient that increased joint pain may occur for 1 to 2 days after injection but usually subsides after a few injections.

● Advise patient to report rashes or skin problems immediately. Pruritus often precedes dermatitis; pruritic skin eruptions that develop while patient is receiving gold salt therapy should be considered a reaction to therapy until proven otherwise. Advise patient to stop therapy until reaction subsides and to notify prescriber.

● Advise patient that stomatitis is often preceded by metallic taste, which should be reported to prescriber immediately. Promote careful oral hygiene during therapy.

● Tell patient to avoid sunlight and artificial ultraviolet light to minimize risk of photosensitivity.

● Stress need for medical follow-up and frequent blood and urine tests during therapy.

☑ Evaluation

● Patient's joint stiffness and pain are relieved.

● Patient doesn't experience injury as a result of drug-induced adverse reactions.

● Patient and family state understanding of drug therapy.

azathioprine
(ay-zuh-THIGH-oh-preen)
Azasan, Imuran, Thioprine◇

Pharmacologic class: purine antagonist
Therapeutic class: immunosuppressant
Pregnancy risk category: D

Indications and dosages

▶ **Immunosuppression in kidney transplantation.** *Adults and children:* Initially, 3 to 5 mg/kg P.O. or I.V. daily, usually beginning on day of transplantation. Maintain at 1 to 3 mg/kg daily depending on patient response.

▶ **Severe, refractory rheumatoid arthritis.** *Adults:* Initially, 1 mg/kg (about 50 mg to 100 mg) P.O. daily as single dose or as two doses. If patient response isn't satisfactory after 6 to 8 weeks, increase dosage by 0.5 mg/kg daily (up to maximum of 2.5 mg/kg daily) at 4-week intervals.

▼ I.V. administration

● Reconstitute 100-mg vial with 10 ml of sterile water for injection. Visually inspect for particles before giving.

● Drug may be given by direct I.V. injection or further diluted in normal saline solution or D_5W and infused over 30 to 60 minutes.

● Use only for patient who can't tolerate P.O. medications.

Contraindications and precautions

● Contraindicated in patients hypersensitive to drug.

● Use cautiously in patients with hepatic or renal dysfunction.

● **Lifespan:** In pregnant women, don't use drug to treat rheumatoid arthritis. In breast-feeding women, drug isn't recommended.

Adverse reactions

GI: nausea, vomiting, esophagitis, anorexia, *pancreatitis,* steatorrhea, mouth ulceration.
Hematologic: LEUKOPENIA, *bone marrow suppression,* anemia, *pancytopenia,* THROMBOCYTOPENIA.
Hepatic: *hepatotoxicity,* jaundice.
Musculoskeletal: arthralgia, muscle wasting.
Skin: rash, alopecia, pruritus.

Other: *immunosuppression,* infections, *neoplasia.*

Interactions

Drug-drug. *ACE inhibitors:* May cause severe leukopenia. Monitor patient closely.
Allopurinol: May impair inactivation of azathioprine. Decrease azathioprine dose to one-fourth or one-third normal dose.
Co-trimoxazole and other drugs that interfere with myelopoiesis: Severe leukopenia, especially in renal transplant patients. Use together cautiously.
Cyclosporine: May decrease cyclosporine level. Monitor level.
Methotrexate: May increase 6-MP metabolite level. Monitor patient for increased adverse effects.
Nondepolarizing neuromuscular blockers: May decrease or reverse effects of these agents. Monitor patient for clinical effects.
Vaccines: May decrease immune response. Postpone routine immunization.
Warfarin: May inhibit anticoagulant effect of warfarin. Monitor PT and INR.

Effects on lab test results

- May increase AST, ALT, alkaline phosphatase, and bilirubin levels. May decrease uric acid levels.
- May decrease hemoglobin, hematocrit, and WBC, RBC, and platelet counts.

Pharmacokinetics

Absorption: Good.
Distribution: Distributed throughout body; I.V. and P.O. forms are 30% protein-bound.
Metabolism: Primarily metabolized to mercaptopurine.
Excretion: Small amounts of azathioprine and mercaptopurine are excreted intact in urine; most of given dose is excreted in urine as secondary metabolites. *Half-life:* About 5 hours.

Route	Onset	Peak	Duration
P.O., I.V.	4-8 wk	1-2 hr	Unknown

Action

Chemical effect: Unknown.
Therapeutic effect: Suppresses immune system activity.

Available forms

Injection: 100 mg
Tablets: 25 mg, 50 mg, 75 mg, 100 mg

NURSING PROCESS

⚕ Assessment
- Obtain history of patient's immune status before therapy.
- Monitor effectiveness by observing patient for signs of organ rejection. Therapeutic response usually occurs within 8 weeks.
- Be alert for adverse reactions and drug interactions.
- Monitor hemoglobin, hematocrit, and WBC and platelet counts at least once monthly—more often at beginning of treatment.
- Evaluate patient's and family's knowledge of drug therapy.

⊞ Nursing diagnoses
- Ineffective protection related to threat of organ rejection
- Risk for infection related to drug-induced immunosuppression
- Deficient knowledge related to drug therapy

⊁ Planning and implementation
- Give in divided doses or after meals to minimize adverse GI effects.
- Benefits must be weighed against risks with systemic viral infections, such as chickenpox and herpes zoster.
- Patients with rheumatoid arthritis previously treated with alkylating drugs, such as cyclophosphamide, chlorambucil, and melphalan, may have prohibitive risk of neoplasia if treated with azathioprine.
- To prevent irreversible bone marrow suppression, stop drug immediately when WBC count is less than 3,000/mm^3. Notify prescriber.
- To prevent bleeding, avoid I.M. injections when platelet count is below 100,000/mm^3.
- ⓢ **ALERT:** Don't confuse azathioprine with azidothymidine, Azulfidine, or azatadine. Don't confuse Imuran with Inderal.
Patient teaching
- Warn patient to report even mild infections (colds, fever, sore throat, and malaise) because drug is a potent immunosuppressant.
- Instruct woman to avoid conception during therapy and for 4 months after stopping therapy.
- Warn patient that thinning of hair is possible.

• Tell patient taking this drug for refractory rheumatoid arthritis that it may take up to 12 weeks to be effective.

☑ **Evaluation**
• Patient exhibits no signs of organ rejection.
• Patient demonstrates no signs and symptoms of infection.
• Patient and family state understanding of drug therapy.

azelastine hydrochloride
(ah-zuh-LAST-een high-droh-KLOR-ighd)
Astelin, Optivar

Pharmacologic class: H$_1$-receptor agonist
Therapeutic class: antihistamine
Pregnancy risk category: C

Indications and dosages

▶ **Seasonal allergic rhinitis, such as rhinorrhea, sneezing, and nasal pruritus.** *Adults and children age 12 and older:* 2 sprays (274 mcg/ 2 sprays) per nostril b.i.d.
Children ages 5 to 11 years: 1 spray (137 mcg/ spray) per nostril b.i.d.
▶ **Vasomotor rhinitis, such as rhinorrhea, nasal congestion, and postnasal drip.** *Adults and children age 12 and older:* 2 sprays (274 mcg/2 sprays) per nostril b.i.d.
▶ **Allergic conjunctivitis.** *Adults and children older than age 3:* Give 1 drop into affected eye b.i.d.

Contraindications and precautions

• Contraindicated in patients hypersensitive to drug.
⚕ **Lifespan:** In pregnant women, drug should be used only if benefit justifies risk to fetus. Breast-feeding women shouldn't take drug. In children younger than age 5, safety and efficacy of drug haven't been established for treatment of seasonal allergic rhinitis. In children younger than age 12, don't use drug for vasomotor rhinitis.

Adverse reactions

CNS: fatigue, *headaches, somnolence,* dysesthesia, dizziness.
EENT: transient eye burning, stinging, nasal burning, conjunctivitis, eye pain, pharyngitis, rhinitis, paroxysmal sneezing, temporary eye blurring, epistaxis, sinusitis.
GI: *bitter taste,* dry mouth, nausea.
Metabolic: weight increase.
Respiratory: *asthma,* dyspnea.
Skin: pruritus.
Other: flulike symptoms.

Interactions

Drug-drug. *Cimetidine:* May increase azelastine level. Avoid using together.
CNS depressants: May reduce alertness and impair CNS performance. Avoid using together.
Drug-lifestyle. *Alcohol use:* May reduce alertness and cause CNS impairment if using the nasal spray. Discourage using together.

Effects on lab test results

None reported.

Pharmacokinetics

Absorption: Ophthalmic solution has low absorption.
Distribution: Systemic bioavailability is 40%.
Metabolism: After dosing to a steady state, level ranges from 20% to 50%.
Excretion: Oral drug is 75% excreted in feces. Less than 10% remains unchanged. *Half-life:* 22 hours.

Route	Onset	Peak	Duration
Nasal	Unknown	2-3 hr	12 hr
Ophthalmic	3 min	Unknown	8 hr

Action

Chemical effect: Exhibits histamine H$_1$-receptor agonist activity.
Therapeutic effect: Relieves seasonal allergic rhinitis.

Available forms

Nasal solution: 1 mg/ml (137 mcg/spray)
Ophthalmic solution: 0.05%

NURSING PROCESS

☡ **Assessment**
• Obtain history of patient's allergy condition before therapy begins and reassess regularly thereafter.
• Be alert for adverse reactions and drug interactions.

- Evaluate patient's and family's knowledge of drug therapy.

⊞ Nursing diagnoses
- Ineffective health maintenance related to underlying allergic condition
- Deficient knowledge related to drug therapy

⟩ Planning and implementation
- Don't contaminate eye dropper tip or solution.
- Make sure patient removes contact lenses before giving eyedrops. Tell patient to wait at least 10 minutes before reinserting them.
- When using nasal spray, avoid spraying into patient's eyes.

Patient teaching
- Warn patient not to drive or perform hazardous activities if somnolence occurs.
- Advise patient not to use alcohol, CNS depressants, or other antihistamines while taking drug.
- Teach patient proper use of nasal spray. Instruct patient to replace child-resistant screw top on bottle with pump unit. Prime delivery system with four sprays or until a fine mist appears. If 3 or more days have elapsed since last use, reprime system with two sprays or until a fine mist appears. Store bottle upright at room temperature with pump closed tightly. Keep unit away from children.
- Tell patient to avoid getting spray in eyes.

☑ Evaluation
- Patient's allergic symptoms are relieved with drug therapy.
- Patient and family state understanding of drug therapy.

azithromycin
(uh-zith-roh-MIGH-sin)
Zithromax

Pharmacologic class: azalide macrolide
Therapeutic class: antibiotic
Pregnancy risk category: B

Indications and dosages

▶ **Acute bacterial exacerbations of chronic obstructive pulmonary disease caused by** *Haemophilus influenzae, Moraxella (Branhamella) catarrhalis,* **or** *Streptococcus pneumoniae;* **uncomplicated skin and skin-** structure infections caused by *Staphylococcus aureus, Streptococcus pyogenes,* **or** *Streptococcus agalactiae;* **and second-line therapy for pharyngitis or tonsillitis caused by** *S. pyogenes. Adults and children age 16 and older:* Initially, 500 mg P.O. as a single dose on day 1, followed by 250 mg daily on days 2 through 5. Total cumulative dose is 1.5 g. Alternatively, for COPD exacerbations, 500 mg P.O. daily for 3 days.

▶ **Community-acquired pneumonia caused by** *Chlamydia pneumoniae, H. influenzae, Mycoplasma pneumoniae, S. pneumoniae;* **I.V. form is also used for** *Legionella pneumophila, M. catarrhalis,* **and** *S. aureus. Adults and children age 16 and older:* 500 mg P.O. as a single dose on day 1, followed by 250 mg daily on days 2 through 5. Total dose is 1.5 g. For patients requiring initial I.V. therapy, 500 mg I.V. as a single daily dose for 2 days, followed by 500 mg P.O. as a single daily dose to complete a 7- to 10-day course of therapy. Switch from I.V. to P.O. therapy should be done at prescriber's discretion and based on patient's clinical response.
Children age 6 months and older: 10 mg/kg P.O. as a single dose on day 1, followed by 5 mg/kg daily on days 2 through 5.

▶ **Nongonococcal urethritis or cervicitis caused by** *Chlamydia trachomatis. Adults and children age 16 and older:* 1 g P.O. as a single dose.

▶ **Prevention of disseminated** *Mycobacterium avium* **complex (MAC) disease in patients with advanced HIV infection.** *Adults:* 1,200 mg P.O. once weekly, as indicated. *Infants and children‡:* 20 mg/kg P.O. (maximum dose of 1.2 g) weekly or 5 mg/kg (maximum dose of 250 mg) can be given P.O. daily. Children 6 years and older may also receive rifabutin 300 mg P.O. daily.

▶ **Disseminated Mycobacterium avium complex in patients with advanced HIV infection.** *Adults:* 600 mg P.O. daily with ethambutol 15 mg/kg daily.

▶ **Urethritis and cervicitis caused by** *Neisseria gonorrhoeae. Adults:* 2 g P.O. as a single dose.

▶ **Pelvic inflammatory disease caused by** *C. trachomatis, N. gonorrhoeae,* **or** *Mycoplasma hominis* **in patients who require initial I.V. therapy.** *Adults and adolescents age 16 and older:* 500 mg I.V. as a single daily dose for 1 to

2 days, followed by 250 mg P.O. daily to complete a 7-day course of therapy. Switch from I.V. to P.O. therapy should be done at prescriber's discretion and based on patient's clinical response.

▶ **Prophylaxis for sexual assault victims‡.**
Adults: 1 g P.O. as a single dose with metronidazole and ceftriaxone.

▶ **Genital ulcer disease caused by** *Haemophilus ducreyi* **(chancroid) in men.**
Adults: 1 g P.O. as a single dose.

▶ **Acute otitis media.** *Children older than age 6 months:* 30 mg/kg P.O. as a single dose. Or, 10 mg/kg P.O. once daily for 3 days. Or 10 mg/kg P.O. on day 1; then 5 mg/kg once daily on days 2 to 5.

▶ **Pharyngitis, tonsillitis cause by** *S. pyogenes. Children age 2 and older:* 12 mg/kg (maximum, 500 mg) P.O. daily for 5 days.

▶ **Chancroid.** *Adults:* 1 g P.O. as a single dose. *Children and infants‡:* 20 mg/kg (maximum, 1 g) P.O.as a single dose.

▶ **Prophylaxis of bacterial endocarditis in penicillin-allergic patients at moderate-to-high risk‡.** *Adults:* 500 mg P.O. 1 hour before the procedure.
Children: 15 mg/kg P.O. 1 hour before the procedure. Don't exceed adult dose.

▶ **Chlamydial ophthalmia neonatorum‡.** *Infants:* 20 mg/kg once daily P.O. for 3 days.

▼ I.V. administration

• Reconstitute drug by adding 4.8 ml sterile water for injection to 500-mg vial and shake until all the drug is dissolved. Further dilute in 250 to 500 ml D_5W, normal saline solution, or other compatible solution.
• Infuse over 1 to 3 hours.
• Reconstituted solution is stable for 7 days if stored in refrigerator (41° F [5° C]).

Contraindications and precautions

• Contraindicated in patients hypersensitive to erythromycin or other macrolides.
• Use cautiously in patients with impaired hepatic function.
≰ **Lifespan:** In pregnant or breast-feeding women, use cautiously.

Adverse reactions

CNS: dizziness, vertigo, headache, fatigue, somnolence.
CV: palpitations, chest pain.

GI: *nausea, vomiting, diarrhea, abdominal pain,* dyspepsia, flatulence, melena, cholestatic jaundice, *pseudomembranous colitis.*
GU: candidiasis, vaginitis, nephritis.
Skin: rash, photosensitivity.
Other: *angioedema.*

Interactions

Drug-drug. *Antacids containing aluminum and magnesium:* May lower peak azithromycin level. Separate administration times by at least 2 hours.
Digoxin: May elevate digoxin level. Monitor patient closely.
Dihydroergotamine, ergotamine: May cause acute ergot toxicity. Avoid using together.
Drugs metabolized by CYP system: May elevate carbamazepine, cyclosporine, hexobarbital, and phenytoin levels. Monitor patient closely.
Theophylline: May increase theophylline level with other macrolides; effect of azithromycin is unknown. Monitor theophylline level carefully.
Triazolam: May increase pharmacologic effect of triazolam. Use cautiously.
Warfarin: May increase PT with other macrolides; effect of azithromycin is unknown. Monitor PT and INR carefully.
Drug-food. *Any food:* May decrease absorption. Give at least 1 hour before or 2 hours after a meal.
Drug-lifestyle. *Sun exposure:* May cause photosensitivity reactions. Advise against prolonged or unprotected sun exposure.

Effects on lab test results

None reported.

Pharmacokinetics

Absorption: Rapid. Food decreases both maximum level and amount of drug absorbed.
Distribution: Rapid throughout body and readily penetrates cells; drug doesn't readily enter CNS. Drug concentrates in fibroblasts and phagocytes. Significantly higher levels are reached in tissues compared with plasma.
Metabolism: None.
Excretion: Mostly in feces after excretion into bile. Less than 10% in urine. *Terminal elimination half-life:* 68 hours.

Route	Onset	Peak	Duration
P.O.	Unknown	2½-4½ hr	Unknown
I.V.	Unknown	Unknown	Unknown

Rapid onset   *Liquid form contains alcohol.   ◆Canada   ◇ Australia   †OTC   ‡Off-label use

Action

Chemical effect: Binds to 50S subunit of bacterial ribosomes, blocking protein synthesis; bacteriostatic or bactericidal, depending on concentration.

Therapeutic effect: Hinders or kills susceptible bacteria, including many gram-positive and gram-negative aerobic and anaerobic bacteria.

Available forms

Injection: 500 mg
Powder for oral suspension: 100 mg/5 ml, 200 mg/5 ml; 1,000 mg/packet
Tablets: 250 mg, 500 mg, 600 mg

NURSING PROCESS

🔧 Assessment

• Obtain history of patient's infection before therapy and reassess regularly thereafter.
• Obtain specimen for culture and sensitivity tests before first dose. Therapy may begin pending test results.
• Be alert for adverse reactions and drug interactions.
• Evaluate patient's and family's knowledge of drug therapy.

⊕ Nursing diagnoses

• Infection related to presence of susceptible bacteria
• Ineffective protection related to drug-induced superinfection
• Deficient knowledge related to drug therapy

▷ Planning and implementation

• Give with or without food.
• Don't give with antacids.
Patient teaching
• Tell patient that tablets or oral suspension may be taken with or without food.
• Tell patient to take all medication as prescribed, even after he feels better.
• Instruct patient to use sunblock and avoid prolonged exposure to the sun to decrease risk of photosensitivity reactions.

✔️ Evaluation

• Patient's infection is eliminated.
• Patient doesn't experience superinfection during therapy.
• Patient and family state understanding of drug therapy.

aztreonam
(az-TREE-oh-nam)
Azactam

Pharmacologic class: monobactam
Therapeutic class: antibiotic
Pregnancy risk category: B

Indications and dosages

▶ **UTI, lower respiratory tract infections, septicemia, skin and skin-structure infections, intra-abdominal infections, surgical infections, gynecologic infections caused by various aerobic organisms; or as adjunct therapy to pelvic inflammatory disease‡ or gonorrhea‡.** *Adults:* 500 mg to 2 g I.V. or I.M. q 8 to 12 hours. For severe systemic or life-threatening infection, 2 g q 6 to 8 hours. Maximum dosage is 8 g daily.

▽ I.V. administration

• Inject bolus dose drug over 3 to 5 minutes directly into vein or I.V. tubing.
• Give infusion over 20 minutes to 1 hour.

Contraindications and precautions

• Contraindicated in patients hypersensitive to drug.
• Use cautiously in patients with impaired renal function. Dosage adjustment may be needed.
🔥 **Lifespan:** In breast-feeding women, drug isn't recommended. In children, safety of drug hasn't been established. In elderly patients, use cautiously; dosage adjustment may be needed.

Adverse reactions

CNS: *seizures,* headache, insomnia, confusion.
CV: hypotension.
EENT: halitosis, altered taste.
GI: diarrhea, nausea, vomiting.
Hematologic: *neutropenia,* anemia, ***thrombocytopenia, pancytopenia.***
Other: hypersensitivity reactions (rash, ***anaphylaxis***); rash, thrombophlebitis at I.V. site; discomfort, swelling at I.M. injection site.

Interactions

Drug-drug. *Aminoglycosides, beta-lactam antibiotics, other anti-infective drugs:* May have synergistic effect. Monitor patient closely.

Reactions may be *common,* uncommon, *life-threatening*, or COMMON AND LIFE-THREATENING.

Cefoxitin, imipenem: May have antagonistic effect. Avoid using together.
Furosemide, probenecid: May increase aztreonam level. Avoid using together.

Effects on lab test results

• May increase BUN, creatinine, ALT, AST, and LDH levels.
• May increase PT, APTT, and INR. May decrease hemoglobin, hematocrit, and neutrophil and RBC counts. May increase or decrease WBC and platelet counts.

Pharmacokinetics

Absorption: Rapid and complete.
Distribution: Rapid and wide to all body fluids and tissues, including bile, breast milk, and CSF.
Metabolism: From 6% to 16% metabolized to inactive metabolites by nonspecific hydrolysis of beta-lactam ring; 56% to 60% protein-bound, less if renal impairment is present.
Excretion: Primarily unchanged in urine by glomerular filtration and tubular secretion; 1.5% to 3.5% excreted unchanged in feces. *Half-life:* Average 1.7 hours.

Route	Onset	Peak	Duration
I.V.	Immediate	Immediate	Unknown
I.M.	Unknown	½ -1¼ hr	Unknown

Action

Chemical effect: Inhibits bacterial cell-wall synthesis, ultimately causing cell-wall destruction; bactericidal.
Therapeutic effect: Kills susceptible bacteria.

Available forms

Injection: 500-mg, 1-g, 2-g vials

NURSING PROCESS

⬛ Assessment

• Obtain history of patient's infection before therapy, and reassess regularly thereafter.
• Obtain urine specimen for culture and sensitivity tests before giving first dose. Therapy may begin pending test results.
• Be aware of adverse reactions and drug interactions.
• Patients who are allergic to penicillins or cephalosporins may not be allergic to this drug. However, closely monitor patients who have had an immediate hypersensitivity reaction to these antibiotics.
• Evaluate patient's and family's knowledge of drug therapy.

🔷 Nursing diagnoses

• Infection related to presence of susceptible bacteria
• Ineffective protection related to drug-induced superinfection
• Deficient knowledge related to drug therapy

⬛ Planning and implementation

• Give I.M. injection deep into large muscle mass, such as upper, outer quadrant of gluteus maximus or lateral aspect of thigh. Give doses larger than 1 g by I.V. route.
Patient teaching
• Tell patient to report pain or discomfort at I.V. site.
• Warn patient receiving drug I.M. that pain and swelling may develop at injection site.
• Instruct patient to report signs or symptoms that suggest superinfection.

⬛ Evaluation

• Patient is free from infection.
• Patient doesn't develop superinfection as a result of therapy.
• Patient and family state understanding of drug therapy.

bacillus Calmette-Guérin (BCG), live intravesical

(bah-SIL-us kal-MET geh-RAN, in-trah-VES-ih-kal)
ImmuCyst♦, Pacis, TheraCys, TICE BCG

Pharmacologic class: bacterial agent, biological response modifier
Therapeutic class: antineoplastic, antituberculotic
Pregnancy risk category: C

Indications and dosages

▶ **In situ carcinoma of urinary bladder (primary and relapsed).** *Adults:* Wait 7 to 14 days after bladder biopsy or transurethral resection. Instill 1 diluted vial (81 mg) TheraCys into bladder via catheter once weekly for 6 weeks, followed by maintenance therapy consisting of 1 dose given at 3, 6, 12, 18, and 24 months after initial treatment. Or, instill 1 diluted vial (50 mg) TICE BCG into bladder via catheter once weekly for 6 weeks. If tumor remission isn't achieved, repeat schedule. Follow with 1 dose q month for 6 to 12 months or longer. Or, instill 120 mg Pacis into bladder via catheter once a week for 6 weeks. If tumor remission hasn't been achieved, repeat schedule. Maintenance dosing for Pacis hasn't been studied.

▶ **Tuberculosis prevention.** *Adults and children age 1 month and older:* 0.2 to 0.3 ml TICE BCG injected percutaneously using a multiple-puncture device.

Neonates younger than age 1 month: Decrease dose by 50% by reconstituting the vaccine with 2 ml instead of 1 ml sterile water for injection without preservatives.

Contraindications and precautions

● Contraindicated in immunocompromised patients, in those receiving immunosuppressive therapy (because of risk of bacterial infection), in those with UTI (because of risk of increased bladder irritation or disseminated BCG infection), and in those with fever of unknown origin. If fever is caused by an infection, withhold drug until patient has recovered.

⚱ Lifespan: In pregnant or breast-feeding women, use cautiously. In children, safety of drug hasn't been established.

Adverse reactions

CNS: fever above 101° F (38.3° C), *malaise,* headache, dizziness, fatigue.
GI: *nausea, vomiting,* anorexia, diarrhea, mild abdominal pain, constipation.
GU: *dysuria, urinary frequency, hematuria, cystitis, urinary urgency,* urinary incontinence, UTI, cramps, pain, decreased bladder capacity, tissue in urine, local infection, **nephrotoxicity,** *genital pain.*
Hematologic: anemia, **leukopenia, thrombocytopenia, DIC.**
Metabolic: *renal toxicity.*
Musculoskeletal: myalgia, arthralgia.
Skin: ulceration, scarring, and lymphangitis at injection site; rash.

Other: hypersensitivity reaction, *chills,* flulike symptoms, systemic infection, **disseminated sepsis.**

Interactions

Drug-drug. *Antibiotics:* May attenuate response to BCG intravesical. Avoid using together.
Bone marrow suppressants, immunosuppressants, radiation therapy: May impair response to BCG intravesical by decreasing immune response; also may increase risk of osteomyelitis or disseminated BCG infection. Avoid using together.

Effects on lab test results

● May increase liver enzyme levels.
● May decrease hemoglobin, hematocrit, and WBC and platelet counts.

Pharmacokinetics

Absorption: Unknown.
Distribution: Unknown.
Metabolism: Unknown.
Excretion: Unknown. *Half-life:* Unknown.

Route	Onset	Peak	Duration
Intravesical, percutaneous	Unknown	Unknown	Unknown

Action

Chemical effect: Causes local inflammatory response. Local infiltration of histiocytes and leukocytes is followed by decrease in superficial tumors in bladder. *Mycobacterium bovis* present in the vaccine is immunologically similar to *M. tuberculosis.* Vaccination stimulates natural infection with *M. tuberculosis* and promotes cell-mediated immunity.
Therapeutic effect: Decreases risk of superficial bladder tumors. Immunizes against *M. tuberculosis.*

Available forms

Powder for suspension: 50-mg vial, 81-mg vial, 120-mg single-dose ampule

NURSING PROCESS

🔎 **Assessment**
● Obtain history of patient's bladder cancer.
● Monitor drug's effectiveness by regularly checking tumor size and growth rate through appropriate studies and by noting results of

follow-up diagnostic tests and overall physical status.
• Be alert for adverse reactions and drug interactions.
• Closely monitor patient for evidence of systemic BCG infection. Such infections are seldom detected by positive cultures.
• Evaluate patient's and family's understanding of drug therapy.

🔁 **Nursing diagnoses**
• Risk for injury related to underlying condition
• Risk for trauma related to instillation procedure for drug therapy
• Deficient knowledge related to drug therapy

▶ **Planning and implementation**
• For 4 hours before each dose, don't allow patient any fluids. Have him empty his bladder.
• Don't use as an immunizing agent to prevent cancer or tuberculosis; don't confuse with BCG vaccine.
⊛ **ALERT:** Don't give BCG intravesical within 7 to 14 days of transurethral resection or biopsy. Fatal disseminated BCG infection may occur after traumatic catheterization.
• To give TheraCys or ImmuCyst, reconstitute with 1 ml of provided diluent per vial, just before use. Don't remove rubber stopper to prepare solution. Use immediately. Add contents of three reconstituted vials to 50 ml of sterile, preservative-free saline solution (final volume, 53 ml). Instill urethral catheter into bladder under aseptic conditions, drain bladder, and infuse 53 ml of prepared solution by gravity feed. Remove catheter and properly dispose of unused drug.
• To give TICE BCG, add 1 ml of preservative-free saline injection to 50 mg vial to resuspend. Leave drug and diluent in contact for 1 minute. Then mix the suspension by withdrawing it into the syringe and expelling it gently back into the vial two or three times. Avoid producing foam—don't shake. Use this reconstituted solution for the tuberculosis vaccine dose. To prepare the carcinoma solution, further dilute the reconstituted product in an additional 49 ml of saline solution, bringing the total volume to 50 ml.
• Give vaccine using a multiple-puncture disc. Keep area dry for at least 24 hours after administration.
• After percutaneous administration, the skin lesion usually appears at the site within 10 to

14 days. Quicker results occur if the patient has tuberculosis.
• Handle drug and all materials used for instillation of drug as biohazardous material because they contain live attenuated mycobacteria. Dispose of syringes, catheters, and containers as biohazardous waste.
• Use strict aseptic technique when giving drug to minimize trauma to GU tract and to prevent introduction of other contaminants.
• If patient has evidence of traumatic catheterization, don't give drug, and alert prescriber. Treatment may resume after 1 week.
• If patient has a short-term fever above 103° F (39.4° C), persistent fever above 101° F (38.3° C) longer than 2 days, or severe malaise, suspect systemic infection and withhold drug. Contact an infectious disease specialist to start fast-acting antituberculosis therapy.
• For symptoms of bladder irritation, give phenazopyridine, acetaminophen, and propantheline. For systemic hypersensitivity, give diphenhydramine. To minimize risk of systemic infection, give isoniazid for 3 days starting on first day of treatment.
Patient teaching
• Tell patient to retain drug in bladder for 2 hours after instillation (if possible). For the first hour, have patient lie prone for 15 minutes, supine for 15 minutes, and on each side for 15 minutes; the second hour may be spent in sitting position.
• Instruct patient to sit when voiding to avoid splashing of urine.
• Instruct patient to disinfect urine for 6 hours after instillation of drug. Tell him to add undiluted household bleach in equal volume to voided urine in toilet and let stand for 15 minutes before flushing.
• Tell patient to call prescriber if symptoms worsen or if the following symptoms develop: blood in urine, frequent urge to urinate, painful urination, fever and chills, nausea, vomiting, joint pain, or rash.
• Tell patient to notify prescriber immediately if cough develops after therapy because it may indicate life-threatening BCG infection.

☑ **Evaluation**
• Patient exhibits no further evidence of superficial bladder tumors.
• Patient doesn't experience trauma as result of drug use.

• Patient and family state understanding of drug therapy.

baclofen
(BAH-kloh-fen)
Clofen◇, Kemstro, Lioresal, Lioresal Intrathecal

Pharmacologic class: chlorophenyl derivative (GABA derivative)
Therapeutic class: skeletal muscle relaxant
Pregnancy risk category: C

Indications and dosages

▶ **Spasticity in multiple sclerosis, spinal cord injury.** *Adults:* Initially, 5 mg P.O. t.i.d. for 3 days. Increase dosage based on response at 3-day intervals by 15 mg (5 mg/dose) daily up to maximum of 80 mg daily (20 mg q.i.d.).
▶ **Management of severe spasticity in patients who don't respond to or cannot tolerate oral baclofen therapy.** *Adults (screening phase):* After test dose, give drug by an implantable infusion pump. The test dose is 50 mcg in 1 ml dilution given into intrathecal space by barbotage over 1 minute or longer. Significantly decreased severity or frequency of muscle spasm or reduced muscle tone should be evident in 4 to 8 hours. If response is inadequate, give second test dose of 75 mcg/1.5 ml 24 hours after the first. If response is still inadequate, give final test dose of 100 mcg/2 ml 24 hours later. Patients unresponsive to 100-mcg dose shouldn't be considered candidates for implantable pump. *Adults (maintenance therapy):* Adjust initial dose based on screening dose that elicits an adequate response. This effective dose is doubled and given over 24 hours. If screening-dose efficacy is maintained for 8 hours or longer, dosage isn't doubled. After first 24 hours, increase dose slowly, as needed and tolerated, by 10% to 30% daily until desired effects occur.
Children younger than age 12: Testing dose is the same as for adults (50 mcg); but for very small children, an initial dose of 25 mcg may be given.

Contraindications and precautions

• Contraindicated in patients hypersensitive to drug. Orally disintegrating tablets are contraindicated in patients hypersensitive to aspartame.

• Use cautiously in patients with impaired renal function or seizure disorder or when spasticity is used to maintain motor function.
⚞ **Lifespan:** In pregnant or breast-feeding women, use cautiously. In children younger than age 12, safety of oral use of drug hasn't been established. In children younger than age 4, safety of intrathecal drug hasn't been established.

Adverse reactions

CNS: drowsiness, dizziness, *headache,* weakness, fatigue, *hypotonia, confusion, somnolence,* paresthesias, **CONVULSIONS.**
CV: ankle edema, hypotension.
EENT: nasal congestion, blurred vision.
GI: nausea, constipation, vomiting.
GU: urinary frequency, urinary incontinence.
Metabolic: hyperglycemia, weight gain.
Musculoskeletal: *muscle rigidity or spasticity,* dysarthria, *rhabdomyolysis,* dysarthria.
Respiratory: dyspnea.
Skin: rash, pruritus, excessive perspiration.
Other: sexual dysfunction, impotence, *high fever, multiple organ-system failure.*

Interactions

Drug-drug. *CNS depressants:* Increases CNS depression. Avoid using together.
MAO inhibitors, tricyclic antidepressants: CNS and respiratory depression, hypotension may occur. Avoid using together.
Drug-lifestyle. *Alcohol use:* Increases CNS depression. Discourage using together.

Effects on lab test results

• May increase AST, alkaline phosphatase, and glucose levels.

Pharmacokinetics

Absorption: Rapid and extensive with P.O. administration; may vary.
Distribution: Widely distributed throughout body, with small amounts crossing blood-brain barrier. It's about 30% protein–bound.
Metabolism: About 15% metabolized in liver by deamination.
Excretion: 70% to 80% in urine unchanged or as metabolites; remainder in feces. *Half-life:* 2½ to 4 hours.

Route	Onset	Peak	Duration
P.O.	Hr-wk	2-3 hr	Unknown
Intrathecal	½-1 hr	4 hr	4-8 hr

Action

Chemical effect: Unknown; appears to reduce transmission of impulses from spinal cord to skeletal muscle.
Therapeutic effect: Relieves muscle spasms.

Available forms

Intrathecal injection: 500 mcg/ml, 2,000 mcg/ml
Orally disintegrating tablets: 10 mg, 20 mg
Tablets: 10 mg, 20 mg, 25 mg

NURSING PROCESS

⚕ Assessment
• Obtain history of patient's pain and muscle spasms from underlying condition before therapy, and reassess regularly thereafter.
• Be alert for adverse reactions and drug interactions.
• Watch for increased risk of seizures in patient with seizure disorder. Seizures have been reported during overdose and withdrawal of intrathecal baclofen as well as in patients maintained on therapeutic doses of intrathecal baclofen. Monitor patient carefully and institute seizure precautions.
• Evaluate patient's and family's understanding of drug therapy.

⚕ Nursing diagnoses
• Acute pain related to spasticity
• Risk for injury related to drug-induced adverse CNS reactions
• Deficient knowledge related to drug therapy

▶ Planning and implementation
• Give with meals or milk to prevent GI distress.
• Don't give orally to treat muscle spasm caused by rheumatic disorders, cerebral palsy, Parkinson's disease, or CVA because efficacy hasn't been established.
• Treatment for oral overdose is supportive; don't induce emesis or use respiratory stimulant in an unconscious patient.
• Implantable pump or catheter failure can result in sudden loss of effectiveness of intrathecal baclofen.
⚠ **ALERT:** Don't give intrathecal injection by I.V., I.M., S.C., or epidural route.
• The amount of relief determines whether dose (and drowsiness) can be reduced.

• Avoid abrupt discontinuation of intrathecal baclofen. Early symptoms of baclofen withdrawal may include return of baseline spasticity, pruritus, hypotension, and paresthesias. Symptoms that have occurred include high fever, altered mental status, exaggerated rebound spasticity, and muscle rigidity that in rare cases has advanced to rhabdomyolysis, multiple organ-system failure, and death. Treat intrathecal baclofen withdrawal by restoring intrathecal baclofen at or near the same dosage as before therapy was stopped. However, if delayed, treat with P.O. or enteral baclofen, or P.O., enteral, or I.V. benzodiazepines to prevent potentially fatal sequelae. P.O. or enteral baclofen alone shouldn't be relied upon to halt the progression of intrathecal baclofen withdrawal.
• About 10% of patients may develop tolerance to drug. In some cases, this may be treated by hospitalizing patient and by slowly withdrawing drug over 2-week period.
Patient teaching
• Tell patient to avoid activities that require alertness until drug's CNS effects are known. Drowsiness usually is transient.
• Tell patient to avoid alcohol while taking drug.
• Advise patient to follow prescriber's orders about rest and physical therapy.
• Advise patient to take drug with food or milk to prevent GI distress.

✓ Evaluation
• Patient reports that pain and muscle spasms have ceased with drug therapy.
• Patient doesn't experience injury as a result of drug-induced drowsiness.
• Patient and family state understanding of drug therapy.

balsalazide disodium
(bal-SAL-a-zide digh-SOH-dee-um)
Colazal

Pharmacologic class: GI agent
Therapeutic class: anti-inflammatory
Pregnancy risk category: B

Indications and dosages

▶ **Ulcerative colitis.** *Adults:* 2.25 g P.O. (three 750-mg capsules) t.i.d. for a total of 6.75 g daily for 8 to 12 weeks.

Contraindications and precautions

• Contraindicated in patients hypersensitive to salicylates or to any component of balsalazide metabolites.
• Use cautiously in patients with history of renal disease or renal dysfunction.
• Use judiciously in patients with pyloric stenosis because of prolonged retention of drug. Safety and effectiveness beyond 12 weeks haven't been established.

⚖ **Lifespan:** In breast-feeding women, use cautiously because it's unknown whether drug appears in breast milk. In children, safety and effectiveness of drug haven't been established.

Adverse reactions

CNS: fever, dizziness, fatigue, headache, insomnia.
EENT: pharyngitis, rhinitis, sinusitis.
GI: abdominal pain, anorexia, constipation, cramps, diarrhea, dyspepsia, flatulence, frequent stools, nausea, rectal bleeding, vomiting, dry mouth.
GU: UTI.
Hepatic: *hepatotoxicity.*
Musculoskeletal: arthralgia, back pain, myalgia.
Respiratory: cough, respiratory infection.
Other: flulike symptoms.

Interactions

Drug-drug. *Azathioprine and 6 mercaptopurine:* Balsalazide may interfere with the metabolism of these drugs. Use with caution.
Oral antibiotics and anti-infectives: May interfere with release of mesalamine in the colon. Monitor patient for worsening of symptoms.

Effects on lab test results

• May increase AST, ALT, LDH, alkaline phosphatase, and bilirubin levels.

Pharmacokinetics

Absorption: Very low and variable in healthy patients. 60 times greater in patients with ulcerative colitis.
Distribution: 99% or more protein-bound.
Metabolism: Metabolized to mesalamine (5-aminosalicylic acid), the active component of the drug.
Excretion: Excreted by the kidneys. Less than 1% recovered in urine. *Half-life:* Unknown.

Route	Onset	Peak	Duration
P.O.	Unknown	Unknown	Unknown

Action

Chemical effect: Balsalazide is converted in the colon to mesalamine, which is then converted to 5-aminosalicylic acid. The mechanism of action is unknown, but it appears to be local rather than systemic. In patients with chronic inflammatory bowel disease, the production of arachidonic acid metabolites is increased. Balsalazide likely blocks the production of arachidonic acid metabolites in the colon.
Therapeutic effect: Decreases inflammation in the colon.

Available forms

Capsules: 750 mg

NURSING PROCESS

Assessment
• Assess patient's underlying condition and note frequency of bowel movements before starting drug therapy.
• Hepatotoxicity, including elevated liver function test results, jaundice, cirrhosis, liver necrosis, and liver failure, has occurred with other products containing or metabolized to mesalamine. Although no signs of hepatotoxicity have been reported with balsalazide disodium, monitor patient closely for evidence of hepatic dysfunction.
• Evaluate patient's and family's knowledge of drug therapy and ulcerative colitis.

Nursing diagnoses
• Diarrhea related to underlying disease process
• Risk of imbalanced nutrition: less than body requirements related to frequent bowel movements due to ulcerative colitis
• Deficient knowledge related to balsalazide disodium therapy

Planning and implementation
• Notify prescriber if drug has been given for 8 to 12 weeks or longer.
Patient teaching
• Advise patient not to take drug if allergic to aspirin or salicylate derivatives.
• Advise patient to report adverse reactions promptly to prescriber.

☑ **Evaluation**
• Patient states that diarrhea has improved.
• Because of decreasing symptoms of ulcerative colitis, patient is able to tolerate and absorb a balanced diet.
• Patient and family state understanding of balsalazide disodium therapy.

basiliximab
(ba-sil-IK-si-mab)
Simulect

Pharmacologic class: recombinant chimeric human monoclonal antibody IgG_{1k}
Therapeutic class: immunosuppressant
Pregnancy risk category: B

Indications and dosages

▶ **Prevention of acute organ rejection in renal transplant patients when used as part of immunosuppressive regimen including cyclosporine and corticosteroids.** *Adults and children weighing 35 kg (77 lb) or more:* 20 mg I.V. given within 2 hours before transplant surgery and 20 mg I.V. given 4 days after transplantation.
Children weighing less than 35 kg: 10 mg I.V. given within 2 hours before transplant and 10 mg I.V. given 4 days post-transplantation.

▼ I.V. administration

• Reconstitute with 5 ml sterile water for injection. Shake vial gently to dissolve powder. Dilute reconstituted solution to volume of 50 ml with normal saline solution or D_5W for infusion. When mixing solution, gently invert bag to avoid foaming. Don't shake.
• Infuse over 20 to 30 minutes by a central or peripheral vein. Don't add or infuse other drugs simultaneously through same I.V. line.
• Use reconstituted solution immediately; may be refrigerated between 36° and 46° F (2° and 8° C) for up to 24 hours or kept at room temperature for 4 hours.

Contraindications and precautions

• Contraindicated in patients hypersensitive to drug or its components.
⚕ **Lifespan:** In pregnant women, use only if potential benefits outweigh risks to fetus. Breast-feeding women should stop nursing or

the drug because of potential for adverse effects; it's unknown whether drug appears in breast milk. In elderly patients, use cautiously.

Adverse reactions

CNS: *fever,* agitation, anxiety, asthenia, depression, *dizziness, headache,* hypoesthesia, *insomnia,* neuropathy, paresthesia, *tremor,* fatigue.
CV: *hemorrhage,* angina pectoris, *arrhythmias,* atrial fibrillation, *heart failure,* chest pain, abnormal heart sounds, *aggravated hypertension, hypertension, leg or peripheral edema,* general edema, hypotension, tachycardia.
EENT: abnormal vision, cataract, conjunctivitis, *rhinitis,* sinusitis, *pharyngitis.*
GI: *abdominal pain, candidiasis, constipation, diarrhea, dyspepsia,* esophagitis, enlarged abdomen, flatulence, gastroenteritis, GI disorder, *GI hemorrhage,* gum hyperplasia, melena, *nausea,* ulcerative stomatitis, *vomiting.*
GU: abnormal renal function, albuminuria, bladder disorder, *dysuria,* frequent micturition, genital edema, hematuria, *increased nonprotein nitrogen,* oliguria, *renal tubular necrosis,* ureteral disorder, *UTI,* urine retention, impotence.
Hematologic: *anemia,* hematoma, *polycythemia, purpura, thrombocytopenia, thrombosis.*
Metabolic: *acidosis,* dehydration, *diabetes mellitus,* fluid overload, hypercalcemia, *hypercholesterolemia, hyperglycemia,* HYPERKALEMIA, hyperlipemia, *hyperuricemia, hypocalcemia, hypokalemia,* hypomagnesemia, *hypophosphatemia,* hypoproteinemia, *weight gain.*
Musculoskeletal: arthralgia, arthropathy, *back pain,* bone fracture, cramps, hernia, *leg pain,* myalgia.
Respiratory: abnormal chest sounds, bronchitis, *bronchospasm, cough, dyspnea,* pneumonia, pulmonary disorder, *pulmonary edema, upper respiratory tract infection.*
Skin: acne, cyst, herpes simplex, herpes zoster, hypertrichosis, pruritus, rash, skin disorder or ulceration.
Other: accidental trauma, *viral infection,* infection, *sepsis, surgical wound complications.*

Interactions

None significant.

Effects on lab test results

• May increase calcium, cholesterol, glucose, lipid, and uric acid levels. May decrease magne-

sium, phosphorus, and protein levels. May increase or decrease potassium level.
• May increase RBC count. May decrease hemoglobin, hematocrit, and platelet count.

Pharmacokinetics

Absorption: Administered I.V.
Distribution: Unknown.
Metabolism: Unknown.
Excretion: Unknown. *Half-life:* About 7.2 days in adults, 9.5 days in children, 9.1 days in adolescents.

Route	Onset	Peak	Duration
I.V.	Unknown	Immediate	Unknown

Action

Chemical effect: Binds specifically to and blocks the interleukin (IL)-2 receptor alpha chain on the surface of activated T lymphocytes, inhibiting IL-2–mediated activation of lymphocytes, a critical pathway in the cellular immune response involved in allograft rejection.
Therapeutic effect: Prevents organ rejection.

Available forms

Injection: 20-mg vials

NURSING PROCESS

▓ Assessment
• Monitor patient for anaphylactoid reactions. Be sure that drugs for treating severe hypersensitivity reactions are available for immediate use.
• Check for electrolyte imbalances and acidosis.
• Monitor patient's intake and output, vital signs, hemoglobin, and hematocrit.
• Be alert for signs and symptoms of opportunistic infections.
• Evaluate patient's and family's knowledge of drug therapy.

⊕ Nursing diagnoses
• Risk for injury related to potential for organ rejection
• Ineffective protection related to drug-induced immunosuppression
• Deficient knowledge related to drug therapy

▷ Planning and implementation
• Use drug only under supervision of prescriber experienced in this type of therapy and management of organ transplantation.

Patient teaching
• Inform patient of potential benefits and risks of therapy, including decreased risk of graft loss or acute rejection. Advise patient that therapy increases risks of developing lymphoproliferative disorders and opportunistic infections. Tell him to report signs and symptoms of infection promptly.
• Tell women of childbearing age to use effective contraception before therapy starts and for 4 months after therapy ends.
• Instruct patient to report adverse effects to prescriber immediately.
• Explain that drug is used with cyclosporine and corticosteroids.

☑ Evaluation
• Patient doesn't experience organ rejection while taking this drug.
• Patient is free from infection and serious bleeding episodes throughout drug therapy.
• Patient and family state understanding of drug therapy.

becaplermin
(be-KAP-ler-min)
Regranex

Pharmacologic class: recombinant human platelet-derived growth factor (rh-PDGF-BB)
Therapeutic class: wound repair agent
Pregnancy risk category: C

Indications and dosages

▶ **Diabetic neuropathic leg ulcers that extend into S.C. tissue or beyond and have adequate blood supply.** *Adults:* Apply daily in ½-inch even thickness to entire surface of wound and cover with a saline solution–moistened dressing for 12 hours. Use the following table to calculate the length of gel to apply in inches or centimeters, which depends on wound size and tube size.

Tube size	Inches	Centimeters
2 g	Ulcer length × ulcer width × 1.3	Ulcer length × ulcer width ÷ 2
7.5 g, 15 g	Ulcer length × ulcer width × 0.6	Ulcer length × ulcer width ÷ 4

Contraindications and precautions

- Contraindicated in patients hypersensitive to drug and in those with neoplasms at application site.
- Don't use in wounds that are sutured.
- ☙ **Lifespan:** In pregnant women, give only when clearly needed. In breast-feeding women, use cautiously. In children younger than age 16, safety and efficacy of drug haven't been established.

Adverse reactions

Musculoskeletal: osteomyelitis.
Skin: erythematous rash.
Other: cellulitis, infection.

Interactions

None significant.

Effects on lab test results

None reported.

Pharmacokinetics

Absorption: Minimal systemic absorption.
Distribution: Unknown.
Metabolism: Unknown.
Excretion: Unknown. *Half-life:* Unknown.

Route	Onset	Peak	Duration
Topical	Unknown	Unknown	Unknown

Action

Chemical effect: Thought to promote chemotactic recruitment and proliferation of cells involved in wound repair and formation of new granulation tissue.
Therapeutic effect: Wound repair.

Available forms

Gel: 100 mcg/g in tubes of 2 g, 7.5 g, 15 g

NURSING PROCESS

☛ Assessment

- Obtain history of patient's underlying condition before therapy, and reassess regularly thereafter.
- Monitor wound size and healing; recalculate amount of drug to be applied at least once weekly. If ulcer doesn't decrease in size by about one-third after 10 weeks, or if complete healing hasn't occurred within 20 weeks, reassess treatment.

- Watch for application site reactions. Sensitization or irritation caused by parabens or m-cresol should be considered.
- Evaluate patient's and family's knowledge of drug therapy.

☷ Nursing diagnoses

- Impaired skin integrity related to leg ulcer
- Acute pain related to presence of skin wound
- Deficient knowledge related to drug therapy

⟩ Planning and implementation

- When using the dosage formula, measure ulcer at its greatest length and width. Squeeze the gel onto clean measuring surface such as waxed paper. Use cotton swab or other application aid to transfer and spread drug over entire ulcer area in a ¹⁄₁₆-inch continuous layer. Place a saline solution–moistened dressing over site and leave in place for about 12 hours. After 12 hours, remove dressing and rinse away residual gel with normal saline solution or water, and apply a fresh moist dressing, without becaplermin, for rest of day.
- Drug is for external use only.
- ⊛ **ALERT:** Don't use drug in wounds that close by primary intention.
- Treatment efficacy hasn't been evaluated for diabetic neuropathic ulcers that don't extend through the dermis into S.C. tissue or for ischemic diabetic ulcers.
- Drug facilitates complete healing of diabetic ulcers when used as an adjunct to good ulcer care practices, which include initial sharp debridement, infection control, and pressure relief.

Patient teaching
- Instruct patient to wash hands thoroughly before applying gel.
- Advise patient not to touch tip of tube against ulcer or any other surfaces.
- Instruct patient on proper procedure for wound care, including applying gel and changing dressings.
- Stress need to keep area covered with a wet dressing at all times.
- Tell patient to store drug in refrigerator (36° to 46° F [2° to 8° C]).
- Instruct patient not to use drug after expiration date.

☑ Evaluation

- Patient's ulcer heals.
- Patient doesn't experience pain.

• Patient and family state understanding of drug therapy.

beclomethasone dipropionate
(bek-loh-METH-eh-sohn digh-proh-PIGH-uh-nayt)
Beclodisk◆, Becloforte Inhaler◇, QVAR, Vanceril, Vanceril Double Strength

Pharmacologic class: glucocorticoid
Therapeutic class: anti-inflammatory, anti-asthmatic
Pregnancy risk category: C

Indications and dosages

▶ **Asthma.** *Adults and children age 12 and older:* For regular strength, 2 inhalations t.i.d. or q.i.d. or 4 inhalations b.i.d.; for patients with severe asthma, start with 12 to 16 sprays per day and then reduce the dosage to the lowest effective level. For double strength, 2 inhalations b.i.d.; for severe asthma, start with 6 to 8 inhalations per day and adjust down. Maximum dosage is 10 inhalations (840 mcg) daily. For QVAR, when used with bronchodilators alone, 40 to 80 mcg b.i.d., initially. When used with inhaled corticosteroids, 40 to 160 mcg b.i.d., initially. Adjust dosage p.r.n. up to a maximum dose of 320 mcg b.i.d.
Children ages 5 to 11: 40 mcg b.i.d. initially, when used with bronchodilators alone, or as adjunct to inhaled corticosteroids. Adjust dosage, p.r.n., up to a maximum dose of 80 mcg b.i.d.

Contraindications and precautions

• Contraindicated in patients hypersensitive to drug or its components (fluorocarbons, oleic acid) and in those with status asthmaticus. Don't use in patients with asthma controlled by bronchodilators or other noncorticosteroids alone or in those with nonasthmatic bronchial diseases.
• Use cautiously, if at all, in patients with tuberculosis, fungal or bacterial infections, ocular herpes simplex, or systemic viral infections. Use with caution in patients receiving systemic corticosteroid therapy.
☀ Lifespan: In pregnant or breast-feeding women, use cautiously. In children younger than age 5, safety and efficacy of QVAR haven't been established.

Adverse reactions

EENT: hoarseness, fungal infections of throat, throat irritation, irritation of nasal mucosa.
GI: dry mouth, fungal infections of mouth.
Respiratory: *bronchospasm.*
Other: *angioedema,* adrenal insufficiency.

Interactions

None significant.

Effects on lab test results

None reported.

Pharmacokinetics

Absorption: Rapid from lungs and GI tract.
Distribution: No evidence of tissue storage of beclomethasone or its metabolites. About 10% to 25% of an orally inhaled dose is deposited in respiratory tract. The remainder, deposited in mouth and oropharynx, is swallowed. When absorbed, it's 87% protein-bound.
Metabolism: Mostly in liver.
Excretion: Unknown, although when drug is given systemically, its metabolites are excreted mainly in feces and, to a lesser extent, in urine. *Half-life:* Average 15 hours.

Route	Onset	Peak	Duration
Inhalation	1-4 wk	Unknown	Unknown

Action

Chemical effect: Decreases inflammation, mainly by stabilizing leukocyte lysosomal membranes.
Therapeutic effect: Helps alleviate asthma symptoms.

Available forms

Oral inhalation aerosol: 40 mcg/metered spray, 50 mcg/metered spray◆, 80 mcg/metered spray

NURSING PROCESS

⚡ Assessment
• Obtain history of patient's asthma before therapy and reassess regularly thereafter.
• Be alert for adverse reactions.
• Monitor patient closely during times of stress (trauma, surgery, or infection) because systemic corticosteroids may be needed to prevent adrenal insufficiency in previously steroid-dependent patients.

• Periodic measurement of growth and development may be necessary during high-dose or prolonged therapy in children.
• Check for irritation of nasal mucosa.
• Evaluate patient's and family's understanding of drug therapy.

🔷 Nursing diagnoses
• Impaired gas exchange related to asthma
• Impaired oral mucous membranes related to drug-induced fungal infections
• Deficient knowledge related to drug therapy

❯ Planning and implementation
🖐 **ALERT:** Never give drug to relieve an emergency asthma attack because onset of action is too slow.
• Give prescribed bronchodilators several minutes before beclomethasone.
• Have patient hold breath for a few seconds after each puff and rest 1 minute between puffs to enhance drug action.
• Spacer device may help ensure delivery of proper dose, although use of such a device with Becloforte Inhaler isn't recommended.
• Taper oral glucocorticoid therapy slowly. Acute adrenal insufficiency and death have occurred in patients with asthma who changed abruptly from oral corticosteroids to beclomethasone.
• Notify prescriber if decreased response is noted after giving drug.
• Have patient gargle and rinse mouth with water after inhalations to help prevent oral fungal infections.
• Keep inhaler clean and unobstructed by washing it with warm water and drying it thoroughly after each use.
Patient teaching
• Inform patient that drug doesn't relieve acute asthma attacks.
• Tell patient who needs a bronchodilator to use it several minutes before drug.
• Instruct patient to wear or carry medical identification indicating need for supplemental systemic glucocorticoid during stress.
• Instruct patient to contact prescriber if response to therapy decreases or if symptoms don't improve within 3 weeks; dosage may need to be adjusted. Tell patient not to exceed recommended dose on his own.

• Tell patient to keep inhaler clean and unobstructed by washing it with warm water and drying it thoroughly.
• Tell patient to prevent oral fungal infections by gargling or rinsing mouth with water after each use but not to swallow water.
• Tell patient to report symptoms of corticosteroid withdrawal, including fatigue, weakness, arthralgia, orthostatic hypotension, and dyspnea.
• Instruct patient to store drug between 36° and 86° F (2° and 30° C). Advise him to ensure delivery of proper dose by gently warming canister to room temperature before using. He may carry canister in pocket to keep it warm.

✅ Evaluation
• Patient's lungs are clear, and breathing and skin color are normal.
• Patient doesn't exhibit an oral fungal infection during therapy.
• Patient and family state understanding of drug therapy.

beclomethasone dipropionate monohydrate
(bek-loh-METH-eh-sohn digh-proh-PIGH-uh-nayt mon-oh-HIGH-drayt)
Beconase AQ Nasal Spray, Vancenase AQ 84 mcg Double Strength, Vancenase Pockethaler

Pharmacologic class: glucocorticoid
Therapeutic class: anti-inflammatory
Pregnancy risk category: C

Indications and dosages
▶ **Symptoms of seasonal or perennial rhinitis; prevention of recurrence of nasal polyps after surgical removal.** *Adults and children age 12 and older:* For 42 mcg/metered spray, give 1 or 2 inhalations in each nostril, b.i.d. Maximum dosage, 336 mcg daily. For 84 mcg/metered spray, give 1 or 2 inhalations in each nostril daily. Maximum dosage, 336 mcg daily. *Children ages 6 to 11:* 1 inhalation in each nostril t.i.d. (252 mcg daily).

Contraindications and precautions

• Contraindicated in patients hypersensitive to drug and in those experiencing status asthmaticus or other acute episodes of asthma.

• Use cautiously, if at all, in patients with active or quiescent respiratory tract tubercular infections or untreated fungal, bacterial, systemic viral, or ocular herpes simplex infections. Also use cautiously in patients who've recently had nasal septal ulcers, nasal surgery, or trauma.

⚹ Lifespan: In pregnant or breast-feeding women, use cautiously. In children younger than age 6, safety of drug hasn't been established.

Adverse reactions

CNS: headache.
EENT: *mild, transient nasal burning and stinging;* nasal congestion; sneezing; epistaxis; watery eyes; nasopharyngeal fungal infections; irritation of nasal mucosa.
GI: nausea, vomiting.

Interactions

None significant.

Effects on lab test results

None reported.

Pharmacokinetics

Absorption: Primarily through nasal mucosa with minimal systemic absorption.
Distribution: Unknown.
Metabolism: Most of drug is metabolized in liver.
Excretion: Unknown, although when drug is given systemically, its metabolites are excreted mainly in feces and, to a lesser extent, in urine. *Biological half-life:* Average 15 hours.

Route	Onset	Peak	Duration
Inhalation	5-7 days	≤ 3 wk	Unknown

Action

Chemical effect: Decreases nasal inflammation, mainly by stabilizing leukocyte lysosomal membranes.
Therapeutic effect: Helps relieve nasal allergy symptoms.

Available forms

Nasal aerosol: 42 mcg/metered spray

Nasal spray: 42 mcg/metered spray, 84 mcg/metered spray

NURSING PROCESS

⏱ Assessment

• Obtain history of patient's allergy symptoms and nasal congestion before therapy, and reassess regularly thereafter.
• Be alert for adverse reactions.
• Monitor patient's hydration status if adverse GI reactions occur.
• Check for irritation of nasal mucosa.
• Evaluate patient's and family's understanding of drug therapy.

⊕ Nursing diagnoses

• Ineffective health maintenance related to allergy-induced nasal congestion
• Risk for deficient fluid volume related to drug-induced adverse GI reactions
• Deficient knowledge related to drug therapy

❯ Planning and implementation

• Drug isn't effective for acute exacerbations of rhinitis. Decongestants or antihistamines may be needed.
• Shake container and invert. Have patient clear his nasal passages and then tilt his head backward. Insert nozzle (pointed away from septum) into nostril, holding other nostril closed. Deliver spray while patient inhales. Shake container and repeat in other nostril.
• Notify prescriber if relief isn't obtained or signs of infection appear.
Patient teaching
• Teach patient how to give himself nasal spray.
• Advise patient to pump new nasal spray three or four times before first use and then once or twice before first use each day thereafter. Also tell patient to clean cap and nosepiece of activator in warm water every day and then air-dry them.
• Advise patient to use drug regularly, as prescribed, because its effectiveness depends on regular use.
• Explain that drug's therapeutic effects, unlike those of decongestants, aren't immediate. Most patients achieve benefit within a few days, but some may require 2 to 3 weeks.
• Warn patient not to exceed recommended doses because of risk of hypothalamic-pituitary-adrenal function suppression.

Reactions may be *common,* uncommon, *life-threatening,* or **COMMON AND LIFE-THREATENING.**

• Tell patient to notify prescriber if symptoms don't improve within 3 weeks or if nasal irritation persists.
• Teach patient good nasal and oral hygiene.

☑ **Evaluation**
• Patient's nasal congestion subsides with therapy.
• Patient maintains adequate hydration throughout therapy.
• Patient and family state understanding of drug therapy.

benazepril hydrochloride
(ben-AY-zuh-pril high-droh-KLOR-ighd)
Lotensin

Pharmacologic class: ACE inhibitor
Therapeutic class: antihypertensive
Pregnancy risk category: C (D in second and third trimesters)

Indications and dosages

▶ **Hypertension.** *Adults not taking diuretics:* Initially, 10 mg P.O. daily. Dosage adjusted, as needed and tolerated; usually, 20 to 40 mg daily, equally divided into one or two doses. Maximum, 80 mg daily.
Adults taking diuretics: Stop diuretic 2 to 3 days before starting benazepril hydrochloride to minimize hypotension. If unable to stop diuretic, start dose at 5 mg daily.
◨ **Adjust-a-dose:** For patients with renal impairment, if creatinine clearance is less than 20 ml/minute, start dose at 5 mg daily. Don't exceed 40 mg P.O. daily.

Contraindications and precautions

• Contraindicated in patients hypersensitive to ACE inhibitors.
• Use cautiously in patients with impaired hepatic or renal function.
⚠ **Lifespan:** In pregnant women, use only if absolutely necessary and then cautiously. With breast-feeding women, use cautiously. In children, safety of drug hasn't been established.

Adverse reactions

CNS: asthenia, headache, dizziness, lightheadedness, anxiety, amnesia, depression, in-

somnia, nervousness, neuralgia, neuropathy, paresthesia, somnolence, syncope.
CV: *symptomatic hypotension,* angina, *arrhythmias,* palpitations, edema.
GI: nausea, vomiting, abdominal pain, constipation, dyspepsia, gastritis, dysphagia, increased salivation.
GU: impotence.
Metabolic: *hyperkalemia,* weight gain.
Musculoskeletal: arthralgia, arthritis, myalgia.
Respiratory: dry, persistent, tickling, nonproductive cough; dyspnea.
Skin: rash, dermatitis, increased diaphoresis, pruritus, photosensitivity, purpura.
Other: *angioedema,* hypersensitivity reactions.

Interactions

Drug-drug. *ACE inhibitors, diuretics, other antihypertensives:* Risk of excessive hypotension. Stop diuretic or lower dose of benazepril, if needed.
Digoxin: May increase digoxin level. Monitor patient for toxicity.
Indomethacin: May reduce hypotensive effects. Monitor blood pressure.
Lithium: Increases lithium level and lithium toxicity. Avoid using together.
Potassium-sparing diuretics, potassium supplements: Risk of hyperkalemia. Monitor patient closely.
Drug-herb. *Capsicum:* May aggravate or cause ACE-induced cough. Discourage using together.
Licorice: May cause sodium retention, thus decreasing ACE effects. Discourage using together.
Drug-food. *Foods, especially those high in fat:* May impair drug absorption. Instruct patient to take drug on an empty stomach.
Sodium substitutes containing potassium: Risk of hyperkalemia. Monitor patient closely.

Effects on lab test results

• May increase BUN, creatinine, and potassium levels.

Pharmacokinetics

Absorption: At least 37%.
Distribution: Protein-binding of benazepril is about 96.7%; that of benazeprilat, 95.3%.
Metabolism: Almost completely metabolized in liver to benazeprilat, which has much greater ACE inhibitory activity than benazepril, and to

glucuronide conjugates of benazepril and benazeprilat.

Excretion: Primarily in urine. *Half-life:* Benazepril, 0.6 hours; benazeprilat, 10 to 12 hours.

Route	Onset	Peak	Duration
P.O.	≤ 1 hr	2-4 hr	24 hr

Action

Chemical effect: Inhibits ACE, preventing conversion of angiotensin I to angiotensin II, a potent vasoconstrictor. Reduced formation of angiotensin II decreases peripheral arterial resistance, thus decreasing aldosterone secretion. This reduces sodium and water retention and lowers blood pressure. Benazepril also has antihypertensive activity in patients with low-renin hypertension.

Therapeutic effect: Lowers blood pressure.

Available forms

Tablets: 5 mg, 10 mg, 20 mg, 40 mg

NURSING PROCESS

Assessment

• Obtain history of patient's blood pressure before therapy and reassess regularly thereafter. Measure blood pressure when drug levels are at peak (2 to 6 hours after dose) and at trough (just before dose) to verify adequate blood pressure control.
• Be alert for adverse reactions and drug interactions.
• Monitor patient's ECG.
• Monitor renal and hepatic function periodically. Also monitor potassium levels.
• Monitor patient's CBC with differential every 2 weeks for first 3 months of therapy and periodically thereafter. Other ACE inhibitors have been linked to agranulocytosis and neutropenia.
• Evaluate patient's and family's understanding of drug therapy.

Nursing diagnoses

• Risk for injury related to hypertension
• Decreased cardiac output related to drug-induced arrhythmias
• Deficient knowledge related to drug therapy

Planning and implementation

• If patient is taking a diuretic, dose should be lower than if patient isn't taking a diuretic; excessive hypotension can occur when drug is given with diuretics.
• Dosage adjustment may be necessary in patients with renal impairment.
• Give drug at about the same time every day to maintain consistent effect on blood pressure.
• Give drug when patient's stomach is empty.

Patient teaching

• Instruct patient to take drug on an empty stomach; meals, particularly those high in fat, can impair absorption.
• Tell patient to avoid sodium substitutes; such products may contain potassium, which can cause hyperkalemia in patients taking drug.
• Tell patient to rise slowly to minimize risk of dizziness, which may occur during first few weeks of therapy. Advise patient to stop taking drug and call prescriber immediately if dizziness occurs.
• Tell patient to use caution in hot weather and during exercise. Inadequate fluid intake, vomiting, diarrhea, and excessive perspiration can lead to light-headedness and syncope.
• Urge patient to report signs of infection, such as fever and sore throat. Also tell him to call prescriber if the following signs or symptoms occur: easy bruising or bleeding; swelling of tongue, lips, face, eyes, mucous membranes, or limbs; difficulty swallowing or breathing; and hoarseness.
• Tell women to notify prescriber if pregnancy occurs. Drug will need to be stopped.

Evaluation

• Patient's blood pressure is normal.
• Patient maintains adequate cardiac output during drug therapy.
• Patient and family state understanding of drug therapy.

benztropine mesylate

(BENZ-troh-peen MES-ih-layt)
Apo-Benztropine ♦, Cogentin

Pharmacologic class: anticholinergic
Therapeutic class: antiparkinsonian
Pregnancy risk category: C

Reactions may be *common*, uncommon, *life-threatening*, or **COMMON AND LIFE-THREATENING.**

Indications and dosages

▶ **Drug-induced extrapyramidal disorders (except tardive dyskinesia).** *Adults:* 1 to 4 mg P.O. or I.M. once or twice daily.
▶ **Acute dystonic reaction.** *Adults:* 1 to 2 mg I.V. or I.M., followed by 1 to 2 mg P.O. b.i.d. to prevent recurrence.
▶ **Parkinsonism.** *Adults:* 0.5 to 6 mg P.O. daily. Initial dose is 0.5 to 1 mg. I.M. or P.O. Because of cumulative action, initiate at a low dose and increase by 0.5 mg q 5 to 6 days. Adjust dosage to meet individual requirements. Maximum daily dose is 6 mg.

▼ I.V. administration

• Drug is seldom used I.V. because of small difference in onset compared with I.M. route.

Contraindications and precautions

• Contraindicated in patients hypersensitive to drug or its components and those with acute angle-closure glaucoma.
• Use cautiously in patients exposed to hot weather, those with mental disorders, and those with Alzheimer's disease.
⚹ Lifespan: In pregnant women, use cautiously. In breast-feeding women and children younger than age 3, drug is contraindicated. In children age 3 and older and patients older than age 60, use cautiously.

Adverse reactions

CNS: disorientation, restlessness, irritability, incoherence, hallucinations, headache, sedation, depression, nervousness, confusion.
CV: palpitations, tachycardia, *paradoxical bradycardia,* flushing.
EENT: dilated pupils, blurred vision, photophobia, difficulty swallowing.
GI: dry mouth, *constipation,* nausea, vomiting, epigastric distress.
GU: urinary hesitancy, urine retention.
Musculoskeletal: muscle weakness.

Interactions

Drug-drug. *Amantadine, phenothiazines, tricyclic antidepressants:* May cause additive anticholinergic adverse reactions, such as hyperthermia or heat intolerance. Notify prescriber immediately if adverse GI effects, fever, or heat intolerance occurs.

Anticholinergics and other antiparkinsonians: May increase anticholinergic effects and may be fatal. Use cautiously.
Cholinesterase inhibitors: May decrease efficacy of cholinesterase inhibitors.

Effects on lab test results

None reported.

Pharmacokinetics

Absorption: Unknown.
Distribution: Largely unknown; however, drug crosses blood-brain barrier.
Metabolism: Unknown.
Excretion: Excreted in urine as unchanged drug and metabolites. After P.O. therapy, small amounts may be excreted in feces as unabsorbed drug.

Route	Onset	Peak	Duration
P.O.	1-2 hr	Unknown	24 hr
I.V., I.M.	≤ 15 min	Unknown	24 hr

Action

Chemical effect: Unknown; thought to block central cholinergic receptors, helping to balance cholinergic activity in basal ganglia.
Therapeutic effect: Improves capability for voluntary movement.

Available forms

Injection: 1 mg/ml in 2-ml ampules
Tablets: 0.5 mg, 1 mg, 2 mg

NURSING PROCESS

Assessment
• Obtain history of patient's dyskinetic movements and underlying condition before therapy.
• Monitor effectiveness by regularly checking body movements for signs of improvement; full effect of drug may take 2 to 3 days.
• Be alert for adverse reactions and drug interactions. Some adverse reactions may result from atropine-like toxicity and are dose-related.
• Evaluate patient's and family's understanding of drug therapy.

Nursing diagnoses
• Impaired physical mobility related to dyskinetic movements

• Risk for injury related to drug-induced adverse CNS reactions
• Deficient knowledge related to drug therapy

≽ Planning and implementation
• Give drug after meals to help prevent GI distress.
• The I.M. route is preferred for parenteral administration.
• Give drug h.s. if patient is to receive single daily dose.
⊛ **ALERT:** Never stop drug abruptly; reduce dose gradually.

Patient teaching
• Warn patient to avoid activities requiring alertness until CNS effects of drug are known.
• If patient is to receive single daily dose, tell him to take it h.s.
• If patient is to receive drug orally, tell him to take it after meals.
• Advise patient to report signs of urinary hesitancy or urine retention.
• Tell patient to relieve dry mouth with cool drinks, ice chips, sugarless gum, or hard candy.
• Advise patient to limit activities during hot weather because drug-induced anhidrosis may result in hyperthermia.

☑ Evaluation
• Patient exhibits improved mobility with reduction in muscle rigidity, akinesia, and tremors.
• Patient doesn't experience injury as a result of drug-induced adverse CNS reactions.
• Patient and family state understanding of drug therapy.

---

beractant (natural lung surfactant)
(beh-RAK-tant)
Survanta

Pharmacologic class: bovine lung extract
Therapeutic class: lung surfactant
Pregnancy risk category: NR

Indications and dosages

▶ **Prevention and rescue treatment of respiratory distress syndrome (RDS) or hyaline membrane disease in premature neonates weighing 1,250 g (2.75 lb) or less at birth or having symptoms of surfactant deficiency.**

Neonates: 4 ml/kg given by intratracheal instillation through a #5 French end-hole catheter inserted into the neonate's endotracheal tube with the tip of the catheter protruding just beyond the end of the tube above the carina. Length of catheter should be shortened before inserting it through the tube. Don't instill into a mainstem bronchus. Give up to four doses in the first 48 hours of life, but no more frequently than q 6 hours. Use the following dosing table.

BERACTANT DOSING TABLE

Weight (g)	Total dose (ml)
600-650	2.6
651-700	2.8
701-750	3
751-800	3.2
801-850	3.4
851-900	3.6
901-950	3.8
951-1,000	4
1,001-1,050	4.2
1,051-1,100	4.4
1,101-1,150	4.6
1,151-1,200	4.8
1,201-1,250	5
1,251-1,300	5.2
1,301-1,350	5.4
1,351-1,400	5.6
1,401-1,450	5.8
1,451-1,500	6
1,501-1,550	6.2
1,551-1,600	6.4
1,601-1,650	6.6
1,651-1,700	6.8
1,701-1,750	7
1,751-1,800	7.2
1,801-1,850	7.4
1,851-1,900	7.6
1,901-1,950	7.8
1,951-2,000	8

Contraindications and precautions

❋ **Lifespan:** For use in premature neonates only.

Adverse reactions

CV: *bradycardia,* vasoconstriction, hypotension.
Respiratory: *endotracheal tube reflux or blockage, apnea,* decreased oxygen saturation, hypocapnia, hypercapnia.
Other: pallor.

Interactions

None significant.

Effects on lab test results

● May decrease oxygen saturation levels. May increase or decrease carbon dioxide levels.

Pharmacokinetics

Absorption: Most of dose becomes lung-associated within hours.
Distribution: Across alveolar surface.
Metabolism: Lipids enter endogenous surfactant pathway of recycling and reutilization.
Excretion: Alveolar clearance of lipid components is rapid.

Route	Onset	Peak	Duration
Intratracheal	½-2 hr	Unknown	2-3 days

Action

Chemical effect: Lowers surface tension of alveoli during respiration and stabilizes alveoli against collapse. An extract of bovine lung containing neutral lipids, fatty acids, surfactant-associated proteins, and phospholipids that mimics naturally occurring surfactant; palmitic acid, tripalmitin, and colfosceril palmitate are added to standardize solution's composition.
Therapeutic effect: Prevents RDS in premature neonates with specific characteristics.

Available forms

Suspension for intratracheal instillation: 25 mg/ml

NURSING PROCESS

Assessment

● Obtain history of neonate's respiratory status before therapy.
● Continuously monitor neonate before, during, and after beractant administration for effectiveness.
● Continuously monitor ECG and transcutaneous oxygen saturation; also, frequently monitor arterial blood pressure and sample arterial blood gas. Transient bradycardia and oxygen desaturation are common after dosing.
● Evaluate parents' understanding of drug therapy.

Nursing diagnoses

● Risk for injury related to potential for RDS
● Deficient knowledge related to drug therapy

Planning and implementation

ALERT: Beractant should be given only by personnel experienced in care of clinically unstable premature neonates. Such personnel should have knowledge of neonatal intubation and airway management.
● Accurate determination of weight is essential to ensure proper measurement of dose.
● Endotracheal tube may be suctioned before giving drug.
● Allow neonate to stabilize before proceeding with administration; however, it's preferable to give drug within 15 minutes of birth to prevent RDS.
● Refrigerate drug at 36° to 46° F (2° to 8° C). Warm before giving by allowing drug to stand at room temperature for at least 20 minutes or by holding in hand for at least 8 minutes. Don't use artificial warming methods. Unopened vials that have been warmed to room temperature may be returned to refrigerator within 8 hours; warm and return drug to refrigerator only once. Vials are for single use only; discard unused drug once vial has been opened.
● Beractant doesn't need sonication or reconstitution before use. Inspect contents before giving; ensure that color is off-white to light brown and that contents are uniform. If settling occurs, swirl vial gently; don't shake. Some foaming is normal.
● Homogeneous distribution of drug is important. In clinical trials, each dose of drug was given in four quarter-doses, with patient positioned differently after each administration. Each quarter-dose was given over 2 to 3 seconds; the catheter was removed and patient ventilated between quarter-doses. With head and body inclined slightly downward, first quarter-dose was given with head turned to right; second quarter-dose with head turned to left. Then head and body were inclined slightly upward; third quarter-dose was given with head turned to

right; fourth quarter-dose with head turned to left.

- Moist breath sounds and crackles can occur immediately after administration. Don't suction neonate for 1 hour unless other signs of airway obstruction are evident.
- Transient episodes of bradycardia and decreased oxygen saturation have occurred. Monitor patient carefully.
- Audiovisual materials that describe dose and administration procedures are available from manufacturer.
- Beractant can rapidly affect oxygenation and lung compliance. Peak ventilator inspiratory pressures may need to be adjusted if chest expansion improves substantially with therapy. Notify prescriber and adjust immediately, as directed, because lung overdistention and fatal pulmonary air leakage may result.
- For active rescue treatment, give first dose within 8 hours of birth.

Patient teaching

- Teach parents about beractant therapy.
- Reassure parents that neonate will be monitored at all times.

☑ **Evaluation**

- Patient doesn't develop RDS.
- Parents state understanding of drug therapy.

---

17 beta-estradiol and norgestimate

(17 bay-ta-eh-stray-DYE-ol nor-JES-ti-mate)
Ortho-Prefest

Pharmacologic class: combined synthetic estrogen and progestin
Therapeutic class: hormone replacement
Pregnancy risk category: X

Indications and dosages

▶ **Moderate-to-severe vasomotor symptoms and vulvar and vaginal atrophy caused by menopause; prevention of osteoporosis in women with an intact uterus.** *Women:* 1 mg estradiol (pink tablet) P.O. daily for 3 days; then 1 mg estradiol/0.09 mg norgestimate (white tablet) P.O. daily for 3 days. Repeat cycle until blister card is empty.

Contraindications and precautions

- Contraindicated in patients hypersensitive to any component of Ortho-Prefest and in patients with cancer of the breast, estrogen-dependent neoplasia, undiagnosed abnormal vaginal bleeding, or active or previous thrombophlebitis or thromboembolic disorders. Hormone replacement therapy is contraindicated for cardiac disease prevention.
- Use cautiously in women who have had a hysterectomy, are overweight, or have abnormal lipid profiles, gallbladder disease, or impaired liver function.

⚠ **Lifespan:** In women who are or may be pregnant, drug is contraindicated.

Adverse reactions

CNS: depression, dizziness, fatigue, pain, *headache.*
CV: edema.
EENT: pharyngitis, sinusitis.
GI: flatulence, nausea, *abdominal pain, weight gain.*
GU: dysmenorrhea, vaginal bleeding, vaginitis, decreased libido.
Musculoskeletal: arthralgia, myalgia, *back pain.*
Respiratory: cough, *upper respiratory tract infection.*
Other: *flulike symptoms,* viral infection, *breast pain,* tooth disorder.

Interactions

None reported.

Effects on lab test results

- May increase thyroid-binding globulin; factors II, VII antigen, VIII antigen, VIII coagulant activity, IX, X, XII, VII-X complex, and II-VII-X complex; beta-thromboglobulin; HDL, triglyceride, corticosteroid, sex steroid, angiotensin and renin substrate, alpha$_1$-antitrypsin, ceruloplasmin, fibrinogen, and plasminogen antigen levels. May decrease folate, metyrapone, LDL, anti-factor Xa, and antithrombin III levels.
- May increase PT, PTT, platelet aggregation time, and platelet count. May decrease T$_3$ resin uptake and glucose tolerance.

Pharmacokinetics

Absorption: Estradiol reaches peak levels about 7 hours after a dose. The metabolite of norgesti-

---

Reactions may be *common,* uncommon, *life-threatening,* or COMMON AND LIFE-THREATENING.

mate, 17-deacetylnorgestimate, reaches peak levels about 2 hours after a dose. When given with a high-fat meal, peak levels of estrone and estrone sulfate increase by 14% and 24% respectively; peak level of 17-deacetylnorgestimate decreases by 16%.

Distribution: Wide. Estradiol is bound mainly to sex hormone–binding globulin and to albumin. The primary active metabolite of norgestimate, 17-deacetylnorgestimate, is about 99% protein-bound.

Metabolism: Mainly metabolized in the liver. Estradiol is converted reversibly to estrone, and both can be converted to estriol, which is the major urinary metabolite. Norgestimate is extensively metabolized by first-pass metabolism to 17-deacetylnorgestimate in the GI tract or liver.

Excretion: Estradiol, estrone, and estriol are excreted in the urine. Norgestimate metabolites are eliminated in the urine or feces. *Half-life:* About 16 hours for estradiol and 37 hours for 17-deacetylnorgestimate in postmenopausal women.

Route	Onset	Peak	Duration
P.O.	Unknown	7 hr (estradiol), 2 hr (norgestimate)	Unknown

Action

Chemical effect: Estradiol mimics the action of endogenous estrogen and natural progesterone. Circulating estrogens modulate pituitary secretion of gonadotropins, luteinizing hormone, and follicle-stimulating hormone. Estrogen replacement therapy reduces elevated levels of these hormones in postmenopausal women. Estrogens also contribute to the reduction of the rate of bone turnover.

Norgestimate mimics the natural hormone progesterone. Progestins counter estrogenic effects by decreasing the number of nuclear estradiol receptors and suppressing epithelial DNA synthesis in endometrial tissue.

Therapeutic effect: Relieves menopausal vasomotor symptoms and vaginal dryness; reduces the severity of osteoporosis.

Available forms

Tablets: Blister card of 15 pink and 15 white tablets. Pink tablets are 1 mg estradiol; white tablets are 1 mg estradiol and 0.09 mg norgestimate.

NURSING PROCESS

🔍 Assessment

• Obtain history of patient's underlying condition before therapy and reassess regularly thereafter.
• Make sure patient has a thorough physical examination before starting drug therapy.
• Assess patient's risks for venous thromboembolism.
• Assess patient's risk for cancer; hormone replacement therapy may increase the risk of breast cancer in postmenopausal women.
• Be alert for adverse reactions.
• Evaluate patient's and family's knowledge of drug therapy.

🔧 Nursing diagnoses

• Ineffective peripheral tissue perfusion related to drug-induced thromboembolism
• Ineffective health maintenance related to underlying condition
• Deficient knowledge related to drug therapy

▶ Planning and implementation

• Reassess patient at 6-month intervals to make sure treatment is still needed.
• Monitor patient for hypercalcemia if she has breast cancer and bone metastases. If severe hypercalcemia occurs, notify the prescriber and stop the drug; take the appropriate measures to reduce calcium level.

Patient teaching

• Explain the risks of taking estrogen therapy, including breast cancer, cancer of the uterus, abnormal blood clotting, gallbladder disease, heart disease, and CVA.
• Tell patient to immediately report any undiagnosed, persistent, or recurring abnormal vaginal bleeding.
• Instruct women to perform monthly breast examinations. Also, recommend a mammogram if patient is older than age 50.
• Tell patient to immediately report pain in the calves or chest, sudden shortness of breath, coughing blood, severe headache, vomiting, dizziness, faintness, changes in vision or speech, and weakness or numbness in arms or legs. These are warning signals of blood clots.
• Urge patient to report evidence of liver problems, such as yellowing of skin or eyes and upper right quadrant pain.

• Instruct patient to report pain, swelling, or tenderness in abdomen, which may indicate gallbladder problems.

• Tell patient to store drug at room temperature away from excessive heat and moisture. It remains stable for 18 months.

☑ **Evaluation**

• Patient has no thromboembolic event during therapy.

• Patient's underlying condition improves.

• Patient and family state understanding of drug therapy.

betamethasone
(bay-tuh-METH-uh-sohn)
Betnesol ◆ , Celestone*

betamethasone acetate and betamethasone sodium phosphate
Celestone Chronodose ◇ , Celestone Soluspan

betamethasone sodium phosphate
Celestone Phosphate, Selestoject

Pharmacologic class: glucocorticoid
Therapeutic class: anti-inflammatory
Pregnancy risk category: NR

Indications and dosages

▶ **Conditions of severe inflammation or that need immunosuppression.** *Adults:* 0.6 to 7.2 mg betamethasone P.O. daily. Or, 0.25 to 2 ml betamethasone sodium phosphate-acetate suspension injected into joint or soft tissue q 1 to 2 weeks, p.r.n. Or, 0.5 to 9 mg betamethasone sodium phosphate I.V., I.M., or injected into joint or soft tissue daily.
Children: 0.0175 to 0.25 mg/kg betamethasone P.O. daily.

▶ **Hyaline membrane disease‡.** *Pregnant women:* Give 2 ml I.M. daily for 2 to 3 days before delivery.

▼ I.V. administration

• Drug is compatible with normal saline solution, D₅W, lactated Ringer's injection, dextrose 5% in lactated Ringer's injection, and dextrose 5% in Ringer's injection. Suspension for injection isn't for I.V. use.

Contraindications and precautions

• Contraindicated in patients hypersensitive to drug and in those with viral or bacterial infections (except in life-threatening situations) or systemic fungal infections.

• Use cautiously and only in life-threatening situations in patients with recent MI or peptic ulcer.

• Use cautiously in patients with renal disease, hypertension, osteoporosis, diabetes mellitus, hypothyroidism, cirrhosis, diverticulitis, nonspecific ulcerative colitis, recent intestinal anastomoses, thromboembolic disorders, seizures, myasthenia gravis, heart failure, tuberculosis, ocular herpes simplex, emotional instability, or psychotic tendencies. Because some formulations contain sulfite preservatives, use cautiously in patients sensitive to sulfites.

⚖ **Lifespan:** In pregnant women, use cautiously. Breast-feeding women should stop breast-feeding if taking drug. In children younger than age 12, safety of drug hasn't been established.

Adverse reactions

CNS: *euphoria, insomnia,* psychotic behavior, pseudotumor cerebri, *seizures.*
CV: *heart failure,* hypertension, edema, *thromboembolism.*
EENT: cataracts, glaucoma.
GI: *peptic ulceration,* GI irritation, increased appetite, *pancreatitis.*
Metabolic: hypokalemia, hyperglycemia, carbohydrate intolerance.
Musculoskeletal: muscle weakness, osteoporosis (long-term use), growth suppression in children.
Skin: hirsutism, delayed wound healing, acne, various skin eruptions.
Other: susceptibility to infections, *acute adrenal insufficiency* after stress (infection, surgery, or trauma) or abrupt withdrawal after long-term therapy.

Interactions

Drug-drug. *Aspirin, indomethacin, other NSAIDs:* May increase risk of GI distress and bleeding. Give together cautiously.
Barbiturates, phenytoin, rifampin: Decreases corticosteroid effect. Corticosteroid dosage may need to be increased.

Oral anticoagulants: Alters dosage requirements. Monitor PT and INR closely.
Potassium-depleting drugs (such as thiazide diuretics): Enhances potassium-depleting effects of betamethasone. Monitor potassium levels.
Skin test antigens: Decreases response. Defer skin testing until therapy is completed.
Toxoids, vaccines: Decreases antibody response and increases risk of neurologic complications. Avoid using together. Delay vaccines, if possible.

Effects on lab test results

• May increase glucose and cholesterol levels. May decrease potassium and calcium levels.

Pharmacokinetics

Absorption: Absorbed readily after P.O. administration. Systemic absorption occurs slowly after intra-articular injections.
Distribution: Removed rapidly from blood and distributed to muscle, liver, skin, intestines, and kidneys. Bound weakly to protein. Only unbound portion is active.
Metabolism: Metabolized in liver to inactive glucuronide and sulfate metabolites.
Excretion: Inactive metabolites and small amounts of drug are excreted in urine. Insignificant quantities of drug are also excreted in feces. *Half-life:* 36 to 54 hours.

Route	Onset	Peak	Duration
P.O.	Unknown	1-2 hr	3¼ days
I.V., I.M., intra-articular	Rapid	Unknown	7-14 days

Action

Chemical effect: Not completely defined. Decreases inflammation, mainly by stabilizing leukocyte lysosomal membranes; suppresses immune response; stimulates bone marrow; and influences protein, fat, and carbohydrate metabolism.
Therapeutic effect: Causes immunosuppression.

Available forms

betamethasone
Syrup: 600 mcg/5 ml
Tablets: 600 mcg
Tablets (effervescent): 500 mcg

betamethasone acetate and betamethasone sodium phosphate
Injection (suspension): betamethasone acetate 3 mg and betamethasone sodium phosphate (equivalent to 3-mg base) per ml
betamethasone sodium phosphate
Injection: 4 mg (equivalent to 3-mg base)/ml in 5-ml vials

NURSING PROCESS

⚕ Assessment

• Obtain history of patient's underlying condition and current health status, including vital signs and weight.
• Be alert for adverse reactions and drug interactions. Most adverse reactions are dose- or duration-dependent.
• Monitor patient's weight, blood pressure, and glucose and potassium levels regularly.
• Monitor patient for early signs of adrenal insufficiency or cushingoid symptoms. Adrenal suppression may last up to 1 year after drug is stopped.
• Monitor patient's stress level. Stress (fever, trauma, surgery, or emotional problems) may increase adrenal insufficiency.
• Evaluate patient's and family's understanding of drug therapy.

Nursing diagnoses

• Ineffective health maintenance related to underlying condition
• Risk for injury related to drug-induced adverse reactions
• Deficient knowledge related to drug therapy

➤ Planning and implementation

• Give drug with milk or food to reduce GI irritation.
• Give I.M. injection deeply to prevent muscle atrophy. Rotate injection sites.
• Prepare drug for prescriber to give by intra-articular route.
• Don't use for alternate-day therapy.
• Give once-daily dose in the morning for best results and least toxicity.
• Adjust to lowest effective dose.
• **ⓧ ALERT:** Gradually reduce drug dosage after long-term therapy. After abrupt withdrawal, patient may experience rebound inflammation, fatigue, weakness, arthralgia, fever, dizziness, lethargy, depression, fainting, orthostatic hypo-

tension, dyspnea, anorexia, and hypoglycemia. After prolonged use, sudden withdrawal may be fatal.

• Expect to increase dose during times of physiologic stress (surgery, trauma, or infection).

• Potassium supplements may be necessary for patients receiving long-term therapy.

Patient teaching

• Tell patient not to stop drug abruptly or without prescriber's consent.

• Tell patient using effervescent tablets to dissolve them in water immediately before ingestion.

• Teach patient about drug's effects. Warn patient receiving long-term therapy about cushingoid symptoms; instruct him to report sudden weight gain or swelling to prescriber.

• Instruct patient to report symptoms of corticosteroid withdrawal, including fatigue, weakness, arthralgia, orthostatic hypotension, and dyspnea.

• Tell patient to contact prescriber if symptoms worsen or drug is no longer effective. Also tell him not to increase dose without prescriber's consent.

• Advise elderly patient receiving long-term therapy to consider exercise or physical therapy. Tell him to ask prescriber about vitamin D or calcium supplements.

• Advise patient receiving prolonged therapy to have periodic ophthalmic examinations.

• Tell patient to report slow healing.

• Instruct patient to wear or carry medical identification indicating his need for supplemental corticosteroids during stress.

☑ **Evaluation**

• Patient's underlying condition improves.

• Patient doesn't experience injury as a result of drug-induced adverse reactions.

• Patient and family state understanding of drug therapy.

---

bethanechol chloride
(beh-THAN-eh-kol KLOR-ighd)
Duvoid

Pharmacologic class: cholinergic agonist
Therapeutic class: urinary tract stimulant
Pregnancy risk category: C

Indications and dosages

▶ **Acute postoperative and postpartum nonobstructive (functional) urinary retention, neurogenic atony of urinary bladder with urinary retention.** *Adults:* 10 to 50 mg P.O. b.i.d. to q.i.d. When used for urine retention, some patients may need 50 to 100 mg P.O. per dose. Use such doses with extreme caution. Or, 2.575 mg S.C. initially, followed by repeat dose q 15 to 30 minutes up to a maximum of 4 doses to determine minimal effective dose. Then, use minimal effective dose q 6 to 8 hours. All doses must be adjusted individually.

▶ **To restore bladder function in patients with chronic neurogenic bladder.** *Adults:* 7.5 to 10 mg S.C. q 4 hours around-the-clock. Dosage adjustments are based on residual urine measurements.

▶ **Bladder dysfunction caused by phenothiazines‡.** *Adults:* 50 to 100 mg P.O. q.i.d.

▶ **To diagnose flaccid or atonic neurogenic bladder‡.** *Adults:* 2.5 mg. S.C. as a single dose.

Contraindications and precautions

• Contraindicated when increased muscle activity of GI or urinary tract is harmful. Also contraindicated in patients hypersensitive to drug or its components and in those with hyperthyroidism, peptic ulceration, latent or active bronchial asthma, pronounced bradycardia or hypotension, vasomotor instability, cardiac or coronary artery disease, seizure disorder, Parkinson's disease, spastic GI disturbances, acute inflammatory lesions of GI tract, peritonitis, mechanical obstruction of GI or urinary tract, marked vagotonia, or uncertain strength or integrity of bladder wall.

⚕ **Lifespan:** In pregnant women, use cautiously. Breast-feeding should be avoided. In children, safety of drug hasn't been established.

Adverse reactions

CNS: headache, malaise.
CV: *bradycardia,* hypotension, flushing, reflex tachycardia.
EENT: lacrimation, miosis.
GI: *abdominal cramps, diarrhea,* excessive salivation, nausea, vomiting, belching, borborygmi, esophageal spasms.
GU: urinary urgency.
Respiratory: *bronchoconstriction,* increased bronchial secretions.
Skin: sweating.

Interactions

Drug-drug. *Anticholinergics, atropine, procainamide, quinidine:* May reverse cholinergic effects. Watch for lack of drug effect.
Anticholinesterases, cholinergic agonists: May cause additive effects or increase toxicity. Avoid using together.
Ganglionic blockers: May cause severe abdominal pain followed by a critical drop in blood pressure. Avoid using together.

Effects on lab test results

• May increase liver enzyme, amylase, and lipase levels.

Pharmacokinetics

Absorption: Poor after P.O. administration; unknown after S.C. administration.
Distribution: Unknown.
Metabolism: Unknown.
Excretion: Unknown.

Route	Onset	Peak	Duration
P.O.	30-90 min	1 hr	1-6 hr
S.C.	5-15 min	5-30 min	2 hr

Action

Chemical effect: Directly stimulates cholinergic receptors, mimicking action of acetylcholine.
Therapeutic effect: Relieves urinary retention.

Available forms

Injection: 5.15 mg/ml
Tablets: 5 mg, 10 mg, 25 mg, 50 mg

NURSING PROCESS

✎ Assessment

• Obtain history of patient's bladder condition before therapy, and reassess regularly throughout therapy.
• Be alert for adverse reactions and drug interactions.
• Evaluate patient's and family's understanding of drug therapy.

✦ Nursing diagnoses

• Impaired urinary elimination related to underlying bladder condition
• Ineffective breathing pattern related to drug-induced bronchoconstriction
• Deficient knowledge related to drug therapy

▷ Planning and implementation

• Give P.O. drug on empty stomach to prevent nausea and vomiting.
• **⚡ ALERT:** Never give I.V. or I.M.
• **⚡ ALERT:** Always have atropine injection readily available and be prepared to give 0.5 mg S.C. or slow I.V. push. Provide respiratory support, p.r.n.
Patient teaching
• Advise patient to take oral dose on an empty stomach.
• Tell patient to report breathing difficulty immediately.

✓ Evaluation

• Patient is able to void without urine retention.
• Patient's respiratory function remains normal during therapy.
• Patient and family state understanding of drug therapy.

bexarotene

(bex-AHR-oh-teen)
Targretin

Pharmacologic class: retinoid (selective retinoid X receptor activator)
Therapeutic class: tumor cell growth inhibitor
Pregnancy risk category: X

Indications and dosages

▶ **Cutaneous effects of cutaneous T-cell lymphoma in patients refractory to at least one previous systemic therapy.** *Adults:* 300 mg/m² P.O. daily as a single dose with a meal. If no response after 8 weeks, increase to 400 mg/m² daily. Adjust dosage to 200 mg/m² daily, and then to 100 mg/m² daily if toxicity occurs, or drug may be temporarily suspended. When toxicity is controlled, dosage may be carefully readjusted upward. Or, for topical application, apply a sufficient amount of 1% gel and rub into the affected areas once q other day, for the first week. Allow gel to dry before applying a dressing. Then, increase at weekly intervals to b.i.d., t.i.d., and q.i.d., according to the individual skin response.
⊠ Adjust-a-dose: For patients with hepatic insufficiency, lower doses may be needed. If toxicity occurs, dosage may be adjusted to 200 mg/m² daily, then to 100 mg/m² daily, or

drug may be temporarily suspended. When toxicity is controlled, readjust upward carefully.

Contraindications and precautions

• Contraindicated in patients hypersensitive to drug or its components.

• Drug isn't recommended for patients taking drugs that increase triglyceride levels or cause pancreatic toxicity, or for those who have risk factors for pancreatitis, such as prior pancreatitis, uncontrolled hyperlipidemia, excessive alcohol consumption, uncontrolled diabetes mellitus, or biliary tract disease.

• Use cautiously in patients with hepatic insufficiency, and in patients hypersensitive to retinoids.

⚖ Lifespan: In pregnant women, drug is contraindicated. In women of childbearing potential, use cautiously.

Adverse reactions

CNS: fever, *headache,* insomnia, *asthenia,* fatigue, syncope, depression, agitation, ataxia, **CVA,** confusion, dizziness, hyperesthesia, hypoesthesia, neuropathy.

CV: *peripheral edema,* chest pain, *hemorrhage,* hypertension, angina, *heart failure,* tachycardia.

EENT: cataracts, pharyngitis, rhinitis, dry eyes, conjunctivitis, ear pain, blepharitis, corneal lesion, keratitis, otitis externa, visual field defect.

GI: *nausea,* diarrhea, vomiting, anorexia, *pancreatitis,* abdominal pain, constipation, dry mouth, flatulence, colitis, dyspepsia, cheilitis, gastroenteritis, gingivitis, melena.

GU: albuminuria, hematuria, incontinence, UTI, urinary urgency, dysuria, abnormal kidney function.

Hematologic: *leukopenia,* anemia, eosinophilia, thrombocythemia, lymphocytosis, *thrombocytopenia.*

Hepatic: bilirubinemia, *liver failure.*

Metabolic: *hyperlipemia, hypercholesteremia, hypothyroidism,* hyperglycemia, hypoproteinemia, hypocalcemia, hyponatremia, weight change.

Musculoskeletal: arthralgia, myalgia, back pain, bone pain, myasthenia, arthrosis.

Respiratory: pneumonia, dyspnea, hemoptysis, pleural effusion, bronchitis, cough, *lung edema, hypoxia.*

Skin: **(P.O.)** *rash, dry skin, exfoliative dermatitis, alopecia, photosensitivity,* pruritus, cellulitis, acne, skin ulcer, skin nodule; **(Topical)** *contact dermatitis, pain, skin disorders, pruritus, rash.*
Other: breast pain, *infection,* chills, flulike syndrome, *sepsis.*

Interactions

Drug-drug. *Diethyltoluamide (DEET):* May increase DEET toxicity with gel form. Avoid using together.

Erythromycin, gemfibrozil, itraconazole, ketoconazole, other inhibitors of CYP 3A4: May increase level of bexarotene. Avoid using together.

Insulin, sulfonylureas: May enhance hypoglycemic action of these drugs, resulting in hypoglycemia in patients with diabetes mellitus. Use together cautiously.

Phenobarbital, phenytoin, rifampin, other inducers of CYP 3A4: May decrease level of bexarotene. Avoid using together.

Vitamin A preparations: May increase potential for vitamin A toxicity. Avoid vitamin A supplements.

Drug-food. *Any food:* Enhances drug absorption. Give with food.

Grapefruit juice: May inhibit CYP 3A4. Don't give together.

Drug-lifestyle. *Sun exposure:* Retinoids may cause photosensitivity. Advise patient to minimize exposure to sunlight and artificial ultraviolet light.

Effects on lab test results

• May increase creatinine, LDH, AST, ALT, bilirubin, amylase, lipid, cholesterol, glucose, and thyroid-stimulating hormone (TSH) levels. May decrease protein, calcium, and sodium levels.

• May increase eosinophil count. May decrease hemoglobin, hematocrit, and WBC and lymphocyte counts. May alter platelet count.

• Bexarotene therapy may increase CA 125 assay values in patients with ovarian cancer.

Pharmacokinetics

Absorption: Increased if given with a meal that contains fat when given P.O. Unknown for topical use.

Distribution: More than 99% protein-bound. Low level with topical use.

Metabolism: Metabolized through oxidative pathways, primarily by the cytochrome P450 3A4 system, to four metabolites. These may maintain retinoid receptor activity.
Excretion: Thought to be eliminated primarily through the hepatobiliary system. *Terminal half-life:* 7 hours.

Route	Onset	Peak	Duration
P.O., topical	Unknown	Unknown	Unknown

Action

Chemical effect: Selectively binds and activates retinoid X receptor subtypes. Once activated, these receptors function as transcription factors that regulate the expression of genes that control cellular differentiation and proliferation. In vitro, bexarotene inhibits the growth of some tumor cell lines of hematopoietic and squamous cell origin; in vivo, it induces tumor cell regression in some animal models. The exact mechanism of action in the treatment of cutaneous T-cell lymphoma is unknown.
Therapeutic effect: Inhibits tumor growth in cutaneous T-cell lymphoma.

Available forms

Capsules: 75 mg
Topical gel: 1%

NURSING PROCESS

Assessment
• Assess women of childbearing potential carefully. A negative pregnancy test should be obtained within 1 week before therapy starts and monthly during therapy.
• Men with sexual partners who are pregnant, who could be pregnant, or who could become pregnant must use condoms during sexual intercourse during therapy and for at least 1 month after therapy ends.
• Obtain total cholesterol, HDL, and triglyceride levels when therapy starts, weekly until the lipid response is established (2 to 4 weeks) and at 8-week intervals thereafter. Elevated triglycerides during treatment should be treated with antilipemic therapy and the dose of bexarotene reduced or suspended, p.r.n.
• Obtain baseline thyroid function tests, and monitor results during treatment.

• Monitor WBC with differential at baseline and periodically during treatment.
• Monitor liver function test results at baseline and after 1, 2, and 4 weeks of treatment. If patient is stable, monitor test results every 8 weeks during treatment. The prescriber may consider suspending treatment if results are three times the upper limit of normal.
• Monitor TSH levels and patient for signs and symptoms of hypothyroidism.
• Obtain ophthalmologic evaluation for cataracts in patients who experience visual difficulties.
• Evaluate patient's and family's knowledge of drug therapy.

Nursing diagnoses
• Ineffective health maintenance related to underlying condition
• Risk for injury related to drug-induced adverse reactions
• Deficient knowledge related to drug therapy

Planning and implementation
• Lower doses may be needed for patients with hepatic insufficiency.
• Give drug with food for better absorption, although not with grapefruit or grapefruit juice.
• Start therapy on the second or third day of a normal menstrual period.
• No more than a 1-month supply of bexarotene should be given to a patient of childbearing potential so the results of pregnancy testing can be assessed regularly and the patient can be reminded to avoid pregnancy.
Patient teaching
• Advise patient to minimize unprotected or prolonged exposure to sunlight or artificial ultraviolet light.
• Teach patient that it may take several capsules to make the necessary dose and that these capsules should all be taken at the same time and with a meal.
• Teach women of childbearing potential the dangers of becoming pregnant while taking bexarotene and the need for monthly pregnancy tests.
• Explain the need for obtaining baseline laboratory tests and for periodic monitoring of these tests.
• Tell patient to report any visual changes.

- Advise patient to wait at least 20 minutes after bathing before applying the gel and to avoid the use of occlusive dressings.
- Tell patient to avoid gel contact with healthy skin or mucous membranes.
- Tell patient to allow the gel to dry for 5 to 10 minutes before covering area with clothing.
- Tell patient to use effective contraception at least 1 month before therapy starts, during therapy, and for at least 1 month after therapy stops. Tell patient to use two reliable forms of contraception simultaneously during therapy unless abstinence is the chosen method.

☑ Evaluation
- Patient exhibits positive response to therapy.
- Patient has no injury as a result of drug-induced adverse reactions.
- Patient and family state understanding of drug therapy.

bimatoprost
(by-MAT-oh-prost)
Lumigan

Pharmacologic class: prostaglandin analogue
Therapeutic class: antiglaucoma drug, ocular antihypertensive
Pregnancy risk category: C

Indications and dosages

▶ **To reduce elevated intraocular pressure (IOP) in patients with open-angle glaucoma or ocular hypertension who are intolerant of or unresponsive to other IOP-lowering drugs.** *Adults:* Instill 1 drop in the conjunctival sac of the affected eye or eyes once daily in the evening.

Contraindications and precautions

- Contraindicated in patients hypersensitive to bimatoprost, benzalkonium chloride, or other ingredients of this product. Also contraindicated in patients with angle-closure glaucoma, inflammatory glaucoma, or neovascular glaucoma.
- Use cautiously in patients with renal or hepatic impairment, active intraocular inflammation (iritis or uveitis), aphakic patients, pseudophakic patients with a torn posterior lens capsule, or patients at risk for macular edema.

🜲 **Lifespan:** In pregnant women, drug isn't recommended. In breast-feeding women, use cautiously because it's unknown whether drug appears in breast milk. In children, safety and efficacy of drug haven't been established.

Adverse reactions

CNS: headache, asthenia.
EENT: *conjunctival hyperemia, growth of eyelashes, ocular pruritus,* ocular dryness, visual disturbance, ocular burning, foreign body sensation, eye pain, pigmentation of the periocular skin, blepharitis, cataract, superficial punctate keratitis, eyelid erythema, ocular irritation, eyelash darkening, eye discharge, tearing, photophobia, allergic conjunctivitis, asthenopia, increased iris pigmentation, conjunctival edema, gradual change in eye color.
Respiratory: *upper respiratory tract infection.*
Skin: hirsutism.
Other: *infection.*

Interactions

None significant.

Effects on lab test results

- May cause abnormal liver function test values.

Pharmacokinetics

Absorption: Absorbed through the cornea.
Distribution: Moderately distributed into tissues. About 12% remains unbound.
Metabolism: Mainly metabolized by oxidation.
Excretion: Metabolites are 67% eliminated in urine; 25% are eliminated in feces.

Route	Onset	Peak	Duration
Ophthalmic	4 hr	10 min	1½ hr

Action

Chemical effect: Drug is a prostamide, which is a synthetic analogue of prostaglandin. It selectively mimics the effects of naturally occurring prostaglandins. Bimatoprost is believed to lower IOP by increasing the outflow of aqueous humor through the trabecular meshwork and uveoscleral routes.
Therapeutic effect: Reduces IOP.

Available forms

Ophthalmic solution: 0.03%

⚖ Assessment

⑤ **ALERT:** Perform complete medication history. If more than one ophthalmic drug is being used, give drugs at least 5 minutes apart.
• Assess patient's underlying condition and eyes before giving eyedrops.
• Monitor patient for excessive ocular irritation and evaluate the success of treatment.
• Evaluate patient's and family's knowledge of drug therapy and administration.

🗐 Nursing diagnoses

• Risk for injury to the eye related to improper administration of drug
• Impaired visual perception related to underlying condition
• Deficient knowledge related to bimatoprost therapy

▶ Planning and implementation

⑤ **ALERT:** Contact lenses must be removed before using solution. Lenses may be reinserted 15 minutes after administration.
• Don't touch the tip of the dropper to the eye. Avoid contamination to the dropper.
• Apply light pressure on lacrimal sac for 1 minute after instillation to minimize systemic absorption of the drug.
• Store drug in original container at 59° to 77° F (15° to 25°C).
• Be aware that an increase in pigmentation of the iris, eyelid, and eyelashes may occur, as well as growth of the eyelashes.

Patient teaching

• Explain to patients receiving treatment in only one eye the possibility for increased brown pigmentation of iris, eyelid skin darkening, and increased length, thickness, pigmentation, or number of lashes in the treated eye.
• Teach patient to instill drops properly and advise him to wash hands before and after instilling solution. Warn him not to touch tip of dropper to eye or surrounding tissue.
• If eye trauma or infection occurs or if eye surgery is needed, tell patient to seek immediate medical advice before continuing to use multidose container.
• Urge patient to immediately report conjunctivitis or lid reactions to prescriber.

☑ Evaluation

• Patient demonstrates proper administration of the drug, and no injury occurs.
• Patient's underlying eye condition responds positively to drug.
• Patient and family state understanding of drug therapy.

bisacodyl

(bigh-suh-KOH-dil)
Bisac-Evac†, Bisacodyl Uniserts†, Bisacolax ♦ †, Bisalax ◇ , Bisco-Lax†, Carter's Little Pills†, Correctol†, Dacodyl†, Deficol†, Dulcolax†, Durolax ◇ , Feen-a-Mint†, Fleet Bisacodyl†, Fleet Laxative†, Fleet Prep Kit†, Laxit ♦ †, Modane†, Theralax†

Pharmacologic class: diphenylmethane derivative
Therapeutic class: stimulant laxative
Pregnancy risk category: NR

Indications and dosages

▶ **Chronic constipation; preparation for childbirth, surgery, or rectal or bowel examination.** *Adults and children age 12 and older:* 10 to 15 mg P.O. in evening or before breakfast; maximum 30 mg P.O. For evacuation before examination or surgery, 10 mg P.R.
Children ages 6 to 11: 5 mg P.O. or P.R. h.s. or before breakfast.

Contraindications and precautions

• Contraindicated in patients hypersensitive to drug and in those with rectal bleeding, gastroenteritis, intestinal obstruction, or symptoms of appendicitis or acute surgical abdomen, such as abdominal pain, nausea, or vomiting.
⚠ Lifespan: In pregnant women, use cautiously.

Adverse reactions

CNS: tetany.
GI: *nausea, vomiting, abdominal cramps,* diarrhea (with high doses), *burning sensation in rectum* (with suppositories), protein-losing enteropathy (with excessive use), laxative dependence (with long-term or excessive use).
Metabolic: *alkalosis,* hypokalemia, fluid and electrolyte imbalance.

Musculoskeletal: muscle weakness (with excessive use).

Interactions

Drug-drug. *Antacids:* May cause gastric irritation or dyspepsia from premature dissolution of enteric coating. Avoid using together.
Drug-food. *Milk:* May cause gastric irritation or dyspepsia from premature dissolution of enteric coating. Avoid using together.

Effects on lab test results

• May increase phosphate and sodium levels. May decrease calcium, magnesium, and potassium levels.

Pharmacokinetics

Absorption: Minimal.
Distribution: Distributed locally.
Metabolism: Up to 15% of P.O. dose may enter enterohepatic circulation.
Excretion: Excreted primarily in feces; some excreted in urine.

Route	Onset	Peak	Duration
P.O.	6-12 hr	Variable	Variable
P.R.	15-60 min	Variable	Variable

Action

Chemical effect: Increases peristalsis, probably by acting directly on smooth muscle of intestine. Thought to irritate musculature or stimulate colonic intramural plexus. Also promotes fluid accumulation in colon and small intestine.
Therapeutic effect: Relieves constipation.

Available forms

Enema: 0.33 mg/dl†, 10 mg/5 ml (microenema) ◊, 10 mg/30 ml
Powder for rectal solution (bisacodyl tannex): 1.5 mg bisacodyl and 2.5 g tannic acid
Suppositories: 10 mg†
Tablets (enteric-coated): 5 mg†

NURSING PROCESS

Assessment

• Obtain history of bowel disorder, GI status, fluid intake, nutritional status, exercise habits, and normal patterns of elimination.
• Monitor effectiveness by checking frequency and characteristics of stools.

• Be alert for adverse reactions and drug interactions.
• Auscultate bowel sounds at least once per shift. Check for pain and cramping.
• Evaluate patient's and family's understanding of drug therapy.

Nursing diagnoses

• Constipation related to interruption of normal pattern of elimination
• Acute pain related to drug-induced abdominal cramps
• Deficient knowledge related to drug therapy

Planning and implementation

• Don't give tablets within 60 minutes of milk or antacid.
• Insert suppository as high as possible into rectum, and try to position suppository against rectal wall. Avoid embedding within fecal material because this may delay onset of action.
• Time administration of drug so as not to interfere with scheduled activities or sleep. Soft, formed stool usually is produced 15 to 60 minutes after P.R. administration.
• Tablets and suppositories are used together to clean colon before and after surgery and before barium enema.
• Store tablets and suppositories below 86° F (30° C).
Patient teaching
• Advise patient to swallow enteric-coated tablet whole to avoid GI irritation. Tell him not to take tablet within 1 hour of milk or antacid.
• Advise patient to report adverse effects to prescriber.
• Teach patient about dietary sources of fiber, including bran and other cereals, fresh fruit, and vegetables.
• Warn patient against excessive use of drug.

Evaluation

• Patient reports return of normal bowel pattern of elimination.
• Patient is free from abdominal pain and cramping.
• Patient and family state understanding of drug therapy.

---

bismuth subgallate

(BIS-muth sub-GAL-ayt)
Devrom

bismuth subsalicylate

Children's Kaopectate†, Extra Strength
Kaopectate†, Kaopectate (Regular)†,
Maximum Strength Pepto-Bismol†,
Pepto-Bismol†

Pharmacologic class: adsorbent
Therapeutic class: antidiarrheal
Pregnancy risk category: NR

Indications and dosages

▶ **To control fecal odors in colostomy,
ileostomy, or incontinence.** *Adults:*1 to
2 tablets subgallate P.O. t.i.d. with meals. Tablet
can be chewed or swallowed whole.
▶ **Mild, nonspecific diarrhea.** *Adults and children age 12 and older:* 30 ml or 2 tablets subsalicylate P.O. q 30 minutes to 1 hour up to a
maximum of 8 doses in 24 hours and for no
longer than 2 days.
Children ages 3 to 5: 5 ml or ½ tablet subsalicylate P.O. q 30 minutes to 1 hour up to a maximum of 8 doses in 24 hours and for no longer
than 2 days.
Children ages 6 to 8: 10 ml or ⅔ tablet subsalicylate P.O. q 30 minutes to 1 hour up to a maximum of 8 doses in 24 hours and for no longer
than 2 days.
Children ages 9 to 11: 15 ml or 1 tablet subsalicylate P.O. q 30 minutes to 1 hour up to a maximum of 8 doses in 24 hours and for no longer
than 2 days.

Contraindications and precautions

• Contraindicated in patients hypersensitive to
salicylates.
• Use cautiously in patients already taking aspirin.
⚹ Lifespan: In pregnant or breast-feeding
women, use cautiously.

Adverse reactions

GI: temporary darkening of tongue and stools.
Other: salicylism (with high doses).

Interactions

Drug-drug. *Aspirin, other salicylates:* May increase risk of salicylate toxicity. Monitor patient
closely.
Oral anticoagulants, oral antidiabetics: Theoretical risk of increased effects of these drugs
after high doses of bismuth subsalicylate. Monitor patient closely.
Probenecid: May be risk of decreased uricosuric effects after high doses of bismuth subsalicylate. Monitor patient closely.
Tetracycline: Decreases tetracycline absorption.
Give drugs at least 2 hours apart.

Effects on lab test results

• May increase lipid levels.

Pharmacokinetics

Absorption: Poor; significant salicylate absorption may occur after using bismuth subsalicylate.
Distribution: Distributed locally in gut.
Metabolism: Metabolized minimally.
Excretion: Bismuth subsalicylate is excreted in
urine.

Route	Onset	Peak	Duration
P.O.	1 hr	Unknown	Unknown

Action

Chemical effect: Unknown; has mild water-binding capacity. Also may adsorb toxins and
provide protective coating for mucosa.
Therapeutic effect: Relieves diarrhea.

Available forms

bismuth subgallate
Tablets (chewable): 200 mg†
bismuth subsalicylate
Caplet: 262 mg
Liquid (Children's): 87 mg/5 ml
Liquid (Extra Strength): 175 mg/5 ml
Liquid (Regular): 87.3 mg/ml
Oral suspension: 130 mg/15 ml, 262.5 mg/
15 ml†, 525 mg/15 ml†
Tablets (chewable): 262.5 mg†

NURSING PROCESS

📑 **Assessment**
• Obtain history of patient's bowel disorder, GI
status, and frequency of loose stools before therapy.

• Monitor drug's effectiveness by checking frequency and characteristics of stools.
• Be alert for adverse reactions and drug interactions.
• Check patient's hearing if he takes drug in large doses.
• Evaluate patient's and family's understanding of drug therapy.

Nursing diagnoses
• Diarrhea related to underlying GI condition
• Disturbed sensory perception (auditory) related to drug-induced salicylism
• Deficient knowledge related to drug therapy

Planning and implementation
• Avoid use before GI radiologic procedures because bismuth is radiopaque and may interfere with X-rays.
• Read label carefully because dosage varies with form of drug.
• If tinnitus occurs, stop drug and notify prescriber.
Patient teaching
• Advise patient that drug contains large amount of salicylate. Each tablet contains 102 mg; regular-strength liquid contains 130 mg/15 ml, and extra-strength liquid contains 230 mg/15 ml.
• Instruct patient to chew tablets well or to shake liquid before measuring dose.
• Tell patient to report diarrhea that persists for longer than 2 days or is accompanied by high fever.
• Tell patient to consult with prescriber before giving bismuth subsalicylate to children or teenagers who have or are recovering from flu or chickenpox.
• Inform patient that both liquid and tablet forms of Pepto-Bismol are effective against traveler's diarrhea. Tablets may be more convenient to carry.
• Tell patient that any darkening of stool or the tongue is temporary.

☑ Evaluation
• Patient reports decrease or absence of loose stools.
• Patient remains free from signs and symptoms of salicylism.
• Patient and family state understanding of drug therapy.

bisoprolol fumarate
(bis-OP-roh-lol FYOO-muh-rayt)
Zebeta

Pharmacologic class: beta blocker
Therapeutic class: antihypertensive
Pregnancy risk category: C

Indications and dosages
▶ **Hypertension.** *Adults:* Initially, 5 mg P.O. once daily. If response is inadequate, increase to 10 mg or 20 mg P.O. daily; 20 mg is maximum recommended dosage.
Adjust-a-dose: For patients with renal impairment or a creatinine clearance of less than 40 ml/minute or hepatic dysfunction, cirrhosis, or hepatitis, start with 2.5 mg P.O. daily. Subsequent dosage adjustment is done cautiously.
▶ **Heart failure‡.** *Adults:* 1.25 mg P.O. daily for 2 to 4 weeks. This low-dose strength isn't available in the U.S. If dose is tolerated, increase dose to 2.5 mg daily for 2 to 4 weeks. Subsequent doses can be doubled q 2 to 4 weeks, if tolerated.

Contraindications and precautions
• Contraindicated in patients hypersensitive to drug and in those with cardiogenic shock, overt cardiac failure, marked sinus bradycardia, or second- or third-degree AV block.
• Use cautiously in patients with bronchospastic disease. These patients should avoid beta blockers because blockade of beta$_1$ receptors isn't absolute and blockage of pulmonary beta$_2$-receptors may result in worsening of symptoms. If avoiding beta blockers is impossible, have a bronchodilator available. Also use cautiously in patients with diabetes, peripheral vascular disease, or thyroid disease; and in those with history of heart failure.
⚖ Lifespan: In pregnant or breast-feeding women, use cautiously. In children, safety of drug hasn't been established.

Adverse reactions
CNS: asthenia, fatigue, dizziness, headache, hypoesthesia, vivid dreams, depression, insomnia.
CV: *bradycardia,* peripheral edema, chest pain, *heart failure.*
EENT: pharyngitis, rhinitis, sinusitis.
GI: nausea, vomiting, diarrhea, dry mouth.

Reactions may be *common,* uncommon, *life-threatening,* or COMMON AND LIFE-THREATENING.

Musculoskeletal: arthralgia.
Respiratory: cough, dyspnea.
Skin: sweating.

Interactions

Drug-drug. *Beta blockers:* May cause extreme hypotension. Don't use together.
Calcium channel blockers: May cause myocardial depression and AV conductive inhibition. Monitor ECG closely.
Guanethidine, reserpine: Can cause hypotension. Monitor patient closely.
NSAIDs: May decrease antihypertensive effect. Monitor blood pressure and adjust dosage.
Rifampin: May increase metabolic clearance of bisoprolol. Monitor patient.

Effects on lab test results

None reported.

Pharmacokinetics

Absorption: Bioavailability after 10-mg dose is about 80%.
Distribution: About 30% protein-bound.
Metabolism: First-pass metabolism of drug is about 20%.
Excretion: Excreted equally by renal and non-renal pathways, with about 50% of dose appearing unchanged in urine and remainder appearing as inactive metabolites. Less than 2% of dose is excreted in feces. *Half-life:* 9 to 12 hours.

Route	Onset	Peak	Duration
P.O.	Unknown	2-4 hr	24 hr

Action

Chemical effect: Not defined. Decreases myocardial contractility, heart rate, and cardiac output; lowers blood pressure; and reduces myocardial oxygen consumption.
Therapeutic effect: Decreases blood pressure.

Available forms

Tablets: 5 mg, 10 mg

NURSING PROCESS

Assessment
• Obtain history of patient's hypertensive status before therapy, and check blood pressure regularly throughout therapy.
• Be alert for adverse reactions and drug interactions.

• Monitor patient's hydration status if adverse GI reactions occur.
• Closely monitor glucose level in patient with diabetes. Beta blockers may mask some evidence of hypoglycemia, such as tachycardia.
• Evaluate patient's and family's understanding of drug therapy.

Nursing diagnoses
• Risk for injury related to presence of hypertension
• Risk for deficient fluid volume related to drug-induced adverse GI reactions
• Deficient knowledge related to drug therapy

Planning and implementation
• Have a beta$_2$ agonist (bronchodilator) available for patients with bronchospastic disease.
ALERT: Don't stop drug abruptly because angina may occur in patients with unrecognized coronary artery disease.
ALERT: Don't confuse Zebeta with Zetia, Zestril, or Zyrtec.
Patient teaching
• Tell patient to take drug as prescribed, even when he's feeling better. Warn him that abruptly discontinuing drug can worsen angina and precipitate MI. Explain that drug must be withdrawn gradually over 1 to 2 weeks.
• Instruct patient to call prescriber if adverse reactions occur.
• Tell patient with diabetes to closely monitor glucose levels.
• Tell patient to check with prescriber or pharmacist before taking OTC medications or herbal remedies.

Evaluation
• Patient's blood pressure is normal.
• Patient maintains adequate fluid balance throughout therapy.
• Patient and family state understanding of drug therapy.

bivalirudin
(bye-VAL-ih-roo-din)
Angiomax

Pharmacologic class: direct thrombin inhibitor
Therapeutic class: anticoagulant
Pregnancy risk category: B

Indications and dosages

▶ **Decrease risk of acute ischemic complications in patients with unstable angina who are undergoing percutaneous transluminal coronary angioplasty (PTCA), given with aspirin.** *Adults:* 1 mg/kg I.V. bolus just before PTCA; then begin 4-hour I.V. infusion at 2.5 mg/kg per hour. After the first 4-hour infusion, another I.V. infusion at 0.2 mg/kg per hour for up to 20 hours may be given, p.r.n. Give with 300 to 325 mg of aspirin.

▧ **Adjust-a-dose:** For patients with renal impairment, if GFR is 30 to 59 ml/minute, reduce dosage by 20%. If GFR is 10 to 29 ml/minute, reduce dosage by 60%.

For dialysis-dependent patients (off dialysis), reduce dosage by 90%.

▽ I.V. administration

● Reconstitute each 250-mg vial with 5 ml of sterile water for injection. Further dilute each reconstituted vial in 50 ml D₅W or normal saline solution to yield a final concentration of 5 mg/ml.
● To prepare low-rate infusion, further dilute each reconstituted vial in 500 ml D₅W or normal saline solution to yield a final concentration of 0.5 mg/ml.
● Don't mix other drugs with bivalirudin before or during administration.
● The prepared solution is stable and may be stored for up to 24 hours at 36° to 46° F (2° to 8° C).

Contraindications and precautions

● Contraindicated in patients hypersensitive to drug or its components and in patients with active major bleeding. Don't use drug in patients with unstable angina who aren't undergoing PTCA or in patients with other acute coronary conditions, or who aren't taking aspirin.
● Use cautiously in patients with heparin-induced thrombocytopenia or heparin-induced thrombocytopenia-thrombosis syndrome and in patients with an increased risk of bleeding.
※ Lifespan: In breast-feeding women, use cautiously; it isn't known whether drug appears in breast milk. In children, safety and efficacy of drug haven't been established. Elderly patients are more likely to have puncture site hemorrhage and catheterization site hematoma.

Adverse reactions

CNS: *cerebral ischemia,* anxiety, *headache,* insomnia, nervousness, fever, *pain,* confusion.
CV: *bradycardia,* hypertension, *hypotension, syncope, ventricular fibrillation,* vascular anomaly.
GI: abdominal pain, dyspepsia, *nausea,* vomiting.
GU: urinary retention, **kidney failure,** oliguria.
Hematologic: *severe, spontaneous bleeding (cerebral, retroperitoneal, GU, GI), arterial site hemorrhage.*
Musculoskeletal: *back pain,* pelvic pain, facial paralysis.
Respiratory: *lung edema.*
Other: pain at injection site, infection, *sepsis.*

Interactions

Drug-drug. *Glycoprotein IIb/IIIa platelet inhibitors:* Safety and effectiveness haven't been established. Avoid using together.
Heparin, warfarin, other oral anticoagulants: Increases risk of bleeding. Use together cautiously. If using low–molecular-weight heparin, stop it at least 8 hours before giving bivalirudin.
Alteplase, amiodarone, amphotericin B, chlorpromazine, diazepam, prochlorperazine edisylate, reteplase, streptokinase, vancomycin: Incompatible with bivalirudin and causes haze formation, microparticulate formation, or gross precipitation. Avoid giving in the same I.V. line.

Effects on lab test results

● May increase ACT, APTT, thrombin time, and PT.

Pharmacokinetics

Absorption: Administered I.V.
Distribution: Binds rapidly to thrombin and has a rapid onset of action.
Metabolism: Rapidly cleared by a combination of renal mechanisms and proteolytic cleavage.
Excretion: Eliminated renally. Total body clearance is similar in patients with normal renal function and mild renal impairment. Clearance is reduced about 20% in patients with moderate and severe renal impairment and is reduced about 80% in dialysis-dependent patients. Bivalirudin is hemodialyzable. *Half-life:* 25 minutes in patients with normal renal function.

Route	Onset	Peak	Duration
I.V.	Rapid	Immediate	Duration of infusion

Action

Chemical effect: Highly specific for thrombin and directly inhibits both clot-bound and circulating thrombin. By inhibiting thrombin, bivalirudin prevents generation of fibrin and further activation of the clotting cascade and inhibits thrombin-induced platelet activation, granule release, and aggregation. Bivalirudin doesn't require the presence of antithrombin to produce an anticoagulant effect.

Therapeutic effect: Prevents blood clots.

Available forms

Injection: 250-mg vial

NURSING PROCESS

✎ Assessment

• Obtain and monitor baseline coagulation tests and hemoglobin and hematocrit before and throughout drug therapy.
• Monitor effectiveness by measuring APTT, PT, and thrombin time values regularly.
• Monitor venipuncture sites for bleeding, hematoma, or inflammation.
• Be alert for adverse reactions.
• **ALERT:** If the patient has an unexplained drop in hematocrit, blood pressure, or other unexplained symptom, consider the possibility of hemorrhage.
• Assess access site for bleeding regularly.
• Evaluate patient's and family's knowledge of drug therapy.

Nursing diagnoses

• Risk for injury related to potential acute ischemic event caused by impaired CV status
• Ineffective protection related to increased risk of bleeding from anticoagulant therapy
• Deficient knowledge related to drug therapy

Planning and implementation

• Patients with renal failure require reduced dosage.
• Don't give by I.M. route.
Patient teaching
• Advise patient that drug can cause bleeding. Urge patient to report immediately to prescriber any unusual bruising or bleeding (nosebleeds,

bleeding gums, petechiae, and hematuria) or tarry or bloody stools.
• Warn patient to avoid other aspirin-containing drugs and drugs used to treat swelling or pain (such as Motrin, Naprosyn, Aleve).
• Advise patient to avoid activities that carry a risk of injury, and instruct patient to use a soft toothbrush and electric razor while taking drug.

☑ Evaluation

• Patient doesn't suffer acute ischemic event after PTCA.
• Patient doesn't suffer drug-induced adverse reactions or bleeding.
• Patient and family state understanding of drug therapy.

bleomycin sulfate
(blee-oh-MIGH-sin SUL-fayt)
Blenoxane

Pharmacologic class: antibiotic, antineoplastic (specific to G2 and M phases of cell cycle)
Therapeutic class: antineoplastic
Pregnancy risk category: D

Indications and dosages

▶ **Hodgkin's lymphoma, squamous cell carcinoma, non-Hodgkin's lymphoma, testicular cancer.** *Adults:* 10 to 20 units/m^2 (0.25 to 0.5 units/kg) I.V., I.M., or S.C. once or twice weekly. After 50% response in patients with Hodgkin's disease, maintenance dosage is 1 unit I.V. or I.M. daily or 5 units I.V. or I.M. weekly.
▶ **Malignant pleural effusion, prevention of recurrent pleural effusions or to manage pneumothorax related to AIDS or *Pneumocystis carinii* pneumonia.** *Adults:* Give 60 units as a single-dose bolus in 50 to 100 ml of normal saline solution by intrapleural injection through a thoracostomy tube. Leave in for 4 hours, then drain and resume suction. Maximum dose is 1 unit/kg.
Elderly patients receiving intrapleural injection: Don't exceed 40 units/m^2.
▶ **AIDS-related Kaposi's sarcoma‡.** *Adults:* 20 units/m^2 daily I.V. continuously over 72 hours q 3 weeks.

▼ I.V. administration

• Reconstitute drug with 5 ml or more of normal saline solution for injection.
• For I.V. infusion, dilute with 50 to 100 ml of normal saline solution for injection. Infuse slowly over 10 minutes. Bleomycin may adsorb to plastic I.V. bags. For prolonged stability, use glass containers.

Contraindications and precautions

• Contraindicated in patients hypersensitive to drug.
• Use cautiously in patients with renal or pulmonary impairment.
⚖ Lifespan: In pregnant or breast-feeding women and in children, safety of drug hasn't been established.

Adverse reactions

CNS: hyperesthesia of scalp and fingers, headache, fever.
GI: *stomatitis, prolonged anorexia, nausea, vomiting,* diarrhea.
Hematologic: leukocytosis.
Musculoskeletal: swelling of interphalangeal joints.
Respiratory: PNEUMONITIS, *pulmonary fibrosis, fine crackles, dyspnea, nonproductive cough.*
Skin: *reversible alopecia; erythema; vesiculation; hardening and discoloration of palmar and plantar skin;* desquamation of hands, feet, and pressure areas; *hyperpigmentation; acne.*
Other: *hypersensitivity reactions (fever up to 106° F [41.1° C] with chills up to 5 hours after injection, anaphylaxis).*

Interactions

Drug-drug. *Digoxin:* May decrease digoxin level. Monitor patient closely for loss of therapeutic effect.
Phenytoin: May decrease phenytoin level. Monitor patient closely.

Effects on lab test results

• May increase uric acid level.
• May increase WBC count.

Pharmacokinetics

Absorption: I.M. administration results in lower levels than those produced by equivalent I.V. doses.

Distribution: Distributed widely into total body water, mainly in skin, lungs, kidneys, peritoneum, and lymphatic tissue.
Metabolism: Unknown; however, extensive tissue inactivation occurs in liver and kidneys, with much less in skin and lungs.
Excretion: Drug and its metabolites excreted primarily in urine. *Half-life:* 2 hours.

Route	Onset	Peak	Duration
I.V., I.M., S.C., intra-pleural	Unknown	Unknown	Unknown

Action

Chemical effect: Unknown; thought to inhibit DNA synthesis and cause scission of single- and double-stranded DNA.
Therapeutic effect: Kills selected types of cancer cells.

Available forms

Injection: 15- and 30-unit vials (1 unit = 1 mg)

NURSING PROCESS

🔍 Assessment

• Obtain history of patient's overall physical status (especially respiratory status, CBC, and pulmonary and renal function tests) before therapy and reassess regularly thereafter.
• Be alert for adverse reactions and drug interactions.
• Adverse pulmonary reactions are common in patients older than age 70. Fatal pulmonary fibrosis occurs in 1% of patients, especially when cumulative dose exceeds 400 units.
• Monitor patient for bleomycin-induced fever, which is common and usually occurs within 3 to 6 hours after giving drug.
• Watch for hypersensitivity reactions, which may be delayed for several hours, especially in patients with lymphoma.
• Assess patient for development of fine crackles and dyspnea.
• Evaluate patient's and family's understanding of drug therapy.

📋 Nursing diagnoses

• Risk for injury related to underlying neoplastic condition
• Impaired gas exchange related to drug-induced adverse pulmonary reactions

---

• Deficient knowledge related to drug therapy

▶ Planning and implementation
• Follow institutional policy for administration of drug to reduce risks. Preparation and administration of parenteral form of this drug cause carcinogenic, mutagenic, and teratogenic risks for personnel.
• Dilute drug in 1 to 5 ml of sterile water for injection, bacteriostatic water for injection, or normal saline solution for injection.
• Follow manufacturer's guidelines for giving S.C. bleomycin.
• For intrapleural use, dissolve drug in 50 to 100 ml normal saline solution for injection. Give through a thoracotomy tube after excess intrapleural fluid has been drained and complete lung expansion has been confirmed.
• Refrigerate unopened vials containing dry powder.
• Refrigerated, reconstituted solution is stable for 4 weeks; at room temperature, it's stable for 2 weeks.
• If pulmonary function test shows a marked decline, stop drug.
• To prevent linear streaking from drug concentrating in keratin of squamous epithelium, don't use adhesive dressings on skin.
• In patients susceptible to post-treatment fever, give acetaminophen before treatment and for 24 hours after treatment.
• If ordered after treatment, give supplemental oxygen at a fraction of inspired oxygen no higher than 25% to avoid potential lung damage.

Patient teaching
• Explain the risks of drug therapy, especially the danger of serious pulmonary reactions in high-risk patients.
• Explain the need for monitoring and the type of monitoring to be done.
• Tell patient that alopecia may occur, but that it's usually reversible.

☑ Evaluation
• Patient exhibits positive response to therapy, as evidenced by follow-up diagnostic test results.
• Patient's gas exchange remains normal throughout therapy.
• Patient and family state understanding of drug therapy.

bortezomib
(bore-TEHZ-uh-mihb)
Velcade

Pharmacologic class: proteosome inhibitor
Therapeutic class: antineoplastic
Pregnancy risk category: D

Indications and dosages

▶ **Multiple myeloma that's progressing after at least two therapies.** *Adults:* 1.3 mg/m^2 by I.V. bolus twice weekly for 2 weeks (days 1, 4, 8, and 11) followed by a 10-day rest period (days 12-21). This 3-week period is a treatment cycle.

◲ **Adjust-a-dose:** Withhold drug if patient develops a grade 3 non-hematologic or a grade 4 hematologic toxicity (excluding neuropathy). When toxicity resolves, restart at a 25% reduced dose. If patient has neuropathic pain, peripheral neuropathy, or both, use this table.

Severity of neuropathy	Dosage
Grade 1 (paresthesias, loss of reflexes, or both) without pain or loss of function	No change
Grade 1 with pain or grade 2 (function altered but not activities of daily living)	No change
Grade 2 with pain or grade 3 (interference with activities of daily living)	Reduce to 1 mg/m^2. Hold drug until toxicity resolves; then start at 0.7 mg/m^2 once weekly.
Grade 4 (permanent sensory loss that interferes with function)	Stop drug

▼ I.V. administration
• Reconstitute with 3.5 ml of normal saline solution. Use caution and aseptic technique when preparing and handling drug. Wear gloves and protective clothing to prevent skin contact.
• Give by I.V. bolus within 8 hours of reconstitution.
• Drug may be stored up to 3 hours in a syringe, but total storage time for reconstituted solution must not exceed 8 hours when exposed to normal indoor lighting.

Rapid onset   *Liquid form contains alcohol.   ◆Canada   ◇ Australia   †OTC   ‡Off-label use

• Store unopened vials at a controlled room temperature, in original packaging, and protect from light.

Contraindications and precautions

• Contraindicated in patients hypersensitive to bortezomib, boron, or mannitol.
• Use cautiously if patient is dehydrated, is receiving other drugs known to cause hypotension, or has a history of syncope.
• Use cautiously, and only after careful assessment of risks and benefits, in patients with severe neuropathy.
⚹ **Lifespan:** In pregnant women, avoid use. Women should avoid becoming pregnant during drug therapy. Women should avoid breastfeeding. In children, safety and efficacy of drug haven't been established.

Adverse reactions

CNS: *anxiety, asthenia, dizziness, dysesthesia, fever, headache, insomnia, paresthesia, peripheral neuropathy, rigors.*
CV: *edema, orthostatic and postural hypotension.*
EENT: *blurred vision.*
GI: *abdominal pain, constipation, decreased appetite, diarrhea, dysgeusia, dyspepsia, nausea, vomiting.*
GU: *dehydration.*
Hematologic: *anemia,* NEUTROPENIA, THROMBOCYTOPENIA.
Musculoskeletal: *arthralgia, back pain, bone pain, limb pain, muscle cramps, myalgia.*
Respiratory: *cough, dyspnea, pneumonia, upper respiratory tract infection.*
Skin: *rash, pruritus.*
Other: *herpes zoster.*

Interactions

Drug-drug. *Antihypertensives:* May cause hypotension. Monitor patient's blood pressure closely.
Inhibitors or inducers of CYP 3A4: Monitor patient closely for either toxicity or reduced effects.
Drugs linked to peripheral neuropathy, such as amiodarone, antivirals, isoniazid, nitrofurantoin, statins: May worsen neuropathy. Use together cautiously.
Oral antidiabetics: May cause hypoglycemia or hyperglycemia. Monitor glucose levels closely.

Effects on lab test results

• May decrease hemoglobin and neutrophil and platelet counts.

Pharmacokinetics

Absorption: Administered I.V.
Distribution: 83% is protein-bound.
Metabolism: Mainly in the liver by CYP enzymes.
Excretion: Unknown. *Half-life:* 9 to 15 hours.

Route	Onset	Peak	Duration
I.V.	Unknown	Unknown	Unknown

Action

Chemical effect: Disrupts intracellular homeostatic mechanisms by inhibiting the 26S proteosome, which regulates intracellular levels of certain proteins, thereby causing cells to die.
Therapeutic effect: Destroys cancer cells.

Available forms

Injection: 3.5 mg

NURSING PROCESS

⏣ Assessment

• Assess patient's condition before therapy and regularly thereafter.
• Assess patient's nutrition and hydration status before and during therapy.
• Evaluate patient's and family's knowledge of drug therapy.

⏣ Nursing diagnoses

• Risk for injury related to potential neuropathy as an adverse effect
• Risk for hypotension related to dehydration
• Risk for imbalanced nutrition: less than body requires related to underlying disease and drug adverse effects

⏵ Planning and implementation

• Patient may need an antiemetic, an antidiarrheal, or both because drug may cause nausea, vomiting, diarrhea, and constipation.
• Adjust antihypertensive dosage, maintain hydration status, and give mineralocorticoids to manage orthostatic hypotension.
• Watch for evidence of neuropathy, such as a burning sensation, hyperesthesia, hypoesthesia, paresthesia, discomfort, or neuropathic pain.

Reactions may be *common*, uncommon, *life-threatening*, or COMMON AND LIFE-THREATENING.

• If patient develops new or worsening peripheral neuropathy, change dose and schedule.

Patient teaching

• Tell patient to notify prescriber about new or worsening peripheral neuropathy.

• Urge women to use effective contraception during treatment.

• Teach patient how to avoid dehydration, and stress the need to tell prescriber about dizziness, light-headedness, or fainting spells.

• Tell patient to use caution when driving or performing potentially hazardous activities because drug may cause fatigue, dizziness, faintness, light-headedness, and double or blurred vision.

▶ **Evaluation**

• Patient has no serious drug reactions.

• Patient maintains adequate nutritional status.

• Patient maintains adequate hydration status.

• Patient and family state understanding of drug therapy.

bosentan
(bow-SEN-tan)
Tracleer

Pharmacologic class: nonselective endothelin receptor antagonist
Therapeutic class: antihypertensive
Pregnancy risk category: X

Indications and dosages

▶ **Pulmonary arterial hypertension in patients with World Health Organization class III or IV symptoms to improve exercise ability and decrease clinical worsening.** *Adults:* 62.5 mg P.O. b.i.d. for 4 weeks. Increase to maintenance dose of 125 mg P.O. b.i.d. In patients weighing less than 40 kg (88 lb), the initial and maintenance dose is 62.5 mg b.i.d.

Contraindications and precautions

• Contraindicated in patients hypersensitive to drug. Don't use in patients with moderate-to-severe liver impairment or in those with elevated aminotransferase levels more than 3 times upper limit of normal.

• Use cautiously in patients with mild liver impairment.

⚠ **Lifespan:** In pregnant women, drug is contraindicated. In breast-feeding women, drug isn't recommended because it's unknown whether drug appears in breast milk. In children, safety and efficacy of drug haven't been established. In elderly patients, select dose cautiously because of greater likelihood of decreased organ function.

Adverse reactions

CNS: *headache,* fatigue.
CV: hypotension, palpitations, flushing, edema, lower leg edema.
EENT: *nasopharyngitis.*
GI: dyspepsia.
Hematologic: anemia.
Hepatic: *liver failure.*
Skin: pruritus.

Interactions

Drug-drug. *Cyclosporin A:* May increase concentrations of bosentan and decrease levels of cyclosporine. Avoid using together.
Glyburide: May increase risk of elevated liver enzyme levels and decrease levels of both drugs. Avoid using together.
Hormonal contraceptives: May cause contraceptive failure. Advise use of an additional method of birth control.
Ketoconazole: May increase bosentan level. Monitor patient for increased effects of bosentan.
Simvastatin, other statins: May decrease levels of these drugs. Monitor cholesterol levels to assess need for statin dosage adjustment.

Effects on lab test results

• May increase liver aminotransferase levels, such as AST, ALT, and bilirubin levels.
• May decrease hemoglobin and hematocrit.

Pharmacokinetics

Absorption: 50% bioavailability after oral administration.
Distribution: More than 98% protein-bound, primarily albumin.
Metabolism: Hepatically metabolized into three metabolites. Bosentan induces CYP 2C9 and CYP 3A4, and possibly CYP 2C19.
Excretion: Eliminated by biliary excretion. Less than 3% of oral dose is recovered in urine.

Route	Onset	Peak	Duration
P.O.	Unknown	3-5 hr	Unknown

Action

Chemical effect: Antagonizes endothelin-1 (ET-1). ET-1 levels are elevated in patients with pulmonary arterial hypertension, suggesting a pathogenic role for ET-1 in this disease.
Therapeutic effect: Increases exercise capacity and cardiac index. Decreases blood pressure, pulmonary arterial pressure, vascular resistance, and mean right arterial pressure.

Available forms

Tablets: 62.5 mg, 125 mg

NURSING PROCESS

🔍 Assessment

• Assess patient's underlying condition before therapy and reassess regularly thereafter.
• Make sure patient isn't pregnant. Obtain monthly pregnancy tests.
• Serious liver injury may occur. Measure aminotransferase levels before treatment and monthly thereafter, and adjust dosage accordingly.
• This drug may cause hematologic changes. Monitor hemoglobin after 1 and 3 months of therapy and then every 3 months thereafter.
• Be alert for adverse events.
• Evaluate patient's and family's knowledge of drug therapy.

🔲 Nursing diagnoses

• Risk of injury related to drug-induced liver enzyme elevations
• Ineffective tissue perfusion (cardiopulmonary) related to underlying condition
• Deficient knowledge related to drug therapy

🔷 Planning and implementation

• To decrease the possibility of potential serious liver injury and to limit the chance for fetal exposure, Tracleer may be prescribed only through the Tracleer access program at 1-866-228-3546 (option 1). Adverse effects also may be reported through this number.
• For patients who develop aminotransferase abnormalities, the dosage may need to be decreased or stopped until aminotransferase levels return to normal. If liver function abnormalities are accompanied by symptoms of liver injury, such as nausea, vomiting, fever, abdominal pain, jaundice, or unusual lethargy or fatigue, or if bilirubin level is greater than or equal to 2 times

upper limit of normal, stop treatment and don't restart.
• Overdose may cause headache, nausea and vomiting, mildly decreased blood pressure, and increased heart rate. Massive overdose may cause severe hypotension requiring CV support. Treatment is symptomatic and supportive.
• To avoid the potential for clinical deterioration, gradual dosage reduction is recommended before discontinuation of drug.

Patient teaching

• Advise patient to take drug only as prescribed.
• Warn patient to avoid becoming pregnant while taking this drug. Reliable contraception must be used and a monthly pregnancy test performed.
• Advise patient to have liver tests and blood counts performed regularly.
• Tell patient not to use hormonal contraceptives, including oral, implantable, and injectable, as her only means of contraception because failure may occur. Major birth defects may result with fetal exposure.

🔲 Evaluation

• Patient doesn't suffer from adverse reactions or liver damage from drug therapy.
• Patient's pulmonary artery pressure decreases, and patient reaches pulmonary hemodynamic stability.
• Patient and family state understanding of drug therapy.

bretylium tosylate

(breh-TIL-ee-um TOH-si-layt)
Bretylate ◇

Pharmacologic class: adrenergic blocker
Therapeutic class: ventricular antiarrhythmic
Pregnancy risk category: C

Indications and dosages

▶ **Ventricular fibrillation or hemodynamically unstable ventricular tachycardia unresponsive to other antiarrhythmics.** *Adults:* 5 mg/kg by I.V. push over 1 minute. If necessary, increase dose to 10 mg/kg and repeat q 15 to 30 minutes until 35 to 40 mg/kg have been given. For continuous suppression, give diluted solution at 1 to 2 mg/minute continuously, or give 5 to 10 mg/kg diluted solution over longer than 8 minutes q

---

6 hours. If unable to obtain I.V. access, may give 5 to 10 mg/kg undiluted I.M. q 1 to 2 hours if the arrhythmia persists or q 6 to 8 hours for maintenance therapy.

▼ I.V. administration

• For maintenance therapy, dilute with dextrose or saline solution for injection before giving.
• When giving as direct I.V. injection, use 20G to 22G needle and inject over 1 minute into vein or I.V. line containing free-flowing compatible solution.
• Keep patient in supine position until tolerance to hypotension develops. Have patient avoid sudden position changes.

Contraindications and precautions

• Contraindicated in patients taking a cardiac glycoside unless arrhythmia is life-threatening, not caused by digitalis, and unresponsive to other antiarrhythmics.
• Use cautiously in patients with fixed cardiac output (aortic stenosis and pulmonary hypertension). Drug may cause severe and sudden drop in blood pressure.
⚠ Lifespan: In pregnant or breast-feeding women, use cautiously. In children, safety and efficacy of drug haven't been established.

Adverse reactions

CNS: *vertigo, dizziness, light-headedness, syncope.*
CV: SEVERE HYPOTENSION (especially orthostatic), *bradycardia,* angina, *transient arrhythmias,* transient hypertension.
GI: severe nausea, vomiting (with rapid infusion).
Musculoskeletal: muscle atrophy, tissue necrosis (with repeated injections).

Interactions

Drug-drug. *Antihypertensives:* May potentiate hypotension. Monitor blood pressure.
Other antiarrhythmics: May have additive or antagonistic antiarrhythmic effects. Monitor patient for additive toxicity.
Sympathomimetics: Bretylium may potentiate effects of drugs given to correct hypotension. Monitor blood pressure.

Effects on lab test results

None reported.

Pharmacokinetics

Absorption: Administered I.V.
Distribution: Distributed widely throughout body. Only about 1% to 10% is protein-bound.
Metabolism: No metabolites have been identified.
Excretion: In urine. *Half-life:* 5 to 10 hours (longer in patients with renal impairment).

Route	Onset	Peak	Duration
I.V.	3 min-2 hr	6-9 hr	6-24 hr

Action

Chemical effect: Unknown; considered a class III antiarrhythmic that initially exerts transient adrenergic stimulation through release of norepinephrine. Subsequent depletion of norepinephrine causes adrenergic blocking actions to predominate, prolonging repolarization and increasing duration of action potential and effective refractory period.
Therapeutic effect: Abolishes ventricular arrhythmias.

Available forms

Injection: 50 mg/ml

NURSING PROCESS

◪ Assessment

• Obtain history of patient's heart rate and rhythm before therapy.
• Monitor drug's effectiveness by evaluating continuous ECG recordings, blood pressure, and heart rate. Initial drug-induced release of norepinephrine may cause transient hypertension and arrhythmias.
• Be alert for adverse reactions and drug interactions.
• Evaluate patient's and family's understanding of drug therapy.

⊞ Nursing diagnoses

• Decreased cardiac output related to presence of ventricular arrhythmia
• Ineffective cerebral tissue perfusion related to drug-induced severe hypotension
• Deficient knowledge related to drug therapy

▷ Planning and implementation

• Drug is used with other cardiac life-support measures, such as cardiopulmonary resuscita-

tion, defibrillation, epinephrine, sodium bicarbonate, and lidocaine.
• To prevent nausea and vomiting, follow dosage directions carefully.
• If supine systolic blood pressure falls below 75 mm Hg, prescriber may order norepinephrine, dopamine, or volume expanders to raise blood pressure.

Patient teaching
• Tell patient to report chest pain or dyspnea immediately.
• Tell patient to avoid sudden position changes.

☑ **Evaluation**
• Patient's ECG reveals that arrhythmia has been corrected.
• Patient's blood pressure remains normal throughout therapy.
• Patient and family state understanding of drug therapy.

bromocriptine mesylate
(broh-moh-KRIP-teen MES-ih-layt)
Parlodel, Parlodel SnapTabs

Pharmacologic class: dopamine receptor agonist
Therapeutic class: semisynthetic ergot alkaloid, dopaminergic agonist, antiparkinsonian, inhibitor of prolactin and growth hormone release
Pregnancy risk category: NR

Indications and dosages

▶ **Parkinson's disease.** *Adults:* 1.25 to 2.5 mg P.O. b.i.d. with meals. Increase dosage q 14 to 28 days, up to 100 mg daily, p.r.n. Usual dosage is 10 to 40 mg daily.
▶ **Acromegaly.** *Adults:* 1.25 to 2.5 mg P.O. h.s. with snack for 3 days. An additional 1.25 to 2.5 mg may be added q 3 to 7 days until patient receives therapeutic benefit. Maximum dosage is 100 mg daily.
▶ **Amenorrhea and galactorrhea related to hyperprolactinemia; infertility or hypogonadism in women.** *Adults:* 1.25 to 2.5 mg P.O. daily. Increase by 2.5 mg daily at 3- to 7-day intervals until desired effect is achieved. Maintenance dosage is usually 5 to 7.5 mg daily, but may be 2.5 to 15 mg daily.

▶ **Premenstrual syndrome‡.** *Adults:* 2.5 to 7.5 mg P.O. b.i.d. from day 10 of menstrual cycle until onset of menstruation.
▶ **Cushing's syndrome‡.** *Adults:* 1.25 to 2.5 mg P.O. b.i.d. to q.i.d.
▶ **Hepatic encephalopathy‡.** *Adults:* 1.25 mg P.O. daily, increase by 1.25 mg q 3 days until 15 mg is reached.
▶ **Neuroleptic malignant syndrome related to neuroleptic drug therapy‡.** *Adults:* 2.5 to 5 mg P.O. 2 to 6 times daily.

Contraindications and precautions

• Contraindicated in patients hypersensitive to ergot derivatives and in those with uncontrolled hypertension and toxemia of pregnancy.
• Use cautiously in patients with renal or hepatic impairment or history of MI with residual arrhythmias.
⚘ **Lifespan:** In breast-feeding women, avoid use because it inhibits lactation. In children younger than age 15, safety of drug hasn't been established.

Adverse reactions

CNS: confusion, hallucinations, uncontrolled body movements, *dizziness, headache,* fatigue, mania, delusions, nervousness, insomnia, depression, *seizures, CVA, syncope.*
CV: *hypotension,* orthostatic hypotension, hypertension, *acute MI.*
EENT: nasal congestion, tinnitus, blurred vision.
GI: *nausea,* vomiting, *abdominal cramps,* constipation, diarrhea.
GU: urine retention, urinary frequency.
Skin: coolness and pallor of fingers and toes.

Interactions

Drug-drug. *Antihypertensives:* May increase hypotensive effects. Dosage adjustment of antihypertensive may be needed.
Ergot alkaloids, estrogens, hormonal contraceptives, progestins: May interfere with effects of bromocriptine. Don't use together.
Erythromycin: May increase bromocriptine levels. Adjustment of bromocriptine may be needed.
Haloperidol, loxapine, MAO inhibitors, methyldopa, metoclopramide, phenothiazines, reserpine: May interfere with effects of bromocriptine. Increase of bromocriptine dosage may be needed.
Levodopa: May have additive effects. Adjustment of levodopa dosage may be needed.

Reactions may be *common,* uncommon, *life-threatening,* or **COMMON AND LIFE-THREATENING.**

Drug-lifestyle. *Alcohol use:* May cause disulfiram-like reaction. Discourage use together.

Effects on lab test results

• May increase BUN, alkaline phosphatase, uric acid, AST, ALT, and CK levels.

Pharmacokinetics

Absorption: 28% absorbed.
Distribution: 90% to 96% bound to albumin.
Metabolism: First-pass metabolism occurs with more than 90% of absorbed dose. Drug is metabolized completely in liver.
Excretion: Major route of excretion is through bile. Only 2.5% to 5.5% of dose excreted in urine. *Half-life:* 15 hours.

Route	Onset	Peak	Duration
P.O.	½ -2 hr	1-3 hr	12-24 hr

Action

Chemical effect: Inhibits secretion of prolactin and acts as dopamine-receptor agonist by activating postsynaptic dopamine receptors.
Therapeutic effect: Reverses amenorrhea and galactorrhea caused by hyperprolactinemia, increases fertility in women, improves voluntary movement, and inhibits prolactin and growth hormone release.

Available forms

Capsules: 5 mg
Tablets: 2.5 mg

NURSING PROCESS

Assessment

• Obtain history of patient's underlying condition before therapy and reassess regularly thereafter.
• Perform baseline and periodic evaluations of cardiac, hepatic, renal, and hematopoietic functions during prolonged therapy.
• Be alert for adverse reactions and drug interactions. Risk of adverse reactions is high (about 68%), particularly at beginning of therapy; most are mild to moderate, with nausea being most common. Adverse reactions are more frequent when drug is used for Parkinson's disease.
• Evaluate patient's and family's knowledge of drug therapy.

Nursing diagnoses

• Ineffective health maintenance related to underlying condition
• Risk for injury related to drug-induced adverse CNS or CV reactions
• Deficient knowledge related to drug therapy

Planning and implementation

• Patients with impaired renal function may require dosage adjustments.
• Give drug with meals.
• Gradually adjust doses to effective levels to minimize adverse reactions.
• For Parkinson's disease, bromocriptine usually is given with either levodopa or carbidopa-levodopa.
Patient teaching
• Advise patient to use contraceptive methods other than oral contraceptives or subdermal implants during treatment.
• Advise patient to rise slowly to an upright position and avoid sudden position changes to avoid dizziness and fainting.
• Advise patient that resumption of menses and suppression of galactorrhea may take 6 weeks or longer.
• Warn patient to avoid hazardous activities that require alertness until CNS and CV effects of drug are known.
• Tell patient to take drug with meals to minimize GI distress.

Evaluation

• Patient exhibits improvement in underlying condition.
• Patient doesn't experience injury as a result of drug-induced adverse reactions.
• Patient and family state understanding of drug therapy.

brompheniramine maleate
(brom-fen-IR-ah-meen MAL-ee-ayt)
Bromphen*†, Dimetane*†, Dimetapp Allergy†, Nasahist B, ND-Stat

Pharmacologic class: alkylamine antihistamine
Therapeutic class: antihistamine (H_1-receptor antagonist)
Pregnancy risk category: C

Indications and dosages

▶ **Rhinitis, allergy symptoms.** *Adults:* 4 to 8 mg P.O. t.i.d. or q.i.d. Or, 8 to 12 mg extended-release P.O. b.i.d. or t.i.d. Or, 5 to 20 mg q 6 to 12 hours I.V., I.M., or S.C. Maximum dosage is 40 mg daily.
Children age 6 and older: 2 to 4 mg P.O. t.i.d. or q.i.d. Or, 8 to 12 mg extended-release P.O. q 12 hours. Or, 0.5 mg/kg I.V., I.M., or S.C. daily in divided doses t.i.d. or q.i.d.
Children younger than age 6: 0.5 mg/kg P.O., I.V., I.M., or S.C. daily in divided doses t.i.d. or q.i.d.

▽ I.V. administration

• Injectable form containing 10 mg/ml can be given diluted or undiluted very slowly I.V. Don't give 100 mg/ml injection I.V.

Contraindications and precautions

• Contraindicated in patients hypersensitive to drug's ingredients and in those with acute asthmatic attacks, severe hypertension, coronary artery disease, angle-closure glaucoma, urine retention, or peptic ulcer. Also contraindicated within 14 days of MAO inhibitor therapy.
• Use cautiously in patients with increased intraocular pressure, diabetes, ischemic heart disease, hyperthyroidism, hypertension, bronchial asthma, or prostatic hyperplasia.
⚘ Lifespan: In pregnant women, use cautiously. In breast-feeding women, drug is contraindicated. In neonates, drug isn't recommended. Children, especially those younger than age 6, may experience paradoxical hyperexcitability. In children age 11 and younger, extended-release tablets aren't recommended. In elderly patients, use cautiously.

Adverse reactions

CNS: dizziness, tremors, irritability, insomnia, syncope, *drowsiness, stimulation* (especially in elderly patients).
CV: hypotension, palpitations.
GI: anorexia, nausea, vomiting, *dry mouth and throat.*
GU: urine retention.
Hematologic: *thrombocytopenia, agranulocytosis.*
Skin: urticaria, rash, diaphoresis.
Other: local stinging.

Interactions

Drug-drug. *CNS depressants:* May increase sedation. Use together cautiously.
MAO inhibitors: May increase anticholinergic effects. Don't use together.

Effects on lab test results

• May decrease platelet and granulocyte counts.

Pharmacokinetics

Absorption: After oral administration, absorbed readily from GI tract; unknown for parenteral administration.
Distribution: Distributed widely throughout body.
Metabolism: About 90% to 95% metabolized by liver.
Excretion: Drug and its metabolites excreted primarily in urine; small amount excreted in feces. *Half-life:* 12 to 34½ hours.

Route	Onset	Peak	Duration
P.O., I.V., I.M., S.C.	15-60 min	2-5 hr (longer for P.O. extended-release)	4-8 hr

Action

Chemical effect: Competes with histamine for H_1-receptor sites on effector cells. Prevents but doesn't reverse histamine-mediated responses.
Therapeutic effect: Relieves allergy symptoms.

Available forms

Elixir: 2 mg/5 ml*†
Injection: 10 mg/ml
Tablets: 4 mg†
Tablets (extended-release): 12 mg†

NURSING PROCESS

📋 **Assessment**
• Assess patient's allergy symptoms before therapy and regularly thereafter.
• Be alert for adverse reactions and drug interactions.
• Monitor CBC during long-term therapy; watch for signs of blood dyscrasias.
• Monitor patient's hydration status if adverse GI reactions occur.
• Evaluate patient's and family's knowledge of drug therapy.

⊞ Nursing diagnoses
- Ineffective health maintenance related to allergy symptoms
- Risk for deficient fluid volume related to drug-induced adverse GI reactions
- Deficient knowledge related to drug therapy

⊠ Planning and implementation
- Give drug with food or milk to reduce GI distress.
- Alert prescriber if patient appears to be developing tolerance to drug. A different antihistamine may need to be substituted.

Patient teaching
- Tell patient to reduce GI distress by taking drug with food or milk.
- Warn patient to avoid alcohol and activities that require alertness until CNS effects of drug are known.
- Tell patient that coffee or tea may reduce drug-induced drowsiness, although drug causes less drowsiness than some other antihistamines.
- Tell patient to relieve dry mouth with ice chips, sugarless gum, or hard candy.
- Instruct patient to notify prescriber if tolerance develops because different antihistamine may need to be ordered.
- Instruct patient to stop drug 4 days before skin tests to preserve accuracy of tests.
- If patient operates machinery or motor vehicles, explain that drug has sedative effects.

☑ Evaluation
- Patient's allergy symptoms are relieved.
- Patient maintains adequate hydration throughout therapy.
- Patient and family state understanding of drug therapy.

budesonide (inhalation)
(byoo-DES-oh-nighd)
Pulmicort Respules, Pulmicort Turbuhaler, Rhinocort Aqua

Pharmacologic class: glucocorticoid
Therapeutic class: anti-inflammatory
Pregnancy risk category: B (C for Rhinocort)

Indications and dosages

▶ **Symptoms of seasonal or perennial allergic rhinitis and non-allergic perennial rhinitis.**
Adults and children age 6 and older: 2 sprays (64 mcg) in each nostril in morning and evening or 4 sprays (128 mcg) in each nostril in morning. Maintenance dosage is fewest number of sprays needed to control symptoms.
▶ **Chronic asthma.** *Adults:* 200 to 400 mcg oral inhalation b.i.d. when patient previously used bronchodilators alone or inhaled corticosteroids; 400 to 800 mcg oral inhalation b.i.d. when patient previously used oral corticosteroids.
Children age 6 and older: Initially, 200 mcg oral inhalation b.i.d. Maximum dosage is 400 mcg b.i.d.
Children ages 1 to 8: 0.25 mg Pulmicort Respules by jet nebulizer with compressor once daily. Increase to 0.5 mg once daily or 0.25 mg b.i.d. in child not receiving systemic or inhaled corticosteroids or 1 mg daily or 0.5 mg b.i.d. if child is receiving oral corticosteroids.

Contraindications and precautions

- Contraindicated in patients hypersensitive to drug or its components and in those who have had recent septal ulcers, nasal surgery, or nasal trauma, until total healing has occurred. Pulmicort Turbuhaler and Pulmicort Respules are contraindicated in the primary treatment of status asthmaticus.
- Use cautiously in patients with tuberculous infections, ocular herpes simplex, or untreated fungal, bacterial, or systemic viral infections.
- ⚠ **Lifespan:** In pregnant or breast-feeding women, use cautiously. In children younger than age 1, Pulmicort Respules aren't indicated. In children younger than age 6, safety of drug hasn't been established.

Adverse reactions

CNS: nervousness, *headache.*
CV: facial edema.
EENT: nasal irritation, epistaxis, pharyngitis, sinusitis, reduced sense of smell, nasal pain, hoarseness.
GI: bad taste, dry mouth, dyspepsia, nausea, vomiting.
Metabolic: weight gain.
Musculoskeletal: myalgia.
Respiratory: cough, candidiasis, wheezing, dyspnea.
Skin: rash, pruritus, contact dermatitis.
Other: hypersensitivity reactions.

Interactions

Drug-drug. *Alternate-day prednisone therapy, inhaled corticosteroids:* May increase risk of hypothalamic-pituitary-adrenal suppression. Monitor patient closely.
Ketoconazole: May increase budesonide level. Use together cautiously.

Effects on lab test results

None reported.

Pharmacokinetics

Absorption: Amount of intranasal dose that reaches systemic circulation is typically low (about 20%).
Distribution: 88% protein-bound.
Metabolism: Rapidly and extensively metabolized in liver.
Excretion: About 67% in urine and about 33% in feces. *Half-life:* About 2 hours.

Route	Onset	Peak	Duration
Nasal inhalation	10 hr	Unknown	Unknown
Oral inhalation	24 hr	1-2 wk	Unknown

Action

Chemical effect: Unknown; probably decreases nasal and pulmonary inflammation, mainly by inhibiting activities of specific cells and mediators involved in allergic response.
Therapeutic effect: Decreases nasal and pulmonary congestion.

Available forms

Inhalation suspension: 0.25 mg/2 ml, 0.5 mg/2 ml
Nasal spray: 32 mcg/metered spray (7-g canister)
Oral inhalation powder: 200 mcg/dose

NURSING PROCESS

⬛ Assessment

● Obtain history of patient's condition before therapy and reassess regularly thereafter.
● Be alert for adverse reactions.
● Evaluate patient's and family's knowledge of drug therapy.

⬛ Nursing diagnoses

● Ineffective health maintenance related to allergy-induced nasal congestion
● Impaired gas exchange related to drug-induced wheezing
● Deficient knowledge related to drug therapy

⬛ Planning and implementation

● Before using nasal inhaler, shake container and invert. Have patient clear his nasal passages and then tilt his head back. Insert nozzle (pointed away from septum) into nostril, holding other nostril closed. Deliver spray while patient inhales. Repeat in other nostril.
● Notify prescriber if relief isn't obtained or signs of infection appear.
● Obtain specimen for culture if signs of nasal infection occur.
Patient teaching
● Teach patient how to use nasal inhaler himself.
● Instruct patient to hold the inhaler upright when loading Pulmicort Turbuhaler, not to blow or exhale into the inhaler, not to shake it while loaded, and to hold the inhaler upright while orally inhaling the dose. Tell patient to place the mouthpiece between the lips and inhale forcefully and deeply.
● Pulmicort Respules can be given only by jet nebulizer connected to an air compressor with satisfactory airflow. System should be equipped with a mouthpiece or face mask.
● Inform patient that use of an oral inhaler results in improvement in asthma control within 24 hours, with maximum benefit at 1 to 2 weeks, or possibly longer.
● Advise parent that antihistamines can cause paradoxical excitement in small children.
⬥ **ALERT:** Advise patient that Pulmicort Turbuhaler and Pulmicort Respules aren't indicated for relief of acute asthma attacks.
● Tell patient that product should be used by only one person to prevent spread of infection.
● Advise patient not to break, incinerate, or store canister in extreme heat; contents are under pressure.
● Warn patient not to exceed prescribed dose or use for long periods because of risk of hypothalamic-pituitary-adrenal axis suppression.
● Tell patient to report worsened condition or symptoms that don't improve in 3 weeks.
● Teach patient good nasal and oral hygiene.

☑ Evaluation

• Patient's nasal congestion subsides.
• Patient has adequate gas exchange.
• Patient and family state understanding of drug therapy.

budesonide (oral)
(byoo-DES-oh-nighd)
Entocort EC

Pharmacologic class: corticosteroid
Therapeutic class: anti-inflammatory
Pregnancy risk category: B

Indications and dosages

▶ **Mild-to-moderate active Crohn's disease involving the ileum or the ascending colon.**
Adults: 9 mg P.O. once daily in the morning for up to 8 weeks. For recurrent episodes of active Crohn's disease, a repeat 8-week course may be given. Taper to 6 mg P.O. daily for 2 weeks before complete cessation.

Contraindications and precautions

• Contraindicated in patients hypersensitive to drug.
• Use cautiously in patients with tuberculosis, hypertension, diabetes mellitus, osteoporosis, peptic ulcer disease, glaucoma, or cataracts. Also use cautiously in patients with a family history of diabetes or glaucoma and those with any other condition in which glucocorticosteroids may have unwanted effects.
⚠ Lifespan: In pregnant women, use only if potential benefit justifies risks. In breast-feeding women, the decision to breast-feed should be based on importance of drug to the mother; glucocorticoids appear in breast milk and infants may have adverse reactions. In children, safety and efficacy of drug haven't been established. In elderly patients, give drug cautiously, starting at the lower end of the dosage range.

Adverse reactions

CNS: *headache,* dizziness, asthenia, hyperkinesia, paresthesia, syncope, tremor, vertigo, fatigue, malaise, agitation, confusion, insomnia, nervousness, somnolence, migraine, fever, pain, sleep disorder.
CV: chest pain, dependent edema, facial edema, hypertension, palpitations, tachycardia, flushing.

EENT: *pharyngitis,* ear infection, eye abnormality, abnormal vision, sinusitis, voice alteration, neck pain.
GI: *nausea,* dyspepsia, abdominal pain, flatulence, vomiting, anus disorder, aggravated Crohn's disease, gastroenteritis, epigastric pain, fistula, glossitis, hemorrhoids, intestinal obstruction, tongue edema, dry mouth, tooth disorder, taste perversion, increased appetite, oral candidiasis.
GU: dysuria, micturition frequency, nocturia, intermenstrual bleeding, menstrual disorder.
Hematologic: leukocytosis, anemia.
Metabolic: *hypercorticism,* hypokalemia, weight gain, ADRENAL INSUFFICIENCY.
Musculoskeletal: back pain, aggravated arthritis, cramps, myalgia, arthralgia, hypotonia.
Respiratory: *respiratory tract infection,* bronchitis, dyspnea, cough.
Skin: acne, alopecia, dermatitis, eczema, skin disorder, increased sweating, ecchymosis.
Other: flulike syndrome, infection.

Interactions

Drug-drug. *CYP3A4 inhibitors (erythromycin, ketoconazole, indinavir, itraconazole, ritonavir, saquinavir):* May increase the effects of budesonide. If drugs must be given together, monitor patient for signs of hypercorticism and consider reducing budesonide dosage.
Drug-food. *Grapefruit or grapefruit juice:* May increase drug effects. Discourage using together.

Effects on lab test results

• May increase alkaline phosphatase and C-reactive protein levels. May increase or decrease potassium level.
• May increase erythrocyte sedimentation rate and atypical neutrophil and WBC counts. May decrease hemoglobin and hematocrit.

Pharmacokinetics

Absorption: Complete.
Distribution: Drug is 85% to 90% protein-bound.
Metabolism: Drug has extensive first-pass metabolism and is rapidly and extensively biotransformed by CYP 3A4 to two major metabolites that have very little glucocorticoid activity.

Excretion: Excreted in urine and feces as metabolites, which primarily are excreted renally.

Route	Onset	Peak	Duration
P.O.	10 hr	½-10 hr	Unknown

Action

Chemical effect: Drug has significant glucocorticoid effects because of its high affinity for glucocorticoid receptors, which leads to improvement of Crohn's disease.
Therapeutic effect: Alleviates symptoms of Crohn's disease.

Available forms

Capsules: 3 mg

NURSING PROCESS

☜ Assessment
• Assess patient's underlying condition before starting therapy and reassess regularly thereafter.
• Monitor patient's laboratory values regularly. Monitor patient for adverse effects.
• Be alert for signs and symptoms of hypercorticism.
• Evaluate patient's and family's knowledge of drug therapy.

☷ Nursing diagnoses
• Diarrhea caused by underlying Crohn's disease
• Imbalanced nutrition: less than body requirements related to underlying Crohn's disease
• Deficient knowledge related to drug therapy

☰ Planning and implementation
• Patients undergoing surgery or other stressful situations may need systemic glucocorticoid supplementation in addition to budesonide therapy.
• When patients are transferred from systemic glucocorticoid therapy to budesonide, monitor them carefully for signs and symptoms of steroid withdrawal. Taper glucocorticoid therapy when budesonide treatment starts.
• Watch for immunosuppression, especially in patients who haven't had diseases such as chickenpox or measles; these diseases can be fatal in patients who are immunosuppressed or receiving glucocorticoids. Monitor adrenocortical function carefully and reduce dosage cautiously.

• Prevent patient exposure to chickenpox or measles. If patient is exposed to measles, consider therapy with pooled intravenous immunoglobulin (IVIG). If patient develops chickenpox, antiviral treatment and varicella zoster immune globulin (VZIG) may be considered.
• Acute toxicity after overdose is rare.
• Prolonged use of drug may cause hypercorticism (symptoms include swelling of the face and neck, acne, bruising, hirsutism, buffalo hump, and skin striae) and adrenal suppression. Treat with immediate gastric lavage or emesis, followed by supportive and symptomatic therapy. For chronic overdose in serious disease requiring continuous steroid therapy, dosage may be reduced temporarily. Dosage may need to be reduced in patients with moderate-to-severe liver disease if they have increased signs or symptoms of hypercorticism.
Patient teaching
• Tell patient to swallow capsules whole and not to chew or break them.
• Advise patient not to drink grapefruit juice while taking drug.
• Tell patient to notify prescriber immediately if exposed to chickenpox or measles.

☑ Evaluation
• Patient's symptoms of Crohn's disease, including diarrhea and abdominal pain, are relieved.
• Patient's nutrition improves as symptoms improve.
• Patient and family state understanding of drug therapy.

bumetanide
(byoo-MEH-tuh-nighd)
Bumex, Burinex ◇

Pharmacologic class: loop diuretic
Therapeutic class: diuretic
Pregnancy risk category: C

Indications and dosages

▶ **Edema in postoperative edema‡, premenstrual syndrome‡, disseminated cancer‡, heart failure, and hepatic or renal disease.**
Adults: 0.5 to 2 mg P.O. once daily. If diuretic response isn't adequate, give second or third dose at 4- to 5-hour intervals. Maximum dosage

is 10 mg daily. Give parenterally if P.O. use isn't feasible. Usual initial dose is 0.5 to 1 mg given I.V. over 1 to 2 minutes or I.M. If response isn't adequate, give second or third dose at 2- to 3-hour intervals. Maximum dosage is 10 mg daily.

⑤ **Adjust-a-dose:** For patients with severe chronic renal insufficiency, a continuous infusion of 12 mg over 12 hours may be more effective and less toxic than intermittent bolus therapy.

▶ **Hypertension‡.** *Adults:* 0.5 mg P.O. daily. Oral maintenance dose is 1 to 4 mg daily, not to exceed 5 mg P.O. daily.

▶ **Heart failure‡.** *Children:* 0.015 mg/kg every other day to 0.1 mg/kg daily. Use with extreme caution in neonates.

▼ I.V. administration

• Give I.V. doses directly using 21G or 23G needle over 1 to 2 minutes.
• For intermittent infusion, give diluted drug through an intermittent infusion device or piggyback into an I.V. line containing free-flowing compatible solution. Infuse at ordered rate. Continuous infusion not recommended.

Contraindications and precautions

• Contraindicated in patients hypersensitive to drug or sulfonamides (possible cross-sensitivity), in those with anuria or hepatic coma, and in those with severe electrolyte depletion.
• Use cautiously in patients with depressed renal function or hepatic cirrhosis or ascites.
🜄 **Lifespan:** In pregnant women, use cautiously. In breast-feeding women, drug is contraindicated. In children, safety of drug hasn't been established.

Adverse reactions

CNS: dizziness, headache.
CV: volume depletion and dehydration, orthostatic hypotension, ECG changes.
EENT: transient deafness.
GI: nausea.
GU: *renal failure,* nocturia, polyuria, azotemia, frequent urination, oliguria.
Hematologic: *thrombocytopenia.*
Metabolic: hypokalemia; hypochloremic alkalosis; asymptomatic hyperuricemia; fluid and electrolyte imbalances, including dilutional hyponatremia, hypocalcemia, and hypomagne-

semia; hyperglycemia; impaired glucose tolerance.
Musculoskeletal: muscle pain and tenderness.
Skin: rash.

Interactions

Drug-drug. *Aminoglycoside antibiotics:* May potentiate ototoxicity. Use together cautiously.
Antihypertensives: May increase risk of hypotension. Use together cautiously.
Chlorothiazide, chlorthalidone, hydrochlorothiazide, indapamide, metolazone: May cause excessive diuretic response resulting in serious electrolyte abnormalities or dehydration. Adjust dosages carefully while monitoring the patient for excessive diuretic responses.
Digoxin: May increase risk of digitalis toxicity from bumetanide-induced hypokalemia. Monitor potassium and digoxin levels.
Indomethacin, NSAIDs, probenecid: May inhibit diuretic response. Use together cautiously.
Lithium: May decrease lithium clearance, increasing risk of lithium toxicity. Monitor lithium level.
Other potassium-wasting drugs: May increase risk of hypokalemia. Use together cautiously.
Drug-herb. *Licorice:* May contribute to excessive potassium loss. Discourage using together.

Effects on lab test results

• May increase creatinine, urine urea, glucose, and cholesterol levels. May decrease potassium, magnesium, sodium, and calcium levels.
• May decrease platelet count.

Pharmacokinetics

Absorption: After P.O. administration, 85% to 95%; food delays absorption of P.O. dose. Complete after I.M. administration.
Distribution: About 92% to 96% protein-bound; unknown whether drug enters CSF.
Metabolism: Metabolized by liver to at least five metabolites.
Excretion: Excreted in urine (80%) and feces (10% to 20%). *Half-life:* 1 to 1½ hours.

Route	Onset	Peak	Duration
P.O.	30-60 min	1-2 hr	4-6 hr
I.V.	3 min	15-30 min	3½-4 hr
I.M.	40 min	Unknown	Unknown

Action

Chemical effect: Inhibits sodium and chloride reabsorption at ascending portion of loop of Henle.
Therapeutic effect: Promotes sodium and water excretion.

Available forms

Injection: 0.25 mg/ml
Tablets: 0.5 mg, 1 mg, 2 mg

NURSING PROCESS

⚕ Assessment
• Obtain history of patient's urine output, vital signs, electrolyte levels, breath sounds, peripheral edema, and weight before therapy and reassess regularly thereafter.
• Be alert for adverse reactions and drug interactions.
• Evaluate patient's and family's knowledge of drug therapy.

⊞ Nursing diagnoses
• Excess fluid volume related to underlying condition
• Impaired urinary elimination related to therapeutic effect of drug therapy
• Deficient knowledge related to drug therapy

▷ Planning and implementation
• Give P.O. dose with food to prevent GI upset.
• To prevent nocturia, give in morning. If second dose is needed, give in early afternoon.
• The safest and most effective dosage schedule for control of edema is intermittent dosage either given on alternate days or given for 3 to 4 days with 1- or 2-day rest periods.
• Drug can be used safely in patients allergic to furosemide; 1 mg of bumetanide equals 40 mg of furosemide. Bumetanide may be less ototoxic than furosemide, but clinical relevance hasn't been determined.
• If oliguria or azotemia develops or increases, anticipate that prescriber may stop drug.
• Notify prescriber if drug-related hearing changes occur.
Patient teaching
• Advise patient to stand up slowly to prevent dizziness; also, tell him to limit alcohol intake and strenuous exercise in hot weather to avoid exacerbating orthostatic hypotension.

• Teach patient to monitor fluid volume by measuring weight and fluid intake and output daily.
• Advise patient to take drug early in day to avoid sleep interruption caused by nocturia.
• Tell patient with diabetes receiving bumetanide to monitor glucose levels closely.

☑ Evaluation
• Patient is free from edema.
• Patient demonstrates adjustment of lifestyle to deal with altered patterns of urinary elimination.
• Patient and family state understanding of drug therapy.

buprenorphine hydrochloride
(byoo-preh-NOR-feen high-droh-KLOR-ighd)
Buprenex, Subutex

buprenorphine hydrochloride and naloxone hydrochloride dihydrate
Suboxone

Pharmacologic class: opioid agonist-antagonist, opioid partial agonist
Therapeutic class: analgesic
Pregnancy risk category: C
Controlled substance schedule: Buprenex: V; Subutex, Suboxone: III

Indications and dosages

▶ **Moderate to severe pain.** *Adults and children age 13 and older:* 0.3 mg I.M. or slow I.V. q 6 hours, p.r.n., or around-the-clock. May repeat 0.3 mg or increase to 0.6 mg, if needed, 30 to 60 minutes after initial dose.
Children ages 2 to 12: 2 to 6 mcg/kg I.V. or I.M. q 4 to 6 hours.
▶ **Opioid dependence.** *Adults:* 12 to 16 mg Suboxone or Subutex S.L. daily. Maintenance therapy with Suboxone is preferred; target dose is 16 mg/day. Increase or decrease in increments of 2 mg or 4 mg according to withdrawal effects, usual range is 4 to 24 mg.
▶ **Postoperative pain‡.** *Adults:* 25 to 250 mcg/hour I.V. infusion over 48 hours.
▶ **Pain‡.** *Adults:* 60 to 80 mcg epidural injection.
▶ **Circumcision‡.** *Children ages 9 months to 9 years:* 3 mg/kg I.M. with surgical anesthesia.

Reactions may be *common*, uncommon, *life-threatening*, or COMMON AND LIFE-THREATENING.

▼ I.V. administration

● Give by direct I.V. injection into vein or through tubing of free-flowing compatible I.V. solution over at least 2 minutes.

Contraindications and precautions

● Contraindicated in patients hypersensitive to drug.
● Use cautiously in debilitated patients and patients with head injury, intracranial lesions, increased intracranial pressure, or severe respiratory, liver, or kidney impairment. Also use cautiously in patients with CNS depression or coma, thyroid irregularities, adrenal insufficiency, prostatic hyperplasia, urethral stricture, acute alcoholism, alcohol withdrawal syndrome, or kyphoscoliosis.
≋ Lifespan: In pregnant and breast-feeding women and in elderly patients, use cautiously.

Adverse reactions

CNS: *dizziness, sedation,* headache, confusion, nervousness, euphoria, *vertigo,* **increased intracranial pressure,** fatigue, weakness, depression, dreaming, psychosis, slurred speech, paresthesia.
CV: *hypotension,* **bradycardia,** tachycardia, hypertension, Wenckebach block, **cyanosis,** flushing.
EENT: *miosis,* blurred vision, diplopia, visual abnormalities, tinnitus, conjunctivitis.
GI: *nausea,* vomiting, constipation, dry mouth.
GU: urine retention.
Respiratory: **respiratory depression,** hypoventilation, dyspnea.
Skin: *pruritus, diaphoresis.*
Other: *injection site reactions,* chills, withdrawal syndrome.

Interactions

Drug-drug. *CNS depressants, MAO inhibitors:* May have additive effects. Monitor patient.
Opioid analgesics: Possible decreased analgesic effect. Avoid using together.
Drug-lifestyle. *Alcohol use:* May have additive effects. Discourage using together.

Effects on lab test results

● May decrease alkaline phosphatase level.
● May decrease hemoglobin, hematocrit, erythrocyte count, and sedimentation rate.

Pharmacokinetics

Absorption: Rapid.
Distribution: About 96% protein-bound.
Metabolism: Metabolized in liver.
Excretion: Excreted primarily in feces. *Half-life:* 1 to 7 hours. *Combination drug half-life:* Buprenorphine, 37 hours; naloxone, 1 hour.

Route	Onset	Peak	Duration
I.V., I.M.	15 min	1 hr	6 hr
S.L.	Unknown	Unknown	2-8 hr

Action

Chemical effect: Binds with opiate receptors in CNS, altering perception of and emotional response to pain.
Therapeutic effect: Relieves pain.

Available forms

Injection: 0.324 mg (0.3 mg base/ml)
Sublingual: 2 mg, 8 mg
Sublingual (combination): 2 mg buprenorphine and 0.5 mg naloxone, 8 mg buprenorphine and 2 mg naloxone

NURSING PROCESS

⊡ Assessment
● Obtain history of patient's pain.
● Monitor respiratory status frequently for at least 1 hour after administration. Notify prescriber if respiratory depression occurs.
● Evaluate patient's and family's knowledge of drug therapy.

⊞ Nursing diagnoses
● Acute pain related to underlying condition
● Ineffective breathing pattern related to drug-induced respiratory depression
● Deficient knowledge related to drug therapy

▷ Planning and implementation
● Data are insufficient to give single I.M. doses greater than 0.6 mg for long-term use.
● Analgesic potency of 0.3 mg buprenorphine is equal to that of 10 mg morphine and 75 mg meperidine, but buprenorphine has a longer duration of action.
● Notify prescriber if pain isn't relieved.
● If patient's respiratory rate falls below 8 breaths per minute, withhold dose, rouse patient to stimulate breathing, and notify prescriber.

• Naloxone won't completely reverse respiratory depression caused by buprenorphine overdose; mechanical ventilation may be necessary. Doxapram and larger-than-usual doses of naloxone also may be ordered.

• Drug may precipitate withdrawal syndrome in narcotic-dependent patients.

• If dependence occurs, withdrawal symptoms may appear up to 14 days after drug is stopped.

Patient teaching

• Warn ambulatory patient about getting out of bed or walking because of dizziness or hypotension.

• When drug is used postoperatively, encourage patient to turn, cough, and deep-breathe to prevent atelectasis.

• Teach patient to avoid activities that require full alertness.

• Instruct patient to avoid alcohol and other CNS depressants.

☑ Evaluation

• Patient reports pain relief.

• Patient's respiratory status is within normal limits.

• Patient and family state understanding of drug therapy.

---

bupropion hydrochloride

(byoo-PROH-pee-on high-droh-KLOR-ighd)
Wellbutrin, Wellbutrin SR, Wellbutrin XL, Zyban

Pharmacologic class: aminoketone
Therapeutic class: antidepressant, aid to smoking cessation
Pregnancy risk category: B

Indications and dosages

▶ **Depression.** *Adults:* 100 mg immediate-release P.O. b.i.d. initially, increased after 3 days to 100 mg P.O. t.i.d., if needed. If no response occurs after several weeks of therapy, dosage increased to 150 mg t.i.d. Don't exceed 150 mg for a single dose. Allow at least 6 hours between successive doses. Maximum, 450 mg daily. Or, initially, 150 mg sustained-release P.O. q morning; increased to target dose of 150 mg P.O. b.i.d. as tolerated as early as day 4 of dosing. Allow at least 8 hours between successive doses. Maximum, 400 mg daily. Or, initially,

150 mg extended-release P.O. q morning; increased to target dose of 300 mg P.O. daily as tolerated as early as day 4 of dosing. Allow at least 24 hours between successive doses. Maximum, 450 mg daily.

⎆ Adjust-a-dose: For patients with mild to moderate hepatic cirrhosis or renal impairment, reduce dosage. For patients with severe hepatic cirrhosis, don't exceed 75 mg immediate-release P.O. daily; 100 mg sustained-release P.O. daily; 150 mg sustained release P.O. q other day; or 150 mg extended-release P.O. q other day.

▶ **Aid to smoking cessation.** *Adults:* 150 mg Zyban P.O. daily for 3 days; increase to 150 mg P.O. b.i.d. (at least 8 hours apart) (maximum dose). Start therapy while patient is still smoking.

▶ **Attention deficit hyperactivity disorder‡.** *Adults:* 150 mg Wellbutrin P.O. daily with regular-release tablets. Adjust dosage to a maximum of 450 mg P.O. daily.

Contraindications and precautions

• Contraindicated in patients hypersensitive to drug, in those who have taken MAO inhibitors during previous 14 days, and in those with seizure disorders, a history of bulimia, or anorexia nervosa because of a higher risk of seizures. Also contraindicated in patients undergoing abrupt discontinuation of alcohol or sedatives (including benzodiazepines). Don't use Wellbutrin with Zyban or other drugs containing bupropion that are used for smoking cessation.

• Use cautiously in patients with renal or hepatic impairment, and in patients with recent MI or unstable heart disease.

⚖ **Lifespan:** In pregnant women, use cautiously. If drug must be given to breast-feeding woman, breast-feeding should be stopped. In children, safety of drug hasn't been established.

Adverse reactions

CNS: fever, *headache*, akathisia, *seizures*, *agitation*, anxiety, *confusion*, delusions, euphoria, hostility, impaired sleep quality, insomnia, sedation, sensory disturbance, syncope, tremor.
CV: *arrhythmias*, hypertension, hypotension, palpitations, tachycardia.
EENT: auditory disturbance, blurred vision.
GI: dry mouth, taste disturbance, increased appetite, constipation, dyspepsia, nausea, vomiting, anorexia.

Reactions may be *common*, uncommon, *life-threatening*, or COMMON AND LIFE-THREATENING.

GU: impotence, menstrual complaints, urinary frequency.
Metabolic: hyperglycemia, weight gain or loss.
Musculoskeletal: arthritis.
Skin: pruritus, rash, cutaneous temperature disturbance, diaphoresis.
Other: chills, decreased libido.

Interactions

Drug-drug. *Carbamazepine:* May decrease bupropion levels. Monitor patient for loss of therapeutic effect.
Levodopa, MAO inhibitors, phenothiazines, tricyclic antidepressants; recent and rapid withdrawal of benzodiazepines: May increase risk of adverse reactions, including seizures. Monitor patient closely.
Nicotine replacement drugs: May cause hypertension. Monitor blood pressure.
Ritonavir: May increase bupropion levels, increasing toxicity risk. Monitor patient closely.
Drug-lifestyle. *Alcohol use:* May alter seizure threshold. Discourage using together.
Sun exposure: Photosensitivity reactions may occur. Advise patient to wear protective clothing and sunblock and avoid sun exposure.

Effects on lab test results

• May increase or decrease glucose level.
• May decrease platelet count, hemoglobin, and hematocrit. May increase or decrease WBC count.

Pharmacokinetics

Absorption: Unknown.
Distribution: About 80% protein-bound.
Metabolism: Probably metabolized in liver; several active metabolites have been identified.
Excretion: Primarily excreted in urine. *Half-life:* 8 to 24 hours.

Route	Onset	Peak	Duration
P.O.	1-3 wk	2 hr	Unknown
Wellbutrin SR	Unknown	3 hr	Unknown
Wellbutrin XL	Unknown	5 hr	Unknown

Action

Chemical effect: Unknown. Drug isn't a tricyclic antidepressant, doesn't inhibit MAO, and is a weak inhibitor of norepinephrine, dopamine, and serotonin reuptake. May work through noradrenergic, dopaminergic, or both mechanisms.

Therapeutic effect: Relieves depression; smoking deterrent.

Available forms

Tablets (extended-release): 150 mg, 300 mg
Tablets (immediate-release): 75 mg, 100 mg
Tablets (sustained-release): 100 mg, 150 mg, 200 mg

NURSING PROCESS

⚕ Assessment

• Obtain history of patient's condition before therapy and reassess regularly thereafter.
• Be alert for adverse reactions and drug interactions.
• Monitor patient with history of bipolar disorder closely. Antidepressants can cause manic episodes during depressed phase of bipolar disorder.
• Evaluate patient's and family's knowledge of drug therapy.

⊕ Nursing diagnoses

• Ineffective individual coping related to underlying condition
• Risk for injury related to drug-induced adverse CNS reactions
• Deficient knowledge related to drug therapy

▷ Planning and implementation

③ **ALERT:** Risk of seizure may be minimized by not exceeding 450 mg/day (immediate-release) and by giving drug daily in three equally divided doses. Increases in doses shouldn't exceed 100 mg/day in a 3-day period. For sustained-release formulations, don't exceed 400 mg/day and give drug daily in two equally divided doses. Increases in doses shouldn't exceed 200 mg/day in a 3-day period. Patients who experience seizures often have predisposing factors, including history of head trauma, prior seizures, or CNS tumors, or they may be taking a drug that lowers seizure threshold.
③ **ALERT:** Don't confuse bupropion with buspirone.
• Make sure patient has swallowed dose.
• Patient may experience period of increased restlessness, agitation, insomnia, and anxiety, especially at beginning of therapy.
• For smoking cessation, begin therapy while patient is still smoking; about 1 week is needed to achieve steady state levels of drug. Patient

should stop smoking during the second week of treatment. Course of treatment is usually 7 to 12 weeks.

Patient teaching
• Advise patient to take drug as scheduled and to take each day's dose in three divided doses (immediate-release) or two divided doses (sustained-release) to minimize risk of seizures.
• Tell patient to avoid alcohol while taking drug because alcohol may contribute to development of seizures.
• Advise patient to avoid hazardous activities that require alertness and good psychomotor coordination until CNS effects of drug are known.
⑤ **ALERT:** Advise patient not to take Wellbutrin with Zyban and to seek medical advice before taking other prescription drugs, OTC medications, or herbal remedies.
• Tell patient not to crush, chew, or divide sustained-release tablets.

☑ Evaluation
• Patient's behavior and communication indicate improvement of depression.
• Patient doesn't experience injury from drug-induced adverse CNS reactions.
• Patient and family state understanding of drug therapy.

buspirone hydrochloride
(byoo-SPEER-ohn high-droh-KLOR-ighd)
BuSpar

Pharmacologic class: azaspirodecanedione derivative
Therapeutic class: anxiolytic
Pregnancy risk category: B

Indications and dosages

▶ **Anxiety disorders, short-term relief of anxiety.** *Adults:* Initially, 5 mg P.O. t.i.d. Increase dosage at 2- to 4-day intervals in 5-mg/day increments. Usual maintenance dosage is 15 to 30 mg daily in two or three divided doses. Don't exceed 60 mg daily.
Ⓢ **Adjust-a-dose:** When given with a CYP 3A4 inhibitor, lower initial dosage to 2.5 mg P.O. b.i.d. Subsequent dosage adjustment of either drug also may be needed.

Contraindications and precautions

• Contraindicated in patients hypersensitive to drug and in those who have taken an MAO inhibitor within 14 days.
• Use cautiously in patients with hepatic or renal failure.
⚖ **Lifespan:** In pregnant women, use cautiously. In breast-feeding women, avoid use. In children, safety of drug hasn't been established.

Adverse reactions

CNS: *dizziness, drowsiness,* nervousness, excitement, insomnia, headache, fatigue.
GI: dry mouth, nausea, diarrhea.

Interactions

Drug-drug. *CNS depressants:* May increase CNS depression. Avoid using together.
MAO inhibitors: May elevate blood pressure. Avoid using together.
Drug-lifestyle. *Alcohol use:* May increase CNS depression. Discourage using together.

Effects on lab test results

• May increase aminotransferase level.
• May decrease WBC and platelet counts.

Pharmacokinetics

Absorption: Rapidly and completely absorbed, but extensive first-pass metabolism limits absolute bioavailability to between 1% and 13% of P.O. dose. Food slows absorption but increases amount of unchanged drug in systemic circulation.
Distribution: 95% protein-bound; doesn't displace other highly protein-bound medications.
Metabolism: In liver.
Excretion: 29% to 63% excreted in urine in 24 hours, primarily as metabolites; 18% to 38% excreted in feces. *Half-life:* 2 to 3 hours.

Route	Onset	Peak	Duration
P.O.	Unknown	40-90 min	Unknown

Action

Chemical effect: Unknown; may inhibit neuronal firing and reduce serotonin turnover in cortical, amygdaloid, and septohippocampal tissue.
Therapeutic effect: Relieves anxiety.

Available forms

Tablets: 5 mg, 10 mg, 15 mg

Assessment
• Obtain history of patient's anxiety before therapy and reassess regularly thereafter.
• Signs of improvement usually appear within 7 to 10 days; optimal results occur after 3 to 4 weeks of therapy.
• Be alert for adverse reactions and drug interactions.
• Evaluate patient's and family's knowledge of drug therapy.

Nursing diagnoses
• Anxiety related to underlying condition
• Fatigue related to drug-induced adverse reactions
• Deficient knowledge related to drug therapy

Planning and implementation
• Although drug has shown no potential for abuse and hasn't been classified as a controlled substance, it isn't recommended for relief from everyday stress.
• Before starting therapy in patient already being treated with a benzodiazepine, make sure he doesn't stop benzodiazepine abruptly; withdrawal reaction may occur.
• Give drug with food or milk.
• Dosage may be increased in 2- to 4-day intervals.
Patient teaching
• Tell patient to take drug with food.
• Warn patient to avoid hazardous activities that require alertness and psychomotor coordination until CNS effects of drug are known.
• Review energy-saving measures with patient and family.
• If patient is already being treated with a benzodiazepine, warn him not to abruptly stop it because withdrawal reaction can occur. Teach him how and when benzodiazepine can be withdrawn safely.

Evaluation
• Patient's anxiety is reduced.
• Patient states that energy-saving measures help combat fatigue caused by therapy.
• Patient and family state understanding of drug therapy.

busulfan
(byoo-SUL-fan)
Busulfex, Myleran

Pharmacologic class: alkylating agent (not specific to cell cycle phase)
Therapeutic class: antineoplastic
Pregnancy risk category: D

Indications and dosages

▶ **Palliative treatment of chronic myelocytic (granulocytic) leukemia (CML).** *Adults:* For remission induction, 4 to 8 mg P.O. daily (0.06 mg/kg or 1.8 mg/m^2). For maintenance therapy, 1 to 3 mg P.O. daily. Dosages may vary. *Children:* 0.06 mg/kg or 1.8 mg/m^2 P.O. daily. Dosages may vary.
▶ **For use with cyclophosphamide as a conditioning regimen before allogeneic hematopoietic progenitor cell transplantation for CML.** *Adults:* 0.8 mg/kg of ideal body weight or actual body weight (whichever is lower) by central venous catheter as a 2-hour infusion q 6 hours for 4 consecutive days for a total of 16 doses. Give phenytoin for seizure prophylaxis. Dosages may vary.
▶ **Myelofibrosis‡.** *Adults:* Initially, give 2 to 4 mg P.O. daily, then followed by the same dose 2 to 3 times weekly. Dosages may vary.

Contraindications and precautions

• Contraindicated in patients with drug-resistant CML.
• Use cautiously in patients recently given other myelosuppressive drugs or radiation therapy and in those with depressed neutrophil or platelet count. Because high-dose therapy has been linked to seizures, use such therapy cautiously in patients with history of head trauma or seizures and in patients receiving other drugs that lower seizure threshold.
⚖ **Lifespan:** In pregnant women, use cautiously, if at all. In breast-feeding women, drug is contraindicated.

Adverse reactions

CNS: *fever, headache, asthenia, pain, insomnia, anxiety, dizziness, depression,* delirium, agitation, *encephalopathy, confusion,* hallucination, lethargy, somnolence, *seizures.*

CV: *edema, chest pain, tachycardia, hypertension, hypotension,* **thrombosis,** *vasodilation, heart rhythm abnormalities,* cardiomegaly, *ECG* **abnormalities, heart failure, pericardial effusion.**

EENT: *rhinitis, epistaxis, pharyngitis,* sinusitis, ear disorder, cataracts.

GI: *cheilosis (P.O.); nausea, stomatitis, mucositis, vomiting, anorexia, diarrhea, abdominal pain and enlargement, dyspepsia, constipation, dry mouth, rectal disorder,* **pancreatitis.**

GU: dysuria, *oliguria,* hematuria, hemorrhagic cystitis.

Hematologic: *granulocytopenia,* **thrombocytopenia, leukopenia,** anemia.

Hepatic: *jaundice,* **hepatic necrosis,** hepatomegaly.

Metabolic: *hypomagnesemia, hyperglycemia, hypokalemia, hypocalcemia, hypervolemia, weight gain, hypophosphatemia, hyponatremia.*

Musculoskeletal: *back pain, myalgia, arthralgia.*

Respiratory: *lung disorder, cough, dyspnea,* **irreversible pulmonary fibrosis, alveolar hemorrhage, asthma,** atelectasis, pleural effusion, **hypoxia,** hemoptysis.

Skin: *rash, pruritus, alopecia,* exfoliative dermatitis, erythema nodosum, acne, skin discoloration, *hyperpigmentation,* anhidrosis.

Other: *inflammation at injection site,* Addison-like wasting syndrome, gynecomastia (P.O.); *chills, allergic reaction,* **graft versus host disease, infection,** hiccup.

Interactions

Drug-drug. *Acetaminophen within 72 hours:* May decrease busulfan clearance. Use together cautiously.

Anticoagulants, aspirin: May increase risk of bleeding. Avoid using together.

Cyclophosphamide: May increase risk of cardiac tamponade in patients with thalassemia. Monitor patient.

Itraconazole: May decrease busulfan clearance. Use together cautiously.

Myelosuppressives: May cause increased myelosuppression. Monitor patient.

Other cytotoxic agents that cause pulmonary injury: Additive pulmonary toxicity. Avoid using together.

Phenytoin: May decrease busulfan level. Monitor busulfan levels.

Thioguanine: May cause hepatotoxicity, esophageal varices, or portal hypertension. Use together cautiously.

Effects on lab test results

- May increase glucose, ALT, bilirubin, alkaline phosphatase, creatinine and BUN levels. May decrease magnesium, calcium, potassium, phosphorus, and sodium levels.
- May decrease hemoglobin and WBC and platelet counts.

Pharmacokinetics

Absorption: Well absorbed from GI tract.
Distribution: Unknown.
Metabolism: Metabolized in liver.
Excretion: Cleared rapidly and excreted in urine. *Half-life:* About 2½ hours.

Route	Onset	Peak	Duration
P.O.	1-2 wk	Unknown	Unknown
I.V.	Unknown	Unknown	Unknown

Action

Chemical effect: Unknown; thought to cross-link strands of cellular DNA and interfere with RNA transcription, causing an imbalance of growth that leads to cell death.
Therapeutic effect: Kills selected type of cancer cell.

Available forms

Injection: 6 mg/ml
Tablets: 2 mg

NURSING PROCESS

⌚ Assessment

- Obtain history of patient's underlying neoplastic disease.
- Monitor WBC and platelet counts weekly while patient is receiving drug. WBC count falls about 10 days after the start of therapy and continues to fall for 2 weeks after stopping drug.
- Monitor uric acid level.
- **⚠ ALERT:** Be alert for adverse reactions and drug interactions. Pulmonary fibrosis may occur as late as 4 to 6 months after treatment.
- Evaluate patient's and family's knowledge of drug therapy.

⊕ Nursing diagnoses
• Ineffective health maintenance related to presence of neoplastic disease
• Risk for infection related to drug-induced immunosuppression
• Deficient knowledge related to drug therapy

⊠ Planning and implementation
• Premedicate patient with Dilantin to decrease risk of seizures that can occur with I.V. infusion.
• Follow facility policy regarding preparation and handling of drug. Label as hazardous drug.
• Give drug at same time each day.
• Make sure patient is adequately hydrated.
• Adjust dosage based on patient's weekly WBC counts and temporarily stop drug therapy if severe leukocytopenia develops. Therapeutic effects are often accompanied by toxicity.
• Give with allopurinol in addition to adequate hydration to prevent hyperuricemia with resulting uric acid nephropathy.
Patient teaching
• Warn patient to watch for signs of infection (fever, sore throat, fatigue) and bleeding (easy bruising, nosebleeds, bleeding gums, melena) and to take temperature daily.
ⓢ **ALERT:** Instruct patient to report symptoms of toxicity so that dosage adjustments can be made. Symptoms include persistent cough and progressive dyspnea with alveolar exudate, suggestive of pneumonia.
• Instruct patient to avoid OTC products that contain aspirin.
• Advise woman of childbearing age to avoid becoming pregnant during therapy. Recommend that patient consult with prescriber before becoming pregnant.
• Advise breast-feeding woman to stop breast-feeding because of possible risk of toxicity in infant.

☑ Evaluation
• Patient exhibits positive response to drug therapy.
• Patient remains free from infection.
• Patient and family state understanding of drug therapy.

butorphanol tartrate
(byoo-TOR-fah-nohl TAR-trayt)
Stadol, Stadol NS

Pharmacologic class: opioid agonist-antagonist; opioid partial agonist
Therapeutic class: analgesic, adjunct to anesthesia
Pregnancy risk category: C

Indications and dosages
▶ **Moderate to severe pain.** *Adults:* 0.5 to 2 mg I.V. q 3 to 4 hours, p.r.n. or around-the-clock. Or, 1 to 4 mg I.M. q 3 to 4 hours, p.r.n. or around-the-clock. Maximum 4 mg per dose. Alternatively, 1 mg by nasal spray q 3 to 4 hours (1 spray in one nostril); repeat in 60 to 90 minutes if pain relief is inadequate.
▶ **Labor for pregnant women at full term and in early labor.** *Adults:* 1 to 2 mg I.V. or I.M., repeated after 4 hours, p.r.n.
▶ **Preoperative anesthesia or preanesthesia.** *Adults:* 2 mg I.M. 60 to 90 minutes before surgery.
▶ **Adjunct to balanced anesthesia.** *Adults:* 2 mg I.V. shortly before induction or 0.5 to 1 mg I.V. in increments during anesthesia.
Ⓢ **Adjust-a-dose:** For patients with hepatic or renal impairment and elderly patients, reduce dosage to 50% of the usual parenteral adult dose at 6-hour intervals p.r.n. For nasal spray, the initial dose (1 spray in one nostril) is the same, but repeat dose is in 90 to 120 minutes, if needed. Repeat doses thereafter q 6 hours, p.r.n.

⩔ I.V. administration
• Give drug by direct I.V. injection into vein or into I.V. line containing free-flowing compatible solution.

Contraindications and precautions
• Contraindicated in patients with narcotic addiction; may precipitate withdrawal syndrome. Also contraindicated in patients hypersensitive to drug or to preservative (benzethonium chloride).
• Use cautiously in patients with head injury, increased intracranial pressure, acute MI, ventricular dysfunction, coronary insufficiency, respiratory disease or depression, or renal or hepatic dysfunction. Also use cautiously in patients who

have recently received repeated doses of narcotic analgesic.

⚘ **Lifespan:** In pregnant women, use cautiously, if at all. In breast-feeding women, drug is contraindicated. In children, use cautiously; drug may cause paradoxical excitement.

Adverse reactions

CNS: *sedation, headache, vertigo, floating sensation,* lethargy, *confusion,* nervousness, unusual dreams, agitation, euphoria, hallucinations, flushing, **increased intracranial pressure.**
CV: palpitations, fluctuation in blood pressure.
EENT: diplopia, blurred vision, *nasal congestion* (with nasal spray).
GI: nausea, vomiting, constipation, *dry mouth.*
Respiratory: **respiratory depression.**
Skin: rash, urticaria, *clamminess, excessive sweating.*

Interactions

Drug-drug. *CNS depressants:* May have additive effects. Use together cautiously.
Opioid analgesics: Possible decreased analgesic effect. Avoid using together.
Drug-lifestyle. *Alcohol use:* May have additive depressant effects. Discourage using together.

Effects on lab test results

None reported.

Pharmacokinetics

Absorption: Well absorbed after I.M. administration; unknown after nasal administration.
Distribution: About 80% protein-bound. After I.V. administration, mean volume of distribution is about 500 L. Drug rapidly crosses placenta, and neonatal levels are 0.4 to 1.4 times maternal levels.
Metabolism: Extensively metabolized in liver to inactive metabolites.
Excretion: Excreted in inactive form, mainly by kidneys. About 11% to 14% of parenteral dose excreted in feces. *Half-life:* About 2 to 9¼ hours.

Route	Onset	Peak	Duration
I.V.	2-3 min	½-1 hr	2-4 hr
I.M.	10-30 min	½-1 hr	3-4 hr
Intranasal	≤15 min	1-2 hr	4-5 hr

Action

Chemical effect: Binds with opiate receptors in CNS, altering both perception of and emotional response to pain through unknown mechanism.
Therapeutic effect: Relieves pain and enhances anesthesia.

Available forms

Injection: 1 mg/ml, 2 mg/ml
Nasal spray: 10 mg/ml

NURSING PROCESS

⧉ Assessment
● Obtain history of patient's pain before and after therapy.
● Be alert for adverse reactions and drug interactions.
● Periodically monitor postoperative vital signs and bladder function. Because drug decreases both rate and depth of respirations, monitoring arterial oxygen saturation may aid in assessing respiratory depression.
● Evaluate patient's and family's knowledge of drug therapy.

⧉ Nursing diagnoses
● Acute pain related to underlying condition
● Risk for injury related to drug-induced adverse CNS reactions
● Deficient knowledge related to drug therapy

⧉ Planning and implementation
● For intranasal use, have patient clear nasal passages before giving drug. Shake container. Tilt patient's head slightly backward; insert nozzle into nostril, pointing away from septum. Have patient hold other nostril closed, and then spray while patient inhales gently.
● S.C. route isn't recommended.
● Psychological and physical addiction may occur.
● Notify prescriber and discuss increasing dose or frequency if pain persists.
● Keep opioid antagonist (naloxone) and resuscitative equipment available.
Patient teaching
● Caution ambulatory patient about getting out of bed or walking. Warn outpatient to refrain from driving and performing other activities that require mental alertness until drug's CNS effects are known.

Reactions may be *common,* uncommon, *life-threatening,* or COMMON AND LIFE-THREATENING.

• Warn patient that drug can cause physical and psychological dependence. Tell him to use drug only as directed and that abrupt withdrawal after prolonged use produces intense withdrawal symptoms.

☑ **Evaluation**
• Patient reports relief from pain.
• Patient doesn't experience injury as a result of therapy.
• Patient and family state understanding of drug therapy.

calcitonin (salmon)
(kal-sih-TOH-nin)
Miacalcin, Salmonine

Pharmacologic class: thyroid hormone, calcium and bone metabolism regulator
Therapeutic class: hypocalcemic, bone resorption inhibitor
Pregnancy risk category: C

Indications and dosages

▶ **Paget's disease of bone (osteitis deformans).** *Adults:* Initially, 100 IU daily I.M. or S.C.; maintenance dosage is 50 to 100 IU daily or every other day.
▶ **Hypercalcemia.** *Adults:* 4 IU/kg q 12 hours I.M. or S.C. If response is inadequate after 1 or 2 days, increase dosage to 8 IU/kg I.M. q 12 hours. If response remains unsatisfactory after 2 more days, increase dosage to maximum of 8 IU/kg q 6 hours.
▶ **Postmenopausal osteoporosis.** *Adults:* 100 IU daily I.M. or S.C. Or, 200 IU (one activation) daily intranasally, alternating nostrils daily. Patients should receive adequate vitamin D and calcium supplements.
▶ **Osteogenesis imperfecta‡.** *Adults:* 2 IU/kg S.C. or I.M. three times weekly with daily calcium supplementation.

Contraindications and precautions

• Contraindicated in patients hypersensitive to drug.

☝ **Lifespan:** In pregnant women, use cautiously. In breast-feeding women, don't use because drug may inhibit lactation. In children, safety and efficacy of drug haven't been established.

Adverse reactions

CNS: headache, weakness, dizziness, paresthesia.
CV: facial flushing.
EENT: nasal symptoms (irritation, redness, sores) with intranasal use, *rhinitis,* epistaxis.
GI: transient nausea, unusual taste, diarrhea, anorexia, *nausea with or without vomiting.*
GU: transient diuresis, urinary frequency, nocturia.
Metabolic: hypocalcemia, hyperglycemia, hyperthyroidism.
Musculoskeletal: back pain, arthralgia.
Skin: rash.
Other: hand swelling, tingling, and tenderness; hypersensitivity reactions, *inflammation at injection site,* **anaphylaxis.**

Interactions

None significant.

Effects on lab test results

• May increase glucose level. May decrease calcium level.

Pharmacokinetics

Absorption: Rapid with intranasal use.
Distribution: Unknown; however, calcitonin doesn't cross the placenta.
Metabolism: Rapidly metabolized in kidneys; additional activity in blood and peripheral tissues.
Excretion: Excreted in urine as inactive metabolites. *Half-life:* Calcitonin human, 60 minutes; calcitonin salmon, 43 to 60 minutes.

Route	Onset	Peak	Duration
I.V.	Immediate	Unknown	12 hr
I.M., S.C.	≤ 15 min	≤ 4 hr	8-24 hr
Intranasal	Rapid	30 min	1 hr

Action

Chemical effect: Decreases osteoclastic activity by inhibiting osteocytic osteolysis; decreases mineral release and matrix or collagen breakdown in bone.
Therapeutic effect: Prohibits bone and kidney (tubular) resorption of calcium.

Available forms

Injection: 200 IU/ml, 2-ml ampules
Nasal spray: 200 IU/activation in 2-ml bottle (0.09 ml/dose)

NURSING PROCESS

⚕ Assessment

• Assess patient's calcium level before therapy and regularly thereafter.
• If using nasal spray, assess nasal passages before beginning treatment and periodically thereafter.
• Monitor alkaline phosphatase and 24-hour urine hydroxyproline levels to evaluate drug effectiveness.
• Examine urine sediment periodically.
• Be alert for adverse reactions.
• Evaluate patient's and family's knowledge of drug therapy.

⊕ Nursing diagnoses

• Risk for trauma related to patient's underlying bone condition
• Ineffective protection related to potential for drug-induced anaphylaxis
• Deficient knowledge related to drug therapy

❯ Planning and implementation

• Perform skin test before therapy.
• Give drug h.s. when possible to minimize nausea and vomiting.
• If dose is larger than 2 ml, give it I.M.
• Alternate nostrils daily when using drug intranasally.
• Use freshly reconstituted solution within 2 hours.
• Keep parenteral calcium available during first doses in case hypocalcemic tetany occurs.
• Refrigerate calcitonin salmon at 36° to 46° F (2° to 8° C). Store open nasal spray at room temperature.
• In patients who relapse after a positive initial response, evaluate for antibody response to hormone protein.
• Keep epinephrine handy; systemic allergic reactions may occur because hormone is protein.
• If symptoms have been relieved after 6 months, stop drug until symptoms or radiologic signs recur.
• ⚠ **ALERT:** Don't confuse calcitonin with calcifediol or calcitriol.

Patient teaching

• Teach patient how to take drug S.C., the preferred route for outpatient self-administration.
• Teach patient to activate nasal spray before first use. He should hold bottle upright and depress side arms six times until a faint mist occurs. This signifies that pump is primed and ready for use. He doesn't need to reprime the pump before each use.
• Instruct patient to report signs of nasal irritation with nasal spray.
• Tell patient to handle missed doses as follows: With daily dosing, take as soon as possible, but don't double the dose. With alternate-day dosing, take missed dose as soon as possible, and then restart alternate days from this dose.
• Remind patient with postmenopausal osteoporosis to take adequate calcium and vitamin D supplements.

☑ Evaluation

• Patient's calcium level is normal.
• Patient doesn't experience anaphylaxis.
• Patient and family state understanding of drug therapy.

calcitriol (1,25-dihydroxycholecalciferol)
(kal-SIH-try-ohl)
Calcijex, Rocaltrol

Pharmacologic class: vitamin D analogue
Therapeutic class: antihypocalcemic
Pregnancy risk category: C

Indications and dosages

❯ **Hypocalcemia in patients undergoing long-term dialysis.** *Adults:* Initially, 0.25 mcg P.O. daily. Increase by 0.25 mcg daily at 4- to 8-week intervals. Maintenance dosage is 0.25 mcg q other day up to 1.25 mcg daily, or 1 to 2 mcg I.V. three times weekly about q other day. Dosages from 0.5 to 4 mcg three times weekly have been used initially. If response to initial dose is inadequate, may increase by 0.5 to 1 mcg at 2- to 4-week intervals. Maintenance dosage is 0.5 to 3 mcg I.V. three times weekly.

► **Hypoparathyroidism and pseudohypoparathyroidism.** *Adults and children age 6 and older:* Initially, 0.25 mcg P.O. daily. Increase dosage at 2- to 4-week intervals. Maintenance dosage is 0.25 to 2 mcg daily.

► **Hypoparathyroidism.** *Children and infants ages 1 to 5:* 0.25 to 0.75 mcg P.O. daily.

► **Management of secondary hyperparathyroidism and resulting metabolic bone disease in predialysis patients (moderate-to-severe chronic renal impairment with creatinine clearance of 15 to 55 ml/minute).** *Adults and children age 3 and older:* Initially, 0.25 mcg P.O. daily. Increase dosage to 0.5 mcg daily, if needed.

Children age 3 and younger: Initially, 10 to 15 mcg/kg P.O. daily.

▼ I.V. administration

• For hypocalcemic patients with chronic renal impairment who are undergoing hemodialysis, give I.V. dose by rapid injection via dialysis catheter at end of hemodialysis treatment.
• Store injection at room temperature; avoid excessive heat or freezing.
• Discard unused portions because drug contains no preservatives.

Contraindications and precautions

• Contraindicated in patients with hypercalcemia or vitamin D toxicity.
⚖ Lifespan: In pregnant or breast-feeding women, use cautiously.

Adverse reactions

CNS: headache, somnolence.
EENT: conjunctivitis, photophobia, rhinorrhea.
GI: nausea, vomiting, constipation, metallic taste, dry mouth, anorexia.
GU: polyuria.
Musculoskeletal: weakness, bone and muscle pain.

Interactions

Drug-drug. *Digoxin:* May increase risk of arrhythmias. Avoid using together.
Cholestyramine, colestipol, excessive use of mineral oil: May decrease absorption of orally administered vitamin D analogues. Avoid using together.
Corticosteroids: Counteracts vitamin D analogue effects. Avoid using together.

Ketoconazole: May decrease endogenous calcitriol level. Monitor patient.
Magnesium-containing antacids: May induce hypermagnesemia, especially in patients with chronic renal impairment. Avoid using together.
Phenytoin, phenobarbital: May reduce plasma calcitriol levels. Higher doses of calcitriol may be needed.
Thiazides: May induce hypercalcemia. Monitor calcium levels and patient closely.
Verapamil: May cause atrial fibrillation due to increased risk of hypercalcemia. Monitor levels and patient closely.

Effects on lab test results

• May increase BUN, ALT, AST, albumin, and cholesterol levels.

Pharmacokinetics

Absorption: Absorbed readily.
Distribution: Distributed widely; protein-bound.
Metabolism: Metabolized in liver and kidneys.
Excretion: Excreted primarily in feces. *Half-life:* 3 to 6 hours.

Route	Onset	Peak	Duration
P.O.	2-6 hr	3-6 hr	3-5 days
I.V.	Immediate	Unknown	3-5 days

Action

Chemical effect: Stimulates calcium absorption from GI tract; promotes calcium secretion from bone to blood.
Therapeutic effect: Raises calcium levels.

Available forms

Capsules: 0.25 mcg, 0.5 mcg
Injection: 1 mcg/ml, 2 mcg/ml
Oral solution: 1 mcg/ml

NURSING PROCESS

⬤ Assessment

• Assess patient's calcium level before therapy and reassess regularly thereafter to monitor drug effectiveness; calcium level times phosphate level shouldn't be more than 70. During dosage adjustment, determine calcium level twice weekly.
• Be alert for adverse reactions and drug interactions.

• Evaluate patient's and family's knowledge of drug therapy.

Nursing diagnoses
• Risk for injury related to patient's underlying condition
• Ineffective protection related to potential for drug-induced vitamin D intoxication
• Deficient knowledge related to drug therapy

Planning and implementation
• Keep drug away from heat and light.
• Give drug at same time daily.
• If hypercalcemia occurs, stop drug and notify prescriber; resume drug after calcium level returns to normal. Patient should receive adequate intake of calcium daily.
• Vitamin D intoxication may cause headache, somnolence, weakness, irritability, hypertension, arrhythmias, conjunctivitis, photophobia, rhinorrhea, nausea, vomiting, constipation, polydipsia, pancreatitis, metallic taste, dry mouth, anorexia, nephrocalcinosis, polyuria, nocturia, weight loss, bone and muscle pain, pruritus, hyperthermia, and decreased libido.
ALERT: Don't confuse calcitriol with calcifediol or calcitonin.

Patient teaching
• Tell patient to immediately report early symptoms of vitamin D intoxication, such as weakness, nausea, vomiting, dry mouth, constipation, muscle or bone pain, or metallic taste.
• Instruct patient to adhere to diet and calcium supplements and to avoid OTC drugs and magnesium-containing antacids.
• Warn patient that calcitriol is most potent form of vitamin D available; severe toxicity can occur if ingested by anyone for whom it wasn't prescribed.
• Tell patient to protect medication from light.

Evaluation
• Patient's calcium level is normal.
• Patient doesn't experience injury from drug-induced vitamin D toxicity.
• Patient and family state understanding of drug therapy.

calcium acetate
(KAL-see-um AS-ih-tayt)
Phos-Lo

calcium carbonate
Apo-Cal ◆ †, Cal-Carb-HD†, Calci-Chew†, Calciday 667†, Calci-Mix†, Calcite 500 ◆ †, Calcium 600†, Cal-Plus†, Calsan ◆ †, Caltrate†, Caltrate 600 ◆ †, Chooz†, Fem Cal†, Florical†, Gencalc 600†, Mallamint†, Nephro-Calci ◆, Nu-Cal† ◆, Os-Cal ◆ †, Os-Cal 500†, Os-Cal Chewable ◆ †, Oysco†, Oysco 500 Chewable†, Oyst-Cal 500†, Oystercal 500†, Oyster Shell Calcium-500†, Rolaids Calcium Rich†, Super Calcium 1200†, Titralac†, Tums†, Tums 500 ◆, Tums E-X†

calcium chloride†
Calciject ◆

calcium citrate†
Citrical†, Citrical Liquitabs ◆ †

calcium glubionate†
Calcium-Sandoz ◆, Neo-Calglucon

calcium gluconate

calcium lactate†

calcium phosphate, dibasic†

calcium phosphate, tribasic
Posture†

Pharmacologic class: mineral, cardiotonic
Therapeutic class: calcium supplement
Pregnancy risk category: C

Indications and dosages

▶ **Hypocalcemic emergency.** *Adults:* 7 to 14 mEq calcium I.V. May be given as 10% calcium gluconate solution or 2% to 10% calcium chloride solution.
Children: 1 to 7 mEq calcium I.V.
Infants: Up to 1 mEq calcium I.V.
▶ **Hypocalcemic tetany.** *Adults:* 4.5 to 16 mEq calcium I.V. Repeat until tetany is controlled.
Children: 0.5 to 0.7 mEq/kg calcium I.V. t.i.d. or q.i.d. until tetany is controlled.

Neonates: 2.4 mEq/kg I.V. daily in divided doses.

▶ **Adjunct in cardiac arrest.** *Adults:* 0.027 to 0.054 mEq/kg calcium chloride I.V., or 2.3 to 3.7 mEq calcium gluconate I.V. *Children:* 0.27 mEq/kg calcium chloride I.V., repeated in 10 minutes if needed. Determine calcium levels before giving further doses.

▶ **Adjunct in magnesium intoxication.** *Adults:* Initially, 7 mEq I.V. Base subsequent doses on patient's response.

▶ **During exchange transfusions.** *Adults:* 1.35 mEq with each 100 ml citrated blood. *Neonates:* 0.45 mEq after each 100 ml citrated blood.

▶ **Hyperphosphatemia in end-stage renal failure.** *Adults:* 2 to 4 tablets calcium acetate P.O. with each meal.

▶ **Dietary supplement.** *Adults:* 800 mg to 1.2 g P.O. daily.

▼ I.V. administration

⚠ **ALERT:** Calcium salts aren't interchangeable; verify preparation before use.

• Give calcium chloride and calcium gluconate only by I.V. route.

• When adding calcium chloride to parenteral solutions that contain other additives (especially phosphorus or phosphate), observe solution closely for precipitate. Use in-line filter.

• Monitor ECG when giving calcium I.V. Stop if patient complains of discomfort, and notify prescriber. After injection, make sure patient remains recumbent for 15 minutes.

⚠ **ALERT:** Severe necrosis and tissue sloughing can occur after extravasation. Calcium gluconate is less irritating to veins and tissues than calcium chloride.

Direct injection

• Warm solutions to body temperature before administration.

• Give direct injection slowly through small needle into large vein or through I.V. line containing free-flowing, compatible solution at no more than 1 ml/minute (1.5 mEq/minute) for calcium chloride or 0.5 to 2 ml/minute for calcium gluconate. Don't use scalp veins in children.

Intermittent infusion

• When giving intermittent infusion, infuse diluted solution through I.V. line containing compatible solution. Maximum, 200 mg/minute calcium gluconate.

• Precipitate will form if drug is given I.V. with sodium bicarbonate or other alkaline drugs. Use an in-line filter.

Contraindications and precautions

• Contraindicated in patients with ventricular fibrillation, hypercalcemia, hypophosphatemia, or renal calculi.

• Use all calcium products cautiously in digitalized patients and in patients with sarcoidosis and renal or cardiac disease.

• Use calcium chloride cautiously in patients with cor pulmonale, respiratory acidosis, and respiratory impairment.

⚖ **Lifespan:** In children, use I.V. drug cautiously.

Adverse reactions

CNS: pain, tingling sensations, sense of oppression or heat waves with I.V. use; syncope with rapid I.V. injection.

CV: mild decrease in blood pressure; vasodilation, *bradycardia, arrhythmias,* and *cardiac arrest* with rapid I.V. injection.

GI: irritation, *hemorrhage,* constipation with oral use; chalky taste with I.V. use; hemorrhage, nausea, vomiting, thirst, abdominal pain with oral calcium chloride.

GU: hypercalcemia, polyuria, renal calculi.

Skin: local reactions including burning, necrosis, tissue sloughing, cellulitis, soft-tissue calcification with I.M. use.

Other: irritation (with S.C. injection); *vein irritation* with I.V. use.

Interactions

Drug-drug. *Atenolol, tetracyclines:* May decrease bioavailability of these drugs and calcium when oral forms are taken together. Separate administration times.

Calcium channel blockers: May decrease calcium effectiveness. Avoid using together.

Digoxin: May increase digitalis toxicity. Give calcium cautiously (if at all) to digitalized patients.

Ciprofloxacin, gatifloxacin, levofloxacin, lomefloxacin, moxifloxacin, norfloxacin, ofloxacin: Calcium carbonate may decrease effects of quinolone. Give antacid at least 6 hours before or 2 hours after the quinolone.

Sodium polystyrene sulfonate: May increase risk of metabolic acidosis in patients with renal disease. Avoid using together in patients with renal disease.

Thiazide diuretics: May increase risk of hypercalcemia. Avoid using together.

Thyroid hormone: Calcium may inhibit the absorption of thyroid drugs. Separate administration times by at least 2 hours.

Drug-food. *Foods containing oxalic acid (rhubarb, spinach), phytic acid (bran, whole cereals), or phosphorus (milk, dairy products):* May interfere with calcium absorption. Tell patient to avoid these foods.

Effects on lab test results

• May increase calcium and 11-hydroxycorticosteroid levels.

• May produce false-negative values for serum and urinary magnesium as measured by the Titan yellow method.

Pharmacokinetics

Absorption: Absorbed actively in GI tract. Pregnancy and reduced calcium intake may enhance absorption. Vitamin D in active form is required for absorption.

Distribution: Enters extracellular fluid and is incorporated rapidly into skeletal tissue. Bone contains 99% of total calcium; 1% is distributed equally between intracellular and extracellular fluids. Levels in CSF are about half those in serum.

Metabolism: Insignificant.

Excretion: Excreted mainly in feces, minimally in urine. *Half-life:* Unknown.

Route	Onset	Peak	Duration
P.O.	Unknown	Unknown	Unknown
I.V.	Immediate	Immediate	½-2 hr

Action

Chemical effect: Replaces and maintains calcium.

Therapeutic effect: Raises calcium level.

Available forms

calcium acetate
Contains 253 mg or 12.7 mEq of elemental calcium/g
Injection: 0.5 mEq Ca‡ per ml
Tablets: 250 mg†, 500 mg†, 667 mg, 668 mg†, 1,000 mg†

calcium carbonate
Contains 400 mg or 20 mEq of elemental calcium/g
Capsules: 364 mg†, 1.25 g†
Oral suspension: 1.25 g/5 ml†
Powder packets: 6.5 g (2,400 mg calcium) per packet†
Tablets: 650 mg†, 667 mg†, 750 mg†, 1.25 g†, 1.5 g†
Tablets (chewable): 350 mg†, 420 mg†, 500 mg†, 625 mg†, 750 mg†, 850 mg†, 1.25 g†

calcium chloride
Contains 270 mg or 13.5 mEq of elemental calcium/g
Injection: 10% solution in 10-ml ampules, vials, and syringes

calcium citrate
Contains 211 mg or 10.6 mEq of elemental calcium/g
Effervescent tablets: 2,376 mg†
Tablets: 950 mg†

calcium glubionate
Contains 64 mg or 3.2 mEq of elemental calcium/g
Syrup: 1.8 g/5 ml

calcium gluconate
Contains 90 mg or 4.5 mEq of elemental calcium/g
Injection: 10% solution in 10-ml ampules and vials, 10-ml or 50-ml vials
Tablets: 500 mg†, 650 mg†, 975 mg†, 1 g†

calcium lactate
Contains 130 mg or 6.5 mEq of elemental calcium/g
Tablets: 325 mg, 650 mg

calcium phosphate, dibasic
Contains 230 mg or 11.5 mEq of elemental calcium/g
Tablets: 468 mg†

calcium phosphate, tribasic
Contains 400 mg or 20 mEq of elemental calcium/g
Tablets: 600 mg†

NURSING PROCESS

🖎 Assessment

• Assess patient's calcium level before therapy and reassess frequently thereafter to monitor drug effectiveness. Hypercalcemia may result after large doses in patients with chronic renal impairment.

- Be alert for adverse reactions and drug interactions.
- Evaluate patient's and family's knowledge of drug therapy.

⊞ Nursing diagnoses
- Ineffective protection related to calcium deficiency
- Risk for injury related to drug-induced adverse reactions
- Deficient knowledge related to drug therapy

▶ Planning and implementation
- If GI upset occurs, give oral calcium products 1 to 1½ hours after meals.
- If hypercalcemia occurs, withhold drug and notify prescriber. Provide emergency supportive care as needed until calcium level returns to normal.
- Signs and symptoms of severe hypercalcemia may include stupor, confusion, delirium, and coma. Signs and symptoms of mild hypercalcemia may include anorexia, nausea, and vomiting.
- ⊛ **ALERT:** Make sure prescriber specifies which calcium form to administer because code carts usually contain both calcium gluconate and calcium chloride.

Patient teaching
- Tell patient to take oral calcium 1 to 1½ hours after meals if GI upset occurs.
- ⊛ **ALERT:** Warn patient to avoid oxalic acid (found in rhubarb and spinach), phytic acid (in bran and whole cereals), and phosphorus (in milk and dairy products) because these substances may interfere with calcium absorption.
- Teach patient to recognize and report signs and symptoms of hypercalcemia.
- Stress importance of follow-up care and regular blood samples to monitor calcium level.

✓ Evaluation
- Patient's calcium level is normal.
- Patient doesn't experience injury from calcium-induced adverse reactions.
- Patient and family state understanding of drug therapy.

calcium carbonate
(KAL-see-um KAR-buh-nayt)
Alka-Mints†, Amitone†, Cal-Sup ◊, Chooz†, Equilet†, Mallamint†, Rolaids Calcium Rich†, Titralac†,Titralac Extra Strength†, Titralac Plus†, Tums†, Tums E-X†, Tums Extra Strength†

Pharmacologic class: electrolyte, calcium supplement
Therapeutic class: antacid
Pregnancy risk category: NR

Indications and dosages
▶ **Antacid, calcium supplement.** *Adults:* 350 mg to 1.5 g P.O. or two pieces of chewing gum 1 hour after meals and h.s. p.r.n.

Contraindications and precautions
- Contraindicated in patients with ventricular fibrillation or hypercalcemia.
- Use cautiously, if at all, in patients receiving digoxin and in patients with sarcoidosis and renal or cardiac disease.

Adverse reactions
GI: constipation, gastric distention, flatulence, rebound hyperacidity, nausea.

Interactions
Drug-drug. *Antibiotics (including tetracyclines), hydantoins, iron, isoniazid, salicylates:* May decrease effects of these drugs because of possible impaired absorption. Separate administration times.
Ciprofloxacin, gatifloxacin, levofloxacin, lomefloxacin, moxifloxacin, norfloxacin, ofloxacin: Calcium carbonate may decrease effects of quinolone. Give antacid at least 6 hours before or 2 hours after the quinolone.
Enteric-coated drugs: May release prematurely in stomach. Separate doses by at least 1 hour.
Thyroid hormone: Calcium may inhibit the absorption of thyroid drugs. Separate administration times by at least 2 hours.
Drug-food. *Milk, other foods high in vitamin D:* Possible milk-alkali syndrome (headache, confusion, distaste for food, nausea, vomiting, hy-

percalcemia, hypercalciuria, calcinosis, and hypophosphatemia). Discourage using together.

Effects on lab test results

• May increase calcium level. May decrease phosphate level.

Pharmacokinetics

Absorption: Absorbed actively in small intestine. Pregnancy and reduced calcium intake may enhance absorption. Vitamin D in its active form is required for absorption.
Distribution: Enters extracellular fluid and is incorporated rapidly into skeletal tissue. Bone contains 99% of total calcium; 1% is distributed equally between intracellular and extracellular fluids. Levels in CSF are about half those of serum.
Metabolism: Insignificant.
Excretion: Excreted mainly in feces, minimally in urine. *Half-life:* Unknown.

Route	Onset	Peak	Duration
P.O.			
fasting	≤ 20 min	Unknown	20-60 min
nonfasting	≤ 20 min	Unknown	3 hr

Action

Chemical effect: Reduces total acid load in GI tract, elevates gastric pH to reduce pepsin activity, strengthens gastric mucosal barrier, and increases esophageal sphincter tone.
Therapeutic effect: Raises calcium level and relieves mild gastric discomfort.

Available forms

Contains 40% calcium; 20 mEq calcium/g.
Chewing gum: 500 mg/piece
Lozenges: 600 mg†
Oral suspension: 250 mg/5 ml, 1 g/5 ml†
Tablets: 500 mg†, 600 mg†, 650 mg†, 1,000 mg†, 1,250 mg†
Tablets (chewable): 350 mg†, 420 mg†, 500 mg†, 750 mg, 850 mg, 1,000 mg, 1,250 mg ◊

NURSING PROCESS

Assessment

• Assess patient's underlying condition before therapy and regularly thereafter.

• Monitor calcium level, especially in patient with mild renal impairment.
• Be alert for adverse reactions and drug interactions.
• Evaluate patient's and family's knowledge of drug therapy.

Nursing diagnoses

• Imbalanced nutrition: less than body requirements related to insufficient calcium intake
• Risk for injury related to calcium-induced hypercalcemia
• Deficient knowledge related to drug therapy

Planning and implementation

• Give 1 hour after meals, as needed.
• Make sure patient with calcium deficiency is receiving adequate calcium in diet.
• Give daily oral calcium supplements in 3 or 4 divided doses.
Patient teaching
• Advise patient not to take calcium carbonate indiscriminately or to switch antacids without consulting prescriber.
• Tell patient to take drug 1 hour after meals and at bedtime, as needed.

Evaluation

• Patient's symptoms are alleviated.
• Patient's calcium level is normal.
• Patient and family state understanding of drug therapy.

calcium polycarbophil

(KAL-see-um pah-lee-KAR-boh-fil)
Equalactin†, Fiberall†, FiberCon†, Fiber-Lax†, FiberNorm†, Mitrolan†

Pharmacologic class: hydrophilic drug
Therapeutic class: bulk laxative, antidiarrheal
Pregnancy risk category: NR

Indications and dosages

▶ **Constipation.** *Adults and children age 12 and older:* 1 g P.O. q.i.d. as required. Maximum dosage is 6 g daily.
Children ages 6 to 11: 500 mg P.O. one to three times daily. Maximum dosage is 3 g daily.
Children ages 3 to 5: 500 mg P.O. b.i.d. Maximum dosage is 1.5 g daily. Use must be directed by prescriber.

▶ **Diarrhea related to irritable bowel syndrome; acute nonspecific diarrhea.** *Adults and children age 12 and older:* 1 g P.O. q.i.d. Maximum dosage is 6 g daily.
Children ages 6 to 11: 500 mg P.O. t.i.d. Maximum dosage is 3 g daily.
Children ages 2 to 5: 500 mg P.O. b.i.d. Maximum dosage is 1.5 g daily. Use must be directed by prescriber.

Contraindications and precautions

• Contraindicated in patients with signs of GI obstruction.

Adverse reactions

GI: abdominal fullness, increased flatus, intestinal obstruction.
Other: laxative dependence with long-term or excessive use.

Interactions

Drug-drug. *Tetracyclines:* May impair tetracycline absorption. Avoid using together.

Effects on lab test results

None reported.

Pharmacokinetics

Absorption: None.
Distribution: None.
Metabolism: None.
Excretion: In feces. *Half-life:* Unknown.

Route	Onset	Peak	Duration
P.O.	12-24 hr	≤ 3 days	Varies

Action

Chemical effect: As a laxative, absorbs water and expands to increase bulk and moisture content of stool, which encourages peristalsis and bowel movement. As an antidiarrheal, absorbs free fecal water, thereby producing formed stools.
Therapeutic effect: Relieves constipation; relieves diarrhea caused by irritable bowel syndrome.

Available forms

Tablets: 500 mg†, 625 mg†, 1,250 mg†
Tablets (chewable): 500 mg†

NURSING PROCESS

⚕ Assessment
• Assess patient's bowel condition.
• Before giving drug for constipation, determine whether patient has adequate fluid intake, exercise, and diet.
• Monitor drug effectiveness by evaluating frequency and characteristics of patient's stools.
• Be alert for adverse reactions and drug interactions.
• Evaluate patient's and family's knowledge of drug therapy.

Nursing diagnoses
• Constipation related to underlying condition
• Diarrhea related to irritable bowel syndrome
• Deficient knowledge related to drug therapy

▶ Planning and implementation
• Give drug with full glass of water when used to treat constipation. Don't give drug with water when used for diarrhea.
• Repeat dose every 30 minutes for severe diarrhea, but don't exceed maximum daily dosage.
• Don't give to patient who has signs of GI obstruction.
Patient teaching
• Advise patient to chew Equalactin or Mitrolan tablets thoroughly before swallowing and to drink a full glass of water with each dose. If drug is used as an antidiarrheal, tell patient not to drink water with dose.
• Teach patient about dietary sources of bulk, including bran and other cereals, fresh fruit, and vegetables.
• For severe diarrhea, advise patient to repeat dose every 30 minutes, but tell him not to exceed maximum daily dosage.

✓ Evaluation
• Patient's elimination pattern returns to normal.
• Patient reports improvement of diarrhea.
• Patient and family state understanding of drug therapy.

calfactant
(kal-FAK-tant)
Infasurf

Pharmacologic class: surfactant
Therapeutic class: respiratory distress syndrome (RDS) agent
Pregnancy risk category: NR

Indications and dosages

▶ **Confirmed RDS in neonates less than 72 hours old who need endotracheal intubation, prevention of RDS in premature infants less than 29 weeks' gestational age at high risk for RDS.** *Neonates:* 3 ml/kg body weight at birth intratracheally, given in two aliquots of 1.5 ml/kg each, q 12 hours for total of three doses.

Contraindications and precautions

• None reported.
⚘ **Lifespan:** Indicated for premature infants only.

Adverse reactions

CV: BRADYCARDIA.
Respiratory: AIRWAY OBSTRUCTION, APNEA, *reflux of drug into endotracheal tube, dislodgment of endotracheal tube, hypoventilation, cyanosis.*

Interactions

None significant.

Effects on lab test results

None reported.

Pharmacokinetics

Absorption: Unknown.
Distribution: Unknown.
Metabolism: Unknown.
Excretion: Unknown. *Half-life:* Unknown.

Route	Onset	Peak	Duration
Intratracheal	24-48 hr	Unknown	Unknown

Action

Chemical effect: Nonpyrogenic lung surfactant that modifies alveolar surface tension, thereby stabilizing the alveoli.

Therapeutic effect: Prevents RDS in premature infants or neonates with specific characteristics.

Available forms

Intratracheal suspension: 35 mg phospholipids and 0.65 mg proteins/ml; 6-ml vial

NURSING PROCESS

🔍 Assessment
• Obtain history of patient's underlying condition before therapy and reassess regularly thereafter.
• Monitor patient for reflux of drug into endotracheal tube, cyanosis, bradycardia, or airway obstruction during the dosing procedure. If these developments occur, stop drug and stabilize infant. After infant is stable, resume dosing with appropriate monitoring.
• After giving drug, carefully monitor infant so that oxygen therapy and ventilatory support can be modified in response to improvements in oxygenation and lung compliance.
• Evaluate parents' knowledge of drug therapy.

🔲 Nursing diagnoses
• Risk for injury related to potential for RDS
• Impaired gas exchange related to presence of RDS
• Deficient knowledge related to drug therapy

▷ Planning and implementation
• Give drug under supervision of a prescriber experienced in the acute care of neonates with respiratory impairment who need intubation.
• Drug is intended only for intratracheal use; give for prophylaxis of RDS as soon as possible after birth, preferably within 30 minutes.
• Suspension settles during storage. Gently swirl or agitate the vial to redisperse, but don't shake. Visible flecks in the suspension and foaming at the surface are normal.
• Withdraw dose into a syringe from single-use vial using a 20G or larger needle; avoid excessive foaming.
• Each single-use vial should be used only once; discard unused material after use.
• Give through a side-port adapter into the endotracheal tube. Have two medical personnel present. Give dose in two aliquots of 1.5 ml/kg each. Give while ventilation continues over 20 to 30 breaths for each aliquot, with small bursts timed to occur only during the inspiratory

cycles. Evaluate respiratory status and reposition infant between each aliquot.
- Store drug at 36° to 46° F (2° to 8° C). Don't warm drug before use; it's not needed. Unopened, unused vials that have warmed to room temperature can be returned to refrigerated storage within 24 hours for future use. Avoid repeated warming to room temperature.

Patient teaching
- Explain to parents the reason for using drug to prevent or treat RDS.
- Notify parents that, although infant may improve rapidly after treatment, he may continue to need intubation and mechanical ventilation.
- Notify parents of the potential adverse effects of drug, including bradycardia, reflux into endotracheal tube, airway obstruction, cyanosis, dislodgment of endotracheal tube, and hypoventilation.
- Reassure parents that infant will be carefully monitored.

☑ **Evaluation**
- Premature infant doesn't develop RDS.
- Patient's gas exchange improves because of oxygenation and increased lung compliance.
- Parents state understanding of drug therapy.

candesartan cilexetil
(kan-dih-SAR-ten se-LEKS-ih-til)
Atacand

Pharmacologic class: angiotensin II receptor antagonist
Therapeutic class: antihypertensive
Pregnancy risk category: C (D in second and third trimesters)

Indications and dosages

▶ **Hypertension (alone or with other antihypertensives).** *Adults:* Initially, 16 mg P.O. once daily when used as monotherapy; usual dosage is 8 to 32 mg P.O. daily as single dose or divided b.i.d.

Contraindications and precautions

- Contraindicated in patients hypersensitive to drug or its components.
- Use cautiously in patients whose renal function depends on the renin-angiotensin-aldosterone system (such as patients with heart failure) because of risk of oliguria and progressive azotemia with acute renal impairment or death. Also use cautiously in patients who are volume- or salt-depleted because of risk of symptomatic hypotension.

⚖ **Lifespan:** In pregnant women, don't use because drug acts directly on the renin-angiotensin system and may cause fetal and neonatal harm and death. If drug is absolutely necessary, limit to first trimester. If pregnancy is suspected, stop drug. Breast-feeding women should either stop breast-feeding or the drug.

Adverse reactions

CNS: dizziness, fatigue, headache.
CV: chest pain, peripheral edema.
EENT: pharyngitis, rhinitis, sinusitis.
GI: abdominal pain, diarrhea, nausea, vomiting.
GU: albuminuria.
Musculoskeletal: arthralgia, back pain.
Respiratory: cough, bronchitis, upper respiratory tract infection.

Interactions

None reported.

Effects on lab test results

- May decrease hemoglobin and hematocrit.

Pharmacokinetics

Absorption: Absolute bioavailability is about 15%.
Distribution: More than 99% binds to plasma protein and doesn't penetrate RBCs.
Metabolism: Rapidly and completely bioactivated by ester hydrolysis to candesartan.
Excretion: About 33% is recovered in urine (26% unchanged) and 67% in feces. *Half-life:* 9 hours.

Route	Onset	Peak	Duration
P.O.	Unknown	3-4 hr	24 hr

Action

Chemical effect: Inhibits the vasoconstrictive action of angiotensin II by blocking the angiotensin II receptor on the surface of vascular smooth muscle and other tissue cells.
Therapeutic effect: Dilates blood vessels and decreases blood pressure.

Available forms

Tablets: 4 mg, 8 mg, 16 mg, 32 mg

Rapid onset   *Liquid form contains alcohol.   ◆ Canada   ◇ Australia   †OTC   ‡Off-label use

🗟 Assessment
• Monitor patient's electrolytes, and assess patient for volume or salt depletion (as from vigorous diuretic use) before starting drug.
• Carefully monitor therapeutic response and adverse reactions, especially in elderly patients and patients with renal impairment.
• Evaluate patient's and family's knowledge of drug therapy.

🔁 Nursing diagnoses
• Decreased cardiac output related to risk for symptomatic hypotension in volume- or salt-depleted patients
• Risk for imbalanced fluid volume in patients with impaired renal function related to drug-induced oliguria
• Deficient knowledge related to drug therapy

⧁ Planning and implementation
• Make sure patient is adequately hydrated before starting therapy.
• Observe patient for hypotension. If it occurs after a dose, place patient in supine position and, if needed, give an I.V. infusion of normal saline solution.
• Most of antihypertensive effect occurs within 2 weeks. Maximal antihypertensive effect is obtained within 4 to 6 weeks. If blood pressure isn't controlled by drug alone, add diuretic.
• Drug can't be removed by hemodialysis.
Patient teaching
• Advise woman of childbearing age about risk of second- and third-trimester exposure to drug. If pregnancy is suspected, tell her to notify prescriber immediately.
• Tell patient to report adverse reactions promptly.
• Instruct patient to take drug exactly as directed.
• Tell patient that drug may be taken without regard to meals.

🗹 Evaluation
• Patient's volume or salt depletion is corrected so that symptomatic hypotension doesn't occur.
• Patient maintains fluid balance.
• Patient and family state understanding of drug therapy.

capecitabine
(kape-SITE-a-been)
Xeloda

Pharmacologic class: fluoropyrimidine carbamate
Therapeutic class: antineoplastic
Pregnancy risk category: D

Indications and dosages

▶ **Metastatic breast cancer resistant to both paclitaxel and an anthracycline-containing chemotherapy regimen or resistant to paclitaxel when further anthracycline therapy isn't indicated; first-line therapy for patients with metastatic colorectal cancer when treatment with fluoropyrimidine therapy alone is preferred; metastatic breast cancer, given with docetaxel after failure of prior anthracycline-containing chemotherapy.**
Adults: 2,500 mg/m² P.O. daily in two divided doses, taken about 12 hours apart and after a meal, for 2 weeks; followed by 1-week rest period. Repeat as an q 3-week cycle. Adjust dosage, based on toxicity. See manufacturer's insert for details on specific dosage reduction.
⧄ **Adjust-a-dose:** For patients with renal impairment, if creatinine clearance is 30 to 50 ml/minute, reduce starting dose by 75%.

Contraindications and precautions
• Contraindicated in patients hypersensitive to 5-fluorouracil (5-FU).
⚖ Lifespan: In pregnant women, use only in life-threatening situations or severe disease for which safer drugs can't be used or are ineffective. Breast-feeding should be stopped during therapy. In children, safety and effectiveness haven't been established. In patients older than age 80, use cautiously because they may have a greater risk of GI adverse effects.

Adverse reactions

CNS: fever, dizziness, fatigue, headache, insomnia, paresthesia, peripheral neuropathy.
CV: edema.
EENT: eye irritation.
GI: diarrhea, nausea, vomiting, stomatitis, abdominal pain, constipation, anorexia, *intestinal obstruction,* dyspepsia.

Hematologic: *neutropenia, thrombocytopenia, leukopenia,* anemia, *lymphopenia.*
Hepatic: hyperbilirubinemia.
Musculoskeletal: myalgia, limb pain, back pain.
Skin: hand-and-foot syndrome, dermatitis, nail disorder, alopecia.
Other: dehydration.

Interactions

Drug-drug. *Leucovorin:* May increase levels of 5-FU with enhanced toxicity. Monitor patient carefully.
Warfarin: May increase risk of bleeding and death. Avoid this combination, monitor PT and INR levels frequently, and adjust warfarin dose, if needed.

Effects on lab test results

• May increase bilirubin level.
• May decrease hemoglobin, hematocrit, and platelet, lymphocyte, and neutrophil counts.

Pharmacokinetics

Absorption: Readily absorbed from the GI tract. Level peaks in 1½ hours; active metabolite level peaks in 2 hours. Food decreases rate and extent of absorption.
Distribution: About 60% is bound to plasma proteins.
Metabolism: Extensively metabolized to 5-FU, an active metabolite.
Excretion: 70% excreted in urine. *Half-life:* About 45 minutes.

Route	Onset	Peak	Duration
P.O.	Unknown	1½-2 hr	Unknown

Action

Chemical effect: Drug is converted to active drug 5-FU, which is metabolized by both normal and tumor cells to metabolites that cause cellular injury via two mechanisms: interference with DNA synthesis to inhibit cell division and interference with RNA processing and protein synthesis.
Therapeutic effect: Inhibits cell growth of selected cancer.

Available forms

Tablets: 150 mg, 500 mg

NURSING PROCESS

⚗ Assessment
• Obtain history of patient's underlying condition before therapy and reassess regularly thereafter.
• Assess patient for coronary artery disease, mild-to-moderate hepatic impairment caused by liver metastases, hyperbilirubinemia, renal insufficiency.
• Monitor PT and INR in patients also taking warfarin; there's an increased risk of bleeding. Patients older than age 60 are also at risk for coagulopathies, even if they aren't on warfarin.
• Monitor patient for severe diarrhea, and notify prescriber if it occurs.
• Monitor patient for hand-and-foot syndrome (numbness, paresthesia, tingling, painless or painful swelling, erythema, desquamation, blistering, and severe pain of hands or feet), hyperbilirubinemia, and severe nausea. If these reactions occur, adjust therapy immediately.
• Evaluate patient's and family's knowledge of drug therapy.

⊕ Nursing diagnoses
• Risk for infection related to adverse effects of drug
• Risk for impaired skin integrity related to potential for hand-and-foot syndrome
• Deficient knowledge related to drug therapy

▷ Planning and implementation
• If diarrhea occurs and patient becomes dehydrated, give fluid and electrolyte replacement. Stop drug immediately until diarrhea resolves or decreases in intensity.
• If hyperbilirubinemia occurs, stop drug.
• Monitor patient carefully for toxicity. To manage toxicity, treat symptoms, interrupt dose, and adjust dosage.
Patient teaching
• Inform patient and family of expected adverse effects of drug, especially nausea, vomiting, diarrhea, and hand-and-foot syndrome (pain, swelling, and redness of hands or feet). Explain that dose will be adjusted.
⚠ **ALERT:** Instruct patient to stop taking drug and to contact prescriber immediately if he develops diarrhea (more than four bowel movements daily or diarrhea at night), vomiting (two to five episodes in 24 hours), nausea, appetite loss or decrease in amount of food taken each day,

stomatitis (pain, redness, swelling or sores in mouth), hand-and-foot syndrome, fever of 100.5° F (38° C) or more, or other evidence of infection.

• Tell patient that most adverse effects improve within 2 or 3 days after stopping drug and that if they don't, he should contact prescriber.

• Tell patient how to take drug. Dosage cycle is usually to take drug for 14 days followed by 7-day rest period. Prescriber determines number of treatment cycles.

• Instruct patient to take drug with water within 30 minutes after breakfast and after dinner.

• If a combination of tablets is prescribed, teach patient importance of correctly identifying the tablets to avoid error.

• For missed doses, instruct patient not to take the missed dose and not to double the next one. Instead, he should continue with regular dosing schedule and check with prescriber.

• Instruct patient to inform prescriber if he's taking folic acid.

☑ **Evaluation**
• Patient doesn't develop infection.
• Patient doesn't develop hand-and-foot syndrome.
• Patient and family state understanding of drug therapy.

captopril
(KAP-toh-pril)
Capoten

Pharmacologic class: ACE inhibitor
Therapeutic class: antihypertensive, adjunct treatment of heart failure and diabetic nephropathy
Pregnancy risk category: C (D in second and third trimesters)

Indications and dosages

▶ **Hypertension.** *Adults:* Initially, 25 mg P.O. b.i.d. or t.i.d. If blood pressure isn't controlled in 1 to 2 weeks, increase dosage to 50 mg b.i.d. or t.i.d. If not controlled after another 1 to 2 weeks, add thiazide diuretic. If blood pressure needs to be reduced further, raise dosage as high as 150 mg t.i.d. while continuing diuretic. Maximum daily dose, 450 mg.

▶ **Heart failure; to reduce risk of death and to slow development of heart failure after MI.** *Adults:* 6.25 to 12.5 mg P.O. t.i.d. initially. Gradually increased to 50 to 100 mg t.i.d. as needed. Maximum daily dose, 450 mg.
▶ **Prevention of diabetic nephropathy.** *Adults:* 25 mg P.O. t.i.d.
▶ **Left ventricular dysfunction after MI.** *Adults:* 6.25 mg P.O. as a single dose 3 days after an MI; then 12.5 mg t.i.d., increasing dosage to 25 mg t.i.d. Target dosage is 50 mg t.i.d.

Contraindications and precautions

• Contraindicated in patients hypersensitive to drug or other ACE inhibitors.
• Use cautiously in patients with renal impairment or serious autoimmune disease (particularly systemic lupus erythematosus), and in patients exposed to other drugs known to affect WBC counts or immune response.
🌑 Lifespan: In pregnant women, use cautiously. If patient becomes pregnant, drug usually is stopped. In breast-feeding women, use cautiously. In children, safety and efficacy of drug haven't been established.

Adverse reactions

CNS: fever, dizziness, fainting.
CV: tachycardia, hypotension, angina pectoris, *heart failure,* pericarditis.
GI: anorexia, dysgeusia.
GU: proteinuria, nephrotic syndrome, membranous glomerulopathy, *renal impairment* (in patients with renal disease or those receiving high dosages), urinary frequency.
Hematologic: *leukopenia, agranulocytosis, pancytopenia, thrombocytopenia.*
Metabolic: *hyperkalemia.*
Respiratory: dry, persistent, tickling, nonproductive cough.
Skin: urticarial rash, maculopapular rash, pruritus.
Other: *angioedema of face and limbs.*

Interactions

Drug-drug. *Antacids:* May decrease captopril effect. Separate administration times.
Digoxin: May increase digoxin level by 15% to 30%. Monitor patient for digitalis toxicity.
Diuretics, other antihypertensives: May increase risk of excessive hypotension. Stop diuretic or lower captopril dosage.

Insulin, oral antidiabetics: May increase risk of hypoglycemia when captopril therapy starts. Monitor patient closely.

Lithium: May increase lithium level and cause lithium toxicity. Monitor patient closely.

NSAIDs: May reduce antihypertensive effect. Monitor blood pressure.

Potassium supplements, potassium-sparing diuretics: May increase risk of hyperkalemia. Avoid these drugs unless hypokalemic levels are confirmed.

Probenecid: May increase captopril level. Avoid using together.

Drug-herb. *Black catechu:* May have additional hypotensive effects of catechu. Discourage using together.

Capsaicin: May worsen cough associated with captopril use. Discourage herb use.

Licorice: May cause sodium retention, which counteracts ACE effects. Monitor blood pressure.

Drug-food. *Any food:* May reduce absorption of drug. Give drug 1 hour before meals.

Effects on lab test results

- May increase alkaline phosphatase, bilirubin, and potassium levels and may cause a transient increase in hepatic enzyme levels.
- May decrease hemoglobin, hematocrit, and WBC, granulocyte, RBC, and platelet counts.

Pharmacokinetics

Absorption: Absorbed through GI tract; food may reduce absorption by up to 40%.

Distribution: Distributed into most body tissues except CNS; 25% to 30% protein-bound.

Metabolism: About 50% metabolized in liver.

Excretion: Excreted primarily in urine, minimally in feces. *Half-life:* Less than 2 hours.

Route	Onset	Peak	Duration
P.O.	15-60 min	30-90 min	6-12 hr

Action

Chemical effect: Thought to inhibit ACE, preventing conversion of angiotensin I to angiotensin II. Reduced formation of angiotensin II decreases peripheral arterial resistance, thus decreasing aldosterone secretion.

Therapeutic effect: Reduces sodium and water retention, lowers blood pressure, and helps improve renal function adversely affected by diabetes.

Available forms

Tablets: 12.5 mg, 25 mg, 50 mg, 100 mg

NURSING PROCESS

✐ Assessment

- Assess patient's underlying condition before therapy and regularly thereafter.
- Monitor blood pressure and pulse rate frequently.
- Monitor WBC and differential counts before therapy, every 2 weeks for first 3 months of therapy, and periodically thereafter.
- Monitor potassium level and renal function (BUN and creatinine clearance levels, urinalysis).
- Be alert for adverse reactions and drug interactions.
- Evaluate patient's and family's knowledge of drug therapy.

🗱 Nursing diagnoses

- Risk for injury related to patient's underlying condition
- Ineffective protection related to drug-induced blood disorder
- Deficient knowledge related to drug therapy

▷ Planning and implementation

- Give 1 hour before meals because food may reduce absorption.
- Because antacids decrease drug's effect, separate administration times.
- If patient develops fever, sore throat, leukopenia, hypotension, or tachycardia, withhold dose and notify prescriber.
- Notify prescriber of abnormal laboratory studies.

Patient teaching

- Instruct patient to take drug 1 hour before meals.
- Inform patient that light-headedness may occur, especially during first few days of therapy. Tell patient to rise slowly to minimize this effect and to report symptoms to prescriber. Tell patient who experiences syncope to stop taking drug and call prescriber immediately.
- Tell patient to use caution in hot weather and during exercise. Inadequate fluid intake, vomiting, diarrhea, and excessive perspiration can lead to light-headedness and syncope.
- Advise patient to report signs of infection, such as fever and sore throat.

• Tell woman to notify prescriber if she becomes pregnant because drug will be stopped.

☑ **Evaluation**
• Patient's underlying condition improves.
• Patient's WBC and differential counts are normal.
• Patient and family state understanding of drug therapy.

carbamazepine
(kar-buh-MEH-zuh-peen)
Apo-Carbamazepine ◆, Atretol, Carbatrol, Epitol, Novo-Carbamaz ◆, Tegretol, Tegretol CR ◆, Tegretol-XR, Teril

Pharmacologic class: iminostilbene derivative
Therapeutic class: anticonvulsant, analgesic
Pregnancy risk category: D

Indications and dosages

▶ **Generalized tonic-clonic and complex partial seizures, mixed seizure patterns.**
Adults and children older than age 12: Initially, 200 mg P.O. b.i.d. for tablets or 100 mg of suspension P.O. q.i.d. Increase at weekly intervals by 200 mg P.O. daily, in divided doses at 6- to 8-hour intervals. Adjust to minimum effective level when control is achieved. Maximum daily dosage, 1 g in children ages 12 to 15, or 1.2 g in patients older than age 15.
Children ages 6 to 12: Initially, 100 mg P.O. b.i.d., or 50 mg of suspension P.O. q.i.d. Increase at weekly intervals by 100 mg P.O. daily. Maximum daily dose is 1 g.
Children younger than age 6: 10 to 20 mg/kg P.O. daily in 2 to 3 divided doses (tablets) or 4 divided doses (suspension). Increase weekly to achieve optimal response. Maximum, 35 mg/kg/day.
▶ **Trigeminal neuralgia.** *Adults:* Initially, 100 mg P.O. b.i.d. or 50 mg of suspension P.O. q.i.d. with meals. Increase by 100 mg q 12 hours for tablets or 50 mg of suspension q.i.d. until pain is relieved. Maximum daily dose is 1,200 mg. Maintenance dosage, 200 to 1,200 mg P.O. daily. Decrease dose to minimum effective level, or stop drug at least once q 3 months.
▶ **Bipolar effective disorder, intermittent explosive disorder‡.** *Adults:* Initially, 200 mg P.O. b.i.d.; increase p.r.n. q 3 to 4 days. Mainte-

nance dosage may range from 600 to 1,600 mg daily.
▶ **Restless leg syndrome‡.** *Adults:* 100 to 300 mg P.O. q h.s.
▶ **Chorea‡.** *Children:* 15 to 25 mg/kg P.O. daily.

Contraindications and precautions

• Contraindicated in patients hypersensitive to drug or tricyclic antidepressants, in patients with previous bone marrow suppression, and within 14 days of MAO inhibitor therapy.
• Use cautiously in patients with mixed seizure disorders because these patients may have increased risk of seizures, usually atypical absence or generalized.
❧ **Lifespan:** In pregnant women, use cautiously. If breast-feeding women must use drug, breast-feeding should be stopped.

Adverse reactions

CNS: fever, dizziness, vertigo, drowsiness, fatigue, ataxia, *worsening of seizures* (usually in patients with mixed seizure disorders, including atypical absence seizures).
CV: *heart failure*, hypertension, hypotension, aggravation of coronary artery disease.
EENT: conjunctivitis, dry mouth and pharynx, blurred vision, diplopia, nystagmus.
GI: nausea, vomiting, abdominal pain, diarrhea, anorexia, stomatitis, glossitis.
GU: urinary frequency, urine retention, impotence, albuminuria, glycosuria.
Hematologic: *aplastic anemia, agranulocytosis,* eosinophilia, leukocytosis, *thrombocytopenia.*
Hepatic: *hepatitis.*
Respiratory: pulmonary hypersensitivity.
Skin: excessive sweating, rash, urticaria, *erythema multiforme, Stevens-Johnson syndrome.*
Other: chills, *water intoxication.*

Interactions

Drug-drug. *Atracurium, cisatracurium, doxacurium, mivacurium, pancuronium, rocuronium, tubocurarine, vecuronium:* May decrease the effects of nondepolarizing muscle relaxant, causing it to be less effective. May need to increase the dose of the nondepolarizing muscle relaxant.
Cimetidine, danazol, diltiazem, macrolides, isoniazid, propoxyphene, valproic acid, verapamil:

May increase carbamazepine level. Use together cautiously.

Clarithromycin, erythromycin, troleandomycin: Metabolism of carbamazepine may be inhibited causing increased levels and risk of toxicity. Avoid using together.

Doxycycline, haloperidol, hormonal contraceptives, phenytoin, tiagabine, theophylline, topiramate, valproate, warfarin: May decrease levels of these drugs. Monitor patient for decreased effect.

Lithium: May increase risk of CNS toxicity of lithium. Avoid using together.

MAO inhibitors: May increase depressant and anticholinergic effects. Don't use together.

Phenobarbital, phenytoin, primidone: May decrease carbamazepine level. Monitor patient for decreased effect.

Drug-herb. *Plantains:* Psyllium seeds may inhibit GI absorption. Discourage using together.

Effects on lab test results

• May increase BUN levels.
• May increase eosinophil count and liver function test values. May decrease hemoglobin, hematocrit, thyroid function test values, and granulocyte, WBC, and platelet counts.

Pharmacokinetics

Absorption: Absorbed slowly from GI tract.
Distribution: Distributed widely throughout body; about 75% protein-bound.
Metabolism: Metabolized by liver to active metabolite; may also induce its own metabolism.
Excretion: 70% in urine and 30% in feces.
Half-life: 25 to 65 hours with single dose; 8 to 29 hours with long-term dosing.

Route	Onset	Peak	Duration
P.O.			
suspension	1 hr-days	1½ hr	Unknown
tablets	1 hr-days	4-12 hr	Unknown

Action

Chemical effect: May stabilize neuronal membranes and limit seizure activity by increasing efflux or decreasing influx of sodium ions across cell membranes in motor cortex during generation of nerve impulses.
Therapeutic effect: Prevents seizure activity; eliminates pain caused by trigeminal neuralgia.

Available forms

Capsules (extended-release): 200 mg, 300 mg
Oral suspension: 100 mg/5 ml
Tablets: 200 mg
Tablets (chewable): 100 mg, 200 mg
Tablets (extended-release): 100 mg, 200 mg, 400 mg

NURSING PROCESS

Assessment

• Assess patient's seizure disorder or trigeminal neuralgia before therapy and regularly thereafter.
• Obtain baseline determinations of urinalysis, BUN level, liver function, CBC, platelet and reticulocyte counts, and iron level. Reassess regularly.
• Monitor drug level and effects closely. Therapeutic level is 4 to 12 mcg/ml.
• Be alert for adverse reactions and drug interactions.
• Evaluate patient's and family's knowledge of drug therapy.

Nursing diagnoses

• Risk for injury related to seizure disorder
• Acute pain related to trigeminal neuralgia
• Deficient knowledge related to drug therapy

Planning and implementation

• Give drug in divided doses, when possible, to maintain consistent blood level.
• Give drug with food to minimize GI distress.
• Shake oral suspension well before measuring dose.
• When giving by NG tube, mix dose with equal volume of water, normal saline solution, or D₅W. Flush tube with 100 ml of diluent after giving dose.
⊛ **ALERT:** When treating seizures or status epilepticus, never stop drug suddenly. If adverse reactions occur, notify prescriber immediately. Increase dosage gradually to minimize adverse reactions.
Patient teaching
• Tell patient to take drug with food to minimize GI distress.
• Tell patient to keep tablets in original container, tightly closed, and away from moisture. Some formulations may harden when exposed to excess moisture, resulting in decreased bioavailability and loss of seizure control.

• Inform patient with trigeminal neuralgia that prescriber may attempt to decrease dosage or withdraw drug every 3 months.

Ⓢ **ALERT:** Tell patient to notify prescriber immediately about fever, sore throat, mouth ulcers, or easy bruising or bleeding.

• Warn patient that drug may cause mild-to-moderate dizziness and drowsiness at first. Advise patient to avoid hazardous activities until effects disappear (usually within 3 to 4 days).

• Advise patient to have periodic eye examinations.

☑ **Evaluation**

• Patient remains free from seizures.

• Patient reports pain relief.

• Patient and family state understanding of drug therapy.

carbidopa and levodopa
(kar-bih-DOH-puh and LEE-vuh-doh-puh)
Sinemet, Sinemet CR

Pharmacologic class: decarboxylase inhibitor–dopamine precursor combination
Therapeutic class: antiparkinsonian
Pregnancy risk category: C

Indications and dosages

▶ **Idiopathic Parkinson's disease, postencephalitic parkinsonism, and symptomatic parkinsonism resulting from carbon monoxide or manganese intoxication.** *Adults:* 1 tablet of 25 mg carbidopa/100 mg levodopa or carbidopa 10 mg/levodopa 100 mg P.O. daily t.i.d. followed by increase of 1 tablet daily or every other day as needed; maximum daily dosage, 8 tablets. 25 mg carbidopa/250 mg levodopa or 10 mg carbidopa/100 mg levodopa tablets are substituted as required to obtain maximum response. Optimum daily dosage must be determined by careful adjustment for each patient. Patients treated with conventional tablets may receive extended-release tablets; dosage is calculated on current levodopa intake. Initially, extended-release tablets given equal to 10% more levodopa per day, increased as needed and tolerated to 30% more levodopa per day. Give in divided doses at intervals of 4 to 8 hours.

Contraindications and precautions

• Contraindicated in patients hypersensitive to drug; in patients with acute angle-closure glaucoma, melanoma, or undiagnosed skin lesions; and within 14 days of MAO inhibitor therapy.

• Use cautiously in patients with severe CV, renal, hepatic, endocrine, or pulmonary disorders; history of peptic ulcer; psychiatric illness; MI with residual arrhythmias; bronchial asthma; emphysema; or well-controlled, chronic, open-angle glaucoma.

⚖ **Lifespan:** In pregnant women, use cautiously. In breast-feeding women, drug is contraindicated. In children, safety and efficacy of drug haven't been established.

Adverse reactions

CNS: choreiform, dystonic, dyskinetic movements; involuntary grimacing, head movements, myoclonic body jerks, ataxia, tremors, muscle twitching; bradykinetic episodes; psychiatric disturbances, memory loss, nervousness, anxiety, disturbing dreams, euphoria, malaise, fatigue, *severe depression, suicidal tendencies,* dementia, delirium, hallucinations.
CV: orthostatic hypotension, *cardiac irregularities,* flushing, hypertension.
EENT: blepharospasm, blurred vision, diplopia, mydriasis or miosis, widening of palpebral fissures, activation of latent Horner's syndrome, oculogyric crises, nasal discharge, excessive salivation.
GI: dry mouth, bitter taste, nausea, vomiting, anorexia, and weight loss at start of therapy; constipation; flatulence; diarrhea; epigastric pain.
GU: urinary frequency, urine retention, urinary incontinence, darkened urine, priapism.
Hematologic: hemolytic anemia.
Hepatic: *hepatotoxicity.*
Respiratory: hyperventilation, hiccups.
Skin: dark perspiration, phlebitis.
Other: excessive and inappropriate sexual behavior.

Interactions

Drug-drug. *Antacids:* May increase absorption of levodopa components. Monitor patient closely.
Antihypertensives: May have additive hypotensive effects. Use together cautiously; monitor blood pressure.

Reactions may be *common,* uncommon, *life-threatening,* or COMMON AND LIFE-THREATENING.

Iron salts: Decreases bioavailability of levodopa and carbidopa. Give iron 1 hour before or 2 hours after giving levodopa and carbidopa.
MAO inhibitors: Increases risk of severe hypertension. Don't use together.
Papaverine, phenytoin: Antagonism of antiparkinsonian actions. Avoid using together.
Phenothiazines, other antipsychotics: May antagonize antiparkinsonian actions. Use together cautiously; monitor for decreased effect.
Drug-herb. *Kava:* Could interfere with action of levodopa and natural dopamine, worsening Parkinson's symptoms. Discourage using together.
Octacosanol: May worsen dyskinesia. Discourage using together.
Drug-food. *Foods high in protein:* May decrease absorption of levodopa. Warn against taking drug with high-protein foods.

Effects on lab test results

• May decrease hemoglobin, hematocrit, and platelet, granulocyte, and WBC counts.
• May falsely increase levels of uric acid, urine ketones, urine catecholamines, and urine vanillylmandelic acid, depending on reagent and test method used.

Pharmacokinetics

Absorption: 40% to 70%.
Distribution: Distributed widely in body tissues except CNS.
Metabolism: Carbidopa isn't metabolized extensively. It inhibits metabolism of levodopa in GI tract, thus increasing its absorption from GI tract and its concentration in plasma.
Excretion: 30% of dose excreted unchanged in urine within 24 hours. When given with carbidopa, amount of levodopa excreted unchanged in urine is increased by about 6%. *Half-life:* 1 to 2 hours.

Route	Onset	Peak	Duration
P.O.			
regular-release	Unknown	40 min	Unknown
extended-release	Unknown	2½ hr	Unknown

Action

Chemical effect: Unknown for levodopa. May be decarboxylated to dopamine, countering depletion of striatal dopamine in extrapyramidal

centers. Carbidopa inhibits peripheral decarboxylation of levodopa without affecting levodopa's metabolism within CNS. Therefore, more levodopa is available to be decarboxylated to dopamine in brain.
Therapeutic effect: Improves voluntary movement.

Available forms

Tablets: carbidopa 10 mg with levodopa 100 mg (Sinemet 10-100), carbidopa 25 mg with levodopa 100 mg (Sinemet 25-100), carbidopa 25 mg with levodopa 250 mg (Sinemet 25-250)
Tablets (extended-release): carbidopa 25 mg with levodopa 100 mg, carbidopa 50 mg with levodopa 200 mg (Sinemet CR)

NURSING PROCESS

⫶ Assessment

• Assess patient's underlying condition before therapy and regularly thereafter; therapeutic response usually follows each dose and disappears within 5 hours; may vary considerably.
• Be alert for adverse reactions and drug interactions.
⊗ **ALERT:** Immediately report muscle twitching and blepharospasm, which may be early signs of drug overdose.
• Test patients receiving long-term therapy regularly for diabetes and acromegaly and perform periodic tests of liver, renal, and hematopoietic function.
• Evaluate patient's and family's knowledge of drug therapy.

⫶ Nursing diagnoses

• Impaired physical mobility related to underlying parkinsonian syndrome
• Disturbed thought processes related to drug-induced CNS adverse reactions
• Deficient knowledge related to drug therapy

⫶ Planning and implementation

• If patient is being treated with levodopa, stop this drug at least 8 hours before starting carbidopa and levodopa.
• Give drug with food to minimize adverse GI reactions.
• Adjust dosage according to patient's response and tolerance.

• If vital signs or mental status change significantly, withhold dose and notify prescriber, then reduce dosage or stop the drug, as needed.
• Be aware of patients with open-angle glaucoma and treat with caution. Monitor patient closely. Watch for change in intraocular pressure and arrange for periodic eye exams.

Patient teaching
• Tell patient to take drug with food to minimize GI upset.
• Caution patient and family not to increase dosage without prescriber's orders.
• Warn patient of possible dizziness and orthostatic hypotension, especially at start of therapy. Tell patient to change positions slowly and to dangle legs before getting out of bed. Elastic stockings may control this adverse reaction in some patients.
• Instruct patient to report adverse reactions and therapeutic effects.
• Inform patient that pyridoxine (vitamin B$_6$) doesn't reverse beneficial effects of carbidopa-levodopa. Multivitamins can be taken without losing control of symptoms.

☑ Evaluation
• Patient exhibits improved mobility with reduction of muscular rigidity and tremor.
• Patient remains mentally alert.
• Patient and family state understanding of drug therapy.

carbidopa, levodopa, and entacapone
(kar-bih-DOH-puh, LEE-vuh-doh-puh, and en-TAH-kah-pohn)
Stalevo

Pharmacologic class: decarboxylase, COMT inhibitor, and dopamine precursor combination
Therapeutic class: antiparkinsonian
Pregnancy risk category: C

Indications and dosages

▶ **Idiopathic parkinsonism.** *Adults:* The optimum daily dosage must be individualized and adjusted according to response by careful adjustment in each patient. For maintenance dosing, reduce the total daily dosage by either decreasing the strength of this drug or by decreasing the frequency by extending the time between doses. When more levodopa is required, give the next higher strength of this drug or increase the frequency, up to the maximum of 8 doses daily, not to exceed the maximum daily dose.

Contraindications and precautions

• Contraindicated in patients hypersensitive to drug or its components and in patients with narrow-angle glaucoma, suspicious undiagnosed skin lesions, or a history of melanoma. Also contraindicated within 14 days of MAO inhibitor therapy.
• Use cautiously in patients with liver, renal, or endocrine disease or biliary obstruction. Also use cautiously in patients with past or current psychosis, severe CV or pulmonary disease, bronchial asthma, or history of MI with residual arrhytmias.
• Patients with chronic wide-angle glaucoma may be treated if the intraocular pressure is well controlled.
▲ **Lifespan:** In pregnant women, use only if the potential benefit justifies the risk to the fetus. In breast-feeding women, use cautiously. In children, safety and efficacy haven't been established.

Adverse reactions

CNS: hallucinations, agitation, anxiety, asthenia, dizziness, *dyskinesia*, fatigue, *hyperkinesia*, hypokinesia, **neuroleptic malignant syndrome**, somnolence, syncope.
CV: hypotension, chest pain.
GI: *nausea, diarrhea,* abdominal pain, constipation, vomiting, dry mouth, dyspepsia, flatulence, gastritis, gastrointestinal disorder, taste.
GU: *urine discoloration,* **nephrotoxicity.**
Hematologic: anemia, *agranulocytosis, thrombocytopenia, leukopenia.*
Musculoskeletal: back pain.
Respiratory: dyspnea.
Skin: sweating.
Other: bacterial infection.

Interactions

Drug-drug. *Antihypertensives:* May cause postural hypotension. Adjust antihypertensive dose, as needed.
Dopamine D2 receptor antagonists (such as phenothiazines, butyrophenones, risperidone, metoclopramide, and isoniazid): May reduce

---

the therapeutic effects of levodopa. Avoid using together.

Drugs that interfere with the biliary excretion, glucuronidation, and intestinal beta-glucuronidase, including probenecid, cholestyramine, and some antibiotics (erythromycin, rifampicin, ampicillin, and chloramphenicol): May interfere with entacapone excretion. Use together cautiously.

Drugs metabolized by COMT, such as isoproterenol, epinephrine, norepinephrine, dopamine, dobutamine, alpha-methyldopa, apomorphine, isoetharine, and bitolterol: May cause increased heart rate, arrhythmias, and excessive changes in blood pressure. Use together cautiously.

Iron salts: May reduce the bioavailability of drug. Adjust dose as needed.

Metoclopramide: May increase bioavailability of carbidopa and levodopa by increasing gastric emptying. Adjust dose as necessary.

Nonselective MAO inhibitor: May cause a hypertensive reaction. Don't use within 14 days of each other.

Phenytoin and papaverine: May reduce the effects of carbidopa and levodopa. Avoid using together.

Selegiline: May cause severe hypotension. Avoid using together.

Tricyclic antidepressants: May cause hypertension and dyskinesia. Use together cautiously.

Drug-food. *Foods high in protein, such as legumes, red meat, and liquid protein shakes:* May delay and reduce the absorption of levodopa. Give drug on an empty stomach.

Effects on lab test results

• May increase growth hormone level. May increase or decrease BUN and bilirubin levels.
• May increase liver function test results. May decrease prolactin secretion.
• May cause a positive Coombs' test. May cause a false-positive reaction for urinary ketone bodies when using a test tape.

Pharmacokinetics

Absorption: Varies. Carbidopa level peaks within 2½ to 3½ hours. Levodopa level peaks in 1 and 1½ hours. Entacapone level peaks within 1½ hours.

Distribution: Levodopa and carbidopa are minimally bound to plasma protein. Entacapone is 98% bound to albumin.

Metabolism: Carbidopa is metabolized to two main metabolites. Levodopa is extensively metabolized to various metabolites. Entacapone is almost completely metabolized.

Excretion: Carbidopa, primarily in urine unchanged; entacapone, 10% in urine, 90% in feces; levodopa, unknown. *Half-life:* 1½ to 2 hours, 1 to 5 hours, and 1 to 4 hours, respectively.

Route	Onset	Peak	Duration
P.O.	< 1 hr	1-1½ hr	Unknown

Action

Chemical effect: Levodopa, a dopamine precursor, converts to dopamine in the brain. Carbidopa inhibits the decarboxylation of peripheral levodopa. When given with levodopa, carbidopa permits more intact levodopa to be transported into the brain. Entacapone is a selective and reversible inhibitor of COMT.

Therapeutic effect: Decreases symptoms of Parkinson's disease.

Available forms

Tablets: 12.5 mg carbidopa, 50 mg levodopa, and 200 mg entacapone; 25 mg carbidopa, 100 mg levodopa, and 200 mg entacapone; 37.5 mg carbidopa, 150 mg levodopa, and 200 mg entacapone.

NURSING PROCESS

✒ Assessment

• Periodically evaluate hepatic, hematopoietic, CV, and renal function.
• Monitor patient for mental disturbances such as depression with suicidal tendencies or hallucinations.
• Be alert for adverse reactions and interactions.
• Evaluate patient's and family's knowledge of drug therapy.

⊕ Nursing diagnoses

• Impaired physical mobility related to underlying parkinsonism.
• Risk for injury related to drug-induced adverse reactions.
• Deficient knowledge related to drug therapy.

▷ Planning and implementation

• Patients taking 200 mg entacapone tablet with each dose of standard release carbidopa and levodopa can be switched to the corresponding strength of this drug containing the same amount of levodopa and carbidopa.

• Patients who experience the signs and symptoms of end-of-dose "wearing off" on standard-release carbidopa and levodopa and have a history of moderate or severe dyskinesia or take more than 600 mg of levodopa per day are likely to require a reduction in daily levodopa dose when entacapone is added to their treatment. Adjust dosage individually with carbidopa and levodopa (1:4 ratio) and entacapone and then transfer to a corresponding dose of this drug once the patient is stabilized.

• Don't cut or break tablets.

• If dyskinesia occurs, reduce dosage.

⊗ **ALERT:** If abruptly reducing or stopping drug, especially in a patient also receiving an antipsychotic, observe him carefully for a syndrome resembling neuroleptic malignant syndrome (elevated temperature, muscle rigidity, involuntary movements, altered consciousness, hyperpyrexia, confusion, tachycardia, tachypnea, sweating, and hyper- or hypotension, leukocytosis, myoglobinuria, and increased myoglobin level). Provide symptomatic treatment as needed.

⊗ **ALERT:** Check for overdose by monitoring respiratory, renal, and CV functions. Use supportive measures along with repeated doses of charcoal over time. Also, give I.V. fluids and ensure adequate airway.

Patient teaching

• Advise patient to take drug with food but not with high-protein meals, to minimize GI upset.

• Tell patient to take drug exactly as prescribed.

• Tell patient not to cut or break tablets.

• Warn patient of adverse reactions, such as hallucinations, diarrhea, nausea, and discolored urine and instruct him to notify prescriber if they occur.

• Instruct patient to notify prescriber of any and all drugs taken to prevent any drug interactions.

✓ **Evaluation**

• Patient has improved physical mobility.

• Patient doesn't suffer any injury from adverse reactions.

• Patient and family state understanding of drug therapy.

carboplatin
(KAR-boh-plat-in)
Paraplatin, Paraplatin-AQ ◆

Pharmacologic class: alkylating drug (not specific to cell cycle phase)
Therapeutic class: antineoplastic
Pregnancy risk category: D

Indications and dosages

▶ **Palliative treatment of ovarian cancer.**
Adults: 360 mg/m^2 I.V. on day 1 q 4 weeks; don't repeat doses until platelet count exceeds 100,000/mm^3 and neutrophil count exceeds 2,000/mm^3. Base later doses on blood counts.
⧄ **Adjust-a-dose:** For patients with renal impairment, starting dose is 250 mg/m^2 I.V. in patients with creatinine clearance of 41 to 59 ml/minute or 200 mg/m^2 in those with creatinine clearance of 16 to 40 ml/minute. Recommended dosage adjustments aren't available for patients with creatinine clearance of 15 ml/minute or less.
▶ **Initial treatment of advanced ovarian cancer with cyclophosphamide.** *Adults:* Initial dose is 300 mg/m^2 I.V. on day 1 q 4 weeks for six cycles. Don't repeat cycles until the neutrophil count is greater than or equal to 2,000/mm^3 and the platelet count is greater than or equal to 100,000/mm^3.

▼ I.V. administration

⊗ **ALERT:** Have epinephrine, corticosteroids, and antihistamines available when giving drug because anaphylactoid reactions may occur within minutes of administration.

• Preparing and giving I.V. form is linked to mutagenic, teratogenic, and carcinogenic risks for personnel. Follow facility policy to reduce risks.

• Reconstitute powder for injection with D$_5$W, normal saline solution, or sterile water for injection to make 10 mg/ml. Add 5 ml of diluent to 50-mg vial, 15 ml of diluent to 150-mg vial, or 45 ml of diluent to 450-mg vial. Then, further dilute for infusion with normal saline solution or D$_5$W. Concentration as low as 0.5 mg/ml can be prepared.

• Give drug by continuous or intermittent infusion over at least 15 minutes.

• Don't use needles or I.V. administration sets that contain aluminum to administer carbo-

---

*Reactions may be common, uncommon, **life-threatening**, or **COMMON AND LIFE-THREATENING**.*

platin; precipitation and loss of drug's potency may occur.
• Store unopened vials at room temperature. Once reconstituted and diluted, drug is stable at room temperature for 8 hours; discard unused drug at this time.

Contraindications and precautions

• Contraindicated in patients hypersensitive to cisplatin, platinum-containing compounds, or mannitol. Also contraindicated in patients with severe bone marrow suppression or bleeding.
≈ **Lifespan:** In pregnant women, drug is contraindicated. In breast-feeding women and in children, safety and efficacy of drug haven't been established. In patients older than age 65, use cautiously because they're at greater risk for neurotoxicity.

Adverse reactions

CNS: dizziness, confusion, *peripheral neuropathy, ototoxicity,* CENTRAL NEUROTOXICITY, *CVA.*
CV: *heart failure, embolism.*
GI: constipation, diarrhea, nausea, vomiting.
Hematologic: THROMBOCYTOPENIA, *leukopenia,* NEUTROPENIA, *anemia,* BONE MARROW SUPPRESSION.
Hepatic: *hepatotoxicity.*
Skin: *alopecia.*
Other: *hypersensitivity reactions.*

Interactions

Drug-drug. *Bone marrow depressants, including radiation therapy:* May increase hematologic toxicity. Monitor hematologic studies.
Nephrotoxic agents: May enhance nephrotoxicity of carboplatin. Monitor renal function tests.

Effects on lab test results

• May increase BUN, creatinine, bilirubin, AST, and alkaline phosphatase levels. May decrease magnesium, calcium, potassium, and sodium levels.
• May decrease hemoglobin, hematocrit, and neutrophil, WBC, RBC, and platelet counts.

Pharmacokinetics

Absorption: Administered I.V.
Distribution: Volume distributed is about equal to that of total body water; no significant protein binding occurs.

Metabolism: Hydrolyzed to form hydroxylated and aquated types.
Excretion: 65% excreted by kidneys within 12 hours, 71% within 24 hours. *Half-life:* 5 hours.

Route	Onset	Peak	Duration
I.V.	Unknown	Unknown	Unknown

Action

Chemical effect: Probably produces cross-linking of DNA strands.
Therapeutic effect: Impairs ovarian cancer cell replication.

Available forms

Powder for injection: 50-mg, 150-mg, 450-mg vials
Solution for injection: 50 mg/5 ml, 150 mg/ 15 ml, 450 mg/45 ml

NURSING PROCESS

☑ Assessment
• Assess patient's condition before therapy and regularly thereafter.
• Determine electrolyte, creatinine, and BUN levels; creatinine clearance; CBC; and platelet count before first infusion and before each course of treatment. Lowest WBC and platelet counts usually occur by day 21. Levels usually return to baseline by day 28.
• Be alert for adverse reactions and drug interactions.
• Evaluate patient's and family's knowledge of drug therapy.

⊞ Nursing diagnoses
• Ineffective health maintenance related to ovarian cancer
• Ineffective protection related to drug-induced adverse reactions
• Deficient knowledge related to drug therapy

▷ Planning and implementation
• Check dose against laboratory test results carefully. Only increase dosage once. Don't exceed 125% of starting dose in subsequent doses.
• Bone marrow suppression may be more severe in patients with creatinine clearance below 60 ml/minute; adjust dosage in these patients.
⑤ **ALERT:** Don't repeat dose unless platelet count exceeds 100,000/mm³.

• Provide antiemetic therapy. Carboplatin can produce severe vomiting.

⊛ **ALERT:** Don't confuse carboplatin with cisplatin.

Patient teaching
• Warn patient to watch for signs of infection (fever, sore throat, fatigue) and bleeding (easy bruising, nosebleeds, bleeding gums, melena). Tell patient to take his own temperature daily.
• Instruct patient to avoid OTC products that contain aspirin.
• Advise woman of childbearing age to avoid pregnancy during therapy and to consult prescriber before becoming pregnant.
• Advise breast-feeding patient to stop breast-feeding because of risk of toxicity to infant.

☑ **Evaluation**
• Patient has positive response to carboplatin as evidenced by follow-up diagnostic tests.
• Patient doesn't experience injury from drug therapy.
• Patient and family state understanding of drug therapy.

carboprost tromethamine
(KAR-boh-prost troh-METH-ah-meen)
Hemabate

Pharmacologic class: prostaglandin
Therapeutic class: oxytocic
Pregnancy risk category: C

Indications and dosages

▶ **Abortion between 13th and 20th weeks of gestation.** *Women:* Initially, 250 mcg deep I.M. Give subsequent doses of 250 mcg at intervals of 1½ to 3½ hours, depending on uterine response. Increase dosage in increments to 500 mcg if contractility is inadequate after several 250-mcg doses. Total dose shouldn't exceed 12 mg.

▶ **Postpartum hemorrhage caused by uterine atony not managed by conventional methods.** *Women:* 250 mcg by deep I.M. injection. Give repeat doses at 15- to 90-minute intervals, p.r.n. Maximum total dose, 2 mg.

Contraindications and precautions

• Contraindicated in women hypersensitive to drug and in those with acute pelvic inflammatory disease or active cardiac, pulmonary, renal, or hepatic disease.

• Use cautiously in women with history of asthma; hypotension; hypertension; CV, adrenal, renal, or hepatic disease; anemia; jaundice; diabetes; seizure disorders; or previous uterine surgery.

⚝ **Lifespan:** No contraindications or precautions reported.

Adverse reactions

CNS: *fever,* headache, anxiety, paresthesia, syncope, weakness.
CV: *arrhythmias,* flushing.
GI: *vomiting, diarrhea,* nausea.
GU: *uterine rupture.*
Skin: rash, diaphoresis.
Other: chills.

Interactions

Drug-drug. *Other oxytocics:* May potentiate action. Avoid using together.

Effects on lab test results

None reported.

Pharmacokinetics

Absorption: Unknown.
Distribution: Unknown.
Metabolism: Enzymatic deactivation occurs in maternal tissues.
Excretion: Excreted primarily in urine. *Half-life:* None.

Route	Onset	Peak	Duration
I.M.	Unknown	15-60 min	16-24 hr

Action

Chemical effect: Produces strong, prompt contractions of uterine smooth muscle, possibly mediated by calcium and cAMP.
Therapeutic effect: Aborts fetus and stops postpartum hemorrhage.

Available forms

Injection: 250 mcg/ml

NURSING PROCESS

▨ **Assessment**
• Assess patient's pregnancy status before therapy.

- Monitor drug effectiveness by evaluating uterine contractions, expulsion of products of conception, or cessation of postpartum hemorrhage.
- Be alert for adverse reactions.
- Evaluate patient's and family's knowledge of drug therapy.

⊕ Nursing diagnoses
- Impaired adjustment related to pregnancy
- Risk for altered body temperature related to drug-induced fever
- Deficient knowledge related to drug therapy

▷ Planning and implementation
- Unlike other prostaglandin abortifacients, drug is given I.M. Injection avoids risk of expelling vaginal suppositories, which may occur with profuse vaginal bleeding.
- Drug should be used only by trained personnel in hospital setting.
- If uterine contractions are ineffective or postpartum bleeding persists, consult prescriber.
Patient teaching
- Explain importance of follow-up care.
- Tell patient to report adverse reactions immediately.

☑ Evaluation
- Patient aborts successfully.
- Patient's temperature remains normal.
- Patient and family state understanding of drug therapy.

carisoprodol
(kar-ih-soh-PROH-dol)
Soma

Pharmacologic class: carbamate derivative
Therapeutic class: skeletal muscle relaxant
Pregnancy risk category: NR

Indications and dosages

▶ **Adjunct in acute, painful musculoskeletal conditions.** *Adults:* 350 mg P.O. t.i.d. and h.s.

Contraindications and precautions

- Contraindicated in patients hypersensitive to related compounds (such as meprobamate) and in patients with intermittent porphyria.
- Use cautiously in patients with hepatic or renal impairment. Prolonged use may lead to

dependence; thus, use cautiously in addiction-prone patients.
⚖ **Lifespan:** In pregnant or breast-feeding women and in children younger than age 12, safety and efficacy of drug haven't been established.

Adverse reactions

CNS: fever, *drowsiness, dizziness,* vertigo, ataxia, tremor, agitation, irritability, headache, depressive reactions, insomnia.
CV: orthostatic hypotension, tachycardia, facial flushing.
GI: nausea, vomiting, increased bowel activity, epigastric distress.
Hematologic: eosinophilia.
Respiratory: *asthmatic episodes,* hiccups.
Skin: rash, *erythema multiforme,* pruritus.
Other: *angioedema, anaphylaxis.*

Interactions

Drug-drug. *CNS depressants:* May increase CNS depression. Avoid using together.
Drug-lifestyle. *Alcohol use:* May increase CNS depression. Discourage using together.

Effects on lab test results

- May increase eosinophil count.

Pharmacokinetics

Absorption: Unknown.
Distribution: Widely distributed throughout body.
Metabolism: Metabolized in liver.
Excretion: Excreted in urine mainly as metabolites; less than 1% of dose excreted unchanged.
Half-life: 8 hours.

Route	Onset	Peak	Duration
P.O.	≤ 30 min	≤ 4 hr	4-6 hr

Action

Chemical effect: Appears to modify central perception of pain without modifying pain reflexes. Blocks interneuronal activity in descending reticular activating system and in spinal cord.
Therapeutic effect: Relieves musculoskeletal pain.

Available forms

Tablets: 350 mg

NURSING PROCESS

⚗ Assessment

- Assess patient's pain before and after giving drug.
- Monitor drug effectiveness by regularly assessing severity and frequency of muscle spasms.
- Be alert for adverse reactions and drug interactions.
- ⊛ **ALERT:** Watch for idiosyncratic reactions after first to fourth doses (weakness, ataxia, visual and speech difficulties, fever, skin eruptions, and mental changes) and for severe reactions (bronchospasm, hypotension, and anaphylaxis).
- Assess patient for history of drug addiction. Prolonged use of drug may lead to dependence.
- Evaluate patient's and family's knowledge of drug therapy.

🖐 Nursing diagnoses

- Acute pain related to patient's underlying condition
- Risk for injury related to drug-induced drowsiness
- Deficient knowledge related to drug therapy

▷ Planning and implementation

- Give drug with meals or milk to prevent GI distress.
- Once adequate amount of pain is relieved, reduce dosage.
- Withhold dose and notify prescriber immediately if unusual reactions occur.
- Don't stop drug abruptly as mild withdrawal effects (such as insomnia, headache, nausea, and abdominal cramps) may result.

Patient teaching

- Warn patient to avoid activities that require alertness or physical dexterity, such as operating machinery or a motor vehicle until drug's CNS effects are known.
- Advise patient to avoid combining drug with alcohol or other CNS depressants.
- Advise patient to follow prescriber's orders about rest and physical therapy.
- Tell patient to take drug with meals or milk to prevent GI distress.

☑ Evaluation

- Patient reports pain has ceased.
- Patient doesn't experience injury from drug-induced CNS adverse reactions.

- Patient and family state understanding of drug.

carmustine (BCNU)
(kar-MUHS-teen)
BiCNU, Gliadel

Pharmacologic class: alkylating drug, nitrosourea (not specific to cell cycle phase)
Therapeutic class: antineoplastic
Pregnancy risk category: D

Indications and dosages

▶ **Hodgkin's disease, non-Hodgkin's lymphoma, and multiple myeloma.** *Adults:* 150 to 200 mg/m² I.V. by slow infusion as single dose; repeat q 6 weeks. Or, 75 to 100 mg/m² I.V. by slow infusion daily for 2 days; repeat q 6 weeks if platelet count is above 100,000/mm³ and WBC count is above 4,000/mm³.
◩ **Adjust-a-dose:** Reduce dosage by 30% when WBC count is 2,000 to 3,000/mm³ and platelet count is 25,000 to 75,000/mm³. Reduce dosage by 50% when WBC count is below 2,000/mm³ and platelet count is below 25,000/mm³.
▶ **Recurrent glioblastoma and metastatic brain tumors (adjunct to surgery to prolong survival); newly diagnosed high-grade malignant glioma patients (adjunct to surgery and radiation).** *Adults:* 8 wafers implanted into resection cavity as size of cavity allows.
▶ **Brain‡, breast‡, GI tract‡, lung‡, and hepatic cancer‡ ; malignant melanomas‡.** *Adults:* 75 to 100 mg/m² I.V. by slow infusion daily for 2 consecutive days; repeat q 6 weeks if platelet count is above 100,000/mm³ and WBC count is above 4,000/mm³.

▼ I.V. administration

- To reconstitute, dissolve 100 mg of drug in 3 ml of absolute alcohol provided by manufacturer. Dilute solution with 27 ml of sterile water for injection. Resulting solution contains 3.3 mg of drug/ml in 10% alcohol. Dilute in normal saline solution or D₅W for I.V. infusion.
- If powder liquefies or appears oily, discard drug because decomposition has occurred.
- Give only in glass containers. Solution is unstable in plastic I.V. bags.

• Give at least 250 ml over 1 to 2 hours. To reduce pain of infusion, dilute further or slow infusion rate.
• Don't mix with other drugs during administration.
• Avoid contact with skin because drug will cause brown stain. If drug contacts skin, wash off thoroughly.
• Store reconstituted solution in refrigerator for 48 hours. May decompose at temperatures above 80° F (27° C).

Contraindications and precautions

• Contraindicated in patients hypersensitive to drug.
≉ Lifespan: In pregnant or breast-feeding women, use is contraindicated. In children, safety and efficacy of drug haven't been established.

Adverse reactions

CNS: ataxia, drowsiness, *brain edema, seizures.*
CV: facial flushing.
EENT: ocular toxicities.
GI: *nausea* beginning in 2 to 6 hours (can be severe), *vomiting, anorexia, dysphagia, esophagitis, diarrhea.*
GU: *nephrotoxicity, renal impairment.*
Hematologic: *cumulative bone marrow suppression* (delayed 4 to 6 weeks, lasting 1 to 2 weeks), *leukopenia, thrombocytopenia, acute leukemia or bone marrow dysplasia* (may occur after long-term use).
Hepatic: *hepatotoxicity.*
Metabolic: possible hyperuricemia (in lymphoma patients when rapid cell lysis occurs).
Respiratory: *pulmonary fibrosis.*
Skin: hyperpigmentation (if drug contacts skin).
Other: *intense pain* (at infusion site from venous spasm).

Interactions

Drug-drug. *Anticoagulants, aspirin, NSAIDs:* May increase risk of bleeding. Avoid using together.
Cimetidine: May increase carmustine's bone marrow toxicity. Avoid using together, if possible.
Digoxin, phenytoin: May reduce levels of these drugs. Use together cautiously; monitor serum levels.
Mitomycin: Increases corneal and conjunctival damage with high doses. Monitor patient.

Myelosuppressives: May increase risk of myelosuppression. Monitor patient's CBC periodically.

Effects on lab test results

• May increase urine urea, AST, bilirubin, and alkaline phosphatase levels.
• May decrease hemoglobin, hematocrit, and WBC and platelet counts.

Pharmacokinetics

Absorption: Administered I.V.
Distribution: Distributed rapidly into CSF.
Metabolism: Metabolized extensively in liver.
Excretion: 60% to 70% excreted in urine within 96 hours, 6% to 10% excreted as carbon dioxide by lungs, and 1% excreted in feces.
Half-life: 15 to 30 minutes.

Route	Onset	Peak	Duration
I.V., wafer	Unknown	Unknown	Unknown

Action

Chemical effect: Inhibits enzymatic reactions involved with DNA synthesis, cross-links strands of cellular DNA, and interferes with RNA transcription, causing growth imbalance that leads to cell death.
Therapeutic effect: Kills selected cancer cells.

Available forms

Injection: 100-mg vial (lyophilized), with 3-ml vial of absolute alcohol supplied as diluent
Wafer: 7.7 mg

NURSING PROCESS

⚖ **Assessment**
• Assess patient's neoplastic disorder before therapy and regularly thereafter.
• Obtain baseline pulmonary function tests before therapy because pulmonary toxicity appears to be related to dose. Evaluate results of liver, renal, and pulmonary function tests periodically thereafter.
• Monitor CBC and uric acid levels.
• Be alert for adverse reactions and drug interactions.
• Evaluate patient's and family's knowledge of drug therapy.

⊕ Nursing diagnoses
• Ineffective health maintenance related to neoplastic disease
• Risk for injury related to drug-induced adverse reactions
• Deficient knowledge related to drug therapy

❯ Planning and implementation
• Preparing and giving drug is linked to carcinogenic, mutagenic, and teratogenic risks; follow facility policy to reduce risks.
• To reduce nausea, give antiemetic before giving drug.
• Unopened foil packs containing wafers are stable at room temperature for 6 hours. Store below -4° F (-20° C).
• If handling wafer in operating room, use double gloves.
• Allopurinol may be used with adequate hydration to prevent hyperuricemia and uric acid nephropathy.
Patient teaching
• Warn patient to watch for signs of infection (fever, sore throat, fatigue) and bleeding (easy bruising, nosebleeds, bleeding gums, melena). Tell patient to take temperature daily.
• Instruct patient to avoid OTC products containing aspirin.
• Advise breast-feeding women to stop breast-feeding because of possible toxicity to infant.
• Advise women of childbearing age to avoid pregnancy during therapy and to consult prescriber before becoming pregnant.

✓ Evaluation
• Patient shows positive response to drug therapy as evidenced by follow-up diagnostic studies.
• Patient doesn't experience injury from drug-induced adverse reactions.
• Patient and family state understanding of drug therapy.

---

carvedilol
(kar-VAY-deh-lol)
Coreg

Pharmacologic class: alpha$_1$ and beta blocker
Therapeutic class: antihypertensive, adjunct treatment for heart failure
Pregnancy risk category: C

Indications and dosages
▶ **Hypertension.** *Adults:* Dosage highly individualized. Initially, 6.25 mg P.O. b.i.d. with food. Obtain a standing blood pressure 1 hour after initial dose. If tolerated, continue dosage for 7 to 14 days. May increase to 12.5 mg P.O. b.i.d. for 7 to 14 days, following blood pressure monitoring protocol noted above. Maximum dosage, 25 mg P.O. b.i.d. as tolerated.
▶ **Mild-to-severe heart failure.** *Adults:* Dosage highly individualized and adjusted carefully. Initially, 3.125 mg P.O. b.i.d. with food for 2 weeks; if tolerated, increase to 6.25 mg P.O. b.i.d. Dosage may be doubled q 2 weeks as tolerated. At start of new dosage, observe patient for dizziness or light-headedness for 1 hour. Maximum dosage for patients weighing less than 85 kg (187 lb) is 25 mg P.O. b.i.d.; for those weighing over 85 kg, maximum dosage is 50 mg P.O. b.i.d.
▶ **Left ventricular dysfunction following MI.** *Adults:* Dosage highly individualized. Start therapy after patient is hemodynamically stable and fluid retention has been minimized. Initially, 6.25 mg P.O. b.i.d. Increase after 3 to 10 days to 12.5 mg b.i.d., then again to a target dose of 25 mg b.i.d. Or start with 3.25 mg b.i.d. or titrate dosage slower if indicated.
⊠ Adjust-a-dose: In patients with pulse rate below 55 beats/minute, reduce dosage.

Contraindications and precautions
• Contraindicated in patients hypersensitive to drug and in those with New York Heart Association class IV decompensated heart failure requiring I.V. inotropic therapy, bronchial asthma or related bronchospastic conditions, second- or third-degree AV block, sick sinus syndrome (unless a permanent pacemaker is in place), cardiogenic shock, or severe bradycardia.
• Drug isn't recommended for patients with symptomatic hepatic impairment.
• Use cautiously in hypertensive patients with left ventricular failure, perioperative patients who receive anesthetics that depress myocardial function, patients with diabetes who receive insulin or oral antidiabetics, and patients subject to spontaneous hypoglycemia. Also use cautiously in patients with thyroid disease, pheochromocytoma, Prinzmetal's variant angina, bronchospastic disease, or peripheral vascular disease.

≛ **Lifespan:** Breast-feeding should be stopped during drug therapy. In children, safety and efficacy of drug haven't been established. In elderly patients, levels are about 50% higher; monitor these patients closely.

Adverse reactions

CNS: *asthenia, fatigue,* pain, *dizziness,* headache, malaise, fever, hypesthesia, paresthesia, syncope, vertigo, somnolence, *CVA,* depression, insomnia.

CV: *hypotension, postural hypertension,* edema, *bradycardia,* angina pectoris, peripheral edema, hypovolemia, fluid overload, *AV block,* hypertension, palpitation, peripheral vascular disorder, chest pain.

EENT: sinusitis, abnormal vision, blurred vision, pharyngitis, rhinitis.

GI: *diarrhea,* vomiting, nausea, melena, periodontitis, abdominal pain, dyspepsia.

GU: impotence, abnormal renal function, albuminuria, hematuria, UTI.

Hematologic: purpura, anemia, *thrombocytopenia.*

Metabolic: *hyperglycemia, weight gain,* weight loss, hypercholesterolemia, hyperuricemia, *hypoglycemia,* hyponatremia, glycosuria, hypervolemia, diabetes mellitus, *hyperkalemia,* gout, hypertriglyceridemia.

Musculoskeletal: arthralgia, back pain, muscle cramps, hypotonia, arthritis.

Respiratory: bronchitis, *upper respiratory tract infection,* cough, rales, dyspnea, *lung edema.*

Other: hypersensitivity reactions, infection, flu-like syndrome, viral infection, injury.

Interactions

Drug-drug. *Calcium channel blockers:* May cause isolated conduction disturbances. Monitor patient's heart rhythm and blood pressure.
Catecholamine-depleting drugs (such as MAO inhibitors, reserpine): May cause bradycardia or severe hypotension. Monitor patient closely.
Cimetidine: May increase bioavailability of carvedilol. Monitor vital signs carefully.
Clonidine: May potentiate blood pressure and heart rate–lowering effects. Monitor vital signs closely.
Digoxin: May increase digoxin level by about 15% during therapy. Monitor digoxin levels and vital signs carefully.
Fluoxetine, paroxetine, propafenone, quinidine: Increases level of R (+) enantiomer of

carvedilol. Monitor patient for hypotension and dizziness.
Insulin, oral antidiabetics: May enhance hypoglycemic properties. Monitor glucose levels.
Rifampin: May reduce levels of carvedilol by 70%. Monitor vital signs closely.
Drug-food. *Any food:* Delays carvedilol absorption but doesn't alter extent of bioavailability. Advise patient to take drug with food to minimize orthostatic effects.

Effects on lab test results

• May increase creatinine, BUN, ALT, AST, GGT, cholesterol, triglyceride, alkaline phosphatase, sodium, uric acid, potassium, and nonprotein nitrogen levels. May increase or decrease glucose levels.
• May decrease PT, INR, and platelet counts.

Pharmacokinetics

Absorption: Rapidly and extensively absorbed with absolute bioavailability of 25% to 35% because of significant first-pass metabolism.
Distribution: Extensively distributed into extravascular tissues; about 98% bound to plasma proteins.
Metabolism: Primarily metabolized by aromatic ring oxidation and glucuronidation.
Excretion: Metabolites are primarily excreted via bile in the feces. Less than 2% is excreted unchanged in urine. *Half-life:* 7 to 10 hours.

Route	Onset	Peak	Duration
P.O.	Unknown	1-2 hr	7-10 hr

Action

Chemical effect: Causes significant reductions in systemic blood pressure, pulmonary arterial pressure, pulmonary capillary wedge pressure, and heart rate.
Therapeutic effect: Lowers blood pressure and heart rate.

Available forms

Tablets: 3.125 mg, 6.25 mg, 12.5 mg, 25 mg

NURSING PROCESS

𝌆 **Assessment**

• Monitor patient for decreased PT and increased alkaline phosphatase, BUN, ALT, and AST levels.

- Assess patient with heart failure for worsened condition, renal impairment, or fluid retention; add or increase diuretics as needed.
- Monitor patient with diabetes closely; drug may mask signs of hypoglycemia or worsen hyperglycemia.
- Monitor elderly patients carefully; drug levels are about 50% higher in elderly patients than in younger patients.
- Observe patient for dizziness or lightheadedness for 1 hour after giving each dose.
- Evaluate patient's and family's knowledge of drug therapy.

🔲 Nursing diagnoses
- Ineffective health maintenance related to underlying disorder
- Ineffective cerebral tissue perfusion secondary to therapeutic action of drug
- Deficient knowledge related to drug therapy

▶ Planning and implementation
- Before therapy begins, stabilize dosages of digoxin, diuretics, and ACE inhibitors.
- **ALERT:** Patients receiving beta blockers who have a history of severe anaphylactic reaction to several allergens may be more reactive to repeated challenge (accidental, diagnostic, or therapeutic). These patients may be unresponsive to dosages of epinephrine typically used to treat allergic reactions.
- Give drug with food to reduce risk of orthostatic hypotension.
- If pulse drops below 55 beats/minute, notify prescriber and reduce dosage.

Patient teaching
- Tell patient not to interrupt or stop drug without medical approval. Drug should be withdrawn gradually over 1 to 2 weeks.
- Advise heart failure patient to call prescriber if weight gain or shortness of breath occurs.
- Inform patient that he may experience low blood pressure when standing. If he's dizzy or faints, advise him to sit or lie down.
- Warn patient not to drive or perform hazardous tasks until CNS effects of drug are known.
- Tell patient to notify prescriber if dizziness or faintness occurs; dosage may need to be adjusted.
- Advise patient with diabetes to report changes in glucose level promptly.

- Inform patient who wears contact lenses that decreased lacrimation may occur.

🔲 Evaluation
- Patient responds well to therapy.
- Patient doesn't experience dizziness or lightheadedness.
- Patient and family state understanding of drug therapy.

caspofungin acetate
(kas-poh-FUN-jin AS-ih-tayt)
Cancidas

Pharmacologic class: glucan synthesis inhibitor
Therapeutic class: antifungal antibiotic
Pregnancy risk category: C

Indications and dosages

▶ **Invasive aspergillosis in patients refractory to or intolerant of other drugs, such as amphotericin B, lipid formulations of amphotericin B, itraconazole.** *Adults:* A single 70-mg loading dose on day 1, followed by 50 mg daily thereafter. Give by slow I.V. infusion over about 1 hour. Duration of treatment based on severity of patient's underlying disease, recovery from immunosuppression, and response.
Adjust-a-dose: For patients with moderate hepatic impairment and a Child-Pugh score of 7 to 9, give 35 mg daily after initial 70 mg loading dose.

▼ I.V. administration
- Allow refrigerated vial to warm to room temperature before diluting.
- Dilute all doses (70-mg, 50-mg, 35-mg) in 250 ml of normal saline solution. In patients with fluid restrictions, dilute the 50-mg and 35-mg doses in 100 ml of normal saline solution.
- **ALERT:** Never mix or dilute caspofungin acetate with any dextrose solution.
- Give drug by slow I.V. infusion of about 1 hour.
- Don't mix or infuse caspofungin acetate with any other drugs.
- Use reconstituted vials within 1 hour or discard.
- Diluted solutions may be stored at 77° F (25° C) for up to 24 hours.

Contraindications and precautions

• Contraindicated in patients hypersensitive to any components of drug.

≋ Lifespan: In breast-feeding women, use cautiously because it's not known whether drug appears in breast milk. In children, safety and efficacy of drug haven't been established.

Adverse reactions

CNS: *headache*, paresthesia, *fever*, chills.
CV: *tachycardia*, *thrombophlebitis*.
GI: nausea, vomiting, diarrhea, abdominal pain, anorexia.
GU: proteinuria, hematuria.
Hematologic: eosinophilia, anemia.
Musculoskeletal: pain, myalgia.
Respiratory: *tachypnea*.
Skin: histamine-mediated symptoms (including rash, facial swelling, phlebitis, pruritus, sensation of warmth, erythema, and sweating).

Interactions

Drug-drug. *Carbamazepine, dexamethasone, efavirenz, nelfinavir, nevirapine, phenytoin, rifampin:* May decrease caspofungin levels. Consider increasing caspofungin dosage to 70 mg daily if patient doesn't respond.
Cyclosporine: Significantly increases AST and ALT levels. Avoid using together unless potential benefit outweighs potential risk.
Tacrolimus: Decreased tacrolimus levels. Monitor tacrolimus levels and adjust tacrolimus dosage accordingly.

Effects on lab test results

• May increase ALT, AST, and alkaline phosphatase levels. May decrease potassium level.
• May increase eosinophil count, urine protein, and urine RBC. May decrease hemoglobin and hematocrit.

Pharmacokinetics

Absorption: Administered I.V.
Distribution: Extensively bound to albumin (about 97%).
Metabolism: Slowly metabolized in the liver.
Excretion: 35% of drug and metabolites is excreted in feces and 41% in urine. Renal clearance of parent drug is very low. *Half-life:* Unknown.

Route	Onset	Peak	Duration
I.V.	Unknown	Unknown	Unknown

Action

Chemical effect: Inhibits synthesis of beta (1,3)-D-glucan, an integral component of the cell walls of susceptible filamentous fungi that isn't found in mammal cells.
Therapeutic effect: Prevents fungi formation.

Available forms

Lyophilized powder for injection: 50-mg, 70-mg single-use vials

NURSING PROCESS

☑ Assessment
• Assess patient's hepatic function before starting drug therapy.
• Observe patient for histamine-mediated reactions (rash, facial swelling, pruritus, sensation of warmth).
• Monitor I.V. site carefully for phlebitis.
• Monitor patient's lab test results carefully during drug therapy for any increase in liver function test values.
• Evaluate patient's and family's knowledge of drug therapy.

⊕ Nursing diagnoses
• Risk for infection and impaired skin integrity related to adverse effects of intravenous drug administration
• Ineffective health maintenance related to underlying disease process and immunocompromised state
• Deficient knowledge related to aspergillosis infection and caspofungin acetate drug therapy

▷ Planning and implementation
• An increase in dosage to 70 mg daily hasn't been studied but may be well tolerated.
• A long course of therapy hasn't been studied but may be well tolerated.
• Adjust dosage in a patient with moderate hepatic insufficiency.
Patient teaching
• Instruct patient to report signs and symptoms of phlebitis.
• Tell patient to report any adverse events during drug therapy.

☑ Evaluation
• Patient doesn't experience any adverse reactions during drug therapy.

Rapid onset   *Liquid form contains alcohol.   ◆Canada   ◇ Australia   †OTC   ‡Off-label use

• Patient responds positively to antifungal drug therapy.
• Patient and family state understanding of drug therapy.

cefaclor
(SEH-fuh-klor)
Ceclor, Ceclor CD

Pharmacologic class: second-generation cephalosporin
Therapeutic class: antibiotic
Pregnancy risk category: B

Indications and dosages

▶ **Respiratory, urinary tract, skin, and soft-tissue infections and otitis media caused by** *Haemophilus influenzae, Streptococcus pneumoniae, S. pyogenes, Escherichia coli, Proteus mirabilis, Klebsiella sp.,* **and** *staphylococci.*
Adults: 250 to 500 mg P.O. q 8 hours. Maximum total daily dosage, 4 g. For extended-release forms, 500 mg P.O. q 12 hours for 7 days for bronchitis. For pharyngitis or skin and skin-structure infections, 375 mg P.O. q 12 hours for 10 days and 7 to 10 days, respectively.
Children: 20 mg/kg P.O. daily divided q 8 hours. For pharyngitis or otitis media, b.i.d. q 12 hours. For more serious infections, 40 mg/kg daily are recommended, not to exceed 1 g daily.
▶ **Acute uncomplicated UTI‡.** *Adults:* 2 g P.O. as a single dose.

Contraindications and precautions

• Contraindicated in patients hypersensitive to other cephalosporins.
• Use cautiously in patients with a history of sensitivity to penicillin because of reports of partial cross-allergenicity. Also use cautiously in patients with renal impairment.
 Lifespan: In pregnant and breast-feeding women, use cautiously. In children younger than age 1 month, safety and effectiveness of oral suspension haven't been established. In children younger than age 16, safety and efficacy of extended-release tablets and capsules haven't been established.

Adverse reactions

CNS: dizziness, headache, somnolence, malaise, fever.

GI: nausea, vomiting, diarrhea, anorexia, dyspepsia, abdominal cramps, *pseudomembranous colitis,* oral candidiasis.
GU: red and white cells in urine, vaginal candidiasis, vaginitis.
Hematologic: *transient leukopenia,* lymphocytosis, anemia, eosinophilia, *thrombocytopenia.*
Skin: *maculopapular rash,* dermatitis.
Other: *hypersensitivity reactions* (serum sickness, *anaphylaxis*).

Interactions

Drug-drug. *Aminoglycosides:* Increases risk of nephrotoxicity. Avoid using together.
Antacids: Decreases absorption of extended-release tablets. Separate administration times by at least 1 hour.
Anticoagulant: Increases anticoagulant effects. Monitor coagulation studies.
Chloramphenicol: May have an antagonistic effect. Avoid using together.
Probenecid: May inhibit excretion and increase levels of cefaclor. Monitor patient.

Effects on lab test results

• May increase ALT, AST, alkaline phosphatase, bilirubin, GGT, and LDH levels.
• May increase eosinophil count. May decrease hemoglobin, hematocrit, and WBC and platelet counts.
• May cause false-positive urine glucose determinations with copper sulfate tests (Clinitest).

Pharmacokinetics

Absorption: Well absorbed from GI tract. Food will delay but not prevent complete GI tract absorption.
Distribution: Distributed widely into most body tissues and fluids; CSF penetration is poor. Drug is 25% protein-bound.
Metabolism: None.
Excretion: Excreted primarily in urine by renal tubular secretion and glomerular filtration. *Half-life:* ½ to 1 hour.

Route	Onset	Peak	Duration
P.O.	Unknown	30-60 min	Unknown

Action

Chemical effect: Inhibits cell-wall synthesis, promoting osmotic instability; usually bactericidal.

Reactions may be *common,* uncommon, *life-threatening,* or COMMON AND LIFE-THREATENING.

Therapeutic effect: Hinders or kills susceptible bacteria.

Available forms

Capsules: 250 mg, 500 mg
Oral suspension: 125 mg/5 ml, 250 mg/5 ml, 187 mg/5 ml, 375 mg/5 ml
Tablets: (extended-release): 375 mg, 500 mg

NURSING PROCESS

🔧 Assessment
• Assess patient's infection before therapy and regularly thereafter.
• Obtain specimen for culture and sensitivity tests before first dose. Therapy may begin pending test results.
• Ask patient about previous reactions to cephalosporins or penicillin before administering first dose.
• Be alert for adverse reactions and drug interactions.
• Monitor patient's hydration status if adverse GI reactions occur.
• Evaluate patient's and family's knowledge of drug therapy.

📋 Nursing diagnoses
• Infection related to bacteria susceptible to drug
• Risk for deficient fluid volume related to drug-induced adverse GI reactions
• Deficient knowledge related to drug therapy

▶ Planning and implementation
• Give drug with food to prevent or minimize GI upset.
• Store reconstituted suspension in refrigerator where it will remain stable for 14 days. Keep tightly closed and shake well before using.
⚠ ALERT: Don't confuse with other cephalosporins with similar-sounding names.
Patient teaching
• Tell patient that drug may be taken with meals.
• Advise patient to take drug exactly as prescribed, even after he feels better.
• Instruct patient to call prescriber if rash develops.
• Teach patient how to store drug.

✓ Evaluation
• Patient is free from infection.
• Patient maintains adequate hydration.

• Patient and family state understanding of drug therapy.

cefadroxil monohydrate
(seh-fuh-DROKS-il MON-oh-HIGH-drayt)
Duricef

Pharmacologic class: first-generation cephalosporin
Therapeutic class: antibiotic
Pregnancy risk category: B

Indications and dosages

▶ **UTIs caused by *Escherichia coli, Proteus mirabilis,* and *Klebsiella sp.*; skin and soft-tissue infections; and streptococcal pharyngitis.** *Adults:* 1 to 2 g P.O. daily, depending on infection treated, usually as a single dose or in 2 divided doses.
Children: 30 mg/kg P.O. daily in two divided doses. Course of treatment is usually at least 10 days.
Ⓢ Adjust-a-dose: For adults with renal impairment, give initial dosage of 1 g P.O. daily. Reduce maintenance dosage based on creatinine clearance. If creatinine clearance is 25 to 50 ml/minute, give 500 mg q 12 hours. If clearance is 10 to 25 ml/minute, give 500 mg q 24 hours. If creatinine clearance is less than 10 ml/minute, give 500 mg q 36 hours.

Contraindications and precautions

• Contraindicated in patients hypersensitive to drug or other cephalosporins.
• Use cautiously in patients with renal impairment or a history of sensitivity to penicillin.
⚖ Lifespan: In pregnant or breast-feeding women, use cautiously.

Adverse reactions

CNS: dizziness, headache, malaise, paresthesia, *seizures.*
GI: *pseudomembranous colitis, nausea,* anorexia, vomiting, diarrhea, glossitis, dyspepsia, abdominal cramps, anal pruritus, tenesmus, oral candidiasis.
GU: genital pruritus, candidiasis.
Hematologic: *transient neutropenia,* eosinophilia, *leukopenia,* anemia, *agranulocytosis, thrombocytopenia.*
Respiratory: dyspnea.

Skin: *maculopapular and erythematous rashes.*
Other: *hypersensitivity reactions* (serum sickness, *anaphylaxis*).

Interactions

Drug-drug. *Probenecid:* May inhibit excretion and increase levels of cefadroxil. Monitor patient.

Effects on lab test results

• May increase ALT, AST, alkaline phosphatase, bilirubin, GGT, and LDH levels.
• May increase eosinophil count. May decrease hemoglobin, hematocrit, and neutrophil, WBC, granulocyte, and platelet counts.
• May cause false-positive urine glucose determinations with copper sulfate tests (Clinitest).

Pharmacokinetics

Absorption: Rapid and complete.
Distribution: Distributed widely into most body tissues and fluids; CSF penetration is poor. Drug is 20% protein-bound.
Metabolism: None.
Excretion: Excreted primarily unchanged in urine. *Half-life:* About 1 to 2 hours.

Route	Onset	Peak	Duration
P.O.	Unknown	1-2 hr	Unknown

Action

Chemical effect: Inhibits cell-wall synthesis, promoting osmotic instability; usually bactericidal.
Therapeutic effect: Hinders or kills susceptible bacteria.

Available forms

Capsules: 500 mg
Oral suspension: 125 mg/5 ml, 250 mg/5 ml, 500 mg/5 ml
Tablets: 1 g

NURSING PROCESS

⚕ Assessment

• Assess patient's infection before therapy and regularly thereafter.
• Obtain specimen for culture and sensitivity tests before first dose. Therapy may begin pending test results.
• Be alert for adverse reactions and drug interactions.

• Monitor patient's hydration status if adverse GI reactions occur.
• Evaluate patient's and family's knowledge of drug therapy.

🔁 Nursing diagnoses

• Infection related to bacteria susceptible to drug
• Risk for deficient fluid volume related to drug-induced adverse GI reactions
• Deficient knowledge related to drug therapy

▷ Planning and implementation

• Drug's half-life permits once- or twice-daily dosing.
• Expect prescriber to lengthen dosage interval to prevent drug accumulation if creatinine clearance is below 50 ml/minute.
• Store reconstituted suspension in refrigerator. Keep container tightly closed and shake well before using.
• About 40% to 75% of patients receiving cephalosporins show false-positive direct Coombs' test.
⚠ ALERT: Don't confuse with other cephalosporins with similar-sounding names.
Patient teaching
• Tell patient to take drug exactly as prescribed, even after he feels better.
• Advise patient to take drug with food or milk to lessen GI discomfort.
• Tell patient to call prescriber if rash develops.
• Inform patient using oral suspension to shake it well before using and to refrigerate mixture in tightly closed container.

✓ Evaluation

• Patient is free from infection.
• Patient maintains adequate hydration.
• Patient and family state understanding of drug therapy.

cefazolin sodium
(sef-EH-zoh-lin SOH-dee-um)
Ancef, Zolicef

Pharmacologic class: first-generation cephalosporin
Therapeutic class: antibiotic
Pregnancy risk category: B

Indications and dosages

▶ **Serious infections of respiratory, biliary, and GU tracts; skin, soft-tissue, bone, and joint infections; septicemia; endocarditis caused by** *Escherichia coli, Enterobacteriaceae,* **gonococci,** *Haemophilus influenzae, Klebsiella, Proteus mirabilis, Staphylococcus aureus, Streptococcus pneumoniae,* **and group A beta-hemolytic streptococci; perioperative prophylaxis‡.** *Adults:* 250 mg I.V. or I.M. q 8 hours to 1 g q 6 hours. Maximum 12 g daily in life-threatening situations.
Children and infants older than 1 month: 25 to 100 mg/kg daily I.V. or I.M. in three or four divided doses.

▶ **Perioperative prophylaxis in contaminated surgery.** *Adults:* 1 g I.V. or I.M. 30 to 60 minutes before surgery; then 0.5 to 1 g I.V. or I.M. q 6 to 8 hours for 24 hours. In operations lasting over 2 hours, another 0.5- to 1-g dose may be given intraoperatively. In cases where infection would be devastating, prophylaxis may be continued for 3 to 5 days.

⧄ **Adjust-a-dose:** For patients with renal impairment, after initial dose, adjust dosage as follows. If creatinine clearance is 35 to 54 ml/minute, give full dose q 8 hours; if creatinine clearance is 11 to 34 ml/minute, give 50% of usual dose q 12 hours; if creatinine clearance is below 10 ml/minute, give 50% of usual dose q 18 to 24 hours.

▼ I.V. administration

• Reconstitute with sterile water, bacteriostatic water, or normal saline solution as follows: 2 ml to 500-mg vial to yield 225 mg/ml or 2.5 ml to 1-g vial to yield 330 mg/ml. Shake well until dissolved.
• For direct injection, further dilute Ancef with 5 ml of sterile water. Inject into large vein or into tubing of free-flowing I.V. solution over 3 to 5 minutes. For intermittent infusion, add reconstituted drug to 50 to 100 ml of compatible solution or use premixed solution. Give frozen solutions of drug in D_5W only by intermittent or continuous I.V. infusion.
• Alternate injection sites if I.V. therapy lasts longer than 3 days. Use of small I.V. needles in larger available veins may be preferable.
• Reconstituted drug is stable for 24 hours at room temperature and 96 hours if refrigerated.

Contraindications and precautions

• Contraindicated in patients hypersensitive to other cephalosporins.
• Use cautiously in patients with a history of sensitivity to penicillin because of cross-allergenicity and in patients with renal impairment.
⚖ **Lifespan:** In pregnant and breast-feeding women, use cautiously.

Adverse reactions

CNS: dizziness, headache, malaise, paresthesia.
GI: *pseudomembranous colitis,* nausea, anorexia, vomiting, *diarrhea,* glossitis, dyspepsia, abdominal cramps, anal pruritus, tenesmus, oral candidiasis.
GU: genital pruritus and candidiasis, vaginitis.
Hematologic: *transient neutropenia, leukopenia,* eosinophilia, anemia, *thrombocytopenia.*
Respiratory: dyspnea.
Skin: *maculopapular and erythematous rashes,* urticaria, *Stevens-Johnson syndrome.*
Other: *hypersensitivity reactions* (serum sickness, *anaphylaxis*).

Interactions

Drug-drug. *Probenecid:* May inhibit excretion and increase levels of cefazolin. Monitor patient.

Effects on lab test results

• May increase ALT, AST, alkaline phosphatase, bilirubin, GGT, and LDH levels.
• May increase eosinophil count. May decrease neutrophil, WBC, and platelet counts.
• May cause false-positive urine glucose determinations with copper sulfate tests (Clinitest).

Pharmacokinetics

Absorption: Unknown after I.M. administration.
Distribution: Distributed widely into most body tissues and fluids; CSF penetration is poor; 74% to 86% protein-bound.
Metabolism: None.
Excretion: Excreted primarily in urine. *Half-life:* About 1 to 2 hours.

Route	Onset	Peak	Duration
I.V.	Immediate	Immediate	Unknown
I.M.	Unknown	1-2 hr	Unknown

Action

Chemical effect: Inhibits cell-wall synthesis, promoting osmotic instability; usually bactericidal.
Therapeutic effect: Hinders or kills susceptible bacteria.

Available forms

Infusion: 500 mg/50-ml or 100-ml vial, 1 g/ 50-ml or 100-ml vial, 500 mg or 1 g RediVials, Faspaks, or ADD-Vantage vials
Injection (parenteral): 250 mg, 500 mg, 1 g

NURSING PROCESS

🔎 Assessment
• Assess patient's infection before therapy and reassess regularly thereafter.
• Obtain specimen for culture and sensitivity tests. Therapy may begin pending test results.
• Ask patient about previous reactions to cephalosporins or penicillin before administering first dose.
• Be alert for adverse reactions and drug interactions.
• Monitor patient's hydration status if adverse GI reactions occur.
• Evaluate patient's and family's knowledge of drug therapy.

🔲 Nursing diagnoses
• Infection related to bacteria susceptible to drug
• Risk for deficient fluid volume related to drug-induced adverse GI reactions
• Deficient knowledge related to drug therapy

📄 Planning and implementation
• Because of long duration of effect, most infections can be treated with dose every 8 hours.
• After reconstitution, inject I.M. drug without further dilution (not as painful as other cephalosporins). Inject deep into large muscle mass, such as gluteus maximus or lateral aspect of thigh.
⚠ **ALERT:** Don't confuse with other cephalosporins with similar-sounding names.
Patient teaching
• Tell patient to report adverse reactions.

☑ Evaluation
• Patient is free from infection.
• Patient maintains adequate hydration.

• Patient and family state understanding of drug therapy.

cefdinir
(SEF-dih-neer)
Omnicef

Pharmacologic class: third-generation cephalosporin
Therapeutic class: antibiotic
Pregnancy risk category: B

Indications and dosages

▶ **Mild to moderate infections caused by susceptible strains of microorganisms for conditions of community-acquired pneumonia and uncomplicated skin and skin-structure infections.** *Adults and children older than age 12:* 300 mg P.O. q 12 hours for 10 days.
Children ages 6 months to 12 years: For uncomplicated skin and skin-structure infections, 7 mg/kg P.O. q 12 hours for 10 days; maximum daily dose 600 mg.
▶ **Acute exacerbations of chronic bronchitis; acute bacterial otitis media; pharyngitis; tonsillitis.** *Adults and children older than age 12:* 300 mg P.O. q 12 hours for 5 to 10 days or 600 mg P.O. q 24 hours for 10 days.
Children ages 6 months to 12 years: 7 mg/kg P.O. q 12 hours for 5 to 10 days or 14 mg/kg P.O. q 24 hours for 10 days, up to a maximum dose of 600 mg daily.
▶ **Acute maxillary sinusitis.** *Adults and children older than age 12:* 300 mg P.O. q 12 hours for 10 days or 600 mg P.O. q 24 hours for 10 days.
Children ages 6 months to 12 years: 7mg/kg P.O. q 12 hours for 10 days or 14 mg/kg P.O. q 24 hours for 10 days.
🔲 **Adjust-a-dose:** For patients with renal impairment, if creatinine clearance is below 30 ml/ minute, reduce dosage to 300 mg P.O. once daily for adults and 7 mg/kg up to 300 mg P.O. once daily for children. In patients receiving long-term hemodialysis, dosage is 300 mg or 7 mg/kg P.O. at end of each dialysis session and subsequently every other day.

Contraindications and precautions

• Contraindicated in patients hypersensitive to cephalosporins.

Reactions may be *common,* uncommon, *life-threatening,* or COMMON AND LIFE-THREATENING.

• Use cautiously in patients hypersensitive to penicillin because of risk of cross-sensitivity with other beta-lactam antibiotics. Also use cautiously in patients with history of colitis or renal impairment.

⚞ **Lifespan:** In breast-feeding women, use cautiously. In children younger than age 6 months, safety and efficacy of drug haven't been established.

Adverse reactions

CNS: headache.
GI: abdominal pain, *diarrhea*, nausea, vomiting.
GU: vaginal candidiasis, vaginitis.
Skin: rash.

Interactions

Drug-drug. *Antacids (aluminum- and magnesium-containing), iron supplements, multivitamins containing iron:* May decrease cefdinir's absorption and bioavailability. Give such preparations 2 hours before or after cefdinir dose.
Probenecid: Inhibits the renal excretion of cefdinir. Monitor patient.

Effects on lab test results

• May increase GGT and alkaline phosphatase levels.
• May increase RBC count and urine protein.

Pharmacokinetics

Absorption: Bioavailability of drug is about 21% after 300-mg capsule dose, 16% after 600-mg capsule dose, and 25% for suspension.
Distribution: 60% to 70% bound to plasma proteins.
Metabolism: Not appreciably metabolized; activity results mainly from parent drug.
Excretion: Eliminated primarily by renal excretion. *Half-life:* 1¾ hours.

Route	Onset	Peak	Duration
P.O.	Unknown	2-4 hr	Unknown

Action

Chemical effect: Kills bacteria by inhibition of cell-wall synthesis.
Therapeutic effect: Is stable in the presence of some beta-lactamase enzymes, causing some microorganisms resistant to penicillins and cephalosporins to be susceptible to this drug.

Available forms

Capsules: 300 mg
Suspension: 125 mg/5 ml

NURSING PROCESS

⚕ Assessment
• Ask patient about previous reactions to cephalosporins or penicillin before giving first dose.
• Obtain specimen for culture and sensitivity tests before giving first dose.
• Monitor patient for symptoms of superinfection.
• Assess patient with diarrhea carefully; pseudomembranous colitis has been reported with drug.
• Evaluate patient's and family's knowledge of drug therapy.

⚑ Nursing diagnoses
• Infection related to susceptible bacteria
• Risk for deficient fluid volume related to drug-induced adverse GI reactions
• Deficient knowledge related to drug therapy

▶ Planning and implementation
• Begin therapy pending culture and sensitivity test results.
• In patients with renal impairment, reduce dosage.
• If allergic reaction is suspected, notify prescriber; stop drug and give emergency treatment as needed.
⚠ ALERT: Don't confuse with other cephalosporins with similar-sounding names.
Patient teaching
• If patient is taking antacids or iron supplements, instruct him to take them 2 hours before or after dose of cefdinir.
• Inform patient with diabetes that each teaspoon of suspension contains 2.86 g of sucrose.
• Tell patient that drug may be taken without regard to meals.
• Advise patient to report severe diarrhea or diarrhea accompanied by abdominal pain.
• Tell patient to report adverse reactions or symptoms of superinfection promptly.

☑ Evaluation
• Patient is free from infection.
• Patient maintains adequate hydration.
• Patient and family state understanding of drug therapy.

cefditoren pivoxil
(sef-da-TOR-en pa-VOX-ill)
Spectracef

Pharmacologic class: semisynthetic third-generation cephalosporin
Therapeutic class: antibiotic
Pregnancy risk category: B

Indications and dosages

▶ **Acute bacterial exacerbation of chronic bronchitis caused by** *Haemophilus influenzae, H. parainfluenzae, Streptococcus pneumoniae* **(penicillin-susceptible strains only), or** *Moraxella catarrhalis. Adults and children age 12 and older:* 400 mg P.O. b.i.d. with meals for 10 days.

▶ **Pharyngitis, tonsillitis, and uncomplicated skin and skin-structure infections caused by** *S. pyogenes. Adults and children age 12 and older:* 200 mg P.O. b.i.d. with meals for 10 days.

Adjust-a-dose: For patients with renal impairment, if creatinine clearance is 30 to 49 ml/minute, don't give more than 200 mg b.i.d. If creatinine clearance is less than 30 ml/minute, give 200 mg daily.

Contraindications and precautions

• Contraindicated in patients hypersensitive to drug, other cephalosporins, and penicillins. Also contraindicated in patients with carnitine deficiency or inborn errors of metabolism that may result in significant carnitine deficiency. Because tablets contain sodium caseinate, a milk protein, don't give them to patients hypersensitive to milk protein (distinct from those with lactose intolerance).
• Use cautiously in patients with renal impairment. Drug is dialyzable.
⚠ **Lifespan:** In breast-feeding women, use cautiously because cephalosporins appear in breast milk. In children younger than age 12, safety and efficacy of drug haven't been established.

Adverse reactions

CNS: headache.
GI: abdominal pain, dyspepsia, *diarrhea*, nausea, vomiting, *colitis*, hepatic dysfunction (including cholestasis).
GU: vaginal candidiasis, hematuria, *nephrotoxicity.*
Hematologic: anemia.
Metabolic: hyperglycemia.
Skin: *Stevens-Johnson syndrome, toxic epidermal necrolysis.*
Other: hypersensitivity reactions (including serum sickness, rash, fever, *anaphylaxis*).

Interactions

Drug-drug. *Aluminum antacids, H₂-receptor antagonists, magnesium:* Reduces cefditoren absorption. Avoid using together. If used together, separate administration times.
Oral anticoagulants: May increase bleeding time. Monitor PT levels and patient closely for unusual bleeding or bruising.
Probenecid: Increases plasma cefditoren level. Avoid using together.
Drug-food. *Moderate- to high-fat meals:* Increases drug bioavailability. Advise patient to take drug with meals.

Effects on lab test results

• May increase liver enzyme levels. May decrease plasma carnitine level.
• May decrease hematocrit, hemoglobin, and PT.
• May cause a false-positive direct Coombs' test result and false-positive reaction for glucose in urine, using copper reduction tests (those involving Benedict's solution, Fehling's solution, or Clinitest tablets).

Pharmacokinetics

Absorption: Absorbed from the GI tract and hydrolyzed by esterases to cefditoren. Giving drug with a meal increases its absolute bioavailability.
Distribution: Distributed widely into most body tissues and fluids based on volume of distribution. CSF penetration is unknown. Drug is about 88% protein-bound.
Metabolism: Not appreciably metabolized.
Excretion: Excreted unchanged mainly in urine by glomerular filtration and tubular secretion.
Half-life: 1¼ to 2 hours in patients with normal renal function.

Route	Onset	Peak	Duration
P.O.	Unknown	1½-3 hr	Unknown

Action

Chemical effect: Primarily bactericidal. Drug acts by adhering to bacterial penicillin-binding proteins, thereby inhibiting cell-wall synthesis. Active against many gram-positive and gram-negative organisms.
Therapeutic effects: Kills susceptible bacteria.

Available forms

Tablets: 200 mg

NURSING PROCESS

Assessment
• Assess patient's history for hypersensitivity to cefditoren, cephalosporins, penicillins, or other contraindications for drug therapy.
• Monitor patient for overgrowth or recurrence of resistant organisms with prolonged or repeated drug therapy.
• Because cefditoren has been linked to *Clostridium difficile*-associated colitis, monitor patient for diarrhea during therapy.
• Monitor patient for hypersensitivity reactions during drug therapy as well as any unusual bleeding or bruising.
• Evaluate patient's and family's knowledge of drug therapy.

Nursing diagnoses
• Noncompliance related to completion of 10-day antibiotic regimen
• Risk for infection with nonsusceptible bacteria or fungi related to prolonged or repeated drug therapy
• Deficient knowledge related to cephalosporin therapy

Planning and implementation
• Give drug with a meal to increase its bioavailability.
• If patient develops diarrhea after receiving cefditoren, keep in mind that this drug may cause pseudomembranous colitis. Notify prescriber immediately, as colitis may be fatal.
• Don't use this drug if patient needs prolonged treatment.
• Signs and symptoms of overdose may include nausea, vomiting, epigastric distress, diarrhea, and seizures. Treatment is symptomatic and supportive.
• If hypersensitivity or allergic reaction occurs, stop drug and provide emergency measures.

• Adjust dosage in patients with renal impairment.
Patient teaching
• Instruct patient to take drug with food to increase its absorption.
• Caution patient not to take drug with an H_2 antagonist or an antacid because they may reduce cefditoren absorption. If an H_2 antagonist or antacid must be used, instruct patient to take them 2 hours before or after drug, despite feeling better.
• Explain to patient the importance of taking drug for the entire treatment duration to prevent any future drug resistance.
• Instruct patient to immediately stop taking drug and call prescriber if any adverse reactions develop, such as rash, hives, difficulty breathing, unusual bleeding or bruising, or diarrhea.
• Encourage patient to contact prescriber if signs and symptoms of infection don't improve after several days of therapy.
• Urge patient not to miss any doses. However, if patient misses a dose, instruct him to take the missed dose immediately and wait 12 hours before taking the next dose. Tell him not to double the dose.

Evaluation
• Patient completes prescribed 10-day therapy.
• Patient doesn't experience any adverse reactions during drug therapy.
• Patient and family state understanding of drug therapy and importance of completing entire drug regimen as prescribed.

cefoperazone sodium
(sef-oh-PER-ah-zohn SOH-dee-um)
Cefobid

Pharmacologic class: third-generation cephalosporin
Therapeutic class: antibiotic
Pregnancy risk category: B

Indications and dosages

▶ **Serious infections of respiratory tract; intra-abdominal, gynecologic, and skin infections; bacteremia; and septicemia.** Susceptible microorganisms include *Streptococcus pneumoniae* and *S. pyogenes; Staphylococcus aureus* (penicillinase- and non-penicillinase–producing) and *S. epidermidis; enterococci; Escherichia coli; Klebsiella; Haemophilus influenzae; Enterobacter; Citrobacter; Proteus;* some *Pseudomonas,* including *P. aeruginosa;* and *Bacteroides fragilis.*

Adults: Usual dosage is 1 to 2 g q 12 hours I.V. or I.M. In severe infections or those caused by less sensitive organisms, total daily dosage may be increased to 16 g.

⧠ **Adjust-a-dose:** For patients with hepatic or biliary obstruction, give doses of 4 g daily cautiously. Higher dosages require monitoring of serum levels.

For patients with hepatic and substantial renal impairment, maximum total daily dose is 2 g daily. Because the drug's half-life is slightly reduced during hemodialysis, give dose after a hemodialysis session.

▼ I.V. administration

• Reconstitute 1- or 2-g vial with minimum of 2.8 ml of compatible I.V. solution; manufacturer recommends using 5 ml/g.

• Give by direct injection into large vein or into tubing of free-flowing I.V. solution over 3 to 5 minutes.

• When giving by intermittent infusion, add reconstituted drug to 20 to 40 ml of compatible I.V. solution and infuse over 15 to 30 minutes.

• Before reconstituting, protect sterile powder from light and store at 77° F (25° C) or below. After reconstituting, don't protect drug from light; it isn't necessary.

Contraindications and precautions

• Contraindicated in patients hypersensitive to drug or other cephalosporins.

• Use cautiously in patients with renal impairment and in patients with a history of sensitivity to penicillin.

⚘ **Lifespan:** In pregnant or breast-feeding women, use cautiously. In children younger than age 12, safety and efficacy of drug haven't been established.

Adverse reactions

CNS: headache, malaise, paresthesia, dizziness.
GI: *pseudomembranous colitis,* nausea, anorexia, vomiting, *diarrhea,* glossitis, dyspepsia, abdominal cramps, tenesmus, anal pruritus, oral candidiasis.
GU: genital pruritus and candidiasis.

Hematologic: *transient neutropenia,* eosinophilia, hemolytic anemia, *hypoprothrombinemia, bleeding.*
Respiratory: dyspnea.
Skin: *maculopapular and erythematous rashes, urticaria.*
Other: *hypersensitivity reactions* (serum sickness, *anaphylaxis*); *pain, induration, sterile abscesses, warmth, tissue sloughing* at injection site; *phlebitis, thrombophlebitis* with I.V. injection.

Interactions

Drug-drug. *Aminoglycosides:* May increase risk of nephrotoxicity. Monitor patient's renal status closely.
Anticoagulants: May increase anticoagulant effects. Use with caution and monitor patient for bleeding.
Probenecid: May inhibit excretion and increase levels of cefoperazone. Monitor patient.
Drug-lifestyle. *Alcohol:* May cause a disulfiram-like reaction including flushing, tachycardia, bronchospasm, sweating, nausea, and vomiting. Strongly discourage alcohol use with these drugs. This reaction could also occur after several days.

Effects on lab test results

• May increase BUN, creatinine, ALT, AST, alkaline phosphatase, bilirubin, GGT, and LDH levels.

• May increase INR and eosinophil count. May decrease hemoglobin, hematocrit, and neutrophil count. May increase or decrease PT.

• May cause false-positive urine glucose determinations with copper sulfate tests (Clinitest).

Pharmacokinetics

Absorption: Unknown after I.M. administration.
Distribution: Distributed widely into most body tissues and fluids; CSF penetration in patients with inflamed meninges; 82% to 93% protein-bound.
Metabolism: Insignificant.
Excretion: Excreted primarily in urine. *Half-life:* About 1½ to 2½ hours.

Route	Onset	Peak	Duration
I.V.	Immediate	Immediate	Unknown
I.M.	Unknown	1-2 hr	Unknown

Reactions may be *common,* uncommon, *life-threatening,* or **COMMON AND LIFE-THREATENING.**

Action

Chemical effect: Inhibits cell-wall synthesis, promoting osmotic instability; usually bactericidal.
Therapeutic effect: Hinders or kills susceptible bacteria.

Available forms

Infusion: 1-g, 2-g piggyback
Parenteral: 1 g, 2 g

NURSING PROCESS

⚕ Assessment

• Assess patient's infection before therapy and reassess regularly thereafter.
• Obtain specimen for culture and sensitivity tests before first dose. Therapy may begin pending test results.
• Ask patient about previous reactions to cephalosporins or penicillin before administering first dose.
• Be alert for adverse reactions and drug interactions.
• Monitor hydration status if patient develops adverse GI reactions. Cefoperazone may increase risk of diarrhea more than other cephalosporins.
• Evaluate patient's and family's knowledge of drug therapy.

⊕ Nursing diagnoses

• Infection related to bacteria susceptible to drug
• Risk for deficient fluid volume related to drug-induced adverse GI reactions
• Deficient knowledge related to drug therapy

⟩ Planning and implementation

• To prepare drug for I.M. injection, using 1-g vial, dissolve drug with 2 ml of sterile water for injection; add 0.6 ml of 2% lidocaine hydrochloride for final concentration of 333 mg/ml. Or, dissolve drug with 2.8 ml of sterile water for injection; then add 1 ml of 2% lidocaine hydrochloride for final concentration of 250 mg/ml. When using 2-g vial, dissolve drug with 3.8 ml of sterile water for injection; then add 1.2 ml of 2% lidocaine hydrochloride for final concentration of 333 mg/ml. Or, dissolve drug with 5.4 ml of sterile water for injection; then add 1.8 ml of 2% lidocaine hydrochloride for final concentration of 250 mg/ml.

• Inject deeply into large muscle mass, such as gluteus maximus or lateral aspect of thigh.
Ⓢ **ALERT:** Don't confuse with other cephalosporins with similar-sounding names.
Patient teaching
• Tell patient to report adverse reactions.

☑ Evaluation

• Patient is free from infection.
• Patient maintains adequate hydration.
• Patient and family state understanding of drug therapy.

cefotaxime sodium
(sef-oh-TAKS-eem SOH-dee-um)
Claforan

Pharmacologic class: third-generation cephalosporin
Therapeutic class: antibiotic
Pregnancy risk category: B

Indications and dosages

▶ **Perioperative prophylaxis in contaminated surgery.** *Adults:* 1 g I.V. or I.M. 30 to 60 minutes before surgery. In patients undergoing cesarean section, give dose as soon as umbilical cord is clamped, followed by 1 g I.V. or I.M. 6 and 12 hours later.
▶ **Serious infections of lower respiratory and urinary tracts, CNS, skin, bone, and joints; gynecologic and intra-abdominal infections; bacteremia; and septicemia. Susceptible microorganisms include streptococci, including** *Streptococcus pneumoniae* **and** *S. pyogenes;* *Staphylococcus aureus* **(penicillinase- and non-penicillinase–producing) and** *S. epidermidis; Escherichia coli; Klebsiella; Haemophilus influenzae; Enterobacter; Proteus;* **and** *Peptostreptococcus;* **and pelvic inflammatory disease‡.** *Adults:* Usual dosage is 1 g I.V. or I.M. q 6 to 12 hours. Up to 12 g daily can be given in life-threatening infections.
Children weighing at least 50 kg (110 lb): Usual adult dose but don't exceed 12 g daily.
Children ages 1 month to 12 years weighing less than 50 kg: 50 to 180 mg/kg I.V. or I.M. daily in four to six divided doses.
Neonates ages 1 to 4 weeks: 50 mg/kg I.V. q 8 hours.

Neonates up to age 1 week: 50 mg/kg I.V. q 12 hours.

▶ **Disseminated gonococcal infection‡.**
Adults: 1 g I.V. q 8 hours.
Neonates and infants: 25 to 50 mg/kg I.V. q 8 to 12 hours for 7 days, or 50 to 100 mg/kg I.M or I.V. q 12 hours for 7 days.

▶ **Gonococcal ophthalmia‡.** *Adults: 500 mg* I.V. q.i.d.
Neonates: 100 mg I.V. or I.M. for one dose; may continue until ocular cultures are negative at 48 to 72 hours.

▶ **Gonorrheal meningitis or arthritis‡.**
Neonates and infants: 25 to 50 mg/kg I.V. q 8 to 12 hours for 10 to 14 days. Or, 50 to 100 mg/kg I.M. or I.V. q 12 hours for 10 to 14 days.

◩ **Adjust-a-dose:** For patients with renal impairment, if creatinine clearance is below 20 ml/ minute, give half the usual dose at the usual interval.

▼ I.V. administration

• For direct injection, reconstitute 500-mg, 1-g, or 2-g vials with 10 ml sterile water for injection. Solutions containing 1 g/14 ml are isotonic.
• Inject drug into large vein or into tubing of free-flowing I.V. solution over 3 to 5 minutes.
• For I.V. infusion, reconstitute infusion vials with 50 to 100 ml D₅W or normal saline solution.
• Infuse drug over 20 to 30 minutes. Interrupt flow of primary I.V. solution during infusion.

Contraindications and precautions

• Contraindicated in patients hypersensitive to drug or other cephalosporins.
• Use cautiously in patients with history of sensitivity to penicillin and in patients with renal impairment.
⚘ **Lifespan:** In pregnant or breast-feeding women, use cautiously.

Adverse reactions

CNS: headache, malaise, paresthesia, dizziness, elevated temperature.
GI: *pseudomembranous colitis,* nausea, anorexia, vomiting, *diarrhea,* glossitis, dyspepsia, abdominal cramps, tenesmus, anal pruritus, oral candidiasis.
GU: genital pruritus and candidiasis.
Hematologic: *transient neutropenia,* eosinophilia, hemolytic anemia, *thrombocytopenia, agranulocytosis.*

Respiratory: dyspnea.
Skin: *maculopapular and erythematous rashes, urticaria.*
Other: hypersensitivity reactions (serum sickness, *anaphylaxis*); *pain, induration, sterile abscesses, warmth, tissue sloughing* at injection site; *phlebitis, thrombophlebitis* with I.V. injection.

Interactions

Drug-drug. *Aminoglycosides:* May increase risk of nephrotoxicity. Monitor renal function closely.
Probenecid: May inhibit excretion and increase levels of cefotaxime. Use together cautiously.

Effects on lab test results

• May increase ALT, AST, alkaline phosphatase, bilirubin, GGT, and LDH levels.
• May increase eosinophil count. May decrease hemoglobin, hematocrit, and neutrophil, platelet, and granulocyte counts.
• May cause false-positive urine glucose determinations with copper sulfate tests (Clinitest).

Pharmacokinetics

Absorption: Unknown after I.M. administration.
Distribution: Distributed widely into most body tissues and fluids; adequate CSF penetration when meninges are inflamed; 13% to 38% protein-bound.
Metabolism: Partially metabolized to active metabolite.
Excretion: Excreted primarily in urine. *Half-life:* 1 to 2 hours.

Route	Onset	Peak	Duration
I.V.	Immediate	Immediate	Unknown
I.M.	Unknown	30 min	Unknown

Action

Chemical effect: Inhibits cell-wall synthesis, promoting osmotic instability; usually bactericidal.
Therapeutic effect: Hinders or kills susceptible bacteria.

Available forms

Infusion: 1 g, 2 g
Injection: 500 mg, 1 g, 2 g

Reactions may be *common,* uncommon, *life-threatening,* or COMMON AND LIFE-THREATENING.

NURSING PROCESS

Assessment
- Assess patient's infection before therapy and reassess regularly thereafter.
- Obtain specimen for culture and sensitivity tests. Therapy may begin before test results are known.
- Ask patient about previous reactions to cephalosporins or penicillin before administering first dose.
- Be alert for adverse reactions and drug interactions.
- Monitor patient's hydration status if adverse GI reactions occur.
- Evaluate patient's and family's knowledge of drug therapy.

Nursing diagnoses
- Infection related to bacteria susceptible to drug
- Risk for deficient fluid volume related to drug-induced adverse GI reactions
- Deficient knowledge related to drug therapy

Planning and implementation
- For I.M. use, inject deeply into large muscle mass, such as gluteus maximus or lateral aspect of thigh.
- **ALERT:** Don't confuse with other cephalosporins with similar-sounding names.

Patient teaching
- Tell patient to report adverse reactions.
- Teach patient to report decrease in urinary output. May have to decrease total daily dosage.

Evaluation
- Patient is free from infection.
- Patient maintains adequate hydration.
- Patient and family state understanding of drug therapy.

cefotetan disodium
(SEF-oh-teh-tan die-SOH-dee-um)
Apatef ◊ , Cefotan

Pharmacologic class: second-generation cephalosporin
Therapeutic class: antibiotic
Pregnancy risk category: B

Indications and dosages

▶ **Serious UTIs, lower respiratory tract infections, and gynecologic, skin and skin-structure, intra-abdominal, and bone and joint infections caused by susceptible streptococci, *Staphylococcus aureus* and *S. epidermidis*, *Escherichia coli*, *Klebsiella*, *Enterobacter*, *Proteus*, *Haemophilus influenzae*, *Neisseria gonorrhoeae*, and *Bacteroides*, including *B. fragilis*.** *Adults:* 1 to 2 g I.V. or I.M. q 12 hours for 5 to 10 days. In life-threatening infections, up to 6 g daily.
Children‡: 40 to 60 mg/kg daily I.V. divided in equally divided doses q 12 hours.
▶ **Perioperative prophylaxis; used in contaminated surgery.** *Adults:* 1 to 2 g I.V. given once 30 to 60 minutes before surgery. In cesarean section, give dose as soon as umbilical cord is clamped.
Adjust-a-dose: For patients with renal impairment, if creatinine clearance is 10 to 30 ml/minute, give usual dose q 24 hours; if creatinine clearance is less than 10 ml/minute, give usual dose q 48 hours.

I.V. administration
- Reconstitute drug with sterile water for injection. Then may be mixed with 50 to 100 ml of D_5W or normal saline solution.
- Interrupt flow of primary I.V. solution during drug infusion. Infuse over 20 to 60 minutes.
- For direct injection, give solutions containing 1 or 2 g of solution over 3 to 5 minutes.

Contraindications and precautions
- Contraindicated in patients hypersensitive to drug or other cephalosporins.
- Use cautiously in patients with history of sensitivity to penicillin and in patients with renal impairment.
Lifespan: In pregnant and breast-feeding women, use cautiously. In children, safety and efficacy of drug haven't been established.

Adverse reactions
CNS: headache, malaise, paresthesia, dizziness.
GI: *pseudomembranous colitis,* nausea, anorexia, vomiting, *diarrhea,* glossitis, dyspepsia, abdominal cramps, tenesmus, anal pruritus.
GU: genital pruritus and candidiasis, ***nephrotoxicity.***
Hematologic: *transient neutropenia,* eosinophilia, hemolytic anemia, hypoprothrombine-

mia, bleeding, *agranulocytosis, thrombocytopenia.*
Respiratory: dyspnea.
Skin: *maculopapular and erythematous rashes, urticaria.*
Other: *hypersensitivity reactions* (serum sickness, *anaphylaxis*); elevated temperature; *pain, induration, sterile abscesses,* tissue sloughing at injection site; *phlebitis, thrombophlebitis* with I.V. injection.

Interactions

Drug-drug. *Aminoglycosides:* May have synergistic effect and increase risk of nephrotoxicity. Use with caution; monitor renal function tests if used together.
Anticoagulants: May increase anticoagulants effects. Use with caution and monitor patient for bleeding.
Probenecid: May inhibit excretion and increase levels of cefotetan. Sometimes used for this effect.
Drug-lifestyle. *Alcohol use:* May cause a disulfiram-like reaction, including flushing, tachycardia, bronchospasm, sweating, nausea, and vomiting. Strongly discourage alcohol use with these drugs. This reaction could also occur after several days.

Effects on lab test results

• May increase ALT, AST, alkaline phosphatase, bilirubin, creatinine, and LDH levels.
• May increase PT and INR and eosinophil count. May decrease hemoglobin, hematocrit, and neutrophil and granulocyte counts. May increase or decrease platelet count.
• May cause false-positive urine glucose determinations with copper sulfate tests (Clinitest).

Pharmacokinetics

Absorption: Unknown after I.M. administration.
Distribution: Distributed widely into most body tissues and fluids; CSF penetration is poor; 75% to 90% protein-bound.
Metabolism: None.
Excretion: Excreted primarily in urine. *Half-life:* About 3 to 4½ hours.

Route	Onset	Peak	Duration
I.V.	Immediate	Immediate	Unknown
I.M.	Unknown	1½-2 hr	Unknown

Action

Chemical effect: Inhibits cell-wall synthesis, promoting osmotic instability; usually bactericidal.
Therapeutic effect: Hinders or kills susceptible bacteria.

Available forms

Infusion: 1-g, 2-g piggyback
Injection: 1 g, 2 g

NURSING PROCESS

⚗ Assessment
• Assess patient's infection before therapy and reassess regularly thereafter.
• Obtain specimen for culture and sensitivity tests before first dose. Therapy may begin pending test results.
• Ask patient about previous reactions to cephalosporins or penicillin before giving first dose.
• Be alert for adverse reactions and drug interactions.
• Monitor patient's hydration status if adverse GI reactions occur.
• Evaluate patient's and family's knowledge of drug therapy.

⊞ Nursing diagnoses
• Infection related to bacteria susceptible to drug
• Risk for deficient fluid volume related to drug-induced adverse GI reactions
• Deficient knowledge related to drug therapy

▷ Planning and implementation
• Reconstitute I.M. injection with sterile water or bacteriostatic water for injection, normal saline solution for injection, or 0.5% or 1% lidocaine hydrochloride. Shake to dissolve and let stand until clear.
• Reconstituted solution remains stable for 24 hours at room temperature or 96 hours if refrigerated.
⊛ **ALERT:** Don't confuse with other cephalosporins with similar-sounding names.
Patient teaching
• Tell patient to report adverse reactions.
• Alert patient to signs of superinfection. Careful observation by patient is essential.

☑ **Evaluation**
- Patient is free from infection.
- Patient maintains adequate hydration.
- Patient and family state understanding of drug therapy.

cefoxitin sodium

(sef-OKS-ih-tin SOH-dee-um)
Mefoxin

Pharmacologic class: second-generation cephalosporin
Therapeutic class: antibiotic
Pregnancy risk category: B

Indications and dosages

▶ **Serious infections of respiratory and GU tracts; skin, soft-tissue, bone, and joint infections; bloodstream and intra-abdominal infections caused by susceptible** *Escherichia coli* **and other coliform bacteria,** *Staphylococcus aureus* **(penicillinase- and nonpenicillinase–producing),** *S. epidermidis, streptococci, Klebsiella, Haemophilus influenzae,* **and** *Bacteroides,* **including** *B. fragilis;* **and perioperative prophylaxis.** *Adults:* 1 to 2 g I.V. q 6 to 8 hours for uncomplicated forms of infection. In life-threatening infections, up to 12 g daily.
Children and infants age 3 months and older: 80 to 160 mg/kg I.V. or I.M. daily given in four to six equally divided doses. Maximum daily dose is 12 g.
▶ **Prophylactic use in surgery.** *Adults:* 2 g I.V. 30 to 60 minutes before surgery; then 2 g I.M. or I.V. q 6 hours for 24 hours.
Children older than age 3 months: 30 to 40 mg/kg I.M. or I.V. 30 to 60 minutes before surgery; then 30 mg/kg q 6 hours for 24 hours.
🔄 **Adjust-a-dose:** For patients with renal impairment, if creatinine clearance is 30 to 50 ml/minute, give 1 to 2 g q 8 to 12 hours; if clearance is 10 to 29 ml/minute, give 1 to 2 g q 12 to 24 hours; and if clearance is 5 to 10 ml/minute, give 500 mg to 1 g q 12 to 24 hours. If clearance is less than 5 ml/minute, give 500 mg to 1 g q 24 to 48 hours.

▼ I.V. administration

- Reconstitute 1 g with at least 10 ml of sterile water for injection and 2 g with 10 to 20 ml of sterile water for injection. Solutions of D_5W and normal saline solution for injection also can be used.
- For direct injection, inject reconstituted drug into large vein or into tubing of free-flowing I.V. solution over 3 to 5 minutes.
- For intermittent infusion, add reconstituted drug to 50 or 100 ml D_5W, $D_{10}W$, or normal saline solution for injection. Interrupt flow of primary I.V. solution during infusion.
- Assess I.V. site frequently for thrombophlebitis.

Contraindications and precautions

- Contraindicated in patients hypersensitive to drug or other cephalosporins.
- Use cautiously in patients with history of sensitivity to penicillin and in patients with renal impairment.
- 🌣 Lifespan: In pregnant or breast-feeding women, use cautiously.

Adverse reactions

CNS: fever.
CV: hypotension.
GI: *pseudomembranous colitis, diarrhea.*
GU: *acute renal failure.*
Hematologic: *transient neutropenia,* eosinophilia, hemolytic anemia, *thrombocytopenia.*
Respiratory: *dyspnea.*
Skin: *maculopapular and erythematous rashes, urticaria.*
Other: *hypersensitivity reactions* (serum sickness, *anaphylaxis*), *phlebitis, thrombophlebitis* with I.V. injection.

Interactions

Drug-drug. *Nephrotoxic drugs:* May increase risk of nephrotoxicity. Monitor renal function closely.
Probenecid: May inhibit excretion and increase levels of cefoxitin. Sometimes used for this effect.

Effects on lab test results

- May increase ALT, AST, alkaline phosphatase, bilirubin, and LDH levels.
- May increase eosinophil count. May decrease hemoglobin, hematocrit, and neutrophil and platelet counts.
- May cause false-positive urine glucose determinations with copper sulfate tests (Clinitest).

Pharmacokinetics

Absorption: Unknown for I.M. administration.
Distribution: Distributed widely into most body tissues and fluids; CSF penetration is poor; 50% to 80% protein-bound.
Metabolism: Insignificant (about 2%).
Excretion: Excreted primarily in urine. *Half-life:* About ½ to 1 hour.

Route	Onset	Peak	Duration
I.V.	Immediate	Immediate	Unknown
I.M.	Rapid	20–30 min	< 6 hr

Action

Chemical effect: Inhibits cell-wall synthesis, promoting osmotic instability; usually bactericidal.
Therapeutic effect: Hinders or kills susceptible bacteria.

Available forms

Infusion: 1 g, 2 g in 50-ml or 100-ml
Injection: 1 g, 2 g

NURSING PROCESS

🗹 Assessment

• Assess patient's infection before therapy and reassess regularly thereafter.
• Obtain specimen for culture and sensitivity tests before first dose. Therapy may begin pending test results.
• Ask patient about previous reactions to cephalosporins or penicillin before giving first dose.
• Be alert for adverse reactions and drug interactions.
• Monitor patient's hydration status if adverse GI reactions occur.
• Evaluate patient's and family's knowledge of drug therapy.

🔁 Nursing diagnoses

• Infection related to bacteria susceptible to drug
• Risk for deficient fluid volume related to drug-induced adverse GI reactions
• Deficient knowledge related to drug therapy

⊠ Planning and implementation

• Reconstitute I.M. injection by adding 2 ml of sterile water for injection or 0.5 or 1% lidocaine hydrochloride (without epinephrine) to each g of cefoxitin.

• For I.M. use, inject deeply into large muscle mass, such as the upper quadrant of the gluteus maximus.
• Patients with renal impairment require dosage adjustment.
• After reconstitution, drug may be stored for 24 hours at room temperature or refrigerated for 1 week.
⚠ **ALERT:** Don't confuse with other cephalosporins with similar-sounding names.

Patient teaching

• Tell patient to report adverse reactions and signs and symptoms of superinfection promptly.
• Instruct patient to notify prescriber if he experiences loose stools or diarrhea.

🗹 Evaluation

• Patient is free from infection.
• Patient maintains adequate hydration.
• Patient and family state understanding of drug therapy.

cefpodoxime proxetil
(sef-poh-DOKS-eem PROKS-eh-til)
Vantin

Pharmacologic class: third-generation cephalosporin
Therapeutic class: antibiotic
Pregnancy risk category: B

Indications and dosages

▶ **Acute, community-acquired pneumonia caused by non-beta-lactamase–producing strains of *Haemophilus influenzae* or *Streptococcus pneumoniae*.** *Adults and children age 12 and older:* 200 mg P.O. q 12 hours for 14 days.
▶ **Acute bacterial exacerbation of chronic bronchitis caused by *S. pneumoniae*, *H. influenzae* (non-beta-lactamase–producing strains), or *Moraxella catarrhalis*.** *Adults and children age 12 and older:* 200 mg P.O. q 12 hours for 10 days.
▶ **Uncomplicated gonorrhea in men and women; rectal gonococcal infections in women.** *Adults and children age 12 and older:* 200 mg P.O. as single dose. Follow with doxycycline 100 mg P.O. b.i.d. for 7 days.
▶ **Uncomplicated skin and skin-structure infections caused by *S. aureus* or *S. pyogenes*.**

Adults and children age 12 and older: 400 mg P.O. q 12 hours for 7 to 14 days.

▶ **Acute otitis media caused by *S. pneumoniae*, *H. influenzae*, or *M. catarrhalis*.** *Children ages 2 months to 12 years:* 5 mg/kg (not to exceed 200 mg) P.O. q 12 hours or 10 mg/kg (not to exceed 400 mg) P.O. daily for 10 days.

▶ **Pharyngitis or tonsillitis caused by *S. pyogenes*.** *Adults and children age 12 and older:* 100 mg P.O. q 12 hours for 5 to 10 days. *Children ages 2 months to 12 years:* 5 mg/kg (not to exceed 100 mg) P.O. q 12 hours for 10 days.

▶ **Uncomplicated UTIs caused by *E. coli*, *Klebsiella pneumoniae*, *Proteus mirabilis*, or *S. saprophyticus*.** *Adults and children age 12 and older:* 100 mg P.O. q 12 hours for 7 days.

▶ **Mild to moderate acute maxillary sinusitis caused by *H. influenzae*, *S. pneumoniae*, or *M. catarrhalis*.** *Adults and children age 12 and older:* 200 mg P.O. q 12 hours for 10 days. *Children ages 2 months to 12 years:* 5 mg/kg P.O. q 12 hours for 10 days; maximum dose is 200 mg.

⧉ **Adjust-a-dose:** For patients with renal impairment, if creatinine clearance is less than 30 ml/minute increase dosage interval to q 24 hours. Patients receiving dialysis should be given dose three times weekly, after dialysis.

Contraindications and precautions

• Contraindicated in patients hypersensitive to drug or other cephalosporins.
• Use cautiously in patients with history of hypersensitivity to penicillin (risk of cross-sensitivity), and patients receiving nephrotoxic drugs (other cephalosporins have had nephrotoxic potential).
⚖ Lifespan: In pregnant or breast-feeding women, use cautiously.

Adverse reactions

CNS: headache.
GI: *diarrhea*, nausea, vomiting, abdominal pain.
GU: vaginal fungal infections.
Skin: rash.
Other: hypersensitivity reactions *(anaphylaxis)*.

Interactions

Drug-drug. *Antacids, H_2-receptor antagonists:* May decrease absorption of cefpodoxime. Avoid using together.

Probenecid: May decrease excretion of cefpodoxime. Monitor patient for toxicity.
Drug-food. *Any food:* May increase drug absorption. Give drug with food.

Effects on lab test results

• May increase or decrease glucose levels. May increase BUN, creatinine, AST, ALT, GGT, alkaline phosphatase, bilirubin, and LDH levels. May decrease albumin, potassium, and sodium levels.
• May increase eosinophil, WBC and granulocyte, lymphocyte, basophil, and platelet counts. May prolong PT and PTT. May decrease hemoglobin and hematocrit.
• May cause false-positive urine glucose determinations with copper sulfate tests (Clinitest). May cause positive Coombs' test.

Pharmacokinetics

Absorption: Absorbed from GI tract.
Distribution: Distributed widely into most body tissues and fluids except CSF; 22% to 33% protein-bound in serum and 21% to 29% protein-bound in plasma.
Metabolism: Drug is de-esterified to its active metabolite, cefpodoxime.
Excretion: Excreted primarily in urine. *Half-life:* 2 to 2¾ hours.

Route	Onset	Peak	Duration
P.O.	Unknown	2-3 hr	Unknown

Action

Chemical effect: Inhibits cell-wall synthesis, promoting osmotic instability; usually bactericidal.
Therapeutic effect: Hinders or kills susceptible bacteria.

Available forms

Oral suspension: 50 mg/5 ml, 100 mg/5 ml in 100-ml bottles
Tablets (film-coated): 100 mg, 200 mg

NURSING PROCESS

⧫ **Assessment**
• Assess patient's infection before therapy and reassess regularly thereafter.
• Obtain specimen for culture and sensitivity tests before first dose. Therapy may begin pending test results.

- Ask patient about previous reactions to cephalosporins or penicillin before giving first dose.
- Be alert for adverse reactions and drug interactions.
- Monitor patient's hydration status if adverse GI reactions occur.
- Evaluate patient's and family's knowledge of drug therapy.

🖭 Nursing diagnoses
- Infection related to bacteria susceptible to drug
- Risk for deficient fluid volume related to drug-induced adverse GI reactions
- Deficient knowledge related to drug therapy

⟩ Planning and implementation
- Give drug with food to minimize adverse GI reactions. Shake well before using.
- Store suspension in refrigerator (36° to 46° F [2° to 8° C]). Discard unused portion after 14 days.
- ⊛ **ALERT:** Don't confuse with other cephalosporins with similar-sounding names.

Patient teaching
- Advise patient to take drug with meals to minimize adverse GI reactions.
- Tell patient to take drug exactly as prescribed, even after he feels better.
- Instruct patient to notify prescriber if rash develops.
- Teach patient how to store drug.
- Instruct patient to notify prescriber about a reduction in urinary output, especially if patient takes a diuretic.

☑ Evaluation
- Patient is free from infection.
- Patient maintains adequate hydration.
- Patient and family state understanding of drug therapy.

cefprozil
(SEF-pruh-zil)
Cefzil

Pharmacologic class: second-generation cephalosporin
Therapeutic class: antibiotic
Pregnancy risk category: B

Indications and dosages
▶ **Pharyngitis or tonsillitis caused by** *Streptococcus pyogenes. Adults and children older than age 12:* 500 mg P.O. daily for 10 days. *Children ages 2 to 12:* 7.5 mg/kg P.O. q 12 hours for 10 days.
▶ **Otitis media caused by** *Streptococcus pneumoniae, Haemophilus influenzae,* **or** *Moraxella catarrhalis. Infants and children ages 6 months to 12 years:* 15 mg/kg P.O. q 12 hours for 10 days.
▶ **Secondary bacterial infections of acute bronchitis and acute bacterial exacerbation of chronic bronchitis caused by** *S. pneumoniae, H. influenzae,* **and** *M. catarrhalis. Adults and children older than age 12:* 500 mg P.O. q 12 hours for 10 days.
▶ **Uncomplicated skin and skin-structure infections caused by** *Staphylococcus aureus* **or** *S. pyogenes. Adults and children older than age 12:* 250 mg P.O. b.i.d., or 500 mg daily to b.i.d. for 10 days.
Children ages 2 to 12: 20 mg/kg P.O. q 24 hours for 10 days. Maximum dose is 1 g P.O. daily.
▶ **Acute sinusitis caused by** *Streptococcus pneumoniae, Haemophilus influenzae,* **and** *Moraxella (Branhamella) catarrhalis. Adults and children older than age 12:* 250 mg or 500 mg P.O. q 12 hours for 10 days.
Children ages 6 months to 12 years: 7.5 mg/kg P.O. q 12 hours or 15 mg/kg P.O. daily for 10 days.
◲ **Adjust-a-dose:** For patients with renal impairment, if creatinine clearance is less than 30 ml/minute, give 50% of usual dose.

Contraindications and precautions
- Contraindicated in patients hypersensitive to drug or other cephalosporins.
- Use cautiously in patients with history of sensitivity to penicillin and patients with hepatic or renal impairment.
- ⚌ **Lifespan:** In pregnant and breast-feeding women, use cautiously. Children shouldn't receive more than the recommended adult dose.

Adverse reactions
CNS: dizziness, hyperactivity, headache, nervousness, insomnia.
GI: diarrhea, *nausea,* vomiting, abdominal pain.
GU: genital pruritus, vaginitis.
Hematologic: eosinophilia.
Skin: rash, urticaria.

Reactions may be *common,* uncommon, ***life-threatening***, or COMMON AND LIFE-THREATENING.

Other: superinfection, *hypersensitivity reactions* (serum sickness, *anaphylaxis*).

Interactions

Drug-drug. *Aminoglycosides:* May increase risk of nephrotoxicity. Monitor patient closely.
Probenecid: May inhibit excretion and increase levels of cefprozil. Monitor patient.

Effects on lab test results

• May increase BUN, creatinine, ALT, AST, alkaline phosphatase, bilirubin, and LDH levels.
• May increase eosinophil count. May decrease WBC, leukocyte, and platelet counts.
• May cause false-positive urine glucose determinations with copper sulfate tests (Clinitest).

Pharmacokinetics

Absorption: About 95% absorbed from GI tract.
Distribution: About 35% protein-bound; distributed into various body tissues and fluids.
Metabolism: Probably metabolized by the liver.
Excretion: Excreted primarily in urine. *Half-life:* 1¼ hours in patients with normal renal function; 2 hours in patients with impaired hepatic function; and 5¼ to 6 hours in patients with end-stage renal disease.

Route	Onset	Peak	Duration
P.O.	Unknown	Unknown	Unknown

Action

Chemical effect: Inhibits cell-wall synthesis, promoting osmotic instability; usually bactericidal.
Therapeutic effect: Hinders or kills susceptible bacteria.

Available forms

Oral suspension: 125 mg/5 ml, 250 mg/5 ml
Tablets: 250 mg, 500 mg

NURSING PROCESS

Assessment
• Assess patient's infection before therapy and reassess regularly thereafter.
• Obtain specimen for culture and sensitivity tests before first dose. Therapy may begin pending test results.
• Ask patient about previous reactions to cephalosporins or penicillin before giving first dose.

• Be alert for adverse reactions and drug interactions.
• Monitor patient's hydration status if adverse GI reactions occur.
• Monitor patient's renal function.
• Evaluate patient's and family's knowledge of drug therapy.

Nursing diagnoses
• Infection related to bacteria susceptible to drug
• Risk for deficient fluid volume related to drug-induced adverse GI reactions
• Deficient knowledge related to drug therapy

Planning and implementation
• Give drug after hemodialysis treatment is completed; drug is removed by hemodialysis.
• Refrigerate reconstituted suspension (stable for 14 days). Keep tightly closed and shake well before using.
• **ALERT:** Don't confuse with other cephalosporins with similar-sounding names.
Patient teaching
• Tell patient to shake suspension well before measuring dose.
• Advise patient to take drug as prescribed, even after he feels better.
• Inform patient that oral suspensions contain drug in bubble-gum flavor to improve palatability and promote compliance in children. Tell him to refrigerate reconstituted suspension and to discard any unused portion after 14 days.
• Advise elderly patients also receiving diuretic therapy to notify prescriber of decreased urine output.

Evaluation
• Patient is free from infection.
• Patient maintains adequate hydration.
• Patient and family state understanding of drug therapy.

ceftazidime
(sef-TAZ-ih-deem)
Ceptaz, Fortaz, Tazicef, Tazidime

Pharmacologic class: third-generation cephalosporin
Therapeutic class: antibiotic
Pregnancy risk category: B

Indications and dosages

▶ **Serious infections of lower respiratory and urinary tracts; gynecologic, intra-abdominal, CNS, and skin infections; bacteremia; and septicemia.** Among susceptible microorganisms are streptococci, including Streptococcus pneumoniae and *S. pyogenes, Staphylococcus aureus, Escherichia coli, Klebsiella, Proteus, Enterobacter, Haemophilus influenzae, Pseudomonas,* and some strains of *Bacteroides. Adults and children older than age 12:* 1 g I.V. or I.M. q 8 to 12 hours; maximum 6 g daily for life-threatening infections.
Children ages 1 month to 12 years: 25 to 50 mg/kg I.V. q 8 hours. Maximum 6 g daily.
Neonates age 4 weeks or younger: 30 mg/kg I.V. q 12 hours.
▶ **Uncomplicated UTI.** *Adults:* 250 mg I.V. or I.M. q 12 hours.
▶ **Complicated UTI.** *Adults:* 500 mg I.V. or I.M. q 8 to 12 hours.
▶ **Uncomplicated pneumonia or mild skin and skin-structure infection.** *Adults:* 0.5 to 1 g I.V. or I.M. q 8 hours.
▶ **Bone and joint infection.** *Adults:* 2 g I.V. q 12 hours.
▶ **Empiric therapy in febrile neutropenic patients‡.** *Adults:* 100 mg/kg I.V. daily in three divided doses; or 2 g I.V. q 8 hours either alone or with an aminoglycoside, such as amikacin.
⊠ **Adjust-a-dose:** For patients with renal impairment, if creatinine clearance is 31 to 50 ml/minute, give 1 g q 12 hours; if clearance is 16 to 30 ml/minute, give 1 g q 24 hours; if clearance is 6 to 15 ml/minute, give 500 mg q 24 hours; if clearance is less than 5 ml/minute, give 500 mg q 48 hours. Drug is removed by hemodialysis; give a supplemental dose of drug after each dialysis treatment.

▼ I.V. administration

• Each brand of this drug includes instructions for reconstitution. Read and follow these instructions carefully.
• Reconstitute sodium carbonate-containing solutions with sterile water for injection. Add 5 ml to 500-mg vial; 10 ml to 1-g or 2-g vial. Shake well to dissolve drug.
• Carbon dioxide is released during dissolution, and positive pressure will develop in vial.

• Reconstitute arginine-containing solutions with 10 ml sterile water for injection; this formulation won't release gas bubbles.
• Infuse drug over 15 to 30 minutes.

Contraindications and precautions

• Contraindicated in patients hypersensitive to drug or other cephalosporins.
• Use cautiously in patients with history of sensitivity to penicillin and in patients with renal impairment.
⚖ **Lifespan:** In pregnant and breast-feeding women, use cautiously. In children age 12 and younger, safety and efficacy of drug haven't been established.

Adverse reactions

CNS: headache, dizziness, *seizures.*
GI: *pseudomembranous colitis,* nausea, vomiting, diarrhea, dysgeusia, abdominal cramps.
GU: genital pruritus, candidiasis.
Hematologic: eosinophilia, *thrombocytosis, leukopenia, agranulocytosis.*
Respiratory: dyspnea.
Skin: *maculopapular and erythematous rashes, urticaria.*
Other: hypersensitivity reactions (serum sickness, *anaphylaxis*); elevated temperature; *pain, induration, sterile abscesses, tissue sloughing at injection site; phlebitis, thrombophlebitis with I.V. injection.*

Interactions

Drug-drug. *Chloramphenicol:* May have an antagonistic effect. Avoid using together.

Effects on lab test results

• May increase ALT, AST, alkaline phosphatase, bilirubin, and LDH levels.
• May increase eosinophil count. May decrease hemoglobin, hematocrit, and WBC and granulocyte counts. May increase or decrease platelet count.
• May cause false-positive urine glucose determinations with copper sulfate tests (Clinitest).

Pharmacokinetics

Absorption: Unknown with I.M. administration.
Distribution: Distributed widely into most body tissues and fluids, including CSF (unlike most other cephalosporins); 5% to 24% protein-bound.

Metabolism: None.
Excretion: Excreted primarily in urine. *Half-life:* About 1½ to 2 hours.

Route	Onset	Peak	Duration
I.V.	Immediate	Immediate	Unknown
I.M.	Unknown	≤ 1 hr	Unknown

Action

Chemical effect: Inhibits cell-wall synthesis, promoting osmotic instability; usually bactericidal.
Therapeutic effect: Hinders or kills susceptible bacteria.

Available forms

Infusion: 1 g, 2 g in 50-ml and 100-ml vials (premixed)
Injection (with arginine): 1 g, 2 g, 6 g
Injection (with sodium carbonate): 500 mg, 1 g, 2 g

NURSING PROCESS

⚕ Assessment
• Assess patient's infection before therapy and reassess regularly thereafter.
• Obtain specimen for culture and sensitivity tests before first dose. Therapy may begin pending test results.
• Ask patient about previous reactions to cephalosporins or penicillin before giving first dose.
• Be alert for adverse reactions and drug interactions.
• Monitor patient's hydration status if adverse GI reactions occur.
• Evaluate patient's and family's knowledge of drug therapy.

🔯 Nursing diagnoses
• Infection related to bacteria susceptible to drug
• Risk for deficient fluid volume related to drug-induced adverse GI reactions
• Deficient knowledge related to drug therapy

▷ Planning and implementation
• Inject deeply into large muscle mass, such as gluteus maximus or lateral aspect of thigh.
• **ALERT:** Commercially available preparations contain either sodium carbonate (Fortaz, Tazicef, Tazidime) or arginine (Ceptaz) to facilitate dissolution of drug.

• **ALERT:** Don't confuse with other cephalosporins with similar-sounding names.
Patient teaching
• Tell patient to report adverse reactions.
• Instruct patient to report any change in urinary output to prescriber immediately. Dosage may need to be reduced to compensate for decreased excretion.

☑ Evaluation
• Patient is free from infection.
• Patient maintains adequate hydration.
• Patient and family state understanding of drug therapy.

ceftibuten
(sef-tih-BYOO-tin)
Cedax

Pharmacologic class: third-generation cephalosporin
Therapeutic class: antibiotic
Pregnancy risk category: B

Indications and dosages

▶ **Acute bacterial exacerbation of chronic bronchitis caused by** *Haemophilus influenzae,* *Moraxella catarrhalis,* **or penicillin-susceptible strains of** *Streptococcus* **pneumoniae.** *Adults and children age 12 and older:* 400 mg P.O. daily for 10 days.
▶ **Pharyngitis and tonsillitis caused by** *Streptococcus pyogenes,* **acute bacterial otitis media caused by** *H. influenzae, M. catarrhalis,* **or** *S. pyogenes. Adults and children age 12 and older:* 400 mg capsules P.O. daily for 10 days. *Children younger than age 12:* 9 mg/kg capsules P.O. daily for 10 days. Maximum daily dose is 400 mg.
Children weighing more than 45 kg (99 lb): 400 mg oral suspension P.O. daily for 10 days. *Children older than age 6 months and weighing 45 kg or less:* 9 mg/kg oral suspension P.O. daily for 10 days.
☒ **Adjust-a-dose:** For patients with renal impairment, if creatinine clearance is 30 to 49 ml/minute, give 4.5 mg/kg or 200 mg P.O. q 24 hours; if creatinine clearance is 5 to 29 ml/minute, give 2.25 mg/kg or 100 mg P.O. q 24 hours. Give 400 mg P.O. as a single dose to

patients undergoing hemodialysis at the end of each dialysis session.

Contraindications and precautions

• Contraindicated in patients hypersensitive to cephalosporins.
• Use cautiously in patients with history of hypersensitivity to penicillin and in patients with GI disease or renal impairment.
※ **Lifespan:** In breast-feeding women and elderly patients, use cautiously. It's not known whether drug appears in breast milk. Monitor elderly patient's renal function and adjust dosage as needed.

Adverse reactions

CNS: headache, dizziness, aphasia, psychosis.
GI: nausea, vomiting, diarrhea, dyspepsia, abdominal pain, loose stools, *pseudomembranous colitis.*
GU: *toxic nephropathy,* renal dysfunction.
Hematologic: *aplastic anemia,* hemolytic anemia, *hemorrhage, neutropenia, agranulocytosis, pancytopenia.*
Hepatic: hepatic cholestasis.
Skin: *Stevens-Johnson syndrome.*
Other: allergic reaction, *anaphylaxis,* drug fever.

Interactions

Drug-food. *Any food:* Decreases bioavailability of drug. Administer drug 2 hours before or 1 hour after a meal.

Effects on lab test results

• May increase ALT, AST, alkaline phosphatase, bilirubin, and BUN and creatinine levels.
• May increase eosinophil count. May decrease hemoglobin, hematocrit, and leukocyte count. May increase or decrease platelet count.

Pharmacokinetics

Absorption: Rapidly absorbed.
Distribution: 65% bound to plasma proteins.
Metabolism: Metabolized by the kidneys.
Excretion: Excreted mainly in urine.

Route	Onset	Peak	Duration
P.O.	Unknown	2-4 hr	Unknown

Action

Chemical effect: Exerts its bacterial action by binding to essential target proteins of the bacterial cell wall, thus inhibiting cell-wall synthesis.

Therapeutic effect: Hinders or kills susceptible bacteria.

Available forms

Capsules: 400 mg
Oral suspension: 90 mg/5 ml, 180 mg/5 ml

NURSING PROCESS

Assessment

• Obtain specimen for culture and sensitivity tests before starting drug.
• Monitor patient for superinfection.
• Obtain specimen for *Clostridium difficile* in patient who develops diarrhea after therapy.
• Evaluate patient's and family's knowledge of drug therapy.

Nursing diagnoses

• Infection related to bacteria susceptible to drug
• Deficient knowledge related to drug therapy

Planning and implementation

• To prepare oral suspension, tap bottle to loosen powder. Follow chart supplied by manufacturer for mixing instructions. Suspension is stable for 14 days if refrigerated.
• Shake suspension well before use.
• Stop drug and notify prescriber if allergic reaction occurs.
⊛ **ALERT:** Don't confuse with other cephalosporins with similar-sounding names.
Patient teaching
• Instruct patient to take drug as prescribed, even if he feels better.
• Instruct patient using oral suspension to shake bottle before use and to take it at least 2 hours before or 1 hour after a meal.
• Instruct patient to store oral suspension in the refrigerator, with lid tightly closed, and to discard unused drug after 14 days.
• Warn breast-feeding woman that it's unclear whether drug appears in breast milk.
• Tell patient with diabetes that suspension has 1 g sucrose per teaspoon.

Evaluation

• Patient is free from infection.
• Patient and family state understanding of drug therapy.

Reactions may be *common,* uncommon, *life-threatening,* or **COMMON AND LIFE-THREATENING.**

ceftizoxime sodium
(sef-tih-ZOKS-eem SOH-dee-um)
Cefizox

Pharmacologic class: third-generation cephalosporin
Therapeutic class: antibiotic
Pregnancy risk category: B

Indications and dosages

▶ **Serious infections of lower respiratory and urinary tracts, gynecologic infections, bacteremia, septicemia, meningitis, intra-abdominal infections, bone and joint infections, and skin infections. Among susceptible microorganisms are** *Streptococcus pneumoniae* **and** *S. pyogenes, Staphylococcus aureus* **(penicillinase- and non-penicillinase–producing) and** *S. epidermidis, Escherichia coli, Klebsiella, Haemophilus influenzae, Enterobacter, Proteus,* **some** *Pseudomonas,* **and** *Peptostreptococcus. Adults:* 1 to 2 g I.V. or I.M. q 8 to 12 hours. In life-threatening infections, 3 to 4 g I.V. q 8 hours.
Children older than age 6 months: 50 mg/kg I.V. q 6 to 8 hours. For serious infections, up to 200 mg/kg daily in divided doses may be used. Maximum 12 g daily.
▶ **Acute bacterial otitis media.** *Children:* 50 mg/kg (not to exceed 1 g) I.M. as a single dose.
⧄ **Adjust-a-dose:** For patients with renal impairment, if creatinine clearance is 50 to 79 ml/minute, give 500 mg to 1.5 g q 8 hours; if clearance is 5 to 49 ml/minute, give 250 mg to 1 g q 12 hours; if clearance is less than 5 ml/minute or patient undergoes hemodialysis, give 500 mg to 1 g q 48 hours or 250 to 500 mg q 24 hours.

▼ I.V. administration

● To reconstitute powder, add 5 ml sterile water to 500-mg vial, 10 ml to 1-g vial, or 20 ml to 2-g vial.
● Reconstitute piggyback vials with 50 to 100 ml of normal saline solution or D_5W. Shake vial well.
● Inject directly into vein over 3 to 5 minutes or slowly into I.V. tubing with free-flowing compatible solution.
● Infuse drug over 15 to 30 minutes.

● After reconstitution or dilution, solutions are stable for 24 hours at room temperature and 96 hours if refrigerated.

Contraindications and precautions

● Contraindicated in patients hypersensitive to drug or other cephalosporins.
● Use cautiously in patients with history of sensitivity to penicillin and in patients with renal impairment.
⚖ **Lifespan:** In pregnant and breast-feeding women, use cautiously. In infants younger than age 6 months, safety and efficacy of drug haven't been established.

Adverse reactions

CNS: fever; headache, malaise, paresthesia, dizziness.
GI: *pseudomembranous colitis,* nausea, anorexia, vomiting, diarrhea, glossitis, dyspepsia, abdominal cramps, tenesmus, anal pruritus.
GU: genital pruritus and candidiasis.
Hematologic: *transient neutropenia,* eosinophilia, hemolytic anemia, *thrombocytopenia.*
Respiratory: dyspnea.
Skin: *maculopapular and erythematous rashes, urticaria.*
Other: hypersensitivity reactions (serum sickness, *anaphylaxis*); *induration, sterile abscesses, tissue sloughing at injection site; phlebitis, thrombophlebitis* with I.V. injection.

Interactions

Drug-drug. *Probenecid:* May inhibit excretion and increase levels of ceftizoxime. Sometimes used for this effect.

Effects on lab test results

● May increase BUN, creatinine, ALT, AST, alkaline phosphatase, bilirubin, GGT, and LDH levels. May decrease albumin and protein levels.
● May increase eosinophil count. May decrease hemoglobin, hematocrit, PT, and RBC, WBC, platelet, granulocyte, and neutrophil counts.
● May cause false-positive urine glucose determinations with copper sulfate tests (Clinitest).

Pharmacokinetics

Absorption: Unknown with I.M. administration.
Distribution: Distributed widely into most body tissues and fluids; unlike many other cephalosporins, ceftizoxime has good CSF penetration and

---

achieves adequate levels in inflamed meninges. Drug is 28% to 31% protein-bound.
Metabolism: None.
Excretion: Excreted primarily in urine. *Half-life:* About 1½ to 2 hours.

Route	Onset	Peak	Duration
I.V.	Immediate	Immediate	Unknown
I.M.	Unknown	½-1½ hr	Unknown

Action

Chemical effect: Inhibits cell-wall synthesis, promoting osmotic instability; usually bactericidal.
Therapeutic effect: Hinders or kills susceptible bacteria.

Available forms

Infusion: 1 g, 2 g in 100-mg vials or in 50 ml of D_5W
Injection: 500 mg, 1 g, 2 g

NURSING PROCESS

⚡ Assessment

• Assess patient's infection before therapy and reassess regularly thereafter.
• Obtain specimen for culture and sensitivity tests before giving first dose. Therapy may begin pending test results.
• Ask patient about previous reactions to cephalosporins or penicillin before giving first dose.
• Be alert for adverse reactions and drug interactions.
• Monitor patient's hydration status if adverse GI reactions occur.
• Evaluate patient's and family's knowledge of drug therapy.

✛ Nursing diagnoses

• Infection related to bacteria susceptible to drug
• Risk for deficient fluid volume related to drug-induced adverse GI reactions
• Deficient knowledge related to drug therapy

▶ Planning and implementation

• Inject deeply into large muscle mass, such as gluteus maximus or lateral aspect of thigh. Divide doses of 2 g or more and give divided doses at two different sites.
• **ALERT:** Don't confuse with other cephalosporins with similar-sounding names.

Patient teaching

• Tell patient to report adverse reactions and signs and symptoms of superinfection promptly.
• Instruct patient to report discomfort at the I.V. site.
• Tell patient to notify prescriber if loose stools or diarrhea occur.

☑ Evaluation

• Patient is free from infection.
• Patient maintains adequate hydration.
• Patient and family state understanding of drug therapy.

ceftriaxone sodium
(sef-trigh-AKS-ohn SOH-dee-um)
Rocephin

Pharmacologic class: third-generation cephalosporin
Therapeutic class: antibiotic
Pregnancy risk category: B

Indications and dosages

▶ **Uncomplicated gonococcal vulvovaginitis.** *Adults and children older than age 12 or weighing more than 45 kg (99 lb):* 125 to 250 mg I.M. as single dose, followed by either 100 mg of doxycycline P.O. q 12 hours for 7 days, or a single oral dose of azithromycin 1 g.
Children younger than age 12 or weighing less than 45 kg: 125 mg I.M. as a single dose.
▶ **Serious infections of lower respiratory and urinary tracts; gynecologic, bone, joint, intra-abdominal, and skin infections; bacteremia; and septicemia caused by such susceptible microorganisms as** *Streptococcus pneumoniae, S. pyogenes, Staphylococcus aureus, S. epidermidis, Escherichia coli, Klebsiella, Haemophilus influenzae, Neisseria meningitides, N. gonorrhoeae, Enterobacter, Proteus, Pseudomonas, Peptostreptococcus,* **and** *Serratia marcescens. Adults and children older than age 12:* 1 to 2 g I.V. or I.M. daily or in equally divided doses, maximum 4 g.
Children age 12 and younger: 50 to 75 mg/kg, maximum 2 g daily, given in divided doses q 12 hours.
▶ **Meningitis.** *Adults and children:* Initially, 100 mg/kg I.M. or I.V. (maximum 4 g); thereafter, 100 mg/kg I.M. or I.V. given once daily or

in divided doses q 12 hours. Maximum 4 g, for 7 to 14 days.

▶ **Preoperative prophylaxis.** *Adults:* 1 g I.V. as single dose 30 minutes to 2 hours before surgery.
▶ **Acute bacterial otitis media.** *Children:* 50 mg/kg I.M. as a single dose; maximum I.M. dose is 1 g.
▶ **Persisting or relapsing otitis media in children‡.** *Children and infants age 3 months and older:* 50 mg/kg I.M daily for 3 days.
▶ **Sexually transmitted epididymitis, pelvic inflammatory disease‡.** *Adults:* 250 mg I.M. as a single dose; follow up with other antibiotics.
▶ **Anti-infectives for sexual assault victims‡.** *Adults:* 125 mg I.M. as a single dose given with other antibiotics.
▶ **Lyme disease‡.** *Adults:* 1 to 2 g I.M. or I.V. q 12 to 24 hours.

▼ I.V. administration

• Reconstitute with sterile water for injection, normal saline solution for injection, D_5W or $D_{10}W$ injection, or combination of saline solution and dextrose injection and other compatible solutions.
• Reconstitute by adding 2.4 ml of diluent to 250-mg vial, 4.8 ml to 500-mg vial, 9.6 ml to 1-g vial, and 19.2 ml to 2-g vial. All reconstituted solutions yield concentration that averages 100 mg/ml.
• After reconstitution, dilute further for intermittent infusion to desired concentration. I.V. dilutions are stable for 24 hours at room temperature.

Contraindications and precautions

• Contraindicated in patients hypersensitive to drug or other cephalosporins.
• Use cautiously in patients with history of sensitivity to penicillin.
⚖ Lifespan: In pregnant and breast-feeding women, use cautiously.

Adverse reactions

CNS: headache, dizziness, fever.
GI: *pseudomembranous colitis,* nausea, vomiting, diarrhea, dysgeusia.
GU: genital pruritus and candidiasis.
Hematologic: eosinophilia, *thrombocytosis, leukopenia.*
Skin: phlebitis, *rash.*
Other: pain, induration, and tenderness at injection site; hypersensitivity reactions (serum sickness, *anaphylaxis*).

Interactions

Drug-drug. *Aminoglycosides:* May have additive effect. Monitor drug levels and adjust dosage as required.
Probenecid: High doses may shorten half-life of ceftriaxone. Avoid using together.
Quinolones: Has synergistic effect against *S. pneumoniae.* Using together against this organism is recommended.
Drug-lifestyle. *Alcohol use:* May cause disulfiram-like reaction. Discourage use together.

Effects on lab test results

• May increase BUN, ALT, AST, alkaline phosphatase, bilirubin, and LDH levels.
• May increase eosinophil and platelet counts. May decrease WBC count.
• May cause false-positive urine glucose determinations with copper sulfate tests (Clinitest).

Pharmacokinetics

Absorption: Unknown with I.M. administration.
Distribution: Distributed widely into most body tissues and fluids; unlike many other cephalosporins, ceftriaxone has good CSF penetration. Drug is 58% to 96% protein-bound.
Metabolism: Partially metabolized.
Excretion: Excreted primarily in urine, minimally in bile. *Half-life:* About 5½ to 11 hours.

Route	Onset	Peak	Duration
I.V.	Immediate	Immediate	Unknown
I.M.	Unknown	1½-4 hr	Unknown

Action

Chemical effect: Inhibits cell-wall synthesis, promoting osmotic instability; usually bactericidal.
Therapeutic effect: Hinders or kills susceptible bacteria.

Available forms

Infusion: 1 g, 2 g
Injection: 250 mg, 500 mg, 1 g, 2 g

NURSING PROCESS

🖎 Assessment

• Assess patient's infection before therapy and reassess regularly thereafter.

Rapid onset   *Liquid form contains alcohol.   ◆Canada   ◇ Australia   †OTC   ‡Off-label use

• Obtain specimen for culture and sensitivity tests. Therapy may begin before test results are known.

• Ask patient about previous reactions to cephalosporins or penicillin before giving first dose.

• Be alert for adverse reactions and drug interactions.

• Monitor patient's hydration status if adverse GI reactions occur.

• Evaluate patient's and family's knowledge of drug therapy.

⊞ **Nursing diagnoses**

• Infection related to bacteria susceptible to drug

• Risk for deficient fluid volume related to drug-induced adverse GI reactions

• Deficient knowledge related to drug therapy

▶ **Planning and implementation**

• Inject deeply into large muscle mass, such as gluteus maximus or lateral aspect of thigh. May use lidocaine 1% without epinephrine to dilute for I.M. use.

⑨ **ALERT:** Don't confuse with other cephalosporins with similar-sounding names.

Patient teaching

• Tell patient to report adverse reactions and signs and symptoms of superinfection promptly.

• Instruct patient to report pain at the I.V. site.

• Tell patient to notify prescriber if loose stools or diarrhea occur.

☑ **Evaluation**

• Patient is free from infection.

• Patient maintains adequate hydration.

• Patient and family state understanding of drug therapy.

---

cefuroxime axetil

(sef-yoor-OKS-eem AKS-eh-til)
Ceftin

cefuroxime sodium

Zinacef

Pharmacologic class: second-generation cephalosporin
Therapeutic class: antibiotic
Pregnancy risk category: B

Indications and dosages

▶ **Pharyngitis, tonsillitis, infections of urinary and lower respiratory tracts, and skin and skin-structure infections.** Susceptible organisms are *Streptococcus pneumoniae, S. pyogenes, Haemophilus influenzae, Klebsiella, Staphylococcus aureus, Escherichia coli, Moraxella catarrhalis* (including beta-lactamase-producing strains) *Enterobacter,* and *Neisseria gonorrhoeae. Adults and children age 13 and older:* 250 mg P.O. q 12 hours. For severe infections, dosage may be increased to 500 mg q 12 hours.

▶ **Serious infections of lower respiratory and urinary tracts, skin and skin-structure infections, bone and joint infections, septicemia, meningitis, gonorrhea, and perioperative prophylaxis.** *Adults and children age 13 and older:* 750 mg to 1.5 g I.V. or I.M. q 8 hours for 5 to 10 days. For life-threatening infections and infections caused by less-susceptible organisms, 1.5 g I.V. or I.M. q 6 hours; for bacterial meningitis, up to 3 g I.V. q 8 hours.
Children age 3 months to 12 years: 50 to 100 mg/kg daily I.V. or I.M. in equally divided doses q 6 to 8 hours. Use higher doses of 100 mg/kg daily (not to exceed adult maximum dosage) for more severe or serious infections. For bacterial meningitis, 200 to 240 mg/kg I.V. in divided doses q 6 to 8 hours.

▶ **Uncomplicated urinary tract infections.** *Adults and children age 13 and older:* 125 to 250 mg P.O. q 12 hours for 7 to 10 days.

▶ **Otitis media.** *Children ages 3 months to 12 years:* 30 mg/kg oral suspension P.O. daily divided in two doses (maximum dose, 1 g) for children who can't swallow tablets, or 250-mg tablet P.O. b.i.d. for 10 days for children who can swallow tablets whole.

▶ **Pharyngitis and tonsillitis.** *Children ages 3 months to 12 years:* 125 mg P.O. q 12 hours for 10 days, in children who can swallow tablets whole. Or, 20 mg/kg daily of oral suspension (maximum 500 mg) in two divided doses for 10 days, in children who can't swallow tablets.

▶ **Perioperative prophylaxis.** *Adults:* 1.5 g I.V. 30 to 60 minutes before surgery; in lengthy operations, 750 mg I.V. or I.M. q 8 hours. For open-heart surgery, 1.5 g I.V. at induction of anesthesia and q 12 hours; total dosage 6 g.

▶ **Acute bacterial maxillary sinusitis caused by** *S. pneumoniae* or *H. influenzae* (only

---

Reactions may be *common,* uncommon, *life-threatening,* or COMMON AND LIFE-THREATENING.

strains that don't produce beta-lactamase).
Adults and children age 13 and older: 250 mg
(tablet) P.O. b.i.d. for 10 days.

Infants and children ages 3 months to 12 years:
30 mg/kg (suspension) by mouth daily in two
divided doses for 10 days. Maximum daily suspension dose is 1,000 mg. For children who can
swallow tablets whole, give 250 mg (tablet) by
mouth b.i.d. for 10 days.

▶ **Secondary bacterial infection of acute
bronchitis.** *Adults and children age 13 and
older:* 250 mg to 500 mg P.O. b.i.d. for 5 to
10 days.

▶ **Early Lyme disease as manifested by
erythema migrans.** *Adults and children age
13 and older:* 500 mg P.O. b.i.d. for 20 days.

▶ **Gonorrhea.** *Adults and children age 13 and
older:* Give a one-time dose of 1.5 g I.M. (I.M.
dose to be divided and given at two different
sites) with 1 g oral probenecid. Or, 1 g P.O. as a
single dose.

Ŋ Adjust-a-dose: For patients with renal impairment, if creatinine clearance is between 10 and
20 ml/minute give 750 mg I.V. or I.M. q 12
hours; if clearance is less than 10 ml/minute,
give 750 mg I.V. or I.M q 24 hours.

▼ I.V. administration

• For each 750-mg vial of Zinacef, reconstitute
with 8 ml sterile water for injection; for each
1.5-g vial, reconstitute with 16 ml. In each case,
withdraw entire contents of vial for dose.

• To give by direct injection, inject into large
vein or into tubing of free-flowing I.V. solution
over 3 to 5 minutes.

• For intermittent infusion, add reconstituted
drug to 100 ml D$_5$W, normal saline solution for
injection, or other compatible I.V. solution. Infuse over 15 to 60 minutes.

Contraindications and precautions

• Contraindicated in patients hypersensitive to
drug or other cephalosporins.

• Use cautiously in patients with history of sensitivity to penicillin and in patients with renal
impairment.

⚕ **Lifespan:** In pregnant and breast-feeding
women, use cautiously. In infants younger than
age 3 months, safety and efficacy of drug
haven't been established.

Adverse reactions

CNS: headache, malaise, paresthesia, dizziness.
GI: *pseudomembranous colitis,* nausea, anorexia, vomiting, diarrhea, glossitis, dyspepsia,
abdominal cramps, tenesmus, anal pruritus.
GU: genital pruritus and candidiasis.
Hematologic: *transient neutropenia,* eosinophilia, hemolytic anemia, *thrombocytopenia.*
Respiratory: dyspnea.
Skin: *maculopapular and erythematous rashes,*
urticaria.
Other: hypersensitivity reactions (serum sickness, *anaphylaxis*); *pain, induration, sterile abscesses, warmth, tissue sloughing at injection
site; phlebitis, thrombophlebitis* with I.V. injection.

Interactions

Drug-drug. *Diuretics:* May increase risk of adverse renal reactions. Monitor renal function
closely.
Probenecid: May inhibit excretion and increase
levels of cefuroxime. Sometimes used for this
effect.
Drug-food. *Any food:* May increase drug absorption and bioavailability. Give drug with
food.

Effects on lab test results

• May increase ALT, AST, alkaline phosphatase,
bilirubin, and LDH levels.

• May increase PT and INR and eosinophil
count. May decrease hemoglobin, hematocrit,
and neutrophil and platelet counts.

• May cause urine glucose determinations to be
false-positive with copper sulfate tests (Clinitest).

Pharmacokinetics

Absorption: Cefuroxime axetil is absorbed
from GI tract with 37% to 52% of oral dose
reaching systemic circulation. Food appears to
enhance absorption. Cefuroxime sodium isn't
well absorbed from GI tract; absorption from
I.M. administration is unknown.
Distribution: Distributed widely into most
body tissues and fluids; CSF penetration is
greater than that of most first- and second-
generation cephalosporins and achieves adequate therapeutic levels in inflamed meninges.
It's 33% to 50% protein-bound.
Metabolism: None.

Excretion: Excreted primarily in urine. *Half-life:* 1 to 2 hours.

Route	Onset	Peak	Duration
P.O.	Unknown	2 hr	Unknown
I.V.	Unknown	Immediate	Unknown
I.M.	Unknown	15-60 min	Unknown

Action

Chemical effect: Inhibits cell-wall synthesis, promoting osmotic instability; usually bactericidal.
Therapeutic effect: Hinders or kills susceptible bacteria, including many gram-positive organisms and enteric gram-negative bacilli.

Available forms

cefuroxime axetil
Suspension: 125 mg/5 ml, 250 mg/5 ml
Tablets: 125 mg, 250 mg, 500 mg
cefuroxime sodium
Infusion: 750 mg, 1.5 g premixed, frozen solution
Injection: 750 mg, 1.5 g

NURSING PROCESS

🜨 Assessment

• Assess patient's infection before therapy and reassess regularly thereafter.
• Obtain specimen for culture and sensitivity tests before first dose. Therapy may begin pending test results.
• Ask patient about previous reactions to cephalosporins or penicillin before giving first dose.
• Be alert for adverse reactions and drug interactions.
• Monitor patient's hydration status if adverse GI reactions occur.
• Evaluate patient's and family's knowledge of drug therapy.

🜨 Nursing diagnoses

• Infection related to bacteria susceptible to drug
• Risk for deficient fluid volume related to drug-induced adverse GI reactions
• Deficient knowledge related to drug therapy

🜨 Planning and implementation

• Food enhances absorption of cefuroxime axetil.
• Cefuroxime axetil is available only in tablet form, which may be crushed for patients who

can't swallow tablets. Tablets may be dissolved in small amounts of apple, orange, or grape juice or chocolate milk. However, drug has bitter taste that's difficult to mask, even with food.
⏱ ALERT: Cefuroxime tablets and oral suspensions aren't bioequivalent and can't be substituted on a mg-for-mg basis.
• Inject deeply into large muscle mass, such as gluteus maximus or lateral aspect of thigh. Prior to I.M. injection, aspirate to avoid injection into a blood vessel.
• Cefuroxime is not considered the drug of choice for meningitis or gonorrhea infections.
⏱ ALERT: Don't confuse with other cephalosporins with similar-sounding names.
Patient teaching
• Instruct patient to take drug exactly as prescribed, even after he feels better.
• Advise patient to take oral drug with food to enhance absorption. Explain that tablets may be crushed, but drug has bitter taste that's difficult to mask, even with food.
• Tell patient to report adverse reactions.

🗹 Evaluation

• Patient is free from infection.
• Patient maintains adequate hydration.
• Patient and family state understanding of drug therapy.

celecoxib
(sel-eh-COKS-ib)
Celebrex

Pharmacologic class: cyclooxygenase-2 inhibitor
Therapeutic class: anti-inflammatory
Pregnancy risk category: C

Indications and dosages

▶ **Relief of signs and symptoms of osteoarthritis.** *Adults:* 200 mg P.O. daily as a single dose or divided equally b.i.d.
▶ **Relief of signs and symptoms of rheumatoid arthritis.** *Adults:* 100 to 200 mg P.O. b.i.d.
▶ **Adjunct to familial adenomatous polyposis to reduce the number of adenomatous colorectal polyps.** *Adults:* 400 mg P.O. b.i.d. with food for up to 6 months.
▶ **Acute pain and primary dysmenorrhea.** *Adults:* Initially, give 400 mg P.O., followed by

an additional 200-mg dose on the first day, if needed. On subsequent days, 200 mg P.O. b.i.d. p.r.n.

Adjust-a-dose: For patients with hepatic impairment, reduce dose by 50%. For elderly patients who weigh less than 50 kg (110 lb), use the lowest recommended dose.

Contraindications and precautions

• Contraindicated in patients hypersensitive to drug, sulfonamides, aspirin, or other NSAIDs and in patients with severe hepatic or renal impairment.

• Use cautiously in patients with known or suspected history of poor CYP 2C9 metabolism and in patients with history of ulcers, GI bleeding, dehydration, anemia, symptomatic liver disease, hypertension, edema, heart failure, or asthma. Also use cautiously in patients who smoke or drink alcohol frequently, and in those who take oral corticosteroids or anticoagulants.

Lifespan: In women in the third trimester of pregnancy, drug is contraindicated. In children younger than age 18, safety and efficacy of drug haven't been established. In elderly and debilitated patients, use cautiously because of the increased risk of GI bleeding and acute renal impairment.

Adverse reactions

CNS: dizziness, *headache*, insomnia.
CV: peripheral edema.
EENT: pharyngitis, rhinitis, sinusitis.
GI: abdominal pain, diarrhea, dyspepsia, flatulence, nausea.
Metabolic: hyperchloremia, hypophosphatemia.
Musculoskeletal: back pain.
Respiratory: upper respiratory tract infection.
Skin: rash.
Other: accidental injury.

Interactions

Drug-drug. *ACE inhibitors:* May diminish antihypertensive effects. Monitor patient's blood pressure.
Aluminum- and magnesium-containing antacids: May reduce celecoxib levels. Separate administration times.
Aspirin: Increases risk of ulcers; low aspirin dosages can be used safely to prevent CV events. Monitor patient for signs and symptoms of GI bleeding.

Fluconazole: May increase celecoxib levels. Reduce dosage of celecoxib to minimal effective level.
Furosemide: NSAIDs can reduce sodium excretion caused by diuretics, leading to sodium retention. Monitor patient for swelling and increased blood pressure.
Lithium: May increase lithium level. Monitor lithium levels closely during treatment.
Warfarin: May increase PT level and bleeding complications. Monitor PT and INR, and check for signs and symptoms of bleeding.
Drug-herb. *Dong quai, feverfew, garlic, ginger, ginkgo, horse chestnut, red clover:* May increase the risk of bleeding. Discourage use together.
Drug-lifestyle. *Chronic alcohol use, smoking:* Increases risks of GI irritation or bleeding. Check for signs and symptoms of bleeding, and discourage use together.

Effects on lab test results

• May increase BUN, ALT, AST, and chloride levels. May decrease phosphate levels.

Pharmacokinetics

Absorption: Plasma levels peak in about 3 hours. Steady state plasma levels can be expected within 5 days if celecoxib is given in multiple doses. Elderly patients have higher levels than younger adult patients.
Distribution: Drug is highly protein-bound, primarily to albumin. It also is extensively distributed into the tissues.
Metabolism: Metabolized in the liver by CYP 2C9. No active metabolites of celecoxib have been identified.
Excretion: Excreted primarily through hepatic metabolism, with less than 3% as unchanged drug excreted in urine and feces. *Half-life:* About 11 hours.

Route	Onset	Peak	Duration
P.O.	Unknown	3 hr	Unknown

Action

Chemical effect: Celecoxib is thought to selectively inhibit cyclooxygenase-2, resulting in decreased prostaglandin synthesis. Its anti-inflammatory effects along with its analgesic and antipyretic properties are thought to be related to a decrease in prostaglandin synthesis.
Therapeutic effect: Relieves osteoarthritis and rheumatoid arthritis symptoms.

Available forms

Capsules: 100 mg, 200 mg, 400 mg

NURSING PROCESS

🗫 Assessment

• Assess patient for appropriateness of therapy. Drug must be used cautiously in patients with history of ulcers or GI bleeding, advanced renal disease, dehydration, anemia, symptomatic liver disease, hypertension, edema, heart failure, or asthma.
• Obtain accurate list of patient's allergies. Patients may be allergic to celecoxib if they're allergic and have had anaphylactic reactions to sulfonamides, aspirin, or other NSAIDs.
• Assess patients for risk factors for GI bleeding, including treatment with corticosteroids or anticoagulants, longer duration of NSAID treatment, smoking, alcoholism, older age, and poor overall health. Patients with a history of ulcers or GI bleeding are at higher risk for GI bleeding while taking NSAIDs such as celecoxib.
• Celecoxib has been linked to a relatively high risk of heart attacks. Monitor patient closely for any signs or symptoms of a MI.
• Monitor patient for signs and symptoms of overt and occult bleeding.
• Celecoxib may be hepatotoxic; monitor patient for signs and symptoms of liver toxicity.
• Evaluate patient's and family's knowledge of drug therapy.

🖭 Nursing diagnoses

• Acute pain related to underlying condition
• Risk for injury related to drug-induced adverse reactions
• Deficient knowledge related to drug therapy

▶ Planning and implementation

• In patients weighing less than 50 kg (110 lb), start therapy at lowest recommended dosage.
• Although drug can be given without regard to meals, food may decrease GI upset.
• Before starting treatment, rehydrate patient.
• Although celecoxib may be used with low aspirin dosages, the combination may increase the risk of GI bleeding.
• NSAIDs such as celecoxib can cause fluid retention; closely monitor patient who has hypertension, edema, or heart failure while taking this drug.

Patient teaching

• Tell patient to report history of allergic reactions to sulfonamides, aspirin, or other NSAIDs before starting therapy.
• Instruct patient to immediately report to prescriber signs of GI bleeding (such as bloody vomitus, blood in urine or stool, and black, tarry stools).
• **⚠ ALERT:** Advise patient to immediately report to prescriber rash, unexplained weight gain, or edema.
• Tell woman to notify prescriber if she becomes pregnant or is planning to become pregnant while taking this drug.
• Instruct patient to take drug with food if stomach upset occurs.
• Advise patient that all NSAIDs, including celecoxib, may adversely affect the liver. Signs and symptoms of liver toxicity include nausea, fatigue, lethargy, itching, jaundice, right upper quadrant tenderness, and flulike syndrome. Advise patient to stop therapy and seek immediate medical advice if he experiences any of these signs or symptoms.
• Inform patient that it may take several days before he feels consistent pain relief.

🗹 Evaluation

• Patient is free from pain.
• Patient doesn't experience injury as a result of drug-induced adverse reactions.
• Patient and family state understanding of drug therapy.

cephalexin hydrochloride
(sef-uh-LEK-sin high-droh-KLOR-ighd)
Keftab

cephalexin monohydrate
Apo-Cephalex ♦ , Biocef, Keflex, Novo-Lexin ♦ , Nu-Cephalex ◇

Pharmacologic class: first-generation cephalosporin
Therapeutic class: antibiotic
Pregnancy risk category: B

Indications and dosages

▶ **Respiratory tract, GI tract, skin, soft-tissue, bone, and joint infections and otitis media caused by** *Escherichia coli* **and other**

coliform bacteria, group A beta-hemolytic streptococci, *Haemophilus influenzae, Klebsiella, Moraxella catarrhalis, Proteus mirabilis, Streptococcus pneumoniae,* and staphylococci. *Adults:* 250 mg to 1 g P.O. q 6 hours or 500 mg q 12 hours; maximum 4 g daily.
Children: 6 to 12 mg/kg P.O. q 6 hours (monohydrate only); maximum 25 mg/kg q 6 hours or 4 g daily.

◗ Adjust-a-dose: For patients with renal impairment, if creatinine clearance is 11 to 40 ml/minute, give 500 mg q 8 to 12 hours; if clearance is 5 to 10 ml/minute, give 250 mg q 12 hours; if clearance is less than 5 ml/minute, give 250 mg q 12 to 24 hours.

Contraindications and precautions

• Contraindicated in patients hypersensitive to cephalosporins.
• Use cautiously in patients hypersensitive to penicillin and in patients with renal impairment.
⚕ Lifespan: In pregnant and breast-feeding women, use cautiously.

Adverse reactions

CNS: dizziness, headache, malaise, paresthesia.
GI: *pseudomembranous colitis,* nausea, anorexia, vomiting, *diarrhea,* glossitis, dyspepsia, abdominal cramps, anal pruritus, tenesmus, oral candidiasis.
GU: genital pruritus, candidiasis, vaginitis.
Hematologic: *transient neutropenia,* eosinophilia, anemia, *thrombocytopenia.*
Respiratory: dyspnea.
Skin: *maculopapular and erythematous rashes, urticaria.*
Other: hypersensitivity reactions (serum sickness, *anaphylaxis*).

Interactions

Drug-drug. *Probenecid:* May increase levels of cephalosporins. Sometimes used for this effect.

Effects on lab test results

• May increase ALT, AST, alkaline phosphatase, bilirubin, and LDH levels.
• May increase eosinophil count. May decrease hemoglobin, hematocrit, and neutrophil and platelet counts.
• May cause false-positive urine glucose determinations with copper sulfate tests (Clinitest).

Pharmacokinetics

Absorption: Rapid and complete. Food delays but doesn't prevent complete absorption.
Distribution: Distributed widely into most body tissues and fluids; CSF penetration is poor. Drug is 6% to 15% protein-bound.
Metabolism: None.
Excretion: Excreted primarily unchanged in urine. *Half-life:* About 30 minutes to 1 hour.

Route	Onset	Peak	Duration
P.O.	Unknown	≤ 1 hr	Unknown

Action

Chemical effect: Inhibits cell-wall synthesis, promoting osmotic instability; usually bactericidal.
Therapeutic effect: Hinders or kills susceptible bacteria.

Available forms

cephalexin hydrochloride
Tablets: 500 mg
cephalexin monohydrate
Capsules: 250 mg, 500 mg
Oral suspension: 125 mg/5 ml, 250 mg/5 ml
Tablets: 250 mg, 500 mg, 1 g

NURSING PROCESS

▨ Assessment

• Assess patient's infection before therapy and reassess regularly thereafter.
• Obtain specimen for culture and sensitivity tests before giving first dose. Therapy may begin pending test results.
• Ask patient about previous reactions to cephalosporins or penicillin before giving first dose.
• Be alert for adverse reactions and drug interactions.
• Monitor patient's hydration status if adverse GI reactions occur.
• Evaluate patient's and family's knowledge of drug therapy.

▨ Nursing diagnoses

• Infection related to bacteria susceptible to drug
• Risk for deficient fluid volume related to drug-induced adverse GI reactions
• Deficient knowledge related to drug therapy

▷ Planning and implementation

• To prepare oral suspension, first add required amount of water to powder in two portions. Shake well after each addition. After mixing, store in refrigerator (stable for 14 days without significant loss of potency). Keep tightly closed and shake well before using.

• Give drug with food or milk to minimize adverse GI reactions.

• Treat group A beta-hemolytic streptococcal infections for a minimum of 10 days.

• If giving a dosage greater than 4 g daily, give initial treatment with a parenteral cephalosporin.

⊛ **ALERT:** Don't confuse with other cephalosporins with similar-sounding names.

Patient teaching

• Inform patient that drug may be taken with meals.

• Instruct patient to take drug exactly as prescribed, even after he feels better.

• Tell patient to call prescriber if rash develops.

• Teach patient how to store drug.

☑ Evaluation

• Patient is free from infection.

• Patient maintains adequate hydration.

• Patient and family state understanding of drug therapy.

---

cetrorelix acetate
(set-RO-rel-icks AS-ih-tayt)
Cetrotide

Pharmacologic class: gonadotropin-releasing hormone (GnRH) analog
Therapeutic class: infertility agent
Pregnancy risk category: X

Indications and dosages

▶ **Infertility; inhibition of premature luteinizing hormone (LH) surges in women undergoing controlled ovarian stimulation.**
Women: Give 0.25 mg once daily or 3 mg once during the early- to mid-follicular phase. Adjust dose according to patient response. If using the 3-mg dose, give it S.C. once during early- to mid-follicular phase, when the estradiol level indicates an appropriate stimulation response, usually on stimulation day 7 (range, days 5 to 9). If human chorionic gonadotropin (hCG) hasn't been given within 4 days after the 3-mg

injection, give 0.25 mg S.C. once daily until the day of hCG administration. Or, if using the 0.25-mg dose, give 0.25 mg S.C. on either stimulation day 5 (morning or evening) or day 6 (morning) and continue once daily until the day of hCG administration. Give hCG only when ultrasound shows a sufficient number of follicles of adequate size.

Contraindications and precautions

• Contraindicated in patients hypersensitive to cetrorelix acetate, extrinsic peptide hormones, mannitol, GnRH, or any other GnRH analogs.

⚰ **Lifespan:** In pregnant women, drug is contraindicated. Rule out pregnancy before starting treatment. In breast-feeding women, don't use because it's unknown whether drug appears in breast milk. In women older than age 65, drug is contraindicated.

Adverse reactions

CNS: headache.
GI: nausea.
GU: ovarian hyperstimulation syndrome.
Other: *anaphylaxis,* local site reactions (including erythema, bruising, itching, and swelling).

Interactions

None reported.

Effects on lab test results

• May increase ALT, AST, GGT, and alkaline phosphatase levels.

Pharmacokinetics

Absorption: Rapid. Mean absolute bioavailability is 85%.
Distribution: Drug is 86% bound to plasma.
Metabolism: After giving 10 mg, small amounts are found in bile samples over 24 hours.
Excretion: Drug is excreted unchanged in urine and as metabolites in bile. *Half-life:* 3-mg single injection; 64 hours; 0.25-mg single dose, 5 hours; 0.25 mg daily for 14 days, 20½ hours.

Route	Onset	Peak	Duration
S.C.	1-2 hr	1-2 hr	≥ 4 days

Action

Chemical effect: Drug competes with natural GnRH for binding to membrane receptors on

---

the gonadotrophic cells of the anterior pituitary and induces the production and release of LH and follicle-stimulating hormone (FSH).
Therapeutic effect: Results in the LH surge, which induces ovulation, resumes oocyte meiosis, and causes luteinization as indicated by the rising progesterone levels.

Available forms

Powder for injection: 0.25 mg, 3 mg

NURSING PROCESS

⚡ Assessment
• Before giving drug, test patient for pregnancy; it must be ruled out before starting treatment.
• Assess patient's history for any hypersensitivity to drug therapy.
• Evaluate patient's and family's knowledge of infertility treatment.

⊕ Nursing diagnoses
• Ineffective coping related to underlying difficulty and frustration with conception
• Risk for impaired skin integrity related to local skin reaction from drug administration
• Noncompliance related to strict drug regimen and monitoring
• Deficient knowledge related to drug therapy and self-administration

▶ Planning and implementation
• Drug should be prescribed by those experienced in fertility treatment.
• Monitor patient carefully for anaphylaxis after initial dose. Symptoms include cough, rash, difficulty breathing, and hypotension. Provide supportive measures, such as airway management, oxygen, epinephrine, corticosteroids, intravenous fluids, antihistamines, and pressor amines.
Patient teaching
• Instruct patient to store 3-mg form at room temperature. Instruct her to store 0.25-mg form in refrigerator at 36° to 46° F (2° to 8° C).
• Instruct patient to report any adverse effects that become bothersome.
• Educate patient on the importance of following the regimen exactly as prescribed to achieve optimal results.
• Instruct patient on the proper administration technique, as follows: Wash hands thoroughly with soap and water. Flip off the plastic cover of

the vial and wipe the top with an alcohol swab. Attach the needle with the yellow mark to the prefilled syringe. Push the needle through the rubber stopper of the vial and slowly inject the liquid into the vial. Leave the syringe in place and gently swirl the vial until the solution is clear and without residue. Don't shake. Draw liquid from the vial into the syringe. Invert the vial and pull the needle back as far as needed to withdraw the entire contents of the vial. Detach the needle with the yellow mark from the syringe and replace it with the needle with the gray mark. Invert the syringe and push the plunger until all air bubbles are gone.
• Tell patient to choose an injection site on the lower abdomen, around the navel. If she receives a multiple dose (0.25-mg) regimen, tell her to choose a different site each day to minimize local irritation. Instruct her to clean the site with an alcohol swab and gently pinch a skinfold surrounding the site of injection. Instruct her to insert the needle completely into the skin at about a 45-degree angle and, once the needle has been inserted completely, to release her grasp of the skin. Tell her to gently pull back the plunger of the syringe to check for correct positioning of the needle. If no blood appears, tell her to inject the entire solution by slowly pushing the plunger. She should then withdraw the needle and gently press an alcohol swab on the injection site.
• If blood appears when the patient pulls back on the plunger, tell her to withdraw the needle and gently press an alcohol swab on the injection site. Explain that she'll need to discard the syringe and the drug vial and to repeat the procedure using a new pack.
• Instruct patient to use a syringe and needle only once and dispose properly. Suggest that she use a medical waste container for disposal.

☑ Evaluation
• Patient responds positively to drug therapy.
• Patient completes drug regimen as prescribed until administration of hCG.
• Patient doesn't suffer adverse effects from drug therapy.
• Patient and family state understanding of drug therapy and patient properly performs self-administration of subcutaneous injections.

chloral hydrate
(KLOR-ul HIGH-drayt)
Aquachloral Supprettes, Noctec, Novo-Chlorhydrate ♦

Pharmacologic class: general CNS depressant
Therapeutic class: sedative-hypnotic
Pregnancy risk category: C
Controlled substance schedule: IV

Indications and dosages
▶ **Sedation.** *Adults:* 250 mg P.O. or P.R. t.i.d. after meals.
Children: 8.3 mg/kg P.O. or P.R. t.i.d.; maximum 500 mg per dose daily; doses may be divided.
▶ **Insomnia.** *Adults:* 500 mg to 1 g P.O. or P.R. 15 to 30 minutes before bedtime.
Children: 50 mg/kg P.O. or P.R. 15 to 30 minutes before bedtime; maximum single dose 1 g.
▶ **Preoperatively.** *Adults:* 500 mg to 1 g P.O. or P.R. 30 minutes before surgery.
▶ **Premedication for EEG.** *Children:* 20 to 25 mg/kg P.O. or P.R.
▶ **Alcohol withdrawal.** *Adults:* 500 mg to 1 g P.O. or P.R.; repeat at 6-hour intervals, p.r.n. Maximum daily dose is 2 g.

Contraindications and precautions
• Contraindicated in patients hypersensitive to drug and in those with hepatic or renal impairment. Oral administration contraindicated in patients with gastric disorders.
• Use cautiously in patients with severe cardiac disease and in patients with mental depression, suicidal tendencies, or history of drug abuse.
⚱ **Lifespan:** In breast-feeding women, avoid use because small amounts of drug appear in breast milk and may cause drowsiness in infants.

Adverse reactions
CNS: hangover, drowsiness, nightmares, dizziness, ataxia, paradoxical excitement.
GI: nausea, vomiting, diarrhea, flatulence.
Hematologic: eosinophilia, *leukopenia.*
Other: hypersensitivity reactions.

Interactions
Drug-drug. *Alkaline solutions:* Incompatible with aqueous solutions of chloral hydrate. Don't mix together.

CNS depressants, including opioid analgesics: May cause excessive CNS depression or vasodilation reaction. Use together cautiously.
Furosemide I.V.: May cause sweating, flushing, variable blood pressure, and uneasiness. Use together cautiously or use different hypnotic drug.
Oral anticoagulants: May increase risk of bleeding. Monitor patient closely.
Phenytoin: May decrease phenytoin levels. Monitor levels closely.
Drug-lifestyle. *Alcohol use:* May react synergistically, increasing CNS depression, or may cause a disulfiram-like reaction (rarely). Strongly discourage alcohol use.

Effects on lab test results
• May increase BUN level.
• May increase eosinophil count. May decrease WBC count.
• May interfere with fluorometric tests for urine catecholamines and Reddy-Jenkins-Thorn test for urine 17-hydroxycorticosteroids. May cause false-positive tests for urine glucose when using copper sulfate tests (Clinitest).

Pharmacokinetics
Absorption: Well absorbed after oral and rectal administration.
Distribution: Distributed throughout body tissue and fluids; trichloroethanol (the active metabolite) is 35% to 41% protein-bound.
Metabolism: Metabolized rapidly and nearly completely in liver and erythrocytes to trichloroethanol; further metabolized in liver and kidneys to trichloroacetic acid and other inactive metabolites.
Excretion: Inactive metabolites are excreted primarily in urine, minimally in bile. *Half-life:* 8 to 10 hours for trichloroethanol.

Route	Onset	Peak	Duration
P.O.	≤ 30 min	Unknown	4-8 hr
P.R.	Unknown	Unknown	4-8 hr

Action
Chemical effect: Unknown; sedative effects may be caused by trichloroethanol.
Therapeutic effect: Promotes sleep and calmness.

Available forms
Capsules: 250 mg, 500 mg
Suppositories: 324 mg, 500 mg, 648 mg

Syrup: 250 mg/5 ml, 500 mg/5 ml

⚗ Assessment
- Assess patient's underlying condition.
- Evaluate effectiveness of drug.
- Be alert for adverse reactions and drug interactions.
- Evaluate patient's and family's knowledge of drug therapy.

✪ Nursing diagnoses
- Disturbed sleep pattern related to patient's underlying condition
- Risk for trauma related to adverse CNS reactions
- Deficient knowledge related to drug therapy

❯ Planning and implementation
⚠ ALERT: There are two strengths of oral liquid form; double-check dose, especially when giving to children. Fatal overdose may occur.
- To minimize unpleasant taste and stomach irritation, dilute or give drug with liquid and after meals.
- Store rectal suppositories in refrigerator.
- Don't use for long-term therapy; drug loses its efficacy in promoting sleep after 14 days of continued use. Long-term use may also cause drug dependence, and patient may experience withdrawal symptoms if drug is suddenly stopped.
Patient teaching
- Warn patient about performing activities that require mental alertness or physical coordination. For inpatients, supervise walking and raise bed rails, particularly for elderly patients.
- Tell patient to store capsules or syrup in dark container and to store suppositories in refrigerator.
- Explain that drug may cause morning hangover. Encourage patient to report severe hangover or feelings of oversedation so prescriber can be consulted to adjust dosage or change drug.

✔ Evaluation
- Patient states drug effectively induced sleep.
- Patient's safety is maintained.
- Patient and family state understanding of drug therapy.

chlorambucil
(klor-AM-byoo-sil)
Leukeran

Pharmacologic class: alkylating agent (not specific to cell-cycle phase)
Therapeutic class: antineoplastic
Pregnancy risk category: D

Indications and dosages

❯ **Chronic lymphocytic leukemia; malignant lymphomas, including lymphosarcoma, giant follicular lymphoma, non-Hodgkin's lymphoma, Hodgkin's disease, autoimmune hemolytic anemia‡, nephrotic syndrome‡, polycythemia vera‡, and ovarian neoplasms‡.**
Adults: 0.1 to 0.2 mg/kg P.O. daily for 3 to 6 weeks; then adjust for maintenance (usually 4 to 10 mg daily).
Children: 0.1 to 0.2 mg/kg or 3 to 6 mg/m² P.O. as a single daily dose. Reduce initial dosage if given within 4 weeks after a full course of radiation therapy or myelosuppressive drugs or if pretreatment leukocyte or platelet counts are depressed from bone marrow disease.
❯ **Macroglobulinemia‡.** *Adults:* 2 to 10 mg P.O. daily.
❯ **Metastatic trophoblastic neoplasia‡.**
Adults: 6 to 10 mg P.O. daily for 5 days; repeat q 1 to 2 weeks.
❯ **Idiopathic uveitis‡.** *Adults:* 6 to 12 mg P.O. daily for 1 year.
❯ **Rheumatoid arthritis‡.** *Adults:* 0.1 to 0.3 mg/kg P.O. daily.

Contraindications and precautions

- Contraindicated in patients hypersensitive or resistant to previous therapy (those hypersensitive to other alkylating agents also may be hypersensitive to chlorambucil).
- Use cautiously in patients with history of head trauma or seizures and in patients receiving other drugs that lower seizure threshold.
- ☀ **Lifespan:** In pregnant women, use cautiously, if at all; drug may harm fetus. In breastfeeding women, drug is contraindicated. In children, safety and efficacy of drug haven't been established; the potential benefits must be weighed against risks.

Adverse reactions

CNS: *seizures.*
GI: *nausea, vomiting, stomatitis.*
GU: *azoospermia, infertility.*
Hematologic: *neutropenia* (delayed up to 3 weeks, lasting up to 10 days after last dose), *thrombocytopenia, anemia, myelosuppression* (usually moderate, gradual, and rapidly reversible).
Hepatic: *hepatotoxicity.*
Metabolic: hyperuricemia.
Respiratory: interstitial pneumonitis, *pulmonary fibrosis.*
Skin: exfoliative dermatitis, rash, *Stevens-Johnson syndrome.*
Other: *allergic febrile reaction.*

Interactions

Drug-drug. *Anticoagulants, aspirin:* May increase risk of bleeding. Avoid using together, but if drugs must be used together, monitor patient's coagulation studies.

Effects on lab test results

• May increase AST, ALT, and alkaline phosphatase levels. May increase blood and urine uric acid levels.
• May decrease hemoglobin, hematocrit, and neutrophil, platelet, WBC, granulocyte, and RBC counts.

Pharmacokinetics

Absorption: Well absorbed from GI tract.
Distribution: Not well understood; drug and its metabolites are highly bound to plasma and tissue proteins.
Metabolism: Metabolized in liver; primary metabolite, phenylacetic acid mustard, also possesses cytotoxic activity.
Excretion: Metabolites are excreted in urine.
Half-life: 2 hours for parent compound; 2½ hours for phenylacetic acid metabolite.

Route	Onset	Peak	Duration
P.O.	3-4 wk	1 hr	Unknown

Action

Chemical effect: Cross-links strands of cellular DNA and interferes with RNA transcription, causing growth imbalance that leads to cell death.
Therapeutic effect: Kills selected cancer cells.

Available forms

Tablets: 2 mg

NURSING PROCESS

✐ Assessment
• Assess patient's underlying neoplastic disorder before therapy and reassess regularly throughout therapy.
• Monitor CBC and uric acid level.
• Be alert for adverse reactions and drug interactions.
• Evaluate patient's and family's knowledge of drug therapy.

⊕ Nursing diagnoses
• Ineffective health maintenance related to presence of neoplastic disease
• Ineffective protection related to drug-induced hematologic adverse reactions
• Deficient knowledge related to drug therapy

▷ Planning and implementation
• Dose is individualized according to patient's response.
• Give drug 1 hour before breakfast and at least 2 hours after evening meal.
• Nausea and vomiting caused by drug can usually be controlled with antiemetics.
• Allopurinol may be used with adequate hydration to prevent hyperuricemia with resulting uric acid nephropathy.
• Follow institutional policy for infection control in immunocompromised patients if WBC count falls below 2,000/mm³ or granulocyte count falls below 1,000/mm³. Severe neutropenia is reversible up to cumulative dosage of 6.5 mg/kg in single course.
Patient teaching
• Warn patient to watch for signs of infection (fever, sore throat, fatigue) and bleeding (easy bruising, nosebleeds, bleeding gums, melena). Tell him to take temperature daily.
• Instruct patient to avoid OTC products that contain aspirin.
• Tell patient to take drug 1 hour before breakfast and 2 hours after evening meal if bothered by nausea and vomiting.
• Instruct patient to maintain fluid intake of 2,400 to 3,000 ml daily, if not contraindicated.

☑ Evaluation

• Patient shows improvement in underlying neoplastic condition on follow-up diagnostic tests.
• Patient remains infection-free and doesn't bleed abnormally.
• Patient and family state understanding of drug therapy.

chloramphenicol sodium succinate

(klor-am-FEN-eh-kol SOH-dee-um SUK-seh-nayt)
Chloromycetin, Chloromycetin Sodium Succinate, Pentamycetin ♦

Pharmacologic class: dichloroacetic acid derivative
Therapeutic class: antibiotic
Pregnancy risk category: C

Indications and dosages

▶ **Haemophilus influenzae meningitis; acute Salmonella typhi infection; meningitis, bacteremia, or other severe infection caused by sensitive Salmonella sp., Rickettsia, or various sensitive gram-negative organisms; lymphogranuloma; or psittacosis.** Adults and children: 50 to 100 mg/kg P.O. or I.V. daily (depending on the severity of infection), divided q 6 hours. Maximum dosage is 100 mg/kg daily.
Full-term infants older than age 2 weeks with normal metabolic processes: Up to 50 mg/kg I.V. daily, divided q 6 hours.
Premature infants, neonates younger than age 2 weeks, and infants and children with immature metabolic processes: 25 mg/kg I.V. once daily. Use I.V. route to treat meningitis.
▶ **Meningitis and other severe infections caused by Streptococcus pneumoniae.** Children and infants age 1 month and older: 75 mg to 100 mg/kg/day I.V. in divided doses q 6 hours.

▼ I.V. administration

• Reconstitute 1-g vial of powder for injection with 10 ml sterile water for injection. Concentration will be 100 mg/ml.
• Give I.V. slowly over at least 1 minute. Check injection site daily for phlebitis and irritation.
• Stable for 30 days at room temperature, but refrigeration recommended. Don't use cloudy solutions.

Contraindications and precautions

• Contraindicated in patients hypersensitive to drug.
• Use cautiously in patients with impaired hepatic or renal function, acute intermittent porphyria, or G6PD deficiency, and in those taking other drugs that cause bone marrow suppression or blood disorders.
• Indicated only for serious infections that cannot be treated with other antibiotics.
☀ **Lifespan:** In pregnant women, use cautiously. Breast-feeding women should avoid breast-feeding during therapy because drug appears in breast milk, posing risk of bone marrow depression and slight risk of gray syndrome.

Adverse reactions

CNS: headache, mild depression, confusion, delirium; peripheral neuropathy (with prolonged therapy).
EENT: optic neuritis (in patients with cystic fibrosis), glossitis, decreased visual acuity.
GI: nausea, vomiting, stomatitis, diarrhea, enterocolitis.
Hepatic: jaundice.
Hematologic: *aplastic anemia, hypoplastic anemia, thrombocytopenia, agranulocytosis, granulocytopenia.*
Other: infection with nonsusceptible organisms, hypersensitivity reactions (fever, rash, urticaria, *anaphylaxis*), jaundice, *gray syndrome in neonates.*

Interactions

Drug-drug. *Chlorpropamide, dicumarol, phenobarbital, phenytoin, tolbutamide:* May increase drug levels. Monitor patient for toxicity.
Folic acid, iron supplements, vitamin B_{12}: Possible delayed response in patients with anemia. Monitor patient closely.

Effects on lab test results

• May decrease hemoglobin, hematocrit, and RBC, granulocyte, and platelet counts.

Pharmacokinetics

Absorption: Well absorbed from GI tract after oral administration.
Distribution: Distributed widely to most body tissues and fluids. About 50% to 60% bound to plasma protein.

Metabolism: Parent drug is metabolized primarily by hepatic glucuronyl transferase to inactive metabolites.
Excretion: 8% to 12% of dose is excreted by kidneys as unchanged drug; remainder is excreted as inactive metabolites. *Half-life:* About 1½ to 4½ hours.

Route	Onset	Peak	Duration
P.O.	Unknown	1-3 hr	Unknown
I.V.	Immediate	Immediate	Unknown

Action

Chemical effect: Inhibits bacterial protein synthesis by binding to 50S subunit of ribosome; bacteriostatic.
Therapeutic effect: Inhibits growth of susceptible bacteria.

Available forms

Capsules: 250 mg
Injection: 100 mg/ml (as sodium succinate)
Oral suspension: 150 mg/5ml (as palmitate)

NURSING PROCESS

🕮 Assessment
• Assess patient's infection before therapy and reassess regularly throughout therapy.
• Obtain specimen for culture and sensitivity tests before first dose. Therapy may begin pending results.
• Monitor drug level. Therapeutic drug level is 5 to 20 mcg/ml.
• Monitor CBC, platelets, iron, and reticulocytes before and every 2 days during therapy.
• Be alert for adverse reactions and drug interactions.
• **ALERT:** Signs and symptoms of gray syndrome in neonates include abdominal distention, gray cyanosis, vasomotor collapse, and respiratory distress. Gray syndrome can lead to death within a few hours after onset of symptoms.
• Evaluate patient's and family's knowledge about drug therapy.

🕮 Nursing diagnoses
• Infection related to presence of bacteria susceptible to drug
• Impaired protection related to drug-induced aplastic anemia
• Deficient knowledge related to drug therapy

⟩ Planning and implementation
• Give oral drug 1 hour before or 2 hours after meals. If patient develops adverse GI effects, give with food.
• If anemia, reticulocytopenia, leukopenia, or thrombocytopenia develops, stop drug immediately and notify prescriber.
• If patient's drug level exceeds 25 mcg/ml, take bleeding precautions and infection-control measures because bone marrow suppression can occur.
Patient teaching
• Instruct patient to report adverse reactions to prescriber, especially nausea, vomiting, diarrhea, fever, confusion, sore throat, or mouth sores.
• Stress importance of having frequent blood tests to monitor therapeutic effectiveness and adverse reactions.

☑ Evaluation
• Patient is free from infection.
• Patient's hematologic status remains unchanged with drug therapy.
• Patient and family state understanding of drug therapy.

chlordiazepoxide
(klor-digh-eh-zuh-POKS-ighd)
Libritabs

chlordiazepoxide hydrochloride
Apo-Chlordiazepoxide ♦ , Librium, Novo-Poxide ♦

Pharmacologic class: benzodiazepine
Therapeutic class: anxiolytic, sedative-hypnotic
Pregnancy risk category: D
Controlled substance schedule: IV

Indications and dosages

▶ **Mild to moderate anxiety.** *Adults:* 5 to 10 mg P.O. t.i.d. or q.i.d.
Children age 6 and older: 5 mg P.O. b.i.d. to q.i.d. Maximum dosage, 10 mg P.O. b.i.d. or t.i.d.
▶ **Severe anxiety.** *Adults:* 20 to 25 mg P.O. t.i.d. or q.i.d. Or, 50 to 100 mg I.V. initially, followed by 25 to 50 mg I.V. 3 or 4 times daily as needed.

Elderly patients: 5 mg P.O. b.i.d. to q.i.d.

▶ **Withdrawal symptoms of acute alcoholism.** *Adults:* 50 to 100 mg P.O., I.V., or I.M. Repeat in 2 to 4 hours, p.r.n. Maximum dosage is 300 mg daily.

▶ **Preoperative apprehension and anxiety.** *Adults:* 5 to 10 mg P.O. t.i.d. or q.i.d. on day preceding surgery. Or, 50 to 100 mg I.M. 1 hour before surgery.

▼ I.V. administration

• Don't give parenteral form to children age 12 and younger.

• Use 5 ml normal saline solution or sterile water for injection as diluent for an ampule containing 100 mg of drug. Give over 1 minute.

Ⓢ **ALERT:** Don't give packaged diluent I.V. because air bubbles may form.

• Be sure equipment and personnel needed for emergency airway management are available. Monitor respirations every 5 to 15 minutes after I.V. administration and before each repeated I.V. dose.

Contraindications and precautions

• Contraindicated in patients hypersensitive to drug.

• Use cautiously in patients with mental depression, porphyria, or hepatic or renal disease. In debilitated patients, use cautiously and at a reduced dosage.

⚠ **Lifespan:** In pregnant women, drug is contraindicated. Breast-feeding women shouldn't use drug because of risk of adverse effects in infant. In children younger than age 6, safety and efficacy of drug haven't been established. In children younger than age 12, parenteral use isn't recommended. In elderly patients, use smallest effective dose to avoid ataxia and oversedation

Adverse reactions

CNS: *drowsiness, lethargy, hangover,* fainting, restlessness, psychosis, confusion, *suicidal tendencies.*
CV: *thrombophlebitis,* transient hypotension.
EENT: visual disturbances.
GI: nausea, vomiting, constipation, abdominal discomfort.
GU: incontinence, urine retention, menstrual irregularities.
Hematologic: *agranulocytosis.*
Skin: swelling, pain at injection site.

Interactions

Drug-drug. *Cimetidine:* May increase sedation. Monitor patient carefully.
CNS depressants: May increase CNS depression. Avoid using together.
Digoxin: May increase digoxin level and risk of toxicity. Monitor patient closely; monitor levels.
Fluconazole, itraconazole, ketoconazole, miconazole: May increase and prolong levels, CNS depression, and psychomotor impairment. Avoid using together.
Drug-herb. *Kava:* May lead to excessive sedation. Discourage use together.
Drug-lifestyle. *Alcohol use:* May cause additive CNS effects. Strongly discourage alcohol use.
Smoking: May increase clearance of benzodiazepines. Monitor patient for lack of effect.

Effects on lab test results

• May increase liver function test values. May decrease granulocyte count.
• May cause false-positive reaction in Gravindex pregnancy test. May interfere with certain tests for urine 17-ketosteroids.

Pharmacokinetics

Absorption: When given orally, drug is absorbed well through GI tract.
Distribution: Distributed widely throughout body. Drug is 80% to 90% protein-bound.
Metabolism: Metabolized in liver to several active metabolites.
Excretion: Most metabolites of drug are excreted in urine. *Half-life:* 5 to 30 hours.

Route	Onset	Peak	Duration
P.O., I.V., I.M.	Unknown	½-4 hr	Unknown

Action

Chemical effect: Unknown. Probably potentiates the effects of GABA levels of brain and suppresses the spread of seizure activity produced by epileptogenic foci in the cortex, thalamus, and limbic structures.
Therapeutic effect: Relieves anxiety and promotes sleep and calmness.

Available forms

chlordiazepoxide
Tablets: 10 mg, 25 mg

---

chlordiazepoxide hydrochloride
Capsules: 5 mg, 10 mg, 25 mg
Powder for injection: 100 mg/ampule

NURSING PROCESS

Assessment
• Assess patient's underlying condition before therapy and reassess regularly thereafter.
• Monitor liver, renal, and hematopoietic function studies periodically in patients receiving repeated or prolonged therapy.
• Monitor patient for abuse and addiction.
• Be alert for adverse reactions and drug interactions.
• Evaluate patient's and family's knowledge of drug therapy.

Nursing diagnoses
• Anxiety related to patient's underlying condition
• Risk for injury related to drug-induced CNS reactions
• Deficient knowledge related to drug therapy

Planning and implementation
• Don't give drug regularly for everyday stress.
• Make sure patient has swallowed tablets before you leave the bedside.
• **ALERT:** Chlordiazepoxide 5 mg and 25 mg unit-dose capsules may appear similar in color when viewed through the package. Verify contents and read label carefully.
• When using I.M., add 2 ml of diluent to powder and agitate gently until clear. Use immediately. I.M. form may be erratically absorbed.
• Recommended for I.M. use only, but may be given I.V.
• Injectable form (as hydrochloride) comes in two types of ampules: as diluent and as powdered drug. Read directions carefully.
• Don't mix injectable form with any other parenteral drug.
• Refrigerate powder and keep away from light; mix just before use and discard remainder.
• Don't withdraw abruptly after long-term administration; withdrawal symptoms may occur.
Patient teaching
• Warn patient to avoid hazardous activities that require alertness and good psychomotor coordination until CNS effects of drug are known.
• Tell patient to avoid alcohol while taking drug.

• Warn patient to take this drug only as directed and not to stop taking it without prescriber's approval. Inform patient of drug's potential for dependence if taken longer than directed.

Evaluation
• Patient says he's less anxious.
• Patient's safety is maintained.
• Patient and family state understanding of drug therapy.

chloroquine hydrochloride
(KLOR-uh-qwin high-droh-KLOR-ighd)
Aralen HCl

chloroquine phosphate
Chlorquin ◇

Pharmacologic class: 4-amino-quinoline
Therapeutic class: antimalarial, amebicide
Pregnancy risk category: C

Indications and dosages

▶ **Acute malarial attacks caused by** *Plasmodium vivax, P. malariae, P. ovale,* **and susceptible strains of** *P. falciparum.* *Adults:* 1 g (600-mg base) P.O. followed by 500 mg (300-mg base) P.O. after 6 to 8 hours; for next 2 days a single dose of 500 mg (300-mg base) P.O. or 4 to 5 ml (160- to 200-mg base) I.M., repeated in 6 hours, if needed, changing to P.O. as soon as possible.
Children: Initially, 10 mg (base)/kg P.O.; then 5 mg (base)/kg at 6, 24, and 48 hours (don't exceed adult dose). Or, 5 mg (base)/kg I.M. initially; repeated in 6 hours p.r.n. Don't exceed 10 mg (base)/kg/24 hours. Switch to oral therapy as soon as possible.
▶ **Malaria prophylaxis.** *Adults:* 500 mg (300-mg base) P.O. on the same day once weekly, beginning 2 weeks before exposure. Continue for 4 weeks after leaving endemic area.
Children: 5 mg (base)/kg P.O. on the same day once weekly (not to exceed adult dosage), beginning 2 weeks before exposure.
▶ **Extraintestinal amebiasis.** *Adults:* 1 g (600-mg base) chloroquine phosphate P.O. daily for 2 days; then 500 mg (300-mg base) daily for at least 2 to 3 weeks. Treatment usually is combined with intestinal amebicide.

Reactions may be *common,* uncommon, *life-threatening,* or **COMMON AND LIFE-THREATENING.**

▶ **Rheumatoid arthritis‡.** *Adults:* 250 mg P.O. daily (chloroquine phosphate) with evening meal.

▶ **Lupus erythematosus‡.** *Adults:* 250 mg P.O. daily (chloroquine phosphate) with evening meal; reduce dosage gradually over several months when lesions regress.

Contraindications and precautions

• Contraindicated in patients hypersensitive to drug and in patients with retinal changes, visual field changes, or porphyria.
• Use cautiously in patients with severe GI, neurologic, or blood disorders. Also use cautiously in patients with hepatic disease or alcoholism (drug concentrates in liver), and in those with G6PD deficiency or psoriasis (drug may exacerbate these conditions).
⚠ **Lifespan:** In pregnant women, drug isn't recommended except for suppression or treatment of malaria (since malaria poses greater danger to mother and fetus than prophylactic administration) or hepatic amebiasis. In breast-feeding women, use cautiously.

Adverse reactions

CNS: mild and transient headache, neuromyopathy, psychic stimulation, fatigue, irritability, nightmares, *seizures,* dizziness.
CV: hypotension, ECG changes.
EENT: *visual disturbances* (blurred vision; difficulty in focusing; reversible corneal changes; typically irreversible, sometimes progressive or delayed retinal changes, such as narrowing of arterioles; macular lesions; pallor of optic disk; optic atrophy; patchy retinal pigmentation, typically leading to blindness), ototoxicity (nerve deafness, vertigo, tinnitus).
GI: anorexia, abdominal cramps, diarrhea, nausea, vomiting, stomatitis.
Hematologic: *agranulocytosis, aplastic anemia,* hemolytic anemia, *thrombocytopenia.*
Skin: pruritus, lichen planus eruptions, skin and mucosal pigmentary changes, pleomorphic skin eruptions.

Interactions

Drug-drug. *Aluminum salts, kaolin, magnesium:* May decrease GI absorption. Separate administration times.
Cimetidine: May decrease hepatic metabolism of chloroquine. Monitor patient for toxicity.

Drug-lifestyle. *Sun exposure:* May worsen drug-induced dermatomes. Tell patient to avoid excessive sun exposure and wear protective clothing and sunblock.

Effects on lab test results

• May decrease hemoglobin, hematocrit, and granulocyte and platelet counts.

Pharmacokinetics

Absorption: Absorbed readily and almost completely.
Distribution: Distributed in liver, spleen, kidneys, heart, and brain and is strongly bound in melanin-containing cells.
Metabolism: About 30% of dose is metabolized by liver.
Excretion: About 70% of dose is excreted unchanged in urine; unabsorbed drug is excreted in feces. Small amounts of drug may be present in urine for months after drug is stopped. Renal excretion is enhanced by urine acidification. *Half-life:* 1 to 2 months.

Route	Onset	Peak	Duration
P.O.	Unknown	1-3 hr	Unknown
I.M.	Unknown	30 min	Unknown

Action

Chemical effect: Unknown. As antimalarial, chloroquine is thought to bind to and alter properties of DNA in susceptible parasites.
Therapeutic effect: Prevents or eradicates malarial infections; eradicates amebiasis.

Available forms

chloroquine hydrochloride
Injection: 50 mg/ml (40-mg/ml base)
chloroquine phosphate
Tablets: 250 mg (150-mg base), 500 mg (300-mg base)

NURSING PROCESS

📋 **Assessment**
• Assess patient's infection before therapy and reassess regularly throughout therapy.
• Ensure that baseline and periodic ophthalmic examinations are performed. Check periodically for ocular muscle weakness after long-term use.
• Assist patient with obtaining audiometric examinations before, during, and after therapy, especially if long-term.

• Monitor CBC and liver function studies periodically during long-term therapy.
• Be alert for adverse reactions and drug interactions.
• Assess patient for possible overdose, which can quickly lead to toxic symptoms: headache, drowsiness, visual disturbances, CV collapse, and seizures, followed by cardiopulmonary arrest. Children are extremely susceptible to toxicity.
• Evaluate patient's and family's knowledge of drug therapy.

🔱 **Nursing diagnoses**
• Infection related to presence of organisms susceptible to drug
• Disturbed sensory perception (visual or auditory) related to adverse reactions to drug
• Deficient knowledge related to drug therapy

▷ **Planning and implementation**
• Give drug at same time of same day each week.
⊛ **ALERT:** Give missed doses as soon as possible. To avoid doubling doses in regimens requiring more than one dose per day, give missed dose within 1 hour of scheduled time or omit dose altogether.
• Replace I.M. use with oral administration as soon as possible.
• Give drug with milk or meals to minimize GI distress. Tablets may be crushed and mixed with food or chocolate syrup for patients who have trouble swallowing; however, drug has bitter taste and patients may find mixture unpleasant. Crushed tablets may be placed inside empty gelatin capsules, which are easier to swallow.
• Store drug in amber-colored containers to protect from light.
• Begin prophylactic antimalarial therapy 2 weeks before exposure and continue for 4 weeks after patient leaves endemic area.
• Monitor patient's weight for significant changes because dosage is calculated by patient's weight.
• If patient develops severe blood disorder not attributable to disease, notify prescriber and stop drug.
Patient teaching
• Tell patient to take drug with food at same time on same day each week.

• Instruct patient to avoid excessive sun exposure to prevent exacerbation of drug-induced dermatoses.
• Tell patient to report blurred vision, increased sensitivity to light, difficulty hearing or ringing in the ears, and muscle weakness.
• Warn patient to avoid alcohol while taking drug.
• Teach patient how to take missed doses.

☑ **Evaluation**
• Patient is free from infection.
• Patient maintains normal visual and auditory function.
• Patient and family state understanding of drug therapy.

chlorothiazide
(klor-oh-THIGH-uh-zighd)
Chlotride ◇ , Diurigen, Diuril

chlorothiazide sodium

Pharmacologic class: thiazide diuretic
Therapeutic class: diuretic, antihypertensive
Pregnancy risk category: D

Indications and dosages

▶ **Edema, hypertension.** *Adults:* 500 mg to 1 g P.O. or I.V. daily or in divided doses.
▶ **Diuresis, hypertension.** *Children and infants age 6 months and older:* 10 to 20 mg/kg P.O. daily in divided doses, not to exceed 375 mg daily.
Infants age 6 months and younger: May require 30 mg/kg P.O. daily in two divided doses.

▽ I.V. administration

• Reconstitute 500 mg with 18 ml sterile water for injection.
• Inject reconstituted drug directly into vein, through I.V. line containing free-flowing, compatible solution, or through intermittent infusion device. Compatible solutions include dextrose and saline.
• Monitor the patient for signs and symptoms of I.V. infiltration.
• Avoid simultaneous administration with whole blood and its derivatives.
• If hypersensitivity reactions occur, stop drug and notify prescriber.

- Store reconstituted solutions at room temperature up to 24 hours.

Contraindications and precautions

- Contraindicated in patients hypersensitive to other thiazides or other sulfonamide-derived drugs and in patients with anuria.
- Use cautiously in patients with severe renal disease and impaired hepatic function.
- ⚖ Lifespan: In pregnant or breast-feeding women, safety and efficacy of drug haven't been established. In children, I.V. administration isn't recommended.

Adverse reactions

CV: orthostatic hypotension.
GI: anorexia, nausea, *pancreatitis.*
GU: impotence, nocturia, polyuria, frequent urination, *renal impairment.*
Hematologic: *aplastic anemia, agranulocytosis, leukopenia, thrombocytopenia.*
Hepatic: *hepatic encephalopathy.*
Metabolic: asymptomatic hyperuricemia; hypokalemia; hyperglycemia and impaired glucose tolerance; fluid and electrolyte imbalances, including dilutional hyponatremia and hypochloremia, metabolic alkalosis and hyperkalemia; gout.
Skin: dermatitis, photosensitivity, rash.
Other: hypersensitivity reaction.

Interactions

Drug-drug. *Barbiturates, opioids:* May increase risk of orthostatic hypotension. Monitor blood pressure closely.
Chlorthalidone, hydrochlorothiazide, indapamide, metolazone and bumetanide, ethacrynic acid, furosemide, torsemide: May cause excessive diuretic response resulting in serious electrolyte abnormalities or dehydration. Adjust doses carefully while monitoring the patient closely for excessive diuretic responses.
Cholestyramine, colestipol: May decrease intestinal absorption of thiazides. Give doses separately.
Diazoxide: May increase antihypertensive, hyperglycemic, and hyperuricemic effects. Use together cautiously.
Digoxin: May increase risk of digitalis toxicity from chlorothiazide-induced hypokalemia. Monitor potassium and digitalis levels.

Lithium: May decrease lithium clearance, increasing risk of lithium toxicity. Monitor lithium level.
NSAIDs: May increase risk of NSAID-induced renal impairment. Monitor patient for this reaction.
Drug-herb. *Licorice root:* Could worsen the potassium depletion caused by thiazides. Avoid using together.
Drug-lifestyle. *Alcohol use:* May increase orthostatic hypotension. Monitor patient closely and place patient on fall precautions.

Effects on lab test results

- May increase uric acid, glucose, and calcium levels. May decrease potassium, sodium, and chloride levels.
- May decrease hemoglobin, hematocrit, and granulocyte, WBC, and platelet counts.

Pharmacokinetics

Absorption: Absorbed incompletely and variably from GI tract.
Distribution: Unknown.
Metabolism: None.
Excretion: Excreted unchanged in urine. *Half-life:* 1 to 2 hours.

Route	Onset	Peak	Duration
P.O.	≤ 2 hr	4 hr	6-12 hr
I.V.	≤ 15 min	30 min	6-12 hr

Action

Chemical effect: Increases sodium and water excretion by inhibiting sodium reabsorption in nephron's cortical diluting site.
Therapeutic effect: Promotes sodium and water excretion.

Available forms

Injection: 500-mg vial
Oral suspension: 250 mg/5 ml
Tablets: 250 mg, 500 mg

NURSING PROCESS

⚖ Assessment

- Assess patient's underlying condition.
- Monitor effectiveness by regularly checking blood pressure, fluid intake, urine output, blood pressure, and weight.
- Expect that therapeutic response may be delayed several days in patients with hypertension.

- Monitor electrolyte and glucose levels.
- Monitor creatinine and BUN levels regularly. If these levels are more than twice normal, drug isn't as effective.
- Monitor blood uric acid level, especially in patients with history of gout.
- Be alert for adverse reactions and drug interactions.
- Evaluate patient's and family's knowledge of drug therapy.

🔷 **Nursing diagnoses**
- Excessive fluid volume related to patient's underlying condition
- Impaired urinary elimination related to drug therapy
- Deficient knowledge related to drug therapy

▶ **Planning and implementation**
- To prevent nocturia, give drug in the morning.
- Many patients with edema respond to intermittent therapy; with intermittent dosing there is less likelihood of excessive response and electrolyte imbalances.
- ⚠️ **ALERT:** Never inject I.M. or S.C.
- Drug may be used with potassium-sparing diuretic to prevent potassium loss.
- Stop thiazides and thiazide-like diuretics before parathyroid function tests are performed.

Patient teaching
- Teach patient and family to identify and report signs of hypersensitivity and hypokalemia.
- Teach patient to monitor fluid intake and output and daily weight.
- Instruct patient to avoid high-sodium foods and to choose high-potassium foods.
- Tell patient to take drug early in day to avoid nocturia.
- Advise patient to avoid sudden posture changes and to rise slowly to avoid orthostatic hypotension.
- Advise patient to use sunblock to prevent photosensitivity reactions.
- Teach patient the importance of periodic laboratory tests to detect possible electrolyte imbalances.

☑️ **Evaluation**
- Patient is free from edema.
- Patient adjusts lifestyle to cope with altered patterns of urine elimination.
- Patient and family state understanding of drug therapy.

chlorpromazine hydrochloride
(klor-PROH-meh-zeen high-droh-KLOR-ighd)
Chlorpromanyl-20 ◆, **Chlorpromanyl-40** ◆,
Largactil ◆ ◇, **Novo-Chlorpromazine** ◆,
Thorazine

Pharmacologic class: aliphatic phenothiazine
Therapeutic class: antipsychotic, antiemetic
Pregnancy risk category: C

Indications and dosages
▶ **Psychosis.** *Adults:* Initially, 30 to 75 mg P.O. daily in two to four divided doses. Increase dosage by 20 to 50 mg twice weekly until symptoms are controlled. Some patients may need up to 800 mg daily. Switch to oral therapy as soon as possible.
Children age 6 months and older: 0.55 mg/kg P.O. q 4 to 6 hours or I.M. q 6 to 8 hours. Or, 1.1 mg/kg P.R. q 6 to 8 hours. Maximum I.M. dose in children younger than age 5 or weighing less than 22.7 kg (50 lb) is 40 mg. Maximum I.M. dose in children ages 5 to 12 or weighing 22.7 to 45.5 kg (100 lb) is 75 mg.
▶ **Nausea and vomiting.** *Adults:* 10 to 25 mg P.O. q 4 to 6 hours, p.r.n. Or, 50 to 100 mg P.R. q 6 to 8 hours, p.r.n. Or, 25 mg I.M. If no hypotension occurs, give 25 to 50 mg I.M. q 3 to 4 hours p.r.n. until vomiting stops.
Children and infants age 6 months and older: 0.55 mg/kg P.O. q 4 to 6 hours or I.M. q 6 to 8 hours. Or, 1.1 mg/kg P.R. q 6 to 8 hours. Maximum I.M. dose in children younger than age 5 or weighing less than 22.7 kg is 40 mg. Maximum I.M. dose in children ages 5 to 12 or weighing 22.7 to 45.5 kg is 75 mg.
▶ **Intractable hiccups, acute intermittent porphyria.** *Adults:* 25 to 50 mg P.O. t.i.d. or q.i.d. If symptoms persist for 2 to 3 days, 25 to 50 mg I.M. If symptoms still persist, 25 to 50 mg diluted in 500 to 1,000 ml normal saline solution and infused slowly.
▶ **Tetanus.** *Adults:* 25 to 50 mg I.V. or I.M. t.i.d. or q.i.d.
Children and infants age 6 months and older: 0.55 mg/kg I.M. or I.V. q 6 to 8 hours. Maximum parenteral dosage in children weighing less than 22.7 kg is 40 mg daily; in children weighing 22.7 to 45.5 kg, 75 mg daily, except in severe cases.

Reactions may be *common*, uncommon, *life-threatening*, or COMMON AND LIFE-THREATENING.

▶ **Relief of apprehension and nervousness before surgery.** *Adults:* Preoperatively, 25 to 50 mg P.O. 2 to 3 hours before surgery or 12.5 to 25 mg I.M. 1 to 2 hours before surgery. During surgery, 12.5 mg I.M.; repeat after 30 minutes if needed or fractional 2-mg doses I.V. at 2-minute intervals; maximum dose 25 mg. Postoperatively, 10 to 25 mg P.O. q 4 to 6 hours or 12.5 mg to 25 mg I.M.; repeat in 1 hour if needed.

Children and infants age 6 months and older: Preoperatively, 0.55 mg/kg P.O. 2 to 3 hours before surgery or I.M. 1 to 2 hours before surgery. During surgery, 0.275 mg/kg I.M. repeated after 30 minutes, if needed or fractional 1-mg doses I.V. at 2-minute intervals, maximum dose 0.275 mg/kg. May repeat fractional I.V. regimen in 30 minutes, if needed; postoperatively, 0.55 mg/kg P.O. q 4 to 6 hours or 0.55 mg/kg I.M.; repeat in 1 hour if needed and hypotension doesn't occur.

▼ I.V. administration

• Drug is compatible with most common I.V. solutions, including D_5W, Ringer's injection, lactated Ringer's injection, and normal saline solution for injection.

• For direct injection, drug may be diluted with normal saline solution for injection and injected into large vein or through tubing of free-flowing I.V. solution. Don't exceed 1 mg/minute for adults or 0.5 mg/minute for children.

• Drug also may be given as I.V. infusion; dilute with 500 or 1,000 ml normal saline solution and infuse slowly.

Contraindications and precautions

• Contraindicated in patients hypersensitive to drug and in patients with CNS depression, bone marrow suppression, subcortical damage, and coma.

• Use cautiously in debilitated patients and in those with hepatic or renal disease, severe CV disease (may cause sudden drop in blood pressure), exposure to extreme heat or cold (including antipyretic therapy), exposure to organophosphate insecticides, respiratory disorders, hypocalcemia, seizure disorders (may lower seizure threshold), severe reactions to insulin or electroconvulsive therapy, glaucoma, or prostatic hyperplasia.

⚜ **Lifespan:** In pregnant or breast-feeding women, drug isn't recommended. In acutely ill or dehydrated children, use cautiously. In elderly patients, also use cautiously.

Adverse reactions

CNS: *extrapyramidal reactions, sedation, seizures, tardive dyskinesia,* pseudoparkinsonism, dizziness, *neuroleptic malignant syndrome.*
CV: *orthostatic hypotension,* tachycardia, ECG changes.
EENT: ocular changes, blurred vision.
GI: *dry mouth, constipation.*
GU: *erectile dysfunction,* urine retention, menstrual irregularities, inhibited ejaculation.
Hematologic: *transient leukopenia, agranulocytosis,* hyperprolactinemia, *aplastic anemia, thrombocytopenia.*
Hepatic: cholestatic jaundice.
Skin: *mild photosensitivity.*
Other: gynecomastia, allergic reactions, I.M. injection site pain, sterile abscess.

Interactions

Drug-drug. *Antacids:* Inhibits absorption of oral phenothiazines. Separate antacid and phenothiazine doses by at least 2 hours.
Anticholinergics, including antidepressants and antiparkinsonians: May increase anticholinergic activity and aggravate parkinsonian symptoms. Use with caution.
Barbiturates, lithium: May decrease phenothiazine effect. Observe patient.
Centrally acting antihypertensives: May decrease antihypertensive effect. Monitor patient's blood pressure carefully.
CNS depressants: May increase CNS depression. Avoid using together.
Meperidine: May cause excessive sedation and hypotension. Don't use together.
Propranolol: May increase levels of both propranolol and chlorpromazine. Monitor patient.
Warfarin: May decrease effect of oral anticoagulants. Monitor PT and INR.
Drug-herb. *Kava:* Can increase the risk or severity of dystonic reactions. Discourage using together.
Dong quai, St. John's wort: Increased risk of photosensitivity. Advise patient to avoid prolonged or unprotected exposure to sunlight.
Yohimbe: May increase risk of toxicity. Discourage using together.

Drug-lifestyle. *Alcohol use:* May increase CNS depression, particularly psychomotor skills. Strongly discourage alcohol use.
Sun exposure: May increase risk of photosensitivity. Discourage prolonged or unprotected exposure to sun.

Effects on lab test results

• May increase CPK, GGT, and prolactin levels.
• May increase eosinophil count. May decrease hemoglobin, hematocrit, and WBC, granulocyte, and platelet counts.

Pharmacokinetics

Absorption: Erratic and variable for oral administration; rapid for I.M. administration.
Distribution: Distributed widely into body; concentration is usually higher in CNS than plasma. Drug is 91% to 99% protein-bound.
Metabolism: Metabolized extensively by liver and forms 10 to 12 metabolites; some are pharmacologically active.
Excretion: Most of drug is excreted as metabolites in urine; some is excreted in feces. Chlorpromazine may undergo enterohepatic circulation.

Route	Onset	Peak	Duration
P.O.	30-60 min	Unknown	4-6 hr
P.O. controlled-release	30-60 min	Unknown	10-12 hr
I.V., I.M.	Unknown	Unknown	Unknown
P.R.	> 1 hr	Unknown	3-4 hr

Action

Chemical effect: Unknown. Probably blocks postsynaptic dopamine receptors in brain and inhibits medullary chemoreceptor trigger zone.
Therapeutic effect: Relieves nausea and vomiting; hiccups; and signs and symptoms of psychosis, acute intermittent porphyria, and tetanus. Produces calmness and sleep preoperatively.

Available forms

Capsules (controlled-release): 30 mg, 75 mg, 150 mg, 200 mg, 300 mg
Injection: 25 mg/ml
Oral concentrate: 30 mg/ml, 100 mg/ml
Suppositories: 25 mg, 100 mg
Syrup: 10 mg/5 ml
Tablets: 10 mg, 25 mg, 50 mg, 100 mg, 200 mg

NURSING PROCESS

Assessment

• Assess patient's underlying condition and reassess regularly thereafter.
• Be alert for adverse reactions and drug interactions.
• Monitor blood pressure regularly. Watch for orthostatic hypotension, especially with parenteral administration. Monitor blood pressure before and after I.M. administration.
• Monitor patient for tardive dyskinesia, which may occur after prolonged use. It may not appear until months or years later and may disappear spontaneously or persist for life despite discontinuation of drug.
• Watch for symptoms of neuroleptic malignant syndrome. It's rare, but commonly fatal. It isn't necessarily related to length of drug use or type of neuroleptic, but over 60% of affected patients are men.
• Monitor therapy with weekly bilirubin tests during first month, periodic blood tests (CBC and liver function), and ophthalmic tests (long-term use).
• Evaluate patient's and family's knowledge of drug therapy.

Nursing diagnoses

• Ineffective health maintenance related to patient's underlying condition
• Impaired physical mobility related to drug-induced extrapyramidal reactions
• Deficient knowledge related to drug therapy

Planning and implementation

• Wear gloves when preparing solutions and prevent any contact with skin and clothing. Oral liquid and parenteral forms can cause contact dermatitis.
• Slight yellowing of injection or concentrate is common; potency isn't affected. Discard markedly discolored solutions.
• Protect liquid concentrate from light.
• Dilute liquid forms with fruit juice, milk, or semisolid food just before giving.
• Don't crush sustained-release preparations; give them whole instead.
• Shake syrup before giving.
• Give deep I.M. only in upper outer quadrant of buttocks. Massage slowly afterward to prevent sterile abscess. Injection stings.
• Store suppositories in cool place.

Reactions may be *common*, uncommon, *life-threatening*, or COMMON AND LIFE-THREATENING.

• Keep patient supine for 1 hour after parenteral administration and advise him to get up slowly.
• Don't withdraw drug abruptly unless required by severe adverse reactions. After abrupt withdrawal from long-term therapy patient may experience gastritis, nausea, vomiting, dizziness, and tremors.
• Withhold dose and notify prescriber if patient develops jaundice, symptoms of blood dyscrasia (fever, sore throat, infection, cellulitis, weakness), persistent extrapyramidal reactions (longer than a few hours), or any such reaction in pregnancy or in children.
• Dystonic reactions may be treated with diphenhydramine.
⊗ **ALERT:** Don't confuse chlorpromazine with chlorpropamide or clomipramine.

Patient teaching

• Warn patient to avoid activities that require alertness or good psychomotor coordination until CNS effects of drug are known. Drowsiness and dizziness usually subside after first few weeks.
• Instruct patient to avoid alcohol while taking drug.
• Tell patient to notify prescriber if urine retention or constipation occurs.
• Tell patient to use sunblock and wear protective clothing to avoid photosensitivity reactions. Chlorpromazine causes higher risk of photosensitivity than other drugs in its class.
• Tell patient to use sugarless gum or hard candy to relieve dry mouth.
• Tell patient not to stop taking drug suddenly but to take it exactly as prescribed and not to double doses to compensate for missed ones.
• Tell patient which fluids are appropriate for diluting concentrate, and show dropper technique for measuring dose. Warn patient to avoid spilling liquid on skin because it may cause rash and irritation.
• Advise patient that injection stings.

☑ **Evaluation**
• Patient has fewer signs and symptoms.
• Patient maintains physical mobility throughout drug therapy.
• Patient and family state understanding of drug therapy.

chlorzoxazone
(klor-ZOKS-uh-zohn)
Paraflex, Parafon Forte DSC, Remular-S

Pharmacologic class: benzoxazole derivative
Therapeutic class: skeletal muscle relaxant
Pregnancy risk category: C

Indications and dosages

Adjunct in acute, painful musculoskeletal conditions. *Adults:* 250 to 750 mg P.O. t.i.d. or q.i.d.

Contraindications and precautions

• Contraindicated in patients hypersensitive to drug and in those with impaired hepatic function.
• Use cautiously in patients with history of drug allergies.
⚩ **Lifespan:** In pregnant or breast-feeding women, use cautiously.

Adverse reactions

CNS: *drowsiness, dizziness, light-headedness,* malaise, headache, overstimulation, tremor.
GI: anorexia, nausea, vomiting, heartburn, abdominal distress, constipation, diarrhea.
GU: urine discoloration (orange or purple-red).
Hematologic: anemia, *agranulocytosis.*
Hepatic: hepatic dysfunction.
Skin: urticaria, redness, itching, petechiae, bruising.
Other: *anaphylaxis.*

Interactions

Drug-drug. *CNS depressants:* May increase CNS depression. Avoid using together.
Drug-lifestyle. *Alcohol use:* May increase CNS depression. Discourage using together.

Effects on lab test results

• May increase AST, ALT, alkaline phosphatase, and bilirubin levels.
• May decrease hemoglobin, hematocrit, and granulocyte count.

Pharmacokinetics

Absorption: Rapid and complete.
Distribution: Widely distributed in body.
Metabolism: Metabolized in liver to inactive metabolites.

Excretion: Excreted in urine as glucuronide metabolite. *Half-life:* 1 to 2 hours.

Route	Onset	Peak	Duration
P.O.	1 hr	1-2 hr	3-4 hr

Action

Chemical effect: Unknown. Appears to modify central perception of pain without modifying pain reflexes. Blocks interneuronal activity in descending reticular activating system and in spinal cord.
Therapeutic effect: Relaxes skeletal muscles.

Available forms

Caplets: 500 mg
Tablets: 250 mg, 500 mg

NURSING PROCESS

⚚ Assessment
• Assess patient's underlying condition before therapy.
• Monitor drug's effectiveness by regularly assessing severity and frequency of muscle spasms.
• Assess amount of relief drug gives. Reduce dosage based on relief provided and drowsiness.
• Be alert for adverse reactions and drug interactions.
• Evaluate patient's and family's knowledge of drug therapy.

⊕ Nursing diagnoses
• Acute pain related to patient's underlying condition
• Risk for injury related to drug-induced adverse CNS reactions
• Deficient knowledge related to drug therapy

⊠ Planning and implementation
• Give drug with meals or milk to prevent GI distress.
• If severe adverse reactions occur, withhold dose and notify prescriber.
Patient teaching
• Tell patient to avoid activities that require mental alertness, such as driving, until full CNS effects of drug are known.
• Advise patient to avoid combining drug with alcohol or other CNS depressants.
• Instruct patient to take drug with food or milk to prevent GI distress.

• Tell patient that drug may discolor urine orange or purple-red.
• Advise patient to follow prescriber's orders regarding physical activity.

☑ Evaluation
• Patient reports that pain has decreased or ceased as result of drug therapy.
• Patient doesn't experience injury as result of drug-induced adverse CNS reactions.
• Patient and family state understanding of drug therapy.

cholestyramine
(koh-leh-STIGH-ruh-meen)
LoCHOLEST, Prevalite, Questran, Questran Light, Questran Lite ◊

Pharmacologic class: anion exchange resin
Therapeutic class: antilipemic, bile acid sequestrant
Pregnancy risk category: C

Indications and dosages

▶ **Primary hyperlipidemia or pruritus caused by partial bile obstruction; adjunct for reduction of elevated cholesterol level in patients with primary hypercholesterolemia.**
Adults: 4 g P.O. once or twice daily. Maintenance dosage is 8 to 16 g P.O. daily. Maximum daily dosage is 24 g P.O.

Contraindications and precautions

• Contraindicated in patients hypersensitive to bile-acid sequestering resins and in patients with complete biliary obstruction.
• Use cautiously in patients at risk for constipation and those with conditions aggravated by constipation, such as severe, symptomatic coronary artery disease.
⚖ Lifespan: In pregnant and breast-feeding women, use cautiously because of possible interference with fat-soluble vitamin absorption. In children, safety and efficacy of drug haven't been established.

Adverse reactions

GI: *constipation,* fecal impaction, hemorrhoids, *abdominal discomfort,* flatulence, *nausea,* vomiting, steatorrhea.

Metabolic: *vitamin A, D, E, and K deficiency; hyperchloremic acidosis* (with long-term use or very high dosage).
Skin: rash; irritation of skin, tongue, and peri-anal area.

Interactions

Drug-drug. *Acetaminophen, beta blockers, digoxin, corticosteroids, fat-soluble vitamins (A, D, E, and K), iron preparations, thiazide diuretics, thyroid hormones, warfarin and other coumarin derivatives:* Reduces absorption of the drugs listed. Administer at least 2 hours apart.

Effects on lab test results

• May increase alkaline phosphatase and chloride levels.
• May decrease hemoglobin and hematocrit.

Pharmacokinetics

Absorption: Not absorbed.
Distribution: None.
Metabolism: None.
Excretion: Insoluble cholestyramine with bile acid complex is excreted in feces. *Half-life:* Unknown.

Route	Onset	Peak	Duration
P.O.	1-2 wk	Unknown	2-4 wk

Action

Chemical effect: A bile-acid sequestrant that combines with bile acid to form insoluble compound that's excreted. The liver must synthesize new bile acid from cholesterol, which reduces low-density-lipoprotein cholesterol levels.
Therapeutic effect: Lowers cholesterol levels and relieves itching caused by partial bile obstruction.

Available forms

Powder: 210-, 231-, 239-, 378-g cans, 9-g single-dose packets. Each scoop of powder or single-dose packet contains 4 g of cholestyramine resin.

NURSING PROCESS

Assessment

• Assess patient's cholesterol level and pruritus before therapy.

• Monitor drug's effectiveness by checking cholesterol and triglyceride levels every 4 weeks or asking patient whether pruritus has diminished or abated.
• Be alert for adverse reactions and drug interactions.
• Monitor patient for fat-soluble vitamin deficiency because long-term use may be linked to deficiency of vitamins A, D, E, and K and folic acid.
• Evaluate patient's and family's knowledge of drug therapy.

Nursing diagnoses

• Risk for injury related to elevated cholesterol levels
• Constipation related to drug-induced adverse GI reactions
• Deficient knowledge related to drug therapy

Planning and implementation

• To mix powder, sprinkle on surface of preferred beverage or wet food (soup, applesauce, crushed pineapple). Let stand a few minutes, then stir to obtain uniform suspension. Mixing with carbonated beverages may result in excess foaming. Use large glass and mix slowly.
• Give drug before meals and at bedtime.
• If drug therapy is stopped, adjust dosage of digoxin to avoid toxicity.
• If severe constipation develops, decrease dosage, add stool softener, or stop drug.
• Give all other drugs at least 1 hour before or 4 to 6 hours after cholestyramine to avoid blocking their absorption.
Patient teaching
• Instruct patient never to take drug in its dry form; esophageal irritation or severe constipation may result. Tell the patient to sprinkle powder on surface of preferred beverage in a large glass; to let mixture stand a few minutes; then to stir thoroughly. The best diluents are water, milk, and juice (especially pulpy fruit juice). Tell him that mixing with carbonated beverages may result in excess foaming. Tell him to swirl small additional amount of liquid in same glass and then to drink it to ensure ingestion of entire dose.
• Advise patient to take all other drugs at least 1 hour before or 4 to 6 hours after cholestyramine to avoid blocking their absorption.
• Teach patient about proper dietary management of serum lipids (restricting total fat and

cholesterol intake), as well as measures to control other cardiac disease risk factors.
● When appropriate, recommend weight control, exercise, and smoking-cessation programs.

☑ Evaluation
● Patient's cholesterol level is normal with drug therapy.
● Patient maintains normal bowel patterns throughout drug therapy.
● Patient and family state understanding of drug therapy.

cidofovir
(sigh-doh-FOH-veer)
Vistide

Pharmacologic class: inhibitor of viral DNA synthesis
Therapeutic class: antiviral
Pregnancy risk category: C

Indications and dosages

▶ **CMV retinitis in patients with AIDS.**
Adults: 5 mg/kg I.V. infused over 1 hour once weekly for 2 consecutive weeks, followed by maintenance dosage of 5 mg/kg I.V. infused over 1 hour once q 2 weeks. Probenecid and prehydration with normal saline solution I.V. must be given at the same time and may reduce risk of nephrotoxicity.
◁ Adjust-a-dose: For patients with renal impairment, if creatinine level increases 0.3 to 0.4 mg/dl above baseline, reduce dose to 3 mg/kg at same rate and frequency. If creatinine level increases 0.5 mg/dl or more above baseline, stop drug.

▼ I.V. administration
● Because of the risk of increased nephrotoxicity, don't exceed recommended dosages or frequency or rate of administration.
● Because of the mutagenic properties of drug, prepare in a class II laminar flow biological safety cabinet. Wear surgical gloves and a closed front surgical gown with knit cuffs.
● To prepare drug for infusion, remove it from vial using syringe, and transfer dose to an infusion bag containing 100 ml normal saline solution. Infuse entire volume I.V. at constant rate over 1 hour. Use a standard infusion pump.

● Don't add other drugs or supplements to admixture for concurrent administration.
● Compatibility with Ringer's solution, lactated Ringer's solution, or bacteriostatic infusion fluids hasn't been evaluated.
● If drug contacts the skin, wash membranes and flush thoroughly with water. Place excess drug and all other materials used in the admixture preparation and administration in a leak-proof, puncture-proof container. Dispose by high temperature incineration.
● Give admixtures for infusion within 24 hours of preparation; don't store in refrigerator or freezer to extend this 24-hour period.
● If admixtures aren't used immediately, they may be refrigerated at 36° to 46° F (2° to 8° C) for longer than 24 hours. Let drug reach room temperature before use.

Contraindications and precautions
● Contraindicated in patients hypersensitive to drug and in those with history of severe hypersensitivity to probenecid or other sulfa-containing drugs.
● Use cautiously in patients with renal impairment.
※ **Lifespan:** In breast-feeding women, don't give drug as intraocular injection.

Adverse reactions
CNS: *fever, asthenia, headache,* amnesia, anxiety, confusion, **seizures,** depression, dizziness, malaise, abnormal gait, hallucinations, insomnia, neuropathy, paresthesia, somnolence.
CV: hypotension, facial edema, orthostatic hypotension, pallor, syncope, tachycardia, vasodilation.
EENT: amblyopia, conjunctivitis, eye disorders, *ocular hypotony,* iritis, pharyngitis, retinal detachment, rhinitis, sinusitis, uveitis, abnormal vision.
GI: *nausea, vomiting, diarrhea, anorexia, abdominal pain,* dry mouth, taste perversion, colitis, constipation, tongue discoloration, dyspepsia, dysphagia, flatulence, gastritis, melena, oral candidiasis, rectal disorders, stomatitis, aphthous stomatitis, mouth ulcerations.
GU: *nephrotoxicity, proteinuria,* glycosuria, hematuria, urinary incontinence, urinary tract infection.
Hematologic: *neutropenia, thrombocytopenia, anemia.*

Reactions may be *common*, uncommon, ***life-threatening***, or COMMON AND LIFE-THREATENING.

Hepatic: hepatomegaly.
Metabolic: fluid imbalance, hyperglycemia, hyperlipemia, hypocalcemia, hypokalemia, weight loss, decreased bicarbonate level.
Musculoskeletal: arthralgia, myasthenia, myalgia, pain in back, chest, or neck.
Respiratory: *asthma,* bronchitis, cough, *dyspnea,* hiccups, increased sputum, lung disorders, pneumonia.
Skin: *rash, alopecia,* acne, skin discoloration, dry skin, pruritus, sweating, urticaria.
Other: *infections, chills, **sarcoma, sepsis,*** allergic reactions, herpes simplex.

Interactions

Drug-drug. *Nephrotoxic drugs (such as aminoglycosides, amphotericin B, foscarnet, I.V. pentamidine):* May increase nephrotoxicity. Avoid using together.
Probenecid: Interacts with metabolism or renal tubular excretion of many drugs. Monitor patient closely.

Effects on lab test results

• May increase BUN, creatinine, urine glucose, protein, alkaline phosphatase, ALT, AST, and LDH levels. May decrease calcium, potassium, and bicarbonate levels.
• May decrease hemoglobin, hematocrit, creatinine clearance and neutrophil and platelet counts.

Pharmacokinetics

Absorption: Administered I.V.
Distribution: Less than 6% plasma protein-bound.
Metabolism: Metabolized mainly by kidneys.
Excretion: Excreted by renal tubular secretion.
Half-life: Unknown.

Route	Onset	Peak	Duration
I.V.	Unknown	Unknown	Unknown

Action

Chemical effect: Selective inhibition of CMV DNA polymerase; inhibits DNA viral synthesis.
Therapeutic effect: Reduces CMV replication.

Available forms

Injection: 75 mg/ml in 5-ml ampule

NURSING PROCESS

Assessment
• Monitor WBC and neutrophil counts with differential and renal function before each dose.
• Monitor intraocular pressure, visual acuity, and ocular symptoms periodically.
• Don't use drug in patients with baseline creatinine above 1.5 mg/dl or calculated creatinine clearance of 55 ml/minute or below unless potential benefits outweigh risks. Monitor creatinine and urine protein within 48 hours before each dose and adjust dose according to renal function.
• Evaluate patient's and family's knowledge of drug therapy.

Nursing diagnoses
• Infection related to presence of virus
• Ineffective protection related to adverse renal reactions
• Deficient knowledge related to drug therapy

Planning and implementation
• Use I.V. prehydration with normal saline solution, and give probenecid with each cidofovir infusion.
• Give 1 L normal saline solution, usually over 1- to 2-hour period immediately before each cidofovir infusion.
Patient teaching
• Inform patient that drug doesn't cure CMV retinitis and that regular ophthalmologic follow-up examinations are needed.
• Explain that close monitoring of renal function is critical.
• Tell patient to take probenecid with food to reduce drug-related nausea and vomiting.
• Advise men to practice barrier contraception during and for 3 months after drug treatment.

Evaluation
• Patient's infection is eradicated.
• Patient doesn't experience serious renal reactions.
• Patient and family state understanding of drug therapy.

cilostazol
(sil-OS-tah-zol)
Pletal

Pharmacologic class: quinolinone phosphodiesterase inhibitor
Therapeutic class: antiplatelet drug
Pregnancy risk category: C

Indications and dosages

▶ **Reduction of symptoms of intermittent claudication.** *Adults:* 100 mg P.O. b.i.d. taken at least 30 minutes before or 2 hours after breakfast and dinner.
◪ **Adjust-a-dose:** Decrease dosage to 50 mg P.O. b.i.d. during coadministration with CYP 3A4- or CYP 2C19-inhibiting drugs, which may interact to increase cilostazol levels.

Contraindications and precautions

• Contraindicated in patients hypersensitive to drug or its components and in those with heart failure.
• Use cautiously in patients with severe underlying heart disease and with other drugs that have antiplatelet activity.
⚹ **Lifespan:** In breast-feeding women, avoid use. In children, safety and efficacy of drug haven't been established.

Adverse reactions

CNS: *headache, dizziness,* vertigo.
CV: *palpitations,* tachycardia, peripheral edema.
EENT: *pharyngitis, rhinitis.*
GI: *abnormal stools, diarrhea,* dyspepsia, abdominal pain, flatulence, nausea.
Musculoskeletal: back pain, myalgia.
Respiratory: increased cough.
Other: *infection.*

Interactions

Drug-drug. *Diltiazem:* Increases cilostazol levels. Reduce cilostazol dosage to 50 mg b.i.d.
Erythromycin, other macrolides: Increases levels of cilostazol and one of the metabolites. Reduce cilostazol dosage to 50 mg b.i.d.
Omeprazole: May increase levels of active cilostazol metabolite. Reduce cilostazol dosage to 50 mg b.i.d.
Strong inhibitors of CYP 3A4, such as fluconazole, fluoxetine, fluvoxamine, itraconazole, keto-
conazole, miconazole, nefazodone, sertraline: Possible increased levels of cilostazol and its metabolites. Reduce cilostazol dosage to 50 mg b.i.d.
Drug-food. *Grapefruit juice:* May increase cilostazol levels. Tell patient to avoid grapefruit juice during therapy.
Drug-lifestyle. *Smoking:* May decrease cilostazol exposure by about 20%. Monitor patient closely and discourage patient from smoking.

Effects on lab test results

• May increase HDL level. May decrease triglyceride level.

Pharmacokinetics

Absorption: Absorption is increased by 90% when given with a high-fat meal. Absolute bioavailability is unknown.
Distribution: Drug is highly protein-bound, primarily to albumin.
Metabolism: In the liver, extensively by primarily CYP 3A4. There are two active metabolites, one of which accounts for at least 50% of pharmacologic activity.
Excretion: 74% through urine. 20% in feces.
Half-life: 11 to 13 hours.

Route	Onset	Peak	Duration
P.O.	Unknown	2-4 hr	Unknown

Action

Chemical effect: Not fully understood. Drug is thought to inhibit the enzyme phosphodiesterase III, causing an increase of cAMP in platelets and blood vessels, thus inhibiting platelet aggregation. Drug reversibly inhibits the aggregation of platelets induced by various stimuli. Drug also has a vasodilating effect that's greatest in the femoral vascular beds.
Therapeutic effect: Reduces symptoms of intermittent claudication.

Available forms

Tablets: 50 mg, 100 mg

NURSING PROCESS

📖 **Assessment**
• Obtain history of patient's underlying condition before therapy and reassess regularly thereafter.

• This drug and similar drugs that inhibit the enzyme phosphodiesterase decrease the likelihood of survival in patients with class III and IV heart failure. Contraindicated in patients with heart failure of any severity.

• Make sure patient has a thorough physical examination before therapy starts.

• Be alert for adverse reactions and drug interactions.

• Evaluate patient's and family's knowledge of drug therapy.

⊕ **Nursing diagnoses**
• Acute pain related to underlying disease
• Ineffective peripheral tissue perfusion secondary to underlying disease
• Deficient knowledge related to drug therapy

▶ **Planning and implementation**
• Give drug at least 30 minutes before or 2 hours after breakfast and dinner.
• Beneficial effects may not be apparent for up to 12 weeks.
• Dosage can be reduced or stopped without such rebound effects as platelet hyperaggregability. Notify prescriber of coagulation study results.

Patient teaching
• Advise patient to read the patient package insert carefully before starting therapy.
• Instruct patient to take cilostazol on an empty stomach, at least 30 minutes before or 2 hours after breakfast and dinner.
• Tell patient that the beneficial effect of drug on intermittent claudication isn't likely to be noticed for 2 to 4 weeks and that it may take as long as 12 weeks.
• Instruct patient not to drink grapefruit juice while taking drug.
• Inform patient that CV risk is unknown in patients who use the drug on a long-term basis and in patients who have severe underlying heart disease.
• Tell patient that drug may cause dizziness. Warn patient not to drive or perform other activities that require alertness until response to drug is known.

☑ **Evaluation**
• Patient experiences a decrease in pain.
• Patient has adequate tissue perfusion.
• Patient and family state understanding of drug therapy.

cimetidine
(sih-MEH-tih-deen)
Tagamet, Tagamet HB†

Pharmacologic class: H$_2$-receptor antagonist
Therapeutic class: antiulcer agent
Pregnancy risk category: B

Indications and dosages

▶ **Prevention of upper GI bleeding in critically ill patients.** *Adults:* 50 mg/hour by continuous I.V. infusion for up to 7 days.
◩ **Adjust-a-dose:** For patients with renal impairment, if creatinine clearance is less than 30 ml/minute, give 25 mg/hour by continuous I.V. infusion.

▶ **Duodenal ulcer (short-term therapy).** *Adults and children age 16 and older:* 800 mg P.O. h.s. Or, 400 mg P.O. b.i.d. or 300 mg q.i.d. (with meals and h.s.). Treatment continued for 4 to 6 weeks unless endoscopy shows healing. For maintenance therapy, 400 mg h.s.

▶ **Active benign gastric ulceration.** *Adults:* 800 mg P.O. h.s., or 300 mg P.O. q.i.d., with meals and h.s., for up to 8 weeks.

▶ **Pathologic hypersecretory conditions (such as Zollinger-Ellison syndrome, systemic mastocytosis, and multiple endocrine adenomas).** *Adults and children age 16 and older:* 300 mg P.O. q.i.d. with meals and h.s.; adjust to patient's needs. Maximum oral daily dosage is 2,400 mg.

▶ **Hospitalized patients with intractable ulcers or hypersecretory conditions or patients who can't take oral medication.** *Adults:* 300 mg diluted to 20 ml with normal saline solution or other compatible solution by I.V. push over 5 minutes q 6 to 8 hours. Or 300 mg diluted in 50 ml dextrose 5% solution or other compatible solution by I.V. infusion over 15 to 20 minutes q 6 to 8 hours. Or 300 mg I.M. q 6 to 8 hours (no dilution is needed). To increase dosage, give 300-mg doses more frequently to maximum daily dose of 2,400 mg. Or, 37.5 mg/hour (900 mg/day) I.V. continuous infusion diluted in 100 to 1,000 ml compatible solution.

▶ **Gastroesophageal reflux disease.** *Adults:* 800 mg P.O. b.i.d. or 400 mg q.i.d. before meals and h.s. for up to 12 weeks.

▶ **Heartburn.** *Adults:* 200 mg (Tagamet HB only) P.O. with water as symptoms occur, or as directed, up to b.i.d. Maximum 400 mg daily. Don't give daily for more than 2 weeks.

▶ **Active upper GI bleeding, peptic esophagitis, stress ulcers‡.** *Adults:* 1 to 2 g I.V. or P.O. daily in four divided doses.

◪ **Adjust-a-dose:** For patients with renal impairment, decrease dosage to 300 mg P.O. or I.V. q 12 hours. If patient also has liver impairment, may need to further reduce dosage. May increase cautiously to q 8 hours.

▼ I.V. administration

- Dilute I.V. solutions with normal saline solution, D₅W, dextrose 10% in water (and combinations of these), lactated Ringer's solution, or 5% sodium bicarbonate injection. Don't dilute with sterile water for injection. Cimetidine is also commonly added to total parenteral nutrition solutions with or without fat emulsion.
- Give direct injection over 5 minutes. Rapid I.V. injection may result in arrhythmias and hypotension.
- Infuse drug over at least 30 minutes to minimize risk of adverse cardiac effects. If giving continuous I.V. infusion, use infusion pump to give a total volume of 250 ml over 24 hours or less.

Contraindications and precautions

- Contraindicated in patients hypersensitive to drug.
- Use cautiously in debilitated patients because they may be more susceptible to drug-induced confusion.

⚖ **Lifespan:** In pregnant women, use cautiously. In breast-feeding women, drug is contraindicated. In patients younger than age 16, safety and efficacy of drug haven't been established. In elderly patients, use cautiously.

Adverse reactions

CNS: confusion, dizziness, headaches, peripheral neuropathy.
CV: *bradycardia.*
GI: mild and transient diarrhea.
Hematologic: *agranulocytosis, neutropenia, thrombocytopenia, aplastic anemia.*
Hepatic: jaundice.
Musculoskeletal: muscle pain.
Skin: acnelike rash, urticaria.
Other: hypersensitivity reactions, mild gynecomastia (if used longer than 1 month).

Interactions

Drug-drug. *Antacids:* May interfere with cimetidine absorption. Separate administration by at least 1 hour.
Lidocaine (I.V.): May decrease clearance of lidocaine, increasing the risk of toxicity. Consider using a different H₂ antagonist. Monitor lidocaine level closely.
Metoprolol, propranolol, timolol: May increase the pharmacologic effects of beta blocker. Consider using another H₂ antagonist or decrease the dose of beta blocker.
Phenytoin, some benzodiazepines, sulfonylureas, theophylline, tacrine, calcium channel blockers, pentoxifylline, carbamazepine, labetalol, valproic acid, warfarin: May inhibit hepatic microsomal enzyme metabolism of these drugs. Monitor levels of these drugs.
Procainamide: May increase procainamide level. Avoid this combination. Monitor procainamide level closely and adjust the dose p.r.n.
Drug-herb. *Pennyroyal:* May change the rate at which toxic metabolites of pennyroyal form. Discourage use while on drug therapy.
Yerba maté: May decrease clearance of yerba maté methylxanthines and cause toxicity. Tell patient to use together cautiously.

Effects on lab test results

- May increase creatinine, alkaline phosphatase, AST, and ALT levels.
- May decrease hemoglobin, hematocrit, and neutrophil, granulocyte, leukocyte, and platelet counts.

Pharmacokinetics

Absorption: 60% to 75% of oral dose is absorbed. Absorption rate but not extent may be affected by food. Degree of absorption unknown after I.M. administration.
Distribution: Distributed to many body tissues. About 15% to 20% of drug is protein-bound.
Metabolism: 30% to 40% of dose is metabolized in liver.
Excretion: Excreted primarily in urine (48% of oral dose, 75% of parenteral dose); 10% of oral dose excreted in feces. *Half-life:* 2 hours.

Route	Onset	Peak	Duration
P.O.	Unknown	45-90 min	4-5 hr
I.V.	Unknown	Immediate	Unknown
I.M.	Unknown	Unknown	Unknown

Reactions may be *common,* uncommon, *life-threatening,* or COMMON AND LIFE-THREATENING.

Action

Chemical effect: Competitively inhibits action of H_2 at receptor sites of parietal cells, decreasing gastric acid secretion.
Therapeutic effect: Lessens upper GI irritation caused by increased gastric acid secretion.

Available forms

Injection: 150 mg/ml; 300 mg in 50 ml normal saline solution for injection
Oral liquid: 300 mg/5 ml
Tablets: 200 mg†, 300 mg, 400 mg, 800 mg

NURSING PROCESS

🔍 Assessment
• Assess patient's underlying upper GI condition before therapy and reassess regularly throughout therapy.
• Be alert for adverse reactions and drug interactions.
• Identify tablet strength when obtaining drug history.
• Monitor patient's CV status during I.V. administration; drug can cause profound bradycardia and other cardiotoxic effects when given too rapidly I.V.
• Evaluate patient's and family's knowledge of drug therapy.

🔷 Nursing diagnoses
• Impaired tissue integrity related to patient's underlying condition
• Diarrhea related to drug-induced adverse reaction
• Deficient knowledge related to drug therapy

🔷 Planning and implementation
• Give tablets with meals to ensure more consistent therapeutic effect.
• I.M. administration may be painful.
• Hemodialysis reduces levels of cimetidine. Schedule cimetidine dose at end of hemodialysis treatment. Adjust dosage in patients with renal impairment.
🔷 ALERT: Don't confuse cimetidine with simethicone.
Patient teaching
• Remind patient taking drug once daily to take it at bedtime for best results.
• Instruct patient to take drug as directed and to continue taking it even after pain subsides, to allow for adequate healing.

• Remind patient not to take antacid within 1 hour of taking drug.
• Advise patient to tell prescriber if he's taking other drugs.
• Urge patient to avoid cigarette smoking because it may increase gastric acid secretion and worsen disease.
• Instruct patient to immediately report black tarry stools, diarrhea, confusion, or rash.

✅ Evaluation
• Patient experiences decrease in or relief of upper GI symptoms with drug therapy.
• Patient maintains normal bowel habits throughout drug therapy.
• Patient and family state understanding of drug therapy.

ciprofloxacin
(sih-proh-FLOKS-uh-sin)
Cipro, Cipro I.V., Ciproxin ◇, Cipro XR

Pharmacologic class: fluoroquinolone antibiotic
Therapeutic class: antibiotic
Pregnancy risk category: C

Indications and dosages

▶ **Mild to moderate UTI.** *Adults:* 250 mg P.O. or 200 mg I.V. q 12 hours.
▶ **Severe or complicated UTI; mild to moderate bone and joint infections; mild to moderate respiratory tract infections; mild to moderate skin and skin-structure infections; infectious diarrhea, intra-abdominal infection.** *Adults:* 500 mg P.O. or 400 mg I.V. q 12 hours.
▶ **Severe or complicated bone or joint infections; severe respiratory tract infections; severe skin and skin-structure infections.** *Adults:* 750 mg P.O. q 12 hours. Or, 400 mg I.V. q 8 hours.
▶ **Mild to moderate acute sinusitis caused by** *Haemophilus influenzae, Streptococcus pneumoniae,* **or** *Moraxella catarrhalis;* **mild-to-moderate chronic bacterial prostatitis caused by** *Escherichia coli* **or** *Proteus mirabilis.* *Adults:* 400 mg I.V. infusion given over 60 minutes q 12 hours.
▶ **Febrile neutropenia.** *Adults:* 400 mg I.V. q 8 hours (given in conjunction with piperacillin

sodium [50 mg/kg I.V. q 4 hours, not to exceed 24 g daily]) for 7 to 14 days.

▶ **Inhalation anthrax (post-exposure).**
Adults: 400 mg I.V. q 12 hours initially until susceptibility tests are known, then switch to 500 mg P.O. b.i.d. when patient's condition improves.
Children: 10 mg/kg I.V. q 12 hours, then switch to 15 mg/kg P.O. q 12 hours when patient's condition improves. Don't exceed 800 mg I.V. daily or 1 g P.O. daily.
For all patients: Also use one or two additional antimicrobials. Treat for a total of 60 days (I.V. and P.O. combined).

▶ **Acute uncomplicated cystitis.** *Adults:* 100 or 250 mg P.O. q 12 hours for 3 days.

▶ **Cutaneous anthrax‡.** *Adults:* 500 mg P.O. b.i.d. for 60 days.
Children: 10 to 15 mg/kg q 12 hours, not to xceed 1 g daily, for 60 days.

▶ **Uncomplicated urethral, endocervical, rectal‡, or pharyngeal‡ gonorrhea.** *Adults:* 500 mg P.O. as a single dose.

▶ *Neisseria meningitidis* **in nasal passages‡.** *Adults:* 500 to 750 mg P.O. as a single dose, or 250 mg P.O. b.i.d. for 2 days, or 500 mg P.O. b.i.d. for 5 days.

🔋 **Adjust-a-dose:** For patients with renal impairment, if creatinine clearance is 30 to 50 ml/minute, give 250 to 500 mg P.O. q 12 hours or the usual I.V. dose; if clearance is 5 to 29 ml/minute, give 250 to 500 mg q 18 hours or 200 to 400 mg I.V. q 18 to 24 hours. If patient is on hemodialysis, give 250 to 500 mg P.O. q 24 hours after dialysis.

▶ **UTI.** *Adults:* If uncomplicated, 500 mg (extended-release) P.O. once daily for 3 days. If complicated, 1 g (extended-release) P.O. once daily for 3 days.

🔋 **Adjust-a-dose:** For patients with renal impairment, if creatinine clearance is less than 30 ml/minute, give 500 mg (extended-release) P.O. daily. For dialysis patients, give dose after dialysis session.

▼ I.V. administration

● Dilute drug using D_5W or normal saline solution for injection to final concentration of 1 to 2 mg/ml. Infuse over 1 hour into large vein.
● If giving drug through a Y-type set, stop the other I.V. solution during infusion.

Contraindications and precautions

● Contraindicated in patients hypersensitive to fluoroquinolones.
● Use cautiously in patients with CNS disorders, such as severe cerebral arteriosclerosis or seizure disorders, and in those at increased risk for seizures. May cause CNS stimulation.
● Immunocompromised patients may receive the usual doses and regimens for anthrax.
🔅 Lifespan: In pregnant women, use cautiously. Pregnant women may receive the usual doses and regimens for anthrax. In breast-feeding women, drug is contraindicated. Drug appears in breast milk. In children, safety and efficacy of drug for indications other than anthrax haven't been established. In children younger than age 18, safety and efficacy of Cipro XR haven't been established; avoid use.

Adverse reactions

CNS: headache, restlessness, tremor, lightheadedness, confusion, hallucinations, *seizures,* paresthesia.
CV: thrombophlebitis.
GI: nausea, diarrhea, vomiting, abdominal pain or discomfort, oral candidiasis.
GU: crystalluria, interstitial nephritis.
Hematologic: eosinophilia, *leukopenia, neutropenia, thrombocytopenia.*
Musculoskeletal: arthralgia, joint or back pain, joint inflammation, joint stiffness, achiness, neck or chest pain.
Skin: rash, photosensitivity, *Stevens-Johnson syndrome.*
Other: burning, pruritus, erythema, swelling with I.V. administration.

Interactions

Drug-drug. *Aluminum hydroxide, aluminum-magnesium hydroxide, calcium carbonate, magnesium hydroxide:* May decrease effects of ciprofloxacin. Give antacid at least 6 hours before or 2 hours after ciprofloxacin.
Iron salts: May decrease absorption of ciprofloxacin, reducing anti-infective response. Give at least 2 hours apart.
Probenecid: May elevate level of ciprofloxacin. Monitor patient for toxicity.
Sucralfate: May decrease absorption of ciprofloxacin, reducing anti-infective response. If use together can't be avoided, give at least 6 hours apart.

Theophylline: May increase theophylline levels and prolong theophylline half-life. Monitor levels of theophylline and observe patient for adverse effects.

Warfarin: May enhance anticoagulant effects. Monitor PT closely.

Drug-herb. *Yerba maté:* May decrease clearance of yerba maté methylxanthines and cause toxicity. Discourage using together.

Drug-food. *Orange juice fortified with calcium:* May decrease GI absorption of drug, reducing effects. Advise patient to avoid taking drug with calcium-fortified orange juice.

Drug-lifestyle. *Caffeine:* May increase effect of caffeine. Monitor patient.

Effects on lab test results

● May increase BUN, creatinine, ALT, AST, alkaline phosphatase, bilirubin, LDH, and GGT levels.
● May increase eosinophil count. May decrease WBC, neutrophil, and platelet counts.

Pharmacokinetics

Absorption: About 70%. Food delays rate of absorption but not extent. Approximately 35% of Cipro XR is an immediate-release formulation, while 65% is a slow-release matrix.

Distribution: Drug is 20% to 40% protein-bound. CSF levels are only about 10% of plasma levels.

Metabolism: Unknown but probably hepatic. Four metabolites have been identified; each has less antimicrobial activity than parent compound.

Excretion: Primarily renal. *Half-life:* About 4 hours. *Half-life of Cipro XR:* About 6 hours in adults with normal renal function.

Route	Onset	Peak	Duration
P.O.	Unknown	1-2 hr	Unknown
P.O. extended-release	Unknown	1-4 hr	Unknown
I.V.	Immediate	Immediate	Unknown

Action

Chemical effect: Unknown. Bactericidal effects may result from inhibition of bacterial DNA gyrase and prevention of replication in susceptible bacteria.

Therapeutic effect: Kills susceptible bacteria.

Available forms

Infusion (premixed): 200 mg in 100 ml D_5W, 400 mg in 200 ml D_5W
Injection: 200 mg, 400 mg
Tablets: 100 mg, 250 mg, 500 mg, 750 mg
Tablets (extended-release, film-coated): 500 mg
Oral suspension: 250 mg/5 ml; 500 mg/5 ml

NURSING PROCESS

⚚ Assessment

● Assess patient's infection before therapy and reassess regularly throughout therapy.
● Obtain specimen for culture and sensitivity tests before first dose. Therapy may begin pending results.
● Be alert for adverse reactions and drug interactions.
● If adverse GI reactions occur, monitor patient's hydration status.
● Evaluate patient's and family's knowledge of drug therapy.

⊞ Nursing diagnoses

● Infection related to presence of bacteria susceptible to drug
● Risk for deficient fluid volume related to drug-induced adverse GI reactions
● Deficient knowledge related to drug therapy

▶ Planning and implementation

● Give oral form 2 hours after meal or 2 hours before or 6 hours after taking antacids, sucralfate, or products that contain iron (such as vitamins with mineral supplements). Food doesn't affect absorption but may delay peak levels.
● Adjust dosage in patients with renal impairment.
● Have patient drink plenty of fluids to reduce risk of crystalluria.
● Additional antimicrobials for anthrax multidrug regimens can include rifampin, vancomycin, penicillin, ampicillin, chloramphenicol, imipenem, clindamycin, and clarithromycin.
● Steroids may be considered as adjunctive therapy for anthrax patients with severe edema and for meningitis, based on experience with bacterial meningitis of other etiologies.
● Ciprofloxacin and doxycycline are first-line therapy for anthrax. Amoxicillin 500 mg P.O. t.i.d. for adults and 80 mg/kg daily divided q

8 hours for children is an option for completion of therapy after improvement.
• Follow current Centers for Disease Control recommendations for anthrax.

Patient teaching
• Tell patient to take drug 2 hours after meal and to take prescribed antacids at least 2 hours after taking drug.
• Advise patient not to crush, split, or chew the extended-release tablets, but to swallow the tablet whole.
• Advise patient to drink plenty of fluids to reduce risk of crystalluria.
• Warn patient to avoid hazardous tasks that require alertness, such as driving, until CNS effects of drug are known.
• Advise patient to avoid caffeine while taking drug because of potential for cumulative caffeine effects.
• Advise patient that hypersensitivity reactions may occur even after first dose. If he notices rash or other allergic reactions, tell him to stop drug immediately and notify prescriber.
• Instruct patient either to stop breast-feeding or to take a different drug.

☑ Evaluation
• Patient is free from infection.
• Patient maintains adequate hydration throughout drug therapy.
• Patient and family state understanding of drug therapy.

cisplatin (cis-platinum)
(sis-PLAH-tin)
Platinol-AQ

Pharmacologic class: alkylating agent (not specific to cell-cycle phase)
Therapeutic class: antineoplastic
Pregnancy risk category: D

Indications and dosages

▶ **Adjunct therapy in metastatic testicular cancer.** *Adults:* 20 mg/m² I.V. daily for 5 days. Repeat q 3 weeks for three cycles or longer.
▶ **Adjunct therapy in metastatic ovarian cancer.** *Adults:* 100 mg/m² I.V.; repeat q 4 weeks. Or, 50 to 100 mg/m² I.V. once q 4 weeks with cyclophosphamide.

▶ **Advanced bladder cancer.** *Adults:* 50 to 70 mg/m² I.V. q 3 to 4 weeks. Give 50 mg/m² q 4 weeks to patients who have received other antineoplastics or radiation therapy.
▶ **Head and neck cancer‡.** *Adults:* 80 to 120 mg/m² I.V. once q 3 weeks.
▶ **Cervical cancer‡.** *Adults:* 50 mg/m² I.V. once q 3 weeks.
▶ **Non-small-cell lung cancer‡.** *Adults:* 75 to 100 mg/m² I.V. q 3 to 4 weeks with other drugs.
▶ **Brain tumor‡.** *Children:* 60 mg/m² I.V. for 2 days q 3 to 4 weeks.
▶ **Osteogenic sarcoma or neuroblastoma‡.** *Children:* 90 mg/m² I.V. q 3 weeks.
▶ **Advanced esophageal cancer‡.** *Adults:* 50 to 120 mg/m² I.V. once q 3 to 4 weeks when used alone, or 75 to 100 mg/m² I.V. once q 3 to 4 weeks when used with chemotherapy.

▼ I.V. administration

• Preparing and giving drug is linked to carcinogenic, mutagenic, and teratogenic risks. Follow facility policy to reduce risks.
• Give mannitol or furosemide boluses or infusions before and with infusion to maintain diureses of 100 to 400 ml/hour during and for 24 hours after therapy.
• Hydrate patient with normal saline solution before giving drug. Maintain urine output of at least 100 ml/hour for 4 consecutive hours before therapy and for 24 hours after therapy. Prehydration and diuresis may reduce renal toxicity and ototoxicity significantly.
• Reconstitute powder using sterile water for injection. Add 10 ml to 10-mg vial or 50 ml to 50-mg vial to make a solution containing 1 mg/ml. Further dilute with D₅W in one-third normal saline solution for injection or dextrose 5% in half-normal saline solution for injection. Solutions are stable for 20 hours at room temperature. Don't refrigerate.
• Infusions are most stable in chloride-containing solutions (such as normal, half-normal, and one-quarter saline solution). Don't use D₅W alone.
• Give as I.V. infusion in 2 L dextrose 5% in half-normal saline solution or dextrose 5% in 0.33% sodium chloride solution with 37.5 g mannitol over 6 to 8 hours.
• Don't use needles or I.V. administration sets that contain aluminum because it will displace platinum, causing loss of potency and formation of black precipitate.

• Don't administer drug through same I.V. line as mesna, sodium bicarbonate, or sodium thiosulfate due to cisplatin inactivation.
• To prevent hypokalemia, potassium chloride (10 to 20 mEq/L) is commonly added to I.V. fluids before and after therapy. Magnesium sulfate may be added to prevent hypomagnesemia.

Contraindications and precautions

• Contraindicated in patients hypersensitive to drug or other platinum-containing compounds. Also contraindicated in patients with severe renal disease, hearing impairment, or myelosuppression.
🡆 Lifespan: In pregnant women, use cautiously and only when absolutely needed because fetal harm may occur. In breast-feeding women, drug isn't recommended. In children, safety and efficacy of drug haven't been established.

Adverse reactions

CNS: *peripheral neuritis, seizures.*
EENT: *tinnitus, hearing loss.*
GI: *nausea and vomiting beginning 1 to 4 hours after dose and lasting 24 hours,* diarrhea, loss of taste, metallic taste.
GU: more prolonged and *severe renal toxicity* with repeated courses of therapy.
Hematologic: MILD MYELOSUPPRESSION, *leukopenia, thrombocytopenia, anemia,* nadirs in circulating platelet and WBC counts on days 18 to 23 with recovery by day 39.
Metabolic: *hypomagnesemia,* hypokalemia, hypocalcemia.
Other: *anaphylactoid reaction.*

Interactions

Drug-drug. *Aminoglycoside antibiotics:* May cause additive nephrotoxicity. Monitor renal function studies carefully.
Bumetanide, furosemide: May cause additive ototoxicity. Avoid using together.
Phenytoin: May decrease phenytoin levels. Monitor serum levels.

Effects on lab test results

• May increase uric acid levels. May decrease magnesium, potassium, calcium, sodium, and phosphate levels.
• May decrease hemoglobin, hematocrit, and WBC, RBC, and platelet counts.

Pharmacokinetics

Absorption: Administered I.V.
Distribution: Distributed widely into tissues, with highest levels in kidneys, liver, and prostate. Drug doesn't readily cross blood-brain barrier. Drug is extensively and irreversibly bound to plasma and tissue proteins.
Metabolism: Unknown.
Excretion: Excreted primarily unchanged in urine. *Half-life:* Initial phase, 25 to 79 minutes; terminal phase, 58 to 78 hours.

Route	Onset	Peak	Duration
I.V.	Unknown	Unknown	Several days

Action

Chemical effect: Probably cross-links strands of cellular DNA and interferes with RNA transcription, causing imbalance of growth that leads to cell death.
Therapeutic effect: Kills selected cancer cells.

Available forms

Injection: 0.5 mg/ml, 1 mg/ml

NURSING PROCESS

⚗ Assessment
• Assess patient's underlying neoplastic disease before therapy and reassess regularly throughout therapy.
• Monitor CBC, electrolyte levels (especially potassium and magnesium), platelet count, and renal function studies before initial and subsequent dosages.
• To detect permanent hearing loss, obtain audiometry test results before initial dose and subsequent courses.
• Be alert for adverse reactions and drug interactions.
• Evaluate patient's and family's knowledge of drug therapy.

⊞ Nursing diagnoses
• Ineffective health maintenance related to presence of neoplastic disease
• Ineffective protection related to drug-induced adverse reactions
• Deficient knowledge related to drug therapy

▶ Planning and implementation

• Renal toxicity is cumulative. Renal function must return to normal before next dose can be given.

• Don't repeat dosage unless platelet count is over 100,000/mm³, WBC count is over 4,000/mm³, creatinine level is under 1.5 mg/dl, or BUN level is under 25 mg/dl.

• Check current protocol. Some clinicians use I.V. sodium thiosulfate to minimize toxicity.

• Nausea and vomiting may be severe and protracted (up to 24 hours). Provide I.V. hydration until patient can tolerate adequate oral intake.

• Antiemetics such as ondansetron, granisetron, and high-dose metoclopramide have been used effectively to prevent and treat nausea and vomiting. Some clinicians combine metoclopramide with dexamethasone and antihistamines, or ondansetron or granisetron with dexamethasone.

• Delayed-onset vomiting (3 to 5 days after treatment) has been reported. Patients may need prolonged antiemetic treatment.

• Immediately give epinephrine, corticosteroids, or antihistamines for anaphylactoid reactions.

③ **ALERT:** Don't confuse cisplatin with carboplatin.

Patient teaching

• Warn patient to watch for signs of infection (fever, sore throat, fatigue) and bleeding (easy bruising, nosebleeds, bleeding gums, melena). Tell him to take his temperature daily.

• Tell patient to report tinnitus immediately.

• Instruct patient to avoid OTC products that contain aspirin.

• Teach patient to record intake and output on daily basis and to report edema or decrease in urine output.

• Encourage patient to notify prescriber if any concerns arise during drug therapy.

☑ Evaluation

• Patient exhibits positive response to cisplatin therapy according to follow-up diagnostic studies.

• Patient doesn't experience permanent injury as a result of drug-induced adverse reactions.

• Patient and family state understanding of drug therapy.

citalopram hydrobromide
(sih-TAL-oh-pram high-droh-BROH-mighd)
Celexa

Pharmacologic class: SSRI
Therapeutic class: antidepressant
Pregnancy risk category: C

Indications and dosages

▶ **Depression.** *Adults:* Initially, 20 mg P.O. once daily, increasing to maximum dose of 40 mg daily after no less than 1 week.

▶ **Panic disorder‡.** *Adults:* 20 to 30 mg P.O. once daily.

ⓢ **Adjust-a-dose:** For elderly patients and patients with hepatic impairment, give 20 mg P.O. once daily, increased to 40 mg daily only for patients not responding to therapy.

Contraindications and precautions

• Contraindicated within 14 days of MAO inhibitor therapy. Also contraindicated in patients hypersensitive to drug, its ingredients, or escitalopram.

• Use cautiously in patients with history of mania, seizures, suicidal ideation, hepatic impairment, or renal impairment.

⚝ **Lifespan:** In breast-feeding women, avoid using drug; drug appears in breast milk and there is a potential for serious adverse reactions in infants. In children, safety and efficacy of drug haven't been established. In elderly patients, reduce dosage.

Adverse reactions

CNS: fever, tremor, somnolence, insomnia, anxiety, agitation, dizziness, paresthesia, migraine, impaired concentration, amnesia, depression, apathy, *suicide attempt,* confusion, fatigue.
CV: tachycardia, orthostatic hypotension, hypotension.
EENT: rhinitis, sinusitis, abnormal accommodation.
GI: nausea, dry mouth, diarrhea, anorexia, dyspepsia, vomiting, abdominal pain, increased saliva, taste perversion, flatulence, weight changes, increased appetite.
GU: dysmenorrhea, amenorrhea, ejaculation disorder, impotence, polyuria.
Musculoskeletal: arthralgia, myalgia.

Respiratory: upper respiratory tract infection, cough.
Skin: rash, pruritus, increased sweating.
Other: yawning, decreased libido.

Interactions

Drug-drug. *Carbamazepine:* May increase citalopram clearance. Monitor patient for effects.
CNS drugs: May increase CNS effects. Use together cautiously.
Drugs that inhibit CYP 3A4 (such as fluconazole) and CYP 2C19 (such as omeprazole): May decrease citalopram clearance. Monitor patient for toxicity.
Imipramine, other tricyclic antidepressants: May increase level of imipramine metabolite desipramine by about 50%. Use together cautiously.
Lithium: May enhance serotonergic effect of citalopram. Use cautiously and monitor lithium levels.
Phenelzine, selegiline, tranylcypromine: May cause "serotonin syndrome" involving CNS irritability, shivering, and altered consciousness. Don't give together. Wait at least 2 weeks after stopping an MAOI before giving any SSRI.
Sumatriptan: May cause weakness, hyperreflexia, and incoordination. Monitor patient closely.
Warfarin: PT increases by 5%. Monitor patient carefully; monitor PT and INR.
Drug-herb. *St. John's wort:* Serotonin levels may rise too high, causing serotonin syndrome. Discourage using together.

Effects on lab test results

None reported.

Pharmacokinetics

Absorption: Absolute bioavailability is 80%.
Distribution: About 80% bound to plasma proteins.
Metabolism: Metabolized primarily by the liver.
Excretion: About 10% of drug is recovered in urine. *Half-life:* 35 hours.

Route	Onset	Peak	Duration
P.O.	Unknown	4 hr	Unknown

Action

Chemical effect: Probably enhances serotonergic activity in CNS resulting from its inhibition of CNS neuronal reuptake of serotonin.
Therapeutic effect: Relieves depression.

Available forms

Oral solution: 10 mg/5 ml
Tablets: 10 mg, 20 mg, 40 mg

NURSING PROCESS

Assessment
• Assess patient's underlying condition before therapy and reassess regularly thereafter.
• Check vital signs regularly for decreased blood pressure or tachycardia.
• Closely supervise high-risk patients at start of drug therapy.
• Evaluate patient's and family's knowledge of drug therapy.

Nursing diagnoses
• Risk for injury related to patient's underlying condition
• Ineffective coping related to patient's underlying condition
• Deficient knowledge related to drug therapy

Planning and implementation
ALERT: Don't start citalopram therapy within 14 days of MAO inhibitor therapy.
• For patient with hepatic impairment, reduce dosage.
• May increase risk of suicide. Don't stop drug abruptly.
ALERT: Don't confuse Celexa with Celebrex or Cerebyx.
Patient teaching
• Inform patient to continue therapy as prescribed even if he improves within 1 to 4 weeks.
• Instruct patient to exercise caution when operating hazardous machinery, including automobiles, because psychoactive drugs can impair judgment, thinking, and motor skills.
• Warn patient that drug may cause photosensitivity; advise patient to take protective measures until tolerance is determined.
• Advise patient to consult prescriber before taking other prescription drugs, OTC medicines, or herbal remedies.
ALERT: If patient wishes to switch from an SSRI to St. John's wort, tell him to wait a few weeks for the SSRI to leave his system before he starts the herb. Urge him to ask his prescriber for advice.
• Warn patient not to consume alcohol during therapy.

• Instruct woman of childbearing age to use birth control during drug therapy and to notify prescriber immediately if she suspects pregnancy.

✓ Evaluation
• Patient's safety is maintained.
• Patient's condition is improved with drug.
• Patient and family state understanding of drug therapy.

clarithromycin
(klah-rith-roh-MIGH-sin)
Biaxin, Biaxin XL

Pharmacologic class: macrolide
Therapeutic class: antibiotic
Pregnancy risk category: C

Indications and dosages

▶ **Pharyngitis or tonsillitis caused by *Streptococcus pyogenes.*** *Adults:* 250 mg P.O. q 12 hours for 10 days. *Children:* 15 mg/kg P.O. daily divided q 12 hours for 10 days.
▶ **Acute maxillary sinusitis caused by *Streptococcus pneumoniae, Haemophilus influenzae,* or *Moraxella catarrhalis.*** *Adults:* 500 mg P.O. q 12 hours for 14 days. Or, two 500-mg extended-release tablets P.O. daily for 14 days. *Children:* 15 mg/kg P.O. daily divided q 12 hours for 10 days.
▶ **Acute exacerbations of chronic bronchitis caused by *M. catarrhalis, S. pneumoniae, H. influenzae,* or *H. parainfluenzae.*** *Adults:* 250 mg P.O. q 12 hours for 7 to 14 days (for *M. catarrhalis* and *S. pneumoniae* only), or 500 mg P.O. q 12 hours for 7 days (up to 14 days for *H. influenzae*). Or, two 500-mg extended-release tablets P.O. daily for 7 days.
▶ **Uncomplicated skin and skin-structure infections caused by *Staphylococcus aureus* or *S. pyogenes.*** *Adults:* 250 mg P.O. q 12 hours for 7 to 14 days.
▶ **Prophylaxis and treatment of disseminated infection from *Mycobacterium avium* complex.** *Adults:* 500 mg P.O. b.i.d.. *Children:* 7.5 mg/kg P.O. b.i.d. up to 500 mg b.i.d.
▶ **Acute otitis media caused by *H. influenzae, M. catarrhalis,* or *S. pneumoniae.*** *Children:* 7.5 mg/kg P.O. q 12 hours, up to 500 mg b.i.d.

▶ ***Helicobacter pylori* eradication to reduce risk of duodenal ulcer recurrence.** *Adults:* For triple-therapy, 500 mg clarithromycin with 30 mg lansoprazole and 1 g amoxicillin, all given q 12 hours for 10 to 14 days; or 500 mg clarithromycin with 20 mg omeprazole and 1 g amoxicillin, all given q 12 hours for 10 days; or rabeprazole 20 mg P.O. b.i.d. in combination with amoxicillin 1,000 mg P.O. b.i.d. and clarithromycin 500 mg P.O. b.i.d. for 7 days. For dual therapy, 500 mg clarithromycin q 8 hours and 40 mg omeprazole once daily for 14 days. *Children:* 15 mg/kg/day divided q 12 hours for 10 days.
▶ **Community-acquired pneumonia due to *Chlamydia pneumoniae, Mycoplasma pneumoniae, Streptococcus pneumoniae, Haemophilus influenzae, H. parainfluenzae, Moraxella catarrhalis.*** *Adults:* 250 mg P.O. q 12 hours for 7 to 14 days (for *H. influenzae,* duration of therapy is 7 days). Don't use conventional tablets to treat pneumonia caused by *H. parainfluenzae* or *M. catarrhalis.* Or, two 500-mg extended-release tablets P.O. daily for 7 days for all listed organisms. *Children:* 15 mg/kg P.O. daily divided q 12 hours for 10 days (for *C. pneumoniae, M. pneumoniae,* or *S. pneumoniae* only).
✎ **Adjust-a-dose:** For patients with renal impairment, if creatinine clearance is less than 30 ml/minute, reduce dose by 50% or double frequency interval.

Contraindications and precautions

• Contraindicated in patients hypersensitive to drug and other macrolides. Coadministration is contraindicated with pimozide or other drugs that prolong QT interval or cause cardiac arrhythmias.
• Use cautiously in patients with hepatic or renal impairment.
⚖ **Lifespan:** In pregnant or breast-feeding women, use cautiously. In infants younger than age 6 months, safety and efficacy of drug haven't been established.

Adverse reactions

CNS: headache.
CV: *arrhythmias.*
GI: *pseudomembranous colitis,* diarrhea, nausea, abnormal taste, dyspepsia, abdominal pain or discomfort, vomiting (pediatric).

Hematologic: coagulation abnormalities, *leukopenia.*
Skin: rash (pediatric).

Interactions

Drug-drug. *Alprazolam, midazolam, triazolam:* May decrease clearance of these drugs, causing CNS adverse reactions. Use together cautiously.
Carbamazepine: May inhibit metabolism of carbamazepine and increase level and risk of toxicity. Avoid using together.
Digoxin: May increase level. Monitor level for digoxin toxicity.
Dihydroergotamine, ergotamine: May cause acute ergot toxicity. Avoid using together.
Disopyramide, pimozide, quinidine: May cause torsades de pointes. Monitor ECG for prolonged QT. Avoid using together.
Fluconazole: May increase clarithromycin levels. Monitor patient.
HMG-CoA reductase inhibitors: May increase levels of these drugs, and cause rare occurrences of rhabdomyolysis.
Oral anticoagulants: May increase effects of anticoagulant. Monitor PT and INR closely.
Ritonavir: May prolong absorption of clarithromycin. Don't adjust dosage in patients with normal renal function; if creatinine clearance is 30 to 60 ml/minute, give 50% of clarithromycin dose; if less than 30 ml/minute, give 25% of clarithromycin dose.
Sildenafil: May prolong absorption of sildenafil. Reduce sildenafil dosage.
Theophylline: May increase level of theophylline. Monitor level carefully.
Zidovudine: May alter zidovudine levels. Monitor patient closely.

Effects on lab test results

• May increase AST, ALT, GGT, alkaline phosphatase, LDH, total bilirubin, creatinine, and BUN levels.
• May increase PT and INR. May decrease WBC counts.

Pharmacokinetics

Absorption: Rapid.
Distribution: Widely distributed.
Metabolism: Drug's major metabolite has significant antimicrobial activity.
Excretion: Excreted in urine. *Half-life:* 5 to 6 hours with 250 mg q 12 hours; 7 hours with 500 mg q 12 hours.

Route	Onset	Peak	Duration
P.O.	Unknown	2-3 hr	Unknown
P.O. extended-release	Unknown	5-6 hr	Unknown

Action

Chemical effect: Binds to 50S subunit of bacterial ribosomes, blocking protein synthesis; bacteriostatic or bactericidal, depending on concentration.
Therapeutic effect: Hinders or kills susceptible bacteria.

Available forms

Suspension: 125 mg/5 ml, 250 mg/5 ml
Tablets: 250 mg, 500 mg
Tablets (extended-release): 500 mg

NURSING PROCESS

⚕ Assessment

• Assess patient's infection before therapy and reassess regularly throughout therapy.
• Obtain urine specimen for culture and sensitivity tests before first dose. Therapy may begin pending results.
• Be alert for adverse reactions and drug interactions.
• If adverse GI reactions occur, monitor patient's hydration status.
• Evaluate patient's and family's knowledge of drug therapy.

⚕ Nursing diagnoses

• Infection related to presence of bacteria susceptible to drug
• Risk for deficient fluid volume related to drug-induced adverse GI reactions
• Deficient knowledge related to drug therapy

⟩ Planning and implementation

• Give drug without regard to meals; it may be taken with milk.
• There have been reported interactions with drugs metabolized by CYP 3A, and also with hexobarbital, phenytoin, and valproate.
• Drug may cause allergic reactions including anaphylaxis, Steven-Johnson syndrome, and toxic epidermal necrolysis; GI effects; CNS effects; thrombocytopenia, neutropenia; hepatic dysfunction; and QT prolongation and ventricular arrhythmias.

Rapid onset   *Liquid form contains alcohol.*   ◆Canada   ◇ Australia   †OTC   ‡Off-label use

ⓧ **ALERT:** Don't confuse or interchange Biaxin XL (extended-release) with Biaxin (immediate release).

Patient teaching
• Tell patient to take all of drug, as prescribed, even after he feels better.
• Tell patient to notify prescriber if adverse reactions occur.
• Tell patient not to chew or crush extended-release tablets.

☑ **Evaluation**
• Patient is free from infection.
• Patient maintains adequate hydration throughout drug therapy.
• Patient and family state understanding of drug therapy.

clindamycin hydrochloride
(klin-duh-MIGH-sin high-droh-KLOR-ighd)
Cleocin, Dalacin C♦ ◊

clindamycin palmitate hydrochloride
Cleocin Pediatric

clindamycin phosphate

Pharmacologic class: lincomycin derivative
Therapeutic class: antibiotic
Pregnancy risk category: B

Indications and dosages
▶ **Infections caused by sensitive staphylococci, streptococci, pneumococci, *Bacteroides, Fusobacterium, Clostridium perfringens,* and other sensitive aerobic and anaerobic organisms.** *Adults:* 150 to 450 mg P.O. q 6 hours. Or, 600 to 2,700 mg I.M. or I.V. daily divided into 2 to 4 doses. Don't exceed 600 mg in a single I.M. dose. Don't give more than 1.2 g I.V. in a 1-hour period. Maximum adult I.V. dose is 4.8 g daily.
Children ages 1 month to 16 years: 8 to 25 mg/kg P.O. daily in three or four equally divided doses. Or, 20 to 40 mg/kg I.M. or I.V. daily, in 3 or 4 equally divided doses, or 350 to 450 mg/m² daily.

Neonates younger than age 1 month: 15 to 20 mg/kg I.V. daily in three or four equally divided doses.
▶ **Endocarditis prophylaxis for dental procedures in patients allergic to penicillin.** *Adults:* 600 mg P.O. 1 hour before procedure or 600 mg I.V. 30 minutes before procedure.
Children ages 1 month to 16 years: 20 mg/kg P.O. 1 hour before procedure or 20 mg/kg I.V. 30 minutes before procedure (not to exceed adult dosage).
▶ **Acne vulgaris.** *Adults:* Apply a thin film of topical solution, gel, or lotion to affected areas b.i.d.
▶ ***Pneumocystis carinii* pneumonia‡.** *Adults:* 600 mg I.V. q 6 hours. Or, 300 to 450 mg P.O. q.i.d. With primaquine, give 15 to 30 mg P.O. daily.
▶ **Toxoplasmosis (cerebral or ocular) in immunocompromised patients‡.** *Adults:* 300 to 450 mg P.O. q 6 to 8 hours with pyrimethamine (25 to 75 mg once daily) and leucovorin (10 to 25 mg once daily).
Infants and children age 16 and younger: 20 to 30 mg/kg P.O. daily in 4 divided doses with oral pyrimethamine (1 mg/kg daily) and oral leucovorin (5 mg once q 3 days).

▼ I.V. administration
• For I.V. infusion, dilute each 300 mg in 50 ml solution, and give no faster than 30 mg/minute (over 10 to 60 minutes). Never give undiluted as bolus.
• Check I.V. site daily for phlebitis and irritation.

Contraindications and precautions
• Contraindicated in patients hypersensitive to antibiotic containing clindamycin or lincomycin.
• Use cautiously in patients with renal or hepatic disease, asthma, history of GI disease, or significant allergies.
⚖ **Lifespan:** Breast-feeding women should stop breast-feeding. In neonates, use cautiously.

Adverse reactions
CV: thrombophlebitis.
GI: unpleasant or bitter taste, **nausea,** vomiting, abdominal pain, ***diarrhea, pseudomembranous colitis,*** esophagitis, flatulence, anorexia, *bloody or tarry stools, dysphagia.*

Hematologic: *transient leukopenia,* eosinophilia, *thrombocytopenia.*
Skin: *maculopapular rash,* urticaria.
Other: *anaphylaxis; pain,* induration, *sterile abscess* (I.M. injection); erythema, pain (I.V. administration).

Interactions

Drug-drug. *Erythromycin:* May block clindamycin site of action. Avoid using together.
Kaolin: May decrease absorption of oral clindamycin. Separate administration times.
Neuromuscular blockers: May potentiate neuromuscular blockade. Monitor patient closely.
Drug-food. *Diet foods with sodium cyclamate:* May decrease drug level. Discourage using together.

Effects on lab test results

• May increase bilirubin, AST, and alkaline phosphatase levels.
• May increase eosinophil count. May decrease WBC and platelet counts.

Pharmacokinetics

Absorption: Rapid and almost complete when administered P.O. Drug is absorbed well after I.M. administration.
Distribution: Distributed widely to most body tissues and fluids (except CSF). Drug is about 93% bound to plasma proteins.
Metabolism: Metabolized partially to inactive metabolites.
Excretion: About 10% of clindamycin dose is excreted unchanged in urine; rest is excreted as inactive metabolites. *Half-life:* 2½ to 3 hours.

Route	Onset	Peak	Duration
P.O.	Unknown	45-60 min	Unknown
I.V.	Immediate	Immediate	Unknown
I.M.	Unknown	3 hr	Unknown

Action

Chemical effect: Inhibits bacterial protein synthesis by binding to 50S subunit of ribosome.
Therapeutic effect: Hinders or kills susceptible bacteria.

Available forms

clindamycin hydrochloride
Capsules: 75 mg, 150 mg, 300 mg
clindamycin palmitate hydrochloride
Oral solution: 75 mg/5 ml

clindamycin phosphate
Injection: 150 mg/ml

NURSING PROCESS

≋ Assessment
• Assess patient's infection before therapy and reassess regularly throughout therapy.
• Obtain urine specimen for culture and sensitivity tests before first dose. Therapy may begin pending results.
• Monitor renal, hepatic, and hematopoietic functions during prolonged therapy.
• Be alert for adverse reactions and drug interactions.
• If adverse GI reactions occur, monitor patient's hydration status.
• Evaluate patient's and family's knowledge of drug therapy.

⊞ Nursing diagnoses
• Infection related to presence of bacteria susceptible to drug
• Risk for deficient fluid volume related to drug-induced adverse GI reactions
• Deficient knowledge related to drug therapy

▶ Planning and implementation
• Don't refrigerate reconstituted oral solution because it will thicken. Drug is stable for 2 weeks at room temperature.
• Give capsule form with full glass of water to prevent dysphagia.
• For I.M. injection, inject drug deeply. Rotate sites. Warn patient that I.M. injection may be painful. Doses over 600 mg per injection aren't recommended.
• I.M. injection may raise CK in response to muscle irritation.
⚛ ALERT: Don't give opioid antidiarrheals to treat drug-induced diarrhea; they may prolong and worsen diarrhea.
⚛ ALERT: Because of an association with severe and even fatal colitis, reserve clindamycin for serious infections only.
Patient teaching
• Advise patient taking capsule form to take with full glass of water to prevent dysphagia.
• Teach patient how to store oral solution.
• Instruct patient to take drug for as long as prescribed, exactly as directed.
• Tell patient to take entire amount prescribed even after he feels better.

- Warn patient that I.M. injection may be painful.
- Instruct patient to report diarrhea and to avoid self-treatment because of the risk of life-threatening pseudomembranous colitis.
- Tell patient receiving drug I.V. to report discomfort at infusion site.

☑ Evaluation
- Patient is free from infection after drug therapy.
- Patient maintains adequate hydration during drug therapy.
- Patient and family state understanding of drug therapy.

clobetasol propionate
(kloh-BAY-tah-sol PRO-pee-uh-nayt)
Cormax, Dermovate*, Embeline E, Temovate, Temovate Emollient, Olux

Pharmacologic class: topical adrenocorticoid
Therapeutic class: anti-inflammatory
Pregnancy risk category: C

Indications and dosages

▶ **Inflammation and pruritus from moderate to severe corticosteroid-responsive dermatoses.** *Adults:* Apply a thin layer to affected skin areas b.i.d., once in the morning and once at night. Limit treatment to 14 days, with no more than 50 g cream or ointment or 50 ml lotion (25 mg total) weekly.
▶ **Inflammation and pruritus from moderate to severe corticosteroid-responsive dermatoses of the scalp; short-term topical therapy for mild to moderate plaque-type psoriasis of nonscalp regions, excluding the face and intertriginous areas.** *Adults:* Apply a small amount of Olux foam, up to a maximum of a golf-ball-size dollop, to affected skin b.i.d., once in the morning and once at night. Limit treatment to 14 days, with no more than 50 g of foam weekly.

Contraindications and precautions

- Contraindicated in patients hypersensitive to corticosteroids. Also contraindicated for the treatment of acne, rosacea, perioral dermatitis, or as monotherapy for the treatment of widespread plaque psoriasis.

- Use caution when applying drug to face, groin, or axillae, because these areas are at an increased risk for atrophic changes.
- Use cautiously in patients with glaucoma and diabetes.
- ⚠ **Lifespan:** In pregnant women, avoid use because of possibility of teratogenic effects. In breast-feeding women, use cautiously and avoid applying to breasts because it's unknown whether drug appears in breast milk. In patients younger than age 12, drug isn't recommended. In elderly patients, begin at the low end of the dosage range and adjust carefully.

Adverse reactions

GU: glucosuria.
Metabolic: hyperglycemia.
Skin: burning and stinging sensation, pruritus, irritation, dryness and cracking, erythema, folliculitis, perioral dermatitis, allergic contact dermatitis, hypopigmentation, hypertrichosis, acneiform eruptions, skin atrophy, telangiectasia (dilatation of capillaries), striae.
Other: *hypothalamic-pituitary-adrenal axis suppression,* Cushing's syndrome, numbness of fingers.

Interactions

None reported.

Effects on lab test results

- May increase glucose level.
- May cause false-positive results with the adrenocorticotropic hormone (ACTH) stimulation, a.m. plasma cortisol, and urine-free cortisol tests.

Pharmacokinetics

Absorption: Dependent on the potency of the preparation, the amount applied, the nature of the skin at the application site, and the use of occlusive dressings. Absorption increases in areas of skin damage, inflammation, or occlusion. Some systemic absorption of topical steroids occurs, especially through the oral mucosa.
Distribution: After topical application, drug is distributed throughout the local skin. Any drug absorbed into the circulation is rapidly removed from the blood and distributed into muscle, liver, skin, intestines, and kidneys.
Metabolism: After topical administration, drug is metabolized primarily in the skin. The small amount absorbed into systemic circulation is

metabolized primarily in the liver to inactive compounds.

Excretion: Drug and active metabolites, in the liver and bile. Inactive metabolites, by the kidneys, primarily as glucuronides and sulfates, but also as unconjugated products. Small amounts of the metabolites are also excreted in the urine and feces. *Half-life:* Unknown.

Route	Onset	Peak	Duration
Topical	Unknown	Unknown	Unknown

Action

Chemical effect: Unknown. Drug is a high-potency group I fluorinated corticosteroid that's usually reserved for the management of severe dermatoses that haven't responded satisfactorily to a less potent formulation.

Therapeutic effect: Decreases inflammation and itching.

Available forms

Cream: 0.05%
Foam: 0.05%
Gel: 0.05%
Ointment: 0.05%
Solution: 0.05%

NURSING PROCESS

Assessment

• Assess patient before and during therapy. Topical corticosteroid therapy may adversely affect and exacerbate symptoms in patients with diabetes or glaucoma.
• Monitor patient for adverse effects of corticosteroid therapy.
• If applied to face, groin, or axillae, observe frequently for skin atrophy.
• During long-term use, obtain ACTH stimulation, a.m. plasma cortisol, and urine-free cortisol tests to monitor patient for hypothalmic-pituitary-adrenal (HPA) axis suppression.
• Evaluate patient's and family's knowledge of drug therapy.

Nursing diagnoses

• Risk of infection related to prolonged and very potent corticosteroid therapy.
• Impaired skin integrity related to underlying skin disease process
• Situational low self-esteem due to underlying skin disease process

• Deficient knowledge related to topical corticosteroid therapy

Planning and implementation

• When applying foam to a hairy area, move the hair away from the affected area of the scalp so that the foam can be applied to each affected area.
• Don't use longer than 2 weeks.
• Drug is for external use only. Avoid rubbing eyes during and after application. If drug gets into the eyes, flush affected eye with copious amounts of water.
• Don't dispense directly onto hand because cream and foam will begin to melt immediately upon contact with warm skin. When using foam, invert can and dispense foam into cap of can or directly onto the lesion.
• Apply sparingly in light film; then massage into skin gently until foam disappears.
• Don't use occlusive dressings or bandages. Don't cover or wrap treated area unless instructed by prescriber.
• If skin infection develops, institute appropriate antifungal or antibacterial treatment. If infection does not respond promptly to treatment, stop drug until infection is under control.
• If irritation, skin infection, striae, or atrophy occurs, stop drug and notify prescriber.
• Drug can suppress HPA axis at doses as low as 2 g daily. If HPA axis suppression occurs, attempt to withdraw drug, reduce dosage, or substitute a less potent steroid.
• If no improvement within 2 weeks, reassess diagnoses.
• Don't refrigerate. Store drug at room temperature.

Patient teaching

• Advise patient that drug is for external use only and to avoid contact with eyes.
• Instruct patient to use medication only as prescribed and only for the indications specified.
• Teach patient proper application of the topical steroid to affected area(s). Explain that occlusive dressings aren't recommended and may increase absorption and skin atrophy.
• Inform patient of potential adverse reactions and signs and symptoms of infection and impaired healing; urge patient to notify prescriber immediately.
• Warn patient not to use drug for longer than 14 days.

• Caution patient that drug is flammable and to avoid flames or smoking during and immediately after application.
• Instruct patients using Olux foam that the contents are under pressure and container shouldn't be punctured or incinerated. Also, tell patient not to expose to heat or store at temperatures above 120° F (49° C).

☑ Evaluation

• Patient doesn't suffer from any infection caused by drug therapy.
• Patient is relieved of symptoms and remains free from any adverse effects of drug therapy.
• Patient's self-esteem increases as patient's skin improves.
• Patient and family state understanding of drug therapy.

clomiphene citrate

(KLOH-meh-feen SIGH-trayt)
Clomid, Milophene, Serophene

Pharmacologic class: chlorotrianisene derivative
Therapeutic class: ovulation stimulant
Pregnancy risk category: X

Indications and dosages

▶ **Induction of ovulation.** *Women:* 50 mg P.O. daily for 5 days starting on day 5 of menstrual cycle if bleeding occurs (first day of menstrual flow is day 1), or at any time if woman hasn't had recent uterine bleeding. If ovulation doesn't occur, may increase dose to 100 mg P.O. daily for 5 days as soon as 30 days after previous course. Repeat until conception occurs or until three courses of therapy are completed.
▶ **Infertility‡.** *Men:* 50 to 400 mg P.O. daily for 2 to 12 months.

Contraindications and precautions

• Contraindicated in patients with undiagnosed abnormal genital bleeding, ovarian cyst not caused by polycystic ovarian syndrome, hepatic disease or dysfunction, uncontrolled thyroid or adrenal dysfunction, or organic intracranial lesion (such as pituitary tumor).
⚠ **Lifespan:** In pregnant women, drug is contraindicated.

Adverse reactions

CNS: headache, restlessness, insomnia, dizziness, light-headedness, depression, fatigue, tension, *vasomotor flushes.*
CV: hypertension.
EENT: blurred vision, diplopia, scotoma, photophobia.
GI: nausea, vomiting, bloating, distention.
GU: urinary frequency and polyuria; *ovarian enlargement and cyst formation,* which regress spontaneously when drug is stopped.
Metabolic: *hyperglycemia,* increased appetite, weight gain.
Skin: reversible alopecia, urticaria, rash, dermatitis.
Other: *breast discomfort.*

Interactions

None significant.

Effects on lab test results

• May increase glucose level.

Pharmacokinetics

Absorption: Absorbed readily from GI tract.
Distribution: May undergo enterohepatic recirculation or may be stored in body fat.
Metabolism: Metabolized by liver.
Excretion: Excreted principally in feces via biliary elimination. *Half-life:* About 5 days.

Route	Onset	Peak	Duration
P.O.	Unknown	Unknown	Unknown

Action

Chemical effect: Appears to stimulate release of pituitary gonadotropins, follicle-stimulating hormone, and luteinizing hormone. This results in maturation of ovarian follicle, ovulation, and development of corpus luteum.
Therapeutic effect: Causes women to ovulate.

Available forms

Tablets: 50 mg

NURSING PROCESS

℞ Assessment

• Assess patient's underlying condition before therapy.
• Monitor drug's effectiveness by assessing ovulation through biphasic body temperature measurement, postovulatory urinary levels of

pregnanediol, estrogen excretion, and changes in endometrial tissues.
• Be alert for adverse reactions.
• Evaluate patient's and family's knowledge of drug therapy.

⊞ **Nursing diagnoses**
• Excess fluid volume related to drug-induced fluid retention
• Sexual dysfunction related to underlying condition
• Deficient knowledge related to drug therapy

▶ **Planning and implementation**
• Prepare administration instructions for patient: Begin daily dosage on fifth day of menstrual flow for 5 consecutive days.
• Don't give more than three courses of therapy to attempt conception.
Patient teaching
• Tell patient about risk of multiple births with drug use; risk increases with higher doses.
• Teach patient how to take and chart basal body temperature and to ascertain whether ovulation has occurred.
• Reassure woman that ovulation typically occurs after first course of therapy. If pregnancy doesn't occur, course of therapy may be repeated twice.
⊛ **ALERT:** Advise woman to stop drug and contact prescriber immediately if pregnancy is suspected because drug may have teratogenic effect on fetus.
• Advise woman to stop drug and contact prescriber immediately if abdominal symptoms or pain occurs because these may indicate ovarian enlargement or ovarian cyst.
• Tell patient to immediately report signs of impending visual toxicity, such as blurred vision, diplopia, scotoma, or photophobia.
• Warn patient to avoid hazardous activities until CNS effects of drug are known. Drug may cause dizziness or visual disturbances.

☑ **Evaluation**
• Patient is free from fluid retention at end of therapy.
• Woman ovulates with drug therapy.
• Patient and family state understanding of drug therapy.

clomipramine hydrochloride
(kloh-MIH-pruh-meen high-droh-KLOR-ighd)
Anafranil

Pharmacologic class: tricyclic antidepressant (TCA)
Therapeutic class: antiobsessive drug
Pregnancy risk category: C

Indications and dosages

▶ **Obsessive-compulsive disorder.** *Adults:* Initially, 25 mg P.O. daily in divided doses with meals, gradually increase to 100 mg daily during first 2 weeks. Then, increase to maximum dosage of 250 mg daily in divided doses with meals as needed. After adjusting dosage, give total daily dosage h.s.
Adolescents and children: Initially, 12.5 mg P.O. b.i.d. with meals, gradually increase to daily maximum of 3 mg/kg or 100 mg P.O., whichever is smaller. Give maximum daily dosage of 3 mg/kg or 200 mg, whichever is smaller; h.s. after adjusting dosage. Reassess and adjust periodically.

Contraindications and precautions

• Contraindicated in patients hypersensitive to drug or other TCAs, in patients in acute recovery period after MI, and within 14 days of MAO inhibitor therapy.
• Use cautiously in patients with history of seizure disorders or with brain damage; in those receiving other seizure threshold-lowering drugs; in patients at risk for suicide; in patients with history of urine retention or angle-closure glaucoma, increased intraocular pressure, CV disease, impaired hepatic or renal function, or hyperthyroidism; in patients with tumors of the adrenal medulla; in patients receiving thyroid drug or electroconvulsive therapy; and in those undergoing elective surgery.
⚠ **Lifespan:** In pregnant and breast-feeding women, use cautiously.

Adverse reactions

CNS: *somnolence, tremors, dizziness,* headache, insomnia, *nervousness, myoclonus, fatigue, EEG changes, **seizures,*** extrapyramidal reactions, asthenia, aggressiveness.
CV: orthostatic hypotension, palpitations, tachycardia.

EENT: otitis media in children, abnormal vision, laryngitis, pharyngitis, rhinitis.
GI: dry mouth, constipation, *nausea,* dyspepsia, diarrhea, anorexia, abdominal pain, eructation.
GU: *urinary hesitancy,* UTI, dysmenorrhea, *impaired ejaculation,* impotence.
Hematologic: anemia, bone marrow suppression.
Metabolic: increased appetite, *weight gain.*
Musculoskeletal: *myalgia.*
Skin: *diaphoresis,* rash, pruritus, photosensitivity, dry skin.
Other: *altered libido.*

Interactions

Drug-drug. *Barbiturates:* May decrease TCA levels. Monitor patient for decreased antidepressant effect.
Cimetidine, methylphenidate: May increase TCA levels. Monitor patient for enhanced antidepressant effect.
CNS depressants: Enhances CNS depression. Avoid using together.
Clonidine: May cause loss of blood pressure control and potentially life-threatening elevations in blood pressure. Avoid using together.
Epinephrine, norepinephrine: May increase hypertensive effect. Use with caution and monitor blood pressure.
MAO inhibitors: May cause hyperpyretic crisis, seizures, coma, or death. Don't use together.
Drug-herb. *St. John's wort:* Serotonin levels may rise too high, causing serotonin syndrome. Discourage using together.
Drug-lifestyle. *Alcohol use:* May enhance CNS depression. Discourage using together.
Sun exposure: Photosensitivity may occur. Urge patient to avoid sun exposure and wear protective clothing and sunblock.

Effects on lab test results

- May decrease hemoglobin and hematocrit.

Pharmacokinetics

Absorption: Well absorbed from the GI tract, but extensive first-pass metabolism limits bioavailability to about 50%.
Distribution: Distributed well into lipophilic tissues; about 98% bound to plasma proteins.
Metabolism: Primarily hepatic. Several metabolites have been identified.

Excretion: About 66% is excreted in urine; remainder in feces. *Half-life:* Parent compound, about 36 hours; active metabolite, 4 to 233 days.

Route	Onset	Peak	Duration
P.O.	≥ 2 wk	Unknown	Unknown

Action

Chemical effect: Selectively inhibits reuptake of serotonin.
Therapeutic effect: Reduces obsessive-compulsive behaviors.

Available forms

Capsules: 25 mg, 50 mg, 75 mg

NURSING PROCESS

🔲 Assessment
- Assess patient's underlying condition before therapy and regularly thereafter.
- Evaluate patient's and family's knowledge of drug therapy.

🔲 Nursing diagnoses
- Ineffective coping related to patient's underlying condition
- Risk for injury related to drug-induced adverse reactions
- Deficient knowledge related to drug therapy

🔲 Planning and implementation
- After dosage adjustment, give total daily dose h.s. During dosage adjustment, divide dose and give with meals to minimize GI effects.
- Don't withdraw drug abruptly.
- Because hypertensive episodes may occur during surgery, taper off drug several days before surgery.
- 🔹 **ALERT:** Don't confuse clomipramine with chlorpromazine or clomiphene; don't confuse Anafranil with enalapril, nafarelin, or alfentanil.
Patient teaching
- Warn patient to avoid hazardous activities requiring alertness and good psychomotor coordination, especially during dosage adjustment. Daytime sedation and dizziness may occur.
- Tell patient to avoid alcohol while taking drug.
- Warn patient not to withdraw drug suddenly.
- Advise patient to use sunblock, wear protective clothing, and avoid prolonged exposure to strong sunlight.

☑ Evaluation

- Patient's behavior and communication indicate improvement of obsessive-compulsive pattern.
- Patient doesn't experience injury from drug-induced adverse CNS reactions.
- Patient and family state understanding of drug therapy.

clonazepam
(kloh-NEH-zuh-pam)
Klonopin, Rivotril ♦ ◇

Pharmacologic class: benzodiazepine
Therapeutic class: anticonvulsant
Pregnancy risk category: D
Controlled substance schedule: IV

Indications and dosages

▶ **Lennox-Gastaut syndrome; atypical absence seizures; akinetic and myoclonic seizures.** *Adults:* Initially, not to exceed 1.5 mg P.O. t.i.d. May be increased by 0.5 to 1 mg q 3 days until seizures are controlled. If given in unequal doses, give largest dose h.s. Maximum daily dosage is 20 mg.
Children age 10 and younger or weighing 30 kg (66 lb) or less: Initially, 0.01 to 0.03 mg/kg P.O. daily (maximum 0.05 mg/kg daily), in two or three divided doses. Increase by 0.25 to 0.5 mg q third day to maximum maintenance dosage of 0.1 to 0.2 mg/kg daily as needed.
▶ **Status epilepticus (where parenteral form is available).** *Adults:* 1 mg by slow I.V. infusion.
Children: 0.5 mg by slow I.V. infusion.
▶ **Panic disorder.** *Adults:* Initially, 0.25 mg P.O. b.i.d.; increase to target dose of 1 mg daily after 3 days. Some patients may benefit from doses up to maximum of 4 mg daily. To achieve 4 mg daily, increase dosage in increments of 0.125 to 0.25 mg b.i.d. q 3 days as tolerated until panic disorder is controlled. Stop drug gradually by decreases of 0.125 mg b.i.d. q 3 days until stopped.
▶ **Restless legs syndrome; adjunct in schizophrenia‡.** *Adults:* 0.5 to 2 mg P.O. q h.s.
▶ **Parkinsonian dysarthria‡.** *Adults:* 0.25 to 0.5 mg P.O. daily.
▶ **Acute manic episodes‡.** *Adults:* 0.75 to 16 mg P.O. daily.

▶ **Multifocal tic disorders‡.** *Adults:* 1.5 to 12 mg P.O. daily.
▶ **Neuralgia‡.** *Adults:* 2 to 4 mg P.O. daily.

▽ I.V. administration

- Drug may be diluted with D_5W, dextrose 2.5% in water, normal saline solution, or half-normal saline solution.
- Mix solutions in glass bottles because drug binds to polyvinyl chloride plastics. If polyvinyl chloride infusion bags are used, give immediately and infuse at 60 ml/hour or greater.
- Give slowly by direct injection or by slow I.V. infusion.

Contraindications and precautions

- Contraindicated in patients hypersensitive to benzodiazepines and in those with acute angle-closure glaucoma or significant hepatic disease.
- Use cautiously in patients with mixed type of seizure because drug may precipitate generalized tonic-clonic seizures. Also, use cautiously in patients with chronic respiratory disease or open-angle glaucoma.
- **♨ Lifespan:** In breast-feeding women, safety and efficacy of drug haven't been established. In children, use cautiously.

Adverse reactions

CNS: *drowsiness, ataxia, behavioral disturbances* (especially in children), slurred speech, tremor, confusion, psychosis, agitation.
EENT: *increased salivation,* diplopia, nystagmus, abnormal eye movements, sore gums.
GI: constipation, gastritis, nausea, abnormal thirst.
GU: dysuria, enuresis, nocturia, urine retention.
Hematologic: *leukopenia, thrombocytopenia,* eosinophilia.
Metabolic: change in appetite.
Musculoskeletal: muscle weakness or pain.
Respiratory: *respiratory depression.*
Skin: rash.

Interactions

Drug-drug. *CNS depressants:* May increase CNS depression. Monitor patient closely.
Fluconazole, ketoconazole, itraconazole, miconazole: May increase and prolong levels, CNS depression, and psychomotor impairment. Don't use together.
Drug-herb. *Catnip, kava, lady's slipper, lemon balm, passion flower, sassafras, skullcap, valer-*

ian: May enhance sedative effects of clonazepam. Discourage using together.
Drug-lifestyle. *Alcohol use:* May cause additive CNS effects. Strongly discourage alcohol use.

Effects on lab test results

• May increase liver function test values and eosinophil count. May decrease WBC and platelet counts.

Pharmacokinetics

Absorption: Well absorbed from GI tract.
Distribution: Distributed widely throughout body; about 85% protein-bound.
Metabolism: Metabolized by liver to several metabolites.
Excretion: Excreted in urine. *Half-life:* 18 to 50 hours.

Route	Onset	Peak	Duration
P.O.	Unknown	1-2 hr	Unknown
I.V.	Unknown	Unknown	Unknown

Action

Chemical effect: Unknown. It probably acts by facilitating effects of inhibitory neurotransmitter GABA.
Therapeutic effect: Prevents or stops seizure activity.

Available forms

Injection: 1 mg/ml ◆
Tablets: 0.5 mg, 1 mg, 2 mg

NURSING PROCESS

ⓩ Assessment

• Assess patient's seizure condition before therapy and reassess regularly thereafter.
• Monitor blood level. Therapeutic blood level is 20 to 80 mg/ml.
• Monitor CBC and liver function tests.
• Be alert for adverse reactions and drug interactions.
• Evaluate patient's and family's knowledge of drug therapy.

⊞ Nursing diagnoses

• Risk for injury related to potential for seizure activity
• Activity intolerance related to drug-induced sedation
• Deficient knowledge related to drug therapy

⊳ Planning and implementation

• Increase oral dosage gradually.
• ⓢ **ALERT:** Never withdraw therapy suddenly because seizures may worsen. If adverse reactions develop, call prescriber at once.
• Withdrawal symptoms are similar to those of barbiturates.
• Maintain seizure precautions.
Patient teaching
• Advise patient to avoid driving or other potentially hazardous activities until CNS effects of drug are known.
• Instruct parents to monitor child's school performance because drug may interfere with attentiveness.
• Instruct patient and family never to stop drug abruptly because seizures may occur.
• Instruct patient or family to notify prescriber if oversedation or other adverse reactions develop or questions arise about drug therapy.

☑ Evaluation

• Patient is free from seizure activity during drug therapy.
• Patient is able to meet daily activity needs.
• Patient and family state understanding of drug therapy.

clonidine hydrochloride
(KLON-uh-deen high-droh-KLOR-ighd)
**Catapres, Catapres-TTS, Dixarit ◆ ◇
Duraclon**

Pharmacologic class: centrally acting sympatholytic
Therapeutic class: antihypertensive
Pregnancy risk category: C

Indications and dosages

▶ **Essential, renal, and malignant hypertension.** *Adults:* Initially, 0.1 mg P.O. b.i.d. Then, increase by 0.1 to 0.2 mg daily q week. Usual dosage range is 0.1 to 0.3 mg b.i.d.; infrequently, dosages as high as 2.4 mg daily are used. Or, transdermal patch applied to nonhairy area of intact skin on upper arm or torso q 7 days. Start with 0.1-mg system and adjust after 1 to 2 weeks with another 0.1-mg system or larger system if increases are needed to maintain normal blood pressure.

▶ **Severe pain.** *Adults:* Starting dosage for continuous epidural infusion is 30 mcg/hour. Titrate according to patient's response.

▶ **Prophylaxis for vascular headache‡.** *Adults:* 0.025 mg P.O. b.i.d. to q.i.d., up to 0.15 mg P.O. daily in divided doses.

▶ **Adjunctive therapy for nicotine withdrawal‡.** *Adults:* Initially, 0.1 mg P.O. b.i.d., then gradually increase dose by 0.1 mg daily q week, up to 0.75 mg P.O. daily, as tolerated. Alternatively, apply transdermal patch (0.1 to 0.2 mg/24 hours) and replace weekly for the first 2 or 3 weeks after smoking cessation.

▶ **Adjunct in opiate withdrawal‡.** *Adults:* 5 to 17 mcg/kg P.O. daily in divided doses for up to 10 days. Adjust dosage to avoid hypotension and excessive sedation, and slowly withdraw drug.

▶ **Adjunct in menopausal symptoms‡.** *Adults:* 0.025 to 0.2 mg P.O. b.i.d. Alternatively, apply transdermal patch (0.1 mg/24 hours) and replace weekly.

▶ **Dysmenorrhea‡.** *Adults:* 0.025 mg P.O. b.i.d. for 14 days before onset of menses and during menses.

▶ **Ulcerative colitis‡.** *Adults:* 0.3 mg P.O. t.i.d.

▶ **Diabetic diarrhea‡.** *Adults:* 0.15 to 1.2 mg P.O. daily. Or, 1 to 2 patches q week (0.3mg/24 hours).

▶ **Neuralgia‡.** *Adults:* 0.2 mg P.O. daily.

▶ **Growth delay in children‡.** *Children:* 0.0375 to 0.15 mg/m^2 P.O. daily.

▶ **Attention deficit hyperactivity disorder (ADHD)‡.** *Children:* Initially, 0.05 mg P.O. q h.s. Increase dose cautiously over 2 to 4 weeks to reach maintenance dosage of 0.05 to 0.4 mg daily depending on the patient's weight and tolerance.

Contraindications and precautions

• Contraindicated in patients hypersensitive to drug. Transdermal form is contraindicated in patients hypersensitive to any component of adhesive layer. Injectable form is contraindicated in patients receiving anti-coagulation therapy and patients with a bleeding diathesis or injection-site infection.

• Use cautiously in patients with severe coronary insufficiency, recent MI, cerebrovascular disease, and chronic renal or hepatic impairment.

⚠ Lifespan: In pregnant women, safety and efficacy of drug haven't been established. In breast-feeding women, use cautiously. In children, safety and efficacy of drug haven't been established.

In children with severe intractable pain from malignancy that is unresponsive to epidural or spinal opiates or other conventional analgesic techniques, injectable form is restricted.

Adverse reactions

CNS: *anxiety, somnolence, confusion, drowsiness, dizziness,* fatigue, sedation, nervousness, headache, vivid dreams.

CV: orthostatic hypotension, *hypotension, bradycardia, severe rebound hypertension.*

GI: *constipation, dry mouth, nausea, vomiting.*

GU: urine retention, impotence, UTI.

Metabolic: transient glucose intolerance.

Skin: *pruritus and dermatitis* with transdermal patch.

Interactions

Drug-drug. *Amitriptyline, amoxapine, clomipramine, desipramine, doxepin, imipramine, nortriptyline, protriptyline, trimipramine:* May cause loss of blood pressure control with potentially life-threatening elevations in blood pressure. Don't use together.

CNS depressants: May enhance CNS depression. Use together cautiously.

MAO inhibitors: May decrease antihypertensive effect. Use together cautiously.

Propranolol, other beta blockers: May cause severe rebound hypertension. Monitor patient carefully.

Drug-herb. *Capsicum, yohimbe:* May reduce antihypertensive effectiveness. Discourage using together.

Effects on lab test results

• May increase glucose and CK levels.

Pharmacokinetics

Absorption: Absorbed well when given P.O. Also absorbed well percutaneously after transdermal topical administration.

Distribution: Distributed widely into body.

Metabolism: Metabolized in liver, where nearly 50% is transformed to inactive metabolites.

Excretion: About 65% of drug is excreted in urine; 20% in feces. *Half-life:* 6 to 20 hours.

Route	Onset	Peak	Duration
P.O.	15-30 min	1½-2½ hr	6-8 hr
Epidural	Immediate	19 min	Unknown
Transdermal	2-3 days	2-3 days	Several days

Action

Chemical effect: Thought to inhibit central vasomotor centers, thereby decreasing sympathetic outflow to heart, kidneys, and peripheral vasculature; this results in decreased peripheral vascular resistance, decreased systolic and diastolic blood pressure, and decreased heart rate.
Therapeutic effect: Lowers blood pressure.

Available forms

Injectable: 100 mg/ml
Tablets: 0.025 mg, 0.1 mg, 0.2 mg, 0.3 mg
Transdermal: TTS-1 (releases 0.1 mg/24 hours), TTS-2 (releases 0.2 mg/24 hours), TTS-3 (releases 0.3 mg/24 hours)

NURSING PROCESS

🔲 Assessment

● Assess patient's blood pressure before therapy and reassess regularly thereafter.
● Antihypertensive effects of transdermal clonidine may take 2 to 3 days to become apparent. Oral antihypertensive therapy may have to be continued in interim.
● Be alert for adverse reactions and drug interactions.
● Observe patient for tolerance to drug's therapeutic effects; patient may require increased dosage.
● Periodic eye examinations are recommended.
● Monitor site of transdermal patch for dermatitis. Ask patient about pruritus.
● Evaluate patient's and family's knowledge of drug therapy.

🔲 Nursing diagnoses

● Risk for injury related to presence of hypertension
● Ineffective protection related to severe rebound hypertension caused by abrupt cessation of drug
● Deficient knowledge related to drug therapy

▶ Planning and implementation

● Drug may be given to lower blood pressure rapidly in some hypertensive emergency situations.
● Adjust dosage to patient's blood pressure and tolerance.
● Give last dose of day at bedtime.
● Epidural clonidine is more likely to be effective in patients with neuropathic pain than somatic or visceral pain.

⑤ **ALERT:** The injection form is for epidural use only. The injection form for epidural use concentrate containing 500 mcg/ml must be diluted before use in normal saline injection to provide a final concentration of 100 mcg/ml.
● When giving by epidural route, carefully monitor infusion pump and inspect catheter tubing for obstruction or dislodgement.
● Monitor patient closely, especially during the first few days of therapy; respiratory depression or deep sedation may occur.
● To improve adherence of patch, apply adhesive overlay. Place patch at different site each week.
● Remove transdermal patch before defibrillation to prevent arcing.
● When stopping therapy in patients receiving both clonidine and beta blocker, gradually withdraw beta blocker first to minimize adverse reactions.
● Discontinuation of clonidine for surgery isn't recommended.
⑤ **ALERT:** Don't confuse clonidine with quinidine or clomiphene; or Catapres with Cetapred or Combipres.

Patient teaching

● Advise patient that abrupt discontinuation of drug may cause severe rebound hypertension. Reduce dosage gradually over 2 to 4 days.
● Tell patient to take last dose of day immediately before bedtime.
● Reassure patient that transdermal patch usually adheres despite showering and other routine daily activities. Instruct him on use of adhesive overlay to improve skin adherence if needed. Also tell patient to place patch at different site each week.
● Caution patient that drug can cause drowsiness, but that tolerance to this adverse effect will develop.
● Inform patient that orthostatic hypotension can be minimized by rising slowly and avoiding sudden position changes.

☑ Evaluation

● Patient's blood pressure is normal with drug therapy.
● Patient states understanding of need to not stop drug abruptly.
● Patient and family state understanding of drug therapy.

Reactions may be *common*, uncommon, *life-threatening*, or COMMON AND LIFE-THREATENING.

clopidogrel bisulfate

(kloh-PIH-doh-grel bigh-SUL-fayt)
Plavix

Pharmacologic class: inhibitor of adenosine diphosphate (ADP)-induced platelet aggregation
Therapeutic class: antiplatelet
Pregnancy risk category: B

Indications and dosages

▶ **To reduce atherosclerotic events in patients with atherosclerosis documented by recent CVA, MI, or peripheral arterial disease.**
Adults: 75 mg P.O. daily.

▶ **To reduce atherosclerotic events in patients with acute coronary syndrome (unstable angina, non–Q-wave MI), including those managed medically and those who are to be managed with percutaneous coronary intervention (with or without stent) or coronary artery bypass graft.** *Adults:* Start therapy with a single 300-mg P.O. loading dose, then continue at 75 mg P.O. once daily. Also, give 75 to 325 mg aspirin once daily during therapy.

Contraindications and precautions

• Contraindicated in patients hypersensitive to drug or its components and in those with pathologic bleeding, such as peptic ulcer or intracranial hemorrhage.
• Use cautiously in patients with hepatic impairment and in those at risk for increased bleeding from trauma, surgery, or other conditions.
⚹ **Lifespan:** In breast-feeding women, drug is contraindicated. In children, safety and efficacy of drug haven't been established.

Adverse reactions

CNS: headache, dizziness, fatigue, depression, pain.
CV: chest pain, edema, hypertension.
EENT: epistaxis, rhinitis.
GI: *hemorrhage,* abdominal pain, dyspepsia, gastritis, constipation, diarrhea, ulcers.
GU: UTI.
Hematologic: purpura.
Musculoskeletal: arthralgia, back pain.
Respiratory: bronchitis, cough, dyspnea, upper respiratory tract infection.
Skin: rash, pruritus.
Other: flulike symptoms.

Interactions

Drug-drug. *Aspirin, NSAIDs:* May increase risk for GI bleeding. Monitor patient for signs of GI bleeding, such as abdominal pain or blood in vomitus or stool.
Heparin, warfarin: Safety hasn't been established. Use together cautiously and monitor patient for bleeding.
Drug-herb. *Dong quai, feverfew, garlic, ginger, horse chestnut, red clover:* Possible increased risk of bleeding. Monitor patient closely.

Effects on lab test results

• May decrease platelet count.

Pharmacokinetics

Absorption: Rapid.
Distribution: Highly bound to plasma protein.
Metabolism: Extensively metabolized by the liver.
Excretion: About 50% is excreted in urine and 46% in feces. *Half-life:* 8 hours.

Route	Onset	Peak	Duration
P.O.	2 hr	Unknown	5 days

Action

Chemical effect: Inhibits binding of ADP to its platelet receptor, which inhibits ADP-mediated activation and subsequent platelet aggregation. Because clopidogrel acts by irreversibly modifying the platelet ADP receptor, platelets exposed to drug are affected for their lifespan.
Therapeutic effect: Prevents clot formation.

Available forms

Tablets: 75 mg

NURSING PROCESS

Assessment
• Assess current use of OTC drugs, such as aspirin or NSAIDs, and herbal remedies.
• Assess patient for increased bleeding or bruising tendencies before and during drug therapy.
• Evaluate patient's and family's knowledge of drug therapy.

Nursing diagnoses
• Risk for injury related to potential for atherosclerotic events from underlying condition

- Ineffective protection related to increased risk of bleeding
- Deficient knowledge related to drug therapy

> **Planning and implementation**

- Five days after stopping drug, expect platelet aggregation to return to normal.
- Withhold drug from patients with hepatic impairment and those at increased risk for bleeding from trauma, surgery, or other pathologic conditions.

⊛ **ALERT:** Don't confuse Plavix (clopidogrel bisulfate) with Paxil (paroxetine).

Patient teaching

- Inform patient it may take longer than usual to stop bleeding. Tell him to refrain from activities in which trauma and bleeding may occur; encourage use of seat belt when in a car.
- Instruct patient to notify prescriber if unusual bleeding or bruising occurs.
- Tell patient to inform prescriber or dentist that he's taking drug before having surgery or starting new drug therapy.
- Inform patient that drug may be taken without regard to meals.

☑ **Evaluation**

- Patient has less risk of CVA, MI, and vascular death.
- Patient states appropriate bleeding precautions to take.
- Patient and family state understanding of drug therapy.

---

clorazepate dipotassium
(klor-AYZ-eh-payt digh-po-TAH-see-um)
Apo-Clorazepate ♦, ClorazeCaps, Gen-Xene, Novoclopate ♦, Tranxene, Tranxene-SD, Tranxene T-Tab

Pharmacologic class: benzodiazepine
Therapeutic class: anxiolytic, anticonvulsant, sedative-hypnotic agent
Pregnancy risk category: D
Controlled substance schedule: IV

Indications and dosages

▶ **Acute alcohol withdrawal.** *Adults:* Day 1 dose is 30 mg P.O. initially, followed by 30 to 60 mg P.O. in divided doses; day 2 dose is 45 to 90 mg P.O. in divided doses; day 3 dose is

22.5 to 45 mg P.O. in divided doses; day 4 dose is 15 to 30 mg P.O. in divided doses; then gradually reduce dosage to 7.5 to 15 mg daily. Maximum daily dose is 90 mg.

▶ **Anxiety.** *Adults:* 15 to 60 mg P.O. daily. *Elderly patients:* Initially, 7.5 to 15 mg daily in divided doses or as a single dose.

▶ **Adjunct in partial seizure disorder.** *Adults and children older than age 12:* Maximum recommended initial dosage is 7.5 mg P.O. t.i.d. Maximum dosage increase is 7.5 mg weekly; maximum dosage is 90 mg daily.
Children ages 9 to 12: Maximum recommended initial dosage is 7.5 mg P.O. b.i.d. Maximum dosage increase is 7.5 mg weekly; maximum dosage is 60 mg daily.

Contraindications and precautions

- Contraindicated in patients hypersensitive to drug and in those with acute angle-closure glaucoma.
- Use cautiously in patients with suicidal tendencies, renal or hepatic impairment, or history of drug abuse.
- Reduce dosage in debilitated patients.

⚘ **Lifespan:** Pregnant women, especially those in their first trimester, should avoid drug. For children younger than age 9, safety and efficacy of drug haven't been established. In elderly patients, reduce dosage.

Adverse reactions

CNS: *drowsiness, lethargy, hangover,* fainting, restlessness, psychosis.
CV: transient hypotension.
EENT: visual disturbances.
GI: nausea, vomiting, abdominal discomfort, dry mouth.
GU: urine retention, incontinence.

Interactions

Drug-drug. *Cimetidine:* May increase sedation. Monitor patient carefully.
CNS depressants: May increase CNS depression. Avoid using together.
Digoxin: May increase levels of digoxin, increasing digoxin toxicity. Monitor digoxin levels.
Drug-herb. *Catnip, kava, lady's slipper, lemon balm, passion flower, sassafras, skullcap, valerian:* Sedative effects may be enhanced. Avoid using together.

Reactions may be *common*, uncommon, *life-threatening*, or COMMON AND LIFE-THREATENING.

Drug-lifestyle. *Alcohol use:* May cause additive CNS effects. Strongly discourage alcohol use with these drugs.
Smoking: May increase clearance of benzodiazepines. Monitor patient for lack of effect and discourage patient from smoking.

Effects on lab test results

• May increase liver function test values.

Pharmacokinetics

Absorption: Complete and rapid after being hydrolyzed in stomach.
Distribution: Distributed widely throughout body. About 80% to 95% of drug is bound to plasma protein.
Metabolism: Metabolized in liver to oxazepam.
Excretion: Inactive glucuronide metabolites are excreted in urine. *Half-life:* 30 to 200 hours.

Route	Onset	Peak	Duration
P.O.	Unknown	½-2 hr	Unknown

Action

Chemical effect: May facilitate action of inhibitory neurotransmitter GABA. Depresses CNS at limbic and subcortical levels of brain and suppresses spread of seizure activity produced by epileptogenic foci in cortex, thalamus, and limbic structures.
Therapeutic effect: Relieves anxiety, prevents seizure activity, and promotes sleep and calmness.

Available forms

Capsules: 3.75 mg, 7.5 mg, 15 mg
Tablets: 3.75 mg, 7.5 mg, 11.25 mg, 15 mg, 22.5 mg

NURSING PROCESS

Assessment

• Assess patient's underlying condition before therapy and reassess regularly thereafter.
• Monitor liver, renal, and hematopoietic function studies periodically in patients receiving repeated or prolonged therapy.
• Be alert for adverse reactions and drug interactions.
• Evaluate patient's and family's knowledge of drug therapy.

Nursing diagnoses

• Anxiety related to patient's underlying condition
• Risk of injury related to drug-induced adverse CNS reactions
• Deficient knowledge related to drug therapy

Planning and implementation

• Possibility of abuse and addiction exists.
Don't withdraw drug abruptly after prolonged use; withdrawal symptoms may occur.
ALERT: Don't confuse clorazepate with clofibrate.
Patient teaching
• Warn patient to avoid activities that require alertness and good psychomotor coordination until CNS effects of drug are known.
• Tell patient to avoid alcohol while taking drug.
• Suggest sugarless chewing gum or hard candy to relieve dry mouth.
• Warn patient to take drug only as directed and not to stop without prescriber's approval. Inform patient of drug's potential for dependence if taken longer than directed.

Evaluation

• Patient says he's less anxious after taking drug.
• Patient doesn't experience injury as a result of drug-induced adverse CNS reactions.
• Patient and family state understanding of drug therapy.

clozapine
(KLOH-zuh-peen)
Clozaril

Pharmacologic class: tricyclic dibenzodiazepine derivative
Therapeutic class: antipsychotic
Pregnancy risk category: B

Indications and dosages

▶ **Schizophrenia in severely ill patients unresponsive to other therapies; Reduction in risk of recurrent suicidal behavior in schizophrenia or schizoaffective disorder.** *Adults:* Initially, 12.5 mg P.O. once daily or b.i.d.; increase by 25 to 50 mg daily (if tolerated) to 300 to 450 mg daily by end of 2 weeks. Base dosage on response, patient tolerance, and adverse reactions. Don't increase dosage more than once or twice weekly and don't exceed 100 mg. Many patients respond to 300 to 600 mg daily, but some may need as much as 900 mg daily. Don't exceed 900 mg daily.

⊠ Adjust-a-dose: Use lowest recommended dose when starting therapy in geriatric patients.

Contraindications and precautions

• Contraindicated in patients with uncontrolled epilepsy, history of drug-induced agranulocytosis, myelosuppressive disorders, severe CNS depression or coma, or WBC count below 3,500/mm^3; and in those taking other drugs that suppress bone marrow function.

• Use cautiously in patients with prostatic hyperplasia or angle-closure glaucoma because clozapine has potent anticholinergic effects. Also use cautiously in patients receiving general anesthesia and in those with hepatic, renal, or cardiac disease.

⚠ Lifespan: In pregnant women, use cautiously. In breast-feeding women, drug is contraindicated. In children, safety and efficacy of drug haven't been established; it is not recommended for children younger than age 12. In elderly patients, use cautiously and at lowest recommended dose.

Adverse reactions

CNS: fever, *drowsiness, sedation, seizures, dizziness, syncope, vertigo,* headache, tremor, disturbed sleep or nightmares, restlessness, hypokinesia or akinesia, agitation, rigidity, akathisia, confusion, fatigue, insomnia, hyperkinesia, weakness, lethargy, ataxia, slurred speech, depression, myoclonus, anxiety.
CV: tachycardia, hypotension, hypertension, chest pain, ECG changes, orthostatic hypotension, *cardiomyopathy.*
GI: dry mouth, constipation, nausea, vomiting, *excessive salivation,* heartburn, constipation.
GU: urinary frequency, urinary urgency, urine retention, incontinence, abnormal ejaculation.
Hematologic: *leukopenia, agranulocytosis.*
Metabolic: weight gain, *severe hyperglycemia.*
Musculoskeletal: muscle pain or spasm, muscle weakness.
Skin: rash.

Interactions

Drug-drug. *Anticholinergics:* May potentiate anticholinergic effects of clozapine. Avoid using together.

Antihypertensives: May potentiate hypotensive effects. Monitor blood pressure.
Bone marrow suppressants: May increase bone marrow toxicity. Don't use together.
Digoxin, warfarin, other highly protein-bound drugs: May increase levels of these drugs. Monitor patient closely for adverse reactions.
Psychoactive drugs: May produce additive effects. Use together cautiously.
Drug-herb. *St. John's wort:* May reduce drug levels causing a loss of symptom control in patients taking an antipsychotic. Discourage using together.
Drug-food. *Caffeine:* May increase levels of clozapine. Large fluctuations in caffeine consumption may affect therapeutic response to drug. Advise patient to limit caffeine.
Drug-lifestyle. *Alcohol use:* May increase CNS depression. Discourage using together.

Effects on lab test results

• May decrease glucose level.
• May decrease WBC and granulocyte counts.

Pharmacokinetics

Absorption: Thought to be absorbed from GI tract.
Distribution: About 95% bound to serum proteins.
Metabolism: Nearly complete.
Excretion: About 50% of drug appears in urine and 30% in feces, mostly as metabolites. *Half-life:* Appears proportional to dose and may range from 8 to 12 hours.

Route	Onset	Peak	Duration
P.O.	Unknown	2½ hr	4-12 hr

Action

Chemical effect: Unknown. Binds to dopaminergic receptors (both D1 and D2) within limbic system of CNS and may interfere with adrenergic, cholinergic, histaminergic, and serotoninergic receptors.
Therapeutic effect: Relieves psychotic signs and symptoms.

Available forms

Tablets: 12.5 mg, 25 mg, 100 mg

NURSING PROCESS

Assessment
- Assess patient's psychotic condition before therapy and reassess regularly thereafter.
- Baseline WBC and differential counts are required before therapy and weekly thereafter.
- Be alert for adverse reactions and drug interactions.
- After stopping drug, monitor WBC counts weekly for at least 4 weeks and monitor patient closely for recurrence of psychotic symptoms.
- Evaluate patient's and family's knowledge of drug therapy.

Nursing diagnoses
- Disturbed thought processes related to patient's underlying condition
- Risk of infection related to potential for drug-induced agranulocytosis
- Deficient knowledge related to drug therapy

Planning and implementation
- Drug carries significant risk of agranulocytosis. If possible, give at least two trials of a standard antipsychotic before giving this drug.
- **ALERT:** Watch for signs and symptoms of cardiomyopathy, including exertional dyspnea, fatigue, orthopnea, paroxysmal nocturnal dyspnea, and peripheral edema, and report them immediately.
- Use WBC count to help determine safety of therapy. If WBC count drops below 3,500/mm³ after therapy starts or count drops substantially from baseline, monitor patient closely for signs of infection. If WBC count is 3,000 to 3,500/mm³ and granulocyte count is above 1,500/mm³, obtain WBC and differential counts twice weekly as directed. If WBC count drops below 3,000/mm³ and granulocyte count drops below 1,500/mm³, interrupt therapy, notify prescriber, and monitor patient for signs of infection. If WBC count returns to above 3,000/mm³ and granulocyte count returns to above 1,500/mm³, restart therapy cautiously. Continue monitoring WBC and differential counts twice weekly until WBC count exceeds 3,500/mm³.
- If WBC count drops below 2,000/mm³ and granulocyte count drops below 1,000/mm³, patient may require protective isolation. If patient develops infection, prepare cultures according to institutional policy and give antibiotics. Some clinicians may perform bone marrow aspiration

to assess bone marrow function. Future therapy is contraindicated in such patients.
- **ALERT:** Drug is linked to an increased risk of fatal myocarditis, especially during, but not limited to the first month of therapy. In patients in whom myocarditis is suspected (unexplained fatigue, dyspnea, tachypnea, chest pain, tachycardia, fever, palpitations, and other signs or symptoms of heart failure or ECG abnormalities such as ST-T wave abnormalities or arrhythmias), stop therapy immediately and don't rechallenge.
- **ALERT:** If drug must be stopped, withdraw gradually over 1- to 2-week period. However, changes in patient's medical condition (including development of leukopenia) may require drug to be stopped abruptly. Abrupt withdrawal of long-term therapy may cause an abrupt recurrence of psychotic symptoms.
- If therapy is reinstated in patients withdrawn from drug, follow usual guidelines for dosage increase. However, reexposure of patient to drug may increase severity and risk of adverse reactions. If therapy was withdrawn for WBC counts below 2,000/mm³ or granulocyte counts below 1,000/mm³, don't expect drug to be continued.
- **ALERT:** If dose is adjusted for a patient already taking St. John's wort, stopping the herb could cause drug level to rise and cause dangerous toxic symptoms.
- Severe hypoglycemia may occur in patients without a history of hypoglycemia. Drug may also cause hyperglycemia. Monitor diabetic patient regularly.
- Give patient no more than a 1-week supply of drug.

Patient teaching
- Warn patient about risk of agranulocytosis. Tell him drug is available only through special monitoring program that requires weekly blood tests to monitor patient for agranulocytosis. Advise patient to report flulike symptoms, fever, sore throat, lethargy, malaise, or other signs of infection.
- Warn patient to avoid hazardous activities that require alertness and good psychomotor coordination while taking drug.
- Tell patient to rise slowly to avoid orthostatic hypotension.
- Advise patient to check with prescriber before taking OTC medicines, herbal remedies, or alcohol.

Rapid onset   *Liquid form contains alcohol.   ◆Canada   ◇ Australia   †OTC   ‡Off-label use

• Recommend ice chips or sugarless candy or gum to help relieve dry mouth.

☑ Evaluation
• Patient demonstrates reduction in psychotic symptoms with drug therapy.
• Patient doesn't develop infection throughout drug therapy.
• Patient and family state understanding of drug therapy.

codeine phosphate
(KOH-deen FOS-fayt)
Paveral ◆

codeine sulfate

Pharmacologic class: opioid
Therapeutic class: analgesic, antitussive
Pregnancy risk category: C
Controlled substance schedule: II

Indications and dosages

▶ **Mild-to-moderate pain.** *Adults:* 15 to 60 mg P.O. or 15 to 60 mg phosphate S.C., I.M., or I.V. q 4 to 6 hours, p.r.n.
Children older than age 1: 0.5 mg/kg P.O., I.M., or S.C. q 4 hours, p.r.n.
▶ **Nonproductive cough.** *Adults:* 10 to 20 mg P.O. q 4 to 6 hours. Maximum daily dosage is 120 mg.
Children ages 6 to 12: 5 to 10 mg P.O. q 4 to 6 hours. Maximum daily dosage is 60 mg.
Children ages 2 to 6: 2.5 to 5 mg P.O. q 6 hours. Maximum daily dosage is 30 mg.

▼ I.V. administration

• Keep opioid antagonist (naloxone) and resuscitative equipment available.
• Give drug very slowly by direct injection into large vein. Don't mix with other solutions because codeine phosphate is incompatible with many drugs.
• **ALERT:** Don't give drug to children by I.V. route.

Contraindications and precautions

• Contraindicated in patients hypersensitive to drug.
• Use cautiously in debilitated patients and in patients with head injury, increased intracranial

pressure, increased CSF pressure, hepatic or renal disease, hypothyroidism, Addison's disease, acute alcoholism, seizures, severe CNS depression, bronchial asthma, COPD, respiratory depression, and shock.
⚠ **Lifespan:** In pregnant and breast-feeding women, in children, and in elderly patients, use cautiously.

Adverse reactions

CNS: *sedation, clouded sensorium, euphoria,* dizziness, *seizures.*
CV: hypotension, flushing, *bradycardia.*
GI: *nausea, vomiting, constipation, dry mouth,* ileus.
GU: urine retention.
Respiratory: *respiratory depression.*
Skin: pruritus.
Other: physical dependence.

Interactions

Drug-drug. *CNS depressants, general anesthetics, hypnotics, MAO inhibitors, other narcotic analgesics, sedatives, tranquilizers, tricyclic antidepressants:* May have additive effects. Use together cautiously. Monitor patient response.
Drug-lifestyle. *Alcohol use:* May have additive effects. Discourage using together.

Effects on lab test results

• May increase amylase and lipase levels.

Pharmacokinetics

Absorption: Well absorbed after oral or parenteral administration. About two-thirds as potent orally as parenterally.
Distribution: Distributed widely throughout body.
Metabolism: Metabolized mainly in liver.
Excretion: Excreted mainly in urine. *Half-life:* 2½ to 4 hours.

Route	Onset	Peak	Duration
P.O.	30-45 min	1-2 hr	4-6 hr
I.V.	Immediate	Immediate	4-6 hr
I.M.	10-30 min	½-1 hr	4-6 hr
S.C.	10-30 min	Unknown	4-6 hr

Action

Chemical effect: Binds with opiate receptors in CNS, altering both perception of and emotional response to pain through unknown mechanism.

Reactions may be *common*, uncommon, *life-threatening*, or COMMON AND LIFE-THREATENING.

Also suppresses cough reflex by direct action on cough center in medulla.
Therapeutic effect: Relieves pain and cough.

Available forms

codeine phosphate
Injection: 15 mg/ml, 30 mg/ml, 60 mg/ml
Oral solution: 15 mg/5 ml, 10 mg/ml ◆
Soluble tablets: 30 mg, 60 mg
codeine sulfate
Tablets: 15 mg, 30 mg, 60 mg

NURSING PROCESS

⚕ Assessment
• Assess patient's pain or cough before and after drug therapy.
• Be alert for adverse reactions and drug interactions.
• Evaluate patient's and family's knowledge of drug therapy.

⚕ Nursing diagnoses
• Acute pain related to patient's underlying condition
• Fatigue related to presence of cough
• Deficient knowledge related to drug therapy

▶ Planning and implementation
• For full analgesic effect, give drug before patient has intense pain.
• ⓘ **ALERT:** Codeine is metabolized to morphine by CYP 2D6; this gene may be absent in 7% of the population, who experience reduced analgesic effect.
• Don't use drug when cough is valuable diagnostic sign or is beneficial (as after thoracic surgery).
• Give drug with food or milk to minimize adverse GI reactions.
• Don't give discolored injection solution.
• Codeine is often prescribed with aspirin or acetaminophen to provide enhanced pain relief.
• Codeine's abuse potential is much lower than that of morphine.
• If patient doesn't experience pain or cough relief, notify prescriber.
• ⓘ **ALERT:** Don't confuse codeine with Cardene, Lodine, or Cordran.
Patient teaching
• Advise patient to take drug with milk or meals to minimize GI distress caused by oral administration.

• Advise patient to ask for or take drug (if at home) before pain becomes severe.
• Warn ambulatory patient about getting out of bed or walking. Tell outpatient to avoid driving and other hazardous activities until CNS effects of drug are known.
• Tell patient to report adverse drug reactions.

☑ Evaluation
• Patient is free of pain after drug administration.
• Patient's cough is suppressed after drug administration.
• Patient and family state understanding of drug therapy.

colchicine
(KOHL-chih-seen)
Colgout ◇

Pharmacologic class: *Colchicum autumnale* alkaloid
Therapeutic class: antigout agent
Pregnancy risk category: C (P.O.), D (I.V.)

Indications and dosages

▶ **Prevention of acute gout attacks as prophylactic or maintenance therapy.** *Adults:* 0.5 or 0.6 mg P.O. daily. Give drug 1 to 4 days per week to patients who normally have one attack per year or fewer; give drug daily to patients who have more than one attack per year. In severe cases, 1 to 1.8 mg daily.
▶ **Prevention of gout attacks in patients undergoing surgery.** *Adults:* 0.5 to 0.6 mg P.O. t.i.d. 3 days before and 3 days after surgery.
▶ **Acute gout, acute gouty arthritis.** *Adults:* Initially, 0.5 to 1.2 mg P.O.; then 0.5 or 0.6 mg q 1 to 2 hours until pain is relieved; nausea, vomiting, or diarrhea ensues; or a maximum dose of 8 mg is reached. Or, 2 mg I.V. followed by 0.5 mg I.V. q 6 hours if needed. Or, a single injection of 3 mg I.V. (Some prescribers prefer to give a single injection of 3 mg I.V.) Total I.V. dosage over 24 hours (one course of treatment) shouldn't exceed 4 mg. Don't give any further drug (I.V. or P.O.) for 7 days or more.
▶ **Familial Mediterranean fever‡.** *Adults:* 1 to 2 mg P.O. daily in divided doses.
▶ **Hepatic cirrhosis‡.** *Adults:* 1 mg P.O. 5 days weekly.

Rapid onset   *Liquid form contains alcohol.   ◆ Canada   ◇ Australia   †OTC   ‡Off-label use

§ **Adjust-a-dose:** For patients with hepatic impairment or creatinine clearance of 10 to 50 ml/minute, decrease dosage by 50%.

▼ I.V. administration

• Give drug by slow I.V. push over 2 to 5 minutes. Monitor patient for signs of extravasation.
• Don't dilute injection with D_5W injection or other fluids that might change pH of solution. If lower concentration is needed, dilute with normal saline solution or sterile water for injection and give over 2 to 5 minutes by direct injection. Preferably, inject into tubing of free-flowing I.V. solution. If diluted solution becomes turbid, don't inject.

Contraindications and precautions

• Contraindicated in patients with serious cardiac disease, renal disease, or GI disorders.
• Use cautiously in debilitated patients and in patients with early evidence of cardiac, renal, or GI disease.
※ **Lifespan:** In pregnant women, use cautiously, if at all, because fetal harm may occur. In breast-feeding women and in children, safety and efficacy of drug haven't been established. In elderly patients, use cautiously.

Adverse reactions

CNS: peripheral neuritis.
GI: *nausea, vomiting, abdominal pain, diarrhea.*
Hematologic: *aplastic anemia, thrombocytopenia, agranulocytosis* (with prolonged use); nonthrombocytopenic purpura.
Hepatic: *hepatic necrosis.*
Skin: alopecia, urticaria, dermatitis.
Other: severe local irritation (if extravasation occurs), *hypersensitivity reactions, anaphylaxis.*

Interactions

Drug-drug. *Loop diuretics:* May decrease efficacy of colchicine prophylaxis. Avoid using together.
Phenylbutazone: May increase risk of leukopenia or thrombocytopenia. Don't use together.
Vitamin B_{12}: May impair absorption of vitamin B_{12}. Avoid using together.
Drug-lifestyle. *Alcohol use:* May impair efficacy of drug prophylaxis. Discourage using together.

Effects on lab test results

• May increase alkaline phosphatase, AST, and ALT levels. May decrease carotene and cholesterol levels.
• May decrease hemoglobin, hematocrit, and platelet and granulocyte counts.
• May cause false-positive results in urine tests for hemoglobin and erythrocytes. May interfere with urinary determinations of 17-hydroxycorticosteroids using the Reddy, Jenkins, and Thorn procedure.

Pharmacokinetics

Absorption: Rapid. Unchanged drug may be reabsorbed from intestine by biliary processes.
Distribution: Distributed rapidly into various tissues. Concentrated in leukocytes and distributed into kidneys, liver, spleen, and intestinal tract, but absent in heart, skeletal muscle, and brain.
Metabolism: Metabolized partially in liver and also slowly metabolized in other tissues.
Excretion: Drug and its metabolites are excreted primarily in feces, with lesser amounts excreted in urine. *Half-life:* 1 to 10½ hours.

Route	Onset	Peak	Duration
P.O.	≤ 12 hr	½-2 hr	Unknown
I.V.	6-12 hr	½-2 hr	Unknown

Action

Chemical effect: As antigout agent, apparently decreases WBC motility, phagocytosis, and lactic acid production, decreasing urate crystal deposits and reducing inflammation. As antiosteolytic drug, apparently inhibits mitosis of osteoprogenitor cells and decreases osteoclast activity.
Therapeutic effect: Relieves gout signs and symptoms.

Available forms

Injection: 0.5 mg/ml
Tablets: 0.5 mg (½₂₀ grain), 0.6 mg (½₀₀ grain) as sugar-coated granules

NURSING PROCESS

⚖ Assessment

• Assess patient's underlying condition before therapy and reassess regularly thereafter.

• Obtain baseline laboratory studies, including CBC and uric acid levels, before therapy and repeat regularly.
• Be alert for adverse reactions and drug interactions.
• Evaluate patient's and family's knowledge of drug therapy.

⊞ Nursing diagnoses
• Acute pain related to presence of gout
• Ineffective protection related to drug-induced hematologic adverse reactions
• Deficient knowledge related to drug therapy

⊠ Planning and implementation
• Give drug with meals to reduce GI effects as maintenance therapy. May be used with uricosurics.
• **⊛ ALERT:** After a full course of 4 mg I.V., don't give drug by any other route for at least 7 days. Drug is toxic and death can result from overdose.
• Don't give I.M. or S.C.; severe local irritation occurs.
• Store drug in tightly closed, light-resistant container.
• Stop drug as soon as gout pain is relieved or at first sign of GI symptoms.
• Force fluids to maintain output at 2,000 ml daily.
Patient teaching
• Teach patient how to take drug.
• Advise patient to report rash, sore throat, fever, unusual bleeding, bruising, fatigue, weakness, numbness, or tingling.
• Tell patient when to stop drug.
• Tell patient to avoid alcohol during drug therapy because it may inhibit drug action.
• Advise patient to avoid all drugs containing aspirin because they may precipitate gout.

☑ Evaluation
• Patient becomes pain-free after drug therapy.
• Patient's CBC and platelet counts remain normal throughout drug therapy.
• Patient and family state understanding of drug therapy.

colesevelam hydrochloride
(koh-leh-SEV-eh-lam high-droh-KLOR-ighd)
Welchol

Pharmacologic class: polymeric bile acid sequestrant
Therapeutic class: antilipemic
Pregnancy risk category: B

Indications and dosages

▶ **Reduction of elevated LDL cholesterol in patients with primary hypercholesterolemia (Frederickson Type IIa). May be given either alone or with an HMG-CoA reductase inhibitor.** *Adults:* If given alone, give three tablets (1,875 mg) P.O. twice daily with meals and liquid or six tablets (3,750 mg) once daily with a meal and liquid. Maximum dose is seven tablets (4,375 mg). If used with an HMG-CoA reductase inhibitor, recommended dose is four to six tablets P.O. daily.

Contraindications and precautions

• Contraindicated in patients hypersensitive to drug or any of its components and in patients with bowel obstruction.
• Use cautiously in patients susceptible to vitamin K deficiency or deficiencies of fat-soluble vitamins. Also use cautiously in patients with dysphagia, swallowing disorders, severe GI motility disorders, and major GI tract surgery. Use cautiously in patients with triglyceride levels above 300 mg/dl because effects aren't known.
⚠ **Lifespan:** In pregnant women, use only if needed. In breast-feeding women, safety and efficacy of drug haven't been established; use only if needed. In children, safety and efficacy haven't been established.

Adverse reactions

CNS: headache, pain, asthenia.
EENT: pharyngitis, rhinitis, sinusitis.
GI: abdominal pain, *constipation,* diarrhea, *dyspepsia, flatulence,* nausea.
Musculoskeletal: myalgia, back pain.
Respiratory: increased cough.
Other: accidental injury, *infection,* flulike syndrome.

Interactions

None reported.

Effects on lab test results

- May increase HDL cholesterol and triglyceride levels. May decrease total cholesterol, LDL cholesterol, and apolipoprotein B levels.

Pharmacokinetics

Absorption: Not absorbed.
Distribution: None.
Metabolism: None.
Excretion: Mainly excreted in feces as a complex bound to bile acids. Less than 0.05% of drug is excreted in urine.

Route	Onset	Peak	Duration
P.O.	Unknown	2 wk	Unknown

Action

Chemical effect: Following oral intake, drug binds to bile acids in the intestines and forms a nonabsorbable complex that is eliminated in feces. Partial removal of bile acids from the enterohepatic circulation results in an increased conversion of cholesterol to bile acids in the liver in an attempt to restore the depleted bile acids. The resulting increase in cholesterol causes systemic clearance of circulating LDL level.
Therapeutic effect: Lowers LDL and total cholesterol levels.

Available forms

Tablets: 625 mg

NURSING PROCESS

Assessment

- Rule out secondary causes of hypercholesterolemia before starting drug, such as poorly controlled diabetes, hypothyroidism, nephrotic syndrome, dysproteinemias, obstructive liver disease, other drug therapy, and alcoholism.
- Monitor total cholesterol, LDL, and triglyceride levels before and periodically during therapy.
- Monitor patient's bowel habits. If severe constipation develops, decrease dosage, add a stool softener, or stop drug.
- Assess patient's compliance with restricted diet and exercise program adjunctive to antilipemic therapy.

- Evaluate patient's and family's knowledge of drug therapy and importance of diet and exercise regimen.

Nursing diagnoses

- Imbalanced nutrition: more than body requirements of saturated fat and cholesterol related to dietary intake and lack of exercise program
- Risk for constipation related to drug-induced adverse gastrointestinal reactions
- Risk for injury related to presence of elevated LDL cholesterol levels
- Deficient knowledge related to antilipemic drug therapy

Planning and implementation

- Give drug with a meal and a liquid.
- Discuss with prescriber adding antilipemic agent (for example, statins) for maximum additive antilipemic effect.

Patient teaching

- Instruct patient to take drug with a meal and a liquid.
- Teach patient to monitor bowel habits. Encourage a diet high in fiber and fluids. Instruct patient to notify prescriber promptly if severe constipation develops.
- Encourage patient to follow prescribed diet that is restricted in saturated fat and cholesterol and high in vegetables and fiber. Also discuss and encourage an exercise program that is appropriate for patient.
- Discuss with patient the importance of regular monitoring of lipid levels.
- Tell patient to notify prescriber if she's pregnant or breast-feeding.

Evaluation

- Patient begins a balanced diet and exercise regimen that's approved by his prescriber.
- Patient doesn't suffer adverse GI effect from drug therapy.
- Patient's LDL cholesterol and total cholesterol levels are within normal limits.
- Patient and family state understanding of drug therapy.

corticotropin (adrenocorticotropic hormone, ACTH)

(kor-teh-koh-TROH-pin)
ACTH, Acthar

repository corticotropin

Pharmacologic class: anterior pituitary hormone
Therapeutic class: diagnostic aid, replacement hormone
Pregnancy risk category: C

Indications and dosages

▶ **Diagnostic test of adrenocortical function.**
Adults: 40 units repository form I.M. or S.C. q 12 hours for 1 to 2 days. Or, 10 to 25 units aqueous form in 500 ml D_5W I.V. over 8 hours, between blood samplings. Individual dosages vary with adrenal glands' sensitivity to stimulation and with specific disease. Infants and younger children require larger doses per kilogram than older children and adults.
▶ **Inflammation, immunosuppression.**
Adults: 20 units aqueous form S.C. or I.M. in four divided doses. Or, 40 to 80 units q 24 to 72 hours (repository form).

▼ I.V. administration

• Use only aqueous form for I.V. administration. Dilute in 500 ml D_5W and infuse over 8 hours.

Contraindications and precautions

• Contraindicated in patients hypersensitive to pork and pork products and in patients with peptic ulcer, scleroderma, osteoporosis, systemic fungal infections, ocular herpes simplex, peptic ulceration, heart failure, hypertension, adrenocortical hyperfunction or primary insufficiency, or Cushing's syndrome. Also contraindicated in those who have had recent surgery.
• Use cautiously in patients being immunized and in those with latent tuberculosis or tuberculin reactivity, hypothyroidism, cirrhosis, acute gouty arthritis, psychotic tendencies, renal insufficiency, diverticulitis, nonspecific ulcerative colitis, thromboembolic disorders, seizures, uncontrolled hypertension, or myasthenia gravis.
⚘ Lifespan: In pregnant women and women of childbearing age, use cautiously. In breast-feeding women, safety and efficacy of drug haven't been established. In children, use cautiously because prolonged use of drug will inhibit skeletal growth; intermittent administration is recommended.

Adverse reactions

CNS: *seizures, dizziness, papilledema,* headache, *euphoria, insomnia,* mood swings, personality changes, depression, psychosis, *increased intracranial pressure.*
CV: *hypertension, heart failure, shock.*
EENT: cataracts, glaucoma.
GI: peptic ulceration (*with perforation and hemorrhage*), *pancreatitis,* abdominal distention, ulcerative esophagitis, nausea, vomiting.
GU: menstrual irregularities.
Metabolic: *activation of latent diabetes mellitus,* suppression of growth in children, *sodium and fluid retention,* calcium and potassium loss, hypokalemic alkalosis, negative nitrogen balance.
Musculoskeletal: muscle weakness, steroid myopathy, loss of muscle mass, osteoporosis, vertebral compression fractures.
Skin: impaired wound healing, thin and fragile skin, petechiae, ecchymoses, facial erythema, diaphoresis, acne, hyperpigmentation, allergic skin reactions, hirsutism.
Other: cushingoid symptoms, progressive increase in antibodies, loss of corticotropin stimulatory effect, *hypersensitivity reactions* (rash, *bronchospasm*).

Interactions

Drug-drug. *Anticonvulsants, barbiturates, rifampin:* May increase metabolism of corticotropin and decrease effectiveness. Monitor patient for lack of effect.
Estrogens: May potentiate effects of cortisol. Adjust dosage as needed.
NSAIDs, salicylates: May increase risk of GI bleeding. Avoid using together.
Oral anticoagulants: May alter PT. Monitor PT and INR. Adjust dosage as needed.
Potassium-wasting diuretics: May increase risk of hypokalemia. Monitor potassium levels.

Effects on lab test results

• May increase glucose level. May decrease potassium and calcium levels.

Pharmacokinetics

Absorption: Rapid after I.M. administration; unknown for S.C. administration.

Distribution: Unknown.
Metabolism: Unknown.
Excretion: Excreted by kidneys. *Half-life:* About 15 minutes.

Route	Onset	Peak	Duration
I.V., I.M., S.C.			
aqueous	Rapid	Varies	2 hr
repository	Rapid	Varies	≤ 3 days

Action

Chemical effect: By replacing body's own tropic hormone, drug stimulates secretion of adrenal cortex hormones.
Therapeutic effect: Diagnoses or treats adrenocortical hormonal deficiency.

Available forms

Aqueous injection: 25 units/vial, 40 units/vial
Repository injection: 40 units/ml, 80 units/ml

NURSING PROCESS

⚕ Assessment

• Assess patient's underlying condition before therapy and reassess regularly during therapy.
• Verify adrenal responsiveness and test for hypersensitivity and allergic reactions before treatment.
• Be alert for adverse reactions and drug interactions.
• Note and record weight changes, fluid exchange, and resting blood pressures until minimal effective dosage is achieved.
• Watch neonates of corticotropin-treated mothers for signs of hypoadrenalism.
• Monitor patient for stress.
• Evaluate patient's and family's knowledge of drug therapy.

🔲 Nursing diagnoses

• Ineffective protection related to underlying condition
• Risk for injury related to drug-induced adverse reactions
• Deficient knowledge related to drug test or therapy

▶ Planning and implementation

• Use as adjunct, not sole, therapy. Use oral form in long-term therapy.
• If giving gel, warm it to room temperature, draw into large needle, and give slowly as deep

I.M. injection with 21G or 22G needle. Warn patient that injection is painful.
Ⓢ **ALERT:** Check product label to be certain medication is for I.V. use; corticotropin repository injection is for I.M. or S.C. use only.
• Refrigerate reconstituted solution and use within 24 hours.
• Counteract edema with low-sodium, high-potassium intake; nitrogen loss with a high-protein diet; and psychotic changes with a reduction in corticotropin dosage or use of sedatives.
• Unusual stress may require additional use of rapidly acting corticosteroids. When possible, gradually reduce corticotropin dosage to smallest effective dose to minimize induced adrenocortical insufficiency. If stressful situation (trauma, surgery, severe illness) occurs shortly after stopping drug, restart therapy.
Ⓢ **ALERT:** Don't confuse corticotropin with cosyntropin.
Patient teaching
• Instruct patient to tell physicians and health care professionals besides the prescriber about corticotropin use because stressful situations, such as trauma, surgery, or severe illness, may necessitate adding rapidly-acting corticosteroids.
• Tell patient to restrict sodium intake and consume high-protein, high-potassium diet.
• Advise patient to have close follow-up care.
• Warn patient that injections, especially I.M. injections, are painful.

☑ Evaluation

• Patient's underlying condition improves with drug therapy.
• Patient doesn't experience injury as a result of drug-induced adverse reactions.
• Patient and family state understanding of drug therapy.

cortisone acetate
(KOR-tih-sohn AS-ih-tayt)
Cortone Acetate

Pharmacologic class: glucocorticoid, mineralocorticoid
Therapeutic class: anti-inflammatory, replacement therapy
Pregnancy risk category: NR

Indications and dosages

▶ **Adrenal insufficiency, allergy, inflammation.** *Adults:* 25 to 300 mg P.O. or 20 to 300 mg I.M. daily or on alternate days. Dosages are individualized, depending on severity of disease.

Contraindications and precautions

• Contraindicated in patients hypersensitive to drug or its ingredients and in those with systemic fungal infections.

• Use cautiously in patients with recent MI and in those with GI ulcer, renal disease, hypertension, osteoporosis, diabetes mellitus, hypothyroidism, cirrhosis, diverticulitis, nonspecific ulcerative colitis, recent intestinal anastomoses, thromboembolic disorders, seizures, myasthenia gravis, heart failure, tuberculosis, ocular herpes simplex, emotional instability, and psychotic tendencies.

⚠ Lifespan: In pregnant and breast-feeding women, use cautiously. In children, long-term use of drug isn't recommended because growth and maturation may be delayed.

Adverse reactions

CNS: *euphoria, insomnia,* psychotic behavior, pseudotumor cerebri, *seizures.*
CV: *arrhythmias, heart failure, thromboembolism,* hypertension, edema.
EENT: cataracts, glaucoma.
GI: *peptic ulceration,* GI irritation, increased appetite, *pancreatitis.*
Metabolic: possible hypokalemia, growth suppression in children, hyperglycemia, and carbohydrate intolerance.
Musculoskeletal: muscle weakness, osteoporosis.
Skin: hirsutism, delayed wound healing, acne, various skin eruptions.
Other: susceptibility to infections, *acute adrenal insufficiency* following increased stress (infection, surgery, or trauma) or abrupt withdrawal after long-term therapy, atrophy at I.M. injection site.

Interactions

Drug-drug. *Aspirin, indomethacin, other NSAIDs:* May increase risk of GI distress and bleeding. Give together cautiously; monitor patient for abdominal pain or blood in vomitus or stool.

Barbiturates, phenytoin, rifampin: May decrease corticosteroid effect. Increase corticosteroid dosage.
Live-attenuated virus vaccines, other toxoids and vaccines: May decrease antibody response and increase risk of neurologic complications. Don't use together.
Oral anticoagulants: May alter dosage requirements. Monitor PT and INR closely and monitor patient for bleeding.
Potassium-depleting drugs (such as thiazide diuretics): Enhanced potassium-wasting effects of cortisone. Monitor potassium levels.
Skin-test antigens: Decreases response. Defer skin testing until therapy is completed.
Drug-lifestyle. *Alcohol use:* May increase risk of GI irritation. Discourage using together.

Effects on lab test results

• May increase glucose and cholesterol levels. May decrease potassium, calcium, T_3, and T_4 levels.

Pharmacokinetics

Absorption: Absorbed readily after oral administration; unknown for I.M. administration.
Distribution: Distributed rapidly to muscle, liver, skin, intestines, and kidneys. Cortisone is extensively bound to plasma proteins. Only unbound portion is active.
Metabolism: Metabolized in liver to active metabolite hydrocortisone, which is metabolized to inactive glucuronide and sulfate metabolites.
Excretion: Inactive metabolites and small amounts of unmetabolized drug are excreted by kidneys. Insignificant quantities of drug also excreted in feces. *Half-life:* 8 to 12 hours.

Route	Onset	Peak	Duration
P.O.	Rapid	2 hr	30-36 hr
I.M.	Slow	20-48 hr	Varies

Action

Chemical effect: Not completely defined. Decreases inflammation, mainly by stabilizing leukocyte lysosomal membranes; suppresses immune response; stimulates bone marrow; and influences protein, fat, and carbohydrate metabolism.
Therapeutic effect: Reduces inflammation; raises corticosteroid therapy.

Available forms

Injection (suspension): 50 mg/ml
Tablets: 5 mg, 10 mg, 25 mg

NURSING PROCESS

⚖ Assessment
• Assess patient's underlying condition before therapy and reassess regularly thereafter.
• Monitor electrolyte and glucose levels. Check patient's weight and vital signs regularly.
• Monitor patient's stress level.
• Be alert for adverse reactions and drug interactions; most adverse reactions are dose- or duration-dependent.
• Evaluate patient's and family's knowledge of drug therapy.

⊕ Nursing diagnoses
• Ineffective protection related to underlying condition
• Risk for injury related to drug-induced adverse reactions
• Deficient knowledge related to drug therapy

▶ Planning and implementation
• Give drug with milk or food to reduce GI irritation.
• Give once-daily dose in morning for best results and least toxicity.
• I.M. route causes slow onset of action. Don't use in acute conditions where rapid effect is needed. May be used on twice-daily schedule matching diurnal variation. Rotate injection sites to prevent muscle atrophy.
• Mixing or diluting parenteral suspension may alter absorption and decrease drug's effectiveness.
• Drug isn't for I.V. use.
• Always adjust to lowest effective dose.
• Gradually reduce drug dosage after long-term therapy.
• If signs of adrenal insufficiency increase, notify prescriber. Unusual stress may require additional use of rapidly acting corticosteroids.
Patient teaching
⚫ **ALERT:** Tell patient not to stop drug abruptly or without prescriber's consent. Abrupt withdrawal may cause rebound inflammation, fatigue, weakness, arthralgia, fever, dizziness, lethargy, depression, fainting, orthostatic hypotension, dyspnea, anorexia, and hypoglycemia.

After prolonged use, sudden withdrawal may be fatal.
• Advise patient receiving long-term therapy to consider exercise or physical therapy. Also tell him to ask prescriber about vitamin D or calcium supplements.
• Tell patient to restrict sodium intake and consume high-protein, high-potassium diet.
• Tell patient to report slow healing.
• Warn patient receiving long-term therapy about cushingoid symptoms and the need to report sudden weight gain or swelling to prescriber.
• Instruct patient to wear or carry medical identification indicating his need for supplemental glucocorticoids during stress.

✓ Evaluation
• Patient shows improvement in underlying condition with drug therapy.
• Patient doesn't experience injury as a result of drug-induced adverse reactions.
• Patient and family state understanding of drug therapy.

co-trimoxazole
(sulfamethoxazole-trimethoprim)
(koh-trigh-MOX-uh-zohl)
Apo-Sulfatrim ◆, Apo-Sulfatrim DS ◆, Bactrim*, Bactrim DS, Bactrim I.V., Cotrim, Cotrim DS, Novo-Trimel ◆, Novo-Trimel D.S. ◆, Resprim ◇, Roubac ◆, Septra*, Septra DS, Septra-I.V., Septrin ◇, SMZ-TMP

Pharmacologic class: sulfonamide and folate antagonist
Therapeutic class: antibiotic
Pregnancy risk category: C (X at term)

Indications and dosages

▶ **UTI, shigellosis.** *Adults:* 160 mg trimethoprim/800 mg sulfamethoxazole (double-strength tablet) P.O. q 12 hours for 10 to 14 days in urinary tract infections and for 5 days in shigellosis. If indicated, I.V. infusion is given at 8 to 10 mg/kg daily (based on trimethoprim component) in two to four divided doses q 6, 8, or 12 hours for up to 14 days. Maximum dose is 960 mg daily trimethoprim.

Reactions may be *common*, uncommon, *life-threatening*, or **COMMON AND LIFE-THREATENING**.

Children age 2 months and older: 8 mg/kg trimethoprim/40 mg/kg sulfamethoxazole P.O. daily, in two divided doses q 12 hours (10 days for urinary tract infections; 5 days for shigellosis). If indicated, I.V. infusion is given at 8 to 10 mg/kg daily (based on trimethoprim component) in two to four divided doses q 6, 8, or 12 hours. Don't exceed adult dose.

▶ **Otitis media in patients with penicillin allergy or penicillin-resistant infections.** *Children and infants age 2 months and older:* 8 mg/kg daily (based on trimethoprim component) P.O., in two divided doses q 12 hours for 10 days.

▶ *Pneumocystis carinii* **pneumonia.** *Adults, children, and infants age 2 months and older:* 20 mg/kg trimethoprim/100 mg/kg sulfamethoxazole P.O. daily, in equally divided doses q 6 hours for 14 days. If indicated, I.V. infusion may be given 15 to 20 mg/kg daily (based on trimethoprim component) in three or four divided doses q 6 to 8 hours for up to 14 days.

▶ **Chronic bronchitis.** *Adults:* 160 mg trimethoprim/800 mg sulfamethoxazole P.O. q 12 hours for 10 to 14 days.

▶ **Traveler's diarrhea.** *Adults:* 160 mg trimethoprim/800 mg sulfamethoxazole P.O. b.i.d. for 3 to 5 days. Some patients may require 2 days of therapy or less.

▶ **UTIs in men with prostatitis.** *Adults:* 160 mg trimethoprim/800 mg sulfamethoxazole P.O. b.i.d. for 3 to 6 months.

▶ **Chronic UTIs.** *Adults:* 40 mg trimethoprim/200 mg sulfamethoxazole (½ tablet) or 80 mg trimethoprim/400 mg sulfamethoxazole P.O. daily or three times weekly for 3 to 6 months.

▶ **Septic agranulocytosis‡.** *Adults:* 2.5 mg/kg I.V. q.i.d.; for prophylaxis, 80 to 160 mg b.i.d.

▶ **Nocardia infection‡.** *Adults:* 640 mg P.O. daily for 7 months.

▶ **Pharyngeal gonococcal infections‡.** *Adults:* 720 mg P.O. daily for 5 days.

▶ **Chancroid‡.** *Adults:* 160 mg P.O. b.i.d. for 7 days.

▶ **Pertussis‡.** *Adults:* 320 mg P.O. daily in two divided doses. *Children:* 40 mg/kg P.O. daily in two divided doses.

▶ **Cholera‡.** *Adults:* 160 mg P.O. b.i.d. for 3 days.

◪ **Adjust-a-dose:** For patients with renal impairment, if creatinine clearance is 15 to 30 ml/minute, reduce daily dose by 50%. Don't use in patients with creatinine clearance less than 15 ml/minute.

▼ I.V. administration

• Dilute contents of 5-ml ampule of drug in 125 ml D_5W before giving. If patient is on a fluid restriction, dilute 5 ml of drug in 75 ml D_5W. Don't mix with other drugs or solutions.
• Infuse slowly over 60 to 90 minutes. Don't give by rapid infusion or bolus injection.
• Don't refrigerate; use within 6 hours if diluted in 125 ml and within 2 hours if diluted in 75 ml. If cloudiness or evidence of crystallization is noted after mixing, discard solution.

Contraindications and precautions

• Contraindicated in patients with megaloblastic anemia caused by folate deficiency, porphyria, severe renal impairment (creatinine clearance less than 15 ml/minute), or hypersensitivity to trimethoprim or sulfonamides.
• Use cautiously and reduce dosages in patients with hepatic impairment, a creatinine clearance of 15 to 30 ml/minute, severe allergy or bronchial asthma, G6PD deficiency, and blood dyscrasia.
⚖ **Lifespan:** In pregnant women at term and in breast-feeding women, drug is contraindicated. In infants younger than age 2 months, safety and efficacy of drug haven't been established.

Adverse reactions

CNS: headache, mental depression, *seizures,* hallucinations, ataxia, nervousness, fatigue, vertigo, insomnia.
CV: thrombophlebitis.
GI: *nausea, vomiting, diarrhea,* abdominal pain, anorexia, stomatitis.
GU: *toxic nephrosis with oliguria and anuria,* crystalluria, hematuria.
Hematologic: *agranulocytosis,* aplastic anemia, megaloblastic anemia, *thrombocytopenia, leukopenia,* hemolytic anemia.
Hepatic: jaundice, *hepatic necrosis.*
Musculoskeletal: muscle weakness.
Skin: *erythema multiforme, Stevens-Johnson syndrome, generalized skin eruption, epidermal necrolysis,* exfoliative dermatitis, photosensitivity, urticaria, pruritus.
Other: *hypersensitivity reactions* (serum sickness, drug fever, *anaphylaxis*).

Interactions

Drug-drug. *Oral anticoagulants:* May increase anticoagulant effect. Monitor patient for bleeding.
Oral antidiabetics: May increase hypoglycemic effect. Monitor glucose level.
Hormonal contraceptives: Decreases contraceptive effectiveness and increases risk of breakthrough bleeding. Suggest nonhormonal form of contraception.
Phenytoin: May inhibit hepatic metabolism of phenytoin. Monitor phenytoin levels.
Drug-herb. *Dong quai, St. John's wort:* Increases risk of photosensitivity. Advise patient to avoid unprotected exposure to sunlight.
Drug-lifestyle. *Sun exposure:* Photosensitivity reactions may occur. Urge patient to avoid sun exposure and wear protective clothing and sunblock.

Effects on lab test results

- May increase BUN, creatinine, aminotransferase, and bilirubin levels.
- May decrease hemoglobin, hematocrit, and granulocyte, platelet, and WBC counts.

Pharmacokinetics

Absorption: Well absorbed from GI tract after oral administration.
Distribution: Distributed widely into body tissues and fluids, including middle ear fluid, prostatic fluid, bile, aqueous humor, and CSF. Protein binding is 44% for trimethoprim, 70% for sulfamethoxazole.
Metabolism: Both components of drug are metabolized by liver.
Excretion: Both components of drug are excreted primarily in urine. *Half-life:* Trimethoprim, 8 to 11 hours; sulfamethoxazole, 10 to 13 hours.

Route	Onset	Peak	Duration
P.O.	Unknown	1-4 hr	Unknown
I.V.	Immediate	Immediate	Unknown

Action

Chemical effect: Sulfamethoxazole component inhibits formation of dihydrofolic acid from PABA; trimethoprim component inhibits dihydrofolate reductase. Both decrease bacterial folic acid synthesis.
Therapeutic effect: Inhibits susceptible bacteria, including *Escherichia coli, Klebsiella, Enterobacter, Proteus mirabilis, Haemophilus in-*

fluenzae, Streptococcus pneumoniae, Staphylococcus aureus, Acinetobacter, Salmonella, Shigella, and *P. carinii.*

Available forms

Injection: trimethoprim 16 mg and sulfamethoxazole 80 mg/ml (5 ml/ampule)
Oral suspension: trimethoprim 40 mg and sulfamethoxazole 200 mg/5 ml
Tablets: trimethoprim 80 mg and sulfamethoxazole 400 mg; trimethoprim 160 mg and sulfamethoxazole 800 mg

NURSING PROCESS

⚗ Assessment

- Assess patient's infection before therapy and reassess regularly thereafter.
- Obtain specimen for culture and sensitivity tests before first dose. Therapy may begin pending results.
- Be alert for adverse reactions and drug interactions.
- If adverse GI reactions occur, monitor patient's hydration status.
- Monitor intake and output. Make sure urine output is at least 1,500 ml daily to ensure proper hydration. Inadequate urine output can lead to crystalluria or tubular deposits of drug.
- Evaluate patient's and family's knowledge of drug therapy.

⊞ Nursing diagnoses

- Infection related to presence of bacteria susceptible to drug
- Risk for deficient fluid volume related to drug-induced adverse GI reactions
- Deficient knowledge related to drug therapy

▶ Planning and implementation

- Give drug with full glass of water at least 1 hour before or 2 hours after meals for maximum absorption. Shake oral suspension thoroughly before giving.
- Never give I.M.
- ⊛ **ALERT:** Double-check dosage, which may be written as trimethoprim component.
- Note that DS in product name means double strength.
- ⊛ **ALERT:** Adverse reactions, especially hypersensitivity reactions, rash, and fever, occur more frequently in patients with AIDS.

Reactions may be *common,* uncommon, *life-threatening,* or COMMON AND LIFE-THREATENING.

Patient teaching
• Tell patient to take entire amount of medication exactly as prescribed, even if he feels better.
• Tell patient to take drug with full glass of water and to drink at least 3 to 4 L of water daily.
• Advise patient to avoid exposure to direct sunlight because of risk of photosensitivity reaction.
• Tell patient to report signs of rash, sore throat, fever, or mouth sores because drug may need to be stopped.

☑ Evaluation
• Patient is free from infection after drug therapy.
• Patient maintains adequate hydration after drug therapy.
• Patient and family state understanding of drug therapy.

cyanocobalamin (vitamin B$_{12}$)
(sigh-an-oh-koh-BAH-luh-meen)
Anacobin♦, Bedoz♦, Crystamine, Crysti 1000, Cyanocobalamin, Cyanoject, Cyomin

hydroxocobalamin (vitamin B$_{12}$)
Hydro-Cobex, LA-12

Pharmacologic class: water-soluble vitamin
Therapeutic class: vitamin, nutrition supplement
Pregnancy risk category: A (C if used in doses above RDA)

Indications and dosages

▶ **RDA for cyanocobalamin.** *Adults and children ages 11 and older:* 2 mcg.
Pregnant women: 2.2 mcg.
Breast-feeding women: 2.6 mcg.
Children ages 7 to 10: 1.4 mcg.
Children ages 4 to 6: 1 mcg.
Children ages 1 to 3: 0.7 mcg.
Infants ages 6 months to 1 year: 0.5 mcg.
Neonates and infants younger than age 6 months and younger: 0.3 mcg.
▶ **Vitamin B$_{12}$ deficiency caused by inadequate diet, subtotal gastrectomy, or any other condition, disorder, or disease except malabsorption related to pernicious anemia or other GI disease.** *Adults:* 30 mcg hydroxocobal-

amin I.M. daily for 5 to 10 days, depending on severity of deficiency. Maintenance dosage is 100 to 200 mcg I.M. once monthly. For subsequent prophylaxis, advise adequate nutrition and daily RDA vitamin B$_{12}$ supplements.
Children: 1 to 5 mg hydroxocobalamin spread over 2 or more weeks in doses of 100 mcg I.M., depending on severity of deficiency. Maintenance dosage is 30 to 50 mcg I.M. monthly. For subsequent prophylaxis, advise adequate nutrition and daily RDA vitamin B$_{12}$ supplements.
▶ **Pernicious anemia or vitamin B$_{12}$ malabsorption.** *Adults:* Initially, 100 mcg cyanocobalamin I.M. or S.C. daily for 6 to 7 days; then 100 mcg I.M. or S.C. once monthly.
Children: 30 to 50 mcg I.M. or S.C. daily over 2 or more weeks; then 100 mcg I.M. or S.C. monthly for life.
▶ **Methylmalonic aciduria.** *Neonates:* 1,000 mcg cyanocobalamin I.M. daily.
▶ **Schilling test flushing dose.** *Adults and children:* 1,000 mcg hydroxocobalamin I.M. as a single dose.

Contraindications and precautions

• Contraindicated in patients with early Leber's disease or hypersensitivity to vitamin B$_{12}$ or cobalt.
• Use cautiously in anemic patients with cardiac, pulmonary, or hypertensive disease and in those with severe vitamin B$_{12}$-dependent deficiencies.
⚠ Lifespan: In premature infants, use cautiously; some products contain benzyl alcohol, which may cause gasping syndrome.

Adverse reactions

CV: peripheral vascular thrombosis, *pulmonary edema, heart failure.*
GI: transient diarrhea.
Skin: itching, transitory exanthema, urticaria.
Other: *anaphylaxis, anaphylactoid reactions* (with parenteral administration); pain, burning (at S.C. or I.M. injection sites).

Interactions

Drug-drug. *Aminoglycosides, chloramphenicol, colchicine, para-aminosalicylic acid and salts:* May cause malabsorption of vitamin B$_{12}$. Don't use together.
Drug-lifestyle. *Alcohol use:* May cause malabsorption of vitamin B$_{12}$. Discourage using together.

Effects on lab test results

• May decrease potassium level.
• May cause false-positive results for intrinsic factor antibody test.

Pharmacokinetics

Absorption: After oral administration, absorbed irregularly from distal small intestine. Depends on sufficient intrinsic factor and calcium. Rapid after I.M. and S.C. administration sites. Vitamin B_{12} is protein-bound.
Distribution: Distributed into liver, bone marrow, and other tissues.
Metabolism: Metabolized in liver.
Excretion: Amount of vitamin B_{12} needed by body is reabsorbed; excess is excreted in urine.
Half-life: About 6 days.

Route	Onset	Peak	Duration
P.O.	Unknown	8-12 hr	Unknown
I.M.	Unknown	60 min	Unknown
S.C.	Unknown	Unknown	Unknown

Action

Chemical effect: Acts as a coenzyme that stimulates metabolic functions. Needed for cell replication, hematopoiesis, and nucleoprotein and myelin synthesis.
Therapeutic effect: Increases vitamin B_{12} level.

Available forms

cyanocobalamin
Injection: 1,000 mcg/ml
Tablets: 25 mcg†, 50 mcg†, 100 mcg†, 250 mcg†, 500 mcg†, 1,000 mcg†
hydroxocobalamin
Injection: 1,000 mcg/ml

NURSING PROCESS

▨ Assessment
• Assess patient's vitamin B_{12} deficiency before therapy.
• Determine reticulocyte count, hematocrit, and B_{12}, iron, and folate levels before beginning therapy.
• Monitor drug's effectiveness by assessing patient for improvement in signs and symptoms of vitamin B_{12} deficiency. Also monitor reticulocyte count, hematocrit, and B_{12}, iron, and folate levels between fifth and seventh day of therapy and periodically thereafter.

• Infection, tumors, and renal, hepatic, and other debilitating diseases may reduce therapeutic response.
• Closely monitor potassium levels for first 48 hours. Be alert for adverse reactions and drug interactions.
• Evaluate patient's and family's knowledge of drug therapy.

⊞ Nursing diagnoses
• Ineffective health maintenance related to underlying vitamin B_{12} deficiency
• Risk for injury related to parenteral administration and drug-induced hypersensitivity reactions
• Deficient knowledge related to drug therapy

▷ Planning and implementation
• Don't mix parenteral liquids in same syringe with other medications.
• Drug is physically incompatible with dextrose solutions, alkaline or strongly acidic solutions, oxidizing or reducing agents, heavy metals, chlorpromazine, phytonadione, prochlorperazine, and many other drugs.
• Hydroxocobalamin is approved for I.M. or deep S.C. use only. Its only advantage over cyanocobalamin is its longer duration.
• Don't give large oral doses of vitamin B_{12} routinely because drug is lost through excretion.
• Protect vitamin from light. Don't refrigerate or freeze.
• Give potassium supplement, if needed.
Patient teaching
• Stress need for patient with pernicious anemia to return for monthly injections. Although total body stores may last 3 to 6 years, anemia will recur without monthly treatment.
• Emphasize importance of well-balanced diet.
• Tell patient to store oral tablets in tightly closed container at room temperature.

☑ Evaluation
• Patient's vitamin B_{12} deficiency is resolved with drug therapy.
• Patient doesn't experience hypersensitivity reactions following parenteral administration of drug.
• Patient and family state understanding of drug therapy.

Reactions may be *common,* uncommon, *life-threatening*, or COMMON AND LIFE-THREATENING.

cyclobenzaprine hydrochloride
(sigh-kloh-BEN-zah-preen high-droh-KLOR-ighd)
Flexeril

Pharmacologic class: tricyclic antidepressant (TCA) derivative
Therapeutic class: skeletal muscle relaxant
Pregnancy risk category: B

Indications and dosages

▶ **Adjunct to rest and physical therapy for relief of muscle spasm associated with acute, painful musculoskeletal conditions.** *Adults:* 5 mg P.O. t.i.d. Based on response, the dose may be increased to 10 mg t.i.d. Use of cyclobenzaprine for periods longer than two or three weeks is not recommended.
Ⓢ **Adjust-a-dose:** In elderly patients and in patients with mild hepatic impairment, start with 5 mg; increase slowly. In patients with moderate to severe hepatic impairment, drug isn't recommended.
▶ **Fibrositis‡.** *Adults:* 10 to 40 mg P.O. daily.

Contraindications and precautions

• Contraindicated in patients hypersensitive to drug; in patients in the acute recovery phase of MI; in patients with hyperthyroidism, heart block, arrhythmias, conduction disturbances, or heart failure; and within 14 days of MAO inhibitor therapy.
• Use cautiously in debilitated patients and in patients with history of urine retention, acute angle-closure glaucoma, or increased intraocular pressure. Also use cautiously in patients taking anticholinergics.
⚖ **Lifespan:** In pregnant and breast-feeding women and in children younger than age 15, safety and efficacy of drug haven't been established. In elderly patients, use cautiously.

Adverse reactions

CNS: *drowsiness,* euphoria, weakness, headache, insomnia, nightmares, paresthesia, *dizziness,* depression, visual disturbances, **seizures.**
CV: tachycardia, **arrhythmias.**
EENT: blurred vision.
GI: *dry mouth,* abdominal pain, dyspepsia, abnormal taste, constipation.
GU: urine retention.
Skin: rash, urticaria, pruritus.

Interactions

Drug-drug. *Anticholinergics:* May have additive anticholinergic effects. Avoid using together.
CNS depressants: May cause additive CNS depression. Avoid using together.
MAO inhibitors: May exacerbate CNS depression or anticholinergic effects. Don't give within 14 days after discontinuing MAO inhibitors.
Drug-lifestyle. *Alcohol use:* May cause additive CNS depression. Discourage using together.

Effects on lab test results

None reported.

Pharmacokinetics

Absorption: Almost complete during first pass through GI tract.
Distribution: 93% plasma protein-bound.
Metabolism: During first pass through GI tract and liver, drug and metabolites undergo enterohepatic recycling.
Excretion: Excreted primarily in urine as conjugated metabolites; also in feces via bile as unchanged drug. *Half-life:* 1 to 3 days.

Route	Onset	Peak	Duration
P.O.	≤ 1 hr	3-8 hr	12-24 hr

Action

Chemical effect: Unknown.
Therapeutic effect: Relieves muscle spasms.

Available forms

Tablets: 5 mg, 10 mg

NURSING PROCESS

🔍 **Assessment**
• Assess patient's underlying condition before therapy.
• Monitor drug's effectiveness by assessing severity and frequency of patient's muscle spasms.
• If drug is stopped abruptly after long-term use, watch for nausea, headache, and malaise.
• Evaluate patient's and family's knowledge of drug therapy.

💠 **Nursing diagnoses**
• Acute pain related to presence of muscle spasms

• Risk for injury related to potential for drug-induced CNS adverse reactions
• Deficient knowledge related to drug therapy

▷ Planning and implementation
⚠ **ALERT:** Watch for symptoms of overdose, including cardiac toxicity. If you suspect toxicity, keep physostigmine available, and notify prescriber immediately.
• Don't give drug with other CNS depressants.
• With high doses, watch for adverse reactions similar to those of other TCAs.
Patient teaching
• Advise patient to report urinary hesitancy or urine retention. If constipation occurs, tell patient to increase fluid intake and suggest use of a stool softener.
• Advise patient not to attempt to split the generic 10-mg tablets because it may cause dosing inconsistencies.
• Warn patient to avoid activities that require alertness until drug's CNS effects are known.
• Warn patient to avoid combining drug with alcohol or other CNS depressants.
• Suggest sugarless chewing gum or hard candy to relieve dry mouth.

☑ Evaluation
• Patient is free from pain with drug therapy.
• Patient doesn't experience injury as a result of drug-induced adverse CNS reactions.
• Patient and family state understanding of drug therapy.

cyclophosphamide
(sigh-kloh-FOS-fuh-mighd)
Cycloblastin ◇ , Cytoxan, Cytoxan Lyophilized, Endoxan-Asta ◇ , Neosar, Procytox ♦

Pharmacologic class: alkylating agent (not specific to cell-cycle phase)
Therapeutic class: antineoplastic
Pregnancy risk category: D

Indications and dosages
▷ **Breast, head, neck, prostate, lung, and ovarian cancers; Hodgkin's disease; chronic lymphocytic leukemia; chronic myelocytic leukemia; acute lymphoblastic leukemia; acute myelocytic leukemia; neuroblastoma;** **retinoblastoma; non-Hodgkin's lymphoma; multiple myeloma; mycosis fungoides; sarcoma.** *Adults and children:* Initially, 40 to 50 mg/kg I.V. in divided doses over 2 to 5 days. Or, 10 to 15 mg/kg I.V. q 7 to 10 days, 3 to 5 mg/kg I.V. twice weekly, or 1 to 5 mg/kg P.O. daily, based on patient tolerance. Adjust subsequent dosage according to evidence of antitumor activity or leukopenia.
▷ **"Minimal change" nephrotic syndrome in children.** *Children:* 2.5 to 3 mg/kg P.O. daily for 60 to 90 days.
▷ **Polymyositis** ‡. *Adults:* 1 to 2 mg/kg P.O. daily.
▷ **Rheumatoid arthritis**‡. *Adults:* 1.5 to 3 mg/kg P.O. daily.
▷ **Wegener's granulomatosis**‡. *Adults:* 1 to 2 mg/kg P.O. daily (usually given with prednisone).

▼ I.V. administration
• Preparing and giving I.V. form of drug are linked to carcinogenic, mutagenic, and teratogenic risks. Follow facility policy to reduce risks.
• Reconstitute powder using sterile water for injection or bacteriostatic water for injection that contains only parabens. For nonlyophilized product, add 5 ml to 100-mg vial, 10 ml to 200-mg vial, 25 ml to 500-mg vial, 50 ml to 1-g vial, or 100 ml to 2-g vial to produce solution containing 20 mg/ml. Shake to dissolve; this may take up to 6 minutes and it may be difficult to completely dissolve drug. Lyophilized preparation is much easier to reconstitute; check package insert for quantity of diluent needed to reconstitute drug.
• Give by direct I.V. injection or infusion. For I.V. infusion, further dilute with D_5W, dextrose 5% in normal saline solution, dextrose 5% in Ringer's injection, lactated Ringer's injection, sodium lactate injection, or half-normal saline solution for injection.
• Check reconstituted solution for small particles. Filter solution if needed.
• Reconstituted solution is stable for 6 days refrigerated or 24 hours at room temperature. However, use stored solutions cautiously because drug contains no preservatives.

Contraindications and precautions
• Contraindicated in patients with severe bone marrow depression.

• Use cautiously in patients who have recently undergone radiation therapy or chemotherapy and in patients with leukopenia, thrombocytopenia, malignant cell infiltration of bone marrow, or hepatic or renal disease.

⚥ **Lifespan:** In pregnant women, use cautiously, if at all, because fetal harm may occur. In breast-feeding women, drug is contraindicated.

Adverse reactions

CV: *cardiotoxicity* (with very high doses and with doxorubicin).

GI: anorexia, *nausea and vomiting* beginning within 6 hours, stomatitis, mucositis.

GU: gonadal suppression (may be irreversible), STERILE HEMORRHAGIC CYSTITIS, bladder fibrosis.

Hematologic: *leukopenia,* nadir between days 8 and 15, recovery in 17 to 28 days; *thrombocytopenia; anemia.*

Metabolic: hyperuricemia.

Respiratory: *pulmonary fibrosis* (with high doses).

Skin: *reversible alopecia* in 50% of patients, especially with high doses.

Other: *secondary malignancies, anaphylaxis,* SIADH (with high doses), *sterility, gonadal suppression.*

Interactions

Drug-drug. *Barbiturates:* May increase pharmacologic effect and enhance cyclophosphamide toxicity caused by induction of hepatic enzymes. Avoid using together.

Cardiotoxic drugs: Additive adverse cardiac effects. Avoid using together.

Chloramphenicol, corticosteroids: Reduces activity of cyclophosphamide. Use cautiously and monitor patient.

Digoxin: May decrease digoxin levels. Monitor levels closely and adjust dosage as needed.

Succinylcholine: Prolongs neuromuscular blockade. Avoid using together.

Effects on lab test results

• May increase uric acid level. May decrease pseudocholinesterase level.

• May decrease hemoglobin, hematocrit, and WBC, RBC, and platelet counts.

Pharmacokinetics

Absorption: Almost complete with P.O. doses of 100 mg or less. Higher doses (300 mg) are about 75% absorbed.

Distribution: Distributed throughout body, although only minimal amounts have been found in saliva, sweat, and synovial fluid. Active metabolites are about 50% bound to plasma proteins.

Metabolism: Metabolized to its active form by hepatic microsomal enzymes. Activity of these metabolites is terminated by metabolism to inactive forms.

Excretion: Drug and its metabolites are eliminated primarily in urine, with 15% to 30% excreted as unchanged drug. *Half-life:* 3 to 12 hours.

Route	Onset	Peak	Duration
P.O., I.V.	Unknown	Unknown	Unknown

Action

Chemical effect: Cross-links strands of cellular DNA and interferes with RNA transcription, causing imbalance of growth that leads to cell death.

Therapeutic effect: Kills specific types of cancer cells; improves renal function in mild nephrotic syndrome in children.

Available forms

Injection: 100-mg, 200-mg, 500-mg, 1-g, 2-g vials

Tablets: 25 mg, 50 mg

NURSING PROCESS

⚕ Assessment

• Assess patient's underlying condition before therapy and reassess regularly during therapy.

• Monitor CBC, uric acid levels, and renal and liver function tests.

• If corticosteroid therapy is stopped, monitor patient for cyclophosphamide toxicity.

• Be alert for adverse reactions and drug interactions.

• Evaluate patient's and family's knowledge of drug therapy.

⚕ Nursing diagnoses

• Ineffective health maintenance related to underlying condition

• Risk for injury related to drug-induced adverse reactions

• Deficient knowledge related to drug therapy

⮞ Planning and implementation

• Tablets are used for children with "minimal change" nephrotic syndrome and not to treat neoplastic disease.

• To prevent hyperuricemia with resulting uric acid nephropathy, allopurinol may be used with adequate hydration.

Patient teaching

• Warn patient that alopecia is likely to occur but that it's reversible.

• Warn patient to watch for signs of infection (fever, sore throat, fatigue) and bleeding (easy bruising, nosebleeds, bleeding gums, melena) and to take temperature daily.

• Instruct patient to avoid OTC products that contain aspirin.

• Encourage patient to void every 1 to 2 hours while awake and to drink at least 3 L of fluid daily to minimize risk of hemorrhagic cystitis. Tell patient not to take drug at bedtime; infrequent urination during night may increase possibility of cystitis. If cystitis occurs, tell patient to stop drug and notify prescriber. Cystitis can occur months after therapy ends. Mesna may be given to lower risk and severity of bladder toxicity.

• Advise both men and women to practice contraception while taking drug and for 4 months after; drug is potentially teratogenic.

• Advise women of childbearing age to avoid becoming pregnant during therapy. Also recommend consulting with prescriber before becoming pregnant.

☑ Evaluation

• Patient shows positive response to drug therapy.

• Patient doesn't experience injury as a result of drug-induced adverse reactions.

• Patient and family state understanding of drug therapy.

cycloserine
(sigh-kloh-SER-een)
Seromycin

Pharmacologic class: isoxizolidone, d-alanine analogue
Therapeutic class: antituberculotic
Pregnancy risk category: C

Indications and dosages

▶ **Adjunct in pulmonary or extrapulmonary tuberculosis.** *Adults:* Initially, 250 mg P.O. q 12 hours for 2 weeks; then, if levels are below 25 to 30 mcg/ml and no toxicity has developed, 250 mg q 8 hours for 2 weeks. If optimum blood levels aren't achieved and no toxicity has developed, increase to 250 mg q 6 hours. Maximum dosage is 1 g daily. If CNS toxicity occurs, stop drug for 1 week and then resume at 250 mg daily for 2 weeks. If no serious toxic effects occur, increase by 250-mg increments q 10 days until level is 25 to 30 mcg/ml.

Contraindications and precautions

• Contraindicated in patients hypersensitive to drug; in patients who consume excessive amounts of alcohol; and in patients with seizure disorders, depression, severe anxiety, psychosis, or severe renal insufficiency.

• Use cautiously in patients with renal impairment and reduce dosage.

⚖ Lifespan: In pregnant and breast-feeding women, use cautiously. In children, safety and efficacy of drug haven't been established.

Adverse reactions

CNS: *seizures,* drowsiness, headache, tremor, dysarthria, vertigo, confusion, loss of memory, *possible suicidal tendencies* and other psychotic symptoms, *nervousness, hallucinations, depression,* hyperirritability, paresthesia, paresis, hyperreflexia, *coma.*
Other: hypersensitivity reactions (allergic dermatitis).

Interactions

Drug-drug. *Ethionamide, isoniazid:* Increases risk of CNS toxicity (seizures, dizziness, or drowsiness). Monitor patient closely.
Drug-lifestyle. *Alcohol use:* Increases risk of CNS toxicity. Advise patient to refrain from alcohol consumption during therapy.

Effects on lab test results

• May increase transaminase level.

Pharmacokinetics

Absorption: About 80%.
Distribution: Distributed widely into body tissues and fluids, including CSF. It doesn't bind to plasma proteins.
Metabolism: May be metabolized partially.

Excretion: Excreted primarily in urine. *Half-life:* 10 hours.

Route	Onset	Peak	Duration
P.O.	Unknown	3-4 hr	Unknown

Action

Chemical effect: Inhibits cell-wall biosynthesis by interfering with bacterial use of amino acids (bacteriostatic).
Therapeutic effect: Aids in eradicating tuberculosis.

Available forms

Capsules: 250 mg

NURSING PROCESS

⚙ Assessment
• Assess patient's underlying condition before therapy.
• Obtain specimen for culture and sensitivity tests before therapy begins and periodically thereafter to detect possible resistance.
• Monitor drug's effectiveness by evaluating culture and sensitivity results; watch for improvement in patient's underlying condition.
• Monitor cycloserine levels periodically, especially in patients receiving high doses (more than 500 mg daily) because toxic reactions may occur with blood levels above 30 mcg/ml.
• Monitor results of hematologic tests and renal and liver function studies.
• Be alert for adverse reactions and drug interactions.
• Evaluate patient's and family's knowledge of drug therapy.

⊞ Nursing diagnoses
• Ineffective health maintenance related to presence of tuberculosis
• Risk for injury related to drug-induced CNS adverse reactions
• Deficient knowledge related to drug therapy

▷ Planning and implementation
• Always give with other antituberculotics to prevent development of resistant organisms. Drug is considered second-line drug in treatment of tuberculosis
• Adjust dosage according to levels, toxicity, or ineffectiveness.

• Give pyridoxine, anticonvulsants, tranquilizers, or sedatives to relieve adverse reactions.
• Pyridoxine may prevent neurotoxicity.
Patient teaching
• Warn patient to avoid alcohol, which may cause serious neurologic reactions.
• Instruct patient to take drug exactly as prescribed; warn against discontinuing drug without prescriber's approval.
• Stress importance of having laboratory studies done to monitor drug effectiveness and toxicity.

☑ Evaluation
• Patient maintains health after drug therapy.
• Patient has no injury as a result of drug-induced adverse reactions.
• Patient and family state understanding of drug therapy.

cyclosporine (cyclosporin)
(sigh-kloh-SPOOR-een)
Neoral, Sandimmun◇, Sandimmune

cyclosporine, modified
Gengraf

Pharmacologic class: polypeptide antibiotic
Therapeutic class: immunosuppressant
Pregnancy risk category: C

Indications and dosages

▶ **Prevention of organ rejection in kidney, liver, or heart transplantation.** *Adults and children:* 15 mg/kg P.O. 4 to 12 hours before transplantation and continued daily postoperatively for 1 to 2 weeks. Reduce dosage by 5% each week to maintenance level of 5 to 10 mg/kg daily. Or, 5 to 6 mg/kg I.V. concentrate 4 to 12 hours before transplantation. Postoperatively, dosage repeated daily until patient can tolerate P.O. forms.
    When converting from Sandimmune to Gengraf, use same daily dose as previously used for Sandimmune. Monitor levels q 4 to 7 days after converting, and monitor blood pressure and creatinine level q 2 weeks during the first 2 months.
▶ **Severe, active rheumatoid arthritis that hasn't adequately responded to methotrexate.** *Adults:* 1.25 mg/kg Gengraf or Neoral P.O. b.i.d. Increase dosage by 0.5 to 0.75 mg/kg daily after 8 weeks and again after 12 weeks to a

maximum of 4 mg/kg daily. If no response is seen after 16 weeks, stop therapy.

▶ **Recalcitrant, plaque psoriasis that isn't adequately responsive to at least one systemic therapy or in patients for whom other systemic therapy is contraindicated or isn't tolerated.** *Adults:* Initially, 2.5 mg/kg Gengraf or Neoral P.O. daily divided b.i.d. Maintain initial dose for 4 weeks. Increase by 0.5 mg/kg daily to a maximum of 4 mg/kg daily at 2-week intervals, p.r.n.

◩ **Adjust-a-dose:** For patients with hypertension, a creatinine level 30% above pretreatment level, or abnormal CBC or liver function test results, decrease dosage by 25% to 50%. If creatinine level is 25% above pretreatment levels, repeat creatinine measurement within 2 weeks. If creatinine level stays 25% to 50% above baseline, reduce dosage by 25% to 50%. If creatinine level is 50% above baseline, reduce dosage by 25% to 50%. If creatinine level isn't reversed after two dosage modifications, stop therapy.

▽ I.V. administration

- Protect I.V. solution from light.
- Dilute each ml of concentrate in 20 to 100 ml of D$_5$W or normal saline solution for injection. Dilute immediately before infusion; infuse over 2 to 6 hours.
- Give I.V. concentrate at one-third oral dose and dilute before use.
- Give drug I.V. to patients who can't tolerate oral drugs.

Contraindications and precautions

- Contraindicated in patients hypersensitive to drug or to polyoxyethylated castor oil (found in injectable form). Neoral and Gengraf are contraindicated in patients with psoriasis or rheumatoid arthritis who also have renal impairment, uncontrolled hypertension, or malignancies.

⚠ **Lifespan:** In pregnant women, use cautiously. In breast-feeding women, safety and efficacy of drug haven't been established.

Adverse reactions

CNS: *tremor,* headache, *seizures.*
CV: flushing, hypertension.
EENT: sinusitis.
GI: *gum hyperplasia,* oral thrush, nausea, vomiting, diarrhea.
GU: NEPHROTOXICITY.

Hematologic: anemia, LEUKOPENIA, THROMBOCYTOPENIA.
Hepatic: *hepatotoxicity.*
Skin: *hirsutism,* acne.
Other: *infections, anaphylaxis.*

Interactions

Drug-drug. *Aminoglycosides, amphotericin B, co-trimoxazole, NSAIDs:* May increase risk of nephrotoxicity. Monitor patient for toxicity.
Amphotericin B, cilastatin, cimetidine, diltiazem, erythromycin, imipenem, ketoconazole, metoclopramide, prednisolone: May increase levels of cyclosporine. Monitor patient for increased toxicity.
Azathioprine, corticosteroids, cyclophosphamide, verapamil: Increase immunosuppression. Monitor patient closely for infection.
Carbamazepine, isoniazid, phenobarbital, phenytoin, rifampin: Possible decreased immunosuppressant effect. May need to increase cyclosporine dosage.
Vaccines: Decrease immune response. Postpone routine immunization.
Drug-herb. *Pill-bearing spurge:* May inhibit CYP 3A enzymes affecting drug metabolism. Discourage using together.
St. John's wort: May significantly lower drug level and contribute to organ rejection. Discourage using together.
Drug-food. *Grapefruit:* May increase drug level and cause toxicity. Discourage using together.

Effects on lab test results

- May increase BUN, creatinine, LDL, bilirubin, AST, ALT, and glucose levels.
- May decrease hemoglobin, hematocrit, and WBC and platelet counts.

Pharmacokinetics

Absorption: Varies widely. Only 30% of Sandimmune oral dose reaches systemic circulation, while 60% of Neoral reaches systemic circulation.
Distribution: Distributed widely outside blood volume. About 90% is protein-bound.
Metabolism: Extensive, in liver.
Excretion: Primarily in feces with 6% in urine.
Half-life: 10 to 27 hours.

Route	Onset	Peak	Duration
P.O.	Unknown	1½-3 hr	Unknown
I.V.	Unknown	Unknown	Unknown

Action

Chemical effect: Inhibits proliferation of T lymphocytes.
Therapeutic effect: Prevents organ rejection.

Available forms

Capsules: 25 mg, 50 mg, 100 mg
Capsules for microemulsion: 25 mg, 100 mg
Injection: 50 mg/ml
Oral solution: 100 mg/ml

NURSING PROCESS

⚕ Assessment

• Assess patient's organ transplant before therapy.
• Monitor effectiveness by evaluating patient for signs and symptoms of organ rejection.
• Monitor drug level at regular intervals.
• Monitor BUN and creatinine levels because nephrotoxicity may develop 2 to 3 months after transplant surgery and require reduced dosage.
• Monitor liver function tests for hepatotoxicity, which usually occurs during first month after transplant.
• Monitor CBC and platelet counts regularly.
• Be alert for adverse reactions and drug interactions.
• Evaluate patient's and family's knowledge of drug therapy.

⊕ Nursing diagnoses

• Risk for injury related to potential for organ rejection
• Ineffective protection related to drug-induced immunosuppression
• Deficient knowledge related to drug therapy

▶ Planning and implementation

• Don't give psoralen plus ultraviolet A (PUVA) or ultraviolet B (UVB) therapy, methotrexate, other immunosuppressants, coal, tar, and radiation therapy to psoriasis patients taking Neoral or Gengraf.
• Always give drug with adrenal corticosteroids.
• Measure oral doses carefully in oral syringe. To increase palatability, mix with whole milk, chocolate milk, or fruit juice (except grapefruit juice). Oral solution for emulsion is less palatable when mixed with milk. Use glass container to minimize adherence to container walls.
• Give drug with meals to minimize GI distress.

⊛ **ALERT:** Sandimmune and Neoral aren't bioequivalent and can't be used interchangeably without prescriber supervision. Convert from Neoral to Sandimmune with increased monitoring to avoid underdosing. Gengraf is bioequivalent to and interchangeable with Neoral capsules.
• Before starting treatment in patients with rheumatoid arthritis, measure blood pressure at least twice and obtain two creatinine levels to estimate baseline. Evaluate blood pressure and creatinine level every 2 weeks during first 3 months, then monthly if patient is stable. Monitor blood pressure and creatinine level after an increase in NSAID dosage or introduction of a new NSAID. If hypertension occurs, decrease dosage of Gengraf or Neoral by 25% to 50%. If hypertension persists, decrease dosage further or control blood pressure with antihypertensives.
• If patient also receives methotrexate, monitor CBC and liver function tests monthly.
• For psoriasis patients, evaluate patient for occult infection and tumors initially and throughout treatment.
• Before starting therapy in psoriasis patients, take blood pressure at least twice and obtain two creatinine levels. Also obtain CBC and BUN, magnesium, uric acid, potassium, and lipid levels. Evaluate blood pressure, CBC, and uric acid, creatinine, BUN, potassium, lipid, and magnesium levels every 2 weeks for the first 3 months, then monthly if patient is stable, or more frequently when adjusting dosage. Reduce dosage by 25% to 50% in case of significant abnormality.
• Monitor blood pressure and creatinine level after an increase in NSAID dosage or introduction of a new NSAID.
⊛ **ALERT:** Don't confuse cyclosporine with cyclophosphamide or cycloserine.
⊛ **ALERT:** Don't confuse Sandimmune with Sandoglobulin or Sandostatin.

Patient teaching

• Encourage patient to take drug at same time each day.
• Advise patient to take Neoral on an empty stomach and not to mix with grapefruit juice.
• Advise patient to take with meals if drug causes nausea. Anorexia, nausea, and vomiting are usually transient and most frequently occur at start of therapy.
• Tell patient not to stop drug without prescriber's approval.

• Instruct patient to swish and swallow nystatin four times daily to prevent oral thrush.
• Instruct patient on infection control and bleeding precautions, as indicated by CBC and platelet count results.

☑ Evaluation
• Patient doesn't experience organ rejection while taking drug.
• Patient is free from infection and serious bleeding episodes throughout drug therapy.
• Patient and family state understanding of drug therapy.

cyproheptadine hydrochloride
(sigh-proh-HEP-tah-deen high-droh-KLOR-ighd)
Periactin

Pharmacologic class: piperidine-derivative antihistamine
Therapeutic class: antihistamine (H$_1$-receptor antagonist), antipruritic
Pregnancy risk category: B

Indications and dosages
▶ **Allergy symptoms, pruritus.** *Adults:* 4 to 20 mg P.O. daily in divided doses. Maximum dosage is 0.5 mg/kg daily.
Children ages 7 to 14: 4 mg P.O. b.i.d. or t.i.d. Maximum dosage is 16 mg daily.
Children ages 2 to 6: 2 mg P.O. b.i.d. or t.i.d. Maximum dosage is 12 mg daily.
▶ **Cushing's syndrome‡.** *Adults:* 8 to 24 mg P.O. daily in divided doses.

Contraindications and precautions
• Contraindicated in debilitated patients; in patients hypersensitive to drug or other drugs of similar chemical structure; in those with acute asthmatic attacks, angle-closure glaucoma, stenosing peptic ulcer, symptomatic prostatic hypertrophy, bladder-neck obstruction, and pyloroduodenal obstruction; and in patients taking MAO inhibitors.
• Use cautiously in patients with increased intraocular pressure, hyperthyroidism, CV disease, hypertension, or bronchial asthma.
☀ **Lifespan:** In pregnant women, use cautiously. In breast-feeding women, neonates, premature infants, and elderly patients, drug is contraindicated.

Adverse reactions
CNS: *drowsiness,* dizziness, headache, fatigue, *seizures* (especially in elderly patients).
GI: nausea, vomiting, epigastric distress, *dry mouth.*
GU: urine retention.
Hematologic: *agranulocytosis, thrombocytopenia.*
Metabolic: weight gain.
Skin: rash.
Other: *anaphylaxis.*

Interactions
Drug-drug. *CNS depressants:* May increase sedation. Use together cautiously.
MAO inhibitors: May increase anticholinergic effects. Don't use together.
Drug-lifestyle. *Sun exposure:* Photosensitivity reactions may occur. Urge patient to avoid sun exposure and wear protective clothing and sunblock.

Effects on lab test results
• May decrease hemoglobin, hematocrit, and WBC, platelet, and granulocyte counts.

Pharmacokinetics
Absorption: Well absorbed from GI tract.
Distribution: Unknown.
Metabolism: Appears to be almost completely metabolized in liver.
Excretion: Metabolites are excreted primarily in urine; unchanged drug isn't excreted in urine, but small amounts of unchanged cyproheptadine and metabolites are excreted in feces. *Half-life:* Unknown.

Route	Onset	Peak	Duration
P.O.	15-60 min	6-9 hr	8 hr

Action
Chemical effect: Competes with histamine for H$_1$-receptor sites on effector cells. Prevents, but doesn't reverse, histamine-mediated responses.
Therapeutic effect: Relieves allergy symptoms and itching.

Available forms
Syrup: 2 mg/5 ml
Tablets: 4 mg

NURSING PROCESS

☑ Assessment
• Assess patient's underlying condition before therapy and reassess regularly during therapy.
• Be alert for adverse reactions and drug interactions.
• Evaluate patient's and family's knowledge of drug therapy.

☺ Nursing diagnoses
• Ineffective health maintenance related to underlying condition
• Risk for injury related to potential for drug-induced adverse CNS reactions
• Deficient knowledge related to drug therapy

⟩ Planning and implementation
• Reduce GI distress by giving drug with food or milk.
• If tolerance is suspected, notify prescriber and use another antihistamine.
Patient teaching
• Instruct patient to take drug with food or milk to reduce GI distress.
• Warn patient to avoid alcohol and hazardous activities until CNS effects of drug are known.
• Tell patient that coffee or tea may reduce drowsiness. Sugarless gum, hard candy, or ice chips may relieve dry mouth.
• Advise patient to stop drug 4 days before allergy skin tests to preserve accuracy of tests.
• Instruct patient to notify prescriber if tolerance develops; different antihistamine may be needed.

☑ Evaluation
• Patient is free from allergy symptoms or pruritus with drug therapy.
• Patient has no injury as result of drug-induced CNS adverse reactions.
• Patient and family state understanding of drug therapy.

cytarabine (ara-C, cytosine arabinoside)
(sigh-TAR-uh-been)
Cytosar ♦ , Cytosar-U

Pharmacologic class: antimetabolite (specific to S phase of cell cycle)

Therapeutic class: antineoplastic
Pregnancy risk category: D

Indications and dosages
▶ **Acute nonlymphocytic leukemia, acute lymphocytic leukemia, blast phase of chronic myelocytic leukemia.** *Adults and children:* 100 mg/m^2 daily by continuous I.V. infusion or 100 mg/m^2 I.V. q 12 hours, given for 5 days and repeated q 2 weeks. For maintenance, 1 mg/kg S.C. once or twice weekly.
▶ **Meningeal leukemia.** *Adults and children:* Highly variable from 5 to 75 mg/m^2 intrathecally. Frequency also varies from once a day for 4 days to once q 4 days. Most common dosage is 30 mg/m^2, q 4 days until CSF is normal, followed by one more dose.

▼ I.V. administration
• Preparing and giving I.V. form are linked to carcinogenic, mutagenic, and teratogenic risks. Follow facility policy to reduce risks.
• To reduce nausea, give antiemetic before drug. Nausea and vomiting are more frequent when large doses are given rapidly by I.V. push. These reactions are less frequent when given by infusion. Dizziness may occur with rapid infusion.
• Reconstitute drug using provided diluent, which is bacteriostatic water for injection containing benzyl alcohol. Avoid this diluent when preparing drug for neonates or for intrathecal use. Reconstitute 100-mg vial with 5 ml of diluent or 500-mg vial with 10 ml of diluent. Reconstituted solution is stable for 48 hours. Discard cloudy reconstituted solution.
• For I.V. infusion, further dilute using normal saline solution for injection, D$_5$W, or sterile water for injection.

Contraindications and precautions
• Contraindicated in patients hypersensitive to drug.
• Use cautiously in patients with hepatic disease.
⚘ **Lifespan:** In pregnant women, drug isn't recommended because fetal harm may occur. In breast-feeding women, drug is contraindicated.

Adverse reactions
CNS: neurotoxicity, including ataxia and cerebellar dysfunction (with high doses).
EENT: keratitis, nystagmus.

GI: *nausea, vomiting,* diarrhea, *constipation, anorexia, anal ulceration,* dysphagia; reddened area at juncture of lips, followed by sore mouth and oral ulcers in 5 to 10 days; high dose given by rapid I.V. may cause projectile vomiting.

GU: urate nephropathy.

Hematologic: *leukopenia,* with initial WBC count nadir 7 to 9 days after drug is stopped and second (more severe) nadir 15 to 24 days after drug is stopped; anemia; reticulocytopenia; *thrombocytopenia,* with platelet count nadir occurring on day 10; *megaloblastosis.*

Hepatic: *hepatotoxicity* (usually mild and reversible).

Metabolic: hyperuricemia.

Skin: *rash.*

Other: flu syndrome, *anaphylaxis.*

Interactions

Drug-drug. *Digoxin:* May decrease digoxin levels. Monitor digoxin levels.
Flucytosine: Decreases flucytosine activity. Monitor patient closely.
Gentamicin: May decrease activity against *Klebsiella pneumoniae.* Avoid using together.

Effects on lab test results

• May increase uric acid level.
• May increase megaloblasts. May decrease hemoglobin, hematocrit, and WBC, RBC, platelet, and reticulocyte counts.

Pharmacokinetics

Absorption: Unknown.
Distribution: Rapidly distributed widely throughout body. About 13% of drug is bound to plasma proteins. Drug penetrates the blood-brain barrier only slightly after rapid I.V. dose; however, when drug is given by continuous I.V. infusion, CSF levels achieve 40% to 60% of that of plasma levels.
Metabolism: Metabolized primarily in liver but also in kidneys, GI mucosa, and granulocytes.
Excretion: Drug and its metabolites are excreted in urine. Less than 10% of dose is excreted as unchanged drug in urine. *Half-life:* Elimination of cytarabine is biphasic, with initial half-life of 8 minutes and terminal phase half-life of 1 to 3 hours.

Route	Onset	Peak	Duration
I.V., intrathecal	Unknown	Unknown	Unknown
S.C.	Unknown	20-60 min	Unknown

Action

Chemical effect: Inhibits DNA synthesis.
Therapeutic effect: Kills selected cancer cells.

Available forms

Injection: 100-mg, 500-mg, 1-g, 2-g vials

NURSING PROCESS

⬚ Assessment
• Assess patient's underlying condition before therapy and reassess regularly throughout therapy.
• Monitor uric acid level, hepatic and renal function studies, and CBC.
• Be alert for adverse reactions and drug interactions.
• If patient receives high doses, watch for neurotoxicity, which may first appear as nystagmus but can progress to ataxia and cerebellar dysfunction.
• Evaluate patient's and family's knowledge of drug therapy.

⬚ Nursing diagnoses
• Ineffective health maintenance related to underlying condition
• Risk for injury related to drug-induced adverse hematologic reactions
• Deficient knowledge related to drug therapy

⬚ Planning and implementation
• When giving intrathecally, use preservative-free normal saline solution. Add 5 ml to 100-mg vial or 10 ml to 500-mg vial. Use immediately after reconstitution. Discard unused drug.
• Maintain high fluid intake and give allopurinol to avoid urate nephropathy in leukemia induction therapy.
• If granulocyte count is below 1,000/mm³ or if platelet count is below 50,000/mm³, modify or stop therapy.
• Corticosteroid eyedrops are prescribed to prevent drug-induced keratitis.
• Prescriber must judge possible benefit against known adverse effects.

Patient teaching

• Warn patient to watch for signs of infection (fever, sore throat, fatigue) and bleeding (easy bruising, nosebleeds, bleeding gums, melena). Tell patient to take temperature daily.

• Instruct patient on infection control and bleeding precautions.

• Advise woman of childbearing age to avoid becoming pregnant during therapy. Also recommend consulting with prescriber before becoming pregnant.

• Encourage patient to drink at least 3 L of fluids daily.

• Instruct patient about need for frequent oral hygiene.

☑ Evaluation

• Patient demonstrates positive response to drug therapy.

• Patient doesn't experience injury as result of drug therapy.

• Patient and family state understanding of drug therapy.

---

cytomegalovirus immune globulin, intravenous (CMV-IGIV)

(sigh-toh-meh-GEH-loh-VIGH-rus ih-MYOON GLOH-byoo-lin)
CytoGam

Pharmacologic class: immune globulin
Therapeutic class: immune serum
Pregnancy risk category: C

Indications and dosages

▶ **To attenuate primary CMV disease in seronegative kidney transplant recipients who receive kidney from a CMV seropositive donor.** *Adults:* Give I.V. based on time after transplantation:
within 72 hours: 150 mg/kg
2 weeks after: 100 mg/kg
4 weeks after: 100 mg/kg
6 weeks after: 100 mg/kg
8 weeks after: 100 mg/kg
12 weeks after: 50 mg/kg
16 weeks after: 50 mg/kg.
Give first dose at 15 mg/kg/hour. Increase to 30 mg/kg/hour after 30 minutes if no adverse reactions occur, then increase to 60 mg/kg/hour

after another 30 minutes if no adverse reactions occur. Don't exceed 75 ml/hour. Subsequent doses may be given at 15 mg/kg/hour for 15 minutes, increasing at 15-minute intervals in stepwise fashion to 60 mg/kg/hour.

▶ **Prophylaxis of CMV disease related to lung, liver, pancreas, and heart transplants.** *Adults:* Use with ganciclovir in organ transplants from CMV seropositive donors into seronegative recipients. Maximum total dose per infusion is 150 mg/kg I.V. Given as follows based on time after transplantation:
within 72 hours: 150 mg/kg
2 weeks after: 150 mg/kg
4 weeks after: 150 mg/kg
6 weeks after: 150 mg/kg
8 weeks after: 150 mg/kg
12 weeks after: 100 mg/kg
16 weeks after: 100 mg/kg.
Give first dose at 15 mg/kg/hour. If no adverse reactions occur after 30 minutes, increase rate to 30 mg/kg/hour. If no adverse reactions occur after another 30 minutes, increase infusion to 60 mg/kg/hour. (Don't exceed 75 ml/hour.) Subsequent doses may be given at 15 mg/kg/hour for 15 minutes, increasing every 15 minutes in a stepwise fashion to a maximum of 60 mg/kg/hour. (Don't exceed 75 ml/hour.) Monitor patient closely during and after each rate change.

▼ I.V. administration

• Remove tab portion of vial cap and clean rubber stopper with 70% alcohol or equivalent. Don't shake vial; avoid foaming. Don't infuse if the solution has color or particulate matter, or is turbid. Don't pre-dilute.

• If possible, give through separate I.V. line using constant infusion pump. Filters are unneeded. If unable to give through separate line, piggyback into existing line of saline solution injection or one of the following dextrose solutions with or without saline solution: dextrose 2.5% in water, D_5W, dextrose 10% in water, or dextrose 20% in water. Don't dilute more than 1:2 with any of these solutions.

• Begin infusion within 6 hours of entering vial; finish within 12 hours.

• Refrigerate drug at 36° to 46° F (2° to 8° C).

Contraindications and precautions

• Contraindicated in patients with selective IgA deficiency or history of sensitivity to other human immunoglobulin preparations.

⚖ **Lifespan:** In pregnant women, use cautiously. In breast-feeding women and in children, safety and efficacy of drug haven't been established.

Adverse reactions

CNS: fever.
CV: flushing, hypotension.
GI: nausea, vomiting.
Musculoskeletal: muscle cramps, back pain.
Respiratory: wheezing.
Other: *anaphylaxis*, chills.

Interactions

Drug-drug. *Live-virus vaccines:* Drug may interfere with immune response to live-virus vaccines. Defer vaccination for at least 3 months.

Effects on lab test results

None reported.

Pharmacokinetics

Absorption: Administered I.V.
Distribution: Unknown.
Metabolism: Unknown.
Excretion: Unknown. *Half-life:* Immediately after transplantation, 8 days; 60 or more days after transplantation, 13 to 15 days.

Route	Onset	Peak	Duration
I.V.	Unknown	Unknown	Unknown

Action

Chemical effect: Supplies relatively high concentration of immunoglobulin G (IgG) antibodies against CMV. Increasing these antibody levels in CMV-exposed patients may reduce risk of serious CMV disease.
Therapeutic effect: Provides passive immunity to CMV.

Available forms

Solution for injection: 50 (± 10) mg (of protein) per ml

NURSING PROCESS

⚗ Assessment
• Assess patient's kidney transplant before therapy.
• Take vital signs before starting therapy and then mid-infusion, post-infusion, and before any increase in infusion rate.

• Monitor drug's effectiveness by evaluating kidney function.
• Be alert for adverse reactions and drug interactions.
• Evaluate patient's and family's knowledge of drug therapy.

⊞ Nursing diagnoses
• Risk for injury related to potential for organ rejection
• Decreased cardiac output related to drug-induced hypotension
• Deficient knowledge related to drug therapy

⟩ Planning and implementation
• If patient develops anaphylaxis or if blood pressure drops, stop infusion, notify prescriber, and administer CPR and drugs, such as diphenhydramine and epinephrine.
Patient teaching
• Teach patient about drug therapy.
• Instruct patient to notify prescriber immediately if adverse reactions develop.

☑ Evaluation
• Patient doesn't reject transplanted kidney during drug therapy.
• Patient maintains normal cardiac output throughout drug therapy.
• Patient and family state understanding of drug therapy.

dacarbazine (DTIC)
(deh-KAR-buh-zeen)
DTIC ♦ , DTIC-Dome

Pharmacologic class: alkylating drug (cell-cycle-phase–nonspecific)
Therapeutic class: antineoplastic
Pregnancy risk category: C

Indications and dosages

▶ **Metastatic malignant melanoma.** *Adults:* 2 to 4.5 mg/kg I.V. daily for 10 days; then q 4 weeks, as tolerated. Or, 250 mg/m² I.V. daily for 5 days; repeat at 3-week intervals.

▶ **Hodgkin's disease.** *Adults:* 150 mg/m² I.V. daily (combined with other drugs) for 5 days; repeat q 4 weeks. Or, 375 mg/m² on first day of combination regimen; repeat q 15 days.

▼ I.V. administration

• Preparing and giving drug raises risk of carcinogenic, mutagenic, and teratogenic effects. Follow facility policy to reduce risks.
• Give antiemetics before giving dacarbazine to help decrease nausea. Nausea and vomiting may subside after several doses.
• Reconstitute drug with sterile water for injection. Add 9.9 ml to 100-mg vial or 19.7 ml to 200-mg vial. The resulting solution should be colorless to clear yellow. For infusion, further dilute, using up to 250 ml of normal saline injection or D₅W. Infuse over 30 minutes.
• During infusion, protect bag from direct sunlight to avoid drug breakdown. Solution may be diluted further or infusion slowed to decrease pain at infusion site.
• If infiltration occurs, stop infusion immediately, apply ice to area for 24 to 48 hours, and notify prescriber.
• Reconstituted solutions are stable for 8 hours at room temperature under normal lighting conditions and up to 3 days if refrigerated. Diluted solutions are stable for 8 hours at room temperature under normal light and up to 24 hours if refrigerated. If solutions turn pink, this is a sign of decomposition; discard drug.

Contraindications and precautions

• Contraindicated in patients hypersensitive to drug.
• Use cautiously if patient's bone marrow function is impaired.
≜ **Lifespan:** In pregnant women, use cautiously and only when absolutely needed because fetal harm may occur. In breast-feeding women, drug is contraindicated. In children, safety and efficacy of drug haven't been established.

Adverse reactions

GI: *severe nausea and vomiting, anorexia.*
Hematologic: *leukopenia, thrombocytopenia* (nadir at 3 to 4 weeks).
Metabolic: hyperuricemia.
Skin: alopecia, phototoxicity.
Other: *flulike syndrome* (fever, malaise, myalgia beginning 7 days after treatment and possibly lasting 7 to 21 days), *anaphylaxis,* severe

pain with concentrated solution or extravasation, tissue damage.

Interactions

Drug-drug. *Allopurinol:* May have additive hypouricemic effects. Monitor patient closely.
Anticoagulants, aspirin: May increase risk of bleeding. Avoid using together.
Bone marrow suppressants: May increase toxicity. Monitor hematologic studies closely.
Phenobarbital, phenytoin, and other drugs that induce hepatic metabolism: May enhance dacarbazine metabolism. Dosage adjustment may be needed.
Drug-lifestyle. *Sun exposure:* May cause photosensitivity reactions, especially during the first 2 days of therapy. Advise patient to avoid prolonged sun exposure and to wear protective clothing and sunblock.

Effects on lab test results

• May increase BUN and liver enzyme levels.
• May decrease WBC, RBC, and platelet counts.

Pharmacokinetics

Absorption: Administered I.V.
Distribution: Thought to localize in body tissues, especially the liver; minimally bound to plasma proteins.
Metabolism: Rapidly metabolized in liver to several compounds, some of which may be active.
Excretion: About 30% to 45% of dose excreted in urine. *Half-life:* Initial, 19 minutes; terminal, 5 hours.

Route	Onset	Peak	Duration
I.V.	Unknown	Unknown	Unknown

Action

Chemical effect: Probably cross-links strands of cellular DNA and interferes with RNA transcription, causing imbalance of growth that leads to cell death.
Therapeutic effect: Kills selected cancer cells.

Available forms

Injection: 100-mg, 200-mg vials

NURSING PROCESS

✍ Assessment
• Obtain history of patient's underlying disease before therapy, and reassess regularly throughout therapy.
• Monitor CBC, platelet count, and liver enzyme levels.
• Be alert for adverse reactions and drug interactions.
• Evaluate patient's and family's knowledge of drug therapy.

🔁 Nursing diagnoses
• Ineffective health maintenance related to presence of neoplastic disease
• Risk for injury related to risk of drug-induced adverse reactions
• Deficient knowledge related to drug therapy

⟫ Planning and implementation
• For Hodgkin's disease, drug usually is given with bleomycin, vinblastine, and doxorubicin.
• To prevent bleeding, avoid all I.M. injections when platelet count is below 50,000/mm³.
• Anticipate need for blood transfusions to combat anemia. Patient may receive injections of RBC colony-stimulating factors to promote RBC production and decrease need for blood transfusions.
⑤ **ALERT:** Don't confuse dacarbazine with Dicarbosil, carbamazepine, or procarbazine.
Patient teaching
• Warn patient to watch for signs of infection (fever, sore throat, fatigue) and bleeding (easy bruising, nosebleeds, bleeding gums, melena). Tell patient to take temperature daily.
• Instruct patient to avoid OTC products containing aspirin.
• Advise patient to avoid sunlight and sunlamps for first 2 days after treatment.
• Reassure patient that flulike syndrome may be treated with mild antipyretics, such as acetaminophen.

☑ Evaluation
• Patient exhibits positive response to therapy, as evidenced on follow-up diagnostic studies and overall physical status.
• Patient has no injury from drug-induced adverse reactions.
• Patient and family state understanding of drug therapy.

daclizumab
(da-KLIZ-yoo-mab)
Zenapax

Pharmacologic class: humanized immunoglobulin G₁ monoclonal antibody
Therapeutic class: immunosuppressant
Pregnancy risk category: C

Indications and dosages

▶ **Prevention of acute organ rejection in patients receiving renal transplants with an immunosuppressive regimen that includes cyclosporine and corticosteroids.** *Adults:* 1 mg/kg I.V. Standard course of therapy is five doses. Give first dose no more than 24 hours before transplantation; give remaining four doses at 14-day intervals.

▼ I.V. administration

• Don't use drug as a direct I.V. injection. Dilute in 50 ml of sterile normal saline solution before administration. To avoid foaming, don't shake. Inspect for particulates or discoloration before use; don't use if either occurs.
• Infuse over 15 minutes via a central or peripheral line. Don't add or infuse other drugs simultaneously through the same line.
• Drug may be refrigerated at 36° to 46° F (2° to 8° C) for 24 hours and is stable at room temperature for 4 hours. Discard solution if not used within 24 hours.
• Protect undiluted solution from direct light.

Contraindications and precautions

• Contraindicated in patients hypersensitive to drug and its components.
⚕ **Lifespan:** In pregnant or breast-feeding women, use cautiously. Women of childbearing age should use contraception before beginning drug therapy, during therapy, and for 4 months after ending therapy.

Adverse reactions

CNS: tremors, headache, dizziness, insomnia, generalized weakness, prickly sensation, fever, pain, fatigue, depression, anxiety.
CV: tachycardia, hypertension, hypotension, aggravated hypertension, edema, fluid overload, chest pain.
EENT: blurred vision, pharyngitis, rhinitis.

Reactions may be *common*, uncommon, *life-threatening*, or COMMON AND LIFE-THREATENING.

GI: constipation, nausea, diarrhea, vomiting, abdominal pain, dyspepsia, pyrosis, abdominal distention, epigastric pain, flatulence, gastritis, hemorrhoids.

GU: *oliguria,* dysuria, *renal tubular necrosis,* renal damage, urine retention, hydronephrosis, urinary tract bleeding, urinary tract disorder, renal insufficiency.

Hematologic: lymphocele, bleeding.

Metabolic: diabetes mellitus, dehydration.

Musculoskeletal: musculoskeletal or back pain, arthralgia, myalgia, leg cramps.

Respiratory: dyspnea, coughing, atelectasis, congestion, *hypoxia,* rales, abnormal breath sounds, pleural effusion, *pulmonary edema.*

Skin: acne, impaired wound healing without infection, pruritus, hirsutism, rash, night sweats, increased sweating.

Other: shivering, limb edema.

Interactions

Drug-drug. *Corticosteroids, cyclosporine, mycophenolate mofetil:* May increase risk of death, especially in those taking antilymphocyte antibodies and in those with severe infections. Avoid using together.

Effects on lab test results

● May increase BUN and creatinine levels.

Pharmacokinetics

Absorption: Administered I.V.
Distribution: Unknown.
Metabolism: Unknown.
Excretion: Unknown. *Half-life:* 20 days.

Route	Onset	Peak	Duration
I.V.	Unknown	Unknown	Unknown

Action

Chemical effect: Inhibits IL-2 binding to prevent IL-2–mediated activation of lymphocytes, a critical pathway in the cellular immune response against allografts. Once in circulation, drug impairs response of immune system.

Therapeutic effect: Prevents organ rejection.

Available forms

Injection: 25 mg/5 ml

⚐ Assessment
● Obtain history of patient's underlying condition before therapy, and reassess regularly.
● Check for opportunistic infections.
● Monitor patient for anaphylactoid reactions.
● Evaluate patient's and family's knowledge of drug therapy.

⊕ Nursing diagnoses
● Risk for injury related to potential for organ rejection
● Ineffective protection related to drug-induced immunosuppression
● Deficient knowledge related to drug therapy

❯ Planning and implementation
● Use only under supervision of a prescriber experienced in immunosuppressant therapy and management of organ transplantation.
● Drug is used as part of an immunosuppressant regimen that includes corticosteroids and cyclosporine.
● Keep drugs used to treat anaphylactic reactions immediately available.

Patient teaching
● Tell patient to consult prescriber before taking other drugs during therapy.
● Advise patient to take precautions against infection.
● Inform patient that neither he nor any household member should receive vaccinations unless medically approved.
● Tell patient to immediately report wounds that fail to heal, unusual bruising or bleeding, or fever.
● Advise patient to drink plenty of fluids during therapy and to report painful urination, blood in the urine, or a decrease in urine amount.
● Instruct women of childbearing age to use effective contraception before starting therapy and to continue until 4 months after completing therapy.

☑ Evaluation
● Patient doesn't experience organ rejection while taking drug.
● Patient is free from infection and serious bleeding episodes throughout drug therapy.
● Patient and family state understanding of drug therapy.

dalteparin sodium
(dal-TEH-peh-rin SOH-dee-um)
Fragmin

Pharmacologic class: low–molecular-weight heparin
Therapeutic class: anticoagulant
Pregnancy risk category: B

Indications and dosages

▶ **Prevention of deep vein thrombosis (DVT) in patients undergoing abdominal or hip replacement surgery who are at risk for thromboembolism.** *Adults:* 2,500 IU S.C. daily. Start 1 to 2 hours before surgery and repeat once daily for 5 to 10 days after surgery until patient is mobile. Or, 5,000 IU S.C. the evening before surgery. Repeat q evening for 5 to 10 days until patient is mobile.

▶ **To decrease risk of thromboembolism in patients with severely restricted mobility.** *Adults:* 5,000 IU S.C. daily for 12 to 14 days.

▶ **Unstable angina, non-Q wave MI.** *Adults:* 120 IU/kg up to 10,000 IU S.C. q 12 hours with oral aspirin (75 to 165 mg/day) therapy. Continue until patient is stable.

Contraindications and precautions

● Contraindicated in patients hypersensitive to drug, heparin, or pork products and in those with major bleeding or thrombocytopenia with positive in vitro tests for antiplatelet antibody in presence of drug.

● Use cautiously in patients with a history of heparin-induced thrombocytopenia; in patients with an increased risk of hemorrhage, such as those with severe uncontrolled hypertension, bacterial endocarditis, congenital or acquired bleeding disorders, active ulceration, angiodysplastic GI disease, or hemorrhagic CVA; and in those who recently underwent brain, spinal, or ophthalmologic surgery.

● Also use cautiously in patients with bleeding diathesis, thrombocytopenia, platelet defects, severe liver or kidney insufficiency, hypertensive or diabetic retinopathy, or recent GI bleeding.

☀ Lifespan: In pregnant or breast-feeding women, use cautiously. In children, safety and efficacy of drug haven't been established.

Adverse reactions

CNS: fever.
Hematologic: *hemorrhage,* bleeding complications, *thrombocytopenia.*
Skin: pruritus, ecchymosis, rash.
Other: *anaphylaxis, hematoma at injection site* (when given with heparin), pain at injection site.

Interactions

Drug-drug. *Antiplatelet drugs, oral anticoagulants:* May increase risk of bleeding. Use together cautiously; monitor patient for bleeding.

Effects on lab test results

● May increase ALT and AST levels.
● May decrease platelet count.

Pharmacokinetics

Absorption: Absolute bioavailability of anti-factor Xa is 87%.
Distribution: Volume of distribution is 40 to 60 ml/kg.
Metabolism: Unknown.
Excretion: Excreted in urine. *Half-life:* 3 to 5 hours.

Route	Onset	Peak	Duration
S.C.	Unknown	4 hr	Unknown

Action

Chemical effect: Enhances inhibition of factor Xa and thrombin by antithrombin.
Therapeutic effect: Prevents DVT.

Available forms

Multidose vial: 10,000 anti-factor Xa IU/ml
Syringe: 2,500 anti-factor Xa IU/0.2 ml; 5,000 anti-factor Xa IU/0.2 ml

NURSING PROCESS

⚗ Assessment
● Obtain history of patient's underlying condition before starting therapy.
● Monitor effectiveness by assessing patient for evidence of DVT.
● Routine CBCs (including platelet count) and fecal occult blood tests are recommended during treatment.
● Be alert for adverse reactions and drug interactions.
● Evaluate patient's and family's knowledge of drug therapy.

⊕ Nursing diagnoses

• Risk for injury related to risk of DVT as result of underlying condition
• Ineffective protection related to drug-induced adverse hematologic reactions
• Deficient knowledge related to drug therapy

⧁ Planning and implementation

• Candidates for therapy are those at risk for DVT. Risk factors include being older than age 40, being obese, and having surgery under general anesthesia lasting longer than 30 minutes. Additional risk factors include cancer and a history of DVT or pulmonary embolism.
• Place patient in sitting or supine position when giving drug. Give S.C. injection deeply. Injection sites include U-shaped area below navel, upper outer side of thigh, and upper outer quadrangle of buttock. Rotate sites daily.
⊛ **ALERT:** Drug should never be given I.M. or I.V.
• Don't mix with other injections or infusions unless specific compatibility data are available that support such mixing.
⊛ **ALERT:** Drug isn't interchangeable (unit for unit) with unfractionated heparin or other low–molecular-weight heparin derivatives.
• Stop drug and notify prescriber if a thromboembolism occurs despite therapy.
Patient teaching
• Instruct patient and family to watch for signs of bleeding and notify prescriber immediately.
• Tell patient to avoid OTC medications containing aspirin or other salicylates.

☑ Evaluation

• Patient doesn't develop DVT.
• Patient maintains stable hematologic function.
• Patient and family state understanding of drug therapy.

---

dantrolene sodium
(DAN-troh-leen SOH-dee-um)
Dantrium, Dantrium Intravenous

Pharmacologic class: hydantoin derivative
Therapeutic class: skeletal muscle relaxant
Pregnancy risk category: C

Indications and dosages

▶ **Spasticity and sequelae from severe chronic disorders (such as multiple sclerosis, cerebral palsy, spinal cord injury, CVA).** *Adults:* 25 mg P.O. daily. Increase in 25-mg increments up to 100 mg b.i.d. to q.i.d. Maximum, 400 mg daily. Maintain each dosage level for 4 to 7 days to determine response.
Children: Initially, 0.5 mg/kg P.O. b.i.d., increase to t.i.d. and then to q.i.d. Increase dose as needed by 0.5 mg/kg daily to 3 mg/kg b.i.d. to q.i.d. Maximum, 100 mg q.i.d.
▶ **Management of malignant hyperthermic crisis.** *Adults and children:* 1 mg/kg I.V. initially, then repeat as needed up to a total dose of 10 mg/kg.
▶ **Prevention or attenuation of malignant hyperthermia in susceptible patients who need surgery.** *Adults:* 4 to 8 mg/kg P.O. daily in three or four divided doses for 1 or 2 days before procedure. Final dose 3 to 4 hours before procedure. Or, 2.5 mg/kg I.V. infused over 1 hour about 1 hour before anesthesia. Additional doses, which must be individualized, may be given intraoperatively, if needed.
▶ **Prevention of recurrence of malignant hyperthermia.** *Adults:* 4 to 8 mg/kg P.O. daily in four divided doses for up to 3 days after hyperthermic crisis.
▶ **To reduce succinylcholine-induced muscle fasciculations and postoperative muscle pain‡.** *Adults weighing less than 45 kg (99 lb):* 100 mg P.O. 2 hours before succinylcholine. *Adults weighing more than 45 kg:* 150 mg P.O. 2 hours before succinylcholine.

▽ I.V. administration

• Give as soon as malignant hyperthermia reaction is recognized.
• Reconstitute each vial with 60 ml of sterile water for injection, and shake vial until clear. Don't use diluent that contains bacteriostatic agent.
• Protect contents from light and use within 6 hours.
• Monitor patient for extravasation.

Contraindications and precautions

• Contraindicated in patients whose spasticity is used to maintain motor function and in patients with upper motor neuron disorders, spasms from rheumatic disorders, or active hepatic disease.

• Use cautiously in women and in patients with hepatic disease or severely impaired cardiac or pulmonary function.

⚖ **Lifespan:** In pregnant women and patients older than age 35, use cautiously. In breast-feeding women, drug is contraindicated.

Adverse reactions

CNS: *muscle weakness, drowsiness, dizziness,* light-headedness, *malaise,* headache, confusion, nervousness, insomnia, hallucinations, *seizures,* fever.
CV: tachycardia, blood pressure changes.
EENT: excessive tearing, auditory or visual disturbances.
GI: anorexia, constipation, cramping, dysphagia, metallic taste, severe diarrhea, drooling, *bleeding.*
GU: urinary frequency, hematuria, incontinence, nocturia, dysuria, crystalluria, difficulty achieving erection.
Hepatic: *hepatitis.*
Musculoskeletal: myalgia.
Respiratory: pleural effusion.
Skin: diaphoresis, abnormal hair growth, eczematous eruption, pruritus, urticaria, photosensitivity.
Other: chills.

Interactions

Drug-drug. *CNS depressants:* May increase CNS depression. Avoid using together.
Estrogens: May increase risk of hepatotoxicity. Use together cautiously.
I.V. verapamil: May cause CV collapse. Never give together. Stop verapamil before giving I.V. dantrolene.
Drug-lifestyle. *Alcohol use:* May increase CNS depression. Avoid using together.
Sunlight: Photosensitivity may occur. Urge patient to avoid prolonged and unprotected sun exposure.

Effects on lab test results

• May increase BUN, ALT, AST, and bilirubin levels.

Pharmacokinetics

Absorption: 35% of P.O. dose absorbed through GI tract.
Distribution: Substantially bound to plasma protein, mainly albumin.

Metabolism: Metabolized in liver to its less active 5-hydroxy derivatives and to its amino derivative by reductive pathways.
Excretion: Excreted in urine as metabolites.
Half-life: P.O., 9 hours; I.V., 4 to 8 hours.

Route	Onset	Peak	Duration
P.O.	≤ 1 week	5 hr	Unknown
I.V.	Unknown	Unknown	Unknown

Action

Chemical effect: Acts directly on skeletal muscle to interfere with intracellular calcium movement.
Therapeutic effect: Relieves muscle spasms.

Available forms

Capsules: 25 mg, 50 mg, 100 mg
Injection: 20 mg/vial

NURSING PROCESS

⚗ Assessment
• Obtain history of patient's spasticity disorder before therapy.
• Obtain liver function tests at start of therapy.
• Monitor effectiveness by evaluating severity of spasticity.
• Be alert for adverse reactions and drug interactions.
• Evaluate patient's and family's knowledge of drug therapy.

⊞ Nursing diagnoses
• Acute pain related to presence of spasticity disorder
• Risk for injury related to drug-induced adverse reactions
• Deficient knowledge related to drug therapy

▷ Planning and implementation
• For optimum drug effect, give daily amount in four divided doses.
• Give drug with meals or milk to prevent GI distress.
• Prepare oral suspension for single dose by dissolving capsule contents in juice or other suitable liquid. For multiple doses, use acid vehicle, such as citric acid in USP syrup. Refrigerate, and use within several days.
• Amount of relief determines whether dosage can be reduced.

Reactions may be *common*, uncommon, *life-threatening*, or COMMON AND LIFE-THREATENING.

• If hepatitis, severe diarrhea, severe weakness, or sensitivity reactions occur, withhold dose and immediately notify prescriber.

⑤ **ALERT:** Don't confuse Dantrium with Daraprim.

Patient teaching

• Tell patient to use caution when eating to avoid choking. Some patients may have trouble swallowing during therapy.

• Warn patient to avoid hazardous activities until full CNS effects of drug are known.

• Advise patient to avoid combining dantrolene with alcohol or other CNS depressants.

• Tell patient to use sunblock and wear protective clothing, to report GI problems immediately, and to follow prescriber's orders regarding rest and physical therapy.

☑ **Evaluation**

• Patient states that pain from muscle spasticity has lessened.

• Patient has no injury from drug-induced adverse reactions.

• Patient and family state understanding of drug therapy.

dapsone (DDS)
(DAP-sohn)
Avlosulfon ♦ , Dapsone 100 ◇

Pharmacologic class: synthetic sulfone
Therapeutic class: antileprotic, antimalarial
Pregnancy risk category: C

Indications and dosages

▶ **Multibacillary leprosy.** *Adults:* 100 mg P.O. daily given with rifampin and clofazimine for 12 months.
Children ages 10 to 14: 50 mg P.O. daily given with rifampin and clofazimine for 12 months.
▶ **Paucibacillary leprosy.** *Adults:* 100 mg P.O. daily given with rifampin for 6 months.
Children ages 10 to 14: 50 mg P.O. daily given with rifampin for 6 months.
Children younger than age 10: 25 mg P.O. daily given with rifampin for 6 months.
▶ **Dermatitis herpetiformis.** *Adults:* Initially, 50 mg P.O. daily; increase to 300 mg daily if symptoms aren't completely controlled. Reduce dose to lowest effective level as soon as possible.

▶ **Malaria suppression or prophylaxis‡.**
Adults: 100 mg P.O. weekly, given with pyrimethamine 12.5 mg P.O. weekly.
Children: 2 mg/kg P.O. weekly given with pyrimethamine 0.25 mg/kg weekly. Continue prophylaxis throughout exposure and for 6 months after exposure.
▶ *Pneumocystis carinii* **pneumonia‡.** *Adults:* 100 mg P.O. daily. Usually given with trimethoprim 20 mg/kg daily, for 21 days.
▶ **Prophylaxis of** *P. carinii* **pneumonia‡.** *Adults:* 50 mg P.O. b.i.d. or 100 mg P.O. daily.
▶ **Prophylaxis of toxoplasmosis in HIV-infected patients‡.** *Adults and adolescents:* 50 mg P.O. daily given with pyrimethamine 50 mg P.O. once weekly and leucovorin 25 mg P.O. once weekly.
Children older than age 1 month: 2 mg/kg or 15 mg/m² (maximum 25 mg) P.O. once daily given with pyrimethamine and leucovorin.

Contraindications and precautions

• Contraindicated in patients hypersensitive to drug.

• Use cautiously in patients with chronic renal, hepatic, or CV disease; refractory types of anemia; or G6PD deficiency.

⚖ **Lifespan:** In pregnant women, use cautiously. In breast-feeding women, drug is contraindicated.

Adverse reactions

CNS: fever, insomnia, psychosis, headache, dizziness, lethargy, severe malaise, paresthesia, peripheral neuropathy, vertigo.
CV: tachycardia.
EENT: tinnitus, blurred vision, allergic rhinitis.
GI: anorexia, abdominal pain, *pancreatitis,* nausea, vomiting.
GU: albuminuria, nephrotic syndrome, renal papillary necrosis, male infertility.
Hematologic: *aplastic anemia, agranulocytosis,* hemolytic anemia, *methemoglobinemia, leukopenia.*
Hepatic: *hepatitis,* cholestatic jaundice.
Respiratory: pulmonary eosinophilia.
Skin: allergic dermatitis, lupus erythematosus, phototoxicity, exfoliative dermatitis, toxic erythema, *erythema multiforme, toxic epidermal necrolysis,* morbilliform and scarlatiniform reactions, urticaria, erythema nodosum.
Other: infectious mononucleosis-like syndrome, *sulfone syndrome,* lymphadenopathy.

Interactions

Drug-drug. *Activated charcoal:* Decreases GI absorption of dapsone. Monitor patient.
Folic acid antagonists (such as methotrexate): May increase risk of adverse hematologic reactions. Monitor patient carefully.
Didanosine: May increase dapsone absorption, leading to therapeutic failure and an increase in infection. Give drug at least 2 hours before or after didanosine.
Rifampin: May increase hepatic metabolism and renal excretion of dapsone. Monitor patient closely.
PABA: May antagonize effect of dapsone by interfering with the primary mechanism of action. Monitor patient.
Probenecid: Decreases urinary excretion of dapsone metabolites, increasing plasma levels. Monitor patient.
Trimethoprim: Increases levels of both drugs, increasing pharmacologic and toxic effects. Monitor patient closely for toxicity.
Drug-lifestyle. *Sunlight:* Photosensitivity may occur. Advise patient to avoid sun exposure and wear protective clothing and sunblock.

Effects on lab test results

• May increase liver enzyme levels.
• May decrease hemoglobin, hematocrit, and WBC, RBC, and granulocyte counts.

Pharmacokinetics

Absorption: Rapid and almost complete.
Distribution: Distributed widely in most body tissues and fluids; 70% to 90% is plasma protein-bound.
Metabolism: Undergoes acetylation by liver enzymes; rate varies and is genetically determined. Almost 50% of Blacks and Whites are slow acetylators, whereas more than 80% of Chinese, Japanese, and Eskimos are fast acetylators. Dosage adjustment may be needed.
Excretion: Dapsone and metabolites excreted primarily in urine; small amounts excreted in feces. *Half-life:* 10 to 50 hours.

Route	Onset	Peak	Duration
P.O.	Unknown	4-8 hr	Unknown

Action

Chemical effect: Unknown; may inhibit folic acid biosynthesis in susceptible organisms (bacteriostatic).

Therapeutic effect: Hinders or kills selected bacteria.

Available forms

Tablets: 25 mg, 100 mg

NURSING PROCESS

⚕ Assessment

• Obtain history of patient's underlying infection and CBC before therapy.
• Monitor effectiveness by assessing for improvement of infection and evaluating culture and sensitivity test results.
• Monitor CBC weekly for first month, monthly for 6 months, and semiannually thereafter.
• Be alert for adverse reactions and drug interactions.
• Evaluate patient's and family's knowledge of drug therapy.

🔷 Nursing diagnoses

• Infection related to presence of susceptible bacteria
• Risk of impaired skin integrity related to drug-induced adverse dermatologic reactions
• Deficient knowledge related to drug therapy

▶ Planning and implementation

• Reduce dosage or temporarily stop drug if hemoglobin falls below 9 g/dl, if WBC count falls below 5,000/mm^3, or if RBC count falls below 2.5 million/mm^3 or remains low.
• If generalized diffuse dermatitis occurs, notify prescriber and prepare to interrupt therapy regimen.
• Give antihistamines to combat drug-induced allergic dermatitis.
• In severe erythema nodosum, therapy should be stopped and glucocorticoids given cautiously.
• Evidence of sulfone syndrome includes fever, malaise, and jaundice with hepatic necrosis. If symptoms occur, immediately stop drug therapy and notify prescriber.
Patient teaching
• Inform patient of need for periodic laboratory studies.
• Teach patient to watch for and promptly report adverse dermatologic changes because such reactions may necessitate stopping drug.
• Warn patient to avoid hazardous activities that require alertness if adverse CNS reactions occur.

Reactions may be *common*, uncommon, *life-threatening*, or COMMON AND LIFE-THREATENING.

☑ Evaluation

• Patient is free from infection.
• Patient maintains normal skin integrity throughout therapy.
• Patient and family state understanding of drug therapy.

daptomycin
(dap-toh-MY-sin)
Cubicin

Pharmacologic class: cyclic lipopeptide antibacterial
Therapeutic class: antibiotic
Pregnancy risk category: B

Indications & dosages

▶ **Complicated skin and skin structure infections caused by susceptible strains of** *Staphylococcus aureus* **(including methicillin-resistant strains),** *Streptococcus pyogenes,* *Streptococcus agalactiae, Streptococcus dysgalactiae,* **and** *Enterococcus faecalis* **(vancomycin-susceptible strains only).** *Adults:* 4 mg/kg by I.V. infusion over 30 minutes q 24 hours for 7 to 14 days.
🔲 **Adjust-a-dose:** For patients renal impairment including those receiving hemodialysis or continuous ambulatory peritoneal dialysis, if creatinine clearance is below 30 ml/minute, give 4 mg/kg I.V. q 48 hours. When possible, give drug after hemodialysis.

▼ I.V. administration

• Reconstitute 250-mg vial with 5 ml of normal saline solution and 500-mg vial with 10 ml. Further dilute admixture with normal saline solution. Vials are for single use; discard excess.
• Drug is incompatible with dextrose solutions and other drugs. Drug is compatible with normal saline solution and lactated Ringer's injection. If a line is used for several drugs, flush it with compatible fluids between drugs.
• For intermittent infusion, give drug over 30 minutes.
• Refrigerate vials at 36° to 46° F (2° to 8° C). Reconstituted and diluted solutions are stable 12 hours at room temperature or 48 hours at 36° to 46° F (2° to 8° C).

Contraindications and precautions

▶ Contraindicated in patients hypersensitive to drug.
▶ Use cautiously in those with renal insufficiency.
🌡 **Lifespan:** In pregnant and breast-feeding women, use cautiously. In children, safety and efficacy haven't been established. In patients over age 65, drug may provide less-successful treatment and cause more adverse reactions. Use cautiously in these patients.

Adverse reactions

CNS: anxiety, confusion, dizziness, fever, headache, insomnia.
CV: *heart failure,* chest pain, edema, hypertension, hypotension.
EENT: sore throat.
GI: abdominal pain, constipation, decreased appetite, diarrhea, nausea, *pseudomembranous colitis,* vomiting.
GU: *renal failure,* UTI.
Hematologic: anemia.
Metabolic: hyperglycemia, *hypoglycemia,* hypokalemia.
Musculoskeletal: limb and back pain.
Respiratory: cough, dyspnea.
Skin: cellulitis, pruritus, rash.
Other: injection site reactions, fungal infections.

Interactions

Drug-drug. *HMG-CoA reductase inhibitors:* May increase risk of myopathy. Consider stopping these drugs while giving daptomycin. *Tobramycin:* May affect levels of both drugs. Use together cautiously. *Warfarin:* May alter anticoagulant activity. Monitor PT and INR for the first several days of daptomycin therapy.

Effects on lab test results

• May increase CPK and alkaline phosphatase levels. May decrease potassium level. May increase or decrease glucose level.
• May increase liver function test values. May decrease hemoglobin and hematocrit.

Pharmacokinetics

Absorption: Administered I.V.
Distribution: 92% protein bound, primarily to albumin.
Metabolism: Unknown.

Excretion: Primarily by the kidney. *Half-life:* About 8 hours.

Route	Onset	Peak	Duration
I.V.	Rapid	< 1 hr	Unknown

Action

Chemical effect: Binds to and depolarizes bacterial membranes to inhibit protein, DNA, and RNA synthesis.
Therapeutic effect: Kills bacteria in susceptible organisms.

Available forms

Powder for injection: 250-mg vial, 500-mg vial

NURSING PROCESS

⚗ Assessment
• Monitor CBC and renal and liver function tests periodically.
• Monitor patient for superinfection because drug may cause overgrowth of nonsusceptible organisms.
• Watch for evidence of pseudomembranous colitis and treat accordingly.
• Evaluate patient's and family's knowledge of drug therapy.

⊕ Nursing diagnoses
• Risk for infection related to bacteria
• Impaired urine elimination related to daptomycin-induced renal failure.
• Deficient knowledge related to drug therapy.

▶ Planning and implementation
• Obtain specimen for culture and sensitivity tests before giving first dose.
⊛ **ALERT:** Because drug may increase the risk of myopathy, monitor CPK levels weekly. If CPK levels rise, monitor them more often. Stop drug in patients with evidence of myopathy and CPK levels over 1,000 units/L. Also stop drug in patients with CPK levels more than 10 times the upper limit of normal. Consider stopping all other drugs linked with myopathy (such as HMG-CoA reductase inhibitors).
Patient teaching
• Advise patient to immediately report muscle weakness and infusion site irritation.
• Tell patient to report severe diarrhea, rash, and infection.

• Inform patient about possible adverse reactions.

☑ Evaluation
• Patient's infection is eradicated.
• Patient's renal function test values remain unchanged.
• Patient and family state understanding of drug therapy.

darbepoetin alfa
(dar-be-POE-e-tin AL-fa)
Aranesp

Pharmacologic class: hematopoietic
Therapeutic class: antianemic
Pregnancy risk category: C

Indications and dosages

▶ **Anemia related to chronic renal failure (CRF) for patient on or off dialysis.** *Adults:* Initially, 0.45 mcg/kg I.V. or S.C. once weekly. Titrate dose to achieve and maintain a target hemoglobin not exceeding 12 g/dl. Don't increase dose more often than monthly. In patients being converted from epoetin alfa, starting dose should be based on the previous epoetin alfa dose, according to this table.

Previous weekly epoetin alfa dose (units/wk)	Weekly darbepoetin alfa dose (mcg/wk)
< 2,500	6.25
2,500-4,999	12.5
5,000-10,999	25
11,000-17,999	40
18,000-33,999	60
34,000-89,999	100
> 90,000	200

⊛ **ALERT:** Give drug less often than epoetin alfa because its half-life is 3 times longer. If patient was receiving epoetin alfa two to three times weekly, he should receive darbepoetin alfa once weekly. If patient was receiving epoetin alfa once weekly, he should receive darbepoetin alfa once every 2 weeks.
◪ **Adjust-a-dose:** If hemoglobin is increasing and approaching 12 g/dl, reduce dose by 25%. If hemoglobin continues to increase, withhold dose until hemoglobin begins to decrease, and

---

restart at a dose 25% below the previous dose. If hemoglobin increases by more than 1 g/dl over 2 weeks, decrease dose by 25%. If increase is less than 1 g/dl over 4 weeks and iron stores are adequate, increase the dose by 25% of previous dose. Further increases can be made at 4-week intervals until target hemoglobin is reached.

Patients who don't need dialysis may need lower maintenance doses because predialysis patients may be more responsive to the effects of darbepoetin alfa and need close monitoring of blood pressure, hemoglobin, renal function, and electrolyte balance.

Drug decreases plasma volume, thereby reducing dialysis efficiency. Thus, patients who are on dialysis may need adjustments in their dialysis prescription.

▶ **Anemia related to chemotherapy in patients with nonmyeloid malignancies.**
Adults: 2.25 mcg/kg S.C. once weekly.
◪ **Adjust-a-dose:** If hemoglobin increases less than 1 g/dl after 6 weeks of therapy, increase dose to 4.5 mcg/kg. If hemoglobin increases by more than 1 g/dl in a 2-week period or if it exceeds 12 g/dl, reduce dose by 25%. If hemoglobin exceeds 13 g/dl, withhold drug until hemoglobin drops to 12 g/dl and restart dose at 25% below the previous dose.

▽ I.V. administration

● Don't shake drug because doing so can denature it.
● Drug is provided in single-dose vials without a preservative. Don't pool or retain unused portions.
● If drug has particulate matter or is discolored, don't use.
● Give undiluted by I.V. injection.
● Don't give with other drug solutions.
● Store drug in refrigerator; don't freeze. Protect drug from light.

Contraindications and precautions

● Contraindicated in patients hypersensitive to drug or its components and in patients with uncontrolled hypertension.
● Use cautiously in patients with underlying hematologic disease, such as hemolytic anemia, sickle cell anemia, thalassemia, or porphyria, because safety and efficacy haven't been established.
☀ Lifespan: In pregnant women and children, safety and efficacy of drug haven't been estab-

lished. With breast-feeding women, use cautiously because it's unknown whether drug appears in breast milk. Elderly patients may have greater sensitivity to the drug.

Adverse reactions

CNS: *headache, dizziness, fatigue, fever,* asthenia, *seizures.*
CV: *hypertension, hypotension,* CARDIAC ARRHYTHMIA, CARDIAC ARREST, angina, *heart failure, thrombosis, edema,* chest pain, fluid overload, *acute MI.*
GI: *diarrhea, vomiting, nausea, abdominal pain,* constipation.
Metabolic: dehydration.
Musculoskeletal: *myalgia, arthralgia, limb pain,* back pain.
Respiratory: *upper respiratory tract infection, dyspnea, cough,* bronchitis, pneumonia, *pulmonary embolism.*
Skin: hemorrhage at access site, pruritus, rash.
Other: *infection,* flulike symptoms.

Interactions

None reported.

Effects on lab test results

● May decrease ferritin level.
● May increase hemoglobin, hematocrit, and RBC count.

Pharmacokinetics

Absorption: Slow and rate-limiting. Bioavailability ranges from 30% to 50% (mean: 37%).
Distribution: Predominantly confined to the vascular space.
Metabolism: Unknown.
Excretion: Steady-state levels occur within 4 weeks. *Half-life:* 21 hours for I.V. route; 49 hours for S.C. injection.

Route	Onset	Peak	Duration
I.V.	Unknown	Unknown	21 hr
S.C.	Unknown	34 hr	49 hr

Action

Chemical effect: Stimulates erythropoiesis, which increases hemoglobin, by the same mechanism as endogenous erythropoietin. Endogenous erythropoietin, produced by the kidneys, is released into the bloodstream in response to hypoxia and increases RBC production. Production of endogenous erythropoietin is impaired in patients with chronic renal impairment, and erythropoietin deficiency is the primary cause of anemia.

Therapeutic effect: Increases RBC production and corrects anemia in patients with chronic renal impairment.

Available forms

Injection (albumin solution): 25 mcg/ml, 40 mcg/ml, 60 mcg/ml, 100 mcg/ml, 200 mcg/ml single-dose vials
Injection (polysorbate solution): 25 mcg/ml, 40 mcg/ml, 60 mcg/ml, 100 mcg/ml, 200 mcg/ml single-dose vials

NURSING PROCESS

⚡ Assessment

• Drug may increase blood pressure. Blood pressure should be adequately controlled before starting therapy. Obtain baseline blood pressure before initiating therapy, and carefully monitor and control patient's blood pressure during drug therapy.
• Monitor renal function and electrolytes in predialysis patients.
• **ALERT:** Hemoglobin may not increase until 2 to 6 weeks after therapy starts. Monitor hemoglobin weekly until stabilized. Don't exceed the target level of 12 g/dl in patients with chronic renal impairment.
• Drug may increase risk of CV events; carefully monitor and assess patient.
• Patient may have seizures. Follow patient closely, especially during the first several months of therapy.

⊕ Nursing diagnoses

• Risk for injury related to drug-induced adverse cardiac events
• Fatigue related to underlying anemia
• Deficient knowledge related to darbepoetin alfa therapy

▷ Planning and implementation

• **ALERT:** Decrease dose if hemoglobin increases 1 g/dl in any 2-week period. Any increase greater than 1 g/dl within a 2-week period will increase the risk of adverse CV reactions, such as seizures, CVA, exacerbation of hypertension, heart failure, acute MI, fluid overload, edema, or vascular thrombosis, infarction, or ischemia. If symptoms occur, decrease drug dose by 25%.

• Monitor iron before and during treatment. Provide supplemental iron if ferritin level is less than 100 mcg/L and transferrin saturation is less than 20%.
• Serious allergic reactions, including rash and urticaria, may occur. If an anaphylactic reaction occurs, stop drug and give appropriate therapy.
• The maximum safe dosage isn't known. Although doses greater than 3 mcg/kg/week for up to 28 weeks can be given, an excessive rise or rate of rise of hemoglobin leads to adverse reactions. If patient has polycythemia, don't give drug.
• If patient doesn't respond to drug therapy, reevaluate patient for other etiologies that may inhibit erythropoiesis, such as folic acid or vitamin B_{12} deficiencies, infections, inflammatory or malignant processes, osteofibrosis cystica, occult blood loss, hemolysis, severe aluminum toxicity, and bone marrow fibrosis.

Patient teaching
• Teach patient how to give drug properly, including how to use and dispose of needles.
• Advise patient of possible adverse effects and allergic reactions.
• Inform patient of need to frequently monitor blood pressure, hemoglobin, and hematocrit. Also, advise patient to comply with any prescribed antihypertensive drug therapy and dietary restrictions to keep blood pressure under control. Uncontrolled blood pressure is believed to cause seizures and hypertensive encephalopathy in patients with chronic renal failure.

☑ Evaluation

• Patient's hemoglobin increases to no more than 12 g/dl.
• Patient's blood pressure remains adequately controlled and patient doesn't suffer any adverse reactions related to drug therapy.
• Patient and family state understanding of drug therapy.

daunorubicin citrate liposomal

(daw-noh-roo-BYE-sin SIH-trayt li-po-SOE-mul)
DaunoXome

Pharmacologic class: anthracycline
Therapeutic class: antineoplastic
Pregnancy risk category: D

Indications and dosages

▶ **First-line cytotoxic therapy for advanced HIV-related Kaposi's sarcoma.** *Adults:* 40 mg/m² I.V. over 60 minutes once q 2 weeks. Treatment should continue unless patient shows signs of progressive disease or until other complications of HIV prevent continuing.

🔲 **Adjust-a-dose:** For patients with renal or hepatic impairment, if bilirubin is 1.2 to 3 mg/dl, give ¾ of normal dose; if bilirubin or creatinine is greater than 3 mg/dl, give ½ the normal dose.

▼ I.V. administration

• Drug should be diluted with D₅W—and only D₅W—before administration. Withdraw the calculated volume of drug from the vial, and transfer it into an equivalent amount of D₅W. The recommended concentration after dilution is 1 mg/ml.

• Don't mix with other drugs, saline solution, bacteriostatic agents, or any other solution.

• After dilution, immediately administer I.V. over 60 minutes. If unable to use drug immediately, refrigerate at 36° to 46° F (2° to 8° C) for a maximum of 6 hours.

• Don't use in-line filters for I.V. infusion.

• Because local tissue necrosis is possible, monitor I.V. site closely to avoid extravasation. If extravasation occurs, stop I.V., apply ice, and notify prescriber.

🔆 **ALERT:** Monitor patient for adverse reactions. A triad of back pain, flushing, and chest tightness may occur within the first 5 minutes of the infusion. These symptoms subside after stopping the infusion and typically don't recur when the infusion resumes at a slower rate.

• Follow facility policy for handling and disposing of antineoplastics.

Contraindications and precautions

• Contraindicated in patients hypersensitive to drug or its constituents.

• Use cautiously in patients with myelosuppression, cardiac disease, previous radiotherapy involving the heart, previous anthracycline use (doxorubicin > 300 mg/m² or equivalent), or hepatic or renal impairment.

⚠ **Lifespan:** In pregnant women, avoid use; may harm fetus. In children and elderly patients, safety and effectiveness haven't been established.

Adverse reactions

CNS: *fever, headache, neuropathy,* depression, dizziness, insomnia, amnesia, anxiety, ataxia, confusion, *seizures,* hallucinations, tremor, hypertonia, meningitis, *fatigue,* malaise, emotional lability, abnormal gait, hyperkinesia, somnolence, abnormal thinking, syncope.

CV: *cardiomyopathy,* chest pain, hypertension, palpitations, *arrhythmias, pericardial effusion, cardiac tamponade, cardiac arrest,* angina pectoris, *pulmonary hypertension,* flushing, edema, tachycardia, *MI.*

EENT: *rhinitis,* sinusitis, abnormal vision, conjunctivitis, tinnitus, eye pain, deafness, taste disturbances, earache, gingival bleeding, tooth caries, dry mouth.

GI: *nausea, diarrhea, abdominal pain, vomiting, anorexia,* constipation, *GI hemorrhage,* gastritis, dysphagia, stomatitis, increased appetite, melena, hemorrhoids, tenesmus.

GU: dysuria, nocturia, polyuria.

Hematologic: NEUTROPENIA, splenomegaly, lymphadenopathy.

Hepatic: hepatomegaly.

Metabolic: dehydration.

Musculoskeletal: *rigors, back pain,* arthralgia, myalgia.

Respiratory: *cough, dyspnea, rhinitis,* hemoptysis, hiccups, pulmonary infiltration, increased sputum.

Skin: alopecia, pruritus, *increased sweating,* dry skin, seborrhea, folliculitis.

Other: *opportunistic infections, allergic reactions,* flulike symptoms, thirst, injection site inflammation.

Interactions

None reported.

Effects on lab test results

• May decrease neutrophil and platelet counts.

Pharmacokinetics

Absorption: Administered I.V.
Distribution: May be distributed primarily in the vascular fluid volume.
Metabolism: Metabolized by the liver into active metabolites.
Excretion: Unknown. *Half-life:* 4½ hours.

Route	Onset	Peak	Duration
I.V.	Unknown	Unknown	Unknown

Action

Chemical effect: Exerts cytotoxic effects by intercalating between DNA base pairs and uncoiling the DNA helix. This inhibits DNA synthesis and DNA-dependent RNA synthesis. Also inhibits polymerase activity. The liposomal preparation maximizes the selectivity of daunorubicin for solid tumors in situ.
Therapeutic effect: Decreases tumor growth for advanced HIV-related Kaposi's sarcoma.

Available forms

Injection: 2 mg/ml (equivalent to 50 mg daunorubicin base)

NURSING PROCESS

Assessment

• Obtain history of patient's underlying condition before therapy, and reassess regularly thereafter.
• Obtain hepatic and renal studies before therapy.
• Monitor cardiac function regularly and before giving each dose because of the risk of cardiac toxicity and heart failure. Left ventricular ejection fraction should be determined at a total cumulative dose of 320 mg/m² and every 160 mg/m² thereafter.
• Monitor patient closely for signs of opportunistic infections because HIV-infected patients are immunocompromised.
• Be alert for adverse reactions and drug interactions.
• Evaluate patient's and family's knowledge of drug therapy.

Nursing diagnoses

• Risk for injury related to drug-induced adverse reactions
• Risk for infection related to myelosuppression
• Deficient knowledge related to drug therapy

Planning and implementation

• Drug causes less nausea, vomiting, alopecia, neutropenia, thrombocytopenia, and potentially less cardiotoxicity than conventional daunorubicin.
• Give only under the supervision of a prescriber specializing in cancer chemotherapy.
• **ALERT:** Monitor hematologic status closely because severe myelosuppression may occur. Obtain and check blood counts before each dose. Withhold treatment if absolute granulocyte count is below 750 cells/mm³.

• **ALERT:** Drug has unique kinetic properties that are different from the conventional daunorubicin hydrochloride. Don't substitute or interchange the drugs on a mg-to-mg basis.
Patient teaching
• Inform patient that alopecia may occur but it's usually reversible.
• Tell patient to notify prescriber about sore throat, fever, or other signs of infection. Tell patient to avoid exposure to people with infections.
• Advise patient to report suspected or known pregnancy during therapy.
• Tell patient to report back pain, flushing, and chest tightness during the infusion.

Evaluation

• Patient has no injury as a result of drug-induced adverse reactions.
• Patient remains free of infection.
• Patient and family state understanding of drug therapy.

daunorubicin hydrochloride
(daw-noh-ROO-buh-sin high-droh-KLOR-ighd)
Cerubidine

Pharmacologic class: antibiotic antineoplastic (cell-cycle-phase–nonspecific)
Therapeutic class: antineoplastic
Pregnancy risk category: D

Indications and dosages

▶ **Remission induction in acute nonlymphocytic (myelogenous, monocytic, erythroid) leukemia.** *Adults:* When given with other drugs, 30 to 45 mg/m² I.V. daily on days 1, 2, and 3 of first course and on days 1 and 2 of subsequent courses with cytarabine infusions.
▶ **Remission induction in acute lymphocytic leukemia.** *Adults:* 45 mg/m² I.V. daily on days 1, 2, and 3.
Children age 2 and older: 25 mg/m² I.V. on day 1 q week for up to 6 weeks, if needed.
Children younger than age 2 or with body surface area of less than 0.5 mg/m²: Calculate dose based on body weight (mg/kg).
▶ **Adjust-a-dose:** For patients with impaired hepatic or renal function, reduce dosage as follows: If bilirubin level is 1.2 to 3 mg/dl, give ¾ of normal dose; if bilirubin or creatinine level exceeds 3 mg/dl, give ½ of the normal dose.

▼ I.V. administration

• Preparing and giving drug have carcinogenic, mutagenic, and teratogenic risks. Follow institutional policy to reduce risks.

• Reconstitute drug using 4 ml of sterile water for injection to produce a 5-mg/ml solution.

• Withdraw desired dose into syringe containing 10 to 15 ml of normal saline solution for injection. Inject into I.V. line containing free-flowing compatible solution of D₅W or normal saline solution for injection over 2 to 3 minutes.

• Monitor I.V. site for extravasation. If it occurs, stop I.V. infusion immediately, notify prescriber, and apply ice to area for 24 to 48 hours.

⊛ ALERT: Don't infuse with dexamethasone or heparin; a precipitate may form.

• Ideally, use within 8 hours of preparation. Reconstituted solution is stable 24 hours at room temperature, 48 hours if refrigerated.

Contraindications and precautions

• Use cautiously in patients with myelosuppression and in those with impaired cardiac, renal, or hepatic function.

🕱 **Lifespan:** In pregnant women, use cautiously, if at all. Breast-feeding isn't recommended during therapy.

Adverse reactions

CNS: fever.
CV: *irreversible cardiomyopathy,* ECG changes, *arrhythmias,* pericarditis, *myocarditis.*
GI: *nausea, vomiting, stomatitis, esophagitis,* anorexia, diarrhea.
GU: red urine.
Hematologic: *bone marrow suppression.*
Hepatic: *hepatotoxicity.*
Metabolic: hyperuricemia.
Skin: rash, pigmentation of fingernails and toenails, *generalized alopecia, tissue sloughing* with extravasation.
Other: *severe cellulitis,* chills, *anaphylaxis.*

Interactions

Drug-drug. *Bone marrow suppressants:* May increase risk of myelosuppression. Monitor patient closely.
Cyclophosphamide: Increases risk of cardiotoxicity. Monitor patient closely.
Doxorubicin: May increase risk of cardiotoxicity. Monitor patient closely.
Hepatotoxic drugs: May increase risk of hepatotoxicity. Monitor hepatic function closely.

Effects on lab test results

• May increase uric acid level.

Pharmacokinetics

Absorption: Administered I.V.
Distribution: Widely distributed in body tissues; drug doesn't cross blood-brain barrier.
Metabolism: Extensively metabolized in liver. One of metabolites has cytotoxic activity.
Excretion: Drug and its metabolites primarily excreted in bile, with small portion excreted in urine. *Half-life:* Initial, 45 minutes; terminal, 18½ hours.

Route	Onset	Peak	Duration
I.V.	Unknown	Unknown	Unknown

Action

Chemical effect: May interfere with DNA-dependent RNA synthesis by intercalation.
Therapeutic effect: Kills selected cancer cells.

Available forms

Injection: 20 mg/vial

NURSING PROCESS

🗲 Assessment

• Obtain history of patient's underlying disease before therapy, and reassess regularly throughout therapy.

• Check ECG before treatment.

• Monitor CBC and liver function tests; monitor ECG every month (or more, if needed) during therapy.

• Monitor pulse rate closely.

• Be alert for adverse reactions and drug interactions.

• Monitor patient for nausea and vomiting, which may be severe and may last 24 to 48 hours. Monitor patient's hydration status during episodes of nausea and vomiting.

• Evaluate patient's and family's knowledge of drug therapy.

🖾 Nursing diagnoses

• Risk for injury related to presence of neoplastic disease

• Risk for deficient fluid volume related to drug-induced nausea and vomiting

• Deficient knowledge related to drug therapy

▷ Planning and implementation

✪ **ALERT:** Never give drug I.M. or S.C.

• Cumulative dosage is limited to 500 to 600 mg/m² (450 mg/m² if patient also receives or has received cyclophosphamide or radiation therapy to cardiac area).

✪ **ALERT:** Color is similar to that of doxorubicin. Don't confuse these two drugs.

• Notify prescriber if adverse cardiac reactions occur. Stop drug immediately and notify prescriber if signs of heart failure or cardiomyopathy develop.

✪ **ALERT:** The risk of myocardial toxicity increases after a total cumulative dose exceeding 400 to 550 mg/m² in adults, 300 mg/m² in children older than age 2, and 10 mg/kg in children younger than age 2.

• Give antiemetics to help control nausea and vomiting.

Patient teaching

• Warn patient to watch for signs of infection and bleeding.

• Advise patient that red urine for 1 to 2 days is normal and doesn't indicate blood in urine.

• Inform patient that alopecia may occur but that it's usually reversible.

• Advise women of childbearing age to avoid becoming pregnant during therapy.

• Instruct patient about need for protective measures, including conservation of energy, balanced diet, adequate rest, personal hygiene, clean environment, and avoidance of people with infections.

☑ Evaluation

• Patient shows positive response to therapy as evidenced by reports of follow-up diagnostic tests and improved physical status.

• Patient maintains adequate hydration throughout therapy.

• Patient and family state understanding of drug therapy.

---

delavirdine mesylate

(deh-luh-VEER-deen MES-ih-layt)
Rescriptor

Pharmacologic class: nonnucleoside reverse transcriptase inhibitor
Therapeutic class: antiviral
Pregnancy risk category: C

Indications and dosages

▶ **HIV-1 infection.** *Adults:* 400 mg P.O. t.i.d. with other appropriate antiretrovirals.

Contraindications and precautions

• Contraindicated in patients hypersensitive to drug's formulation.

• Use cautiously in patients with impaired hepatic function.

⚘ **Lifespan:** In pregnant women, use only if potential benefits outweigh risks to fetus. Breast-feeding women should avoid breast-feeding to reduce risk of transmitting HIV to infant. In children younger than age 16, safety hasn't been established.

Adverse reactions

CNS: *asthenia, fatigue, headache,* anxiety, depression, insomnia, fever, localized pain.
EENT: pharyngitis, sinusitis.
GI: *nausea,* vomiting, diarrhea, *abdominal pain (generalized or localized).*
Respiratory: upper respiratory tract infection, bronchitis, cough.
Skin: *rash.*
Other: flu syndrome.

Interactions

Drug-drug. *Antacids:* Reduces absorption of delavirdine. Separate doses by at least 1 hour.
Amphetamine, antihistamines (nonsedating), benzodiazepines, calcium channel blockers, clarithromycin, dapsone, ergot alkaloids, indinavir, quinidine, rifabutin, sedative hypnotics, warfarin: Increases or prolongs therapeutic and adverse effects of these drugs. Avoid using together; however, reduced doses of indinavir and clarithromycin may be used.
Carbamazepine, phenobarbital, phenytoin: Decreases delavirdine levels; use together cautiously.
Clarithromycin, fluoxetine, ketoconazole: Causes a 50% increase in delavirdine bioavailability. Monitor patient. Reduce dose of clarithromycin.
Didanosine: Decreases absorption of both drugs 20%. Separate doses by at least 1 hour.
H₂-receptor antagonists: Increased gastric pH reduces absorption of delavirdine. Long-term use isn't recommended.
HMG-CoA reductase inhibitors, such as atorvastatin, lovastatin, and simvastatin: Increases levels of these drugs, raising risk for myopathy, including rhabdomyolysis. Avoid using together.

Reactions may be *common,* uncommon, *life-threatening*, or COMMON AND LIFE-THREATENING.

Rifabutin, rifampin: Decreases delavirdine levels. Rifabutin levels are increased by 100%. Avoid using together.

Saquinavir: Increases bioavailability of saquinavir fivefold. Monitor AST and ALT levels frequently when used together.

Sildenafil: Increases sildenafil plasma concentrations and may increase risk for sildenafil-associated adverse events, including hypotension, visual changes, and priapism. Do not exceed 25 mg of sildenafil in a 48-hour period.

Effects on lab test results

• May increase ALT, GGT, amylase, bilirubin, and AST levels. May increase or decrease glucose level.

• May increase PT, PTT and eosinophil count. May decrease hemoglobin, hematocrit, and granulocyte, neutrophil, WBC, RBC, and platelet counts.

Pharmacokinetics

Absorption: Rapidly absorbed after oral administration.

Distribution: 98% bound to plasma protein.

Metabolism: Extensively converted to inactive metabolites. Primarily metabolized in liver by cytochrome enzyme systems.

Excretion: 51% excreted in the urine (less than 5% unchanged), 44% excreted in the feces.

Half-life: 5¾ hours.

Route	Onset	Peak	Duration
P.O.	Unknown	1 hr	Unknown

Action

Chemical effect: Drug binds directly to reverse transcriptase and blocks RNA- and DNA-dependent DNA polymerase activities.

Therapeutic effect: Inhibits HIV replication.

Available forms

Tablets: 100 mg, 200 mg

NURSING PROCESS

Assessment

• Assess patient's underlying condition before therapy and regularly thereafter.

• Be alert for adverse reactions and drug interactions.

• Monitor patient for drug-induced rash.

• Evaluate patient's and family's knowledge of drug therapy.

Nursing diagnoses

• Risk for impaired skin integrity related to potential adverse effects of medication

• Risk for infection related to patient's underlying condition

• Deficient knowledge related to drug therapy

Planning and implementation

• If rash develops, give diphenhydramine, hydroxyzine, or topical corticosteroids to relieve symptoms.

• Resistance develops rapidly when drug is used as monotherapy. Always give with appropriate antiretroviral therapy.

• Drug may be dispersed in water before ingestion. Add tablets to at least 3 oz (89 ml) of water, let stand for a few minutes, then stir well. Have patient drink promptly, rinse glass, and swallow the rinse to make sure entire dose is consumed.

Patient teaching

• Tell patient to stop drug and call prescriber if he develops severe rash or rash accompanied by symptoms such as fever, blistering, oral lesions, conjunctivitis, swelling, or muscle or joint aches.

• Tell patient that drug doesn't cure HIV-1 infection and that he may continue to acquire illnesses related to HIV-1 infection.

• Urge patient to remain under medical supervision when taking drug because long-term effects aren't known.

• Advise patient to take drug as prescribed and not to alter doses without prescriber's approval. If a dose is missed, tell him to take the next dose as soon as possible but not to double the next dose.

• Inform patient that drug may be taken without regard to food.

• Tell patient with achlorhydria to take drug with an acidic beverage, such as orange or cranberry juice.

• Advise patient taking sildenafil of increased risk for sildenafil-associated adverse events, including hypotension, visual changes, and priapism. Tell patient to promptly report any symptoms to prescriber. Tell him not to exceed 25 mg of sildenafil in a 48-hour period.

- Advise patient to report use of other prescription drugs, OTC medicines, or herbal remedies.

☑ **Evaluation**
- Patient's skin integrity is maintained.
- Patient is free from opportunistic infections.
- Patient and family state understanding of drug therapy.

desipramine hydrochloride
(deh-SIP-rah-meen high-droh-KLOR-ighd)
Norpramin

Pharmacologic class: dibenzazepine tricyclic antidepressant (TCA)
Therapeutic class: antidepressant
Pregnancy risk category: C

Indications and dosages

▶ **Depression.** *Adults:* Initially, 100 to 200 mg P.O. daily in divided doses; increase to maximum of 300 mg daily. Or, entire dose can be given h.s.
Elderly patients and adolescents: 25 to 100 mg P.O. daily in divided doses; increase gradually to maximum of 150 mg daily, if needed.

Contraindications and precautions

- Contraindicated in patients hypersensitive to drug, in those in acute recovery phase of MI, and within 14 days of MAO inhibitor therapy.
- Use cautiously in patients taking thyroid medication and in those with CV disease, seizure disorder, glaucoma, thyroid disorder, or history of urine retention.
⚘ **Lifespan:** In pregnant and breast-feeding women, use cautiously. In children younger than age 12, safety and efficacy of drug haven't been established.

Adverse reactions

CNS: *drowsiness, dizziness,* excitation, tremors, weakness, confusion, headache, nervousness, EEG changes, *seizures,* extrapyramidal reactions.
CV: orthostatic hypotension, *tachycardia, ECG changes,* hypertension.
EENT: *blurred vision,* tinnitus, mydriasis.
GI: *dry mouth, constipation,* nausea, vomiting, anorexia, paralytic ileus.
GU: *urine retention.*

Skin: rash, urticaria, *diaphoresis,* photosensitivity.
Other: *sudden death,* hypersensitivity reaction.

Interactions

Drug-drug. *Anticholinergics:* May enhance anticholinergic effects. Monitor patient closely.
Barbiturates, CNS depressants: May enhance CNS depression. Avoid using together.
Cimetidine, methylphenidate: May increase desipramine levels. Monitor patient for adverse reactions.
Clonidine: May cause loss of blood pressure control with potentially life threatening elevations in blood pressure. Don't use together.
Epinephrine, norepinephrine: May increase hypertensive effect. Use together cautiously.
MAO inhibitors: May cause severe excitation, hyperpyrexia, or seizures, usually with high dosage. Use together cautiously.
SSRIs: May inhibit the metabolism of TCAs, causing toxicity. Symptoms of TCA toxicity may persist for several weeks after stopping SSRI. At least 5 weeks may be needed when switching from fluoxetine to a tricyclic antidepressant because of the long half-life of the active and parent metabolite.
Drug-lifestyle. *Alcohol use:* May enhance CNS depression. Discourage using together.
Smoking: May lower desipramine level. Monitor patient for lack of effect; encourage smoking cessation.
Sun exposure: Increases risk of photosensitivity. Advise against unprotected or prolonged sun exposure.

Effects on lab test results

- May increase or decrease glucose levels.
- May increase liver function test values.

Pharmacokinetics

Absorption: Rapid.
Distribution: Distributed widely throughout body, including CNS; 90% protein-bound.
Metabolism: By liver; significant first-pass effect may explain different levels in patients taking same dosage.
Excretion: Primarily in urine. *Half-life:* Unknown.

Route	Onset	Peak	Duration
P.O.	2-4 wk	4-6 hr	Unknown

Reactions may be *common,* uncommon, *life-threatening*, or COMMON AND LIFE-THREATENING.

Action

Chemical effect: May increase amount of norepinephrine, serotonin, or both in the CNS by blocking their reuptake by neurons.
Therapeutic effect: Relieves depression.

Available forms

Tablets: 10 mg, 25 mg, 50 mg, 75 mg, 100 mg, 150 mg

NURSING PROCESS

Assessment

• Obtain history of patient's depression before therapy, and reassess regularly.
• Be alert for adverse reactions and drug interactions.
• Evaluate patient's and family's knowledge of drug therapy.

Nursing diagnoses

• Ineffective individual coping related to depression
• Risk for injury related to drug-induced adverse reactions
• Deficient knowledge related to drug therapy

Planning and implementation

• Don't stop drug abruptly. Abrupt withdrawal of long-term therapy may cause nausea, headache, and malaise.
• Because drug produces fewer anticholinergic effects than other TCAs, it's prescribed often for patients with cardiac problems.
• Because hypertensive episodes may occur during surgery, stop drug gradually several days before surgery.
• **ALERT:** This drug may cause sudden death in children, although the cause isn't clearly defined.
• If signs of psychosis occur or increase, reduce dosage.
Patient teaching
• Warn patient to avoid hazardous activities until CNS effects of drug are known. Drowsiness and dizziness usually subside after a few weeks.
• Tell patient to avoid alcohol during therapy because it may antagonize drug effects.
• Warn patient not to stop drug suddenly.
• Advise patient to consult prescriber before taking other prescription drugs, OTC medications, or herbal remedies.

• Instruct patient to use sunblock, wear protective clothing, and avoid prolonged exposure to strong sunlight.

Evaluation

• Patient behavior and communication indicate improvement of depression.
• Patient has no injury as a result of drug-induced adverse reactions.
• Patient and family state understanding of drug therapy.

desloratadine

(des-lor-AT-a-deen)
Clarinex, Clarinex Reditabs

Pharmacologic class: selective H_1-receptor antagonist
Therapeutic class: antihistamine
Pregnancy risk category: C

Indications and dosages

▶ **Relief of nasal and non-nasal symptoms of allergic rhinitis (seasonal and perennial); symptomatic relief of pruritus and reduction in the number and size of hives in patients with chronic idiopathic urticaria.** *Adults and children age 12 and older:* 5 mg P.O. daily.
Adjust-a-dose: In patients with hepatic or renal impairment, start dosage at 5 mg P.O. every other day.

Contraindications and precautions

• Contraindicated in patients hypersensitive to drug, its components, or loratadine. Drug can't be eliminated by hemodialysis.
Lifespan: Breast-feeding patients should stop nursing or stop taking the drug because drug appears in breast milk. In children younger than age 12, safety and efficacy of drug haven't been established. In elderly patients, use cautiously because of possible decreased hepatic, renal, or cardiac function and because they may have other diseases and be taking other drugs.

Adverse reactions

CNS: headache, somnolence, fatigue, dizziness.
CV: tachycardia.
EENT: pharyngitis.
GI: nausea, dry mouth, dyspepsia.
GU: dysmenorrhea.

Musculoskeletal: myalgia.
Other: flulike symptoms, *hypersensitivity reaction* (including rash, edema, or *anaphylaxis*).

Interactions

None reported.

Effects on lab test results

• May increase liver enzyme and bilirubin levels.

Pharmacokinetics

Absorption: Level peaks in about 3 hours. Drug doesn't cross the blood-brain barrier.
Distribution: Drug is 82% to 87% bound to plasma proteins. Active metabolite is 85% to 89% protein bound.
Metabolism: Extensively metabolized in the liver to active metabolite.
Excretion: It's equally eliminated in the urine and feces, primarily as metabolites. *Half-life:* 1 day.

Route	Onset	Peak	Duration
P.O.	Unknown	3 hr	Unknown
P.O. orally disintegrating	Unknown	2½-4 hours	Unknown

Action

Chemical effect: Inhibits histamine release from human mast cells *in vitro*.
Therapeutic effect: Relieves allergy symptoms.

Available forms

Orally disintegrating tablets (Reditabs): 5 mg
Tablets: 5 mg

NURSING PROCESS

Assessment
• Assess patient's condition before therapy and regularly thereafter.
• Be alert for adverse reactions.
• Evaluate patient's and family's knowledge of drug therapy.

Nursing diagnoses
• Ineffective health maintenance related to underlying allergic condition
• Fatigue related to drug-induced reaction
• Deficient knowledge related to drug therapy

Planning and implementation
• Drug may be taken with or without food.
• Overdose may cause somnolence and increased heart rate. If these symptoms occur, consider removing unabsorbed drug through standard measures and provide symptomatic and supportive treatment.
Patient teaching
• Advise patient not to exceed recommended dosage. Doses of more than 5 mg don't increase effectiveness and may cause somnolence.
• Tell patient to report adverse effects.
• Store tablets at 36° to 86°F (2° to 30°C); store orally disintegrating tablets at 59° to 86°F (15° to 30° C)
• Instruct patient to remove orally disintegrating tablet from blister pack and immediately place on the tongue.
• Inform patient that orally disintegrating tablet may be taken with or without water.

Evaluation
• Patient's allergic symptoms are relieved.
• Patient doesn't suffer any drug-induced adverse effects.
• Patient and family state understanding of drug therapy.

desmopressin acetate
(dez-moh-PREH-sin AS-ih-tayt)
DDAVP, Stimate

Pharmacologic class: posterior pituitary hormone
Therapeutic class: antidiuretic, hemostatic
Pregnancy risk category: B

Indications and dosages

▶ **Nonnephrogenic diabetes insipidus, temporary polyuria, and polydipsia from pituitary trauma.** *Adults:* 10 to 40 mcg intranasally daily in one to three divided doses. Adjust morning and evening doses separately for adequate diurnal rhythm of water turnover. Or, 0.05 mg P.O. b.i.d. Adjust each dose separately for an adequate diurnal rhythm of water turnover. Total oral daily dosage should be increased or decreased as needed to achieve desired response. Doses may range from 0.1 to 1.2 mg, divided into two or three daily doses. Oral therapy should start 12 hours after last intranasal

dose. Or, give 2 to 4 mcg I.V. or S.C. daily, usually in two equally divided doses.
Children ages 3 months to 12 years: 0.05 to 0.3 ml intranasally daily in one or two doses.
Children age 4 and older: Begin with 0.05 mg oral form P.O. b.i.d. Adjust each dose separately for an adequate diurnal rhythm of water turnover. Increase or decrease total oral daily dosage to achieve desired response. Doses may range from 0.1 to 1.2 mg, divided into two or three daily doses. Start oral therapy 12 hours after the last intranasal dose.
Children younger than age 4: Adjust dosage of oral form individually to prevent an excessive decrease in plasma osmolality.
▶ **Hemophilia A and von Willebrand's disease.** *Adults and children:* 0.3 mcg/kg diluted in normal saline solution and infused I.V. over 15 to 30 minutes. May repeat dose, if necessary, based on laboratory response and patient's condition. Intranasal dose is 1 spray (of solution containing 1.5 mg/ml) into each nostril to provide total of 300 mcg.
Adults and children weighing less than 50 kg (110 lb): 1 spray into a single nostril (150 mcg).
▶ **Primary nocturnal enuresis.** *Children age 6 and older:* Initially, 20 mcg intranasally h.s. Adjust dosage according to response. Maximum recommended dosage is 40 mcg daily. Or, 0.2 mg P.O. h.s. Adjust dose up to 0.6 mg P.O. to achieve desired response. Oral therapy may start 24 hours after last intranasal dose.

▼ I.V. administration

• For adults and children weighing more than 10 kg (22 lb), dilute with 50 ml sterile physiologic saline solution. For children weighing 10 kg or less, 10 ml of diluent is recommended.
• Inspect for particulate matter and discoloration before infusing drug.
• Monitor blood pressure and pulse during infusion.

Contraindications and precautions

• Contraindicated in patients hypersensitive to drug and in those with type IIB von Willebrand's disease.
• Use cautiously in patients with coronary artery insufficiency or hypertensive CV disease and in those with conditions linked to fluid and electrolyte imbalance, such as cystic fibrosis, because these patients are prone to hyponatremia.

⚖ **Lifespan:** In pregnant and breast-feeding women, use cautiously. In infants younger than age 3 months, use of drug isn't recommended because of their increased tendency to develop fluid imbalance. In children younger than age 12, safety of parenteral form of drug hasn't been established for management of diabetes insipidus.

Adverse reactions

CNS: headache.
CV: slight rise in blood pressure.
EENT: nasal congestion, rhinitis, epistaxis, sore throat.
GI: nausea, abdominal cramps.
GU: vulvar pain.
Respiratory: cough.
Other: flushing, local erythema, swelling or burning after injection.

Interactions

Drug-drug. *Demeclocycline, epinephrine, heparin, lithium:* Decreases response to desmopressin. Monitor patient closely.
Drug-lifestyle. *Alcohol use:* May increase risk of adverse effects. Discourage using together.

Effects on lab test results

None reported.

Pharmacokinetics

Absorption: After intranasal administration, 10% to 20% of dose through nasal mucosa. After S.C. administration, unknown. After P.O. administration, minimal.
Distribution: Unknown.
Metabolism: Unknown.
Excretion: Unknown. *Half-life:* Fast phase, about 8 minutes; slow phase, 114 hours.

Route	Onset	Peak	Duration
P.O.	1 hr	4-7 hr	8-12 hr
I.V.	15-30 min	1½-2 hr	4-12 hr
S.C.	Unknown	Unknown	Unknown
Intranasal	≤ 1 hr	1-5 hr	8-12 hr

Action

Chemical effect: Increases permeability of renal tubular epithelium to adenosine monophosphate and water; epithelium promotes reabsorption of water and produces concentrated urine (ADH effect). Desmopressin also increases factor VIII activity by releasing endogenous factor VIII from plasma storage sites.

Therapeutic effect: Decreases diuresis and promotes clotting.

Available forms

Injection: 4 mcg/ml
Nasal solution: 0.1 mg/ml, 1.5 mg/ml
Tablets: 0.1 mg, 0.2 mg

NURSING PROCESS

⚗ Assessment
- Obtain history of patient's underlying condition before therapy.
- Monitor effectiveness by checking patient's fluid intake and output, serum and urine osmolality, and urine specific gravity for treatment of diabetes insipidus or relief of symptoms of other disorders.
- Be alert for adverse reactions and drug interactions.
- Monitor patient carefully for hypertension during high-dose treatment.
- Evaluate patient's and family's knowledge of drug therapy.

⊞ Nursing diagnoses
- Deficient fluid volume related to underlying condition
- Acute pain related to drug-induced headache
- Deficient knowledge related to drug therapy

▷ Planning and implementation
- When giving S.C., rotate injection sites.
- Follow manufacturer's instructions exactly for intranasal administration.
- Ensure nasal passages are intact, clean, and free of obstruction prior to intranasal use.
- Intranasal use can cause changes in nasal mucosa, resulting in erratic, unreliable absorption. Report worsening condition to prescriber, who may prescribe injectable DDAVP.
- Don't use drug to treat severe cases of von Willebrand's disease or hemophilia A with factor VIII levels of 0% to 5%.
- Patients may be switched from intranasal to S.C. form, such as during episodes of rhinorrhea. Give ¹⁄₁₀ or ¼ of their usual nasal dose S.C.
- When drug is used to treat diabetes insipidus, adjust dosage according to patient's fluid output. Adjust morning and evening doses separately for adequate diurnal rhythm of water turnover.
- ⊛ **ALERT:** Don't confuse desmopressin with vasopressin.

Patient teaching
- Instruct patient to clear nasal passages before using drug intranasally.
- Patient may have trouble measuring and inhaling drug into nostrils. Teach patient and caregiver correct method of administration.
- Advise patient to report conditions such as nasal congestion, allergic rhinitis, or upper respiratory tract infection; dosage adjustment may be required.
- Teach patient using S.C. desmopressin to rotate injection sites to avoid tissue damage.
- Warn patient to drink only enough water to satisfy thirst.
- Inform patient that when treating hemophilia A and von Willebrand's disease, giving desmopressin may avoid hazards of using blood products.
- Advise patient to wear or carry medical identification indicating use of drug.

☑ Evaluation
- Patient achieves normal fluid and electrolyte balance.
- Patient states that headache is relieved with mild analgesic.
- Patient and family state understanding of drug therapy.

dexamethasone
(deks-ah-METH-uh-sohn)
Decadron*, DexaMeth, Dexamethasone Intensol*, Dexasone ♦ , Dexone 0.5, Dexone 0.75, Dexone 1.5, Dexone 4, Hexadrol*, Mymethasone*, Oradexon ♦

dexamethasone acetate
Cortostat LA, Dalalone D.P., Decaject-L.A., Dexasone-L.A., Dexone L.A., Solurex-LA

dexamethasone sodium phosphate
AK-Dex, Cortastat, Cortastat 10, Dalalone, Decadrol, Decadron Phosphate, Decaject, Dexacen-4, Dexacorten, Dexone, Hexadrol Phosphate, Primethasone, Solurex

Pharmacologic class: glucocorticoid
Therapeutic class: anti-inflammatory, immunosuppressant
Pregnancy risk category: NR

Reactions may be *common*, uncommon, *life-threatening*, or COMMON AND LIFE-THREATENING.

Indications and dosages

▶ **Cerebral edema.** *Adults:* Initially, 10 mg dexamethasone sodium phosphate I.V. Then, 4 mg I.M. q 6 hours until symptoms subside (usually 2 to 4 days). Then, taper down over 5 to 7 days.

▶ **Inflammatory conditions, allergic reactions, neoplasias.** *Adults:* 4 mg dexamethasone sodium phosphate I.M. as a single dose. Continue maintenance therapy with dexamethasone tablets, 1.5 mg P.O. b.i.d. for 2 days; then, 0.75 mg P.O. b.i.d. for 1 day; then, 0.75 mg P.O. once daily for 2 days; then, stop drug. Or, 4 to 16 mg dexamethasone acetate I.M. into joint or soft tissue q 1 to 3 weeks. Or, 0.8 to 1.6 mg into lesions q 1 to 3 weeks.

▶ **Shock.** *Adults:* 1 to 6 mg/kg dexamethasone sodium phosphate I.V. as single dose or 40 mg I.V. q 2 to 6 hours, p.r.n. Or, 20 mg I.V. as a single dose, followed by continuous infusion of 3 mg/kg q 24 hours.

▶ **Dexamethasone suppression test for Cushing's syndrome.** *Adults:* After determining baseline 24-hour urine levels of 17-hydroxycorticosteroids, 0.5 mg P.O. q 6 hours for 48 hours; 24-hour urine collection made for determination of 17-hydroxycorticosteroid excretion again during second 24 hours of dexamethasone administration. Or, 1 mg P.O. as a single dose at 11 p.m. Draw plasma cortisol level at 8 a.m. the following day.

▶ **Prevention of hyaline membrane disease in premature infants‡.** *Adults:* 5 mg dexamethasone sodium phosphate I.M. t.i.d. to mother for 2 days before delivery.

▶ **Prevention of chemotherapy-induced nausea and vomiting‡.** *Adults:* 10 to 20 mg I.V. before giving chemotherapy. Additional doses (individualized for each patient and usually lower than initial dose) may be given I.V. or P.O. for 24 to 72 hours following cancer chemotherapy, if needed.

▼ I.V. administration

• When giving as direct injection, inject undiluted over at least 1 minute.

• When giving as intermittent or continuous infusion, dilute solution according to manufacturer's instructions and give over prescribed duration. For continuous infusion, change solution every 24 hours.

Contraindications and precautions

• Contraindicated in patients hypersensitive to drug or its components and in those with systemic fungal infections.

• Use cautiously in patients with recent MI and in those with GI ulcer, renal disease, hypertension, osteoporosis, diabetes mellitus, hypothyroidism, cirrhosis, diverticulitis, nonspecific ulcerative colitis, recent intestinal anastomoses, thromboembolic disorders, seizures, myasthenia gravis, heart failure, tuberculosis, ocular herpes simplex, emotional instability, or psychotic tendencies. Because some forms contain sulfite preservatives, use cautiously in patients sensitive to sulfites.

⚖ **Lifespan:** In pregnant women, use cautiously. In breast-feeding women, drug isn't recommended. In children and adolescents, long-term use of drug may delay growth and maturation.

Adverse reactions

CNS: *euphoria, insomnia,* psychotic behavior, pseudotumor cerebri, *seizures.*
CV: *heart failure,* hypertension, edema, *arrhythmias, thromboembolism.*
EENT: cataracts, glaucoma.
GI: *peptic ulceration,* GI irritation, increased appetite, *pancreatitis.*
GU: menstrual irregularities.
Metabolic: hypokalemia, hyperglycemia, carbohydrate intolerance.
Musculoskeletal: muscle weakness, osteoporosis, growth suppression in children.
Skin: hirsutism, delayed wound healing, acne, skin eruptions, atrophy at I.M. injection sites.
Other: cushingoid state (moonface, buffalo hump, central obesity), susceptibility to infections, *acute adrenal insufficiency may follow increased stress (infection, surgery, or trauma) or abrupt withdrawal after long-term therapy.*

Interactions

Drug-drug. *Antidiabetics, including insulin:* May decrease corticosteroid response. May need dosage adjustment.
Aspirin, indomethacin, other NSAIDs: May increase risk of GI distress and bleeding. Give together cautiously.
Barbiturates, phenytoin, rifampin: May decrease corticosteroid effect. Increase corticosteroid dosage.
Digoxin: May increase risk of arrhythmia from hypokalemia. May need dosage adjustment.

Oral anticoagulants: May alter dosage requirements. Monitor PT and INR closely.
Potassium-depleting drugs: May enhance potassium-wasting effects of dexamethasone. Monitor potassium levels.
Salicylates: May decrease salicylate levels. Monitor patient for lack of therapeutic effects.
Skin-test antigens: May decrease response of skin test antigens. Defer skin testing until therapy is completed.
Toxoids, vaccines: May decrease antibody response and increased risk of neurologic complications. Avoid using together.
Drug-lifestyle. *Alcohol use:* Increases risk of gastric irritation and GI ulceration. Discourage using together.

Effects on lab test results

• May increase glucose and cholesterol levels. May decrease potassium, calcium, T_3, and T_4 levels.

Pharmacokinetics

Absorption: Absorbed readily after P.O. administration. Absorption of suspension for injection depends on whether it's injected into an intra-articular space, a muscle, or blood supply to a muscle.
Distribution: Distributed to muscle, liver, skin, intestines, and kidneys. Drug is bound weakly to plasma proteins (transcortin and albumin). Only unbound portion is active.
Metabolism: Metabolized in liver to inactive glucuronide and sulfate metabolites.
Excretion: Inactive metabolites and small amounts of unmetabolized drug excreted by kidneys. Insignificant quantities of drug are also excreted in feces. *Half-life:* About 1 to 2 days.

Route	Onset	Peak	Duration
P.O.	1-2 hr	1-2 hr	2½ days
I.V., I.M.	≤ 1 hr	1 hr	2 days-3 wk

Action

Chemical effect: Not clearly defined; decreases inflammation, mainly by stabilizing leukocyte lysosomal membranes; suppresses immune response; stimulates bone marrow; and influences protein, fat, and carbohydrate metabolism.
Therapeutic effect: Relieves cerebral edema, reduces inflammation and immune response, and reverses shock.

Available forms

dexamethasone
Elixir: 0.5 mg/5 ml*
Oral solution: 0.5 mg/5 ml, 1 mg/ml*
Tablets: 0.25 mg, 0.5 mg, 0.75 mg, 1 mg, 1.5 mg, 2 mg, 4 mg, 6 mg
dexamethasone acetate
Injection: 8 mg/ml, 16 mg/ml suspension
dexamethasone sodium phosphate
Injection: 4 mg/ml, 10 mg/ml, 20 mg/ml, 24 mg/ml

NURSING PROCESS

Assessment

• Obtain history of patient's underlying condition before therapy.
• Monitor patient's weight, blood pressure, glucose level, and electrolyte levels.
• Be alert for adverse reactions and drug interactions. Most adverse reactions to corticosteroids are dose- or duration-dependent.
• Watch for depression or psychotic episodes, especially in high-dose therapy.
• Evaluate patient's and family's knowledge of drug therapy.

Nursing diagnoses

• Ineffective health maintenance related to underlying condition
• Risk for injury related to drug-induced adverse reactions
• Deficient knowledge related to drug therapy

Planning and implementation

• For better results and less toxicity, give once-daily dose in morning.
• Give with food when possible.
• Give I.M. injection deeply into gluteal muscle. Rotate injection sites to prevent muscle atrophy.
• Avoid S.C. injection because atrophy and sterile abscesses may occur.
• Always adjust to lowest effective dose.
ALERT: Gradually reduce dosage after long-term therapy. Abrupt withdrawal may cause rebound inflammation, fatigue, weakness, arthralgia, fever, dizziness, lethargy, depression, fainting, orthostatic hypotension, dyspnea, anorexia, and hypoglycemia. After prolonged use, abrupt withdrawal may be fatal.
ALERT: Unless contraindicated, give patient low-sodium diet high in potassium and protein. Also, give potassium supplements as directed.

• If patient's stress level (physical or psychological) increases, notify prescriber because dosage may need to be increased.

• If patient has adverse reaction, notify prescriber and provide supportive and symptomatic treatment.

⊛ ALERT: Don't confuse dexamethasone with desoximetasone.

Patient teaching
• Tell patient not to stop drug abruptly or without prescriber's consent because abrupt withdrawal may be fatal.

• Teach patient signs of early adrenal insufficiency (fatigue, muscle weakness, joint pain, fever, anorexia, nausea, dyspnea, dizziness, and fainting).

• Instruct patient to wear or carry medical identification that indicates need for supplemental systemic glucocorticoids during stress, especially as dosage is decreased.

• Warn patient receiving long-term therapy about cushingoid symptoms and the need to notify prescriber about sudden weight gain or swelling.

• Warn patient about easy bruising.

• Advise patient receiving long-term therapy to consider exercise or physical therapy. Give vitamin D or calcium supplements.

• Advise patient receiving long-term therapy to have periodic ophthalmologic examinations.

☑ Evaluation
• Patient's condition improves with drug therapy.
• Patient has no injury as a result of drug therapy.
• Patient and family state understanding of drug therapy.

dexmedetomidine hydrochloride
(DEX-meh-dih-TOE-mih-deen high-droh-KLOR-ighd)
Precedex

Pharmacologic class: selective alpha$_2$-adrenoreceptor agonist with sedative properties
Therapeutic class: sedative
Pregnancy risk category: C

Indications and dosages

▶ Sedation of initially intubated and mechanically ventilated patients in ICU setting.

Adults: Loading infusion of 1 mcg/kg I.V. over 10 minutes; then a maintenance infusion of 0.2 to 0.7 mcg/kg/hour for up to 24 hours; adjust to achieve the desired level of sedation.

◲ **Adjust-a-dose:** In elderly patients and those with renal or hepatic failure, reduce dosage.

▼ I.V. administration

• Dilute in normal saline solution. To prepare the infusion, withdraw 2 ml of drug and add to 48 ml of normal saline injection to a total of 50 ml. Shake gently to mix well.

• Don't give through the same I.V. line with blood or plasma because physical compatibility hasn't been established.

• Infusion is compatible with lactated Ringer's solution, D$_5$W, normal saline solution, and 20% mannitol. It's also compatible with thiopental sodium, etomidate, vecuronium bromide, pancuronium bromide, succinylcholine, atracurium besylate, mivacurium chloride, glycopyrrolate bromide, phenylephrine hydrochloride, atropine sulfate, midazolam, morphine sulfate, fentanyl citrate, and plasma substitute.

⊛ **ALERT:** Don't give infusion for longer than 24 hours.

Contraindications and precautions

• Use cautiously in patients with advanced heart block or renal or hepatic impairment.

☀ **Lifespan:** In pregnant women, use only if benefits outweigh risks; may be toxic to fetus. In breast-feeding women, use cautiously. In children, use isn't recommended. In elderly patients, use cautiously.

Adverse reactions

CNS: pain.
CV: hypotension, *bradycardia, arrhythmias.*
GI: *nausea,* thirst.
GU: oliguria.
Hematologic: anemia, leukocytosis.
Respiratory: *hypoxia,* pleural effusion, *pulmonary edema.*
Other: infection.

Interactions

Drug-drug. *Anesthetics, hypnotics, opioids, sedatives:* May enhance effects. May need to reduce dexmedetomidine dose.

Effects on lab test results

● May increase WBC count. May decrease hemoglobin and hematocrit.

Pharmacokinetics

Absorption: Administered I.V.
Distribution: Rapid and wide. 94% protein-bound.
Metabolism: Almost complete.
Excretion: 95% in urine and 4% in feces. *Half-life:* About 2 hours.

Route	Onset	Peak	Duration
I.V.	Unknown	Unknown	Unknown

Action

Chemical effect: Selectively stimulates alpha$_2$-adrenoceptor in the CNS.
Therapeutic effect: Produces sedation of initially intubated and mechanically ventilated patients.

Available forms

Injection: 100 mcg/ml in 2-ml vials and 2-ml ampules

NURSING PROCESS

Assessment

● Assess renal and hepatic function before administration, particularly in elderly patients.
● Assess patient's response to drug. Some patients receiving drug may stir and be alert when stimulated. Don't consider this evidence of lack of efficacy in the absence of other signs and symptoms.
● Be alert for adverse reactions and drug interactions.
● Evaluate patient's and family's knowledge of drug therapy.

Nursing diagnoses

● Risk for injury related to drug-induced adverse reactions
● Impaired spontaneous ventilation related to underlying disease process
● Deficient knowledge related to drug therapy

Planning and implementation

⊛ **ALERT:** Use a controlled infusion device at the rate calculated for body weight.
● Continuously monitor cardiac status.

● Drug can be continuously infused in mechanically ventilated patients before, during, and after extubation. Drug doesn't need to be stopped before extubation.

Patient teaching

● Tell patient that he'll be sedated while the drug is given, but that he may awake when stimulated.
● Tell patient that he'll be closely monitored and attended while sedated.

☑ Evaluation

● Patient has no injury as a result of drug-induced adverse reactions.
● Patient regains spontaneous ventilation.
● Patient and family state understanding of drug therapy.

dexmethylphenidate hydrochloride
(dex-meth-il-FEN-uh-date high-droh-KLOR-ighd)
Focalin

Pharmacologic class: CNS stimulant
Therapeutic class: CNS stimulant
Pregnancy risk category: C
Controlled substance schedule: II

Indications and dosages

▶ **Attention deficit hyperactivity disorder (ADHD).** *Children age 6 and older:* For patients who aren't taking racemic methylphenidate or are taking another stimulant, starting dosage is 2.5 mg P.O. twice daily, spaced at least 4 hours apart. For patients who are being switched from methylphenidate, starting dose is one-half of the current methylphenidate dosage. Additionally, adjust dosage weekly in increments of 2.5 to 5 mg daily, up to a maximum dosage of 20 mg daily in divided doses.

Contraindications and precautions

● Contraindicated in patients hypersensitive to drug or its components. Also contraindicated in patients with severe anxiety, tension, agitation, or glaucoma and in those who have motor tics or a family history or diagnosis of Tourette syndrome. Also contraindicated within 14 days of MAO inhibitor therapy because hypertensive crisis may occur. Don't use to treat severe depression or to prevent or treat normal fatigue states.

• Use cautiously in patients with a history of drug abuse, alcoholism, psychosis, seizures, hypertension, hyperthyroidism, heart failure, or recent MI.

⚖ Lifespan: In pregnant women, use only if benefits outweigh risks. With breast-feeding women, use cautiously because it's unknown whether drug appears in breast milk. For children younger than age 6, don't give drug.

Adverse reactions

CNS: fever, insomnia, nervousness, growth suppression, psychosis, blurred vision.
CV: tachycardia, hypertension.
GI: anorexia, *abdominal pain,* nausea.
Hematologic: *leukopenia,* anemia.
Metabolic: weight loss.
Musculoskeletal: twitching (motor or vocal tics), arthralgia.

Interactions

Drug-drug. *Anticoagulants, anticonvulsants, and SSRIs, tricyclics:* Inhibits metabolism of these drugs. May need to decrease dosage of these drugs; monitor drug levels.
Antihypertensives: Decreases effectiveness of these drugs. Use together cautiously; monitor blood pressure.
Clonidine, other centrally acting alpha-2 agonists: May cause serious adverse effects. Use together cautiously.
MAO inhibitors: Increases risk of hypertensive crisis. Avoid using together or within 14 days after stopping MAO inhibitor.

Effects on lab test results

• May increase liver function test results. May decrease hemoglobin, hematocrit, and WBC count.

Pharmacokinetics

Absorption: Rapid. Level peaks in 1 to 1½ hours. Food delays rate of peak level but doesn't affect the amount absorbed.
Distribution: Rapid.
Metabolism: Extensive via de-esterification. Doesn't inhibit the CYP system. No active metabolites.
Excretion: 90% in urine. *Half-life:* About 2 hours.

Route	Onset	Peak	Duration
P.O.	Unknown	1-1½ hr	Unknown

Action

Chemical effect: May block presynaptic reuptake of norepinephrine and dopamine and increase the release of these neurotransmitters.
Therapeutic effect: Increases attention span and decreases hyperactivity and impulsiveness related to ADHD.

Available forms

Tablets: 2.5 mg, 5 mg, 10 mg

NURSING PROCESS

⚗ Assessment

• Diagnosis of ADHD must be based on complete history and evaluation of the child with consultation of psychological, educational, and social resources.
• Monitor blood pressure and pulse routinely during drug therapy.
• Be alert for drug-induced adverse reactions.
• Check CBC with differential and platelet counts with long-term use.

⊞ Nursing diagnoses

• Ineffective health maintenance related to underlying condition
• Ineffective coping by family of patient's underlying hyperactivity condition
• Deficient knowledge of drug therapy

❯ Planning and implementation

• Drug is meant to be an adjunct to comprehensive treatment program that includes psychological, educational, and social support.
• The drug contains only the active isomer required to effectively manage the symptoms of ADHD, at half the dose of Ritalin.
• Growth may be suppressed with long-term stimulant use. Monitor children for growth and weight gain. If growth is suppressed or if weight gain is lower than expected, stop drug.
• Reduce dosage or stop treatment if symptoms are aggravated or adverse reactions occur.
• If seizures occur, stop treatment.
• Symptoms of overdose include vomiting, agitation, tremors, hyperreflexia, muscle twitching, convulsions, euphoria, confusion, hallucinations, delirium, sweating, flushing, headache, hyperpyrexia, tachycardia, palpitations, cardiac arrhythmias, hypertension, mydriasis, and dry mucous membranes. Primary treatment is sup-

portive care and protection against self-injury and additional overstimulation.
- Stop treatment if symptoms don't improve after 1 month of treatment.

Patient teaching
- Advise parents to monitor child's height and weight and to tell prescriber if they suspect any growth suppression.
- Advise patient to take drug at the same time every day at the prescribed dose. Tell patient to report any adverse reactions to prescriber immediately.

☑ Evaluation
- Patient responds positively with drug therapy.
- Patient and family are effectively coping with patient's underlying condition.
- Patient and family state understanding of drug therapy.

dextran, high–molecular-weight (dextran 70, dextran 75)
(DEKS-tran, high moh-LEH-kyoo-ler wayt)
Dextran 70, Dextran 75, Gentran 70, Gendex 75, Macrodex

Pharmacologic class: glucose polymer
Therapeutic class: plasma volume expander
Pregnancy risk category: C

Indications and dosages

▶ **Plasma expander.** *Adults:* 30 g (500 ml of 6% solution) I.V. In emergencies, may give 1.2 to 2.4 g (20 to 40 ml)/minute. In normovolemic or nearly normovolemic patients, don't infuse faster than 240 mg (4 ml)/minute. Don't give more than 1.2 g/kg during the first 24 hours of therapy. Actual dosage depends on amount of fluid loss and resulting hemoconcentration and must be determined for each patient.

▼ I.V. administration

- Use D$_5$W instead of normal saline solution because drug is hazardous for patients with heart failure, especially when given in normal saline solution.
- Prescriber may order dextran 1, a dextran adjunct, to protect against drug-induced anaphylaxis. Give 20 ml of dextran 1 (containing

150 mg/ml) I.V. over 60 seconds 1 to 2 minutes before I.V. infusion of dextran.
- Observe patient closely during early phase of infusion, when most anaphylactic reactions occur.
- Store drug at constant 77° F (25° C). Precipitate may form in storage; heat to dissolve.

Contraindications and precautions

- Contraindicated in patients hypersensitive to drug and in those with marked hemostatic defects, marked cardiac decompensation, renal disease with severe oliguria or anuria, hypervolemic conditions, or severe bleeding disorders.
- Use cautiously in patients with active hemorrhage, thrombocytopenia, impaired renal clearance, chronic liver disease, or abdominal conditions and in patients undergoing bowel surgery.
≋ **Lifespan:** In pregnant women, use cautiously. Breast-feeding women should stop nursing or stop the drug. In children, safety and efficacy of drug haven't been established.

Adverse reactions

CNS: fever.
CV: fluid overload, thrombophlebitis.
EENT: nasal congestion.
GI: nausea, vomiting.
GU: increased specific gravity and viscosity of urine, tubular stasis and blocking, oliguria, anuria.
Musculoskeletal: arthralgia.
Skin: urticaria.
Other: hypersensitivity reactions, *anaphylaxis*.

Interactions

Drug-drug. *Abciximab, aspirin, heparin, thrombolytics, warfarin:* May increase bleeding. Use together cautiously; monitor patient for bleeding.

Effects on lab test results

- May increase ALT and AST levels.
- May increase bleeding time. May decrease hemoglobin and hematocrit. May significantly suppress platelet function with doses of 15 ml/kg.

Pharmacokinetics

Absorption: Administered I.V.
Distribution: Distributed throughout vascular system.

Metabolism: Drug molecules with molecular weights above 50,000 are enzymatically degraded by dextranase to glucose at rate of about 70 to 90 mg/kg/day.

Excretion: Drug molecules with molecular weights below 50,000 are eliminated by urine.

Half-life: Unknown.

Route	Onset	Peak	Duration
I.V.	Immediate	Immediate	Unknown

Action

Chemical effect: Expands plasma volume by way of colloidal osmotic effect, drawing fluid from interstitial to intravascular space, providing fluid replacement.

Therapeutic effect: Expands plasma volume.

Available forms

Injection: dextran 70 in normal saline solution or D_5W; 6% dextran 75 in normal saline solution or D_5W

NURSING PROCESS

📑 Assessment

• Obtain history of patient's underlying condition and hydration before therapy, and reassess regularly. Frequently assess vital signs, fluid intake and output, and urine or serum osmolarity levels.

• Be alert for adverse reactions.

• Watch for circulatory overload and rise in central venous pressure. Plasma expansion is slightly greater than volume infused.

• Check hemoglobin and hematocrit.

• Evaluate patient's and family's knowledge of drug therapy.

⊕ Nursing diagnoses

• Decreased cardiac output related to underlying condition

• Risk for injury related to potential for drug-induced hypersensitivity reaction

• Deficient knowledge related to drug therapy

▷ Planning and implementation

• If oliguria or anuria occurs or isn't relieved by infusion, stop dextran and give loop diuretic.

• If hematocrit values fall below 30% by volume, notify prescriber.

• Drug may interfere with analyses of blood grouping, crossmatching, and bilirubin, glucose, and protein levels.

• ⊛ **ALERT:** Low– and high–molecular-weight dextrans aren't interchangeable. Verify preparation before use.

Patient teaching

• Inform patient, if alert, and family about dextran therapy.

• Instruct patient to notify prescriber if adverse reactions occur, such as itching.

☑ Evaluation

• Patient's vital signs and urine output return to normal.

• Patient doesn't develop hypersensitivity reaction to drug.

• Patient and family state understanding of drug therapy.

---

dextran, low–molecular-weight (dextran 40)

(DEKS-tran, loh moh-LEH-kyoo-ler wayt)

Dextran 40, Gentran 40, 10% LMD, Rheomacrodex

Pharmacologic class: glucose polymer
Therapeutic class: plasma volume expander
Pregnancy risk category: C

Indications and dosages

▶ **Plasma volume expansion.** *Adults:* Dosage by I.V. infusion depends on amount of fluid loss. Initially, 10 ml/kg of dextran infused rapidly with central venous pressure monitoring; remainder of dose given slowly. Total dosage not to exceed 20 ml/kg in the first 24 hours. If therapy is continued longer than 24 hours, don't exceed 10 ml/kg daily. Continue for no longer than 5 days.

▶ **Prevention of venous thrombosis.** *Adults:* 10 ml/kg (500 to 1,000 ml) I.V. on day of procedure; 500 ml on days 2 and 3.

▶ **Hemodiluent in extracorporeal circulation.** *Adults:* 10 to 20 ml/kg added to perfusion circuit. Total dosage not to exceed 20 ml/kg.

▽ I.V. administration

• Prescriber may order dextran 1, a dextran adjunct, to protect against drug-induced anaphylaxis. Give 20 ml of dextran 1 (containing 150 mg/ml) I.V. over 60 seconds, 1 to 2 minutes before I.V. infusion of dextran.

- Use D$_5$W solution instead of normal saline solution because drug is hazardous for patients with heart failure, especially when given in normal saline solution.
- Observe patient closely during early phase of infusion, when most anaphylactic reactions occur.
- Store at constant 77° F (25° C). Precipitate may form during storage; heat to dissolve.
- Discard partially used containers.

Contraindications and precautions

- Contraindicated in patients hypersensitive to drug and in those with marked hemostatic defects, marked cardiac decompensation, and renal disease with severe oliguria or anuria.
- Use cautiously in patients with active hemorrhage, thrombocytopenia, or diabetes mellitus.
▲ Lifespan: In pregnant women, use cautiously. Breast-feeding women should stop breast-feeding or not use drug. In children, safety and efficacy of drug haven't been established.

Adverse reactions

CV: thrombophlebitis.
GI: nausea, vomiting.
GU: tubular stasis and blocking, increased urine viscosity.
Hematologic: anemia.
Skin: urticaria.
Other: hypersensitivity reactions, *anaphylaxis.*

Interactions

None significant.

Effects on lab test results

- May increase ALT and AST levels.
- May increase bleeding time. May decrease hemoglobin and hematocrit.

Pharmacokinetics

Absorption: Administered I.V.
Distribution: Distributed throughout vascular system.
Metabolism: Drug molecules with molecular weights above 50,000 are enzymatically degraded by dextranase to glucose at about 70 to 90 mg/kg/day.

Excretion: By kidneys for drug molecules with molecular weights below 50,000. *Half-life:* Unknown.

Route	Onset	Peak	Duration
I.V.	Immediate	Immediate	≤ 3 hr

Action

Chemical effect: Expands plasma volume by colloidal osmotic effect, drawing fluid from interstitial to intravascular space, providing fluid replacement.
Therapeutic effect: Expands plasma volume.

Available forms

Injection: 10% dextran 40 in D$_5$W or normal saline solution

NURSING PROCESS

🔍 Assessment
- Obtain history of patient's underlying condition and hydration before therapy, and reassess regularly. Frequently assess vital signs, fluid intake and output, and urine or serum osmolarity levels.
- Be alert for adverse reactions.
- Watch for circulatory overload and rise in central venous pressure. Plasma expansion is slightly greater than volume infused.
- Check hemoglobin and hematocrit.
- Evaluate patient's and family's knowledge of drug therapy.

🔷 Nursing diagnoses
- Decreased cardiac output related to underlying condition
- Risk for injury related to potential for drug-induced hypersensitivity reaction
- Deficient knowledge related to drug therapy

▶ Planning and implementation
- If oliguria or anuria occurs or isn't relieved by infusion, stop dextran and give loop diuretic.
- If hematocrit falls below 30% by volume, notify prescriber.
- Drug may interfere with analyses of blood grouping, crossmatching, and bilirubin, glucose, and protein levels.
⊛ ALERT: Low– and high–molecular-weight dextrans aren't interchangeable. Verify preparation before use.

Reactions may be *common,* uncommon, *life-threatening,* or COMMON AND LIFE-THREATENING.

Patient teaching
- Tell patient and family about therapy.
- Instruct patient to notify prescriber if adverse reactions, such as itching, occur.

☑ Evaluation
- Patient's vital signs and urine output return to normal.
- Patient has no hypersensitivity reaction to drug.
- Patient and family state understanding of drug therapy.

dextroamphetamine sulfate
(deks-troh-am-FET-uh-meen SUL-fayt)
Dexedrine*, Dexedrine Spansule, Dextrostat, Ferndex, Oxydess II, Spancap #1

Pharmacologic class: amphetamine
Therapeutic class: CNS stimulant
Pregnancy risk category: C
Controlled substance schedule: II

Indications and dosages

▶ **Narcolepsy.** *Adults:* 5 to 60 mg P.O. daily in divided doses.
Children age 12 and older: 10 mg P.O. daily; increase by 10-mg increments weekly until desired response occurs or adult dose is reached.
Children ages 6 to 11: 5 mg P.O. daily; increase by 5-mg increments weekly until desired response occurs. Give first dose on awakening, additional doses (one or two) at intervals of 4 to 6 hours.
▶ **Attention deficit hyperactivity disorder (ADHD).** *Children age 6 and older:* 5 mg P.O. once daily or b.i.d.; increase by 5-mg increments weekly, p.r.n.
Children ages 3 to 5: 2.5 mg P.O. daily; increase by 2.5-mg increments weekly, p.r.n. Rarely, it's necessary to exceed 40 mg daily.
▶ **Short-term adjunct in exogenous obesity‡.**
Adults: 5 to 30 mg P.O. daily 30 to 60 minutes before meals in divided doses of 5 to 10 mg. Or, one 10- or 15-mg sustained-released capsule daily as a single dose in the morning.

Contraindications and precautions

- Contraindicated in patients hypersensitive to sympathomimetic amines, patients with idiosyncratic reactions to them, patients who took an MAO inhibitor within 14 days, and patients with hyperthyroidism, moderate-to-severe hypertension, symptomatic CV disease, glaucoma, advanced arteriosclerosis, or a history of drug abuse.
- Use cautiously in patients with motor and phonic tics, Tourette syndrome, and agitated states.
≜ Lifespan: In pregnant women, use cautiously. In breast-feeding women, safety and efficacy of drug haven't been established.

Adverse reactions

CNS: *restlessness,* tremors, *insomnia,* dizziness, headache, overstimulation, dysphoria.
CV: *tachycardia, palpitations,* hypertension, *arrhythmias.*
GI: dry mouth, unpleasant taste, diarrhea, constipation, anorexia, weight loss, and other GI disturbances.
GU: impotence.
Skin: urticaria.
Other: altered libido, chills.

Interactions

Drug-drug. *Acetazolamide, alkalizing agents, antacids, sodium bicarbonate:* May increase renal reabsorption. Monitor patient for enhanced amphetamine effects.
Acidifying agents, ammonium chloride, ascorbic acid: May decrease level and increase renal clearance of dextroamphetamine. Monitor patient for decreased amphetamine effects.
Adrenergic blockers: Adrenergic blockers are inhibited by amphetamines. Avoid using together.
Antihistamines: Amphetamines may counteract sedative effects of antihistamines. Monitor patient for loss of therapeutic effects.
Chlorpromazine: Inhibits central stimulant effects of amphetamines; may be used to treat amphetamine poisoning. Monitor patient closely.
Haloperidol, phenothiazines, tricyclic antidepressants: Decreases amphetamine effect. Increase dose as needed.
Insulin, oral antidiabetics: May decrease antidiabetic requirement. Monitor glucose levels.
Lithium carbonate: May inhibit antiobesity and stimulating effects of amphetamines. Monitor patient closely.
MAO inhibitors: May cause severe hypertension; possibly hypertensive crisis. Don't use within 14 days of MAO inhibitor therapy.

Meperidine: Amphetamines potentiate analgesic effect. Use together cautiously.

Methenamine: Increases urinary excretion and reduces efficacy of amphetamines. Monitor effects.

Norepinephrine: May enhance adrenergic effect of norepinephrine. Monitor patient closely.

Phenobarbital, phenytoin: May delay absorption of dextroamphetamine. Monitor patient closely.

Propoxyphene: In cases of propoxyphene overdose, amphetamine CNS stimulation is potentiated and fatal seizures can occur. Don't use together.

Drug-food. *Caffeine:* May increase amphetamine and related amine effects. Monitor patient closely.

Effects on lab test results

• May increase corticosteroid level.

Pharmacokinetics

Absorption: Rapid; sustained-release capsules more slowly.
Distribution: Distributed widely throughout body.
Metabolism: Unknown.
Excretion: Excreted in urine. *Half-life:* 10 to 12 hours.

Route	Onset	Peak	Duration
P.O.	Unknown	Unknown	Unknown

Action

Chemical effect: Unknown; probably promotes nerve impulse transmission by releasing stored norepinephrine from nerve terminals in brain. Main sites of activity appear to be the cerebral cortex and reticular activating system.
Therapeutic effect: Helps prevent sleep and calms hyperactive children.

Available forms

Capsules (sustained-release): 5 mg, 10 mg, 15 mg
Tablets: 5 mg, 10 mg

NURSING PROCESS

☑ Assessment

• Obtain history of patient's underlying condition before therapy, and reassess regularly throughout therapy.

• Be alert for adverse reactions and drug interactions.
• Monitor sleeping pattern, and observe patient for signs of excessive stimulation.
• Evaluate patient's and family's knowledge of drug therapy.

🔷 Nursing diagnoses

• Ineffective health maintenance related to underlying condition
• Disturbed sleep pattern related to drug-induced insomnia
• Deficient knowledge related to drug therapy

▶ Planning and implementation

• Give at least 6 hours before bedtime to avoid sleep interference.
• Prolonged use may cause psychological dependence or habituation, especially in patients with history of drug addiction. After prolonged use, reduce dosage gradually to prevent acute rebound depression.

Patient teaching

• Warn patient to avoid hazardous activities until CNS effects of drug are known.
• Tell patient to avoid drinks containing caffeine, which increases effects of amphetamines and related amines.
• Inform patient that fatigue may result as drug effects wear off.
• Instruct patient to report signs of excessive stimulation.
• Inform patient that when tolerance to anorexigenic effect develops, he should stop drug, not increase dose. Tell him to report decreased effectiveness of drug. Warn patient against stopping drug abruptly.

☑ Evaluation

• Patient shows improvement in underlying condition.
• Patient can sleep without difficulty.
• Patient and family state understanding of drug therapy.

Reactions may be *common*, uncommon, *life-threatening*, or COMMON AND LIFE-THREATENING.

dextromethorphan hydrobromide

(deks-troh-meth-OR-fan high-droh-BROH-mighd)
Balminil D.M. ◆, Benylin DM†, Broncho-Grippol-DM ◆, Children's Hold†, DexAlone†, Hold†, Koffex ◆, Pertussin Cough Suppressant†, Pertussin CS†, Pertussin ES*†, Robitussin Pediatric†, St. Joseph Cough Suppressant for Children†, Sucrets Cough Control Formula†, Trocal†, Vicks Formula 44 Pediatric Formula†

More commonly available in combination products such as: Anti-Tuss DM Expectorant†, Cheracol D Cough†, Extra Action Cough†, Glycotuss DM†, Guiamid D.M. Liquid†, Guiatuss-DM†, Halotussin-DM Expectorant†, Kolephrin GG/DM†, Mytussin DM†, Naldecon Senior DX†, Pertussin All-Night CS†, Rhinosyn-DMX Expectorant†, Robitussin-DM†, Silexin Cough†, Tolu-Sed DM†, Tuss-DM†, Unproco†, Vicks Children's Cough Syrup†, Vicks DayQuil Liquicaps†

Pharmacologic class: levorphanol derivative (dextrorotatory methyl ether)
Therapeutic class: antitussive (nonnarcotic)
Pregnancy risk category: C

Indications and dosages

▶ **Nonproductive cough.** *Adults and children older than age 12:* 10 to 30 mg P.O. q 4 hours, or 30 mg gelcaps q 6 to 8 hours. Or, 60 mg extended-release liquid b.i.d. Maximum, 120 mg daily.
Children ages 6 to 12: 5 to 10 mg P.O. q 4 hours, or 15 mg q 6 to 8 hours. Or, 30 mg extended-release liquid b.i.d. Maximum, 60 mg daily.
Children ages 2 to 5: 2.5 to 5 mg P.O. q 4 hours, or 7.5 mg q 6 to 8 hours. Or, 15 mg extended-release liquid b.i.d. Maximum, 30 mg daily. Dosages for children younger than age 2 must be individualized.

Contraindications and precautions

• Contraindicated within 14 days of MAO inhibitor therapy.
• Use cautiously in sedated or debilitated patients and in patients confined to supine position. Also, use cautiously in patients with aspirin sensitivity.

⚖ **Lifespan:** In pregnant women, use cautiously. In breast-feeding women, safety and efficacy of drug haven't been established. In atopic children, use cautiously.

Adverse reactions

CNS: drowsiness, dizziness.
GI: nausea, vomiting, stomach pain.

Interactions

Drug-drug. *MAO inhibitors:* May increase risk of hypotension, coma, hyperpyrexia, and death. Don't use within 2 weeks of dextromethorphan hydrobromide therapy.
Selegiline: May increase risk of confusion, coma, hyperpyrexia. Avoid using together.
Drug-herb. *Parsley:* May cause serotonin syndrome. Discourage using together.

Effects on lab test results

None reported.

Pharmacokinetics

Absorption: Absorbed readily from GI tract.
Distribution: Unknown.
Metabolism: Metabolized extensively by liver.
Excretion: Small amount excreted unchanged. Metabolites excreted primarily in urine; about 7% to 10% excreted in feces. *Half-life:* About 11 hours.

Route	Onset	Peak	Duration
P.O.	≤ 30 min	Unknown	3-12 hr

Action

Chemical effect: Suppresses cough reflex by direct action on cough center in medulla.
Therapeutic effect: Prevents cough.

Available forms

Gelcaps: 30 mg†
Liquid (extended-release): 30 mg/5 ml
Lozenges: 2.5 mg, 5 mg†, 7.5 mg†, 15 mg†
Solution: 3.5 mg/5 ml, 5 mg/5 ml*†, 7.5 mg/5 ml*†, 10 mg/5 ml*†, 15 mg/5 ml*†, 10 mg/15 ml*

NURSING PROCESS

🔎 **Assessment**
• Obtain history of patient's cough before and after giving drug.

• Be alert for adverse reactions and drug interactions.
• Evaluate patient's and family's knowledge of drug therapy.

🔤 **Nursing diagnoses**
• Fatigue related to presence of nonproductive cough
• Risk for injury related to drug-induced adverse CNS reactions
• Deficient knowledge related to drug therapy

▷ **Planning and implementation**
• Don't use drug when cough is valuable diagnostic sign or is beneficial (such as after thoracic surgery).
• As an antitussive, 15 to 30 mg of dextromethorphan is equivalent to 8 to 15 mg of codeine.
• Use drug with chest percussion and vibration.
• Notify prescriber if cough isn't relieved by drug.

Patient teaching
• Instruct patient to follow directions on medication bottle exactly; stress importance of not taking more drug than directed.
• Tell patient to call prescriber if cough persists more than 7 days.
• Suggest sugarless throat lozenges to decrease throat irritation and resulting cough.
• Advise patient to use humidifier to moisten air and ionizer or air filter to filter dust, smoke, and air pollutants.

✔ **Evaluation**
• Patient's cough is relieved.
• Patient has no injury as a result of therapy.
• Patient and family state understanding of drug therapy.

dextrose (d-glucose)
(DEKS-trohs)

Pharmacologic class: carbohydrate
Therapeutic class: total parenteral nutrition (TPN) component, caloric agent, fluid volume replacement
Pregnancy risk category: C

Indications and dosages

▷ **Fluid replacement and calorie supplement in patients who can't maintain adequate oral intake or who are restricted from doing so.**
Adults and children: Dosage depends on fluid and calorie requirements. Peripheral I.V. infusion of 2.5%, 5%, or 10% solution or central I.V. infusion of 20% solution is used for minimal fluid needs; 25% solution is used to treat acute hypoglycemia in neonate or older infant; 50% solution is used to treat insulin-induced hypoglycemia; 10%, 20%, 30%, 40%, 50%, 60%, and 70% solutions diluted in admixtures, normally amino acid solutions, for TPN are given through the central vein.

▼ I.V. administration

• Control infusion rate carefully; maximal rate is 0.8 g/kg/hour. Use infusion pump when infusing with amino acids for TPN.
⚠ ALERT: Never infuse concentrated solutions rapidly; this may cause hyperglycemia and fluid shift.
⚠ ALERT: Use central veins to infuse dextrose solutions with concentrations greater than 10%.
• Check injection site frequently to prevent irritation, tissue sloughing, necrosis, and phlebitis.

Contraindications and precautions

• Contraindicated in patients in diabetic coma while glucose level remains excessively high. Use of concentrated solutions is contraindicated in patients with intracranial or intraspinal hemorrhage, in dehydrated patients with delirium tremens, and in patients with severe dehydration, anuria, hepatic coma, or glucose-galactose malabsorption syndrome.
• Use cautiously in patients with cardiac or pulmonary disease, hypertension, renal insufficiency, urinary obstruction, or hypovolemia.
⚖ Lifespan: In pregnant women, use only if necessary. In breast-feeding women and in children (especially infants of diabetic mothers), use cautiously.

Adverse reactions

CNS: confusion, *unconsciousness in hyperosmolar hyperglycemic nonketotic syndrome.*
CV: *pulmonary edema, worsened hypertension, heart failure* (with fluid overload in susceptible patients), *phlebitis, venous sclerosis.*
GU: glycosuria, osmotic diuresis.

Reactions may be *common*, uncommon, *life-threatening*, or COMMON AND LIFE-THREATENING.

Metabolic: hyperglycemia, hypervolemia, hyperosmolarity (with rapid infusion of concentrated solution or prolonged infusion), *hypoglycemia* from rebound hyperinsulinemia (rapid termination of long-term infusions).
Skin: sloughing, tissue necrosis with prolonged or concentrated infusions or extravasation, especially with peripheral administration.

Interactions

None significant.

Effects on lab test results

- May increase or decrease glucose level.

Pharmacokinetics

Absorption: Administered I.V.
Distribution: Distributed throughout plasma volume.
Metabolism: Metabolized to carbon dioxide and water.
Excretion: Excess excreted in urine. *Half-life:* Unknown.

Route	Onset	Peak	Duration
I.V.	Immediate	Immediate	Unknown

Action

Chemical effect: Simple water-soluble sugar that minimizes glyconeogenesis and promotes anabolism in patient who can't receive sufficient oral caloric intake.
Therapeutic effect: Provides supplemental calories and fluid.

Available forms

Injection: 3-ml ampule (10%); 5-ml ampule (10%); 10 ml (25%); 50 ml (5% and 50% available in vial, ampule, and Bristoject); 70-ml pintop vial (70% for additive use only); 100 ml (5%); 250 ml (5%, 10%); 500 ml (5%, 10%, 20%, 30%, 40%, 50%, 60%, 70%); 1,000 ml (2.5%, 5%, 10%, 20%, 30%, 40%, 50%, 60%, 70%)

NURSING PROCESS

⚕ Assessment

- Obtain history of patient's underlying condition before therapy, and reassess regularly throughout therapy.
- Be alert for adverse reactions.

- Evaluate patient's and family's knowledge of drug therapy.

⚙ Nursing diagnoses

- Imbalanced nutrition: less than body requirements related to underlying condition
- Ineffective health maintenance related to drug-induced hyperglycemia
- Deficient knowledge related to drug therapy

⧯ Planning and implementation

⑨ ALERT: Verify percentage before giving. Concentrations aren't interchangeable.
⑨ ALERT: Never stop hypertonic solutions abruptly. If rebound hyperinsulinemia occurs, have $D_{10}W$ available to treat hypoglycemia.
Patient teaching

- Inform patient of the need for dextrose therapy, the method by which it will be given, and the adverse reactions that should be reported.

☑ Evaluation

- Patient shows improvement of underlying condition.
- Patient maintains normal glucose level throughout therapy.
- Patient and family state understanding of drug therapy.

diazepam
(digh-AZ-uh-pam)
Diastat, Apo-Diazepam ♦ , Diazemuls ♦ ◇ , Diazepam Intensol, Novo-Dipam ♦ , PMS-Diazepam ♦ , Valium, Vivol ♦

Pharmacologic class: benzodiazepine
Therapeutic class: anxiolytic, skeletal muscle relaxant, anticonvulsant, sedative-hypnotic
Pregnancy risk category: D
Controlled substance schedule: IV

Indications and dosages

▶ **Anxiety.** *Adults:* Depending on severity, 2 to 10 mg P.O. b.i.d. to q.i.d. Or, 2 to 10 mg I.M. or I.V. q 3 to 4 hours, if needed.
Elderly patients: 2 to 2.5 mg P.O. once or twice daily; increase gradually, as needed.
Children age 6 months and older: 1 to 2.5 mg P.O. t.i.d. or q.i.d.; increase gradually, as needed and tolerated.

▶ **Acute alcohol withdrawal.** *Adults:* 10 mg P.O. t.i.d. or q.i.d. for the first 24 hours and reduce to 5 mg P.O. t.i.d. or q.i.d., p.r.n. Or, initially, 10 mg I.M. or I.V.; then 5 to 10 mg I.M. or I.V. in 3 to 4 hours, if needed.

▶ **Before endoscopic procedures.** *Adults:* I.V. dose titrated to desired sedative response (up to 20 mg). Or, 5 to 10 mg I.M. 30 minutes before procedure.

▶ **Muscle spasm.** *Adults:* 2 to 10 mg P.O. b.i.d. to q.i.d. daily. Or, 5 to 10 mg I.M. or I.V. initially; then 5 to 10 mg I.M. or I.V. in 3 to 4 hours, p.r.n. For tetanus, larger doses may be required. *Elderly patients:* 2 to 2.5 mg I.M. or I.V. once or twice daily; increase, as needed. *Children age 5 and older:* 5 to 10 mg I.M. or I.V. q 3 to 4 hours, p.r.n. *Infants older than age 30 days and children younger than age 5:* 1 to 2 mg I.M. or I.V. slowly repeated q 3 to 4 hours, p.r.n.

▶ **Preoperative sedation.** *Adults:* 10 mg I.M. (preferred) or I.V. before surgery.

▶ **Cardioversion.** *Adults:* 5 to 15 mg I.V. 5 to 10 minutes before procedure.

▶ **Adjunct in seizure disorders.** *Adults:* 2 to 10 mg P.O. b.i.d. to q.i.d. *Elderly patients:* 2 to 2.5 mg P.O. once or twice daily, increased as needed. *Children and infants age 6 months and older:* 1 to 2.5 mg P.O. t.i.d. or q.i.d. initially; increased as tolerated and needed.

▶ **Status epilepticus.** *Adults:* 5 to 10 mg I.V. (preferred) or I.M. initially. Repeat q 10 to 15 minutes, p.r.n., up to maximum dose of 30 mg. Repeat in 2 to 4 hours, p.r.n. *Children age 5 and older:* 1 mg I.V. q 2 to 5 minutes up to maximum of 10 mg. Repeat in 2 to 4 hours, p.r.n. *Infants older than age 30 days and children younger than age 5:* 0.2 to 0.5 mg I.V. slowly q 2 to 5 minutes up to maximum of 5 mg. Repeat in 2 to 4 hours, p.r.n.

▶ **Control of acute repetitive seizure activity in patients already taking anticonvulsants.** *Adults and children age 12 and older:* 0.2 mg/kg P.R. using applicator. A second dose may be given 4 to 12 hours after the first dose, if needed. *Children ages 6 to 11:* 0.3 mg/kg P.R. using applicator. A second dose may be given 4 to 12 hours after the first dose, if needed. *Children ages 2 to 5:* 0.5 mg/kg P.R. using applicator. A second dose may be given 4 to 12 hours after the first dose, if needed.

▼ I.V. administration

- Give drug I.V. at no more than 5 mg/minute.
- When injecting, give directly into vein. If this is impossible, inject slowly through infusion tubing as near to venous insertion site as possible. Watch closely for phlebitis at injection site.
- To avoid extravasation, don't inject into small veins.

Ⓢ **ALERT:** Monitor respirations every 5 to 15 minutes and before each repeated I.V. dose. Have emergency resuscitation equipment and oxygen at bedside when giving drug I.V.

Contraindications and precautions

- Contraindicated in patients hypersensitive to drug and in those with angle-closure glaucoma, shock, coma, or acute alcohol intoxication (parenteral form).
- Use cautiously in patients with hepatic or renal impairment, depression, or chronic open-angle glaucoma.

⚖ **Lifespan:** In pregnant women (especially during the first trimester) and in breast-feeding women, avoid use of drug. In infants younger than age 6 months, oral form of drug is contraindicated. In elderly and debilitated patients, use cautiously. Reduce dosage because these patients may be more susceptible to adverse CNS effects of drug.

Adverse reactions

CNS: *pain, drowsiness, lethargy, hangover, ataxia,* fainting, depression, restlessness, anterograde amnesia, psychosis, slurred speech, tremors, headache, insomnia.
CV: transient hypotension, **bradycardia, CV collapse.**
EENT: diplopia, blurred vision, nystagmus.
GI: nausea, vomiting, abdominal discomfort, constipation.
GU: incontinence, urine retention.
Respiratory: *respiratory depression.*
Skin: rash, urticaria, desquamation.
Other: physical or psychological dependence, *acute withdrawal syndrome* after sudden discontinuation in physically dependent people, *phlebitis at injection site.*

Interactions

Drug-drug. *Cimetidine:* May increase sedation. Monitor patient carefully.
CNS depressants: May increase CNS depression. Avoid using together.

Reactions may be *common,* uncommon, *life-threatening,* or COMMON AND LIFE-THREATENING.

Diltiazem: May increase CNS depression and prolong effects of diazepam. Use lower dose of diazepam.

Fluconazole, ketoconazole, itraconazole, miconazole: May increase and prolong levels, CNS depression, and psychomotor impairment. Don't use together.

Digoxin: May increase level of digoxin, increasing toxicity. Monitor digoxin level.

Phenobarbital: May increase effects of both drugs. Use together cautiously.

Phenytoin: May increase level of phenytoin. Monitor patient for toxicity.

Ranitidine: May decrease absorption. Monitor patient for decreased effect.

Drug-herb. *Kava, sassafras, valerian:* Sedative effects may be enhanced. Discourage using together.

Drug-lifestyle. *Alcohol use:* May cause additive CNS effects. Strongly discourage alcohol use with these drugs.

Smoking: May increase benzodiazepine clearance. Monitor patient for lack of drug effect.

Effects on lab test results

● May increase liver function test values. May decrease neutrophil count.

Pharmacokinetics

Absorption: I.M. administration results in erratic absorption.

Distribution: Distributed widely throughout body; about 85% to 95% bound to plasma protein.

Metabolism: Metabolized in liver to active metabolite, desmethyldiazepam.

Excretion: Most metabolites of diazepam excreted in urine, with only small amount excreted in feces. *Half-life:* About 1 to 12 days.

Route	Onset	Peak	Duration
P.O.	30 min	½-2 hr	3-8 hr
I.V.	1-5 min	≤ 15 min	15-60 min
I.M.	Unknown	2 hr	Unknown
P.R.	Unknown	1-5 hr	Unknown

Action

Chemical effect: Unknown; probably depresses CNS at limbic and subcortical levels of brain; suppresses spread of seizure activity produced by epileptogenic foci in cortex, thalamus, and limbic structures.

Therapeutic effect: Relieves anxiety, muscle spasms, and seizures (parenteral form); promotes calmness and sleep.

Available forms

Injection: 5 mg/ml
Oral solution: 5 mg/ml, 5 mg/5 ml
Rectal gel: 2.5 mg*, 5 mg*, 10 mg*, 15 mg*, 20 mg*
Sterile emulsion for injection: 5 mg/ml
Tablets: 2 mg, 5 mg, 10 mg

NURSING PROCESS

⚰ Assessment

● Obtain history of patient's underlying condition before therapy, and reassess regularly thereafter.

● Periodically monitor liver, kidney, and hematopoietic function studies in patient receiving repeated or prolonged therapy.

● Be alert for adverse reactions and drug interactions.

● Evaluate patient's and family's knowledge of drug therapy.

🔁 Nursing diagnoses

● Ineffective health maintenance related to underlying condition

● Risk for injury related to drug-induced adverse CNS reactions

● Deficient knowledge related to drug therapy

▶ Planning and implementation

● When oral concentrate solution is used, dilute dose just before giving. Use water, juice, or carbonated beverages, or mix with semisolid food such as applesauce or pudding.

● Avoid P.R. use of Diastat for more than 5 episodes per month or one episode every 5 days.

⚠ **ALERT:** Diastat rectal gel should be given only by caregivers who can distinguish the distinct cluster of seizures or events from the patient's ordinary seizure activity, who have been instructed and can give the treatment competently, who understand which seizure characteristics may or may not be treated with Diastat, and who can monitor the patient's response and recognize when immediate professional help is needed.

● I.M. administration isn't recommended because absorption is variable and injection is painful. Used only when I.V. route and P.O. route aren't applicable.

• Don't mix injectable form with other drugs because diazepam is incompatible with most drugs.

• Don't store parenteral solution in plastic syringes.

• Parenteral emulsion—a stabilized oil-in-water emulsion—should appear milky white and uniform. Avoid mixing with any other drugs or solutions, and avoid infusion sets or containers made from polyvinyl chloride. If diluting, mix drug with I.V. fat emulsion. Use admixture within 6 hours.

• Possibility of abuse and addiction exists. Don't withdraw drug abruptly after long-term use; withdrawal symptoms may occur.

⊛ **ALERT:** Don't confuse diazepam with diazoxide.

Patient teaching
• Warn patient to avoid hazardous activities until CNS effects of drug are known.

• Tell patient to avoid alcohol during drug therapy.

• Warn patient to take drug only as directed and not to stop it without prescriber's approval.

• Warn patient about risk of physical and psychological dependence.

☑ Evaluation
• Patient shows improvement in underlying condition.

• Patient has no injury as result of drug-induced adverse CNS reactions.

• Patient and family state understanding of drug therapy.

diazoxide
(digh-uz-OKS-ighd)
Hyperstat IV, Proglycem

Pharmacologic class: peripheral vasodilator
Therapeutic class: antihypertensive
Pregnancy risk category: C

Indications and dosages

▶ **Hypertensive crisis.** *Adults and children:* 1 to 3 mg/kg by I.V. bolus (maximum, 150 mg) q 5 to 15 minutes until adequate response occurs. Repeat at 4- to 24-hour intervals, p.r.n.

▶ **Hypoglycemia from hyperinsulinism.**
Adults and children: 3 to 8 mg/kg P.O. daily in 2 or 3 divided doses q 8 to 12 hours.
Infants and neonates: 8 to 15 mg/kg P.O. daily in 2 or 3 divided doses q 8 to 12 hours.

▼ I.V. administration

• Protect I.V. solutions from light. Don't use darkened I.V. solutions because they aren't potent.

• Give drug through peripheral vein only. Don't give I.M., S.C., or into body cavities.

• Place patient in supine or Trendelenburg position during and for 1 hour after infusion.

• Monitor blood pressure and ECG continuously.

• Watch for infiltration and irritation; extravasation can cause tissue damage and necrosis.

• Notify prescriber immediately if severe hypotension develops, and keep norepinephrine available.

Contraindications and precautions

• Contraindicated in patients hypersensitive to drug, other thiazides, or other sulfonamide-derived drugs. Also contraindicated in treatment of compensatory hypertension (as in coarctation of the aorta or arteriovenous shunt).

• Use cautiously in patients with impaired cerebral or cardiac function or uremia.

⚘ Lifespan: In pregnant women, use cautiously. In breast-feeding women, drug isn't recommended.

Adverse reactions

CNS: *headache,* dizziness, light-headedness, euphoria, *cerebral ischemia, paralysis.*
CV: *orthostatic hypotension,* flushing, warmth, angina, *myocardial ischemia, arrhythmias,* ECG changes, *shock, MI.*
GI: *nausea, vomiting,* abdominal discomfort, dry mouth, constipation, diarrhea.
Hematologic: *thrombocytopenia.*
Metabolic: *sodium and water retention, hyperglycemia,* hyperuricemia.
Skin: diaphoresis.
Other: inflammation, pain (with extravasation).

Interactions

Drug-drug. *Antihypertensives:* May cause severe hypotension. Use together cautiously; monitor blood pressure closely.

Hydantoins: May decrease levels of hydantoins, resulting in decreased anticonvulsant action. Monitor patient closely.

Sulfonylureas: May cause hyperglycemia. Monitor glucose level.

Thiazide diuretics: May increase diazoxide effects. Use together cautiously.

Insulin and oral antidiabetics: May alter insulin and oral antidiabetic requirements in previously stable patients. Monitor glucose level.

Effects on lab test results

• May increase glucose and uric acid levels.
• May decrease platelet count.

Pharmacokinetics

Absorption: After oral administration, hyperglycemic effect begins in 1 hour. After I.V. administration, blood pressure should decrease promptly with maximum effect in 1 hour.
Distribution: Distributed throughout body; about 90% protein-bound.
Metabolism: Metabolized partially in liver.
Excretion: Diazoxide and its metabolites excreted slowly by kidneys. *Half-life:* 21 to 36 hours.

Route	Onset	Peak	Duration
P.O.	≤ 1 hr	Unknown	< 8 hr
I.V.	≤ 1 min	2-5 min	2-12 hr

Action

Chemical effect: Directly relaxes arteriolar smooth muscle and decreases peripheral vascular resistance. Increases glucose levels by inhibiting pancreatic release of insulin, stimulating catecholamine release or increasing hepatic release of glucose.
Therapeutic effect: Lowers blood pressure; increases blood sugar.

Available forms

Capsules: 50 mg
Injection: 15 mg/ml
Oral suspension: 50 mg/ml

NURSING PROCESS

🔳 Assessment

• Obtain history of patient's blood pressure before therapy.
• Weigh patient daily.

• Monitor glucose levels daily; watch closely for signs of severe hyperglycemia or hyperosmolar nonketotic syndrome.
• Check patient's uric acid levels frequently.
• Be alert for adverse reactions and drug interactions.
• Evaluate patient's and family's knowledge of drug therapy.

🔳 Nursing diagnoses

• Risk for injury related to presence of hypertension
• Excess fluid volume related to drug-induced fluid retention
• Deficient knowledge related to drug therapy

▷ Planning and implementation

• Check patient's standing blood pressure before stopping drug.
• If fluid or sodium retention develops, prescriber may order diuretics.
⑤ ALERT: Don't confuse diazoxide with Dyazide or diazepam, Hyperstat with Nitrostat, Hyper-Tet, or HyperHep.
Patient teaching
• Inform patient that orthostatic hypotension can be minimized by rising slowly and avoiding sudden position changes.
• Instruct patient to remain in supine position for 30 minutes after injection.

☑ Evaluation

• Patient's blood pressure returns to normal.
• Patient maintains normal fluid and electrolyte balance during therapy.
• Patient and family state understanding of drug therapy.

diclofenac potassium
(digh-KLOH-fen-ek poh-TAH-see-um)
Cataflam

diclofenac sodium
Solaraze, Voltaren, Voltaren SR ♦ , Voltaren-XR

Pharmacologic class: NSAID
Therapeutic class: antiarthritic, antiinflammatory
Pregnancy risk category: B

Indications and dosages

▶ **Ankylosing spondylitis.** *Adults:* 25 mg delayed-release tablets P.O. q.i.d. (and h.s., p.r.n.).

▶ **Osteoarthritis.** *Adults:* 50 mg immediate- or delayed-release tablets P.O. b.i.d. or t.i.d. Or, 75 mg P.O. b.i.d. Or, 100 mg extended-release tablets P.O. daily.

▶ **Rheumatoid arthritis.** *Adults:* 50 mg immediate- or delayed-release tablets P.O. t.i.d. or q.i.d. Or, 75 mg P.O. b.i.d. Or, 50 to 100 mg P.R. (where available) h.s. as substitute for last P.O. dose of day. Not to exceed 225 mg daily. Or, 100 mg extended-release tablets P.O. daily or b.i.d.

▶ **Analgesia and primary dysmenorrhea.** *Adults:* 50 mg diclofenac potassium P.O. t.i.d. If needed, 100 mg may be given for first dose only.

▶ **Actinic keratosis.** *Adults:* Apply gel to lesion b.i.d.

Contraindications and precautions

• Contraindicated in patients hypersensitive to drug and in those with hepatic porphyria or a history of asthma, urticaria, or other allergic reactions after taking aspirin or other NSAIDs.
• Use cautiously in patients with history of peptic ulcer disease, hepatic dysfunction, cardiac disease, hypertension, conditions that cause fluid retention, or impaired kidney function.
⚖ Lifespan: During late pregnancy or while breast-feeding, drug isn't recommended. In children, safety and efficacy of drug haven't been established.

Adverse reactions

CNS: anxiety, depression, dizziness, drowsiness, insomnia, irritability, myoclonus, migraine, headache.
CV: *heart failure,* hypertension, edema, fluid retention.
EENT: tinnitus, *laryngeal edema,* swelling of lips and tongue, blurred vision, eye pain, night blindness, epistaxis, reversible hearing loss.
GI: taste disorder, *abdominal pain or cramps, constipation, diarrhea, indigestion, nausea,* abdominal distention, flatulence, peptic ulceration, *bleeding,* melena, bloody diarrhea, appetite change, colitis.
GU: azotemia, proteinuria, *acute renal failure,* oliguria, interstitial nephritis, papillary necrosis, nephrotic syndrome, *fluid retention.*
Hepatic: jaundice, *hepatitis, hepatotoxicity.*

Metabolic: *hypoglycemia,* hyperglycemia.
Musculoskeletal: back, leg, or joint pain.
Respiratory: asthma.
Skin: rash, pruritus, urticaria, eczema, dermatitis, alopecia, photosensitivity, bullous eruption, *Stevens-Johnson syndrome,* allergic purpura.
Other: *anaphylaxis, angioedema.*

Interactions

Drug-drug. *Anticoagulants, including warfarin:* May increase risk of bleeding. Monitor patient closely for bleeding.
Aspirin: May increase risk of bleeding. Don't use together.
Beta blockers: Antihypertensive effect may be blunted. Monitor blood pressure closely.
Cyclosporine, digoxin, lithium, methotrexate: Diclofenac may reduce renal clearance of these drugs and increase risk of toxicity. Monitor patient closely; monitor drug levels if appropriate.
Diuretics: May decrease effectiveness of diuretics. Monitor patient for fluid retention.
Insulin, oral antidiabetics: Diclofenac may alter antidiabetic requirement. Monitor glucose levels.
Potassium-sparing diuretics: Enhances potassium retention and increased potassium levels. Monitor patient for hyperkalemia.
Drug-herb. *Dong quai, feverfew, garlic, ginger, horse chestnut, red clover:* May increase risk of bleeding. Discourage using together.
St. John's wort: May increase risk of photosensitivity. Advise patient to avoid unprotected and prolonged exposure to sunlight.
Drug-lifestyle. *Sun exposure:* May cause photosensitivity reactions. Urge patient to wear protective clothing and sunblock.

Effects on lab test results

• May increase ALT, AST, alkaline phosphatase, bilirubin, BUN, creatinine, and LDH levels. May increase or decrease glucose level.

Pharmacokinetics

Absorption: After P.O. or P.R. administration, rapidly and almost completely absorbed. Absorption is delayed by food.
Distribution: Highly (nearly 100%) protein-bound.
Metabolism: Undergoes first-pass metabolism, with 60% of unchanged drug reaching systemic circulation.

Reactions may be *common,* uncommon, *life-threatening*, or COMMON AND LIFE-THREATENING.

Excretion: About 40% to 60% excreted in urine; balance is excreted in bile. *Half-life:* About 1 to 2 hours after P.O. dose.

Route	Onset	Peak	Duration
P.O., P.R.	30 min	Unknown	8 hr
P.O. enteric-coated	30 min	2-3 hr	8 hr

Action

Chemical effect: Produces anti-inflammatory, analgesic, and antipyretic effects, possibly by inhibiting prostaglandin synthesis.
Therapeutic effect: Relieves inflammation, pain, and fever.

Available forms

diclofenac potassium
Tablets: 50 mg
diclofenac sodium
Suppositories: 50 mg ◆, 100 mg ◆
Tablets (delayed-release/enteric-coated): 25 mg, 50 mg, 75 mg
Tablets (extended-release): 100 mg ◆

NURSING PROCESS

Assessment
- Obtain history of patient's underlying condition before therapy.
- Monitor effectiveness by assessing patient for pain relief.
- Liver function test results may become elevated during therapy. Monitor transaminase level, especially ALT level, periodically in a patient undergoing long-term therapy. Take first level within the first 8 weeks of therapy.
- Be alert for adverse reactions and drug interactions.
- Evaluate patient's and family's knowledge of drug therapy.

Nursing diagnoses
- Acute pain related to underlying condition
- Risk for injury related to drug-induced adverse reactions
- Deficient knowledge related to drug therapy

Planning and implementation
- Give drug with milk or food if GI distress occurs.

- Notify prescriber immediately if patient develops signs of GI bleeding, hepatotoxicity, or other adverse reactions.
- Rectal preparation is not commercially available in the United States. May be substituted for the last oral dose of the day.

Patient teaching
- Tell patient to take drug with milk or food to minimize GI distress.
- Instruct patient not to crush, break, or chew enteric-coated tablets.
- Teach patient signs and symptoms of GI bleeding, and tell him to contact prescriber immediately if they occur.
- Teach patient signs and symptoms of hepatotoxicity, including nausea, fatigue, lethargy, pruritus, jaundice, right upper quadrant tenderness, and flulike symptoms. Tell him to contact prescriber immediately if these symptoms appear.

Evaluation
- Patient is free from pain.
- Patient has no injury as result of drug-induced adverse reactions.
- Patient and family state understanding of drug therapy.

dicyclomine hydrochloride
(digh-SIGH-kloh-meen high-droh-KLOR-ighd)
**Antispas, Bemote, Bentyl, Bentylol ◆,
Byclomine, Dibent, Dilomine, Di-Spaz,
Formulex ◆, Lomine ◆, Merbentyl ◇,
Or-Tyl, Spasmoban ◆**

Pharmacologic class: anticholinergic
Therapeutic class: antimuscarinic, GI antispasmodic
Pregnancy risk category: B

Indications and dosages

▶ **Irritable bowel syndrome and other functional GI disorders.** *Adults:* Initially, 20 mg P.O. q.i.d.; increase to 40 mg q.i.d. Or, 20 mg I.M. q 4 to 6 hours.
Children age 2 and older: 10 mg P.O. t.i.d. or q.i.d.
Infants ages 6 months to 2 years: 5 to 10 mg P.O. t.i.d. or q.i.d.
▶ **Infant colic‡.** *Infants age 6 months and older:* 5 to 10 mg P.O. t.i.d. or q.i.d. Adjust dosage according to patient's needs and response.

Contraindications and precautions

• Contraindicated in patients hypersensitive to anticholinergics and in those with obstructive uropathy, obstructive disease of GI tract, reflux esophagitis, severe ulcerative colitis, myasthenia gravis, unstable CV status in acute hemorrhage, or glaucoma.

• Use cautiously in patients with autonomic neuropathy, hyperthyroidism, coronary artery disease, arrhythmias, heart failure, hypertension, hiatal hernia, hepatic or renal disease, prostatic hypertrophy, or ulcerative colitis.

⚠ Lifespan: In pregnant patients, use cautiously. In breast-feeding women and infants younger than age 6 months, drug is contraindicated.

Adverse reactions

CNS: fever, *headache, dizziness,* insomnia, drowsiness; nervousness, confusion, excitement (in elderly patients).
CV: *palpitations,* tachycardia.
EENT: blurred vision, increased intraocular pressure, mydriasis.
GI: nausea, vomiting, *constipation, dry mouth,* abdominal distention, heartburn, paralytic ileus.
GU: *urinary hesitancy, urine retention,* impotence.
Skin: urticaria, decreased sweating or possibly anhidrosis, other dermal changes.
Other: allergic reactions.

Interactions

Drug-drug. *Amantadine, antihistamines, antiparkinsonians, disopyramide, glutethimide, meperidine, phenothiazines, procainamide, quinidine, tricyclic antidepressants:* May cause additive adverse effects. Avoid using together.
Antacids: May decrease absorption of oral anticholinergics. Separate administration times by 2 to 3 hours.
Ketoconazole: Anticholinergics may interfere with ketoconazole absorption. Give at least 2 hours after ketoconazole.

Effects on lab test results

None reported.

Pharmacokinetics

Absorption: About 67% of P.O. dose absorbed from GI tract; unknown after I.M. administration.
Distribution: Unknown.
Metabolism: Unknown.

Excretion: After P.O. administration, 80% excreted in urine and 10% in feces; unknown after I.M. administration. *Half-life:* Initial, about 2 hours; secondary, 9 to 10 hours.

Route	Onset	Peak	Duration
P.O.	Unknown	1-1½ hr	Unknown
I.M.	Unknown	Unknown	Unknown

Action

Chemical effect: Appears to exert nonspecific, indirect spasmolytic action on smooth muscle. Dicyclomine also possesses local anesthetic properties that may be partly responsible for spasmolysis.
Therapeutic effect: Relieves GI spasms.

Available forms

Capsules: 10 mg, 20 mg
Injection: 10 mg/ml
Syrup: 5 mg/5 ml ◊, 10 mg/5 ml
Tablets: 10 mg ◊, 20 mg

NURSING PROCESS

⬛ Assessment
• Obtain history of patient's underlying condition before therapy.
• Monitor effectiveness by regularly assessing patient for pain relief and improvement of underlying condition.
• Be alert for adverse reactions and drug interactions.
• Evaluate patient's and family's knowledge of drug therapy.

⬛ Nursing diagnoses
• Acute pain related to underlying condition
• Risk for injury related to drug-induced adverse CNS reactions
• Deficient knowledge related to drug therapy

⬛ Planning and implementation
• Drug is synthetic tertiary derivative that may cause atropine-like adverse reactions. Overdose may cause curare-like effects such as respiratory paralysis.
• High environmental temperatures may induce heatstroke during drug use. If symptoms occur, stop drug.
• Give 30 to 60 minutes before meals and at bedtime. Bedtime dose can be larger; give at least 2 hours after last meal of day.

Reactions may be *common,* uncommon, *life-threatening,* or COMMON AND LIFE-THREATENING.

⊙ **ALERT:** Don't give by S.C. or I.V. route.
• Adjust dosage according to patient's needs and response. Doses up to 40 mg P.O. q.i.d. may be used in adults, but safety and efficacy for more than 2 weeks haven't been established.
⊙ **ALERT:** The dicyclomine label may be misleading. The ampule label reads 10 mg/ml, but doesn't indicate that the ampule contains 2 ml of solution (20 mg of drug).
⊙ **ALERT:** Don't confuse dicyclomine with dyclonine or doxycycline; don't confuse Bentyl with Aventyl or Benadryl.

Patient teaching
• Instruct patient to refrain from driving and performing other hazardous activities if he's drowsy or dizzy or has blurred vision.
• Tell him to drink plenty of fluids to help prevent constipation.
• Urge patient to report rash or skin eruption.
• Tell patient to use sugarless gum or hard candy to relieve dry mouth.

☑ **Evaluation**
• Patient is free from pain.
• Patient doesn't experience injury as a result of drug-induced adverse CNS reactions.
• Patient and family state understanding of drug therapy.

didanosine (ddI)
(digh-DAN-uh-zeen)
Videx, Videx EC

Pharmacologic class: purine analogue
Therapeutic class: antiviral
Pregnancy risk category: B

Indications and dosages

▶ **HIV infection when antiretroviral therapy is warranted.** *Adults weighing 60 kg (132 lb) and over:* 200 mg tablets P.O. q 12 hours or 400 mg tablets P.O. daily. Or, 250 mg buffered powder q 12 hours. Or, 400 mg delayed-release capsules P.O. daily.
Adults weighing less than 60 kg: 125 mg P.O. q 12 hours or 250 mg P.O. once daily. Or, 167 mg buffered powder q 12 hours. Or, 250 mg delayed-release capsules P.O. daily.
Children older than age 8 months: 120 mg/m² P.O. q 12 hours.

Children ages 2 weeks to 8 months: 100 mg/m² P.O. q 12 hours.
⊠ **Adjust-a-dose:** In adults who weigh 60 kg or more with creatinine clearance of 30 to 59 ml/minute, give 100-mg tablet b.i.d., 200-mg tablet or 200-mg delayed-release capsule once daily, or 100-mg buffered powder b.i.d; for clearance of 10 to 29 ml/minute, give 150-mg tablet, 125-mg delayed-release capsule, or 167-mg buffered powder once daily. For clearance less than 10 ml/minute, give 100-mg tablet, 125-mg delayed-release capsule, or 100-mg buffered powder once daily.
In adults who weigh less than 60 kg and have a clearance of 30 to 59 ml/minute, give 75-mg tablet b.i.d., 150-mg tablet or 125-mg delayed-release capsule once daily, or 100-mg buffered powder b.i.d; for clearance of 10 to 29 ml/minute, give 100-mg tablet, 125-mg delayed-release capsule, or 100-mg buffered powder once daily. For clearance less than 10 ml/minute or patients on dialysis, give 75-mg tablet or 100-mg buffered powder once daily. Capsules aren't indicated for these patients. No additional dose is needed after hemodialysis.

Contraindications and precautions
• Contraindicated in patients hypersensitive to drug or its components.
• Use cautiously in patients with a history of pancreatitis and in patients with peripheral neuropathy, renal or hepatic impairment, or hyperuricemia.
≋ **Lifespan:** In pregnant women, use cautiously. In breast-feeding women, drug isn't recommended.

Adverse reactions
CNS: *headache, fever,* insomnia, *dizziness, seizures,* confusion, anxiety, nervousness, hypertonia, abnormal thinking, twitching, depression, asthenia, pain, *peripheral neuropathy.*
CV: hypertension, edema, hyperlipemia, **heart failure.**
GI: *diarrhea, nausea, vomiting, abdominal pain, pancreatitis,* dry mouth, dyspepsia, flatulence.
Hematologic: *thrombocytopenia, leukopenia,* granulocytosis, anemia.
Hepatic: liver abnormalities, *hepatic failure, severe hepatomegaly.*
Metabolic: *lactic acidosis.*
Musculoskeletal: myalgia, arthritis, myopathy.

Respiratory: cough, dyspnea, pneumonia.
Skin: rash, pruritus, alopecia.
Other: infection, sarcoma, *anaphylactoid reaction, chills.*

Interactions

Drug-drug. *Amprenavir, delavirdine, indinavir, nelfinavir, ritonavir, saquinavir:* May alter pharmacokinetics of didanosine or these drugs. Separate dosing times.
Antacids containing magnesium or aluminum hydroxides: Enhances adverse effects of antacid component (including diarrhea or constipation) when given with didanosine tablets or pediatric suspension. Avoid using together.
Dapsone, ketoconazole, drugs that require gastric acid for adequate absorption: Decreases absorption from buffering action. Give these drugs 2 hours before didanosine.
Fluoroquinolones, tetracyclines: May decrease absorption from buffering agents in didanosine tablets or antacids in pediatric suspension. Monitor patient for decreased effectiveness.
Itraconazole: May decrease levels of itraconazole. Avoid using together.
Tenofovir with lamivudine: May cause early failure or resistance. Avoid this combination.
Drug-herb. *St. John's wort:* Decreases drug levels, decreasing therapeutic effect. Discourage using together.
Drug-food. *Any food:* Increases rate of absorption. Give drug on an empty stomach.

Effects on lab test results

• May increase uric acid, AST, ALT, alkaline phosphatase, and bilirubin levels.
• May decrease hemoglobin, hematocrit, WBC, granulocyte, and platelet counts.

Pharmacokinetics

Absorption: Degrades rapidly in gastric acid. Commercially available preparations contain buffers to raise stomach pH. Bioavailability averages 33%; tablets may exhibit better bioavailability than buffered powder for oral solution. Food can decrease absorption by 50%.
Distribution: Widely distributed; drug penetration into CNS varies, but CSF levels average 46% of plasma levels.
Metabolism: Not fully understood; probably similar to that of endogenous purines.
Excretion: In urine. *Half-life:* 48 minutes.

Route	Onset	Peak	Duration
P.O.	Unknown	30 min-1 hr	Unknown

Action

Chemical effect: Unknown; appears to inhibit replication of HIV by preventing DNA replication.
Therapeutic effect: Inhibits replication of HIV.

Available forms

Delayed-release capsules: 125 mg, 200 mg, 250 mg, 400 mg
Powder for oral solution (buffered): 100 mg/packet, 167 mg/packet, 250 mg/packet
Powder for oral solution (pediatric): 10 mg/ml in 2- and 4-g bottles
Tablets (chewable): 25 mg, 50 mg, 100 mg, 150 mg, 200 mg

NURSING PROCESS

Assessment
• Obtain history of patient's underlying condition before therapy, and reassess regularly thereafter.
• Be alert for adverse reactions and drug interactions.
• Evaluate patient's and family's knowledge of drug therapy.

Nursing diagnoses
• Infection related to presence of HIV infection
• Diarrhea related to drug-induced adverse effect on bowel
• Deficient knowledge related to drug therapy

Planning and implementation
• Give on empty stomach at least 30 minutes before or 2 hours after meals, regardless of dosage form used; giving drug with meals can decrease absorption by 50%.
• Give patient two tablets of the appropriate strength at each dose to provide adequate buffering.
• Give once-daily dosing only to adults whose disease requires it.
• To give single-dose packets containing buffered powder for oral solution, pour contents into 4 oz of water. Don't use fruit juice or other beverages that may be acidic. Stir for 2 to 3 minutes until powder dissolves completely. Give immediately.

• Use care when preparing powder or crushing tablets to avoid excessive dispersal of powder into air.

• Pharmacist must prepare pediatric powder for oral solution before dispensing. It must be constituted with purified water, USP, and then diluted with antacid (either Mylanta Double Strength Liquid or Maalox TC Suspension) to final concentration of 10 mg/ml. The admixture is stable for 30 days if refrigerated (at 36° to 46° F [2° to 8° C]). Shake solution well before measuring dose.

• If pancreatitis is suspected, stop drug and don't continue until pancreatitis is ruled out.

• If patient has diarrhea while using powdered form, consider switching to tablet form.

Patient teaching

• Instruct patient to chew tablets thoroughly before swallowing and to drink at least 1 oz of water with each dose because tablets contain buffers that raise stomach pH to levels that prevent degradation of active drug. If tablets are manually crushed, stir them thoroughly in 1 oz of water to disperse particles uniformly; then have patient drink mixture immediately.

• Inform patient on sodium-restricted diet that each two-tablet dose of didanosine contains 529 mg of sodium; each single packet of buffered powder for oral solution contains 1.38 g of sodium.

• Warn patient about adverse CNS reactions, and tell patient to take safety precautions.

• Tell patient to notify prescriber if adverse GI reactions occur.

☑ Evaluation

• Patient improves with therapy.
• Patient regains normal bowel pattern.
• Patient and family state understanding of drug therapy.

---

diflunisal

(digh-FLOO-neh-sol)
Dolobid

Pharmacologic class: NSAID, salicylic acid derivative
Therapeutic class: nonopioid analgesic, antipyretic, anti-inflammatory
Pregnancy risk category: C

Indications and dosages

▶ **Mild to moderate pain.** *Adults:* Initially, 500 mg to 1 g P.O., followed by 250 to 500 mg q 8 to 12 hours.

▶ **Osteoarthritis, rheumatoid arthritis.** *Adults:* 500 mg to 1 g P.O. daily in two divided doses, usually q 12 hours. Maximum, 1,500 mg daily.

⧐ Adjust-a-dose: For patients older than age 65, give half the usual adult dose.

Contraindications and precautions

• Contraindicated in patients hypersensitive to drug and in those who develop acute asthmatic attacks, urticaria, or rhinitis after taking aspirin or other NSAIDs.

• Use cautiously in patients with GI bleeding, history of peptic ulcer disease, renal impairment, compromised cardiac function, hypertension, or other conditions predisposing patient to fluid retention.

⚖ Lifespan: In breast-feeding women, drug isn't recommended. In children and teenagers with chickenpox or flulike illness, salicylates aren't recommended because of epidemiologic connection to Reye's syndrome.

Adverse reactions

CNS: *dizziness,* somnolence, insomnia, *headache,* fatigue.
EENT: *tinnitus,* visual disturbances.
GI: *nausea, dyspepsia, GI pain, diarrhea,* vomiting, constipation, flatulence.
GU: renal impairment, hematuria, interstitial nephritis.
Skin: rash, pruritus, sweating, stomatitis, *erythema multiforme, Stevens-Johnson syndrome.*
Other: dry mucous membranes.

Interactions

Drug-drug. *Acetaminophen, hydrochlorothiazide, indomethacin:* Diflunisal may substantially increase levels of these drugs, increasing risk of toxicity. Avoid using together.
Antacids: May decrease diflunisal level. Monitor patient for possible decreased therapeutic effect.
Aspirin: May increase adverse effects. Monitor patient closely.
Cyclosporine: Diflunisal may increase nephrotoxicity of cyclosporine. Avoid using together.
Methotrexate: May increase toxicity of methotrexate. Avoid using together.

Oral anticoagulants, thrombolytics: May enhance effects of these drugs. Use together cautiously.
Sulindac: Diflunisal may decrease level of sulindac's active metabolite. Monitor patient for decreased effect.
Drug-herb. *Dong quai, feverfew, garlic, ginger, horse chestnut, red clover:* May increase risk of bleeding. Discourage using together.

Effects on lab test results

None reported.

Pharmacokinetics

Absorption: Rapid and complete.
Distribution: Highly protein-bound.
Metabolism: In liver.
Excretion: In urine. *Half-life:* 8 to 12 hours.

Route	Onset	Peak	Duration
P.O.	1 hr	2-3 hr	8-12 hr

Action

Chemical effect: May inhibit prostaglandin synthesis.
Therapeutic effect: Relieves inflammation and pain; reduces body temperature.

Available forms

Tablets: 250 mg, 500 mg

NURSING PROCESS

Assessment
● Obtain history of patient's underlying condition before therapy, and reassess regularly thereafter.
● Be alert for adverse reactions and drug interactions.
● Evaluate patient's and family's knowledge of drug therapy.

Nursing diagnoses
● Acute pain related to underlying condition
● Risk for deficient fluid volume related to drug-induced adverse reactions
● Deficient knowledge related to drug therapy

Planning and implementation
● Give drug with milk or food to minimize adverse GI reactions.
● **ALERT:** Don't confuse Dolobid with Slo-bid.

Patient teaching
● Advise patient to take with water, milk, or meals.
● Warn patient to check with prescriber or pharmacist before taking OTC medications or herbal remedies to avoid possible interactions with drugs, such as those containing aspirin or salicylates.

Evaluation
● Patient is free from pain.
● Patient maintains adequate hydration throughout therapy.
● Patient and family state understanding of drug therapy.

digoxin
(dih-JOKS-in)
Digitek, Digoxin, Lanoxicaps, Lanoxin*

Pharmacologic class: cardiac glycoside
Therapeutic class: antiarrhythmic, inotropic
Pregnancy risk category: C

Indications and dosages

▶ **Heart failure, atrial fibrillation and flutter, paroxysmal atrial tachycardia.** *Adults:* For rapid digitalization, give 0.75 to 1.25 mg tablets or elixir P.O. over 24 hours in two or more divided doses q 6 to 8 hours. Or, give 0.4 to 0.6 mg capsules P.O. initially, followed by 0.1 to 0.3 mg q 6 to 8 hours, as needed and tolerated, for 24 hours. Or, give 0.4 to 0.6 mg I.V. initially, followed by 0.1 to 0.3 mg I.V. q 4 to 8 hours, as needed and tolerated, for 24 hours. For slow digitalization, give 0.125 to 0.5 tablets or elixir mg daily for 5 to 7 days. Maintenance dose is 0.125 to 0.5 mg daily. Or, give 0.05 to 0.35 mg capsules daily in two divided doses for 7 to 22 days, as needed, until therapeutic level is reached. Maintenance dose is 0.05 to 0.35 mg daily in one or two divided doses. Or, give appropriate daily maintenance dose for 7 to 22 days as needed until therapeutic levels are reached. Maintenance dose is 0.125 to 0.5 mg I.V. daily in one or two divided doses.
Children age 10 and older: 10 to 15 mcg/kg tablets or elixir P.O. over 24 hours in two or more divided doses q 6 to 8 hours. Maintenance dose is 25% to 35% of total digitalizing dose. For rapid digitalization, give 8 to 12 mcg/kg

capsules P.O. over 24 hours, divided as above. Maintenance dose is 25% to 35% of total digitalizing dose, given daily as a single dose. Or, give 8 to 12 mcg/kg I.V. over 24 hours, divided as above. Maintenance dose is 25% to 35% of total digitalizing dose, given daily as a single dose.

Children ages 5 to 10: 20 to 35 mcg/kg tablets or elixir P.O. over 24 hours in two or more divided doses q 6 to 8 hours. Maintenance dose is 25% to 35% of total digitalizing dose. For rapid digitalization, give 15 to 30 mcg/kg capsules P.O. over 24 hours, divided as above. Maintenance dose is 25% to 35% of total digitalizing dose, divided and given in two or three equal portions daily. Or, give 15 to 30 mcg/kg I.V. over 24 hours, divided as above. Maintenance dose is 25% to 35% of total digitalizing dose, divided and given in two or three equal portions daily.

Children ages 2 to 5: 30 to 40 mcg/kg tablets or elixir P.O. over 24 hours in two or more divided doses q 6 to 8 hours. Maintenance dose is 25% to 35% of total digitalizing dose. For rapid digitalization, give 25 to 35 mcg/kg capsules P.O. over 24 hours, divided as above. Maintenance dose is 25% to 35% of total digitalizing dose, divided and given in two or three equal portions daily. Or, give 25 to 35 mcg/kg I.V. over 24 hours, divided as above. Maintenance dose is 25% to 35% of total digitalizing dose, divided and given in two or three equal portions daily.

Infants ages 1 month to 2 years: 35 to 60 mcg/kg tablets or elixir P.O. over 24 hours in two or more divided doses q 6 to 8 hours. Maintenance dose is 25% to 35% of total digitalizing dose. For rapid digitalization, give 30 to 50 mcg/kg I.V. over 24 hours, divided as above. Maintenance dose is 25% to 35% of total digitalizing dose, divided and given in two or three equal portions daily.

Neonates: 25 to 35 mcg/kg tablets or elixir P.O. over 24 hours in two or more divided doses q 6 to 8 hours. Maintenance dose is 25% to 35% of total digitalizing dose. For rapid digitalization, give 20 to 30 mcg/kg I.V. over 24 hours, divided as above. Maintenance dose is 25% to 35% of the total digitalizing dose, divided and given in two or three equal portions daily.

Premature infants: 20 to 30 mcg/kg tablets or elixir P.O. over 24 hours in two or more divided doses q 6 to 8 hours. Maintenance dose is 20% to 30% of total digitalizing dose. For rapid digitalization, give 15 to 25 mcg/kg I.V. over 24 hours, divided as above. Maintenance dose is 20% to 30% of the total digitalizing dose, divided and given in two or three equal portions daily.

⊠ **Adjust-a-dose:** For children, digitalizing dose is based on child's age and is given in three or more divided doses over the first 24 hours. Initial dose is 50% of the total dose; subsequent doses are given q 4 to 8 hours as needed and tolerated.

For patients with renal impairment, decrease dosage. For patients with hyperthyroidism, may need to increase dosage.

▼ I.V. administration

• Digoxin may be diluted fourfold with D_5W, normal saline solution, or sterile water for injection to reduce the chance of precipitation.
• Infuse drug slowly over at least 5 minutes.
• Protect preparations from light.

Contraindications and precautions

• Contraindicated in patients hypersensitive to drug and in those with digitalis-induced toxicity, ventricular fibrillation, or ventricular tachycardia unless caused by heart failure.
• Use cautiously in patients with acute MI, incomplete AV block, sinus bradycardia, PVCs, chronic constrictive pericarditis, hypertrophic cardiomyopathy, renal insufficiency, severe pulmonary disease, or hypothyroidism.
⚖ Lifespan: In pregnant and breast-feeding women and in elderly patients, use cautiously.

Adverse reactions

CNS: fatigue, generalized muscle weakness, agitation, hallucinations, headache, malaise, dizziness, vertigo, stupor, paresthesia.
CV: *arrhythmias, heart failure,* hypotension.
EENT: yellow-green halos around visual images, blurred vision, light flashes, photophobia, diplopia.
GI: anorexia, nausea, vomiting, diarrhea.

Interactions

Drug-drug. *Amiloride:* Inhibits digoxin effect and increases digoxin excretion. Monitor patient for altered digoxin effect.
Amiodarone, diltiazem, nifedipine, quinidine, verapamil: Increases digoxin levels. Monitor patient for digoxin toxicity.

Amphotericin B, carbenicillin, corticosteroids, diuretics (including loop diuretics, chlorthalidone, metolazone, and thiazides), ticarcillin: May decrease potassium level, predisposing patient to digitalis toxicity. Monitor potassium levels.

Antacids, kaolin-pectin: May decrease digoxin absorption. Schedule doses as far as possible from P.O. digoxin administration.

Cholestyramine, colestipol, metoclopramide: May decrease absorption of P.O. digoxin. Monitor patient for decreased effect and low blood levels. Increase dosage.

Parenteral calcium, thiazides: May increase calcium level and decrease magnesium level, predisposing patient to digitalis toxicity. Monitor calcium and magnesium levels.

Drug-herb. Betel palm, fumitory, goldenseal, lily of the valley, motherwort, rue, shepherd's purse: Possible increased cardiac effect. Discourage using together.

Horsetail, licorice: May deplete potassium stores, leading to digitalis toxicity. Monitor potassium level closely.

Oleander, Siberian ginseng, squill: Possible enhanced toxicity. Discourage using together.

St. John's wort: May reduce therapeutic effect of digoxin, requiring an increased dosage. Monitor patient for loss of therapeutic effect, and advise patient to avoid this herb.

Drug-lifestyle. Alcohol use: May increase CNS effects. Discourage using together.

Effects on lab test results

None reported.

Pharmacokinetics

Absorption: With tablet or elixir form, 60% to 85% of dose is absorbed. With capsule form, bioavailability increases, with about 90% to 100% of dose absorbed.

Distribution: Distributed widely in body tissues; about 20% to 30% bound to plasma proteins.

Metabolism: Small amount of digoxin is thought to be metabolized in liver and gut by bacteria. This metabolism varies and may be substantial in some patients. Drug undergoes some enterohepatic recirculation (also variable). Metabolites have minimal cardiac activity.

Excretion: Most of dose excreted by kidneys as unchanged drug, although a substantial amount of metabolized or reduced drug may be excret-

ed. In patients with renal impairment, biliary excretion is more important excretion route. *Half-life:* 30 to 40 hours.

Route	Onset	Peak	Duration
P.O.	30 min-2 hr	2-6 hr	3-4 days
I.V.	5-30 min	1-4 hr	3-4 days

Action

Chemical effect: Inhibits sodium-potassium-activated adenosine triphosphatase, thereby promoting movement of calcium from extracellular to intracellular cytoplasm and strengthening myocardial contraction. Also acts on CNS to enhance vagal tone, slowing conduction through SA and AV nodes and providing antiarrhythmic effect.

Therapeutic effect: Strengthens myocardial contractions and slows conduction through SA and AV nodes.

Available forms

Capsules: 0.05 mg, 0.1 mg, 0.2 mg
Elixir: 0.05 mg/ml
Injection: 0.05 mg/ml, 0.1 mg/ml (pediatric), 0.25 mg/ml
Tablets: 0.125 mg, 0.25 mg

NURSING PROCESS

🔖 Assessment

• Obtain history of patient's underlying condition before therapy.
• Monitor effectiveness by taking apical pulse for 1 full minute before each dose. Evaluate ECG and regularly assess patient's cardiopulmonary status for signs of improvement.
• Monitor drug level. Therapeutic level ranges from 0.5 to 2 ng/ml. Take level 8 hours after last P.O. dose.
• Monitor potassium level carefully.
• Be alert for adverse reactions and drug interactions.
• Evaluate patient's and family's knowledge of drug therapy.

🔖 Nursing diagnoses

• Decreased cardiac output related to underlying condition
• Ineffective protection related to digoxin toxicity caused by drug
• Deficient knowledge related to drug therapy

Planning and implementation

• Hypothyroid patients are extremely sensitive to glycosides; hyperthyroid patients may need larger doses. Reduce dosage in patients with renal impairment.

• Before giving loading dose, obtain baseline data (heart rate and rhythm, blood pressure, and electrolyte levels) and question patient about use of drug within 2 to 3 weeks.

• Loading dose is always divided over first 24 hours unless patient's condition indicates otherwise.

• Before giving drug, take apical pulse for 1 full minute. Record and report to prescriber significant changes (sudden increase or decrease in pulse rate, pulse deficit, irregular beats, and regularization of previously irregular rhythm). If these changes occur, check blood pressure and obtain 12-lead ECG.

⊛ **ALERT:** Withhold drug and notify prescriber if pulse rate slows to 60 beats/minute or less.

• Because absorption of digoxin from parenteral route and from liquid-filled capsules is superior to absorption from tablets or elixir, expect dosage reduction of 20% to 25% when changing from tablets or elixir to liquid-filled capsules or parenteral therapy.

• For digoxin toxicity, give agents that bind drug in intestine (for example, colestipol or cholestyramine). Treat arrhythmias with phenytoin I.V. or lidocaine I.V. and potentially life-threatening toxicity with specific antigen-binding fragments (such as digoxin immune Fab).

• Withhold drug for 1 to 2 days before elective cardioversion. Adjust dose after cardioversion.

⊛ **ALERT:** Be careful when calculating doses. Tenfold errors can easily occur with children's dosages.

⊛ **ALERT:** Don't confuse digoxin with doxepin.

Patient teaching

• Instruct patient and caregiver about drug action, dosage regimen, pulse taking, reportable signs, and follow-up plans.

• Instruct patient not to substitute one brand of digoxin for another.

• Tell patient to eat potassium-rich foods.

☑ Evaluation

• Patient has adequate cardiac output.

• Patient has no digoxin toxicity.

• Patient and family state understanding of drug therapy.

digoxin immune Fab (ovine)
(dih-JOKS-in ih-MYOON Fab)
Digibind, DigiFab

Pharmacologic class: antibody fragment
Therapeutic class: cardiac glycoside antidote
Pregnancy risk category: C

Indications and dosages

▶ **Potentially life-threatening digoxin toxicity.** *Adults and children:* Dosage based on ingested amount or level of digoxin. When calculating amount of antidote, round up to the nearest whole number.

For digoxin tablets, find the number of antidote vials by multiplying the ingested amount by 0.8; divide answer by 0.5. For example, if patient takes 25 tablets of 0.25-mg digoxin, the ingested amount is 6.25 mg. Multiply 6.25 mg by 0.8 and divide answer by 0.5 to obtain 10 vials of antidote.

For digoxin capsules, find the number of antidote vials by dividing the ingested dose in mg by 0.5. For example, if patient takes 50 of 0.2-mg capsules, the ingested amount is 10 mg. Divide 10 mg by 0.5 to obtain 20 vials of antidote.

If the digoxin level is known, determine the number of antidote vials as follows: multiply the digoxin level in ng/ml by patient's weight in kg, divide by 100. For example, if digoxin is 4 ng/ml, and patient weighs 60 kg, multiply together to obtain 240. Divide by 100 to obtain 2.4 vials; then round up to 3 vials.

▶ **Acute toxicity, or if estimated ingested amount or digoxin level is unknown.** *Adults and children:* Consider administering 10 vials of digoxin immune Fab and observing patient's response. Follow with another 10 vials if indicated. Dose is effective in most life-threatening ingestions in adults and children, but may cause volume overload in young children.

▼ I.V. administration

• Reconstitute with 4 ml of sterile water for injection. For infusion, further dilute solution with normal saline. For children or other patients who need small doses, reconstitute Digibind in 38-mg vial with 34 ml of normal saline for 1 mg/ml concentration; reconstitute DigiFab in 40-mg vial with 36 ml of normal saline for 1 mg/ml concentration.

• Infuse over 30 minutes; if cardiac arrest is imminent, may give as a bolus injection. Infuse via a 0.22-micron membrane filter to ensure no undissolved particulate matter is infused.
• Use reconstituted solution promptly. If not used immediately, refrigerate for up to 4 hours.

Contraindications and precautions

• Use cautiously in patients allergic to ovine proteins. In these high-risk patients, skin testing is recommended because drug is derived from digoxin-specific antibody fragments obtained from immunized sheep.
⚘ Lifespan: In pregnant or breast-feeding women, use cautiously.

Adverse reactions

CV: *heart failure,* rapid ventricular rate.
Metabolic: hypokalemia.
Other: *hypersensitivity reactions, anaphylaxis.*

Interactions

None reported.

Effects on lab test results

• May decrease potassium level.

Pharmacokinetics

Absorption: Administered I.V.
Distribution: Unknown.
Metabolism: Unknown.
Excretion: Excreted in urine. *Half-life:* 15 to 20 hours.

Route	Onset	Peak	Duration
I.V.	Varies	End of dose	2-6 hr

Action

Chemical effect: Binds molecules of digoxin, making them unavailable for binding at site of action on cells.
Therapeutic effect: Reverses digitalis toxicity.

Available forms

Injection: 38-mg vial (Digibind) and 40-mg vial (DigiFab)

NURSING PROCESS

Assessment

• Obtain history of patient's digitalis intoxication before therapy.

• Monitor effectiveness by watching for decreased signs and symptoms of digitalis toxicity; in most patients, signs of digitalis toxicity disappear within a few hours.
• Because drug interferes with digitalis immunoassay measurements, standard digoxin levels are misleading until drug is cleared from body (about 2 days).
• Be alert for adverse reactions.
• Evaluate patient's and family's knowledge of drug therapy.

Nursing diagnoses

• Ineffective health maintenance related to digitalis intoxication
• Decreased cardiac output related to drug-induced heart failure
• Deficient knowledge related to drug therapy

Planning and implementation

• Drug is used only for life-threatening overdose in patients with shock or cardiac arrest; ventricular arrhythmias, such as ventricular tachycardia or fibrillation; progressive bradycardia, such as severe sinus bradycardia; or second- or third-degree AV block not responsive to atropine.
• Give oxygen. Keep resuscitation equipment nearby.
Patient teaching
• Instruct patient to report respiratory difficulty, chest pain, or dizziness immediately.

Evaluation

• Patient exhibits improved health with alleviation of digitalis toxicity.
• Patient demonstrates adequate cardiac output through normal vital signs and urine output and clear mental status.
• Patient and family state understanding of drug therapy.

diltiazem hydrochloride
(dil-TIGH-uh-zem high-droh-KLOR-ighd)
Cardizem, Cardizem CD, Cardizem LA, Cardizem SR, Cartia XT, Dilacor XR, Diltia XT, Tiazac

Pharmacologic class: calcium channel blocker
Therapeutic class: antianginal
Pregnancy risk category: C

Indications and dosages

▶ **Vasospastic angina (Prinzmetal's [variant] angina), classic chronic stable angina pectoris.** *Adults:* 30 mg P.O. t.i.d. or q.i.d. before meals and h.s. Dosage increased gradually to maximum of 360 mg daily in divided doses. Or, 120 to 180 mg extended-release capsules P.O. once daily. Adjust dosage up to 480 mg once daily.

▶ **Hypertension.** *Adults:* 60 to 120 mg sustained-release capsules P.O. b.i.d. Adjust to effect. Maximum recommended dosage is 360 mg daily. Or, 180 to 240 mg extended-release capsules daily initially. Adjust dosage as needed. For Cardizem LA, dosage is individualized. As monotherapy, 120 to 240 mg Cardizem LA P.O. once daily at the same time each day, either in the morning or at bedtime. Adjust dosage about every 14 days. Maximum, 540 mg daily.

▶ **Atrial fibrillation or flutter; paroxysmal supraventricular tachycardia.** *Adults:* 0.25 mg/kg as I.V. bolus injection over 2 minutes. If response is inadequate, 0.35 mg/kg I.V. after 15 minutes, followed with continuous infusion of 10 mg/hour. May be increased in increments of 5 mg/hour. Maximum, 15 mg/hour.

▼ I.V. administration

● For direct I.V. injection, no dilution of 5 mg/ml injection is needed.

● For continuous I.V. infusion, add 5 mg/ml injection to 100, 200, or 500 ml of normal saline solution, D_5W, or 5% dextrose and half-normal saline solution to produce a final concentration of 1, 0.83, or 0.45 mg/ml, respectively.

● Reconstitute drug in monovials labeled as containing 100 mg according to manufacturer's directions.

● For direct injection or continuous infusion, give slowly while continuously monitoring ECG and blood pressure.

● Don't give infusions lasting longer than 24 hours.

⊕ **ALERT:** Furosemide forms a precipitate when mixed with diltiazem injection. Give through separate I.V. lines.

Contraindications and precautions

● Contraindicated in patients hypersensitive to drug and in those with sick sinus syndrome, second- or third-degree AV block in absence of artificial pacemaker, hypotension (systolic blood pressure below 90 mm Hg), acute MI, or pulmonary congestion (documented by X-ray).

● Use cautiously in patients with heart failure and those with impaired liver or kidney function.

⚖ **Lifespan:** With pregnant women, use cautiously. Breast-feeding should be stopped during drug use. In children, safety and efficacy of drug haven't been established. With elderly patients, use cautiously.

Adverse reactions

CNS: *headache,* somnolence, dizziness, insomnia, asthenia.
CV: *edema,* **arrhythmias,** flushing, **bradycardia,** hypotension, conduction abnormalities, **heart failure, AV block,** abnormal ECG.
GI: nausea, constipation, vomiting, diarrhea, abdominal discomfort.
GU: nocturia, polyuria.
Skin: rash, pruritus, photosensitivity.

Interactions

Drug-drug. *Anesthetics:* Effects may be potentiated. Monitor patient.
Cimetidine: May inhibit diltiazem metabolism. Monitor patient for toxicity.
Cyclosporine: Diltiazem may increase cyclosporine levels, possibly by decreasing its metabolism, leading to increased risk of cyclosporine toxicity. Avoid using together.
Digoxin: Diltiazem may increase levels of digoxin. Monitor patient and digoxin levels.
Diazepam, midazolam, triazolam: May increase CNS depression and prolong effects of these drugs. Use lower dose of these benzodiazepines.
Propranolol, other beta blockers: May precipitate heart failure or prolong cardiac conduction time. Use together cautiously.
Drug-lifestyle. *Sunlight:* Photosensitivity may occur. Advise patient to avoid unprotected or prolonged sun exposure.

Effects on lab test results

● May cause transient elevation of liver enzyme levels.

Pharmacokinetics

Absorption: About 80% of dose is absorbed rapidly from GI tract. Only about 40% of drug enters systemic circulation because of significant first-pass effect in liver.

Distribution: About 70% to 85% of circulating diltiazem is bound to plasma proteins.
Metabolism: Metabolized in liver.
Excretion: About 35% excreted in urine and about 65% in bile as unchanged drug and inactive and active metabolites. *Half-life:* 3 to 9 hours.

Route	Onset	Peak	Duration
P.O.	30 min-4 hr	2-18 hr	6-24 hr
I.V.			
bolus	3 min	Immediate	1-3 hr
infusion	3 min	Immediate	< 10 hr

Action

Chemical effect: Inhibits calcium ion influx across cardiac and smooth muscle cells, decreasing myocardial contractility and oxygen demand; also dilates coronary arteries and arterioles.
Therapeutic effect: Relieves anginal pain, lowers blood pressure, and restores normal sinus rhythm.

Available forms

Cardizem
Injection: 5 mg/ml (25 mg and 50 mg)
Tablets: 30 mg, 60 mg, 90 mg, 120 mg
Cardizem CD
Capsules (extended-release): 120 mg, 180 mg, 240 mg, 300 mg, 360 mg
Cardizem SR
Capsules (sustained-release): 60 mg, 90 mg, 120 mg
Cardizem LA
Tablets (extended-release): 120 mg, 180 mg, 240 mg, 300 mg, 360 mg, 420 mg
Cartia XT
Capsules (extended-release): 120 mg, 180 mg, 240 mg, 300 mg
Dilacor XR
Capsules (extended-release) containing multiple units of 60 mg: 120 mg, 180 mg, 240 mg
Diltia XT
Capsules (extended-release) containing multiple units of 60 mg: 120 mg, 180 mg, 240 mg
Tiazac
Capsules (sustained-release): 120 mg, 180 mg, 240 mg, 300 mg, 360 mg, 420 mg

NURSING PROCESS

⚚ Assessment
• Obtain history of patient's underlying condition before therapy, and reassess regularly thereafter.
• Monitor blood pressure when therapy starts and when dosage changes.
• Monitor patient's ECG and heart rate and rhythm regularly.
• Be alert for adverse reactions and drug interactions.
• Evaluate patient's and family's knowledge of drug therapy.

⊕ Nursing diagnoses
• Ineffective health maintenance related to underlying condition
• Decreased cardiac output related to drug-induced adverse reactions
• Deficient knowledge related to drug therapy

▶ Planning and implementation
• Give tablets before meals and at bedtime.
• Patients controlled on diltiazem alone or with other medications may be switched to Cardizem LA tablets once a day at the nearest equivalent total daily dose.
⚕ **ALERT:** If systolic blood pressure is below 90 mm Hg or heart rate is below 60 beats/minute, withhold dose and notify prescriber.
• Assist patient with ambulation during start of therapy because dizziness may occur.
• Restrict patient's fluid and sodium intake to minimize edema.
⚕ **ALERT:** Don't confuse Cardizem SR with Cardene SR.
Patient teaching
• If nitrate therapy is prescribed during adjustment of diltiazem dosage, urge patient compliance. Tell patient that S.L. nitroglycerin may be taken as needed and as directed when angina is acute.
• Instruct patient to call prescriber if he experiences chest pain, shortness of breath, dizziness, palpitations, or swelling of the limbs.
• Tell patient to swallow extended- and sustained-release capsules whole and not to open, crush, or chew them.
• Instruct patient to take drug exactly as prescribed, even when feeling better.
• Advise patient to minimize exposure to direct sunlight and to take precautions when in sun because of drug-induced photosensitivity.

Reactions may be *common*, uncommon, *life-threatening*, or **COMMON AND LIFE-THREATENING**.

- Instruct patient to limit fluid and sodium intake to minimize edema.

✅ Evaluation
- Patient exhibits improvement in underlying condition.
- Patient maintains adequate cardiac output throughout therapy.
- Patient and family state understanding of drug therapy.

dimercaprol
(digh-mer-KAP-rohl)
BAL in Oil

Pharmacologic class: chelating agent
Therapeutic class: heavy metal antagonist
Pregnancy risk category: C

Indications and dosages

▶ **Severe arsenic or gold poisoning.** *Adults and children:* 3 mg/kg deep I.M. q 4 hours for 2 days; then q.i.d. on third day; then b.i.d. for 10 days.

▶ **Mild arsenic or gold poisoning.** *Adults and children:* 2.5 mg/kg deep I.M. q.i.d. for 2 days; then b.i.d. on third day; then once daily for 10 days.

▶ **Mercury poisoning.** *Adults and children:* Initially, 5 mg/kg deep I.M.; then 2.5 mg/kg daily or b.i.d. for 10 days.

▶ **Acute lead encephalopathy or lead level exceeding 100 mcg/dl.** *Adults and children:* 4 mg/kg deep I.M.; then q 4 hours with edetate calcium disodium (250 mg/m² I.M.). Use separate sites. Maximum, 5 mg/kg per dose.

Contraindications and precautions

- Contraindicated in patients with hepatic dysfunction (except postarsenical jaundice).
- Use cautiously in patients with hypertension or oliguria.
- ⚜ Lifespan: In pregnant and breast-feeding women, safety and efficacy of drug haven't been established.

Adverse reactions

CNS: *fever,* headache, paresthesia.
CV: *transient increase in blood pressure,* tachycardia.

EENT: blepharospasm, conjunctivitis, lacrimation, rhinorrhea, excessive salivation.
GI: *halitosis; nausea; vomiting; burning sensation in lips, mouth, and throat; abdominal pain.*
GU: *dysuria,* renal damage.
Musculoskeletal: muscle pain or weakness.
Skin: diaphoresis, sterile abscess.
Other: *pain at injection site,* pain or tightness in throat, chest, or hands; decreased iodine uptake; pain in teeth.

Interactions

Drug-drug. *Iron:* Toxic metal complex formed; use together is contraindicated. Wait 24 hours after last dimercaprol dose.

Effects on lab test results

None reported.

Pharmacokinetics

Absorption: Unknown.
Distribution: Distributed to all tissues, mainly intracellular space.
Metabolism: Uncomplexed drug is metabolized rapidly to inactive products.
Excretion: Most metal complexes and inactive metabolites are excreted in urine and feces.
Half-life: Unknown.

Route	Onset	Peak	Duration
I.M.	Unknown	30-60 min	4 hr

Action

Chemical effect: Forms complexes with heavy metals.
Therapeutic effect: Treats heavy metal intoxication.

Available forms

Injection: 100 mg/ml

NURSING PROCESS

📋 Assessment
- Obtain history of patient's toxicity before therapy.
- Assess effectiveness by monitoring level of substance ingested and for improvement in patient's condition.
- Be alert for adverse reactions and drug interactions.
- Monitor patient's hydration status if adverse GI reactions occur.

- Observe injection site for local reaction.
- Evaluate patient's and family's knowledge of drug therapy.

⊞ Nursing diagnoses
- Risk for poisoning related to exposure to toxic substance
- Risk for deficient fluid volume related to drug-induced nausea and vomiting
- Deficient knowledge related to drug therapy

⊅ Planning and implementation
⊛ **ALERT:** Don't give I.V.; give by deep I.M. route only. Massage injection site after administration.
- Be careful not to let drug come in contact with skin because it may cause skin reaction.
- Don't schedule patient for ^{131}I uptake thyroid tests during therapy because drug decreases results.
- Solution with slight sediment is usable.
- Drug is ineffective in arsine gas poisoning.
⊛ **ALERT:** Don't use for iron, cadmium, or selenium toxicity. Complex form is highly toxic, even fatal.
- Use ephedrine or antihistamine to prevent or relieve mild adverse reactions.
- Keep urine alkaline to prevent renal damage; give oral sodium bicarbonate.
- Apply ice or cold compresses to injection site to alleviate local discomfort.

Patient teaching
- Warn patient that drug has unpleasant garlic-like odor.
- Advise patient that drug may cause pain at injection site.
- Instruct patient to report changes in urine output, fever, pain, nausea, or vomiting immediately.

☑ Evaluation
- Patient's toxicity is eliminated.
- Patient maintains adequate hydration throughout therapy.
- Patient and family state understanding of drug therapy.

diphenhydramine hydrochloride
(digh-fen-HIGH-drah-meen high-droh-KLOR-ighd)
Allerdryl ♦ †, AllerMax Caplets†, Allermed†, Banophen†, Banophen Caplets†, Beldin†, Belix†, Benadryl†, Benadryl 25†, Benadryl Kapseals, Benylin Cough†, Bydramine Cough†, Compoz†, Diphenadryl†, Diphen Cough†, Diphenhist†, Diphenhist Captabs†, Genahist†, Hyrexin-50, Nytol Maximum Strength†, Nytol with DPH†, Sleep-Eze 3†, Sominex Formula 2†, Tusstat†, Twilite Caplets†, Uni-Bent Cough†

Pharmacologic class: ethanolamine derivative antihistamine
Therapeutic class: antihistamine (H_1-receptor antagonist), antiemetic, antivertigo agent, antitussive, sedative-hypnotic, antidyskinetic (anticholinergic)
Pregnancy risk category: B

Indications and dosages

▶ **Rhinitis, allergy symptoms, motion sickness, Parkinson's disease.** *Adults and children age 12 and older:* 25 to 50 mg P.O. t.i.d. or q.i.d. Or, 10 to 50 mg deep I.M. or I.V. Maximum I.M. or I.V. dosage is 400 mg daily.
Children younger than age 12: 5 mg/kg daily P.O., deep I.M., or I.V. in divided doses q.i.d. Maximum, 300 mg daily.
▶ **Sedation.** *Adults:* 25 to 50 mg P.O. or deep I.M., p.r.n.
▶ **Nighttime sleep aid.** *Adults:* 50 mg P.O. h.s.
▶ **Nonproductive cough.** *Adults:* 25 mg P.O. q 4 to 6 hours (up to 150 mg daily).
Children ages 6 to 11: 12.5 mg P.O. q 4 to 6 hours (up to 75 mg daily).
Children ages 2 to 5: 6.25 mg P.O. q 4 to 6 hours (up to 25 mg daily).

▼ I.V. administration

- Make sure I.V. site is patent. Drug given perivascularly may cause tissue irritation.
- Don't give I.V. faster than 25 mg/minute.

Contraindications and precautions

- Contraindicated in patients hypersensitive to drug and in patients having acute asthmatic attacks.
- Use cautiously in patients with angle-closure glaucoma, prostatic hyperplasia, pyloroduode-

nal and bladder-neck obstruction, asthma or COPD, increased intraocular pressure, hyperthyroidism, CV disease, hypertension, or stenosing peptic ulcer.

⚶ **Lifespan:** In pregnant women, use cautiously. In neonates, premature neonates, and breastfeeding women, drug is contraindicated. Children younger than age 12 should use only as directed by prescriber.

Adverse reactions

CNS: *drowsiness,* confusion, insomnia, headache, vertigo, *sedation, sleepiness, dizziness,* incoordination, fatigue, restlessness, tremor, nervousness, *seizures.*
CV: palpitations, hypotension, tachycardia.
EENT: diplopia, blurred vision, nasal congestion, tinnitus.
GI: *nausea,* vomiting, diarrhea, *dry mouth,* constipation, *epigastric distress,* anorexia.
GU: dysuria, urine retention, urinary frequency.
Hematologic: hemolytic anemia, *thrombocytopenia, agranulocytosis.*
Respiratory: thickening of bronchial secretions.
Skin: urticaria, photosensitivity, rash.
Other: *anaphylactic shock.*

Interactions

Drug-drug. *CNS depressants:* May increase sedation. Use together cautiously; monitor patient for increased sedation.
MAO inhibitors: May increase anticholinergic effects. Don't use together.
Other products containing diphenhydramine, including topical forms: May increase risk of adverse reactions. Avoid using together.
Drug-lifestyle. *Alcohol use:* May increase adverse CNS effects. Discourage using together.
Sun exposure: Photosensitivity reactions may occur. Urge patient to wear protective clothing and sunblock.

Effects on lab test results

• May decrease hemoglobin, hematocrit, and platelet and granulocyte counts.

Pharmacokinetics

Absorption: Well absorbed from GI tract after P.O. administration; unknown after I.M. administration.
Distribution: Distributed widely throughout body, including CNS; about 82% protein-bound.

Metabolism: Metabolized in liver.
Excretion: Drug and metabolites excreted primarily in urine. *Half-life:* About 3½ hours.

Route	Onset	Peak	Duration
P.O.	≤15 min	1-4 hr	6-8 hr
I.V.	Immediate	1-4 hr	6-8 hr
I.M.	Unknown	1-4 hr	6-8 hr

Action

Chemical effect: Competes with histamine for H_1-receptor sites on effector cells. Prevents but doesn't reverse histamine-mediated responses, particularly histamine's effects on smooth muscle of bronchial tubes, GI tract, uterus, and blood vessels. Provides local anesthesia by preventing initiation and transmission of nerve impulses and suppresses cough reflex by direct effect in medulla of brain.
Therapeutic effect: Relieves allergy symptoms, motion sickness, and cough; improves voluntary movement; and promotes sleep and calmness.

Available forms

Capsules: 25 mg†, 50 mg†
Chewable tablets: 12.5 mg†
Elixir: 12.5 mg/5 ml*†
Injection: 10 mg/ml, 50 mg/ml
Syrup: 12.5 mg/5 ml†, 6.25 mg/5 ml†
Tablets: 25 mg†, 50 mg†

NURSING PROCESS

⚕ Assessment
• Obtain history of patient's underlying condition before therapy, and reassess regularly thereafter.
• Be alert for adverse reactions and drug interactions.
• Evaluate patient's and family's knowledge of drug therapy.

⊕ Nursing diagnoses
• Ineffective health maintenance related to underlying condition
• Risk for injury related to drug-induced adverse CNS reactions
• Deficient knowledge related to drug therapy

❯ Planning and implementation
• Reduce GI distress by giving drug with food or milk.

- Alternate injection sites to prevent irritation. Give I.M. injection deep into large muscle.
- Notify prescriber if tolerance is observed because another antihistamine may need to be substituted.

⊛ **ALERT:** Do not confuse diphenhydramine with dicyclomine, or Benadryl with Bentyl or Benylin.

Patient teaching
- Instruct patient to take drug 30 minutes before travel to prevent motion sickness.
- Warn patient to avoid alcohol and to refrain from driving or performing other hazardous activities that require alertness.
- Tell patient that coffee or tea may reduce drowsiness.
- Inform patient that ice chips, sugarless gum, or hard candy may relieve dry mouth.
- Advise patient to stop drug 4 days before allergy skin tests to preserve accuracy of tests.
- Tell patient to notify prescriber if tolerance develops because different antihistamine may need to be prescribed.
- Warn patient of possible photosensitivity. Advise use of sunblock or protective clothing.
- Warn patient to avoid using other products containing diphenhydramine, including topical forms because of risk of adverse reactions.

☑ **Evaluation**
- Patient shows improvement in underlying condition.
- Patient has no injury as result of therapy.
- Patient and family state understanding of drug therapy.

diphenoxylate hydrochloride and atropine sulfate
(digh-fen-OKS-ul-ayt high-droh-KLOR-ighd and AH-troh-peen SUL-fayt)
Logen, Lomanate, Lomotil*, Lonox

Pharmacologic class: opioid
Therapeutic class: antidiarrheal
Pregnancy risk category: C
Controlled substance schedule: V

Indications and dosages

▶ **Acute, nonspecific diarrhea.** *Adults:* Initially, 5 mg P.O. q.i.d.; then reduce dosage as soon as initial control is achieved. Maximum, 20 mg P.O. daily.
Children ages 2 to 12: 0.3 to 0.4 mg/kg liquid form P.O. daily in four divided doses. Maintenance dose may be as low as ¼ of initial dose. Maximum, 20 mg P.O. daily.

Contraindications and precautions

- Contraindicated in patients hypersensitive to drugs and in those with acute diarrhea from poison (until toxic material is eliminated from GI tract), acute diarrhea caused by organisms that penetrate the intestinal mucosa, or diarrhea from antibiotic-induced pseudomembranous enterocolitis. Also contraindicated in jaundiced patients.
- Use cautiously in patients with hepatic disease, narcotic dependence, or acute ulcerative colitis. Stop therapy immediately if abdominal distention or other signs of toxic megacolon develop, and notify prescriber.
☀ **Lifespan:** In pregnant women, use cautiously. In breast-feeding women, drug isn't recommended. In children ages 2 to 12, use cautiously and in liquid form only. In children younger than age 2, drug is contraindicated.

Adverse reactions

CNS: *sedation, dizziness,* headache, drowsiness, lethargy, restlessness, depression, euphoria, malaise, confusion, numbness in limbs.
CV: tachycardia.
EENT: mydriasis.
GI: *dry mouth,* nausea, vomiting, abdominal discomfort or distention, paralytic ileus, anorexia, fluid retention in bowel, *pancreatitis.*
GU: urine retention.
Respiratory: *respiratory depression.*
Skin: pruritus, rash.
Other: *angioedema, anaphylaxis,* possible physical dependence with long-term use.

Interactions

Drug-drug. *Barbiturates, CNS depressants, opioids, tranquilizers:* May enhance CNS depression. Monitor patient closely for increased sedation.
MAO inhibitors: May cause a hypertensive crisis. Don't use together.
Drug-lifestyle. *Alcohol use:* May enhance CNS depression. Discourage using together.

Effects on lab test results
None reported.

Pharmacokinetics
Absorption: About 90% absorbed.
Distribution: Unknown.
Metabolism: Metabolized extensively by liver.
Excretion: Metabolites excreted mainly in feces with lesser amounts excreted in urine.
Half-life: Diphenoxylate, 2½ hours; its major metabolite, diphenoxylic acid, 4½ hours; atropine, 2½ hours.

Route	Onset	Peak	Duration
P.O.	45-60 min	3 hr	3-4 hr

Action

Chemical effect: Unknown; probably increases smooth-muscle tone in GI tract, inhibits motility and propulsion, and diminishes secretions.
Therapeutic effect: Relieves diarrhea.

Available forms

Liquid: 2.5 mg/5 ml (with atropine sulfate 0.025 mg/5 ml)*
Tablets: 2.5 mg (with atropine sulfate 0.025 mg)

NURSING PROCESS

Assessment
• Assess patient's diarrhea before and regularly during therapy.
• Be alert for adverse reactions and drug interactions.
• Evaluate patient's and family's knowledge of drug therapy.

Nursing diagnoses
• Diarrhea related to underlying condition
• Ineffective breathing pattern related to drug-induced respiratory depression
• Deficient knowledge related to drug therapy

Planning and implementation
• Fluid retention in the bowel may mask depletion of extracellular fluid and electrolytes, especially in young children treated for acute gastroenteritis. Correct fluid and electrolyte disturbances before starting drug. Dehydration may increase risk of delayed toxicity.
• Keep in mind that 2.5-mg dose is as effective as 5 ml of camphorated opium tincture.

• Drug isn't indicated for treating antibiotic-induced diarrhea.
• Drug is unlikely to be effective if no response occurs within 48 hours.
• Risk of physical dependence increases with high dosage and long-term use. Atropine sulfate helps discourage abuse.
• Use naloxone to treat respiratory depression caused by overdose.
ALERT: Don't confuse Lomotil (diphenoxylate hydrochloride and atropine sulfate) with Lamictal (lamotrigine).

Patient teaching
• Tell patient not to exceed recommended dosage.
• Warn patient not to use drug to treat acute diarrhea for longer than 2 days. Encourage him to seek medical attention if diarrhea persists.
• Advise patient to avoid hazardous activities, such as driving, until CNS effects of drug are known.

Evaluation
• Patient regains normal bowel pattern.
• Patient maintains normal breathing pattern throughout therapy.
• Patient and family state understanding of drug therapy.

dipyridamole
(digh-peer-IH-duh-mohl)
Apo-Dipyridamole ♦ , Novo-Dipiradol ♦ , Persantin ◊ , Persantin 100 ◊ , Persantine

Pharmacologic class: pyrimidine analogue
Therapeutic class: coronary vasodilator, platelet aggregation inhibitor
Pregnancy risk category: B

Indications and dosages

▶ **Inhibition of platelet adhesion in prosthetic heart valves.** *Adults:* 75 to 100 mg P.O. q.i.d. (with warfarin or aspirin).
▶ **Alternative to exercise in evaluation of coronary artery disease during thallium-201 myocardial perfusion scintigraphy.** *Adults:* 0.57 mg/kg as I.V. infusion at constant rate over 4 minutes (0.142 mg/kg/minute).
▶ **Chronic angina pectoris‡.** *Adults:* 50 mg P.O. t.i.d. at least 1 hour before meals; 2 to 3

months of therapy may be required to achieve therapeutic response.

▶ **Prevention of thromboembolic complications in patients with various thromboembolic disorders other than prosthetic heart valves‡.** *Adults:* 150 to 400 mg P.O. daily (with warfarin or aspirin).

▽ I.V. administration

• If giving drug as diagnostic agent, dilute in half-normal or normal saline solution or D_5W in at least a 1:2 ratio for total volume of 20 to 50 ml.
• Inject thallium-201 within 5 minutes after completing 4-minute dipyridamole infusion.
• Avoid freezing and protect from direct light.

Contraindications and precautions

• Use cautiously in patients with hypotension.
⚕ **Lifespan:** In pregnant women, use cautiously. In breast-feeding women and in children, safety and efficacy of drug haven't been established.

Adverse reactions

CNS: headache, dizziness, weakness.
CV: flushing, fainting, hypotension, chest pain, ECG abnormalities, blood pressure lability, hypertension (with I.V. infusion).
GI: nausea, vomiting, diarrhea, abdominal distress.
Skin: rash, irritation (with undiluted injection), pruritus.

Interactions

Drug-drug. *Heparin:* May cause increased bleeding. Monitor patient closely for increased bleeding; monitor PTT.
Theophylline: May prevent coronary vasodilation by I.V. dipyridamole. Avoid using together.
Drug-herb. *Dong quai, feverfew, garlic, ginger, horse chestnut, red clover:* May increase risk of bleeding. Discourage using together.

Effects on lab test results

None reported.

Pharmacokinetics

Absorption: Variable and slow; bioavailability ranges from 27% to 59%.
Distribution: Wide distribution in body tissues. Protein binding ranges from 91% to 97%.
Metabolism: Metabolized by liver.

Excretion: Elimination occurs by way of biliary excretion of glucuronide conjugates. Some dipyridamole and conjugates may undergo enterohepatic circulation and fecal excretion; small amount is excreted in urine. *Half-life:* 1 to 12 hours.

Route	Onset	Peak	Duration
P.O.	Unknown	45-150 min	Unknown
I.V.	Unknown	2 min after therapy stops	Unknown
I.M.	Unknown	Unknown	Unknown

Action

Chemical effect: May involve its ability to increase adenosine, which is a coronary vasodilator and platelet aggregation inhibitor.
Therapeutic effect: Dilates coronary arteries and helps prevent clotting.

Available forms

Injection: 10 mg/2 ml
Tablets: 25 mg, 50 mg, 75 mg

NURSING PROCESS

⚖ Assessment

• Obtain history of patient's underlying condition before therapy, and reassess regularly thereafter.
• Be alert for adverse reactions and drug interactions.
• Evaluate patient's and family's knowledge of drug therapy.

⊞ Nursing diagnoses

• Ineffective cardiopulmonary tissue perfusion related to underlying condition
• Acute pain related to drug-induced headache
• Deficient knowledge related to drug therapy

▷ Planning and implementation

• Give drug 1 hour before meals. If patient develops adverse GI reactions, give drug with meals.
• The value of dipyridamole as part of an antithrombotic regimen is controversial; its use may not provide significantly better results than aspirin alone.
⚠ **ALERT:** Don't confuse dipyridamole with disopyramide; or Persantine with Periactin.

Patient teaching

- Instruct patient when to take drug.
- Tell patient to have his blood pressure checked frequently.
- Advise patient to take mild analgesic if headache occurs.
- Instruct patient to notify prescriber if chest pain occurs.

✓ Evaluation

- Patient maintains adequate tissue perfusion and cellular oxygenation.
- Patient obtains relief from drug-induced headache with use of mild analgesic.
- Patient and family state understanding of drug therapy.

disopyramide
(digh-so-PEER-uh-mighd)
Rythmodan ♦ ◇

disopyramide phosphate
Norpace, Norpace CR, Rythmodan LA ♦

Pharmacologic class: pyridine derivative
Therapeutic class: antiarrhythmic
Pregnancy risk category: C

Indications and dosages

▶ **Symptomatic PVCs (unifocal, multifocal, or coupled); ventricular tachycardia not severe enough to require cardioversion.**
Adults: For parenteral use, initially give 2 mg/kg I.V. slowly (over not less than 15 minutes). Give drug until arrhythmia is gone or patient has received 150 mg. Repeat dosage if conversion is successful but arrhythmia returns. Total I.V. dosage shouldn't exceed 300 mg in first hour. Follow with I.V. infusion of 0.4 mg/kg/hour (usually 20 to 30 mg/hour) to maximum of 800 mg daily.
Adults weighing over 50 kg (110 lb): Initial loading dose: 300 mg P.O. for rapid control of ventricular arrhythmia. Follow with 150 mg q 6 hours, then 150 mg q 12 hours with controlled-release capsules.
Adults weighing 50 kg or less: Initial loading dose is 200 mg P.O., then 100 mg P.O. q 6 hours as conventional capsules or 200 mg P.O. q 12 hours with controlled-release capsules.

Children ages 12 to 18: 6 to 15 mg/kg P.O. daily, divided into equal amounts and given q 6 hours.
Children ages 4 to 12: 10 to 15 mg/kg P.O. daily, divided into equal amounts and given q 6 hours.
Children ages 1 to 4: 10 to 20 mg/kg P.O. daily, divided into equal amounts and given q 6 hours.
Children younger than age 1: 10 to 30 mg/kg P.O. daily, divided into equal amounts and given q 6 hours.
⊠ **Adjust-a-dose:** For patients with renal impairment, if creatinine clearance is 30 to 40 ml/minute, give 100 mg q 8 hours; if creatinine clearance is 15 to 30 ml/minute, give 100 mg q 12 hours; if creatinine clearance is less than 15 ml/minute, give 100 mg q 24 hours.

▽ I.V. administration

- Add 200 mg to 500 ml of compatible solution, such as normal saline solution or D_5W.
- Use an infusion pump to give drug. Don't mix with other drugs.
- Give slowly, over at least 15 minutes.
- Switch to P.O. therapy as soon as possible.

Contraindications and precautions

- Contraindicated in patients hypersensitive to drug and in those with cardiogenic shock or second- or third-degree heart block without an artificial pacemaker.
- Use cautiously and avoid, if possible, in patients with heart failure.
- Use cautiously in patients with underlying conduction abnormalities, urinary tract diseases (especially prostatic hypertrophy), hepatic or renal impairment, myasthenia gravis, or acute angle-closure glaucoma.
- ⚘ **Lifespan:** In pregnant women, use cautiously. In breast-feeding women, drug isn't recommended.

Adverse reactions

CNS: dizziness, agitation, depression, syncope, fatigue, headache, acute psychosis.
CV: *hypotension, heart failure, heart block,* edema, *arrhythmias,* chest pain.
EENT: blurred vision, dry eyes, dry nose.
GI: nausea, vomiting, anorexia, bloating, abdominal pain, constipation, dry mouth, diarrhea.
GU: urine retention, urinary hesitancy.
Hepatic: cholestatic jaundice.
Metabolic: weight gain.
Musculoskeletal: aches, pain, muscle weakness.

Respiratory: shortness of breath.
Skin: rash, pruritus, dermatosis.

Interactions

Drug-drug. *Antiarrhythmics:* May cause additive or antagonized antiarrhythmic effects. Monitor patient ECG closely.
Erythromycin: May increase disopyramide levels may occur, causing arrhythmias and prolonged QTc interval. Monitor ECG closely.
Phenytoin: May increase metabolism of disopyramide. Monitor patient for decreased antiarrhythmic effect.
Rifampin: Disopyramide levels may be decreased. Monitor patient for decreased effectiveness.
Drug-herb. *Jimson weed:* May adversely affect CV function. Discourage using together.

Effects on lab test results

None reported.

Pharmacokinetics

Absorption: Rapidly and well absorbed from GI tract with P.O. administration.
Distribution: Well distributed throughout extracellular fluid but not extensively bound to tissues. Protein-binding varies but generally ranges from about 50% to 65%.
Metabolism: Metabolized in liver.
Excretion: Excreted in urine. *Half-life:* About 7 hours.

Route	Onset	Peak	Duration
P.O.	30 min-3½ hr	2-2½ hr	1½-8½ hr
I.V.	Unknown	Unknown	Unknown

Action

Chemical effect: Unknown; considered class Ia antiarrhythmic that depresses phase 0 and prolongs action potential. All class I drugs have membrane-stabilizing effects.
Therapeutic effect: Restores normal sinus rhythm.

Available forms

disopyramide
Capsules: 100 mg ♦ , 150 mg ♦
disopyramide phosphate
Capsules: 100 mg, 150 mg
Capsules (controlled-release): 100 mg, 150 mg

Injection: 10 mg/ml ♦ ◊
Tablets (sustained-release): 150 mg ♦

NURSING PROCESS

⬛ Assessment
• Obtain history of patient's arrhythmia before therapy.
• Monitor effectiveness by assessing patient's ECG pattern and apical pulse rate.
• Be alert for adverse reactions and drug interactions.
• Evaluate patient's and family's knowledge of drug therapy.

⬛ Nursing diagnoses
• Decreased cardiac output related to underlying arrhythmia
• Ineffective protection related to drug-induced proarrhythmias
• Deficient knowledge related to drug therapy

▶ Planning and implementation
• Correct any underlying electrolyte abnormalities before therapy begins.
• Check apical pulse before giving drug. Notify prescriber if pulse rate is slower than 60 beats/minute or faster than 120 beats/minute.
• Don't use sustained- and controlled-release preparations for rapid control of ventricular arrhythmias, when therapeutic blood levels must be rapidly attained; in patients with cardiomyopathy or possible cardiac decompensation; or in those with severe renal impairment.
• For administration to young children, pharmacist may prepare disopyramide suspension from 100-mg capsules using cherry syrup. Suspension should be dispensed in amber glass bottles and protected from light.
• Stop drug if heart block develops, if QRS complex widens by more than 25%, or if QT interval is prolonged by more than 25% above baseline; also notify prescriber.
Patient teaching
• When switching patient from immediate- to sustained-release capsules, advise him to take sustained-release capsule 6 hours after last immediate-release capsule was taken.
• Teach patient importance of taking drug on time and exactly as prescribed. This may require use of alarm clock for night doses.
• Advise patient to chew gum or hard candy to relieve dry mouth.

- Tell patient not to crush or chew extended-release tablets.

☑ Evaluation
- Patient's ECG reveals that arrhythmia has been corrected.
- Patient develops no new arrhythmias as result of therapy.
- Patient and family state understanding of drug therapy.

disulfiram
(digh-SUL-fih-ram)
Antabuse

Pharmacologic class: aldehyde dehydrogenase inhibitor
Therapeutic class: alcohol deterrent
Pregnancy risk category: NR

Indications and dosages

▶ **Adjunct in management of chronic alcoholism.** *Adults:* 250 to 500 mg P.O. as single dose in morning for 1 to 2 weeks. Can be taken in evening if drowsiness occurs. Maintenance dosage is 125 to 500 mg P.O. daily (average dosage 250 mg) until permanent self-control is established. Treatment may continue for months or years.

Contraindications and precautions

- Contraindicated during alcohol intoxication and within 12 hours of alcohol ingestion. Also contraindicated in patients hypersensitive to disulfiram or thiram derivatives used in pesticides and rubber vulcanization; patients with psychoses, myocardial disease, or coronary occlusion; and patients receiving metronidazole, paraldehyde, alcohol, or alcohol-containing preparations.
- Use cautiously in patients receiving phenytoin therapy and in patients with diabetes mellitus, hypothyroidism, seizure disorder, cerebral damage, nephritis, or hepatic cirrhosis or insufficiency.
- ⚖ Lifespan: In pregnant women, don't use. In breast-feeding women, use cautiously. In children, safety and efficacy of drug haven't been established.

Adverse reactions
CNS: drowsiness, headache, fatigue, delirium, depression, neuritis, peripheral neuritis, polyneuritis, restlessness, and psychotic reactions.
EENT: optic neuritis.
GI: metallic or garlic aftertaste.
GU: impotence.
Skin: acneiform or allergic dermatitis.
Other: *disulfiram reaction.*

Interactions
Drug-drug. *Alfentanil:* May prolong duration of effect. Monitor patient closely.
Anticoagulants: May increase anticoagulant effect. Adjust dosage of anticoagulant accordingly; monitor patient for bleeding.
CNS depressants: Increases CNS depression. Use together cautiously.
Isoniazid: May cause ataxia or marked change in behavior. Avoid using together.
Metronidazole: Will cause psychotic reaction. Avoid using together; wait for 2 weeks following disulfiram.
Midazolam: May increase plasma levels of midazolam. Use together cautiously.
Paraldehyde: Will cause toxic levels of acetaldehyde. Don't use together.
Phenytoin: May increase toxic effects of phenytoin. Monitor phenytoin levels closely and adjust dose.
Tricyclic antidepressants, especially amitriptyline: May cause transient delirium. Monitor patient closely.
Drug-herb. *Passion flower, pill-bearing spurge, pokeweed, squaw vine, squill, sundew, sweet flag, tormentil, valerian, yarrow:* Disulfiram reaction may occur if herb form contains alcohol. Discourage using together.
Drug-lifestyle. *Alcohol use:* May cause disulfiram reaction including flushing, tachycardia, bronchospasm, sweating, nausea, and vomiting. Death may also occur. Warn patients against using products containing alcohol or drinking alcohol.

Effects on lab test results
- May increase cholesterol level.

Pharmacokinetics
Absorption: Absorbed completely from GI tract.
Distribution: Highly lipid-soluble and initially localized in adipose tissue.

Metabolism: Mostly oxidized in liver.
Excretion: Primarily excreted in urine; 5% to
20% eliminated in feces. *Half-life:* Unknown.

Route	Onset	Peak	Duration
P.O.	1-2 hr	Unknown	< 14 days

Action

Chemical effect: Blocks oxidation of ethanol at
acetaldehyde stage. Excess acetaldehyde produces highly unpleasant reaction in presence of
even small amounts of ethanol.
Therapeutic effect: Deters alcohol consumption.

Available forms

Tablets: 250 mg, 500 mg

NURSING PROCESS

Assessment
• Obtain history of patient's alcoholism before
therapy.
• Complete physical examination and laboratory studies, including CBC, chemistry panel, and
transaminase determination, should precede
therapy. Repeat physical examination and laboratory studies regularly.
• Monitor effectiveness by assessing patient's
abstinence from alcohol.
• Measure serum alcohol level weekly.
• Be alert for adverse reactions and drug interactions. Disulfiram reaction is precipitated by
alcohol use and may include flushing, throbbing
headache, dyspnea, nausea, copious vomiting,
diaphoresis, thirst, chest pain, palpitations, hyperventilation, hypotension, syncope, anxiety,
weakness, blurred vision, and confusion. In severe reactions patient may experience respiratory depression, CV collapse, arrhythmias, MI,
acute heart failure, seizures, unconsciousness,
and death.
• Mild reactions may occur in sensitive patients
with blood alcohol levels of 5 to 10 mg/dl;
symptoms are fully developed at 50 mg/dl;
unconsciousness typically occurs at 125- to
150-mg/dl level. Reaction may last from 30
minutes to several hours or as long as alcohol
remains in blood.
• Evaluate patient's and family's knowledge of
drug therapy.

Nursing diagnoses
• Ineffective health maintenance related to alco-
holism
• Acute pain related to drug-induced headache
• Deficient knowledge related to drug therapy

Planning and implementation
• Use only under close medical and nursing supervision. Only give drug to patient who hasn't
used alcohol for at least 12 hours. Patient should
clearly understand consequences of therapy and
give permission for its use. Use drug only if patient is cooperative, well-motivated, and receiving supportive psychiatric therapy.
• Drug is usually given during the day, although
it may be given at night if drowsiness occurs.
Establish lowered maintenance dose until permanent self-control is practiced. Keep in mind
that treatment may continue for months or
years.

Patient teaching
• Caution patient's family that drug should never be given to the patient without his knowledge; severe reaction or death could result if the
patient ingests alcohol.
• Warn patient to avoid all sources of alcohol
(for example, sauces and cough syrups). Even
external application of liniments, shaving lotion,
and back-rub preparations may precipitate disulfiram reaction. Tell patient that alcohol reaction
may occur as long as 2 weeks after single dose
of disulfiram; the longer patient remains on
drug, the more sensitive he becomes to alcohol.
• Tell patient to wear or carry medical identification identifying him as a disulfiram user.
• Reassure patient that drug-induced adverse reactions (unrelated to alcohol use), such as
drowsiness, fatigue, impotence, headache, peripheral neuritis, and metallic or garlic taste,
subside after about 2 weeks of therapy.

Evaluation
• Patient abstains from alcohol consumption.
• Patient's headache is relieved with mild anal-
gesic therapy.
• Patient and family state understanding of drug
therapy.

dobutamine hydrochloride
(doh-BYOO-tuh-meen high-droh-KLOR-ighd)
Dobutrex

Pharmacologic class: adrenergic, beta$_1$ agonist
Therapeutic class: inotropic agent
Pregnancy risk category: B

Indications and dosages

▶ **To increase cardiac output in short-term treatment of cardiac decompensation caused by depressed contractility, such as during refractory heart failure, and as adjunct in cardiac surgery.** *Adults:* 2 to 20 mcg/kg/minute I.V. infusion. Rarely, rates up to 40 mcg/kg/minute may be needed; however, such doses may worsen ischemia.

▽ I.V. administration

● Dilute concentrate for injection before administration. Compatible solutions include D$_5$W, half-normal saline solution injection, normal saline solution injection, and lactated Ringer's injection. The contents of one vial (250 mg) diluted with 1,000 ml of solution yield 250 mcg/ml; diluted with 500 ml, 500 mcg/ml; diluted with 250 ml, 1,000 mcg/ml. Concentration shouldn't exceed 5 mg/ml.
● Oxidation of drug may slightly discolor admixtures containing dobutamine. This doesn't indicate significant loss of potency, provided drug is used within 24 hours of reconstitution.
● Give drug using central venous catheter or large peripheral vein. Titrate infusion according to prescriber's orders and patient's condition. Use infusion pump.
● Don't mix with sodium bicarbonate injection because drug is incompatible with alkaline solutions.
⑤ **ALERT:** Don't give in same I.V. line with other drugs. Drug is incompatible with heparin, hydrocortisone sodium succinate, cefazolin, neutral cephalothin, penicillin, and ethacrynate sodium.
● I.V. solutions remain stable for 24 hours.
● Watch for irritation and infiltration; extravasation can cause inflammation, tissue damage and necrosis. Change I.V. sites regularly to avoid phlebitis.

Contraindications and precautions

● Contraindicated in patients hypersensitive to drug or its components and in those with idiopathic hypertrophic subaortic stenosis.
● Use cautiously in patients with history of hypertension. Drug may cause exaggerated pressor response.
☀ **Lifespan:** In pregnant and breast-feeding women and in children, safety and efficacy of drug haven't been established.

Adverse reactions

CNS: headache.
CV: *increased heart rate, hypertension,* PVCs, angina, nonspecific chest pain, phlebitis, *hypotension.*
GI: nausea, vomiting.
Musculoskeletal: mild leg cramps or tingling sensation.
Respiratory: shortness of breath, *asthma attacks.*
Other: *anaphylaxis.*

Interactions

Drug-drug. *Beta blockers:* May antagonize dobutamine effects. Don't use together.
Bretylium: May potentiate action of vasopressors on adrenergic receptors; arrhythmias may result. Monitor ECG closely.
General anesthetics: Greater risk of ventricular arrhythmias. Monitor patient closely.
Tricyclic antidepressants: May potentiate the pressor response and cause arrhythmias. Use with caution.
Drug-herb. *Rue:* Increases inotropic potential. Monitor vital signs closely.

Effects on lab test results

● May decrease potassium level.

Pharmacokinetics

Absorption: Administered I.V.
Distribution: Widely distributed throughout body.
Metabolism: Metabolized by liver.
Excretion: Excreted mainly in urine with minor amounts in feces. *Half-life:* About 2 minutes.

Route	Onset	Peak	Duration
I.V.	1-2 min	≤ 10 min after therapy stops	< 5 min

Action

Chemical effect: Directly stimulates beta$_1$ receptors to increase myocardial contractility and stroke volume. At therapeutic dosages, drug decreases peripheral vascular resistance (afterload), reduces ventricular filling pressure (preload), and may facilitate AV node conduction.
Therapeutic effect: Increases cardiac output.

Available forms

Injection: 12.5 mg/ml in 20-ml vials
Premixed: 0.5 mg/ml (125 mg or 250 mg) in D$_5$W, 1 mg/ml (250 mg or 500 mg) in D$_5$W, 2 mg/ml (500 mg) in D$_5$W, 4 mg/ml (1000 mg) in D$_5$W

NURSING PROCESS

Assessment

• Assess patient's condition before therapy and regularly thereafter.
• Continuously monitor ECG, blood pressure, pulmonary capillary wedge pressure, cardiac condition, and urine output.
• Monitor electrolyte level.
• Be alert for adverse reactions and drug interactions.
• Evaluate patient's and family's knowledge of drug therapy.

Nursing diagnoses

• Decreased cardiac output related to underlying condition
• Acute pain related to headache
• Deficient knowledge related to drug therapy

Planning and implementation

• Before starting dobutamine, correct hypovolemia with plasma volume expanders.
• Give digoxin before drug. Because drug increases AV node conduction, patients with atrial fibrillation may develop rapid ventricular rate.
⊛ **ALERT:** Don't confuse dobutamine with dopamine.
Patient teaching
• Tell patient to report chest pain, shortness of breath, and headache.

Evaluation

• Patient regains adequate cardiac output exhibited by stable vital signs, normal urine output, and clear mental status.

• Patient's headache is relieved with analgesic administration.
• Patient and family state understanding of drug therapy.

docetaxel
(doks-uh-TAKX-ul)
Taxotere

Pharmacologic class: taxoid antineoplastic
Therapeutic class: antineoplastic
Pregnancy risk category: D

Indications and dosages

▶ **Locally advanced or metastatic breast cancer for which prior chemotherapy has failed.** *Adults:* 60 to 100 mg/m^2 I.V. over 1 hour q 3 weeks.
◨ **Adjust-a-dose:** If patient initially receives 100 mg/m^2 and experiences febrile neutropenia, neutrophils less than 500 cells/mm^3 for more than 1 week, or severe or cumulative cutaneous reactions, decrease dose to 75 mg/m^2. If reactions continue, decrease dose to 55 mg/m^2 or stop therapy.

If patient receives 60 mg/m^2 initially and doesn't experience febrile neutropenia, neutrophils less than 500 cells/mm^3, severe or cumulative cutaneous reactions, or severe peripheral neuropathy, dosage may be increased. Stop therapy in patient who develops grade 3 peripheral neuropathy.
▶ **Locally advanced or metastatic non–small-cell lung cancer after failure of platinum-based chemotherapy.** *Adults:* 75 mg/m^2 I.V. over 1 hour q 3 weeks.
◨ **Adjust-a-dose:** For patients with febrile neutropenia, neutrophils less than 500 cells/mm^3 for more than 1 week, severe or cumulative cutaneous reactions, or other grade 3 or 4 nonhematologic toxicity, stop drug until toxicity is resolved; then restart at 55 mg/m^2. For patients who develop grade 3 or higher peripheral neuropathy, stop drug entirely.
▶ **Unresectable, locally advanced, or metastatic non–small-cell lung cancer in patient who has not previously received chemotherapy for this condition, with cisplatin.** *Adults:* 75 mg/m^2 docetaxel I.V. over 1 hour immediately followed by cisplatin 75 mg/m^2 I.V. over 30 to 60 minutes every 3 weeks.

◨ **Adjust-a-dose:** For patients whose lowest platelet count during the previous course of therapy was less than 25,000 cells/mm³, those with febrile neutropenia, and those with serious nonhematologic toxicities, decrease docetaxel dosage to 65 mg/m². In patients who require a further dose reduction, a dose of 50 mg/m² is recommended. For cisplatin dosage adjustments, see manufacturers' prescribing information.

▼ I.V. administration

ⓢ **ALERT:** Premedicate with oral corticosteroids for 3 days, starting 1 day before treatment to reduce fluid retention and hypersensitivty reactions.

• Wear gloves during drug preparation and administration. If solution contacts skin, wash immediately and thoroughly with soap and water. If drug contacts mucous membranes, flush thoroughly with water. Mark all waste materials with chemotherapy hazard labels.

• Prepare and store infusion solutions in bottles (glass or polypropylene) or plastic bags, and administer through polyethylene-lined administration sets.

• Dilute drug with diluent supplied. Allow drug and diluent to stand at room temperature for 5 minutes before mixing. After adding diluent contents to vial, rotate vial gently for 15 seconds. Let solution stand for a few minutes for foam to dissipate.

• To prepare solution for infusion, withdraw required amount of premixed solution from vial and add it to 250 ml normal saline solution or D₅W to yield 0.3 to 0.9 mg/ml. Doses exceeding 240 mg need a larger volume of infusion solution to stay below 0.9 mg/ml of docetaxel. Mix infusion thoroughly by manual rotation.

• Administer drug as a 1-hour infusion; store unopened vials in the refrigerator.

• Discard solution if it isn't clear or it contains precipitates. Use infusion solution within 8 hours.

Contraindications and precautions

• Contraindicated in patients hypersensitive to drug or to other polysorbate 80-containing drugs and in those with neutrophil counts below 1,500 cells/mm³.

☀ **Lifespan:** In pregnant and breast-feeding women, drug is contraindicated. In children younger than age 16, safety and efficacy of drug haven't been established.

Adverse reactions

CNS: pain, *asthenia,* paresthesia, dysesthesia, weakness.
CV: *fluid retention,* hypotension.
GI: *stomatitis, nausea, vomiting, diarrhea.*
Hematologic: *anemia,* NEUTROPENIA, FEBRILE NEUTROPENIA, MYELOSUPPRESSION, LEUKOPENIA, THROMBOCYTOPENIA, *septic and nonseptic death.*
Musculoskeletal: back pain, *myalgia,* arthralgia.
Respiratory: dyspnea.
Skin: *alopecia,* skin eruptions, desquamation, nail pigmentation alterations, nail pain, flushing, rash.
Other: HYPERSENSITIVITY REACTIONS, infection, chest tightness, drug fever, chills.

Interactions

Drug-drug. *Agents that are induced, inhibited, or metabolized by CYP 3A4 (cyclosporin, ketoconazole, erythromycin, troleandomycin):* May modify docetaxel metabolism when given together. Use together cautiously.

Effects on lab test results

• May increase ALT, AST, bilirubin, and alkaline phosphatase levels.
• May decrease hemoglobin, hematocrit, and WBC and platelet counts.

Pharmacokinetics

Absorption: Administered I.V.
Distribution: 94% is protein-bound.
Metabolism: Partly by liver.
Excretion: Mainly in feces. *Half-life:* About 12 hours.

Route	Onset	Peak	Duration
I.V.	Immediate	Unknown	Unknown

Action

Chemical effect: Disrupts the microtubular network essential for mitotic and interphase cellular functions.
Therapeutic effect: Inhibits mitosis, producing antineoplastic effect.

Available forms

Injection: 20 mg, 80 mg

⚕ Assessment
• Monitor blood count frequently during therapy.
• Evaluate patient's and family's knowledge of drug therapy.

⚕ Nursing diagnoses
• Ineffective health maintenance related to neoplastic disease
• Deficient knowledge related to drug therapy

▷ Planning and implementation
• Don't give drug to patients with bilirubin levels exceeding upper limit of normal. Also, avoid use of drug in patients with ALT or AST levels above 1.5 times upper limit of normal and alkaline phosphatase levels over 2.5 times upper limit of normal or in patients with baseline neutrophil count less than 1,500/mm³.
⚠ ALERT: Don't confuse Taxotere with Taxol.
Patient teaching
• Warn patient that alopecia occurs in almost 80% of patients.
• Tell patient to promptly report sore throat, fever, unusual bruising or bleeding, or signs of fluid retention.

☑ Evaluation
• Patient shows positive response to drug.
• Patient and family state understanding of drug therapy.

docosanol
(doe-KOE-san-ole)
Abreva

Pharmacologic class: topical antiviral
Therapeutic class: antiviral
Pregnancy risk category: B

Indications and dosages

▶ Recurrent oral-facial herpes simplex (cold sores). *Adults and children age 12 and older:* Apply topically 5 times daily to affected area.

Contraindications and precautions

• Contraindicated in patients hypersensitive to drug or any of its components.

☙ Lifespan: In breast-feeding women, use cautiously because it's unknown whether drug appears in breast milk. In children younger than age 12, safety and efficacy of drug haven't been established.

Adverse reactions

CNS: *headache.*
Other: reaction at application site.

Interactions

None reported.

Effects on lab test results

None reported.

Pharmacokinetics

Absorption: Not absorbed.
Distribution: Not distributed.
Metabolism: Not metabolized.
Excretion: Not excreted.

Route	Onset	Peak	Duration
Topical	Unknown	Unknown	Unknown

Action

Chemical effect: Inhibits the fusion between the cell's plasma membrane and the herpes simplex virus lipid envelope, thereby blocking the viral entry into cells and the subsequent replication of the virus.
Therapeutic effect: Shortens healing time and relieves pain from the herpes simplex lesions.

Available forms

Cream: 10%

⚕ Assessment
• Assess patient before and during therapy.
• Monitor patient for any adverse drug effects.

⚕ Nursing diagnoses
• Acute pain related to underlying lesions
• Deficient knowledge related to drug therapy

▷ Planning and implementation
• Use drug only to treat oral-facial herpes simplex. Avoid application in or near patient's eyes.
• Start treatment as early as possible after symptoms start and continue until lesions have healed.

- Enforce strict handwashing before and after application.

Patient teaching
- Advise patient to start treatment as soon as symptoms appear and continue until the lesions heal.
- Notify patient that lesions are considered contagious until completely healed.
- Urge patient to report worsening condition or any adverse reactions to drug therapy.
- Urge patient to wash hands with soap and warm water before and immediately after application.

☑ Evaluation
- Patient's symptoms are relieved with drug therapy.
- Patient and family state understanding of drug therapy.

---

docusate calcium (dioctyl calcium sulfosuccinate)
(DOK-yoo-sayt KAL-see-um)
DC Softgels , Pro-Cal-Sof , Surfak

docusate potassium (dioctyl potassium sulfosuccinate)
Diocto-K†, Kasof†

docusate sodium (dioctyl sodium sulfosuccinate)
Colace†, Coloxyl ◇ , Coloxyl Enema Concentrate ◇ , Dialose†, Diocto†, Dioeze†, Disonate†, DOK†, DOS Softgels†, Doxinate†, D-S-S†, Modane Soft†, Pro-Sof†, Regulax SS†, Regulex ♦ †, Regutol†, Therevac Plus†, Therevac-SB†

Pharmacologic class: surfactant
Therapeutic class: emollient laxative
Pregnancy risk category: C

Indications and dosages

▶ **Stool softener.** *Adults and children age 12 and older:* 50 to 300 mg P.O. daily until bowel movements are normal. Or, give enema (where available). Dilute 1:24 with sterile water before administration, and give 100 to 150 ml (reten-

tion enema), 300 to 500 ml (evacuation enema), or 0.5 to 1.5 liters (flushing enema).
Children ages 6 to 12: 40 to 120 mg docusate sodium P.O. daily.
Children ages 3 to 6: 20 to 60 mg docusate sodium P.O. daily.
Children younger than age 3: 10 to 40 mg docusate sodium P.O. daily. Higher dosages used for initial therapy. Adjust dosage to individual response.
Adults and children: Usual dosage 240 mg docusate calcium P.O. daily until bowel movements are normal.

Contraindications and precautions

- Contraindicated in patients hypersensitive to drug and in those with intestinal obstruction, undiagnosed abdominal pain, signs of appendicitis, fecal impaction, or acute surgical abdomen.
- ⚖ Lifespan: In pregnant women, use cautiously.

Adverse reactions

EENT: throat irritation.
GI: bitter taste, mild abdominal cramping, diarrhea, laxative dependence with long-term or excessive use.

Interactions

Drug-drug. *Mineral oil:* May increase mineral oil absorption and cause toxicity and lipoid pneumonia. Separate administration times.

Effects on lab test results

None reported.

Pharmacokinetics

Absorption: Absorbed minimally in duodenum and jejunum.
Distribution: Distributed primarily locally, in gut.
Metabolism: None.
Excretion: In feces. *Half-life:* Unknown.

Route	Onset	Peak	Duration
P.O.	Varies	Varies	24-72 hr
P.R.	Unknown	Unknown	Unknown

Action

Chemical effect: Reduces surface tension of interfacing liquid contents of bowel. This detergent activity promotes incorporation of additional liquid into stool, thus forming softer mass.

Therapeutic effect: Softens stool.

Available forms

docusate calcium
Capsules: 50 mg†, 240 mg†
docusate potassium
Capsules: 100 mg†, 240 mg†
docusate sodium
Capsules: 50 mg†, 60 mg†, 100 mg†, 240 mg†, 250 mg†
Enema concentrate: 18 g/100 ml (must be diluted) ◊
Oral liquid: 150 mg/15 ml†
Oral solution: 50 mg/ml†
Syrup: 20 mg/5ml*†, 50 mg/15 ml†, 60 mg/15 ml†, 100 mg/30 ml†
Tablets: 100 mg†

NURSING PROCESS

⁂ Assessment
• Obtain history of patient's bowel patterns before therapy, and reassess regularly thereafter.
• Before giving drug for constipation, determine if patient has adequate fluid intake, exercise, and diet.
• Be alert for adverse reactions and drug interactions.
• Evaluate patient's and family's knowledge of drug therapy.

⊕ Nursing diagnoses
• Constipation related to underlying condition
• Diarrhea related to prolonged or excessive use of drug
• Deficient knowledge related to drug therapy

⊠ Planning and implementation
• Give liquid in milk, fruit juice, or infant formula to mask bitter taste.
• Drug is laxative of choice for patients who shouldn't strain during defecation, including patients recovering from MI or rectal surgery, for those with rectal or anal disease that makes passage of firm stool difficult, and for those with postpartum constipation.
• Store drug at 59° to 86° F (15° to 30° C), and protect liquid from light.
• If abdominal cramping occurs, stop drug and notify prescriber.

• Drug doesn't stimulate intestinal peristaltic movements.
⊛ **ALERT:** Don't confuse Colace and Calan.

Patient teaching
• Teach patient about dietary sources of bulk, which include bran and other cereals, fresh fruit, and vegetables.
• Instruct patient to use only occasionally and not to use for more than 1 week without prescriber's knowledge.
• Tell patient to stop drug if severe cramping occurs and notify prescriber.

☑ Evaluation
• Patient's constipation is relieved.
• Patient remains free from diarrhea during therapy.
• Patient and family state understanding of drug therapy.

dofetilide
(doh-FET-eh-lighd)
Tikosyn

Pharmacologic class: antiarrhythmic
Therapeutic class: class III antiarrhythmic
Pregnancy risk category: C

Indications and dosages

▶ **Maintenance of normal sinus rhythm in patients with symptomatic atrial fibrillation or atrial flutter for longer than 1 week who have been converted to normal sinus rhythm; conversion of atrial fibrillation and atrial flutter to normal sinus rhythm.** *Adults:* Dosage is individualized and is based on creatinine clearance and QT interval, which must be obtained before first dose. (If pulse is less than 60 beats/minute, use QT interval.) Usual dosage is 500 mcg P.O. b.i.d. for patients with creatinine clearance above 60 ml/minute.
⊠ **Adjust-a-dose:** For patients with renal impairment, if creatinine clearance is 40 to 60 ml/minute, give 250 mcg P.O. b.i.d. If creatinine clearance is 20 to 39 ml/minute, give 125 mcg P.O. b.i.d. If creatinine clearance is less than 20 ml/minute, drug is contraindicated.

For patients who develop prolonged QT interval, adjust dosage or stop drug.

Contraindications and precautions

• Contraindicated in patients with congenital or acquired prolonged-QT interval syndromes. Also contraindicated in patients with baseline QTc interval greater than 440 msec (500 msec in patients with ventricular conduction abnormalities). Also contraindicated in patients with creatinine clearance below 20 ml/min and in patients hypersensitive to drug and in those receiving verapamil, cimetidine, trimethoprim (alone or with sulfamethoxazole), or ketoconazole.
• Use cautiously in patients with severe hepatic impairment.
⚝ Lifespan: In pregnant women, use cautiously. In breast-feeding women, drug is not recommended. In children, safety and efficacy of drug haven't been established.

Adverse reactions

CNS: *headache,* dizziness, insomnia, anxiety, migraine, *cerebral ischemia, CVA,* asthenia, paresthesia, syncope.
CV: *ventricular fibrillation, ventricular tachycardia, torsades de pointes, AV block,* bundle branch block, *heart block,* chest pain, angina, atrial fibrillation, peripheral edema, hypertension, palpitations, *bradycardia,* edema, *cardiac arrest, MI.*
EENT: facial paralysis.
GI: nausea, diarrhea, abdominal pain.
GU: UTI.
Hepatic: *liver damage.*
Musculoskeletal: back pain, arthralgia.
Respiratory: respiratory tract infection, dyspnea, increased cough.
Skin: rash, sweating.
Other: flulike syndrome, *angioedema.*

Interactions

Drug-drug. *Cimetidine, ketoconazole, sulfamethoxazole, trimethoprim, verapamil:* Increases plasma levels of dofetilide. Don't use together.
Inhibitors of renal cationic secretion (prochlorperazine, megestrol): May increase dofetilide levels. Avoid using together.
Inhibitors of CYP 3A4 (macrolide antibiotics, azole antifungals, protease inhibitors, serotonin reuptake inhibitors, amiodarone, cannabinoids, diltiazem, nefazodone, norfloxacin, quinine, zafirlukast): May decrease metabolism and increase dofetilide levels. Use together cautiously; monitor patient for toxicity.

Triamterene, metformin, amiloride: May increase dofetilide levels. Use together cautiously.
Drug-food. *Grapefruit juice:* May decrease drug's hepatic metabolism and increase its level. Avoid using together.

Effects on lab test results

None reported.

Pharmacokinetics

Absorption: Greater than 90%; levels peak at 2 to 3 hours. Steady-state levels are achieved in 2 to 3 days. Unaffected by food or antacid.
Distribution: Widely distributed throughout the body and has a volume of distribution of 3 L/kg. Protein-binding is 60% to 70%.
Metabolism: Metabolized to a small extent by the CYP 3A4 isoenzyme of the CYP system of the liver.
Excretion: About 80% is excreted in the urine, of which 80% is excreted as unchanged drug with the remaining 20% consisting of inactive or minimally active metabolites. *Half-life:* 10 hours.

Route	Onset	Peak	Duration
P.O.	Unknown	2-3 hr	Unknown

Action

Chemical effect: Prolongs repolarization without affecting conduction velocity by blocking the cardiac ion channel carrying potassium current.
Therapeutic effect: Maintains normal sinus rhythm in patients with symptomatic atrial fibrillation or atrial flutter who have been converted to normal sinus rhythm; converts atrial fibrillation and atrial flutter to normal sinus rhythm.

Available forms

Distributed only to hospitals and other institutions with applicable dosing and treatment initiation programs. Inpatient and subsequent outpatient discharge and refills of prescriptions are allowed only upon confirmation that prescriber has access to these programs.
Capsules: 125 mcg (0.125 mg), 250 mcg (0.25 mg), 500 mcg (0.5 mg)

NURSING PROCESS

☝ **Assessment**
• Obtain accurate medication list from patient before starting drug; stop antiarrhythmic under

careful monitoring for at least three half-lives. Don't give drug within 3 months of amiodarone unless level is below 0.3 mcg/ml.
• Assess patient's QTc interval, cardiac rhythm, and vital signs before starting medication. Prolongation of the QTc interval requires subsequent dosage adjustments or discontinuation. Continuous ECG monitoring is required for a minimum of 3 days.
• Obtain potassium level before starting therapy and then regularly thereafter. Hypokalemia and hypomagnesemia may occur when giving potassium-depleting diuretics, increasing the risk of torsades de pointes. Achieve and maintain normal potassium level.
• Monitor patient for prolonged diarrhea, sweating, and vomiting; report them to prescriber because electrolyte imbalance may increase the risk of arrhythmias.
• Monitor renal function and QTc interval every 3 months.
• Evaluate patient's and family's knowledge of drug therapy.

⊕ Nursing diagnoses
• Decreased cardiac output related to underlying arrhythmia
• Risk for injury related to drug-induced adverse reactions
• Deficient knowledge related to drug therapy

❯ Planning and implementation
• If patient doesn't convert to normal sinus rhythm within 24 hours after starting drug, use electrical conversion.
• Don't discharge patient within 12 hours of conversion to normal sinus rhythm.
• If drug must be stopped to allow administration of other interacting drugs, allow washout period of at least 2 days before starting other drug.
Patient teaching
• Instruct patient to notify prescriber about any change in prescription drugs, OTC medications, or herbal remedies.
• Urge patient to immediately report excessive or prolonged diarrhea, sweating, vomiting, or loss of appetite or thirst to prescriber.
• Inform patient that dofetilide can be taken without regard to meals or antacids.
• Tell patient not to take drug with grapefruit juice.
• Warn patient not to use OTC Tagamet-HB for ulcers or heartburn. Explain that antacids and

OTC acid reducers such as Zantac 75 mg, Pepcid, Axid, and Prevacid are acceptable.
• Instruct woman to notify prescriber about planned, suspected, or known pregnancy.
• Advise patient not to breast-feed while taking dofetilide.
• If patient misses a dose, tell him to skip it and wait for the next scheduled dose. Caution against doubling the dose.

☑ Evaluation
• Patient maintains normal sinus rhythm.
• Patient has no injury as a result of drug-induced adverse reactions.
• Patient and family state understanding of drug therapy.

dolasetron mesylate
(doh-LEH-seh-trohn MES-ih layt)
Anzemet

Pharmacologic class: selective serotonin (5-HT₃) receptor antagonist
Therapeutic class: antiemetic
Pregnancy risk category: B

Indications and dosages

▶ **Prevention of nausea and vomiting from cancer chemotherapy.** *Adults:* 100 mg P.O. given as a single dose 1 hour before chemotherapy. Or, 1.8 mg/kg (or a fixed dose of 100 mg) as a single I.V. dose given 30 minutes before chemotherapy.
Children ages 2 to 16: 1.8 mg/kg P.O. 1 hour before chemotherapy. Or, 1.8 mg/kg as single I.V. dose 30 minutes before chemotherapy. Injectable form can be mixed with apple juice and given P.O. Maximum dose is 100 mg.
▶ **Prevention of postoperative nausea and vomiting.** *Adults:* 100 mg P.O. within 2 hours before surgery. Or, 12.5 mg as single I.V. dose about 15 minutes before cessation of anesthesia.
Children ages 2 to 16: 1.2 mg/kg P.O. given within 2 hours before surgery, up to maximum of 100 mg. Or, 0.35 mg/kg (up to 12.5 mg) as single I.V. dose about 15 minutes before cessation of anesthesia. Injectable form can be mixed with apple juice and given P.O.
▶ **Postoperative nausea and vomiting.** *Adults:* 12.5 mg as a single I.V. dose as soon as nausea or vomiting begins.

Reactions may be *common*, uncommon, *life-threatening*, or COMMON AND LIFE-THREATENING.

Children ages 2 to 16: 0.35 mg/kg, up to maximum dose of 12.5 mg, as a single I.V. dose as soon as nausea or vomiting begins.

▼ I.V. administration

• Injection can be infused as rapidly as 100 mg/30 seconds, or diluted in 50 ml of compatible solution and infused over 15 minutes.
• Stop drug and notify prescriber immediately if arrhythmia develops.
• After dilution, solution is stable for 24 hours at room temperature or 48 hours if refrigerated.

Contraindications and precautions

• Contraindicated in patients hypersensitive to drug.
• Give cautiously to patients who have or may develop prolonged cardiac conduction intervals, such as those with electrolyte abnormalities, history of arrhythmias, and cumulative high-dose anthracycline therapy.
≛ Lifespan: In breast-feeding women, use cautiously. In infants, drug isn't recommended.

Adverse reactions

CNS: fever, *headache,* dizziness, drowsiness, fatigue.
CV: *arrhythmias, bradycardia,* ECG changes, hypotension, hypertension, tachycardia.
GI: *diarrhea,* dyspepsia, abdominal pain, constipation, anorexia.
GU: oliguria, urine retention.
Skin: pruritus, rash.
Other: chills, pain at injection site.

Interactions

Drug-drug. *Drugs that prolong ECG intervals (such as antiarrhythmics):* May increase risk of arrhythmia. Monitor patient closely.
Drugs that inhibit CYP enzymes (such as cimetidine): May increase hydrodolasetron levels. Monitor patient for adverse effects.
Drugs that induce CYP enzymes (such as rifampin): May decrease hydrodolasetron levels. Monitor patient for decreased efficacy of drug.

Effects on lab test results

• May increase ALT and AST levels.

Pharmacokinetics

Absorption: Rapid for hydrodolasetron, an active metabolite that has an absolute bioavailability of 75%. Absorption of the parent compound is rarely seen.
Distribution: Widely distributed with 69% to 77% bound to plasma protein.
Metabolism: To an active metabolite, hydrodolasetron, by carbonyl reductase. Rarely detected in plasma because of rapid and complete metabolism.
Excretion: About two-thirds of hydrodolasetron is recovered in urine; one-third in feces. *Half-life:* 8 hours.

Route	Onset	Peak	Duration
P.O.	Rapid	1 hr	8 hr
I.V.	Rapid	36 min	7 hr

Action

Chemical effect: Blocks the action of serotonin, thereby preventing serotonin from stimulating the vomiting reflex.
Therapeutic effect: Prevents nausea and vomiting.

Available forms

Injection: 20 mg/ml as 12.5 mg/0.625 ml ampule or 100 mg/5 ml vial
Tablets: 50 mg, 100 mg

NURSING PROCESS

▨ Assessment

• Assess patient for history of nausea and vomiting related to chemotherapy or postoperative recovery.
• Be alert for potential adverse reactions and drug interactions.
• Monitor ECG carefully in patients who have or may develop prolonged cardiac conduction intervals.
• Evaluate patient's and family's knowledge of drug therapy.

▨ Nursing diagnoses

• Imbalanced nutrition: less than body requirements, related to nausea and vomiting
• Risk for injury related to drug-induced adverse CNS reaction
• Deficient knowledge related to drug therapy

▨ Planning and implementation

• Injection for P.O. administration is stable in apple juice for 2 hours at room temperature.

⊛ **ALERT:** Don't confuse Avandamet with Anzemet.

Patient teaching
• Tell patient about potential adverse effects.
• Instruct patient not to mix injection in juice for P.O. use until just before dosing.
• Tell patient to report nausea or vomiting.

☑ **Evaluation**
• Patient has no nausea and vomiting.
• Patient is free from injury.
• Patient and family state understanding of drug therapy

donepezil hydrochloride
(doh-NEH-peh-zil high-droh-KLOR-ighd)
Aricept

Pharmacologic class: reversible inhibitor of acetylcholinesterase
Therapeutic class: psychotherapeutic agent for Alzheimer's disease
Pregnancy risk category: C

Indications and dosages

▶ **Mild to moderate dementia of the Alzheimer's type.** *Adults:* Initially, 5 mg P.O. daily h.s. After 4 to 6 weeks, may increase dosage to 10 mg daily.

Contraindications and precautions

• Contraindicated in patients hypersensitive to drug or to piperidine derivatives.
• Use cautiously in patients with history of ulcer disease, CV disease, asthma or obstructive pulmonary disease, or urinary outflow impairment. Also use cautiously in patients currently taking NSAIDs.
⚘ **Lifespan:** In pregnant women, use only if benefit justifies risk to fetus. Breast-feeding women shouldn't breast-feed during therapy. In children, safety and efficacy of drug haven't been established.

Adverse reactions

CNS: syncope, pain, *headache,* insomnia, dizziness, depression, abnormal dreams, somnolence, *seizures,* tremor, irritability, paresthesia, aggression, vertigo, ataxia, restlessness, abnormal crying, fatigue, nervousness, aphasia.

CV: chest pain, hypertension, vasodilation, atrial fibrillation, hypotension.
EENT: cataracts, sore throat, blurred vision, eye irritation.
GI: *nausea, diarrhea,* vomiting, anorexia, fecal incontinence, *GI bleeding,* bloating, epigastric pain.
GU: frequent urination.
Metabolic: weight decrease, dehydration.
Musculoskeletal: muscle cramps, arthritis, toothache, bone fracture.
Respiratory: *dyspnea, bronchitis.*
Skin: pruritus, urticaria, diaphoresis, ecchymosis.
Other: hot flushes, increased libido, accident, influenza.

Interactions

Drug-drug. *Anticholinergics:* May interfere with anticholinergic activity. Monitor patient for effects.
Bethanechol, succinylcholine: May have additive effects. Monitor patient closely.
Carbamazepine, dexamethasone, phenytoin, phenobarbital, rifampin: May increase rate of donepezil elimination. Monitor patient for effects.
Cholinomimetics, cholinesterase inhibitors: Synergistic effect. Monitor patient closely.
Drug-herb. *Jaborandi tree, pill-bearing spurge:* Additive effect may occur when combined, and risk of toxicity may be increased. Discourage using together.

Effects on lab test results

None reported.

Pharmacokinetics

Absorption: Well absorbed.
Distribution: 96% plasma protein-bound, mainly to albumin.
Metabolism: Extensively metabolized.
Excretion: Excreted in urine and feces. *Half-life:* About 70 hours.

Route	Onset	Peak	Duration
P.O.	Unknown	3-4 hr	Unknown

Action

Chemical effect: Reversibly inhibits acetylcholinesterase in the CNS, thereby increasing the acetylcholine level.

Reactions may be *common,* uncommon, *life-threatening*, or COMMON AND LIFE-THREATENING.

Therapeutic effect: Temporarily improves cognitive function in patients with Alzheimer's disease.

Available forms

Tablets: 5 mg, 10 mg

NURSING PROCESS

Assessment
• Monitor patient for symptoms of active or occult GI bleeding.
• Evaluate patient's and family's knowledge of drug therapy.

Nursing diagnoses
• Risk for injury related to adverse effects of drug
• Deficient knowledge related to drug therapy

Planning and implementation
• Give drug h.s. and without regard to food.
• If cholinergic crisis (severe nausea, vomiting, salivation, sweating, bradycardia, hypotension, respiratory depression, convulsions, and collapse) occurs, treat with an anticholinergic such as atropine.
Patient teaching
• Explain that drug doesn't alter underlying degenerative disease but can alleviate symptoms.
• Tell caregiver to give drug in the evening, just before bedtime.
• Advise patient and caregiver to immediately report significant adverse effects or changes in overall health status.
• Tell caregiver to inform health care team that patient is taking drug before patient receives anesthesia.

Evaluation
• Patient remains free from injury.
• Patient and family state understanding of drug therapy.

dopamine hydrochloride
(DOH-puh-meen high-droh-KLOR-ighd)
Intropin, Revimine ◆

Pharmacologic class: adrenergic
Therapeutic class: inotropic, vasopressor
Pregnancy risk category: C

Indications and dosages

▶ To treat shock and correct hemodynamic imbalances; to improve perfusion to vital organs; to increase cardiac output; to correct hypotension. *Adults:* Initially, 1 to 5 mcg/kg/minute by I.V. infusion. Adjust dosage to desired hemodynamic or renal response, increase by 1 to 4 mcg/kg/minute at 10- to 30-minute intervals.

I.V. administration
• Dilute with D_5W, normal saline solution, or combination of D_5W and normal saline solution. Mix just before use.
• Use continuous infusion pump to regulate flow rate.
• Use central line or large vein, such as in antecubital fossa, to minimize risk of extravasation. If extravasation occurs, stop infusion immediately and call prescriber. Extravasation may require treatment by infiltration of area with 5 to 10 mg of phentolamine and 10 to 15 ml of normal saline solution.
• Don't mix other drugs in I.V. container with dopamine. Don't give alkaline drugs (for example, sodium bicarbonate or phenytoin sodium), oxidizing drugs, or iron salts through I.V. line containing dopamine.
• Discard after 24 hours or earlier if solution is discolored.

Contraindications and precautions
• Contraindicated in patients with uncorrected tachyarrhythmias, pheochromocytoma, or ventricular fibrillation.
• Use cautiously in patients with occlusive vascular disease, cold injuries, diabetic endarteritis, and arterial embolism; and in those taking MAO inhibitors.
Lifespan: With pregnant women, use cautiously. In breast-feeding women and children, safety and efficacy of drug haven't been established.

Adverse reactions
CNS: headache.
CV: *arrhythmias,* ectopic beats, tachycardia, anginal pain, palpitations, *hypotension,* **bradycardia, widening of QRS complex,** conduction disturbances, vasoconstriction, hypertension.
GI: nausea, vomiting.
GU: azotemia.
Respiratory: *asthma attacks,* dyspnea.

Skin: necrosis, tissue sloughing with extravasation, piloerection.
Other: *anaphylaxis.*

Interactions

Drug-drug. *Alpha-adrenergic blockers, beta blockers:* May antagonize dopamine effects. Monitor patient for effect.
Phenelzine, tranylcypromine: May cause severe headache, hypertension, fever, and hypertensive crisis. Avoid using together.
Ergot alkaloids: May cause elevations in blood pressure. Don't use together.
Inhaled anesthetics: Increases risk of arrhythmias or hypertension. Monitor vital signs and ECG closely.
Oxytocic drugs: May potentiate pressor effect resulting in severe hypertension. Avoid using together, if possible.
Phenytoin: May lower blood pressure of dopamine-stabilized patients. Monitor blood pressure carefully.
Tricyclic antidepressants: May decrease pressor response. Monitor patient closely.

Effects on lab test results

• May increase glucose and urea levels.

Pharmacokinetics

Absorption: Administered I.V.
Distribution: Widely distributed throughout body; doesn't cross blood-brain barrier.
Metabolism: Metabolized to inactive compounds in liver, kidneys, and plasma.
Excretion: Excreted in urine, mainly as its metabolites. *Half-life:* About 9 minutes.

Route	Onset	Peak	Duration
I.V.	≤ 5 min	Unknown	≤ 10 min after therapy stops

Action

Chemical effect: Stimulates dopaminergic, beta-adrenergic, and alpha-adrenergic receptors of sympathetic nervous system.
Therapeutic effect: Increases cardiac output and blood pressure.

Available forms

Injection: 40 mg/ml, 80 mg/ml, 160 mg/ml as concentrate for injection for I.V. infusion; 0.8 mg/ml (200 or 400 mg) in D_5W; 1.6 mg/ml (400 or 800 mg) in D_5W; 3.2 mg/ml (800 mg) in D_5W as parenteral injection for I.V. infusion.

NURSING PROCESS

Assessment
• Obtain history of patient's underlying condition before therapy.
• During infusion, frequently monitor ECG, blood pressure, cardiac output, central venous pressure, pulmonary capillary wedge pressure, pulse rate, urine output, and color and temperature of limbs.
• Be alert for adverse reactions and drug interactions.
• Be aware that acidosis decreases effectiveness of dopamine.
• After drug is stopped, watch closely for sudden drop in blood pressure.
• Evaluate patient's and family's knowledge of drug therapy.

Nursing diagnoses
• Ineffective tissue perfusion (cerebral, cardiopulmonary, and renal) related to underlying condition
• Risk for injury related to drug-induced adverse reactions
• Deficient knowledge related to drug therapy

Planning and implementation
• Dosages of 0.5 to 2 mcg/kg/minute mainly stimulate dopamine receptors and dilate renal vasculature. Dosages of 2 to 10 mcg/kg/minute stimulate beta-adrenergic receptors for positive inotropic effect. Higher dosages also stimulate alpha-adrenergic receptors, causing vasoconstriction and increased blood pressure. Most patients are satisfactorily maintained on dosages below 20 mcg/kg/minute.
• Drug isn't used to treat blood or fluid volume deficit. If deficit exists, replace fluid before giving vasopressors.
• Taper dosage slowly to evaluate stability of blood pressure.
• If disproportionate rise in diastolic pressure (a marked decrease in pulse pressure) is observed in patient receiving dopamine, decrease infusion rate and watch carefully for further evidence of predominant vasoconstrictor activity, unless such effect is desired.
• If adverse reactions develop, notify prescriber, who will adjust or stop dosage. Also, if urine

---

flow decreases without hypotension, notify prescriber; reduce dosage.

⚠ **ALERT:** Don't confuse dopamine with dobutamine.

Patient teaching

• Emphasize importance of reporting discomfort at I.V. site immediately.

• Explain to patient the need for drug therapy.

✔ **Evaluation**

• Patient regains adequate cerebral, cardiopulmonary, and renal tissue perfusion.

• Patient doesn't experience injury as result of drug-induced adverse reactions.

• Patient and family state understanding of drug therapy.

---

dorzolamide hydrochloride
(dor-ZOLE-uh-mighd high-droh-KLOR-ighd)
Trusopt

Pharmacologic class: carbonic anhydrase inhibitor, sulfonamide
Therapeutic class: antiglaucoma agent
Pregnancy risk category: C

Indications and dosages

▶ **Increased intraocular pressure (IOP) in patients with ocular hypertension or open-angle glaucoma.** *Adults:* Instill 1 drop in the conjunctival sac of affected eye t.i.d.

Contraindications and precautions

• Contraindicated in patients hypersensitive to any component of drug or in those with renal impairment.

• Use cautiously in patients with impaired hepatic function.

⚠ **Lifespan:** In pregnant women, use only if potential benefits outweigh risks to fetus. In breast-feeding women, drug isn't recommended because it's unknown if it appears in breast milk. In children, safety and efficacy of drug haven't been established. In elderly patients, use cautiously because they may have greater sensitivity to drug.

Adverse reactions

CNS: asthenia, fatigue, headache, dizziness, paresthesia.
EENT: *ocular burning, stinging, discomfort; superficial punctate keratitis; ocular allergic re-*actions *(including conjunctivitis, itching, and lid reactions);* blurred vision; lacrimation; dryness; photophobia; iridocyclitis; redness; transient myopia; eyelid crusting; ocular pain; throat irritation.
GI: *bitter taste,* nausea.
GU: urolithiasis.
Respiratory: *bronchospasm,* dyspnea.
Skin: rash, pruritus, urticaria, contact dermatitis.
Other: *angioedema.*

Interactions

Drug-drug. *Oral carbonic anhydrase inhibitors:* May cause additive effects. Don't use together.
Topical beta blockers: May cause additive effects. Give drugs 10 minutes apart.

Effects on lab tests results

• May decrease potassium and pH levels.

Pharmacokinetics

Absorption: Reaches the systemic circulation when applied topically.
Distribution: 33% bound to plasma proteins. Accumulates in RBCs during chronic dosing as a result of binding to carbonic anhydrase II.
Metabolism: Metabolized in the liver by CYP isoenzymes.
Excretion: Primarily excreted unchanged in urine. *Half-life:* 4 months.

Route	Onset	Peak	Duration
Ophthalmic	1-2 hr	2-3 hr	8 hr

Action

Chemical effect: Inhibits carbonic anhydrase in the ciliary processes of the eye. This action reduces aqueous humor secretion, presumably by slowing the formation of bicarbonate ions with subsequent reduction in sodium and fluid transport.
Therapeutic effect: Reduces IOP.

Available forms

Ophthalmic solution: 2%

NURSING PROCESS

▨ **Assessment**

• Assess patient before starting therapy.

• Because drug is a sulfonamide and is absorbed systemically, the adverse allergic reac-

---

tions caused by sulfonamides, such as Stevens-Johnson syndrome, agranulocytosis, and aplastic anemia, may occur. Although these symptoms haven't been shown with this drug, be alert for any signs and symptoms of them during therapy.
• Overdose may result in electrolyte imbalance, acidosis, and possible CNS effects. Monitor electrolyte levels (especially potassium) and pH levels. Treatment is supportive.
• Evaluate patient's and family's understanding of drug therapy.

⊕ **Nursing diagnoses**
• Risk for infection to the eyes related to inadvertent contamination of the multidose container
• Disturbed visual perception related to underlying ocular condition
• Deficient knowledge related to drug therapy

▷ **Planning and implementation**
• If patient is wearing contact lenses, remove lenses before administration. Contact lenses may be reinserted 15 minutes after administration.
• Apply light finger pressure on lacrimal sac for 1 minute after instillation to minimize systemic absorption of drug.
• If more than one topical ophthalmic drug is being used, give drugs at least 10 minutes apart.
Patient teaching
• Teach patient how to instill drops properly. Advise him to wash hands before and after instilling solution, and warn him not to touch dropper or tip to eye or surrounding tissue to prevent contamination to the dropper.
• Instruct patient to remove contact lenses, if any, before administration and to reinsert 15 minutes after dosage.
• Advise patient to report ocular reactions, particularly conjunctivitis and lid reactions, immediately to prescriber and to stop drug.

☑ **Evaluation**
• Patient doesn't suffer from any infection related to drug administration.
• Patient's underlying condition is resolved with drug therapy.
• Patient and family state understanding of drug therapy.

doxacurium chloride
(doks-uh-KYOO-ree-um KLOR-ighd)
Nuromax

Pharmacologic class: nondepolarizing neuromuscular blocker
Therapeutic class: skeletal muscle relaxant
Pregnancy risk category: C

Indications and dosages

▶ **To provide skeletal muscle relaxation during surgery as adjunct to general anesthesia.**
Dosage is highly individualized. All times of onset and duration of neuromuscular blockade are averages, and considerable individual variation is normal.
Adults: 0.05 mg/kg rapid I.V. produces adequate conditions for endotracheal intubation in 5 minutes in about 90% of patients when used as part of thiopental-narcotic induction technique. Lower doses may require longer delay before intubation is possible. Neuromuscular blockade at this dose lasts for average of 100 minutes.
Children older than age 2: Initial dose of 0.03 mg/kg I.V. given during halothane anesthesia produces effective blockade in 7 minutes with duration of 30 minutes. Under same conditions, 0.05 mg/kg produces blockade in 4 minutes with duration of 45 minutes.
▶ **Maintenance of neuromuscular blockade during long procedures.** *Adults and children:* After initial dose of 0.05 mg/kg I.V., maintenance doses of 0.005 to 0.01 mg/kg prolong neuromuscular blockade for an average of 30 minutes. Children usually require more frequent administration of maintenance doses.
⊠ **Adjust-a-dose:** Patients with renal or hepatic insufficiency may need dosage adjustment. Adjust dosage to ideal body weight in patients 30% or more above their ideal weight to avoid prolonged neuromuscular blockade. Patients with severe burns and some patients with severe liver disease may need higher initial doses. Doses of 0.8 mg/kg or more cause intubating conditions within 4 minutes with neuromuscular blockade lasting 160 minutes or longer. Consequently, reserve higher doses for long procedures. If giving drug during steady-state anesthesia with enflurane, halothane, or isoflurane, reduce dose 33%.

▼ I.V. administration

• Use drug only under direct medical supervision by personnel skilled in use of neuromuscular blockers and techniques for maintaining patent airway. Don't use unless facilities and equipment for intubation, mechanical ventilation, oxygen therapy, and drug antagonist are within reach.
• To avoid distress to patient, don't give drug until patient's consciousness is obtunded by general anesthetic. Drug has no effect on consciousness or pain threshold.
• Prepare drug for I.V. use with D_5W, normal saline solution injection, dextrose 5% in normal saline solution injection, lactated Ringer's injection, or dextrose 5% in lactated Ringer's injection.
• When diluted, drug is compatible with alfentanil, fentanyl, and sufentanil.
• Give immediately after reconstitution. Discard unused solutions after 8 hours.

Contraindications and precautions

• Contraindicated in patients hypersensitive to drug. Drug isn't recommended during prolonged mechanical ventilation in ICU, before or after administration of nondepolarizing neuromuscular blocking agents, or during cesarean delivery.
• Use cautiously and reduce dosage in debilitated patients, in patients in whom neuromuscular blockade may be difficult to initiate or reverse, and in patients with metastatic cancer, severe electrolyte disturbances, or neuromuscular diseases. Patients with myasthenia gravis or myasthenic syndrome (Eaton-Lambert syndrome) are particularly sensitive to effects of nondepolarizing relaxants. Shorter-acting drugs are recommended for such patients.
⚖ Lifespan: In breast-feeding women, use cautiously. In infants younger than age 2, safety and efficacy of drug haven't been established. In neonates, drug is contraindicated because drug contains benzyl ethanol, which has been linked to fatalities in neonates.

Adverse reactions

Musculoskeletal: prolonged muscle weakness.
Respiratory: dyspnea, *respiratory depression, respiratory insufficiency or apnea.*

Interactions

Drug-drug. *Bacitracin, colistimethate, colistin, kanamycin, polymyxin B, tetracyclines:* May po-

tentiate neuromuscular blockade, leading to increased skeletal muscle relaxation and prolongation of effect. Use together cautiously.
Amikacin, gentamicin, neomycin, streptomycin, tobramycin: May increase the effects of nondepolarizing muscle relaxant, including prolonged respiratory depression. Use together only when necessary. Reduce dose of nondepolarizing muscle relaxant.
Carbamazepine, phenytoin: May decrease the effects of doxacurium, causing it to be less effective. May need to increase the dose of the doxacurium.
Inhaled anesthetics, quinidine: May enhance activity or prolong action of nondepolarizing neuromuscular blockers. Monitor patient closely.
Magnesium salts: May enhance neuromuscular blockade. Monitor patient for excessive weakness.

Effects on lab test results

None reported.

Pharmacokinetics

Absorption: Administered I.V.
Distribution: Protein-binding is about 30% in human plasma.
Metabolism: Thought not to be metabolized.
Excretion: Eliminated primarily unchanged in urine and bile. *Half-life:* About 1½ to 2 minutes.

Route	Onset	Peak	Duration
I.V.	≤ 5 min	3-9 min	1-4 hr

Action

Chemical effect: Competes with acetylcholine for receptor sites at motor end plate. Because cholinesterase inhibitors may antagonize this action, doxacurium is considered a competitive antagonist.
Therapeutic effect: Relaxes skeletal muscles.

Available forms

Injection: 1 mg/ml

NURSING PROCESS

✏ Assessment
• Obtain history of patient's underlying condition before therapy.

• Monitor patient continuously throughout drug administration.
• Be alert for adverse reactions and drug interactions.
• Because drug has minimal vagolytic action, watch for bradycardia, which may occur during anesthesia.
• Monitor respirations closely until patient is fully recovered from neuromuscular blockade, as evidenced by tests of muscle strength (hand grip, head lift, and ability to cough).
• Evaluate patient's and family's knowledge of drug therapy.

Nursing diagnoses
• Ineffective health maintenance related to underlying condition
• Impaired spontaneous ventilation related to drug's effects on respiratory muscles
• Deficient knowledge related to drug therapy

Planning and implementation
• Acid-base and electrolyte balance may influence actions of nondepolarizing neuromuscular blockers. Alkalosis may counteract paralysis, and acidosis may enhance it.
• Nerve stimulator and train-of-four monitoring are recommended to document antagonism of neuromuscular blockade and recovery of muscle strength. Before attempting pharmacologic reversal with neostigmine, have some evidence of spontaneous recovery.
• Provide respiratory support as needed.
• Give pain medication regularly if pain is thought to be present; patient may experience pain but not be able to show it.
ALERT: Careful dosage calculation is essential. Always verify dosage with another health care professional.
ALERT: Don't confuse doxacurium with doxapram or doxorubicin.
Patient teaching
• If patient isn't under influence of anesthesia, talk to him and keep him informed of surroundings because drug doesn't affect consciousness. Reassure him that all his vital needs are being met and that he's being monitored constantly.

Evaluation
• Patient shows improvement in underlying condition.
• Patient regains ability to maintain spontaneous ventilation after effects of drug have subsided.

• Patient and family state understanding of drug therapy.

doxapram hydrochloride
(DOKS-uh-prahm high-droh-KLOR-ighd)
Dopram

Pharmacologic class: analeptic
Therapeutic class: CNS and respiratory stimulant
Pregnancy risk category: B

Indications and dosages

▶ **Postanesthesia respiratory stimulation, drug-induced CNS depression, chronic pulmonary disease with acute hypercapnia.**
Adults: 0.5 to 1 mg/kg of body weight (up to 2 mg/kg in CNS depression) by I.V. injection or infusion. Repeated q 5 minutes, if needed. Maximum, 4 mg/kg, up to 3 g daily
▶ **COPD.** *Adults:* 1 to 2 mg/minute by I.V. infusion. Maximum, 3 mg/minute for maximum duration of 2 hours.

I.V. administration
• For I.V. infusion, add 250 mg of drug to 250 ml of 5% or 10% dextrose or normal saline solution injection; concentration equals 1 mg/ml.
• For acute hypercapnia related to COPD, add 400 mg of drug to 180 ml of dextrose or normal saline solution to equal 2mg/ml. Infuse at 1 to 3 mg/minute.
• Give drug slowly; rapid infusion may cause hemolysis. Drug is incompatible with strongly alkaline drugs such as thiopental sodium, aminophylline, and sodium bicarbonate.
• Watch for irritation and infiltration; extravasation can cause tissue damage and necrosis.

Contraindications and precautions
• Contraindicated in patients with seizure disorders; head injury; CV disorders; frank, uncompensated heart failure; severe hypertension; CVA; respiratory failure or incompetence secondary to neuromuscular disorders, muscle paresis, flail chest, obstructed airway, pulmonary embolism, pneumothorax, restrictive respiratory disease, acute bronchial asthma, or dyspnea; or hypoxia not related to hypercapnia.

• Don't use in patients with severe hypotension. If sudden hypotension occurs, stop drug.

• Use cautiously in patients with bronchial asthma, severe tachycardia or arrhythmias, cerebral edema or increased CSF pressure, hyperthyroidism, pheochromocytoma, or metabolic disorders.

☖ Lifespan: With pregnant women, use cautiously. In breast-feeding women and children, safety and efficacy of drug haven't been established.

Adverse reactions

CNS: *seizures, headache,* dizziness, apprehension, disorientation, pupillary dilation, bilateral Babinski's signs, paresthesia, fever.
CV: *chest pain and tightness, increase in blood pressure, variations in heart rate,* depressed T waves, *arrhythmias,* flushing.
EENT: sneezing, *laryngospasm.*
GI: nausea, vomiting, diarrhea.
GU: urine retention, bladder stimulation with incontinence.
Musculoskeletal: muscle spasms.
Respiratory: hiccups, rebound hypoventilation, cough, *bronchospasm,* dyspnea.
Skin: pruritus, diaphoresis.

Interactions

Drug-drug. *MAO inhibitors, sympathomimetics:* May potentiate adverse CV effects. Use together cautiously.

Effects on lab test results

• May increase BUN levels.
• May decrease hemoglobin, hematocrit, and erythrocyte, WBC, and RBC counts.

Pharmacokinetics

Absorption: Administered I.V.
Distribution: Distributed throughout body.
Metabolism: 99% metabolized by liver.
Excretion: Excreted in urine. *Half-life:* 2½ to 4 hours.

Route	Onset	Peak	Duration
I.V.	20-40 sec	1-2 min	5-12 min

Action

Chemical effect: Not clearly defined; acts either directly on central respiratory centers in medulla or indirectly on chemoreceptors.
Therapeutic effect: Stimulates respirations.

Available forms

Injection: 20 mg/ml (benzyl alcohol 0.9%)

NURSING PROCESS

☑ Assessment

• Obtain history of patient's underlying condition before therapy.
• Assess blood pressure, heart rate, deep tendon reflexes, and arterial blood gases before giving drug, and closely throughout therapy.
• Monitor effectiveness by observing patient for improvement in CNS and respiratory function.
• Be alert for adverse reactions and drug interactions.
• Evaluate patient's (if appropriate) and family's knowledge of drug therapy.

🔁 Nursing diagnoses

• Ineffective breathing pattern related to underlying condition
• Risk for trauma related to potential for drug-induced seizure activity
• Deficient knowledge related to drug therapy

▷ Planning and implementation

• Don't use in patients with severe hypotension. If sudden hypotension occurs or dyspnea develops, stop drug.
• Establish adequate airway before giving drug. Prevent patient from aspirating vomitus by placing him on his side. Have suction equipment nearby.
• Drug is used only in surgical- or emergency-department situations.
• Stop drug and notify prescriber if patient shows signs of increased arterial carbon dioxide or oxygen tension, or if mechanical ventilation is started.
(⑤ **ALERT:** Don't confuse doxapram with doxorubicin, doxepin, doxacurium, or doxazosin.
Patient teaching
• If patient is alert, instruct him to report chest pain or tightness immediately.

☑ Evaluation

• Patient regains normal respiratory pattern.
• Patient has no seizures as result of therapy.
• Patient and family state understanding of drug therapy.

doxazosin mesylate

(doks-AY-zoh-sin MES-ih-layt)

Cardura

Pharmacologic class: alpha-adrenergic blocker
Therapeutic class: antihypertensive
Pregnancy risk category: C

Indications and dosages

▶ **Essential hypertension.** *Adults:* Initially,
1 mg P.O. daily. Increase to 2 mg daily, then
4 mg daily, then to 8 mg. Maximum, 16 mg
daily, but dosage above 4 mg daily increases
risk of adverse reactions. To minimize adverse
reactions, adjust dosage slowly (typically increased only q 2 weeks).
▶ **BPH.** *Adults:* Initially, 1 mg P.O. once daily
morning or evening; may increase to 2 mg and,
thereafter, to 4 mg and to 8 mg once daily p.r.n.
Recommended adjustment interval is 1 to 2
weeks.

Contraindications and precautions

• Contraindicated in patients hypersensitive to
drug and to quinazoline derivatives (including
prazosin and terazosin).
• Use cautiously in patients with impaired liver
function.
⚜ **Lifespan:** In pregnant women, use cautiously. In breast-feeding women, drug isn't recommended because it appears in breast milk at levels about 20 times greater than those in maternal
plasma. In children, safety and efficacy of drug
haven't been established.

Adverse reactions

CNS: *dizziness,* vertigo, *asthenia, headache,*
somnolence, drowsiness, pain.
CV: *orthostatic hypotension,* hypotension, ede-
ma, palpitations, **arrhythmias,** tachycardia.
EENT: rhinitis, pharyngitis, abnormal vision.
GI: nausea, vomiting, diarrhea, constipation.
Musculoskeletal: arthralgia, myalgia.
Respiratory: dyspnea.
Skin: rash, pruritus.

Interactions

Drug-drug. *Clonidine:* May decrease clonidine
effects. Adjust dosage.
Drug-herb. *Butcher's broom:* May reduce effects of drug. Discourage using together.

Effects on lab test results

• May decrease WBC and neutrophil counts.

Pharmacokinetics

Absorption: Readily absorbed from GI tract.
Distribution: 98% protein-bound.
Metabolism: Extensively metabolized in liver.
Excretion: 63% excreted in bile and feces; 9%
excreted in urine. *Half-life:* 19 to 22 hours.

Route	Onset	Peak	Duration
P.O.	1-2 hr	5-6 hr	24 hr

Action

Chemical effect: Acts on peripheral vasculature
to produce vasodilation.
Therapeutic effect: Lowers blood pressure.

Available forms

Tablets: 1 mg, 2 mg, 4 mg, 8 mg

NURSING PROCESS

📝 Assessment

• Obtain history of patient's blood pressure before therapy, and reassess regularly thereafter.
• Determine effect on standing and supine
blood pressure at 2 to 6 hours and 24 hours after
administration.
• Be alert for adverse reactions.
• Monitor patient's ECG for arrhythmias.
• Evaluate patient's and family's knowledge of
drug therapy.

🔬 Nursing diagnoses

• Risk for injury related to presence of hypertension
• Decreased cardiac output related to drug-
induced adverse CV reactions
• Deficient knowledge related to drug therapy

▷ Planning and implementation

• Dosage must be increased gradually, with adjustments every 2 weeks for hypertension and
every 1 to 2 weeks for BPH.
• If syncope occurs, place patient in recumbent
position and treat supportively. A transient hypotensive response isn't considered a con-
traindication to continued therapy.
Ⓢ **ALERT:** Don't confuse doxazosin with
doxapram, doxorubicin, or doxepin.
Ⓢ **ALERT:** Don't confuse Cardura with
Coumadin, K-Dur, Cardene, or Cordarone.

Reactions may be *common,* uncommon, *life-threatening,* or COMMON AND LIFE-THREATENING.

Patient teaching

• Advise patient that he's susceptible to a first-dose effect similar to that produced by other alpha-adrenergic blockers—marked orthostatic hypotension accompanied by dizziness or syncope. Orthostatic hypotension is most common after first dose, but it can also occur when stopping therapy or adjusting dosage.
• Warn patient that dizziness or fainting may occur. Advise patient to refrain from driving and performing other hazardous activities until drug's adverse CNS effects are known.
• Stress importance of regular follow-up visits.

☑ Evaluation

• Patient's blood pressure becomes normal.
• Patient maintains adequate cardiac output throughout therapy.
• Patient and family state understanding of drug therapy.

doxepin hydrochloride
(DOKS-eh-pin high-droh-KLOR-ighd)
Novo-Doxepin ◆ , Sinequan, Triadapin ◆

Pharmacologic class: tricyclic antidepressant
Therapeutic class: antidepressant
Pregnancy risk category: C

Indications and dosages

▶ **Depression, anxiety.** *Adults:* Initially, 25 to 75 mg P.O. daily in divided doses to maximum of 300 mg daily. Or, entire maintenance dose may be given once daily with maximum dose of 150 mg P.O.
§ **Adjust-a-dose:** Reduce dosage in elderly or debilitated patients, adolescents, and those receiving other drugs (especially anticholinergics).

Contraindications and precautions

• Contraindicated in patients hypersensitive to drug and in those with glaucoma or a tendency for urine retention.
≛ **Lifespan:** In pregnant women and in children younger than age 12, safety and efficacy of drug haven't been established. In breast-feeding women, drug isn't recommended.

Adverse reactions

CNS: *drowsiness, dizziness,* excitation, tremors, weakness, confusion, headache, nervousness, EEG changes, *seizures,* extrapyramidal reactions, ataxia, paresthesia, hallucinations.
CV: *orthostatic hypotension, tachycardia, ECG changes,* hypertension.
EENT: *blurred vision,* tinnitus, mydriasis.
GI: *dry mouth, glossitis, constipation,* nausea, vomiting, anorexia.
GU: *urine retention.*
Hematologic: eosinophilia, *bone marrow depression, including leukopenia, thrombocytopenia, aplastic anemia, and agranulocytosis.*
Skin: *diaphoresis,* rash, urticaria, photosensitivity.
Other: *hypersensitivity reaction.*

Interactions

Drug-drug. *Barbiturates, CNS depressants:* May enhance CNS depression. Avoid using together.
Cimetidine, fluoxetine, sertraline, methylphenidate: May increase doxepin levels. Monitor patient for increased adverse reactions.
Clonidine: May cause loss of blood pressure control with potentially life-threatening elevations in blood pressure. Don't use together.
Epinephrine, norepinephrine: May increase hypertensive effect. Use cautiously; monitor blood pressure closely.
MAO inhibitors: May cause severe excitation, hyperpyrexia, or seizures, usually with high dosage. Avoid using together.
Drug-herb. *St. John's wort, SAMe, yohimbe:* May elevate serotonin level. Discourage using together.
Drug-food. *Carbonated beverages, grape juice:* Incompatible. Avoid using together.
Drug-lifestyle. *Alcohol use:* May enhance CNS depression. Discourage using together.
Sun exposure: Increases risk of photosensitivity reactions. Discourage unprotected or prolonged exposure to the sun.

Effects on lab test results

• May increase or decrease glucose level.
• May increase liver function test values and eosinophil count. May decrease hemoglobin, hematocrit, and RBC, WBC, granulocyte, and platelet counts.

Pharmacokinetics

Absorption: Absorbed rapidly from GI tract.
Distribution: Distributed widely in body, including CNS; 90% protein-bound.
Metabolism: Metabolized by liver. A significant first-pass effect may explain variability of serum levels in different patients taking same dosage.
Excretion: Most of drug excreted in urine.

Route	Onset	Peak	Duration
P.O.	Unknown	≤ 2 hr	Unknown

Action

Chemical effect: Unknown; increases amount of norepinephrine, serotonin, or both in CNS by blocking their reuptake by presynaptic neurons.
Therapeutic effect: Relieves depression and anxiety.

Available forms

Capsules: 10 mg, 25 mg, 50 mg, 75 mg, 100 mg, 150 mg
Oral concentrate: 10 mg/ml

NURSING PROCESS

✒ Assessment

• Assess patient's depression or anxiety before and during therapy.
• Be alert for adverse reactions and drug interactions.
• Evaluate patient's and family's knowledge of drug therapy.

🔅 Nursing diagnoses

• Ineffective individual coping related to underlying condition
• Risk for injury related to drug-induced adverse CNS reactions
• Deficient knowledge related to drug therapy

▷ Planning and implementation

• Dilute oral concentrate with 120 ml of water, milk, or juice (except grape juice). Don't mix with carbonated beverages because of incompatibility.
• Don't withdraw drug abruptly. Abrupt withdrawal of long-term therapy may cause nausea, headache, and malaise, which don't indicate addiction.
• Stop drug gradually several days before surgery because hypertensive episodes may occur.

• If signs of psychosis occur or increase, notify prescriber and reduce dosage.
• **⑤ ALERT:** Don't confuse doxepin with doxazosin, digoxin, doxapram, or Doxidan; don't confuse Sinequan with saquinavir.

Patient teaching

• Tell patient to dilute oral concentrate with 120 ml of water, milk, or juice (orange, grapefruit, tomato, prune, or pineapple). Drug is incompatible with carbonated beverages and grape juice.
• Advise patient to take full dose at bedtime, but warn of possible morning orthostatic hypotension.
• Warn patient to avoid hazardous activities that require alertness and good psychomotor coordination until CNS effects of drug are known. Drowsiness and dizziness usually subside after a few weeks.
• Tell patient to avoid alcohol during drug therapy.
• Warn patient not to stop drug therapy suddenly.
• Advise patient to consult prescriber before taking prescription drugs, OTC medications, or herbal remedies.
• Advise patient to use sunblock, wear protective clothing, and avoid prolonged exposure to strong sunlight.

☑ Evaluation

• Patient behavior and communication indicate improvement of depression or anxiety.
• Patient has no injury as result of drug-induced adverse CNS reactions.
• Patient and family state understanding of drug therapy.

doxercalciferol
(dox-er-kal-SIF-eh-rol)
Hectorol

Pharmacologic class: synthetic vitamin D analogue
Therapeutic class: parathyroid hormone antagonist
Pregnancy risk category: B

Indications and dosages

▶ **Reduction of elevated intact parathyroid hormone (PTH) levels in the management of secondary hyperparathyroidism in patients**

---

undergoing long-term renal dialysis. *Adults:* Initially, 10 mcg P.O. three times weekly at dialysis. Adjust dosage as needed to lower intact PTH levels to 150 to 300 pg/ml. Increase dosage by 2.5 mcg at 8-week intervals if the intact PTH level doesn't go down by 50% and fails to reach target range. Maximum, 20 mcg P.O. three times weekly. If intact PTH levels fall below 100 pg/ml, stop drug for 1 week and then resume at a dose that's at least 2.5 mcg lower than the last dose.

Contraindications and precautions

• Contraindicated in patients with a recent history of hypercalcemia, hyperphosphatemia, or vitamin D toxicity.
• Use cautiously in patients with hepatic insufficiency, and frequently monitor calcium, phosphorus, and intact PTH levels in these patients.
⚖ Lifespan: In breast-feeding women and in children younger than age 12, drug isn't recommended. In elderly patients, use cautiously because adverse CNS reactions, orthostatic hypotension, and GI and GU distresses are more likely to develop.

Adverse reactions

CNS: *dizziness, headache, malaise,* sleep disorder.
CV: *bradycardia,* edema.
GI: anorexia, dyspepsia, *nausea, vomiting,* constipation.
Metabolic: weight gain or loss.
Musculoskeletal: arthralgia.
Respiratory: *dyspnea.*
Skin: pruritus.
Other: abscess.

Interactions

Drug-drug. *Cholestyramine, mineral oil:* Reduces intestinal absorption of doxercalciferol. Avoid using together.
Glutethimide, phenobarbital, and other enzyme inducers; phenytoin and other enzyme inhibitors: May affect doxercalciferol metabolism. Adjust dosage as directed.
Magnesium-containing antacids: May cause hypermagnesemia. Monitor patient for toxicity.
Calcium-containing or non-aluminum-containing phosphate binders: May cause hypercalcemia or hyperphosphatemia and decrease effectiveness of doxercalciferol. Use to-

gether cautiously, and adjust dosage of phosphate binders as directed.
Vitamin D supplements: May cause additive effects and hypercalcemia. Monitor patient for toxicity.
Orlistat: May interfere with intestinal absorption of vitamin D analogues. Give drug at least 2 hours before or 2 hours after Orlistat administration.

Effects on lab test results

None reported.

Pharmacokinetics

Absorption: Absorbed from the GI tract.
Distribution: Unknown.
Metabolism: Metabolized to its active forms in the liver.
Excretion: Major metabolite of doxercalciferol attains peak blood levels at 11 to 12 hours after repeated oral doses. *Half-life:* 32 to 37 hours, with a range of up to 96 hours.

Route	Onset	Peak	Duration
P.O.	Unknown	11-12 hr	Unknown

Action

Chemical effect: Once activated, doxercalciferol and other biologically active vitamin D metabolites regulate calcium levels required for essential body functions. Doxercalciferol acts directly on the parathyroid glands to suppress PTH synthesis and secretion.
Therapeutic effect: Reduces elevated intact PTH levels.

Available forms

Capsules: 2.5 mcg

NURSING PROCESS

⏳ Assessment
• Assess hepatic function before starting therapy.
• Monitor calcium, phosphorus, and intact PTH levels. Monitor them more frequently in patients with hepatic insufficiency.
• Be alert for adverse reactions and drug interactions.
• Evaluate patient's and family's knowledge of drug therapy.

🔹 Nursing diagnoses
- Imbalanced nutrition: less than body requirements related to adverse GI effects
- Risk for injury related to adverse CNS effects
- Deficient knowledge related to drug therapy

▶ Planning and implementation
- Give doxercalciferol with dialysis (about every other day). Dosing must be individualized and based on intact PTH levels, with monitoring of calcium and phosphorus levels before doxercalciferol therapy and weekly thereafter.
- If patient has hypercalcemia or hyperphosphatemia, or if the calcium level multiplied by the phosphorus level (Ca × P) is greater than 70, immediately stop doxercalciferol until these values decrease.
- Progressive hypercalcemia from vitamin D overdose may require emergency attention. Acute hypercalcemia may worsen arrhythmias and seizures and affects the action of digoxin. Chronic hypercalcemia can lead to vascular and soft-tissue calcification.
- Calcium-based or non-aluminum-containing phosphate binders and a low-phosphate diet are used to control phosphorus levels in patients undergoing dialysis. Expect dosage adjustments in doxercalciferol and concurrent therapies, such as dietary phosphate binders, to sustain PTH suppression and to maintain calcium and phosphorus levels within acceptable ranges.

Patient teaching
- Inform patient that dosage must be adjusted over several months to achieve satisfactory PTH suppression.
- Tell patient to adhere to a low-phosphorus diet and to follow instructions regarding calcium supplementation.
- Tell patient to obtain prescriber's approval before using OTC drugs, including antacids and vitamin preparations containing calcium or vitamin D.
- Inform patient that early signs and symptoms of hypercalcemia include weakness, headache, somnolence, nausea, vomiting, dry mouth, constipation, muscle pain, bone pain, and metallic taste. Late signs and symptoms include polyuria, polydipsia, anorexia, weight loss, nocturia, conjunctivitis, pancreatitis, photophobia, rhinorrhea, pruritus, hyperthermia, decreased libido, hypertension, and arrhythmias.

☑ Evaluation
- Patient has no nausea and vomiting.
- Patient remains free from injury.
- Patient and family state understanding of drug therapy.

---

doxorubicin hydrochloride
(doks-oh-ROO-bih-sin high-droh-KLOR-ighd)
Adriamycin◇, Adriamycin PFS, Adriamycin RDF, Rubex

Pharmacologic class: antineoplastic antibiotic (cell-cycle-phase–nonspecific)
Therapeutic class: antineoplastic
Pregnancy risk category: D

Indications and dosages

▶ **Bladder, breast, lung, ovarian, stomach, testicular, and thyroid cancers; Hodgkin's disease; acute lymphoblastic and myeloblastic leukemia; Wilms' tumor; neuroblastoma; lymphoma; sarcoma.** *Adults:* 60 to 75 mg/m² I.V. as single dose q 3 weeks; or 30 mg/m² I.V. in single daily dose on days 1 through 3 of 4-week cycle. Alternatively, 20 mg/m² I.V. once weekly. Maximum cumulative dose is 550 mg/m².

🔋 **Adjust-a-dose:** In elderly patients and those with myelosuppression or impaired cardiac or hepatic function, dosage may need adjustment.

Decrease dosage if bilirubin level increases: 50% of dosage when bilirubin level is 1.2 to 3 mg/dl; 25% of dosage when bilirubin level is greater than 3 mg/dl.

▼ I.V. administration
- Preparing and giving I.V. drug carry carcinogenic, mutagenic, and teratogenic risks. Follow facility policy to reduce risks.
- Reconstitute using preservative-free normal saline solution injection. Add 5 ml to 10-mg vial, 10 ml to 20-mg vial, or 25 ml to 50-mg vial. Shake vial, and allow drug to dissolve; final concentration is 2 mg/ml. Give by direct injection into I.V. line of free-flowing compatible I.V. solution containing D_5W or normal saline solution injection in no less than 3 minutes.
- Drug is a severe vesicant; extravasation may cause tissue necrosis. To avoid extravasation,

---

don't place I.V. line over joints or in limbs with poor venous or lymphatic drainage.
• If extravasation occurs, stop I.V. infusion immediately, notify prescriber, and apply ice to area for 24 to 48 hours. Monitor area closely because extravasation reaction may be progressive. Early consultation with plastic surgeon may be advisable.
• If vein streaking occurs, slow administration rate. If welts occur, stop administration and notify prescriber.
• Precipitate may form if drug is mixed with aminophylline, cephalothin, dexamethasone, fluorouracil, heparin, or hydrocortisone.
• Refrigerated, reconstituted solution is stable for 48 hours; at room temperature, it's stable for 24 hours.

Contraindications and precautions

• Contraindicated in patients with marked myelosuppression induced by previous treatment with other antitumor drugs or radiotherapy and in those who have received lifetime cumulative dose of 550 mg/m^2.
⚜ Lifespan: In pregnant and breast-feeding women, drug isn't recommended. In children, safety and efficacy of drug haven't been established.

Adverse reactions

CV: cardiac depression, seen in such ECG changes as sinus tachycardia, T-wave flattening, ST-segment depression, voltage reduction; *arrhythmias; irreversible cardiomyopathy.*
EENT: conjunctivitis.
GI: *nausea, vomiting,* diarrhea, *stomatitis,* esophagitis, anorexia.
GU: transient red urine.
Hematologic: *leukopenia* during days 10 through 15, with recovery by day 21; *thrombocytopenia;* MYELOSUPPRESSION.
Skin: *complete alopecia;* urticaria; facial flushing; *hyperpigmentation of nails, dermal creases, or skin* (especially in previously irradiated areas).
Other: *severe cellulitis or tissue sloughing if drug extravasates,* hyperuricemia, *anaphylaxis.*

Interactions

Drug-drug. *Calcium channel blockers:* May potentiate cardiotoxic effects. Monitor patient closely.

Digoxin: May decrease digoxin levels. Monitor patient closely.
Paclitaxel: Decreases doxorubicin clearance. Monitor patient for toxicity.
Phenobarbital: Increases doxorubicin clearance. Monitor patient closely.
Phenytoin: Decreases levels of phenytoin. Check levels.
Streptozocin: May increase and prolong blood levels. Dosage may need adjustment.
Drug-herb. *Green tea:* May enhance antitumor effects of drug. Urge patient to discuss with prescriber before using together.

Effects on lab test results

• May increase bilirubin and glucose levels. May decrease calcium levels.
• May decrease hemoglobin, hematocrit, and WBC, neutrophil, and platelet counts.

Pharmacokinetics

Absorption: Administered I.V.
Distribution: Distributed widely in body tissues; doesn't cross blood-brain barrier.
Metabolism: Extensively metabolized by hepatic microsomal enzymes to several metabolites, one of which possesses cytotoxic activity.
Excretion: Excreted primarily in bile, minimally in urine. *Half-life:* Initial, 30 minutes; terminal, 16½ hours.

Route	Onset	Peak	Duration
I.V.	Unknown	Unknown	Unknown

Action

Chemical effect: Unknown; thought to interfere with DNA-dependent RNA synthesis by intercalation.
Therapeutic effect: Hinders or kills certain cancer cells.

Available forms

Injection (preservative-free): 2 mg/ml
Powder for injection: 10-mg, 20-mg, 50-mg, 100-mg, 150-mg vials

NURSING PROCESS

🝢 **Assessment**
• Obtain history of patient's neoplastic disorder before therapy, and reassess regularly thereafter.
• Assess ECG before treatment.

- Monitor CBC and liver function tests; monitor ECG monthly during therapy.
- Be alert for adverse reactions and drug interactions.
- Evaluate patient's and family's knowledge of drug therapy.

🔯 Nursing diagnoses
- Ineffective health maintenance related to presence of neoplastic disease
- Decreased cardiac output related to drug-induced cardiotoxicity
- Deficient knowledge related to drug therapy

▶ Planning and implementation
- To reduce nausea, premedicate with antiemetic.
- If skin or mucosal contact occurs, immediately wash area with soap and water.
- In case of leak or spill, inactivate drug with 5% sodium hypochlorite solution (household bleach).
- Never give drug by I.M. or S.C. route.
- If tachycardia develops, stop drug or slow rate of infusion; notify prescriber.
- Stop drug immediately if signs of heart failure develop, and notify prescriber. Limit cumulative dosage to 550 mg/m² (400 mg/m² when patient also receives or has received cyclophosphamide or radiation therapy to cardiac area) to prevent heart failure.
- Alternative dosage schedule (once-weekly dosing) causes a lower risk of cardiomyopathy.
- Provide adequate hydration; alkalinizing urine or giving allopurinol may prevent or minimize uric acid nephropathy.
- Report adverse reactions to prescriber and provide supportive care.
- **⚡ ALERT:** Red color of doxorubicin is similar to that of daunorubicin. Take care to avoid confusing these two drugs.
- **⚡ ALERT:** Liposomal doxorubicin and conventional doxorubicin aren't interchangable. Clearance of liposomal form is significantly less than with the conventional form. Decrease liposomal doxorubicin dose.

Patient teaching
- Warn patient to watch for signs of infection (fever, sore throat, fatigue) and bleeding (easy bruising, nosebleeds, bleeding gums, melena). Have patient take temperature daily.

- Advise patient that orange to red urine for 1 to 2 days is normal and doesn't indicate presence of blood in urine.
- Tell patient that total alopecia may occur within 3 to 4 weeks. Hair may regrow 2 to 5 months after drug is stopped.
- Instruct patient to report symptoms of heart failure and other cardiac signs and symptoms promptly to prescriber.
- Tell patient to use safety precautions to prevent injury.

✅ Evaluation
- Patient exhibits positive response to therapy, as noted on improved follow-up studies.
- Patient maintains adequate cardiac output throughout therapy.
- Patient and family state understanding of drug therapy.

---

doxorubicin hydrochloride liposomal
(doks-oh-ROO-bih-sin high-droh-KLOR-ighd li-po-SOE-mal)
Doxil

Pharmacologic class: anthracycline
Therapeutic class: antineoplastic
Pregnancy risk category: D

Indications and dosages

▶ **Metastatic carcinoma of the ovary in patients with disease refractory to paclitaxel- and platinum-based chemotherapy regimens.** *Adults:* 50 mg/m² (doxorubicin hydrochloride equivalent) I.V. at an initial infusion rate of 1 mg/minute once q 4 weeks for at least 4 courses. Continue treatment as long as patient doesn't progress, shows no evidence of cardiotoxicity, and continues to tolerate treatment. If no infusion-related adverse events are observed, increase infusion rate to complete administration over 1 hour.
▶ **AIDS-related Kaposi's sarcoma in patients with disease that has progressed with previous combination chemotherapy or in patients who are intolerant to such therapy.** *Adults:* 20 mg/m² (doxorubicin hydrochloride equivalent) I.V. over 30 minutes, once q 3 weeks, for

as long as patient responds satisfactorily and tolerates treatment.

◩ **Adjust-a-dose:** For patients with impaired hepatic function, if bilirubin level is 1.2 to 3 mg/dl, give ½ of the normal dose; if bilirubin level is more than 3 mg/dl, give ¼ of the normal dose. Consult package insert for dose modifications for palmar-plantar erythrodysesthesia, hematologic toxicity, and stomatitis.

▼ I.V. administration

• Follow facility procedures for proper handling and disposal of antineoplastics.
• Dilute dose (maximum, 90 mg) in 250 ml of D₅W using aseptic technique.
⊛ **ALERT:** Carefully check label on the I.V. bag before giving drug. Accidentally substituting Doxil for conventional doxorubicin hydrochloride can cause severe adverse effects.
• Infuse I.V. over 30 to 60 minutes, depending on the dose. Don't use with in-line filters.
• Monitor patient carefully during infusion. Acute infusion reactions (flushing, shortness of breath, facial swelling, headache, chills, back pain, tightness in the chest or throat, or hypotension) may occur. These reactions resolve over several hours to a day once the infusion is stopped. The reaction may resolve by slowing the infusion rate.
• If extravasation occurs, stop infusion immediately and restart in another vein. Applying ice over the extravasation site for about 30 minutes may help to alleviate the local reaction.
• Refrigerate diluted solution at 36° to 46° F (2° to 8° C), and give within 24 hours.

Contraindications and precautions

• Contraindicated in patients hypersensitive to the conventional form of doxorubicin hydrochloride or any component in the liposomal form. Also, contraindicated in patients with marked myelosuppression or those who have received a lifetime cumulative dose of 550 mg/m² (400 mg/m² if patient received radiotherapy to the mediastinal area or simultaneous therapy with other cardiotoxic drugs, such as cyclophosphamide).
• Use in patients with a history of cardiovascular disease only when benefit of drug outweighs risk to patient.
• Use cautiously in patients who have received another anthracycline.

⚥ **Lifespan:** In breast-feeding women, drug isn't recommended because it's unknown if it appears in breast milk. In children, safety and efficacy of drug haven't been established. In elderly patients, use cautiously because of a possible greater sensitivity to the drug.

Adverse reactions

CNS: fever, *asthenia,* paresthesia, headache, somnolence, dizziness, depression, insomnia, anxiety, malaise, emotional lability, fatigue.
CV: chest pain, hypotension, tachycardia, peripheral edema, *cardiomyopathy, heart failure, arrhythmias,* pericardial effusion.
EENT: mucous membrane disorder, mouth ulceration, pharyngitis, rhinitis, conjunctivitis, retinitis, optic neuritis.
GI: *nausea,* vomiting, constipation, anorexia, diarrhea, abdominal pain, taste perversion, dyspepsia, oral candidiasis, enlarged abdomen, esophagitis, dysphagia, *stomatitis,* glossitis.
GU: albuminuria.
Hematologic: *leukopenia,* NEUTROPENIA, THROMBOCYTOPENIA, *anemia.*
Hepatic: hyperbilirubinemia.
Metabolic: dehydration, weight loss, hypocalcemia, hyperglycemia.
Musculoskeletal: myalgia, back pain.
Respiratory: dyspnea, increased cough, pneumonia.
Skin: *rash, alopecia,* dry skin, pruritus, skin discoloration, skin disorder, exfoliative dermatitis, herpes zoster, sweating, *palmar-plantar erythrodysesthesia.*
Other: *allergic reaction,* chills, *infection, sepsis,* infusion-related reactions.

Interactions

No drug interactions have been reported; however, doxorubicin hydrochloride liposomal may interact with drugs known to interact with the conventional form of doxorubicin hydrochloride.

Effects on lab test results

• May increase bilirubin and glucose levels. May decrease calcium level.
• May increase PT. May decrease hemoglobin, hematocrit, and WBC, neutrophil, and platelet counts.

Pharmacokinetics

Absorption: Administered I.V.

Distribution: Distributed mostly to vascular fluid. Plasma protein-binding hasn't been determined; however, plasma protein-binding of doxorubicin is about 70%.

Metabolism: Doxorubicinol, the major metabolite of doxorubicin, is detected at very low levels in plasma.

Excretion: Plasma elimination is slow and biphasic. *Half-life:* About 5 hours in the first phase, 55 hours in the second phase at doses of 10 to 20 mg/m^2.

Route	Onset	Peak	Duration
I.V.	Unknown	Unknown	Unknown

Action

Chemical effect: Doxil is doxorubicin hydrochloride encapsulated in liposomes that, because of their small size and persistence in circulation, can penetrate the altered vasculature of tumors. The mechanism of action of doxorubicin hydrochloride is probably related to its ability to bind DNA and inhibit nucleic acid synthesis.

Therapeutic effect: Hinders or kills certain cancer cells in patients with ovarian cancer or AIDS-related Kaposi's sarcoma.

Available forms

Injection: 2 mg/ml

NURSING PROCESS

⬛ Assessment

• Obtain an accurate medication list from patient, including previous or current chemotherapeutic drugs.

• Evaluate patient's hepatic function before therapy, and adjust dosage accordingly.

• Monitor cardiac function closely by endomyocardial biopsy, echocardiography, or gated radionuclide scans. If results indicate possible cardiac injury, the benefit of continued therapy must be weighed against the risk of myocardial injury.

• Be alert for adverse reactions.

• Evaluate patient's and family's knowledge of drug therapy.

⊞ Nursing diagnoses

• Risk for infection related to myelosuppression

• Risk for injury related to drug-induced adverse reactions

• Deficient knowledge related to drug therapy

▶ Planning and implementation

• Don't give drug by I.M. or S.C. route.

• **ALERT:** Don't substitute on a mg-by-mg basis with conventional doxorubicin hydrochloride.

• Drug may potentiate the toxicity of other antineoplastic therapies.

• The total dose should also take into account any previous or simultaneous therapy with related compounds, such as daunorubicin. Heart failure and cardiomyopathy may occur after therapy stops.

• Monitor CBC, including platelets, before each dose and frequently throughout therapy. Leukopenia is usually transient. Hematologic toxicity may require dosage reduction or suspension or delay of therapy. Persistent severe myelosuppression may result in superinfection or hemorrhage. Patient may need granulocyte colony-stimulating factor (or granulocyte-macrophage colony-stimulating factor) to support blood counts.

Patient teaching

• Tell patient to notify prescriber about symptoms of hand-foot syndrome, such as tingling or burning, redness, flaking, bothersome swelling, small blisters, or small sores on the palms of hands or soles of feet.

• Advise patient to report symptoms of stomatitis, such as painful redness, swelling, or sores in the mouth.

• Advise patient to avoid exposure to people with infections. Tell patient to report fever of 100.5° F (38° C) or higher.

• Urge patient to report nausea, vomiting, tiredness, weakness, rash, or mild hair loss.

• Advise woman of childbearing age to avoid pregnancy during therapy.

☑ Evaluation

• Patient has no infection.

• Patient has no injury as a result of drug-induced adverse reactions.

• Patient and family state understanding of drug therapy.

Reactions may be *common,* uncommon, *life-threatening*, or COMMON AND LIFE-THREATENING.

doxycycline

doxycycline hyclate
Apo-Doxy ♦, Doryx, Doxy-100, Doxy-200, Doxycin ♦, Doxytec ♦, Novo-Doxylin ♦, Nu-Doxycycline ♦, Periostat, Vibramycin, Vibra-Tabs

doxycycline hydrochloride ◇
Doryx ◇, Doxsig ◇, Doxylin ◇, Doxy Tablets ◇ Vibramycin ◇ Vibra-Tabs ◇

doxycycline monohydrate
Adoxa, Monodox, Vibramycin

Pharmacologic class: tetracycline
Therapeutic class: antibiotic
Pregnancy risk category: D

Indications and dosages

▶ **Infections caused by sensitive gram-negative and gram-positive organisms, *Chlamydia*, *Mycoplasma*, *Rickettsia*, and organisms that cause trachoma.** *Adults and children weighing more than 45 kg (99 lb):* 100 mg P.O. q 12 hours on first day; then 100 mg P.O. daily. Or, 200 mg I.V. on first day in one or two infusions; then 100 to 200 mg I.V. daily. For severe infections 100 mg P.O. q 12 hours may be used.
Children older than age 8 and weighing less than 45 kg: 4.4 mg/kg P.O. or I.V. daily in divided doses q 12 hours on first day, then 2.2 to 4.4 mg/kg daily.

▶ **Gonorrhea in patients allergic to penicillin.** *Adults:* 100 mg P.O. b.i.d. for 7 days. Or, 300 mg P.O. initially; repeat dose in 1 hour.

▶ **Primary or secondary syphilis in patients allergic to penicillin.** *Adults and children older than age 8:* 100 mg P.O. b.i.d. for 2 weeks (early detection) or for 4 weeks (if more than 1 year's duration).

▶ **Uncomplicated urethral, endocervical, or rectal infection caused by *Chlamydia trachomatis* or *Ureaplasma urealyticum*.** *Adults:* 100 mg P.O. b.i.d. for at least 7 days.

▶ **Prevention of malaria.** *Adults:* 100 mg P.O. daily.
Children older than age 8: 2 mg/kg P.O. once daily. Dosage shouldn't exceed adult dose. Begin 1 to 2 days before travel to malarious area

and continue throughout travel and for 4 weeks thereafter.

▶ **Adjunct to scaling and root planing to promote attachment level gain and to reduce pocket depth in patients with adult periodontitis.** *Adults:* 20 mg Periostat P.O. b.i.d. more than 1 hour before or 2 hours after the morning and evening meals and after scaling and root planing. Effective for 9 months.

▶ **Adjunct to other antibiotics for inhalation, GI, and oropharyngeal anthrax.** *Adults:* 100 mg I.V. q 12 hours initially until susceptibility test are known. Switch to 100 mg P.O. b.i.d. when clinically appropriate. Treat for 60 days total.
Children older than age 8 and weighing more than 45 kg: 100 mg I.V. q 12 hours, then switch to 100 mg P.O. b.i.d. when clinically appropriate. Treat for 60 days total.
Children older than age 8 and weighing 45 kg or less: 2.2 mg/kg I.V. q 12 hours, then switch to 2.2 mg/kg P.O. b.i.d. when clinically appropriate. Treat for 60 days total.
Children age 8 and younger: 2.2 mg/kg I.V. q 12 hours, then switch to 2.2 mg/kg P.O. b.i.d. when clinically appropriate. Treat for 60 days total.

▶ **Cutaneous anthrax.** *Adults:* 100 mg P.O. b.i.d. for 60 days.
Children older than age 8 and weighing more than 45 kg: 100 mg P.O. q 12 hours for 60 days.
Children older than age 8 and weighing 45 kg or less: 2.2 mg/kg P.O. q 12 hours for 60 days.
Children age 8 and younger: 2.2 mg/kg P.O. q 12 hours for 60 days.

▶ **Adjunct to severe acne.** *Adults:* 200 mg Adoxa P.O. on day 1 (give as 100 mg q 12 hours or 50 mg q 6 hrs); follow with a maintenance dose of 100 mg P.O. daily, or 50 mg P.O. b.i.d.

▶ **Prevention of traveler's diarrhea commonly caused by enterotoxigenic *E. coli*‡.** *Adults:* 100 mg P.O. daily for up to 3 days.

▶ **Prophylaxis for rape victims‡.** *Adults and adolescents:* 100 mg Adoxa P.O. b.i.d. for 7 days after a single 2-g oral dose of metronidazole is given with a single 125-mg I.M. dose of ceftriaxone.

▶ **Lyme disease‡.** *Adults and children older than age 9:* 100 mg Adoxa P.O. b.i.d. or t.i.d. for 10 to 30 days.

▶ **Pleural effusions related to cancer‡.** *Adults:* 500 mg of doxycycline diluted in

250 ml of normal saline solution and instilled into pleural space via chest tube.

▼ I.V. administration

● Reconstitute powder for injection with sterile water for injection. Use 10 ml in 100-mg vial and 20 ml in 200-mg vial. Dilute solution to 100 to 1,000 ml for I.V. infusion. Avoid extravasation. Don't infuse solutions that are more concentrated than 1 mg/ml.
● Depending on the dose, duration of infusion is typically 1 to 4 hours. Infusion must be completed within 12 hours.
● Monitor I.V. infusion site for signs of thrombophlebitis, which may occur with I.V. administration.
● Don't expose drug to light or heat. Protect it from sunlight during infusion.
● Reconstituted injectable solution is stable for 72 hours if refrigerated.

Contraindications and precautions

● Contraindicated in patients hypersensitive to drug or other tetracyclines.
● Use cautiously in patients with impaired kidney or liver function.
● **Lifespan:** In breast-feeding women, avoid use of drug. Pregnant women and immunocompromised patients should receive the usual doses and regimens for anthrax. During last half of pregnancy and in children younger than age 8, use of these drugs may cause permanent discoloration of teeth, enamel defects, and bone growth retardation. These effects are dose-limited; therefore, drug may be used for a short time (7 to 14 days) before 6 months of gestation.

Adverse reactions

CNS: *intracranial hypertension (pseudotumor cerebri).*
CV: pericarditis, thrombophlebitis.
EENT: glossitis, dysphagia.
GI: anorexia, *epigastric distress, nausea,* vomiting, *diarrhea,* oral candidiasis, enterocolitis, anogenital inflammation.
Hematologic: *neutropenia,* eosinophilia, *thrombocytopenia,* hemolytic anemia.
Musculoskeletal: bone growth retardation if used in children under age 8.
Skin: *maculopapular and erythematous rash, photosensitivity, increased pigmentation, urticaria.*

Other: hypersensitivity reactions, *anaphylaxis,* superinfection, permanent discoloration of teeth, enamel defects.

Interactions

Drug-drug. Antacids *(including sodium bicarbonate) and laxatives containing aluminum, magnesium, or calcium; antidiarrheals:* May decrease antibiotic absorption. Give antibiotic 1 hour before or 2 hours after these drugs.
Carbamazepine, phenobarbital: May decrease antibiotic effect. Avoid using together, if possible.
Ferrous sulfate and other iron products, zinc: May decrease antibiotic absorption. Give drug 3 hours after or 2 hours before iron administration.
Hormonal contraceptives: Decreases contraceptive effectiveness and increased risk of breakthrough bleeding. Recommend nonhormonal form of birth control.
Methoxyflurane: May cause nephrotoxicity with tetracyclines. Avoid using together.
Oral anticoagulants: May increase anticoagulant effect. Monitor PT and INR, and adjust dosage.
Penicillins: May interfere with bactericidal action of penicillins. Avoid using together.
Drug-lifestyle. *Alcohol use:* Decreases antibiotic effect. Avoid using together.
Sun exposure: Photosensitivity reactions may occur. Urge patient to avoid unprotected and prolonged sun exposure.

Effects on lab test results

● May increase BUN and liver enzyme levels.
● May increase eosinophil count. May decrease hemoglobin, hematocrit, and platelet, neutrophil, and WBC counts.
● Parenteral form may cause false-positive reading of copper sulfate tests (Clinitest). All forms may cause false-negative reading of glucose oxidase reagent (Diastix or Chemstrip uG).

Pharmacokinetics

Absorption: 90% to 100% absorbed after P.O. administration; milk or other dairy products insignificantly alter absorption.
Distribution: Distributed widely in body tissues and fluids. Poor penetration in CSF. Drug is 25% to 93% protein-bound.
Metabolism: Insignificantly metabolized; some hepatic degradation occurs.

Reactions may be *common,* uncommon, *life-threatening,* or **COMMON AND LIFE-THREATENING.**

Excretion: Excreted primarily unchanged in urine; some drug is excreted in feces. *Half-life:* About 1 day after multiple dosing.

Route	Onset	Peak	Duration
P.O.	Unknown	1½-4 hr	Unknown
I.V.	Immediate	Unknown	Unknown

Action

Chemical effect: May exert bacteriostatic effect by binding to 30S ribosomal subunit of microorganisms, thus inhibiting protein synthesis.
Therapeutic effect: Hinders bacterial growth.

Available forms

doxycycline calcium
Syrup: 50 mg/5 ml
doxycycline hyclate
Capsules: 20 mg, 50 mg, 100 mg
Capsules (coated pellets): 75 mg, 100 mg
Injection: 100 mg, 200 mg
Tablets: 20 mg, 100 mg
doxycycline hydrochloride ◊
Capsules: 50 mg ◊, 100 mg ◊
Tablets: 50 mg ◊, 100 mg ◊
doxycycline monohydrate
Capsules: 50 mg, 100 mg
Oral suspension: 25 mg/5 ml
Tablets: 50 mg, 75 mg, 100 mg

NURSING PROCESS

Assessment
• Obtain history of patient's infection before therapy, and reassess regularly thereafter.
• Obtain specimen for culture and sensitivity tests before first dose. Therapy may begin pending test results.
• Be alert for adverse reactions and drug interactions.
• Monitor patient's hydration status if adverse GI reactions occur.
• Evaluate patient's and family's knowledge of drug therapy.

Nursing diagnoses
• Infection related to presence of susceptible bacteria
• Risk for deficient fluid volume related to drug-induced adverse GI reactions
• Deficient knowledge related to drug therapy

Planning and implementation
• Check expiration date. Outdated or deteriorated tetracyclines may cause reversible nephrotoxicity (Fanconi's syndrome).
• Give drug with milk or food if adverse GI reactions develop.
• Follow current CDC recommendations for anthrax.
• Ciprofloxacin and doxycycline are first-line therapy for anthrax. 500 mg amoxicillin P.O. t.i.d. for adults and 80 mg/kg/day divided every 8 hours for children is an option for completing therapy after improvement.
• Cutaneous anthrax with signs of systemic involvement, extensive edema, or lesions on the head or neck requires I.V. therapy and a multidrug approach.
• Additional antimicrobials for anthrax multidrug regimens can include rifampin, vancomycin, penicillin, ampicillin, chloramphenicol, imipenem, clindamycin, and clarithromycin.
• Steroids may be considered as adjunctive therapy for anthrax patients with severe edema and for meningitis, based on experience with bacterial meningitis of other etiologies.
• If meningitis is suspected, doxycycline would be less optimal because of poor CHS penetration.
• Notify prescriber of adverse reactions. Some adverse reactions, such as superinfection, may necessitate substitution of another antibiotic.
⑤ **ALERT:** Don't confuse doxycycline with doxylamine or dicyclomine.

Patient teaching
• Tell patient to take entire amount of medication exactly as prescribed, even after he feels better.
• Instruct patient to take oral doxycycline with milk or food but not antacids if adverse GI reactions develop. Tell patient to take drug no less than 1 hour before bedtime to prevent irritation from esophageal reflux.
• Advise parent giving drug to a child that tablets may be crushed and mixed with lowfat milk, lowfat chocolate milk, regular (whole) chocolate milk, chocolate pudding, or with apple juice that is mixed with sugar in equal proportions. Store mixtures in refrigerator, except apple juice mixture (which can be stored at room temperature), and discard after 24 hours.
• Tell patient to use sunscreen and avoid strong sunlight during therapy to prevent photosensitivity reactions.

Rapid onset   *Liquid form contains alcohol.   ◆Canada   ◊ Australia   †OTC   ‡Off-label use

• Stress good oral hygiene.
• Tell patient to check expiration dates and to discard outdated doxycycline because it may become toxic.
• Advise patient taking hormonal contraceptive to use alternative means of contraception within 1 week of therapy.

☑ **Evaluation**
• Patient is free from infection.
• Patient maintains adequate hydration throughout therapy.
• Patient and family state understanding of drug therapy.

dronabinol (delta-9-tetrahydrocannabinol)
(droh-NAB-eh-nohl)
Marinol

Pharmacologic class: cannabinoid
Therapeutic class: antiemetic, appetite stimulant
Pregnancy risk category: C
Controlled substance schedule: III

Indications and dosages

▶ **Nausea and vomiting from chemotherapy.** *Adults:* 5 mg/m² P.O. 1 to 3 hours before administration of chemotherapy. Then, same dose q 2 to 4 hours after chemotherapy for total of four to six doses daily. If needed, dosage increased in increments of 2.5 mg/m² to maximum of 15 mg/m² per dose.

▶ **Anorexia and weight loss in patients with AIDS.** *Adults:* 2.5 mg P.O. b.i.d. before lunch and dinner, increase p.r.n. to maximum of 20 mg daily.

Contraindications and precautions

• Contraindicated in patients hypersensitive to sesame oil or cannabinoids.
• Use cautiously in patients with heart disease, psychiatric illness, or history of drug abuse.
⚠ **Lifespan:** In breast-feeding women, drug isn't recommended. In children, safety and efficacy of drug haven't been established. In elderly patients, use cautiously.

Adverse reactions

CNS: *dizziness, drowsiness, euphoria,* ataxia, depersonalization, disorientation, hallucinations, *somnolence,* headache, muddled thinking, asthenia, amnesia, confusion, *paranoia.*
CV: tachycardia, orthostatic hypotension, palpitations, vasodilation.
EENT: visual disturbances.
GI: dry mouth, *nausea, vomiting, abdominal pain,* diarrhea.

Interactions

Drug-drug. *CNS depressants, psychotomimetic substances, sedatives:* May have additive effects. Avoid using together.
Drug-lifestyle. *Alcohol use:* May have additive effects. Discourage using together.

Effects on lab test results

None reported.

Pharmacokinetics

Absorption: Almost 95% absorbed.
Distribution: Distributed rapidly in many tissue sites; 97% to 99% protein-bound.
Metabolism: Undergoes extensive metabolism in liver. Metabolite activity is unknown.
Excretion: Excreted primarily in feces. *Half-life:* About 1 to 1½ days.

Route	Onset	Peak	Duration
P.O.	Unknown	2-4 hr	4-6 hr

Action

Chemical effect: Unknown.
Therapeutic effect: Relieves nausea and vomiting caused by chemotherapy and stimulates appetite.

Available forms

Capsules: 2.5 mg, 5 mg, 10 mg

NURSING PROCESS

🔲 **Assessment**
• Obtain history of patient's underlying condition before therapy.
• Monitor effectiveness by assessing for nausea, vomiting, or weight gain. Drug effects may persist for days after therapy ends.
• Be alert for adverse reactions and drug interactions.

Reactions may be common, uncommon, *life-threatening*, or COMMON AND LIFE-THREATENING.

• Monitor patient for dependence. Dronabinol is the principal active substance in *Cannabis sativa* (marijuana). It can produce physical and psychological dependence and has high potential for abuse.
• Monitor patient's hydration status, weight, and nutritional status regularly.
• Evaluate patient's and family's knowledge of drug therapy.

⊞ Nursing diagnoses
• Risk for deficient fluid volume related to nausea and vomiting from chemotherapy
• Disturbed thought processes related to drug-induced adverse CNS reactions
• Deficient knowledge related to drug therapy

▶ Planning and implementation
• Give drug only to patients who haven't responded satisfactorily to other antiemetics.
• Give drug 1 to 3 hours before chemotherapy starts and again 2 to 4 hours after chemotherapy.
Patient teaching
• Inform patient that drug may cause unusual changes in mood or other adverse behavioral effects.
• Caution patient to avoid hazardous activities until full CNS effects of drug are known.
• Warn family members to make sure patient is supervised by a responsible person during and immediately after treatment.

✓ Evaluation
• Patient maintains adequate hydration.
• Patient regains normal thought processes after effects of drug therapy have dissipated.
• Patient and family state understanding of drug therapy.

drotrecogin alfa (activated)
(droh-truh-KO-jin al-fa)
Xigris

Pharmacologic class: recombinant protease of human activated protein C
Therapeutic class: antithrombotic
Pregnancy risk category: C

Indications and dosages

▶ **Reduction of mortality in patients with severe sepsis (sepsis from acute organ dysfunction) who are at a high risk of dying.**
Adults: 24 mcg/kg/hour I.V. infusion for a total of 96 hours.

▼ I.V. administration
• Reconstitute 5-mg vials with 2.5 ml sterile water for injection, USP and 20-mg vials with 10 ml of sterile water for injection, USP. The resulting concentration is about 2 mg/ml. Gently swirl each vial until powder is completely dissolved; avoid inverting or shaking the vial.
• Prepare the I.V. solution immediately after reconstitution because drug contains no preservative. If the reconstituted vial isn't used immediately, it may be held at controlled room temperature of 59° to 86° F (15° to 30° C) but must be used within 3 hours.
• Further dilute the reconstituted solution with sterile normal saline injection. Withdraw appropriate amount of reconstituted drug into a prepared infusion bag of sterile normal saline solution. When adding the drug, direct the stream to the side of the bag to minimize agitation of the solution.
• Gently invert the infusion bag to obtain a homogenous solution. Don't transport the infusion bag between locations using mechanical delivery systems.
• Inspect for particle matter and discoloration before administration.
• Give drug within 12 hours of preparing.
• When using an I.V. pump to give the drug, the solution of reconstituted drug is typically diluted into an infusion bag containing sterile normal saline solution to a final concentration between 100 mcg/ml and 200 mcg/ml.
• When using a syringe pump to give the drug, the reconstituted solution is typically diluted with sterile normal saline solution to a final concentration between 100 mcg/ml and 1,000 mcg/ml. When giving at low concentrations (less than about 200 mcg/ml) at low flow rates (less than about 5 ml/hr), the infusion set must be primed for about 15 minutes at a flow rate of about 5 ml/hour.
⑤ **ALERT:** Give via a dedicated I.V. line or lumen of a multilumen central venous catheter. The only other solutions that can be given through the same line are normal saline solution, lactated Ringer's injection, dextrose, or dextrose and saline mixtures.
• Store in a refrigerator at 35° to 46° F (2° to 8° C). Don't freeze. Avoid heat or direct sunlight.

Rapid onset   *Liquid form contains alcohol.   ♦ Canada   ◊ Australia   †OTC   ‡Off-label use

Contraindications and precautions

• Contraindicated in patients with active internal bleeding, hemorrhagic CVA within 3 months, intracranial or intraspinal surgery within 2 months, severe head trauma, trauma with an increased risk of life-threatening bleeding, an epidural catheter, intracranial neoplasm or mass lesion, or evidence of cerebral herniation. Drug is also contraindicated in patients hypersensitive to drotrecogin alfa (activated) or any of its components.

• Use cautiously in patients with an increased risk of bleeding, such as those who are taking heparin (15 units/kg/hour or more); those with a platelet count of less than 30,000 × 10⁶/L (even if the platelet count is increased after transfusions), those with an INR greater than 3; those who have experienced GI bleeding within 6 weeks; those who have had thrombolytic therapy within 3 days; those who have been given oral anticoagulants, glycoprotein IIb/IIIa inhibitors, aspirin (more than 650 mg/day) or other platelet inhibitors within 7 days; those who have had ischemic CVA within 3 months; those who have had intracranial arteriovenous malformation or aneurysm, bleeding diathesis, chronic severe hepatic disease, or any other condition in which bleeding constitutes a significant hazard or would be particularly difficult to manage because of its location.

⚱ Lifespan: In pregnant women, drug should be used only if clearly needed. Breast-feeding women should stop nursing or stop taking the drug, taking into account the importance of the drug to the mother; it's unknown whether drug appears in breast milk. In children, safety and efficacy of drug haven't been established.

Adverse reactions

Hematologic: HEMORRHAGE.

Interactions

Drug-drug. *Drugs that affect hemostasis:* Increases risk of bleeding. Use together cautiously; monitor patient for bleeding.

Effects on lab test results

• May increase APTT and PT. May interfere with APTT and one-stage coagulation assays based on APTT (such as factors VIII, IX, and XI assays).

Pharmacokinetics

Absorption: Administered I.V.
Distribution: Steady-state levels attained within 2 hours after starting infusion.
Metabolism: Unknown.
Excretion: Unknown. *Half-life:* Unknown.

Route	Onset	Peak	Duration
I.V.	Rapid	Unknown	Unknown

Action

Chemical effect: Antisepsis action is unknown. May produce dose-dependent reductions in D-dimer and IL-6. Activated Protein C exerts an anti-thrombotic effect by inhibiting factors Va and VIIIa. May exert an anti-inflammatory effect by inhibiting human tumor necrosis factor production by monocytes, by blocking leukocyte adhesion to selectins, and by limiting the thrombin-induced inflammatory responses.
Therapeutic effect: Prevents clots and blocks cell death.

Available forms

Injection: 5 mg; 20 mg

NURSING PROCESS

⚕ Assessment
• Assess patient before starting and during drug therapy for risk of bleeding or contraindications.
• Monitor patient closely for bleeding. If significant bleeding occurs, immediately stop the infusion.
• Because drug may prolong APTT, it can't be used to reliably assess the status of the coagulopathy during infusion. Because drug has minimal effect on PT, PT may be used to monitor the status of the coagulopathy in these patients.

⚕ Nursing diagnoses
• Risk for injury caused by increased bleeding potential related to drug therapy.
• Deficient knowledge related to drug therapy.

⚕ Planning and implementation
• If the infusion is interrupted, restart at the 24-mcg/kg/hour infusion rate. Dose escalation, bolus doses, and dose adjustment based on clinical or laboratory parameters aren't recommended.
• Stop drug 2 hours before an invasive surgical procedure with a risk of bleeding. After hemo-

stasis is reached, drug may be restarted 12 hours after major invasive procedures or surgery or immediately after uncomplicated, less-invasive procedures.

Patient teaching

• Inform patient of potential adverse reactions.

• Instruct patient to promptly report signs of bleeding.

• Advise patient that bleeding may occur for up to 28 days after treatment.

☑ Evaluation

• Patient doesn't experience any hemorrhaging during and 28 days after drug therapy.

• Patient and family state understanding of drug therapy.

dutasteride

doo-TAS-teer-ighd

Avodart

Pharmacologic class: 5-alpha-reductase enzyme inhibitor
Therapeutic class: BPH drug
Pregnancy risk category: X

Indications & dosages

▶ **BPH.** *Adults:* 0.5 mg P.O. once daily.

Contraindications & precautions

• Contraindicated in patients hypersensitive to drug, its components, or other 5-alpha-reductase inhibitors.

• Use cautiously in patients with hepatic disease and in those taking long-term potent CYP 3A4 inhibitors.

≛ **Lifespan:** In women and children, drug is contraindicated. It's unknown whether drug appears in breast milk.

Adverse reactions

GU: impotence, decreased libido, ejaculation disorder.
Other: gynecomastia.

Interactions

Drug-drug. *CYP 3A4 inhibitors (cimetidine, diltiazem, itraconazole, ketoconazole, macrolide antibiotics, protease inhibitors, ritonavir, verapamil):* May increase dutasteride level. Use together cautiously.

Effects on lab test results

• May decrease prostate-specific antigen (PSA) level.

Pharmacokinetics

Absorption: Bioavailability is about 60%.
Distribution: Drug is 99% bound to albumin and 96.6% bound to alpha$_1$-acid glycoprotein.
Metabolism: Extensively metabolized by CYP 3A4.
Excretion: Mainly in feces, 5% unchanged and 40% as metabolites, trace amounts in urine.
Half-life: 5 weeks.

Route	Onset	Peak	Duration
P.O.	Unknown	2-3 hr	Unknown

Action

Chemical effect: Inhibits the conversion of testosterone to dihydrotestosterone (DHT), the androgen primarily responsible for the initial development and subsequent enlargement of the prostate gland.
Therapeutic effect: Resolves BPH.

Available forms

Capsules: 0.5 mg

NURSING PROCESS

☜ Assessment

• Before therapy, assess patient to rule out other urological diseases.

• Carefully monitor patients with a large residual urinary volume or severely diminished urinary flow, or both, for obstructive uropathy.

• Perform digital rectal examinations and other evaluations for prostate cancer on patients with BPH before starting therapy and periodically thereafter.

• Be alert for adverse effects.

• Evaluate patient's and family's knowledge of drug therapy.

☷ Nursing diagnoses

• Impaired urinary elimination related to underlying condition

• Sexual dysfunction related to adverse effects of medication

• Deficient knowledge related to drug therapy

ⓘ Planning and implementation
- Because drug may be absorbed through the skin, women who are or may become pregnant shouldn't handle the drug.
- If capsule leaks onto skin, wash the area immediately with soap and water.
- Patients taking drug shouldn't donate blood within 6 months of last dose.
- Establish new baseline PSA level in men treated for 3 to 6 months and use it to assess potentially cancer-related changes in PSA level.
- To interpret PSA level in men treated for 6 months or more, double the PSA level for comparison with normal levels in untreated men.

Patient teaching
- Tell patient to swallow the capsule whole and to take with or without food.
- Inform patient that ejaculate volume may decrease, but sexual function will remain normal.
- Tell patient that pregnant women shouldn't handle drug. A boy born to a woman who was exposed to the drug during pregnancy may have abnormal sex organs.
- Tell patient not to donate blood within 6 months of his final dose.

☑ Evaluation
- Patient has normal urinary flow without urinary residual volume.
- Patient doesn't experience adverse effects.
- Patient and family state understanding of drug therapy.

E

edetate calcium disodium (calcium EDTA)
(ED-eh-tayt KAL-see-um digh-SOH-dee-um)
Calcium Disodium Versenate

Pharmacologic class: chelating agent
Therapeutic class: heavy metal antagonist
Pregnancy risk category: B

Indications and dosages

▶ **Acute lead encephalopathy or lead levels above 70 mcg/dl.** *Adults and children:* 1.5 g/m²

I.V. or I.M. daily in divided doses at 12-hour intervals for 3 to 5 days, usually with dimercaprol. Give a second course in 5 to 7 days.
▶ **Lead poisoning without encephalopathy, or asymptomatic patient with lead levels below 70 mcg/dl.** *Children:* 1 g/m² I.V. or I.M. daily in divided doses.

▼ I.V. administration
- Dilute drug with D_5W or normal saline injection to 2 to 4 mg/ml.
- Infuse half of daily dose over 1 hour in asymptomatic patients or 2 hours in symptomatic patients. Give rest of infusion at least 6 hours later. Or, give by slow infusion over at least 8 hours.
- ⓧ **ALERT:** Because I.V. use may increase intracranial pressure, don't give by that route to treat lead encephalopathy. Give by I.M. route instead.

Contraindications and precautions
- Contraindicated in patients with anuria, acute renal disease, or hepatitis.
- Use cautiously in patients with mild renal disease. Reduce dosages.
- ≜ **Lifespan:** In pregnant women, use cautiously.

Adverse reactions
CNS: sudden fever, headache, paresthesia, numbness, fatigue.
CV: *arrhythmias,* hypotension.
EENT: sneezing and nasal congestion.
GI: anorexia, nausea, vomiting.
GU: proteinuria, hematuria, *nephrotoxicity with renal tubular necrosis leading to fatal nephrosis.*
Metabolic: hypercalcemia, zinc deficiency.
Musculoskeletal: arthralgia, myalgia.
Other: chills, excessive thirst.

Interactions
Drug-drug. *Zinc insulin:* Interferes with action of insulin by binding with zinc. Monitor patient closely.
Zinc supplements: May decrease effectiveness of edetate calcium disodium and zinc supplements because of chelation. Withhold zinc supplements until therapy is complete.

Effects on lab test results
• May increase AST, ALT, and calcium levels.
• May decrease hemoglobin and hematocrit.

Pharmacokinetics
Absorption: Well absorbed after I.M. administration.
Distribution: Primarily in extracellular fluid.
Metabolism: None.
Excretion: In urine. *Half-life:* 20 minutes to 1½ hours.

Route	Onset	Peak	Duration
I.V., I.M.	1 hr	24-48 hr	Unknown

Action
Chemical effect: Forms stable, soluble complexes with metals, particularly lead.
Therapeutic effect: Abolishes effects of lead poisoning.

Available forms
Injection: 200 mg/ml

NURSING PROCESS

⚗ Assessment
• Obtain history of patient's underlying condition before therapy.
• Monitor effectiveness by checking lead level and observing for decreasing signs and symptoms of lead poisoning.
• Monitor fluid intake and output, urinalysis, BUN, and ECG daily.
• Be alert for adverse reactions.
• Evaluate patient's and family's knowledge of drug therapy.

Nursing diagnoses
• Risk for injury related to lead poisoning
• Ineffective renal tissue perfusion related to drug-induced fatal nephrosis
• Deficient knowledge related to drug therapy

Planning and implementation
• When giving I.M., add procaine hydrochloride to I.M. solution to minimize pain. Watch for local reactions.
• Use I.M., especially for children and patients with lead encephalopathy.
• Force fluids to facilitate lead excretion, except in patients with lead encephalopathy.
• To avoid toxicity, use with dimercaprol.

• Apply ice or cold compresses to injection site to ease local reaction.
⊛ ALERT: Don't confuse edetate calcium with edetate disodium, which is used to treat hypercalcemia.
Patient teaching
• Warn patient that some adverse reactions—such as fever, chills, thirst, and nasal congestion—may occur 4 to 8 hours after administration.
• Encourage patient and family to identify and remove source of lead in home.

☑ Evaluation
• Patient sustains no injury as result of lead poisoning.
• Patient has no signs of altered renal tissue perfusion.
• Patient and family state understanding of drug therapy.

edetate disodium
(ED-eh-tayt digh-SOH-dee-um)
Disodium EDTA, Edathamil Disodium, Endrate, Sodium Edetate

Pharmacologic class: chelating agent
Therapeutic class: heavy metal antagonist
Pregnancy risk category: C

Indications and dosages
▶ **Hypercalcemic crisis.** *Adults:* 50 mg/kg by slow I.V. infusion. Maximum dose is 3 g I.V. daily.
Children: 40 to 70 mg/kg by slow I.V. infusion. Maximum dose is 70 mg/kg I.V. daily.
▶ **Digoxin-induced arrhythmias.** *Adults and children:* 15 mg/kg/hour I.V. daily. Maximum dose is 60 mg/kg I.V. daily.

▼ I.V. administration
• Dilute before use. For adults, add dose to 500 ml of D_5W or normal saline solution and give over 3 or more hours. For children, dilute to maximum of 30 mg/ml in D_5W or normal saline solution and give over 3 or more hours.
⊛ ALERT: Don't exceed recommended dose or rate of administration.
• Avoid rapid I.V. infusion; profound hypocalcemia may occur, leading to tetany, seizures, ar-

rhythmias, and respiratory arrest. Drug isn't recommended for direct or intermittent injection.
• Watch for irritation and infiltration; extravasation can cause tissue damage and necrosis.
• Record I.V. site used and avoid repeated use of same site to decrease likelihood of thrombophlebitis.
• Keep I.V. calcium available to treat hypocalcemia.
• Keep patient in bed for 15 minutes after infusion to avoid orthostatic hypotension.

Contraindications and precautions

• Contraindicated in patients hypersensitive to drug and in those with anuria, known or suspected hypocalcemia, significant renal disease, active or healed tubercular lesions, or a history of seizures or intracranial lesions.
• Use cautiously in patients with limited cardiac reserve, heart failure, or hypokalemia.
≉ **Lifespan:** In pregnant and breast-feeding women, use cautiously.

Adverse reactions

CNS: circumoral paresthesia, numbness, headache.
CV: hypertension, thrombophlebitis, orthostatic hypotension.
GI: nausea, vomiting, diarrhea, anorexia, abdominal cramps.
GU: *nephrotoxicity* with urinary urgency, nocturia, dysuria, polyuria, proteinuria, renal insufficiency, *renal failure, tubular necrosis.*
Metabolic: *severe hypocalcemia, hypomagnesia.*
Skin: dermatitis, erythema.
Other: infusion site pain.

Interactions

Drug-drug. *Digoxin:* Sudden drop in calcium caused by edetate disodium may reverse effects of digoxin. Monitor patient closely.
Insulin: Decreases glucose and may cause possible chelation of zinc in insulin. Dosage adjustments of insulin may be required.

Effects on lab test results

• May decrease calcium and magnesium levels.

Pharmacokinetics

Absorption: Administered I.V.

Distribution: Distributed widely throughout body but doesn't enter CSF in significant amounts.
Metabolism: None.
Excretion: In urine. *Half-life:* Unknown.

Route	Onset	Peak	Duration
I.V.	Unknown	Unknown	Unknown

Action

Chemical effect: Chelates with metals, such as calcium, to form stable, soluble complex.
Therapeutic effect: Lowers calcium level.

Available forms

Injection: 150 mg/ml

NURSING PROCESS

⚖ Assessment

• Obtain history of patient's calcium level before therapy.
• Monitor effectiveness by obtaining calcium level after each dose. If used to treat digoxin-induced arrhythmias, evaluate patient's ECG frequently.
• Monitor kidney function tests frequently.
• Be alert for adverse reactions.
• Evaluate patient's and family's knowledge of drug therapy.

⊞ Nursing diagnoses

• Risk for injury related to hypercalcemia
• Ineffective protection related to drug-induced hypocalcemia
• Deficient knowledge related to drug therapy

▶ Planning and implementation

• If generalized systemic reactions (fever, chills, back pain, emesis, muscle cramps, urinary urgency) occur 4 to 8 hours after infusion, report them to prescriber. Treatment is usually supportive. Symptoms usually subside within 12 hours.
• Other drug treatments for hypercalcemia are safer and more effective than edetate disodium.
⊛ **ALERT:** Don't confuse edetate disodium with edetate calcium disodium, which is used to treat lead toxicity.
Patient teaching
• Instruct patient to report immediately respiratory difficulty, dizziness, and muscle cramping.

• Advise patient to move from sitting or lying position slowly to avoid dizziness.
• Reassure patient that generalized systemic reaction usually subsides within 12 hours.

☑ **Evaluation**
• Patient sustains no injury as result of hypercalcemia.
• Patient's calcium level doesn't fall below normal after edetate disodium therapy.
• Patient and family state understanding of drug therapy.

edrophonium chloride
(ed-roh-FOH-nee-um KLOR-ighd)
Enlon, Reversol, Tensilon

Pharmacologic class: cholinesterase inhibitor
Therapeutic class: cholinergic agonist, diagnostic drug
Pregnancy risk category: NR

Indications and dosages

▶ **As curare antagonist to reverse nondepolarizing neuromuscular blockade.** *Adults:* 10 mg I.V. given slowly over 30 to 45 seconds. Repeat dose as needed to maximum of 40 mg. Larger dosages may potentiate effect of curare.
▶ **Diagnostic aid in myasthenia gravis (Tensilon test).** *Adults:* 1 to 2 mg I.V. over 15 to 30 seconds; then 8 mg if no response (increase in muscle strength) occurs. Or, 10 mg I.M. If cholinergic reaction occurs, 2 mg I.M. is given 30 minutes later to rule out false-negative response.
Children weighing more than 34 kg (75 lb): 2 mg I.V. If no response within 45 seconds, 1 mg q 45 seconds to maximum of 10 mg. Or, 5 mg I.M.
Children weighing less than 34 kg: 1 mg I.V. If no response within 45 seconds, 1 mg q 45 seconds to maximum of 5 mg. Or, 2 mg I.M. (Use I.M. route in children because of difficulty with I.V. route.) Same reactions may occur as with I.V. test, but they appear after 2- to 10-minute delay.
Infants: 0.5 mg to 1 mg I.M. or S.C.
▶ **To differentiate myasthenic crisis from cholinergic crisis.** *Adults:* 1 mg I.V. If no response in 1 minute, may repeat dose once. Increased muscle strength confirms myasthenic

crisis; no increase or exaggerated weakness confirms cholinergic crisis.

▼ I.V. administration

• For easier administration, use tuberculin syringe with I.V. needle.

Contraindications and precautions

• Contraindicated in patients hypersensitive to anticholinesterases and in those with mechanical obstruction of intestine or urinary tract.
• Use cautiously in patients with bronchial asthma or arrhythmias.
⚠ Lifespan: In pregnant and breast-feeding women, safety of drug hasn't been established.

Adverse reactions

CNS: *seizures,* weakness, dysarthria.
CV: hypotension, *bradycardia, AV block, cardiac arrest.*
EENT: excessive lacrimation, diplopia, *laryngospasm,* miosis, conjunctival hyperemia, dysphagia.
GI: nausea, vomiting, *diarrhea, abdominal cramps,* excessive salivation.
GU: urinary frequency, incontinence.
Musculoskeletal: muscle cramps, muscle fasciculation.
Respiratory: *respiratory paralysis, bronchospasm,* increased bronchial secretions.
Skin: diaphoresis.

Interactions

Drug-drug. *Aminoglycosides, anesthetics:* May prolong or enhance muscle weakness. Monitor patient closely.
Cholinergics: May increase effects. Stop all other cholinergics before giving drug.
Corticosteroids, magnesium, procainamide, quinidine: May antagonize cholinergic effects. Observe patient for lack of drug effect.
Digoxin: May increase heart's sensitivity to edrophonium. Use together cautiously.
Drug-herb. *Jaborandi tree, pill-bearing spurge:* Possible additive effect with risk of toxicity. Discourage using together.

Effects on lab test results

None reported.

Pharmacokinetics

Absorption: Administered I.M. or I.V.
Distribution: Unknown.

Metabolism: Unknown.
Excretion: Unknown. *Half-life:* Unknown.

Route	Onset	Peak	Duration
I.V.	30-60 sec	Unknown	5-10 min
I.M.	2-10 min	Unknown	5-30 min

Action

Chemical effect: Inhibits destruction of acetylcholine released from parasympathetic and somatic efferent nerves. Acetylcholine accumulates, promoting increased stimulation of receptor.
Therapeutic effect: Reverses nondepolarizing neuromuscular blocker.

Available forms

Injection: 10 mg/ml in 1-ml ampules and in 10- or 15-ml vials

NURSING PROCESS

⬛ Assessment
• Obtain history of patient's underlying condition before therapy.
• Monitor effectiveness by evaluating reduction of symptoms of underlying condition. When giving drug to differentiate myasthenic crisis from cholinergic crisis, observe patient's muscle strength closely.
• Be alert for adverse reactions and drug interactions.
• Evaluate patient's and family's knowledge of drug therapy.

⬛ Nursing diagnoses
• Ineffective health maintenance related to underlying condition
• Impaired gas exchange related to drug-induced bronchospasm
• Deficient knowledge related to drug therapy

⬛ Planning and implementation
• Stop all other cholinergics before giving drug.
• Use I.M. route to give drug to children because of difficulty with I.V. insertion in children.
• ⚕ **ALERT:** Keep atropine injection readily available, and give 0.5 to 1 mg S.C. or slow I.V. push, if needed. Provide respiratory support.
Patient teaching
• Tell patient to report adverse reactions immediately, especially difficulty breathing.

☑ Evaluation
• Patient shows improvement in underlying condition.
• Patient maintains adequate gas exchange throughout therapy.
• Patient and family state understanding of drug therapy.

efalizumab
(eh-fah-LEE-zoo-mab)
Raptiva

Pharmacologic class: immunosuppressant
Therapeutic class: antipsoriatic
Pregnancy risk category: C

Indications and dosages

▶ **Chronic moderate to severe plaque psoriasis when systemic therapy or phototherapy is appropriate.** *Adults:* Single dose of 0.7 mg/kg S.C.; follow with weekly doses of 1 mg/kg S.C. Maximum single dose, 200 mg.

Contraindications and precautions

• Contraindicated in patients hypersensitive to drug or its components and in patients with significant infection.
• Use cautiously in patients with chronic infection or a history of recurrent infection. Also use cautiously in patients with a history of or high risk for malignancy.
⚖ **Lifespan:** In pregnant women, give the drug only when clearly needed; it isn't known whether drug harms fetus. In breast-feeding women, avoid breast-feeding during therapy; it isn't known whether drug appears in breast milk. In children, safety and efficacy haven't been established. In elderly patients, use cautiously because of the increased likelihood of infection.

Adverse reactions

CNS: *CVA,* fever, *headache, pain.*
GI: *nausea.*
Musculoskeletal: back pain, myalgia.
Skin: acne.
Other: *chills,* flu syndrome, ***hypersensitivity reaction, infection.***

Reactions may be *common,* uncommon, *life-threatening*, or **COMMON AND LIFE-THREATENING.**

Interactions

Drug-drug. *Other immunosuppressants:* Increased risk of infection and malignancy. Avoid using together.
Vaccines: Decreased or absent immune response to vaccine. Avoid using together.

Effects on lab test results

- May increase alkaline phosphatase level.
- May increase lymphocyte and leukocyte counts. May decrease platelet count.

Pharmacokinetics

Absorption: 50% bioavailable.
Distribution: Unknown.
Metabolism: Unknown.
Excretion: Unknown. *Half-life:* Unknown.

Route	Onset	Peak	Duration
S.C.	1-2 days	Unknown	25 days

Action

Chemical effect: Binds to a leukocyte function antigen and decreases its expression, thus inhibiting the action of T-lymphocytes at sites of inflammation, including psoriatic skin.
Therapeutic effect: Decreases inflammation of psoriatic skin.

Available forms

Injection: 125-mg single-use vial

NURSING PROCESS

⚡ Assessment

- Monitor for thrombocytopenia. Check the patient's platelet count monthly during initial treatment and then every three months.
- Monitor the patient for worsening of psoriasis during or after therapy.
- Evaluate patient's and family's knowledge of drug therapy.

🔷 Nursing diagnoses

- Impaired skin integrity related to underlying condition
- Ineffective protection related to drug-induced thrombocytopenia
- Deficient knowledge related to drug therapy

▶ Planning and implementation

- To reconstitute, inject 1.3 ml of sterile water for injection into the vial. Swirl gently to dissolve the powder, which takes less than 5 minutes. Don't shake the vial.
- Reconstitute the drug immediately before use.
- Don't use any other diluent besides sterile water, and use a vial only once.
- The reconstituted solution should be colorless to pale yellow and free of particulates. Don't use the solution if it contains particulates or is discolored.
- If you don't use the reconstituted solution immediately, store it at room temperature and use it within 8 hours of reconstitution.
- Rotate injection sites.
- Don't add other drugs to the solution.
- Keep powder refrigerated, and protect vials from light.
- Stop the drug if the patient develops a severe infection or malignancy.
- Don't give vaccines to patients taking this drug because the immune response may be inadequate.

Patient teaching

- Tell the patient to take the drug exactly as prescribed.
- Explain that platelet counts will be monitored during therapy.
- Urge the patient to immediately report evidence of severe thrombocytopenia, such as bleeding gums, bruising, or petechiae.
- Tell the patient to report weight changes because the dose may need to be changed.
- Advise the patient to report any newly diagnosed infection or malignancy.
- Tell the patient to report worsening psoriasis.
- Caution the patient to immediately report pregnancy or suspected pregnancy.

☑ Evaluation

- Patient's underlying condition improves with drug therapy.
- Patient develops no serious complications from drug-induced thrombocytopenia.
- Patient and family state understanding of drug therapy.

efavirenz

(eh-fah-VEER-enz)
Sustiva

Pharmacologic class: nonnucleoside, reverse transcriptase inhibitor

Therapeutic class: antiretroviral agent
Pregnancy risk category: C

Indications and dosages

▶ **HIV-1 infection.** *Adults:* 600 mg P.O. daily with a protease inhibitor or nucleoside analogue reverse transcriptase inhibitors.
Children age 3 and older weighing 10 to less than 15 kg (22 to less than 33 lb): 200 mg P.O. daily.
Children weighing 15 to less than 20 kg (33 to less than 44 lb): 250 mg P.O. daily.
Children weighing 20 to less than 25 kg (44 to less than 55 lb): 300 mg P.O. daily.
Children weighing 25 to less than 32.5 kg (55 to less than 72 lb): 350 mg P.O. daily.
Children weighing 32.5 to less than 40 kg (72 to less than 88 lb): 400 mg P.O. daily.
Children weighing 40 kg (88 lb) or more: 600 mg P.O. once daily.
Give above doses with protease inhibitor or nucleoside analogue reverse transcriptase inhibitors.

Contraindications and precautions

• Contraindicated in patients hypersensitive to drug or its components.
• Use cautiously in patients with hepatic impairment or in those receiving hepatotoxic drugs.
⚖ **Lifespan:** In pregnant and breast-feeding women, drug is contraindicated. In children and elderly patients, use cautiously.

Adverse reactions

CNS: abnormal dreams or thinking, agitation, amnesia, confusion, depersonalization, depression, *dizziness,* euphoria, fatigue, hallucinations, headache, hypoesthesia, impaired concentration, insomnia, somnolence, nervousness, fever.
GI: abdominal pain, anorexia, *diarrhea,* dyspepsia, flatulence, *nausea,* vomiting.
GU: hematuria, renal calculi.
Skin: increased sweating, *erythema multiforme, Stevens-Johnson syndrome, toxic epidermal necrolysis, rash,* pruritus.

Interactions

Drug-drug. *Ergot derivatives, midazolam, and triazolam:* Competition for CYP enzyme system may result in inhibition of the metabolism of these drugs and cause serious or life-threatening adverse events (such as arrhythmias, prolonged sedation, or respiratory depression). Avoid using together.
Clarithromycin and indinavir, amprenavir, lopinavir and ritonavir: May decrease levels of these drugs. Consider alternative therapy or dosage adjustment.
Drugs that induce the CYP enzyme system (such as phenobarbital, rifampin): Increase clearance of efavirenz, resulting in lower level. Avoid using together.
Ethinyl estradiol and ritonavir: May increase levels of ethinyl estradiol and ritonavir. Monitor patient.
Hormonal contraceptives: May increase levels of ethinyl estradiol, no data on progesterone component. Advise use of a reliable method of barrier contraception in addition to use of hormonal contraceptive.
Psychoactive drugs: May cause additive CNS effects. Avoid use together.
Rifabutin: Decreases rifabutin concentrations. Increase the dose to 450 to 600 mg once daily or 600 mg two to three times a week.
Ritonavir: Increases levels of both drugs. Monitor patient closely.
Saquinavir: May significantly decrease saquinavir level. Also decreases exposure of efavirenz. Don't use with saquinavir as sole protease inhibitor.
Warfarin: Level and effects of warfarin may increase or decrease. Monitor INR.
Drug-herb. *St. John's wort:* Decreases efavirenz levels. Discourage using together.
Drug-food. *High-fat meals:* May increase absorption of drug, increasing risk of side effects. Instruct patient to maintain a proper low-fat diet.
Drug-lifestyle. *Alcohol use:* Enhances CNS effects. Discourage alcohol use.

Effects on lab test results

• May increase ALT, AST, and cholesterol levels.

Pharmacokinetics

Absorption: Steady-state levels reached in 6 to 10 days. Food increases amount of drug in body.
Distribution: Highly bound to proteins, predominantly albumin.
Metabolism: Primarily by CYP system to metabolites that are inactive against HIV-1.
Excretion: Primarily in feces with a small number of metabolites excreted in urine. *Half-life:* 40 to 76 hours.

Route	Onset	Peak	Duration
P.O.	Unknown	3-5 hr	Unknown

Action

Chemical effect: A nonnucleoside, reverse transcriptase inhibitor that inhibits the transcription of HIV-1 RNA to DNA, a critical step in the viral replication process.

Therapeutic effect: Lowers amount of HIV in the blood (viral load) and increases CD4 lymphocytes.

Available forms

Capsules: 50 mg, 100 mg, 200 mg
Tablets: 600 mg

NURSING PROCESS

▓ Assessment

• Monitor liver function test results in patients with history of hepatitis B or C and in those taking ritonavir.
• Monitor cholesterol levels.
• Children may be more prone to adverse reactions, especially diarrhea, nausea, vomiting, and rash.
• Evaluate patient's and family's knowledge of drug therapy.

⊞ Nursing diagnoses

• Risk for infection related to patient's underlying condition
• Risk for impaired skin integrity related to potential adverse effects of drug
• Deficient knowledge related to drug therapy

▷ Planning and implementation

• Use drug with other antiretrovirals because resistant viruses emerge rapidly when used alone. Don't use as monotherapy or add on as a single drug to a failing regimen.
• Using drug with ritonavir may cause a higher occurrence of adverse effects (such as dizziness, nausea, paresthesia, and elevated liver enzyme levels).
• Give drug on an empty stomach, preferably at bedtime.
• Pregnancy must be ruled out before starting therapy in women of child-bearing age.
• Give drug h.s. to decrease noticeable CNS adverse effects.

Patient teaching

• Instruct patient to take drug on an empty stomach, preferably at bedtime, and to take it with water, juice, milk, or soda.
• Inform patient about need for scheduled blood tests to monitor liver function and cholesterol levels.
• Tell patient to use reliable method of barrier contraception in addition to hormonal contraceptives and to notify prescriber immediately if pregnancy is suspected.
• Inform patient that drug doesn't cure HIV infection and that it won't affect the complications of HIV. Explain that it doesn't reduce the risk of HIV transmission through sexual contact or blood contamination.
• Instruct patient to take drug at same time daily and always with other antiretrovirals.
• Tell patient to take drug exactly as prescribed and not to stop without medical approval.
• Inform patient that rash is most common adverse effect. Tell patient to report it, or any other adverse effects, immediately; rash may be serious in rare cases.
• Instruct patient to report use of other medications.
• Advise patient that dizziness, difficulty sleeping or concentrating, drowsiness, or unusual dreams may occur the first few days of therapy. Reassure patient that these symptoms typically resolve after 2 to 4 weeks and that it may help to take drug h.s.
• Tell patient to avoid alcoholic beverages, driving, or operating machinery until drug's effects are known.

☑ Evaluation

• Patient is free from opportunistic infections.
• Patient's skin integrity is maintained.
• Patient and family state understanding of drug therapy.

eflornithine hydrochloride
(ee-FLOR-ni-theen high-droh-KLOR-ighd)
Vaniqa

Pharmacologic class: ornithine decarboxylase (ODC) inhibitor
Therapeutic class: hair growth retardant
Pregnancy risk category: C

Indications and dosages

▶ **To reduce unwanted facial hair.** *Women and girls age 12 and older:* Apply a thin layer to affected areas of the face and adjacent areas under chin and rub in thoroughly twice daily, at least 8 hours apart.

Contraindications and precautions

• Contraindicated in patients hypersensitive to drug or any of its ingredients.

❀ **Lifespan:** In breast-feeding women, use cautiously because it's unknown whether drug appears in breast milk. In girls younger than age 12, drug is contraindicated.

Adverse reactions

CNS: headache, dizziness, asthenia, vertigo, numbness.
CV: facial edema.
GI: dyspepsia, anorexia, nausea.
Skin: *acne, pseudofolliculitis barbae,* dry skin, pruritus, erythema, skin irritation, rash, alopecia, folliculitis, ingrown hair, bleeding, cheilitis, contact dermatitis, swollen lips, herpes simplex, rosacea, stinging, tingling, or burning sensation.

Interactions

None reported.

Effects on lab test results

• May increase ALT and AST levels.

Pharmacokinetics

Absorption: Less than 1% of the radioactive dose is absorbed.
Distribution: Reaches steady state in 4 days with twice-daily application.
Metabolism: None.
Excretion: Unchanged in urine. *Half-life:* About 8 hours.

Route	Onset	Peak	Duration
Topical	Unknown	8 hr	Unknown

Action

Chemical effect: Thought to irreversibly inhibit skin ODC activity. ODC is an enzyme that synthesizes polyamines.
Therapeutic effect: Decreases facial hair growth rate.

Available forms

Cream: 13.9%

✍ Assessment

• Assess patient's affected areas before and during treatment.
• Be alert for any adverse skin reactions.

⊕ Nursing diagnoses

• Disturbed body image related to unwanted facial hair
• Impaired skin integrity related to drug-induced adverse skin reactions

▶ Planning and implementation

🚫 **ALERT:** Drug reduces unwanted facial hair in women only. Apply only to affected areas on the face and chin.
• If adverse effects become bothersome, instruct patient to limit use to once a day. If side effects persist, tell patient to consult prescriber.
• Store at room temperature.
Patient teaching
• Tell patient to apply cream to face and chin only.
• Instruct patient to apply in a thin layer to affected areas twice daily, at least 8 hours apart. Avoid washing treated area for at least 4 hours.
• If skin irritation or intolerance develops, tell patient to temporarily reduce the frequency of application to once a day. If irritation continues, tell her to stop using drug.
• Advise patient that drug isn't a depilatory, but rather is believed to retard hair growth. She will likely need to continue using a hair-removal method with drug. Tell her not to apply cream within 5 minutes of other hair-removal method.
• Tell patient that improvement may be seen in as little as 4 to 8 weeks of initial treatment. The condition may return to pretreatment levels 8 weeks after stopping treatment.

☑ Evaluation

• Patient's rate of facial hair growth decreases and skin improves in response to drug therapy.
• Patient doesn't suffer any adverse reactions from drug therapy.

---

eletriptan hydrobromide

(el-eh-TRIP-tan high-dro-BRO-mighd)

Relpax

Pharmacologic class: serotonin 5-HT₁ receptor agonist
Therapeutic class: antimigraine drug
Pregnancy risk category: C

Indications and dosages

▶ **Acute migraine with or without aura.**
Adults: 20 to 40 mg P.O. at the first migraine symptom. If headache recurs after initial relief, repeat dose at least 2 hours later to a maximum of 80 mg daily.

Contraindications and precautions

• Contraindicated in patients hypersensitive to drug or its components and in those with severe hepatic impairment; ischemic heart disease, such as angina pectoris, a history of MI, or silent ischemia; coronary artery vasospasm, including Prinzmetal's variant angina; and other CV conditions. Also contraindicated in patients with cerebrovascular disorders, such as CVA or transient ischemic attack; peripheral vascular disease, including ischemic bowel disease; uncontrolled hypertension; or hemiplegic or basilar migraine.
• Avoid use within 24 hours of another 5-HT₁ agonist or an ergotamine-containing or ergot-type drug.
🔺 **Lifespan:** In pregnant women, use drug only if potential benefit justifies risk to the fetus. In breast-feeding women, use cautiously; drug appears in breast milk. In children, safety and effectiveness haven't been established. In elderly patients, use cautiously because they may have 15% lower drug clearance, the half-life of the drug is prolonged to about 6 hours, and these patients may develop higher blood pressure than younger patients.

Adverse reactions

CNS: *asthenia,* dizziness, headache, hypertonia, hypesthesia, pain, paresthesia, somnolence, vertigo.
CV: chest tightness, pain, and pressure; flushing; palpitations.
GI: abdominal pain, discomfort, or cramps; dry mouth; dyspepsia; dysphagia; nausea.

Musculoskeletal: back pain.
Respiratory: pharyngitis.
Skin: increased sweating.
Other: chills.

Interactions

Drug-drug. *CYP 3A4 inhibitors, such as clarithromycin, itraconazole, ketoconazole, nefazodone, nelfinavir, ritonavir, and troleandomycin:* Decreases eletriptan metabolism. Avoid use within 72 hours of these drugs.
Ergotamine-containing or ergot-type drugs (such as dihydroergotamine or methysergide), other 5-HT₁ agonists: May prolong vasospastic reactions. Avoid use within 24 hours of these drugs.
Propranolol: Increases bioavailability of eletriptan. No dosage adjustment is needed.

Effects on lab test results

None reported.

Pharmacokinetics

Absorption: Oral bioavailability is 50%. Drug level peaks in 1.5 to 2 hours.
Distribution: About 85% protein bound.
Metabolism: Primarily by the CYP 3A4 enzyme. The metabolite of eletriptan is active but without therapeutic effect.
Excretion: Clearance is 10% renal and 90% nonrenal. *Half-life:* About 4 hours.

Route	Onset	Peak	Duration
P.O.	½ hr	1½-2 hr	Unknown

Action

Chemical effect: Binds to 5-HT₁ receptors and may constrict intracranial blood vessels and inhibit proinflammatory neuropeptide release.
Therapeutic effect: Relieves migraine symptoms.

Available forms

Tablets: 20 mg, 40 mg

NURSING PROCESS

📝 **Assessment**
• Obtain history of patient's underlying condition before therapy.
• Assess patient for medical history or risk factors for liver disease, heart disease, cerebrovas-

cular disease, peripheral vascular disease, ischemic bowel, or uncontrolled hypertension.
• Be alert for adverse reactions.
• Evaluate patient's and family's knowledge of drug therapy.

🔚 Nursing diagnoses
• Recurrent acute pain related to migraine headaches
• Risk for injury related to adverse reactions
• Deficient knowledge related to drug therapy

⏩ Planning and implementation
• Drug isn't intended for migraine prevention. Use only in patients with a clear diagnosis of migraine. If the first use produces no response, reconsider diagnosis. A second dose will probably not be effective if the first dose causes no response.
• The safety of treating more than three migraines in 30 days hasn't been established.
ⓧ **ALERT:** Serious cardiac events, including acute MI, arrhythmias, and death, occur rarely within a few hours after use.
• Don't use in patients with risk factors for coronary artery disease (hypertension, hypercholesterolemia, smoking, obesity, diabetes, strong family history of coronary artery disease), in postmenopausal women, or in men older than age 40, unless evaluation proves that patient is reasonably free of underlying CV disease. If drug is used in these patients, give the first dose under medical supervision.
• Ophthalmologic effects may occur with long-term use.
Patient teaching
• Instruct patient to take dose at the first sign of a migraine headache. If the headache returns after the first dose, he may take a second dose after 2 hours. Caution patient not to take more than 80 mg in 24 hours.
• Warn patient to avoid driving and operating machinery if he feels dizzy or fatigued after taking drug.
• Tell patient to immediately report pain, tightness, heaviness, or pressure in the chest, throat, neck, or jaw.

☑ Evaluation
• Patient experiences relief from migraine headache.
• Patient has no signs of adverse reaction to the drug.

• Patient and family state understanding of drug therapy and conditions which are contraindications for use of this drug.

emtricitabine
(em-trih-SIGH-tah-been)
Emtriva

Pharmacologic class: nucleoside reverse transcriptase inhibitor
Therapeutic class: antiretroviral
Pregnancy risk category: B

Indications and dosages
▶ **HIV-1 infection.** *Adults:* 200 mg P.O. daily with other antiretrovirals.
⬛ **Adjust-a-dose:** If baseline creatinine clearance is 30 to 49 ml/minute, give 200 mg q 48 hours; if creatinine clearance is 15 to 29 ml/minute, give 200 mg q 72 hours; if clearance is less than 15 ml/minute (including patients requiring dialysis), give 200 mg q 96 hours. For patients on hemodialysis, if dosing on day of dialysis, give dose after dialysis.

Contraindications and precautions
• Contraindicated in patients hypersensitive to drug or any of its components.
• Use cautiously in patients with renal impairment. Reduce dose in these patients.
• Drug isn't indicated for treatment of chronic hepatitis B virus (HBV) infection, and the safety and effectiveness of the drug has not been established in patients infected with HBV and HIV.
⚘ **Lifespan:** In pregnant women, use cautiously; there are no adequate and well-controlled studies in pregnant women. Mothers should avoid breast-feeding to prevent transmitting HIV to infants. In children, safety and effectiveness haven't been established.

Adverse reactions
CNS: *headache, asthenia,* nightmares, depression, insomnia, peripheral neuropathy, neuritis, paresthesia.
EENT: *rhinitis.*
GI: *diarrhea, nausea,* abdominal pain, dyspepsia, vomiting.
Hepatic: *severe hepatomegaly steatosis.*
Metabolic: *lactic acidosis.*

Musculoskeletal: arthralgia, myalgia.
Respiratory: *cough.*
Skin: *rash (skin discoloration, maculopapular rash, pruritus, urticarial and purpuric lesions, vesiculobullous rash).*

Interactions

None reported.

Effects on lab test results

• May increase ALT, AST, bilirubin, triglyceride, amylase, lipase, creatine kinase, and glucose levels.

Pharmacokinetics

Absorption: Rapid.
Distribution: At peak level, the mean plasma-to-blood ratio is approximately 1 and the mean semen-to-plasma ratio is about 4.
Metabolism: Not metabolized by CYP enzymes. Less than 15% undergoes oxidation and glucuronidation by the liver.
Excretion: Primarily in urine. *Half-life:* About 10 hours.

Route	Onset	Peak	Duration
P.O.	Unknown	1-2 hr	Unknown

Action

Chemical effect: Inhibits the activity of HIV-1 reverse transcriptase by competing with a natural substrate and by being incorporated into new viral DNA chains, which results in their destruction.
Therapeutic effect: Helps block HIV replication.

Available forms

Capsule: 200 mg

NURSING PROCESS

▣ Assessment

• Monitor liver and renal function tests.
• Test all HIV-positive patients for chronic HBV infection before starting therapy.
• In patients infected with both HBV and HIV, exacerbations of hepatitis B may occur after stopping drug. Closely monitor these patients for at least several months after stopping treatment.
• Evaluate patient's and family's knowledge of drug therapy.

▣ Nursing diagnoses

• Risk for infection related to patient's underlying condition
• Risk for disturbed body image related to redistribution of body fat due to antiretroviral therapy
• Deficient knowledge related to drug therapy

▣ Planning and implementation

• If patient develops symptoms of lactic acidosis or pronounced hepatotoxicity, stop drug.
• Redistribution or accumulation of body fat, including central obesity, dorsocervical fat enlargement (buffalo hump), peripheral wasting, facial wasting, breast enlargement, and cushingoid appearance may occur.
• The effects of higher doses aren't known. Hemodialysis treatment removes approximately 30% of the dose over a 3-hour dialysis period starting within 1½ hours of treatment.
Patient teaching
• Tell patient that drug is not a cure for HIV infection, and it does not reduce the risk of transmitting HIV to others through sexual contact or blood contamination.
• Tell patient that drug has to be taken for life.
• Stress the importance of compliance and planning compliance strategies in advance.
• Inform patient of potential adverse reactions, including lactic acidosis, hepatotoxicity, and the redistribution or accumulation of body fat.
• Tell patient to contact prescriber immediately if she suspects she is pregnant.

▣ Evaluation

• Patient remains free of opportunistic infection.
• Patient experiences no adverse drug effects.
• Patient and family state understanding of drug therapy.

enalaprilat
(eh-NAH-leh-prel-at)

enalapril maleate
Amprace†, Renitec†, Vasotec

Pharmacologic class: ACE inhibitor
Therapeutic class: antihypertensive
Pregnancy risk category: C (D in second and third trimesters)

Indications and dosages

▶ **Hypertension.** *Adults:* For patient not taking a diuretic, initially 5 mg P.O. once daily; adjust according to response. Usual dosage range is 10 to 40 mg daily as single dose or two divided doses. Or, 1.25 mg I.V. over 5 minutes q 6 hours. For patient taking a diuretic, initially 2.5 mg P.O. once daily. Or, 0.625 mg I.V. over 5 minutes, repeat in 1 hour if needed, followed by 1.25 mg I.V. q 6 hours.

▶ **To convert from I.V. to P.O. therapy.** *Adults:* Initially, 5 mg P.O. once daily; if patient was receiving 0.625 mg I.V., then 2.5 mg P.O. once daily. Adjust dosage to response.

▶ **To convert from P.O. to I.V. therapy.** *Adults:* 1.25 mg I.V. over 5 minutes q 6 hours. Higher amounts haven't shown greater effectiveness.

▶ **Heart failure.** *Adults:* Initially, 2.5 mg P.O. once daily. Increase dosage after a few days or weeks according to response. Recommended range is 2.5 to 20 mg twice daily.

▶ **Asymptomatic left ventricular dysfunction.** *Adults:* 2.5 mg P.O. b.i.d., adjust as tolerated to target of 20 mg P.O. daily in divided doses.

◨ **Adjust-a-dose:** In patients with renal insufficiency or hyponatremia, start at 2.5 mg P.O. daily; adjust slowly.

▼ I.V. administration

• Compatible solutions include D_5W, normal saline solution injection, dextrose 5% in lactated Ringer's injection, and D_5W in normal saline solution injection.

• Inject drug slowly over at least 5 minutes, or dilute in 50 ml of compatible solution and infuse over 15 minutes.

Contraindications and precautions

• Contraindicated in patients hypersensitive to drug and those with history of angioedema from previous treatment with ACE inhibitor.

• Use cautiously in patients with renal impairment, especially those with bilateral renal artery stenosis or unilateral renal artery stenosis in a solitary functioning kidney.

⚖ Lifespan: In pregnant women, use cautiously and only when absolutely needed because fetal harm may occur. In breast-feeding women and in children, safety hasn't been established.

Adverse reactions

CNS: *headache, dizziness, fatigue,* vertigo, asthenia, syncope.
CV: *hypotension,* chest pain.
GI: diarrhea, nausea, abdominal pain, vomiting.
GU: decreased renal function (in patients with bilateral renal artery stenosis or heart failure).
Hematologic: *neutropenia, thrombocytopenia, agranulocytosis.*
Metabolic: *hyperkalemia.*
Respiratory: *dry, persistent, tickling, nonproductive cough;* dyspnea.
Skin: rash.
Other: *angioedema.*

Interactions

Drug-drug. *Diuretics:* May cause excessive reduction of blood pressure. Monitor patient.
Insulin, oral antidiabetics: May increase risk of hypoglycemia, especially at start of enalapril therapy. Monitor patient and glucose levels closely.
Lithium: May increase risk of lithium toxicity. Monitor lithium levels.
NSAIDs: May reduce antihypertensive effect. Monitor blood pressure.
Potassium supplements, potassium-sparing diuretics: May increase risk of hyperkalemia. Avoid these drugs unless hypokalemic blood levels are confirmed.
Drug-herb. *Licorice:* May cause sodium retention and increase blood pressure, interfering with therapeutic effects of ACE inhibitors. Discourage licorice intake during drug therapy.
Drug-lifestyle. *Alcohol use:* May produce additive hypotensive effect. Discourage using together.
Sun exposure: Photosensitivity reaction may occur. Urge patient to avoid unprotected or prolonged sun exposure.

Effects on lab test results

• May increase ALT, AST, bilirubin, BUN, creatinine, and potassium levels. May decrease sodium level.
• May decrease hemoglobin, hematocrit, and neutrophil, granulocyte, and platelet counts.

Pharmacokinetics

Absorption: About 60% of P.O. dose absorbed from GI tract.
Distribution: Unknown.

Metabolism: Metabolized extensively to active metabolite.
Excretion: About 94% in urine and feces as enalaprilat and enalapril. *Half-life:* 12 hours.

Route	Onset	Peak	Duration
P.O.	1 hr	4-6 hr	24 hr
I.V.	15 min	1-4 hr	6 hr

Action

Chemical effect: Unknown; inhibits ACE, which prevents conversion of angiotensin I to angiotensin II, a potent vasoconstrictor. Reduced formation of angiotensin II decreases peripheral arterial resistance, thus decreasing aldosterone secretion.
Therapeutic effect: Lowers blood pressure.

Available forms

Injection: 1.25 mg/ml
Tablets: 2.5 mg, 5 mg, 10 mg, 20 mg

NURSING PROCESS

▓ Assessment
• Obtain history of patient's blood pressure before therapy and reassess regularly.
• Monitor CBC with differential counts before therapy, every 2 weeks for first 3 months of therapy, and periodically thereafter.
• Monitor potassium intake and potassium level.
• Be alert for adverse reactions and drug interactions.
• Evaluate patient's and family's knowledge of drug therapy.

⊕ Nursing diagnoses
• Risk for injury related to presence of hypertension
• Risk for infection related to drug-induced adverse hematologic reactions
• Deficient knowledge related to drug therapy

▷ Planning and implementation
• If patient has hypotension after first dose, adjust dose as long as patient is under medical supervision.
• If CBC becomes abnormal or if evidence of infection arises, notify prescriber immediately.
• Angioedema (including laryngeal edema) may occur, especially after first dose. If it occurs, notify prescriber and stop treatment immediately.

Institute appropriate therapy (epinephrine solution 1:1,000 [0.3 to 0.5 ml] S.C.), and take measures to ensure patent airway.
Patient teaching
• Advise patient to report evidence of angioedema, such as breathing difficulty and swelling of face, eyes, lips, or tongue.
• Instruct patient to report signs of infection, such as fever and sore throat.
• Advise patient that light-headedness can occur, especially during first few days of therapy. Tell patient to rise slowly to minimize this effect and to report symptoms to prescriber. If patient experiences syncope, tell him to stop taking drug and to call prescriber immediately.
• Tell patient to use caution in hot weather and during exercise. Inadequate fluid intake, vomiting, diarrhea, and excessive perspiration can lead to light-headedness and syncope.
• Advise patient to avoid sodium substitutes; these products may contain potassium, which can cause hyperkalemia.
• Tell patient to notify prescriber if pregnancy occurs. Drug will need to be stopped.

☑ Evaluation
• Patient's blood pressure becomes normal.
• Patient's CBC remains normal throughout therapy.
• Patient and family state understanding of drug therapy.

enfuvirtide
(ehn-FOO-ver-tighd)
Fuzeon

Pharmacologic class: HIV-1/CD4 fusion inhibitor
Therapeutic class: anti-HIV drug, antiviral
Pregnancy risk category: B

Indications and dosages

▶ **HIV-1 infection with other antiretrovirals, in patients with continued HIV-1 replication despite antiretroviral therapy.** *Adults:* 90 mg/ml S.C. b.i.d., injected into the upper arm, anterior thigh, or abdomen.
Children ages 6 to 16: 2 mg/kg S.C. b.i.d.; maximum 90 mg per dose.

Contraindications and precautions

• Contraindicated in patients hypersensitive to drug.

♨ **Lifespan:** In pregnant women, use only if clearly needed. Breast-feeding women should stop breast-feeding to prevent transmitting HIV to infants. In children younger than age 6, safety and effectiveness haven't been established.

Adverse reactions

CNS: anxiety, asthenia, depression, *insomnia*, peripheral neuropathy.
EENT: conjunctivitis, sinusitis, taste disturbance.
GI: abdominal pain, constipation, *diarrhea, nausea, pancreatitis.*
Hematologic: lymphadenopathy.
Metabolic: anorexia, weight decrease.
Musculoskeletal: myalgia.
Respiratory: *bacterial pneumonia,* cough.
Skin: pruritus, skin papilloma, *ecchymosis.*
Other: herpes simplex, influenza, flulike illness, *injection site reactions.*

Interactions

None reported.

Effects on lab test results

• May increase triglyceride, amylase, lipase, ALT, AST, CPK, and GGT levels.
• May decrease hemoglobin, hematocrit, and eosinophil count.

Pharmacokinetics

Absorption: Absorbed well after S.C. administration into arm, thigh, or abdomen.
Distribution: 92% protein bound.
Metabolism: May undergo catabolism to its constituent amino acids; hydrolyzed to a metabolite detectable in plasma.
Excretion: Unknown. *Half-life:* 4 hours.

Route	Onset	Peak	Duration
S.C.	Unknown	4-8 hr	Unknown

Action

Chemical effect: Interferes with entry of HIV-1 into cells by inhibiting fusion of HIV-1 to cell membranes.
Therapeutic effect: Controls symptoms of HIV infection.

Available forms

Injection: 108-mg single-use vials (90 mg/1 ml after reconstitution)

NURSING PROCESS

⚕ Assessment
• Confirm that patient is infected with HIV. Use drug only in patients who are HIV-positive.
• Assess patient for evidence of bacterial pneumonia.
• Observe injection site for local reaction.
• Evaluate patient's and family's knowledge of drug therapy.

⊞ Nursing diagnoses
• Risk for infection related to underlying condition
• Deficient knowledge related to drug therapy

⊳ Planning and implementation
• Reconstitute vial with 1.1 ml sterile water for injection. Tap vial for 10 seconds and then gently roll it between hands to prevent foaming. Let drug stand for up to 45 minutes to ensure reconstitution. Or, gently roll vial between hands until product is completely dissolved. Then draw up correct dose and inject drug.
• If drug isn't used immediately after reconstitution, refrigerate in original vial and use within 24 hours. Don't inject drug until it's at room temperature.
• Store unreconstituted vials at room temperature.
• Vial is for single use; discard unused portion.
⊛ ALERT: Drug is available only through a progressive distribution program. Information may be obtained by calling 866-694-6670.
• Rotate injection sites. Don't inject into the same site for two consecutive doses, and don't inject into moles, scar tissue, bruises, or the navel.
• Injection site reactions (pain, discomfort, induration, erythema, pruritus, nodules, cysts, ecchymosis) are common and may require analgesics or rest.
⊛ ALERT: Monitor patient closely for bacterial pneumonia. Patients at high risk include those with a low initial CD4 count or high initial viral load, those who use I.V. drugs or smoke, and those with history of lung disease.
• Hypersensitivity may occur with the first dose or later doses. If symptoms occur, stop drug.

- Register pregnant women in the Antiretroviral Pregnancy Registry by phoning 1-800-258-4263.

Patient teaching

- Teach patient how to prepare and give drug and how to safely dispose of used needles and syringes.
- Tell patient to rotate injection sites and to watch for cellulitis or local infection.
- Urge patient to immediately report evidence of pneumonia, such as cough with fever, rapid breathing, or shortness of breath.
- Tell patient to stop taking drug and seek medical attention if evidence of hypersensitivity develops, such as rash, fever, nausea, vomiting, chills, rigors, and hypotension.
- Inform patient that drug doesn't cure HIV infection and that it must be taken with other antiretrovirals.
- Tell patient to inform prescriber if she's pregnant, plans to become pregnant, or is breastfeeding while taking this drug.
- Tell patient that drug may impair the ability to drive or operate machinery.

☑ Evaluation

- Patient is free from opportunistic infections.
- Patient and family state understanding of drug therapy.

enoxaparin sodium
(eh-NOKS-uh-pah-rin SOH-dee-um)
Lovenox

Pharmacologic class: low–molecular-weight heparin derivative
Therapeutic class: anticoagulant
Pregnancy risk category: B

Indications and dosages

▶ **Prevention of deep vein thrombosis (DVT), which may lead to pulmonary embolism, following hip or knee replacement surgery.** *Adults:* 30 mg S.C. q 12 hours for 7 to 10 days. Initial dose given 12 to 24 hours after surgery, provided hemostasis has been established. Or, for hip replacement surgery, 40 mg S.C. once daily given initially 12 hours before surgery. May continue with 40 mg S.C. once daily or 30 mg S.C. q 12 hours for 3 weeks.

▶ **Prevention of DVT, which may lead to pulmonary embolism, following abdominal surgery.** *Adults:* 40 mg S.C. once daily for 7 to 10 days with initial dose given 2 hours before surgery.

▶ **Prevention of ischemic complications of unstable angina and non–Q-wave MI.** *Adults:* 1 mg/kg S.C. q 12 hours for 2 to 8 days together with oral aspirin therapy (100 to 325 mg/day).

▶ **Inpatient with acute DVT with and without pulmonary embolism.** *Adults:* 1 mg/kg S.C. q 12 hours. Or, 1.5 mg/kg S.C. once daily (at same time every day) for 5 to 7 days until therapeutic oral anticoagulant effect (INR of 2 to 3) is achieved. Warfarin therapy usually starts within 72 hours of enoxaparin injection.

▶ **Outpatient with acute DVT without pulmonary embolism.** *Adults:* 1 mg/kg S.C. q 12 hours for 5 to 7 days until INR of 2 to 3 is achieved. Warfarin sodium therapy is usually started within 72 hours of enoxaparin injection.

▶ **Patients during acute illness who are at risk of embolism because of decreased mobility.** *Adults:* 40 mg S.C. once daily for 6 to 11 days. Up to 14 days may be tolerated.

Contraindications and precautions

- Contraindicated in patients hypersensitive to drug, heparin, or pork products; in those with active major bleeding or thrombocytopenia; and in those who demonstrate antiplatelet antibodies in presence of drug.
- Not recommended for thromboprophylaxis in patients with prosthetic heart valves.
- Use cautiously in patients with postoperative indwelling epidural catheters or patients who have had epidural or spinal anesthesia. Epidural and spinal hematomas may result in long-term or permanent paralysis. Also use cautiously in patients with history of heparin-induced thrombocytopenia, in patients with conditions that put them at increased risk for hemorrhage (such as bacterial endocarditis), and in patients with congenital or acquired bleeding disorders, ulcer disease, angiodysplastic GI disease, hemorrhagic CVA, or recent spinal, eye, or brain surgery.
- ☀ Lifespan: In pregnant women, use only if clearly needed. In breast-feeding women, use cautiously. In children, safety hasn't been established.

Adverse reactions

CNS: fever, pain, confusion, *neurologic injury* (when used with spinal or epidural puncture).
CV: edema, peripheral edema, *CV toxicity.*
GI: nausea.
Hematologic: hypochromic anemia, *thrombocytopenia, hemorrhage, bleeding complications.*
Skin: irritation, pain, hematoma, or erythema at injection site; *rash; urticaria,* ecchymosis.
Other: *angioedema.*

Interactions

Drug-drug. *Anticoagulants, antiplatelet drugs, NSAIDs:* May increase risk of bleeding. Don't use together.
Plicamycin, valproic acid: May cause hypoprothrombinemia and inhibit platelet aggregation. Monitor patient closely.

Effects on lab test results

• May increase ALT and AST levels.
• May decrease hemoglobin, hematocrit, and platelet count.

Pharmacokinetics

Absorption: Unknown.
Distribution: Unknown.
Metabolism: Unknown.
Excretion: Unknown. *Half-life:* 4½ hours.

Route	Onset	Peak	Duration
S.C.	Unknown	3-5 hr	< 24 hr

Action

Chemical effect: Accelerates formation of antithrombin IIIB–thrombin complex and deactivates thrombin, preventing conversion of fibrinogen to fibrin. Enoxaparin has higher antifactor Xa–antifactor IIa activity ratio.
Therapeutic effect: Prevents pulmonary embolism and DVT.

Available forms

Ampules: 30 mg/0.3 ml
Syringes (prefilled): 30 mg/0.3 ml, 40 mg/0.4 ml
Syringes (graduated prefilled): 60 mg/0.6 ml, 80 mg/0.8 ml, 100 mg/ml, 120 mg/0.8 ml, 150 mg/ml
Vial (multi-dose): 300 mg/3 ml (contains 15 mg/ml of benzyl alcohol)

☞ Assessment

• Obtain history of patient's coagulation parameters before therapy.
• Monitor effectiveness by evaluating patient for signs and symptoms of pulmonary embolism or DVT.
• Monitor platelet counts regularly. Patient with normal coagulation doesn't require regular monitoring of PT, INR, and PTT.
• Frequently monitor neurological status in patients who have had spinal or epidural anesthesia. If abnormalities are discovered, alert prescriber immediately.
• Be alert for adverse reactions and drug interactions.
• Evaluate patient's and family's knowledge of drug therapy.

⊞ Nursing diagnoses

• Risk for injury related to risk for pulmonary embolism or DVT after knee or hip replacement surgery
• Ineffective protection related to drug-induced bleeding complications
• Deficient knowledge related to drug therapy

▶ Planning and implementation

⊛ **ALERT:** To avoid drug loss, don't expel air bubble from 30- or 40-mg prefilled syringes.
⊛ **ALERT:** Never give drug I.M.
• Don't massage after S.C. injection. Rotate sites among the left and right enterolateral and the left and right posterolateral abdominal walls.
⊛ **ALERT:** Drug can't be used interchangeably (unit for unit) with unfractionated heparin or other low–molecular-weight heparins.
• Avoid excessive I.M. injections of other drugs to prevent or minimize hematomas. If possible, don't give I.M. injections when patient is anticoagulated.
• To treat severe overdose, give protamine sulfate (a heparin antagonist) by slow I.V. infusion at concentration of 1% to equal dosage of enoxaparin injected.
Patient teaching
• Instruct patient and family to watch for signs of bleeding and notify prescriber immediately.
• Tell patient to avoid OTC drugs that contain aspirin or other salicylates.

Reactions may be *common,* uncommon, *life-threatening,* or **COMMON AND LIFE-THREATENING.**

- Tell pregnant women and women of child-bearing potential about the potential hazard to fetus and mother if drug is used during pregnancy.

☑ **Evaluation**

- Patient doesn't develop pulmonary embolism or DVT.
- Patient has no bleeding complications during therapy.
- Patient and family state understanding of drug therapy.

entacapone
(en-TAK-uh-pohn)
Comtan

Pharmacologic class: COMT inhibitor
Therapeutic class: antiparkinsonian
Pregnancy risk category: C

Indications and dosages

▶ **Adjunct to levodopa and carbidopa in idiopathic Parkinson's disease in patients who experience end-of-dose wearing-off.**
Adults: 200 mg P.O. with each dose of levodopa-carbidopa to maximum of eight times daily. Maximum dosage is 1,600 mg daily. Reducing daily levodopa dose or extending the interval between doses may be needed to optimize patient's response.

Contraindications and precautions

- Contraindicated in patients hypersensitive to drug.
- Use cautiously in patients with hepatic impairment, biliary obstruction, or orthostatic hypotension.
⚘ **Lifespan:** In pregnant women, use only if potential benefits justify risk to fetus. In breast-feeding women, use cautiously.

Adverse reactions

CNS: *dyskinesia, hyperkinesia,* hypokinesia, dizziness, anxiety, somnolence, agitation, fatigue, asthenia, hallucinations.
GI: *nausea, diarrhea,* abdominal pain, constipation, vomiting, dry mouth, dyspepsia, flatulence, gastritis, taste perversion.
GU: *urine discoloration.*

Hematologic: purpura.
Musculoskeletal: back pain.
Respiratory: dyspnea.
Skin: sweating.
Other: bacterial infection.

Interactions

Drug-drug. *Ampicillin, chloramphenicol, cholestyramine, erythromycin, probenecid, rifampin:* May block biliary excretion, resulting in higher levels of entacapone. Use cautiously.
CNS depressants: May have additive effects. Use cautiously.
Drugs metabolized by COMT (bitolterol, dobutamine, dopamine, epinephrine, isoetharine, isoproterenol, norepinephrine): May cause higher levels of these drugs, resulting in increased heart rate, changes in blood pressure, or possibly arrhythmias. Use cautiously.
Nonselective MAO inhibitors (such as phenelzine, tranylcypromine): May inhibit normal catecholamine metabolism. Don't use together.
Drug-lifestyle. *Alcohol use:* May cause additive CNS effects. Discourage using together.

Effects on lab test results

None reported.

Pharmacokinetics

Absorption: Rapid, with level peaking in about 1 hour. Food doesn't affect absorption.
Distribution: About 98% protein-bound, mainly to albumin, and doesn't distribute widely into tissues.
Metabolism: Almost completely metabolized by glucuronidation before elimination.
Excretion: About 10% in urine; the remainder in bile and feces. *Half-life:* 0.4 to 0.7 hours for first phase and 2.4 hours for second phase.

Route	Onset	Peak	Duration
P.O.	1 hr	1 hr	6 hr

Action

Chemical effect: Drug is a reversible inhibitor of peripheral COMT, which is responsible for elimination of various catecholamines, including dopamine. Blocking this pathway when giving levodopa-carbidopa may result in higher levels of levodopa, thereby allowing greater dopaminergic stimulation in the CNS and leading to a greater effect on parkinsonian symptoms.

Therapeutic effect: Controls idiopathic Parkinson's disease signs and symptoms.

Available forms

Tablets: 200 mg

NURSING PROCESS

⚡ Assessment
● Assess hepatic and biliary function before starting therapy.
● Monitor blood pressure closely. Watch for orthostatic hypotension.
● Monitor patient for hallucinations.
● Evaluate patient's and family's knowledge of drug therapy.

⊞ Nursing diagnoses
● Impaired physical mobility related to presence of parkinsonism
● Disturbed thought processes related to drug-induced adverse reactions
● Deficient knowledge related to drug therapy

▷ Planning and implementation
● Use with levodopa-carbidopa; not effective when drug is given as monotherapy.
● Drug may be given with immediate- or sustained-release levodopa-carbidopa and may be taken with or without food.
● Lower levodopa-carbidopa dose or increase dosing interval to avoid adverse effects.
● Drug may cause or worsen dyskinesia despite reduction of levodopa dosage.
● Watch for diarrhea. It usually begins 4 to 12 weeks after therapy starts, but may begin as early as first week or as late as many months after therapy starts.
● Rapid withdrawal or abrupt reduction in dose could lead to signs and symptoms of Parkinson's disease; it may also lead to hyperpyrexia and confusion, a symptom complex resembling neuroleptic malignant syndrome. Discontinue drug slowly and monitor patient closely. Adjust other dopaminergic treatments.
● Observe for urine discoloration.
● Rarely, rhabdomyolysis has occurred with drug use.

Patient teaching
● Instruct patient not to crush or break tablet and to take it at same time as levodopa-carbidopa.
● Warn patient to avoid hazardous activities until CNS effects of drug are known.
● Advise patient to avoid alcohol during treatment.
● Instruct patient to use caution when standing after a prolonged period of sitting or lying down because dizziness may occur. This effect is more common early in therapy.
● Warn patient that hallucinations, increased dyskinesia, nausea, and diarrhea may occur.
● Inform patient that drug may cause urine to turn brownish orange.
● Advise patient to notify prescriber if she's pregnant or breast-feeding or if she plans to become pregnant.

☑ Evaluation
● Patient exhibits improved physical mobility.
● Patient maintains normal thought process.
● Patient and family state understanding of drug therapy.

ephedrine sulfate
(eh-FED-rin SUL-fayt)
Kondon's Nasal†, Pretz-D†

Pharmacologic class: adrenergic
Therapeutic class: bronchodilator, vasopressor (parenteral form), nasal decongestant
Pregnancy risk category: C

Indications and dosages

▶ **Hypotension.** *Adults:* 25 to 50 mg I.M. or S.C., or 10 to 25 mg I.V., p.r.n., to maximum of 150 mg/24 hours.
Children: 3 mg/kg or 100 mg/m² S.C. or I.V. daily in four to six divided doses.
▶ **Bronchodilation, nasal decongestion.**
Adults and children older than age 12: 25 to 50 mg P.O. q 3 to 4 hours p.r.n. For patient use as a bronchodilator, 12.5 to 25 mg P.O. q 4 hr. Maximum, 150 mg in 24 hours. As a nasal decongestant, 0.5% solution applied topically to nasal mucosa as drops or on nasal pack. Instill no more often than q 4 hours.
Children ages 2 to 12: 2 to 3 mg/kg P.O. daily in four to six divided doses.

▼ I.V. administration

- Compatible with most common I.V. solutions.
- Give 10 to 25 mg by I.V. injection slowly; repeat in 5 to 10 minutes, if needed.

Contraindications and precautions

- Contraindicated in patients hypersensitive to drug and other sympathomimetic drugs; in those with porphyria, severe coronary artery disease, arrhythmias, angle-closure glaucoma, psychoneurosis, angina pectoris, substantial organic heart disease, or CV disease; and in those taking MAO inhibitors.
- Use cautiously in patients with hypertension, hyperthyroidism, nervous or excitable states, diabetes, or prostatic hyperplasia.

⚑ Lifespan: In pregnant women and in children and older men, use cautiously. Breastfeeding should be avoided during drug therapy.

Adverse reactions

CNS: *insomnia, nervousness,* dizziness, headache, euphoria, confusion, delirium.
CV: *palpitations,* tachycardia, hypertension, precordial pain.
EENT: dryness of nose and throat.
GI: nausea, vomiting, anorexia.
GU: urine retention, painful urination from visceral sphincter spasm.
Musculoskeletal: muscle weakness.
Skin: diaphoresis.

Interactions

Drug-drug. *Acetazolamide:* Increases ephedrine levels. Monitor patient for toxicity.
Alpha-adrenergic blockers: Doesn't counteract beta blocker effects, resulting in hypotension. Monitor blood pressure.
Antihypertensives: Decreases effects. Monitor blood pressure.
Beta blockers: Doesn't counteract alpha-adrenergic effects, resulting in hypertension. Monitor blood pressure.
Digoxin, general anesthetics (halogenated hydrocarbons): Increases risk of ventricular arrhythmias. Monitor patient closely.
Ergot alkaloids: Enhances vasoconstrictor activity. Monitor patient closely.
Guanadrel, guanethidine: Enhances pressor effects of ephedrine. Monitor patient closely.
Isocarboxazid: When given with sympathomimetics, may cause hypertensive crisis. Don't use together.

Methyldopa, reserpine: May inhibit effects of ephedrine. Use together cautiously.
Phenelzine, tranylcypromine: May cause severe headache, hypertension, fever, and hypertensive crisis. Avoid using together.
Tricyclic antidepressants: May decrease pressor response. Monitor patient's blood pressure closely.

Effects on lab test results

None reported.

Pharmacokinetics

Absorption: Rapid and complete after P.O., I.M., or S.C. administration; unknown after nasal administration.
Distribution: Widely distributed throughout body.
Metabolism: Slow, in liver.
Excretion: Unchanged in urine. Rate of excretion depends on urine pH. *Half-life:* 3 to 6 hours.

Route	Onset	Peak	Duration
P.O.	15-60 min	Unknown	3-5 hr
I.V.	≤ 5 min	Unknown	Unknown
I.M.	10-20 min	Unknown	30 min-1 hr
S.C.	Unknown	Unknown	30 min-1 hr
Intranasal	Unknown	Unknown	Unknown

Action

Chemical effect: Stimulates alpha-adrenergic and beta blocker receptors; direct- and indirect-acting sympathomimetic.
Therapeutic effect: Raises blood pressure, causes bronchodilation, and relieves nasal congestion.

Available forms

Capsules: 25 mg, 50 mg
Injection: 25 mg/ml, 50 mg/ml
Nasal solution: 0.25%†, 0.5%†, 1%†
Tablets: 30 mg†

NURSING PROCESS

▓ Assessment

- Obtain history of patient's underlying condition before therapy, and reassess regularly.
- Be alert for adverse reactions and drug interactions.

Rapid onset   *Liquid form contains alcohol.*   ♦ Canada   ◊ Australia   †OTC   ‡Off-label use

- Evaluate patient's and family's knowledge of drug therapy.

Nursing diagnoses
- Ineffective health maintenance related to underlying condition
- Risk for deficient fluid volume related to drug-induced adverse GI reactions
- Deficient knowledge related to drug therapy

Planning and implementation
- Hypoxia, hypercapnia, and acidosis, which may reduce drug effectiveness or increase adverse reactions, must be identified and corrected before or during ephedrine administration.
- Volume deficit must be corrected before giving vasopressors. This drug isn't a substitute for blood or fluid volume replenishment.
- To prevent insomnia, avoid giving within 2 hours before bedtime.
- When effectiveness decreases, notify prescriber. Effectiveness decreases after 2 to 3 weeks, as tolerance develops. Increase dosage if needed; drug isn't addictive.

Patient teaching
- Warn patient not to take OTC drugs that contain ephedrine without consulting prescriber.
- Teach patient how to instill nose drops and warn him not to exceed recommended dosage.
- Advise patient to notify prescriber if effectiveness decreases because dosage may need to be adjusted.
- Instruct patient to notify prescriber if adverse reactions occur.
- Caution patient not to perform hazardous activities if adverse CNS reactions occur.

Evaluation
- Patient exhibits improvement in underlying condition.
- Patient maintains adequate hydration throughout therapy.
- Patient and family state understanding of drug therapy.

---

epinastine hydrochloride
(eh-pin-AH-stein high-droh-KLOR-ighd)
Elestat

Pharmacologic class: histamine (H_1-receptor) antagonist and mast cell stabilizer

Therapeutic class: ophthalmic antihistamine
Pregnancy risk category: C

Indications and dosages

▶ **To prevent itching in allergic conjunctivitis.** *Adults and children age 3 and older:* Instill 1 drop into each eye twice daily. Continue treatment as long as allergen is present, even if patient has no symptoms.

Contraindications and precautions
- Contraindicated in patients hypersensitive to drug or its components.
- **Lifespan:** In pregnant or breast-feeding women, use cautiously. In children under age 3, safety and effectiveness haven't been established.

Adverse reactions

CNS: headache.
EENT: burning eyes, hyperemia, increased lymph nodes near eyes, pharyngitis, pruritus, rhinitis, sinusitis.
Respiratory: increased cough, *upper respiratory tract infection.*
Other: *infection (cold symptoms).*

Interactions

None reported.

Effects on lab test results

None reported.

Pharmacokinetics

Absorption: Immediate.
Distribution: 64% bound to plasma proteins.
Metabolism: Less than 10% of drug.
Excretion: Mainly unchanged in urine. *Half-life:* About 12 hours.

Route	Onset	Peak	Duration
Ophthalmic	Immediate	Unknown	8 hr

Action

Chemical effect: By antagonizing H_1-receptors and stabilizing mast cells, drug inhibits release of mediators from cells involved in hypersensitivity reactions.
Therapeutic effect: Temporarily prevents eye itching.

Available forms

Ophthalmic solution: 0.05% in 5-and 10-ml bottles

NURSING PROCESS

Assessment

• Drug is for ophthalmic use only. Don't inject or give orally.
• Monitor patient for infection.
• Evaluate patient's and family's knowledge of drug therapy.

Nursing diagnoses

• Ineffective health maintenance related to underlying condition
• Risk for infection related to adverse effects of drug.
• Deficient knowledge related to drug therapy

Planning and implementation

• Drug shouldn't be used for contact lens-related eye irritation.
• Preservative in drug may be absorbed by soft contact lenses. If patient wears soft lenses, have him wait at least 10 minutes after dose to insert lenses.

Patient teaching

• Teach patient proper instillation technique. To avoid contaminating the drops, warn patient not to touch the dropper tip to eyelids, skin around the eyes, or anything else.
• Caution patient not to use drops to treat contact lens-related eye irritation and not to wear contact lenses if eyes are red.
• Advise patient to report adverse reactions.
• Tell patient to keep bottle tightly closed when not in use.

Evaluation

• Patient responds well to therapy.
• Patient remains free from infection during drug therapy.
• Patient and family state understanding of drug therapy.

epinephrine (adrenaline)
(eh-pih-NEF-rin)
Adrenalin†, Bronkaid Mist†, Bronkaid Mistometer♦, Primatene Mist†

epinephrine bitartrate
AsthmaHaler Mist†, Bronitin Mist†, Bronkaid Mist Suspension†, Medihaler-Epi†, Primatene Mist Suspension†

epinephrine hydrochloride
Adrenalin Chloride†, Ana-Guard, EpiPen Auto-Injector, EpiPen Jr. Auto-Injector, Sus-Phrine

Pharmacologic class: adrenergic
Therapeutic class: bronchodilator, vasopressor, cardiac stimulant, local anesthetic, topical anti-hemorrhagic
Pregnancy risk category: C

Indications and dosages

▶ **Bronchospasm, hypersensitivity reactions, anaphylaxis.** *Adults:* 0.1 to 0.5 ml of 1:1,000 S.C. or I.M.; repeat q 10 to 15 minutes, p.r.n. Or, 0.1 to 0.25 ml of 1:1,000 (1 to 2.5 ml of commercially available 1:10,000 injection or of 1:10,000 dilution prepared by diluting 1 ml of commercially available 1:1,000 injection with 10 ml of water for injection or normal saline injection) I.V. slowly over 5 to 10 minutes.
Children: 0.01 ml (10 mcg) of 1:1,000/kg S.C.; repeat q 20 minutes to 4 hours, p.r.n. Or, 0.005 ml/kg of 1:200 of Sus-Phrine S.C.; repeat q 8 to 12 hours, p.r.n.
▶ **Hemostasis.** *Adults:* 1:50,000 to 1:1,000 applied topically.
▶ **Acute asthma attacks.** *Adults and children age 4 and older:* 160 to 250 mcg (metered aerosol), which is equivalent to one inhalation, repeat once if needed after at least 1 minute; don't give subsequent doses for at least 3 hours. Or, give 1% (1:100) solution of epinephrine or 2.25% solution of racepinephrine by hand-bulb nebulizer as one to three deep inhalations; repeat q 3 hours, p.r.n.
▶ **Prolonging local anesthetic effect.** *Adults and children:* Mix 1:500,000 to 1:50,000 with local anesthetic.

▶ **Restoring cardiac rhythm in cardiac arrest.** *Adults:* 1 mg I.V. or 2 to 2.5 mg into endotracheal tube. If no I.V. route or intratracheal route is available, give drug intracardiac. Intracardiac dose is 0.3 to 0.5 mg (1:10,000 solution). Up to 5 mg may be given, especially in patients who don't respond to usual I.V. dose. After initial I.V. administration, drug may be infused I.V. at 1 to 4 mcg/minute.
Children: 10 mcg/kg I.V., or 5 to 10 mcg (0.05 to 0.1 ml of 1:10,000)/kg intracardiac.

▽ I.V. administration

● Don't mix with alkaline solutions. Use D₅W, normal saline injection, lactated Ringer's injection, or combinations of dextrose in sodium chloride. Mix just before use.
● Discard solution after 24 hours or if solution is discolored or contains precipitate. Keep solution in light-resistant container, and don't remove before use.

Contraindications and precautions

● Contraindicated in patients with angle-closure glaucoma, shock (other than anaphylactic shock), organic brain damage, cardiac dilation, arrhythmias, coronary insufficiency, or cerebral arteriosclerosis. Also contraindicated in patients receiving general anesthesia with halogenated hydrocarbons or cyclopropane and in patients in labor (may delay second stage).
● Some commercial products contain sulfites and are contraindicated in patients with sulfite allergies except when epinephrine is being used for treatment of serious allergic reactions or in other emergency situations.
● In conjunction with local anesthetics, epinephrine is contraindicated for use in fingers, toes, ears, nose, or genitalia.
● Use cautiously in patients with long-standing bronchial asthma or emphysema who have developed degenerative heart disease and in those with hyperthyroidism, CV disease, hypertension, psychoneurosis, or diabetes.
🕮 **Lifespan:** In pregnant women not in labor and in children and elderly patients, use cautiously. In breast-feeding women, avoid breast-feeding during drug therapy.

Adverse reactions

CNS: *nervousness, tremors,* euphoria, anxiety, cold limbs, vertigo, *headache, drowsiness,* diaphoresis, disorientation, agitation, fear, weakness, *cerebral hemorrhage, CVA,* increased rigidity and tremors (in patients with Parkinson's disease).
CV: *palpitations,* widened pulse pressure, *hypertension, tachycardia,* **ventricular fibrillation,** *shock,* anginal pain, ECG changes (including decreased T-wave amplitude).
GI: *nausea,* vomiting.
Metabolic: hyperglycemia, glycosuria.
Respiratory: dyspnea.
Skin: urticaria, pain.
Other: pallor, *hemorrhage at injection site.*

Interactions

Drug-drug. *Alpha-adrenergic blockers:* May cause hypotension from unopposed beta blocker effects. Monitor blood pressure.
Antihistamines, thyroid hormones: When given with sympathomimetics, may cause severe adverse cardiac effects. Avoid giving together.
Carteolol, nadolol, penbutolol, pindolol, propranolol, timolol: May cause an initial hypertensive episode followed by bradycardia. Stop the beta blocker 3 days before anticipated epinephrine use. Monitor patient closely.
Digoxin, general anesthetics (halogenated hydrocarbons): May increase risk of ventricular arrhythmias. Monitor patient closely.
Doxapram, methylphenidate: May enhance CNS stimulation or pressor effects. Monitor patient closely.
Ergot alkaloids: May enhance vasoconstrictor activity. Monitor patient closely.
Guanadrel, guanethidine: Enhances pressor effects of epinephrine. Monitor patient closely.
Levodopa: Enhances risk of cardiac arrhythmias. Monitor patient closely.
MAO inhibitors: Increases risk of hypertensive crisis. Don't use together.
Tricyclic antidepressants: May increase the pressor response and cause arrhythmias. Use cautiously.

Effects on lab test results

● May increase BUN, glucose, and lactic acid levels.

Pharmacokinetics

Absorption: Well absorbed after S.C. or I.M. injection. Rapidly absorbed after inhalation administration.
Distribution: Distributed widely throughout body.

Metabolism: Metabolized at sympathetic nerve endings, liver, and other tissues to inactive metabolites.

Excretion: Excreted in urine, mainly as its metabolites and conjugates. *Half-life:* Unknown.

Route	Onset	Peak	Duration
I.V.	Immediate	≤ 5 min	1-4 hr
I.M.	Varies	Unknown	1-4 hr
S.C.	6-15 min	≤ 30 min	1-4 hr
Inhalation	3-5 min	Unknown	1-3 hr

Action

Chemical effect: Stimulates alpha-adrenergic and beta blocker receptors in sympathetic nervous system.

Therapeutic effect: Relaxes bronchial smooth muscle, causes cardiac stimulation, relieves allergic signs and symptoms, stops local bleeding, and decreases pain sensation.

Available forms

Aerosol inhaler: 160 mcg†, 200 mcg†, 220mcg†, 250 mcg/metered spray†
Injection: 0.01 mg/ml (1:100,000), 0.1 mg/ml (1:10,000), 0.5 mg/ml (1:2,000), 1 mg/ml (1:1,000) parenteral; 5 mg/ml (1:200) parenteral suspension
Nebulizer inhaler: 0.5%†, 1% (1:100) ◆ †, 2.25% (racepinephrine) ◊ †

NURSING PROCESS

📋 Assessment

• Obtain history of patient's underlying condition before therapy, and reassess regularly.
• When administering I.V., monitor blood pressure, heart rate, and ECG when therapy starts and frequently thereafter.
• Be alert for adverse reactions and drug interactions.
• Evaluate patient's and family's knowledge of drug therapy.

🔖 Nursing diagnoses

• Ineffective health maintenance related to underlying condition
• Decreased cardiac output related to drug-induced adverse CV effects
• Deficient knowledge related to drug therapy

▶ Planning and implementation

• Keep in mind that 1 mg of epinephrine is equal to 1 ml of 1:1,000 or 10 ml of 1:10,000.
• Epinephrine is drug of choice in emergency treatment of acute anaphylactic reactions.
• Avoid I.M. administration of parenteral suspension into buttocks. Gas gangrene may occur because epinephrine reduces oxygen tension of tissues, encouraging growth of contaminating organisms.
• Massage site after I.M. injection to counteract possible vasoconstriction. Repeated local injection can cause necrosis, resulting from vasoconstriction at injection site.
• Wait 2 minutes between bronchodilator inhalations. Always give bronchodilator first and wait 5 minutes before giving a different inhalant. Don't give patient more than 12 bronchodilator inhalations in 24 hours.
• Giving medication on time is important.
• If adverse reactions develop, notify prescriber; adjust dosage or stop the drug, as needed. Also notify prescriber if patient's pulse increases by 20% or more when drug is given.
• If blood pressure rises sharply, rapid-acting vasodilators, such as nitrites or alpha-adrenergic blockers, can be given to counteract marked pressor effect of large doses of epinephrine.
• Epinephrine is destroyed rapidly by oxidizing agents, such as iodine, chromates, nitrates, nitrites, oxygen, and salts of easily reducible metals (such as iron).

Patient teaching

• Tell patient to take drug exactly as prescribed and to take it around the clock.
• Teach patient to perform oral inhalation correctly. Give the following instructions for using metered-dose inhaler:
– Clear nasal passages and throat.
– Breathe out, expelling as much air from lungs as possible.
– Place mouthpiece well into mouth and inhale deeply as dose from inhaler is released.
– Hold breath for several seconds, remove mouthpiece, and exhale slowly.
• Tell patient to wait at least 2 minutes between inhalations.
• Tell patient who also is using corticosteroid inhaler to use bronchodilator first, then wait about 5 minutes before using corticosteroid. This allows bronchodilator to open air passages for maximum effectiveness.

Rapid onset   *Liquid form contains alcohol.   ◆ Canada   ◊ Australia   †OTC   ‡Off-label use

• Instruct patient who has acute hypersensitivity reactions, such as to bee stings, to self-inject epinephrine at home.
• Tell patient to reduce intake of foods containing caffeine, such as coffee, colas, and chocolates, when taking bronchodilator.
• Instruct patient to contact prescriber immediately if he experiences fluttering of heart, rapid beating of heart, shortness of breath, or chest pain.
• Tell patient to obtain approval from prescriber before taking OTC medicines or herbal remedies.
• Show patient how to check pulse. Instruct him to check pulse before and after using bronchodilator and to call prescriber if pulse rate increases by more than 20 beats/minute.

☑ **Evaluation**
• Patient shows improvement in underlying condition.
• Patient maintains adequate cardiac output throughout therapy.
• Patient and family state understanding of drug therapy.

epirubicin hydrochloride
(ep-uh-ROO-bih-sin high-droh-KLOR-ighd)
Ellence

Pharmacologic class: anthracycline
Therapeutic class: antineoplastic
Pregnancy risk category: D

Indications and dosages

▶ **Adjuvant therapy in patients with evidence of axillary node tumor involvement following resection of primary breast cancer.**
Adults: 100 to120 mg/m^2 I.V. infusion over 3 to 5 minutes via a free-flowing I.V. solution on day 1 of each cycle q 3 to 4 weeks; or divided equally in two doses on days 1 and 8 of each cycle. Maximum cumulative (lifetime) dose is 900 mg/m^2.
◙ **Adjust-a-dose:** Dosage change after the first cycle is based on toxicity. For patient with platelet count below 50,000/mm^3, absolute neutrophil count (ANC) below 250/mm^3, neutropenic fever, or grade 3 or 4 nonhematologic toxicity, reduce day-1 dose in subsequent cycles to 75% of the day-1 dose in the current cycle.

Delay day-1 therapy in subsequent cycles until platelet count is 100,000/mm^3 or above, ANC is 1,500/mm^3 or above, and nonhematologic toxicities recover to grade 1.
For patients receiving divided doses (days 1 and 8), give 75% of the day-1 dose on day 8 if platelet count is 75,000 to 100,000/mm^3 and ANC is 1,000 to 1,499/mm^3. If day-8 platelet count is below 75,000/mm^3, ANC is below 1,000/mm^3, or grade 3 or 4 nonhematologic toxicity occurs, skip the day-8 dose.
Give lower dosages to patients with bone marrow, hepatic, or severe renal impairment.

▼ **I.V. administration**
⑤ **ALERT:** Drug is a vesicant. Never give I.M. or S.C. Always give through free-flowing I.V. solution of normal saline solution or D$_5$W over 3 to 5 minutes.
• Don't mix in same syringe with other drugs.
• Don't mix drug with heparin or fluorouracil because precipitation may result.
• Give prophylactic antibiotic therapy with trimethoprim and sulfamethoxazole or a fluoroquinolone to patients receiving 120 mg/m^2 dose.
• Give antiemetics before giving drug to reduce nausea and vomiting.
• Avoid veins over joints or in limbs with compromised venous or lymphatic drainage.
• If burning or stinging occurs, immediately stop infusion, and restart in another vein.
• Facial flushing and local erythematous streaking along the vein may indicate too-rapid administration.
• Discard unused solution in vial 24 hours after vial penetrated.

Contraindications and precautions

• Contraindicated in patients hypersensitive to drug, other anthracyclines, or anthracenediones. Also contraindicated in patients with baseline neutrophil counts below 1,500 cells/mm^3, in those with severe myocardial insufficiency or recent MI, in those previously treated with anthracyclines to total cumulative doses, and in those with severe hepatic dysfunction.
• Use cautiously in patients with active or dormant cardiac disease, previous or simultaneous radiotherapy to the mediastinal and pericardial area, or previous therapy with other anthracyclines or anthracenediones. Also use cautiously with other cardiotoxic drugs.

✲ **Lifespan:** In pregnant and breast-feeding women, drug is contraindicated. In children, safety of drug hasn't been established. In elderly patients, especially women older than age 70, use cautiously because of greater chance of toxicity.

Adverse reactions

CNS: *lethargy,* fever.
CV: *cardiomyopathy, heart failure.*
EENT: *conjunctivitis, keratitis.*
GI: *nausea, vomiting, diarrhea,* anorexia, *mucositis.*
GU: *amenorrhea.*
Hematologic: LEUKOPENIA, NEUTROPENIA, *febrile neutropenia, anemia,* THROMBOCY-TOPENIA.
Skin: *alopecia,* rash, itch, skin changes.
Other: *infection, local toxicity, hot flushes.*

Interactions

Drug-drug. *Cytotoxic drugs:* Additive toxicities (especially hematologic and GI) may occur. Monitor patient closely.
Calcium channel blockers, other cardioactive compounds: May increase risk of heart failure. Monitor cardiac function closely.
Cimetidine: Increases epirubicin level (by 50%) and decreases clearance. Avoid using together.
Radiation therapy: Effects may be enhanced. Monitor patient carefully.

Effects on lab test results

• May decrease hemoglobin, hematocrit, and WBC, neutrophil, and platelet counts.

Pharmacokinetics

Absorption: Administered I.V.
Distribution: Rapid and widely distributed into tissues. Protein-binding is about 77%, mainly to albumin, and appears to concentrate in RBCs.
Metabolism: Extensive and rapid. Several metabolites form with little to no cytotoxic activity.
Excretion: Mostly biliary and, to a lesser extent, urinary. *Half-life:* 31 to 35 hours.

Route	Onset	Peak	Duration
I.V.	Unknown	Unknown	Unknown

Action

Chemical effect: The precise mechanism of epirubicin's cytotoxic effects isn't completely known. It's thought to form a complex with DNA by intercalation between nucleotide base pairs, thereby inhibiting DNA, RNA, and protein synthesis. DNA cleavage occurs, resulting in cytocidal activity. Drug may also interfere with replication and transcription of DNA, and it generates cytotoxic free radicals.
Therapeutic effect: Kills certain cancer cells.

Available forms

Injection: 2 mg/ml

NURSING PROCESS

⚕ **Assessment**
• Obtain baseline total bilirubin, AST, creatinine, and CBC (including ANC), and evaluate cardiac function by measuring left ventricular ejection fraction (LVEF) before therapy.
• Monitor LVEF regularly during therapy, and stop drug at the first sign of cardiac impairment. Monitor patient for early signs of cardiac toxicity, including sinus tachycardia, ECG abnormalities, tachyarrhythmias, bradycardia, AV block, and bundle branch block.
• Obtain total and differential WBC, RBC, and platelet counts before and during each cycle of therapy.
• Evaluate patient's and family's knowledge of drug therapy.

⚕ **Nursing diagnoses**
• Risk for injury related to drug-induced adverse reactions
• Risk for infection related to myelosuppression
• Deficient knowledge related to drug therapy

▶ **Planning and implementation**
• Give drug under the supervision of a prescriber experienced in the use of cancer chemotherapy. Pregnant women shouldn't handle this drug.
• Wear protective clothing (goggles, gown, disposable gloves) when handling this drug.
• Delayed cardiac toxicity may occur 2 to 3 months after completion of treatment. It causes reduced LVEF, evidence of heart failure (tachycardia, dyspnea, pulmonary edema, dependent edema, hepatomegaly, ascites, pleural effusion, and gallop rhythm). Delayed cardiac toxicity is dependent upon the cumulative dose of epirubicin. Don't exceed a cumulative dose of 900 mg/m^2.

• Monitor uric acid, potassium, calcium phosphate, and creatinine immediately after initial chemotherapy administration in patients susceptible to tumor lysis syndrome. Hydration, urine alkalinization, and prophylaxis with allopurinol may prevent hyperuricemia and minimize complications of tumor lysis syndrome.

• Lowest WBC usually occurs 10 to 14 days after drug administration and returns to normal by day 21.

• Anthracycline-induced leukemia may occur.

• Administration of drug after previous radiation therapy may induce an inflammatory cell reaction at the site of irradiation.

Patient teaching

• Advise patient to report nausea, vomiting, stomatitis, dehydration, fever, evidence of infection, symptoms of heart failure (tachycardia, dyspnea, edema), or injection site pain.

• Inform patient of the risk of cardiac damage and treatment-related leukemia.

• Tell women of childbearing age not to become pregnant and men to use effective contraception during treatment.

• Advise women that irreversible amenorrhea or premature menopause may occur.

• Advise patient about probable hair loss. Tell patient that hair regrowth usually occurs 2 to 3 months after therapy is stopped.

• Advise patient that urine may appear red 1 to 2 days after administration of the drug.

☑ **Evaluation**

• Patient sustains no injury from drug-induced adverse reactions.

• Patient remains free of infection.

• Patient and family state understanding of drug therapy.

eplerenone
(eh-PLAIR-eh-nown)
Inspra

Pharmacologic class: aldosterone receptor antagonist
Therapeutic class: antihypertensive
Pregnancy risk category: B

Indications and dosages

▶ **Hypertension.** *Adults:* 50 mg P.O. once daily. If response is inadequate after 4 weeks, in-

crease dosage to 50 mg P.O. b.i.d. Maximum, 100 mg daily.

▶ **Heart failure post-MI.** *Adults:* Initially, 25 mg P.O. daily. Increase to 50 mg P.O. daily as tolerated within 4 weeks and according to potassium level.

Contraindications and precautions

• Contraindicated in patients with potassium greater than 5.5 mEq/L, type 2 diabetes with microalbuminuria, creatinine level greater than 2 mg/dl in men or greater than 1.8 mg/dl in women, or creatinine clearance less than 50 ml/minute. Also contraindicated in patients treated simultaneously with potassium supplements, potassium-sparing diuretics (amiloride, spironolactone, or triamterene), or strong CYP 3A4 inhibitors such as ketoconazole and itraconazole.

• Use cautiously in patients with mild to moderate hepatic impairment.

⚕ **Lifespan:** In pregnant women, use only if the potential benefits justify the risk to the fetus. In breast-feeding women, use cautiously; it's unknown whether drug appears in breast milk. In children, safety and effectiveness haven't been established.

Adverse reactions

CNS: dizziness, fatigue.
GI: diarrhea, abdominal pain.
GU: albuminuria, abnormal vaginal bleeding.
Metabolic: *hyperkalemia.*
Respiratory: cough.
Other: flu syndrome, gynecomastia.

Interactions

Drug-drug. *ACE inhibitors, angiotensin II receptor antagonists:* Increases risk of hyperkalemia. Use together cautiously.
Lithium: Increases risk of lithium toxicity. Monitor lithium level.
NSAIDs: May reduce the antihypertensive effect and cause severe hyperkalemia in patients with renal impairment. Monitor blood pressure and potassium level.
Potassium supplements, potassium-sparing diuretics (amiloride, spironolactone, triamterene): Increases risk of hyperkalemia and sometimes fatal arrhythmias. Avoid using together.

Strong CYP 3A4 inhibitors (itraconazole, keto-conazole): Increases eplerenone level. Avoid using together.

Weak CYP 3A4 inhibitors (erythromycin, fluconazole, saquinavir, verapamil): Increases eplerenone level. Reduce eplerenone starting dose to 25 mg P.O. once daily.

Drug-herb. *St. John's wort:* May decrease eplerenone level over time. Discourage using together.

Effects on lab test results

• May increase potassium, creatinine, BUN, triglyceride, cholesterol, ALT, and GGT levels. May decrease sodium level.

Pharmacokinetics

Absorption: Bioavailability of drug is unknown.
Distribution: Protein binding is about 50%, primarily to alpha$_1$-acid glycoproteins.
Metabolism: Predominantly by CYP 3A4 pathway. No active metabolites have been identified.
Excretion: Less than 5% of dose is recovered unchanged in the urine and feces. *Half-life:* 4 to 6 hours.

Route	Onset	Peak	Duration
P.O.	Unknown	1½ hr	Unknown

Action

Chemical effect: Binds to mineralocorticoid receptors and blocks aldosterone. Aldosterone increases blood pressure through induction of sodium reabsorption and possibly other mechanisms.
Therapeutic effect: Lowers blood pressure.

Available forms

Tablets: 25 mg, 50 mg, 100 mg

NURSING PROCESS

Assessment

• Obtain history of patient's underlying condition before therapy.
• Obtain patient's baseline blood pressure and potassium levels and reassess regularly.
• Evaluate patient's and family's understanding of drug therapy.

Nursing diagnoses

• Risk for ineffective health maintenance related to hypertension
• Risk for injury related to the presence of hypertension
• Deficient knowledge related to drug therapy

Planning and implementation

• Drug may be used alone or with other antihypertensives.
• Full therapeutic effect of the drug occurs within 4 weeks.
• Monitor patient for signs and symptoms of hyperkalemia.
• Overdose may cause hypotension and hyperkalemia. Treat symptoms and provide support. Drug binds extensively to charcoal but can't be removed by hemodialysis.
Patient teaching
• Tell patient drug can be taken with or without food.
• Advise patient to avoid potassium supplements and salt substitutes during treatment.
• Tell patient to report adverse reactions.

Evaluation

• Patient's blood pressure remains within normal limits.
• Patient's potassium remains within normal limits.
• Patient and family state understanding of drug therapy.

epoetin alfa (erythropoietin)
(ee-POH-eh-tin AL-fah)
Epogen, Eprex†, Procrit

Pharmacologic class: glycoprotein
Therapeutic class: hematopoietic
Pregnancy risk category: C

Indications and dosages

▶ **Anemia from reduced production of endogenous erythropoietin caused by end-stage renal disease.** *Adults:* Dosage is individualized. Starting dosage is 50 to 100 units/kg I.V. three times weekly. (Patients with chronic renal impairment who are not on dialysis or patients receiving continuous peritoneal dialysis may receive drug S.C. or I.V.) Reduce dosage when target hematocrit is reached or if hematocrit rises more than 4% in any 2-week period. If hematocrit doesn't increase by 5 to 6 points after 8 weeks of therapy, increase dosage. Maintenance dosage is individualized.

▶ **Anemia in children with chronic renal impairment who are undergoing dialysis.** *Infants and children ages 1 month to 16 years:* 50 units/kg I.V. or S.C. three times weekly. Reduce dosage when target hematocrit is reached or if hematocrit rises more than 4 points in a 2-week period. Increase dosage if hematocrit doesn't rise by 5 to 6 points after 8 to 12 weeks of therapy and is below target range. Maintenance dose is highly individualized to maintain hematocrit in target range.

▶ **Adjunct treatment for HIV-infected patients with anemia secondary to zidovudine therapy.** *Adults:* 100 units/kg I.V. or S.C. three times weekly for 8 to 12 weeks or until target hematocrit is reached.

▶ **Anemia secondary to chemotherapy.** *Adults:* 150 units/kg S.C. three times weekly for 8 weeks or until target hematocrit is reached. Increase up to 300 units/kg S.C. three times weekly, if needed.

▶ **Anemia related to rheumatoid arthritis and rheumatic disease‡.** *Adults:* 50 to 200 units/kg S.C. three times weekly.

▶ **Anemia related to prematurity‡.** *Neonates:* 25 to 100 units/kg S.C. three times weekly.

▽ I.V. administration

• Give drug by direct injection without dilution.
• Don't mix with other drugs.
• Solution contains no preservatives. Discard unused portion.

Contraindications and precautions

• Contraindicated in patients with uncontrolled hypertension, hypersensitivity to mammal-cell–derived products or albumin.

☀ **Lifespan:** In pregnant and breast-feeding women, use cautiously. In children younger than age 1 month, safety hasn't been established.

Adverse reactions

CNS: *headache, seizures, paresthesia, fatigue, fever,* dizziness, *asthenia.*
CV: *increased clotting of arteriovenous grafts, hypertension, edema.*
GI: *nausea, vomiting, diarrhea.*
Hematologic: iron deficiency, thrombocytosis.
Musculoskeletal: *arthralgia.*

Respiratory: *cough, shortness of breath.*
Skin: *rash, urticaria.*
Other: *injection site reaction.*

Interactions

None significant.

Effects on lab test results

• May increase BUN, creatinine, uric acid, potassium, and phosphate levels.
• May increase platelet count.

Pharmacokinetics

Absorption: After S.C. administration, systemic absorption is delayed, incomplete, and variable compared with I.V. administration.
Distribution: Unknown.
Metabolism: Unknown.
Excretion: Unknown. *Half-life:* 4 to 13 hours for patient with chronic renal failure.

Route	Onset	Peak	Duration
I.V.	1-6 wk	Immediate	Unknown
S.C.	1-6 wk	5-24 hr	Unknown

Action

Chemical effect: Mimics effects of erythropoietin, a naturally occurring hormone produced by the kidneys. Drug acts on erythroid tissues in bone marrow, stimulating mitotic activity of erythroid progenitor cells and early precursor cells. It functions as both growth and differentiating factors, enhancing rate of RBC production.
Therapeutic effect: Corrects anemia.

Available forms

Injection: 2,000 units/ml, 3,000 units/ml, 4,000 units/ml, 10,000 units/ml, 20,000 units/ml, 40,000 units/ml

NURSING PROCESS

⚏ Assessment

• Assess patient's CBC and blood pressure before therapy.
• Assess effectiveness by monitoring CBC results. Hematocrit may rise and cause excessive clotting. Watch for evidence of blood clot formation such as shortness of breath and cold, swollen, or pulseless limb.
• Patient's response depends on amount of endogenous erythropoietin. Patients with

500 units/L or more usually have transfusion-dependent anemia and probably won't respond to drug. Those with levels below 500 units/L usually respond well.

• Before and during therapy, monitor patient's iron status. Most patients will require supplemental iron to support erythropoiesis.

• Monitor blood pressure closely. Up to 80% of patients with chronic renal impairment have hypertension. Blood pressure may rise, especially when hematocrit is increasing in early part of therapy.

• After injection (usually within 2 hours), some patients complain of pain or discomfort in their limbs (long bones) and pelvis and of coldness and sweating. Symptoms may persist for up to 12 hours and then disappear.

• If adverse GI reactions occur, monitor patient's hydration status.

• Evaluate patient's and family's knowledge of drug therapy.

🔲 Nursing diagnoses
• Ineffective protection related to reduced production of endogenous erythropoietin
• Risk for deficient fluid volume related to drug-induced adverse GI reactions
• Deficient knowledge related to drug therapy

▶ Planning and implementation
• When used in HIV-infected patient, individualize dosage based on response. Dosage recommendations are for patients with endogenous erythropoietin levels of 500 units/L or less and cumulative zidovudine doses of 4.2 g/week or less.

• Patient may need additional heparin to prevent clotting during dialysis.

• Start diet restrictions or drug therapy to control blood pressure.

Patient teaching
• Advise patient that blood specimens will be drawn weekly for blood counts and that dosage adjustments may be made based on results.

• Warn patient to avoid hazardous activities, such as driving or operating heavy machinery, early in therapy. Excessively rapid rise in hematocrit may increase the risk of seizures.

• Tell patient to notify prescriber if adverse reactions occur.

☑ Evaluation
• Patient's blood count is normal.

• Patient maintains adequate hydration throughout therapy.
• Patient and family state understanding of drug therapy.

eprosartan mesylate
(eh-proh-SAR-ten MEH-sih-layt)
Teveten

Pharmacologic class: angiotensin II receptor antagonist
Therapeutic class: antihypertensive
Pregnancy risk category: C (D in second and third trimesters)

Indications and dosages
▶ **Hypertension.** *Adults:* Initially, 600 mg P.O. daily. Daily dosage ranges from 400 to 800 mg given as single daily dose or two divided doses. Drug can be given alone or with other antihypertensives.

Contraindications and precautions
• Contraindicated in patients hypersensitive to drug or its components.
• Use cautiously in patients with an activated renin-angiotensin system, such as volume- or salt-depleted patients, and in patients whose renal function may depend on the activity of the renin-angiotensin-aldosterone system, such as patients with severe heart failure.
• Use cautiously in patients with renal artery stenosis.
☬ **Lifespan:** In pregnant and breast-feeding women, drug is contraindicated. In children, safety and effectiveness haven't been established. In elderly patients, use cautiously because of decreased response to drug.

Adverse reactions
CNS: depression, fatigue, headache, dizziness.
CV: chest pain, dependent edema, hypertriglyceridemia.
EENT: pharyngitis, rhinitis, sinusitis.
GI: abdominal pain, dyspepsia, diarrhea.
GU: UTI.
Hematologic: *neutropenia.*
Musculoskeletal: arthralgia, myalgia.
Respiratory: cough, upper respiratory tract infection, bronchitis.
Other: injury, viral infection.

Interactions

None significant.

Effects on lab test results

- May increase BUN and triglyceride levels.
- May decrease neutrophil count.

Pharmacokinetics

Absorption: Absolute bioavailability of single oral dose is about 13%. Level peaks in 1 to 2 hours.
Distribution: Protein-binding is about 98%.
Metabolism: No active metabolites.
Excretion: Eliminated by biliary and renal excretion, primarily as unchanged drug; about 90% is recovered in feces and about 7% in urine. *Half-life:* 5 to 9 hours.

Route	Onset	Peak	Duration
P.O.	1-2 hr	1-3 hr	24 hr

Action

Chemical effect: Blocks vasoconstrictor and aldosterone-secreting effects of angiotensin II by selectively blocking binding of angiotensin II to its receptor sites in many tissues, such as vascular smooth muscle and the adrenal gland.
Therapeutic effect: Lowers blood pressure.

Available forms

Tablets: 400 mg, 600 mg

NURSING PROCESS

☑ Assessment

- Monitor blood pressure closely during start of treatment. If hypotension occurs, place patient in supine position and, if needed, give I.V. infusion of normal saline solution.
- Determine patient's fluid balance status and sodium level before starting drug therapy.
- Elderly patients have a slightly decreased response to drug.
- Be alert for adverse reactions.
- Evaluate patient's and family's knowledge of drug therapy.

⊕ Nursing diagnoses

- Risk for injury related to presence of hypertension
- Risk for infection related to neutropenia
- Deficient knowledge related to drug therapy

▷ Planning and implementation

- Correct hypovolemia and hyponatremia before starting therapy to reduce risk of symptomatic hypotension.
- A transient episode of hypotension doesn't contraindicate continued treatment. Drug may be restarted once patient's blood pressure has stabilized.
- Drug may be used alone or with other antihypertensives, such as diuretics and calcium channel blockers. Maximum blood pressure response may take 2 to 3 weeks.
- Monitor patient for facial or lip swelling because angioedema has occurred with other angiotensin II antagonists.

Patient teaching

- Advise woman of childbearing age to use reliable form of contraception and to notify prescriber immediately if pregnancy is suspected. Stop drug under medical supervision.
- Advise patient to report facial or lip swelling and signs and symptoms of infection, such as fever or sore throat.
- Tell patient to notify prescriber before taking OTC product to treat a dry cough.
- Inform patient that drug may be taken without regard to meals.
- Tell patient to store drug at a controlled room temperature (68° to 77° F [20° to 25° C]).

☑ Evaluation

- Patient's blood pressure is well controlled, and patient remains free of injury.
- WBC count is normal.
- Patient and family state understanding of drug therapy.

eptifibatide

(ep-tih-FY-beh-tide)
Integrilin

Pharmacologic class: glycoprotein IIb/IIIa (GP IIb/IIIa) inhibitor
Therapeutic class: antiplatelet drug
Pregnancy risk category: B

Indications and dosages

▶ **Acute coronary syndrome (unstable angina or non–Q-wave MI) in patients being managed medically and in those undergoing percutaneous coronary intervention (PCI).**

Adults with creatinine less than 2 mg/dl: 180 mcg/kg I.V. bolus as soon as possible following diagnosis, followed by a continuous I.V. infusion of 2 mcg/kg per minute until hospital discharge or initiation of coronary artery bypass graft surgery, up to 72 hours. If undergoing PCI, continue infusion until hospital discharge, or for up to 18 to 24 hours after the procedure, whichever comes first, up to 96 hours. Give patients weighing more than 121 kg (266 lb) a maximum bolus of 22.6 mg followed by a maximum infusion rate of 15 mg/hour.

Adults with creatinine between 2 and 4 mg/dl: 180 mcg/kg I.V. bolus as soon as possible following diagnosis, followed by an infusion rate of 1 mcg/kg per minute. For patients weighing more than 121 kg (266 lb), the maximum bolus dose is 22.6 mg and the maximum infusion rate is 7.5 mg/hour.

▶ **Patients undergoing PCI.** *Adults with creatinine less than 2 mg/dl initiated at the time of PCI:* 180 mcg/kg I.V. bolus given immediately before the procedure, immediately followed by an infusion of 2 mcg/kg/minute and a second IV bolus of 180 mcg/kg given 10 minutes after the first bolus. Continue infusion until hospital discharge or for up to 18 to 24 hours, whichever comes first; a minimum of 12 hours of eptifibatide infusion is recommended. Give patients weighing more than 121 kg a maximum bolus of 22.6 mg/bolus followed by a maximum of 15 g/hour.

Adults with creatinine between 2 and 4 mg/dl initiated at the time of PCI: 180 mcg/kg given immediately before the procedure, immediately followed by an infusion of 1 mcg/kg per minute and a second bolus of 180 mcg/kg given 10 minutes after the first bolus. Give patients weighing more than 121 kg a maximum of 22.6 mg/bolus followed by a maximum rate of 7.5 mg/hour.

▼ I.V. administration

● Inspect solution for particulate matter before use. If particles are visible, the sterility is suspect; discard solution.
● Withdraw bolus dose from 10-ml vial into a syringe and give by I.V. push over 1 to 2 minutes. Give I.V. infusion undiluted directly from 100-ml vial using an infusion pump.
● Drug may be given in same I.V. line with normal saline solution or normal saline and 5%

dextrose; main infusion may also contain up to 60 mEq/L of potassium chloride.
● Drug may be given in same I.V. line as alteplase, atropine, dobutamine, heparin, lidocaine, meperidine, metoprolol, midazolam, morphine, nitroglycerin, or verapamil.
● **⊛ ALERT:** Don't give drug in same I.V. line as furosemide.
● When obtaining I.V. access, avoid use of noncompressible sites (such as subclavian or jugular veins).
● Drug is intended for use with heparin and aspirin.
● Refrigerate vials at 36° to 46° F (2° to 8° C). Protect from light until administration.

Contraindications and precautions

● Contraindicated in patients hypersensitive to drug or its ingredients and in those with history of bleeding diathesis, evidence of active abnormal bleeding within previous 30 days, severe hypertension (systolic blood pressure over 200 mm Hg or diastolic blood pressure over 110 mm Hg) not adequately controlled with antihypertensives, major surgery within previous 6 weeks, history of CVA within 30 days, history of hemorrhagic CVA, current or planned use of another parenteral GP IIb/IIIa inhibitor, or platelet count below 100,000/mm3. Also contraindicated in patients whose creatinine level is 2 mg/dl or higher (for the 180-mcg/kg bolus and 2-mcg/kg/minute infusion) or 4 mg/dl or higher (for the 135-mcg/kg bolus and 0.5-mcg/kg/ minute infusion) and in patients dependent on dialysis.
⚜ **Lifespan:** In breast-feeding women, use cautiously. In children, safety hasn't been established.

Adverse reactions

CV: hypotension.
GU: hematuria.
Hematologic: BLEEDING, *thrombocytopenia.*
Other: *bleeding at femoral artery access site.*

Interactions

Drug-drug. *Clopidogrel, dipyridamole, NSAIDs, oral anticoagulants (warfarin), thrombolytics, ticlopidine:* May increase risk of bleeding. Monitor patient closely.
Other inhibitors of platelet receptor IIb/IIIa: May have potential for serious bleeding. Don't give together.

Effects on lab test results

• May decrease platelet count.

Pharmacokinetics

Absorption: Administered I.V.
Distribution: 25% bound to proteins.
Metabolism: None reported. No major metabolites are detected.
Excretion: Most of drug is excreted in urine.
Half-life: 2½ hours.

Route	Onset	Peak	Duration
I.V.	Immediate	Immediate	4-6 hr after therapy stops

Action

Chemical effect: Drug reversibly binds to the glycoprotein IIb/IIIa (GP IIb/IIIa) receptor on human platelets and inhibits platelet aggregation.
Therapeutic effect: Prevents clot formation.

Available forms

Injection: 10-ml (2 mg/ml), 100-ml (0.75 mg/ml) vials

NURSING PROCESS

📖 Assessment

• Obtain history of patient's underlying medical conditions, especially conditions that put patient at increased risk for bleeding.
• Obtain accurate patient weight. Use drug cautiously in patients weighing more than 143 kg (315 lb).
• Perform baseline laboratory tests before start of drug therapy; also determine hemoglobin, hematocrit, platelet count, and PT, INR, PTT, and creatinine levels.
• Monitor patient for bleeding.
• Evaluate patient's and family's knowledge of drug therapy.

🌐 Nursing diagnoses

• Ineffective cardiopulmonary tissue perfusion related to presence of acute coronary syndrome
• Risk for injury related to increased bleeding tendencies
• Deficient knowledge related to drug therapy

⊠ Planning and implementation

• Stop this drug and heparin, and achieve sheath hemostasis by standard compressive techniques at least 4 hours before hospital discharge.
• In patients undergoing coronary artery bypass graft surgery, stop infusion before surgery.
• Minimize use of arterial and venous punctures, I.M. injections, urinary catheters, and nasotracheal and nasogastric tubes.
• If patient's platelet count is below 100,000/mm^3, notify prescriber and stop this drug and heparin.
Patient teaching
• Explain that drug is a blood thinner used to prevent heart attack.
• Explain that the benefits of the drug far outweigh the risk of serious bleeding.
• Instruct patient to report chest discomfort or other adverse events immediately.

☑ Evaluation

• Patient maintains adequate cardiopulmonary tissue perfusion.
• Patient has no life-threatening bleeding episode.
• Patient and family state understanding of drug therapy.

ertapenem sodium
(er-ta-PEN-uhm SOH-dee-um)
Invanz

Pharmacologic class: 1-beta methyl-carbapenem
Therapeutic class: anti-infective
Pregnancy risk category: B

Indications and dosages

▶ **Complicated intra-abdominal infections caused by** *Escherichia coli, Clostridium clostridiiforme, Eubacterium lentum, Peptostreptococcus* **species,** *Bacteroides fragilis, B. distasonis, B. ovatus, B. thetaiotaomicron, B. uniformis.* *Adults:* 1 g I.V. or I.M. once daily for 5 to 14 days.
▶ **Complicated skin and skin-structure infections caused by** *Staphylococcus aureus* **(methicillin-susceptible strains),** *Streptococcus pyogenes, E. coli, Peptostreptococcus* **species.** *Adults:* 1 g I.V. or I.M. once daily for 7 to 14 days.

▶ **Community-acquired pneumonia caused by** *S. pneumoniae* **(penicillin-susceptible strains),** *Haemophilus influenzae* **(beta-lactamase–negative strains),** *Moraxella catarrhalis*. *Adults:* 1 g I.V. or I.M. once daily for 10 to 14 days. If improvement occurs after at least 3 days of treatment, appropriate oral therapy may be used to complete the full course of therapy.

▶ **Complicated UTI, including pyelonephritis caused by** *E. coli, Klebsiella pneumoniae*. *Adults:* 1 g I.V. or I.M. once daily for 10 to 14 days. After at least 3 days of treatment, if improvement occurs, appropriate oral therapy may be used to complete the full course of therapy.

▶ **Acute pelvic infections including postpartum endomyometritis, septic abortion, and postsurgical gynecologic infections caused by** *S. agalactiae, E. coli, B. fragilis, Porphyromonas asaccharolyticus, Peptostreptococcus species, Prevotella bivia*. *Adults:* 1 g I.V. or I.M. once daily for 3 to 10 days.

Adjust-a-dose: If creatinine clearance is 30 ml/minute or less, give 500 mg daily. A supplementary dose of 150 mg is recommended after a hemodialysis session only in patients who are given the recommended daily ertapenem dose of 500 mg within 6 hours before hemodialysis.

▼ I.V. administration

● Reconstitute the contents of a 1-g drug vial with 10 ml of water for injection, normal saline injection, or bacteriostatic water for injection. Shake well to dissolve, and immediately transfer contents of the reconstituted vial to 50 ml of normal saline injection.

ALERT: Don't use diluents containing dextrose.

● Infuse over 30 minutes. Complete the infusion within 6 hours of reconstitution.

● Don't store lyophilized powder above 77° F (25° C). The reconstituted solution, immediately diluted in normal saline injection, may be stored at room temperature and used within 6 hours or stored for 24 hours under refrigeration (41° F [5° C]) and used within 4 hours after removal from refrigeration. Don't freeze solutions of ertapenem.

Contraindications and precautions

● Contraindicated in patients hypersensitive to any component of the drug or to other drugs in the same class and in patients who have had anaphylactic reactions to beta-lactams. I.M. use is contraindicated in patients hypersensitive to local anesthetics of the amide type (because lidocaine hydrochloride is the diluent). Methicillin-resistant *Staphylococci* and *Enterococci* sp. are resistant to ertapenem.

● Use cautiously in patients with CNS disorders or compromised renal function, as seizures may occur. Ertapenem sodium may be removed by hemodialysis, if needed.

Lifespan: In pregnant women, use only if clearly needed. In breast-feeding women, use only if potential benefit outweighs the risk because drug appears in breast milk. In children, safety and effectiveness haven't been established. In elderly patients with renal impairment, select dose carefully and monitor renal function.

Adverse reactions

CNS: asthenia, fatigue, anxiety, altered mental status, dizziness, headache, insomnia, *seizures*, fever, pain.

CV: edema, swelling, chest pain, hypertension, hypotension, tachycardia.

EENT: pharyngitis.

GI: abdominal pain, acid regurgitation, oral candidiasis, constipation, *diarrhea*, dyspepsia, nausea, vomiting, abdominal distention, *C. difficile* infection, *pseudomembranous colitis*.

GU: vaginitis, renal dysfunction, hematuria, urinary retention.

Hematologic: coagulation abnormalities, eosinophilia, anemia, *neutropenia, leukopenia, thrombocytopenia, thrombocytosis*.

Hepatic: jaundice.

Metabolic: hyperglycemia, *hyperkalemia*, hypernatremia.

Musculoskeletal: leg pain.

Respiratory: cough, dyspnea, rales, rhonchi, *respiratory distress*.

Skin: erythema, pruritus, rash, extravasation, infused vein complication, phlebitis, thrombophlebitis.

Other: *septicemia, death*, chills, *hypersensitivity reactions*.

Interactions

Drug-drug. *Probenecid:* Reduces renal clearance and increases half-life. Avoid using together.

Effects on lab test results

● May increase ALT, AST, alkaline phosphatase, BUN, creatinine, glucose, potassium, sodium,

and bilirubin levels. May decrease albumin and sodium bicarbonate level.
- May increase PT, PTT, eosinophil count, and urinary RBC and WBC counts. May decrease hemoglobin, hematocrit, and segmented neutrophil and WBC counts. May increase or decrease platelet count.

Pharmacokinetics

Absorption: Almost completely absorbed after I.M. administration. Mean bioavailability of 90%.
Distribution: Highly bound to proteins, primarily albumin.
Metabolism: Doesn't inhibit metabolism mediated by any of the following CYP isoforms: 1A2, 2C9, 2C19, 2D6, 2E1, and 3A4. Stable against hydrolysis by a variety of beta-lactamases, including penicillinase, cephalosporinase, and extended-spectrum beta-lactamase. Hydrolyzed by metallo-beta-lactamases.
Excretion: Primarily by the kidneys. *Half-life:* 4 hours.

Route	Onset	Peak	Duration
I.V.	Immediate	30 min	24 hr
I.M.	Unknown	2 hr	24 hr

Action

Chemical effect: The bactericidal activity of ertapenem results from the inhibition of cell wall synthesis and is mediated through ertapenem binding to penicillin-binding proteins
Therapeutic effect: Kills susceptible bacteria.

Available forms

Injection: 1 g

NURSING PROCESS

⚗ Assessment
- Check for previous penicillin, cephalosporin, or other beta-lactam hypersensitivity.
- If giving I.M., check for hypersensitivity to local, amide-type anesthetics.
- Obtain specimens for culture and sensitivity testing before giving first dose. Therapy may start before results are available.
- Monitor renal, hepatic, and hematopoietic function during prolonged therapy.
- Be alert for adverse reactions, particularly diarrhea, seizures, and superinfection.

- Evaluate patient's and family's knowledge of drug therapy.

⚗ Nursing diagnoses
- Diarrhea related to drug-induced adverse reaction
- Ineffective health maintenance related to underlying infectious disease process
- Deficient knowledge related to anti-infective therapy

▷ Planning and implementation
⊛ ALERT: Don't mix or infuse together with other medications.
⊛ ALERT: Don't confuse Avinza (morphine sulfate) with Invanz (ertapenem)
- When giving I.M., reconstitute the contents of a 1-g vial of drug with 3.2 ml of 1% lidocaine hydrochloride injection (without epinephrine). Refer to prescribing information for lidocaine hydrochloride. Shake vial thoroughly to form solution. Immediately withdraw the contents of the vial and give by deep I.M. injection into a large muscle, such as the gluteal muscles or lateral part of the thigh. Use reconstituted I.M. solution within 1 hour of preparing. Don't give reconstituted solution I.V.
- Avoid inadvertent injection into a blood vessel during I.M. administration.
- If diarrhea persists during therapy, stop drug and collect stool specimen for culture to rule out pseudomembranous colitis.
- If allergic reaction occurs, stop drug immediately. Serious anaphylactic reactions require immediate emergency treatment with airway management, epinephrine, oxygen, and I.V. steroids.
- Continue anticonvulsants in patients with known seizure disorders. If focal tremors, myoclonus, or seizures occur, evaluate patients neurologically and give anticonvulsants if not done earlier. Decrease or stop drug after reexamining dosage.
- Signs and symptoms of overdose may include nausea, diarrhea, and dizziness. If an overdose occurs, stop drug and treat supportively until drug has been eliminated from the body.
Patient teaching
- Inform patient of potential adverse reactions and urge him to notify prescriber immediately if they occur.
- Tell patient to alert prescriber if he develops diarrhea.

☑ Evaluation
- Patient tolerates and responds well to drug therapy.
- Patient doesn't develop colitis or any other adverse reactions from drug therapy.
- Patient and family state understanding of drug therapy.

erythromycin base
(eh-rith-roh-MIGH-sin bays)
Apo-Erythro ♦ , E-Base, E-Mycin, Erybid ♦ , ERYC, Ery-Tab, Erythromycin Base Filmtab, Erythromycin Delayed-Release, PCE Dispertab

erythromycin estolate
Ilosone, Ilosone Pulvules

erythromycin ethylsuccinate
Apo-Erythro-ES ♦ , EES, EES Granules ◇ , EryPed, EryPed 200, EryPed 400

erythromycin lactobionate
Erythrocin

erythromycin stearate
Apo-Erythro-S ♦ , Erythrocin Stearate

Pharmacologic class: erythromycin
Therapeutic class: antibiotic
Pregnancy risk category: B

Indications and dosages

▶ **Acute pelvic inflammatory disease caused by *Neisseria gonorrhoeae*.** *Adults:* 500 mg erythromycin lactobionate I.V. q 6 hours for 3 days; then 250 mg erythromycin base, estolate, or stearate. Or 400 mg ethylsuccinate P.O. q 6 hours for 7 days.

▶ **Endocarditis prophylaxis for dental procedures in patients allergic to penicillin.** *Adults:* Initially, 800 mg ethylsuccinate or 1 g stearate P.O. 2 hours before procedure; then 400 mg ethylsuccinate or 500 mg stearate P.O. 6 hours later.
Children: Initially, 20 mg/kg ethylsuccinate or stearate P.O. 2 hours before procedure; then one-half initial dose 6 hours later.

▶ **Intestinal amebiasis.** *Adults:* 250 mg base, estolate, or stearate, or 400 mg ethylsuccinate, P.O. q 6 hours for 10 to 14 days.
Children: 30 to 50 mg/kg base, estolate, ethylsuccinate, or stearate P.O. daily in divided doses q 6 hours for 10 to 14 days.

▶ **Mild to moderately severe respiratory tract, skin, and soft-tissue infections caused by sensitive group A beta-hemolytic streptococci, *Bordetella pertussis*, *Corynebacterium diphtheriae*, *Diplococcus pneumoniae*, *Listeria monocytogenes*, *Mycoplasma pneumoniae*.** *Adults:* 250 to 500 mg base, estolate, or stearate P.O. q 6 hours; or 400 to 800 mg erythromycin ethylsuccinate P.O. q 6 hours; or 15 to 20 mg/kg I.V. daily as continuous infusion or in divided doses q 6 hours.
Children: 30 to 50 mg/kg oral erythromycin salts P.O. daily in divided doses q 6 hours; or 15 to 20 mg/kg I.V. daily in divided doses q 4 to 6 hours.

▶ **Syphilis.** *Adults:* 500 mg base, estolate, or stearate P.O. q.i.d. for 15 days.

▶ **Legionnaires' disease.** *Adults:* 1 to 4 g P.O. or I.V. daily in divided doses for 10 to 21 days.

▶ **Uncomplicated urethral, endocervical, or rectal infections when tetracyclines are contraindicated.** *Adults:* 500 mg base, estolate, or stearate or 800 mg ethylsuccinate P.O. q.i.d. for at least 7 days.

▶ **Urogenital *Chlamydia trachomatis* infections during pregnancy.** *Adults:* 500 mg base, estolate, or stearate P.O. q.i.d. for at least 7 days, or 250 mg base, estolate, or stearate or 400 mg ethylsuccinate P.O. q.i.d. for at least 14 days.

▶ **Conjunctivitis caused by *C. trachomatis* in neonates.** *Neonates:* 50 mg/kg P.O. daily in four divided doses for 10 to 14 days.

▶ **Pneumonia of infancy caused by *C. trachomatis*.** *Infants:* 50 mg/kg P.O. daily in four divided doses for at least 3 weeks; a second course may be needed.

▶ **Early form of Lyme disease in persons allergic to penicillins and cephalosporins and in whom tetracyclines are contraindicated‡.** *Adults:* 250 to 500 mg base P.O. t.i.d. or q.i.d. Or, 30 to 40 mg/kg P.O. daily in divided doses for 10 to 30 days.
Children younger than age 8: 30 to 40 mg/kg base P.O. daily in divided doses (not to exceed adult dose) for 10 to 30 days.

▶ **Early Lyme disease manifested as erythema migrans‡.** *Adults:* 500 mg base P.O. q.i.d. for 14 to 21 days.
Children: 12.5 mg/kg base P.O. q.i.d. (maximum dose 500 mg/dose) for 14 to 21 days.

▼ I.V. administration

- Reconstitute drug according to manufacturer's directions, and dilute each 250 mg in at least 100 ml of normal saline solution.
- Infuse over 1 hour.
- Don't give erythromycin lactobionate with other drugs.

Contraindications and precautions

- Contraindicated in patients hypersensitive to drug or other macrolides and in patients taking pimozide. Erythromycin estolate is contraindicated in patients with hepatic disease.
- Use other erythromycin salts cautiously in patients with impaired liver function.
- ⚖ **Lifespan:** In pregnant and breast-feeding women, use cautiously. In neonates, avoid drug because it may contain benzyl alcohol.

Adverse reactions

CNS: fever.
CV: *ventricular arrhythmias, venous irritation or thrombophlebitis* after I.V. injection.
EENT: hearing loss with high I.V. doses.
GI: *abdominal pain and cramping, nausea, vomiting, diarrhea.*
Hepatic: cholestatic jaundice (erythromycin estolate).
Skin: urticaria, rash, eczema.
Other: overgrowth of nonsusceptible bacteria or fungi, *anaphylaxis.*

Interactions

Drug-drug. *Carbamazepine:* Increases carbamazepine levels and increases risk of toxicity. Avoid using together.
Clindamycin, lincomycin: May be antagonistic. Don't use together.
Cyclosporine: Increases cyclosporine levels. Monitor patient closely for toxicity.
Digoxin: Increases digoxin levels. Monitor patient for digoxin toxicity.
Disopyramide: Increases disopyramide level, resulting, in some cases, in arrhythmias and prolonged QT intervals. Monitor ECG.
Ergot alkaloids: May cause acute ergot toxicity. Monitor carefully.

HMG-CoA reductase inhibitors: May increase risk of myopathy and rhabdomyolysis. Avoid using together.
Midazolam, triazolam: Increases effects of these drugs. Monitor patient closely.
Oral anticoagulants: Increases anticoagulant effects. Monitor PT and INR closely; monitor patient for bleeding.
Tacrolimus: Increases tacrolimus levels and increases risk of adverse reactions, such as nephrotoxicity. Use together cautiously.
Theophylline: Decreases erythromycin level and increases risk of theophylline toxicity. Use together cautiously.
Vinblastine: Increases risk of vinblastine toxicity. Use together cautiously.
Drug-herb. *Pill-bearing spurge:* May inhibit CYP 3A enzymes and alter drug metabolism. Discourage use together.

Effects on lab test results

- May falsely elevate urinary catecholamines, 17-hydroxycorticosterone, and 17-ketosteroids. May interfere with colorimetric assays, resulting in falsely elevated AST and ALT levels.

Pharmacokinetics

Absorption: Most erythromycin salts are absorbed in duodenum. Because erythromycin base is acid-sensitive, it must be buffered or have enteric coating to prevent destruction by gastric acid. Acid salts and esters (estolate, ethylsuccinate, and stearate) aren't affected by gastric acidity and, therefore, are well absorbed; they're unaffected or possibly even enhanced by presence of food. Give base and stearate preparations on empty stomach.
Distribution: Widely distributed in most body tissues and fluids except CSF, where it appears at low levels. About 80% of erythromycin base and 96% of erythromycin estolate are protein-bound.
Metabolism: Partially metabolized in liver to inactive metabolites.
Excretion: Mainly unchanged in bile; small amount (less than 5%) in urine. *Half-life:* About 1.6 hours.

Route	Onset	Peak	Duration
P.O.	Unknown	1-4 hr	Unknown
I.V.	Immediate	Immediate	Unknown

Reactions may be *common,* uncommon, *life-threatening,* or COMMON AND LIFE-THREATENING.

Action

Chemical effect: Inhibits bacterial protein synthesis by binding to 50S subunit of ribosome.
Therapeutic effect: Inhibits bacterial growth.

Available forms

erythromycin base
Capsules (delayed-release): 250 mg
Tablets (enteric-coated): 250 mg, 333 mg, 500 mg
Tablets (filmtabs): 250 mg, 500 mg
erythromycin estolate
Capsules: 250 mg
Oral suspension: 125 mg/5 ml, 250 mg/5 ml
Tablets: 500 mg
erythromycin ethylsuccinate
Oral suspension: 100 mg/2.5 ml, 200 mg/5 ml, 400 mg/5 ml
Powder for oral suspension: 200 mg/5 ml, 400 mg/5ml
Tablets: 400 mg
erythromycin lactobionate
Injection: 500-mg, 1-g vials
erythromycin stearate
Tablets (film-coated): 250 mg, 500 mg

NURSING PROCESS

Assessment

• Obtain history of patient's infection before therapy and reassess regularly.
• Obtain urine specimen for culture and sensitivity tests. Therapy may begin, pending results.
• Be alert for adverse reactions and drug interactions.
• If adverse GI reactions occur, monitor patient's hydration status.
• Monitor liver function (increased levels of alkaline phosphatase, ALT, AST, and bilirubin may occur). Erythromycin estolate may cause serious hepatotoxicity in adults (reversible cholestatic jaundice). Other erythromycin salts cause hepatotoxicity to lesser degree. Patients who develop hepatotoxicity from estolate may react similarly to treatment with other erythromycin preparations.
• Evaluate patient's and family's knowledge of drug therapy.

Nursing diagnoses

• Infection related to presence of susceptible bacteria

• Risk for deficient fluid volume related to potential for drug-induced adverse GI reactions
• Deficient knowledge related to drug therapy

Planning and implementation

ALERT: American Heart Association no longer recommends using erythromycins to prevent bacterial endocarditis. However, practitioners who have successfully used the drug as prophylaxis in individual patients may continue to do so.
• When giving suspension, note concentration.
• For best absorption, give oral form with full glass of water 1 hour before or 2 hours after meals. Coated tablets may be taken with meals. Tell patient not to drink fruit juice with drug.
• Coated tablets or encapsulated pellets cause less GI upset; they may be more tolerable in patients who can't tolerate drug.
Patient teaching
• Tell patient how to take oral drug.
• Tell patient to take entire amount of drug exactly as prescribed, even after he feels better.
• Instruct patient to notify prescriber if adverse reactions occur, especially nausea, abdominal pain, and fever.

Evaluation

• Patient is free from infection.
• Patient maintains adequate hydration with therapy.
• Patient and family state understanding of drug therapy.

escitalopram oxalate
(ES-sigh-TAL-uh-pram ocks-UH-layt)
Lexapro

Pharmacologic class: SSRI
Therapeutic class: antidepressant
Pregnancy risk category: C

Indications and dosages

▶ **Major depressive disorder.** *Adults:* Initially, 10 mg P.O. daily, increasing to 20 mg if needed after at least 1 week.
Adjust-a-dose: For elderly patients and those with hepatic impairment, 10 mg P.O. daily, initially and as maintenance dosage.
▶ **Short-term treatment of generalized anxiety disorder.** *Adults:* Initially, 10 mg P.O.

daily. May increase to 20 mg daily after at least 1 week. Don't use for more than 8 weeks.

Contraindications and precautions

● Contraindicated in patients hypersensitive to drug, citalopram, or its active ingredients. Also contraindicated within 14 days of MAO inhibitor therapy.
● Use cautiously in patients with suicidal ideation, a history of mania, seizure disorders, or renal or hepatic impairment. Also use cautiously in patients with diseases that produce altered metabolism or hemodynamic responses.
☙ Lifespan: In pregnant women, use drug only if benefits outweigh risks. Breast-feeding women should stop breast-feeding or stop taking drug; drug appears in breast milk. In children, safety and effectiveness haven't been established. In elderly patients, use cautiously because they may have greater sensitivity to drug.

Adverse reactions

CNS: fever, *headache, insomnia,* dizziness, *somnolence,* paresthesia, light-headedness, migraine, tremor, vertigo, abnormal dreams, irritability, impaired concentration, fatigue, lethargy.
CV: palpitations, hypertension, flushing, chest pain.
EENT: rhinitis, sinusitis, blurred vision, tinnitus, earache.
GI: *nausea,* diarrhea, constipation, indigestion, abdominal pain, vomiting, increased or decreased appetite, dry mouth, flatulence, heartburn, cramps, gastroesophageal reflux.
GU: *ejaculation disorder,* impotence, anorgasmia, menstrual cramps, UTI, urinary frequency.
Metabolic: weight gain or loss.
Musculoskeletal: arthralgia, myalgia, muscle cramps, extremity pain.
Respiratory: bronchitis, cough.
Skin: rash, increased sweating.
Other: decreased libido, yawning, flulike symptoms, toothache.

Interactions

Drug-drug. *Carbamazepine:* May increase escitalopram clearance caused by P450 induction. Monitor patient for expected antidepressant effect and adjust dose as needed.
Cimetidine: May increase escitalopram level. Monitor patient for increased adverse reactions to escitalopram.

Citalopram: Causes additive effects. Avoid using together.
CNS drugs: Causes additive effects. Use together cautiously.
Desipramine, other drugs metabolized by CYP 2D6: May increase levels of these drugs. Use together cautiously.
Lithium: May enhance serotonergic effect of escitalopram. Use together cautiously, and monitor lithium level.
MAO inhibitors: May cause serious, sometimes fatal, reactions. Avoid using drug within 14 days of MAO inhibitor.
Sumatriptan: May increase serotonergic effects, leading to weakness, enhanced reflex response, and incoordination. Use together cautiously.
Drug-lifestyle. *Alcohol use:* May increase CNS effects. Discourage using together.

Effects on lab test results

None reported.

Pharmacokinetics

Absorption: Absolute bioavailability is 80%.
Distribution: Protein binding is about 56%.
Metabolism: Extensive, primarily by CYP 3A4 and CYP 2C19 to inactive metabolites.
Excretion: About 8% unchanged in urine. *Half-life:* 27 to 32 hours.

Route	Onset	Peak	Duration
P.O.	Unknown	5 hr	Unknown

Action

Chemical effect: May increase serotonergic activity in the CNS resulting from inhibition of neuronal reuptake of serotonin. Drug is the S-enantiomer of the racemic compound citalopram, which may be the active component.
Therapeutic effect: Relieves depressive symptoms and anxiety.

Available forms

Oral solution: 5 mg/5 ml
Tablets: 5 mg, 10 mg, 20 mg

NURSING PROCESS

☙ Assessment
● Obtain history of patient's medical condition before therapy.
● Closely monitor patients at high risk of suicide.

Reactions may be *common,* uncommon, *life-threatening*, or COMMON AND LIFE-THREATENING.

• Evaluate patient for history of drug abuse and observe for signs of misuse or abuse.
• Evaluate patient's and family's understanding of drug therapy.

🔷 Nursing diagnoses
• Ineffective individual coping related to underlying condition
• Risk for interrupted family processes related to underlying condition
• Deficient knowledge related to drug therapy

⟫ Planning and implementation
• In case of overdose, establish and maintain an airway, induce vomiting, and give activated charcoal. Closely observe and monitor vital signs and cardiac status, and maintain supportive care. Dialysis isn't effective; no known antidote exists.

Patient teaching
• Inform patient that symptoms will improve gradually over several weeks, rather than immediately.
• Tell patient to continue taking drug as prescribed even though improvement may occur within 1 to 4 weeks.
• Tell patient to use caution while driving or operating hazardous machinery because of drug's potential to impair judgment, thinking, or motor skills.
• Advise patient to consult prescriber before taking other prescription or OTC drugs.
• Tell patient that drug may be taken in the morning or evening without regard to meals.
• Encourage patient to avoid alcohol while taking drug.
• Tell patient to notify prescriber provider if she's pregnant or breast-feeding

☑ Evaluation
• Patient is able to carry out activities vital to usual role performance.
• Patient doesn't experience interrupted family processes.
• Patient and family state understanding of drug therapy.

---

esmolol hydrochloride
(EZ-moh-lohl high-droh-KLOR-ighd)
Brevibloc

Pharmacologic class: beta blocker
Therapeutic class: antiarrhythmic
Pregnancy risk category: C

Indications and dosages

▶ **Supraventricular tachycardia; control of ventricular rate in patients with atrial fibrillation or flutter in perioperative, postoperative, or other emergent circumstances; noncompensatory sinus tachycardia when heart rate requires specific interventions.** *Adults:* Loading dose is 500 mcg/kg/minute by I.V. infusion over 1 minute, followed by 4-minute maintenance infusion of 50 mcg/kg/minute. If adequate response doesn't occur within 5 minutes, loading dose is repeated and followed by maintenance infusion of 100 mcg/kg/minute for 4 minutes. Loading dose is repeated and maintenance infusion increased in stepwise manner, p.r.n. Maximum maintenance infusion for tachycardia is 200 mcg/kg/minute.
▶ **Management of perioperative and postoperative tachycardia or hypertension.** *Adults:* For perioperative treatment, 80 mg (about 1 mg/kg) I.V. bolus over 30 seconds, followed by 150 mcg/kg/minute I.V., if needed. Adjust infusion rate, p.r.n., to maximum of 300 mcg/kg/minute. Postoperative treatment is same as for supraventricular tachycardia, although dosages adequate for control may be as high as 300 mcg/kg/minute.

▽ I.V. administration
• Don't give by I.V. push; use infusion-control device. The 10-mg/ml single-dose vial may be used without diluting, but injection concentrate (250 mg/ml) must be diluted to no more than 10 mg/ml before infusion. Remove 20 ml from 500 ml of D_5W, lactated Ringer's solution, or half-normal or normal saline solution, and add two ampules of drug.
⚠ **ALERT:** Drug isn't compatible with 5% sodium bicarbonate injection, diazepam, furosemide, or thiopental sodium.
• Doses greater than 200 mcg/kg/minute aren't recommended.

• When patient's heart rate becomes stable, replace drug with a longer-acting antiarrhythmic, such as propranolol, digoxin, or verapamil; 30 minutes after giving first dose of replacement, reduce infusion rate of this drug by 50%. Monitor patient response, and if pulse is controlled for 1 hour after giving second dose of replacement, stop infusion.

• If local reaction develops at infusion site, change to another site. Avoid using butterfly needles.

• Don't abruptly stop drug because withdrawal effects may occur following chronic use. If immediate withdrawal is needed, use caution.

• Drug is intended for short-term use, no longer than 48 hours.

• Watch for irritation and infiltration; extravasation may cause tissue damage or necrosis.

Contraindications and precautions

• Contraindicated in patients with sinus bradycardia, heart block greater than first-degree, cardiogenic shock, or overt heart failure.

• Use cautiously in patients with impaired kidney function, diabetes, or bronchospasm.

⚖ **Lifespan:** In pregnant and breast-feeding women, use cautiously. In children, safety hasn't been established.

Adverse reactions

CNS: dizziness, somnolence, headache, agitation, fatigue, confusion.
CV: HYPOTENSION, peripheral ischemia.
EENT: nasal congestion.
GI: *nausea*, vomiting.
Respiratory: *bronchospasm,* wheezing, dyspnea.
Other: inflammation, induration at infusion site.

Interactions

Drug-drug. *Digoxin:* Esmolol may increase digoxin levels by 10% to 20%. Monitor digoxin levels.
Morphine: May increase esmolol levels. Adjust esmolol carefully.
Prazosin: May increase the risk of orthostatic hypotension in the early phases of use together. Assist patient to stand slowly until effects are known.

Reserpine, other catecholamine-depleting drugs: May cause additive bradycardia and hypotension. Adjust esmolol carefully.
Succinylcholine: Esmolol may prolong neuromuscular blockade. Monitor patient.
Verapamil: May increase the effects of both drugs. Monitor cardiac function closely and decrease dosages as needed.

Effects on lab test results

None reported.

Pharmacokinetics

Absorption: Administered I.V.
Distribution: Rapid; 55% protein-bound.
Metabolism: Rapid.
Excretion: By kidneys as metabolites. *Half-life:* About 9 minutes.

Route	Onset	Peak	Duration
I.V.	Immediate	30 min	< 30 min

Action

Chemical effect: Decreases heart rate, myocardial contractility, and blood pressure.
Therapeutic effect: Restores normal sinus rhythm.

Available forms

Injection: 10 mg/ml, 250 mg/ml

NURSING PROCESS

🕮 **Assessment**
• Obtain history of patient's arrhythmias before therapy.
• Monitor ECG and blood pressure continuously during infusion. Up to 50% of patients treated with esmolol develop hypotension. Monitor patient closely, especially if pretreatment blood pressure was low.
• Be alert for adverse reactions and drug interactions.
• Evaluate patient's and family's knowledge of drug therapy.

🕮 **Nursing diagnoses**
• Decreased cardiac output related to presence of arrhythmias
• Ineffective cerebral tissue perfusion related to drug-induced hypotension
• Deficient knowledge related to drug therapy

⫸ Planning and implementation

• If patient develops severe dose-related hypotension, decrease dose or stop infusion and immediately notify prescriber. Hypotension will reverse within 30 minutes.

• If patient develops symptoms of heart failure (shortness of breath, night cough, swelling of the limbs), notify prescriber.

Patient teaching

• Inform patient of need for continuous ECG, blood pressure, and heart rate monitoring to assess effectiveness of drug and detect adverse reactions.

☑ Evaluation

• Patient regains normal cardiac output with correction of arrhythmias.

• Patient's blood pressure remains normal throughout therapy.

• Patient and family state understanding of drug therapy.

esomeprazole magnesium
(e-soh-MEP-rah-zohl mag-NEEZ-ee-uhm)
Nexium

Pharmacologic class: proton pump inhibitor, s-isomer of omeprazole
Therapeutic class: gastroesophageal drug
Pregnancy risk category: B

Indications and dosages

▶ **Gastroesophageal reflux disease (GERD), healing of erosive esophagitis.** *Adults:* 20 or 40 mg P.O. daily for 4 to 8 weeks. If symptoms persist, treatment may be extended for an additional 4 to 8 weeks.

▶ **Long-term maintenance of healing in erosive esophagitis.** *Adults:* 20 mg P.O. daily for no more than 6 months.

▶ **Eradication of** *Helicobacter pylori* **to reduce duodenal ulcer recurrence.** *Adults:* Combination triple therapy with esomeprazole magnesium 40 mg P.O. daily plus amoxicillin 1,000 mg P.O. b.i.d. and clarithromycin 500 mg P.O. b.i.d., all for 10 days.

🜹 **Adjust-a-dose:** For patients with severe hepatic impairment, the maximum dose is 20 mg P.O. daily.

Contraindications and precautions

• Contraindicated in patients hypersensitive to any component of esomeprazole or omeprazole. Combination triple therapy for the eradication of *H. pylori* is contraindicated in patients hypersensitive to clarithromycin, macrolide antibiotics, amoxicillin, or penicillin.

• Use cautiously in patients with severe hepatic insufficiency.

⚖ **Lifespan:** In pregnant women, use only if clearly needed. In breast-feeding women, use cautiously because it's unknown whether drug appears in breast milk. In children, safety and effectiveness haven't been established.

Adverse reactions

CNS: headache.
GI: diarrhea, abdominal pain, nausea, flatulence, dry mouth, vomiting, constipation.

Interactions

Drug-drug. *Amoxicillin, clarithromycin:* Increases esomeprazole levels. Monitor patient for toxicity. Don't give clarithromycin and pimozide together.
Diazepam: Decreases diazepam clearance and increases levels of diazepam. Monitor patient for diazepam toxicity.
Digoxin, iron salts, ketoconazole: May interfere with drug absorption. Monitor patient closely.
Other drugs metabolized by CYP 2C19: Alters esomeprazole clearance. Monitor patient closely, especially elderly patient or patient with hepatic insufficiency.
Drug-food. *Any food:* Reduces bioavailability. Advise patient to take drug 1 hour before eating.

Effects on lab test results

• May increase creatinine, uric acid, bilirubin, alkaline phosphatase, ALT, AST potassium, sodium, thyroxine, and TSH levels.
• May increase hemoglobin, hematocrit, and WBC and platelet counts.

Pharmacokinetics

Absorption: Level peaks in 1½ hours. The level following a 40-mg dose is three times higher than after a 20-mg dose. Repeated daily dosing of 40 mg yields systemic bioavailability of 90% compared with a single 40-mg dose, which yields 64%. Giving drug with food reduces mean level by 33% to 53%.

Distribution: About 97% protein-bound.
Metabolism: Extensive in the liver by CYP 2C19 to form hydroxy and desmethyl metabolites. CYP 2C19 exhibits polymorphism. About 3% of whites and 15% to 20% of Asians who lack CYP 2C19 have decreased levels. CYP 3A4 metabolizes the remaining amount.
Excretion: Less than 1% of active parent drug is excreted in urine. About 80% of the drug is excreted as inactive metabolites in urine. Remaining inactive metabolites are excreted in feces. Systemic clearance of esomeprazole decreases with multiple-dose administration. *Half-life:* 1 to 1½ hours.

Route	Onset	Peak	Duration
P.O.	Unknown	1½ hr	13-17 hr

Action

Chemical effect: Suppresses gastric secretion through proton pump inhibition. Inhibits the H^+-K^+-ATPase pump in gastric parietal cells, thereby reducing gastric acidity by blocking the final step in acid production.
Therapeutic effect: Decreases gastric acid.

Available forms

Capsules (delayed-release containing enteric-coated pellets): 20 mg, 40 mg

NURSING PROCESS

Assessment

• Assess patient's condition before and during drug therapy.
• Monitor liver function test results because drug is extensively metabolized by cytochrome P450-2C19. Patients with hepatic insufficiency have a risk of increased liver function test results.
• Long-term therapy with omeprazole has caused atrophic gastritis. Be alert for adverse reactions.
• Evaluate patient's and family's knowledge of drug therapy.

Nursing diagnoses

• Impaired tissue integrity related to underlying gastroesophageal condition
• Imbalanced nutrition: Less than body requirements related to decreased oral intake due to underlying gastroesophageal disorder
• Deficient knowledge related to drug therapy

Planning and implementation

• Food decreases the extent of absorption; give esomeprazole at least 1 hour before meals.
• Overdosage may result in confusion, drowsiness, blurred vision, tachycardia, nausea, diaphoresis, dry mouth, and headache. Because drug isn't dialyzable, supportive care is recommended.
• Urge patient to avoid alcohol and foods that increase gastric secretions.
Patient teaching
• Tell patient to take drug exactly as prescribed and at least 1 hour before meals.
• If patient has trouble swallowing capsule, suggest that he open it, sprinkle contents into applesauce, and swallow applesauce immediately. Warn against crushing or chewing the drug pellets.
• Tell patient to report continued or worsened symptoms or any adverse reactions.

Evaluation

• Patient responds positively to drug therapy.
• Patient is able to tolerate liquids and foods orally without any nausea or vomiting.
• Patient and family state understanding of drug therapy.

estazolam
(eh-STAZ-uh-lam)
ProSom

Pharmacologic class: benzodiazepine
Therapeutic class: hypnotic
Pregnancy risk category: X
Controlled substance schedule: IV

Indications and dosages

▶ **Insomnia.** *Adults:* 1 mg P.O. h.s. Some patients may need 2 mg.
Elderly patients: 1 mg P.O. h.s. Use higher doses with care. Frail elderly or debilitated patients may take 0.5 mg, but this low dose may be only marginally effective.

Contraindications and precautions

• Contraindicated in patients hypersensitive to drug.
• Use cautiously in patients with hepatic, renal, or pulmonary disease; depression; or suicidal tendencies.

Reactions may be *common,* uncommon, *life-threatening*, or COMMON AND LIFE-THREATENING.

❄ **Lifespan:** In pregnant or breast-feeding women, drug is contraindicated. In children, safety hasn't been established.

Adverse reactions

CNS: fatigue, dizziness, *daytime drowsiness, somnolence, asthenia, hypokinesia,* headache, abnormal thinking.
GI: dyspepsia, abdominal pain.
Musculoskeletal: back pain, stiffness.

Interactions

Drug-drug. *Cimetidine, disulfiram, isoniazid, hormonal contraceptives:* May impair metabolism and clearance of benzodiazepines and prolong their half-life. Monitor patient for increased CNS depression.
CNS depressants, including antihistamines, opioid analgesics, and benzodiazepines: Increases CNS depression. Avoid using together.
Digoxin, phenytoin: Increases levels of these drugs, resulting in toxicity. Monitor levels closely.
Fluconazole, ketoconazole, itraconazole, miconazole: May increase and prolong drug level, CNS depression, and psychomotor impairment. Don't use together.
Rifampin: May increase metabolism and clearance and decrease half-life. Watch for decreased effectiveness.
Theophylline: May act as a drug antagonist. Watch for decreased effectiveness.
Drug-herb. *Catnip, kava, lady's slipper, lemon balm, passionflower, sassafras, skullcap, valerian:* Sedative effects may be enhanced. Discourage using together.
Drug-lifestyle. *Alcohol use:* Increases CNS and respiratory depression. Strongly discourage using together.
Smoking: May increase drug metabolism and clearance and decrease half-life. Monitor patient for decreased effectiveness.

Effects on lab test results

• May increase ALT and AST levels.

Pharmacokinetics

Absorption: Rapid and complete.
Distribution: 93% protein-bound.
Metabolism: Extensive.
Excretion: Metabolites excreted primarily in urine. Less than 5% excreted in urine as unchanged drug; 4% of 2-mg dose excreted in feces. *Half-life:* 10 to 24 hours.

Route	Onset	Peak	Duration
P.O.	Unknown	1-3 hr	Unknown

Action

Chemical effect: May act on limbic system and thalamus of CNS by binding to specific benzodiazepine receptors.
Therapeutic effect: Promotes sleep.

Available forms

Tablets: 1 mg, 2 mg

NURSING PROCESS

🔖 **Assessment**
• Obtain history of patient's sleep pattern before therapy and reassess regularly.
• Monitor liver and kidney function and CBC periodically during long-term therapy.
• Be alert for adverse reactions and drug interactions.
• Watch for possible withdrawal symptoms. Patients who receive 6 weeks of continuous therapy may experience withdrawal symptoms if drug is stopped suddenly.
• Evaluate patient's and family's knowledge of drug therapy.

✦ **Nursing diagnoses**
• Disturbed sleep pattern related to underlying condition
• Risk for trauma related to drug-induced adverse CNS reactions
• Deficient knowledge related to drug therapy

▷ **Planning and implementation**
• Before leaving bedside, make sure patient has swallowed drug.
• Take precautions to prevent hoarding by depressed, suicidal, or drug-dependent patient or patient who has history of drug abuse.
Patient teaching
• Tell patient not to increase dosage of drug but to inform prescriber if he thinks that drug is no longer effective.
• Warn patient to avoid hazardous activities that require mental alertness or physical coordination. For inpatient (particularly elderly patient), supervise walking and raise side rails.

• Warn patient that additive depressant effects can occur if alcohol is consumed while taking drug or within 24 hours afterward.

• If patient uses a hormonal contraceptive, recommend an alternative birth-control method during therapy because drug may enhance contraceptive hormone metabolism and decrease its effect.

☑ **Evaluation**

• Patient is able to sleep.

• Patient's safety is maintained.

• Patient and family state understanding of drug therapy.

estradiol (oestradiol)

(eh-struh-DIGH-ol)
Alora, Climara, Dermestril ◇ **, Esclim, Estrace, Estrace Vaginal Cream, Estraderm, Estraderm MX** ◇ **, Estring, FemPatch, Femtran** ◇ **, Gynodiol, Menorest** ◇ **, Oesclim** ♦ **, Vivelle, Vivelle-Dot**

estradiol acetate
Femring Vaginal Ring

estradiol cypionate
Depo-Estradiol

estradiol hemihydrate
Estrasorb, Vagifem

estradiol valerate (oestradiol valerate)
Delestrogen

Pharmacologic class: estrogen
Therapeutic class: estrogen replacement, antineoplastic
Pregnancy risk category: X

Indications and dosages

▶ **Vasomotor symptoms, vulvar and vaginal atrophy, hypoestrogenism from hypogonadism, castration, or primary ovarian failure.** *Adults:* 1 to 2 mg estradiol P.O. daily in cycles of 21 days on and 7 days off or cycles of 5 days on and 2 days off. Or, 0.025-mg/day Esclim system applied to a clean, dry area of the trunk twice weekly. Adjust dose, if needed, after the first 2 or 3 weeks of therapy, then 3 to 6 months p.r.n. Or, 1 Estraderm transdermal system delivering 0.05 mg/24 hours applied twice weekly. Or, as a Vivelle system delivering either 0.05 mg/24 hours or 0.0375 mg/24 hours applied twice weekly. Or, as a Climara system delivering 0.05 mg/24 hours or 0.1 mg/24 hours applied once weekly in cycles of 3 weeks on and 1 week off. Or, 1 to 5 mg estradiol cypionate I.M. q 3 to 4 weeks. Or, 10 to 20 mg estradiol valerate I.M. q 4 weeks, p.r.n.

▶ **Atrophic vaginitis, kraurosis vulvae.** *Women:* 2 to 4 g estradiol intravaginal applications of cream daily for 1 to 2 weeks. When vaginal mucosa is restored, maintenance dosage of 1 g one to three times weekly in cyclic regimen. Or, 0.05 mg/24 hours Climara applied weekly in a cyclic regimen. Or, 0.05 mg/24 hours Estraderm applied twice weekly in a cyclic regimen. Or, 10 to 20 mg estradiol valerate I.M. q 4 weeks, p.r.n.

▶ **Palliative treatment for advanced, inoperable breast cancer.** *Men and postmenopausal women:* 10 mg estradiol P.O. t.i.d. for 3 months.

▶ **Palliative treatment for advanced inoperable prostate cancer.** *Men:* 1 to 2 mg estradiol P.O. t.i.d. Or, 30 mg estradiol valerate I.M. q 1 to 2 weeks.

▶ **Prevention of postmenopausal osteoporosis in high-risk patients.** *Women:* 0.025 mg/day Vivelle, Vivelle-Dot, or Alora or 0.5 mg/day Estraderm applied to a clean, dry area of the trunk twice weekly. Or, 0.025 mg/day Climara patch applied once weekly in a continuous regimen.

▶ **Vasomotor symptoms.** *Adults:* 0.05 mg/day Climara patch applied once weekly in a continuous regimen.

Contraindications and precautions

• Contraindicated in patients with thrombophlebitis, thromboembolic disorders, estrogen-dependent neoplasia, breast or reproductive organ cancer (except as palliative treatment), or undiagnosed abnormal genital bleeding. Also contraindicated in patients with history of thrombophlebitis or thromboembolic disorders linked to estrogen use (except as palliative treatment of breast and prostate cancer).

• Use cautiously in patients with cerebrovascular or coronary artery disease, asthma, bone diseases, migraine, seizures, or cardiac, hepatic, or renal dysfunction and in women with strong family history of breast cancer or who have breast nodules, fibrocystic disease, or abnormal mammogram findings.

⚡ **Lifespan:** In pregnant and breast-feeding women, drug is contraindicated. In children, drug shouldn't be used.

Adverse reactions

CNS: headache, dizziness, chorea, depression, *seizures.*
CV: thrombophlebitis, *thromboembolism,* hypertension, edema.
EENT: worsening of myopia or astigmatism, intolerance of contact lenses.
GI: *nausea,* vomiting, abdominal cramps, bloating, diarrhea, constipation, *pancreatitis.*
GU: breakthrough bleeding, altered menstrual flow, dysmenorrhea, amenorrhea, *increased risk of endometrial cancer,* cervical erosion, altered cervical secretions, enlargement of uterine fibromas, vaginal candidiasis, testicular atrophy, impotence.
Hepatic: cholestatic jaundice, gallbladder disease, *hepatic adenoma.*
Metabolic: increased appetite, weight changes, hyperglycemia, hypercalcemia.
Skin: melasma, urticaria, erythema nodosum, dermatitis, hair loss.
Other: *possibility of increased risk of breast cancer,* breast changes (tenderness, enlargement, secretion), gynecomastia.

Interactions

Drug-drug. *Bromocriptine:* May cause amenorrhea, interfering with bromocriptine effects. Avoid using together.
Carbamazepine, phenobarbital, rifampin: Decreases effectiveness of estrogen therapy. Monitor patient closely.
Corticosteroids: May enhance effects. Monitor patient closely.
Cyclosporine: Increases risk of toxicity. Use together with caution, and frequently monitor cyclosporine levels.
Dantrolene, other hepatotoxic drugs: Increases risk of hepatotoxicity. Monitor patient closely.
Oral anticoagulants: May decrease anticoagulant effects. Dosage adjustments may be needed. Monitor PT and INR.
Tamoxifen: Estrogens may interfere with effectiveness of tamoxifen. Avoid using together.
Drug-food. *Caffeine:* May increase caffeine levels. Monitor effects.

Drug-lifestyle. *Smoking:* Increases risk of CV effects. If smoking continues, may need alternative therapy; urge patient to stop smoking.

Effects on lab test results

• May increase total T_4, thyroid-binding globulin, triglyceride, and clotting factor VII, VIII, IX, and X levels.
• May increase PT and norepinephrine-induced platelet aggregation.

Pharmacokinetics

Absorption: Well absorbed but substantially inactivated by liver after P.O. use. Rapid and lasts days after I.M. use. Readily into systemic circulation after transdermal use.
Distribution: Highest levels in fat. About 50% to 80% protein-bound.
Metabolism: Primarily in liver.
Excretion: Primarily through kidneys. *Half-life:* Unknown.

Route	Onset	Peak	Duration
P.O., I.M., intravaginal	Unknown	Unknown	Unknown
Transdermal Esclim	Unknown	27-30 hr	Unknown

Action

Chemical effect: Increases synthesis of DNA, RNA, and protein and reduces release of follicle-stimulating hormone and luteinizing hormone from pituitary gland.
Therapeutic effect: Relieves vasomotor menopausal symptoms, provides estrogen replacement, relieves vaginal dryness, and palliates advanced prostate or breast cancer.

Available forms

estradiol
Tablets (micronized): 0.5 mg, 1 mg, 1.5 mg, 2 mg
Transdermal: 0.025 mg/24 hours, 0.0375 mg/24 hours, 0.05 mg/24 hours, 0.06 mg/day, 0.075 mg/24 hours, 0.1 mg/24 hours
Vaginal cream (in nonliquefying base): 0.01%
Vaginal ring: 0.0075 mg/24 hours
estradiol acetate
Vaginal ring: 0.05 mg/24 hours, 0.1 mg/24 hours
estradiol cypionate
Injection (in oil): 5 mg/ml

estradiol hemihydrate
Topical emulsion: 4.35 mg hemihydrate/1.74 g;
3.48 g of emulsion delivers 0.05 mg estradiol/
day
Vaginal tablets: 25 mcg
estradiol valerate
Injection (in oil): 10 mg/ml, 20 mg/ml,
40 mg/ml

NURSING PROCESS

📖 Assessment
• Obtain history of patient's underlying condition before therapy and reassess regularly.
• Make sure patient has thorough physical examination before starting estrogen therapy.
• Ask patient about allergies, especially to foods or plants. Estradiol is available as aqueous solution or as solution in peanut oil; estradiol cypionate, as solution in cottonseed oil or vegetable oil; estradiol valerate, as solution in castor oil, sesame oil, or vegetable oil.
• Patient receiving long-term therapy will have yearly examinations. Periodically monitor lipid level, blood pressure, body weight, and liver function.
• Evaluate patient's and family's knowledge of drug therapy.

🔃 Nursing diagnoses
• Ineffective health maintenance related to underlying condition
• Ineffective tissue perfusion (cerebral, peripheral, pulmonary, or myocardial) related to drug-induced thromboembolism
• Deficient knowledge related to drug therapy

▶ Planning and implementation
• Give oral drug at mealtimes or h.s. (for once-daily dose) to minimize nausea.
• To give as I.M. injection, make sure drug is well-dispersed in solution by rolling vial between palms. Inject deep into large muscle. Rotate injection sites to prevent muscle atrophy. Never give drug I.V.
• Apply transdermal patch to clean, dry, hairless, intact skin on abdomen or buttocks. Don't apply to breasts, waistline, or other areas where clothing can loosen patch. When applying, ensure good contact with skin, especially around edges, and hold in place with palm for about 10 seconds. Rotate application sites.

• Begin transdermal patch 1 week after withdrawal of oral therapy, or sooner if menopausal symptoms appear before end of week.
• Because of risk of thromboembolism, stop therapy at least 1 month before procedures that increase risk of prolonged immobilization or thromboembolism, such as knee or hip surgery. If you suspect thromboembolism, withhold drug and notify prescriber.
⚡ **ALERT:** Estrogen preparations aren't interchangeable.

Patient teaching
• Inform patient about adverse effects of estrogen.
• Emphasize importance of regular physical examinations. Postmenopausal women who use estrogen replacement for more than 5 years may be at increased risk for endometrial cancer. Tell patient that risk is reduced by using cyclic rather than continuous therapy and lowest possible dosages of estrogen. Adding progestins to regimen decreases risk of endometrial hyperplasia; it's unknown if progestins affect risk of endometrial carcinoma. Drug probably doesn't increase risk of breast cancer.
• Teach patient how to use vaginal cream. Tell her to wash vaginal area with soap and water before applying. Tell her to apply drug h.s. or to lie flat for 30 minutes after application to minimize drug loss.
• Warn patient to immediately report abdominal pain; pain, numbness, or stiffness in legs or buttocks; pressure or pain in chest; shortness of breath; severe headaches; visual disturbances, such as blind spots, flashing lights, or blurriness; vaginal bleeding or discharge; breast lumps; swelling of hands or feet; yellow skin or sclera; dark urine; and light-colored stools.
• Explain to patient receiving cyclic therapy for postmenopausal symptoms that, although withdrawal bleeding may occur during week off drug, fertility hasn't been restored. Pregnancy can't occur because she hasn't ovulated.
• Tell diabetic patient to report elevated glucose level and adjust antidiabetic dosage.
• Teach woman how to perform routine breast self-examination.

✅ Evaluation
• Patient shows improvement in underlying condition.
• Patient has no thromboembolic event during therapy.

• Patient and family state understanding of drug therapy.

estrogens, conjugated (estrogenic substances, conjugated; oestrogens, conjugated)
(ES-troh-jenz, KAHN-jih-gayt-ed)
C.E.S. ♦, Cenestin, Premarin, Premarin Intravenous

Pharmacologic class: estrogen
Therapeutic class: estrogen replacement, antineoplastic, antiosteoporotic
Pregnancy risk category: X

Indications and dosages

▶ **Abnormal uterine bleeding caused by hormonal imbalance.** *Women:* 25 mg I.V. or I.M. Repeat dose in 6 to 12 hours, if needed.
▶ **Vulvar or vaginal atrophy.** *Women:* 0.5 to 2 g cream intravaginally once daily in cycles of 3 weeks on, 1 week off. Or, 0.3 mg P.O. daily.
▶ **Castration, primary ovarian failure.** *Adults:* Initially, 1.25 mg P.O. daily in cycles of 3 weeks on, 1 week off. Adjust dose p.r.n.
▶ **Hypogonadism.** *Women:* 0.3 to 0.625 mg P.O. daily, given cyclically 3 weeks on, 1 week off.
▶ **Moderate to severe vasomotor symptoms with or without moderate to severe symptoms of vulvar and vaginal atrophy related to the menopause.** *Women:* 0.3 mg P.O. daily, or cyclically 25 days on, 5 days off.
▶ **Palliative treatment for inoperable prostatic cancer.** *Men:* 1.25 to 2.5 mg P.O. t.i.d.
▶ **Palliative treatment for breast cancer.** *Adults:* 10 mg P.O. t.i.d. for 3 months or more.
▶ **Prevention of osteoporosis.** *Adults:* 0.3 to 0.625 mg P.O. daily, or cyclically, 25 days on, 5 days off.

▽ I.V. administration

• Refrigerate before reconstituting. Agitate gently after adding diluent.
• Withdraw 5 ml of air from vial before adding diluent. Gently agitate to mix drug. Avoid shaking container.
• Reconstitute powder for injection with diluent provided (sterile water for injection with benzyl alcohol).

• Avoid mixing with solutions of acidic pH to prevent incompatibility.
• When giving by direct I.V. injection, give slowly to avoid flushing.

Contraindications and precautions

• Contraindicated in patients with thrombophlebitis, thromboembolic disorders, estrogendependent neoplasia, breast or reproductive organ cancer (except for palliative treatment), or undiagnosed abnormal genital bleeding.
• Use cautiously in patients with cerebrovascular or coronary artery disease, asthma, bone disease, migraine, seizures, or cardiac, hepatic, or renal dysfunction and in women with close family history of breast or genital tract cancer or who have breast nodules, fibrocystic disease, or abnormal mammogram findings.
⑤ **ALERT:** Don't use estrogens and progestins to prevent CV disease. Drug may increase risks of MI, CVA, invasive breast cancer, pulmonary emboli, and deep vein thrombosis in postmenopausal women undergoing 5 years of combination therapy. Because of these risks, drug should be given at the lowest effective doses and for the shortest duration possible.
≝ **Lifespan:** In pregnant and breast-feeding women, drug is contraindicated. In children, drug shouldn't be used.

Adverse reactions

CNS: headache, dizziness, chorea, depression, lethargy, *seizures.*
CV: thrombophlebitis; *thromboembolism;* hypertension; edema; *increased risk of CVA, pulmonary embolism, and MI.*
EENT: worsening of myopia or astigmatism, intolerance of contact lenses.
GI: *nausea,* vomiting, abdominal cramps, bloating, diarrhea, constipation, anorexia, *pancreatitis.*
GU: breakthrough bleeding, altered menstrual flow, dysmenorrhea, amenorrhea, *increased risk of endometrial cancer,* cervical erosion, altered cervical secretions, enlargement of uterine fibromas, vaginal candidiasis, testicular atrophy, impotence.
Hepatic: gallbladder disease, cholestatic jaundice, *hepatic adenoma.*
Metabolic: increased appetite, weight changes, hyperglycemia, hypercalcemia.

Skin: melasma, urticaria, erythema nodosum, dermatitis, flushing (with rapid I.V. administration), hirsutism, hair loss.
Other: breast changes (tenderness, enlargement, secretion), *possibility of increased risk of breast cancer,* gynecomastia.

Interactions

Drug-drug. *Bromocriptine:* May cause amenorrhea, interfering with bromocriptine effects. Avoid using together.
Carbamazepine, phenobarbital, rifampin: Decreases estrogen effectiveness. Monitor patient closely.
Corticosteroids: Possible enhanced effects. Monitor patient closely.
Cyclosporine: Increases risk of toxicity. Use together with caution, and frequently monitor cyclosporine levels.
Dantrolene, other hepatotoxic drugs: Increases risk of hepatotoxicity. Monitor patient closely.
Oral anticoagulants: May decrease anticoagulant effects. Dosage adjustments may be needed. Monitor PT and INR.
Tamoxifen: Estrogens may interfere with effectiveness of tamoxifen. Avoid using together.
Drug-food. *Caffeine:* May increase caffeine levels. Monitor effects.
Drug-lifestyle. *Smoking:* Increases risk of CV effects. If smoking continues, patient may need alternative therapy. Urge patient to stop smoking.

Effects on lab test results

• May increase glucose, calcium, total T_4, thyroid-binding globulin, phospholipid, triglyceride, and clotting factor VII, VII, IX, and X levels.
• May increase PT and norepinephrine-induced platelet aggregation.

Pharmacokinetics

Absorption: Rapid, continuing for days after I.M. use.
Distribution: Highest levels in fat; about 50% to 80% protein-bound.
Metabolism: Primarily in liver.
Excretion: Majority through kidneys. *Half-life:* Unknown.

Route	Onset	Peak	Duration
All routes	Unknown	Unknown	Unknown

Action

Chemical effect: Increases synthesis of DNA, RNA, and protein in responsive tissues; also reduces release of follicle-stimulating hormone and luteinizing hormone from pituitary gland.
Therapeutic effect: Provides estrogen replacement, relieves vasomotor menopausal symptoms and vaginal dryness, helps prevent severity of osteoporosis, and provides palliative action for prostate and breast cancer.

Available forms

Injection: 25 mg/5 ml
Tablets: 0.3 mg, 0.45 mg, 0.625 mg, 0.9 mg, 1.25 mg
Vaginal cream: 0.625 mg/g

NURSING PROCESS

⚕ Assessment
• Obtain history of patient's underlying condition before therapy and reassess regularly.
• Make sure patient has thorough physical examination before starting estrogen therapy.
• Patient receiving long-term therapy will have yearly examinations. Periodically monitor lipid levels, blood pressure, body weight, and liver function.
• Be alert for adverse reactions and drug interactions.
• Evaluate patient's and family's knowledge of drug therapy.

⊕ Nursing diagnoses
• Ineffective health maintenance related to underlying condition
• Ineffective tissue perfusion (cerebral, peripheral, pulmonary, or myocardial) related to drug-induced thromboembolism
• Deficient knowledge related to drug therapy

▷ Planning and implementation
• Give oral forms at mealtimes or h.s. (for once-daily dose) to minimize nausea.
• When giving I.M., inject deep into large muscle. Rotate injection sites to prevent muscle atrophy.
• Use I.M. or I.V. for rapid treatment of dysfunctional uterine bleeding or to reduce surgical bleeding.
• Because of risk of thromboembolism, stop therapy at least 1 month before procedures that may cause prolonged immobilization or throm-

---

Reactions may be *common*, uncommon, *life-threatening*, or COMMON AND LIFE-THREATENING.

boembolism, such as knee or hip surgery. If thromboembolism is suspected, withhold drug, notify prescriber, and provide supportive care.

⑤ **ALERT:** Estrogens aren't interchangeable.

Patient teaching

• Inform patient about adverse effects.

• Emphasize importance of regular physical examinations. Postmenopausal women using drug for more than 5 years may be at increased risk for endometrial carcinoma, which is reduced by using cyclic rather than continuous therapy and lowest possible dosages. Adding progestins to regimen decreases risk of endometrial hyperplasia; it's unknown if progestins decrease or increase risk of endometrial cancer. Drug probably doesn't increase risk of breast cancer.

• Teach patient how to use vaginal cream. Tell her to wash vaginal area with soap and water before applying. Tell her to apply drug h.s. or to lie flat for 30 minutes after application to minimize drug loss.

• Explain to patient on cyclic therapy for postmenopausal symptoms that, although withdrawal bleeding may occur during week off drug, fertility hasn't been restored. Pregnancy can't occur because she hasn't ovulated.

• Warn patient to immediately report abdominal pain; pain, numbness, or stiffness in legs or buttocks; pressure or pain in chest; shortness of breath; severe headaches; visual disturbances, such as blind spots, flashing lights, or blurriness; vaginal bleeding or discharge; breast lumps; swelling of hands or feet; yellow skin or sclera; dark urine; and light-colored stools.

• Tell diabetic patient to report elevated glucose test results so antidiabetic dosage can be adjusted.

• Teach woman how to perform routine breast self-examination.

☑ **Evaluation**

• Patient shows improvement in underlying condition.

• Patient has no thromboembolic event during therapy.

• Patient and family state understanding of drug therapy.

estrogens, esterified
(ES-troh-jenz, ES-ter-eh-fighd)
Estratab, Menest, Neo-Estrone†

Pharmacologic class: estrogen
Therapeutic class: antineoplastic
Pregnancy risk category: X

Indications and dosages

▶ **Inoperable prostate cancer.** *Men:* 1.25 to 2.5 mg P.O. t.i.d.

▶ **Breast cancer.** *Men and postmenopausal women:* 10 mg P.O. t.i.d. for 3 or more months.

▶ **Hypogonadism.** *Women:* 2.5 to 7.5 mg P.O. daily in divided doses in cycles of 20 days on, 10 days off.

▶ **Castration, primary ovarian failure.** *Women:* 2.5 mg P.O. daily to t.i.d. in cycles of 3 weeks on, 1 week off.

▶ **Vasomotor menopausal symptoms.** *Women:* Average dosage is 1.25 mg P.O. daily in cycles of 3 weeks on, 1 week off.

▶ **Atrophic vaginitis or urethritis.** *Women:* 0.3 to 1.25 mg P.O. daily in cycles of 3 weeks on, 1 week off.

▶ **Prevention of osteoporosis.** *Women:* Initially, 0.3 mg P.O. daily; may be increased to maximum 1.25 mg daily.

Contraindications and precautions

• Contraindicated in patients with breast cancer (except metastatic disease), estrogen-dependent neoplasia, active thrombophlebitis or thromboembolic disorders, undiagnosed abnormal genital bleeding, hypersensitivity to drug, or history of thromboembolic disease.

• Use cautiously in patients with history of hypertension, depression, cardiac or renal dysfunction, liver impairment, bone diseases, migraine, seizures, or diabetes mellitus.

⚠ **Lifespan:** In pregnant or breast-feeding women, drug is contraindicated. In children, drug shouldn't be used.

Adverse reactions

CNS: headache, dizziness, chorea, depression, lethargy, *seizures.*

CV: thrombophlebitis; *thromboembolism;* hypertension; edema; *increased risk of CVA, pulmonary embolism, and MI.*

EENT: worsening of myopia or astigmatism, intolerance of contact lenses.
GI: *nausea,* vomiting, abdominal cramps, bloating, diarrhea, constipation, anorexia, ***pancreatitis.***
GU: breakthrough bleeding, altered menstrual flow, dysmenorrhea, amenorrhea, *possibility of increased risk of breast cancer, increased risk of endometrial cancer,* cervical erosion, altered cervical secretions, enlargement of uterine fibromas, vaginal candidiasis, testicular atrophy, impotence.
Hepatic: cholestatic jaundice, *hepatic adenoma,* gallbladder disease.
Metabolic: increased appetite, weight changes, hypercalcemia.
Skin: melasma, rash, erythema nodosum, dermatitis, hirsutism, hair loss.
Other: gynecomastia, breast changes (tenderness, enlargement, secretion).

Interactions

Drug-drug. *Bromocriptine:* May cause amenorrhea, interfering with bromocriptine effects. Avoid using together.
Carbamazepine, phenobarbital, rifampin: Decreases effectiveness of estrogen therapy. Monitor patient closely.
Corticosteroids: Possible enhanced effects. Monitor patient closely.
Cyclosporine: Increases risk of toxicity. Use together with caution and frequently monitor cyclosporine levels.
Dantrolene, other hepatotoxic drugs: Increases risk of hepatotoxicity. Monitor patient closely.
Oral anticoagulants: May increase anticoagulant effect. Dosage adjustments may be needed. Monitor PT and INR and monitor patient for bleeding.
Tamoxifen: Estrogens may interfere with effectiveness of tamoxifen. Avoid using together.
Drug-food. *Caffeine:* May increase caffeine levels. Monitor effects.
Drug-lifestyle. *Smoking:* Increases risk of CV effects. Urge patient to stop smoking. If smoking continues, patient may need alternative therapy.

Effects on lab test results

• May increase calcium and clotting factor VII, VIII, IX, and X levels.
• May increase PT and norepinephrine-induced platelet aggregation.

Pharmacokinetics

Absorption: Well absorbed but substantially inactivated by liver.
Distribution: Highest levels in fat; about 50% to 80% protein-bound.
Metabolism: Primarily in liver.
Excretion: Primarily by kidneys. *Half-life:* Unknown.

Route	Onset	Peak	Duration
P.O.	Unknown	Unknown	Unknown

Action

Chemical effect: Increases synthesis of DNA, RNA, and protein and reduces release of follicle-stimulating hormone and luteinizing hormone from pituitary gland.
Therapeutic effect: Provides estrogen replacement, hinders prostate and breast cancer cell growth, and relieves vasomotor menopausal symptoms and vaginal dryness.

Available forms

Tablets: 0.3 mg, 0.625 mg, 1.25 mg, 2.5 mg
Tablets (film-coated): 0.3 mg, 0.625 mg, 1.25 mg, 2.5 mg

NURSING PROCESS

Assessment

• Obtain history of patient's underlying condition before therapy, and reassess regularly thereafter.
• Make sure patient has thorough physical examination before starting drug therapy.
• Patient receiving long-term therapy will have yearly examinations. Periodically monitor lipid levels, blood pressure, body weight, and liver function.
• Be alert for adverse reactions and drug interactions.
• Evaluate patient's and family's knowledge of drug therapy.

Nursing diagnoses

• Ineffective health maintenance related to underlying condition
• Ineffective tissue perfusion (cerebral, peripheral, pulmonary, or myocardial) related to drug-induced thromboembolism
• Deficient knowledge related to drug therapy

⟩ Planning and implementation

• Give oral forms at mealtimes or bedtime (for once-daily dose) to minimize nausea.

• Because of risk of thromboembolism, stop therapy at least 1 month before procedures that may cause prolonged immobilization or thromboembolism, such as knee or hip surgery. If thromboembolism is suspected, withhold drug, notify prescriber, and provide supportive care.

Ⓧ ALERT: Estrogens aren't interchangeable.

Patient teaching

• Inform patient about adverse effects.

• Emphasize importance of regular physical examinations. Postmenopausal women who use drug for more than 5 years for menopausal symptoms may be at increased risk for endometrial carcinoma, which is reduced by using cyclic rather than continuous therapy and lowest possible dosages of estrogen. Adding progestins to regimen decreases risk of endometrial hyperplasia; it's unknown if progestins increase or decrease risk of endometrial cancer. Drug probably doesn't increase risk of breast cancer.

• Explain to patient on cyclic therapy for postmenopausal symptoms that although withdrawal bleeding may occur during week off drug, fertility hasn't been restored. Pregnancy can't occur because she hasn't ovulated.

• Warn patient to immediately report abdominal pain; pain, numbness, or stiffness in legs or buttocks; pressure or pain in chest; shortness of breath; severe headaches; visual disturbances, such as blind spots, flashing lights, or blurriness; vaginal bleeding or discharge; breast lumps; swelling of hands or feet; yellow skin or sclera; dark urine; and light-colored stools.

• Tell diabetic patient to report elevated glucose test results so antidiabetic dosage can be adjusted.

• Teach woman how to perform routine breast self-examination.

☑ Evaluation

• Patient shows improvement in underlying condition.

• Patient has no thromboembolic event during therapy.

• Patient and family state understanding of drug therapy.

estropipate (piperazine estrone sulfate)
(es-troh-PIH-payt)
Ogen, Ortho-Est

Pharmacologic class: estrogen
Therapeutic class: estrogen replacement
Pregnancy risk category: X

Indications and dosages

⟩ **Management of moderate-to-severe vasomotor symptoms, vulvar and vaginal atrophy.** *Women:* 0.75 to 6 mg P.O. daily 3 weeks on, 1 week off, or 2 to 4 g of vaginal cream daily. Typically, dosage given on cyclic, short-term basis.

⟩ **Primary ovarian failure, castration, hypogonadism.** *Women:* Given on cyclic basis—1.5 to 9 mg P.O. daily for first 3 weeks, followed by rest period of 8 to 10 days. If bleeding doesn't occur by end of rest period, repeat cycle.

⟩ **Prevention of osteoporosis.** *Women:* 0.625 mg P.O. daily for 25 days of 31-day cycle. Regimen may be repeated p.r.n.

Contraindications and precautions

• Contraindicated in patients with active thrombophlebitis, thromboembolic disorders, estrogen-dependent neoplasia, undiagnosed genital bleeding, or breast, reproductive organ, or genital cancer.

• Use cautiously in patients with cerebrovascular or coronary artery disease, asthma, depression, bone disease, migraine, seizures, or cardiac, hepatic, or renal dysfunction and in women with family history (mother, grandmother, sister) of breast or genital tract cancer or who have breast nodules, fibrocystic disease, or abnormal mammogram findings.

☀ Lifespan: In pregnant and breast-feeding women, drug is contraindicated. In children, drug shouldn't be used.

Adverse reactions

CNS: depression, headache, dizziness, migraine, *seizures.*
CV: edema; thrombophlebitis; *increased risk of CVA, pulmonary embolism, thromboembolism, and MI.*

GI: nausea, vomiting, abdominal cramps, bloating.
GU: increased size of uterine fibromas, *increased risk of endometrial cancer, possibility of increased risk of breast cancer,* vaginal candidiasis, cystitis-like syndrome, dysmenorrhea, amenorrhea, breakthrough bleeding.
Hepatic: cholestatic jaundice.
Metabolic: hypercalcemia, weight changes.
Skin: hemorrhagic eruption, erythema nodosum, *erythema multiforme,* hirsutism, melasma, hair loss.
Other: breast engorgement or enlargement, libido changes, aggravation of porphyria.

Interactions

Drug-drug. *Bromocriptine:* May cause amenorrhea, interfering with bromocriptine effects. Avoid using together.
Carbamazepine, phenobarbital, rifampin: Decreases effectiveness of estrogen therapy. Monitor patient closely.
Corticosteroids: Possible enhanced effects. Monitor patient closely.
Cyclosporine: Increases risk of toxicity. Use together with caution and frequently monitor cyclosporine levels.
Dantrolene, other hepatotoxic drugs: Increases risk of hepatotoxicity. Monitor patient closely.
Oral anticoagulants: May decrease anticoagulant effects. Dosage adjustments may be needed. Monitor PT and INR.
Tamoxifen: Estrogens may interfere with effectiveness of tamoxifen. Avoid using together.
Drug-food. *Caffeine:* May increase caffeine levels. Monitor effects.
Drug-lifestyle. *Smoking:* Increases risk of CV effects. Urge patient to stop smoking. If smoking continues, patient may need alternate therapy.

Effects on lab test results

• May increase calcium, total T_4, thyroid-binding globulin, phospholipid, triglyceride, and clotting factor VII, VIII, IX, and X levels.
• May increase PT and norepinephrine-induced platelet aggregation.

Pharmacokinetics

Absorption: Not well characterized after P.O. or intravaginal administration.
Distribution: Highest levels in fat; about 50% to 80% protein-bound.

Metabolism: Primarily in liver.
Excretion: Primarily by kidneys. *Half-life:* Unknown.

Route	Onset	Peak	Duration
P.O., intra-vaginal	Unknown	Unknown	Unknown

Action

Chemical effect: Increases synthesis of DNA, RNA, and protein and reduces release of follicle-stimulating hormone and luteinizing hormone from pituitary gland.
Therapeutic effect: Provides estrogen replacement, relieves vasomotor menopausal symptoms, and helps reduce severity of osteoporosis.

Available forms

Tablets: 0.75 mg, 1.5 mg, 3 mg, 6 mg
Vaginal cream: 1.5 mg/g (0.15%)

NURSING PROCESS

Assessment

• Obtain history of patient's underlying condition before therapy, and reassess regularly.
• Make sure patient has thorough physical examination before starting drug therapy.
• Patient receiving long-term therapy will have yearly examinations. Periodically monitor lipid levels, blood pressure, body weight, and liver function.
• Be alert for adverse reactions and drug interactions.
• Evaluate patient's and family's knowledge of drug therapy.

Nursing diagnoses

• Ineffective health maintenance related to underlying condition
• Ineffective tissue perfusion (cerebral, peripheral, pulmonary, or myocardial) related to drug-induced thromboembolism
• Deficient knowledge related to drug therapy

Planning and implementation

• Give oral forms with meals or h.s. (for once-daily dose) to minimize nausea.
• Because of risk of thromboembolism, stop therapy at least 1 month before procedures that may cause prolonged immobilization or thromboembolism, such as knee or hip surgery. If

---

thromboembolism is suspected, withhold drug, notify prescriber, and provide supportive care.

⊛ **ALERT:** Estrogens aren't interchangeable.

Patient teaching

• Inform patient about adverse effects.

• Emphasize importance of regular physical examinations. Postmenopausal women who use drug for more than 5 years may be at increased risk for endometrial carcinoma, which is reduced by using cyclic rather than continuous therapy and lowest possible dosages. Adding progestins to regimen decreases risk of endometrial hyperplasia; it's unknown if progestins increase or decrease risk of endometrial cancer. Drug probably doesn't increase risk of breast cancer.

• Teach patient how to use vaginal cream. Tell her to wash vaginal area with soap and water before applying. Tell her to use drug h.s. or to lie flat for 30 minutes after application to minimize drug loss.

• Explain to patient on cyclic therapy for postmenopausal symptoms that, although withdrawal bleeding may occur during week off drug, fertility hasn't been restored. Pregnancy can't occur because she hasn't ovulated.

• Explain to patient being treated for hypogonadism that therapy length depends on her endometrial response to drug. If satisfactory withdrawal bleeding doesn't occur, oral progestin may be added to regimen. Explain to patient that despite return of withdrawal bleeding, pregnancy can't occur because she isn't ovulating.

• Warn patient to immediately report abdominal pain; pain, numbness, or stiffness in legs or buttocks; pressure or pain in chest; shortness of breath; severe headaches; visual disturbances, such as blind spots, flashing lights, or blurriness; vaginal bleeding or discharge; breast lumps; swelling of hands or feet; yellow skin or sclera; dark urine; and light-colored stools.

• Tell diabetic patient to report elevated glucose test results so antidiabetic dosage can be adjusted.

• Teach woman how to perform routine self breast examination.

☑ **Evaluation**

• Patient shows improvement in underlying condition.

• Patient has no thromboembolic event during therapy.

• Patient and family state understanding of drug therapy.

etanercept

(ee-TAN-er-sept)

Enbrel

Pharmacologic class: tumor necrosis factor (TNF) blocker
Therapeutic class: antirheumatic
Pregnancy risk category: B

Indications and dosages

▶ **Psoriatic arthritis, ankylosing spondylitis, reducing signs and symptoms and delaying structural damage in patients with moderately to severely active rheumatoid arthritis.**
Adults: 25 mg S.C. twice weekly, on same day or 72 to 96 hours apart. Methotrexate, glucocorticoids, salicylates, NSAIDs, or analgesics may be continued during treatment.

▶ **Reducing signs and symptoms of moderately to severely active polyarticular-course juvenile rheumatoid arthritis in patients who have had an inadequate response to one or more disease-modifying antirheumatic drugs.**
Children ages 4 to 17: 0.4 mg/kg (maximum, 25 mg/dose) S.C. twice weekly, on same day or 72 to 96 hours apart.

Contraindications and precautions

• Contraindicated in patients hypersensitive to drug and in those with sepsis. Stop drug in patients who develop serious infections or sepsis.

• Live vaccines are contraindicated during drug therapy.

• Use cautiously in patients with a history of recurring infections and in those with underlying diseases that predispose them to infection, such as diabetes or heart failure.

⚕ **Lifespan:** In pregnant women, use cautiously. In breast-feeding women and in children younger than age 4, drug isn't recommended.

Adverse reactions

CNS: asthenia, *headache,* dizziness.
EENT: *rhinitis,* pharyngitis, sinusitis.
GI: abdominal pain, dyspepsia.
Respiratory: *upper respiratory tract infections,* cough, respiratory disorder.
Skin: rash.

Other: *infections,* **malignancies,** *injection site reaction.*

Interactions

Drug-drug. *Live-virus vaccinations:* Transmission of infection remains unknown. Avoid using together.

Effects on lab test results

• May cause positive antinuclear antibody or positive anti–double-stranded DNA antibodies measured by radioimmunoassay and *Crithidia luciliae* assay.

Pharmacokinetics

Absorption: Level peaks in 72 hours.
Distribution: Unknown.
Metabolism: Unknown.
Excretion: Unknown. *Half-life:* 115 hours.

Route	Onset	Peak	Duration
S.C.	Unknown	72 hr	Unknown

Action

Chemical effect: Binds specifically to TNF and blocks its action, reducing inflammatory and immune responses found in rheumatoid arthritis.
Therapeutic effect: Reduces signs and symptoms of rheumatoid arthritis.

Available forms

Injection: 25 mg single-use vial

NURSING PROCESS

Assessment

• Obtain history of patient's underlying condition before therapy, and reassess regularly.
• Obtain accurate immunization history from parents or guardians of juvenile rheumatoid arthritis patients; if possible, patients will be brought up to date with all immunizations before treatment is started.
• Monitor patient for infection.
• Evaluate patient's and family's knowledge of drug therapy.

Nursing diagnoses

• Acute pain related to underlying condition
• Risk for infection related to drug-induced adverse reactions
• Deficient knowledge related to drug therapy

Planning and implementation

• Drug is for S.C. injection only.
• Reconstitute aseptically with 1 ml of supplied sterile bacteriostatic water for injection, USP (0.9% benzyl alcohol). Don't filter reconstituted solution during preparation or administration. Inject diluent slowly into vial. Minimize foaming by gently swirling during dissolution rather than shaking. Dissolution takes less than 5 minutes.
• Inspect solution for particulates and discoloration before use. Reconstituted solution should be clear and colorless. Don't use solution if it's discolored, cloudy, or if particulates exist.
• Don't add other drugs or diluents to reconstituted solution.
• Use reconstituted solution as soon as possible; may be refrigerated in vial for up to 6 hours at 36° to 46° F (2° to 8° C).
• Injection sites should be at least 1 inch apart; don't use areas where skin is tender, bruised, red, or hard. Recommended sites include the thigh, abdomen, and upper arm. Rotate sites regularly.
• Don't give live vaccines during therapy.
• Drug may affect defenses against infection. If serious infection occurs, notify prescriber and stop therapy.
• Needle cover of diluent syringe contains dry natural rubber (latex) and shouldn't be handled by persons sensitive to latex.

Patient teaching
• If patient will be administering drug, teach mixing and injection techniques, including rotation of injection sites.
• Instruct patient to use puncture-resistant container to dispose of needles and syringes.
• Tell patient that injection site reactions typically occur within first month of therapy and decrease thereafter.
• Urge patient to avoid live vaccines during therapy. Stress importance of alerting other health care providers of etanercept use.
• Instruct patient to promptly report evidence of infection to prescriber.
• Advise breast-feeding women to stop breast-feeding during drug therapy.

Evaluation

• Patient has decreased pain.
• Patient is free from infection.
• Patient and family state understanding of drug therapy.

ethacrynate sodium

(eth-uh-KRIH-nayt SOH-dee-um)
Sodium Edecrin

ethacrynic acid

Edecril ◊ , Edecrin

Pharmacologic class: loop diuretic
Therapeutic class: diuretic
Pregnancy risk category: B

Indications and dosages

▶ **Acute pulmonary edema.** *Adults:* 50 mg
or 0.5 to 1 mg/kg I.V. to maximum dose of
100 mg. Usually, only one dose is needed; occasionally, second dose may be required.
▶ **Edema.** *Adults:* 50 to 200 mg P.O. daily. Refractory cases may require up to 200 mg b.i.d.
Children: Initial dose is 25 mg P.O.; increase
cautiously in 25-mg increments daily until desired effect is achieved.
▶ **Hypertension‡.** *Adults:* Initially, 25 mg P.O.
daily. Adjust dosage p.r.n. Maximum maintenance dose is 200 mg P.O. daily in two divided
doses.

▼ I.V. administration

• Reconstitute vacuum vial with 50 ml of D_5W
or normal saline solution.
• Give slowly through I.V. line of running infusion over several minutes.
• Discard unused solution after 24 hours. Don't
use cloudy or opalescent solutions.
• If more than one I.V. dose is needed, use new
injection site to avoid thrombophlebitis.

Contraindications and precautions

• Contraindicated in patients hypersensitive to
drug and in those with anuria.
• Use cautiously in patients with electrolyte abnormalities or hepatic impairment.
☙ **Lifespan:** In pregnant women, use cautiously. In breast-feeding women, drug isn't recommended. In infants, drug is contraindicated.

Adverse reactions

CNS: fever, malaise, confusion, fatigue, vertigo,
headache, nervousness.
CV: volume depletion and dehydration, orthostatic hypotension.

EENT: transient deafness (with too-rapid I.V.
injection), blurred vision, tinnitus, hearing loss.
GI: cramping, diarrhea, anorexia, nausea, vomiting, GI BLEEDING, *pancreatitis.*
GU: nocturia, polyuria, frequent urination, oliguria, hematuria.
Hematologic: *agranulocytosis, neutropenia,
thrombocytopenia,* azotemia.
Metabolic: asymptomatic hyperuricemia; hypochloremic alkalosis; fluid and electrolyte imbalances, including dilutional hyponatremia, hypokalemia, hypocalcemia, hypomagnesemia;
hyperglycemia and impairment of glucose tolerance.
Skin: dermatitis, rash.
Other: chills.

Interactions

Drug-drug. *Aminoglycoside antibiotics:* Potentiated ototoxic adverse reactions of both drugs.
Use together cautiously.
Antihypertensives: Increases risk of hypotension. Use together cautiously.
Chlorothiazide, chlorthalidone, hydrochlorothiazide, indapamide, metolazone: May cause excessive diuretic response, resulting in serious
electrolyte abnormalities or dehydration. Adjust
doses carefully while monitoring patient closely
for excessive diuretic responses.
Cisplatin: Increases risk of ototoxicity. Avoid
using together.
Digoxin: Increases risk of digoxin toxicity from
ethacrynate-induced hypokalemia. Monitor
potassium and digoxin levels.
Lithium: Decreases lithium clearance, increasing risk of lithium toxicity. Monitor lithium
level.
Metolazone: May cause profound diuresis and
enhanced electrolyte loss. Use together cautiously.
NSAIDs: May decrease diuretic effectiveness.
Use together cautiously.
Warfarin: Potentiates anticoagulant effect. Use
together cautiously.
Drug-herb. *Licorice root:* May contribute to
potassium depletion caused by diuretics. Discourage licorice root intake.
Drug-lifestyle. *Sun exposure:* Photosensitivity
may occur. Discourage prolonged or unprotected exposure to sunlight.

Effects on lab test results

- May increase glucose and uric acid levels. May decrease potassium, sodium, calcium, and magnesium levels.
- May decrease granulocyte, neutrophil, and platelet counts.

Pharmacokinetics

Absorption: Ethacrynic acid is absorbed rapidly from GI tract. Ethacrynate sodium is administered I.V.
Distribution: Unknown.
Metabolism: Unknown.
Excretion: Unknown.

Route	Onset	Peak	Duration
P.O.	30 min	2 hr	6-8 hr
I.V.	5 min	15-30 min	2 hr

Action

Chemical effect: Inhibits sodium and chloride reabsorption at renal tubules and ascending loop of Henle.
Therapeutic effect: Promotes sodium and water excretion.

Available forms

Injection: 50 mg (with 62.5 mg of mannitol and 0.1 mg of thimerosal)
Tablets: 25 mg, 50 mg

NURSING PROCESS

📆 Assessment

- Obtain history of patient's underlying condition before therapy.
- Monitor effectiveness by regularly checking urine output, weight, peripheral edema, and breath sounds.
- Monitor fluid intake, blood pressure, and electrolyte levels.
- Monitor uric acid levels, especially in patients with history of gout.
- Be alert for adverse reactions and drug interactions.
- Evaluate patient's and family's knowledge of drug therapy.

🔷 Nursing diagnoses

- Excess fluid volume related to underlying condition
- Impaired urinary elimination related to diuretic therapy

- Deficient knowledge related to drug therapy

▷ Planning and implementation

- Give drug with food or milk because P.O. use may cause GI upset.
- To prevent nocturia, give P.O. doses in morning.
- Don't mix with whole blood or its derivatives.
- Don't give S.C. or I.M. because of local pain and irritation.
- Potassium chloride and sodium supplements may be needed.
- If diarrhea occurs, notify prescriber because severe diarrhea may necessitate stopping drug.

Patient teaching
- Advise patient to avoid sudden posture changes and to rise slowly to avoid orthostatic hypotension.
- Advise diabetic patient to closely monitor glucose levels.
- Teach patient and family to identify and report signs of hypersensitivity or fluid and electrolyte disturbances.
- Teach patient to monitor fluid volume by daily weight and intake and output.
- Tell patient to take oral drug early in day to avoid interruption of sleep by nocturia.

☑ Evaluation

- Patient is free from edema.
- Patient demonstrates adjustment of lifestyle to deal with altered patterns of urinary elimination.
- Patient and family state understanding of drug therapy.

ethambutol hydrochloride
(ee-THAM-byoo-tol high-droh-KLOR-ighd)
Etibi ♦ , Myambutol

Pharmacologic class: semisynthetic antituberculotic
Therapeutic class: antituberculotic
Pregnancy risk category: B

Indications and dosages

▷ **Adjunct therapy for pulmonary tuberculosis.** *Adults and children age 13 and older:* For patients who haven't received previous antitubercular therapy, 15 mg/kg P.O. daily. For patients who have received previous antitubercular therapy, 25 mg/kg P.O. daily for 60 days until cultures are negative; then, decrease to 15 mg/kg P.O. daily.

▶ **Adjunct therapy for pulmonary** *Mycobacterium avium* **complex infections in patients without HIV‡.** *Adults:* 25 mg/kg P.O. daily for 2 months followed by 15 mg/kg P.O. daily until cultures are negative for 1 year.

▶ **Adjunct therapy for disseminated** *Mycobacterium avium* **complex infections‡.** *Adults:* 15 mg/kg P.O. daily for patient's lifetime.

Contraindications and precautions

• Contraindicated in patients hypersensitive to drug and in patients with optic neuritis.
• Use cautiously in patients with impaired kidney function, cataracts, recurrent eye inflammations, gout, and diabetic retinopathy.
⚠ Lifespan: In pregnant and breast-feeding women, use cautiously. In children younger than age 13, drug is contraindicated.

Adverse reactions

CNS: fever, malaise, headache, dizziness, confusion, possibly hallucinations, peripheral neuritis.
EENT: dose-related optic neuritis (vision loss and loss of color discrimination, especially red and green).
GI: anorexia, nausea, vomiting, abdominal pain.
Hematologic: *thrombocytopenia.*
Respiratory: bloody sputum.
Skin: dermatitis, pruritus, *toxic epidermal necrolysis.*
Other: *anaphylactoid reactions,* precipitation of gout.

Interactions

Drug-drug. *Aluminum salts:* May delay and reduce absorption of ethambutol. Separate administrations by several hours.

Effects on lab test results

• May increase ALT, AST, bilirubin, and uric acid levels. May decrease glucose level.
• May decrease platelet count.

Pharmacokinetics

Absorption: Rapid.
Distribution: Wide; 8% to 22% protein-bound.
Metabolism: Undergoes partial hepatic metabolism.

Excretion: After 24 hours, about 50% of unchanged drug and 8% to 15% of its metabolites in urine; 20% to 25% in feces. *Half-life:* About 3½ hours.

Route	Onset	Peak	Duration
P.O.	Unknown	2-4 hr	Unknown

Action

Chemical effect: May interfere with synthesis of one or more metabolites of susceptible bacteria, altering cellular metabolism during cell division (bacteriostatic).
Therapeutic effect: Hinders bacterial growth.

Available forms

Tablets: 100 mg, 400 mg

NURSING PROCESS

Assessment
• Obtain history of patient's infection before therapy.
• Perform visual acuity and color discrimination tests before and during therapy.
• Monitor effectiveness by regularly assessing for improvement in patient's condition and evaluating culture and sensitivity test results.
• Obtain AST and ALT levels before starting therapy. Then, monitor AST and ALT levels every 2 to 4 weeks.
• Monitor uric acid level; observe patient for symptoms of gout.
• Be alert for adverse reactions and drug interactions.
• Evaluate patient's and family's knowledge of drug therapy.

Nursing diagnoses
• Infection related to presence of susceptible bacteria
• Disturbed sensory perception (visual) related to drug-induced adverse reactions
• Deficient knowledge related to drug therapy

Planning and implementation
• Anticipate dosage reduction in patient with impaired kidney function.
• Always give ethambutol with other antituberculotics to prevent development of resistant organisms.

Patient teaching
- Reassure patient that visual disturbances will disappear several weeks to months after drug is stopped.
- Warn patient not to perform hazardous activities if visual disturbances or adverse CNS reactions occur.
- Emphasize need for regular follow-up care.

☑ **Evaluation**
- Patient is free from infection.
- Patient regains pretreatment visual ability after therapy has stopped.
- Patient and family state understanding of drug therapy.

---

ethinyl estradiol and desogestrel

(ETH-uh-nil es-truh-DIGH-ol and DAY-so-jest-rul)
monophasic: Apri, Desogen, Ortho-Cept
biphasic: Mircette, Kariva
triphasic: Cyclessa

ethinyl estradiol and ethynodiol diacetate

monophasic: Demulen 1/35, Demulen 1/50, Zovia 1/35E, Zovia 1/50E

ethinyl estradiol and levonorgestrel

emergency: Preven
monophasic: Levlen, Nordette, Alesse, Aviane, Lessina, Portia
triphasic: Tri-Levlen, Triphasil, Trivora, Enpresse

ethinyl estradiol and norethindrone

monophasic: Brevicon, Genora 0.5/35, Genora 1/35, ModiCon, NEE 1/35, Norethin 1/35E, Norinyl 1+35, Ortho-Novum 1/35, Ovcon-35, Ovcon-50
biphasic: Necon 10/11, Nortrel, Ortho-Novum 10/11
triphasic: Necon 7/7/7, Nortrel 7/7/7, Ortho-Novum 7/7/7, Tri-Norinyl

ethinyl estradiol and norethindrone acetate

monophasic: Junel 21-1/20, Junel 21-1.5/30, Loestrin 21 1/20, Loestrin 21 1.5/30
triphasic: Estrostep

ethinyl estradiol and norgestimate

monophasic: MonoNessa, Ortho-Cyclen, Sprintec
triphasic: Ortho Tri-Cyclen, Ortho Tri-Cyclen Lo, Tri-Sprintec

ethinyl estradiol and norgestrel

monophasic: Cryselle, Lo/Ovral, Ovral, Ogestrel

ethinyl estradiol, norethindrone acetate, and ferrous fumarate

monophasic: Loestrin Fe 1/20, Loestrin Fe 1.5/30, Microgestin Fe 1/20, Microgestin Fe 1.5/30

mestranol and norethindrone

monophasic: Necon, Norinyl 1+50, Ortho-Novum 1/50
triphasic: Estrostep Fe, Estrostep 21

Pharmacologic class: estrogen with progestin
Therapeutic class: hormonal contraceptive
Pregnancy risk category: X

Indications and dosages

▶ **Contraception.** *Women:* 1 monophasic tablet P.O. daily, beginning on day 5 of menstrual cycle (first day of menstrual flow is day 1). With 20- and 21-tablet packages, new dosing cycle begins 7 days after last tablet taken. With 28-tablet packages, dosage is 1 tablet daily without interruption; extra tablets are placebos or contain iron. Or, first-color biphasic tablet P.O. daily for 10 days; then next color tablet for 11 days. Or, 1 triphasic tablet P.O. daily in sequence specified by brand.
▶ **Moderate acne vulgaris in women and girls age 15 and older who have no known contraindications to hormonal contraceptive therapy, desire hormonal contraception, have achieved menarche, and are unresponsive to topical antiacne medications.** *Women and girls age 15 and older:* 1 tablet Estrostep, Ortho Tri-Cyclen, or Tri-Sprintec P.O. daily (21 tablets contain active ingredients and 7 are inert).

Contraindications and precautions

- Contraindicated in patients with thromboembolic disorders, cerebrovascular or coronary artery disease, diplopia or ocular lesion arising from ophthalmic vascular disease, classic migraine, MI, known or suspected breast cancer, known or suspected estrogen-dependent neoplasia, benign or malignant liver tumors, active liver disease or history of cholestatic jaundice with pregnancy or prior use of hormonal contraceptives, or undiagnosed abnormal vaginal bleeding.
- Use cautiously in patients with cardiac, renal, or hepatic insufficiency; hyperlipidemia; hypertension; migraine; seizure disorders; or asthma.

⚠ Lifespan: In adolescents, hormonal contraception isn't advised until after at least 2 years of well-established menstrual cycles and completion of physiologic maturation to avoid later fertility and menstrual problems. In women who are pregnant or suspect they may be pregnant and in breast-feeding women, drug is contraindicated.

Adverse reactions

CNS: *headache, dizziness,* depression, lethargy, migraine.
CV: *thromboembolism,* hypertension, edema, *pulmonary embolism, CVA.*
EENT: worsening of myopia or astigmatism, intolerance of contact lenses, exophthalmos, diplopia.
GI: granulomatous colitis, *nausea,* vomiting, abdominal cramps, bloating, diarrhea, constipation, anorexia, *pancreatitis.*
GU: *breakthrough bleeding,* dysmenorrhea, amenorrhea, cervical erosion or abnormal secretions, enlargement of uterine fibromas, vaginal candidiasis.
Hepatic: gallbladder disease, cholestatic jaundice, *liver tumors.*
Metabolic: changes in appetite, weight gain, hyperglycemia, hypercalcemia.
Skin: rash, acne, *erythema multiforme.*
Other: breast changes (*tenderness,* enlargement, secretion).

Interactions

Drug-drug. *Bromocriptine:* May cause amenorrhea, interfering with bromocriptine effects. Avoid using together.

Carbamazepine, phenobarbital, phenytoin, rifampin: Decreases effectiveness of estrogen therapy. Monitor patient closely.
Corticosteroids: Possibly enhanced effects. Monitor patient closely.
Dantrolene, other hepatotoxic drugs: Increases risk of hepatotoxicity. Monitor patient closely.
Griseofulvin, penicillins, sulfonamides, tetracyclines: May decrease effectiveness of hormonal contraceptives. Avoid using together, if possible, or use barrier contraception for the duration of therapy.
Oral anticoagulants: May decrease anticoagulant effects. Dosage adjustments may be needed. Monitor PT and INR.
Tamoxifen: Estrogens may interfere with effectiveness of tamoxifen. Avoid using together.
Drug-food. *Caffeine:* May increase caffeine levels. Monitor effects.
Drug-lifestyle. *Smoking:* Increases risk of CV effects and thrombosis. Discourage patient from smoking. If smoking continues, may need a different form of contraception.

Effects on lab test results

- May increase glucose, calcium, fibrinogen, triglyceride, total T_4, thyroid-binding globulin, plasminogen, liver enzyme, and clotting factor II, VII, VIII, IX, X, and XII levels.
- May increase PT, phospholipid concentrations, and norepinephrine-induced platelet aggregation.

Pharmacokinetics

Absorption: Mostly well absorbed.
Distribution: Wide; extensively bound to proteins.
Metabolism: Mainly in liver.
Excretion: In urine and feces. *Half-life:* 6 to 20 hours.

Route	Onset	Peak	Duration
P.O.	Unknown	Varies	Unknown

Action

Chemical effect: Inhibits ovulation through negative feedback mechanism directed at hypothalamus. Estrogen suppresses secretion of follicle-stimulating hormone, blocking follicle development and ovulation. Progestin suppresses secretion of luteinizing hormone so ovulation can't occur. Progestin thickens cervical mucus, which interferes with sperm migration, and prevents implantation.

Therapeutic effect: Prevents pregnancy and relieves signs and symptoms of endometriosis.

Available forms

monophasic

ethinyl estradiol and desogestrel
Tablets: ethinyl estradiol 30 mcg and desogestrel 0.15 mg (Apri, Desogen, Ortho-Cept), ethinyl estradiol 25 mcg and desogestrel 0.1 mg

ethinyl estradiol and ethynodiol diacetate
Tablets: ethinyl estradiol 35 mcg and ethynodiol diacetate 1 mg (Demulen 1/35, Zovia 1/35E); ethinyl estradiol 50 mcg and ethynodiol diacetate 1 mg (Demulen 1/50, Zovia 1/50E)

ethinyl estradiol and levonorgestrel
Tablets: ethinyl estradiol 30 mcg and levonorgestrel 0.15 mg (Levlen, Levora, Nordette, Portia); ethinyl estradiol 20 mcg, levonorgestrel 0.1 mg (Alesse, Aviane, Lessina)

ethinyl estradiol and norethindrone
Tablets: ethinyl estradiol 35 mcg and norethindrone 0.4 mg (Ovcon-35); ethinyl estradiol 35 mcg and norethindrone 0.5 mg (Brevicon, Necon, Nortel, ModiCon); ethinyl estradiol 35 mcg and norethindrone 1 mg (Necon 1/35, Nortel 1/35, Norinyl 1+35, Ortho-Novum 1/35); ethinyl estradiol 50 mcg and norethindrone 1 mg (Ovcon-50)

ethinyl estradiol and norethindrone acetate
Tablets: ethinyl estradiol 20 mcg and norethindrone acetate 1 mg (Loestrin 21 1/20); ethinyl estradiol 30 mcg and norethindrone acetate 1.5 mg (Loestrin 21 1.5/30)

ethinyl estradiol and norgestimate
Tablets: ethinyl estradiol 35 mcg and norgestimate 0.25 mg (Ortho Cyclen)

ethinyl estradiol and norgestrel
Tablets: ethinyl estradiol 30 mcg and norgestrel 0.3 mg (Cryselle, Lo/Ovral, Lo/Ovral 28); ethinyl estradiol 50 mcg and norgestrel 0.5 mg (Ovral, Ovral 28, Ogestrel 0.5/50)

ethinyl estradiol, norethindrone acetate, and ferrous fumarate
Tablets: ethinyl estradiol 20 mcg, norethindrone acetate 1 mg, and ferrous fumarate 75 mg (Loestrin Fe 1/20, Microgestin Fe 1/20); ethinyl estradiol 30 mcg, norethindrone acetate 1.5 mg, and ferrous fumarate 75 mg (Loestrin Fe 1.5/30, Microgestin Fe 1.5/30)

mestranol and norethindrone
Tablets: mestranol 50 mcg and norethindrone 1 mg (Necon 1/50, Norinyl 1+50, Ortho-Novum 1/50)

biphasic

ethinyl estradiol and desogestrel
ethinyl estradiol 20 mcg and desogestrel 0.15 mg (Kariva, Mircette)

ethinyl estradiol and norethindrone
Tablets: ethinyl estradiol 35 mcg and norethindrone 0.5 mg during phase 1 [10 days]; ethinyl estradiol 35 mcg and norethindrone 1 mg during phase 2 [11 days] (Necon 10/11, Ortho-Novum 10/11)

triphasic

ethinyl estradiol and desogestrel
Tablets: desogestrel 0.1 mg and ethinyl estradiol 25 mcg (7 tablets); desogestrel 0.125 mg and ethinyl estradiol 25 mcg (7 tablets); desogestrel 0.15 mg and ethinyl estradiol 25 mcg (7 tablets) (Cyclessa)

ethinyl estradiol and levonorgestrel
Tablets: ethinyl estradiol 30 mcg and levonorgestrel 0.05 mg during phase 1 [6 days]; ethinyl estradiol 40 mcg and levonorgestrel 0.075 mg during phase 2 [5 days]; ethinyl estradiol 30 mcg and levonorgestrel 0.125 mg during phase 3 [10 days] (Tri-Levlen, Triphasil, Trivora-28, Enpresse)

ethinyl estradiol and norethindrone
Tablets: ethinyl estradiol 35 mcg and norethindrone 0.5 mg during phase 1 [7 days]; ethinyl estradiol 35 mcg and norethindrone 1 mg during phase 2 [9 days]; ethinyl estradiol 35 mcg and norethindrone 0.5 mg during phase 3 [5 days] (Tri-Norinyl); ethinyl estradiol 35 mcg and norethindrone 0.5 mg during phase 1 [7 days]; ethinyl estradiol 35 mcg and norethindrone 0.75 mg during phase 2 [7 days]; ethinyl estradiol 35 mcg and norethindrone 1 mg during phase 3 [7 days] (Necon 7/7/7, Nortrel 7/7/7, Ortho-Novum 7/7/7)

ethinyl estradiol and norethindrone acetate
Tablets: ethinyl estradiol 0.02 mg and norethindrone acetate 1 mg (5 tablets), ethinyl estradiol 0.03 mg and norethindrone acetate 1 mg (7 tablets), ethinyl estradiol 0.035 mg and norethindrone acetate 1 mg (9 tablets) (Estrostep Fe, Estrostep 21)

ethinyl estradiol and norgestimate
Tablets: ethinyl estradiol 35 mcg and norgestimate 0.18 mg during phase 1 [7 days]; ethinyl estradiol 35 mcg and norgestimate 0.215 mg during phase 2 [7 days]; ethinyl estradiol 35 mcg and norgestimate 0.25 mg during phase 3 [7 days] (Ortho Tri-Cyclen)

Reactions may be *common*, uncommon, *life-threatening*, or COMMON AND LIFE-THREATENING.

NURSING PROCESS

⚖ Assessment
- Obtain history of patient's pregnancy status or underlying endometriosis before therapy.
- Monitor effectiveness by determining if pregnancy test is negative or if patient with endometriosis has diminished signs and symptoms.
- Periodically monitor lipid levels, blood pressure, body weight, and liver function.
- Be alert for adverse reactions and drug interactions.
- Evaluate patient's and family's knowledge of drug therapy.

🔷 Nursing diagnoses
- Health-seeking behavior (prevention of pregnancy) related to family planning
- Acute pain related to drug-induced headache
- Deficient knowledge related to drug therapy

▷ Planning and implementation
- Make sure patient has been properly instructed about prescribed hormonal contraceptive before she takes first dose.
- ⑤ **ALERT:** Make sure patient has negative pregnancy test before therapy starts.
- If patient develops granulomatous colitis, stop therapy and notify prescriber.
- Stop drug at least 1 week before surgery to decrease risk of thromboembolism. Tell patient to use other, nonhormonal method of birth control.
- ⑤ **ALERT:** Don't confuse Nortel 7/7/7 with Nortrel 0.5/35 or Nortrel 1/35.
- ⑤ **ALERT:** Don't confuse Necon 7/7/7 with Nortrel 7/7/7.

Patient teaching
- Tell patient to take tablets at same time each day; nighttime dosing may reduce nausea and headaches.
- Advise patient to use barrier method of birth control for first week of first cycle.
- Tell patient that missed doses in midcycle greatly increase likelihood of pregnancy.
- If one tablet is missed, tell patient to take it as soon as remembered or to take two tablets the next day and continue regular schedule. If patient misses 2 consecutive days, instruct her to take two tablets daily for 2 days and then resume normal schedule. Also advise her to use second method of birth control for 7 days after two missed doses. If she misses three or more

doses, tell her to discard remaining tablets in monthly package and to use another method. If next menstrual period doesn't begin on schedule, warn patient to rule out pregnancy before starting new dosing cycle. If menstrual period begins, have patient start new dosing cycle 7 days after last tablet was taken.
- Warn patient that headache, nausea, dizziness, breast tenderness, spotting, and breakthrough bleeding are common at first. These effects should diminish after 3 to 6 months.
- Instruct patient to weigh herself at least twice weekly and to report sudden weight gain or edema to prescriber.
- Warn patient to avoid exposure to ultraviolet light or prolonged exposure to sunlight.
- ⑤ **ALERT:** Warn patient to immediately report abdominal pain; numbness, stiffness, or pain in legs or buttocks; pressure or pain in chest; shortness of breath; severe headache; visual disturbances, such as blind spots, blurriness, or flashing lights; undiagnosed vaginal bleeding or discharge; two consecutive missed menstrual periods; lumps in breast; swelling of hands or feet; or severe pain in abdomen.
- Advise patient of increased risks of smoking while using hormonal contraceptives.
- Teach patient how to perform breast self-examination.
- If one menstrual period is missed and tablets have been taken on schedule, tell patient to continue taking them. If two consecutive menstrual periods are missed, tell patient to stop drug and have pregnancy test. Progestins may cause birth defects if taken early in pregnancy.
- Advise patient not to take same drug for longer than 12 months without consulting prescriber. Stress importance of Papanicolaou test and annual gynecologic examination.
- Advise patient to check with prescriber about how soon pregnancy may be attempted after hormonal therapy is stopped.
- Warn patient of possible delay in achieving pregnancy when drug is stopped.
- Advise women on prolonged contraceptive therapy to stop drug and use other nonhormonal birth control methods. Periodically reassess patient while off hormone therapy.

✅ Evaluation
- Patient doesn't become pregnant.
- Patient obtains relief from drug-induced headache with administration of mild analgesic.

• Patient and family state understanding of drug therapy.

ethinyl estradiol (EE) and drospirenone (DRSP)
(ETH-in-il es-tra-DIE-ol and droh-SPEER-ih-nohn)
Yasmin

Pharmacologic class: combination, low-dose monophasic hormonal contraceptive
Therapeutic class: hormonal contraceptive
Pregnancy risk category: X

Indications and dosages

▶ **Contraception.** *Women and postpubertal girls:* 1 yellow tablet P.O. daily beginning on day 1 of menstrual cycle (first day of menstruation). Continue taking 1 yellow tablet P.O. daily for 21 consecutive days, at the same time each day, preferably after the evening meal or h.s.; then take 1 white inert tablet P.O. daily on days 22 through 28. Begin the next and all subsequent 28-day regimens on the same day of the week that the first regimen began, following the same schedule. Restart taking yellow tablets on the next day after taking the last white tablet. Or, 1 yellow tablet P.O. daily, beginning on the first Sunday after the onset of menstruation. Continue taking 1 yellow tablet P.O. daily for 21 consecutive days, at the same time each day, preferably after the evening meal or h.s.; then take 1 white inert tablet P.O. daily on days 22 through 28. Begin the next and all subsequent 28-day regimens on the same day of the week that the first regimen began, following the same schedule. Restart taking yellow tablets on the next day after taking the last white tablet.

Contraindications and precautions

• Contraindicated in women with hepatic dysfunction, tumor, or disease; renal or adrenal insufficiency; thrombophlebitis, thromboembolic disorders, or history of deep-vein thrombosis or thromboembolic disorders; cerebrovascular or coronary artery disease; known or suspected breast cancer, endometrial cancer, or other estrogen-dependent neoplasia; unexplained vaginal bleeding; or cholestatic jaundice of pregnancy or jaundice with other contraceptive pill use. Also contraindicated in women older

than age 35 who smoke 15 or more cigarettes daily.
• Use cautiously in patients with risk factors for CV disease, such as hypertension, hyperlipidemias, obesity, and diabetes.
⚠ Lifespan: In women who are pregnant or suspect they may be pregnant, drug is contraindicated. In breast-feeding women, drug is contraindicated because jaundice and breast enlargement may occur in breast-fed infants, and drug decreases the quantity and quality of breast milk. Advise use of other forms of contraception until infant is completely weaned. Don't use in girls before menarche.

Adverse reactions

CNS: asthenia, *cerebral hemorrhage, cerebral thrombosis,* depression, dizziness, emotional lability, headache, migraine nervousness.
CV: *arterial thromboembolism,* hypertension, edema, *mesenteric thrombosis, MI, thrombophlebitis.*
EENT: cataracts, change in corneal curvature (steepening), intolerance to contact lenses, pharyngitis, retinal thrombosis, sinusitis.
GI: abdominal pain, abdominal cramping, bloating, changes in appetite, colitis, diarrhea, gastroenteritis, nausea, vomiting.
GU: amenorrhea, breakthrough bleeding, change in cervical erosion and secretion, change in menstrual flow, cystitis, cystitis-like syndrome, dysmenorrhea, *hemolytic uremic syndrome,* renal impairment, leukorrhea, menstrual disorder, premenstrual syndrome, spotting, temporary infertility after discontinuing treatment, UTI, vaginal candidiasis, vaginitis.
Hepatic: *Budd-Chiari syndrome,* cholestatic jaundice, gallbladder disease, *hepatic adenomas,* benign liver tumors.
Metabolic: reduced tolerance to carbohydrates, porphyria, weight gain.
Musculoskeletal: back pain.
Respiratory: bronchitis, *pulmonary embolism,* upper respiratory tract infection.
Skin: acne, *erythema multiforme,* erythema nodosum, hemorrhagic eruption, hirsutism, loss of scalp hair, melasma, pruritus, rash.
Other: changes in libido, breast changes, decreased lactation.

Interactions

Drug-drug. *ACE inhibitors, aldosterone antagonists, angiotensin-II receptor antagonists,*

NSAIDs, potassium-sparing diuretics, heparin: Increases risk of hyperkalemia. Monitor potassium levels.

Acetaminophen: Decreases acetaminophen level. Adjust acetaminophen dose as needed.

Ampicillin, griseofulvin, tetracycline: Decreases contraceptive effect. Encourage use of additional method of birth control while taking the antibiotic.

Ascorbic acid, atorvastatin: Increases concentrations of contraceptive. Monitor patient for adverse effects.

Carbamazepine, phenobarbital, phenytoin: Increases metabolism of EE and decreased contraceptive effectiveness. Encourage use of alternative method of birth control.

Clofibrate, morphine, salicylic acid, temazepam: Decreases levels and increases clearance of these drugs. Monitor patient for effectiveness.

Cyclosporine, prednisolone, theophylline: Increases levels of these drugs. Monitor patient for adverse effects and toxicity.

Phenylbutazone, rifampin: Decreases contraceptive effectiveness and increases breakthrough bleeding. Encourage use of alternative method of birth control.

Drug-herb. *St. John's wort:* Decreases contraceptive effect and increases breakthrough bleeding. Encourage use of additional method of birth control or avoid using together.

Drug-lifestyle. *Smoking:* Increases risk of CV adverse effects and thromboembolism. Warn patient to avoid smoking and tobacco products while taking hormonal contraceptives.

Effects on lab test results

• May increase circulating total thyroid hormone, triglyceride, other binding protein, sex hormone-binding globulin, total circulating endogenous sex steroid, corticoid, potassium, folate, liver enzyme, and factor VII, VIII, IX, and X levels.

• May increase PT. May decrease glucose tolerance.

Pharmacokinetics

Absorption: Levels peak within 1 to 3 hours. Steady state level of DRSP occurs after 10 days and EE occurs during the second half of the treatment cycle.

Distribution: Wide. DRSP is about 97% bound to nonspecific proteins. EE is about 98% bound to albumin and other nonspecific proteins.

Metabolism: DRSP is metabolized mainly by metabolites in plasma, and to a minor extent in the liver by CYP 3A4 to inactive metabolites. EE is primarily metabolized by hydroxylation and subject to pre-systemic conjugation in the small bowel and the liver.

Excretion: Small amounts of DRSP unchanged in the urine and feces. EE breast as metabolites in the urine and feces. *DRSP half-life:* 30 hours. *EE half-life:* 24 hours.

Route	Onset	Peak	Duration
P.O.	Unknown	1-3 hr	Unknown

Action

Chemical effect: Suppresses gonadotropins follicle-stimulating hormone and luteinizing hormone, thereby preventing ovulation, changing the cervical mucus to increase the difficulty of the sperm to penetrate, and changing the endometrium to increase the difficulty of implantation.

Therapeutic effect: Reduces the opportunity for conception.

Available forms

Tablets: 21 yellow tablets containing 3 mg DRSP and 0.03 mg EE, and 7 inert, white tablets.

NURSING PROCESS

🔲 Assessment

• Determine if patient is pregnant before starting drug.

• Obtain patient's medical history, smoking status, CV status, and potassium level before starting drug.

• Assess and be alert for adverse reactions. The use of contraceptives causes increased risk of MI, thromboembolism, CVA, hepatic neoplasia, gallbladder disease, and hypertension, especially in patients with hypertension, diabetes, hyperlipidemia, and obesity.

• Monitor patients laboratory results during drug therapy.

• Evaluate patient's and family's knowledge of contraception and drug therapy.

🔲 Nursing diagnoses

• Risk for injury related to drug-induced adverse reactions

• Health seeking behavior for the prevention of pregnancy related to family planning
• Deficient knowledge of contraceptive drug therapy

>> **Planning and implementation**

• Because of increased risk of thromboembolism in the postpartum period, don't start drug earlier than 4 to 6 weeks after delivery.
• If patient misses two consecutive periods, tell her to obtain a negative pregnancy test result before continuing contraceptive. If pregnancy test is positive, tell her to immediately stop drug.
• In patients scheduled to have elective surgery that may increase the risk of thromboembolism, stop contraceptive use from at least 4 weeks before until 2 weeks after surgery. Also avoid use during and after prolonged immobilization. Advise patient to use alternative methods of birth control.
• Overdose may cause nausea and withdrawal bleeding. Monitor concentrations of potassium and sodium and watch for signs of metabolic acidosis.
• If loss of vision, proptosis, diplopia, papilledema, or retinal vascular lesions occur, stop use and evaluate patient. Recommend that contact lens wearers be evaluated by an ophthalmologist if they have changes in vision or lens intolerance.
• Evaluate patient who experiences unusual breakthrough bleeding for malignancy or pregnancy.
• If patient suffers from sharp or crushing chest pains, hemoptysis, sudden shortness of breath, calf pain, breast lumps, severe stomach pains, difficulty sleeping, weakness, fatigue, or jaundice, stop drug. Notify prescriber immediately and offer supportive treatment as needed.

Patient teaching

• Inform patient that pills are used to prevent pregnancy and don't protect against HIV and other sexually transmitted diseases.
• Advise patient of the dangers of smoking while taking hormonal contraceptives. Suggest that she choose a different form of birth control if she continues smoking.
• Tell patient to schedule gynecological examinations yearly and perform breast self-examination monthly.
• Inform patient that spotting, light bleeding, or stomach upset may occur during the first one to three packs of pills. Tell her to continue taking

the pills and to notify prescriber if these symptoms persist.
• Tell patient to take the pill at the same time each day, preferably during the evening or h.s.
• Tell patient to immediately report sharp chest pain, coughing of blood, or sudden shortness of breath, pain in the calf, crushing chest pain or chest heaviness, sudden severe headache or vomiting, dizziness or fainting, visual or speech disturbances, weakness, or numbness in an arm or leg, loss of vision, breast lumps, severe stomach pain or tenderness, difficulty sleeping, lack of energy, fatigue, or change in mood, jaundice with fever, fatigue, loss of appetite, dark urine, or light-colored bowel movements.
• Tell patient to notify prescriber if she wears contact lenses and notices a change in vision or has difficulty wearing the lenses.
• Advise patient to use additional method of birth control during the first 7 days of the first cycle of hormonal contraceptive.
• Tell patient that the risk of pregnancy increases with each active yellow tablet she forgets to take.
• If patient misses one tablet, tell her to take it as soon as she remembers and to take the next pill at the regular time.
• If patient misses two tablets during week 1 or 2 of the pack, tell her to use an additional method of birth control for 7 days. Instruct her to take two pills on the day she remembers and two pills the next day, and then to resume the normal schedule.
• If patient misses two tablets during week 3, tell her to use an additional method of birth control for 7 days. If she uses day 1 start, tell her to throw away the rest of the pack and start a new pack the same day. If she uses Sunday start, tell her to keep taking one pill each day until Sunday, then to throw away the pack, and start a new pack that day. Tell patient that she may miss her period this month, but to notify prescriber if she misses it 2 months in a row because it may mean she's pregnant.
• If patient misses three or more tablets during the first 3 weeks, tell her to use an additional method of birth control for 7 days. If she uses day 1 start, tell her to throw away the rest of the pack and start a new pack the same day. If she uses Sunday start, tell her to keep taking one pill each day until Sunday, then to throw away the pack, and start a new pack that day. Tell patient that she may miss her period this month,

---

Reactions may be *common,* uncommon, *life-threatening,* or COMMON AND LIFE-THREATENING.

but to notify prescriber if she misses it 2 months in a row because it may mean she's pregnant.
- If patient misses any of the white tablets, tell her to throw away the missed pills and keep taking one pill each day until the pack is empty. She doesn't need to use an additional method of birth control.
- Tell patient to use an additional method of birth control and notify prescriber if she isn't sure what to do about missed pills.

☑ Evaluation
- Patient doesn't suffer from any drug-induced adverse reactions.
- Patient doesn't become pregnant.
- Patient and family state understanding of drug therapy.

ethinyl estradiol and etonogestrel vaginal ring
(ETH-ih-nil es-tra-DYE-ole and et-oh-noe-JES-trel)
NuvaRing

Pharmacologic class: progestin/estrogen intravaginal contraceptive
Therapeutic class: combination hormonal contraceptive vaginal ring
Pregnancy risk category: X

Indications and dosages
▶ **Contraception.** *Women:* Insert one ring vaginally, and leave in place for 3 weeks. Insert new ring exactly 1 week after the previous ring was removed, even if menstrual bleeding is still present.

Contraindications and precautions
- Contraindicated in patients hypersensitive to any component of drug and patients older than age 35 who smoke 15 or more cigarettes daily. Also contraindicated in patients with thrombophlebitis, thromboembolic disorder, history of deep vein thrombophlebitis, cerebral vascular or coronary artery disease (current or previous), valvular heart disease with complications, severe hypertension, diabetes with vascular complications, headache with focal neurological symptoms, major surgery with prolonged immobilization, known or suspected cancer of the endometrium or breast, estrogen-dependent neo-

plasia, abnormal undiagnosed vaginal bleeding, jaundice related to pregnancy or previous use of hormonal contraceptive, active liver disease, or benign or malignant hepatic tumors.
- Use cautiously in patients with hypertension, hyperlipidemias, obesity, or diabetes. Also use cautiously in patients with conditions that could be aggravated by fluid retention, a history of depression, or impaired liver function.
≵ **Lifespan:** In women who are or may be pregnant, drug is contraindicated. In breast-feeding women, drug isn't recommended. Tell patient to use alternative forms of contraception until baby is weaned. Don't start drug earlier than 4 weeks after delivery in women who choose not to breast-feed. In women who haven't reached menarche, drug is contraindicated. Don't use in postmenopausal women.

Adverse reactions
CNS: *headache,* emotional lability.
EENT: *sinusitis.*
GI: *nausea.*
GU: *vaginitis, leukorrhea,* device-related events (such as foreign body sensation, coital difficulties, device expulsion), vaginal discomfort.
Metabolic: *weight gain.*
Respiratory: *upper respiratory tract infection.*

Interactions
Drug-drug. *Acetaminophen, ascorbic acid, atorvastatin, itraconazole:* Increases ethinyl estradiol levels. Monitor patient for adverse effects.
Ampicillin, barbiturates, carbamazepine, felbamate, griseofulvin, oxcarbazepine, phenylbutazone, phenytoin, rifampin, tetracyclines, topiramate: Decreases contraceptive effectiveness and increased risk of pregnancy, breakthrough bleeding, or both. Tell patient to use an additional form of contraception while taking these drugs.
Anti-HIV protease inhibitors: May increase or decrease the bioavailability of estrogen or progestin. Consider other methods of birth control.
Clofibric acid, morphine, salicylic acid, temazepam: Increases clearance of these drugs. Monitor patient for effectiveness.
Cyclosporine, prednisolone, theophylline: Increases levels of these drugs. Monitor cyclosporine and theophylline levels and adjust dosages as needed.

Drug-herb. *St. John's wort:* May reduce contraceptive effectiveness, increase risk of pregnancy, and increase risk of breakthrough bleeding. Discourage using together.

Drug-lifestyle. *Smoking:* Increases risk of serious CV side effects and thromboembolism, especially in those women age 35 and older and who smoke 15 or more cigarettes daily. Urge patient to quit smoking.

Effects on lab test results

• May increase levels of prothrombin; factor VII, VIII, IX, and X; thyroid-binding globulin (leading to increased circulating total thyroid hormone levels); other binding protein; sex hormone–binding globulin; triglyceride; lipoprotein; and other lipids. May decrease antithrombin III and folate levels.

• May increase norepinephrine-induced platelet aggregation. May decrease T_3 resin uptake and glucose tolerance.

Pharmacokinetics

Absorption: Both hormonal components are rapidly absorbed. Bioavailability of etonogestrel and ethinyl estradiol is 100% and 55.6%, respectively.

Distribution: Etonogestrel is 66% protein-bound and 32% bound to sex hormone–binding globulin. Ethinyl estradiol is about 98% nonspecific protein-bound and increases levels of sex hormone–binding globulin.

Metabolism: Both components of drug are metabolized in the liver by CYP 3A4.

Excretion: Both components are mainly in urine, bile, and feces. *Half-life:* ethinyl estradiol, 45 hours; etonogestrel, 29 hours.

Route	Onset	Peak	Duration
Vaginal	Immediate	Unknown	Unknown

Action

Chemical effect: Suppresses gonadotropins, which inhibits ovulation, increases the viscosity of cervical mucus (decreasing the ability of sperm to enter the uterus), and alters the endometrial lining (reducing potential for implantation).

Therapeutic effect: Decreases risk of pregnancy.

Available forms

Vaginal ring: Delivers 0.120 mg etonogestrel and 0.015 mg ethinyl estradiol daily.

NURSING PROCESS

⚕ Assessment

• Assess patient for pregnancy before starting drug.

• Obtain patient's medical history, smoking status, CV status, and risk factors before starting drug.

• Be alert for adverse reactions.

• The use of contraceptives causes increased risk of MI, thromboembolism, CVA, hepatic neoplasia, gallbladder disease, and hypertension, especially in patients with hypertension, diabetes, hyperlipidemia, and obesity. Monitor patient for signs and symptoms related to these occurrences.

• Monitor patient's laboratory results during drug therapy.

• Evaluate patient's and family's knowledge of contraception and drug therapy.

⊞ Nursing diagnoses

• Risk for injury related to drug-induced adverse reactions

• Health seeking behavior for the prevention of pregnancy related to family planning

• Deficient knowledge of contraceptive drug therapy

▶ Planning and implementation

• Stop drug at least 4 weeks before and for 2 weeks after procedures that may increase the risk of thromboembolism and during and after prolonged immobilization.

• If patient develops unexplained partial or complete loss of vision, proptosis, diplopia, papilledema, or retinal vascular lesions, stop drug.

• If patient has hypertension or renal disease, monitor blood pressure closely. If blood pressure rises, stop drug.

• If migraine begins or worsens or if patient has recurrent, persistent, or severe headaches, stop drug.

• If jaundice occurs, stop drug. The hormones may be poorly metabolized in patients with liver disease.

• If patient has persistent or severe abnormal menstrual bleeding, look for cause. If amenorrhea occurs, rule out pregnancy.

Reactions may be *common*, uncommon, *life-threatening*, or **COMMON AND LIFE-THREATENING**.

• If depression occurs, stop drug to determine whether depression is drug-related.

• If no hormonal contraceptive is used in the preceding month, insert ring on day 5 of the menstrual cycle (counting the first day of menstruation as day 1). For the first cycle of use, use an additional form of birth control within 7 days of inserting ring.

• When switching from other combination (estrogen plus progestin) hormonal contraceptives, insert the ring within 7 days of the last dose of combined hormonal contraceptive, no later than the day that a new cycle of tablets would have begun. No back-up form of contraception is needed.

• When switching from a progestin-only form of contraception, use a back-up form of contraception for the first 7 days of using the ring in any of the following situations: If switching from progestin-only tablets, insert ring on any day of the month; don't skip any days between the last oral dose and insertion of the ring. If switching from progestin-only implants (such as Norplant), insert the vaginal ring on the same day that the implants are removed. If switching from progestin-only intrauterine device (IUD), insert the vaginal ring on the same day that the IUD is removed. If switching from contraceptive injections (such as Depo-Provera), insert the vaginal ring on the same day that the next injection would be due. Begin use within the first 5 days after complete first-trimester abortion, 4 weeks postpartum in women who aren't breast-feeding, or 4 weeks after a second-trimester abortion.

• If the ring is removed or expelled (for example, while removing a tampon or moving the bowels), wash with cool to lukewarm water and reinsert immediately. If the ring stays out for more than 3 hours, contraceptive may not be effective, and a back-up method of contraception is recommended until the newly reinserted ring is used continuously for 7 days.

• Rule out pregnancy if patient hasn't adhered to the prescribed regimen and a menstrual period is missed, if prescribed regimen is adhered to and two periods are missed, or if the patient has retained the ring for longer than 4 weeks.

• Overdose may cause nausea, vomiting, vaginal bleeding, or other menstrual irregularities. Offer supportive treatment.

Patient teaching

• Teach patient or provide patient with instructions for proper placement of vaginal ring. Also encourage proper handwashing before and after ring insertion to prevent vaginal infections.

• Emphasize the importance of having annual physical examinations to check for adverse effects or developing contraindications.

• Tell patient that drug doesn't protect against HIV and other sexually transmitted diseases.

• Advise patient not to smoke while using contraceptive.

• Tell patient not to use a diaphragm if a back-up method of birth control is needed.

• Tell patient who wears contact lenses to contact an ophthalmologist if vision or lens tolerance change.

• Advise patient to wash the ring with cool to lukewarm (not hot) water and reinsert immediately if it's removed or expelled (for example, while removing a tampon, straining, or moving bowels). Stress that contraceptive may not be effective if the ring stays out for more than 3 hours, tell her to use a back-up method of contraception until the newly reinserted ring is used continuously for 7 days.

☑ **Evaluation**

• Patient doesn't suffer from any drug-induced adverse reactions or vaginal infections.

• Patient doesn't become pregnant.

• Patient and family state understanding of drug therapy.

ethinyl estradiol and norelgestromin transdermal system

(ETH-ih-nil es-tra-DYE-ole and nor-el-GES-tro-min)
Ortho Evra

Pharmacologic class: transdermal contraceptive patch
Therapeutic class: combination hormonal contraceptive
Pregnancy risk category: X

Indications and dosages

▶ **Contraception.** *Women:* Apply one patch weekly for 3 weeks. Week 4 is patch-free. On the day after week 4 ends, apply a new patch to start a new 4-week cycle. Apply each new patch on the same day of the week.

Contraindications and precautions

• Contraindicated in patients hypersensitive to any component of drug and in those with a history of deep vein thrombosis or related disorder, current or past history of cerebrovascular or coronary artery disease, past or current known or suspected breast cancer, endometrial cancer or other known or suspected estrogen-dependent neoplasia, hepatic adenoma or carcinoma, or known or suspected pregnancy. Also contraindicated in patients with thrombophlebitis, thromboembolic disorders, valvular heart disease with complications, severe hypertension, diabetes with vascular involvement, headaches with focal neurological symptoms, major surgery with prolonged immobilization, undiagnosed abnormal genital bleeding, cholestatic jaundice of pregnancy or jaundice with previous hormonal contraceptive use, or acute or chronic hepatocellular disease with abnormal liver function.

• Use cautiously in patients with CV disease risk factors, with conditions that might be aggravated by fluid retention, or with a history of depression.

☙ Lifespan: In breast-feeding women, safety and effectiveness haven't been established. Advise them to use alternative methods of birth control. Girls who haven't reached menarche shouldn't use contraceptive patch because safety and effectiveness haven't been evaluated.

Adverse reactions

CNS: *headache*, emotional lability.
CV: *thromboembolic events, MI,* hypertension, edema, **cerebral hemorrhage.**
EENT: contact lens intolerance.
GI: *nausea, abdominal pain,* vomiting.
GU: *menstrual cramps,* changes in menstrual flow, vaginal candidiasis.
Hepatic: *hepatic adenomas,* benign liver tumors, gallbladder disease.
Metabolic: weight changes.
Respiratory: *upper respiratory tract infection.*
Skin: *application site reaction.*
Other: *breast tenderness, enlargement, or secretion.*

Interactions

Drug-drug. *Acetaminophen, clofibric acid, morphine, salicylic acid, temazepam:* Decreases levels or increases clearance of these drugs. Monitor patient for lack of effect.
Ampicillin, barbiturates, carbamazepine, felbamate, griseofulvin, oxcarbazepine, phenylbutazone, phenytoin, rifampin, topiramate: Contraceptive effectiveness may be reduced, resulting in unintended pregnancy or breakthrough bleeding. If used together, encourage back-up method of contraception.
Anti-HIV protease inhibitors: Effectiveness and safety of contraceptives may be affected. Use together cautiously.
Ascorbic acid, atorvastatin, itraconazole, ketoconazole: Increases hormone levels. Use together cautiously.
Cyclosporine, prednisolone, theophylline: Increases levels of these drugs. Monitor patient for adverse effects.
Drug-herb. *St John's wort:* May reduce effectiveness of contraceptive and cause breakthrough bleeding. Discourage using together.
Drug-lifestyle. *Smoking:* Increases risk of serious CV side effects, especially in those older than age 35 who smoke 15 or more cigarettes daily. Urge patient to quit smoking.

Effects on lab test results

• May increase factor VII, VIII, IX, and X; circulating total thyroid hormone; triglyceride; other binding protein; sex hormone-binding globulin; total circulating endogenous sex steroid; and corticoid levels. May decrease antithrombin III and folate levels.
• May increase prothrombin. May decrease free T_3 resin uptake and glucose tolerance.

Pharmacokinetics

Absorption: Rapid with peak at or about 48 hours. Maintained at a steady state while the patch is worn.
Distribution: Norelgestromin and norgestrel (a metabolite) are more than 97% protein bound. Norelgestromin is bound to albumin and not to SHBGs, but norgestrel is bound primarily to SHBG, which limits its biological activity. Ethinyl estradiol is extensively bound to albumin.
Metabolism: In the liver. Ethinyl estradiol is metabolized to various hydroxylated products.
Excretion: Norelgestromin and ethinyl estradiol are eliminated in 28 hours and 17 hours, respectively. The metabolites are eliminated in the

---

Reactions may be common, uncommon, *life-threatening,* or COMMON AND LIFE-THREATENING.

urine and feces. *Ethinyl estradiol half-life:* 6 to 45 hours. *Norelgestromin half-life:* 28 hours.

Route	Onset	Peak	Duration
Transdermal	Rapid	2 days	Unknown

Action

Chemical effect: Suppresses gonadotropins and inhibits ovulation. Changes cervical mucus, complicating entry of sperm into the uterus and changes endometrium, decreasing the likelihood of implantation.

Therapeutic effect: Reduces risk of pregnancy.

Available forms

Transdermal patch: norelgestromin 6 mg and ethinyl estradiol 0.75 mg (releases 150 mcg of norelgestromin and 20 mcg of ethinyl estradiol every 24 hours)

NURSING PROCESS

Assessment
• Rule out pregnancy before starting drug.
• Obtain patient's medical history, smoking status, and CV status before starting drug.
• Be alert for any drug-induced adverse reactions.
• The use of contraceptives causes increased risk of MI, thromboembolism, CVA, hepatic neoplasia, gallbladder disease, and hypertension, especially in patients with hypertension, diabetes, hyperlipidemia, and obesity. Monitor patient for signs and symptoms related to these occurrences.
• Monitor patient's laboratory results during drug therapy.
• Evaluate patient's knowledge of contraception and drug therapy.

Nursing diagnoses
• Risk for injury related to drug-induced adverse reactions
• Health seeking behavior for the prevention of pregnancy related to family planning
• Deficient knowledge of contraceptive drug therapy

Planning and implementation
• Encourage women with a history of hypertension or renal disease to use a different method of contraception. If Ortho Evra is used, monitor blood pressure closely and stop use if hypertension occurs.

• Drug may be less effective in women weighing 90 kg (198 lb) or more.
• Cigarette smoking increases the risk of serious CV adverse effects. This risk increases especially in women age 35 and older who smoke 15 or more cigarettes per day.
• If woman is starting the patch for the first time, she should wait until the day she begins her menstrual period. She will then choose a first-day start or a Sunday start.
• If woman chooses a first-day start, the patch should be applied during the first 24 hours of her menstrual period. If therapy starts after day 1 of the menstrual cycle, a non-hormonal back-up method of birth control should be used for the first week of the first treatment cycle.
• If the woman chooses a Sunday start, the patch should be applied on the first Sunday after her menstrual period starts. She must use back-up contraception for the first week of her cycle. If the woman's menstrual period begins on a Sunday, she should apply the first patch on that day, and no back-up contraception is needed.
• To switch from a hormonal contraceptive, begin treatment on the first day of withdrawal bleeding. If therapy starts later than the first day of withdrawal bleeding, back-up contraception should be used for the first week.
• Therapy should be started no sooner than 4 weeks after childbirth. If the woman hasn't had a menstrual period, pregnancy should be ruled out, and a back-up contraception should be used for the first week.
• After abortion or miscarriage in the first trimester, the patch may be started immediately. If it isn't started within 5 days of a first-trimester abortion, follow directions for a woman starting therapy for the first time.
• Therapy should be started no earlier than 4 weeks after a second-trimester abortion or miscarriage.
• If used postpartum or postabortion, risk of thromboembolic disease increases.
• If breakthrough bleeding occurs for more than a few cycles, stop treatment and evaluate cause.
• If no withdrawal bleeding occurs on patch-free week, resume treatment on the next scheduled patch-change day. If withdrawal bleeding fails to occur for two consecutive cycles, rule out pregnancy.
• If skin becomes irritated, the patch may be removed and a new patch applied at a different site until the next patch-change day.

• Stop use at least 4 weeks before and for 2 weeks after elective surgery that increases risk of thromboembolism and during and after prolonged immobilization.

• If patient has vision loss, proptosis, diplopia, papilledema, retinal vascular lesions, or recurrent, persistent, or severe headaches, stop use.

• If jaundice occurs, stop use.

• If patient becomes severely depressed, stop use and evaluate whether the depression is drug-related.

Patient teaching

• Emphasize the importance of having annual physical examinations to check for adverse effects or developing contraindications.

• Tell patient that the contraceptive patch doesn't protect against HIV and other sexually transmitted diseases.

• Advise patient to immediately apply a new patch once the used patch is removed, on the same day of the week, every 7 days for 3 weeks. Week 4 is patch-free. Tell patient to expect bleeding to occur during this time.

• Advise patient to start a new cycle, applying a new patch on the usual patch-change day, regardless of when the menstrual period starts or ends.

• Teach patient how to properly apply the patch.

• Tell patient to apply each patch to a new clean, dry area of the skin on the buttocks, abdomen, upper outer arm, or upper torso, to avoid irritation. Tell patient not to apply to the breasts or to skin that's red, irritated, or cut. Instruct patient to avoid creams, oils, powder, or makeup on or near the skin where the patch will be placed because it may cause the patch to become loose.

• Tell patient what to do if a patch is partially or completely detached:

– If patch is detached for less than 24 hours, try to reapply it to the same place or replace it with a new patch immediately. No back-up contraception is needed.

– If the patch is detached for 24 hours or more, or if the woman isn't sure how long the patch has been detached, she should stop the current cycle and start a new cycle immediately by applying a new patch. Back-up contraception must be used for the first week of the new cycle because the patient may not be protected from pregnancy.

– Tell patient not to attempt to reapply patch if it's no longer sticky, if it has become stuck to itself or another surface, if it has other material stuck to it, or if it has previously become loose or fallen off. If patient can't reapply a patch, she must apply a new patch immediately. She shouldn't use adhesives or wraps to hold the patch in place.

• Tell patient what to do if she forgets to change her patch:

– At the start of the cycle: Tell patient to apply the first patch of the new cycle as soon as she remembers and to use back-up contraception for the first week of the new cycle.

– In the middle of the patch cycle for 1 or 2 days: Advise patient to apply a new patch immediately. She should apply the next patch on the usual patch-change day. No back-up contraception is needed.

– In the middle of the patch cycle for more than 2 days: Tell patient to stop the current contraceptive cycle and start a new 4-week cycle immediately by applying a new patch. She should use back-up contraception for 1 week.

– At the end of a patch cycle: If patient forgets to take off her patch, tell her to remove it as soon as she remembers. Tell patient to start next cycle on the usual patch-change day, the day after day 28. No back-up contraception is needed.

• If patient wants to change her patch-change day, tell her to complete her current cycle and apply a new patch on the desired day during the patch-free week. There shouldn't be more than 7 consecutive patch-free days.

• Tell patient what to do if she misses a menstrual period:

– If patient hasn't adhered to the prescribed schedule, pregnancy should be ruled out at the time of the first missed period.

– If patient adhered to the prescribed regimen and missed one period, she should continue using the patches. If she adhered to the prescribed regimen and missed two consecutive periods, pregnancy should be ruled out.

• Tell patient to immediately stop drug if pregnancy is confirmed.

• Tell patient who wears contact lenses to contact an ophthalmologist if visual changes or changes in lens tolerance develop.

• Stress that if patient isn't sure what to do about mistakes with patch use, she should use a back-up method of birth control, such as a condom, spermicide, or diaphragm. She should contact her prescriber for further instructions.

☑ **Evaluation**

• Patient doesn't suffer from any drug-induced adverse reactions.

Reactions may be *common*, uncommon, *life-threatening*, or COMMON AND LIFE-THREATENING.

- Patient doesn't become pregnant.
- Patient and family state understanding of drug therapy.

etodolac (ultradol)

(eh-toh-DOH-lak)
Lodine, Lodine XL

Pharmacologic class: NSAID
Therapeutic class: antiarthritic
Pregnancy risk category: C (D in third trimester)

Indications and dosages

▶ **Acute pain.** *Adults:* 200 to 400 mg P.O. of film-coated tablets or capsules q 6 to 8 hours.
▶ **Acute or long-term management of osteoarthritis or rheumatoid arthritis.** *Adults:* 600 to 1,000 mg P.O. daily of film-coated tablets or capsules in two divided doses. For extended-release tablets, usual dosage is 400 to 1,000 mg P.O. once daily.

Contraindications and precautions

- Contraindicated in patients hypersensitive to drug and in those with history of aspirin- or NSAID-induced asthma, rhinitis, urticaria, or other allergic reactions.
- Use cautiously in patients with history of GI bleeding, ulceration, and perforation, in patients with renal or hepatic impairment, heart failure, hypertension, cardiac function impairments, and those who are predisposed to fluid retention.
- Lifespan: During third trimester of pregnancy, drug isn't recommended. In pregnant women during first and second trimesters and breastfeeding women, use cautiously. In children younger than age 18, safety hasn't been established.

Adverse reactions

CNS: *asthenia, malaise, dizziness,* depression, drowsiness, nervousness, insomnia, headache, fever, syncope.
CV: hypertension, *heart failure,* flushing, palpitations, edema, fluid retention.
EENT: blurred vision, tinnitus, photophobia, dry mouth.
GI: *dyspepsia,* flatulence, abdominal pain, diarrhea, nausea, constipation, gastritis, melena, vomiting, anorexia, peptic ulceration with or without *GI bleeding* or *perforation,* ulcerative stomatitis, thirst.
GU: dysuria, urinary frequency, *renal impairment.*
Hematologic: hemolytic anemia, *leukopenia, thrombocytopenia, agranulocytosis.*
Hepatic: *hepatitis.*
Metabolic: weight gain.
Respiratory: *asthma.*
Skin: pruritus, rash, photosensitivity, *Stevens-Johnson syndrome.*
Other: chills.

Interactions

Drug-drug. *Antacids:* May decrease peak levels of drug. Monitor patient for decreased etodolac effect.
Aspirin: Reduces protein-binding of etodolac without altering its clearance. Significance isn't known. Avoid using together.
Beta blockers, diuretics: Effects may be blunted. Monitor patient closely.
Cyclosporine: Impairs elimination and increases risk of nephrotoxicity. Avoid using together.
Digoxin, lithium, methotrexate: Etodolac may impair elimination of these drugs, resulting in increased levels and risk of toxicity. Monitor blood levels.
Phenytoin: Increases levels of phenytoin. Monitor patient and levels for toxicity.
Warfarin: May decrease protein-binding of warfarin but doesn't change its clearance. Although no dosage adjustment is needed, monitor PT and INR closely and watch for bleeding.
Drug-herb. *Dong quai, feverfew, garlic, ginger, horse chestnut, red clover:* May increase risk of bleeding. Discourage using together.
St. John's wort: Increases risk of photosensitivity. Discourage using together.
Drug-lifestyle. *Alcohol use:* Increases chance of adverse effects. Discourage using together.
Sun exposure: Photosensitivity reactions may occur. Urge patient to avoid unprotected or prolonged exposure to sunlight.

Effects on lab test results

- May increase BUN and creatinine levels. May decrease uric acid levels.
- May increase liver function test results. May decrease hemoglobin, hematocrit, and platelet, granulocyte, and WBC counts.
- May cause false-positive test for urinary bilirubin.

Pharmacokinetics

Absorption: Well absorbed from GI tract.
Distribution: To liver, lungs, heart, and kidneys.
Metabolism: Extensive.
Excretion: In urine primarily as metabolites; 16% is excreted in feces. *Half-life:* 7¼ hours.

Route	Onset	Peak	Duration
P.O.	≤ 30 min	1-2 hr	4-12 hr

Action

Chemical effect: May inhibit prostaglandin synthesis.
Therapeutic effect: Relieves inflammation and pain.

Available forms

Capsules: 200 mg, 300 mg
Tablets (extended-release): 400 mg, 500 mg, 600 mg
Tablets (film-coated): 400 mg, 500 mg

NURSING PROCESS

⚞ Assessment

• Obtain history of patient's underlying condition before therapy.
• Evaluate patient for decreased inflammation and pain.
• Be alert for adverse reactions and drug interactions.
• Evaluate patient's and family's knowledge of drug therapy.

⚘ Nursing diagnoses

• Acute pain related to underlying condition
• Risk for injury related to drug-induced adverse reactions
• Deficient knowledge related to drug therapy

⮚ Planning and implementation

• Give drug with milk or meals to minimize GI discomfort.
ⓈALERT: Don't confuse Lodine with iodine.
Patient teaching
• Advise patient that serious GI toxicity, including peptic ulceration and bleeding, can occur as a result of taking NSAIDs, despite absence of GI symptoms. Teach patient the signs and symptoms of GI bleeding, such as dark tarry stools, generalized weakness, coffee ground

emesis, and tell him to contact prescriber immediately if they occur.
• Tell patient to take drug with milk or food.
• Instruct patient to notify prescriber if other adverse reactions occur or if drug doesn't relieve pain.
• Advise patient to use sunblock, wear protective clothing, and avoid prolonged exposure to sunlight to prevent photosensitivity reactions.
• Tell patient not to use drug during last trimester of pregnancy.

✓ Evaluation

• Patient is free from pain.
• Patient has no injury as result of drug-induced adverse reactions.
• Patient and family state understanding of drug therapy.

etoposide (VP-16)

(eh-toh-POH-sighd)
Etopophos, Toposar, VePesid

Pharmacologic class: podophyllotoxin (cell cycle–phase specific, G2 and late S phases)
Therapeutic class: antineoplastic
Pregnancy risk category: D

Indications and dosages

▶ **Testicular cancer.** *Adults:* 50 to 100 mg/m^2 I.V. on 5 consecutive days q 3 to 4 weeks; or 100 mg/m^2 on days 1, 3, and 5 q 3 to 4 weeks for 3 to 4 courses of therapy.
▶ **Small-cell carcinoma of lung.** *Adults:* 35 mg/m^2/day I.V. for 4 days; or 50 mg/m^2/day I.V. for 5 days. P.O. dose is two times I.V. dose rounded to nearest 50 mg.
▶ **AIDS-related Kaposi's sarcoma‡.** *Adults:* 150 mg/m^2 I.V. for 3 consecutive days q 4 weeks. Repeat cycles, p.r.n.

▽ I.V. administration

• Dilute drug for infusion in either D$_5$W or normal saline solution to 0.2 or 0.4 mg/ml. Higher concentrations may crystallize.
• Give drug by slow I.V. infusion (over at least 30 minutes) to prevent severe hypotension.
• Solutions diluted to 0.2 mg/ml are stable 96 hours at room temperature in plastic or glass unprotected from light; solutions diluted to

---

0.4 mg/ml are stable 48 hours under same conditions.

⊛ **ALERT:** If systolic blood pressure falls below 90 mm Hg, stop infusion and notify prescriber.

• Don't give through membrane-type in-line filter because diluent may dissolve filter.

• Keep diphenhydramine, hydrocortisone, epinephrine, and needed emergency equipment available to establish airway in case of anaphylaxis.

Contraindications and precautions

• Contraindicated in patients hypersensitive to drug.

• Use cautiously in patients who have had previous cytotoxic or radiation therapy.

⚞ **Lifespan:** In pregnant women, drug isn't recommended unless absolutely needed because fetal harm may occur. In breast-feeding women, drug isn't recommended. In children, safety of drug hasn't been established.

Adverse reactions

CNS: peripheral neuropathy.
CV: hypotension.
GI: *nausea, vomiting, anorexia, diarrhea*, abdominal pain, *stomatitis*.
Hematologic: *anemia, myelosuppression* (dose-limiting), LEUKOPENIA, THROMBOCYTOPENIA.
Skin: reversible alopecia.
Other: *anaphylaxis*, rash.

Interactions

Drug-drug. *Warfarin:* May further prolong PT. Monitor patient for bleeding and monitor PT and INR.

Effects on lab test results

• May decrease hemoglobin, hematocrit, and WBC, RBC, platelet, and neutrophil counts.

Pharmacokinetics

Absorption: Only moderately absorbed across GI tract after P.O. administration. Bioavailability ranges from 25% to 75%, with average of 50% of dose being absorbed.
Distribution: Distributed widely in body tissues; crosses blood-brain barrier to limited and variable extent. Etoposide is about 94% protein-bound.
Metabolism: Only small portion of dose is metabolized in liver.

Excretion: Excreted primarily in urine as unchanged drug; smaller portion excreted in feces.
Half-life: Initial, 30 minutes to 2 hours; terminal, 5½ to 11 hours.

Route	Onset	Peak	Duration
P.O., I.V.	Unknown	Unknown	Unknown

Action

Chemical effect: Unknown.
Therapeutic effect: Inhibits selected cancer cell growth.

Available forms

Capsules: 50 mg
Injection: 20 mg/ml
Powder for injection: 100 mg

NURSING PROCESS

▓ Assessment

• Obtain history of patient's underlying condition before therapy.

• Obtain baseline blood pressure before therapy, and monitor blood pressure at 30-minute intervals during infusion.

• Monitor effectiveness by noting results of follow-up diagnostic tests and overall physical status and by regularly checking tumor size and rate of growth through appropriate studies. Etoposide has produced complete remission in small-cell lung cancer and testicular cancer.

• Monitor CBC. Observe patient for signs of bone marrow suppression.

• Be alert for adverse reactions and drug interactions.

• Evaluate patient's and family's knowledge of drug therapy.

⊕ Nursing diagnoses

• Ineffective health maintenance related to presence of neoplastic disease

• Ineffective protection related to drug induced adverse hematologic reactions

• Deficient knowledge related to drug therapy

▶ Planning and implementation

• Follow facility policy to reduce risks. Preparation and administration of parenteral form create carcinogenic, mutagenic, and teratogenic risks for staff.

• Store capsules in refrigerator.

Rapid onset   *Liquid form contains alcohol.   ◆Canada   ◇Australia   †OTC   ‡Off-label use

Patient teaching

• Warn patient to watch for signs of infection and bleeding. Teach patient how to take infection-control and bleeding precautions.
• Tell patient that hair loss is possible but reversible.
• Instruct patient to report discomfort, pain, or burning at I.V. insertion site.

☑ Evaluation

• Patient exhibits positive response to therapy.
• Patient's immune function returns to normal with cessation of therapy.
• Patient and family state understanding of drug therapy.

exemestane
(ecks-eh-MES-tayn)
Aromasin

Pharmacologic class: aromatase inhibitor
Therapeutic class: antineoplastic
Pregnancy risk category: D

Indications and dosages

▶ **Advanced breast cancer in postmenopausal women whose disease has progressed after tamoxifen therapy.** *Adults:* 25 mg P.O. once daily after a meal.

Contraindications and precautions

• Contraindicated in patients hypersensitive to drug or its components.
⚹ **Lifespan:** In premenopausal women, drug is contraindicated.

Adverse reactions

CNS: fever, *depression, insomnia, anxiety, fatigue, pain,* dizziness, headache, paresthesia, generalized weakness, asthenia, confusion, hypoesthesia.
CV: *hot flushes,* hypertension, edema, chest pain.
EENT: sinusitis, rhinitis, pharyngitis.
GI: *nausea,* vomiting, abdominal pain, anorexia, constipation, diarrhea, dyspepsia.
GU: UTI.
Metabolic: increased appetite.
Musculoskeletal: pathologic fractures, arthralgia, back pain, skeletal pain.

Respiratory: *dyspnea,* bronchitis, coughing, upper respiratory tract infection.
Skin: rash, increased sweating, alopecia, itching.
Other: infection, flulike syndrome, lymphedema.

Interactions

Drug-drug. *Drugs that induce CYP3A4:* May decrease exemestane level. Monitor patient closely for toxicity.
Estrogen-containing drugs: May affect drug. Don't give together.

Effects on lab test results

None reported.

Pharmacokinetics

Absorption: Rapidly absorbed, with about 42% of dose absorbed from the GI tract following P.O. administration. Level increases by 40% after a high-fat meal.
Distribution: Extensively distributed in tissues and 90% bound to proteins.
Metabolism: Extensively metabolized by the liver. The main liver isoenzyme involved is CYP 3A4.
Excretion: Excreted equally in urine and feces. Less than 1% is excreted unchanged in urine.
Elimination half-life: About 24 hours.

Route	Onset	Peak	Duration
P.O.	Unknown	1-2 hr	Unknown

Action

Chemical effect: Acts as a false substrate for the aromatase enzyme, the principal enzyme that converts androgens to estrogens in premenopausal and postmenopausal women. Drug is then processed to an intermediate that binds irreversibly to the enzyme's active site, causing inactivation. This effect is known as "suicide inhibition" and results in lower levels of circulating estrogens. Deprivation of estrogen is an effective and selective way to treat estrogen-dependent breast cancer in postmenopausal women.
Therapeutic effect: Hinders function of breast cancer cells.

Available forms

Tablets: 25 mg

NURSING PROCESS

☑ Assessment

- Assess patient's breast cancer before therapy and regularly thereafter.
- Monitor patient for adverse reactions.
- If adverse GI reactions occur, monitor patient's hydration status.
- Evaluate patient's and family's knowledge of drug therapy.

🔟 Nursing diagnoses

- Ineffective health maintenance related to presence of breast cancer
- Risk for impaired physical mobility related to potential adverse musculoskeletal effects
- Deficient knowledge related to drug therapy

⊠ Planning and implementation

- Give drug only to postmenopausal women.
- Don't give with estrogen-containing drugs because doing so could interfere with intended action.
- Continue treatment until tumor progression is evident.
- ⓢ **ALERT:** Don't confuse exemestane with estramustine.

Patient teaching

- Tell patient to take drug after a meal.
- Inform patient that she may need to take drug for a long period of time.
- Advise patient to report adverse effects to prescriber.

☑ Evaluation

- Patient responds well to drug.
- Patient has no musculoskeletal adverse reactions.
- Patient and family state understanding of drug therapy.

ezetimibe
(eh-ZET-eh-mighb)
Zetia

Pharmacologic class: selective cholesterol absorption inhibitor
Therapeutic class: antilipemic
Pregnancy risk category: C

Indications and dosages

▶ **Primary hypercholesterolemia, alone or with HMG-CoA reductase inhibitors; adjunct to atorvastatin or simvastatin in patients with homozygous familial hypercholesterolemia; homozygous sitosterolemia to reduce sitosterol and campesterol levels.**
Adults: 10 mg P.O. daily.

Contraindications and Precautions

- Contraindicated in patients allergic to any component of the drug. Use with a HMG-CoA reductase inhibitor is contraindicated in patients with active hepatic disease or unexplained increase in transaminase levels.
- ⚠ **Lifespan:** In pregnant women, use only if the benefits outweigh risk to the fetus. If used in pregnant women, do not give with an HMG-CoA reductase inhibitor. Breast-feeding isn't recommended during therapy; it's unknown whether drug appears in breast milk. In children, safety and effectiveness haven't been established. Elderly patients may have a greater sensitivity to drug.

Adverse reactions

CNS: dizziness, headache, fatigue.
CV: chest pain.
EENT: pharyngitis, sinusitis.
GI: abdominal pain, diarrhea.
Musculoskeletal: back pain, arthralgia, myalgia.
Respiratory: cough, *upper respiratory tract infection.*
Other: viral infection.

Interactions

Drug-drug. *Bile acid sequestrant (cholestyramine):* Decreases ezetimibe level. Give ezetimibe at least 2 hours before or 4 hours after cholestyramine.
Cyclosporine, fenofibrate, gemfibrozil: Increases ezetimibe level. Monitor patient closely for adverse effects.
Fibrates: May increase excretion of cholesterol into the gallbladder bile. Avoid using together.

Effects on lab test results

- May increase liver function test results.

Pharmacokinetics

Absorption: Absorbed and conjugated to an active metabolite.

Distribution: More than 90% bound to proteins.

Metabolism: Primarily and rapidly metabolized in the small intestine and liver via glucuronide conjugation.

Excretion: Biliary and renal. *Half-life:* 22 hours.

Route	Onset	Peak	Duration
P.O.	Unknown	4-12 hr	Unknown

Action

Chemical effect: Inhibits absorption of cholesterol by the small intestine. Decreases hepatic cholesterol stores and increases cholesterol clearance.

Therapeutic effect: Lowers cholesterol levels.

Available forms

Tablets: 10 mg

NURSING PROCESS

Assessment
• Obtain history of patient's underlying condition before therapy.
• Monitor total cholesterol, LDL, HDL, and triglyceride levels before and during therapy.
• Evaluate patient's and family's knowledge of drug therapy.

Nursing Diagnoses
• Risk for injury related to elevated cholesterol levels
• Deficient knowledge related to drug therapy

Planning and Implementation
• Use drug only after diet and other non-drug treatments prove ineffective. Have patient follow a standard low-cholesterol diet before and during therapy.
• Before starting treatment, evaluate patient for secondary causes of dyslipidemia.
• When drug is used with an HMG-CoA reductase inhibitor, check liver function test results at start of therapy and thereafter according to the recommendations relevant to the HMG-CoA reductase inhibitor being used.
• Use with an HMG-CoA reductase inhibitor significantly reduces total cholesterol, LDL, apolipoprotein B, and triglyceride levels and (except with pravastatin) increases HDL level more than use of an HMG-CoA reductase inhibitor alone.

ALERT: Don't confuse Zetia with Zebeta, Zestril, or Zyrtec.

Patient teaching
• Emphasize importance of following a cholesterol-lowering diet during treatment.
• Tell patient he may take drug without regard to meals.
• Advise patient to notify prescriber of unexplained muscle pain, weakness, or tenderness.
• Urge patient to tell prescriber if he's taking herbal or dietary supplements.
• Advise patient to visit his prescriber for routine follow-up and blood tests.
• Tell patient to notify prescriber if she becomes pregnant.

Evaluation
• Patient's cholesterol level is within normal limits.
• Patient and family state understanding of drug therapy.

factor IX complex
(FAK-tor nighn KOM-pleks)
Bebulin VH Immuno, Benefix, Konyne 80, Profilnine SD, Proplex T

factor IX (human)
AlphaNine SD, Mononine

Pharmacologic class: blood derivative
Therapeutic class: systemic hemostatic
Pregnancy risk category: C

Indications and dosages

▶ **Factor IX deficiency (hemophilia B or Christmas disease), anticoagulant overdosage.** *Adults and children:* To calculate approximate units of factor IX needed, use the following equations:

Human product. 1 unit/kg × body weight in kilograms × percentage of desired increase of factor IX level.

Recombinant product. 1 to 1.2 units/kg × body weight in kilograms × percentage of desired increase of factor IX level.

Proplex T. 0.5 units/kg × body weight in kilograms × percentage of desired increase of factor IX level.

Infusion rates vary with product and patient comfort. Dosage is highly individualized, depending on degree of deficiency, level of factor IX desired, patient weight, and severity of bleeding.

▼I.V. administration

• Reconstitute with 20 ml of sterile water for injection for each vial of lyophilized drug. Keep refrigerated until ready to use; warm to room temperature before reconstituting.
• Avoid rapid infusion. If tingling sensation, fever, chills, or headache develop, decrease flow rate and notify prescriber.
• Use within 3 hours of reconstitution. Drug is unstable in solution. Don't shake, refrigerate, or mix solution with other I.V. solutions.
• Store away from heat.

Contraindications and precautions

• Contraindicated in patients with hepatic disease when intravascular coagulation or fibrinolysis is suspected. Mononine is contraindicated in patients hypersensitive to mouse protein. Benefix is contraindicated in patients hypersensitive to hamster protein.
⚖ Lifespan: In pregnant and breast-feeding women and in neonates and infants, use cautiously.

Adverse reactions

CNS: *transient fever,* headache.
CV: *thromboembolic reactions, MI, DIC, pulmonary embolism, flushing,* changes in blood pressure.
GI: nausea, vomiting.
Skin: urticaria.
Other: *chills, tingling,* **hypersensitivity reactions** *(anaphylaxis,* hives, chest tightening, hypotension).

Interactions

Drug-drug. *Aminocaproic acid:* May increase risk of thrombosis. Avoid using together.

Effects on lab test results

None reported.

Pharmacokinetics

Absorption: Administered I.V.

Distribution: Equilibration within extravascular space takes 4 to 6 hours.
Metabolism: Cleared by plasma.
Excretion: Unknown. *Half-life:* About 22 hours.

Route	Onset	Peak	Duration
I.V.	Immediate	10-30 min	Unknown

Action

Chemical effect: Directly replaces deficient clotting factor.
Therapeutic effect: Causes clotting.

Available forms

Injection: Vials, with diluent. Units specified on label.

NURSING PROCESS

🔖 Assessment

• Assess patient's coagulation studies and bleeding disorder before and after therapy.
• Be alert for adverse reactions and drug interactions.
• Monitor vital signs regularly.
• Evaluate patient's and family's knowledge of drug therapy.

🔖 Nursing diagnoses

• Ineffective health maintenance related to underlying disorder
• Ineffective protection related to drug-induced intravascular hemolysis
• Deficient knowledge related to drug therapy

▶ Planning and implementation

• Because of the risk of viral infectivity from human-derived blood products, give hepatitis A and B vaccines before factor IX complex.
• Risk of hepatitis must be weighed against risk of not receiving drug. Because of manufacturing process, risk of HIV transmission is extremely low.
• If signs of hypersensitivity reactions occur, stop drug infusion immediately and notify prescriber.
Patient teaching
• Explain drug action to patient.
• Explain to patient the risks of viral infections from human-derived blood products.
• Tell patient to report adverse reactions promptly.

☑ Evaluation
- Patient is free from bleeding.
- Patient doesn't experience injury.
- Patient and family state understanding of drug therapy.

famciclovir
(fam-SIGH-kloh-veer)
Famvir

Pharmacologic class: synthetic acyclic guanine derivative
Therapeutic class: antiviral
Pregnancy risk category: B

Indications and dosages

▶ **Acute herpes zoster.** *Adults:* 500 mg P.O. q 8 hours for 7 days.
▶ **Recurrent episodes of genital herpes.** *Adults:* 125 mg P.O. b.i.d. for 5 days. Therapy begins as soon as symptoms occur.
▶ **Recurrent herpes simplex virus infections in HIV-infected patients.** *Adults:* 500 mg P.O. b.i.d. for 7 days.
▶ **Long-term suppressive therapy of recurrent episodes of genital herpes.** *Adults:* 250 mg P.O. q 12 hours for up to 1 year.

Contraindications and precautions

- Contraindicated in patients hypersensitive to drug.
- Use cautiously in patients with renal or hepatic impairment. Dosage adjustment may be needed.
- ☕ Lifespan: In pregnant women, use cautiously. Breast-feeding women shouldn't breast-feed during therapy. In children, safety hasn't been established.

Adverse reactions

CNS: *headache,* fatigue, dizziness, paresthesia, somnolence.
EENT: pharyngitis, sinusitis.
GI: diarrhea, *nausea,* vomiting, constipation, anorexia, abdominal pain.
Musculoskeletal: back pain, arthralgia.
Skin: pruritus; zoster-related signs, symptoms, and complications.

Interactions

Drug-drug. *Probenecid:* May increase level of famciclovir. Monitor patient for increased adverse effects.

Effects on lab test results

None reported.

Pharmacokinetics

Absorption: Absolute bioavailability is 77%.
Distribution: Less than 20% is bound to proteins.
Metabolism: Extensive, in liver to active drug, penciclovir, and inactive metabolites.
Excretion: Primarily in urine. *Half-life:* 2 to 3 hours.

Route	Onset	Peak	Duration
P.O.	Unknown	≤ 1 hr	Unknown

Action

Chemical effect: Converted to penciclovir, which enters viral cells and inhibits DNA polymerase and viral DNA synthesis.
Therapeutic effect: Inhibits viral replication. Spectrum of activity includes herpes simplex types 1 and 2 and varicella-zoster viruses.

Available forms

Tablets: 125 mg, 250 mg, 500 mg

NURSING PROCESS

☑ Assessment
- Assess patient's viral infection before therapy, and reassess regularly throughout therapy.
- Be alert for adverse reactions and drug interactions.
- If adverse GI reactions occur, monitor patient's hydration status.
- Evaluate patient's and family's knowledge of drug therapy.

⊕ Nursing diagnoses
- Infection related to presence of virus susceptible to famciclovir
- Risk for deficient fluid volume related to drug's adverse GI reactions
- Deficient knowledge related to drug therapy

▶ Planning and implementation
- Reduce dosage in patients with renal insufficiency.

Reactions may be *common,* uncommon, *life-threatening,* or COMMON AND LIFE-THREATENING.

- Drug may be taken without regard to meals.

Patient teaching

- Teach patient how to prevent spread of infection to others.
- Urge patient to recognize and report early symptoms of herpes infection, such as tingling, itching, or pain.

☑ Evaluation

- Patient is free from infection.
- Patient maintains adequate hydration.
- Patient and family state understanding of drug therapy.

famotidine

(fam-OH-tih-deen)
Pepcid†, Pepcid AC†, Pepcid RPD, Pepcidine ◇

Pharmacologic class: H$_2$-receptor antagonist
Therapeutic class: antiulcer agent
Pregnancy risk category: B

Indications and dosages

▶ **Duodenal ulcer (short-term treatment).**
Adults: For acute therapy, 40 mg P.O. once daily h.s. or 20 mg P.O. b.i.d. Maintenance, 20 mg P.O. once daily h.s.
▶ **Benign gastric ulcer (short-term treatment).** *Adults:* 40 mg P.O. daily h.s. for 8 weeks.
▶ **Pathologic hypersecretory conditions (such as Zollinger-Ellison syndrome).** *Adults:* 20 mg P.O. q 6 hours up to 160 mg q 6 hours.
▶ **Gastroesophageal reflux disease (GERD).**
Adults: 20 mg P.O. b.i.d. for up to 6 weeks. For esophagitis caused by GERD, 20 to 40 mg b.i.d. for up to 12 weeks.
Children ages 1 to 16: 1 mg/kg/day P.O. in divided doses b.i.d. up to 40 mg P.O. twice daily
▶ **Peptic ulcer in children.** *Children ages 1 to 16:* 0.5 mg/kg/day orally h.s. or divided twice daily up to 40 mg/day.
▶ **Heartburn, prevention of heartburn.**
Adults: 10 mg Pepcid AC P.O. 1 hour before meals (prevention) or 10 mg Pepcid AC P.O. with water when symptoms occur. Maximum, 20 mg daily. Drug shouldn't be taken daily for more than 2 weeks.
▶ **Hospitalized patients with intractable ulcerations or hypersecretory conditions or**

patients who can't take oral medication‡.
Adults: 20 mg I.V. q 12 hours.

▽ I.V. administration

- To prepare I.V. injection, dilute 2 ml (20 mg) drug with compatible I.V. solution to total volume of either 5 or 10 ml. Compatible solutions include sterile water for injection, normal saline injection, D$_5$W or dextrose 10% in water injection, 5% sodium bicarbonate injection, and lactated Ringer's injection.
- Inject over at least 2 minutes.
- For intermittent I.V. infusion, dilute 20 mg (2 ml) drug in 100 ml of compatible solution. Solution is stable for 48 hours at room temperature after dilution. Store I.V. injection in refrigerator at 36° to 46° F (2° to 8° C).
- Infuse over 15 to 30 minutes.
- If infiltration or phlebitis occurs, apply warm compresses and use different site for next dose.

Contraindications and precautions

- Contraindicated in patients hypersensitive to drug.
- ⚜ **Lifespan:** In pregnant and breast-feeding women, use cautiously. In children, safety hasn't been established.

Adverse reactions

CNS: *headache,* dizziness, vertigo, malaise, paresthesia, fever.
CV: palpitations, flushing.
EENT: tinnitus, orbital edema.
GI: diarrhea, constipation, anorexia, taste disorder, dry mouth.
Musculoskeletal: musculoskeletal pain.
Skin: acne, dry skin.
Other: transient irritation at I.V. site.

Interactions

None significant.

Effects on lab test results

- May increase BUN, creatinine, and liver enzyme levels.

Pharmacokinetics

Absorption: When given orally, about 40% to 45% is absorbed.
Distribution: Wide.
Metabolism: About 30% to 35% by liver.

Excretion: Mostly unchanged in urine. *Half-life:* 2½ to 3½ hours.

Route	Onset	Peak	Duration
P.O.	≤ 1 hr	1-3 hr	10-12 hr
I.V.	≤ 1 hr	20 min	10-12 hr

Action

Chemical effect: Competitively inhibits action of H_2 at receptor sites of parietal cells, decreasing gastric acid secretion.
Therapeutic effect: Decreases gastric acid levels and prevents heartburn.

Available forms

Gelcaps: 10 mg
Injection: 10 mg/ml, 20 mg/50 ml (premixed)
Powder for oral suspension: 40 mg/5 ml after reconstitution
Tablets: 10 mg, 20 mg†, 40 mg
Tablets, chewable: 10 mg†
Tablets, orally disintegrating: 20 mg, 40 mg

NURSING PROCESS

⚗ Assessment
• Assess patient's GI disorder before therapy and reassess regularly.
• Be alert for adverse reactions.
• Evaluate patient's and family's knowledge of drug therapy.

⊕ Nursing diagnoses
• Impaired tissue integrity related to underlying GI disorder
• Constipation related to drug's adverse effect on GI tract
• Deficient knowledge related to drug therapy

⟩ Planning and implementation
• Give drug h.s. or, if giving more than one daily dose, give last dose of day h.s.
• Store reconstituted oral suspension below 86° F (30° C). Discard after 30 days.
Patient teaching
• Tell patient to take drug with food. Remind him that drug is most effective if taken h.s. Tell patient taking 20 mg b.i.d. to take one dose h.s.
• With prescriber's knowledge, allow patient to take antacids, especially at beginning of therapy when pain is severe.
• Urge patient not to smoke because it may increase gastric acid secretion and worsen disease.

• Advise patient not to take drug for more than 8 weeks unless specifically ordered by prescriber. Tell patient not to self-medicate for heartburn longer than 2 weeks without prescriber's knowledge.

☑ Evaluation
• Patient reports decrease in or relief of GI pain with drug.
• Patient regains normal bowel pattern.
• Patient and family state understanding of drug therapy.

felodipine

(feh-LOH-dih-peen)
Agon◇, Agon SR◇, Plendil, Plendil ER◇, Renedil♦

Pharmacologic class: calcium-channel blocker
Therapeutic class: antihypertensive
Pregnancy risk category: C

Indications and dosages

▶ **Hypertension.** *Adults:* Initially, 5 mg P.O. daily. Adjust dosage based on response, usually at no less than 2-week intervals. Usual dosage is 2.5 to 10 mg daily.
Elderly patients: 2.5 mg P.O. daily, adjust as for adults. Maximum, 10 mg daily.

Contraindications and precautions

• Contraindicated in patients hypersensitive to drug.
• Use cautiously in patients with heart failure, particularly those receiving beta blockers, and in patients with impaired hepatic function.
☀ **Lifespan:** In pregnant women, use cautiously. In breast-feeding women, breast-feeding isn't recommended during therapy. In children, safety hasn't been established.

Adverse reactions

CNS: *headache,* dizziness, paresthesia, asthenia.
CV: *flushing, peripheral edema,* chest pain, palpitations.
EENT: rhinorrhea, pharyngitis, gingival hyperplasia.
GI: abdominal pain, nausea, constipation, diarrhea.
Musculoskeletal: muscle cramps, back pain.

Reactions may be *common,* uncommon, *life-threatening,* or COMMON AND LIFE-THREATENING.

Respiratory: upper respiratory infection, cough.
Skin: rash.

Interactions

Drug-drug. *Anticonvulsants:* May decrease felodipine level. Avoid using together.
Cimetidine, erythromycin, itraconazole, keto-conazole: Decreases felodipine clearance. Give lower doses of felodipine.
Metoprolol: May alter pharmacokinetics of metoprolol. No dosage adjustment necessary. Monitor patient for adverse effects.
Theophylline: May slightly decrease theophylline levels. Monitor patient's response carefully.
Drug-food. *Grapefruit:* May increase drug level. Discourage using together.
Lime: May increase level and adverse effects of drug. Discourage using together.

Effects on lab test results

None reported.

Pharmacokinetics

Absorption: Almost complete, but extensive first-pass metabolism reduces absolute bioavailability to about 20%.
Distribution: More than 99% bound to proteins.
Metabolism: Unknown, although thought to be hepatic.
Excretion: More than 70% of dose appears in urine and 10% in feces as metabolites. *Half-life:* 11 to 16 hours.

Route	Onset	Peak	Duration
P.O.	2-5 hr	2½-5 hr	24 hr

Action

Chemical effect: Unknown; however, drug is a dihydropyridine derivative that prevents entry of calcium ions into vascular smooth muscle and cardiac cells.
Therapeutic effect: Lowers blood pressure.

Available forms

Tablets: 5 mg ◊
Tablets (extended-release): 2.5 mg, 5 mg, 10 mg

NURSING PROCESS

⚡ Assessment
• Assess patient's blood pressure before therapy and reassess regularly.

• Be alert for adverse reactions and drug interactions.
• Evaluate patient's and family's knowledge of drug therapy.

🔷 Nursing diagnoses
• Risk for injury related to presence of hypertension
• Excessive fluid volume related to drug-induced peripheral edema
• Deficient knowledge related to drug therapy

▶ Planning and implementation
• Drug may be given without regard to food.
Patient teaching
• Instruct patient to swallow tablets whole and not to crush or chew them.
• Tell patient to take drug even when he feels better; to watch his diet; and to check with prescriber or pharmacist before taking other medications, including OTC medicines and herbal remedies.
• Advise patient to practice good oral hygiene and to see dentist regularly.

✓ Evaluation
• Patient's blood pressure is normal.
• Patient doesn't develop complications from peripheral edema.
• Patient and family state understanding of drug therapy.

fenofibrate
(feh-noh-FIGH-brayt)
Tricor, Lofibra

Pharmacologic class: fibric acid derivative
Therapeutic class: antilipemic
Pregnancy risk category: C

Indications and dosages

▶ **Adjunct to diet for patients with very high triglyceride levels (type IV and V hyperlipidemia) who are at high risk of pancreatitis and who don't respond adequately to diet alone.** *Adults:* 67- to 200-mg capsule or 54- to 160-mg tablet P.O. daily. Based on response to repeat triglyceride level tests at 4- to 8-week intervals, increase dosage if necessary to maximum of 200-mg capsule or 160-mg tablet daily.

▶ **Adjunct to diet for the reduction of LDL cholesterol, total cholesterol, triglycerides, and apolipoprotein B, and to increase HDL in patients with primary hypercholesterolemia or mixed dyslipidemia (Frederickson types IIa and IIb).** *Adults:* 200-mg capsule or 160-mg tablet P.O. daily.

◙ **Adjust-a-dose:** For patients with renal impairment (creatinine clearance less than 50 ml/minute) and elderly patients, initially give 67-mg capsule or 54-mg tablet daily and increase dose only after effects on renal function and triglyceride levels are evaluated.

Contraindications and precautions

• Contraindicated in patients hypersensitive to drug and in those with gallbladder disease, hepatic dysfunction, primary biliary cirrhosis, severe renal dysfunction, or unexplained persistent liver function abnormalities.
• Use cautiously in patients with history of pancreatitis.
⚘ **Lifespan:** In children, safety and effectiveness haven't been established.

Adverse reactions

CNS: dizziness, pain, asthenia, fatigue, paresthesia, insomnia, headache.
CV: *arrhythmias.*
EENT: eye irritation, eye floaters, earache, conjunctivitis, blurred vision, rhinitis, sinusitis.
GI: dyspepsia, eructation, flatulence, nausea, vomiting, abdominal pain, constipation, diarrhea, *pancreatitis,* increased appetite.
GU: polyuria, vaginitis.
Hepatic: cholelithiasis.
Musculoskeletal: arthralgia.
Respiratory: cough.
Skin: pruritus, rash.
Other: hypersensitivity reaction, *infection,* flu-like syndrome, decreased libido.

Interactions

Drug-drug. *Bile acid sequestrants:* May bind and inhibit absorption of drug. Give drug 1 hour before or 4 to 6 hours after bile acid sequestrants.
Coumarin-type anticoagulants: Potentiation of anticoagulant effect. Monitor PT and INR closely. Reduce anticoagulant dosage p.r.n.
Cyclosporine, immunosuppressants, nephrotoxic agents: May cause renal dysfunction, which may compromise the elimination of drug. Use together cautiously.

HMG-CoA reductase inhibitors: No data available; however, because of risk of myopathy, rhabdomyolysis, and acute renal impairment reported with combined use of HMG-CoA reductase inhibitors and gemfibrozil (another fibrate derivative), don't give the drugs together.
Drug-food. *Any food:* Absorption of drug is increased. Give drug with meals.
Drug-lifestyle. *Alcohol use:* May elevate triglyceride levels. Discourage using together.

Effects on lab test results

• May increase BUN, creatinine, ALT, and AST levels. May decrease uric acid levels.
• May decrease hemoglobin, hematocrit, and WBC count.

Pharmacokinetics

Absorption: Well absorbed from GI tract.
Distribution: About 99% bound to proteins.
Metabolism: Rapidly hydrolyzed by esterases to active metabolite, fenofibric acid.
Excretion: About 60% excreted in urine, mainly as metabolites, and 25% in feces. *Half-life:* 20 hours.

Route	Onset	Peak	Duration
P.O.	Unknown	6-8 hr	Unknown

Action

Chemical effect: Exact mechanism unknown. May inhibit triglyceride synthesis, resulting in a decrease in the quantity of very–low-density lipoproteins released into circulation. Drug also may stimulate breakdown of triglyceride-rich protein.
Therapeutic effect: Decreases triglyceride levels.

Available forms

Micronized capsules: 67 mg, 134 mg, 200 mg
Tablets: 54 mg, 160 mg

NURSING PROCESS

▨ **Assessment**
• Assess baseline lipid levels and liver function test results before therapy and periodically thereafter.
• Be alert for adverse reactions and drug interactions.
• Evaluate patient's and family's knowledge of drug therapy.

⊞ Nursing diagnoses
- Imbalanced nutrition: less than body requirements related to drug-induced adverse GI reactions
- Risk for infection related to adverse drug reactions
- Deficient knowledge related to drug therapy

▶ Planning and implementation
- Stop drug in patients who don't have an adequate response after 2 months of treatment with maximum dose.
- Give tablets with meals to increase bioavailability.
- Patients with severe renal impairment need evaluation of renal function and triglyceride levels before dosage increase.
- Counsel patient on importance of adhering to triglyceride-lowering diet.

Patient teaching
- Advise patient to promptly report symptoms of unexplained muscle weakness, pain, or tenderness, especially if accompanied by malaise or fever.
- Urge patient to take drug with meals to optimize drug absorption.
- Advise patient to continue weight-control measures, including diet and exercise, and to reduce alcohol intake before starting therapy.
- Instruct patient who also takes bile acid resin to take fenofibrate 1 hour before or 4 to 6 hours after bile acid resin.

☑ Evaluation
- Patient maintains adequate nutritional intake.
- Patient remains free from infection.
- Patient and family state understanding of drug therapy.

---

fentanyl citrate
(FEN-tuh-nihl SIGH-trayt)
Sublimaze

fentanyl transdermal system
Duragesic-25, Duragesic-50, Duragesic-75, Duragesic-100

fentanyl transmucosal
Actiq

Pharmacologic class: opioid analgesic

Therapeutic class: analgesic, adjunct to anesthesia, anesthetic
Pregnancy risk category: C
Controlled substance schedule: II

Indications and dosages

▶ **Adjunct to general anesthetic.** *Adults:* For low-dose therapy, 2 mcg/kg I.V. For moderate-dose therapy, 2 to 20 mcg/kg I.V.; then 25 to 100 mcg I.V. or I.M., p.r.n. For high-dose therapy, 20 to 50 mcg/kg I.V.; then 25 mcg to one-half initial loading dose I.V. p.r.n.
Children ages 2 to 12: 2 to 3 mcg/kg I.V. or I.M. during induction and maintenance phases of general anesthesia.
▶ **Adjunct to regional anesthesia.** *Adults:* 50 to 100 mcg I.M. or slow I.V. over 1 to 2 minutes.
▶ **Postoperative pain.** *Adults:* 50 to 100 mcg I.M. q 1 to 2 hours, p.r.n.
▶ **Management of chronic pain.** *Adults:* One transdermal system applied to upper torso on area of skin that isn't irritated and hasn't been irradiated. Start with 25-mcg/hour system; adjust dosage as needed and tolerated. Each system may be worn for up to 72 hours.
▶ **Breakthrough cancer pain in opioid-tolerant patients.** *Adults:* 200 mcg Actiq P.O. transmucosally initially; adjust dose based on response. Each lozenge should be sucked on for 15 minutes. An additional lozenge may be taken 30 minutes after start of the previous dose. Don't use more than 2 units per episode of breakthrough pain.

▼ I.V. administration

- Only staff trained in giving I.V. anesthetics and managing their adverse effects should give drug I.V.
- Keep naloxone and resuscitation equipment available when giving drug I.V.
- Drug is commonly used I.V. with droperidol to produce neuroleptanalgesia.

Contraindications and precautions

- Contraindicated in patients intolerant of drug.
- Use cautiously in debilitated patients and in patients with head injury, increased CSF pressure, COPD, decreased respiratory reserve, potentially compromised respirations, hepatic or renal disease, or bradyarrhythmias.
- ✳ **Lifespan:** In pregnant and breast-feeding women, use cautiously. Actiq isn't indicated for

---

use during labor and delivery. In children younger than age 2, safety hasn't been established. In children younger than age 16, safety of Actiq hasn't been established. In elderly patients, use cautiously.

Adverse reactions

CNS: *sedation, somnolence, clouded sensorium, euphoria,* dizziness, headache, *confusion, asthenia,* nervousness, hallucinations, anxiety, depression.
CV: *hypotension,* hypertension, *arrhythmias,* chest pain, *bradycardia.*
EENT: *dry mouth.*
GI: *nausea, vomiting, constipation,* ileus, abdominal pain.
GU: *urine retention.*
Respiratory: *respiratory depression,* hypoventilation, dyspnea, *apnea.*
Skin: *pruritus, diaphoresis.*
Other: physical dependence, reaction at application site (erythema, papules, edema).

Interactions

Drug-drug. *CNS depressants, general anesthetics, hypnotics, MAO inhibitors, other opioid analgesics, sedatives, tricyclic antidepressants:* May have additive effects. Use together cautiously. Reduce fentanyl dose by one-quarter to one-third. Also, reduce dosages of interacting drugs.
Diazepam: CV depression may occur when given with high doses of fentanyl. Monitor patient closely.
Droperidol: May cause hypotension and decreased pulmonary arterial pressure. Monitor patient closely.
Drug-lifestyle. *Alcohol use:* May have additive effects. Discourage using together.

Effects on lab test results

None reported.

Pharmacokinetics

Absorption: Varies with transmucosal or transdermal use.
Distribution: Accumulates to adipose tissue and skeletal muscle.
Metabolism: In liver.
Excretion: In urine. *Half-life:* About 3½ hours after parenteral use, 5 to 15 hours after transmucosal use, 18 hours after transdermal use.

Route	Onset	Peak	Duration
I.V.	1-2 min	3-5 min	30 min-1 hr
I.M.	7-15 min	20-30 min	1-2 hr
Transmucosal	15 min	20-30 min	Unknown
Transdermal	12-24 hr	1-3 days	Varies

Action

Chemical effect: May bind with opioid receptors in CNS, altering both perception of and emotional response to pain.
Therapeutic effect: Relieves pain.

Available forms

Injection: 50 mcg/ml
Transdermal system: patches designed to release 25, 50, 75, or 100 mcg of fentanyl per hour
Transmucosal: 200 mcg, 400 mcg, 600 mcg, 800 mcg, 1,200 mcg, 1,600 mcg

NURSING PROCESS

⚕ Assessment

• Assess patient's underlying condition before therapy.
• Evaluate degree of pain relief obtained after each administration.
• Periodically monitor postoperative vital signs and bladder function. Because drug decreases both rate and depth of respirations, monitoring of arterial oxygen saturation (SaO_2) may help assess respiratory depression.
• Monitor patient who develops adverse reactions to transdermal system for at least 12 hours after removal. Drug levels may take as long as 17 hours to decline by 50%.
• Be alert for adverse reactions and drug interactions.
• Evaluate patient's and family's knowledge of drug therapy.

Nursing diagnoses

• Acute pain related to underlying condition
• Ineffective breathing pattern related to respiratory depression
• Deficient knowledge related to drug therapy

❯ Planning and implementation

• For better analgesic effect, give drug before patient has intense pain.

Reactions may be *common,* uncommon, *life-threatening,* or COMMON AND LIFE-THREATENING.

• To give Actiq transmucosal lozenge:
– Open child-proof foil package with scissors immediately before use.
– Place lozenge in patient's mouth between the cheek and the lower gums, occasionally switching sides using the handle.
– Make sure patient sucks the lozenge, rather than chewing and swallowing, which may cause lower peak concentrations.
– Make sure patient consumes the lozenge in 15 minutes. Faster or slower consumption may reduce its effects.
– If signs of excess opioid effects appear before the entire lozenge dissolves, remove the lozenge from the patient's mouth and decrease future doses.
– Dispose of Actiq, particularly any unused portions, in the storage container provided in Actiq's welcome kit.
⑤ **ALERT:** Ask patient and caregivers about the presence of children in the home. Actiq lozenges may be fatal to a child. Proper disposal is necessary.
• Transdermal drug isn't recommended for postoperative pain.
• Use dosage equivalency charts to calculate transdermal dose based on daily morphine intake—for example, for every 90 mg of oral morphine or 15 mg of I.M. morphine per 24 hours, 25 mcg/hour of transdermal fentanyl is needed.
• Adjust dosage gradually in patient using transdermal system. Reaching steady-state levels of new dosage may take up to 6 days; delay dosage adjustment until after at least two applications.
• High doses can produce muscle rigidity, which can be reversed with neuromuscular blockers; however, patient must be ventilated artificially.
• Immediately report respiratory rate below 12 breaths/minute or decreased respiratory volume or SaO_2.
• When drug is used postoperatively, encourage patient to turn, cough, and breathe deeply to prevent atelectasis.
• Most patients have good control of pain for 3 days while wearing transdermal system, but a few may need new application after 48 hours. Because level rises for first 24 hours after application, analgesic effect can't be evaluated on the first day. Make sure patient has adequate supplemental analgesic to prevent breakthrough pain.

• When reducing opioid therapy or switching to different analgesic, withdraw transdermal system gradually. Because drug level drops gradually after removal, give half of equianalgesic dose of new analgesic 12 to 18 hours after removal.

Patient teaching
• Teach patient proper application of transdermal patch. Instruct patient to clip hair at application site, but to avoid razor, which may irritate skin. Tell him to wash area with clear water if necessary, but not with soaps, oils, lotions, alcohol, or other substances that may irritate skin or prevent adhesion. Urge him to dry area completely before application.
• Tell patient to remove transdermal system from package just before applying, to hold in place for 10 to 20 seconds, and to be sure edges of patch adhere to the skin.
• Teach patient to dispose of transdermal patch by folding so adhesive side adheres to itself and then flushing it down toilet.
• If patient needs another patch after 72 hours, tell him to apply it to new site.
• Inform patient that heat from fever or environment may increase transdermal delivery and cause toxicity, which requires dosage adjustment. Instruct patient to notify prescriber if fever occurs or if he will be spending time in hot climate.
⑤ **ALERT:** Strongly warn patient to keep drug safely secured, away from children.
• Teach patient how to properly take transmucosal Actiq.
⑤ **ALERT:** Teach patient proper disposal of transmucosal Actiq units because ingestion of Actiq may be fatal in children.

☑ **Evaluation**
• Patient is free from pain.
• Patient maintains adequate ventilation throughout drug therapy.
• Patient and family state understanding of drug therapy.

ferrous fumarate
(FEH-rus FYOO-muh-rayt)
Femiron†, Feostat†, Feostat Drops†,
Ferretts †, Fumasorb†, Fumerin†,
Hemocyte†, Ircon†, Maniron †, Neo-Fer ♦ †,
Nephro-Fer†, Novofumar ♦ †, Palafer ♦ †,
Palafer Pediatric Drops ♦ , Span-FF†

ferrous gluconate
Fergon†, Fertinic ♦ , Novoferrogluc ♦

ferrous sulfate
Apo-Ferrous Sulfate ♦ , Feosol*†, Feratab,
Fer-Gen-Sol Drops†, Fer-In-Sol*†, Fer-Iron
Drops†, Fero-Grad ♦ , Fero-Gradumet†,
Irospan†, Mol-Iron

ferrous sulfate, dried
Feosol, Fer-In-Sol, Fe⁵⁰, Slow-Fe†

Pharmacologic class: oral iron supplement
Therapeutic class: hematinic
Pregnancy risk category: A

Indications and dosages

▶ **Iron deficiency.** *Adults:* 50 to 100 mg ferrous fumarate elemental iron P.O. t.i.d. Or, 325 mg ferrous gluconate P.O. q.i.d., increased to 650 mg q.i.d. if needed and tolerated. Or, 300 mg ferrous sulfate P.O. b.i.d. to q.i.d. Or, 1 extended-release capsule (160 to 525 mg) ferrous sulfate P.O. daily to b.i.d.
Children: 4 to 6 mg/kg ferrous fumarate P.O. daily, divided into three doses.
Children age 2 and older: 3 mg/kg ferrous gluconate P.O. daily in three to four divided doses. Or, 3 mg/kg ferrous sulfate P.O. daily in three or four divided doses.

Contraindications and precautions

• Contraindicated in patients with primary hemochromatosis, hemosiderosis, hemolytic anemia (unless iron deficiency anemia is also present), peptic ulcer disease, regional enteritis, or ulcerative colitis, and in those receiving repeated blood transfusions.
• Use cautiously on long-term basis.
☀ **Lifespan:** In breast-feeding women, iron supplements usually are recommended. In children, use cautiously. Extended-release forms

aren't recommended for children. In elderly patients, may cause constipation.

Adverse reactions

GI: *nausea, epigastric pain, vomiting, constipation,* diarrhea, black stools, anorexia.
Other: suspension and drops may temporarily stain teeth.

Interactions

Drug-drug. *Antacids, cholestyramine resin, fluoroquinolones, levodopa, penicillamine, tetracycline, vitamin E:* Decreases iron absorption. Separate doses by 2 to 4 hours.
Chloramphenicol: Increases iron response. Watch patient carefully.
Fluoroquinolones, penicillamine, tetracyclines: Decreases GI absorption, possibly decreasing levels and effectiveness. Separate doses by 2 to 4 hours.
L-thyroxine: Decreases L-thyroxine absorption. Separate doses by at least 2 hours. Monitor thyroid function.
Levodopa, methyldopa: Decreases absorption and effectiveness of levodopa and methyldopa. Monitor patient for decreased effects of these drugs.
Vitamin C: May increase iron absorption. Suggest patient take vitamin C with drug.
Drug-food. *Cereals, cheese, coffee, eggs, milk, tea, whole-grain breads, yogurt:* May impair oral iron absorption. Advise against using together.

Effects on lab test results

None reported.

Pharmacokinetics

Absorption: Primarily at duodenum and proximal jejunum. Up to 10% is absorbed by healthy people; patients with iron-deficiency anemia may absorb up to 60%. Enteric coating and some extended-release formulas have decreased absorption because they're designed to release mineral past points of highest GI absorption. Food may decrease absorption by 33% to 50%.
Distribution: Binds immediately to carrier protein, transferrin, then to bone marrow for incorporation into hemoglobin. Highly protein-bound.
Metabolism: Liberated by destruction of hemoglobin but is conserved and reused by body.

Excretion: Healthy people lose only small amounts of mineral each day. Men and post-menopausal women lose about 1 mg/day, and premenopausal women about 1.5 mg/day. The loss usually occurs in nails, hair, feces, and urine; trace amounts are lost in bile and sweat. *Half-life:* Unknown.

Route	Onset	Peak	Duration
P.O.	≤ 4 days	7-10 days	2-4 mo

Action

Chemical effect: Provides elemental iron, an essential component in formation of hemoglobin.
Therapeutic effect: Relieves iron deficiency.

Available forms

ferrous fumarate
(Each 100 mg provides 33 mg of elemental iron.)
Drops: 45 mg/0.6 ml†
Oral suspension: 100 mg/5 ml†
Tablets: 200 mg, 324 mg, 325 mg, 350 mg
Tablets (chewable): 100 mg†
ferrous gluconate
(Each 100 mg provides 11.6 mg of elemental iron.)
Capsules: 86 mg†
Tablets: 240 mg, 300 mg†, 320 mg† (contains 37 mg elemental iron), 325 mg†
ferrous sulfate
(About 20% elemental iron; dried and powdered, it's about 32% elemental iron.)
Capsules: 150 mg†, 159 mg (dried), 190 mg (dried), 250 mg†, 390 mg†
Capsules (extended-release): 150 mg (dried), 160 mg (dried)
Drops: 75 mg/0.6 ml, 125 mg/ml
Elixir: 220 mg/5 ml*†
Solution: 75 mg/0.6 ml, 300 mg/5 ml
Syrup: 90 mg/5 ml*†
Tablets: 195 mg†, 300 mg†, 325 mg†, 187 mg (dried), 200 mg (dried)
Tablets (extended-release): 160 mg (dried)†, 525 mg

NURSING PROCESS

⚗ Assessment

• Obtain baseline assessment of patient's iron deficiency before therapy.

• Evaluate hemoglobin, hematocrit, and reticulocyte count during therapy.
• Be alert for adverse reactions and drug interactions.
• Evaluate patient's and family's knowledge of drug therapy.

💠 Nursing diagnoses

• Fatigue related to iron deficiency
• Constipation related to adverse effect of drug therapy on GI tract
• Deficient knowledge related to drug therapy

▶ Planning and implementation

• Give tablets with juice or water, but not with milk or antacids.
• Dilute liquid forms in juice or water, but not in milk or antacids.
• To avoid staining teeth, give suspension or elixir with straw and place drops at back of throat.
• Don't crush or allow patient to chew extended-release forms.
• GI upset may be related to dose. Between-meal dosing is preferable, but iron can be given with some foods, although absorption may be decreased. Enteric-coated products reduce GI upset but also reduce amount of iron absorbed.
• Oral iron may turn stools black. Although this unabsorbed iron is harmless, it could mask presence of melena. Have stools tested for presence of blood.

Patient teaching
🟢 **ALERT:** Inform parents that as few as three tablets can cause poisoning in children.
• If patient misses dose, tell him to take it as soon as he remembers but not to double the dose.
• Advise patient to avoid certain foods that may impair oral iron absorption, including yogurt, cheese, eggs, milk, whole-grain breads and cereals, tea, and coffee.
• Teach dietary measures for preventing constipation.

☑ Evaluation

• Patient reports fatigue is no longer a problem in daily life.
• Patient states appropriate measures to prevent or relieve constipation.
• Patient and family state understanding of drug therapy.

Rapid onset   *Liquid form contains alcohol.*   ♦ Canada   ◊ Australia   †OTC   ‡Off-label use

fexofenadine hydrochloride
(feks-oh-FEN-uh-deen high-droh-KLOR-ighd)
Allegra, Telfast ◆

Pharmacologic class: H₁-receptor antagonist
Pharmacologic class: H_1-receptor antagonist
Therapeutic class: antihistamine
Pregnancy risk category: C

Indications and dosages

▶ **Seasonal allergic rhinitis.** *Adults and children age 12 and older:* 60 mg P.O. b.i.d. or 180 mg P.O. once daily.
Children ages 6 to 11: 30 mg P.O. b.i.d.
▶ **Chronic idiopathic urticaria.** *Children age 12 and older:* 60 mg P.O. b.i.d.
Children ages 6 to 11: 30 mg P.O. b.i.d.
◙ **Adjust-a-dose:** For patients with renal impairment, if creatinine clearance is less than 80 ml/minute, increase dosage interval to q 24 hours.

Contraindications and precautions

• Contraindicated in patients hypersensitive to drug or its components.
• Use cautiously in patients with renal impairment.
⚠ **Lifespan:** In pregnant women, use only if clearly needed and avoid use in the third trimester. In breast-feeding women, use cautiously because it's unknown whether drug appears in breast milk. In children younger than age 6, safety and effectiveness haven't been established.

Adverse reactions

CNS: fatigue, drowsiness.
GI: nausea, dyspepsia.
GU: dysmenorrhea.
Other: viral infection.

Interactions

Drug-drug. *Erythromycin, ketoconazole:* Increases fexofenadine levels. Prolonged QT interval has been seen with other antihistamines. Monitor patient closely.
Drug-food. *Apple:* May decrease drug level. Discourage using together.
Grapefruit: May decrease level, reducing therapeutic effects. Discourage using together.
Orange juice: May decrease GI absorption of drug, reducing effects. Discourage using together.

Effects on lab test results

None reported.

Pharmacokinetics

Absorption: Rapid.
Distribution: Protein-binding is 60% to 70%.
Metabolism: Unknown.
Excretion: About 80% in feces and 11% in urine. *Half-life:* 14½ hours.

Route	Onset	Peak	Duration
P.O.	Unknown	3 hr	14 hr

Action

Chemical effect: Selectively inhibits peripheral H₁-receptors.
Chemical effect: Selectively inhibits peripheral H_1-receptors.
Therapeutic effect: Relieves symptoms of seasonal allergies.

Available forms

Capsules: 180 mg
Tablets: 30 mg, 60 mg, 120 mg ◇, 180 mg

NURSING PROCESS

◪ Assessment
• Assess patient's seasonal allergy symptoms before therapy and thereafter.
• Monitor patient for adverse reactions.
• Evaluate patient's and family's knowledge of drug therapy.

◈ Nursing diagnoses
• Risk for injury related to fatigue and drowsiness caused by drug
• Ineffective health maintenance related to underlying condition
• Deficient knowledge related to drug therapy

▷ Planning and implementation
• Reduce daily dose in patient with renal impairment or currently on dialysis.
• Avoid giving with apple, orange, or grapefruit juice.
Patient teaching
• Instruct patient not to exceed prescribed dosage and to take drug only during seasonal allergy symptoms.
• Warn patient to avoid alcohol and hazardous activities that require alertness until CNS effects of drug are known.

Reactions may be *common*, uncommon, **life-threatening**, or COMMON AND LIFE-THREATENING.

- Tell patient that coffee or tea may reduce drowsiness. Suggest sugarless gum or hard candy or ice chips to relieve dry mouth.
- Tell patient to avoid taking drug with apple, orange, or grapefruit juice.

☑ **Evaluation**
- Patient experiences limited fatigue and drowsiness caused by the drug.
- Patient responds well to the drug.
- Patient and family state understanding of drug therapy.

filgrastim (granulocyte colony-stimulating factor; G-CSF)
(fil-GRAH-stem)
Neupogen

Pharmacologic class: biologic response modifier
Therapeutic class: colony-stimulating factor, hematopoietic
Pregnancy risk category: C

Indications and dosages

▶ **Agranulocytosis‡, pancytopenia with colchine overdose‡, acute leukemia‡, hematologic toxicity with zidovudine therapy‡, decrease risk of infection in patients with nonmyeloid cancers receiving myelosuppressive antineoplastics.** *Adults and children:* 5 mcg/kg I.V. or S.C. daily as single dose. May be increased in increments of 5 mcg/kg for each chemotherapy cycle, depending on duration and severity of nadir of absolute neutrophil count (ANC).

▶ **To decrease risk of infection in patients with nonmyeloid cancers receiving myelosuppressive antineoplastics followed by bone marrow transplant.** *Adults and children:* 10 mcg/kg I.V. or S.C. daily at least 24 hours after cytotoxic chemotherapy and bone marrow infusion. Adjust subsequent dosages according to neutrophil response.

▶ **Congenital neutropenia.** *Adults:* 6 mcg/kg S.C. b.i.d. Adjust dosage based on response.

▶ **Idiopathic or cyclic neutropenia.** *Adults:* 5 mcg/kg S.C. daily. Adjust dosage based on response.

▶ **Peripheral blood progenitor cell collection.** *Adults:* 10 mcg/kg S.C. daily for at least 4 days before first leukapheresis and continuing until the last leukapheresis is completed.

▶ **Myelodysplasia‡.** *Adults:* 0.3 to 10 mcg/kg S.C. daily.

▶ **Neutropenia from HIV infection‡.** *Adults and adolescents:* 5 to 10 mcg/kg S.C. or I.V. daily for 2 to 4 weeks.

▼ I.V. administration

- Dilute in 50 to 100 ml of D_5W. If final concentration will be 2 to 15 mcg/ml, add albumin at 2 mg/ml (0.2%) to minimize binding of drug to plastic containers or tubing.
- Give by intermittent infusion over 15 to 60 minutes or continuous infusion over 24 hours.
- Refrigerate drug at 36° to 46° F (2° to 8° C). Don't freeze; avoid shaking. Store at room temperature for maximum of 6 hours; discard after 6 hours.

Contraindications and precautions

- Contraindicated in patients hypersensitive to proteins derived from *Escherichia coli* or to drug or its components.
- ⚖ **Lifespan:** In pregnant and breast-feeding women, use cautiously.

Adverse reactions

CNS: *fever, fatigue,* headache, weakness.
CV: *MI, arrhythmias,* chest pain.
GI: *nausea, vomiting, diarrhea, mucositis,* stomatitis, constipation.
GU: hematuria, proteinuria.
Hematologic: *thrombocytopenia,* leukocytosis.
Musculoskeletal: *skeletal pain.*
Respiratory: dyspnea, cough.
Skin: *alopecia,* rash, cutaneous vasculitis.
Other: *hypersensitivity reactions.*

Interactions

Drug-drug. *Chemotherapy drugs:* Rapidly dividing myeloid cells are sensitive to cytotoxic drugs. Don't use filgrastim within 24 hours before or after a chemotherapy dose.

Effects on lab test results

- May increase creatinine, uric acid, alkaline phosphatase, and LDH levels.
- May increase WBC count. May decrease platelet count.

Pharmacokinetics

Absorption: Rapid.
Distribution: Unknown.
Metabolism: Unknown.
Excretion: Unknown. *Half-life:* About 3½ hours.

Route	Onset	Peak	Duration
I.V.	5-60 min	24 hr	1-7 days
S.C.	5-60 min	2-8 hr	1-7 days

Action

Chemical effect: Stimulates proliferation and differentiation of hematopoietic cells. Drug is specific for neutrophils.
Therapeutic effect: Raises WBC levels.

Available forms

Injection: 300 mcg/ml

NURSING PROCESS

🔖 Assessment
• Assess patient's underlying condition before therapy.
• Obtain baseline CBC and platelet counts before and during therapy.
• Be alert for adverse reactions and drug interactions.
• Ask patient about skeletal pain.
• Evaluate patient's and family's knowledge of drug therapy.

🔲 Nursing diagnoses
• Ineffective protection related to underlying condition or treatment
• Acute pain related to adverse drug effects on skeletal muscle
• Deficient knowledge related to drug therapy

▷ Planning and implementation
• Don't give drug within 24 hours of cytotoxic chemotherapy.
• Once dose is withdrawn, don't reenter vial. Discard unused portion. Vials are for single-dose use and contain no preservatives.
• Give daily for up to 2 weeks or until ANC has returned to 10,000/mm³ after expected chemotherapy-induced neutrophil nadir.
Patient teaching
• Teach patient how to give drug and how to dispose of used needles, syringes, drug containers, and unused drug.

• Tell patient to report bruising or spontaneous bleeding, such as frequent nosebleeds.
• Teach patient how to manage skeletal pain.

☑ Evaluation
• Patient's WBC count is normal.
• Patient reports skeletal pain is bearable or relieved with analgesic administration and comfort measures.
• Patient and family state understanding of drug therapy.

finasteride
(fin-ES-teh-righd)
Propecia, Proscar

Pharmacologic class: steroid (synthetic 4-azasteroid) derivative
Therapeutic class: androgen synthesis inhibitor
Pregnancy risk category: X

Indications and dosages

▶ **Adjunct therapy after radical prostatectomy‡, first-stage prostate cancer‡, acne‡, or hirsutism‡; to reduce risk of acute urinary retention and need for surgery, including prostatectomy and transurethral resection of prostate; symptomatic BPH.** *Adults:* 5 mg Proscar P.O. daily
▶ **Male pattern baldness.** *Men:* 1 mg Propecia P.O. daily.

Contraindications and precautions

• Contraindicated in patients hypersensitive to drug or to other 5-alpha-reductase inhibitors, such as dutasteride. Use cautiously in patients with liver dysfunction.
⚠ **Lifespan:** In women and children, drug is contraindicated.

Adverse reactions

GU: impotence, decreased volume of ejaculate.
Other: decreased libido.

Interactions

None significant.

Effects on lab test results

• May decrease PSA level.

Pharmacokinetics

Absorption: Not clearly defined, although average bioavailability was 63% in one study.
Distribution: About 90% bound to proteins; crosses blood-brain barrier.
Metabolism: Extensive.
Excretion: 39% excreted in urine as metabolites; 57% in feces. *Half-life:* Unknown.

Route	Onset	Peak	Duration
P.O.	Unknown	1-2 hr	About 2 wk

Action

Chemical effect: Competitively inhibits steroid 5-reductase, an enzyme that forms potent androgen 5-dihydrotestosterone (DHT) from testosterone. Because DHT influences development of prostate gland, lower levels will relieve symptoms of BPH. For male pattern baldness, a balding scalp contains increased amounts of DHT; drug decreases scalp and serum DHT levels.
Therapeutic effect: Relieves symptoms of BPH, reduces hair loss, and promotes hair growth.

Available forms

Tablets: 1 mg, 5 mg

NURSING PROCESS

⚖ Assessment

• Before therapy, assess patient's BPH, and evaluate him for conditions that could mimic BPH, including hypotonic bladder; prostate cancer, infection, or stricture; or relevant neurologic conditions. Carefully monitor patients with large residual urine volume or severely diminished urine flow. These patients may not be candidates for therapy.
• Evaluate patient for improvement in BPH symptoms.
• Perform periodic digital rectal examinations.
• Be alert for adverse reactions and drug interactions.
• Carefully evaluate sustained increases in PSA levels, which could indicate noncompliance.
• Evaluate patient's and family's knowledge of drug therapy.

🔅 Nursing diagnoses

• Impaired urinary elimination related to BPH
• Ineffective sexuality patterns related to drug-induced impotence
• Deficient knowledge related to drug therapy

▷ Planning and implementation

• Because it's impossible to identify which patients will respond to therapy, keep in mind that a minimum of 6 months of therapy may be necessary.

Patient teaching
• Warn woman who is or may become pregnant not to handle crushed or broken tablets because of risk of adverse effects on fetus.
• Reassure patient that although drug may decrease volume of ejaculate, it doesn't appear to impair normal sexual function. Impotence and decreased libido have occurred in less than 4% of patients.
• Tell patient taking drug for male pattern baldness that he may not notice any effects for 3 months or more.
• Warn patient not to donate blood until at least 1 month after final dose.
• Tell patient that drug may be taken without regard to meals.

☑ Evaluation

• Patient's BPH symptoms diminish.
• Patient states appropriate ways to manage sexual dysfunction.
• Patient and family state understanding of drug therapy.

flecainide acetate
(FLEH-kay-nighd AS-ih-tayt)
Tambocor

Pharmacologic class: benzamide derivative
Therapeutic class: antiarrhythmic
Pregnancy risk category: C

Indications and dosages

▶ **Paroxysmal supraventricular tachycardia; paroxysmal atrial fibrillation or flutter in patients without structural heart disease.**
Adults: 50 mg P.O. q 12 hours. Increase in increments of 50 mg b.i.d. q 4 days until efficacy is achieved. Maximum, 300 mg daily.
▶ **Life-threatening ventricular arrhythmias, such as sustained ventricular tachycardia.**
Adults: 100 mg P.O. q 12 hours. Increase in increments of 50 mg b.i.d. q 4 days until efficacy is achieved. Maximum, 400 mg daily for most patients. Or, give 2 mg/kg I.V. push over at least 10 minutes; or dilute dose and give as infusion.

Adjust-a-dose: For patients with renal impairment, if creatinine clearance is 35 ml/minute or less, initial dose is 100 mg once daily or 50 mg b.i.d.; if more than 35 ml/minute, initial dose is 100 mg q 12 hours. Adjust doses cautiously for all renally impaired patients.

▼ I.V. administration ◇

• For I.V. infusion, mix only with D₅W.
• When giving by I.V. push, give over at least 10 minutes.

Contraindications and precautions

• Contraindicated in patients hypersensitive to drug and in those with cardiogenic shock or second- or third-degree AV block or right bundle branch block related to left hemiblock (in absence of artificial pacemaker).
• Use cautiously in patients with heart failure, cardiomyopathy, severe renal or hepatic disease, prolonged QT interval, sick sinus syndrome, or blood dyscrasia.
 Lifespan: In pregnant women, use cautiously. In breast-feeding women, avoid breast-feeding during drug therapy. In children, safety hasn't been established.

Adverse reactions

CNS: *dizziness, headache,* fatigue, tremor, anxiety, insomnia, depression, malaise, paresthesia, ataxia, vertigo, *light-headedness, syncope,* asthenia, fever.
CV: edema, *new or worsened arrhythmias,* chest pain, *heart failure, cardiac arrest,* palpitations, flushing.
EENT: *blurred vision and other visual disturbances.*
GI: nausea, constipation, abdominal pain, dyspepsia, vomiting, diarrhea, anorexia.
Respiratory: *dyspnea.*
Skin: rash.

Interactions

Drug-drug. *Amiodarone, cimetidine:* May alter pharmacokinetics. Watch for toxicity.
Digoxin: May increase digoxin level by 15% to 25%. Monitor digoxin level; watch for toxicity.
Disopyramide, verapamil: Negative inotropic properties may be additive with flecainide. Avoid giving together.
Propranolol, other beta blockers: Increases both flecainide and propranolol levels by 20% to

30%. Monitor patient for propranolol and flecainide toxicity.
Urine acidifying and alkalinizing agents: Extremes of urine pH may substantially alter excretion of flecainide. Monitor patient for flecainide toxicity or decreased effectiveness.
Drug-lifestyle. *Smoking:* May lower drug level. Discourage smoking.

Effects on lab test results

None reported.

Pharmacokinetics

Absorption: Rapid and almost complete; bioavailability is 85% to 90%.
Distribution: May be well distributed throughout body. Only about 40% binds to proteins.
Metabolism: In liver to inactive metabolites. About 30% of oral dose escapes metabolism.
Excretion: In urine. *Half-life:* 12 to 27 hours.

Route	Onset	Peak	Duration
P.O.	Unknown	2-3 hr	Unknown
I.V.	Immediate	Immediate	Unknown

Action

Chemical effect: Decreases excitability, conduction velocity, and automaticity as result of slowed atrial, AV node, His-Purkinje system, and intraventricular conduction and causes slight but significant prolongation of refractory periods in these tissues.
Therapeutic effect: Restores normal sinus rhythm.

Available forms

Injection: 10 mg/ml ◇
Tablets: 50 mg, 100 mg, 150 mg

NURSING PROCESS

 Assessment
• Assess patient's arrhythmia before therapy.
• Monitor effectiveness by continuous ECG monitoring initially; long-term oral administration requires regular ECG readings.
• Monitor level, especially in patient with renal impairment or heart failure. Therapeutic level ranges from 0.2 to 1 mcg/ml. Risk of adverse effects increases when trough level exceeds 1 mcg/ml.
• Monitor potassium level regularly.

- Be alert for adverse reactions and drug inter-actions.
- Evaluate patient's and family's knowledge of drug therapy.

⊞ Nursing diagnoses
- Decreased cardiac output related to underly-ing arrhythmia
- Ineffective protection related to drug-induced new arrhythmias
- Deficient knowledge related to drug therapy

▷ Planning and implementation
- If used to prevent ventricular arrhythmias, give drug only to patient with documented life-threatening arrhythmias.
- If patient has pacemaker, check that pacing threshold was determined 1 week before and af-ter starting therapy because drug can alter endo-cardial pacing thresholds.
- Correct hypokalemia or hyperkalemia before giving drug because these electrolyte distur-bances may alter effect.
- Twice-daily dosing enhances patient compli-ance.
- Because of drug's long half-life, its full effect may take 3 to 5 days. Give I.V. lidocaine with drug for first several days.
- Keep emergency equipment nearby when giv-ing drug.
- If ECG disturbances occur, withhold drug, ob-tain rhythm strip, and notify prescriber immedi-ately.
Patient teaching
- Stress importance of taking oral drug exactly as prescribed.
- Warn patient to avoid hazardous activities that require alertness or good vision if adverse CNS or visual reactions occur.
- Tell patient to limit fluid and sodium intake to minimize heart failure or fluid retention and to weigh himself daily on the same scale at around the same time. Urge him to report promptly sud-den weight gain.

☑ Evaluation
- Patient regains normal cardiac output with abolishment of underlying arrhythmia after drug therapy.
- Patient doesn't develop new arrhythmias.
- Patient and family state understanding of drug therapy.

fluconazole
(floo-KON-uh-zohl)
Diflucan

Pharmacologic class: bis-triazole derivative
Therapeutic class: antifungal
Pregnancy risk category: C

Indications and dosages
▶ **Oropharyngeal and esophageal candidia-sis.** *Adults:* 200 mg P.O. or I.V. on first day, fol-lowed by 100 mg once daily. Higher doses (up to 400 mg daily) have been used for esophageal disease. Continue for 2 weeks after symptoms resolve.
Children: 6 mg/kg P.O. or I.V. on first day, followed by 3 mg/kg once daily for at least 2 weeks.
▶ **Vulvovaginal candidiasis.** *Adults:* 150 mg P.O. as a single dose.
▶ **Systemic candidiasis.** *Adults:* 400 mg P.O. or I.V. on first day, followed by 200 mg once daily. Continue at least 4 weeks or for 2 weeks after symptoms resolve.
Children: 6 to 12 mg/kg P.O. or I.V. daily.
▶ **Cryptococcal meningitis.** *Adults:* 400 mg P.O. or I.V. on first day, followed by 200 mg once daily. Higher doses (up to 400 mg daily) may be used. Continue for 10 to 12 weeks after CSF culture is negative.
Children: 12 mg/kg P.O. or I.V. on first day, fol-lowed by 6 mg/kg P.O. or I.V. daily for 10 to 12 weeks after CSF culture becomes negative.
▶ **Prevention of candidiasis in bone marrow transplant.** *Adults:* 400 mg. P.O. or I.V. once daily. Start prophylaxis several days before an-ticipated granulocytopenia. Continue therapy for 7 days after neutrophil count rises above 1,000 cells/mm³.
▶ **Suppression of relapse of cryptococcal meningitis in patients with AIDS.** *Adults:* 200 mg P.O. or I.V. daily.
Children: 3 to 6 mg/kg P.O. daily.
◩ **Adjust-a-dose:** For patients with renal impair-ment, if creatinine clearance is less than 50 ml/minute, reduce dose by 50% in patients not re-ceiving dialysis. For patients on hemodialysis, give 100% of usual dose after each dialysis ses-sion.

▶ **Candidal infection, long-term suppression in patients with HIV infection‡.** *Adults:* 100 to 200 mg P.O. or I.V. daily.

▶ **Prevention of mucocutaneous candidiasis, cryptococcosis, coccidioidomycosis, or histoplasmosis in patients with HIV infection‡.** *Adults:* 200 to 400 mg P.O. or I.V. daily. *Children and infants:* 2 to 8 mg/kg P.O. daily.

◩ **Adjust-a-dose:** For patients with renal impairment, if creatinine clearance is 21 to 49 ml/minute, give 50% of usual adult dose. If creatinine clearance is 11 to 20 ml/minute, give 25% of usual adult dose. For patients on hemodialysis, give one full dose after each session.

▼ I.V. administration

• Don't remove protective overwrap from I.V. bags of fluconazole until just before use to ensure product sterility. Plastic container may show some opacity from moisture absorbed during sterilization. This is normal, won't affect drug, and will diminish over time.
• Give by continuous infusion at no more than 200 mg/hour. Use infusion pump. To prevent air embolism, don't connect in series with other infusions.
• Don't add any other drugs to solution.

Contraindications and precautions

• Contraindicated in patients hypersensitive to drug.
• Although no information exists regarding cross-sensitivity, use cautiously in patients hypersensitive to other antifungal azole compounds.
⚠ Lifespan: In pregnant women, use cautiously. In breast-feeding women, drug isn't recommended.

Adverse reactions

CNS: headache.
GI: *nausea,* vomiting, abdominal pain, diarrhea.
Hepatic: *hepatotoxicity.*
Skin: rash, *Stevens-Johnson syndrome.*
Other: *anaphylaxis.*

Interactions

Drug-drug. *Alprazolam, chlordiazepoxide, clonazepam, clorazepate, diazepam, estazolam, flurazepam, midazolam, quazepam, triazolam:* May increase and prolong level, CNS depression, and psychomotor impairment. Don't use together.

Amitriptyline: Increases amitriptyline levels. Avoid combination, if possible.
Atorvastatin, fluvastatin, lovastatin, pravastatin, simvastatin: May increase levels and adverse effects of these HMG-CoA reductase inhibitors. Avoid using together. If they must be given together, reduce dose of HMG-CoA reductase inhibitor.
Carbamazepine: Increases carbamazepine levels. Monitor levels closely.
Cyclosporine, phenytoin, tacrolimus: May increase levels of these drugs. Monitor cyclosporine or phenytoin levels and watch for drug toxicity.
Isoniazid, phenytoin, oral sulfonylureas, rifampin, valproic acid: May increase risk of elevated hepatic transaminases. Monitor patient and level closely.
Oral antidiabetics (tolbutamide, glyburide, glipizide): May increase levels of these drugs. Monitor patient for enhanced hypoglycemic effect.
Rifampin: Enhances fluconazole metabolism. Monitor patient for lack of response.
Theophylline: Decreases theophylline clearance. Monitor level.
Warfarin: May increase risk of bleeding. Monitor PT and INR.
Zidovudine: Zidovudine activity may be increased. Monitor patient closely.
Drug-lifestyle. *Alcohol use:* May increase risk of hepatotoxicity. Discourage using together.

Effects on lab test results

• May increase alkaline phosphatase, ALT, AST, bilirubin, and GGT levels.
• May decrease WBC and platelet counts.

Pharmacokinetics

Absorption: Rapid and complete after P.O. administration.
Distribution: Well distributed to various sites, including CNS, saliva, sputum, blister fluid, urine, normal skin, nails, and blister skin. Drug is 12% protein-bound.
Metabolism: Partial.
Excretion: Primarily by kidneys; more than 80% unchanged in urine. *Half-life:* 20 to 50 hours.

Route	Onset	Peak	Duration
P.O.	Unknown	1-2 hr	Unknown
I.V.	Immediate	Immediate	Unknown

Action

Chemical effect: Inhibits fungal CYP, an enzyme responsible for fungal sterol synthesis, and weakens fungal cell walls.
Therapeutic effect: Hinders fungal growth.

Available forms

Injection: 200 mg/100 ml, 400 mg/200 ml
Powder for oral suspension: 10 mg/ml, 40 mg/ml
Tablets: 50 mg, 100 mg, 150 mg, 200 mg

NURSING PROCESS

🔢 Assessment

• Assess patient's fungal infection before therapy and reassess regularly.
• Periodically monitor liver function during prolonged therapy. Although adverse hepatic effects are rare, they can be serious.
• Be alert for adverse reactions and drug interactions.
• If adverse GI reactions occur, monitor patient's hydration status.
• Evaluate patient's and family's knowledge of drug therapy.

🔢 Nursing diagnoses

• Infection related to presence of susceptible fungi
• Risk for deficient fluid volume related to adverse GI reactions
• Deficient knowledge related to drug therapy

🔢 Planning and implementation

• If patient develops mild rash, monitor him closely. If lesions progress, stop drug and notify prescriber.
Patient teaching
• Urge patient to adhere to regimen and to return for follow-up.
• Tell patient to report adverse reactions to prescriber.

🔢 Evaluation

• Patient is free from infection.
• Patient maintains adequate hydration.
• Patient and family state understanding of drug therapy.

flucytosine (5-fluorocytosine, 5-FC)

(floo-SIGH-toh-seen)
Ancobon, Ancotil ◇

Pharmacologic class: fluorinated pyrimidine
Therapeutic class: antifungal
Pregnancy risk category: C

Indications and dosages

▶ Severe fungal infections caused by susceptible strains of *Candida* (including septicemia, endocarditis, urinary tract and pulmonary infections) and *Cryptococcus* (meningitis, pulmonary infection, and possible UTIs). *Adults:* 50 to 150 mg/kg P.O. daily in divided doses given q 6 hours.
▶ Chromomycosis‡. *Adults:* 150 mg/kg P.O. daily.

Contraindications and precautions

• Contraindicated in patients hypersensitive to drug.
• Use cautiously in those with hepatic or renal impairment or bone marrow suppression.
❄ **Lifespan:** In pregnant women, use cautiously. Breast-feeding women should stop breast-feeding or the drug. In children, safety hasn't been established.

Adverse reactions

CNS: dizziness, confusion, headache, vertigo, sedation, fatigue, weakness, hallucinations, psychosis, ataxia, paresthesia, parkinsonism, peripheral neuropathy.
CV: chest pain, *cardiac arrest.*
EENT: hearing loss.
GI: nausea, vomiting, diarrhea, abdominal pain, dry mouth, duodenal ulcer, *hemorrhage,* ulcerative colitis.
GU: azotemia, crystalluria, *renal impairment.*
Hematologic: anemia, eosinophilia, *leukopenia, bone marrow suppression, thrombocytopenia, agranulocytosis, aplastic anemia.*
Hepatic: jaundice.
Metabolic: *hypoglycemia,* hypokalemia.
Respiratory: *respiratory arrest,* dyspnea.
Skin: occasional rash, pruritus, urticaria, photosensitivity.

Interactions

Drug-drug. *Amphotericin B:* May have synergistic effects and enhance toxicity when used together. Monitor patient.

Effects on lab test results

• May increase urine urea, alkaline phosphatase, ALT, AST, bilirubin, creatinine, and BUN levels. May decrease glucose and potassium levels.
• May increase eosinophil count. May decrease hemoglobin, hematocrit, and WBC, platelet, and granulocyte counts.

Pharmacokinetics

Absorption: From 75% to 90% of dose is absorbed; food decreases absorption rate.
Distribution: Wide. CSF levels vary from 60% to 100% of blood levels. 2% to 4% bound to proteins.
Metabolism: Only small amounts of drug are metabolized.
Excretion: About 75% to 95% excreted unchanged in urine; less than 10% excreted unchanged in feces. *Half-life:* 2½ to 6 hours.

Route	Onset	Peak	Duration
P.O.	Unknown	1-2 hr	Unknown

Action

Chemical effect: May penetrate fungal cells, where it's converted to fluorouracil—a known metabolic antagonist—and causes defective protein synthesis.
Therapeutic effect: Hinders fungal growth, including some strains of *Cryptococcus* and *Candida.*

Available forms

Capsules: 250 mg, 500 mg

NURSING PROCESS

Assessment
• Assess patient's fungal infection before therapy and reassess regularly.
• Before therapy, obtain hematologic tests and renal and liver function studies. Make sure susceptibility tests showing that organism is flucytosine-sensitive are on chart.
• Monitor blood, liver, and renal function studies frequently; obtain susceptibility tests weekly to monitor drug resistance.

• If possible, regularly perform blood level assays of drug to maintain flucytosine at therapeutic level (25 to 120 mcg/ml). Higher levels may be toxic.
• Be alert for adverse reactions and drug interactions.
• If adverse GI reactions occur, monitor patient's hydration.
• Evaluate patient's and family's knowledge of drug therapy.

Nursing diagnoses
• Infection related to presence of susceptible fungi
• Risk for deficient fluid volume related to adverse GI reactions
• Deficient knowledge related to drug therapy

Planning and implementation
• Give capsules over 15 minutes to reduce adverse GI reactions.
Patient teaching
• Inform patient that therapeutic response may take weeks or months.
• Tell patient how to take capsules.
• Warn patient to avoid activities requiring mental alertness if adverse CNS reactions occur.

Evaluation
• Patient is free from infection.
• Patient maintains adequate hydration throughout drug therapy.
• Patient and family state understanding of drug therapy.

fludarabine phosphate
(floo-DAR-uh-been FOS-fayt)
Fludara

Pharmacologic class: antimetabolite, purine antagonist
Therapeutic class: antineoplastic
Pregnancy risk category: D

Indications and dosages

▶ **B-cell chronic lymphocytic leukemia in patients who either haven't responded or have responded inadequately to at least one standard alkylating agent regimen, mycosis fungoides‡, hairy cell leukemia‡, and Hodgkin's and malignant lymphoma‡.** *Adults:* 25 mg/m²

I.V. over 30 minutes for 5 consecutive days. Repeat cycle q 28 days.

⛔ **Adjust-a-dose:** For patients with renal impairment, if creatinine clearance is 30 to 70 ml/minute, decrease dose by 20%. Don't give if creatinine clearance is less than 30 ml/minute.

▶ **Chronic lymphocytic leukemia‡.** *Adults:* Usually, 18 to 30 mg/m² I.V. over 30 minutes for 5 consecutive days q 28 days. Therapy is based upon patient's response and tolerance.

▼ I.V. administration

• Preparing and giving drug creates mutagenic, teratogenic, and carcinogenic risks. Follow facility policy to reduce risks.
• To prepare solution, add 2 ml of sterile water for injection to solid cake of drug. Drug will dissolve within 15 seconds; each ml will contain 25 mg of drug. Dilute further in 100 or 125 ml of D₅W or normal saline injection.
• Use within 8 hours of reconstitution.
• Store drug in refrigerator at 36° to 46° F (2° to 8° C).

Contraindications and precautions

• Contraindicated in patients hypersensitive to drug or its components.
• Use cautiously in patients with renal insufficiency.
⚠ **Lifespan:** In pregnant women, use cautiously and only when necessary. In breast-feeding women, and in children, safety of drug hasn't been established.

Adverse reactions

CNS: *fever, fatigue, malaise, weakness, paresthesia,* headache, peripheral neuropathy, sleep disorder, depression, pain, cerebellar syndrome, **CVA,** transient ischemic attack, agitation, *confusion, coma.*
CV: *edema,* angina, phlebitis, **arrhythmias, heart failure, MI, supraventricular tachycardia, deep venous thrombosis, aneurysm, hemorrhage.**
EENT: *visual disturbances,* hearing loss, delayed blindness (with high doses), sinusitis, pharyngitis, epistaxis.
GI: *nausea, vomiting, diarrhea,* constipation, *anorexia,* stomatitis, **GI BLEEDING,** esophagitis, mucositis.
GU: dysuria, *UTIs,* urinary hesitancy, proteinuria, hematuria, **renal impairment.**
Hematologic: *anemia,* MYELOSUPPRESSION, NEUTROPENIA, THROMBOCYTOPENIA.

Hepatic: *liver failure,* cholelithiasis.
Metabolic: hyperglycemia, dehydration, hyperuricemia, hyperphosphatemia.
Musculoskeletal: myalgia.
Respiratory: *cough, pneumonia, dyspnea, upper respiratory infection,* allergic pneumonitis, hemoptysis, **hypoxia,** bronchitis.
Skin: alopecia, diaphoresis, *rash,* pruritus, seborrhea.
Other: *chills,* INFECTION, *tumor lysis syndrome, anaphylaxis.*

Interactions

Drug-drug. *Other myelosuppressants:* May increase toxicity. Avoid using together.
Pentostatin: Increases risk of pulmonary toxicity. Avoid using together.

Effects on lab test results

• May increase glucose, phosphate, potassium, and uric acid levels.
• May decrease hemoglobin, hematocrit, and platelet and neutrophil counts.

Pharmacokinetics

Absorption: Administered I.V.
Distribution: Unknown.
Metabolism: Rapidly dephosphorylated and then phosphorylated intracellularly to its active metabolite.
Excretion: 23% in urine as unchanged active metabolite. *Half-life:* About 10 hours.

Route	Onset	Peak	Duration
I.V.	7-21 hr	Unknown	Unknown

Action

Chemical effect: Unknown; actions may be multifaceted. After conversion to its active metabolite, fludarabine interferes with DNA synthesis by inhibiting DNA polymerase alpha, ribonucleotide reductase, and DNA primase.
Therapeutic effect: Kills susceptible cancer cells.

Available forms

Powder for injection: 50 mg

NURSING PROCESS

⚕ **Assessment**
• Assess patient's underlying condition before therapy and reassess regularly.

• Careful hematologic monitoring is needed, especially of neutrophil and platelet counts. Bone marrow suppression can be severe.
• Be alert for adverse reactions and drug interactions.
• Evaluate patient's and family's knowledge of drug therapy.

⊕ Nursing diagnoses
• Ineffective health maintenance related to presence of leukemia
• Ineffective protection related to drug-induced immunosuppression
• Deficient knowledge related to drug therapy

⊠ Planning and implementation
• Optimal duration of therapy isn't known. Recommendations suggest three additional cycles after achieving maximal response.
Patient teaching
• Warn patient to watch for evidence of infection and bleeding.
• Tell patient to notify prescriber if adverse reactions occur.

☑ Evaluation
• Patient shows positive response to fludarabine therapy.
• Patient develops no serious infections or bleeding complications.
• Patient and family state understanding of drug therapy.

fludrocortisone acetate
(floo-droh-KOR-tuh-sohn AS-ih-tayt)
Florinef

Pharmacologic class: mineralocorticoid, glucocorticoid
Therapeutic class: mineralocorticoid replacement therapy
Pregnancy risk category: C

Indications and dosages
▶ **Adrenal insufficiency (partial replacement), adrenogenital syndrome.** *Adults:* 0.1 to 0.2 mg P.O. daily.
▶ **Orthostatic hypotension‡.** *Adults:* 0.1 to 0.4 mg P.O. daily.

Contraindications and precautions
• Contraindicated in patients hypersensitive to drug and in those with systemic fungal infections.
• Use cautiously in patients with hypothyroidism, cirrhosis, ocular herpes simplex, emotional instability and psychotic tendencies, nonspecific ulcerative colitis, diverticulitis, fresh intestinal anastomoses, active or latent peptic ulcer, renal insufficiency, hypertension, osteoporosis, and myasthenia gravis.
⚖ **Lifespan:** In pregnant women, use only when clearly needed. In breast-feeding women, use cautiously. In children, long-term use may delay growth and maturation.

Adverse reactions
CV: *sodium and water retention,* hypertension, cardiac hypertrophy, edema, ***heart failure.***
Metabolic: hypokalemia.
Skin: bruising, diaphoresis, urticaria, allergic rash.

Interactions
Drug-drug. *Barbiturates, phenytoin, rifampin:* Increases clearance of fludrocortisone acetate. Monitor patient for effect.
Potassium-depleting drugs (such as thiazide diuretics): Enhances potassium-wasting effects of fludrocortisone. Monitor potassium levels.
Drug-food. *Sodium-containing drugs or foods:* May increase blood pressure. Advise patient to avoid these drugs or food and limit sodium intake.

Effects on lab test results
• May decrease potassium level.

Pharmacokinetics
Absorption: Readily from GI tract.
Distribution: To muscle, liver, skin, intestines, and kidneys. Extensively bound to proteins. Only unbound portion is active.
Metabolism: In liver to inactive metabolites.
Excretion: In urine; insignificant amount in feces. *Half-life:* 18 to 36 hours.

Route	Onset	Peak	Duration
P.O.	Varies	Varies	1-2 days

Action

Chemical effect: Increases sodium reabsorption and potassium and hydrogen secretion at distal convoluted tubule of nephron.

Therapeutic effect: Increases sodium levels and decreases potassium and hydrogen levels.

Available forms

Tablets: 0.1 mg

NURSING PROCESS

Assessment
• Assess patient's underlying condition before therapy and reassess regularly.
• Monitor patient's blood pressure, weight, and electrolyte levels.
• Be alert for adverse reactions and drug interactions.
• Evaluate patient's and family's knowledge of drug therapy.

Nursing diagnoses
• Ineffective health maintenance related to underlying adrenal condition
• Excessive fluid volume related to drug-induced adverse reactions
• Deficient knowledge related to drug therapy

Planning and implementation
• Drug is used with cortisone or hydrocortisone in patients with adrenal insufficiency.
• If hypertension occurs, notify prescriber, who may lower dosage by 50%.
• Potassium supplements may be needed for excessive potassium loss.
• Signs of overdosage include excessive weight gain, edema, hypertension, hypokalemia, and increased heart size. Stop treatment for a few days until symptoms subside and then resume drug at a reduced dose.

Patient teaching
• Tell patient to notify prescriber about worsened symptoms, such as hypotension, weakness, cramping, and palpitations.
• Warn patient that mild peripheral edema is common.

Evaluation
• Patient's health is improved.
• Patient develops no sodium and water retention.

• Patient and family state understanding of drug therapy.

flumazenil
(floo-MAZ-ih-nil)
Romazicon

Pharmacologic class: benzodiazepine antagonist
Therapeutic class: antidote
Pregnancy risk category: C

Indications and dosages

▶ **Complete or partial reversal of sedative effects of benzodiazepines after anesthesia or short diagnostic procedures (conscious sedation).** *Adults:* Initially, 0.2 mg I.V. over 15 seconds. If patient doesn't reach desired level of consciousness after 45 seconds, dose is repeated. Repeat at 1-minute intervals until cumulative dose of 1 mg has been given (initial dose plus four more doses), if needed. Most patients respond after 0.6 to 1 mg of drug. In case of resedation, dose may be repeated after 20 minutes; however, don't give more than 1 mg at any one time and no more than 3 mg/hour.

▶ **Suspected benzodiazepine overdose.** *Adults:* Initially, 0.2 mg I.V. over 15 seconds. If patient doesn't reach desired level of consciousness after 30 seconds, give 0.3 mg over 30 seconds. If patient still doesn't respond adequately, give 0.5 mg over 30 seconds; repeat 0.5-mg doses p.r.n. at 1-minute intervals up to a cumulative dose of 3 mg. Most patients with benzodiazepine overdose respond to cumulative doses between 1 and 3 mg; rarely, patients who respond partially after 3 mg may need additional doses. Don't give more than 5 mg over 5 minutes initially. Sedation that persists after this dosage is unlikely to be caused by benzodiazepines. In case of resedation, repeat dose after 20 minutes; however, don't give more than 1 mg at any one time and no more than 3 mg/hour.

I.V. administration
• Compatible solutions include D₅W, lactated Ringer's injection, and normal saline solution.
• Give drug into I.V. line in large vein with free-flowing I.V. solution to minimize pain at injection site.

• Discard within 24 hours any unused drug that has been drawn into syringe or diluted.

Contraindications and precautions

• Contraindicated in patients hypersensitive to drug or benzodiazepines; in patients who show evidence of serious cyclic antidepressant overdose; and in those who received a benzodiazepine to treat a potentially life-threatening condition (such as status epilepticus).
• Use cautiously in patients at high risk for developing seizures; in patients who recently have received multiple doses of parenteral benzodiazepine; in patients displaying signs of seizure activity; in patients who may be at risk for unrecognized benzodiazepine dependence, such as ICU patients; and in patients with head injury, psychiatric, or alcohol-dependent problems.
⚥ Lifespan: In pregnant or breast-feeding women, use cautiously. In children, safety hasn't been established.

Adverse reactions

CNS: *dizziness, headache, seizures,* agitation, emotional lability, tremor, insomnia.
CV: *arrhythmias,* cutaneous vasodilation, palpitations.
EENT: *abnormal or blurred vision.*
GI: *nausea, vomiting.*
Respiratory: dyspnea, hyperventilation.
Skin: *diaphoresis.*
Other: *pain at injection site.*

Interactions

Drug-drug. *Antidepressants, drugs that can cause seizures or arrhythmias:* Seizures or arrhythmias can develop after effect of benzodiazepine overdose is removed. Use with caution, if at all, in cases of mixed overdose.

Effects on lab test results

None reported.

Pharmacokinetics

Absorption: Administered I.V.
Distribution: Redistributes rapidly; 50% bound to proteins.
Metabolism: By liver. Ingestion of food during I.V. infusion enhances metabolism, probably by increasing hepatic blood flow.

Excretion: About 90% to 95% appears in urine as metabolites; remainder excreted in feces.
Half-life: About 54 minutes.

Route	Onset	Peak	Duration
I.V.	Unknown	Unknown	Unknown

Action

Chemical effect: Competitively inhibits actions of benzodiazepines on GABA-benzodiazepine receptor complex.
Therapeutic effect: Awakens patient from sedative effects of benzodiazepines.

Available forms

Injection: 0.1 mg/ml in 5- and 10-ml multiple-dose vials

NURSING PROCESS

🔖 Assessment

• Assess patient's sedation before therapy.
• Assess patient's level of consciousness frequently.
• Be alert for adverse reactions and drug interactions.
⚠ ALERT: Monitor patient closely for resedation that may occur after reversal of benzodiazepine effects; flumazenil's duration of action is shorter than that of all benzodiazepines. Monitor patient closely after long-acting benzodiazepines, such as diazepam, or high doses of short-acting benzodiazepines, such as 10 mg of midazolam. In most cases, severe resedation is unlikely in patient who shows no signs of resedation 2 hours after 1-mg dose of flumazenil.
• Monitor patient's ECG for evidence of arrhythmias.
• Evaluate patient's and family's knowledge of drug therapy.

🔅 Nursing diagnoses

• Ineffective protection related to sedated state
• Decreased cardiac output related to drug-induced seizures
• Deficient knowledge related to drug therapy

▶ Planning and implementation

• If arrhythmias or other adverse reactions occur, notify prescriber and treat accordingly.
Patient teaching
• Warn patient to avoid hazardous activities within 24 hours of procedure.

Reactions may be *common,* uncommon, *life-threatening*, or COMMON AND LIFE-THREATENING.

• Tell patient to avoid alcohol, CNS depressants, and OTC drugs for 24 hours.
• Give family members important instructions, or provide patient with written instructions.

☑ **Evaluation**
• Patient is awake and alert.
• Patient maintains adequate cardiac output.
• Patient and family state understanding of drug therapy.

---

fluorouracil (5-fluorouracil, 5-FU)
(floo-roh-YOOR-uh-sil)
Adrucil, Carac, Efudex, Fluoroplex

Pharmacologic class: antimetabolite (cell cycle–phase specific, S phase)
Therapeutic class: antineoplastic
Pregnancy risk category: D

Indications and dosages

▶ **Colon, rectal, breast, stomach, and pancreatic cancers.** *Adults:* 12 mg/kg I.V. daily for 4 days; if no toxicity, give 6 mg/kg on 6th, 8th, 10th, and 12th day; then begin single weekly maintenance dose of 10 to 15 mg/kg I.V. after toxicity (if any) from initial course subsides. Dosages based on lean body weight. Maximum single dose is 800 mg.
▶ **Palliative treatment of advanced colorectal cancer.** *Adults:* 425 mg/m² I.V. daily for 5 consecutive days. Give with 20 mg/m² of leucovorin I.V. Repeat at 4-week intervals for two additional courses; then repeat at intervals of 4 to 5 weeks, as tolerated.
▶ **Multiple actinic (solar) keratoses; superficial basal cell carcinoma.** *Adults:* Apply cream or topical solution b.i.d.
▶ **Multiple actinic or solar keratosis of the face and anterior scalp.** *Adults:* Apply a thin layer of cream or topical solution to the washed and dried affected area daily for up to 4 weeks.

▼ I.V. administration

• Give antiemetic to reduce nausea before giving drug.
• Preparing and giving I.V drug creates carcinogenic, mutagenic, and teratogenic risks for staff. Follow facility policy to reduce risks.
• Drug may be given by direct injection without dilution.

• For I.V. infusion, drug may be diluted with D₅W, sterile water for injection, or normal saline injection.
• Infuse slowly over 2 to 8 hours. Don't use cloudy solution. If crystals form, redissolve by warming.
• Use plastic I.V. containers for giving continuous infusions. Solution is more stable in plastic I.V. bags than in glass bottles.

Contraindications and precautions

• Contraindicated in patients hypersensitive to drug and in those with poor nutrition, bone marrow suppression (WBC counts of 5,000/mm³ or less or platelet counts of 100,000/mm³ or less), or potentially serious infections, and in those who have had major surgery within previous month.
• Use cautiously after high-dose pelvic radiation therapy and in patients who received alkylating agents, or have impaired hepatic or renal function or widespread neoplastic infiltration of bone marrow.
⚠ **Lifespan:** In pregnant and breast-feeding women, drug isn't recommended. In children, safety hasn't been established.

Adverse reactions

CNS: acute cerebellar syndrome, ataxia, confusion, disorientation, euphoria, headache, nystagmus, *weakness, malaise.*
CV: thrombophlebitis, *myocardial ischemia,* angina.
EENT: epistaxis, photophobia, lacrimation, lacrimal duct stenosis, visual changes.
GI: *stomatitis, GI ulcer (may precede leukopenia), nausea and vomiting, diarrhea, anorexia, GI bleeding.*
Hematologic: *leukopenia; thrombocytopenia; agranulocytosis;* anemia; WBC count nadir 9 to 14 days after first dose; platelet count nadir in 7 to 14 days.
Skin: *reversible alopecia; dermatitis; erythema; scaling; pruritus;* contact dermatitis; nail changes; pigmented palmar creases; erythematous, desquamative rash of hands and feet with long-term use ("hand-foot syndrome"); photosensitivity; *pain, burning,* soreness, suppuration, and swelling with topical use.
Other: *anaphylaxis.*

Interactions

Drug-drug. *Leucovorin calcium, previous treatment with alkylating agents:* Increases fluorouracil toxicity. Use cautiously.
Drug-lifestyle. *Sun exposure:* Photosensitivity reactions may occur. Urge patient to avoid unprotected or prolonged sun exposure.

Effects on lab test results

• May increase alkaline phosphatase, AST, ALT, bilirubin, and LDH levels. May increase 5-hydroxyindoleacetic acid level in urine.
• May decrease hemoglobin, hematocrit, and WBC, RBC, platelet, and granulocyte counts.

Pharmacokinetics

Absorption: Unknown for topical forms.
Distribution: Wide; crosses blood-brain barrier.
Metabolism: Majority of drug degraded in liver; small amount converted in tissues to active metabolite.
Excretion: Metabolites primarily excreted through lungs as carbon dioxide; small portion excreted in urine as unchanged drug. *Half-life:* 20 minutes.

Route	Onset	Peak	Duration
I.V., topical	Unknown	Unknown	Unknown

Action

Chemical effect: Inhibits DNA synthesis.
Therapeutic effect: Inhibits cell growth of selected cancers.

Available forms

Cream: 1%, 5%
Injection: 50 mg/ml
Topical solution: 1%, 2%, 5%

NURSING PROCESS

📖 Assessment

• Assess patient's condition before therapy and reassess regularly.
• Monitor fluid intake and output, CBC, platelet count, and renal and hepatic function tests.
• Be alert for adverse reactions and drug interactions.
• Fluorouracil toxicity may be delayed for 1 to 3 weeks.
• Monitor patient receiving topical form for serious adverse reactions. Ingestion and systemic absorption may cause leukopenia, thrombocy-

topenia, stomatitis, diarrhea, or GI ulceration, bleeding, and hemorrhage. Application to large ulcerated areas may cause systemic toxicity.
• Watch for stomatitis or diarrhea (signs of toxicity).
• Evaluate patient's and family's knowledge of drug therapy.

📖 Nursing diagnoses

• Ineffective health maintenance related to underlying neoplastic condition
• Ineffective protection related to adverse hematologic reactions
• Deficient knowledge related to drug therapy

▶ Planning and implementation

🚫 **ALERT:** Drug sometimes is ordered as 5-fluorouracil or 5-FU. The numeral 5 is part of drug name and shouldn't be confused with dosage units.
• When giving topically, apply cautiously near eyes, nose, and mouth.
• Avoid occlusive dressings because they increase risk of inflammatory reactions in adjacent normal skin.
• Wash hands immediately after handling topical form.
• Wash and dry affected area; wait 10 minutes. Apply thin layer of medication to affected area.
• Use 1% topical form on face. Higher concentrations are used for thicker-skinned areas or resistant lesions.
• Use 5% topical form for superficial basal cell carcinoma confirmed by biopsy.
• May apply sunscreen and moisturizer 2 hours after application.
• Local irritation isn't markedly increased by extending treatment from 2 to 4 weeks, and is generally resolved within 2 weeks of cessation of treatment
• Don't refrigerate fluorouracil.
• Use sodium hypochlorite 5% (household bleach) to inactivate drug in event of spill.
• If diarrhea occurs, stop drug and notify prescriber.
• If WBC count is less than 2,000/mm³, consider protective isolation.
Patient teaching
• Warn patient that alopecia may occur, but it is reversible.
• Advise patient to avoid prolonged exposure to sunlight or ultraviolet light when topical form is used.

Reactions may be *common,* uncommon, *life-threatening,* or COMMON AND LIFE-THREATENING.

• Tell patient to use sunblock to avoid inflammatory erythematous dermatitis. Long-term use of drug may cause erythematous, desquamative rash of hands and feet. May be treated with pyridoxine (50 to 150 mg P.O. daily) for 5 to 7 days.

• Warn patient that topically treated area may be unsightly during therapy and for several weeks after. Full healing may take 1 to 2 months. Local irritation generally resolves after 2 weeks of cessation of drug treatment.

• Inform patient that sunscreen and a moisturizer may be applied 2 hours after drug application.

☑ **Evaluation**

• Patient shows positive response to fluorouracil therapy.

• Patient develops no serious adverse hematologic reactions.

• Patient and family state understanding of drug therapy.

---

fluoxetine hydrochloride
(floo-OKS-eh-teen high-droh-KLOR-ighd)
Prozac, Prozac-20 ◇ **, Prozac Weekly, Sarafem**

Pharmacologic class: SSRI
Therapeutic class: antidepressant
Pregnancy risk category: B

Indications and dosages

▶ **Depression, obsessive-compulsive disorder.** *Adults:* Initially, 20 mg P.O. in morning; dosage increased according to patient response. May be given b.i.d. in morning and at noon. Maximum, 80 mg daily.
Children ages 7 to 17: For obsessive-compulsive disorder, 10 mg P.O. daily. After 2 weeks, increase dose to 20 mg/day to maximum of 60 mg/day. In lower-weight children, increase dose to 20 to 30 mg/day after several weeks. Maximum, 60 mg/day.
Children ages 8 to 18: For depression, 10 to 20 mg P.O. daily. After 1 week, increase to 20 mg daily. Start lower-weight children at 10 mg/day and increase dose to 20 mg/day after several weeks.
▶ **Maintenance therapy for depression in stabilized patients (not for newly diagnosed depression).** *Adults:* 90 mg Prozac Weekly P.O.

once weekly. Start 7 days after the last daily dose of Prozac 20 mg.
▶ **Depression.** *Adults age 65 and older:* Initially, 20 mg P.O. daily in the morning. Increase dosage based on response. Doses may be given twice daily, in the morning and at noon. Maximum, 80 mg daily. As needed, lower or give less-frequent dose to these patients, especially those with systemic illness and those who take multiple drugs for other illnesses.
▶ **Binge eating and vomiting behaviors in patients with moderate-to-severe bulimia nervosa.** *Adults:* 60 mg daily P.O. in the morning.
▶ **Premenstrual dysphoric disorder (PMDD).** *Adults:* 20 mg Sarafem P.O. daily continuously (every day of the menstrual cycle) or intermittently (daily dose starting 14 days prior to the anticipated onset of menstruation through the first full day of menses and repeating with each new cycle). Maximum, 80 mg daily.
▶ **Anorexia nervosa‡.** *Adults:* 40 mg P.O. daily in weight-restored patients.
▶ **Depression linked to bipolar disorder‡.** *Adults:* 20 to 60 mg P.O. daily.
▶ **Panic disorder with or without agoraphobia.** *Adults:* 10 mg P.O. daily. May increase in 10-mg increments at intervals of no less than 1 week to maximum dose of 60 mg.
▶ **Cataplexy‡.** *Adults:* 20 mg P.O. daily or b.i.d. in conjunction with CNS stimulant therapy.
▶ **Alcohol dependence‡.** *Adults:* 60 mg P.O. daily.

Contraindications and precautions

• Contraindicated in patients hypersensitive to drug and in those taking MAO inhibitors within 14 days of starting therapy. Don't give MAO inhibitors or thioridazine within 5 weeks of drug.

• Use cautiously in patients at high risk for suicide and in those with history of mania, seizures, diabetes mellitus, or hepatic, renal, or CV disease.

⚘ **Lifespan:** In pregnant women, use cautiously. In breast-feeding women, drug isn't recommended. In children, safety hasn't been established.

Adverse reactions

CNS: *fever, nervousness, anxiety, insomnia, somnolence, headache, drowsiness,* fatigue, tremor, dizziness, asthenia.
CV: palpitations.

EENT: nasal congestion, pharyngitis, sinusitis.
GI: *nausea, diarrhea, dry mouth, anorexia,* dyspepsia, constipation, abdominal pain, vomiting, flatulence, increased appetite.
Metabolic: weight loss.
Musculoskeletal: muscle pain.
Respiratory: cough, upper respiratory infection, *respiratory distress.*
Skin: rash, pruritus, urticaria.
Other: flulike syndrome, hot flushes, sexual dysfunction.

Interactions

Drug-drug. *Amphetamines, SSRIs, trazodone, dextromethorphan, meperidine, tramadol, sumatriptan, dihydroergotamine:* May increase risk of serotonin syndrome. Avoid use together.
Benzodiazines, lithium, tricyclic antidepressants: Increases CNS effects. Monitor patient and level closely; adjust doses, p.r.n.
Cyproheptadine: May reverse or decrease pharmacologic effect. Monitor patient closely.
Flecainide, carbamazepine, vinblastine: Increases levels of these drugs. Monitor levels and patient for adverse effects.
Insulin, oral antidiabetics: Alters glucose levels and need for antidiabetic. Adjust dosage.
Phenelzine, selegiline, tranylcypromine: May cause serotonin syndrome (CNS irritability, shivering, and altered consciousness). Don't give drug within 2 weeks of an SSRI.
Phenytoin: May increase phenytoin level and risk of toxicity. Monitor phenytoin level and adjust dosage.
Sumatriptan: May cause weakness, hyperreflexia, and incoordination. Monitor patient closely.
Thioridazine: May raise level of thioridazine, leading to an increased risk of serious ventricular arrhythmias and sudden death. Don't give within 5 weeks of each other.
Tryptophan: May increase toxic reaction with agitation, GI distress, and restlessness. Don't use together.
Warfarin, other highly protein-bound drugs: May increase level of fluoxetine or other highly protein-bound drugs. Monitor level closely.
Drug-herb. *St. John's wort:* Increases risk of serotonin syndrome. Discourage use together.
Drug-lifestyle. *Alcohol use:* Increases CNS depression. Discourage use together.

Effects on lab test results

None reported.

Pharmacokinetics

Absorption: Well absorbed.
Distribution: About 95% protein-bound.
Metabolism: Primarily in liver to active metabolites.
Excretion: By kidneys. *Half-life:* 2 to 3 days.

Route	Onset	Peak	Duration
P.O.	1-4 wk	6-8 hr	Unknown

Action

Chemical effect: May inhibit CNS neuronal uptake of serotonin.
Therapeutic effect: Relieves depression and obsessive-compulsive behaviors.

Available forms

Capsules: 90 mg *(Prozac Weekly)*
Oral solution: 20 mg/5 ml
Pulvules: 10 mg, 20 mg, 40 mg
Tablets: 10 mg

NURSING PROCESS

Assessment
● Assess patient's condition before therapy, and reassess regularly.
● Be alert for adverse reactions and drug interactions.
● Evaluate patient's and family's knowledge of drug therapy.

Nursing diagnoses
● Ineffective individual coping related to patient's underlying condition
● Disturbed sleep pattern related to drug-induced insomnia
● Deficient knowledge related to drug therapy

Planning and implementation
● Elderly or debilitated patients and patients with renal or hepatic dysfunction may need lower dosages or less frequent dosing.
● Give drug in morning to prevent insomnia.
● Give antihistamines or topical corticosteroids to treat rashes or pruritus.
● Lower-weight children may need several weeks between dosage increases.
Patient teaching
● Tell patient not to take drug in afternoon or evening because fluoxetine commonly causes nervousness and insomnia.

Reactions may be *common*, uncommon, *life-threatening*, or COMMON AND LIFE-THREATENING.

• Tell patient to take drug without regard to meals or food.

• Warn patient to avoid hazardous activities that require alertness and psychomotor coordination until CNS effects of drug are known.

• Advise patient to consult prescriber before taking any other prescription or OTC medications.

☑ **Evaluation**

• Patient behavior and communication indicate improvement of depression with drug therapy.

• Patient has no insomnia with drug use.

• Patient and family state understanding of drug therapy.

fluphenazine decanoate
(floo-FEN-uh-zeen deh-kuh-NOH-ayt)
Modecate ♦ ◇ , Modecate Concentrate ♦ , Prolixin Decanoate

fluphenazine enanthate
Moditen Enanthate ♦ , Prolixin Enanthate

fluphenazine hydrochloride
Anatensol ◇ * , Apo-Fluphenazine ♦ , Modecate Concentrate ♦ , Moditen HCl ♦ , Permitil*, Permitil Concentrate, Prolixin*, Prolixin Concentrate* ♦

Pharmacologic class: phenothiazine (piperazine derivative)
Therapeutic class: antipsychotic
Pregnancy risk category: C

Indications and dosages

▶ **Psychotic disorders.** *Adults:* Initially, 2.5 to 10 mg hydrochloride P.O. daily in divided doses q 6 to 8 hours; may increase cautiously to 20 mg. Maintenance, 1 to 5 mg P.O. daily. Or, 12.5 to 25 mg decanoate or enanthate I.M. or S.C. q 4 to 6 weeks. Maximum dose, 100 mg.
Elderly patients: Initially, 1 to 2.5 mg P.O. daily. Adjust according to response.

Contraindications and precautions

• Contraindicated in patients hypersensitive to drug and in those with CNS depression, bone marrow suppression, other blood dyscrasia, subcortical damage, liver damage, or coma.

• Use cautiously in debilitated patients, and those with pheochromocytoma, severe CV disease (may cause sudden drop in blood pressure), peptic ulcer, exposure to extreme heat or cold (including antipyretic therapy) or phosphorous insecticides, respiratory disorder, hypocalcemia, seizure disorder (may lower seizure threshold), severe reactions to insulin or electroconvulsive therapy, mitral insufficiency, glaucoma, or prostatic hyperplasia. Use parenteral form cautiously in patients with asthma and patients allergic to sulfites.

⚛ **Lifespan:** In pregnant or breast-feeding women and elderly patients, use cautiously.

Adverse reactions

CNS: *extrapyramidal reactions, tardive dyskinesia,* sedation, pseudoparkinsonism, EEG changes, drowsiness, *seizures,* dizziness, *neuroleptic malignant syndrome.*
CV: orthostatic hypotension, tachycardia, ECG changes.
EENT: *dry mouth,* ocular changes, *blurred vision,* nasal congestion.
GI: *constipation.*
GU: *urine retention,* dark urine, menstrual irregularities, gynecomastia, inhibited ejaculation.
Hematologic: *leukopenia, agranulocytosis, aplastic anemia,* eosinophilia, hemolytic anemia.
Hepatic: cholestatic jaundice.
Metabolic: weight gain, increased appetite.
Skin: *mild photosensitivity.*
Other: allergic reactions.

Interactions

Drug-drug. *Antacids:* Inhibits absorption of oral phenothiazines. Separate doses by at least 2 hours.
Anticholinergics: Increases anticholinergic effects. Avoid using together.
Barbiturates, lithium: May decrease phenothiazine effect. Observe patient.
Centrally acting antihypertensives: Decreases antihypertensive effect. Monitor blood pressure.
CNS depressants: Increases CNS depression. Avoid using together.
Drug-lifestyle. *Alcohol use:* Increases CNS depression, particularly psychomotor skills. Strongly discourage use together.
Sun exposure: Increases risk of photosensitivity. Discourage prolonged or unprotected exposure to sun.

Effects on lab test results

• May increase eosinophil count and liver function test results. May decrease hemoglobin, hematocrit, and WBC, granulocyte, and platelet counts.

Pharmacokinetics

Absorption: Rate and extent vary with route of administration; oral tablet absorption is erratic and variable.
Distribution: Wide. CNS levels are usually higher than those in blood. Drug is 91% to 99% protein-bound.
Metabolism: Extensively by liver, but no active metabolites are formed.
Excretion: Mostly in urine; some in feces through biliary tract. *Half-life:* Hydrochloride, 15 hours; decanoate, 7 to 10 days.

Route	Onset	Peak	Duration
P.O.	≤ 1 hr	30 min	6-8 hr
I.M., S.C.	1-3 days	Unknown	1-6 wk

Action

Chemical effect: Unknown; may block dopamine receptors in brain.
Therapeutic effect: Relieves psychotic signs and symptoms.

Available forms

fluphenazine decanoate
Depot injection: 25 mg/ml, 100 mg/ml ♦
fluphenazine enanthate
Depot injection: 25 mg/ml
fluphenazine hydrochloride
Elixir: 2.5 mg/5 ml*
I.M. injection: 2.5 mg/ml
Oral concentrate: 5 mg/ml*
Tablets: 1 mg, 2.5 mg, 5 mg, 10 mg

NURSING PROCESS

Assessment

• Assess patient's condition before therapy and regularly thereafter.
• Monitor therapy with weekly bilirubin tests during first month, periodic blood tests (CBC and liver function), and periodic renal function and ophthalmic tests (long-term use).
• Be alert for adverse reactions and drug interactions.
• Monitor patient for tardive dyskinesia, which may occur after prolonged use. Reaction may not appear until months or years later and may disappear spontaneously or persist for life despite stopping drug.
• Evaluate patient's and family's knowledge of drug therapy.

Nursing diagnoses

• Impaired thought processes related to psychosis
• Impaired physical mobility related to extrapyramidal reactions
• Deficient knowledge related to drug therapy

Planning and implementation

⚠ ALERT: Prolixin concentrate and Permitil concentrate are 10 times more concentrated than Prolixin elixir (5 mg/ml vs. 0.5 mg/ml). Check dosage order carefully.
• Dilute liquid concentrate with water, fruit juice (except apple), milk, or semisolid food just before administration.
• When giving I.M. or S.C., for long-acting forms (decanoate and enanthate), which are oil preparations, use dry needle of at least 21G. Allow 24 to 96 hours for onset of action. Note and report adverse reactions in patient taking these drug forms.
• Oral liquid and parenteral forms can cause contact dermatitis. Wear gloves when preparing solutions, and avoid contact with skin and clothing.
• Protect drug from light. Slight yellowing of injection or concentrate is common and doesn't affect potency. Discard markedly discolored solutions.
• If patient, especially a pregnant woman or a child, develops symptoms of blood dyscrasia (fever, sore throat, infection, cellulitis, weakness) or extrapyramidal reactions for longer than a few hours, withhold dose and notify prescriber.
• Acute dystonic reactions may be treated with diphenhydramine.
• Don't withdraw drug abruptly unless severe adverse reactions occur. After abrupt withdrawal of long-term therapy, patient may experience gastritis, nausea, vomiting, dizziness, tremor, feeling of warmth or cold, diaphoresis, tachycardia, headache, and insomnia.
Patient teaching
• Warn patient to avoid activities that require alertness and psychomotor coordination until CNS effects of drug are known.

Reactions may be *common*, uncommon, *life-threatening*, or COMMON AND LIFE-THREATENING.

- Tell patient not to mix concentrate with beverages containing caffeine, tannics (such as tea) or pectinates (such as apple juice).
- Tell patient to avoid alcohol during therapy.
- Advise patient to relieve dry mouth with sugarless gum or hard candy.
- Have patient report urine retention or constipation.
- Tell patient to use sunblock and to wear protective clothing.
- Inform patient that drug may discolor urine.
- Stress importance of not stopping drug suddenly.

☑ Evaluation
- Patient demonstrates decrease in psychotic behavior.
- Patient maintains pretreatment physical mobility.
- Patient and family state understanding of drug therapy.

flurazepam hydrochloride
(floo-RAH-zuh-pam high-droh-KLOR-ighd)
Apo-Flurazepam ◆, Dalmane, Novo-Flupam ◆, Somnol ◆

Pharmacologic class: benzodiazepine
Therapeutic class: sedative-hypnotic
Pregnancy risk category: X
Controlled substance schedule: IV

Indications and dosages

▶ **Insomnia.** *Adults:* 15 to 30 mg P.O. h.s. Dose repeated once, p.r.n.

Contraindications and precautions

- Contraindicated in patients hypersensitive to drug.
- Use cautiously in patients with impaired hepatic or renal function, chronic pulmonary insufficiency, mental depression, suicidal tendencies, or history of drug abuse.
- ☆ Lifespan: In pregnant women, drug is contraindicated. In breast-feeding women, drug isn't recommended. In children younger than age 15, safety hasn't been established. In elderly patients, use cautiously and at a lower dose because they're more susceptible to CNS effects from drug.

Adverse reactions

CNS: *daytime sedation, dizziness, drowsiness, disturbed coordination,* lethargy, confusion, *headache,* light-headedness, nervousness, hallucinations, staggering, ataxia, disorientation, *coma.*
GI: nausea, vomiting, heartburn, diarrhea, abdominal pain.
Other: physical or psychological dependence.

Interactions

Drug-drug. *Cimetidine:* May increase sedation due to decreased hepatic metabolism of benzodiazepines. Monitor patient carefully.
CNS depressants, including opioid analgesics: May cause excessive CNS depression. Use together cautiously.
Digoxin: Digoxin levels may increase, resulting in digoxin toxicity. Monitor patient and digoxin levels closely.
Disulfiram, hormonal contraceptives, isoniazid: May decrease metabolism of benzodiazepines, leading to toxicity. Monitor patient closely.
Fluconazole, itraconazole, ketoconazole, miconazole: May increase and prolong level, CNS depression, and psychomotor impairment. Don't use together.
Phenytoin: May increase phenytoin levels. Monitor patient for toxicity.
Rifampin: Enhances metabolism of benzodiazepines. Monitor patient for decreased effectiveness.
Theophylline: May antagonize with flurazepam. Monitor patient for decreased effectiveness.
Drug-herb. *Catnip, kava, lady's slipper, lemon balm, passionflower, sassafras, skullcap, valerian:* Sedative effects may be enhanced. Discourage using together.
Drug-lifestyle. *Alcohol use:* May cause additive CNS and respiratory depression. Strongly discourage using together.
Smoking: Enhances metabolism of benzodiazepines. Discourage using together.

Effects on lab test results
- May increase AST, ALT, total and direct bilirubin, and alkaline phosphatase levels.

Pharmacokinetics

Absorption: Rapid.
Distribution: Wide; about 97% bound to protein.
Metabolism: In liver to active metabolite.

Excretion: Excreted in urine. *Half-life:* 50 to 100 hours.

Route	Onset	Peak	Duration
P.O.	Unknown	30 min-1 hr	Unknown

Action

Chemical effect: Unknown; may act on limbic system, thalamus, and hypothalamus of CNS to produce hypnotic effects.
Therapeutic effect: Promotes sleep and calmness.

Available forms

Capsules: 15 mg, 30 mg
Tablets: 15 mg ♦ , 30 mg ♦

NURSING PROCESS

Assessment
• Assess patient's sleep patterns and CNS status before therapy.
• Evaluate patient's ability to sleep. Drug is more effective on second, third, and fourth nights of use.
• Be alert for adverse reactions and drug interactions.
• Evaluate patient's and family's knowledge of drug therapy.

Nursing diagnoses
• Disturbed sleep pattern related to underlying patient problem
• Risk for trauma related to drug-induced adverse CNS reactions
• Deficient knowledge related to drug therapy

Planning and implementation
• Before leaving bedside, make sure patient has swallowed capsule.
Patient teaching
• Encourage patient to continue drug, even if it doesn't relieve insomnia on first night.
• Warn patient to avoid activities that require alertness or physical coordination. For inpatient, supervise walking and raise bed rails, particularly for elderly patient.
• Advise patient that physical and psychological dependence is possible with long-term use.

Evaluation
• Patient notes drug-induced sleep.
• Patient's safety is maintained.

• Patient and family state understanding of drug therapy.

flutamide
(FLOO-tuh-mighd)
Euflex ♦ , Eulexin

Pharmacologic class: nonsteroidal anti-androgen
Therapeutic class: antineoplastic
Pregnancy risk category: D

Indications and dosages

▶ **Locally advanced (stage B2) or metastatic (stage D2) prostatic carcinoma.** *Adults:* 250 mg P.O. q 8 hours. Used with luteinizing hormone-releasing hormone analogues such as leuprolide acetate.

Contraindications and precautions

• Contraindicated in patients hypersensitive to drug and in those with severe hepatic impairment.
⚖ Lifespan: In women, drug is contraindicated. In male children, safety hasn't been established. In elderly patients, use cautiously because its half-life is prolonged.

Adverse reactions

CNS: drowsiness, confusion, depression, anxiety, nervousness, paresthesia.
CV: peripheral edema, hypertension.
GI: *diarrhea, nausea, vomiting,* anorexia.
GU: *impotence.*
Hematologic: *thrombocytopenia, leukopenia,* anemia, hemolytic anemia.
Hepatic: *hepatitis, hepatic encephalopathy.*
Skin: rash, photosensitivity.
Other: *hot flushes, loss of libido,* gynecomastia.

Interactions

Drug-drug. *Warfarin:* May increase PT. Monitor patient's PT and INR.
Drug-lifestyle. *Sun exposure:* May cause sensitivity reactions. Warn patient to avoid unprotected or prolonged sun exposure.

Effects on lab test results

• May increase BUN, creatinine, and liver enzyme levels.

• May decrease hemoglobin, hematocrit, and WBC and platelet counts.

Pharmacokinetics

Absorption: Rapid and complete.
Distribution: Animal studies show drug concentrates in prostate. Drug and its active metabolite are about 95% protein-bound.
Metabolism: More than 97% metabolized rapidly, with at least six metabolites identified.
Excretion: More than 95% excreted in urine.
Half-life: 6 hours.

Route	Onset	Peak	Duration
P.O.	Unknown	2 hr	Unknown

Action

Chemical effect: Inhibits androgen uptake or prevents androgen binding in cell nuclei in target tissues.
Therapeutic effect: Hinders prostatic cancer cell activity.

Available forms

Capsules: 125 mg
Tablets: 250 mg ◆

NURSING PROCESS

Assessment

• Assess patient's prostatic cancer before therapy.
• Monitor liver function test results periodically.
• Be alert for adverse reactions.
• If adverse GI reactions occur, monitor hydration status.
• Evaluate patient's and family's knowledge of drug therapy.

Nursing diagnoses

• Ineffective health maintenance related to presence of prostatic cancer
• Risk for deficient fluid volume related to adverse GI reactions
• Deficient knowledge related to drug therapy

Planning and implementation

• Drug may be given without regard to meals.
• Give with luteinizing hormone-releasing antagonist (such as leuprolide acetate).
Patient teaching
• Make sure patient knows that flutamide must be taken continuously with drug used for med-

ical castration (such as leuprolide acetate) to allow full benefit of therapy. Leuprolide suppresses testosterone production while flutamide inhibits testosterone action at cellular level. Together they can impair growth of androgen-responsive tumors. Advise patient not to stop either drug.
• Tell patient to notify prescriber if adverse reactions occur.

Evaluation

• Patient responds well to drug.
• Patient maintains adequate hydration throughout drug therapy.
• Patient and family state understanding of drug therapy.

fluticasone propionate
(FLU-tih-ka-sohn proh-PIGH-oh-nayt)
Flonase, Flovent Inhalation Aerosol, Flovent Rotadisk

Pharmacologic class: corticosteroid
Therapeutic class: topical and inhalation anti-inflammatory
Pregnancy risk category: C

Indications and dosages

▶ **Asthma prevention and chronic asthma in patients who need oral corticosteroids.** *Adults and children age 12 and older:* In those previously taking bronchodilators alone, initially, 88 mcg Flovent Inhalation Aerosol b.i.d. to maximum of 440 mcg b.i.d. Or, initially, 100 mcg Flovent Rotadisk b.i.d. to maximum of 500 mcg b.i.d.
Patients previously taking inhaled corticosteroids: Initially, 88 to 220 mcg Flovent Inhalation Aerosol b.i.d. to maximum of 440 mcg b.i.d. Or, initially, 100 to 250 mcg Flovent Rotadisk b.i.d. to maximum of 500 mcg b.i.d.
Patients previously taking oral corticosteroids: 880 mcg Flovent Inhalation Aerosol b.i.d. Or, 1,000 mcg Flovent Rotadisk b.i.d.
Children ages 4 to 11: For patients previously on bronchodilators alone or on inhaled corticosteroids, initially, 50 mcg Flovent Rotadisk b.i.d. to maximum of 100 mcg b.i.d.
Patients starting inhalation aerosol or Rotadisk therapy who are currently receiving oral corticosteroid therapy: Reduce prednisone dose to

---

no more than 2.5 mg/day on a weekly basis, beginning after at least 1 week of therapy with fluticasone.

▶ **Management of nasal symptoms of seasonal and perennial allergic and nonallergic rhinitis.** *Adults:* 2 sprays (100 mcg) Flonase in each nostril once daily or 1 spray (50 mcg) b.i.d. Reduce dosage to 1 spray in each nostril daily for maintenance therapy. Or, for seasonal allergic rhinitis, 2 sprays (100 mcg) in each nostril once daily p.r.n. for symptom control, although greater symptom control maybe achieved with regular use.

Children age 4 and older: Initially, 1 spray (50 mcg) Flonase in each nostril once daily. If patient doesn't respond, increase to 2 sprays (100 mcg) in each nostril daily. Once adequate control is achieved, decrease dose to 1 spray in each nostril daily. Maximum dose is 2 sprays in each nostril daily.

Contraindications and precautions

• Contraindicated in patients hypersensitive to ingredients of these preparations. Also contraindicated as primary treatment of patients with status asthmaticus or other acute episodes of asthma in whom intensive measures are needed.
• Flovent Rotadisk is contraindicated in patients with lactose or milk allergies.
• Use cautiously in patients with ocular herpes simplex or untreated systemic, bacterial, viral, fungal, or parasitic infection, and in those with active or quiescent pulmonary tuberculosis.
⚖ Lifespan: In breast-feeding women, use cautiously. In children younger than age 4, drug isn't recommended.

Adverse reactions

CNS: fever, *headache,* dizziness, migraine, nervousness.
EENT: mouth irritation, *oral candidiasis, pharyngitis,* acute nasopharyngitis, nasal congestion, sinusitis, dysphonia, rhinitis, otitis media, tonsillitis, nasal discharge, earache, laryngitis, epistaxis, sneezing, hoarseness, conjunctivitis, eye irritation.
GI: diarrhea, abdominal pain, viral gastroenteritis, colitis, abdominal discomfort, nausea, vomiting.
GU: dysmenorrhea, candidiasis of vagina, pelvic inflammatory disease, vaginitis, vulvovaginitis, irregular menstrual cycle.

Metabolic: cushingoid features, weight gain.
Musculoskeletal: growth retardation in children, pain in joints, aches and pains, disorder or symptoms of neck sprain or strain, sore muscles.
Respiratory: *upper respiratory tract infection,* bronchitis, chest congestion, dyspnea, irritation from inhalant.
Skin: dermatitis, urticaria.
Other: dental problems, influenza.

Interactions

Drug-drug. *Ketoconazole:* May increase mean fluticasone levels. Use care when giving fluticasone with long-term ketoconazole and other known CYP 3A4 inhibitors.

Effects on lab test results

• May increase glucose level.

Pharmacokinetics

Absorption: Most of the drug delivered to the lungs is absorbed systemically, with an average of about 30% of the delivered dose reaching the lungs. Less than 2% is absorbed from the nasal mucosa.
Distribution: Animal studies show drug concentrates in prostate. Drug and its active metabolite are about 91% protein-bound.
Metabolism: Through the liver via CYP 3A4 pathway.
Excretion: Less than 5% is excreted in the urine as metabolites. Remainder excreted in feces as unchanged drug and metabolites. *Half-life:* 3 hours.

Route	Onset	Peak	Duration
Inhalation	24 hr	1-2 wk	Several days
Nasal	12 hr-3 days	4-7 days	Several days

Action

Chemical effect: Synthetic glucocorticoid with potent anti-inflammatory activity inhibits many cell types and mediator production or secretion involved in asthma. These anti-inflammatory actions may contribute to drug's effectiveness in asthma.
Therapeutic effect: Improves breathing ability by reducing inflammation.

Available forms

Nasal suspension: 50 mcg metered inhaler
Oral inhalation aerosol: 44 mcg, 110 mcg, 220 mcg
Oral inhalation powder: 50 mcg, 100 mcg, 250 mcg

NURSING PROCESS

⚙ Assessment

• Obtain history of patient's underlying condition before therapy, and reassess regularly.
• Because of risk of systemic absorption of inhaled corticosteroids, observe patient carefully for evidence of systemic corticosteroid effects.
• Monitor patient, especially postoperatively or during periods of stress, for evidence of inadequate adrenal response.
• Monitor growth in children closely because growth suppression may occur.
• Evaluate patient's and family's knowledge of drug therapy.

⊕ Nursing diagnoses

• Ineffective breathing pattern related to respiratory condition
• Impaired oral mucous membrane related to potential adverse effect of oral candidiasis
• Deficient knowledge related to drug therapy

❯ Planning and implementation

• During withdrawal from oral corticosteroids, some patients may have symptoms of systemically active corticosteroid withdrawal, such as joint or muscle pain, lethargy, and depression, despite maintenance or even improvement of respiratory function.
• Bronchospasm may occur with an immediate increase in wheezing after dosing. If bronchospasm occurs following inhalation, treat immediately with a fast-acting inhaled bronchodilator.
• Some patients taking high doses may have an abnormal response to the 6-hour cosyntropin stimulation test.
⚠ **ALERT:** Use lowest effective dose in children to minimize growth suppression.
Patient teaching
• Tell patient that drug isn't intended to relieve acute bronchospasm.

• For proper use of drug and to attain maximum improvement, tell patient to use drug at regular intervals as directed.
• Instruct patient not to increase dosage but to contact prescriber if symptoms don't improve or if condition worsens.
• Instruct patient to contact prescriber immediately when episodes of asthma that aren't responsive to bronchodilators occur during course of treatment with fluticasone. During such episodes, patients may need therapy with oral corticosteroids.
• Warn patient to avoid exposure to chickenpox or measles and, if exposed, to consult prescriber immediately.
• Tell patient to carry or wear medical identification indicating that he may need supplementary corticosteroids during stress or a severe asthma attack.
• During periods of stress or a severe asthma attack, instruct patient who has been withdrawn from systemic corticosteroids to resume oral corticosteroids (in large doses) immediately and to contact prescriber for further instruction. Instruct him to rinse his mouth after inhalation.
• Instruct patient to shake canister well before using inhalation aerosol and to avoid spraying inhalation aerosol into eyes.
• Advise patient to store fluticasone powder in a dry place.

☑ Evaluation

• Patient has normal breathing pattern.
• Patient doesn't develop oral candidiasis.
• Patient and family state understanding of drug therapy.

fluticasone propionate and salmeterol inhalation powder

(FLU-tih-ka-sohn proh-PIGH-oh-nayt and sal-MEH-teh-rohl)
Advair Diskus 100/50, Advair Diskus 250/50, Advair Diskus 500/50

Pharmacologic class: corticosteroid, long-acting beta$_2$-adrenergic agonist
Therapeutic class: anti-inflammatory, bronchodilator
Pregnancy risk category: C

Indications and dosages

In all patients, after the control of asthma has been achieved, adjust to lowest effective dose.

▶ **Chronic asthma.** *Adults and children older than age 12:* 1 oral inhalation twice daily, morning and evening, at least 12 hours apart. Maximum oral inhalation of Advair Diskus is 500/50 twice daily.

Adults and children older than age 12 not currently taking an inhaled corticosteroid: 1 oral inhalation of Advair Diskus 100/50 twice daily.

Adults and children older than age 12 currently taking beclomethasone dipropionate: If daily dose of beclomethasone dipropionate is 420 mcg or less, start with 1 oral inhalation of Advair Diskus 100/50 twice daily. If beclomethasone dipropionate daily dose is 462 to 840 mcg, start with one oral inhalation of Advair Diskus 250/50 twice daily.

Adults and children older than age 12 currently taking budesonide: If daily dose of budesonide is 400 mcg or less, start with 1 oral inhalation of Advair Diskus 100/50 twice daily. If budesonide daily dose is 800 to 1,200 mcg, start with 1 oral inhalation of Advair Diskus 250/50 twice daily. If budesonide daily dose is 1,600 mcg, start with 1 oral inhalation of Advair Diskus 500/50 twice daily.

Adults and children older than age 12 currently taking flunisolide: If daily dose of flunisolide is 1,000 mcg or less, start with 1 oral inhalation of Advair Diskus 100/50 twice daily. If flunisolide daily dose is 1,250 to 2,000 mcg, start with 1 oral inhalation of Advair Diskus 250/50 twice daily.

Adults and children older than age 12 currently taking fluticasone propionate inhalation aerosol: If daily dose of fluticasone propionate inhalation aerosol is 176 mcg or less, start with 1 oral inhalation of Advair Diskus 100/50 twice daily. If fluticasone propionate inhalation aerosol daily dose is 440 mcg, start with 1 oral inhalation of Advair Diskus 250/50 twice daily. If fluticasone propionate inhalation aerosol daily dose is 660 to 880 mcg, start with 1 oral inhalation of Advair Diskus 500/50 twice daily.

Adults and children older than age 12 currently taking fluticasone propionate inhalation powder: If fluticasone propionate inhalation powder daily dose is 200 mcg or less, start with 1 oral inhalation of Advair Diskus 100/50 twice daily. If fluticasone propionate inhalation powder daily dose is 500 mcg, start with 1 oral inhalation of Advair Diskus 250/50 twice daily. If fluticas-

one propionate inhalation powder daily dose is 1,000 mcg, start with 1 oral inhalation of Advair Diskus 500/50 twice daily.

Adults and children older than age 12 currently taking triamcinolone acetonide: If triamcinolone acetonide daily dose is 1,000 mcg or less, start with 1 oral inhalation of Advair Diskus 100/50 twice daily. If triamcinolone acetonide daily dose is 1,100 to 1,600 mcg, start with 1 oral inhalation of Advair Diskus 250/50 twice daily.

▶ **Maintenance therapy for airflow obstruction in patients with COPD from chronic bronchitis.** *Adults:* 1 inhalation 250/50 twice daily, about 12 hours apart.

Contraindications and precautions

● Contraindicated in patients hypersensitive to any component of the drug. Also contraindicated as primary treatment of status asthmaticus or other potentially life-threatening acute asthmatic episodes.

● Drug isn't indicated for the treatment of exercise-induced bronchospasms.

● Use cautiously in patients with active or quiescent respiratory tuberculosis infection; untreated systemic fungal, bacterial, viral, or parasitic infection; or ocular herpes simplex. Also use cautiously in patients with CV disorders, especially coronary insufficiency, cardiac arrhythmias, and hypertension; in patients with seizure disorders or thyrotoxicosis; in patients unusually responsive to sympathomimetic amines; and in patients with hepatic impairment (because salmeterol is metabolized mainly in the liver).

⚠ **Lifespan:** In children, safety and effectiveness haven't been established. Closely monitor growth in children because growth suppression may occur. Maintain child on lowest effective dose to minimize potential for growth suppression.

Adverse reactions

CNS: pain, sleep disorder, tremor, hypnagogic effects, fever, compressed nerve syndromes, *headache,* agitation, nervousness.
CV: palpitations, chest pains, fluid retention, rapid heart rate, ***arrhythmias.***
EENT: *pharyngitis,* sinusitis, hoarseness/dysphonia, oral candidiasis, rhinorrhea, rhinitis, sneezing, nasal irritation, blood in nasal mucosa, keratitis, conjunctivitis, eye redness, viral eye infections, congestion.

Reactions may be *common,* uncommon, ***life-threatening***, or **COMMON AND LIFE-THREATENING.**

GI: nausea, vomiting, abdominal pain and discomfort, diarrhea, gastroenteritis, oral discomfort and pain, constipation, oral ulcerations, oral erythema and rashes, appendicitis, dental discomfort and pain, unusual taste.

Musculoskeletal: muscle pain, arthralgia, articular rheumatism, muscle stiffness, tightness, rigidity, bone and cartilage disorders, back pain.

Respiratory: *upper respiratory tract infection,* lower viral respiratory infections, bronchitis, cough, pneumonia, *paradoxical bronchospasms, severe asthma or asthma-related deaths (especially in blacks).*

Skin: viral skin infections, urticaria, skin flakiness, disorders of sweat and sebum, sweating.

Other: bacterial infections, allergies, allergic reactions, influenza.

Interactions

Drug-drug. *Beta blockers:* Blocked pulmonary effect of salmeterol may produce severe bronchospasm in patients with asthma. Avoid using together. If necessary, use a cardioselective beta blocker cautiously.

Ketoconazole, other inhibitors of CYP: May increase fluticasone levels and adverse effects. Use together cautiously.

Loop diuretics, thiazide diuretics: ECG changes or hypokalemia may result from or be worsened by potassium-wasting diuretics. Use together cautiously.

MAO inhibitors, tricyclic antidepressants: May potentiate the action of salmeterol on the vascular system. Avoid use within 2 weeks of taking these drugs.

Effects on lab test results

• May increase or decrease liver function test values.

Pharmacokinetics

Absorption: Most of fluticasone propionate dose is systemically absorbed. Salmeterol acts locally in the lung; therefore, levels don't predict effect. Because of the small therapeutic dose, level of salmeterol is low and undetectable after inhalation. Following long-term therapy of 50 mcg twice daily, salmeterol is found in blood within 5 to 45 minutes and level peaks at 20 minutes.

Distribution: Fluticasone is 91% bound to proteins, is weakly and reversibly bound to erythrocytes, and isn't bound significantly to human transcortin. Salmeterol is 96% bound to proteins.

Metabolism: Mainly in liver by CYP 3A4 isoenzyme, with renal clearance accounting for less than 0.02% of the total. The only circulating metabolite is the 17 beta-carboxylic acid derivative, which is formed via the CYP 3A4 pathway. Salmeterol base extensively metabolized by hydroxylation.

Excretion: Fluticasone has less than 5% of a dose excreted in urine as metabolites, with remainder excreted in feces as an unchanged drug and metabolite. Salmeterol xinafoate is about 25% to 60% eliminated in urine and feces, respectively, over a period of 7 days. No significant amount of unchanged salmeterol base is detected in either urine or feces. *Fluticasone half-life:* About 8 hours; *salmeterol half-life:* 5½ hours.

Route	Onset	Peak	Duration
Inhalation			
salmeterol	Unknown	5 min	Unknown
fluticasone	Unknown	1-2 hr	Unknown

Action

Chemical effect: Fluticasone's action is unknown. Salmeterol xinafoate stimulates intracellular adenyl cyclase, the enzyme that catalyzes conversion of adenosine triphosphate (ATP) to cAMP. Increased cAMP levels relax bronchial smooth muscle and inhibit release of mediators of immediate hypersensitivity from cells, especially mast cells. Inhibits release of mast cell mediators, such as histamine, leukotrienes, and prostaglandin D2, from human lung.

Therapeutic effect: Reduces inflammation in the lungs and opens airways to improve pulmonary function.

Available forms

Inhalation powder: 100 mcg fluticasone/ 50 mcg salmeterol, 250 mcg fluticasone/50 mcg salmeterol, 500 mcg fluticasone/50 mcg salmeterol

NURSING PROCESS

Assessment

• Obtain patient's medical history and assess patient before initiating therapy.

ALERT: Chronic overdose of fluticasone may cause signs and symptoms of hypercorticism. Salmeterol overdose may cause seizures, angina, hypertension, hypotension, tachycardia, arrhythmias, nervousness, headache, tremor, muscle cramps, dry mouth, palpitations, nausea, prolonged QT interval, ventricular arrhythmia, hypokalemia, hyperglycemia, cardiac arrest, and death. Stop drug and give a cardioselective beta blocker. Monitoring cardiac status.

• Monitor patient for urticaria, angioedema, rash, bronchospasm, or other signs of hypersensitivity, which may occur immediately after a dose of Advair Diskus.

• Monitor patient for increased use of inhaled short-acting beta$_2$-agonist. The dose of Advair Diskus may need to be increased.

• Monitor patient for hypercorticism and adrenal suppression. If these occur, reduce dosage slowly.

• Monitor patient for eosinophilia, vasculitic rash, worsening pulmonary symptoms, cardiac complications, or neuropathy, which may be signs of a serious eosinophilic condition.

• Monitor patient for signs or symptoms of thrush.

• Evaluate patient's and family's knowledge of drug therapy.

🔷 Nursing diagnoses

• Ineffective airway clearance related to underlying asthmatic condition

• Risk of impaired gas exchange related to poor pulmonary function

• Activity intolerance related to underlying asthmatic condition

• Deficient knowledge related to proper inhalation with the Diskus device and drug therapy

❯ Planning and implementation

🔹 **ALERT:** Don't switch patient from systemic corticosteroids to Advair Diskus because of hypothalamic-pituitary-adrenal axis suppression. Death can occur from adrenal insufficiency.

• After control of asthma has been achieved, adjust to the lowest effective dosage.

🔹 **ALERT:** Don't start Advair Diskus therapy during rapidly deteriorating or potentially life-threatening episodes of asthma. Serious acute respiratory events, including death, can occur, especially in blacks.

🔹 **ALERT:** Don't use Advair Diskus to treat status asthmaticus. When a patient uses Advair Diskus, make sure the patient has an inhaled, short-acting beta$_2$-agonist (such as albuterol) for

acute symptoms that occur between doses of Advair Diskus.

🔹 **ALERT:** Advair Diskus can produce paradoxical bronchospasm. If it does, treat immediately with a short-acting, inhaled bronchodilator (such as albuterol) and stop Advair Diskus therapy.

• If patient is exposed to chickenpox, give varicella zoster immune globulin as prophylaxis. If chickenpox develops, give an antiviral.

• If patient is exposed to measles, give pooled I.M. immunoglobulin as prophylaxis.

• Store at controlled room temperature (68° F to 77° F [20° to 25° C]) in a dry place away from direct heat or sunlight. Discard the device 1 month after removal from the moisture-protective over-wrap pouch or after every foil-wrapped blister has been used, whichever comes first. Don't attempt to take the device apart.

Patient teaching

• Instruct patient on proper use of Diskus device to provide the most effective treatment.

• Instruct patient to keep the Diskus in a dry place, to avoid washing the mouthpiece or other parts of the device, and to avoid taking the Diskus apart.

• Tell patient to stop taking an oral or inhaled long-acting beta$_2$-agonist simultaneously when beginning treatment with Advair Diskus.

🔹 **ALERT:** Explain to patient that Advair Diskus is used only for long-term maintenance and not for acute symptoms of asthma or for prevention of exercise-induced bronchospasm. Urge patient to use a short-acting beta$_2$-agonist (such as albuterol) for relief of acute symptoms.

• Instruct patient to rinse mouth after each inhalation to prevent oral candidiasis.

• Inform patient that improvement may be seen within 30 minutes after an Advair dose; however, the full benefit may not occur for 1 week or more.

🔹 **ALERT:** Instruct patient not to exceed recommended prescribing dose under any circumstances.

• Instruct patient to report decreasing effects or increasing use of the short-acting beta$_2$-agonist inhaler immediately to his prescriber.

• Instruct patient not to use Advair Diskus with a spacer device.

• Tell patient to report palpitations, chest pain, rapid heart rate, tremor, or nervousness immediately to prescriber. Also instruct patient to avoid stimulants, such as caffeine, while on Advair

Diskus therapy because they may increase these adverse reactions.

• Instruct patient to contact prescriber immediately if exposed to chickenpox or measles.

☑ **Evaluation**

• Patient's activity tolerance increases.

• Patient doesn't suffer from any adverse effects related to fluticasone propionate and salmeterol inhalation powder.

• Patient has a normal breathing pattern and optimal air exchange.

• Patient and family state understanding of drug therapy.

fluvastatin sodium

(floo-vuh-STAH-tin SOH-dee-um)
Lescol, Lescol XL

Pharmacologic class: HMG-CoA reductase inhibitor
Therapeutic class: cholesterol inhibitor
Pregnancy risk category: X

Indications and dosages

▶ **Reduction of LDL and total cholesterol levels in patients with primary hypercholesterolemia (types IIa and IIb) or to slow progression of coronary atherosclerosis in patients with coronary artery disease; elevated triglyceride and apolipoprotein B levels in patients with primary hypercholesterolemia and mixed dyslipidemia whose response to dietary restriction and other nonpharmacologic measures has been inadequate.** *Adults:* Initially, 20 to 40 mg P.O. h.s. Increase dosage p.r.n. to maximum of 80 mg daily (in divided doses).

▶ **To reduce the risk of undergoing coronary revascularization procedures.** *Adults:* For patients requiring LDL cholesterol reduction of 25% or more, initially 40 mg (regular-release) P.O. and 80 mg (extended-release) P.O. as a single dose in the evening. Or, 40 mg (regular-release) P.O. b.i.d. For patients requiring LDL cholesterol reduction of less than 25%, initially 20 mg P.O. daily. The recommended dosing range is 20 to 80 mg daily.

◩ **Adjust-a-dose:** With a persistent increase in ALT or AST levels of at least three times the upper limit of normal, withdraw drug. Drug is pri-

marily cleared hepatically so dosage adjustments for mild to moderate renal impairment aren't necessary. Exercise caution with severe impairment.

Contraindications and precautions

• Contraindicated in patients hypersensitive to drug and in those with active liver disease or conditions that cause unexplained, persistent elevations of transaminase levels.

• Use cautiously in patients with severe renal impairment or with history of liver disease or heavy alcohol use.

⚖ **Lifespan:** In pregnant and breast-feeding women and women of childbearing age, drug is contraindicated. In children, safety hasn't been established.

Adverse reactions

CNS: headache, fatigue, dizziness, insomnia.
EENT: sinusitis, rhinitis, pharyngitis.
GI: dyspepsia, diarrhea, nausea, vomiting, abdominal pain, constipation, flatulence.
Musculoskeletal: arthropathy, myalgia, arthralgia.
Respiratory: *upper respiratory infection,* cough, bronchitis.
Skin: rash.
Other: tooth disorder, hypersensitivity reactions (***thrombocytopenia, leukopenia,*** hemolytic anemia).

Interactions

Drug-drug. *Cholestyramine, colestipol:* May bind with fluvastatin in GI tract and decrease absorption. Separate administration times by at least 4 hours.
Cimetidine, omeprazole, ranitidine: May decrease fluvastatin metabolism. Monitor patient for enhanced effects.
Cyclosporine and other immunosuppressants, erythromycin, gemfibrozil, niacin: May increase risk of polymyositis and rhabdomyolysis. Avoid using together.
Digoxin: May increase digoxin level. Monitor digoxin levels carefully.
Fluconazole, itraconazole, ketoconazole: May increase level and adverse effects of fluvastatin. Avoid using together. If they must be given together, reduce dose of fluvastatin.
Rifampin: Enhances rifampin metabolism and decreases level. Monitor patient for lack of effect.

Drug-herb. *Red yeast rice:* Contains components similar to those of statin drugs, increasing the risk of adverse events or toxicity. Discourage using together.
Drug-lifestyle. *Alcohol use:* May increase risk of hepatotoxicity. Discourage using together.

Effects on lab test results

• May increase ALT, AST, bilirubin, and CK levels.
• May decrease hemoglobin, hematocrit, and platelet and WBC counts.

Pharmacokinetics

Absorption: Rapid and almost complete on empty stomach.
Distribution: More than 98% protein-bound.
Metabolism: Complete.
Excretion: About 5% in urine, 90% in feces as metabolites. *Half-life:* Less than 1 hour.

Route	Onset	Peak	Duration
P.O.	Unknown	30-45 min	Unknown

Action

Chemical effect: Inhibits HMG-CoA reductase, an early (and rate-limiting) step in synthetic pathway of cholesterol.
Therapeutic effect: Lowers blood LDL and cholesterol levels.

Available forms

Capsules: 20 mg, 40 mg
Tablets (extended release): 80 mg

NURSING PROCESS

Assessment
• Assess patient's LDL and total cholesterol levels before therapy and evaluate regularly.
• Perform liver function tests periodically.
• Be alert for adverse reactions and drug interactions.
• Evaluate patient's and family's knowledge of drug therapy.

Nursing diagnoses
• Risk for injury related to elevated LDL and cholesterol blood levels
• Diarrhea related to adverse effect of drug on GI tract
• Deficient knowledge related to drug therapy

Planning and implementation
• Start drug only after diet and other nondrug therapies have proven ineffective.
• Give drug h.s. to enhance effectiveness.
• Maintain standard low-cholesterol diet during therapy.
Patient teaching
• Tell patient that drug may be taken without regard to meals; effectiveness is enhanced if taken in evening.
• Teach patient about proper dietary management, weight control, and exercise. Explain their importance in controlling lipid levels.
• Warn patient to restrict alcohol consumption.
• Tell patient to inform prescriber of any adverse reactions, particularly muscle aches and pains.
• Tell patient to stop drug and notify prescriber about planned, suspected, or known pregnancy.

Evaluation
• Patient's LDL and total cholesterol levels are within normal limits.
• Patient maintains normal bowel pattern.
• Patient and family state understanding of drug therapy.

fluvoxamine maleate
(floo-VOKS-uh-meen MAL-ee-ayt)
Luvox

Pharmacologic class: SSRI
Therapeutic class: antidepressant
Pregnancy risk category: C

Indications and dosages

▶ **Depression‡, obsessive-compulsive disorder.** *Adults:* Initially, 50 mg P.O. daily h.s. Increase in 50-mg increments q 4 to 7 days until maximum benefit occurs. Maximum, 300 mg daily. Give total daily doses exceeding 100 mg in two divided doses.
Children ages 8 to 17‡: 25 mg P.O. daily h.s. Dose may be increased in 25-mg increments q 4 to 7 days as tolerated until maximum benefit achieved. Maximum, 200 mg daily for children ages 8 to 11 and 300 mg for children ages 12 to 17. Give total daily doses exceeding 50 mg in two divided doses.
Adjust-a-dose: For elderly patients and patients with hepatic impairment, initially, 25 mg

P.O. daily, then adjust upward gradually to a maximum daily dose of 200 mg.

Contraindications and precautions

• Contraindicated in patients hypersensitive to SSRIs or any of their ingredients and within 2 weeks of an MAO inhibitor.

• Use with thioridazine or pimozide is contraindicated because ventricular arrhythmias and death may occur.

• Use cautiously in patients with hepatic dysfunction, conditions that may affect hemodynamic responses or metabolism, or history of mania or seizures.

⚕ Lifespan: In pregnant women, use cautiously. In breast-feeding women, drug isn't recommended. In elderly patients, use cautiously and start at a lower dose.

Adverse reactions

CNS: *headache, asthenia, somnolence, insomnia, nervousness, dizziness,* tremor, anxiety, hypertonia, *agitation,* depression, CNS stimulation.
CV: palpitations, vasodilation.
EENT: amblyopia.
GI: *nausea, diarrhea, constipation, dyspepsia,* anorexia, *vomiting,* flatulence, dysphagia, taste perversion, *dry mouth.*
GU: abnormal ejaculation, urinary frequency, impotence, anorgasmia, urine retention.
Respiratory: upper respiratory tract infection, dyspnea, yawning.
Skin: sweating.
Other: decreased libido, flulike syndrome, chills, tooth disorder.

Interactions

Drug-drug. *Benzodiazepines, theophylline, warfarin:* Reduces clearance of these drugs by fluvoxamine. Use together cautiously (except for diazepam, which shouldn't be given with fluvoxamine). Adjust dosage, p.r.n.
Carbamazepine, clozapine, methadone, metoprolol, propranolol, tricyclic antidepressants: Elevates levels of these drugs. Use together cautiously. Monitor patient closely for adverse reactions. Adjust dosage if needed.
Diltiazem: Bradycardia may occur. Monitor heart rate.
Lithium, tryptophan: May enhance fluvoxamine effects. Use together cautiously.

Phenelzine, selegiline, tranylcypromine: May cause serotonin syndrome, which may include CNS irritability, shivering, and altered consciousness. Use together may also cause severe excitation, hyperpyrexia, myoclonus, delirium, and coma. Don't give an MAO inhibitor within 2 weeks of an SSRI.
Pimozide, thioridazine: May prolong QT interval. Avoid using together.
Sumatriptan: May cause weakness, hyperreflexia, and incoordination. Monitor patient closely.
Drug-herb. *St. John's wort:* May cause serotonin syndrome. Discourage using together.
Drug-food. *Caffeine:* Decreases caffeine elimination and increases caffeine effects. Discourage using together.
Drug-lifestyle. *Alcohol use:* May increase CNS effects. Discourage using together.
Smoking: Decreases effectiveness of drug. Discourage patient from smoking.
Sun exposure: May cause photosensitivity. Avoid prolonged or unprotected exposure to sunlight.

Effects on lab test results

None reported.

Pharmacokinetics

Absorption: Well absorbed.
Distribution: 77% protein-bound.
Metabolism: In liver.
Excretion: In urine. *Half-life:* 17 hours.

Route	Onset	Peak	Duration
P.O.	3-10 wk	3-8 hr	Unknown

Action

Chemical effect: May selectively inhibit neuronal uptake of serotonin, which is thought to reduce obsessive-compulsive disorders.
Therapeutic effect: Decreases obsessive-compulsive behavior.

Available forms

Tablets: 25 mg, 50 mg, 100 mg

NURSING PROCESS

⚗ **Assessment**
• Assess patient's condition before therapy, and reassess regularly. Several weeks of therapy may be needed before positive response occurs.

- Be alert for adverse reactions and drug interactions.
- Evaluate patient's and family's knowledge of drug therapy.

🔛 Nursing diagnoses
- Ineffective individual coping related to underlying condition
- Diarrhea related to adverse effect of drug on GI tract
- Deficient knowledge related to drug therapy

⏩ Planning and implementation
- Don't give drug within 14 days of MAO inhibitor therapy.
- Give drug h.s. and without regard to meals.

Patient teaching
- Warn patient to avoid hazardous activities until CNS effects of drug are known.
- Advise patient to avoid alcoholic beverages during drug therapy.
- Inform patient that smoking may decrease effectiveness of drug.
- Tell patient that drug may be taken without regard to food.
- Instruct woman to notify prescriber about planned, suspected, or known pregnancy.
- Tell patient who develops rash, hives, or related allergic reaction to notify prescriber.
- Inform patient that several weeks of therapy may be needed to obtain full antidepressant effect. Once improvement occurs, advise patient not to stop drug unless directed by prescriber.
- Advise patient to check with prescriber before taking OTC medications or herbal remedies; interactions can occur.

☑ Evaluation
- Patient's obsessive-compulsive behaviors are diminished.
- Patient maintains normal bowel patterns.
- Patient and family state understanding of drug therapy.

folic acid (vitamin B)
(FOH-lek AS-id)
Apo-Folic ♦ , Folvite, Novo-Folacid ♦

Pharmacologic class: folic acid derivative
Therapeutic class: vitamin supplement
Pregnancy risk category: A

Indications and dosages

▶ **To maintain health.** *Infants:* Up to 0.1 mg P.O. daily.
Children younger than age 4: Up to 0.3 mg P.O. daily.
Adults and children age 4 and older: 0.4 mg P.O. daily.
Pregnant or lactating women: 0.8 mg P.O. daily.
▶ **Megaloblastic or macrocytic anemia caused by folic acid or other nutritional deficiency, hepatic disease, alcoholism, intestinal obstruction, excessive hemolysis.** *Adults and children age 4 and older:* 0.4 mg to 1 mg P.O., S.C., or I.M. daily. After anemia caused by folic acid deficiency is corrected, proper diet and supplements are needed to prevent recurrence.
Children younger than age 4: Up to 0.3 mg P.O., S.C., or I.M. daily.
Pregnant and breast-feeding women: 0.8 mg P.O., S.C., or I.M. daily.
▶ **Prevention of megaloblastic anemia in pregnancy and fetal damage.** *Adults:* Up to 1 mg P.O., S.C., or I.M. daily throughout pregnancy.
▶ **Nutritional supplement.** *Adults:* 0.1 mg P.O., S.C., or I.M. daily.
Children: 0.05 mg P.O. daily.
▶ **To test folic acid deficiency in patients with megaloblastic anemia without masking pernicious anemia.** *Adults and children:* 0.1 to 0.2 mg P.O. or I.M. for 10 days, with diet low in folate and vitamin B_{12}.
▶ **Tropical sprue.** *Adults:* 3 to 15 mg P.O. daily.

Contraindications and precautions

- Contraindicated in patients with vitamin B_{12} deficiency or undiagnosed anemia.
- ⚖ Lifespan: In pregnant women, folic acid therapy is recommended to prevent neural tube defects.

Adverse reactions

CNS: general malaise.
GI: bitter taste, anorexia, nausea, flatulence.
Respiratory: *bronchospasm.*
Other: allergic reactions (rash, pruritus, erythema).

Interactions

Drug-drug. *Aminosalicylic acid, chloramphenicol, methotrexate, sulfasalazine, trimethoprim:* Antagonism of folic acid. Monitor patient for decreased folic acid effect. Use together cautiously.

Anticonvulsants (such as phenobarbital, phenytoin): May increase anticonvulsant metabolism and decrease anticonvulsant blood levels. Monitor patient closely.

Effects on lab test results

- May decrease RBC count.
- May falsely decrease folate level.

Pharmacokinetics

Absorption: Absorbed rapidly from GI tract, mainly from proximal part of small intestine, when given orally. Absorption unknown after S.C. or I.M. administration.
Distribution: Distributed into all body tissues; liver contains about half of total body folate stores. Folate is concentrated actively in CSF.
Metabolism: Metabolized in liver.
Excretion: Excess folate is excreted unchanged in urine; small amounts of folic acid have been recovered in feces. About 0.05 mg/day of normal body folate stores is lost by combination of urinary and fecal excretion and oxidative cleavage of molecule. *Half-life:* Unknown.

Route	Onset	Peak	Duration
P.O., I.M., S.C.	Unknown	30-60 min	Unknown

Action

Chemical effect: Stimulates normal erythropoiesis and nucleoprotein synthesis.
Therapeutic effect: Nutritional supplement.

Available forms

Injection: 5 mg/ml with 1.5% benzyl alcohol or 10 mg/ml with 1.5% benzyl alcohol and 0.2% EDTA
Tablets: 0.1 mg†, 0.4 mg†, 0.8 mg†, 1 mg

NURSING PROCESS

⟐ Assessment

- Assess patient's folic acid deficiency before therapy.
- Evaluate CBC and assess patient's physical status throughout therapy.
- Be alert for adverse reactions and drug interactions.
- Evaluate patient's and family's knowledge of drug therapy.

⟐ Nursing diagnoses

- Imbalanced nutrition: less than body requirements related to presence of folic acid deficiency
- Deficient knowledge related to drug therapy

⟐ Planning and implementation

- Patient with small-bowel resection and intestinal malabsorption may need parenteral administration.
- Don't mix with other drugs in same syringe for I.M. injections.
- Protect from light and heat; store at room temperature.
- Give vitamin B_{12} with this therapy if needed.
- Make sure patient is getting properly balanced diet.

⚠ **ALERT:** Don't confuse folic acid with folinic acid.

Patient teaching
- Teach patient proper nutrition to prevent recurrence of anemia.
- Tell patient to report hypersensitivity reactions or breathing difficulty.
- Urge patient to avoid alcohol because it increases folic acid requirements.

⟐ Evaluation

- Patient's CBC is normal.
- Patient and family state understanding of drug therapy.

fondaparinux sodium
(fon-duh-PAIR-in-ux SOH-dee-uhm)
Arixtra

Pharmacologic class: inhibitor of activated factor X (Xa)
Therapeutic class: anticoagulant
Pregnancy risk category: B

Indications and dosages

▶ **To prevent deep vein thrombosis, which may lead to pulmonary embolism in patients undergoing surgery for hip fracture, hip replacement, or knee replacement.** *Adults:* 2.5 mg S.C. once daily for 5 to 9 days; maximum 11 days. Give initial dose after hemostasis is established, 6 to 8 hours after surgery. Giving the dose earlier than 6 hours after surgery increases the risk for major bleeding. In patients undergoing hip fracture surgery, an extended prophylaxis course of up to 24 additional days is recommended, and a total of 32 days (perioperative and extended prophylaxis) has been tolerated.

Contraindications and precautions

• Contraindicated in patients with creatinine clearance less than 30 ml/minute; in those who are hypersensitive to the drug or weigh less than 50 kg (110 lb); and in those with active major bleeding, bacterial endocarditis, or thrombocytopenia with a positive test result for antiplatelet antibody while taking drug.
• Use cautiously in patients also being treated with platelet inhibitors and in those at increased risk for bleeding, such as patients with congenital or acquired bleeding disorders, with active ulcerative and angiodysplastic GI disease, with hemorrhagic CVA, or shortly after brain, spinal, or ophthalmologic surgery. Also use cautiously in patients who have had epidural or spinal anesthesia or spinal puncture; they have an increased risk for developing an epidural or spinal hematoma (which may cause permanent paralysis).
• Use caution in patients undergoing elective hip surgery with mild or moderate renal impairment. Also use cautiously in patients with creatinine clearance 30 to 50 ml/minute, with a history of heparin-induced thrombocytopenia, or with a bleeding diathesis, uncontrolled arterial hypertension, or a history of recent GI ulceration, diabetic retinopathy, and hemorrhage.
⚠ Lifespan: In pregnant women, don't use drug unless clearly needed. In breast-feeding women, use cautiously because it's unknown whether drug appears in breast milk. In children, safety and effectiveness of drug haven't been established. In elderly patients, use cautiously because the risk of major bleeding increases with age. In patients older than age 75, total clearance of drug was approximately 25% lower than in patients younger than age 65.

Adverse reactions

CNS: insomnia, dizziness, confusion, pain, headache, *fever,* **spinal and epidural hematomas.**
CV: hypotension, edema.
GI: *nausea,* constipation, vomiting, diarrhea, dyspepsia.
GU: UTI, urinary retention.
Hematologic: **hemorrhage,** *anemia,* hematoma, **postoperative hemorrhage, thrombocytopenia.**
Metabolic: hypokalemia.

Skin: mild local irritation (injection site bleeding, rash, pruritus), bullous eruption, purpura increased wound drainage, rash.

Interactions

Drug-drug. *Drugs that increase risk of bleeding (NSAIDs, platelet inhibitors, anticoagulants):* Increases risk of hemorrhage. Stop use before starting fondaparinux. If must be used together, monitor patient closely for bleeding.

Effects on lab results

• May increase creatinine, AST, ALT, and bilirubin levels. May decrease potassium level.
• May decrease hemoglobin, hematocrit, and platelet count.

Pharmacokinetics

Absorption: Rapid and complete; 100% bioavailability.
Distribution: Mainly in blood. At least 94% bound to AT-III.
Metabolism: In vivo metabolism hasn't been investigated since most of the drug is eliminated unchanged in urine in people with normal kidney function.
Excretion: Up to 77% of a single dose in urine unchanged in 72 hours. Prolonged in patients over age 75, in patients who weigh less than 50 kg (110 lb), and in patients with renal impairment. *Half-life:* 17 to 21 hours.

Route	Onset	Peak	Duration
S.C.	Unknown	2-3 hr	Unknown

Action

Chemical effect: Binds to antithrombin III (AT-III) and potentiates by about 300 times the natural neutralization of factor Xa by AT-III. Neutralization of factor Xa interrupts the coagulation cascade, thereby inhibiting formation of thrombin and thrombus development.
Therapeutic effect: Prevents the formation of blood clots.

Available forms

Injection: 2.5 mg/0.5 ml prefilled syringe

NURSING PROCESS

⚕ Assessment
• Assess patient's underlying condition before initiating therapy.

- Be alert for adverse reactions and drug interactions.
- Patient who has received epidural or spinal anesthesia is at increased risk for developing an epidural or spinal hematoma, which may result in long-term or permanent paralysis. Monitor patient closely for neurological impairment.
- Monitor renal function periodically and stop drug in patient who develops unstable renal function or severe renal impairment.
- Routinely assess patient for signs and symptoms of bleeding, and regularly monitor CBC, platelet count, creatinine level, and stool occult blood test results. If platelet count is less than 100,000/mm^3, stop drug.
- Effect may last for 2 to 4 days after stopping drug in patient with normal renal function.
- Don't use PT and APTT tests to measure effectiveness.
- Evaluate patient's and family's knowledge of drug therapy.

🔲 Nursing diagnoses
- Risk for injury related to potential for thrombosis or pulmonary emboli development from underlying condition
- Increased risk for trauma related to increased risk of bleeding and hemorrhaging due to drug therapy
- Deficient knowledge related to anticoagulant therapy

▶ Planning and implementation
- Give by S.C. injection only. Give the drug S.C. in fatty tissue only, rotating administration injection sites.
- Visually inspect the single-dose, prefilled syringe for particulate matter and discoloration before administration.
- Don't mix with other injections or infusions.
- ⚠ **ALERT:** Don't use interchangeably with heparin, low–molecular-weight heparins, or heparinoids.
- To avoid loss of drug, don't expel air bubble from the syringe.
- If patient begins to overtly bleed during therapy, apply strong pressure to area and notify prescriber immediately.
- Overdosage may lead to hemorrhagic complications. Stop drug and treat bleeding appropriately.

- ⚠ **ALERT:** Don't confuse fondaparinux (Arixtra) with the lab test anti-factor Xa, sometimes written anti-Xa.
- ⚠ **ALERT:** Don't confuse Arixtra with Bextra.

Patient teaching
- Teach patient signs and symptoms of bleeding. If any occur, patient should contact prescriber immediately.
- Instruct patient to avoid OTC products that contain aspirin, other salicylates, or NSAIDs and other prescribed anticoagulants.
- Teach patient the correct way to give drug to himself S.C.
- Show patient the different sites for injection and explain to patient that he must alternate injection sites to prevent hardening of fatty tissues.
- Teach patient the proper disposal of the syringe.

🔲 Evaluation
- Patient doesn't suffer from any pulmonary embolus or thrombus during drug therapy.
- Patient is free from any injury or bleeding.
- Patient and family state understanding of drug therapy.

formoterol fumarate inhalation powder
(for-MOE-tur-all FOO-muh-rayt)
Foradil Aerolizer

Pharmacologic class: long-acting selective beta$_2$-adrenergic agonist
Therapeutic class: bronchodilator
Pregnancy risk category: C

Indications and dosages

▶ **Prevention and maintenance treatment of bronchospasm in patients with reversible obstructive airway disease or nocturnal asthma who usually need short-acting inhaled beta$_2$-adrenergic agonists.** *Adults and children age 5 and older:* One 12-mcg capsule by inhalation via Aerolizer inhaler q 12 hours. Don't give more than one capsule twice daily (24 mcg daily). If symptoms are present between doses, use a short-acting beta$_2$-adrenergic agonist for immediate relief.

▶ **Prevention of exercise-induced bronchospasm.** *Adults and children age 12 and older:*

One 12-mcg capsule by inhalation via Aerolizer inhaler at least 15 minutes before exercise, given occasionally, p.r.n. Avoid giving additional doses within 12 hours of first dose.

▶ **Maintenance of COPD.** *Adults:* One 12-mcg capsule by inhalation via Aerolizer inhaler q 12 hours. Total daily dose of greater than 24 mcg isn't recommended.

Contraindications and precautions

• Contraindicated in patients hypersensitive to drug or its components.

• Use cautiously in patients with CV disease, particularly coronary insufficiency, cardiac arrhythmias, and hypertension; in those who are unusually responsive to sympathomimetic amines; and in those with diabetes mellitus because hyperglycemia and ketoacidosis have occurred rarely with use of beta agonists.

• Use cautiously in patients with lactose or milk allergy, seizure disorders or thyrotoxicosis.

✷ **Lifespan:** In pregnant women, use cautiously because drug may interfere with uterine contractility. In breast-feeding women, use cautiously because it isn't known whether drug appears in breast milk. In children younger than age 5, safety and effectiveness of drug haven't been established for asthma. In children younger than age 12, safety hasn't been established for exercise-induced bronchospasm.

Adverse reactions

CNS: tremor, dizziness, insomnia, nervousness, headache, fatigue, malaise.
CV: chest pain, angina, hypertension, hypotension, tachycardia, *arrhythmias*, palpitations.
EENT: dry mouth, tonsillitis, dysphonia.
GI: nausea.
Metabolic: hypokalemia, hyperglycemia, *metabolic acidosis.*
Musculoskeletal: muscle cramps.
Respiratory: bronchitis, chest infection, dyspnea.
Skin: rash.
Other: viral infection.

Interactions

Drug-drug. *Adrenergics:* May potentiate sympathetic effects of formoterol. Use together cautiously.
Beta blockers: May antagonize effects of beta agonists, causing bronchospasm in asthmatic patients. Avoid use except when benefits out-

weigh risks. Use cardioselective beta blockers cautiously to minimize risk of bronchospasm.
Corticosteroids, diuretics, xanthine derivatives: May potentiate hypokalemic effect of formoterol. Use together cautiously.
Loop or thiazide diuretics: May worsen ECG changes or hypokalemia with beta agonists. Use together cautiously, and monitor patient closely.
MAO inhibitors, tricyclic antidepressants, and other drugs that prolong the QT interval: May increase risk of ventricular arrhythmias. Use together cautiously.

Effects on lab test results

• May decrease potassium level. May increase glucose level.

Pharmacokinetics

Absorption: Rapid. Drug levels peak within 5 minutes after a 120-mcg dose. Most of inhaled dose is probably swallowed and absorbed from the GI tract.
Distribution: 61% to 64% bound to proteins.
Metabolism: Occurs primarily via direct glucuronidation and O-demethylation (involving CYP 2D6, 2C19, 2C9, and 2A6). Doesn't appear to inhibit CYP 450 enzymes at therapeutic levels.
Excretion: 59% to 62% eliminated in urine and 32% to 34% eliminated in feces over 5 days. When 12 to 24 mcg is given to asthma patients, about 10% of total dose is excreted in urine as unchanged drug and 15% to 18% is eliminated in urine as direct glucuronide conjugates of formoterol. *Half-life:* Unknown.

Route	Onset	Peak	Duration
Oral inhalation	1-3 min	½-1½ hr	12 hr

Action

Chemical effect: Relaxes bronchial and cardiac smooth muscle by acting on beta$_2$ adrenergic receptors; stimulates intracellular adenyl cyclase, the enzyme responsible for catalyzing the conversion of adenosine triphosphate (ATP) to cAMP. This increase in cAMP leads to relaxation of bronchial smooth muscle and inhibition of mediator release from mast cells.
Therapeutic effect: Prevents and controls bronchospasm.

Available forms

Capsules for inhalation: 12 mcg

NURSING PROCESS

☞ Assessment

• Assess patient's underlying condition before therapy and reassess regularly.
• Evaluate patient's use of short acting beta$_2$ agonists for immediate relief of bronchospasm. Drug may be used with short-acting beta$_2$ agonists, inhaled corticosteroids, and theophylline therapy to manage asthma.
• Evaluate patient's and family's knowledge of drug therapy.

⚙ Nursing diagnoses

• Impaired gas exchange related to underlying pulmonary condition
• Risk for activity intolerance related to underlying pulmonary condition
• Knowledge deficit related to formoterol fumarate therapy

⟫ Planning and implementation

• For patient using drug twice daily, don't give additional doses to prevent exercise-induced bronchospasm.
• Don't use as a substitute for short-acting beta$_2$ agonists for immediate relief of bronchospasm or as a substitute for inhaled or oral corticosteroids.
• Don't begin use in patients with rapidly deteriorating or significantly worsening asthma.
• If usual dose doesn't control symptoms of bronchoconstriction, and the patient's short-acting beta$_2$ agonist becomes less effective, reevaluate patient and treatment regimen.
• For patients who formerly used regularly scheduled short-acting beta$_2$ agonists, decrease use of these drugs to an as-needed basis when long-acting therapy starts.
• Before dispensing, store drug in refrigerator. Once dispensed to patient, drug may be stored at room temperature. Don't remove capsule from unopened blister until immediately before administration. Give capsules only by oral inhalation and use only with the Aerolizer inhaler; they aren't for oral ingestion. Don't let the patient exhale into the device. Don't use Foradil Aerolizer with a spacer device. Pierce capsules only once. In rare instances, the gelatin capsule may break into small pieces and enter the patient's mouth or throat with inhalation. However, the Aerolizer contains a screen that should catch any broken pieces before they leave the device. To minimize risk of shattering capsule, strictly follow storage and use instructions.

• Drug may cause life-threatening paradoxical bronchospasm. If this occurs, stop drug immediately and use an different drug.
• Monitor patient for tachycardia, hypertension, and other adverse CV effects. If they occur, stop drug.
• Watch for immediate hypersensitivity reactions, such as anaphylaxis, urticaria, angioedema, rash, and bronchospasm.
• Signs and symptoms of overdose include excessive beta blocker stimulation and exaggeration of adverse effects; cardiac arrest and death may result. To treat overdose, stop drug, monitor cardiac status, give appropriate symptomatic relief or supportive therapy, and use cardioselective beta blockers cautiously. It's unknown whether dialysis is beneficial.
ⓢ **ALERT:** Don't confuse Foradil (formoterol fumarate) with Toradol (ketorolac).

Patient teaching

• Tell patient not to increase the dose or frequency of use without medical advice.
• Warn patient not to stop or reduce other medication taken for asthma.
• Advise patient that drug isn't for acute asthmatic episodes; instead, he should use short-acting beta$_2$ agonist.
• Advise patient to report worsening symptoms, less-effective treatment, or increasing use of short-acting beta$_2$ agonist.
• Tell patient to report nausea, vomiting, shakiness, headache, fast or irregular heartbeat, chest pain, or sleeplessness.
• Tell patient being treated for exercise-induced bronchospasm to take drug at least 15 minutes before exercise. Additional doses can't be taken for 12 hours.
• Tell patient not to use the Foradil Aerolizer with a spacer device or to exhale or blow into the inhaler.
• Advise patient to avoid washing the Aerolizer and to always keep it dry. Advise patient to use the new device that comes with each refill.
• Tell patient to avoid exposing capsules to moisture and to handle them only with dry hands.

☑ **Evaluation**
- Patient's pulmonary symptoms improve.
- Patient's activity intolerance improves.
- Patient and family state understanding of drug therapy.

fosamprenavir calcium
(foss-am-PREH-nuh-veer CAL-see-um)
Lexiva

Pharmacologic classification: HIV protease inhibitor
Therapeutic classification: antiretroviral
Pregnancy risk category: C

Indications and dosages
▶ **HIV infection with other antiretrovirals.**
Adults: In patients previously untreated, 1,400 mg P.O. twice daily (without ritonavir). Or, 1,400 mg P.O. once daily and ritonavir 200 mg P.O. once daily. Or, 700 mg P.O. twice daily and ritonavir 100 mg P.O. twice daily. In patients previously treated with a protease inhibitor, 700 mg P.O. twice daily plus ritonavir 100 mg P.O. twice daily.
◩ **Adjust-a-dose:** If the patient receives efavirenz, fosamprenavir, and ritonavir once daily, give an additional 100 mg/day of ritonavir (300 mg total). If the patient has mild or moderate hepatic impairment and takes fosamprenavir without ritonavir, reduce the dosage to 700 mg P.O. twice daily.

Contraindications and precautions

▶ Contraindicated in patients hypersensitive to amprenavir or its components. Also contraindicated with dihydroergotamine, ergonovine, ergotamine, flecainide, methylergonovine, midazolam, pimozide, propafenone, and triazolam.
▶ Use cautiously in patients allergic to sulfonamides and those with mild to moderate hepatic impairment. Avoid use in patients with severe hepatic impairment.
⚖ **Lifespan:** In pregnant women, breastfeeding women, and children, safety and effectiveness haven't been established.

Adverse reactions

CNS: *depression, fatigue, headache, oral paresthesia.*

GI: *abdominal pain, diarrhea, nausea, vomiting.*
Skin: pruritus, *rash.*

Interactions

Drug-drug. *Amitriptyline, cyclosporine, imipramine, tacrolimus:* May increase levels of these drugs. Monitor drug levels.
Antiarrhythmics (amiodarone, lidocaine, quinidine): May increase antiarrhythmic level. Use together cautiously, and monitor antiarrhythmic levels.
Atorvastatin: May increase atorvastatin level. Give 20 mg/day or less of atorvastatin, and monitor patient carefully. Or, consider other HMG-CoA reductase inhibitors, such as fluvastatin, pravastatin, or rosuvastatin.
Benzodiazepines (alprazolam, clorazepate, diazepam, flurazepam): May increase benzodiazepine level. Decrease benzodiazepine dosage as needed.
Bepridil: May increase bepridil level, possibly leading to arrhythmias. Use together cautiously.
Calcium channel blockers (amlodipine, diltiazem, felodipine, isradipine, nicardipine, nifedipine, nimodipine, nisoldipine, verapamil): May increase calcium channel blocker level. Use together cautiously.
Carbamazepine, dexamethasone, H₂-receptor antagonists, phenobarbital, phenytoin, proton-pump inhibitors: May decrease amprenavir level. Use together cautiously.
Delavirdine: May cause loss of virologic response and resistance to delavirdine. Avoid using together.
Dihydroergotamine, ergonovine, ergotamine, flecainide, methylergonovine, midazolam, pimozide, propafenone, triazolam: May cause serious adverse reactions. Avoid using together.
Efavirenz, nevirapine, saquinavir: May decrease amprenavir level. Appropriate combination doses haven't been established.
Efavirenz with ritonavir: May decrease amprenavir level. Increase ritonavir by 100 mg/day (300 mg total) when giving efavirenz, fosamprenavir, and ritonavir once daily. No change needed in ritonavir when giving efavirenz, fosamprenavir, and ritonavir twice daily.
Ethinyl estradiol and norethindrone: May increase ethinyl estradiol/norethindrone levels. Recommend nonhormonal contraception.
Indinavir, nelfinavir: May increase amprenavir level. Appropriate combination doses haven't been established.

Reactions may be *common*, uncommon, *life-threatening*, or COMMON AND LIFE-THREATENING.

Ketoconazole, itraconazole: May increase keto-conazole and itraconazole levels. Reduce keto-conazole or itraconazole dosage as needed if patient receives more than 400 mg daily. More than 200 mg/day isn't recommended.

Lopinavir with ritonavir: May decreased ampre-navir and lopinavir levels. Appropriate combina-tion doses haven't been established.

Lovastatin, simvastatin: May increase risk of myopathy, including rhabdomyolysis. Avoid us-ing together.

Methadone: May decrease methadone level. In-crease methadone dosage as needed.

Rifabutin: May increase rifabutin level. Obtain CBC weekly to watch for neutropenia, and de-crease rifabutin dosage by at least half. If pa-tient receives ritonavir, decrease dosage by at least 75% from the usual 300 mg/day. Maxi-mum, 150 mg every other day or three times weekly.

Rifampin: May decrease amprenavir level and drug effect. Avoid using together.

Sildenafil, vardenafil: May increase sildenafil and vardenafil levels. Recommend cautious use of sildenafil at 25 mg every 48 hours or varde-nafil at no more than 2.5 mg every 24 hours. If patient receives ritonavir, recommend cautious use of vardenafil at no more than 2.5 mg every 72 hours. Tell patient to report adverse events.

Warfarin: May alter warfarin level. Monitor INR.

Drug-herb. *St. John's wort:* May cause loss of virologic response and resistance to fosampre-navir or its class of protease inhibitors. Discour-age use together.

Effects on lab test results

• May increase lipase, triglyceride, AST, and ALT levels.
• May decrease neutrophil count.

Pharmacokinetics

Absorption: Food has no effect.
Distribution: 90% protein-bound.
Metabolism: Rapidly and almost completely hydrolyzed to amprenavir before reaching sys-temic circulation. Amprenavir is metabolized by CYP 3A4 enzyme system.
Excretion: Unknown. *Half-life:* 7¾ hours.

Route	Onset	Peak	Duration
P.O.	Unknown	1½-4 hr	Unknown

Action

Chemical effect: Converts rapidly to ampre-navir, which binds to the active site of HIV-1 protease and causes formation of immature non-infectious viral particles.
Therapeutic effect: Hinders HIV activity.

Available forms

Tablets: 700 mg

Assessment
• Monitor patient with hemophilia for sponta-neous bleeding.
• During initial treatment, monitor patient for such opportunistic infections as mycobacterium avium complex, CMV, *Pneumocystis carinii* pneumonia, and tuberculosis.
• Assess patient for redistribution or accumula-tion of body fat, as in central obesity, dorsocer-vical fat enlargement (buffalo hump), peripheral wasting, facial wasting, breast enlargement, and a cushingoid appearance.
• Evaluate patient's and family's knowledge of drug therapy.

Nursing diagnoses
• Infection related to presence of HIV
• Risk for deficient fluid volume related to ad-verse GI reactions
• Deficient knowledge related to drug therapy

Planning and implementation
• Patients with hepatitis B or C or marked in-crease in transaminase level before treatment may have increased risk of transaminase eleva-tion. Monitor patient closely during treatment.
Patient teaching
• Tell patient that drug doesn't reduce the risk of transmitting HIV to others.
• Inform patient that the drug may reduce the risk of progression to AIDS and death.
• Explain that drug must be used with other an-tiretrovirals.
• Tell patient not to alter the dose or stop taking drug without consulting the health care provider.
• Urge patient to inform health care provider about sulfa allergy.
• Because this drug may interact with many drugs, urge patient to tell health care provider about any prescription or OTC drugs and herbal

products the he takes (especially St. John's wort).

• Explain that body fat may redistribute or accumulate.

☑ Evaluation

• Patient responds well to therapy.
• Patient maintains adequate hydration.
• Patient and family state understanding of drug therapy.

foscarnet sodium (phosphonoformic acid)

(fos-KAR-net SOH-dee-um)

Foscavir

Pharmacologic class: pyrophosphate analogue
Therapeutic class: antiviral
Pregnancy risk category: C

Indications and dosages

▶ **CMV retinitis in patients with AIDS.**
Adults: Initially, 60 mg/kg I.V. over 1 hour q 8 hours for 2 to 3 weeks, depending on response. Or, 90 mg/kg I.V. q 12 hours over 1.5 to 2 hours for 2 to 3 weeks, depending on response. Follow with maintenance infusion of 90 mg/kg I.V. daily over 2 hours; if disease progresses, increase dose as needed and tolerated to 120 mg/kg daily.
☒ Adjust-a-dose: In patients with renal impairment, adjust dosage for creatinine clearance less than 1.5 ml/kg/minute. If creatinine clearance is less than 0.4 ml/kg/minute, stop drug.

▶ **Mucocutaneous acyclovir-resistant herpes simplex virus (HSV) infections.** *Adults:* 40 mg/kg I.V. infused over at least 1 hour, either q 8 or 12 hours for 2 to 3 weeks or until healed.
☒ Adjust-a-dose: In patients with renal impairment, if creatinine clearance is less than 1.5 ml/kg/minute, adjust dosage. If creatinine clearance is less than 0.4 ml/kg/minute, stop drug.

▶ **Varicella zoster infection‡.** *Adults:* 40 mg/kg I.V. q 8 hours for 14 to 21 days.

▼ I.V. administration

• Use infusion pump to give drug over at least 1 hour. To minimize renal toxicity, ensure adequate hydration before and during infusion.

⚡ ALERT: If infusing via central venous access, the standard 24 mg/ml solution may or may not be diluted. When a peripheral vein catheter is used, dilute solution to 12 mg/ml with D_5W or normal saline solution.

• Don't exceed recommended dosage, infusion rate, or frequency of administration. All doses must be individualized based on patient's renal function.
• Use solution within 24 hours of first entry into sealed bottle.

⚡ ALERT: To reduce the risk of nephrotoxicity, give 750 to 1,000 ml of normal saline solution or D_5W before first dose and then concurrently with each subsequent dose.

Contraindications and precautions

• Contraindicated in patients hypersensitive to drug.
• Use cautiously and at reduced doses in patients with abnormal renal function because drug will accumulate and toxicity will increase. Because drug is nephrotoxic, it may worsen renal impairment. Some nephrotoxicity occurs in most patients treated with drug.

☀ Lifespan: In pregnant or breast-feeding women, use cautiously. In children, safety hasn't been established. In elderly patients, use cautiously because they are more likely to have decreased renal function.

Adverse reactions

CNS: *fever,* pain, *headache, seizures, fatigue, malaise, asthenia, paresthesia, dizziness, hypoesthesia, neuropathy,* tremor, ataxia, generalized spasms, dementia, stupor, sensory disturbances, meningitis, aphasia, abnormal coordination, EEG abnormalities, depression, confusion, anxiety, insomnia, somnolence, nervousness, amnesia, agitation, aggressive reaction.
CV: *hypertension, palpitations, ECG abnormalities, sinus tachycardia,* cerebrovascular disorder, *first-degree AV block, hypotension, flushing,* edema, facial edema.
EENT: visual disturbances, eye pain, conjunctivitis, sinusitis, pharyngitis, rhinitis.
GI: taste perversion, dry mouth, *nausea, diarrhea, vomiting, abdominal pain, anorexia,* constipation, dysphagia, *rectal hemorrhage,* melena, flatulence, ulcerative stomatitis, *pancreatitis.*
GU: *abnormal renal function, albuminuria, dysuria, polyuria, urethral disorder, urine reten-*

tion, UTI, acute renal impairment, nephrotoxicity, candidiasis.

Hematologic: anemia, *granulocytopenia, leukopenia, bone marrow suppression, thrombocytopenia, thrombosis,* lymphadenopathy.

Hepatic: abnormal hepatic function.

Metabolic: hypokalemia, hypomagnesemia, hypophosphatemia or hyperphosphatemia, hypocalcemia, hyponatremia.

Musculoskeletal: leg cramps, arthralgia, myalgia.

Respiratory: *cough, dyspnea,* pneumonic respiratory insufficiency, pulmonary infiltration, *stridor, pneumothorax, bronchospasm,* hemoptysis.

Skin: *rash, increased sweating,* pruritus, skin ulceration, erythematous rash, seborrhea, skin discoloration.

Other: *sepsis,* rigors, inflammation, pain at infusion site, lymphoma-like disorder, sarcoma, back or chest pain, bacterial or fungal infections, abscess, flulike symptoms.

Interactions

Drug-drug. *Nephrotoxic drugs (such as aminoglycosides, amphotericin B):* May increase risk of nephrotoxicity. Avoid using together.

Pentamidine: May increase risk of nephrotoxicity and severe hypocalcemia. Don't use together.

Zidovudine: Possible increased risk or severity of anemia. Monitor blood counts.

Effects on lab test results

• May increase BUN, creatinine, phosphate, ALT, AST, alkaline phosphatase, and bilirubin levels. May decrease calcium, magnesium, phosphate, potassium, and sodium levels.

• May decrease hemoglobin, hematocrit, and granulocyte and WBC counts. May increase or decrease platelet count.

Pharmacokinetics

Absorption: Administered I.V.
Distribution: 14 to 17% protein-bound.
Metabolism: Not metabolized.
Excretion: 80% to 90% appears unchanged in urine. *Half-life:* About 3 hours.

Route	Onset	Peak	Duration
I.V.	Immediate	Immediate	Unknown

Action

Chemical effect: Inhibits all known herpes and CMVs in vitro by blocking pyrophosphate binding site on DNA polymerases and reverse transcriptases.

Therapeutic effect: Kills viruses.

Available forms

Injection: 24 mg/ml in 250- and 500-ml bottles

NURSING PROCESS

Assessment

• Assess patient's infection before therapy and regularly thereafter.

• Obtain electrolyte levels and creatinine clearance before beginning therapy, then two or three times weekly during induction and at least once every 1 to 2 weeks during maintenance.

• Drug may cause dose-related transient decrease in ionized calcium, which may not be reflected in laboratory values. Assess for tetany and seizures with abnormal electrolyte levels.

• Monitor patient's hemoglobin and hematocrit. Up to 33% of patients will develop anemia. It may be severe enough that patient needs transfusions.

• Be alert for adverse reactions and drug interactions.

• Evaluate patient's and family's knowledge of drug therapy.

Nursing diagnoses

• Infection related to presence of herpes virus susceptible to drug

• Disturbed sensory perception (tactile) related to drug's adverse effect

• Deficient knowledge related to drug therapy

Planning and implementation

• Because drug is highly toxic and toxicity is probably dose-related, use lowest effective maintenance dose.

Patient teaching

• Advise patient to report circumoral tingling, numbness in limbs, and paresthesia.

Evaluation

• Patient is free from infection.

• Patient has no adverse neurologic reactions.

• Patient and family state understanding of drug therapy.

fosinopril sodium

(foh-SIN-oh-pril SOH-dee-um)
Monopril

Pharmacologic class: ACE inhibitor
Therapeutic class: antihypertensive
Pregnancy risk category: C (D in second and third trimesters)

Indications and dosages

▶ **Hypertension.** *Adults:* Initially, 10 mg P.O. daily. Adjust dosage based on blood pressure at peak and trough levels. Usual dosage is 20 to 40 mg, up to 80 mg daily. Divide dosage, if needed.
Children ages 6 to 16, weighing 50 kg (110 lb) or more: Give 5 to 10 mg P.O. daily.
▶ **Adjunct therapy for heart failure.** *Adults:* Initially, 10 mg P.O. once daily. Increase dosage over several weeks to maximum tolerable, but no more than 40 mg P.O. daily. If possible, stop diuretic therapy.
☒ **Adjust-a-dose:** For patients who have heart failure with moderate-to-severe renal impairment or who are being vigorously diuresed, give initial dose of 5 mg P.O. daily.

Contraindications and precautions

• Contraindicated in patients hypersensitive to drug or other ACE inhibitors. Avoid use in patients with renal artery stenosis.
• Use cautiously in patients with impaired renal or hepatic function.
⚘ **Lifespan:** In pregnant women, use cautiously and only when necessary to prevent fetal harm. In breast-feeding women, drug is contraindicated. In children younger than age 6 or those weighing less than 50 kg, safety of drug hasn't been established.

Adverse reactions

CNS: headache, dizziness, fatigue, syncope, paresthesia, sleep disturbance, *CVA.*
CV: chest pain, angina, *MI,* rhythm disturbances, palpitations, hypotension, orthostatic hypotension.
EENT: tinnitus, sinusitis.
GI: dry mouth, nausea, vomiting, diarrhea, *pancreatitis,* abdominal distention, abdominal pain, constipation.
GU: renal insufficiency.

Hepatic: *hepatitis.*
Metabolic: *hyperkalemia.*
Musculoskeletal: arthralgia, musculoskeletal pain, myalgia.
Respiratory: *dry, persistent, tickling, nonproductive cough; bronchospasm.*
Skin: urticaria, rash, photosensitivity, pruritus.
Other: decreased libido, sexual dysfunction, gout, *angioedema.*

Interactions

Drug-drug. *Antacids:* May impair absorption. Separate administration times by at least 2 hours.
Diuretics, other antihypertensives: May increase risk of excessive hypotension. Stop diuretic or lower fosinopril dosage if needed.
Lithium: May increase lithium levels and lithium toxicity. Avoid using together.
Potassium-sparing diuretics, potassium supplements, sodium substitutes containing potassium: May increase risk of hyperkalemia. Monitor potassium levels.
Drug-herb. *Licorice:* May cause sodium retention and increase blood pressure, interfering with therapeutic effect of ACE inhibitor. Discourage ingestion of licorice during drug therapy.
Drug-food. *Salt substitutes containing potassium:* May increase risk of hyperkalemia. Monitor potassium closely.
Drug-lifestyle. *Alcohol use:* May have additive hypotensive effects. Discourage using together.

Effects on lab test results

• May increase BUN, creatinine, and potassium levels.
• May increase liver function test results. May decrease hemoglobin and hematocrit.

Pharmacokinetics

Absorption: Slow, primarily in proximal small intestine.
Distribution: More than 95% protein-bound.
Metabolism: Hydrolyzed mainly in liver and gut.
Excretion: 50% in urine; remainder in feces.
Half-life: 11½ hours.

Route	Onset	Peak	Duration
P.O.	≤ 1 hr	2-6 hr	24 hr

Reactions may be *common,* uncommon, *life-threatening,* or COMMON AND LIFE-THREATENING.

Action

Chemical effect: Antihypertensive action not clearly defined. Inhibits ACE, preventing conversion of angiotensin I to angiotensin II, a potent vasoconstrictor. Reduced formation of angiotensin II decreases peripheral arterial resistance, thus decreasing aldosterone secretion. **Therapeutic effect:** Lowers blood pressure.

Available forms

Tablets: 10 mg, 20 mg, 40 mg

NURSING PROCESS

Assessment
• Assess blood pressure before therapy and regularly thereafter.
• Assess renal and hepatic function before and during therapy.
• Monitor potassium intake and potassium level. Diabetic patients, those with renal impairment, and those receiving drugs that can increase potassium levels may develop hyperkalemia.
• Other ACE inhibitors have been linked to agranulocytosis and neutropenia. Monitor CBC with differential counts before therapy, every 2 weeks for first 3 months of therapy, and periodically thereafter.
• If adverse GI reactions occur, monitor patient's hydration status.
• Evaluate patient's and family's knowledge of drug therapy.

Nursing diagnoses
• Risk for injury related to presence of hypertension
• Risk for deficient fluid volume related to adverse GI reactions
• Deficient knowledge related to drug therapy

Planning and implementation
• Drug may be taken without regard to meals. However, taking drug with food slows absorption of drug.
Patient teaching
• Tell patient to avoid sodium substitutes; they may contain potassium, which increases the risk of hyperkalemia.
• Urge patient to report signs of infection (such as fever and sore throat); easy bruising or bleeding; swelling of tongue, lips, face, eyes, mucous membranes, or limbs; difficulty swallowing or breathing; and hoarseness.
• Tell patient to use caution in hot weather and during exercise. Inadequate fluid intake, vomiting, diarrhea, and excessive perspiration can lead to light-headedness and syncope.
• Tell woman to notify prescriber about planned, suspected, or known pregnancy. Drug will probably need to be stopped.

Evaluation
• Patient's blood pressure is normal.
• Patient maintains adequate hydration throughout drug therapy.
• Patient and family state understanding of drug therapy.

fosphenytoin sodium
(fahs-FEN-eh-toyn SOH-dee-um)
Cerebyx

Pharmacologic class: prodrug of phenytoin; hydantoin
Therapeutic class: anticonvulsant
Pregnancy risk category: D

indications and dosages

▶ **Status epilepticus.** *Adults:* 15 to 20 mg phenytoin sodium equivalent (PE)/kg I.V. at 100 to 150 mg PE/minute as loading dose; then 4 to 6 mg PE/kg I.V. daily as maintenance dose. (Phenytoin may be used instead of fosphenytoin as maintenance, using the appropriate dose.)
▶ **Prevention and treatment of seizures during neurosurgery (nonemergent loading or maintenance dosing).** *Adults:* Loading dose of 10 to 20 mg PE/kg I.M. or I.V. at infusion rate not exceeding 150 mg PE/minute. Maintenance dose is 4 to 6 mg PE/kg I.V. or I.M. daily.
▶ **Short-term substitution for oral phenytoin therapy.** *Adults:* Same total daily dosage equivalent as oral phenytoin sodium therapy given as a single daily dose I.M. or I.V. at infusion rate not exceeding 150 mg PE/minute. Some patients may need more frequent dosing.

I.V. administration

• Dilute drug in D_5W or normal saline solution for injection to a level ranging from 1.5 to 25 mg PE/ml.
• Don't exceed 150 mg PE/minute.

- Monitor patient's ECG, blood pressure, and respiration throughout period of maximal phenytoin levels—about 10 to 20 minutes after end of fosphenytoin infusion.
- Refrigerate at 36° to 46° F (2° C to 8° C). Don't keep at room temperature for longer than 48 hours.

Contraindications and precautions

- Contraindicated in patients hypersensitive to drug, its components, phenytoin, or other hydantoins. Also, contraindicated in patients with sinus bradycardia, SA block, second- or third-degree AV block, Adams-Stokes syndrome, or acute hepatotoxicity. Drug isn't indicated for absence seizures.
- Use cautiously in patients with renal and hepatic disease or in those with hypoalbuminemia.
- ⚛ Lifespan: In pregnant women, use drug only if nature, frequency, and severity of seizures pose a serious threat to the patient. In breast-feeding women, drug isn't recommended. In children, safety of drug hasn't been established. In elderly patients, reduce dosage because of decreased metabolism and decreased phenytoin clearance.

Adverse reactions

CNS: abnormal thinking, agitation, asthenia, *ataxia,* brain edema, decreased reflexes, *dizziness,* dysarthria, headache, extrapyramidal syndrome, fever, hypesthesia, increased reflexes, incoordination, **intracranial hypertension,** nervousness, paresthesia, speech disorder, *somnolence,* stupor, vertigo.
CV: hypotension, hypertension, tachycardia, tremor, facial edema, vasodilatation, **severe CV reactions (such as ventricular fibrillation).**
EENT: amblyopia, deafness, diplopia, *nystagmus,* tinnitus.
GI: constipation, dry mouth, nausea, taste perversion, tongue disorder, vomiting.
Hepatic: *hepatotoxicity.*
Metabolic: hypokalemia.
Musculoskeletal: back pain, myasthenia, pelvic pain.
Respiratory: pneumonia.
Skin: ecchymosis, *pruritus,* rash.
Other: accidental injury, chills, infection, injection-site reaction and pain.

Interactions

Drug-drug. *Amiodarone, chloramphenicol, chlordiazepoxide, cimetidine, diazepam, dicumarol, disulfiram, estrogens, ethosuximide, fluoxetine, H_2-receptor antagonists, halothane, isoniazid, methylphenidate, phenothiazines, phenylbutazone, salicylates, succinimides, sulfonamides, tolbutamide, trazodone:* May increase phenytoin level and thus its therapeutic effects. Use together cautiously.
Carbamazepine, reserpine: May decrease phenytoin level. Monitor patient.
Coumarin, digitoxin, doxycycline, estrogens, furosemide, hormonal contraceptives, rifampin, quinidine, theophylline, vitamin D: Phenytoin may decrease effectiveness of these drugs because of increased hepatic metabolism. Monitor patient closely.
Phenobarbital, valproic acid, sodium valproate: May increase or decrease phenytoin level. Monitor patient.
Tricyclic antidepressants: May lower seizure threshold and require adjustments in phenytoin dosage. Use cautiously.
Drug-lifestyle. *Acute alcohol use:* May increase phenytoin level and thus its therapeutic effects. Discourage alcohol use.
Chronic alcohol use: May decrease phenytoin level. Monitor patient; discourage alcohol use.

Effects on lab test results

- May increase alkaline phosphatase, GGT, and glucose levels. May decrease potassium and T_4 levels.
- May decrease platelet, WBC, granulocyte, leukocyte, and RBC counts.

Pharmacokinetics

Absorption: Complete.
Distribution: Widely throughout body; 95 to 99% protein-bound.
Metabolism: Metabolized in the liver; undergoes rapid hydrolysis to phenytoin.
Excretion: Excreted in the urine as phenytoin metabolites. *Half-life:* 15 minutes.

Route	Onset	Peak	Duration
I.V.	Unknown	Immediate	Unknown
I.M.	Unknown	30 min	Unknown

Action

Chemical effect: Because fosphenytoin is a prodrug of phenytoin, its anticonvulsant action

---

Reactions may be *common,* uncommon, *life-threatening,* or COMMON AND LIFE-THREATENING.

is the same. Phenytoin is thought to stabilize neuronal membranes and limit seizure activity. **Therapeutic effect:** Prevents and controls seizures.

Available forms

Injection: 2 ml (150 mg fosphenytoin sodium equivalent to 100 mg phenytoin sodium), 10 ml (750 mg fosphenytoin sodium equivalent to 500 mg phenytoin sodium)

NURSING PROCESS

Assessment
• Don't give drug I.M. for status epilepticus because therapeutic phenytoin levels may not occur as rapidly as with I.V. administration.
• Don't monitor phenytoin level until about 2 hours after the end of I.V. infusion or 4 hours after I.M. administration.
• Evaluate patient's and family's knowledge of drug therapy.

Nursing diagnoses
• Risk for trauma related to seizures
• Deficient knowledge related to drug therapy

Planning and implementation
• Drug should always be prescribed and dispensed in PE units. Don't make any adjustments in recommended doses when substituting fosphenytoin for phenytoin, and vice versa.
• I.M. use generates systemic phenytoin levels similar to oral phenytoin sodium, allowing essentially interchangeable use.
③ **ALERT:** Abrupt withdrawal of drug may cause status epilepticus. Gradually withdraw, substitute, or reduce drug dosage.
③ **ALERT:** Don't confuse Cerebyx with Celexa or Celebrex.
Patient teaching
• Warn patient that sensory disturbances may occur with I.V. use.
• Instruct patient to immediately report adverse reactions, especially rash.
• Warn patient not to stop drug abruptly or to adjust dosage without consulting prescriber.

Evaluation
• Patient is free from seizures.
• Patient and family state understanding of drug therapy.

frovatriptan succinate
(froh-vah-TRIP-tan SUK-seh-nayt)
Frova

Pharmacologic class: serotonin $5HT_1$ receptor agonist with high affinity for $5HT_{1B/1D}$ receptors
Therapeutic class: antimigraine drug
Pregnancy risk category: C

Indications and dosages

▶ **Migraine attacks with or without aura.**
Adults: 2.5 mg P.O. taken at the first sign of migraine attack. If the headache recurs after initial relief, a second tablet may be given after waiting for at least 2 hours. Don't give more than three tablets daily.

Contraindications and precautions

• Contraindicated in patients hypersensitive to drug or any of the inactive ingredients. Also contraindicated in patients with ischemic heart disease (such as angina pectoris, history of myocardial infarction, or documented silent ischemia) and in patients who have symptoms or findings consistent with ischemic heart disease, coronary artery vasospasm (including Prinzmetal's variant angina), or other significant underlying CV conditions. Don't use in patients with cerebrovascular syndromes, such as CVA of any type or transient ischemic attacks, or in patients with peripheral vascular disease, including, but not limited to, ischemic bowel disease. Contraindicated in patients with uncontrolled hypertension and in patients with hemiplegic or basilar migraine.
🕭 **Lifespan:** In pregnant women, use drug only if potential benefit justifies risk to the fetus. In breast-feeding women, use cautiously because it's unknown whether drug appears in breast milk. In children, safety and effectiveness haven't been established. In elderly patients, mean blood concentrations are 1½ to 2 times higher. No special dosing is suggested. Experience in older patients is limited.

Adverse reactions

CNS: dizziness, headache, fatigue, pain, paresthesia, insomnia, anxiety, somnolence, dysesthesia, hypoesthesia.
CV: flushing, palpitations, chest pain.

EENT: abnormal vision, tinnitus, sinusitis, rhinitis.
GI: dry mouth, dyspepsia, vomiting, abdominal pain, diarrhea, nausea.
Musculoskeletal: skeletal pain.
Skin: increased sweating.
Other: hot or cold sensation.

Interactions

Drug-drug. *Ergotamine-containing or ergot-type medications (such as dihydroergotamine or methysergide):* May cause prolonged vasospastic reactions. Don't use within 24 hours of each other.
$5HT_{1B/1D}$ agonists: May have additive effects. Use of other $5HT_1$ agonists within 24 hours of frovatriptan isn't recommended.
Hormonal contraceptives, propranolol: Increases bioavailablity of frovatriptan. Monitor patient for adverse effects.
SSRIs (such as citalopram, fluoxetine, fluvoxamine, paroxetine, sertraline): May cause weakness, hyperreflexia, and incoordination. Monitor patient closely.

Effects on lab test results

None reported.

Pharmacokinetics

Absorption: Oral bioavailability of 20% in men and 30% in women. Peak level is achieved in 2 to 4 hours. Food delays the time to peak, but not the bioavailability of the drug.
Distribution: About 15% protein-bound.
Metabolism: Metabolized in the liver by CYP 1A2. Among the minor metabolites, desmethyl frovatriptan has low affinity for $5HT_{1B/1D}$ receptors compared with the active compound. Drug doesn't appear to be an inducer or inhibitor of CYP.
Excretion: Excreted in the urine and feces as unchanged drug and various metabolites (hydroxylated frovatriptan, N-acetyl desmethyl frovatriptan, hydroxylated N-acetyl desmethyl frovatriptan and desmethyl frovatriptan). *Half-life:* 26 hours.

Route	Onset	Peak	Duration
P.O.	Unknown	2-4 hr	Unknown

Action

Chemical effect: May inhibit excessive dilation of extracerebral, intracranial arteries in migraine headaches.
Therapeutic effect: Relieves pain caused by migraines.

Available forms

Tablets: 2.5 mg

NURSING PROCESS

◆ Assessment

• Assess underlying condition before therapy and reassess regularly throughout therapy.
• Obtain complete medical history, paying particular attention to history of CV and cerebrovascular disease.
• Evaluate patient's and family's knowledge of drug therapy.

◆ Nursing diagnoses

• Acute pain related to migraine headache
• Activity intolerance related to migraine headache
• Knowledge deficit related to frovatriptan succinate therapy

◆ Planning and implementation

⑤ **ALERT:** Don't give within 24 hours of treatment with another $5HT_1$ agonist or an ergotamine-containing or ergot-like medication.
⑤ **ALERT:** Serious cardiac events, including acute myocardial infarction, life-threatening cardiac rhythm disturbances, and death have been reported within a few hours of administration of $5HT_1$ agonists.
• Drug may bind to the melanin of the eye and cause ophthalmic effects. No specific ophthalmic monitoring is recommended.
• The safety of treating an average of more than four migraine attacks in a 30-day period hasn't been established.
• If frovatriptan is used in patients with risk factors for unrecognized coronary artery disease (such as hypertension, hypercholesterolemia, smoking, obesity, strong family history of coronary artery disease, female with surgical or physiological menopause, male older than age 40), it's strongly recommended that the first dose be given in prescriber's office or other medically staffed and equipped facility. Consider obtaining an ECG following the first dose.

It's further suggested that intermittent, long-term users of $5HT_1$ agonists or those who have or acquire risk factors undergo periodic cardiac evaluation while using frovatriptan.

Patient teaching

• Instruct patient to take the dose at the first sign of a migraine headache. If the headache comes back after the first dose, a second dose may be taken after 2 hours. Tell patient not to take more than three tablets in a 24-hour period.

• Inform patient that, in rare cases, patients have experienced serious heart problems, CVA, or increased blood pressure after taking the drug.

• Advise patient to take extra care or avoid driving and operating machinery if dizziness or fatigue develops.

• Emphasize importance of immediately reporting pain, tightness, heaviness, or pressure in the chest, throat, neck, or jaw, or rash or itching after taking the drug.

• Instruct patient not to take drug within 24 hours of taking another serotonin receptor agonist or ergotamine-type medication.

☑ Evaluation

• Patient is relieved of pain.

• Patient's activity tolerance returns to baseline.

• Patient and family state understanding of drug therapy.

fulvestrant
(ful-VES-trant)
Faslodex

Pharmacologic class: estrogen receptor antagonist
Therapeutic class: antineoplastic
Pregnancy risk category: D

Indications and dosages

▶ **Hormone-receptor–positive metastatic breast cancer in postmenopausal women with disease progression following anti-estrogen therapy.** *Adults:* 250 mg (one 5-ml syringe or two 2.5-ml syringes) by slow I.M. injection into buttocks once monthly.

Contraindications and precautions

• Use cautiously in patients with moderate or severe hepatic impairment.

☀ Lifespan: Women of childbearing age and potential should avoid getting pregnant while receiving drug. It crosses the placenta after a single I.M. dose and harms the fetus. Breast-feeding women should stop breast-feeding or stop drug; it's unknown whether drug appears in breast milk, and there is a potential for serious adverse reactions in infants. In children, safety and effectiveness haven't been established.

Adverse reactions

CNS: *pain,* dizziness, *asthenia, headache,* insomnia, fever, paresthesia, depression, anxiety.
CV: *vasodilation (hot flashes),* chest pain, peripheral edema.
EENT: *pharyngitis.*
GI: *nausea, vomiting, constipation, abdominal pain, diarrhea,* anorexia.
GU: UTI.
Hematologic: anemia.
Musculoskeletal: *bone pain, back pain, pelvic pain,* arthritis.
Respiratory: *dyspnea, cough.*
Skin: rash, sweating.
Other: accidental injury, flulike syndrome, *injection site pain.*

Interactions

None reported.

Effects on lab test results

• May decrease hemoglobin and hematocrit.

Pharmacokinetics

Absorption: Unknown.
Distribution: Extensive and rapid. 99% bound to proteins.
Metabolism: Extensively via several pathways. Identified metabolites are either less active than or exhibit activity similar to the parent drug.
Excretion: Hepatically cleared; 90% of drug is found in feces. Renal elimination is less than 1%. *Half-life:* 29 to 51 days.

Route	Onset	Peak	Duration
I.M.	Unknown	7 days	1 month

Action

Chemical effect: Competitively binds estrogen receptors and down-regulates estrogen-receptor protein in breast cancer cells.
Therapeutic effect: Fights cancer cells.

Available forms

Injection: 50 mg/ml in 2.5-ml and 5-ml pre-filled syringes

NURSING PROCESS

◪ Assessment

• Monitor hemoglobin and hematocrit before and during therapy.
• Confirm that patient isn't pregnant before therapy begins.
• Observe injection site for local reaction.
• Evaluate patient's and family's understanding of drug therapy.

◲ Nursing diagnoses

• Ineffective health maintenance related to underlying condition
• Risk for imbalanced nutrition: less than body required, related to side effects of therapy
• Risk for acute pain related to side effects of therapy
• Deficient knowledge related to drug therapy

≯ Planning and implementation

• Because drug is given I.M., don't use in patients with bleeding diatheses or thrombocytopenia, or in those taking anticoagulants.
⊛ ALERT: The drug is packaged in one 5-ml prefilled syringe or two 2.5-ml prefilled syringes. If using the 2.5-ml syringes, both syringes must be given to achieve the full 250 mg recommended monthly dose.
• Expel the gas bubble from syringe prior to administration.
• Use in premenopausal women hasn't been studied.

Patient teaching

• Tell patient the most common adverse reactions are GI symptoms, headache, back pain, hot flushes and sore throat.
• Advise women of childbearing age to avoid pregnancy and to report suspected pregnancy immediately. Drug crosses the placenta after a single I.M. dose and harms the fetus.

◪ Evaluation

• Patient maintains adequate nutrition during therapy.
• Patient doesn't experience pain as a side effect of therapy.
• Patient and family state understanding of drug therapy.

furosemide (frusemide ◆)

(fyoo-ROH-seh-mighd)
Apo-Furosemide ◆ , Furoside ◆ , Lasix*,
Lasix Special ◆ , Myrosemide*,
Novosemide ◆ , Uritol ◆

Pharmacologic class: loop diuretic
Therapeutic class: diuretic, antihypertensive
Pregnancy risk category: C

Indications and dosages

▶ **Acute pulmonary edema.** *Adults:* 40 mg I.V. injected slowly over 1 to 2 minutes; then 80 mg I.V. in 1 to 1½ hours, if needed.
Infants and children: 1 mg/kg I.M. or I.V. If desired results don't occur after 2 hours, may increase initial dose by 1 mg/kg. Separate doses by at least 2 hours.
▶ **Edema.** *Adults:* 20 to 80 mg P.O. daily in morning, second dose in 6 to 8 hours; carefully adjust up to 600 mg daily if needed. Or, 20 to 40 mg I.M. or I.V., increased by 20 mg q 2 hours until desired response occurs. Give I.V. dose slowly over 1 to 2 minutes.
Infants and children: 2 mg/kg P.O. daily; increase by 1 to 2 mg/kg in 6 to 8 hours, if needed; carefully adjust up to 6 mg/kg daily, if needed. Or, 1 mg/kg slow IV; increase by 1 mg/kg q 2 hours until desired response.
▶ **Heart failure and chronic renal impairment.** *Adults:* 2 to 2.5 g/day P.O. or I.V. Maximum I.V. injection is 1 g/day given over 30 minutes.
▶ **Hypertension.** *Adults:* 40 mg P.O. b.i.d. Adjust dosage according to response.
▶ **Hypercalcemia‡.** *Adults:* 80 to 100 mg I.V. q 1 to 2 hours; or 120 mg P.O. daily.

▽ I.V. administration

• Give drug by direct injection over 1 to 2 minutes.
• Or, dilute with D_5W, normal saline solution, or lactated Ringer's solution, and infuse no faster than 4 mg/minute to avoid ototoxicity.
• Use prepared infusion solution within 24 hours.

Contraindications and precautions

• Contraindicated in patients hypersensitive to drug and in those with anuria.

• Use cautiously in patients with hepatic cirrhosis.

• Patients with allergy to sulfonamides may also be allergic to furosemide.

⚖ **Lifespan:** In pregnant women, use only if benefits outweigh risks. In breast-feeding women, drug isn't recommended.

Adverse reactions

CNS: fever, vertigo, headache, dizziness, paresthesia, restlessness, weakness.
CV: volume depletion and dehydration, orthostatic hypotension, thrombophlebitis (with I.V. use).
EENT: transient deafness (with too-rapid I.V. injection), blurred or yellow vision.
GI: abdominal discomfort and pain, diarrhea, anorexia, nausea, vomiting, constipation, *pancreatitis.*
GU: azotemia, nocturia, polyuria, frequent urination, oliguria.
Hematologic: *agranulocytosis, leukopenia, thrombocytopenia,* anemia, *aplastic anemia.*
Hepatic: *hepatic dysfunction.*
Metabolic: hypokalemia, hypochloremic alkalosis, asymptomatic hyperuricemia, hyperglycemia and glucose intolerance, fluid and electrolyte imbalances, including dilutional hyponatremia, hypocalcemia, and hypomagnesemia.
Musculoskeletal: muscle spasm.
Skin: dermatitis, purpura, photosensitivity.
Other: gout, transient pain at I.M. injection site.

Interactions

Drug-drug. *Aminoglycoside antibiotics, cisplatin:* Potentiates ototoxicity. Use together cautiously.
Amphotericin B, corticosteroids, corticotropin: May increase risk of hypokalemia. Monitor potassium levels closely.
Antidiabetics: Decreases hypoglycemic effects. Monitor glucose levels.
Antihypertensives: May increase risk of hypotension. Use together cautiously.
Chlorothiazide, chlorthalidone, hydrochlorothiazide, indapamide, metolazone: May cause excessive diuretic response resulting in serious electrolyte abnormalities or dehydration. Adjust doses carefully while monitoring the patient closely for excessive diuretic responses.
Digoxin, neuromuscular blockers: May increase toxicity from furosemide-induced hypokalemia. Monitor potassium levels closely.

Ethacrynic acid: May increase risk of ototoxicity. Don't use together.
Lithium: Decreases lithium excretion, resulting in lithium toxicity. Monitor lithium level.
NSAIDs: Inhibits diuretic response. Use together cautiously.
Salicylates: May cause salicylate toxicity. Use together cautiously.
Drug-herb. *Aloe.* Possible increased drug effects. Monitor patient for dehydration.
Licorice: May cause rapid potassium loss. Monitor patient for hypokalemia; discourage licorice intake.
Drug-lifestyle. *Alcohol use:* Additive hypotensive and diuretic effect. Discourage using together.
Sun exposure: Photosensitivity reactions may occur. Urge patient to avoid unprotected or prolonged sun exposure.

Effects on lab test results

• May increase glucose, cholesterol, and uric acid levels. May decrease potassium, sodium, calcium, and magnesium levels.
• May decrease hemoglobin, hematocrit, and granulocyte, WBC, and platelet counts.

Pharmacokinetics

Absorption: About 60% absorbed from GI tract after P.O. administration; unknown after I.M. use.
Distribution: About 95% protein-bound.
Metabolism: Minimally by liver.
Excretion: About 50% to 80% in urine. *Half-life:* About 30 minutes.

Route	Onset	Peak	Duration
P.O.	20-60 min	1-2 hr	6-8 hr
I.V.	5 min	30 min	2 hr
I.M.	Unknown	Unknown	Unknown

Action

Chemical effect: Inhibits sodium and chloride reabsorption at proximal and distal tubules and ascending loop of Henle.
Therapeutic effect: Promotes water and sodium excretion.

Available forms

Injection: 10 mg/ml
Oral solution: 40 mg/5 ml, 10 mg/ml*
Tablets: 20 mg, 40 mg, 80 mg, 500 mg ◆

NURSING PROCESS

⚙ Assessment
- Assess patient's underlying condition before therapy.
- Monitor weight, peripheral edema, breath sounds, blood pressure, fluid intake and output, and electrolyte, glucose, BUN, and carbon dioxide levels.
- Monitor uric acid level, especially if patient has a history of gout.
- Be alert for adverse reactions and drug interactions.
- Evaluate patient's and family's knowledge of drug therapy.

⊕ Nursing diagnoses
- Excessive fluid volume related to presence of edema
- Impaired urinary elimination related to diuretic therapy
- Deficient knowledge related to drug therapy

❯ Planning and implementation
- Give P.O. and I.M. doses in morning to prevent nocturia. Give second doses in early afternoon.
- Store tablets in light-resistant container to prevent discoloration. Don't use yellowed injectable preparation.
- Refrigerate oral furosemide solution to ensure drug stability.
- If oliguria or azotemia develops or increases, notify prescriber.

Patient teaching
- Advise patient to stand slowly to prevent dizziness, to avoid alcohol, and to minimize strenuous exercise in hot weather.
- Instruct patient to report ringing in ears, severe abdominal pain, or sore throat and fever because they may indicate toxicity.
- Ⓢ **ALERT:** Discourage patient from storing different drugs in same container because this increases risk of errors. The most popular strengths of furosemide and digoxin are white tablets of similar size.
- Tell patient to check with prescriber before taking OTC medications or herbal remedies.

✓ Evaluation
- Patient is free from edema.
- Patient demonstrates adjustment of lifestyle to cope with altered patterns of urinary elimination.

- Patient and family state understanding of drug therapy.

gabapentin
(geh-buh-PEN-tin)
Neurontin

Pharmacologic class: anticonvulsant
Therapeutic class: antiseizure
Pregnancy risk category: C

Indications and dosages

▶ **Adjunct treatment of partial seizures with and without secondary generalization in patients with epilepsy.** *Adults and children older than age 12:* Initially, 300 mg P.O. t.i.d. Increase dosage gradually based on response. Dosages of 900 to 1,800 mg daily in three divided doses are effective for most patients. Dosages up to 3,600 mg daily are well tolerated. *Starting dosage, children ages 3 to 12:* 10 to 15 mg/kg P.O. daily in three divided doses, adjusting over 3 days to reach effective dosage. *Effective dosage, children ages 5 to 12:* 25 to 35 mg/kg P.O. daily in three divided doses. *Effective dosage, children ages 3 to 4:* 40 mg/kg P.O. daily in three divided doses.
Ⓢ **Adjust-a-dose:** For adults and children age 12 and older with renal impairment or undergoing hemodialysis, if creatinine clearance is 30 to 59 ml/minute, give 400 to 1,400 mg P.O. daily, divided b.i.d. If creatinine clearance is 15 to 29 ml/minute, give 200 to 700 mg P.O. daily. If creatinine clearance is less than 15 ml/minute, give 100 to 300 mg P.O. daily; reduce dose in proportion to creatinine clearance (for example, patients with a creatinine clearance of 7.5 ml/minute, give ½ the dose that a patient with 15 ml/minute would receive).
For patients on dialysis, maintenance dosages are based on estimated creatinine clearance. Give supplemental postdialysis dose of 125 to 350 mg after each 4 hours of dialysis.
▶ **Postherpetic neuralgia.** *Adults:* 300 mg P.O. once daily on day 1, then 300 mg b.i.d. on day 2, and 300 mg t.i.d. on day 3. Adjust p.r.n. for

pain relief to a maximum daily dose of 1,800 mg, divided t.i.d.

Contraindications and precautions

• Contraindicated in patients hypersensitive to drug.
≋ **Lifespan:** In pregnant women, use cautiously. In breast-feeding women and in children younger than age 3, safety of drug hasn't been established.

Adverse reactions

CNS: *somnolence, dizziness, ataxia, fatigue, nystagmus, tremor,* nervousness, dysarthria, amnesia, depression, abnormal thinking, twitching, abnormal coordination.
CV: peripheral edema, vasodilation.
EENT: *diplopia, rhinitis,* pharyngitis, dry throat, *amblyopia.*
GI: nausea, vomiting, dyspepsia, dry mouth, constipation.
GU: impotence.
Hematologic: *leukopenia.*
Metabolic: increased appetite, weight gain.
Musculoskeletal: back pain, myalgia, fractures.
Respiratory: cough.
Skin: pruritus, abrasion.
Other: dental abnormalities.

Interactions

Drug-drug. *Antacids:* Decreases gabapentin absorption. Separate administration times by at least 2 hours.
Drug-lifestyle. *Alcohol use:* Increases CNS depression. Discourage use.

Effects on lab test results

• May decrease WBC count.
• May cause false-positive tests for urine protein when Ames-N-Multistix SG dipstick test is used.

Pharmacokinetics

Absorption: Bioavailability isn't dose-proportional but averages 60%.
Distribution: Circulates largely unbound to protein.
Metabolism: Insignificant.
Excretion: Excreted by kidneys as unchanged drug. *Half-life:* 5 to 7 hours.

Route	Onset	Peak	Duration
P.O.	Unknown	2-4 hr	Unknown

Action

Chemical effect: Unknown; although structurally related to GABA, drug doesn't interact with GABA receptors and isn't converted metabolically into GABA or a GABA agonist.
Therapeutic effect: Prevents and treats partial seizures and treats postherpetic neuralgia.

Available forms

Capsules: 100 mg, 300 mg, 400 mg
Solution: 250 mg/5 ml
Tablets (film-coated): 600 mg, 800 mg

NURSING PROCESS

Assessment
• Assess patient's disorder before therapy and regularly thereafter.
• Routine monitoring of level isn't necessary. Drug doesn't appear to alter levels of other anticonvulsants.
• Be alert for adverse reactions and drug interactions.
• Evaluate patient's and family's knowledge of drug therapy.

Nursing diagnoses
• Risk for trauma related to seizures
• Risk for injury related to drug-induced adverse CNS reactions
• Deficient knowledge related to drug therapy

Planning and implementation
• Give first dose h.s. to minimize drowsiness, dizziness, fatigue, and ataxia.
ALERT: If stopping drug or substituting another drug, do so gradually over at least 1 week to minimize risk of seizures. Don't suddenly withdraw other anticonvulsants in patient starting therapy.
• Take seizure precautions.
ALERT: Don't confuse Neurontin (gabapentin) with Noroxin (norfloxacin).
Patient teaching
• Tell patient drug can be taken without regard to meals.
• Warn patient to avoid hazardous activities until CNS effects of drug are known.

Evaluation
• Patient is free from seizures.
• Patient has no injury from adverse CNS reactions.

- Patient and family state understanding of drug therapy.

galantamine hydrobromide
(gah-LAN-tah-meen high-droh-BROH-mide)
Reminyl

Pharmacologic class: reversible, competitive acetylcholinesterase inhibitor
Therapeutic class: cholinomimetic
Pregnancy risk category: B

Indications and dosages

▶ **Mild to moderate dementia of Alzheimer's type.** *Adults:* Initially, 4 mg P.O. b.i.d., preferably with morning and evening meals. If dose is well tolerated after minimum of 4 weeks of therapy, increase to 8 mg b.i.d. A further increase to 12 mg b.i.d. may be attempted only after at least 4 weeks of the previous dose. Recommended dosage range is 16 to 24 mg daily in two divided doses.
⊠ **Adjust-a-dose:** For patients with hepatic impairment with a Child-Pugh score of 7 to 9, don't exceed 16 mg daily. Don't give drug to patients with a Child-Pugh score of 10 to 15. For patients with moderate renal impairment, don't exceed 16 mg daily. Don't give drug to patients with a creatinine clearance less than 9 ml/minute.

Contraindications and precautions

- Contraindicated in patients hypersensitive to drug or its components.
- Use cautiously in patients with supraventricular cardiac conduction disorders and in those taking other drugs that significantly slow the heart rate. Use cautiously before or during procedures involving anesthesia with succinylcholine-type or other similar neuromuscular blockers. Use cautiously in patients with history of peptic ulcer disease and in those taking NSAIDs. Because of the potential for cholinomimetic effects, use cautiously in patients with bladder outflow obstruction, seizures, asthma, or COPD.
- ⚘ **Lifespan:** In breast-feeding women, drug is contraindicated because it's unknown whether drug appears in breast milk. In children, safety and effectiveness of drug haven't been established.

Adverse reactions

CNS: dizziness, headache, tremor, depression, insomnia, somnolence, fatigue, syncope.
CV: *bradycardia.*
EENT: rhinitis.
GI: *nausea, vomiting,* anorexia, *diarrhea,* abdominal pain, dyspepsia.
GU: UTI, hematuria.
Hematologic: anemia.
Metabolic: weight loss.

Interactions

Drug-drug. *Amitriptyline, fluoxetine, fluvoxamine, quinidine:* May decrease galantamine clearance. Monitor patient closely.
Anticholinergics: May antagonize activity of anticholinergics. Monitor patient.
Cholinergics (such as bethanechol, succinylcholine): May have a synergistic effect. Monitor patient closely. May need to avoid use before procedures using general anesthesia with succinylcholine-type neuromuscular blockers.
Cimetidine, erythromycin, ketoconazole, paroxetine: May increase bioavailability of galantamine. Monitor patient closely.

Effects on lab test results

- May decrease hemoglobin and hematocrit.

Pharmacokinetics

Absorption: Rapid and well absorbed, with an oral bioavailability of about 90%. Levels peak in 1 hour. In elderly patients, levels are 30% to 40% higher than in young, healthy people.
Distribution: Primarily to blood. Protein binding isn't significant.
Metabolism: In liver by CYP 2D6 and CYP 3A4 and glucuronidated. Using together with inhibitors of these enzyme systems may result in modest increases in drug bioavailability.
Excretion: In urine, unchanged as glucuronide and metabolites. *Half-life:* About 7 hours.

Route	Onset	Peak	Duration
P.O.	Unknown	1 hr	Unknown

Action

Chemical effect: Unknown; may enhance cholinergic function by increasing the level of acetylcholine in the brain.
Therapeutic effect: Improves cognition in patients with Alzheimer's disease.

Available forms

Oral solution: 4 mg/ml
Tablets: 4 mg, 8 mg, 12 mg
Oral solution and tablets are bioequivalent.

NURSING PROCESS

⚕ Assessment

• Assess underlying condition before therapy and reassess regularly.
• Bradycardia and heart block have been reported in patients with and without underlying cardiac conduction abnormalities. Consider all patients at risk for adverse effects on cardiac conduction.
• Patients are at increased risk for gastric ulcers because of the potential for increased gastric acid secretion. Monitor patient closely for symptoms of active or occult GI bleeding.
• Evaluate patient's and family's knowledge of drug therapy.

🔲 Nursing diagnoses

• Risk for injury due to wandering related to Alzheimer's disease
• Risk for imbalanced fluid volume related to drug-induced adverse GI reactions
• Deficient knowledge related to galantamine hydrobromide therapy

▶ Planning and implementation

• Give drug with food and antiemetics and ensure adequate fluid intake to decrease the risk of nausea and vomiting.
• If drug is stopped for several days, restart dose at the lowest dose and increase, at a minimum of 4-week intervals, to the previous dosage level.
• Use proper technique when dispensing the oral solution with the pipette. Dispense measured amount in a liquid and give right away.
• Don't give more than 16 mg daily in patients with moderate hepatic or renal impairment.
• In case of overdose, contact a poison control center for the latest management recommendations. Treatment is supportive and symptomatic. Atropine I.V. may be used as an antidote. An initial dose of 0.5 to 1 mg is recommended, with subsequent doses based on response. It's unknown if drug is removed by dialysis.
Patient teaching
• Advise patient or caretaker to take drug with morning and evening meals.
• Inform patient or caretaker that dosage increases should occur at no more than 4-week intervals.

• Explain that nausea and vomiting are common adverse effects.
• Advise patient or caretaker that following the recommended dosing and administration schedule can minimize common adverse effects.
• Tell patient or caretaker that, if therapy is interrupted for several days or longer, the drug should be restarted at the lowest dose and increased based on the prescriber's dosing schedule.
• Advise patient or caretaker to report signs and symptoms of bradycardia immediately to the prescriber.
• Advise patient or caretaker that drug is believed to enhance cognitive function, but there's no evidence that it alters the underlying disease process.

☑ Evaluation

• Patient's cognition improves and tendency to wander decreases.
• Patient and family state that drug-induced adverse GI reactions haven't occurred.
• Patient and family state understanding of drug therapy.

ganciclovir (DHPG)
(jan-SIGH-kloh-veer)
Cytovene, Cytovene-IV

Pharmacologic class: synthetic nucleoside
Therapeutic class: antiviral
Pregnancy risk category: C

Indications and dosages

▶ **CMV retinitis in immunocompromised patients, including those with AIDS.** *Adults:* Induction treatment is 5 mg/kg I.V. over 1 hour q 12 hours for 14 to 21 days (normal renal function); maintenance treatment is 5 mg/kg I.V. daily for 7 days weekly, or 6 mg/kg I.V. daily for 5 days weekly. Or, following I.V. induction treatment, give 1,000 mg P.O. t.i.d. with food or 500 mg P.O. 6 times a day q 3 hours with food while awake.
▶ **Prevention of CMV disease in transplant recipients at risk for CMV disease.** *Adults:* 5 mg/kg I.V. over 1 hour q 12 hours for 7 to 14 days, followed by 5 mg/kg I.V. once daily for 7 days weekly, or 6 mg/kg I.V. once daily for 5 days weekly. Alternatively, 1,000 mg P.O. t.i.d. with food. Length of therapy in transplant

Creatinine clearance (ml/min)	Initial I.V. dosage		Maintenance I.V. dosage		P.O. dosage	
	Dose (mg/kg)	Interval	Dose (mg/kg)	Interval	Dose (mg)	Interval
50-69	2.5	12 hours	2.5	24 hours	1,500	24 hours
					500	8 hours
25-49	2.5	24 hours	1.25	24 hours	1,000	24 hours
					500	12 hours
10-24	1.25	24 hours	0.625	24 hours	500	24 hours
< 10 or on hemodialysis	1.25	3 times weekly	0.625	3 times weekly	500	3 times weekly

recipients depends on duration and degree of immunosuppression.

▶ **Prevention of CMV disease in patients with advanced HIV infection at risk for development of CMV disease.** *Adults:* 1,000 mg P.O. t.i.d. with food.

▶ **Other CMV infections‡.** *Adults:* 5 mg/kg I.V. over 1 hour q 12 hours for 14 to 21 days. Or, 2.5 mg/kg I.V. over 1 hour q 8 hours for 14 to 21 days.

⚛ Adjust-a-dose: For patients with renal impairment, adjust dosage according to the table above.

▼ I.V. administration

• Reconstitute with 10 ml sterile water for injection. Shake vial to dissolve drug.
• Further dilute appropriate dose in normal saline solution, D_5W, Ringer's lactate, or Ringer's solutions (typically 100 ml).
⚛ ALERT: Use caution when preparing solution, which is alkaline.
⚛ ALERT: Infuse over 1 hour. Faster infusions will cause increased toxicity. Never exceed recommended infusion rate. Use infusion pump. Don't give as I.V. bolus or by rapid infusion.
• Infusion concentrations greater than 10 mg/ml aren't recommended.

Contraindications and precautions

• Contraindicated in patients hypersensitive to drug and in those with absolute neutrophil count below 500/mm³ or platelet count below 25,000/mm³.
• Use cautiously and at reduced dosage in patients with renal impairment.
• Patients with allergies to acyclovir may also react to ganciclovir.
⚛ Lifespan: In pregnant and breast-feeding women, drug isn't recommended. In children, safety of drug hasn't been established.

Adverse reactions

CNS: pain, altered dreams, confusion, ataxia, dizziness, headache, *seizures, coma,* behavioral changes.
CV: *arrhythmias,* hypotension, hypertension.
EENT: retinal detachment in CMV retinitis patients.
GI: nausea, vomiting, diarrhea, anorexia.
GU: hematuria.
Hematologic: *thrombocytopenia, agranulocytosis, leukopenia, granulocytopenia,* anemia.
Other: inflammation, phlebitis at injection site.

Interactions

Drug-drug. *Cytotoxic drugs:* Increases toxic effects, especially hematologic effects and stomatitis. Monitor patient closely.
Imipenem and cilastatin: Heightens seizure activity. Monitor patient closely.
Immunosuppressants (such as azathioprine, corticosteroids, cyclosporine): Enhances immune and bone marrow suppression. Use together cautiously.
Probenecid: Increases ganciclovir levels. Monitor patient closely.
Zidovudine: Increases risk of granulocytopenia. Monitor patient closely.

Effects on lab test results

• May increase creatinine, ALT, AST, GGT, and alkaline phosphatase levels.
• May decrease hemoglobin, hematocrit, and granulocyte, platelet, neutrophil, and WBC counts.

Pharmacokinetics

Absorption: Poorly absorbed after P.O. administration. Bioavailability is about 5% under fasting conditions.

Distribution: Preferentially concentrates in CMV-infected cells; only 2% to 3% protein-bound.
Metabolism: Over 90% of drug isn't metabolized.
Excretion: Mostly excreted unchanged. *Half-life:* About 3 hours.

Route	Onset	Peak	Duration
P.O.			
fasting	Unknown	1¾ hr	Unknown
with food	Unknown	3 hr	Unknown
I.V.	Immediate	Immediate	Unknown

Action

Chemical effect: Unknown; may inhibit viral DNA synthesis of CMV.
Therapeutic effect: Inhibits CMV.

Available forms

Capsules: 250 mg, 500 mg
Injection: 500 mg/vial

NURSING PROCESS

🔧 Assessment

• Assess patient's condition before therapy and regularly thereafter.
• Obtain CBC, neutrophil, and platelet counts every 2 days during twice-daily ganciclovir dosing and at least weekly thereafter.
• Monitor hydration if adverse GI reactions occur with oral drug.
• Be alert for adverse reactions and drug interactions.
• Evaluate patient's and family's knowledge of drug therapy.

🔷 Nursing diagnoses

• Infection related to CMV retinitis
• Ineffective protection related to adverse hematologic reactions
• Deficient knowledge related to drug therapy

▶ Planning and implementation

• Give oral form of drug with food.
• **⊛ ALERT:** Don't give drug S.C. or I.M. because severe tissue irritation could result.
• **⊛ ALERT:** Encourage fluid intake; ensure adequate hydration during drug infusion.
• Alert prescriber to signs of renal impairment because the dosage will need adjustment.

• Capsules are linked to a risk of rapid rate of CMV retinitis progression. Capsules should not be used for induction treatment; use only as maintenance therapy in patients who benefit from not taking drug I.V.
Patient teaching
• Tell patient to take oral form of drug with food.
• Stress importance of drinking adequate fluids throughout therapy.
• Advise patient to report pain or discomfort at I.V. site.
• Instruct patient about infection-control and bleeding precautions.

☑ Evaluation

• Patient is free from infection.
• Patient has no serious adverse hematologic reactions.
• Patient and family state understanding of drug therapy.

ganirelix acetate
(gan-eh-REL-iks AS-ih-tayt)
Antagon

Pharmacologic class: gonadotropin-releasing hormone (Gn-RH) antagonist
Therapeutic class: fertility drug
Pregnancy risk category: X

Indications and dosages

▶ **Inhibition of premature luteinizing hormone (LH) surges in women undergoing medically supervised, controlled ovarian hyperstimulation.** *Adults:* 250 mcg S.C. once daily during early to midfollicular phase of menstrual cycle. Continue daily until enough follicles of sufficient size are confirmed by ultrasound; human chorionic gonadotropin will then be given to induce final maturation of follicles.

Contraindications and precautions

• Contraindicated in patients hypersensitive to drug or its components or to Gn-RH or Gn-RH analogue.
• Use cautiously in patients with potential hypersensitivity to Gn-RH and in those with latex allergies because the product packaging contains natural rubber latex.

※ **Lifespan:** In pregnant women, drug is contraindicated. In breast-feeding women, avoid using drug.

Adverse reactions

CNS: headache.
GI: abdominal pain, nausea.
GU: vaginal bleeding, gynecologic abdominal pain, ovarian hyperstimulation syndrome, miscarriage.
Other: injection site reaction.

Interactions

None reported.

Effects on lab test results

• May decrease bilirubin levels.
• May increase WBC count. May decrease hemoglobin and hematocrit.

Pharmacokinetics

Absorption: Rapid, with an average of 91% absorbed.
Distribution: 82% bound to proteins.
Metabolism: Drug is found essentially unchanged in urine up to 24 hours after dose. Two metabolites have been detected in feces.
Excretion: Primarily in feces; metabolites can be detected nearly 8 days after a dose. *Half-life:* 13 to 16 hours.

Route	Onset	Peak	Duration
S.C.	Unknown	1 hr	Unknown

Action

Chemical effect: Blocks pituitary Gn-RH receptors and suppresses LH and follicle-stimulating hormone (FSH) secretion. This suppression in the early- to mid- menstrual cycle stops premature gonadotropin surges that could interfere with medically supervised ovarian hyperstimulation.
Therapeutic effect: Increases fertility.

Available forms

Injection: 250 mcg/0.5 ml in prefilled syringes

NURSING PROCESS

🔲 Assessment
• Before starting treatment, make sure patient isn't pregnant.

• Monitor patient who reports previous potential hypersensitivity to Gn-RH carefully; monitor patient closely after first injection.
• Evaluate patient's and family's knowledge of drug therapy.

🔲 Nursing diagnoses
• Disturbed self-esteem related to infertility
• Acute pain secondary to drug-induced adverse reactions
• Deficient knowledge related to drug therapy

▶ Planning and implementation
• Only prescribers experienced in infertility treatments should prescribe this drug.
• Natural rubber latex packaging of this product may cause allergic reactions in a hypersensitive patient.
Patient teaching
• Tell patient that the correct use of drug injection is extremely important to the success of the fertility treatments. Patient must be able to follow strict administration schedule.
• Teach patient proper technique for S.C. administration of drug.
• Advise patient to use the abdomen or upper thigh for injection and to alternate injection sites with each dose.
• Advise patient to store drug at room temperature, away from heat and light, and out of children's reach.

🔲 Evaluation
• Patient becomes pregnant.
• Patient has no adverse reactions.
• Patient and family state understanding of drug therapy.

gatifloxacin
(ga-tih-FLOCKS-ah-sin)
Tequin

Pharmacologic class: fluoroquinolone antibiotic
Therapeutic class: antibiotic
Pregnancy risk category: C

Indications and dosages

▶ **Acute bacterial exacerbation of chronic bronchitis caused by** *Streptococcus pneumoniae, Haemophilus influenzae, Haemophilus*

---

parainfluenzae, Moraxella catarrhalis, or *Staphylococcus aureus. Adults:* 400 mg I.V. or P.O. daily for 5 days.

▶ **Complicated UTI caused by** *Escherichia coli, Klebsiella pneumoniae,* or *Proteus mirabilis;* **acute pyelonephritis caused by** *E. coli. Adults:* 400 mg I.V. or P.O. daily for 7 to 10 days.

▶ **Acute sinusitis caused by** *S. pneumoniae* **or** *H. influenzae. Adults:* 400 mg I.V. or P.O. daily for 10 days.

▶ **Community-acquired pneumonia caused by** *S. pneumoniae, H. influenzae, H. parainfluenzae, M. catarrhalis, S. aureus, Mycoplasma pneumoniae, Chlamydia pneumoniae,* or *Legionella pneumophila. Adults:* 400 mg I.V. or P.O. daily for 7 to 14 days.

▶ **Inhalation anthrax** ‡**, postexposure to inhalation anthrax, prevention or treatment when parenteral regimen not available.** *Adults:* 400 mg P.O. once daily for 60 days.

▶ **Uncomplicated urethral gonorrhea in men and cervical gonorrhea or acute uncomplicated rectal infections in women caused by** *Neisseria gonorrhoeae. Adults:* 400 mg P.O. as single dose.

▶ **Uncomplicated urinary tract infection caused by** *E. coli, K. pneumoniae,* or *P. mirabilis. Adults:* 400 mg I.V. or P.O. as single dose, or 200 mg I.V. or P.O. daily for 3 days.

▶ **Uncomplicated skin and skin-structure infections caused by** *S. aureus* **(methicillin-susceptible strains only) or** *Streptococcus pyogenes. Adults:* 400 mg I.V. or P.O. daily for 7 to 10 days.

ⓝ **Adjust-a-dose:** For patients with renal impairment, if creatinine clearance is less than 40 ml/minute or if the patient is on hemodialysis or continuous peritoneal dialysis, give initial dose of 400 mg P.O., followed by 200 mg P.O. daily.

▼ **I.V. administration**

• Dilute drug in single-use vials with D₅W or normal saline solution to 2 mg/ml before administration. Diluted solutions are stable for 14 days at room temperature or refrigerated. Frozen solutions are stable for up to 6 months, except for 5% sodium bicarbonate solutions. Thaw at room temperature. After being thawed, solutions are stable for 14 days when stored at room temperature or refrigerated. Don't mix with other drugs.
• Infuse over 60 minutes.

• Discard any unused portion of single-dose vials.

Contraindications and precautions

• Contraindicated in patients hypersensitive to fluoroquinolones or in patients with prolonged QTc interval or uncorrected hypokalemia.
• Use cautiously in patients with significant bradycardia, acute myocardial ischemia, known or suspected CNS disorders, or renal insufficiency.
☲ Lifespan: In pregnant women, use only if benefits outweigh risks to fetus. Breast-feeding women should either stop nursing or not take the drug, taking into account the importance of the drug to the mother. In children, safety and effectiveness of drug haven't been established.

Adverse reactions

CNS: headache, dizziness, abnormal dreams, insomnia, paresthesia, tremor, fever, vertigo.
CV: palpitations, chest pain, peripheral edema.
EENT: tinnitus, abnormal vision, pharyngitis.
GI: nausea, diarrhea, abdominal pain, constipation, dyspepsia, oral candidiasis, *pseudomembranous colitis,* glossitis, stomatitis, mouth ulcer, vomiting, disturbed taste.
GU: dysuria, hematuria, vaginitis.
Musculoskeletal: arthralgia, myalgia, back pain.
Respiratory: dyspnea.
Skin: rash, sweating.
Other: *anaphylaxis,* chills, redness at injection site.

Interactions

Drug-drug. *Aluminum hydroxide, aluminum-magnesium hydroxide, calcium carbonate, magnesium hydroxide:* May decrease effects of gatifloxacin. Give antacid at least 6 hours before or 2 hours after gatifloxacin.
Antidiabetics (glyburide, insulin): Possible symptomatic hypoglycemia or hyperglycemia. Monitor glucose level.
Antipsychotics, cisapride, erythromycin, tricyclic antidepressants: May prolong QT interval. Use cautiously.
Class IA antiarrhythmics (quinidine, procainamide), class III antiarrhythmics (amiodarone, sotalol): May prolong QT interval. Avoid using together.
NSAIDs: May increase risk of CNS stimulation and seizures. Use together cautiously.

Probenecid: Increases gatifloxacin levels and prolongs its half-life. Monitor patient closely.
Warfarin: May enhance effects of warfarin. Monitor PT and INR.
Drug-lifestyle. *Sun exposure:* Photosensitivity reactions may occur. Urge patient to avoid unprotected or prolonged sun exposure.

Effects on lab test results

• May increase ALT, AST, and LDH levels.

Pharmacokinetics

Absorption: Well absorbed.
Distribution: Wide. 20% protein-bound.
Metabolism: Limited biotransformation.
Excretion: More than 70% excreted unchanged by the kidneys. *Half-life:* 7 to 14 hours.

Route	Onset	Peak	Duration
P.O.	Unknown	1-2 hr	Unknown
I.V.	Unknown	Unknown	Unknown

Action

Chemical effect: Inhibits DNA gyrase and topoisomerase, preventing cell replication and division. It's active against gram-positive and gram-negative organisms.
Therapeutic effect: Kills susceptible bacteria.

Available forms

Injection: 200 mg/20-ml vial, 400 mg/40-ml vial; 200 mg in 100 ml D$_5$W, 400 mg in 200 ml D$_5$W
Tablets: 200 mg, 400 mg

NURSING PROCESS

🔢 Assessment

• In patient being treated for gonorrhea, test for syphilis and chlamydia at time of diagnosis.
• In patient with renal insufficiency, monitor kidney function.
• In patient with diabetes, monitor glucose level.
• Monitor patient on digoxin for digoxin toxicity.
• Be alert for adverse reactions and drug interactions.
• Evaluate patient's and family's knowledge of drug therapy.

🔢 Nursing diagnoses

• Infection related to presence of bacteria susceptible to drug
• Risk for injury related to drug-induced adverse reactions
• Deficient knowledge related to drug therapy

▶ Planning and implementation

• Give oral form of drug 4 hours before antacids containing aluminum or magnesium, didanosine buffered solution tablets or buffered powder, or products containing zinc, magnesium, or iron.
• If patient has seizures, increased intra-cranial pressure, psychosis, or CNS stimulation leading to tremors, restlessness, light-headedness, confusion, hallucinations, paranoia, depression, nightmares, and insomnia, stop drug and notify prescriber.
• If patient has a skin rash or other signs of hypersensitivity, stop drug and notify prescriber.
• If patient has pain, inflammation, or rupture of a tendon, stop drug and notify prescriber.
• Monitor patient for diarrhea because pseudomembranous colitis may occur in patients taking antibiotics.
⚡ ALERT: Don't confuse Tequin with Ticlid or Tegretol.
Patient teaching
• Tell patient to take drug as prescribed and to finish all of the medication even if symptoms disappear.
• Advise patient to take drug 4 hours before products containing aluminum, magnesium, zinc, or iron.
• Advise patient to use sunblock and protective clothing when exposed to excessive sunlight.
• Warn patient to avoid hazardous tasks until adverse CNS effects of drugs are known.
• Advise diabetic patient to monitor glucose levels and notify prescriber if hypoglycemia occurs.
• Advise patient to report immediately palpitations, fainting spells, skin rash, hives, difficulty swallowing or breathing, swelling of the lips, tongue, face, tightness in throat, hoarseness, or other symptoms of allergic reaction.
• Advise patient to stop drug, refrain from exercise, and notify prescriber if pain, inflammation, or rupture of a tendon occur.

✅ Evaluation

• Patient is free from infection after drug therapy.

Reactions may be *common*, uncommon, *life-threatening*, or COMMON AND LIFE-THREATENING.

• Patient has no injury as a result of drug-induced adverse reactions.
• Patient and family state understanding of drug therapy.

gatifloxacin ophthalmic solution
(gah-ti-FLOCKS-ah-sin off-THAL-mick suh-LOO-shun)
Zymar

Pharmacologic class: fluoroquinolone antibiotic
Therapeutic class: antibiotic
Pregnancy risk category: C

Indications and dosages

▶ **Bacterial conjunctivitis.** *Adults and children age 1 and older:* While patient is awake, instill 1 drop into affected eyes q 2 hours, up to 8 times daily for 2 days. Then, instill 1 drop up to 4 times daily for 5 more days.

Contraindications and precautions

• Contraindicated in patients hypersensitive to drug, quinolones, or their components.
⚘ **Lifespan:** In pregnant and breast-feeding women, use cautiously.

Adverse reactions

CNS: headache.
EENT: chemosis, conjunctival hemorrhage, *conjunctival irritation,* discharge, dry eyes, eye irritation, eyelid edema, *increased lacrimation, keratitis,* pain, *papillary conjunctivitis,* red eyes, reduced visual acuity.
GI: taste disturbance.

Interactions

None reported.

Effects on lab test results

None reported.

Pharmacokinetics

Absorption: Unknown.
Distribution: Unknown.
Metabolism: Unknown.
Excretion: Unknown. *Half-life:* Unknown.

Route	Onset	Peak	Duration
Ophthalmic	Unknown	Unknown	Unknown

Action

Chemical effect: Inhibits DNA gyrase and topoisomerase, preventing cell replication and division.
Therapeutic effect: Clears eye infection from susceptible bacteria.

Available forms

Solution: 0.3% in 2.5- and 5-ml bottles

NURSING PROCESS

Assessment
• Monitor therapy for effectiveness.
• Monitor patient for adverse reactions.
• Evaluate patient's and family's knowledge of drug therapy.

Nursing diagnoses
• Disturbed visual perception related to eye infection
• Deficient knowledge related to drug therapy

Planning and implementation
• Don't inject solution subconjunctivally or into the anterior chamber of the eye.
• Systemic drug causes serious hypersensitivity reactions. If allergic reaction occurs, stop drug and treat symptoms.
• Monitor patient for superinfection.
Patient teaching
• Tell patient to immediately stop drug and seek medical treatment if evidence of a serious allergic reaction develops, such as itching, rash, swelling of the face or throat, or difficulty breathing.
• Tell patient not to wear contact lenses during treatment.
• Warn patient to avoid touching the applicator tip to anything, including eyes and fingers.
• Teach patient that prolonged use may encourage infections with non-susceptible bacteria.

Evaluation
• Patient recovers from infection.
• Patient and family state understanding of drug therapy.

gefitinib
(geh-FIT-eye-nib)
Iressa

Pharmacologic class: tyrosine kinase inhibitor
Therapeutic class: antineoplastic
Pregnancy risk category: D

Indications and dosages

▶ **Locally advanced or metastatic non–small-cell lung cancer after platinum-based and docetaxel chemotherapies have failed.** *Adults:* 250 mg P.O. once daily.

Contraindications and precautions

• Contraindicated in patients hypersensitive to drug or its components.
• Give cautiously to patients with severe renal impairment.
⚠ **Lifespan:** In pregnant women, use only if benefit of drug outweighs risk of harm to the fetus. Breast-feeding women shouldn't breast-feed during drug therapy because of potential harm to infant; it's unknown whether drug appears in breast milk. In children, safety and effectiveness of drug haven't been established.

Adverse reactions

CNS: asthenia.
CV: peripheral edema.
EENT: amblyopia, conjunctivitis.
GI: anorexia, *diarrhea*, mouth ulcers, *nausea, vomiting.*
Metabolic: weight loss.
Respiratory: *dyspnea, interstitial lung disease.*
Skin: *acne, dry skin,* pruritus, *rash.*

Interactions

Drug-drug. *Drugs that increase gastric pH, such as antacids, H_2 blockers, sodium bicarbonate, or ranitidine:* May reduce availability and effectiveness of gefitinib. Monitor patient closely.
Drugs that induce CYP 3A4, such as rifampin and phenytoin: May decrease gefitinib levels. If patient has no severe adverse reactions, increase gefitinib dosage to 500 mg daily.
Drugs that inhibit CYP 3A4, such as ketoconazole and itraconazole: May increase gefitinib levels. Monitor patient closely, and adjust dosage p.r.n.

Warfarin: May increase INR and risk of bleeding. Monitor INR and patient closely.

Effects on lab test results

• May increase liver function test values.

Pharmacokinetics

Absorption: Slow. Level peaks in 3 to 7 hours. Oral bioavailability is 60% and is unchanged by food.
Distribution: 90% protein bound independent of drug level.
Metabolism: Undergoes extensive hepatic metabolism by the CYP 3A4 isoenzyme system. Of five metabolites, only one retains partial activity.
Excretion: 86% in feces and less than 4% in urine. *Half-life:* 48 hours.

Route	Onset	Peak	Duration
P.O.	Unknown	3-7 hr	48 hr

Action

Chemical effect: Inhibits cell growth and replication by binding to and blocking the intracellular enzyme (tyrosine kinase) of the epidermal growth factor receptor present on the surface of many normal and cancer cells.
Therapeutic effect: Kills cancer cells.

Available forms

Tablets: 250 mg

NURSING PROCESS

⚕ Assessment
• Monitor liver function test results before and during therapy.
• Monitor nutritional status and GI side effects of drug.
• Monitor patient for signs of pulmonary toxicity.
• Monitor patient for ocular symptoms.
• Rarely, drug may cause pancreatitis, epidermal necrolysis, and erythema multiforme. Monitor patient carefully.

⚕ Nursing Diagnoses
• Risk for imbalanced nutrition: less than body requires related to side effect of therapy
• Risk for impaired gas exchange related to pulmonary toxicity
• Deficient knowledge related to drug therapy

⧉ Planning and implementation

- In patients who have severe adverse GI or skin reactions, stop drug for up to 14 days, p.r.n.
- Stop drug in patients who develop ocular symptoms (eye pain; corneal erosion, sloughing, or ulceration; abnormal eyelash growth; ocular ischemia or hemorrhage), p.r.n.
- Patients who develop acute dyspnea, cough, and a low-grade fever may have interstitial lung disease, and these effects may worsen quickly. Stop the drug immediately. One-third of patients who develop this form of pulmonary toxicity die.
- Drug may cause allergic reactions that include angioedema and urticaria.
- Drug may cause an asymptomatic increase in liver function test results. Stop drug if changes are severe.

Patient teaching

- Explain ways to avoid dehydration.
- Tell patient to seek medical care right away for severe or persistent diarrhea, nausea, anorexia, or vomiting; new or worsening of pulmonary problems, such as shortness of breath or coughing; eye problems, such as irritation, pain, or altered vision; or a rash.
- Urge women to avoid becoming pregnant.
- Tell pregnant woman that drug may harm the fetus.

☑ Evaluation

- Patient doesn't experience any GI adverse effects.
- Patient doesn't experience pulmonary toxicity.
- Patient and family state understanding of drug therapy.

---

gemfibrozil
(jem-FIGH-broh-zil)
Apo-Gemfibrozil ♦ , Gen-Fibro ♦ , Lopid, Novo-Gemfibrozil ♦ , Nu-Gemfibrozil ♦

Pharmacologic class: fibric acid derivative
Therapeutic class: antilipemic
Pregnancy risk category: C

Indications and dosages

▶ **Type IV and V hyperlipidemia unresponsive to diet and other drugs; reduction of risk of coronary heart disease in patients with type IIb hyperlipidemia who can't tolerate or** who are refractory to treatment with bile acid sequestrants or niacin. *Adults:* 1,200 mg P.O. daily in two divided doses, 30 minutes before morning and evening meals. If no benefit occurs after 3 months, stop drug.

Contraindications and precautions

- Contraindicated in patients hypersensitive to drug and in those with hepatic or severe renal dysfunction (including primary biliary cirrhosis) or gallbladder disease.

☀ **Lifespan:** In pregnant women, use cautiously. In breast-feeding women and in children, safety of drug hasn't been established.

Adverse reactions

CNS: blurred vision, headache, dizziness.
GI: *abdominal and epigastric pain,* diarrhea, nausea, vomiting, flatulence, *dyspepsia.*
Hematologic: *severe anemia, leukopenia, thrombocytopenia, bone marrow hypoplasia.*
Hepatic: bile duct obstruction, gallstones.
Musculoskeletal: painful limbs, *rhabdomyolysis.*
Skin: rash, dermatitis, pruritus.

Interactions

Drug-drug. *Cyclosporine:* May decrease cyclosporine effects. Monitor cyclosporine level.
HMG-CoA reductase inhibitors: Myopathy with rhabdomyolysis may occur. Don't use together.
Oral anticoagulants: May enhance effects of oral anticoagulants. Monitor patient.
Repaglinide: May increase repaglinide level. Avoid using together.

Effects on lab test results

- May increase ALT, AST, and CK levels. May decrease potassium level.
- May decrease hemoglobin, hematocrit, and eosinophil, WBC, and platelet counts.

Pharmacokinetics

Absorption: Well absorbed from GI tract.
Distribution: 95% protein-bound.
Metabolism: By liver.
Excretion: Primarily in urine, with some in feces. *Half-life:* 1¼ hours. Biological half-life is considerably longer, as a result of enterohepatic circulation and reabsorption in the GI tract.

Route	Onset	Peak	Duration
P.O.	2-5 days	> 4 wk	Unknown

Rapid onset   *Liquid form contains alcohol.   ♦ Canada   ◇ Australia   †OTC   ‡Off-label use

Action

Chemical effect: Inhibits peripheral lipolysis and also reduces triglyceride synthesis in liver.
Therapeutic effect: Lowers triglyceride levels and raises HDL levels.

Available forms

Capsules: 300 mg ◆
Tablets: 600 mg

NURSING PROCESS

ᴬᴮ Assessment

• Obtain patient's triglyceride and HDL levels before therapy and regularly thereafter.
• Perform periodic CBCs and liver function tests during first 12 months of therapy.
• Be alert for adverse reactions and drug interactions.
• Evaluate patient's and family's knowledge of drug therapy.

⊕ Nursing diagnoses

• Risk for injury related to elevated blood lipids and cholesterol levels
• Diarrhea related to drug's adverse effect on GI tract
• Deficient knowledge related to drug therapy

▷ Planning and implementation

• Give drug 30 minutes before breakfast and dinner.
• Make sure patient is following standard low-cholesterol diet.
Patient teaching
• Instruct patient to take drug 30 minutes before breakfast and dinner.
• Teach patient dietary management of lipids (restricting total fat and cholesterol intake) and measures to control other cardiac disease risk factors. If appropriate, suggest weight control, exercise, and smoking cessation programs.
• Advise patient to avoid driving or other potentially hazardous activities until drug's CNS effects are known.
• Tell patient to observe bowel movements and to report signs of steatorrhea or bile duct obstruction.

☑ Evaluation

• Patient's triglyceride and cholesterol levels are normal.
• Patient regains normal bowel patterns.

• Patient and family state understanding of drug therapy.

gemifloxacin mesylate

(geh-mih-FLOCKS-a-sin MESS-ih-late)
Factive

Pharmacologic class: fluoroquinolone
Therapeutic class: antibacterial
Pregnancy risk category: C

Indications and dosages

▶ **Acute bacterial exacerbation of chronic bronchitis caused by** *Streptococcus pneumoniae, Haemophilus influenzae, Haemophilus parainfluenzae, Moraxella catarrhalis. Adults:* 320 mg P.O. once daily for 5 days.
▶ **Mild to moderate community-acquired pneumonia caused by** *S. pneumoniae* (including penicillin-resistant strains), *H. influenzae, M. catarrhalis, Mycoplasma pneumoniae, Chlamydia pneumoniae, Klebsiella pneumoniae. Adults:* 320 mg P.O. once daily for 7 days.
◨ **Adjust-a-dose:** For patients with renal impairment, if creatinine clearance is 40 ml/minute or less or if patient receives routine hemodialysis or continuous ambulatory peritoneal dialysis, reduce dosage to 160 mg P.O. once daily.

Contraindications and precautions

• Contraindicated in patients hypersensitive to fluoroquinolones or their components, those with a history of prolonged QT interval, those with uncorrected electrolyte disorders, and those taking a class IA or III antiarrhythmic.
• Use cautiously in patients with epilepsy, predisposition to seizures, or renal impairment.
⚘ **Lifespan:** In pregnant and breast-feeding women, drug is contraindicated. Use only if benefits outweigh risks. In children, safety and effectiveness of drug haven't been established.

Adverse reactions

CNS: headache.
GI: abdominal pain, diarrhea, nausea, *pseudomembranous colitis,* vomiting.
Musculoskeletal: ruptured tendons.
Skin: rash.
Other: *hypersensitivity reactions.*

Reactions may be *common,* uncommon, *life-threatening,* or COMMON AND LIFE-THREATENING.

Interactions

Drug-drug. *Antacids (magnesium or aluminum), didanosine (chewable tablets, buffered tablets, or pediatric powder for oral solution), iron, multivitamins containing metal cations (such as zinc), sucralfate:* May decrease gemifloxacin level. Give gemifloxacin at least 3 hours before or 2 hours after these drugs.
Antiarrhythmics (amiodarone, procainamide, quinidine, sotalol): May increase risk of prolonged QT interval. Avoid using together.
Drugs that affect QT interval, such as antidepressants, antipsychotics, and erythromycin: May increase risk of prolonged QT interval. Use together cautiously.
Probenecid: May increase gemifloxacin levels. Use together cautiously.
Warfarin: May increase anticoagulation effects. Monitor patient's PT and INR.
Drug-lifestyle. *Sun exposure:* May increase risk of photosensitivity. Discourage excessive or unprotected exposure to ultraviolet light or sunlight.

Effects on lab test results

• May increase ALT and AST levels.

Pharmacokinetics

Absorption: Rapid and unaffected by food.
Distribution: Wide, especially to lung tissue and fluids. About 60% to 70% protein-bound.
Metabolism: Limited, mainly hepatic; some minor metabolites formed.
Excretion: In feces and urine as unchanged drug and metabolites. *Half-life:* 4 to 12 hours.

Route	Onset	Peak	Duration
P.O.	Unknown	½-2 hr	Unknown

Action

Chemical effect: Prevents cell growth by inhibiting DNA gyrase and topoisomerase IV, which interferes with DNA synthesis.
Therapeutic effect: Kills susceptible bacteria.

Available forms

Tablets: 320 mg

NURSING PROCESS

Assessment

• Serious, occasionally fatal hypersensitivity reactions may occur; monitor patient carefully.

• Drug may cause CNS effects, such as tremors and anxiety. Monitor patient carefully.
• Carefully monitor patient's liver enzymes levels. Liver enzymes levels may rise during therapy but will resolve afterward.
• Evaluate patient's and family's knowledge of drug therapy.

Nursing diagnoses

• Risk for injury related to adverse effects of drug therapy
• Deficient knowledge related to drug therapy

Planning and implementation

• Rash is more likely to appear in patients younger than age 40, especially women and those taking hormone therapy. Stop drug if rash appears.
• Drug may cause tendon rupture, arthropathy, or osteochondrosis; stop drug if patient reports pain, inflammation, or rupture.
• If patient has a photosensitivity reaction, stop drug.
• Serious diarrhea may indicate pseudomembranous colitis; stop drug if needed.
• Keep patient adequately hydrated to avoid concentration of urine.
• In acute overdose, empty patient's stomach by inducing vomiting or performing gastric lavage. Hydrate patient if needed, and continue treating symptoms. Hemodialysis removes 20% to 30% of a dose.

Patient teaching
• Instruct patient to finish full course of treatment, even if symptoms improve.
• Tell patient to stop drug and seek medical care if evidence of hypersensitivity reaction develops.
• Tell patient to report serious diarrhea.
• Instruct patient to drink fluids liberally during treatment.
• Warn patient against taking OTC medications or dietary supplements with this drug without consulting prescriber.
• Tell patient to avoid excessive exposure to sunlight or ultraviolet light.
• Urge patient to report pain, inflammation, or rupture of tendons.
• Warn patient to avoid driving or other hazardous activities until effects of drug are known.

☑ Evaluation

• Patient remains free from infection and injury from adverse reactions.
• Patient and family state understanding of drug therapy.

gemtuzumab ozogamicin
(gem-TOO-zuh-mab oh-zoh-GAM-ih-sin)
Mylotarg

Pharmacologic class: antibody-cytotoxic antitumor antibiotic conjugate
Therapeutic class: chemotherapeutic drug
Pregnancy risk category: D

Indications and dosage

▶ **Patients with CD33-positive acute myeloid leukemia in first relapse who are not considered candidates for cytotoxic chemotherapy.** *Adults age 60 and older:* 9 mg/m^2 I.V. infusion over 2 hours every 14 days for a total of two doses. Premedicate with diphenhydramine 50 mg P.O., and acetaminophen 650 to 1,000 mg P.O. 1 hour before infusion.

▼ I.V. administration

• Premedicate with diphenhydramine and acetaminophen. Additional doses of acetaminophen 650 to 1,000 mg P.O. can be given every 4 hours, p.r.n.
• **ⓢ ALERT:** Drug is sensitive to light and must be protected from direct and indirect sunlight and unshielded fluorescent light during preparation and administration.
• Administer in 100 ml of normal saline injection. Place the 100-ml I.V. bag into a UV protectant bag. Use drug solution in I.V. bag immediately.
• Use a separate I.V. line equipped with a low–protein-binding 1.2-micron terminal filter for administration of drug. May be infused by central or peripheral line.
• **ⓢ ALERT:** Don't give I.V. push or bolus.
• Monitor vital signs during infusion and for 4 hours after infusion.

Contraindications and precautions

• Contraindicated in patients hypersensitive to drug or its components.
• Use cautiously in patients with hepatic impairment.

🍂 **Lifespan:** Drug is indicated only for adults age 60 and older. In pregnant women, avoid using drug. Advise women of childbearing potential to avoid becoming pregnant. Breast-feeding women should stop nursing or stop taking drug because of the potential for serious adverse reactions in infants; it's unknown whether drug appears in breast milk. In children, safety and effectiveness of drug haven't been established.

Adverse reactions

CNS: *asthenia, depression, dizziness, headache, insomnia, pain, fever.*
CV: hypertension, *hypotension, tachycardia.*
EENT: *epistaxis, pharyngitis, rhinitis.*
GI: *enlarged abdomen, abdominal pain, anorexia, constipation, diarrhea, dyspepsia, nausea, stomatitis, vomiting.*
GU: *hematuria,* VAGINAL HEMORRHAGE.
Hematologic: *anemia,* BLEEDING, LEUKOPENIA, NEUTROPENIA, NEUTROPENIC FEVER, THROMBOCYTOPENIA, SEVERE MYELOSUPPRESSION.
Hepatic: *hepatotoxicity, hyperbilirubinemia.*
Metabolic: hyperglycemia, *hypokalemia, hypomagnesemia.*
Musculoskeletal: *arthralgia, back pain.*
Respiratory: *increased cough,* dyspnea, *hypoxia,* pneumonia.
Skin: *rash.*
Other: *herpes simplex, chills,* SEPSIS.

Interactions

None reported.

Effects on lab test results

• May increase liver enzyme, lactic dehydrogenase, and glucose levels. May decrease potassium and magnesium levels.
• May decrease hemoglobin, hematocrit, and leukocyte, neutrophil, and platelet counts.

Pharmacokinetics

Absorption: Administered I.V.
Distribution: Unknown.
Metabolism: Unknown. Studies suggest that liver microsomal enzymes are involved.
Excretion: Unknown. *Half-life:* Total and unconjugated calicheamicin, 45 and 100 hours, respectively, after the first dose. After the second dose, total calicheamicin, 60 hours.

Route	Onset	Peak	Duration
I.V.	Unknown	Unknown	Unknown

Action

Chemical effect: May bind to the CD33 antigen expressed on the surface of leukemic blasts in patients with acute myeloid leukemia. This results in the formation of a complex that is internalized by the cell. The calicheamicin derivative is then released inside the cell, causing DNA double strand breaks and cell death.
Therapeutic effect: Kills cancer cells.

Available forms

Powder for injection: 5 mg

NURSING PROCESS

☑ Assessment

• Monitor CBC and platelets before and during therapy.
• Monitor liver enzymes before and during therapy.
• Monitor patient for post infusion reactions and tumor lysis syndrome.
• Monitor I.V. site for local reactions.
• Evaluate patient's and family's knowledge of drug therapy.

⊞ Nursing diagnoses

• Risk for injury related to adverse effects of drug
• Risk for infection related to drug induced adverse hematologic reactions
• Deficient knowledge related to drug therapy

≥ Planning and implementation

• Use only under the supervision of a prescriber experienced in the use of cancer chemotherapeutic drugs.
• Drug may produce a postinfusion symptom complex of chills, fever, hypotension, hypertension, hyperglycemia, hypoxia, and dyspnea that may occur during the first 24 hours after administration.
• Tumor lysis syndrome may occur. Provide adequate hydration and treat with allopurinol to prevent hyperuricemia.
• Drug isn't dialyzable.
• Severe myelosuppression will occur in all patients given the recommended dose of this drug. Careful hematologic monitoring is required.

• Monitor electrolytes, hepatic function, CBC, and platelets during therapy.
Patient teaching
• Inform patient about postinfusion symptoms and instruct him to continue to take acetaminophen 650 to 1,000 mg every 4 hours p.r.n.
• Tell patient to watch for signs of infection (fever, sore throat, and fatigue) and bleeding (easy bruising, nosebleeds, bleeding gums, and melena). Tell patient to take temperature daily.

☑ Evaluation

• Patient remains free of infection.
• Patient's lab values remain above critical levels throughout course of therapy.
• Patient and family state understanding of drug therapy.

gentamicin sulfate
(jen-tuh-MIGH-sin SUL-fayt)
Cidomycin ♦ , Garamycin, Gentamicin Sulfate ADD-Vantage, Jenamicin

Pharmacologic class: aminoglycoside
Therapeutic class: antibiotic
Pregnancy risk category: D

Indications and dosages

▶ **Serious infections caused by sensitive strains of** *Pseudomonas aeruginosa, Escherichia coli, Proteus, Klebsiella, Serratia, Enterobacter, Citrobacter, Staphylococcus.*
Adults: 3 mg/kg daily in divided doses I.M. or I.V. infusion q 8 hours (in 50 to 200 ml of normal saline solution or D_5W infused over 30 minutes to 2 hours). For life-threatening infections, patient may receive up to 5 mg/kg daily in three to four divided doses. Reduce dosage to 3 mg/kg daily as soon as clinically indicated.
Children: 2 to 2.5 mg/kg q 8 hours I.M. or by I.V. infusion.
Neonates older than age 1 week and infants: 2.5 mg/kg daily I.M. or I.V. q 8 hours.
Preterm infants and neonates age 1 week and younger: 2.5 mg/kg I.V. q 12 hours.
▶ **Meningitis.** *Adults:* Systemic therapy as above; 4 to 8 mg intrathecally daily also may be used.
Children and infants older than age 3 months: Systemic therapy as above; 1 to 2 mg intrathecally daily may also be used.

▶ **Endocarditis prophylaxis for GI or GU procedure or surgery.** *Adults:* 1.5 mg/kg up to a maximum dose of 80 mg. I.M., or I.V. 30 to 60 minutes before procedure or surgery and then q 8 hours after first dose. Give separately with aqueous penicillin or ampicillin.
Children: 2 mg/kg I.M. or I.V. 30 to 60 minutes before procedure or surgery and then q 8 hours after first doses. Give separately with aqueous penicillin G or ampicillin G.
▶ **Posthemodialysis to maintain therapeutic level.** *Adults:* 1 to 1.7 mg/kg I.M. or by I.V. infusion after each dialysis.
Children: 2 to 2.5 mg/kg I.M. or by I.V. infusion after each dialysis.

▽ I.V. administration

- When giving drug by intermittent I.V. infusion, dilute with 50 to 200 ml of D$_5$W or normal saline injection.
- Infuse over 30 minutes to 2 hours.
- After infusion, flush line with normal saline solution or D$_5$W.

Contraindications and precautions

- Contraindicated in patients hypersensitive to drug or other aminoglycosides.
- Use cautiously in patients with renal impairment or neuromuscular disorders.
- ☼ **Lifespan:** In pregnant women, don't use because drug is teratogenic. In neonates, infants, and the elderly, use cautiously.

Adverse reactions

CNS: headache, lethargy, numbness, paresthesias, twitching, peripheral neuropathy, *seizures, neurotoxicity.*
EENT: *ototoxicity.*
GU: NEPHROTOXICITY.
Hematologic: *thrombocytopenia, leukopenia, agranulocytosis.*
Other: hypersensitivity reactions.

Interactions

Drug-drug. *Acyclovir, amphotericin B, cisplatin, methoxyflurane, other aminoglycosides, vancomycin:* May increase ototoxicity and nephrotoxicity. Use together cautiously.
Atracurium, doxacurium, mivacurium, pancuronium, rocuronium, tubocurarine, vecuronium: May potentiate neuromuscular blockade. Monitor patient closely.

Cephalothin: May increase nephrotoxicity. Use together cautiously; monitor renal function.
Dimenhydrinate: May mask symptoms of ototoxicity. Use with caution.
Diuretics: May increase ototoxicity. Avoid using together.
General anesthetics: May increase the effects of nondepolarizing muscle relaxant including prolonged respiratory depression. Use together only when necessary.
Indomethacin: May decrease renal clearance of gentamicin leading to increased risk of toxicity.
I.V. loop diuretics (such as furosemide): May increase ototoxicity. Use cautiously.
Neurotoxic drugs: May increase neurotoxicity. Avoid using together.
Parenteral penicillins (such as ampicillin, ticarcillin): May inactivate gentamicin in vitro. Don't mix together.

Effects on lab test results

- May increase BUN, creatinine, nonprotein nitrogen, ALT, AST, bilirubin, and LDH levels.
- May increase eosinophil count. May decrease hemoglobin, hematocrit, and WBC, platelet, and granulocyte counts.

Pharmacokinetics

Absorption: Rapid and complete after I.M. administration.
Distribution: Wide. CSF penetration is low even in adults with inflamed meninges. Higher CSF levels are achieved in neonates, compared to adults. Protein binding is minimal.
Metabolism: Not metabolized.
Excretion: Excreted primarily in urine; small amounts may be excreted in bile. *Half-life:* 2 to 3 hours.

Route	Onset	Peak	Duration
I.V.	Immediate	15-30 min	Unknown
I.M.	Unknown	30-90 min	Unknown
Intrathecal	Unknown	Unknown	Unknown

Action

Chemical effect: Inhibits protein synthesis by binding to ribosomes.
Therapeutic effect: Kills susceptible bacteria (many aerobic gram-negative organisms and some aerobic gram-positive organisms). Drug may act against some aminoglycoside-resistant bacteria.

Available forms

Injection: 40 mg/ml (adult), 10 mg/ml (pediatric), 2 mg/ml (intrathecal)
I.V. infusion (premixed): 40 mg, 60 mg, 70 mg, 80 mg, 90 mg, 100 mg, 120 mg, 160 mg, 180 mg available in normal saline solution

NURSING PROCESS

Assessment

• Assess patient's infection and hearing before therapy and regularly thereafter.
• Obtain specimen for culture and sensitivity tests before first dose.
• Weigh patient and review baseline renal function studies before therapy and regularly during therapy. Notify prescriber of any changes; adjust dosage.
• Obtain blood for peak drug level 1 hour after I.M. injection and 30 minutes to 1 hour after I.V. infusion; for trough levels, draw blood just before next dose. Don't collect blood in heparinized tube because heparin is incompatible with aminoglycosides.
• Peak level above 12 mcg/ml and trough level above 2 mcg/ml may increase risk of toxicity.
• Be alert for adverse reactions and drug interactions.
• Evaluate patient's and family's knowledge of drug therapy.

Nursing diagnoses

• Infection related to presence of susceptible bacteria
• Impaired urinary elimination related to nephrotoxicity
• Deficient knowledge related to drug therapy

Planning and implementation

• Give I.M. injection deep into large muscle mass (gluteal or midlateral thigh); rotate injection sites. Don't inject more than 2 g of drug per site.
• Use preservative-free forms of gentamicin for intrathecal route.
• Hemodialysis (8 hours) removes up to 50% of drug.
• Notify prescriber about signs of decreasing renal function or changes in hearing.
• Therapy usually continues for 7 to 10 days. If no response occurs in 3 to 5 days, therapy may be stopped and new specimens obtained for culture and sensitivity testing.

• Therapeutic peak and trough levels are 4 to 12 mcg/ml and less than 2 mcg/ml, respectively.
• Encourage adequate fluid intake; patient should be well hydrated while taking drug to minimize chemical irritation of renal tubules.
Patient teaching
• Instruct patient to notify prescriber about adverse reactions, such as changes in hearing.
• Emphasize importance of drinking at least 2 L of fluids daily, if not contraindicated.

Evaluation

• Patient is free from infection.
• Patient maintains normal renal function throughout drug therapy.
• Patient and family state understanding of drug therapy.

glimepiride
(gligh-MEH-peh-righd)
Amaryl

Pharmacologic class: sulfonylurea
Therapeutic class: antidiabetic
Pregnancy risk category: C

Indications and dosages

▶ **Adjunct to diet and exercise to lower glucose level in patients with type 2 (non–insulin-dependent) diabetes mellitus whose hyperglycemia can't be managed by diet and exercise alone.** *Adults:* Initially, 1 to 2 mg P.O. once daily with first main meal of day. Usual maintenance dosage is 1 to 4 mg P.O. once daily. After reaching 2 mg, dosage increased in increments not exceeding 2 mg q 1 to 2 weeks, based on patient's response. Maximum, 8 mg daily.
▶ **Adjunct to insulin therapy in patients with type 2 (non–insulin-dependent) diabetes mellitus whose hyperglycemia can't be managed by diet and exercise with oral hypoglycemics.** *Adults:* 8 mg P.O. once daily with first main meal of day with low-dose insulin. Adjust insulin upward weekly p.r.n., based on patient's response.
Adjust-a-dose: For patients with renal impairment, initial dose is 1 mg P.O. daily with breakfast, then adjust based on the patient's fasting glucose levels.

Contraindications and precautions

● Contraindicated in patients hypersensitive to drug, in those with diabetic ketoacidosis, and in those with allergies to sulfonamide or thiazide diuretics.

● Use cautiously in debilitated or malnourished patients and in those with adrenal, pituitary, hepatic, or renal insufficiency.

⚠ **Lifespan:** In breast-feeding women, drug is contraindicated. In children, safety and effectiveness of drug haven't been established. In elderly patients, use cautiously because they might be more sensitive to the drug.

Adverse reactions

CNS: dizziness, asthenia, headache.
EENT: changes in accommodation.
GI: nausea.
Hematologic: *leukopenia,* hemolytic anemia, *agranulocytosis, thrombocytopenia, aplastic anemia, pancytopenia.*
Hepatic: cholestatic jaundice.
Metabolic: *hypoglycemia.*
Skin: allergic skin reactions (pruritus, erythema, urticaria, and morbilliform or maculopapular eruptions).

Interactions

Drug-drug. *Beta blockers:* May mask symptoms of hypoglycemia. Monitor glucose levels carefully.
Drugs that produce hyperglycemia, other diuretics: May lead to loss of glucose control. May require dosage adjustment.
Insulin: May increase potential for hypoglycemia. Monitor glucose levels closely.
NSAIDs, other highly protein-bound drugs: May increase hypoglycemic action of sulfonylureas, such as glimepiride. Monitor patient carefully.
Drug-herb. *Aloe, bitter melon, bilberry leaf, burdock, dandelion, fenugreek, garlic, ginseng:* May improve glucose control, which may allow reduction of oral hypoglycemic. Tell patient to discuss herbs with prescriber before use.
Drug-lifestyle. *Alcohol use:* May alter glycemic control, most commonly hypoglycemia. May cause disulfiram-like reaction. Discourage using together.
Sun exposure: May cause photosensitivity. Discourage prolonged or unprotected exposure to the sun.

Effects on lab test results

● May increase BUN, creatinine, alkaline phosphatase, ALT, and AST levels. May decrease glucose and sodium levels.
● May decrease hemoglobin, hematocrit, and WBC, RBC, platelet, and granulocyte counts.

Pharmacokinetics

Absorption: Complete.
Distribution: Almost completely protein-bound.
Metabolism: Complete.
Excretion: In urine and feces. *Half-life:* About 9 hours.

Route	Onset	Peak	Duration
P.O.	≤ 1 hr	2-3 hr	24 hr

Action

Chemical effect: Stimulates release of insulin from pancreatic beta cells; increases sensitivity of peripheral tissues to insulin.
Therapeutic effect: Lowers glucose levels.

Available forms

Tablets: 1 mg, 2 mg, 4 mg

NURSING PROCESS

Assessment
● Monitor fasting glucose periodically to determine therapeutic response. Also monitor glycosylated hemoglobin, usually every 3 to 6 months, to more precisely assess long-term glycemic control.
● Evaluate patient's and family's knowledge of drug therapy.

Nursing diagnoses
● Ineffective health maintenance related to hyperglycemia
● Risk for injury related to drug-induced hypoglycemia
● Deficient knowledge related to drug therapy

Planning and implementation
● Oral hypoglycemic drugs have been linked to an increased risk of CV mortality compared with diet alone or with diet and insulin therapy.
● Give drug with the first meal of the day.
Patient teaching
● Tell patient to take drug with first meal of day.

- Stress importance of adhering to diet, weight-reduction, exercise, and personal hygiene programs. Explain to patient and family how to monitor glucose levels, and teach them signs, symptoms, and treatment of hyperglycemia and hypoglycemia.
- Advise patient to wear or carry medical identification that describes his condition.
- Instruct patient to avoid alcohol consumption during therapy.

☑ Evaluation
- Patient's glucose level is normal.
- Patient recognizes hypoglycemia early and treats it before injury occurs.
- Patient and family state understanding of drug therapy.

glipizide
(GLIGH-peh-zighd)
Glucotrol, Glucotrol XL, Minidiab ◇

Pharmacologic class: sulfonylurea
Therapeutic class: antidiabetic
Pregnancy risk category: C

Indications and dosages

▶ **Adjunct to diet to lower glucose level in patients with type 2 (non–insulin-dependent) diabetes mellitus.** *Adults:* Initially, 5 mg P.O. daily 30 minutes before breakfast. Start elderly patients or those with liver disease at 2.5 mg immediate-release or 5 mg extended-release. Maximum once-daily dose is 15 mg. Maximum recommended total daily dose is 40 mg. Alternatively, 5 mg extended-release tablets P.O. daily. Adjust in 5-mg increments q 3 months depending on level of glycemic control. Maximum daily dose for extended-release tablets, 20 mg.
▶ **To replace insulin therapy.** *Adults:* If insulin dosage is more than 20 units daily, patient is started at usual dosage in addition to 50% of insulin. If insulin dosage is less than 20 units, stop insulin.

Contraindications and precautions

- Contraindicated in patients hypersensitive to drug, in those with diabetic ketoacidosis, and in those with allergies to sulfonamides or thiazide diuretics.

- Use cautiously in patients with renal and hepatic disease and in debilitated or malnourished patients.
- ⚖ Lifespan: In pregnant and breast-feeding women, drug is contraindicated. In children, safety hasn't been established because of the rarity of type 2 diabetes mellitus in this population. In elderly patients, use cautiously.

Adverse reactions

CNS: dizziness.
CV: facial flushing.
GI: nausea, vomiting, constipation.
Hematologic: *agranulocytosis, thrombocytopenia, aplastic anemia.*
Hepatic: cholestatic jaundice.
Metabolic: *hypoglycemia.*
Skin: rash, pruritus.

Interactions

Drug-drug. *Anabolic steroids, chloramphenicol, clofibrate, guanethidine, MAO inhibitors, phenylbutazone, probenecid, salicylates, sulfonamides:* May increase hypoglycemic activity. Monitor glucose level.
Beta blockers: May prolong hypoglycemic effect and mask symptoms of hypoglycemia. Use together cautiously.
Corticosteroids, glucagon, rifampin, thiazide diuretics: May decrease hypoglycemic response. Monitor glucose level.
Hydantoins: May increase levels of hydantoins. Monitor levels.
Oral anticoagulants: May increase hypoglycemic activity or enhanced anticoagulant effect. Monitor glucose level, PT, and INR.
Drug-herb. *Aloe, bilberry leaf, bitter melon, burdock, dandelion, fenugreek, garlic, ginseng:* May improve glucose control, which may allow reduction of oral hypoglycemic. Tell patient to discuss herbs with prescriber before use.
Drug-lifestyle. *Alcohol use:* May alter glycemic control, most commonly hypoglycemia. May also cause disulfiram-like reaction. Discourage using together.
Sun exposure: May cause photosensitivity. Discourage prolonged or unprotected sun exposure.

Effects on lab test results

- May increase BUN, creatinine, alkaline phosphatase, AST, and LDH levels. May decrease glucose levels.

• May decrease hemoglobin, hematocrit, and granulocyte and platelet counts.

Pharmacokinetics

Absorption: Rapid and complete from GI tract.
Distribution: Distributed within extracellular fluid; about 98% to 99% protein-bound.
Metabolism: By liver to inactive metabolites.
Excretion: Primarily in urine; small amounts in feces. *Half-life:* 2 to 4 hours.

Route	Onset	Peak	Duration
P.O.	15-30 min	1-3 hr	10-24 hr

Action

Chemical effect: May stimulate insulin release from pancreas, reduce glucose output by liver, and increase peripheral sensitivity to insulin.
Therapeutic effect: Lowers glucose levels.

Available forms

Tablets: 5 mg, 10 mg
Tablets (extended-release): 2.5 mg, 5 mg, 10 mg

NURSING PROCESS

Assessment

• Assess glucose level before therapy and regularly thereafter.
• Patient transferring from insulin therapy to oral antidiabetic needs glucose monitoring at least three times daily before meals.
• During periods of increased stress, such as from infection, fever, surgery, or trauma, patient may need insulin therapy. Monitor patient closely for hyperglycemia in these situations.
• Be alert for adverse reactions and drug interactions.
• Evaluate patient's and family's knowledge of drug therapy.

Nursing diagnoses

• Ineffective health maintenance related to hyperglycemia
• Risk for injury related to drug-induced hypoglycemia
• Deficient knowledge related to drug therapy

Planning and implementation

• Give drug about 30 minutes before meals.

• Some patients taking drug may attain effective control on once-daily regimen; others show better response with divided dosing.
• Treat hypoglycemic reaction with oral form of rapid-acting carbohydrates or with glucagon or I.V. glucose if patient can't swallow or is comatose. Follow up treatment with complex carbohydrate snack when patient is awake, and determine cause of reaction.
• Make sure adjunct therapies, such as diet and exercise, are being used appropriately.
• **ALERT:** Don't confuse glipizide with glyburide.

Patient teaching

• Teach patient about diabetes and the importance of following therapeutic regimen; adhering to specific diet, weight reduction, exercise, and personal hygiene programs; and avoiding infection. Explain how and when to monitor glucose level, and teach recognition and treatment of hypoglycemia and hyperglycemia.
• Tell patient not to change dosage without prescriber's consent and to report any adverse reactions.
• Advise patient not to take other medications, including OTC drugs or herbal remedies, without first checking with prescriber.
• Instruct patient to avoid alcohol consumption during drug therapy.
• Advise patient to carry medical identification at all times.

Evaluation

• Patient's glucose level is normal with drug therapy.
• Patient doesn't experience hypoglycemia or hyperglycemia.
• Patient and family state understanding of drug therapy.

glipizide and metformin hydrochloride
(GLIP-uh-zighd and met-FOR-min high-droh-KLOR-ighd)
Metaglip

Pharmacologic class: sulfonylurea and biguanide
Therapeutic class: antidiabetic
Pregnancy risk category: C

Indications and dosages

▶ **First-line therapy, as adjunct to diet and exercise, to improve glycemic control in patients with type 2 (non–insulin-dependent) diabetes.** *Adults:* Initially, 2.5 mg/250 mg P.O. once daily with a meal. In patients whose fasting glucose level is 280 to 320 mg/dl, start with 2.5 mg/500 mg P.O. b.i.d. Increase dosage in increments of one tablet per day q 2 weeks, up to a maximum of 10 mg/1,000 mg or 10 mg/2,000 mg daily in divided doses.

▶ **Second-line therapy in type 2 diabetes when diet, exercise, and initial treatment with a sulfonylurea or metformin can't provide adequate glycemic control.** *Adults:* Initially, 2.5 mg/500 mg or 5 mg/500 mg P.O. b.i.d. with the morning and evening meals. Increase in increments of no more than 5 mg/500 mg daily, up to the minimum effective dose needed to adequately control glucose or to a maximum daily dose of 20 mg/2,000 mg.

Contraindications and precautions

• Contraindicated in patients hypersensitive to any components of the drug and in those with renal disease, creatinine level at least 1.5 mg/dl in men and at least 1.4 mg/dl in women, abnormal creatinine clearance, heart failure, shock, acute MI, septicemia, or acute or chronic metabolic acidosis, including diabetic ketoacidosis. Also contraindicated after surgery.
• Use cautiously in patients with hepatic dysfunction, malnourished or debilitated patients, and those with adrenal or pituitary insufficiency. Also use cautiously in patients with abnormal vitamin B_{12} levels or hypoglycemia, and in those who consume alcohol.
⚕ Lifespan: In pregnant women, use only if benefits outweigh the risks to fetus. If the drug is used, stop therapy at least 1 month before delivery. In breast-feeding women, drug isn't recommended. In children, safety and effectiveness of drug haven't been established. In elderly patients, use cautiously because aging causes reduced renal function. Don't start treatment in patients age 80 or older unless renal function is normal. Don't give older patients the maximum dose.

Adverse reactions

CNS: *headache,* dizziness.
CV: hypertension.

GI: nausea, *diarrhea,* vomiting, abdominal pain.
GU: UTI.
Metabolic: *hypoglycemia, lactic acidosis.*
Musculoskeletal: muscle pain.
Respiratory: *upper respiratory tract infection.*

Interactions

Drug-drug. *Azoles, beta blockers, chloramphenicol, coumarins, MAO inhibitors, NSAIDs, probenecid, salicylates, sulfonamides:* May increase the effect of sulfonylureas. Monitor patient closely for hypoglycemia. May increase loss of glucose control when these drugs are withdrawn.
Calcium channel blockers, corticosteroids, estrogens, highly protein-bound drugs, isoniazid, hormonal contraceptives, nicotinic acid, phenytoin, phenothiazines, sympathomimetics, thyroid products, thiazides and other diuretics: May increase risk of hyperglycemia and loss of glucose control. Increases risk of hypoglycemia when these drugs are withdrawn. Monitor glucose level.
Cationic drugs (amiloride, digoxin, morphine, procainamide, quinidine, quinine, ranitidine, triamterene, trimethoprim, vancomycin): May increase metformin level. Monitor patient carefully.
Furosemide: May increase metformin level and decreases furosemide level. Monitor patient closely.
Iodinated contrast material used in radiologic studies: May increase risk of acute renal impairment. Stop the drug for 48 hours before and after such tests.
Nifedipine: May increase metformin level. Decrease metformin dose if needed.
Drug-herb. *Juniper berries, ginseng, garlic, fenugreek, coriander, dandelion root, celery:* May increase risk of hypoglycemia. Discourage use together.
Drug-lifestyle. *Alcohol use:* May increase risk of hypoglycemia and lactic acidosis. Discourage use together.

Effects on lab test results

• May decrease glucose and vitamin B_{12} levels.

Pharmacokinetics

Absorption: Glipizide absorption is rapid and complete. Metformin absorption is delayed by food.

Distribution: Glipizide is extensively protein bound. Metformin is negligibly bound to proteins.
Metabolism: Glipizide is metabolized extensively in the liver. The primary metabolites are inactive. Metformin isn't metabolized.
Excretion: Inactive metabolites and unchanged glipizide are excreted in the urine. Metformin is excreted unchanged in the urine. *Glipizide half-life:* 2 to 4 hours. *Metformin half-life:* About 6 hours.

Route	Onset	Peak	Duration
P.O.			
glipizide	15-30 min	1-3 hr	Unknown
metformin	Unknown	Unknown	Unknown

Action

Chemical effect: Glipizide appears to lower glucose levels by stimulating the pancreas to release insulin. Metformin decreases hepatic glucose production and intestinal absorption of glucose and improves insulin sensitivity.
Therapeutic effect: Lowers glucose levels.

Available forms

Tablets: 2.5 mg glipizide/250 mg metformin hydrochloride; 2.5 mg/500 mg; 5 mg/500 mg

NURSING PROCESS

Assessment
• Monitor CBC and renal function annually.
• Periodically monitor fasting glucose level and glycosylated hemoglobin.
• If laboratory abnormalities or vague, poorly defined illness occurs, evaluate patient for ketoacidosis or lactic acidosis. If acidosis occurs, stop drug immediately.
• Evaluate patient's and family's knowledge of drug therapy

Nursing diagnoses
• Risk for ineffective health maintenance related to underlying disease
• Risk for deficient fluid volume related to high glucose levels
• Deficient knowledge related to drug therapy

Planning and implementation
• Temporarily stop drug in patients undergoing radiological studies involving iodinated contrast materials or any surgical procedure.

• To reduce the risk of lactic acidosis, use the minimum effective dose and monitor renal function regularly during treatment.
• Stop drug in patients with any condition linked to hypoxemia, dehydration, or sepsis.
• Overdose of glipizide may produce hypoglycemia. Patients taking more than 100 g of metformin may develop hypoglycemia and lactic acidosis, but no proof exists that taking the drug causes this.
• Treat mild hypoglycemia with oral glucose and adjustments in drug dosage or meal patterns. Severe hypoglycemia with coma, seizures, or other neurological impairment requires immediate hospitalization. If hypoglycemic coma is diagnosed or suspected, give a rapid I.V. injection of 50% glucose solution, followed by a continuous infusion of a 10% solution at a rate that will maintain a glucose level above 100 mg/dl. Monitor patient closely for 24 to 48 hours because hypoglycemia may recur.
• Hemodialysis may remove metformin but not glipizide.

Patient teaching
• Tell patient to take once daily with breakfast or twice daily with breakfast and dinner.
• Tell patient to immediately report signs of lactic acidosis, including unexplained hyperventilation, myalgia, malaise, unusual drowsiness, suddenly developing a slow or irregular heartbeat, or feeling cold, dizzy, or light-headed.
• Tell patient that GI symptoms are common during initial therapy but should resolve. Tell patient to report persistent or new onset of GI symptoms.
• Advise patient to avoid drinking alcohol.

Evaluation
• Patient's glucose level remains normal during drug therapy.
• Patient doesn't suffer from fluid volume deficit.
• Patient and family state understanding of drug therapy.

glucagon
(GLOO-kuh-gon)

Pharmacologic class: pancreatic hormone
Therapeutic class: antihypoglycemic
Pregnancy risk category: B

Indications and dosages

▶ **Hypoglycemia.** *Adults and children weighing more than 20 kg (44 lb):* 1 mg I.V., I.M., or S.C.
Children weighing 20 kg or less: 0.5 mg I.V., I.M., or S.C.
▶ **Diagnostic aid for radiologic examination.** *Adults:* 0.25 to 2 mg I.V. or I.M. before start of radiologic procedure.

▼ I.V. administration

• Reconstitute drug in 1-unit vial with 1 ml of diluent; reconstitute drug in 10-unit vial with 10 ml of diluent. Use only diluent supplied by manufacturer when preparing doses of 2 mg or less. For larger doses, dilute with sterile water for injection.
• Don't exceed concentration of 1 mg/ml (1 unit/ml).
• For I.V. drip infusion, use dextrose solution, which is compatible with glucagon; drug forms precipitate in chloride solutions.
• Inject directly into vein or into I.V. tubing of free-flowing compatible solution over 2 to 5 minutes. Interrupt primary infusion during glucagon injection if using same I.V. line.
• May repeat in 15 minutes if necessary.
• If patient fails to respond, give I.V. glucose. When patient responds, give supplemental carbohydrate promptly.

Contraindications and precautions

• Contraindicated in patients hypersensitive to drug and in those with pheochromocytoma.
• Use cautiously in patients with history of insulinoma or pheochromocytoma.
※ **Lifespan:** In pregnant women, use only if absolutely necessary. In breast-feeding women, use cautiously. In children, safety and effectiveness of drug as a diagnostic aid haven't been established.

Adverse reactions

GI: nausea, vomiting.
Other: *allergic reactions* (including urticaria, *respiratory distress,* and hypotension).

Interactions

Drug-drug. *Oral anticoagulants:* Anticoagulant effect may be increased. Monitor PT and INR closely; monitor patient for bleeding.

Effects on lab test results

• May decrease potassium level.

Pharmacokinetics

Absorption: Unknown.
Distribution: Unknown.
Metabolism: Extensive by liver, in kidneys and plasma, and at its tissue receptor sites in plasma membranes.
Excretion: By kidneys. *Half-life:* 8 to 18 minutes.

Route	Onset	Peak	Duration
I.V., I.M., S.C.	Almost immediate	≤ 30 min	1-2 hr

Action

Chemical effect: Promotes catalytic depolymerization of hepatic glycogen to glucose.
Therapeutic effect: Raises glucose level.

Available forms

Powder for injection: 1 mg (1 unit)/vial

NURSING PROCESS

✍ Assessment

• Assess patient's glucose level before therapy and after drug administration.
• Be alert for adverse reactions and drug interactions.
• If patient vomits, monitor his hydration.
• Evaluate patient's and family's knowledge of drug therapy.

🔲 Nursing diagnoses

• Risk for injury related to hypoglycemia
• Risk for deficient fluid volume related to drug-induced vomiting
• Deficient knowledge related to drug therapy

▶ Planning and implementation

• For I.M use, reconstitute drug in 1-unit vial with 1 ml of diluent; reconstitute drug in 10-unit vial with 10 ml of diluent. Use only diluent supplied by manufacturer when preparing doses of 2 mg or less. For larger doses, dilute with sterile water for injection.
• Arouse lethargic patient as quickly as possible and give additional carbohydrates orally to prevent secondary hypoglycemic reactions. Notify prescriber that patient's hypoglycemic episode required glucagon use. If patient doesn't re-

spond to glucagon administration, provide emergency intervention. Unstable hypoglycemic diabetic patient may not respond to glucagon; give dextrose I.V. instead.

• If patient can't retain some form of sugar for 1 hour because of nausea or vomiting, notify prescriber.

Patient teaching
• Instruct patient and family in proper drug administration.
• Teach them to recognize signs and symptoms of hypoglycemia, and tell them to notify prescriber immediately in emergencies.

☑ **Evaluation**
• Patient's glucose level returns to normal.
• Patient remains well hydrated.
• Patient and family state understanding of drug therapy.

glyburide (glibenclamide)
(GLIGH-byoo-righd)
Albert Glyburide ♦ , Apo-Glyburide ♦ , DiaBeta, Euglucon ♦ , Gen-Glybe ♦ , Glynase PresTab, Micronase, Novo-Glyburide ♦ , Nu-Glyburide ♦

Pharmacologic class: sulfonylurea
Therapeutic class: antidiabetic
Pregnancy risk category: B (Micronase, Glynase), category C (DiaBeta)

Indications and dosages
▶ **Adjunct to diet to lower glucose level in patients with type 2 (non–insulin-dependent) diabetes mellitus.** *Adults:* Initially, 1.25 to 5 mg regular tablets P.O. once daily with breakfast. For maintenance, 1.25 to 20 mg daily as single dose or in divided doses. Or initially, 0.75 to 3 mg micronized formulation P.O. daily. For maintenance, 0.75 to 12 mg P.O. daily in single or divided doses.
▶ **To replace insulin therapy.** *Adults:* Initially, if insulin dosage is more than 40 units daily, 5 mg regular tablets or 3 mg micronized formulation P.O. once daily in addition to 50% of insulin dosage. If insulin dosage is 20 to 40 units daily, 5 mg regular tablets or 3 mg micronized formulation P.O. once daily with abrupt insulin discontinuation. If insulin dosage is less than 20 units daily, 2.5 to 5 mg regular tablets or

1.5 to 3 mg micronized formulation P.O. once daily with abrupt insulin discontinuation.

Contraindications and precautions
• Contraindicated in patients hypersensitive to drug, in those with diabetic ketoacidosis, and in those with allergies to sulfonamides or thiazide diuretics.
• Use cautiously in patients with hepatic or renal impairment and in debilitated or malnourished patients.
⚠ **Lifespan:** In pregnant and breast-feeding women and in children, drug is contraindicated. In elderly patients, use cautiously.

Adverse reactions
CV: facial flushing.
GI: nausea, epigastric fullness, heartburn.
Hematologic: *agranulocytosis, thrombocytopenia, aplastic anemia.*
Hepatic: cholestatic jaundice.
Metabolic: *hypoglycemia.*
Skin: rash, pruritus.

Interactions
Drug-drug. *Anabolic steroids, chloramphenicol, clofibrate, guanethidine, MAO inhibitors, phenylbutazone, salicylates, sulfonamides:* May increase hypoglycemic activity. Monitor glucose level.
Beta blockers: May prolong hypoglycemic effect and masks symptoms of hypoglycemia. Use together cautiously.
Corticosteroids, glucagon, rifampin, thiazide diuretics: May decrease hypoglycemic response. Monitor glucose level.
Hydantoins: May increase level of hydantoins. Monitor level.
Oral anticoagulants: May increase hypoglycemic activity or enhanced anticoagulant effect. Monitor glucose level, PT, and INR.
Drug-herb. *Aloe, bitter melon, bilberry leaf, burdock, dandelion, fenugreek, garlic, ginseng:* Improvement in glucose control may allow reduction of oral hypoglycemic. Tell patient to discuss herbs with prescriber before use.
Drug-lifestyle. *Alcohol use:* May alter glycemic control, most commonly hypoglycemia. May also cause disulfiram-like reaction. Discourage using together.
Sun exposure: May cause photosensitivity. Discourage prolonged or unprotected exposure to sunlight.

Reactions may be *common*, uncommon, *life-threatening*, or COMMON AND LIFE-THREATENING.

Effects on lab test results

• May increase BUN, alkaline phosphatase, bilirubin, AST, ALT, and LDH levels. May decrease glucose level.

• May decrease hemoglobin, hematocrit, and WBC, platelet, and granulocyte counts.

Pharmacokinetics

Absorption: Almost complete.
Distribution: Unknown, although it's 99% protein-bound.
Metabolism: Metabolized completely by liver to inactive metabolites.
Excretion: Excreted as metabolites in urine and feces in equal proportions. *Half-life:* 10 hours.

Route	Onset	Peak	Duration
P.O.	45-60 min	2-4 hr	24 hr

Action

Chemical effect: Unknown; may stimulate insulin release from pancreas, reduce glucose output by liver, increase peripheral sensitivity to insulin, and cause mild diuresis.
Therapeutic effect: Lowers glucose levels.

Available forms

Tablets: 1.25 mg, 2.5 mg, 5 mg
Tablets (micronized): 1.5 mg, 3 mg, 4.5 mg, 6 mg

NURSING PROCESS

Assessment

• Assess glucose level before therapy and regularly thereafter.

• Patient transferring from insulin therapy to oral antidiabetic needs glucose monitoring at least three times daily before meals.

• During periods of increased stress, such as from infection, fever, surgery, or trauma, patient may need insulin therapy. Monitor patient closely for hyperglycemia in these situations.

• Be alert for adverse reactions and drug interactions.

• Evaluate patient's and family's knowledge of drug therapy.

Nursing diagnoses

• Ineffective health maintenance related to hyperglycemia

• Risk for injury related to drug-induced hypoglycemia

• Deficient knowledge related to drug therapy

Planning and implementation

• Micronized glyburide (Glynase PresTab) contains drug in smaller particle size and isn't bioequivalent to regular tablets. Adjust dosage in patient who has been taking Micronase or DiaBeta.

• Although most patients take drug once daily, patient taking more than 10 mg daily may achieve better results with twice-daily dosage.

• Treat hypoglycemic reaction with oral form of rapid-acting carbohydrates if patient can swallow or with glucagon or I.V. glucose if patient can't swallow or is comatose. Follow up treatment with complex carbohydrate snack when patient is awake, and determine cause of reaction.

• Make sure that adjunct therapy, such as diet and exercise, is appropriate.

ALERT: Don't confuse glyburide with glipizide.

Patient teaching

• Teach patient about diabetes and the importance of following therapeutic regimen; adhering to specific diet, weight reduction, exercise, and personal hygiene programs; and avoiding infection.

• Explain how and when to monitor glucose levels, and teach recognition and treatment of hypoglycemia and hyperglycemia.

• Tell patient not to change dosage without prescriber's consent and to report any adverse reactions.

• Advise patient not to take other medications, including OTC drugs and herbal remedies, without first checking with prescriber.

• Instruct patient to avoid alcohol consumption during drug therapy.

• Advise patient to wear or carry medical identification at all times.

Evaluation

• Patient's glucose level is normal with drug therapy.

• Patient doesn't experience hypoglycemia.

• Patient and family state understanding of drug therapy.

glyburide and metformin hydrochloride

(GLIGH-byoo-righd and met-FOR-min high-droh-KLOR-ighd)
Glucovance

Pharmacologic class: combination sulfonylurea and biguanide
Therapeutic class: antidiabetic
Pregnancy risk category: B

Indications and dosages

▶ **Adjunct to diet and exercise to improve glycemic control in patients with type 2 (non–insulin-dependent) diabetes whose hyperglycemia cannot be controlled with diet and exercise alone.** *Adults:* Initially, 1.25 mg/250 mg P.O. once daily or b.i.d. with meals.
◈ **Adjust-a-dose:** In patients with glycosylated hemoglobin above 9% or a fasting glucose level above 200 mg/dl, start with 1.25 mg/250 mg twice daily with morning and evening meals. Increase daily dose in increments of 1.25 mg/250 mg per day q 2 weeks up to the minimum dose needed to adequately control glucose. Maximum, 20 mg glyburide and 2,000 mg metformin daily.
▶ **Second-line therapy in patients with type 2 diabetes when diet, exercise, and initial treatment with a sulfonylurea or metformin don't provide adequate glycemic control.** *Adults:* Initially 2.5 mg/500 mg or 5 mg/500 mg twice daily with meals. Increase in increments of no more than 5 mg/500 mg up to the minimum effective dose needed to adequately control glucose. Maximum, 20 mg glyburide and 2,000 mg metformin daily.

Contraindications and precautions

• Contraindicated in patients hypersensitive to drugs, and in patients with renal disease, renal dysfunction, or metabolic acidosis (including diabetic ketoacidosis). Also contraindicated in patients receiving drug treatment for heart failure.
• Use cautiously in hepatically impaired, debilitated, or malnourished patients and in those with adrenal or pituitary insufficiency because of increased risk of hypoglycemia.
⚜ **Lifespan:** In breast-feeding women, drug isn't recommended. In children, safety and effectiveness of drug haven't been established. In elderly patients, use cautiously. Monitor their renal function, and don't give the maximum dose of Glucovance. In patients age 80 and older, don't start treatment unless creatinine clearance shows that renal function isn't reduced.

Adverse reactions

CNS: headache, dizziness.
GI: *diarrhea,* nausea, vomiting, abdominal pain.
Metabolic: HYPOGLYCEMIA.
Respiratory: *upper respiratory infection.*

Interactions

Drug-drug. *Beta blockers, chloramphenicol, ciprofloxacin, coumarins, highly protein-bound drugs, MAO inhibitors, miconazole, NSAIDs, probenecid, salicylates, sulfonamides:* May increase hypoglycemic activity of glyburide. Monitor glucose level.
Calcium channel blockers, corticosteroids, estrogens, isoniazid, nicotinic acid, hormonal contraceptives, phenothiazines, phenytoin, sympathomimetics, thiazides and other diuretics, thyroid drugs: May increase risk of hyperglycemia. Monitor patient's glucose level.
Cationic drugs (such as amiloride, cimetidine, digoxin, morphine, procainamide, quinidine, quinine, ranitidine, triamterene, trimethoprim, vancomycin): May increase metformin level. Monitor patient.
Furosemide: May increase metformin level and decreases furosemide level. Monitor patient closely.
Nifedipine: May increase metformin level. Metformin dosage may need to be decreased.
Drug-lifestyle. *Alcohol use:* May alter glycemic control, most commonly hypoglycemia. May also cause disulfiram-like reaction with glyburide component. Also may increase metformin effects on lactate metabolism. Avoid using together.

Effects on lab test results

• May increase lactate levels. May decrease glucose level.

Pharmacokinetics

glyburide
Absorption: Almost complete.
Distribution: Extensively protein-bound.
Metabolism: Metabolized completely by liver to weakly active metabolites.

Excretion: Excreted as metabolites in urine and bile in equal proportions. *Half-life:* 10 hours.
metformin
Absorption: Food decreases extent and slightly delays rate.
Distribution: Negligibly bound to proteins.
Metabolism: Not metabolized.
Excretion: Unchanged in urine. *Half-life:* About 6 hours.

Route	Onset	Peak	Duration
P.O.			
glyburide	1 hr	4 hr	24 hr
metformin	Unknown	Unknown	Unknown

Action

Chemical effect: Glyburide stimulates the release of insulin from the pancreas. Metformin decreases hepatic glucose production and intestinal absorption of glucose and improves insulin sensitivity.
Therapeutic effect: Lowers glucose level.

Available forms

Tablets: 1.25 mg glyburide and 250 mg metformin, 2.5 mg glyburide and 500 mg metformin, 5 mg glyburide and 500 mg metformin

NURSING PROCESS

Assessment
• Assess underlying condition before therapy and reassess regularly.
• Obtain list of current and past medications taken by the patient. For patients previously treated with glyburide or metformin, the starting dose of Glucovance shouldn't exceed the daily dose of the glyburide (or equivalent dose of another sulfonylurea) and metformin already being taken.
• Assess glucose level before therapy and regularly thereafter. Monitor glycosylated hemoglobin to assess long-term therapy.
• Obtain baseline renal function studies and don't start drug if creatinine levels are 1.5 mg/dl or more for men or 1.4 mg/dl or more for women. Monitor renal function at least once yearly while the patient takes drug and more often in those with increased risk of renal dysfunction. If renal impairment is detected, stop drug.
• Monitor patient closely during times of increased stress, such as infection, fever, surgery, or trauma; insulin therapy may be needed.

• Monitor patient's hematologic status for megaloblastic anemia. Patient with inadequate vitamin B_{12} or calcium intake or absorption is predisposed to developing subnormal vitamin B_{12} levels when taking metformin.
• Evaluate patient's and family's knowledge of drug therapy.

Nursing diagnoses
• Ineffective tissue perfusion, peripheral, related to presence of hyperglycemia
• Risk for injury related to drug-induced hypoglycemia
• Deficient knowledge related to glyburide and metformin hydrochloride therapy

Planning and implementation
• Make sure that adjunct therapy, such as diet and exercise, is appropriate.
• Temporarily stop drug in patients undergoing radiologic studies involving intravascular administration of iodinated contrast materials, because use of such products may result in acute alteration of renal function.
• Temporarily stop drug in patient having surgery that requires restricted intake of food and fluids, and don't restart until restriction is lifted.
• Treat mild hypoglycemic symptoms aggressively with oral glucose and by adjusting drug, dosage, and meal patterns. Severe hypoglycemic reactions with coma, seizure, or other neurologic impairment occur infrequently but demand immediate hospitalization. If hypoglycemic coma is diagnosed or suspected, give patient a rapid I.V. injection of 50% glucose solution followed by continuous infusion of 10% glucose solution at a rate that will maintain glucose at a level above 100 mg/dl. Monitor patient with hypoglycemia closely until out of danger and, if the reaction is severe, for a minimum of 24 to 48 hours, because hypoglycemia may recur.
• For patients requiring additional glycemic control, add a thiazolidinedione.
• Lactic acidosis is a rare, but serious, complication that can result from metformin accumulation. The risk of lactic acidosis increases with the degree of renal impairment and patient's age. Early symptoms of lactic acidosis may include malaise, myalgias, respiratory distress, increasing somnolence, and nonspecific abdominal distress. GI symptoms that occur after a patient is stabilized with Glucovance are unlikely to be drug-related and could be from lactic aci-

dosis or other serious disease. Suspect lactic acidosis in any diabetic patient with metabolic acidosis lacking evidence of ketoacidosis.
• If CV collapse, acute heart failure, acute MI, or other conditions characterized by hypoxemia occur, stop drug; these conditions may be related to lactic acidosis and may cause prerenal azotemia.
• Evaluate patient for evidence of ketoacidosis or lactic acidosis, including electrolytes, ketones, glucose, pH, lactate, pyruvate, and metformin levels. If evidence of acidosis occurs, stop drug.

Patient teaching
• Tell patient to take once-daily dose with breakfast or twice-daily doses with breakfast and dinner.
• Teach patient about diabetes and the importance of following therapeutic regimen; adhering to diet, weight reduction, regular exercise, and hygiene programs; and avoiding infection.
• Explain how and when to monitor glucose level and how to differentiate between hypoglycemia and hyperglycemia.
• Tell patient that his vitamin B_{12} level will be tested every 2 to 3 years.
• Instruct patient to stop drug and report unexplained hyperventilation, myalgia, malaise, unusual somnolence, or other symptoms of early lactic acidosis.
• Tell patient that GI symptoms are common early in drug therapy. GI symptoms that occur after prolonged therapy may be related to lactic acidosis or other serious disease and should be reported promptly.
• Advise patient against excessive alcohol intake, either acute or chronic.
• Advise patient not to take any other medications, including OTC drugs, without checking with prescriber.
• Instruct patient to wear or carry medical identification.

☑ **Evaluation**
• Patient's glucose level is normal with drug therapy.
• Patient doesn't experience hypoglycemia.
• Patient and family state understanding of drug therapy.

glycerin
(GLIH-seh-rin)
Fleet†, Fleet Babylax†, Sani-Supp†

Pharmacologic class: trihydric alcohol
Therapeutic class: laxative (osmotic)
Pregnancy risk category: NR

Indications and dosages

▶ **Constipation.** *Adults and children age 6 and older:* 2 to 3 g as rectal suppository or 5 to 15 ml as enema.
Children younger than age 6: 1 to 1.7 g as rectal suppository, or 2 to 5 ml as enema.

Contraindications and precautions

• Contraindicated in patients hypersensitive to drug and in those with intestinal obstruction, undiagnosed abdominal pain, vomiting or other signs of appendicitis, fecal impaction, or acute surgical abdomen.
⚠ Lifespan: In pregnant women, use drug only when potential benefits outweigh risks to fetus.

Adverse reactions

GI: *cramping pain,* rectal discomfort, hyperemia of rectal mucosa.

Interactions

None significant.

Effects on lab test results

None reported.

Pharmacokinetics

Absorption: Poor.
Distribution: Local.
Metabolism: Unknown.
Excretion: In feces. *Half-life:* Unknown.

Route	Onset	Peak	Duration
P.R.	15-60 min	15-60 min	15-60 min

Action

Chemical effect: Draws water from tissues into feces to stimulate evacuation.
Therapeutic effect: Promotes stool evacuation.

Available forms

Enema (pediatric): 4 ml/applicator†
Suppositories: adult, children, and infant sizes†

NURSING PROCESS

🔲 Assessment
- Obtain assessment of patient's constipation before therapy.
- Monitor effectiveness by noting patient's response after administration.
- Be alert for adverse GI reactions.
- Evaluate patient's and family's knowledge of drug therapy.

🔲 Nursing diagnoses
- Constipation related to interruption of normal pattern of elimination
- Acute pain related to abdominal cramping
- Deficient knowledge related to drug therapy

▶ Planning and implementation
- Drug is used mainly to reestablish proper toilet habits in laxative-dependent patient.
- Drug must be retained for at least 15 minutes; usually acts within 1 hour. Entire suppository doesn't need to melt to be effective.
- Make sure that patient has easy and immediate access to a bathroom, bedside commode, or bedpan after giving drug.
- If drug isn't effective, notify prescriber.

Patient teaching
- Warn patient that abdominal cramping may occur but will subside when bowel is emptied.
- Teach patient a proper diet high in fiber and water.

🔲 Evaluation
- Patient reports return of normal bowel pattern of elimination.
- Patient states that abdominal cramping is transient.
- Patient and family state understanding of drug therapy.

goserelin acetate
(GOH-seh-reh-lin AS-ih-tayt)
Zoladex, Zoladex 3-Month

Pharmacologic class: luteinizing hormone-releasing hormone (LH-RH; Gn-RH) analogue
Therapeutic class: antineoplastic
Pregnancy risk category: X (for endometriosis); D (for advanced breast cancer)

Indications and dosages

▶ **Endometriosis, advanced breast cancer.**
Adults: One 3.6-mg implant S.C. q 28 days into upper abdominal wall for 6 months in endometriosis, longer in breast cancer. For endometriosis, maximum duration of therapy is 6 months.
▶ **Palliative treatment of advanced carcinoma of the prostate.** *Men:* One 10.8-mg implant S.C. q 12 weeks into upper abdominal wall, given with radiotherapy and Flutamide.
▶ **Endometrial thinning before endometrial ablation for dysfunctional uterine bleeding.**
Adults: One or two 3.6-mg implants S.C. into upper abdominal wall. Give each implant 4 weeks apart.

Contraindications and precautions

- Contraindicated in patients hypersensitive to LH-RH, LH-RH agonist analogues, or goserelin acetate.
- The 10.8-mg implant is contraindicated for use in women.
- Use cautiously in patients with risk factors for osteoporosis, such as family history of osteoporosis, chronic alcohol or tobacco abuse, or use of drugs that affect bone density.
- ⚠ Lifespan: In pregnant and breast-feeding women and in children, drug is contraindicated.

Adverse reactions

CNS: *CVA,* lethargy, pain (worsened in first 30 days), dizziness, insomnia, anxiety, depression, headache, emotional lability, fever.
CV: edema, *heart failure, arrhythmias,* hypertension, *MI,* peripheral vascular disorder, chest pain.
GI: nausea, vomiting, diarrhea, constipation, ulcer.
GU: *impotence, lower urinary tract symptoms,* renal insufficiency, urinary obstruction, UTI, amenorrhea, vaginal dryness.
Hematologic: anemia.
Metabolic: hyperglycemia, weight increase.
Musculoskeletal: loss of bone mineral density.
Respiratory: COPD, upper respiratory tract infection.
Skin: rash, diaphoresis.
Other: chills, *hot flushes,* breast swelling and tenderness, changes in breast size, *sexual dysfunction,* gout.

Interactions

None reported.

Effects on lab test results

- May increase ALT, AST, LDL, HDL, cholesterol, triglycerides, calcium, and glucose levels.
- May decrease hemoglobin and hematocrit.

Pharmacokinetics

Absorption: Slow.
Distribution: Low protein-binding.
Metabolism: Hydrolysis of C-terminal amino acids.
Excretion: Mostly via the kidneys with approximately 20% unchanged. *Half-life:* About 4 hours.

Route	Onset	Peak	Duration
S.C.	2-4 wk	12-15 days	Throughout therapy

Action

Chemical effect: LH-RH analogue that acts on pituitary to decrease release of follicle-stimulating hormone and LH, resulting in dramatically lowered levels of sex hormones.
Therapeutic effect: Decreases effects of sex hormones on tumor growth in prostate gland and tissue growth in uterus.

Available forms

Implants: 3.6 mg, 10.8 mg

NURSING PROCESS

🔲 Assessment

- Assess patient's condition before therapy and regularly thereafter.
- When used for prostate cancer, LH-RH analogues such as goserelin may initially worsen symptoms because drug initially increases testosterone levels. Some patients may have increased bone pain. Rarely, disease (spinal cord compression or ureteral obstruction) may worsen.
- Be alert for adverse reactions.
- Evaluate patient's and family's knowledge of drug therapy.

🔲 Nursing diagnoses

- Ineffective health maintenance related to underlying condition
- Acute pain related to drug's adverse effect
- Deficient knowledge related to drug therapy

🔲 Planning and implementation

- Give under supervision of prescriber.

- Give drug into upper abdominal wall using aseptic technique. After cleaning area with alcohol swab (and injecting local anesthetic), stretch patient's skin with one hand while grasping barrel of syringe with the other. Insert needle into S.C. fat; then change direction of needle so that it parallels abdominal wall. Push in needle until hub touches patient's skin and then withdraw about 1 cm (this creates gap for drug to be injected) before depressing plunger completely.
- To avoid need for new syringe and injection site, don't aspirate after inserting needle.
- Implant comes in preloaded syringe. If package is damaged, don't use syringe. Make sure drug is visible in translucent chamber.
- After implantation, area requires bandage after needle is withdrawn.
- If implants require removal, schedule patient for ultrasound to locate them.
- Notify prescriber of adverse reactions and provide supportive care.

Patient teaching

- Advise patient to report every 28 days for new implant. A delay of a couple of days is permissible.
- Tell patient to call prescriber if menstruation persists or breakthrough bleeding occurs. Menstruation should stop during treatment.
- After therapy ends, inform patient that she may experience delayed return of menses. Persistent amenorrhea is rare.
- Warn patient that pain may occur.

🔲 Evaluation

- Patient responds well to drug.
- Patient has no pain.
- Patient and family state understanding of drug therapy.

granisetron hydrochloride
(grah-NEEZ-eh-trohn high-droh-KLOR-ighd)
Kytril

Pharmacologic class: selective 5-hydroxy tryptamine (5-HT$_3$) receptor antagonist
Therapeutic class: antiemetic, antinauseant
Pregnancy risk category: B

Indications and dosages

▶ **Prevention of nausea and vomiting caused by emetogenic cancer chemotherapy.** *Adults* *and children age 2 and older:* 10 mcg/kg undiluted by direct injection over 30 seconds, or diluted and infused over 5 minutes. Begin infusion within 30 minutes before chemotherapy starts. Or, for adults, 1 mg P.O. up to 1 hour before chemotherapy and repeated 12 hours later. Or, for adults, 2 mg P.O. daily within 1 hour before chemotherapy.

▶ **Prevention of nausea and vomiting from radiation, including total body irradiation and fractionated abdominal radiation.** *Adults:* 2 mg P.O. once daily within 1 hour of radiation.

▶ **Postoperative nausea and vomiting.** *Adults:* 1 mg I.V. undiluted and given over 30 seconds. For prevention, give before anesthesia induction or immediately before reversal.

▼ I.V. administration

• Dilute drug with normal saline injection or D₅W to make 20 to 50 ml.
• Infuse over 5 minutes beginning within 30 minutes before chemotherapy starts and only on days chemotherapy is given.
• Diluted solutions are stable for 24 hours at room temperature.

Contraindications and precautions

• Contraindicated in patients hypersensitive to drug.
🕭 **Lifespan:** In pregnant and breast-feeding women, use cautiously. In children younger than age 2, safety hasn't been established for treatment of nausea and vomiting from chemotherapy. Safety of oral granisetron hasn't been established in children of any age. In children, safety hasn't been established for the prevention or treatment of postoperative nausea and vomiting.

Adverse reactions

CNS: *headache, asthenia,* somnolence, agitation, anxiety, CNS stimulation, insomnia, *fever, pain, dizziness.*
CV: hypertension, ***hypotension, bradycardia.***
GI: *nausea, vomiting,* diarrhea, *constipation,* taste disorder, abdominal pain, flatulence, dyspepsia, decreased appetite.
GU: UTI, oliguria.
Hematologic: anemia, *leukocytosis, leukopenia, thrombocytopenia.*
Respiratory: cough, sputum increased.
Skin: rash, dermatitis, alopecia.
Other: *hypersensitivity reactions (anaphylaxis, urticaria, dyspnea, hypotension),* infection.

Interactions

Drug-herb. *Horehound:* May enhance serotonergic effects. Discourage using together.

Effects on lab test results

• May increase ALT and AST levels.
• May decrease hemoglobin, hematocrit, and WBC and platelet counts.

Pharmacokinetics

Absorption: Unknown.
Distribution: Distributed freely between plasma and RBCs; protein binding about 65%.
Metabolism: By liver.
Excretion: In urine and feces. *Half-life:* 5 to 9 hours.

Route	Onset	Peak	Duration
P.O., I.V.	Unknown	Unknown	Unknown

Action

Chemical effect: Located in CNS at area postrema (chemoreceptor trigger zone) and in peripheral nervous system on nerve terminals of vagus nerve. Drug's blocking action may occur at both sites.
Therapeutic effect: Prevents nausea and vomiting from chemotherapy.

Available forms

Injection: 1 mg/ml
Oral solution: 1 mg/5 ml
Tablets: 1 mg

NURSING PROCESS

⚷ Assessment
• Assess patient's chemotherapy and GI reactions before therapy.
• Monitor patient for nausea and vomiting.
• Be alert for adverse reactions.
• If drug is ineffective or diarrhea occurs, monitor hydration.
• Evaluate patient's and family's knowledge of drug therapy.

▣ Nursing diagnoses
• Risk for deficient fluid volume related to nausea and vomiting
• Acute pain related to drug-induced headache
• Deficient knowledge related to drug therapy

▶ Planning and implementation
• Give oral form of drug 1 hour before chemotherapy; repeat in 12 hours.
ⓢ **ALERT:** Don't mix with other drugs; compatibility data are limited.
• If patient has nausea or vomits, alert prescriber.
Patient teaching
• Tell patient to notify prescriber if adverse drug reactions occur.

☑ Evaluation
• Patient has no nausea or vomiting with chemotherapy.
• Patient's headache is relieved with mild analgesic.
• Patient and family state understanding of drug therapy.

guaifenesin (glyceryl guaiacolate)
(gwah-FEH-nih-sin)
Anti-Tuss*†, Balminil Expectorant ♦,
Breonesin†, Diabetic Tussin EX, Fenesin,
Ganidin NR, Gee-Gee†, Genatuss, GG-
Cen*†, Glyate*†, Glytuss, Guaifenex G,
Guaifenex LA, Guiatuss*†, Halotussin*,
Humavent LA, Humibid LA, Humibid
Pediatric, Humibid Sprinkle, Hytuss†,
Hytuss-2X†, Mucinex†, Muco-Fen LA,
Mytussin AF, Naldecon Senior EX†,
Organidin NR, Respa-GF, Resyl ♦ †,
Robitussin*†, Touro EX

Pharmacologic class: propanediol derivative
Therapeutic class: expectorant
Pregnancy risk category: C

Indications and dosages
▶ **Expectorant.** *Adults and children age 12
and older:* 200 to 400 mg P.O. q 4 hours, or
600 to 1,200 mg extended-release capsules q
12 hours. Maximum, 2,400 mg daily.
Children ages 6 to 11: 100 to 200 mg P.O. q
4 hours, or 600 mg extended release capsules q
12 hours. Maximum, 1,200 mg daily.
Children ages 2 to 5: 50 to 100 mg P.O. q
4 hours. Maximum, 600 mg daily.

Contraindications and precautions
• Contraindicated in patients hypersensitive to
drug.

☀ **Lifespan:** In pregnant women, use cautiously. In breast-feeding women, safety of drug
hasn't been established.

Adverse reactions
CNS: drowsiness.
GI: stomach pain, diarrhea, vomiting, nausea
(with large doses).
Skin: rash.

Interactions
None significant.

Effects on lab test results
• May cause false 5-hydroxyindoleacetic acid
and vanillylmandelic acid levels.

Pharmacokinetics
Absorption: Readily absorbed.
Distribution: Unknown.
Metabolism: Unknown.
Excretion: Renal, as inactive metabolites. *Half-
life:* Unknown.

Route	Onset	Peak	Duration
P.O.	Unknown	Unknown	Unknown

Action
Chemical effect: Increases production of respiratory tract fluids to help liquefy and reduce viscosity of tenacious secretions.
Therapeutic effect: Thins respiratory secretions for easier removal.

Available forms
Capsules: 200 mg†
Capsules (extended-release): 300 mg
Liquid: 100 mg/5 ml
Solution: 50 mg/ml, 100 mg/5 ml†, 200 mg/
5 ml*†
Syrup: 100 mg/5 ml*†
Tablets: 100 mg†, 200 mg†
Tablets (sustained-release): 575 mg, 600 mg,
800 mg
Tablets (extended-release, film-coated):
600 mg†, 1,200 mg†

NURSING PROCESS

⧫ Assessment
• Assess patient's sputum production before and
after giving drug.
• Be alert for adverse reactions.

• If adverse GI reactions occur, monitor patient's hydration.
• Evaluate patient's and family's knowledge of drug therapy.

⊞ Nursing diagnoses
• Ineffective airway clearance related to underlying condition
• Risk for deficient fluid volume related to adverse GI reactions
• Deficient knowledge related to drug therapy

⊡ Planning and implementation
• Give drug with a full glass of water.
Patient teaching
• Inform patient that persistent cough may indicate a serious condition. Tell him to contact prescriber if cough lasts longer than 1 week, recurs frequently, or accompanies a high fever, rash, or severe headache.
• Advise patient to take each dose with a full glass of water before and after dose; increasing fluid intake may prove beneficial.
• Encourage patient to perform deep-breathing exercises.

☑ Evaluation
• Patient's lungs are clear, and respiratory secretions are normal.
• Patient maintains adequate hydration.
• Patient and family state understanding of drug therapy.

guanfacine hydrochloride
(GWAHN-fuh-seen high-droh-KLOR-ighd)
Tenex

Pharmacologic class: centrally acting sympatholytic
Therapeutic class: antihypertensive
Pregnancy risk category: B

Indications and dosages
▶ **Hypertension.** *Adults:* Initially, 1 mg P.O. daily h.s. Increase to 2 mg P.O. h.s. after 3 to 4 weeks, p.r.n. Further increase to 3 mg P.O. h.s. after another 3 to 4 weeks, p.r.n. Average is 1 to 3 mg daily.

Contraindications and precautions
• Contraindicated in patients hypersensitive to drug.
• Use cautiously in patients with severe coronary insufficiency, cerebrovascular disease, recent MI, or chronic renal or hepatic insufficiency.
⚠ **Lifespan:** In pregnant women, use cautiously. In children and breast-feeding women, safety hasn't been established.

Adverse reactions
CNS: *drowsiness, dizziness,* fatigue, headache, insomnia.
CV: *bradycardia,* orthostatic hypotension, rebound hypertension.
GI: *constipation,* diarrhea, nausea, *dry mouth.*
Skin: dermatitis, pruritus.

Interactions
Drug-drug. *CNS depressants:* May increase sedation. Avoid using together.
Drug-lifestyle. *Alcohol use:* May enhance CNS effect. Discourage use together.

Effects on lab test results
None reported.

Pharmacokinetics
Absorption: Good and complete; about 80% bioavailable.
Distribution: High; about 70% protein-bound.
Metabolism: In liver.
Excretion: In urine. *Half-life:* About 17 hours.

Route	Onset	Peak	Duration
P.O.	Unknown	1-4 hr	24 hr

Action
Chemical effect: Unknown; may inhibit central vasomotor center, decreasing sympathetic outflow to heart, kidneys, and peripheral vasculature.
Therapeutic effect: Lowers blood pressure.

Available forms
Tablets: 1 mg, 2 mg

NURSING PROCESS

⊡ Assessment
• Assess blood pressure before therapy and regularly thereafter.
• Be alert for adverse reactions. Risk and severity increase with higher dosages.

• Evaluate patient's and family's knowledge of drug therapy.

◆ Nursing diagnoses
• Risk for injury related to presence of hypertension
• Constipation related to adverse effects on GI tract
• Deficient knowledge related to drug therapy

▶ Planning and implementation
• Give daily dosage h.s. to minimize daytime drowsiness.
• Drug may be used alone or with diuretic.
Patient teaching
• Tell patient not to stop therapy abruptly. Rebound hypertension is less common than with similar drugs but may occur.
• Advise patient to avoid activities that require alertness until CNS response to drug is known.
• Instruct patient to check with prescriber before taking other OTC medications.

☑ Evaluation
• Patient's blood pressure is normal.
• Patient's bowel pattern is normal.
• Patient and family state understanding of drug therapy.

haloperidol
(hal-oh-PER-uh-dol)
Apo-Haloperidol ◆ , Haldol, Novo-Peridol ◆ , Peridol ◆ , PMS- Haloperidol ◆ , Serenace ◇

haloperidol decanoate
Haldol Decanoate, Haldol LA ◆

haloperidol lactate
Haldol

Pharmacologic class: phenylbutylpiperidine derivative
Therapeutic class: antipsychotic
Pregnancy risk category: C

Indications and dosages
▶ **Psychotic disorders.** *Adults and children age 12 and older:* Initial range is 0.5 to 5 mg P.O. b.i.d. or t.i.d. Or, 2 to 5 mg I.M. q 4 to 8 hours, although hourly administration may be needed until control is obtained. Maximum, 100 mg P.O. daily.
Children ages 3 to 11: 0.05 to 0.15 mg/kg P.O. given b.i.d. or t.i.d. Severely disturbed children may need higher doses.
▶ **Chronically psychotic patients who need prolonged therapy.** *Adults:* Initially, 10 to 20 times previous daily dose of oral haloperidol equivalent up to a maximum of 100 mg decanoate given I.M. q 4 weeks. Usual maintenance dose, 10 to 15 times previous daily dose in oral haloperidol equivalents.
▶ **Nonpsychotic behavior disorders.** *Children ages 3 to 12:* 0.05 to 0.075 mg/kg P.O. b.i.d. or t.i.d. Maximum, 6 mg P.O. daily.
▶ **Tourette syndrome.** *Adults:* 0.5 to 1.5 mg P.O. t.i.d. Some patients may require up to 10 mg/day in two or three divided doses.
Children ages 3 to 12: 0.05 to 0.075 mg/kg P.O. b.i.d. or t.i.d.
▶ **Delirium‡.** *Adults:* 1 to 2 mg I.V. q 2 to 4 hours.

Contraindications and precautions
• Contraindicated in patients hypersensitive to drug and in those with parkinsonism, coma, or CNS depression.
• Use cautiously in debilitated patients; in patients who take anticonvulsants, anticoagulants, antiparkinsonians, or lithium; and in patients with history of seizures or EEG abnormalities, severe CV disorders, allergies, glaucoma, or urine retention.
⚞ Lifespan: In pregnant women, safety of drug hasn't been established. In breast-feeding women, drug isn't recommended. In elderly patients, use cautiously; they need a lower initial dose and a more gradual dose adjustment.

Adverse reactions
CNS: *severe extrapyramidal reactions, tardive dyskinesia*, sedation, **seizures, neuroleptic malignant syndrome.**
CV: tachycardia, ECG changes (including prolonged QT interval and *torsades de pointes*), hypotension, hypertension, **bradycardia.**
EENT: *blurred vision.*
GU: urine retention, menstrual irregularities.

Hematologic: transient *leukopenia* and leukocytosis.
Hepatic: jaundice.
Skin: rash.
Other: gynecomastia.

Interactions

Drug-drug. *Carbamazepine:* May decrease haloperidol level. Monitor patient.
CNS depressants: May increase CNS depression. Avoid using together.
Fluoxetine: May cause severe extrapyramidal reaction. Don't use together.
Lithium: May cause lethargy and confusion with high doses. Monitor patient.
Methyldopa: May cause symptoms of dementia or psychosis to appear. Monitor patient.
Phenytoin: May decrease haloperidol level. Monitor patient.
Drug-herb. *Nutmeg:* May cause loss of symptom control or interference with therapy for psychiatric illness. Discourage using together.
Drug-lifestyle. *Alcohol use:* May increase CNS depression. Discourage using together.

Effects on lab test results

• May increase liver function test values. May increase or decrease WBC count.

Pharmacokinetics

Absorption: About 60% of P.O. dose absorbed; about 70% of I.M. dose absorbed within 30 minutes. I.M. route provides 4 to 10 times more active drug than oral route.
Distribution: Wide, with high levels in adipose tissue; 91% to 99% protein-bound.
Metabolism: Extensive.
Excretion: About 40% in urine within 5 days; about 15% in feces by way of biliary tract. *Half-life:* P.O., 24 hours; I.M., 21 hours.

Route	Onset	Peak	Duration
P.O.	Unknown	3-6 hr	Unknown
I.M.			
lactate	Unknown	10-20 min	Unknown
decanoate	Unknown	3-9 days	Unknown

Action

Chemical effect: May block postsynaptic dopamine receptors in brain.
Therapeutic effect: Decreases psychotic behaviors.

Available forms

haloperidol
Tablets: 0.5 mg, 1 mg, 2 mg, 5 mg, 10 mg, 20 mg
haloperidol decanoate
Injection: 50 mg/ml, 100 mg/ml
haloperidol lactate
Injection: 5 mg/ml
Oral concentrate: 2 mg/ml

NURSING PROCESS

🔖 Assessment

• Assess patient's disorder before therapy and regularly thereafter.
• Be alert for adverse reactions and drug interactions.
• Monitor patient for tardive dyskinesia. It may occur after prolonged use. It may not appear until months or years later and may disappear spontaneously or persist for life despite discontinuation of drug.
• Evaluate patient's and family's knowledge of drug therapy.

🔲 Nursing diagnoses

• Disturbed thought processes related to underlying condition
• Impaired physical mobility related to extrapyramidal effects
• Deficient knowledge related to drug therapy

▶ Planning and implementation

🔵 **ALERT:** Give drug by deep I.M. injection in gluteal region, using a 21G needle. Maximum volume of each injection shouldn't exceed 3 ml.
🔵 **ALERT:** Not recommended I.V.; optimum I.V. dosage has not been established.
• When changing from oral to injection form, give patient 10 to 15 times oral dose once monthly (maximum, 100 mg).
• Protect drug from light. Slight yellowing of injection or concentrate is common and doesn't affect potency. Discard markedly discolored solutions.
• Don't stop drug abruptly unless severe adverse reactions occur.
• Acute dystonic reactions may be treated with diphenhydramine.
Patient teaching
• Warn patient to avoid activities that require alertness and psychomotor coordination until CNS effects of drug are known.

- Tell patient to avoid alcohol while taking drug.
- Tell patient to relieve dry mouth with sugarless gum or hard candy.
- Instruct patient to take drug exactly as prescribed and not to double doses to compensate for missed ones.

☑ **Evaluation**

- Patient demonstrates decreased psychotic behavior and agitation.
- Patient maintains physical mobility.
- Patient and family state understanding of drug therapy.

heparin sodium

(HEH-puh-rin SOH-dee-um)
Hepalean ◆ , Heparin Leo ◆ , Heparin Lock Flush Solution (with Tubex), Hep-Lock, Liquaemin Sodium, Uniparin◇

Pharmacologic class: anticoagulant
Therapeutic class: anticoagulant
Pregnancy risk category: C

Indications and dosages

Heparin dosing is highly individualized, depending upon patient's disease state, age, and renal and hepatic status.

▶ **Deep vein thrombosis, pulmonary embolism.** *Adults:* Initially, 10,000 units I.V. bolus; then adjust according to PTT and give I.V. q 4 to 6 hours (5,000 to 10,000 units). Or, 5,000 units I.V. bolus; then 20,000 to 40,000 units in 24 hours by I.V. infusion pump. Adjust hourly rate 4 to 6 hours after bolus dose according to PTT.
Children: Initially, 50 units/kg I.V. drip. Maintenance dosage is 100 units/kg I.V. drip over 4 hours. Constant infusion: 20,000 units/m² daily. Adjust dosages according to PTT.

▶ **Embolism prevention.** *Adults:* 5,000 units S.C. q 8 to 12 hours. In surgical patients, give first dose 2 hours before procedure; follow with 5,000 units S.C. q 8 to 12 hours for 5 to 7 days or until patient is fully ambulatory.

▶ **Open-heart surgery.** *Adults:* (total body perfusion) 150 to 400 units/kg continuous I.V. infusion.

▶ **DIC.** *Adults:* 50 to 100 units/kg I.V. q 4 hours as a single injection or constant infusion. If no improvement in 4 to 8 hours, stop drug.

Children: 25 to 50 units/kg I.V. q 4 hours, as a single injection or constant infusion. If no improvement in 4 to 8 hours, stop drug.

▶ **Maintaining patency of I.V. indwelling catheters.** *Adults:* 10 to 100 units I.V. flush. Use sufficient volume to fill device. Not intended for therapeutic use.

▶ **Unstable angina‡.** *Adults:* 70 to 80 mg/kg I.V. loading dose; follow by infusion maintaining PTT at 1.5 to 2 times control level during first week of anginal pain.

▶ **Post MI, cerebral thrombosis in evolving CVA, left ventricular thrombi, heart failure, history of embolism, and atrial fibrillation‡.** *Adults:* 5,000 units S.C. q 12 hours empirically. Or, 75 units/kg continuous infusion to maintain PTT at 1.5 to 2 times control value; follow by warfarin sodium.

▼ I.V. administration

- Check order and vial carefully. Heparin comes in various concentrations.
- Give drug I.V. using infusion pump to provide maximum safety because of long-term effect and irregular absorption when given S.C.
- Check constant I.V. infusions regularly, even when pumps are in good working order, to prevent giving too much or too little.

⑤ **ALERT:** Never piggyback other drugs into infusion line while heparin infusion is running. Many antibiotics and other drugs deactivate heparin. Never mix any drug with heparin in syringe when bolus therapy is used.

⑤ **ALERT:** Don't skip dose or "catch up" with I.V. containing heparin. If I.V. is out, restart it as soon as possible, and reschedule bolus dose immediately.

Contraindications and precautions

- Contraindicated in patients hypersensitive to drug.
- Conditionally contraindicated in patients with active bleeding; blood dyscrasia; bleeding tendencies, such as hemophilia, thrombocytopenia, or hepatic disease with hypoprothrombinemia; suspected intracranial hemorrhage; suppurative thrombophlebitis; inaccessible ulcerative lesions (especially of GI tract) and open ulcerative wounds; extensive denudation of skin; ascorbic acid deficiency and other conditions causing increased capillary permeability; subacute bacterial endocarditis; shock; advanced renal disease; threatened abortion; severe hypertension; during

or after brain, eye, or spinal cord surgery; during spinal tap or spinal anesthesia; and during continuous tube drainage of stomach or small intestine. Although heparin is clearly hazardous in these conditions, risk versus benefits must be evaluated.

• Use cautiously in patients with mild hepatic or renal disease, alcoholism, or occupations with risk of physical injury; and in patients with history of allergies, asthma, or GI ulcerations.

⚖ Lifespan: In pregnant women who need anticoagulation, most clinicians use heparin. During menses and immediately postpartum, use cautiously. In elderly patients, use cautiously and at reduced dosage.

Adverse reactions

CNS: fever.
EENT: rhinitis, conjunctivitis, lacrimation.
Hematologic: *hemorrhage* (with excessive dosage), *overly prolonged clotting time, thrombocytopenia.*
Skin: irritation, mild pain, hematoma, ulceration, pruritus, urticaria, cutaneous or subcutaneous necrosis.
Other: *white clot syndrome; hypersensitivity reactions,* chills, burning of feet, *anaphylaxis.*

Interactions

Drug-drug. *Aspirin:* May increase the risk of bleeding. Monitor coagulation tests and patient closely for bleeding.
Oral anticoagulants: May cause additive anticoagulation. Monitor PT, INR, and PTT; monitor patient for bleeding.
Other antiplatelet drugs: May increase anticoagulant effect. Use together cautiously.
Thrombolytics: May increase risk of hemorrhage. Monitor patient closely for bleeding.
Drug-herb. *Dong quai, feverfew, garlic, ginger, horse chestnut, motherwort, red clover:* May increase risk of bleeding. Monitor patient closely for bleeding.

Effects on lab test results

• May increase ALT and AST levels.
• May increase INR, PT, and PTT. May decrease platelet count.

Pharmacokinetics

Absorption: Peak level varies.
Distribution: Extensively bound to lipoprotein, globulins, and fibrinogen.

Metabolism: Thought to be removed by reticuloendothelial system, with some metabolism occurring in liver.
Excretion: Small amount in urine as unchanged drug. *Half-life:* 1 to 2 hours. Half-life is dose-dependent and nonlinear and may be disproportionately prolonged at higher doses.

Route	Onset	Peak	Duration
I.V.	Immediate	Unknown	Unknown
S.C.	20-60 min	2-4 hr	Unknown

Action

Chemical effect: Accelerates formation of antithrombin III–thrombin complex and deactivates thrombin, preventing conversion of fibrinogen to fibrin.
Therapeutic effect: Decreases ability of blood to clot.

Available forms

Products are derived from beef lung or porcine intestinal mucosa.
heparin sodium
Carpuject: 5,000 units/ml
Disposable syringes: 1,000 units/ml, 2,500 units/ml, 5,000 units/ml, 7,500 units/ml, 10,000 units/ml, 15,000 units/ml, 20,000 units/ml, 40,000 units/ml
Premixed I.V. solutions: 1,000 units in 500 ml of normal saline solution; 2,000 units in 1,000 ml of normal saline solution; 12,500 units in 250 ml of half-normal saline solution; 25,000 units in 250 ml of half-normal saline solution; 25,000 units in 500 ml of half-normal saline solution; 10,000 units in 100 ml of D_5W; 12,500 units in 250 ml of D_5W; 25,000 units in 250 ml of D_5W; 25,000 units in 500 ml of D_5W; 20,000 units in 500 ml of D_5W
Unit-dose ampules: 1,000 units/ml, 5,000 units/ml, 10,000 units/ml
Vials: 1,000 units/ml, 2,500 units/ml, 5,000 units/ml, 7,500 units/ml, 10,000 units/ml, 15,000 units/ml, 20,000 units/ml, 40,000 units/ml
heparin sodium flush
Disposable syringes: 10 units/ml, 100 units/ml
Vials: 10 units/ml, 100 units/ml

NURSING PROCESS

📝 Assessment

• Assess patient's underlying condition before therapy.

- Draw blood to establish baseline coagulation values before therapy.
- Monitor effectiveness by measuring PTT carefully and regularly. Anticoagulation present when PTT values are 1½ to 2 times control values.
- During intermittent I.V. therapy, always draw blood 30 minutes before next dose to avoid falsely elevated PTT. Draw blood for PTT 8 hours after start of continuous I.V. heparin therapy. Don't draw blood for PTT from I.V. tubing of heparin infusion or from infused vein; falsely elevated PTT will result. Always draw blood from opposite arm.
- Be alert for adverse reactions and drug interactions.
- Monitor platelet counts regularly. Thrombocytopenia caused by heparin may be linked to a type of arterial thrombosis known as white clot syndrome.
- Solutions more concentrated than 100 units/ml can irritate blood vessels.
- Evaluate patient's and family's knowledge of drug therapy.

😑 Nursing diagnoses
- Risk for injury related to potential for thrombosis or emboli development from underlying condition
- Ineffective protection related to increased bleeding risks
- Deficient knowledge related to drug therapy

▶ Planning and implementation
- Give low-dose injections sequentially between iliac crests in lower abdomen deep into S.C. fat. Inject drug slowly. Leave needle in place for 10 seconds after injection; then withdraw. Don't massage after S.C. injection, and watch for bleeding at injection site. Alternate sites every 12 hours.
- Drug requirements are higher in early phases of thrombogenic diseases and febrile states; lower when patient's condition stabilizes.
- Place notice above patient's bed to inform I.V. team or laboratory staff to apply pressure dressings after taking blood.
- Take bleeding precautions.
- To minimize the risk of hematoma, avoid excessive I.M. injection of other drugs. If possible, don't give I.M. injections at all.
- ⊛ **ALERT:** To treat severe heparin calcium or heparin sodium overdose, use protamine sulfate, a heparin antagonist. Dosage is based on dose of

heparin, its route of administration, and time elapsed since it was given. As a general rule, 1 to 1.5 units of protamine/100 units of heparin are given if only a few minutes have elapsed; 0.5 to 0.75 mg protamine/100 units heparin if 30 to 60 minutes have elapsed; and 0.25 to 0.375 mg protamine/100 units heparin if 2 hours or more have elapsed.
- Abrupt withdrawal may cause increased coagulability, and heparin therapy is usually followed by oral anticoagulants for prophylaxis.
- ⊛ **ALERT:** Don't give heparin with low–molecular-weight heparins (LMWH).
- ⊛ **ALERT:** Don't confuse heparin with Hespan.
- ⊛ **ALERT:** Spell out units instead of abbreviating as "U" to reduce the risk of error by misreading it as a zero (0).

Patient teaching
- Instruct patient and family to watch for signs of bleeding and to notify prescriber immediately if they occur.
- Tell patient to avoid OTC medications containing aspirin, other salicylates, some herbal remedies, and other drugs that may interact with heparin.

✓ Evaluation
- Patient's PTT is reflective of goal of heparin therapy.
- Patient has no injury from bleeding.
- Patient and family state understanding of drug therapy.

hepatitis B immune globulin, human
(hep-uh-TIGH-tus bee ih-MYOON GLOH-byoo-lin, HYOO-mun)
BayHep B, HBIG, Nabi-HB

Pharmacologic class: immunologic drug
Therapeutic class: hepatitis B prophylaxis; immunoglobulin
Pregnancy risk category: C

Indications and dosages
▶ **Hepatitis B exposure in high-risk patients.**
Adults and children: 0.06 ml/kg I.M. within 7 days after exposure (preferably within first 24 hours). If patient refuses hepatitis B vaccine, repeat dosage 28 days after exposure.

Reactions may be *common,* uncommon, *life-threatening,* or **COMMON AND LIFE-THREATENING.**

Neonates born to patients who test positive for hepatitis B surface antigen (HBsAg): 0.5 ml I.M. within 12 hours of birth.

Contraindications and precautions

• Contraindicated in patients with history of anaphylactic reactions to immune serum.
• Use cautiously in patients with severe thrombocytopenia or any coagulation disorder that would contraindicate I.M. injections.
⚥ **Lifespan:** In pregnant and breast-feeding women, use cautiously. It's unknown whether drug appears in breast milk.

Adverse reactions

CNS: *headache.*
Musculoskeletal: *myalgia.*
Skin: urticaria.
Other: *anaphylaxis, angioedema,* injection site reactions (*erythema,* pain).

Interactions

Drug-drug. *Live-virus vaccines:* May interfere with response to live-virus vaccines. Defer routine immunization for 3 months.

Effects on lab test results

None reported.

Pharmacokinetics

Absorption: Slow.
Distribution: Unknown.
Metabolism: Unknown.
Excretion: Unknown. *Half-life:* Antibodies to HBsAg, 21 days.

Route	Onset	Peak	Duration
I.M.	1-6 days	3-11 days	≥ 2 mo

Action

Chemical effect: Provides passive immunity to hepatitis B.
Therapeutic effect: Prevents hepatitis B.

Available forms

Injection: 1-ml, 4-ml, 5-ml vials

NURSING PROCESS

⚗ Assessment
• Assess patient's allergies and reaction to immunizations before therapy.

• Monitor effectiveness by checking patient's antibody titers.
• Be alert for anaphylaxis.
• Evaluate patient's and family's knowledge of drug therapy.

⊕ Nursing diagnoses
• Ineffective protection related to lack of immunity to hepatitis B
• Deficient knowledge related to drug therapy

▷ Planning and implementation
• Inject drug into anterolateral aspect of thigh or deltoid muscle in older children and adults; inject into anterolateral aspect of thigh for neonates and children younger than age 3.
• Make sure epinephrine 1:1,000 is available in case anaphylaxis occurs.
• For postexposure prophylaxis (for example, needle stick, direct contact), drug is usually given with hepatitis B vaccine.
Patient teaching
• Instruct patient to report respiratory difficulty immediately.

☑ Evaluation
• Patient exhibits passive immunity to hepatitis B.
• Patient and family state understanding of drug therapy.

hetastarch
(HET-uh-starch)
Hespan

Pharmacologic class: amylopectin derivative
Therapeutic class: plasma volume expander
Pregnancy risk category: C

Indications and dosages

▶ **Plasma expander.** *Adults:* 500 to 1,000 ml I.V., depending on amount of blood lost and resulting hemoconcentration. Total dosage usually doesn't exceed 1,500 ml daily. Up to 20 ml/kg hourly may be used in hemorrhagic shock.

▽ I.V. administration

• During continuous-flow centrifugation, leukapheresis ratio is usually 1 part hetastarch to 8 parts venous whole blood.
• Discard partially used bottles.

• If allergic or sensitivity reaction occurs, stop drug and notify prescriber. Give antihistamine, if needed.

Contraindications and precautions

• Contraindicated in patients with severe bleeding disorders, severe heart failure, and renal impairment with oliguria and anuria.

⚞ **Lifespan:** In pregnant women, use cautiously. Women shouldn't breast-feed during therapy. In children, safety of drug hasn't been established.

Adverse reactions

CNS: mild fever, headaches.
CV: peripheral edema of legs.
EENT: periorbital edema.
GI: nausea, vomiting.
Respiratory: wheezing.
Skin: urticaria.
Other: *hypersensitivity reactions.*

Interactions

None significant.

Effects on lab test results

None reported.

Pharmacokinetics

Absorption: Administered I.V.
Distribution: In plasma.
Metabolism: Hetastarch molecules larger than 50,000 molecular weight are slowly degraded to molecules that can be excreted.
Excretion: 40% of hetastarch molecules smaller than 50,000 molecular weight are excreted in urine within 24 hours. Those that aren't hydroxyethylated are slowly degraded to glucose. *Half-life:* 17 to 48 days.

Route	Onset	Peak	Duration
I.V.	Immediate	Immediate	Unknown

Action

Chemical effect: Expands plasma volume.
Therapeutic effect: Reverses fluid volume deficit.

Available forms

Injection: 500 ml (6 g/100 ml in normal saline solution)

NURSING PROCESS

🕮 Assessment
• Assess patient's underlying condition before therapy.
• Check for improvement in underlying condition. Assess vital signs and cardiopulmonary status.
• To avoid circulatory overload, monitor patient with renal impairment carefully.
• Monitor CBC, total leukocyte and platelet counts, leukocyte differential count, hemoglobin, hematocrit, PT, INR, PTT, and electrolyte, BUN, and creatinine levels.
• Be alert for adverse reactions.
• Evaluate patient's and family's knowledge of drug therapy.

🔟 Nursing diagnoses
• Deficient fluid volume related to underlying condition
• Ineffective health maintenance related to hypersensitivity reaction
• Deficient knowledge related to drug therapy

▶ Planning and implementation
• Hetastarch isn't a substitute for blood or plasma.
⊛ **ALERT:** Don't confuse Hespan with heparin.
Patient teaching
• Inform patient about need for drug.
• Tell patient to report difficulty breathing.

☑ Evaluation
• Patient regains normal fluid volume after drug therapy.
• Patient doesn't develop hypersensitivity reaction to drug.
• Patient and family state understanding of drug therapy.

hydralazine hydrochloride
(high-DRAL-uh-zeen high-droh-KLOR-ighd)
Alphapress ◇, **Apresoline, Novo-Hylazin** ◆

Pharmacologic class: peripheral vasodilator
Therapeutic class: antihypertensive
Pregnancy risk category: C

Indications and dosages

▶ **Essential hypertension (orally, alone or with other antihypertensives); severe essential hypertension (parenterally, to lower blood pressure quickly).** *Adults:* Initially, 10 mg P.O. q.i.d.; gradually increase to 50 mg q.i.d., p.r.n. Maximum recommended dosage is 200 mg daily, but some patients may need 300 to 400 mg daily. Or, give 10 to 20 mg I.V. slowly and repeat p.r.n. Switch to P.O. antihypertensives as soon as possible. Or, 10 to 50 mg I.M., repeat p.r.n. Switch to P.O. form as soon as possible.

▶ **Management of severe heart failure‡.** *Adults:* Initially 50 to 75 mg P.O., then adjust according to patient's response. Most patients respond to 200 to 600 mg daily, divided q 6 to 12 hours, but doses as high as 3 g daily have been given.

▶ **Management of hypertensive emergencies related to pregnancy (preeclampsia, eclampsia).** *Adults:* 5 to 10 mg I.V.; repeat q 20 to 30 minutes p.r.n. to achieve adequate blood pressure control. Or, infuse at 0.5 to 10 mg/hour.

▼ I.V. administration

• Drug is compatible with normal saline solution, Ringer's and lactated Ringer's solutions, and several other common I.V. solutions. Drug may react with dextrose. Manufacturer doesn't recommend mixing drug in infusion solutions. Check with pharmacist for additional compatibility information.
• Hydralazine changes color in most infusion solutions, but the change doesn't indicate loss of potency.
• Give drug slowly and repeat p.r.n., usually every 4 to 6 hours.
• Monitor blood pressure closely.

Contraindications and precautions

• Contraindicated in patients hypersensitive to drug and in those with coronary artery disease or mitral valvular rheumatic heart disease.
• Use cautiously in patients with suspected cardiac disease, CVA, or severe renal impairment, and in those taking other antihypertensives.
⚠ **Lifespan:** In pregnant women, use cautiously. In breast-feeding women and in children, safety of drug hasn't been established.

Adverse reactions

CNS: peripheral neuritis, *headache,* dizziness.
CV: orthostatic hypotension, tachycardia, *arrhythmias,* angina, palpitations.
GI: nausea, vomiting, diarrhea, anorexia.
Hematologic: *neutropenia, leukopenia, agranulocytopenia.*
Metabolic: *weight gain,* sodium retention.
Skin: rash.
Other: *lupus-like syndrome* (especially with high doses).

Interactions

Drug-drug. *Diazoxide, MAO inhibitors:* May cause severe hypotension. Use together cautiously.
Indomethacin: May decrease hydralazine effects. Monitor patient.
Metoprolol, propranolol: May increase levels and effects of these drugs. Monitor patient closely; adjust dose of either drug p.r.n.

Effects on lab test results

• May decrease hemoglobin, hematocrit, and neutrophil, WBC, RBC, granulocyte, and platelet counts.

Pharmacokinetics

Absorption: Absorbed rapidly from GI tract. Food enhances absorption. Degree of absorption is unknown after I.M. administration.
Distribution: Distributed widely throughout body; about 88% to 90% protein-bound.
Metabolism: Metabolized extensively in GI mucosa and liver.
Excretion: Primarily in urine; about 10% of P.O. dose in feces. *Half-life:* 3 to 7 hours.

Route	Onset	Peak	Duration
P.O.	20-30 min	1-2 hr	2-4 hr
I.V.	≤ 5 min	15-30 min	2-6 hr
I.M.	10-30 min	1 hr	2-6 hr

Action

Chemical effect: Unknown. As a direct-acting vasodilator, its predominant effect relaxes arteriolar smooth muscle.
Therapeutic effect: Lowers blood pressure.

Available forms

Injection: 20 mg/ml
Tablets: 10 mg, 25 mg, 50 mg, 100 mg

NURSING PROCESS

Assessment

- Assess blood pressure before therapy and regularly thereafter.
- Monitor CBC, lupus erythematosus cell preparation, and antinuclear antibody titer determination during long-term therapy.
- Be alert for adverse reactions and drug interactions.
- Evaluate patient's and family's knowledge of drug therapy.

Nursing diagnoses

- Risk for injury related to presence of hypertension
- Excessive fluid volume related to sodium retention
- Deficient knowledge related to drug therapy

Planning and implementation

- Give oral form of drug with meals to increase absorption.
- Some clinicians combine hydralazine therapy with diuretics and beta blockers to decrease sodium retention and tachycardia and to prevent angina.
- Compliance may be improved by giving drug twice daily. Check with prescriber.

ALERT: Don't confuse hydralazine with hydroxyzine.

Patient teaching

- Instruct patient to take oral form with meals.
- Inform patient that orthostatic hypotension can be minimized by rising slowly and avoiding sudden position changes.
- Tell patient not to stop drug suddenly but to call prescriber if unpleasant adverse reactions occur.
- Tell patient to limit sodium intake.

Evaluation

- Patient's blood pressure is normal.
- Fluid retention doesn't develop.
- Patient and family state understanding of drug therapy.

hydrochlorothiazide
(high-droh-klor-oh-THIGH-uh-zighd)
Apo-Hydro ♦, Aquazide-25, Aquazide-H, Dichlotride ◊, Diuchlor H ♦, Esidrix, Ezide, HydroDIURIL, Hydro-Par, Microzide, Neo-Codema ♦, Novo-Hydrazide ♦, Oretic, Urozide ♦

Pharmacologic class: thiazide diuretic
Therapeutic class: diuretic, antihypertensive
Pregnancy risk category: B

Indications and dosages

▶ **Edema.** *Adults:* 25 to 100 mg P.O. daily or intermittently.
▶ **Hypertension.** *Adults:* 12.5 to 50 mg P.O. once daily. May increase or decrease daily dose based on blood pressure.
Children ages 2 to 12: 2.2 mg/kg or 60 mg/m² P.O. daily in two divided doses. Usual dosage range is 37.5 to 100 mg P.O. daily.
Infants and children ages 6 months to younger than 2 years: 2.2 mg/kg or 60 mg/m² P.O. daily in two divided doses. Usual dosage range is 12.5 to 37.5 mg P.O. daily.
Infants younger than age 6 months: Up to 3.3 mg/kg daily in two divided doses.

Contraindications and precautions

- Contraindicated in patients with anuria and in patients hypersensitive to other thiazides or sulfonamide derivatives.
- Use cautiously in patients with severe renal disease, impaired hepatic function, and progressive hepatic disease.

Lifespan: In pregnant women, drug isn't recommended because fetal harm may occur. In breast-feeding women, safety of drug hasn't been established. In elderly patients, use lower initial dose.

Adverse reactions

CV: volume depletion and dehydration, orthostatic hypotension.
GI: anorexia, nausea, *pancreatitis*.
GU: nocturia, polyuria, frequent urination, *renal impairment*.
Hematologic: *aplastic anemia, agranulocytosis, leukopenia, thrombocytopenia*.
Hepatic: *hepatic encephalopathy*.

Metabolic: hypokalemia, asymptomatic hyperuricemia, hyperglycemia and impairment of glucose tolerance, fluid and electrolyte imbalances, including dilutional hyponatremia and hypochloremia, *metabolic alkalosis,* and hypercalcemia.

Skin: dermatitis, photosensitivity, rash.

Other: gout, *anaphylactic reactions,* hypersensitivity reactions, such as pneumonitis and vasculitis.

Interactions

Drug-drug. *Antidiabetics:* May decrease effectiveness of hypoglycemics. Adjust dosage as needed; monitor glucose level.

Antihypertensives: May have additive antihypertensive effect. Use together cautiously; monitor blood pressure closely.

Barbiturates, opioids: May increase orthostatic hypotensive effect. Monitor patient closely.

Bumetanide, ethacrynic acid, furosemide, torsemide: May cause excessive diuretic response resulting in serious electrolyte abnormalities or dehydration. Adjust doses carefully while monitoring patient closely for excessive diuretic responses.

Cholestyramine, colestipol: May decrease intestinal absorption of thiazides. Give drugs separately.

Diazoxide: May increase antihypertensive, hyperglycemic, and hyperuricemic effects. Use together cautiously.

Digoxin: May increase risk of digoxin toxicity from hydrochlorothiazide-induced hypokalemia. Monitor potassium and digoxin levels.

Lithium: May decrease lithium excretion, increasing risk of lithium toxicity; monitor level.

NSAIDs: May increase risk of NSAID-induced renal impairment. Monitor patient closely.

Drug-herb. *Dandelion:* May interfere with diuretic activity. Discourage using together.

Licorice root: May contribute to the potassium depletion caused by thiazides. Discourage using together.

Drug-lifestyle. *Alcohol use:* May increase orthostatic hypotensive effect. Discourage using together.

Sun exposure: May increase photosensitivity. Urge patient to avoid unprotected or prolonged sun exposure.

Effects on lab test results

• May increase glucose, cholesterol, triglyceride, calcium, and uric acid levels. May decrease potassium, sodium, and chloride levels.

• May decrease hemoglobin, hematocrit, and granulocyte, WBC, and platelet counts.

Pharmacokinetics

Absorption: Rate and extent varies with different forms of drug.

Distribution: Protein binding is 40% to 68%.

Metabolism: None.

Excretion: Excreted unchanged in urine. *Half-life:* 5½ to 15 hours.

Route	Onset	Peak	Duration
P.O.	2 hr	4-6 hr	6-12 hr

Action

Chemical effect: Increases sodium and water excretion by inhibiting sodium and chloride reabsorption in the distal segment of the nephron.

Therapeutic effect: Promotes sodium and water excretion and lowers blood pressure.

Available forms

Capsules: 12.5 mg
Oral solution: 50 mg/5 ml
Tablets: 25 mg, 50 mg, 100 mg

NURSING PROCESS

Assessment

• Assess patient's edema or blood pressure before starting therapy.

• Monitor effectiveness by regularly checking blood pressure, urine output, and weight. In patient with hypertension, therapeutic response may be delayed several days.

• Monitor electrolyte levels.

• Monitor creatinine and BUN levels regularly. Drug isn't as effective if these levels are more than twice normal.

• Monitor uric acid levels, especially in patient with history of gout.

• Be alert for adverse reactions and drug interactions.

• Evaluate patient's and family's knowledge of drug therapy.

Nursing diagnoses

• Ineffective health maintenance related to presence of edema or hypertension

- Impaired urinary elimination related to diuretic effect of drug
- Deficient knowledge related to drug therapy

⊠ Planning and implementation
- Give drug in morning to prevent nocturia.
- If nausea occurs, give drug with food.
- Drug may be used with potassium-sparing diuretic to prevent potassium loss.

⊛ **ALERT:** Avoid abbreviating hydrochlorothiazide as HCTZ, which can be misread as HCT (hydrocortisone).

Patient teaching
- Advise patient to take drug with food to minimize GI upset.
- Warn patient to avoid sudden posture changes and to rise slowly to avoid orthostatic hypotension.
- Instruct patient to avoid alcohol consumption during drug therapy.
- Advise patient to use sunblock to prevent photosensitivity reactions.
- Tell patient to check with prescriber before taking OTC medications or herbal remedies.

☑ Evaluation
- Patient's blood pressure is normal, and no edema is present.
- Patient demonstrates adjustment of lifestyle to deal with altered patterns of urinary elimination.
- Patient and family state understanding of drug therapy.

hydrocortisone
(high-droh-KOR-tuh-sohn)
Cortef, Cortenema, Hydrocortone

hydrocortisone acetate
Cortifoam, Hydrocortone Acetate

hydrocortisone cypionate
Cortef

hydrocortisone sodium phosphate
Hydrocortone Phosphate

hydrocortisone sodium succinate
A-hydroCort, Solu-Cortef

Pharmacologic class: adrenocortical steroids

Therapeutic class: adrenocorticoid replacement; glucocorticoid
Pregnancy risk category: NR

Indications and dosages
▶ **Severe inflammation, adrenal insufficiency.**
Adults: 20 to 240 mg hydrocortisone or cypionate P.O. daily. Or, 5 to 75 mg acetate injected into joints or soft tissue. Usually given once every 2 to 3 weeks, although some conditions may require weekly injections. Dosage varies with degree of inflammation and size and location of the joint or soft tissues. Or, 15 to 240 mg phosphate I.V., I.M., or S.C. daily, divided into 12-hour intervals. Or, initially, 100 to 500 mg succinate I.V. or I.M.; may repeat q 2 to 6 hours p.r.n.
▶ **Adjunct for ulcerative colitis and proctitis.**
Adults: 1 enema (100 mg) hydrocortisone or acetate P.R. nightly for 21 days.

▼ I.V. administration
- Hydrocortisone sodium phosphate may be added directly to D₅W or normal saline solution for I.V. administration.
- Reconstitute hydrocortisone sodium succinate with bacteriostatic water or bacteriostatic sodium chloride solution before adding to I.V. solutions. When giving by direct I.V. injection, inject over at least 30 seconds. For infusion, dilute with D₅W, normal saline solution, or D₅W in normal saline solution to 1 mg/ml or less.
- Don't use acetate or suspension form for I.V. use. When giving as direct injection, inject directly into vein or I.V. line containing free-flowing compatible solution over 30 seconds to several minutes. When giving as intermittent or continuous infusion, dilute solution according to manufacturer's instructions and give over prescribed duration. If used for continuous infusion, change solution every 24 hours.

Contraindications and precautions
- Contraindicated in patients allergic to drug or its components and in those with systemic fungal infections. Hydrocortisone sodium succinate is contraindicated in premature infants.
- Use cautiously in patients with recent MI, and in those with GI ulcer, renal disease, hypertension, osteoporosis, diabetes mellitus, hypothyroidism, cirrhosis, diverticulitis, nonspecific ulcerative colitis, recent intestinal anastomoses, thromboembolic disorders, seizures, myasthenia gravis, heart failure, tuberculosis, ocular herpes

simplex, emotional instability, and psychotic tendencies.

⚥ **Lifespan:** In pregnant women, use cautiously. In breast-feeding women, drug isn't recommended in high doses. In children, long-term use may delay growth and maturation.

Adverse reactions

Most adverse reactions are dose- or duration-dependent.
CNS: *euphoria, insomnia,* psychotic behavior, pseudotumor cerebri, *seizures.*
CV: *heart failure,* hypertension, edema, *arrhythmias, thromboembolism.*
EENT: cataracts, glaucoma.
GI: *peptic ulceration,* GI irritation, increased appetite, *pancreatitis.*
Metabolic: hypokalemia, hyperglycemia, carbohydrate intolerance.
Musculoskeletal: muscle weakness, growth suppression in children, osteoporosis.
Skin: hirsutism, delayed wound healing, acne, various skin eruptions, easy bruising.
Other: susceptibility to infections, *acute adrenal insufficiency with increased stress (infection, surgery, or trauma) or abrupt withdrawal after long-term therapy.*

Interactions

Drug-drug. *Aspirin, indomethacin, other NSAIDs:* May increase risk of GI distress and bleeding. Give together cautiously.
Barbiturates, phenytoin, rifampin: May decrease corticosteroid effect; may require increased dosage.
Live-attenuated virus vaccines, other toxoids and vaccines: May decrease antibody response and increases risk of neurologic complications. Avoid using together.
Oral anticoagulants: May alter dosage requirements. Monitor PT and INR closely.
Potassium-depleting drugs (such as thiazide diuretics): May enhance potassium-wasting effects of hydrocortisone. Monitor potassium level.
Skin-test antigens: May decrease skin response. Defer skin testing until therapy is completed.
Drug-lifestyle. *Alcohol use:* May increase risk of GI effects. Discourage using together.

Effects on lab test results

• May increase glucose and cholesterol levels. May decrease potassium and calcium levels.

Pharmacokinetics

Absorption: Rapid after P.O. use. Variable after I.M. or intra-articular injection. Unknown after rectal use.
Distribution: Distributed to muscle, liver, skin, intestines, and kidneys. Extensively protein-bound. Only unbound portion is active.
Metabolism: Metabolized in liver.
Excretion: Inactive metabolites and small amounts of unmetabolized drug excreted in urine; insignificant quantities excreted in feces. *Half-life:* 8 to 12 hours.

Route	Onset	Peak	Duration
P.O., I.V., I.M., P.R.	Varies	Varies	Varies

Action

Chemical effect: Not clearly defined; decreases inflammation, mainly by stabilizing leukocyte lysosomal membranes; suppresses immune response; stimulates bone marrow; and influences nutrient metabolism.
Therapeutic effect: Reduces inflammation, suppresses immune function and raises adrenocorticoid hormonal levels.

Available forms

hydrocortisone
Enema: 100 mg/60 ml
Tablets: 5 mg, 10 mg, 20 mg
hydrocortisone acetate
Enema: 10% aerosol foam (provides 90 mg/application)
Injection: 25 mg/ml*, 50 mg/ml* suspension
Suppositories: 25 mg
hydrocortisone cypionate
Oral suspension: 10 mg/5 ml
hydrocortisone sodium phosphate
Injection: 50 mg/ml solution
hydrocortisone sodium succinate
Injection: 100 mg/vial*, 250 mg/vial*, 500 mg/vial*, 1,000 mg/vial*

NURSING PROCESS

🔍 **Assessment**

• Assess patient's condition before therapy and regularly thereafter.
• Monitor patient's weight, blood pressure, and electrolyte levels.

• Monitor patient for stress. Fever, trauma, surgery, and emotional problems may increase adrenal insufficiency.
• Periodic measurement of growth and development may be needed during high-dose or prolonged therapy in child.
• Be alert for adverse reactions and drug interactions.
• Evaluate patient's and family's knowledge of drug therapy.

🔟 **Nursing diagnoses**
• Ineffective health maintenance related to underlying condition
• Ineffective protection related to immunosuppression
• Deficient knowledge related to drug therapy

▶ **Planning and implementation**
• For better results and less toxicity, give once-daily dose in morning.
• Give oral dose with food.
• Give I.M. injection deep into gluteal muscle. Rotate injection sites to prevent muscle atrophy.
• Rectal suppositories may produce the same systemic effects as other forms of hydrocortisone. If therapy must exceed 21 days, stop gradually by giving every other night for 2 or 3 weeks.
⊛ **ALERT:** Avoid S.C. injection because atrophy and sterile abscesses may occur.
⊛ **ALERT:** Don't confuse Solu-Cortef with Solu-Medrol (methylprednisolone sodium succinate).
• Injectable forms aren't used for alternate-day therapy.
• High-dose therapy usually doesn't continue beyond 48 hours.
• Always adjust to lowest effective dose, and gradually reduce dosage after long-term therapy.
• Give potassium supplements.
• If evidence of adrenal insufficiency appears, notify prescriber and increase dosage.
• Notify prescriber about adverse reactions. Provide supportive care.
⊛ **ALERT:** Avoid abbreviating drug as HCT, which can be misread as HCTZ (hydrochlorothiazide).
Patient teaching
• Teach patient signs of early adrenal insufficiency (fatigue, muscle weakness, joint pain, fever, anorexia, nausea, dyspnea, dizziness, and fainting).

• Instruct patient to carry or wear medical identification that identifies need for supplemental systemic glucocorticoids during stress.
⊛ **ALERT:** Tell patient not to stop drug abruptly or without prescriber's consent. Abrupt withdrawal may lead to rebound inflammation, fatigue, weakness, arthralgia, fever, dizziness, lethargy, depression, fainting, orthostatic hypotension, dyspnea, anorexia, and hypoglycemia. After prolonged use, sudden withdrawal may be fatal.
• Warn patient receiving long-term therapy about cushingoid symptoms and tell him to report sudden weight gain or swelling to prescriber. Also, advise him to consider exercise or physical therapy, to ask his prescriber about vitamin D or calcium supplements, and to have periodic ophthalmic examinations.
• Warn patient about easy bruising.

☑ **Evaluation**
• Patient's condition improves.
• Serious complications related to drug-induced immunosuppression don't develop.
• Patient and family state understanding of drug therapy.

hydromorphone hydrochloride (dihydromorphinone hydrochloride)
(high-droh-MOR-fohn high-droh-KLOR-ighd)
Dilaudid, Dilaudid-HP

Pharmacologic class: opioid
Therapeutic class: opioid analgesic, antitussive
Pregnancy risk category: C
Controlled substance schedule: II

Indications and dosages

▶ **Moderate to severe pain.** *Adults:* 2 to 4 mg P.O. q 4 to 6 hours, p.r.n. Or, 1 to 2 mg I.M., S.C., or I.V. (slowly over at least 2 to 3 minutes) q 4 to 6 hours p.r.n. Or, 3-mg rectal suppository q 6 to 8 hours p.r.n.
▶ **Cough.** *Adults:* 1 mg P.O. q 3 to 4 hours p.r.n. *Children ages 6 to 12:* 0.5 mg P.O. q 3 to 4 hours p.r.n.

▽ I.V. administration

• For infusion, drug may be mixed in D_5W, normal saline solution, D_5W in normal saline solu-

tion, D$_5$W in half-normal saline solution, or Ringer's or lactated Ringer's solutions.
• For direct injection, give over at least 2 minutes.

Contraindications and precautions

• Contraindicated in patients hypersensitive to drug, in patients with intracranial lesions from increased intracranial pressure, and whenever ventilatory function is depressed, as in status asthmaticus, COPD, cor pulmonale, emphysema, or kyphoscoliosis.
• Use cautiously in debilitated patients and in patients with hepatic or renal disease, hypothyroidism, Addison's disease, prostatic hypertrophy, or urethral stricture.
⚠ **Lifespan:** In pregnant and breast-feeding women and in elderly patients, use cautiously.

Adverse reactions

CNS: *sedation, somnolence, clouded sensorium,* dizziness, *euphoria, seizures.*
CV: hypotension, *bradycardia.*
EENT: blurred vision, diplopia, nystagmus.
GI: nausea, vomiting, constipation, ileus.
GU: urine retention.
Respiratory: *respiratory depression, bronchospasm.*
Other: induration with repeated S.C. injections, physical dependence.

Interactions

Drug-drug. *CNS depressants, general anesthetics, hypnotics, MAO inhibitors, other opioid analgesics, sedatives, tranquilizers, tricyclic antidepressants:* May have additive effects. Use together cautiously. Reduce hydromorphone dose, and monitor patient response.
Drug-lifestyle. *Alcohol use:* May have additive effects. Discourage using together.

Effects on lab test results

• May increase amylase and lipase levels.

Pharmacokinetics

Absorption: Well absorbed after oral, rectal, or parenteral administration.
Distribution: Unknown.
Metabolism: Primarily in liver.
Excretion: Primarily in urine. *Half-life:* 2½ to 4 hours.

Route	Onset	Peak	Duration
P.O.	30 min	30 min-2 hr	4-5 hr
I.V.	10-15 min	15-30 min	2-3 hr
I.M.	15 min	30-60 min	4-5 hr
S.C.	15 min	30-90 min	4 hr
P.R.	Unknown	Unknown	4 hr

Action

Chemical effect: Binds with opioid receptors in CNS, altering perception of and emotional response to pain. Suppresses cough reflex by direct action on cough center in medulla.
Therapeutic effect: Relieves pain and cough.

Available forms

Injection: 1 mg/ml, 2 mg/ml, 4 mg/ml, 10 mg/ml
Injection (lyophilized powder): 250 mg/vial
Liquid: 5 mg/5 ml
Suppositories: 3 mg
Tablets: 2 mg, 4 mg, 8 mg

NURSING PROCESS

⚖ Assessment
• Assess patient's pain or cough before and after giving drug.
⊛ ALERT: Respiratory depression and hypotension can occur with I.V. administration. Monitor respiratory and circulatory status frequently.
• Drug may worsen or mask gallbladder pain.
• Drug is a commonly abused opioid. Be alert for addictive behavior or drug abuse.
• Be alert for adverse reactions and drug interactions.
• Evaluate patient's and family's knowledge of drug therapy.

⬡ Nursing diagnoses
• Acute pain related to underlying condition
• Ineffective breathing pattern related to respiratory depression
• Deficient knowledge related to drug therapy

▷ Planning and implementation
• For better analgesic effect, give drug before patient's pain becomes intense.
• Dilaudid-HP, a highly concentrated form (10 mg/ml), may be given in smaller volumes to prevent discomfort caused by large-volume I.M. or S.C. injections. Check dosage carefully.

- Rotate injection sites to avoid induration with S.C. injection.
- Keep resuscitation equipment and opioid antagonist (naloxone) available.
- Postoperatively, encourage patient to turn, cough, and deep-breathe to avoid atelectasis.
- Recommend increased intake of fiber and fluids and a stool softener to prevent constipation during maintenance therapy.

Patient teaching
- Advise ambulatory patient to be careful when getting out of bed or walking. Warn patient to avoid activities that require mental alertness until CNS effects of drug are known.
- Encourage patient to ask for drug before pain becomes severe.
- If patient's respiratory rate decreases, tell patient or caregiver to notify prescriber.
- Instruct patient to avoid alcohol consumption during drug therapy.

☑ Evaluation
- Patient is free from pain.
- Patient maintains adequate breathing patterns.
- Patient and family state understanding of drug therapy.

hydroxychloroquine sulfate
(high-droks-ee-KLOR-oh-kwin SUL-fayt)
Plaquenil

Pharmacologic class: 4-aminoquinoline
Therapeutic class: antimalarial, antiinflammatory
Pregnancy risk category: C

Indications and dosages

▶ **Suppressive prophylaxis of malaria attacks caused by *Plasmodium vivax, P. malariae, P. ovale,* and susceptible strains of *P. falciparum. Adults:* 310 mg base P.O. weekly on same day of week. Begin 1 to 2 weeks before exposure and continue for 4 weeks after leaving endemic areas.
Children: 5 mg base/kg P.O. weekly, not to exceed 310 mg.
Patients untreated before exposure: Initial loading dose is doubled (620 mg for adults, 10 mg/kg for children) P.O. in two divided doses 6 hours apart.

▶ **Acute malarial attacks.** *Adults:* Initially, 620 mg base P.O.; then 310 mg base after 6 hours; then 310 mg base daily for 2 days. *Children:* Initial dose, 10 mg base/kg (up to 620 mg base); second dose, 5 mg base/kg (up to 310 mg base) 6 hours after first dose; third dose, 5 mg base/kg 18 hours after second dose; fourth dose, 5 mg base/kg 24 hours after third dose.
▶ **Lupus erythematosus (chronic discoid and systemic).** *Adults:* 400 mg (sulfate) P.O. daily or b.i.d., continued for several weeks or months, depending on response. Prolonged maintenance dosage: 200 to 400 mg (sulfate) daily.
▶ **Rheumatoid arthritis.** *Adults:* Initially, 400 to 600 mg (sulfate) P.O. daily. When good response occurs (usually in 4 to 12 weeks), reduce dosage by 50% and continue at 200 to 400 mg daily.

Contraindications and precautions

- Contraindicated in patients hypersensitive to drug, and in patients with retinal or visual field changes or porphyria.
- Use cautiously in patients with severe GI, neurologic, or blood disorders, and in patients with hepatic disease or alcoholism because drug concentrates in liver. Also use cautiously in those with G6PD deficiency or psoriasis because drug may worsen these conditions.
☀ **Lifespan:** In pregnant women, use cautiously. In breast-feeding women, safety of drug hasn't been established. In children who need long-term therapy, drug is contraindicated.

Adverse reactions

CNS: irritability, nightmares, ataxia, *seizures,* psychic stimulation, toxic psychosis, vertigo, nystagmus, lassitude, fatigue, dizziness, hypoactive deep tendon reflexes.
EENT: visual disturbances (blurred vision; difficulty in focusing; reversible corneal changes; typically irreversible, sometimes progressive or delayed retinal changes, such as narrowing of arterioles; macular lesions; pallor of optic disk; optic atrophy; visual field defects; patchy retinal pigmentation, commonly leading to blindness), ototoxicity (irreversible nerve deafness, tinnitus, labyrinthitis).
GI: anorexia, abdominal cramps, diarrhea, nausea, vomiting.
Hematologic: *agranulocytosis, leukopenia, thrombocytopenia, aplastic anemia; hemolysis* (in patients with G6PD deficiency).

Reactions may be *common,* uncommon, *life-threatening,* or COMMON AND LIFE-THREATENING.

Metabolic: weight loss.
Musculoskeletal: skeletal muscle weakness.
Skin: pruritus, lichen planus eruptions, skin and mucosal pigmentary changes, pleomorphic skin eruptions, alopecia, bleaching of hair.

Interactions

Drug-drug. *Aluminum and magnesium salts, kaolin:* Decreases GI absorption. Separate administration times.
Cimetidine: Decreases hepatic metabolism of hydroxychloroquine. Monitor patient for toxicity.

Effects on lab test results

● May decrease hemoglobin, hematocrit, and granulocyte, WBC, and platelet counts.

Pharmacokinetics

Absorption: Readily absorbed and almost complete.
Distribution: Concentrates in liver, spleen, kidneys, heart, and brain and is strongly bound in melanin-containing cells. Drug is bound to proteins.
Metabolism: By liver.
Excretion: Most excreted unchanged in urine.
Half-life: 32 to 50 days.

Route	Onset	Peak	Duration
P.O.	Unknown	2-4½ hr	Unknown

Action

Chemical effect: Unknown; may bind to and alter properties of DNA in susceptible organisms.
Therapeutic effect: Prevents or hinders growth of *P. malariae, P. ovale, P. vivax,* and *P. falciparum.* Relieves inflammation.

Available forms

Tablets: 200 mg (equivalent to 155 mg base)

NURSING PROCESS

☑ Assessment
● Assess patient's condition before therapy and regularly thereafter.
● Make sure baseline and periodic ophthalmic examinations are performed. Check periodically for ocular muscle weakness after long-term use.
● Obtain audiometric examinations before, during, and after therapy, especially during long-term therapy.

● Monitor CBC and liver function studies periodically during long-term therapy.
● Assess patient for overdose, which can quickly lead to toxic symptoms, including headache, drowsiness, visual disturbances, CV collapse, and seizures, followed by cardiopulmonary arrest. Children are extremely susceptible to toxicity and shouldn't receive long-term treatment.
● Be alert for adverse reactions and drug interactions.
● Evaluate patient's and family's knowledge of drug therapy.

⊞ Nursing diagnoses
● Infection related to susceptible organisms
● Disturbed sensory perception (visual and auditory) related to adverse reactions to drug
● Deficient knowledge related to drug therapy

▶ Planning and implementation
● Give drug right before or after meals on same day of each week.
● Notify prescriber immediately about severe blood disorder that can't be attributed to disease. Blood reaction may require discontinuation.
Patient teaching
● Advise patient to take drug immediately before or after meals on same day each week to enhance compliance for prophylaxis.
● If adverse CNS or visual disturbances occur, warn patient to avoid hazardous activities.
● Tell patient to promptly report visual or auditory changes.

☑ Evaluation
● Patient is free from infection.
● Patient maintains normal visual and auditory function.
● Patient and family state understanding of drug therapy.

hydroxyurea
(high-droks-ee-yoo-REE-uh)
Droxia, Hydrea

Pharmacologic class: antimetabolite (cell cycle–phase specific, S phase)
Therapeutic class: antineoplastic; antisickling drug
Pregnancy risk category: D

Indications and dosages

Dosage and indications for hydroxyurea may vary. Check current literature for recommended protocol.

▶ **Solid tumors.** *Adults:* 80 mg/kg Hydrea P.O. as a single dose q 3 days; or 20 to 30 mg/kg Hydrea P.O. as a single daily dose.

▶ **Head and neck cancers, excluding the lip.** *Adults:* 80 mg/kg Hydrea P.O. as a single dose q 3 days.

▶ **Resistant chronic myelocytic leukemia.** *Adults:* 20 to 30 mg/kg Hydrea P.O. as a single daily dose.

▶ **To reduce the frequency of painful crises and to reduce the need for blood transfusions in patients with sickle cell anemia with recurrent moderate-to-severe painful crises (generally at least 3 during the preceding 12 months).** *Adults:* Base dosage on the patient's actual or ideal weight, whichever is less. The initial dose is 15 mg/kg Droxia P.O. as a single daily dose. The patient's blood count must be monitored every 2 weeks; see package insert for dosage adjustment.

Contraindications and precautions

● Contraindicated in patients hypersensitive to drug and in those with marked bone marrow depression.
● Use cautiously in patients with renal dysfunction.
⚖ Lifespan: In pregnant and breast-feeding women, drug isn't recommended. In children, safety of drug hasn't been established.

Adverse reactions

CNS: drowsiness, hallucinations, *seizures.*
GI: anorexia, nausea, vomiting, diarrhea, stomatitis.
Hematologic: *leukopenia, thrombocytopenia,* anemia, *megaloblastosis, bone marrow suppression* (dose-limiting and dose-related, with rapid recovery).
Metabolic: hyperuricemia.
Skin: rash, pruritus.

Interactions

Drug-drug. *Cytotoxic drugs, radiation therapy:* May enhance toxicity of hydroxyurea. Use together cautiously.

Effects on lab test results

● May increase BUN, creatinine, and uric acid levels.
● May decrease hemoglobin, hematocrit, and WBC, RBC, and platelet counts.

Pharmacokinetics

Absorption: Well absorbed. Levels is higher with a large, single dose than with divided doses.
Distribution: Crosses blood-brain barrier.
Metabolism: About 50% of dose is degraded in liver.
Excretion: 50% of drug in urine as unchanged drug; metabolites excreted through lungs as carbon dioxide and in urine as urea. *Half-life:* 3 to 4 hours.

Route	Onset	Peak	Duration
P.O.	Unknown	2 hr	Unknown

Action

Chemical effect: Unknown; thought to inhibit DNA synthesis.
Therapeutic effect: Hinders growth of certain cancer cells.

Available forms

Capsules: 200 mg, 300 mg, 400 mg, 500 mg

NURSING PROCESS

⬛ Assessment
● Assess patient's condition before therapy and regularly thereafter.
● Measure CBC, BUN, uric acid, and creatinine levels.
● Auditory and visual hallucinations and hematologic toxicity increase with decreased renal function.
● Radiation therapy may increase risk or severity of GI distress or stomatitis.
● Be alert for adverse reactions and drug interactions.
● Evaluate patient's and family's knowledge of drug therapy.

⬛ Nursing diagnoses
● Ineffective health maintenance related to presence of neoplastic disease
● Ineffective protection related to adverse hematologic reactions
● Deficient knowledge related to drug therapy

Reactions may be *common,* uncommon, *life-threatening,* or COMMON AND LIFE-THREATENING.

⟩⟩ Planning and implementation
- Keep patient hydrated.
- Dosage modification may be needed after chemotherapy or radiation therapy.
- Bone marrow suppression is dose-limited and dose-related with rapid recovery.

Patient teaching
- If patient can't swallow capsules, tell him to empty contents of capsules into water and drink immediately.
- Warn patient to watch for signs of infection (fever, sore throat, fatigue) and bleeding (easy bruising, nosebleeds, bleeding gums, melena). Instruct patient to take infection-control and bleeding precautions. Tell patient to take temperature daily.
- Advise woman of childbearing age to avoid becoming pregnant during therapy and to consult with prescriber before becoming pregnant.

☑ Evaluation
- Patient responds well to drug therapy.
- Serious infections or bleeding complications don't develop.
- Patient and family state understanding of drug therapy.

---

hydroxyzine embonate ◇
(high-DROKS-ih-zeen EM-boh-nayt)
Atarax

hydroxyzine hydrochloride
Anx, Apo-Hydroxyzine ◆, Atarax*, Hydroxacen, Hyzine-50, Multipax ◆, Neucalm, Novo-Hydroxyzin ◆, QYS, Vistacon-50, Vistaject-50, Vistaril

hydroxyzine pamoate
Vistaril

Pharmacologic class: antihistamine (piperazine derivative)
Therapeutic class: anxiolytic, sedative, antipruritic, antiemetic, antispasmodic
Pregnancy risk category: C

Indications and dosages

▶ **Anxiety.** *Adults:* 50 to 100 mg P.O. q.i.d.
Children age 6 and older: 50 to 100 mg P.O. daily in divided doses.

Children younger than age 6: 50 mg P.O. daily in divided doses.
▶ **Preoperative and postoperative adjunct therapy.** *Adults:* 25 to 100 mg I.M. q 4 to 6 hours.
Children: 1.1 mg/kg I.M. q 4 to 6 hours.
▶ **Pruritus from allergies.** *Adults:* 25 mg P.O. t.i.d. or q.i.d.
Children age 6 and older: 50 to 100 mg P.O. daily in divided doses.
Children younger than age 6: 50 mg P.O. daily in divided doses.
▶ **Psychiatric and emotional emergencies, including acute alcoholism.** *Adults:* 50 to 100 mg I.M. q 4 to 6 hours, p.r.n.
▶ **Nausea and vomiting (excluding nausea and vomiting of pregnancy).** *Adults:* 25 to 100 mg I.M.
Children: 1.1 mg/kg I.M.
▶ **Prepartum and postpartum adjunct therapy.** *Adults:* 25 to 100 mg I.M.

Contraindications and precautions

- Contraindicated in patients hypersensitive to drug.
- ⚖ Lifespan: In early pregnancy, drug is contraindicated. In breast-feeding women, safety of drug hasn't been established. In elderly patients, use cautiously and at lower doses.

Adverse reactions

CNS: *drowsiness,* involuntary motor activity.
GI: *dry mouth.*
Other: marked discomfort at I.M. injection site, hypersensitivity reactions (wheezing, dyspnea, chest tightness).

Interactions

Drug-drug. *CNS depressants:* May increase CNS depression. Avoid using together.
MAO inhibitors: May enhance anticholinergic effects. Use together cautiously.
Drug-lifestyle. *Alcohol use:* May increase CNS depression. Discourage using together.
Sun exposure: Photosensitivity may occur. Urge patient to avoid unprotected or prolonged sun exposure.

Effects on lab test results

- Drug may cause false elevations of urine 17-hydroxycorticosteroids, depending on test method used.

Pharmacokinetics

Absorption: Rapid and complete after P.O. administration. Unknown for I.M. administration.
Distribution: Unknown.
Metabolism: Almost complete.
Excretion: Metabolites excreted primarily in urine; small amounts of drug and metabolites excreted in feces. *Half-life:* 3 hours.

Route	Onset	Peak	Duration
P.O.	15-30 min	2 hr	4-6 hr
I.M.	Unknown	Unknown	4-6 hr

Action

Chemical effect: Unknown; may suppress activity in key regions of subcortical area of CNS.
Therapeutic effect: Relieves anxiety and itching, promotes calmness, and alleviates nausea and vomiting.

Available forms

hydroxyzine embonate
Capsules: 25 mg, 50 mg
hydroxyzine hydrochloride
Capsules: 10 mg ♦ ◇ 25 mg ♦ ◇ , 50 mg ♦ ◇
Injection: 25 mg/ml, 50 mg/ml
Syrup: 10 mg/5 ml
Tablets: 10 mg, 25 mg, 50 mg, 100 mg
Tablets (film-coated): 10 mg, 25 mg, 50 mg
hydroxyzine pamoate
Capsules: 25 mg, 50 mg, 100 mg
Oral suspension: 25 mg/5 ml

NURSING PROCESS

🔲 Assessment

• Assess patient's condition before therapy and regularly thereafter.
• Be alert for adverse reactions and drug interactions.
• Evaluate patient's and family's knowledge of drug therapy.

🔲 Nursing diagnoses

• Ineffective health maintenance related to underlying condition
• Risk for injury related to adverse CNS reactions
• Deficient knowledge related to drug therapy

🔲 Planning and implementation

• Reduce dosage in elderly and debilitated patients.

• Parenteral form (hydroxyzine hydrochloride) for I.M. use only; Z-track injection method is preferred. Aspirate I.M. injection carefully to prevent inadvertent intravascular injection. Inject deep into large muscle mass.
🔮 **ALERT:** Never give I.V.
🔮 **ALERT:** Don't confuse hydroxyzine with hydralazine.

Patient teaching
• Warn patient to avoid hazardous activities until CNS effects of drug are known.
• Tell patient to avoid alcohol during drug therapy.
• Suggest sugarless hard candy or gum to relieve dry mouth.

🔲 Evaluation

• Patient exhibits improved health.
• Patient doesn't experience injury.
• Patient and family state understanding of drug therapy.

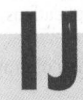

ibuprofen

(igh-byoo-PROH-fen)
ACT-3 ◇ , **Advil**†, **Advil Children's, Advil Infants' Drops**†, **Advil Liqui-Gels**†, **Advil Migraine**†, **Apo-Ibuprofen** ♦ , **Brufen** ◇ , **Genpril Caplets**†, **Genpril Tablets**†, **Haltran**†, **IBU**†, **Ibu-Tab**†, **Junior Strength Motrin**†, **Menadol, Midol Cramp**†, **Midol IB, Motrin, Motrin Children's**†, **Motrin Drops**†, **Motrin IB Caplets**†, **Motrin IB Gelcaps**†, **Motrin IB Tablets**†, **Motrin Infants' Drops**†, **Motrin Migraine Pain Caplets**†, **Novo-Profen** ♦ , **Nurofen** ♦ , **Rafen** ◇ , **Saleto-200**

Pharmacologic class: NSAID
Therapeutic class: nonopioid analgesic, antipyretic, anti-inflammatory
Pregnancy risk category: B

Indications and dosages

▶ **Rheumatoid arthritis, osteoarthritis.**
Adults: 300 to 800 mg P.O. t.i.d. or q.i.d. not to exceed 3.2 g P.O. daily.

Children: 20 to 40 mg/kg P.O. daily, divided into 3 to 4 doses.

▶ **Mild to moderate pain, dysmenorrhea.**
Adults: 400 mg P.O. q 4 to 6 hours, p.r.n.
Children ages 6 months to 12 years: 10 mg/kg/dose P.O. q 6 to 8 hours; maximum, 40 mg/kg daily.

▶ **Fever.** *Adults and children older than age 12:* 200 to 400 mg P.O. q 4 to 6 hours, p.r.n. Don't exceed 1.2 g P.O. daily or give for longer than 3 days.
Children ages 6 months to 12 years: If temperature is below 102.5° F (39.2° C), recommended dosage is 5 mg/kg P.O. q 6 to 8 hours, p.r.n. Treat higher temperatures with 10 mg/kg P.O. q 6 to 8 hours, p.r.n., to maximum dosage of 40 mg/kg daily.

Contraindications and precautions

● Contraindicated in patients hypersensitive to drug and in those with syndrome of nasal polyps, angioedema, and bronchospastic reactivity to aspirin or other NSAIDs.
● Use cautiously in patients with GI disorders, history of peptic ulcer disease, hepatic or renal disease, cardiac decompensation, hypertension, or intrinsic coagulation defects.
⚜ Lifespan: In pregnant and breast-feeding women, drug isn't recommended. In infants younger than age 6 months, safety and effectiveness of drug haven't been established.

Adverse reactions

CNS: *headache, drowsiness, dizziness,* cognitive dysfunction, aseptic meningitis.
CV: *peripheral edema,* edema, hypertension, **heart failure.**
EENT: visual disturbances, *tinnitus.*
GI: *epigastric distress, nausea, occult blood loss, peptic ulceration.*
GU: *reversible renal failure.*
Hematologic: prolonged bleeding time, anemia, **neutropenia, pancytopenia, thrombocytopenia, aplastic anemia, leukopenia, agranulocytosis.**
Respiratory: *bronchospasm.*
Skin: pruritus, rash, urticaria, photosensitivity reactions, *Stevens-Johnson syndrome.*

Interactions

Drug-drug. *Antihypertensives, furosemide, thiazide diuretics:* May decrease effectiveness of diuretics or antihypertensives. Monitor patient.

Aspirin: May decrease drug level and increase risk of adverse GI reactions. Avoid using together.
Corticosteroids: May increase risk of adverse GI reactions. Avoid using together.
Cyclosporine: May increase nephrotoxicity of both drugs. Avoid using together.
Digoxin: May increase digoxin levels. Monitor levels closely for digoxin toxicity.
Lithium, oral anticoagulants: May increase levels or effects of these drugs. Monitor patient for toxicity.
Methotrexate: May increase risk of methotrexate toxicity. Monitor patient closely.
Probenecid: Probenecid may increase level and toxicity of NSAIDs. Monitor patient for signs of toxicity.
Drug-herb. *Dong quai, feverfew, garlic, ginger, horse chestnut, red clover:* May increase risk of bleeding. Monitor patient closely for bleeding.
St. John's wort: May increase risk of photosensitivity reactions. Advise patient to avoid unprotected or prolonged exposure to sunlight.
Drug-lifestyle. *Alcohol use:* May increase risk of adverse GI reactions. Discourage using together.
Smoking: May increase risk for gastric ulceration. Discourage using together.
Sun exposure: May cause photosensitivity reactions. Advise patient to avoid unprotected or prolonged exposure to sunlight.

Effects on lab test results

● May increase BUN, creatinine, ALT, AST, and potassium levels. May decrease glucose level.
● May decrease hemoglobin, hematocrit, and neutrophil, WBC, RBC, platelet, and granulocyte counts.

Pharmacokinetics

Absorption: Rapid and complete from GI tract.
Distribution: Highly protein-bound.
Metabolism: Undergoes biotransformation in liver.
Excretion: Mainly in urine, with some biliary excretion. *Half-life:* 2 to 4 hours.

Route	Onset	Peak	Duration
P.O.	≤ 30 min	2-4 hr	≥ 4 hr

Action

Chemical effect: Unknown; produces anti-inflammatory, analgesic, and antipyretic effects, possibly by inhibiting prostaglandin synthesis.
Therapeutic effect: Relieves pain, fever, and inflammation.

Available forms

Caplets: 200 mg†
Capsules (liquid-filled): 200 mg†
Oral drops: 40 mg/ml†
Oral suspension: 100 mg/5 ml†
Tablets: 100 mg†, 200 mg†, 400 mg, 600 mg, 800 mg
Tablets (chewable): 50 mg†, 100 mg†
Tablets (film-coated): 100 mg†, 200 mg†, 400 mg, 600 mg, 800 mg

NURSING PROCESS

▧ Assessment
• Assess patient's underlying condition before starting drug therapy.
• Evaluate patient for relief from pain, fever, or inflammation. Full effects on arthritis may take 2 to 4 weeks.
• Check renal and hepatic function periodically in long-term therapy.
• Be alert for adverse reactions and drug interactions.
• Evaluate patient's and family's knowledge of drug therapy.

▧ Nursing diagnoses
• Chronic pain related to underlying condition
• Risk for injury related to drug-induced adverse reactions
• Deficient knowledge related to drug therapy

▧ Planning and implementation
• Give with meals or milk to reduce adverse GI reactions.
• If drug is ineffective, notify prescriber.
• If renal or hepatic abnormalities occur, stop drug and notify prescriber.
Patient teaching
• Tell patient to take drug with meals or milk to reduce adverse GI reactions.
• **ALERT:** Tell patient not to exceed 1.2 g daily, not to give drug to children younger than age 12, and not to take drug for extended periods without consulting prescriber.

• Warn patient that using drug with aspirin, alcohol, or corticosteroids may increase risk of adverse GI reactions.
• Serious GI toxicity, including peptic ulceration and bleeding, can occur in patients taking NSAIDs despite absence of GI symptoms.
• Teach patient to recognize and report signs and symptoms of GI bleeding.
• Instruct patient to avoid alcohol during therapy.
• Instruct patient to use sunblock, wear protective clothing, and avoid prolonged exposure to sunlight.

▧ Evaluation
• Patient is free from pain.
• Patient doesn't experience injury from adverse reactions.
• Patient and family state understanding of drug therapy.

ibutilide fumarate
(igh-BYOO-tih-lighd FYOO-muh-rayt)
Corvert

Pharmacologic class: ibutilide derivative
Therapeutic class: class III antiarrhythmic
Pregnancy risk category: C

Indications and dosages

▶ **Rapid conversion of recent atrial fibrillation or atrial flutter to sinus rhythm.** *Adults weighing 60 kg (132 lb) or more:* 1 mg I.V. over 10 minutes.
Adults weighing less than 60 kg: 0.01 mg/kg I.V. over 10 minutes.

▽ I.V. administration
• Give undiluted or diluted in 50 ml of diluent. Add to normal saline solution for injection or D_5W injection before infusion. Add contents of one 10-ml vial (0.1 mg/ml) to a 50-ml infusion bag to form admixture of about 0.017 mg/ml ibutilide fumarate. Use strict aseptic technique. Drug is compatible with polyvinyl chloride plastic bags and polyolefin bags.
• Admixtures with approved diluents are chemically and physically stable for 24 hours at room temperature or 48 hours if refrigerated.
• Inspect parenteral drugs for particles and discoloration before giving.

⏹ ALERT: Stop infusion if arrhythmia stops or if patient develops sustained or nonsustained ventricular tachycardia or significantly prolonged QT interval. If arrhythmia doesn't stop within 10 minutes after infusion ends, give a second 10-minute infusion of equal strength.

Contraindications and precautions

• Contraindicated in patients hypersensitive to drug or its components.

• Drug isn't recommended for use in patients with history of polymorphic ventricular tachycardia, such as torsades de pointes.

• Use cautiously in patients with hepatic or renal dysfunction (usually, no dosage adjustments are needed).

⚠ **Lifespan:** In pregnant women, use cautiously. In breast-feeding women and in children, safety of drug hasn't been established.

Adverse reactions

CNS: headache.
CV: ventricular extrasystoles, *nonsustained ventricular tachycardia*, hypotension, bundle branch block, *sustained polymorphic ventricular tachycardia*, *AV block*, hypertension, QT interval prolongation, *bradycardia*, palpitations, tachycardia.
GI: nausea.

Interactions

Drug-drug. *Class IA antiarrhythmics (such as disopyramide, procainamide, quinidine), other class III drugs (such as amiodarone, sotalol):* May increase risk of prolonged refractory state. Avoid using together.
Digoxin: Supraventricular arrhythmias may mask cardiotoxicity from excessive digoxin levels. Use cautiously.
H₁-receptor antagonist antihistamines, phenothiazines, tetracyclic antidepressants, tricyclic antidepressants, other drugs that prolong QT interval: May increase risk of proarrhythmias. Monitor patient closely.

Effects on lab test results

None reported.

Pharmacokinetics

Absorption: Administered I.V.
Distribution: Highly distributed; about 40% protein-bound.
Metabolism: Not clearly defined.

Excretion: Excreted in urine and feces. *Half-life:* Averages about 6 hours.

Route	Onset	Peak	Duration
I.V.	Unknown	Unknown	Unknown

Action

Chemical effect: Prolongs action potential in isolated cardiac myocyte and increases atrial and ventricular refractoriness; has predominantly class III properties.
Therapeutic effect: Restores normal sinus rhythm.

Available forms

Injection: 0.1 mg/ml

NURSING PROCESS

⚕ Assessment
• Assess patient's arrhythmia before therapy.
⏹ ALERT: Monitor ECG continuously during therapy and for at least 4 hours afterward (or until QT interval returns to baseline) because drug can induce or worsen ventricular arrhythmias. If ECG shows arrhythmic activity, monitor longer.
• Be alert for adverse reactions and drug interactions.
• Evaluate patient's and family's knowledge of drug therapy.

⬚ Nursing diagnoses
• Decreased cardiac output related to arrhythmias
• Risk for injury related to life-threatening arrhythmias
• Deficient knowledge related to drug therapy

▶ Planning and implementation
• Drug should only be given by skilled personnel. During and after administration, have proper equipment and facilities, such as cardiac monitoring, intracardiac pacing, cardioverter/defibrillator, and medication for treatment of sustained ventricular tachycardia, available.
• Correct hypokalemia and hypomagnesemia before therapy to reduce risk of proarrhythmia.
Patient teaching
• Tell patient to promptly report adverse reactions, especially headaches, dizziness, weakness, palpitations, or chest pains.

• Instruct patient to report any discomfort at injection site.

☑ Evaluation

• Patient regains normal sinus rhythm.
• Life-threatening arrhythmia doesn't develop.
• Patient and family state understanding of drug therapy.

idarubicin hydrochloride
(igh-duh-ROO-bih-sin high-droh-KLOR-ighd)
Idamycin, Idamycin PFS

Pharmacologic class: anthracycline antibiotic
Therapeutic class: antineoplastic
Pregnancy risk category: D

Indications and dosages

▶ **Acute myeloid leukemia, including French-American-British classifications M1 through M7, with other approved antileukemic drugs.** *Adults:* 12 mg/m² by slow I.V. injection (over 10 to 15 minutes) daily for 3 days with 100 mg/m² of cytarabine by continuous I.V. infusion daily for 7 days or cytarabine as 25-mg/m² bolus followed by 200 mg/m² by continuous infusion daily for 5 days. Give second course, if needed. If patient develops severe mucositis, don't give until recovery is complete, and reduce dosage by 25%.

🔲 **Adjust-a-dose:** For patients with hepatic or renal impairment, reduce dosage. If bilirubin level is above 5 mg/dl, withhold drug.

▽ I.V. administration

• Follow facility policy to reduce risks. Preparation and administration of parenteral form are linked to carcinogenic, mutagenic, and teratogenic risks for personnel.
• Reconstitute to final concentration of 1 mg/ml using normal saline solution for injection. Add 5 ml to 5-mg vial or 10 ml to 10-mg vial. Don't use bacteriostatic saline solution. Vial is under negative pressure.
• Give over 10 to 15 minutes into free-flowing I.V. infusion of normal saline solution or D₅W that is running into large vein. If extravasation occurs, stop infusion immediately, elevate limb, and notify prescriber. Treat with intermittent ice packs—30 minutes immediately and then 30 minutes q.i.d. for 4 days.

• Reconstituted solutions are stable for 72 hours at 59° to 86°F (15° to 30°C), 7 days if refrigerated. Label unused solutions with chemotherapy hazard label.

Contraindications and precautions

• No known contraindications.
• Use cautiously in patients with bone marrow suppression induced by previous drug therapy or radiotherapy and in patients with impaired hepatic or renal function or pre-existing heart disease and previous therapy with anthracyclines at high cumulative doses or other potentially cardiotoxic drugs.
⚠ **Lifespan:** In pregnant and breast-feeding women, drug isn't recommended. In children, safety of drug hasn't been established.

Adverse reactions

CNS: *fever,* headache, changed mental status, peripheral neuropathy, *seizures.*
CV: *heart failure,* atrial fibrillation, chest pain, *MI, myocardial insufficiency, arrhythmias,* HEMORRHAGE, *myocardial toxicity.*
GI: *nausea, vomiting,* cramps, diarrhea, *mucositis, severe enterocolitis with perforation.*
Hematologic: MYELOSUPPRESSION.
Skin: alopecia, rash, urticaria, bullous erythrodermatous rash on palms and soles, urticaria at injection site, erythema at previously irradiated sites, tissue necrosis at injection site if extravasation occurs.
Other: INFECTION.

Interactions

Drug-drug. *Alkaline solutions, heparin:* Incompatible. Don't mix idarubicin with other drugs unless specific compatibility data are available.

Effects on lab test results

• May increase BUN and creatinine levels.
• May increase liver function test results. May decrease hemoglobin, hematocrit, and RBC, WBC, and platelet counts.

Pharmacokinetics

Absorption: Administered I.V.
Distribution: 97% lipophilic and tissue-bound, with highest levels in nucleated blood and bone marrow cells.
Metabolism: Extensively outside of liver. Metabolite has cytotoxic activity.

Reactions may be *common,* uncommon, *life-threatening,* or COMMON AND LIFE-THREATENING.

Excretion: Primarily biliary, minimal renal.
Half-life: 20 to 22 hours.

Route	Onset	Peak	Duration
I.V.	Unknown	≤ 3 min	Unknown

Action

Chemical effect: May inhibit nucleic acid synthesis by intercalation; interacts with enzyme topoisomerase II.
Therapeutic effect: Hinders growth of susceptible cancer cells.

Available forms

Powder for injection: 1 mg/ml available in 5-, 10-, and 20-mg vials

NURSING PROCESS

⬛ Assessment

• Assess patient's condition before therapy and regularly thereafter.
• Assess patient for systemic infection, and control infection before therapy begins.
• Monitor CBC and hepatic and renal function test results frequently.
• Be alert for adverse reactions and drug interactions, especially signs of heart failure.
• Evaluate patient's and family's knowledge of drug therapy.

⬛ Nursing diagnoses

• Ineffective health maintenance related to presence of underlying condition
• Ineffective protection related to adverse hematologic reactions
• Deficient knowledge related to drug therapy

⬛ Planning and implementation

• Take appropriate preventive measures (including adequate hydration) before starting treatment.
⊛ ALERT: Don't confuse idarubicin with daunorubicin.
⊛ ALERT: Never give drug I.M. or S.C.
• Hyperuricemia may result from rapid destruction of leukemic cells. Give allopurinol.
Patient teaching
• Teach patient to recognize and report signs of extravasation, infection, bleeding, and heart failure, such as shortness of breath and leg swelling.

• Advise patient that red urine for several days is normal and doesn't indicate blood in urine.
• Advise women of child-bearing age to use a reliable contraceptive during therapy and to consult with prescriber before becoming pregnant.

⬛ Evaluation

• Patient responds well to drug.
• Serious adverse hematologic reactions don't develop.
• Patient and family state understanding of drug therapy.

ifosfamide
(igh-FOHS-fuh-mighd)
IFEX

Pharmacologic class: alkylating drug (cell-cycle–phase nonspecific)
Therapeutic class: antineoplastic
Pregnancy risk category: D

Indications and dosages

▶ **Testicular cancer.** *Adults:* 1.2 g/m² I.V. daily for 5 consecutive days. Repeat q 3 weeks or after patient recovers from hematologic toxicity.
▶ **Lung cancer, Hodgkin's and malignant lymphoma, breast cancer, acute lymphocytic leukemia, ovarian cancer, gastric cancer, pancreatic cancer, sarcomas, cervical cancer, and uterine cancer‡.** *Adults:* 1.2 to 2.5 g/m² I.V. daily for 3 to 5 days, with cycles of therapy repeated p.r.n.

▽ I.V. administration

• Follow facility policy to reduce risks. Preparation and administration of parenteral form are linked to carcinogenic, mutagenic, and teratogenic risks for personnel.
• Reconstitute each gram of drug with 20 ml of diluent to yield 50 mg/ml. Use sterile water for injection or bacteriostatic water for injection. Solutions may be further diluted with sterile water, dextrose 2.5% or 5% in water, half-normal or normal saline solution for injection, D₅W and normal saline solution for injection, or lactated Ringer's injection.
• Infuse each dose over at least 30 minutes.
• Ifosfamide and mesna are physically compatible and may be mixed in same I.V. solution.

Rapid onset *Liquid form contains alcohol. ◆Canada ◇ Australia †OTC ‡Off-label use

● Reconstituted solution is stable for 1 week at room temperature or 6 weeks if refrigerated. If drug was reconstituted with sterile water, however, use solution within 6 hours.

Contraindications and precautions

● Contraindicated in patients hypersensitive to drug and in those with severely depressed bone marrow function.

● Use cautiously in patients with renal impairment or compromised bone marrow from leukopenia, granulocytopenia, extensive bone marrow metastases, previous radiation therapy, or previous therapy with cytotoxic drugs.

⚠ Lifespan: In pregnant and breast-feeding women, drug is contraindicated. In children, safety of drug hasn't been established.

Adverse reactions

CNS: *lethargy, somnolence, confusion, depressive psychosis,* **coma, seizures,** *ataxia.*
GI: *nausea, vomiting.*
GU: *hemorrhagic cystitis* (dose-limiting, occurring in up to 50% of patients), *hematuria,* **nephrotoxicity.**
Hematologic: *leukopenia, thrombocytopenia, myelosuppression.*
Skin: *alopecia.*

Interactions

Drug-drug. *Anticoagulants, aspirin:* May increase risk of bleeding. Avoid using together.
Barbiturates, chloral hydrate, phenytoin: May increase ifosfamide toxicity by inducing hepatic enzymes that hasten formation of toxic metabolites. Monitor patient closely.
Mesna: May decrease ifosfamide-induced bladder toxicity. Consult prescriber about using together.
Myelosuppressants: May enhance hematologic toxicity. Dosage adjustment may be needed.

Effects on lab test results

● May increase BUN, creatinine, bilirubin, and liver enzyme levels.
● May decrease hemoglobin, hematocrit, and WBC, RBC, and platelet counts.

Pharmacokinetics

Absorption: Administered I.V.
Distribution: Crosses blood-brain barrier but its metabolites don't; therefore, alkylating activity doesn't occur in CSF.

Metabolism: About 50% of dose is metabolized in liver.
Excretion: Primarily in urine. *Half-life:* About 14 hours.

Route	Onset	Peak	Duration
I.V.	Unknown	Unknown	Unknown

Action

Chemical effect: Cross-links strands of cellular DNA and interferes with RNA transcription, which causes growth imbalance that leads to cell death.
Therapeutic effect: Kills cancer cells.

Available forms

Injection: 1 g (supplied with 200-mg ampule of mesna), 3 g (supplied with 400-mg ampule of mesna)

NURSING PROCESS

▓ Assessment

● Assess patient's condition before therapy and regularly thereafter.
● Obtain urinalysis before each dose. If microscopic hematuria is present, evaluate patient for hemorrhagic cystitis. Adjust dosage of mesna, a protecting agent given with drug, if needed.
● Monitor CBC and renal and liver function test results.
● Be alert for adverse reactions and drug interactions.
● Assess patient for mental status changes; dosage may need to be decreased.
● Evaluate patient's and family's knowledge of drug therapy.

▓ Nursing diagnoses

● Ineffective health maintenance related to presence of cancer
● Ineffective protection related to adverse CNS and hematologic reactions
● Deficient knowledge related to drug therapy

▓ Planning and implementation

● Give antiemetic before giving drug to decrease nausea.
● Give drug with mesna to prevent hemorrhagic cystitis. Give mesna with or before drug to prevent cystitis. Give at least 2 L of fluids daily, either P.O. or I.V.

Reactions may be *common,* uncommon, *life-threatening,* or COMMON AND LIFE-THREATENING.

⊛ **ALERT:** Don't confuse ifosfamide with cyclophosphamide.
• Don't give drug h.s.; infrequent voiding at night may increase risk of cystitis. If cystitis develops, stop drug and notify prescriber.
• Bladder irrigation with normal saline solution may decrease possibility of cystitis.
• Institute infection-control and bleeding precautions.

Patient teaching
• Tell patient to void frequently to minimize contact of drug and its metabolites with bladder mucosa.
• Warn patient to watch for evidence of infection (fever, sore throat, fatigue), CNS effects (somnolence and dizziness), and bleeding (easy bruising, nosebleeds, bleeding gums, melena). Teach patient about infection-control and bleeding precautions, and tell him to report adverse effects. Tell him to take his temperature daily.
• Instruct patient to avoid OTC drugs that contain aspirin.
• Stress importance of adequate fluid intake. Explain that it may help prevent hemorrhagic cystitis.
• Warn patient that hyperpigmentation may occur.

☑ **Evaluation**
• Patient responds well to drug.
• Serious infections and CNS and bleeding complications don't develop.
• Patient and family state understanding of drug therapy.

imatinib mesylate
(i-MAH-tin-nib MES-uh-late)
Gleevec

Pharmacologic class: protein-tyrosine kinase inhibitor
Therapeutic class: antineoplastic
Pregnancy risk category: D

Indications and dosages

▶ **Chronic myeloid leukemia (CML) in blast crisis, in accelerated phase, or in chronic phase after failure of interferon-alpha therapy; newly diagnosed Philadelphia chromosome–positive chronic-phase CML.** *Adults:* For chronic-phase CML, 400 mg P.O.

daily as single dose with a meal and large glass of water. For accelerated-phase CML or blast crisis, 600 mg P.O. daily as single dose with a meal and large glass of water. Continue treatment as long as patient continues to benefit. May increase daily dose to 600 mg P.O. in chronic phase or to 800 mg P.O. (400 mg P.O. b.i.d.) in accelerated phase or blast crisis. Increase dosage only if there is an absence of severe adverse reactions and absence of severe non–leukemia-related neutropenia or thrombocytopenia in the following circumstances: disease progression (at any time), failure to achieve a satisfactory hematologic response after at least 3 months of treatment, or loss of a previously achieved hematologic response.
▶ **Patients with Kit (CD117) positive unresectable or metastatic malignant GI stromal tumors (GIST).** *Adults:* 400 or 600 mg P.O. daily.
▶ **Philadelphia chromosome–positive chronic-phase CML in patients whose disease has recurred after stem cell transplant or who are resistant to interferon-alpha therapy.** *Children age 3 and older:* 260 mg/m² P.O. as single daily dose or divided into two doses, taken with a meal and large glass of water. May increase dosage to 340 mg/m² daily.
◩ **Adjust-a-dose:** For severe nonhematologic adverse reactions (severe hepatotoxicity or severe fluid retention), withhold drug until resolved; resume treatment based on initial severity of reaction. For patient with bilirubin level higher than three times the institutional upper limit of normal (IULN) or liver transaminase levels higher than five times IULN, withhold drug until bilirubin level returns to less than 1½ IULN and transaminase levels to less than 2½ IULN. Then, resume drug at reduced daily dose. (Adult dosages can be decreased from 400 mg to 300 mg or from 600 mg to 400 mg. Children's dosages can be decreased from 260 mg/m² daily to 200 mg/m² daily or from 340 mg/m² daily to 260 mg/m² daily.)
For severe hematologic reactions in patients with chronic-phase CML (starting dose 400 mg or 260 mg/m² in children) or GIST (starting dose 400 mg) and an absolute neutrophil count (ANC) less than 1 × 10⁹/L or platelets less than 50 x 10⁹/L, take these steps:
1. Stop drug until ANC is 1.5 × 10⁹/L or greater and platelets are 75 × 10⁹/L or greater.

2. Resume treatment at original starting dose of 400 mg or 600 mg, or 260 mg/m^2 in children.
3. If recurrence of ANC less than 1 × 10^9/L, and/or platelets less than 50 × 10^9/L, repeat step 1 and resume drug at reduced dose (300 mg if starting dose was 400 mg; 400 mg if starting dose was 600 mg; or in children, 200 mg/m^2 if starting dose was 260 mg/m^2).

For severe hematologic reactions in patients with accelerated phase CML and blast crisis or GIST (starting dose 600 mg) and ANC less than 0.5 × 10^9/L and/or platelets less than 10 × 10^9/L occurring after at least 1 month of treatment, take these steps:
1. Check if cytopenia is related to leukemia via marrow aspirate or biopsy.
2. If cytopenia is unrelated to leukemia, reduce dose of drug to 400 mg.
3. If cytopenia persists 2 weeks, reduce further to 300 mg.
4. If cytopenia persists 4 weeks and is still unrelated to leukemia, stop Gleevec until ANC is 1 × 10^9/L or greater and platelets are 20 × 10^9/L or greater and then resume treatment at 300 mg.

Contraindications and precautions

• Contraindicated in patients hypersensitive to drug or its components.
• Use cautiously in hepatically impaired patients.
≋ Lifespan: In pregnant and breast-feeding women, avoid using drug. It's unknown whether drug appears in breast milk. In children younger than age 3, safety of drug hasn't been established. In elderly patients, use cautiously because they may have an increased risk of edema when taking drug.

Adverse reactions

CNS: *headache,* CEREBRAL HEMORRHAGE, *fatigue, weakness, fever.*
CV: *edema.*
EENT: *nasopharyngitis, epistaxis.*
GI: *anorexia, nausea, diarrhea, abdominal pain, constipation, vomiting, dyspepsia,* GI HEMORRHAGE.
Hematologic: HEMORRHAGE, NEUTROPENIA, THROMBOCYTOPENIA, *anemia.*
Metabolic: *hypokalemia,* weight increase.
Musculoskeletal: *myalgia, muscle cramps, musculoskeletal pain, arthralgia.*

Respiratory: *cough, dyspnea, pneumonia.*
Skin: *rash,* pruritus, *petechiae.*
Other: *night sweats.*

Interactions

Drug-drug. *Acetaminophen:* May increase risk of liver toxicity. Monitor patient.
CYP 3A4 inhibitors (clarithromycin, erythromycin, itraconazole, ketoconazole): May decrease metabolism and increase imatinib level. Monitor patient for toxicity.
CYP 3A4 inducers (carbamazepine, dexamethasone, phenobarbital, phenytoin, rifampin): May increase metabolism and decrease imatinib level. Use cautiously.
Dihydropyridine calcium channel blockers, certain HMG-CoA reductase inhibitors, cyclosporine, pimozide, triazolo-benzodiazepines: May increase levels of these drugs. Monitor patient for toxicity and obtain levels.
Warfarin: May alter metabolism of warfarin. Avoid use together; instead, use standard heparin or a low–molecular-weight heparin.
Drug-herb. *St. John's wort:* May decrease drug effects. Warn patient not to use together.

Effects on lab test results

• May increase creatinine, bilirubin, alkaline phosphatase, AST, and ALT levels. May decrease potassium level.
• May decrease hemoglobin, hematocrit, and neutrophil and platelet counts.

Pharmacokinetics

Absorption: Well absorbed.
Distribution: 98% protein-bound.
Metabolism: Primarily by CYP 3A4.
Excretion: Primarily in feces as metabolites.
Half-life: 18 to 40 hours.

Route	Onset	Peak	Duration
P.O.	Unknown	2-4 hr	Unknown

Action

Chemical effect: Inhibits Bcr-Abl tyrosine kinase, which is the abnormal tyrosine kinase created in CML; in vivo, it inhibits tumor growth of Bcr-Abl–transfected murine myeloid cells and Bcr-Abl–positive leukemia lines derived from CML patients in blast crisis.
Therapeutic effect: Stops tumor growth.

Reactions may be *common,* uncommon, ***life-threatening,*** or COMMON AND LIFE-THREATENING.

Available forms

Capsules: 50 mg, 100 mg
Tablets: 100 mg, 400 mg

NURSING PROCESS

🖊 Assessment

• Assess neoplastic disease before therapy and reassess regularly.
• Obtain baseline weight before beginning therapy then weigh patient daily. Evaluate and treat unexpected and rapid weight gain.
• Evaluate patient's and family's knowledge of drug therapy.
• Monitor patient closely for fluid retention, which can be severe.
• Monitor CBC weekly for first month, then monitor biweekly for second month, and periodically thereafter.
• Monitor liver function test results carefully because severe hepatotoxicity may occur; decrease dosage as needed.
• Because the long-term safety of this drug isn't known, monitor renal and liver toxicity and immunosuppression carefully.

🔟 Nursing diagnoses

• Ineffective health maintenance related to neoplastic disease
• Risk for falls related to drug-induced adverse reactions
• Deficient knowledge related to drug therapy

▶ Planning and implementation

• For CML, increase dosage only if there is an absence of severe adverse reactions and absence of severe non–leukemia-related neutropenia or thrombocytopenia in these circumstances: disease progression (at any time), failure to achieve a satisfactory hematologic response after at least 3 months of treatment, or loss of a previously achieved hematologic response.
• Because GI irritation is common, give drug with food.
Patient teaching
• Instruct patient to take drug with food and a large glass of water.
• Urge patient to report any adverse effects, such as fluid retention, to prescriber.
• Advise patient to have periodic liver and kidney function tests and blood work to determine blood counts.

• Tell patient to avoid OTC products with acetaminophen.

☑ Evaluation

• Patient shows positive response to drug therapy on follow-up studies.
• Patient doesn't experience falls.
• Patient and family state understanding of drug therapy.

imipenem and cilastatin sodium
(im-ih-PEN-em and sigh-luh-STAT-in SO-dee-um)
Primaxin IM, Primaxin IV

Pharmacologic class: carbapenem (thienamycin class); beta-lactam antibiotic
Therapeutic class: antibiotic
Pregnancy risk category: C

Indications and dosages

▶ **Mild to moderate lower respiratory tract, skin, skin-structure, intra-abdominal, and gynecologic infections; serious lower respiratory and urinary tract, intra-abdominal, and gynecologic infections; bacterial septicemia; bone and joint infections; serious soft-tissue infections; endocarditis; polymicrobic infections.** *Adults weighing at least 70 kg (154 lb):* 500 to 750 mg I.M. q 12 hours. Or, 250 mg to 1 g I.V. q 6 to 8 hours. Maximum I.V. dosage is 50 mg/kg or 4 g daily, whichever is less.
Children age 3 months and older: 15 to 25 mg/kg I.V. q 6 hours. Maximum dosage for fully susceptible organisms is 2 g daily and for moderately susceptible organisms, 4 g daily (based on adult studies).
Infants ages 4 weeks to 3 months and weighing at least 1.5 kg (3.3 lb): 25 mg/kg I.V. q 6 hours.
Neonates ages 1 to 4 weeks and weighing at least 1.5 kg: 25 mg/kg I.V. q 8 hours.
Neonates younger than 1 week and weighing at least 1.5 kg: 25 mg/kg I.V. q 12 hours.
▧ **Adjust-a-dose:** For patients who weigh less than 70 kg (154 lb), give lower dose or use longer intervals between doses if needed.
For patients with renal impairment, if creatinine clearance is 6 to 20 ml/minute, give 125 to 250 mg I.V. q 12 hours. If creatinine clearance is less then 5 ml/minute, withhold drug unless hemodialysis is instituted within 48 hours.

▽I.V. administration

• When reconstituting powder, shake until solution is clear. Solutions may range from colorless to yellow, and variations of color within this range don't affect drug's potency. After reconstitution, solution is stable for 10 hours at room temperature and for 48 hours when refrigerated.
• Don't give drug by direct I.V. bolus injection. Give 250- or 500-mg dose by I.V. infusion over 20 to 30 minutes. Infuse each 1-g dose over 40 to 60 minutes. If nausea occurs, slow infusion.

Contraindications and precautions

• Contraindicated in patients hypersensitive to drug.
• Use cautiously in patients allergic to penicillins or cephalosporins, and in those with history of seizure disorders, especially if they also have compromised renal function.
⚘ Lifespan: In pregnant and breast-feeding women, use cautiously. In children younger than age 12, I.M. safety and effectiveness haven't been established. In children with CNS infections, I.V. use isn't recommended because of risk of seizures; in children weighing less than 30 kg (66 lb) with renal impairment, use also isn't recommended. In elderly patients, use cautiously because they may have decreased renal function.

Adverse reactions

CNS: *seizures,* dizziness, somnolence, fever.
CV: hypotension, thrombophlebitis.
GI: nausea, vomiting, diarrhea, *pseudomembranous colitis.*
Skin: rash, urticaria, pruritus.
Other: *hypersensitivity reactions (anaphylaxis),* pain at injection site.

Interactions

Drug-drug. *Beta-lactam antibiotics:* May cause in vitro antagonism. Avoid use together.
Cyclosporine: May increase adverse CNS effects of both drugs, possibly because of additive or synergistic toxicity. Avoid use together.
Ganciclovir: May cause seizures. Avoid use together.
Probenecid: May increase cilastatin levels. Avoid use together.

Effects on lab test results

• May increase BUN, creatinine, ALT, AST, alkaline phosphatase, bilirubin, and LDH levels.
• May increase eosinophil count. May decrease hemoglobin, hematocrit, and WBC and platelet counts.

Pharmacokinetics

Absorption: Imipenem is about 75% bioavailable; cilastatin is about 95% bioavailable.
Distribution: Rapid and wide. About 20% of imipenem is protein-bound; 40% of cilastatin is protein-bound.
Metabolism: Imipenem is metabolized by kidney dehydropeptidase I, resulting in low urine levels. Cilastatin inhibits this enzyme, thereby reducing imipenem metabolism.
Excretion: About 70% excreted unchanged by kidneys. *Half-life:* 1 hour after I.V. dose; 2 to 3 hours after I.M. dose.

Route	Onset	Peak	Duration
I.V.	Unknown	Immediate	Unknown
I.M.	Unknown	1-2 hr	Unknown

Action

Chemical effect: Imipenem is bactericidal and inhibits bacterial cell wall synthesis. Cilastatin inhibits enzymatic breakdown of imipenem in kidneys, making it effective in urinary tract.
Therapeutic effect: Kills susceptible organisms, including many gram-positive, gram-negative, and anaerobic bacteria.

Available forms

Powder for I.M. injection: 500- and 750-mg vials
Powder for I.V. injection: 250- and 500-mg vials

NURSING PROCESS

◼ Assessment

• Assess patient's infection before therapy and regularly thereafter.
• Obtain urine specimen for culture and sensitivity tests before first dose. Therapy may begin pending results.
• Be alert for adverse reactions and drug interactions.
• If adverse GI reactions occur, monitor patient's hydration status.

- Evaluate patient's and family's knowledge of drug therapy.

◘ Nursing diagnoses
- Infection related to presence of susceptible organisms
- Risk for deficient fluid volume related to adverse GI reactions
- Deficient knowledge related to drug therapy

⊠ Planning and implementation
- Reconstitute drug for I.M. injection with 1% lidocaine hydrochloride (without epinephrine) as directed.
⊛ **ALERT:** If seizures develop and persist despite anticonvulsants, notify prescriber, stop drug, and institute seizure precautions and protocols.
Patient teaching
- Instruct patient to report adverse reactions because supportive therapy may be needed.
- Warn patient about pain at injection site.

☑ Evaluation
- Patient is free from infection.
- Patient maintains adequate hydration throughout therapy.
- Patient and family state understanding of drug therapy.

imipramine hydrochloride
(ih-MIP-ruh-meen high-droh-KLOR-ighd)
Apo-Imipramine ◆, Impril ◆,
Melipramine ◇, Norfranil, Novopramine ◆,
Tipramine, Tofranil

imipramine pamoate
Tofranil-PM

Pharmacologic class: dibenzazepine tricyclic antidepressant
Therapeutic class: antidepressant
Pregnancy risk category: D

Indications and dosages
▶ **Depression.** *Adults:* 75 to 100 mg P.O. daily in divided doses, increase in 25- to 50-mg increments to maximum dosage. Or, 25 mg P.O. daily, increase in 25-mg increments every other day. Or, entire dosage may be given h.s. Maximum dosage is 200 mg P.O. daily for outpa-

tients, 300 mg P.O. daily for inpatients, and 100 mg P.O. daily for elderly patients.
▶ **Enuresis.** *Children age 6 and older:* 25 mg P.O. 1 hour before bedtime. If no response within 1 week, increase dosage 50 mg nightly for children younger than age 12 or 75 mg nightly for children age 12 and older. Maximum dosage is 2.5 mg/kg P.O. daily.
▶ **Attention deficit hyperactivity disorder‡.** *Children age 6 and older:* 2 to 5 mg/kg P.O. given in 2 to 3 divided daily doses.

Contraindications and precautions
- Contraindicated in patients hypersensitive to drug, patients receiving MAO inhibitors, and patients in acute recovery phase of MI.
- Use cautiously in patients at risk for suicide; patients receiving thyroid drugs; and patients with history of urine retention or angle-closure glaucoma, increased intraocular pressure, CV disease, impaired hepatic function, hyperthyroidism, seizure disorder, or renal impairment.
⚘ **Lifespan:** In pregnant and breast-feeding women, drug isn't recommended. In children, safety hasn't been established for treating depression. In elderly patients, use lower dose and more gradual dose increases to avoid toxicity.

Adverse reactions
CNS: *drowsiness, dizziness,* excitation, tremor, weakness, confusion, headache, nervousness, EEG changes, *seizures,* extrapyramidal reactions.
CV: *orthostatic hypotension, tachycardia, ECG changes,* hypertension, *MI, CVA, arrhythmias, heart block.*
EENT: *blurred vision,* tinnitus, mydriasis.
GI: *dry mouth, constipation,* nausea, vomiting, anorexia, paralytic ileus.
GU: *urine retention,* impotence, testicular swelling.
Metabolic: *hypoglycemia,* hyperglycemia.
Skin: rash, urticaria, *diaphoresis,* photosensitivity reactions.
Other: hypersensitivity reactions, gynecomastia, galactorrhea and breast enlargement, altered libido, SIADH.

Interactions
Drug-drug. *Barbiturates, CNS depressants:* May enhance CNS depression. Avoid using together.

Cimetidine, methylphenidate: May increase imipramine level. Monitor patient for adverse reactions.

Clonidine: May cause loss of blood pressure control with potentially life-threatening elevations in blood pressure. Don't use together.

Epinephrine, norepinephrine: May cause life-threatening hypertensive effect. Use cautiously; monitor patient's blood pressure.

Fluoxetine: May increase effects of tricyclic antidepressants; symptoms may persist several weeks after fluoxetine therapy stops. Monitor symptoms closely.

MAO inhibitors: May cause hyperpyretic crisis, severe seizures, and death. Don't use together.

Drug-herb. *SAM-e, St. John's wort:* May elevate serotonin level. Discourage use together.

Yohimbe: May increase blood pressure effects. Avoid use together.

Drug-lifestyle. *Alcohol use:* May enhance CNS depression. Discourage using together.

Smoking: May decrease imipramine level. Monitor patient for lack of effect; discourage patient from smoking.

Sun exposure: May increase risk of photosensitivity reactions. Advise patient to avoid unprotected or prolonged exposure to sunlight.

Effects on lab test results

- May increase or decrease glucose level.
- May increase liver function test values.

Pharmacokinetics

Absorption: Rapid and complete.
Distribution: Wide. 90% protein-bound.
Metabolism: By liver. A significant first-pass effect may explain variable level in different patients taking same dose.
Excretion: Mostly in urine. *Half-life:* 11 to 25 hours.

Route	Onset	Peak	Duration
P.O.	Unknown	1-2 hr	Unknown

Action

Chemical effect: Increases amount of norepinephrine, serotonin, or both in CNS by blocking their reuptake by presynaptic neurons.
Therapeutic effect: Relieves depression and childhood enuresis (hydrochloride form).

Available forms

imipramine hydrochloride
Tablets: 10 mg, 25 mg, 50 mg
imipramine pamoate
Capsules: 75 mg, 100 mg, 125 mg, 150 mg

NURSING PROCESS

Assessment
- Assess patient's condition before therapy and regularly thereafter.
- Be alert for adverse reactions and drug interactions.
- Evaluate patient's and family's knowledge of drug therapy.

Nursing diagnoses
- Ineffective individual coping related to depression
- Deficient knowledge related to drug therapy

Planning and implementation
- Reduce dosage in elderly or debilitated patients, adolescents, and patients with aggravated psychotic symptoms.
- **ALERT:** Don't confuse imipramine with desipramine.
- Although doses can be given up to four times daily, patients also may receive entire daily dose at one time because of drug's long action.
- Don't withdraw drug abruptly.
- Drug causes high risk of orthostatic hypotension. Check sitting and standing blood pressures after initial dose.
- Because of hypertensive episodes during surgery in patients receiving tricyclic antidepressants, gradually stop drug over several days before surgery. After abrupt withdrawal of long-term therapy, patient may experience nausea, headache, and malaise. Treat patient symptomatically. These symptoms don't indicate addiction.
- If signs of psychosis occur or increase, notify prescriber, reduce dosage, and institute safety precautions.

Patient teaching
- Advise patient to take full dose h.s. but warn about possible morning orthostatic hypotension.
- Suggest taking drug with food or milk if it causes stomach upset.
- Suggest relieving dry mouth with sugarless chewing gum or hard candy. Encourage good

dental prophylaxis because persistent dry mouth may increase the risk of dental caries.
- Tell patient to avoid alcohol and smoking during therapy.
- Warn patient to avoid hazardous activities until CNS effects of drug are known.
- Warn patient not to stop drug suddenly.
- Advise patient to consult prescriber before taking other prescription drugs, OTC drugs, or herbal remedies.
- Advise patient to use sunblock, wear protective clothing, and avoid prolonged exposure to sunlight to prevent photosensitivity reactions.

☑ **Evaluation**
- Patient behavior and communication show diminished depression.
- Patient and family state understanding of drug therapy.

immune globulin intramuscular (gamma globulin, IG, IGIM)
(ih-MYOON GLOB-yoo-lin in-truh-MUS-kyoo-ler)
BayGam

immune globulin intravenous (IGIV)
Gamimune N, Gammagard S/D, Gammar-P IV, Iveegam EN, Panglobulin, Polygam S/D, Carimune, Venoglobulin-S

Pharmacologic class: immunologic drug
Therapeutic class: immune serum
Pregnancy risk category: C

Indications and dosages

▶ **Primary humoral immunodeficiency (IGIV); treatment of primary defective antibody synthesis such as agammaglobulinemia or hypogammaglobulinemia in patients who are at increased risk of infection.** *Adults and children:* 100 to 200 mg/kg I.V. Gamimune N monthly, at 0.01 to 0.02 ml/kg/minute for 30 minutes. If no discomfort, rate can slowly be increased to a maximum of 0.08 ml/kg/minute. Or, 200 to 400 mg/kg I.V. Gammagard S/D, then monthly doses of 100 mg/kg. Start infusion at 0.5 ml/kg/hour and increase to maximum of 4 ml/kg/hour. Dose is related to patient response. Or, 200 mg/kg I.V. Iveegam EN month-

ly. May increase dose to maximum of 800 mg/ kg or give more frequently to produce desired effect. Infusion rate is 1 to 2 ml/minute for 5% solution. Or, 200 mg/kg I.V. Panglobulin or Carimune monthly. Start with 0.5 to 1 ml/ minute of 3% solution; gradually increase dose to 2.5 ml/minute after 15 to 30 minutes. Or, 200 to 400 mg/kg I.V. Polygam S/D at 0.5 ml/ kg/hour, increasing to a maximum of 4 ml/kg/ hour. Subsequent dose is 100 mg/kg I.V. monthly. Or, 200 mg/kg I.V. Venoglobulin-S monthly. Increase dose to 300 to 400 mg/kg and give more often than once monthly if IgG levels aren't adequate. Infuse at 0.01 to 0.02 ml/ kg/minute for 30 minutes; if tolerated, increase 5% solutions to 0.08 ml/kg/minute and 10% solutions to 0.05 ml/kg/minute. Or, initially, 1.3 ml/kg I.M. Maintenance dose of 0.66 ml/kg (at least 100 mg/kg) q 3 to 4 weeks. Maximum single dose of IGIM is 30 to 50 ml in adults and 20 to 30 ml in infants and small children.
Adults: 200 to 400 mg/kg I.V. Gammar-P IV q 3 to 4 weeks. Infuse at 0.01 ml/kg/minute and increase to 0.02 ml/kg/minute after 15 to 30 minutes if no problems occur. Maximum infusion rate is 0.06 ml/kg/minute.
Adolescents and children: 200 to 400 mg/kg I.V. Gammar-P IV q 3 to 4 weeks.
▶ **Idiopathic thrombocytopenic purpura (IGIV).** *Adults and children:* 400 mg/kg 5% solution I.V. Gamimune N for 5 days; or 1,000 mg/kg 10% solution I.V. for 1 to 2 days with maintenance dose of 10% solution at 400 to 1,000 mg/kg I.V. single infusion to maintain 30,000/mm³ platelet count. Or, 1,000 mg/ kg I.V. Gammagard S/D or Polygam S/D as a single dose. Give up to three doses on alternate days, if needed. Or, 400 mg/kg I.V. Panglobulin or Carimune for 2 to 5 consecutive days, depending on platelet count and immune response. Or, maximum of 2,000 mg/kg I.V. Venoglobulin-S over 5 days or less. Maintenance dose is 1,000 mg/kg given as needed.
▶ **Bone marrow transplant (IGIV).** *Adults older than age 20:* 500 mg/kg 5% or 10% solution I.V. Gamimune N on days 7 and 2 pretransplantation; then weekly until 90 days posttransplantation.
▶ **B-cell chronic lymphocytic leukemia (IGIV).** *Adults:* 400 mg/kg I.V. Gammagard S/D or Polygam S/D q 3 to 4 weeks.

▶ **Pediatric HIV infection (IGIV).** *Children:* 400 mg/kg I.V. Gamimune N q 28 days, at 0.01 to 0.02 ml/kg/minute for 30 minutes; increase to maximum of 0.08 ml/kg/minute.

▶ **Kawasaki syndrome (IGIV).** *Adults:* 400 mg/kg I.V. Iveegam EN daily over 2 hours for 4 consecutive days, or a single dose of 2,000 mg/kg I.V. over 10 to 12 hours. Start within 10 days of disease onset. Treat concurrently with aspirin (80 to 100 mg/kg P.O. daily through day 14; then 3 to 10 mg/kg P.O. daily for 5 weeks). Or, either a single dose of 1g/kg or 400 mg/kg I.V. Gammagard S/D or Polygam S/D daily for 4 days beginning within 7 days of onset of fever. Treat concurrently with aspirin (80 to 100 mg/kg in 4 divided daily doses).

▶ **Hepatitis A exposure (IGIM).** *Adults and children:* 0.02 ml/kg I.M. as soon as possible after exposure. Up to 0.06 ml/kg may be given for prolonged or intense exposure.

▶ **Measles exposure (IGIM).** *Adults and children:* 0.02 ml/kg I.M. within 6 days after exposure.

▶ **Measles postexposure prophylaxis (IGIM).** *Immunocompromised children:* 0.5 ml/kg I.M. (maximum, 15 ml) within 6 days after exposure.

▶ **Chickenpox exposure (IGIM).** *Adults and children:* 0.6 to 1.2 ml/kg I.M. as soon as possible after exposure.

▶ **Rubella exposure in first trimester of pregnancy (IGIM).** *Women:* 0.55 ml/kg I.M. as soon as possible after exposure (within 72 hours).

▽ I.V. administration

● I.V. products aren't interchangeable. Gammagard requires a filter, which is supplied by manufacturer.
● Most adverse effects are related to rapid infusion rate. Infuse slowly.
● If there is a risk of a thrombotic event, don't give an infusion concentration higher than 5%, start infusion rate no faster than 0.5 ml/kg per hour, and speed up slowly only if well tolerated to a maximum rate of 4 ml/kg per hour.

Contraindications and precautions

● Contraindicated in patients hypersensitive to drug and in patients with selective IgA deficiencies.
● I.M. administration contraindicated in patients with severe thrombocytopenia or other coagulation-bleeding disorders.

● Use Gammagard S/D cautiously in patients with a history of CV disease or thrombotic episodes. Use cautiously in patients with renal impairment.
● I.V. drug may cause thrombotic events. The exact cause of this is unknown; therefore, use caution when giving drug to patients with a history of CV disease or thrombotic episodes.
❦ **Lifespan:** In pregnant and breast-feeding women, use cautiously.

Adverse reactions

CNS: *severe headache requiring hospitalization.*
CV: chest pain, *MI, heart failure* (Gammagard S/D).
GI: nausea, vomiting.
GU: nephrotic syndrome, *acute tubular necrosis,* osmotic nephrosis, *acute renal impairment.*
Musculoskeletal: muscle stiffness at injection site.
Respiratory: *pulmonary embolism, transfusion-related acute lung injury.*
Skin: urticaria, erythema.
Other: *anaphylaxis.*

Interactions

Drug-drug. *Live-virus vaccines:* Antibodies in the vaccine may interfere with drug therapy. Don't give within 6 months after giving immune globulin.

Effects on lab test results

● May increase BUN and creatinine.

Pharmacokinetics

Absorption: Slow.
Distribution: Evenly between intravascular and extravascular spaces.
Metabolism: Unknown.
Excretion: Unknown. *Half-life:* 21 to 24 days in immunocompromised patients.

Route	Onset	Peak	Duration
I.V.	Immediate	Immediate	Unknown
I.M.	Unknown	2-5 days	Unknown

Action

Chemical effect: Provides passive immunity by increasing antibody titer. The primary component is IgG.
Therapeutic effect: Helps prevent infections.

Available forms

IGIM
Injection: 2- and 10-ml vials
IGIV
Injection: 5% and 10% in 10-, 50-, 100-, 200-, and 250-ml vials (Gamimune N); 5% and 10% in 50-, 100-, and 200-ml vials (Venoglobulin-S)
Powder for injection: 50 mg protein/ml in 2.5-, 5-, and 10-g vials (Gammagard S/D); 1-, 2.5-, and 5-g vials (Gammar-P IV); 500-mg and 1-, 2.5-, and 5-g vials (Iveegam); 2.5-, 5-, and 10-g vials (Polygam S/D); 3-, 6-, and 12-g vials (Panglobulin, Carimune)

NURSING PROCESS

✍ Assessment
- Obtain history of allergies and reactions to immunizations.
- Observe patient for signs of anaphylaxis or other adverse reactions immediately after injection.
- Inspect injection site for local reactions.
- Monitor effectiveness by checking antibody titers after administration.
- Evaluate patient's and family's knowledge of drug therapy.

🔤 Nursing diagnoses
- Ineffective protection related to lack of or decreased immunity
- Ineffective breathing pattern related to anaphylaxis
- Deficient knowledge related to drug therapy

▷ Planning and implementation
- Give I.M. injection in gluteal region. Divide doses over 10 ml and inject into several muscle sites to reduce local pain and discomfort.
- If 6 weeks or more have passed since exposure or since symptoms have begun, don't give immune globulin to help prevent hepatitis A.
- Make sure epinephrine 1:1,000 is available in case of anaphylaxis.
- ⊛ **ALERT:** I.V. and I.M. products aren't interchangeable.
Patient teaching
- Instruct patient to report respiratory difficulty immediately.
- Tell patient that local reactions may occur at injection site.

- Instruct patient to notify prescriber promptly if adverse reaction persists or becomes severe.

☑ Evaluation
- Patient exhibits increased passive immunity.
- Patient shows no signs of anaphylaxis.
- Patient and family state understanding of drug therapy.

indapamide
(in-DAP-uh-mighd)
Lozide ♦ , Lozol, Natrilix ◇

Pharmacologic class: thiazide-like diuretic
Therapeutic class: diuretic, antihypertensive
Pregnancy risk category: B

Indications and dosages

▶ **Edema.** *Adults:* Initially, 2.5 mg P.O. daily in morning. Increase to 5 mg daily after 1 week, if needed.
▶ **Hypertension.** *Adults:* Initially, 1.25 mg P.O. daily in morning. Increase to 2.5 mg daily after 4 weeks. Increase to 5 mg daily after 4 more weeks.

Contraindications and precautions

- Contraindicated in patients hypersensitive to drug and other sulfonamide-derived drugs and in patients with anuria.
- Use cautiously in patients with severe renal disease, impaired hepatic function, and progressive hepatic disease.
- ☀ **Lifespan:** In pregnant women, use cautiously. In breast-feeding women and in children, safety of drug hasn't been established.

Adverse reactions

CNS: headache, irritability, nervousness, dizziness, light-headedness, weakness.
CV: volume depletion and dehydration, orthostatic hypotension.
GI: nausea, *pancreatitis.*
GU: nocturia, polyuria, frequent urination.
Metabolic: anorexia, hypokalemia, asymptomatic hyperuricemia, *metabolic alkalosis,* hyponatremia, hypochloremia.
Musculoskeletal: muscle cramps and spasms.
Skin: dermatitis, photosensitivity reactions, rash.
Other: gout.

Interactions

Drug-drug. *Antihypertensives:* May cause severe hypotension. Use together cautiously.
Bumetanide, ethacrynic acid, furosemide, torsemide: May cause excessive diuretic response resulting in serious electrolyte abnormalities or dehydration. Adjust doses carefully while monitoring the patient closely for excessive diuretic responses.
Diazoxide: May increase antihypertensive, hyperglycemic, and hyperuricemic effects. Use together cautiously.
Digoxin: May increase risk of digoxin toxicity from indapamide-induced hypokalemia. Monitor potassium and digoxin levels.
Lithium: May decrease lithium clearance and increases risk of lithium toxicity. Use together cautiously.
NSAIDs: May reduce the diuretic, natriuretic, and antihypertensive effects. Monitor patient.
Drug-lifestyle. *Sun exposure:* May cause photosensitivity reactions. Avoid prolonged and unprotected exposure to sunlight.

Effects on lab test results

• May increase glucose, cholesterol, triglyceride, and uric acid levels. May decrease potassium, sodium, and chloride levels.

Pharmacokinetics

Absorption: Complete.
Distribution: Wide because of its lipophilicity; 71% to 79% protein-bound.
Metabolism: Undergoes significant hepatic metabolism.
Excretion: Primarily in urine; smaller amounts in feces. *Half-life:* About 14 hours.

Route	Onset	Peak	Duration
P.O.	1-2 hr	≤ 2 hr	≤ 36 hr

Action

Chemical effect: Unknown; probably inhibits sodium reabsorption in distal segment of nephron. Also has direct vasodilating effect, possibly from calcium channel-blocking action.
Therapeutic effect: Promotes water and sodium excretion and lowers blood pressure.

Available forms

Tablets: 1.25 mg, 2.5 mg

⚡ Assessment

• Assess patient's underlying condition before therapy.
• Monitor effectiveness by assessing fluid intake and output, weight, and blood pressure. In hypertensive patient, therapeutic response may be delayed several days.
• Monitor electrolytes and glucose levels.
• Monitor creatinine and BUN levels regularly. If these levels are more than twice normal, drug is less effective.
• Monitor uric acid level, especially if patient has history of gout.
• Be alert for adverse reactions and drug interactions.
• Evaluate patient's and family's knowledge of drug therapy.

🔲 Nursing diagnoses

• Risk for injury related to presence of hypertension
• Excessive fluid volume related to presence of edema
• Deficient knowledge related to drug therapy

▶ Planning and implementation

• To prevent nocturia, give drug in morning.
• Drug may be used with potassium-sparing diuretic to prevent potassium loss.
Patient teaching
• Advise patient to avoid sudden postural changes and to rise slowly to avoid orthostatic hypotension.
• Advise patient to use sunblock and avoid prolonged exposure to sunlight to prevent photosensitivity reactions.
• Teach patient to monitor fluid volume by recording daily weight and intake and output.
• Tell patient to avoid high-sodium foods and to choose high-potassium foods.
• Advise patient to take drug early in day to avoid nocturia.

☑ Evaluation

• Patient's blood pressure is normal.
• Patient is free from edema.
• Patient and family state understanding of drug therapy.

---

indinavir sulfate

(in-DIH-nuh-veer SUL-fayt)

Crixivan

Pharmacologic class: protease inhibitor
Therapeutic class: antiviral
Pregnancy risk category: C

Indications and dosages

▶ **HIV.** *Adults:* 800 mg P.O. q 8 hours.

◪ **Adjust-a-dose:** For patients with mild to moderate hepatic insufficiency resulting in cirrhosis, reduce dosage to 600 mg P.O. q 8 hours.

Contraindications and precautions

• Contraindicated in patients hypersensitive to drug.
• Use cautiously and at a reduced dosage in patients with hepatic insufficiency.
⚠ **Lifespan:** In breast-feeding women, drug is not recommended. In children, safety and effectiveness of drug haven't been established.

Adverse reactions

CNS: headache, insomnia, dizziness, malaise, somnolence, asthenia, fatigue.
GI: abdominal pain, *nausea,* diarrhea, vomiting, acid regurgitation, anorexia, dry mouth, taste perversion.
GU: nephrolithiasis.
Hematologic: anemia, *neutropenia.*
Hepatic: *hyperbilirubinemia.*
Musculoskeletal: flank pain, back pain.
Other: redistribution and accumulation of body fat.

Interactions

Drug-drug. *Amprenavir, saquinavir:* May increase levels of these drugs. Dosage adjustments probably aren't needed.
Carbamazepine: May decrease indinavir level. Avoid using together.
Clarithromycin: May alter level of clarithromycin. Monitor patient.
Didanosine: May need normal gastric pH for optimal absorption of indinavir. Give these drugs and indinavir at least 1 hour apart on an empty stomach.
Efavirenz, nevirapine: May decrease indinavir level. Increase indinavir to 1,000 mg q 8 hours.

HMG-CoA reductase inhibitors: May increase levels of these drugs and increase risk of myopathy and rhabdomyolysis. Avoid using together.
Ketoconazole, itraconazole, delavirdine: May increase level of indinavir. Consider a dosage reduction of indinavir to 600 mg q 8 hours.
Midazolam, triazolam: Competition for CYP 3A4 by indinavir may inhibit the metabolism of these drugs and create the potential for serious or life-threatening events, such as arrhythmias or prolonged sedation. Don't give together.
Nelfinavir: May increase levels of indinavir by 50% and nelfinavir by 80%. There is limited data on adjusting the dosage to indinavir 1,200 mg b.i.d. and nelfinavir 1,250 mg b.i.d. Monitor patient closely.
Rifabutin: May increase level of rifabutin and decrease level of indinavir. Give indinavir 1,000 mg q 8 hours and decrease the rifabutin dose to either 150 mg daily or 300 mg two to three times a week.
Rifampin: May significantly diminish level of indinavir because rifampin is a potent inducer of CYP 3A4. Avoid using together.
Ritonavir: May increase level of indinavir by 2 to 5 times. Adjust dosage to indinavir 400 mg b.i.d. and ritonavir 400 mg b.i.d., or indinavir 800 mg b.i.d. and ritonavir 100 to 200 mg b.i.d.
Sildenafil: May increase sildenafil level, and increase risk of adverse effects (hypotension, visual changes, and priapism). Don't exceed 25 mg of sildenafil in a 48-hour period.
Drug-herb. *St. John's wort:* May reduce level of indinavir by more than 50%. Discourage use together.
Drug-food. *Any food:* May substantially decrease absorption of oral indinavir. Give drug on an empty stomach.
Grapefruit juice: May decrease level and therapeutic effect of indinavir. Advise patient to take drug with liquid other than grapefruit juice.

Effects on lab test results

• May increase ALT, AST, bilirubin, amylase, triglycerides, cholesterol, and glucose levels.
• May decrease hemoglobin, hematocrit, and neutrophil and platelet counts.

Pharmacokinetics

Absorption: Rapid.
Distribution: 60% bound to proteins.

Metabolism: By liver and kidneys.
Excretion: In urine. *Half-life:* 2 hours.

Route	Onset	Peak	Duration
P.O.	Unknown	< 1 hr	1-8 hr

Action

Chemical effect: Binds to protease active sites and inhibits their activity. Prevents cleavage of viral polyproteins, resulting in formation of immature, noninfectious viral particles.
Therapeutic effect: Reduces symptoms of HIV.

Available forms

Capsules: 100 mg, 200 mg, 333 mg, and 400 mg

NURSING PROCESS

Assessment
• Monitor adverse reactions and drug interactions.
• Evaluate patient's and family's knowledge of drug therapy.

Nursing diagnoses
• Infection related to presence of virus
• Risk for deficient fluid volume related to effect on kidneys
• Deficient knowledge related to drug therapy

Planning and implementation
• Give at least 48 oz (1.5 L) of fluids every 24 hours to maintain adequate hydration.
• Give drug on an empty stomach, 1 hour before or 2 hours after a meal.
Patient teaching
• Instruct patient to use barrier protection during sexual intercourse.
• If patient misses a dose, advise him to take the next dose at regularly scheduled time and not to double the dose.
• Instruct patient to take drug on an empty stomach with water 1 hour before or 2 hours after a meal.
• Instruct patient to store capsules in the original container and to keep the desiccant in the bottle.
• Instruct patient to drink at least 48 oz (1.5 L) of fluid daily.
• Advise HIV-positive women to avoid breastfeeding to prevent transmitting virus to infant.

• Instruct patient to report evidence of nephrolithiasis (flank pain, hematuria) or diabetes (increased thirst, polyuria) promptly.
• Advise patient taking sildenafil that he may be at increased risk for sildenafil-associated adverse reactions, including hypotension, visual changes, and priapism, and he should promptly report any symptoms to prescriber. Patient shouldn't take more than 25 mg of sildenafil in a 48-hour period.

Evaluation
• Patient's health improves and signs and symptoms of underlying condition diminish with use of drug.
• Patient maintains adequate hydration.
• Patient and family state understanding of drug therapy.

indomethacin
(in-doh-METH-uh-sin)
Apo-Indomethacin ♦ , Arthrexin ◇ ,
Indocid ♦ ◇ Indocid SR ♦ , Indocin*,
Indocin SR, Novo-Methacin ♦

indomethacin sodium trihydrate
Apo-Indomethacin ♦ , Indocid PDA ♦ ,
Indocin I.V., Novo-Methacin ♦

Pharmacologic class: NSAID
Therapeutic class: non-opioid analgesic, antipyretic, anti-inflammatory
Pregnancy risk category: B

Indications and dosages

▶ **Moderate to severe rheumatoid arthritis or osteoarthritis, ankylosing spondylitis.**
Adults: 25 mg P.O. b.i.d. or t.i.d. with food or antacids. Increase by 25 mg or 50 mg daily q 7 days up to 200 mg daily. Or, 50 mg P.R. q.i.d. Or, 75 mg sustained-release capsules P.O. to start, in morning or h.s., followed, if needed, by another 75 mg b.i.d.
▶ **Acute gouty arthritis.** *Adults:* 50 mg P.O. t.i.d. Reduce dose as soon as possible, then stop. Don't use sustained-release capsules.
▶ **Acute painful shoulders (bursitis or tendinitis).** *Adults:* 75 to 150 mg P.O. daily t.i.d. or q.i.d. with food or antacids for 7 to 14 days.

▶ **To close hemodynamically significant patent ductus arteriosus in premature infants.** *Neonates less than 48 hours old:* 0.2 mg/kg I.V. followed by two doses of 0.1 mg/kg at 12- to 24-hour intervals. *Neonates ages 2 to 7 days:* 0.2 mg/kg I.V. followed by two doses of 0.2 mg/kg at 12- to 24-hour intervals. *Neonates more than 7 days old:* 0.2 mg/kg I.V. followed by two doses of 0.25 mg/kg at 12- to 24-hour intervals.

▶ **Pericarditis‡.** *Adults:* 75 to 200 mg P.O. daily in three to four divided doses.

▶ **Dysmenorrhea‡.** *Adults:* 25 mg P.O. t.i.d. with food or antacids.

▶ **Bartter's syndrome‡.** *Adults:* 150 mg P.O. daily with food or antacids.
Children: 0.5 to 2 mg/kg P.O. in divided doses.

▼ I.V. administration

• Reconstitute powder for injection with sterile water for injection or normal saline solution. For each 1-mg vial, add 1 ml of diluent to yield 1 mg/ml; add 2 ml of diluent to yield 0.5 mg/ml.

• Give by direct injection over 5 to 10 seconds.

⊛ **ALERT:** Use only preservative-free diluents to prepare I.V. injection. Never use diluents containing benzyl alcohol because it has been linked to fatal gasping syndrome in neonates. Because injection contains no preservatives, reconstitute immediately before administration and discard unused solution.

• If patient has anuria or marked oliguria, don't give second or third scheduled I.V. dose; instead, notify prescriber.

Contraindications and precautions

• Contraindicated in patients hypersensitive to drug and in those with history of aspirin- or NSAID-induced asthma, rhinitis, or urticaria. Suppositories contraindicated in patients with history of proctitis or recent rectal bleeding.

• Because of its high risk of adverse effects during prolonged use, don't use drug routinely as analgesic or antipyretic.

• Use cautiously in patients with epilepsy, parkinsonism, hepatic or renal disease, CV disease, infection, mental illness or depression, or history of GI disease.

☙ **Lifespan:** In pregnant and breast-feeding women, drug is contraindicated. In children age 14 and older, safety and effectiveness of drug

haven't been established and it is not recommended. In infants with untreated infection, active bleeding, coagulation defects, thrombocytopenia, congenital heart disease (in whom patency of ductus arteriosus is needed for satisfactory pulmonary or systemic blood flow), necrotizing enterocolitis, or renal impairment, drug is contraindicated. In elderly patients, use cautiously.

Adverse reactions

P.O. and P.R.

CNS: *headache, dizziness,* depression, drowsiness, confusion, peripheral neuropathy, *seizures,* psychic disturbances, syncope, vertigo.

CV: hypertension, *edema, heart failure.*

EENT: blurred vision, corneal and retinal damage, hearing loss, tinnitus.

GI: *nausea, vomiting,* anorexia, *diarrhea, peptic ulceration, GI bleeding.*

GU: hematuria, *acute renal failure.*

Hematologic: hemolytic anemia, *aplastic anemia, agranulocytosis, leukopenia, thrombocytopenic purpura,* iron-deficiency anemia.

Metabolic: *hyperkalemia.*

Skin: pruritus, urticaria, *Stevens-Johnson syndrome.*

Other: *hypersensitivity reactions* (rash, *respiratory distress, anaphylaxis, angioedema*).

I.V.

GI: *GI bleeding,* vomiting.

GU: *renal dysfunction,* azotemia.

Metabolic: hyponatremia, *hyperkalemia, hypoglycemia.*

Other: *hypersensitivity reactions* (rash, *respiratory distress, anaphylaxis, angioedema*).

Interactions

Drug-drug. *Aminoglycosides, cyclosporine, methotrexate:* Indomethacin may enhance toxicity of these drugs. Avoid using together.

Antihypertensives: May reduce antihypertensive effect. Monitor blood pressure closely.

Aspirin: May decrease indomethacin level and increase the risk of GI toxicity. Avoid using together.

Corticosteroids: May increase risk of GI toxicity. Don't use together.

Diflunisal, probenecid: May decrease indomethacin excretion. Monitor patient for increased adverse reactions to indomethacin.

Digoxin: Indomethacin may prolong half-life of digoxin. Use together cautiously; monitor digoxin level.

Dipyridamole: May enhance fluid retention. Avoid using together.

Furosemide, thiazide diuretics: May impair response to both drugs. Avoid using together, if possible.

Lithium: May increase lithium levels. Monitor patient for lithium toxicity.

Triamterene: May cause nephrotoxicity. Monitor patient closely.

Drug-herb. *Dong quai, feverfew, garlic, ginger, horse chestnut, red clover:* May increase risk of bleeding. Monitor patient closely for bleeding.

St. John's wort: May increase risk of photosensitivity. Advise patient to avoid unprotected or prolonged exposure to sunlight.

Senna: May block laxative effects. Discourage using together.

Drug-lifestyle. *Alcohol use:* May increase risk of GI toxicity. Discourage using together.

Effects on lab test results

• May increase AST, ALT, BUN, creatinine, and potassium levels. May decrease glucose and sodium levels.

• May decrease hemoglobin, hematocrit, and WBC, granulocyte, and platelet counts.

Pharmacokinetics

Absorption: Rapid and complete.
Distribution: Highly protein-bound.
Metabolism: In liver.
Excretion: Mainly in urine, with some biliary excretion. *Half-life:* 4½ hours.

Route	Onset	Peak	Duration
P.O.	30 min	1-4 hr	4-6 hr
I.V.	Immediate	Immediate	Unknown
P.R.	2-4 hr	Unknown	4-6 hr

Action

Chemical effect: Unknown; produces antiinflammatory, analgesic, and antipyretic effects, possibly by inhibiting prostaglandin synthesis.
Therapeutic effect: Relieves pain, fever, and inflammation.

Available forms

indomethacin
Capsules: 25 mg, 50 mg
Capsules (sustained-release): 75 mg

Oral suspension: 25 mg/5 ml
Suppositories: 50 mg
indomethacin sodium trihydrate
Injection: 1-mg vials

Assessment

• Assess patient's condition before therapy and regularly thereafter.

• Monitor patient carefully for bleeding and for reduced urine output during I.V. use.

• Be alert for adverse reactions and drug interactions.

• Evaluate patient's and family's knowledge of drug therapy.

Nursing diagnoses

• Chronic pain related to underlying condition
• Risk for injury related to adverse reactions
• Deficient knowledge related to drug therapy

Planning and implementation

• If GI upset occurs, give oral form of drug with food, milk, or antacid.

• If ductus arteriosus reopens, give second course of one to three doses. If ineffective, surgery may be needed.

• If patient has bleeding or reduced urine output, stop drug and notify prescriber.

• Drug may enhance hypothalamic-pituitary-adrenal axis response to dexamethasone suppression test.

• Notify prescriber if drug is ineffective.

Patient teaching

• Tell patient to take oral form of drug with food, milk, or antacid if GI upset occurs.

• Inform patient that use of oral form with aspirin, alcohol, or corticosteroids may increase risk of adverse GI reactions.

• Teach patient signs and symptoms of GI bleeding, and tell him to report them to prescriber. Serious GI toxicity, including peptic ulceration and bleeding, can occur in patients taking oral NSAIDs despite absence of GI symptoms.

• Instruct patient to avoid alcohol consumption during drug therapy.

• Tell patient to notify prescriber immediately about visual or hearing changes. Patient receiving long-term oral therapy should have regular eye examinations, hearing tests, CBC, and renal function tests to detect toxicity.

Reactions may be *common,* uncommon, *life-threatening*, or **COMMON AND LIFE-THREATENING.**

• Advise patient to avoid hazardous activities if adverse CNS reactions occur.

☑ **Evaluation**

• Patient is free from pain.
• Patient doesn't experience injury from adverse reactions.
• Patient and family state understanding of drug therapy.

infliximab

(in-FLICKS-ih-mab)
Remicade

Pharmacologic class: monoclonal antibody
Therapeutic class: anti-inflammatory
Pregnancy risk category: B

Indications and dosages

▶ **To reduce signs and symptoms and induce and maintain remission in patients with moderately to severely active Crohn's disease who have had an inadequate response to conventional therapy; to reduce the number of draining enterocutaneous and rectovaginal fistulas and maintaining fistula closure in patients with fistulizing Crohn's disease.** *Adults:* 5 mg/kg I.V. infusion (over a period of not less than 2 hours), given as an induction regimen at 0, 2, and 6 weeks followed by a maintenance regimen of 5 mg/kg q 8 weeks thereafter. For patients who respond and then lose their response, consideration may be given to treatment with 10 mg/kg. Patients who don't respond by week 14 are unlikely to respond with continued dosing; consider stopping drug in these patients.
▶ **With methotrexate, to reduce signs and symptoms, inhibit the progression of structural damage, and improve function in patients with moderately to severely active rheumatoid arthritis who haven't responded adequately to methotrexate.** *Adults:* 3 mg/kg I.V. infusion over a period of not less than 2 hours. Give additional doses of 3 mg/kg at 2 and 6 weeks after initial infusion and q 8 weeks thereafter. If response is inadequate, increase up to 10 mg/kg or give q 4 weeks.

▼ I.V. administration

• Drug is incompatible with plasticized polyvinyl chloride equipment or devices; prepare only in glass infusion bottles or polypropylene or polyolefin infusion bags. Give through polyethylene-lined administration sets with an in-line, sterile, nonpyrogenic, low–protein-binding filter (pore size of 1.2 mm or less).
• Vials don't contain antibacterial preservatives; use reconstituted drug immediately. Reconstitute with 10 ml sterile solution for injection using syringe with 21G or smaller needle. Don't shake; gently swirl to dissolve powder. Solution should be colorless to light yellow and opalescent; it may contain a few translucent particles. If you see other particles or discoloration, don't use.
• Dilute total volume of reconstituted drug to 250 ml with normal saline solution for injection. Infusion concentration range is 0.4 to 4 mg/ml. Infuse within 3 hours of preparation and for at least 2 hours after starting.
• Don't infuse drug in same I.V. line with other drugs.
• If an infusion reaction occurs, stop drug, notify prescriber, and give acetaminophen, antihistamines, corticosteroids, and epinephrine.

Contraindications and precautions

• Contraindicated in patients hypersensitive to murine proteins or other components of drug.
• In patients with mild heart failure (New York Heart Association [NYHA] Class I or II), use cautiously. Patients with moderate to severe heart failure (NYHA Class III or IV) shouldn't use this drug.
• Tuberculosis, invasive fungal infections, and other fatal opportunistic infections may occur.
⚖ **Lifespan:** In pregnant women, give only if clearly needed. Breast-feeding women shouldn't breast-feed during drug therapy; it's unknown whether drug appears in breast milk. In children, safety of drug hasn't been established. In elderly patients, use drug cautiously.

Adverse reactions

CNS: pain, *headache, fatigue, fever,* depression, dizziness, malaise, insomnia.
CV: *hypertension,* peripheral edema, hypotension, tachycardia, chest pain, flushing.
EENT: *pharyngitis, rhinitis, sinusitis,* conjunctivitis.
GI: *nausea, abdominal pain,* vomiting, constipation, *dyspepsia, diarrhea,* flatulence, intestinal obstruction, mouth pain, ulcerative stomatitis.
GU: dysuria, increased urinary frequency, *UTI.*

Hematologic: anemia, hematoma.
Musculoskeletal: myalgia, *arthralgia,* arthritis, *back pain.*
Respiratory: *upper respiratory tract infections,* bronchitis, *coughing,* dyspnea.
Skin: *rash,* pruritus, candidiasis, acne, alopecia, eczema, erythema, erythematous rash, maculopapular rash, papular rash, dry skin, increased sweating, urticaria, ecchymosis.
Other: chills, flulike syndrome, hot flushes, abscess, toothache, hypersensitivity reaction, allergic reaction.

Interactions

Drug-drug. *Live vaccines:* No data are available on response to vaccines or on the secondary transmission of infection by live virus vaccines. Don't use together.

Effects on lab test results

• May increase liver enzyme levels.
• May decrease hemoglobin and hematocrit.

Pharmacokinetics

Absorption: Administered I.V.
Distribution: Primarily within the vascular compartment.
Metabolism: Unknown.
Excretion: Unknown. *Half-life:* 9½ days.

Route	Onset	Peak	Duration
I.V.	Unknown	Unknown	Unknown

Action

Chemical effect: Binds to tumor necrosis factor (TNF)-alpha to neutralize its activity and inhibit its binding with receptors, thereby reducing the infiltration of inflammatory cells and production of TNF-alpha in inflamed areas of the intestine.
Therapeutic effect: Relieves inflammation.

Available forms

Injection: 100-mg vials

NURSING PROCESS

⏳ Assessment

• Obtain history of patient's underlying condition before therapy and reassess regularly.
• Observe patient for infusion-related reactions, including fever, chills, pruritus, urticaria, dyspnea, hypotension, hypertension, and chest pain, within 2 hours of infusion.

• Monitor liver function test results.
• Observe patient for development of lymphomas and infection. Patients with chronic Crohn's disease and long-term exposure to immunosuppressants are more likely to develop lymphomas and infections.
• Drug may affect normal immune responses. Monitor patient for development of autoimmune antibodies and lupus-like syndrome; stop drug if symptoms develop. Symptoms should resolve.
• If drug is used in patients with heart failure, monitor patient's cardiac status.
• Evaluate patient's and family's knowledge of drug therapy.

🔲 Nursing diagnoses

• Chronic pain related to inflammation of the GI tract
• Imbalanced nutrition: Less than body requirements related to underlying medical condition
• Deficient knowledge related to drug therapy

▷ Planning and implementation

• If patient develops new or worsening symptoms of heart failure, stop drug.
• Patients may develop tuberculosis, invasive fungal infections, and other, sometimes fatal, opportunistic infections. Test patient for latent tuberculosis infection with a tuberculin skin test. Start treatment of latent tuberculosis infection before therapy.
• Patient may develop histoplasmosis, listeriosis, and pneumocystosis. For patients who have resided in regions where histoplasmosis is endemic, the benefits and risks of therapy should be carefully considered before starting therapy.
Patient teaching
• Tell patient about infusion reaction symptoms, and instruct him to report them.
• Inform patient of postinfusion adverse effects, and tell him to report them promptly.

☑ Evaluation

• Patient is free from pain.
• Patient maintains adequate nutrition.
• Patient and family state understanding of drug therapy.

---

influenza virus vaccine live, intranasal

(inn-floo-EHN-zah VY-russ VACK-zeen LYV, inn-truh-NAZ-ul)

FluMist

Pharmacologic class: neuraminidase inhibitor
Therapeutic class: antiviral
Pregnancy risk category: C

Indications and dosages

▶ **Active immunization for influenza A and B viruses.** *Children ages 5 to 8 (not previously vaccinated with FluMist):* 2 doses of 0.5 ml each, 60 days apart (± 14 days for initial season).
Children ages 5 to 8 (previously vaccinated with FluMist): 0.5 ml per season.
Children and adults ages 9 to 49: 0.5 ml per season.

Contraindications and precautions

• Contraindicated in patients hypersensitive to any component of drug, including eggs or egg products. Also contraindicated in patients who may be immunosuppressed or have altered or compromised immune status as a consequence of treatment with systemic corticosteroids, alkylating drugs, antimetabolites, radiation, or other immunosuppressive therapies. Contraindicated in patients with known or suspected immune deficiency diseases, such as combined immunodeficiency, agammaglobulinemia, or thymic abnormalities; conditions such as HIV infection, malignancy, leukemia, or lymphoma; or a history of Guillain-Barre syndrome or asthma or reactive airway disease.
⚑ **Lifespan:** In pregnant women, drug is contraindicated. In breast-feeding women, use cautiously; it's unknown whether FluMist appears in breast milk. In children ages 5 to 17 receiving aspirin or aspirin-containing products, drug is contraindicated because of the association with Reye syndrome. In children younger than age 5 and adults age 65 and older, safety of drug hasn't been established.

Adverse reactions

CNS: irritability, headache, fever.
EENT: runny nose, nasal congestion, sore throat.
GI: vomiting.
Musculoskeletal: muscle aches.
Respiratory: cough.
Other: chills, decreased activity.

Interactions

Drug-drug. *Aspirin:* May cause Reye syndrome. Avoid using together.
Antivirals active against influenza A or B viruses: May cause synergistic or decreased effect. Wait 48 hours after stopping antiviral therapy before giving vaccine. Don't give antivirals within 2 weeks of vaccine.

Effects on lab test results

None reported.

Pharmacokinetics

Absorption: Unknown.
Distribution: Unknown.
Metabolism: Unknown.
Excretion: Unknown. *Half-life:* Unknown.

Route	Onset	Peak	Duration
Intranasal	Unknown	Unknown	Unknown

Action

Chemical effect: May play a role in prevention and recovery from infection. Induces influenza strain-specific serum antibodies.
Therapeutic effect: Protects against the flu.

Available forms

Intranasal spray: 0.5 ml

NURSING PROCESS

🗒 **Assessment**
• Assess health and immune status of patient.
• To prevent allergic or other adverse reactions, review patient's history for possible sensitivity to influenza vaccine components, including eggs and egg products.
• Be alert for adverse reactions.
• Evaluate patient's and family's knowledge of therapy.

🔖 **Nursing diagnoses**
• Risk for infection related to influenza A and B virus
• Deficient knowledge related to vaccine therapy

▶ Planning and implementation

⚕ **ALERT:** Keep epinephrine injection (1:1,000) or compatible treatment readily available in the event of an acute anaphylactic reaction.

• Don't give drug until at least 72 hours after a patient's fever has started.

• Advise vaccine recipients and the parents of immunized children to avoid close contact within the same household with immunocompromised individuals for at least 21 days.

• Report adverse reactions. The U.S. Department of Health and Human Services has established a Vaccine Adverse Event Reporting System to manage reports of suspected adverse reactions for any vaccine (1-800-822-7967). Reporting forms may also be obtained at the FDA web site (http://www.vaers.org).

• Give drug before exposure to influenza. The peak of influenza activity is variable from year to year, but generally occurs between late December and early March. Because the duration of protection of drug isn't known and yearly variation in the influenza strains is possible, revaccinate annually to increase the likelihood of protection.

• Drug shouldn't be given with other vaccines.

• Drug may not protect 100% of patients.

• Thaw drug before giving. To thaw, hold the sprayer in the palm of the hand and support the plunger rod with the thumb. Give the vaccine immediately. Or, thaw drug in a refrigerator and store at 36° to 46° F (2° to 8° C) for no more than 24 hours before use. When thawed, drug is a colorless to pale yellow liquid that's clear to slightly cloudy; some particulates may be present, but they don't affect use.

• Give approximately 0.25 ml into each nostril while the recipient is in an upright position. Insert the tip of the sprayer just inside the nose and depress the plunger to spray. The dose-divider clip is removed from the sprayer to give the second half of the dose into the other nostril.

Patient teaching

• Inform parents of children ages 5 to 8 that two doses of drug are required the first time it's used.

• Tell patient to avoid close contact within the same household with immunocompromised individuals for at least 21 days.

• Instruct patient to report any suspected adverse reactions to the prescriber or clinic where the vaccine was given.

• Inform patient that annual revaccination may increase the likelihood of protection and that not every person who receives the vaccine will be protected.

☑ Evaluation

• Patient remains free of adverse effects of the therapy.

• Patient does not contract influenza A or B virus.

• Patient and family state understanding of vaccine therapy.

insulin aspart (rDNA origin) injection
(IN-suh-lin AS-part)
NovoLog

insulin aspart (rDNA origin) protamine suspension and insulin aspart (rDNA origin) injection
Novolog 70/30

Pharmacologic class: human insulin analogue
Therapeutic class: antidiabetic
Pregnancy risk category: C

Indications and dosages

▶ **Control of hyperglycemia in diabetes mellitus.** *Adults:* 0.5 to 1 unit/kg S.C. NovoLog daily within 5 to 10 minutes of start of meal. About 50% to 70% of the daily insulin requirement may be provided by this drug and the remainder by intermediate-acting or long-acting insulin. Initially, dose for NovoLog external insulin infusion pumps is based on the total daily insulin dose of the previously used regimen. Give 50% of the total dose as a bolus at mealtime, and the remainder as basal infusion. Adjust dose as needed. Or, give Novolog 70/30 twice daily within 15 minutes of meals.

Contraindications and precautions

• Contraindicated during episodes of hypoglycemia and in patients hypersensitive to NovoLog or one of its excipients.

• Use cautiously in patients prone to hypoglycemia and hypokalemia, such as patients who are fasting, have autonomic neuropathy, or are using potassium-lowering drugs or drugs sensitive to potassium levels.

☀ **Lifespan:** In breast-feeding women, use cautiously; drug may appear in breast milk. In children, safety and effectiveness haven't been established.

Adverse reactions

Metabolic: *hypoglycemia, hyperkalemia.*
Skin: lipodystrophy, pruritus, rash.
Other: allergic reactions, injection site reactions.

Interactions

Drug-drug. *ACE inhibitors, disopyramide, fibrates, fluoxetine, MAO inhibitors, oral antidiabetics, propoxyphene, salicylates, somatostatin analogue (octreotide), and sulfonamide antibiotics:* May enhance the glucose-lowering effects of insulin and may potentiate hypoglycemia. Monitor glucose level and signs of hypoglycemia. May require insulin dose adjustment.
Carteolol, nadolol, pindolol, propanolol, timolol: May mask symptoms of hypoglycemia as a result of beta blockade (such as tachycardia). Use cautiously in patients with diabetes.
Corticosteroids, danazol, diuretics, estrogens, progestogens such as in hormonal contraceptives, isoniazid, niacin, phenothiazine derivatives, somatropin, sympathomimetics such as epinephrine, salbutamol, and terbutaline, and thyroid hormones: May reduce the glucose-lowering effect of insulin and may cause hyperglycemia. Monitor glucose level. May require insulin dosage adjustment.
Guanethidine, reserpine: May mask signs and symptoms of hypoglycemia (may be reduced or absent). Monitor glucose level.
Lithium salts, pentamidine: May enhance or weaken glucose-lowering effect of insulin, causing hypoglycemia or hyperglycemia. Pentamidine may cause hypoglycemia, which may sometimes be followed by hyperglycemia. Monitor glucose level.
Drug-lifestyle. *Alcohol use:* May increase the glucose-lowering effects of insulin. Discourage using together.

Effects on lab test results

• May decrease glucose and potassium levels.

Pharmacokinetics

Absorption: Bioavailable as regular human insulin. Faster absorption and onset and shorter duration of action compared to regular human insulin.
Distribution: 0% to 9% protein-binding, similar to regular insulin.
Metabolism: Unknown.
Excretion: Unknown. *Half-life:* 81 minutes (compare with regular insulin's half-life of 141 minutes).

Route	Onset	Peak	Duration
S.C.			
Novolog	15-30 min	1-3 hr	3-5 hr
Novolog 70/30	Rapid	1-4 hr	24 hr

Action

Chemical effect: Binds to insulin receptors on muscle and fat cells, lowers glucose level, facilitates the cellular uptake of glucose, and inhibits the output of glucose from the liver.
Therapeutic effect: Lowers glucose level.

Available forms

10-ml vial for injection: 100 units of insulin aspart per ml (U-100)
3-ml PenFill cartridges: 100 units/ml

NURSING PROCESS

☜ Assessment

• Assess underlying condition before therapy and reassess regularly.
• Monitor glucose levels before and regularly throughout therapy.
• Monitor patient's glycosylated hemoglobin regularly.
• Monitor urine ketones when glucose level is elevated.
• Monitor patient for injection site reactions.
• Monitor patient with an external insulin pump for erythematous, pruritic, or thickened skin at injection site.
• Evaluate patient's and family's knowledge of drug therapy.

⊞ Nursing diagnoses

• Risk for impaired skin integrity related to adverse drug effects
• Risk for injury related to drug-induced hypoglycemia

• Deficient knowledge related to insulin aspart therapy

⟩ Planning and implementation

• Give NovoLog 5 to 10 minutes before the start of a meal. Give Novolog 70/30 up to 15 minutes before the start of a meal. Because of drug's rapid onset and short duration of action, patients may require the addition of longer-acting insulins to prevent pre-meal hyperglycemia.

• Give S.C. into the abdominal wall, thigh, or upper arm. Rotate sites to minimize lipodystrophies.

• Monitor patient for hypoglycemia, which may occur as a result of an excess of insulin relative to food intake, energy expenditure, or both. The warning signs and symptoms of hypoglycemia include shaking, sweating, dizziness, fatigue, hunger, irritability, confusion, blurred vision, headaches, or nausea and vomiting. Treat mild episodes of hypoglycemia with oral glucose. Adjust drug dosage, meal patterns, or exercise, if needed. Treat more severe episodes involving coma, seizure, or neurologic impairment with I.M. or S.C. glucagon or concentrated I.V. glucose. Sustain carbohydrate intake and observe because hypoglycemia may recur.

• Look at insulin vial before use. NovoLog should appear as a clear, colorless solution. It should never contain particulate matter, appear cloudy or viscous, or be discolored. Novolog 70/30 should appear uniformly white and cloudy and should never contain particulate matter or be discolored.

• Don't use drug after its expiration date. Discard after expiration date.

• Store drug between 36° and 46° F (2° and 8° C). Don't freeze. Don't expose vials to excessive heat or sunlight. Open vials are stable at room temperature for 28 days.

⊛ **ALERT:** Pump or infusion-set malfunctions or insulin degradation can lead to hyperglycemia and ketosis in a short time because of an S.C. depot of fast-acting insulin.

⊛ **ALERT:** Don't confuse Novolog 70/30 with Novolin 70/30.

⊛ **ALERT:** Don't confuse Novolog with Novolin or Humalog.

• Don't dilute or mix insulin aspart with any other insulin when using an external insulin pump.

• Insulin aspart is recommended for use with Disetronic H-TRON plus V100 with Disetronic 3.15 plastic cartridges and Classic or Tender infusion sets, and MiniMed Models 505, 506, and 507 with MiniMed 3-ml syringes and Polyfin or Sof-set infusion sets. The use of insulin aspart in quick-release infusion sets and cartridge adapters has not been assessed.

• Replace infusion sets and insulin aspart in the reservoir and choose a new infusion site every 48 hours or less to avoid insulin degradation and infusion set malfunction.

• Discard drug exposed to temperatures higher than 98.6°F (37°C). The temperature may exceed room temperature when the pump housing, cover, tubing, or sport case is exposed to sunlight or radiant heat.

⊛ **ALERT:** Spell out "units" to reduce the risk of error of misreading "U" as "0" (zero).

Patient teaching

• Inform patient of the possible risks and benefits of drug.

• Teach patient to recognize symptoms of hypoglycemia and hyperglycemia and how to treat them.

• Instruct patient on injection techniques, timing of dose to meals, adherence to meal planning, importance of regular glucose monitoring and periodic glycosylated hemoglobin testing, and proper storage of insulin.

• Tell woman to notify prescriber if she plans to become or becomes pregnant; information on drug in pregnancy or lactation isn't available.

• Instruct patient to report changes at injection site, including redness, itchiness, or thickened skin.

• Tell patient not to dilute or mix insulin aspart with any other insulin when using an external insulin pump.

• Teach patient how to properly use the external insulin pump.

☑ Evaluation

• Patient doesn't experience adverse reactions from drug.

• Patient's glucose level is within the normal range.

• Patient and family state understanding of drug therapy.

---

insulin glargine (rDNA) injection
IN-suh-lin GLAR-gene (rDNA) in-JEK-shun
Lantus

Pharmacologic class: insulin analogue
Therapeutic class: antidiabetic
Pregnancy risk category: C

Indications and dosages

▶ **Management of type 1 or type 2 diabetes mellitus in patients who need basal (long-acting) insulin for the control of hyperglycemia.** *Adults and children age 6 and older:* Individualize dosage and start drug S.C. at the same dose as the current insulin dose at the same time each day.
▶ **Management of type 2 diabetes mellitus in patients previously treated with oral antidiabetics.** *Adults:* 10 units S.C. once daily h.s. Adjust as needed to total daily dosage of 2 units to 100 units S.C. at the same time each day.

Contraindications and precautions

• Contraindicated in patients hypersensitive to insulin glargine or its excipients. Don't use drug during episodes of hypoglycemia.
• Use cautiously in patients with renal or hepatic impairment, and adjust dosage as directed.
⚠ **Lifespan:** In breast-feeding women, use cautiously. In children younger than age 6 years, safety and effectiveness of drug haven't been established. In elderly patients, use conservatively to avoid hypoglycemia.

Adverse reactions

Metabolic: *hypoglycemia.*
Skin: lipodystrophy, pruritus, rash.
Other: allergic reactions, pain at injection site.

Interactions

Drug-drug. *ACE inhibitors, disopyramide, fibrates, fluoxetine, MAO inhibitors, octreotide, oral antidiabetics, propoxyphene, salicylates, sulfonamide antibiotics:* May cause hypoglycemia and increased insulin effect. Monitor glucose level. Insulin glargine dosage may need adjustment.
Carteolol, nadolol, pindolol, propanolol, timolol: May mask symptoms of hypoglycemia as a result of beta blockade (such as tachycardia). Use cautiously in patients with diabetes.

Clonidine: May mask signs of hypoglycemia and may either potentiate or weaken glucose-lowering effect of insulin. Monitor glucose level carefully. Insulin glargine dosage may need adjustment.
Corticosteroids, danazol, diuretics, estrogens, isoniazid, phenothiazines (prochlorperazine, promethazine), progestins (hormonal contraceptives), sympathomimetics (albuterol, epinephrine, terbutaline), thyroid hormones: May reduce the glucose-lowering effect of insulin. Monitor glucose level. Insulin glargine dosage may need adjustment.
Guanethidine, reserpine: May mask signs of hypoglycemia. Avoid using together, if possible. Monitor glucose level carefully.
Lithium: May either enhance or weaken the glucose-lowering effect of insulin. Monitor glucose level. Insulin glargine dosage may need adjustment.
Pentamidine: May cause hypoglycemia, which may be followed by hyperglycemia. Avoid using together, if possible.
Drug-herb. *Aloe, bilberry leaf, bitter melon, burdock, dandelion, fenugreek, garlic, ginseng:* May improve glucose control and allow a reduced antidiabetic dosage. Tell patient to discuss the use of herbal remedies with prescriber before use.
Licorice root: May increase dosage requirements of insulin. Discourage using together.
Drug-lifestyle. *Alcohol use:* May increase the glucose-lowering effects of insulin. Discourage using together.
Emotional stress, exercise: May enhance or weaken the glucose-lowering effect of insulin. Monitor glucose level. Insulin glargine dosage may need adjustment.

Effects on lab test results

• May decrease glucose level.

Pharmacokinetics

Absorption: Slower, more prolonged absorption than NPH insulin and a relatively constant level over 24 hours with no pronounced peak when compared with NPH insulin. After injection into S.C. tissue, the acidic solution is neutralized, leading to formation of microprecipitates. From these microprecipitates, small amounts of insulin glargine are slowly released.
Distribution: Unknown.

Metabolism: Partly metabolized to form two active metabolites with in vitro activity similar to that of insulin.
Excretion: Unknown. *Half-life:* Unknown.

Route	Onset	Peak	Duration
S.C.	Slow	None	10¾-24 hr

Action

Chemical effect: Increases glucose transport across muscle and fat cell membranes to reduce glucose level. Promotes conversion of glucose to its storage form, glycogen. Triggers amino acid uptake and conversion to protein in muscle cells and inhibits protein degradation. Stimulates triglyceride formation and inhibits release of free fatty acids from adipose tissue. Stimulates lipoprotein lipase activity, which converts circulating lipoproteins to fatty acids.
Therapeutic effect: Lowers glucose level.

Available forms

Injection: 10-ml vial

NURSING PROCESS

◪ Assessment
• Obtain history of patient's underlying condition before therapy and reassess regularly. As with any insulin, the desired glucose level and the doses and timing of antidiabetic drug must be determined individually.
• Monitor glucose level closely.
• Monitor patient for hypoglycemia. Early symptoms may be different or less pronounced in patients with longstanding diabetes, diabetic nerve disease, or intensified diabetes control.
• Evaluate patient's and family's knowledge of drug therapy.

⊕ Nursing diagnoses
• Ineffective health maintenance related to hyperglycemia
• Risk for injury related to drug-induced hypoglycemia
• Deficient knowledge related to drug therapy

▷ Planning and implementation
• Drug isn't intended for I.V. use. Its prolonged duration of activity depends on injection into the S.C. space.

• Because of its prolonged duration, insulin glargine isn't the insulin of choice for diabetic ketoacidosis.
• The rate of absorption and onset and the duration of action may be affected by exercise and other circumstances such as illness and emotional stress.
• Don't dilute drug or mix it with any other insulin or solution.
• As with any insulin therapy, lipodystrophy may occur at injection site and delay insulin absorption. Rotate injection sites to reduce lipodystrophy.
⊛ ALERT: Don't confuse Lantus with Lente.
⊛ ALERT: Spell out units to reduce the risk of error by misreading "U" as "0" (zero).
• Store unopened vials at 36° F to 46° F. Don't freeze. Discard opened vials, whether refrigerated or not after 28 days. May store opened vials at room temperature away from direct heat and light.
Patient teaching
• Teach patient proper glucose-monitoring techniques and proper diabetes management.
• Teach diabetic patient signs and symptoms of hypoglycemia, such as fatigue, weakness, confusion, headache, and pale skin.
• Advise patient to treat mild episodes of hypoglycemia with oral glucose tablets. Encourage patient to always carry glucose tablets in case of a hypoglycemic episode.
• Teach patient the importance of maintaining a diabetic diet. Explain that adjustments in drug dosage, meal patterns, and exercise may be needed to regulate blood glucose.
• Tell patient that any change of insulin should be made cautiously and only under medical supervision. Changes in insulin strength, manufacturer, type (regular, NPH, insulin analogs), species (animal, human), or method of manufacture (ribosomal DNA versus animal source) may necessitate a dosage change. Oral antidiabetic treatment may need to be adjusted.
• Tell patient to consult prescriber before using OTC drugs.
• Advise patient not to dilute or mix any other insulin or solution with insulin glargine. Tell patient to discard the vial if the solution is cloudy.
• Instruct patient to store insulin glargine vials in the refrigerator, if possible.

Reactions may be *common,* uncommon, *life-threatening,* or **COMMON AND LIFE-THREATENING.**

☑ Evaluation
● Patient's blood glucose level is normal.
● Patient doesn't experience hypoglycemic reactions.
● Patient and family state understanding of drug therapy.

insulins
(IN-suh-linz)

insulin analog injection (lispro)
Humalog, Humalog mix 75/25, Humalog mix 50/50

insulin injection (regular insulin, crystalline zinc insulin)
Actrapid HM ◇, Actrapid HM Penfill ◇, Actrapid MC ◇, Actrapid MC Penfill ◇, Humulin R†, Hypurin Neutra ◇, Insulin 2 Neutral ◇, Novolin R†, Novolin R PenFill†, Pork Regular Iletin II†, Regular (Concentrated) Iletin II, Regular Purified Pork Insulin†, Velosulin Human ◇, Velosulin Insuject ◇

insulin zinc suspension (lente)
Humulin L†, Lente Iletin II†, Lente Insulin†, Lente MC ◇, Lente Purified Pork Insulin† Monotard HM ◇, Monotard M ◇

insulin zinc suspension, extended (ultralente)
Humulin U†, Ultralente Insulin†, Ultratard HM ◇, Ultratard MC ◇

insulin zinc suspension, prompt (semilente)
Semilente MC ◇

isophane insulin suspension (neutral protamine Hagedorn insulin, NPH)
Humulin N†, Hypurin Isophane ◇, Insulatard ◇, Insulatard Human ◆, Isotard MC ◇ Novolin N†, Novolin N PenFill†, NPH Insulin†, Pork NPH Iletin II†, Protaphane HM ◇, Protaphane HM Penfill ◇, Protaphane MC ◇

isophane insulin suspension with insulin injection
Actraphane HM ◇, Actraphane HM Penfill ◇, Actraphane MC ◇, Humulin 50/50†, Humulin 70/30†, Novolin 70/30, Novolin 70/30 PenFill†

protamine zinc suspension (PZI)
Protamine Zinc Insulin MC ◇

Pharmacologic class: pancreatic hormone
Therapeutic class: antidiabetic
Pregnancy risk category: B

Indications and dosages

▶ **Diabetic ketoacidosis.** *Adults:* 0.15 units/kg regular insulin as I.V. bolus, followed by 0.1 units/kg/hour by continuous infusion. Continue infusion until glucose level drops to 250 mg/dl; then start S.C. insulin with dose and interval adjusted according to patient's glucose level. Or, 0.4 to 0.6 units/kg in two doses, 50% given I.V. and 50% given S.C. or I.M.; then 0.1 units/kg given S.C. or I.M. q 1 hr based on glucose level.
Children: 0.1 unit/kg regular insulin as I.V. bolus; then 0.1 unit/kg hourly by continuous infusion until glucose level drops to 250 mg/dl; then start S.C. insulin.
▶ **Type 1 diabetes mellitus (insulin-dependent), adjunct to type 2 diabetes mellitus (non–insulin-dependent) inadequately controlled by diet and oral antidiabetics.** *Adults and children:* Therapeutic regimen is adjusted based on patient's glucose level.
▶ **Control of hyperglycemia with longer-acting insulin in patients with type 1 diabetes mellitus and with sulfonylureas in patients with type 2 diabetes mellitus.** *Adults and children older than age 3:* Dosage of insulin lispro rDNA origin, Humalog varies and must be determined by a prescriber familiar with patient's metabolic needs, eating habits, and other lifestyle variables. Inject S.C. up to 15 minutes before or immediately after a meal.
▶ **Control of hyperglycemia with Humalog and longer-acting insulin in patients with type 1 diabetes mellitus.** *Adults:* Dosage varies among patients and must be determined by prescriber familiar with patient's metabolic needs, eating habits, and other lifestyle variables. Inject

---

Rapid onset   *Liquid form contains alcohol.   ◆ Canada   ◇ Australia   †OTC   ‡Off-label use

S.C. within 15 minutes before or immediately after a meal.

▶ **Control of hyperglycemia with Humalog and sulfonylureas in patients with type 2 diabetes mellitus.** *Adults and children older than age 3:* Dosage varies among patients and must be determined by prescriber familiar with patient's metabolic needs, eating habits, and other lifestyle variables. Inject S.C. within 15 minutes before or immediately after a meal.

▼ I.V. administration

• Use only regular insulin.
• Inject directly into vein, through intermittent infusion device, or into port close to I.V. access site. Intermittent infusion isn't recommended.
• If given by continuous infusion, infuse drug diluted in normal saline solution at prescribed rate.

Contraindications and precautions

• Contraindicated in hypoglycemia and in patients hypersensitive to insulin or any of its ingredients.
⚠ **Lifespan:** In pregnant and breast-feeding women, insulin is drug of choice to treat diabetes.

Adverse reactions

Metabolic: *hypoglycemia,* hyperglycemia (rebound, or Somogyi, effect).
Skin: urticaria, itching, swelling, redness, stinging, warmth at injection site, rash.
Other: *lipoatrophy, lipohypertrophy,* hypersensitivity reactions, *anaphylaxis,* rash.

Interactions

Drug-drug. *AIDS antivirals, corticosteroids, dextrothyroxine, epinephrine, thiazide diuretics:* May diminish insulin response. Monitor patient for hyperglycemia.
Anabolic steroids, clofibrate, guanethidine, MAO inhibitors, salicylates, tetracyclines: May prolong hypoglycemic effect. Monitor glucose level carefully.
Carteolol, nadolol, pindolol, propanolol, timolol: May mask symptoms of hypoglycemia as a result of beta blockade (such as tachycardia). Use cautiously in patients with diabetes.
Hormonal contraceptives: May decrease glucose tolerance in diabetic patients. Monitor glucose levels and adjust insulin dosage carefully.

Drug-herb. *Basil, bay, bee pollen, burdock, ginseng, glucomannan, horehound, marshmallow, myrrh, sage:* May affect glycemic control. Monitor glucose level carefully.
Drug-lifestyle. *Alcohol use:* May increase the glucose-lowering effects of insulin. Discourage using together.
Marijuana use: May increase glucose level. Tell patient about this interaction.
Smoking: May increase glucose level and decrease response to insulin. Discourage patient from smoking; have patient monitor glucose level closely.

Effects on lab test results

• May decrease glucose, magnesium, and potassium levels.

Pharmacokinetics

Absorption: Highly variable after S.C. administration depending on insulin type and injection site.
Distribution: Wide.
Metabolism: Some is bound and inactivated by peripheral tissues, but most appears to be degraded in liver and kidneys.
Excretion: Filtered by renal glomeruli; undergoes some tubular reabsorption. *Half-life:* About 9 minutes after I.V. administration.

Route	Onset	Peak	Duration
I.V.	≤ 30 min	15-30 min	30 min-1 hr
S.C.	15 min-8 hr	2-30 hr	5-36 hr

Action

Chemical effect: Increases glucose transport across muscle and fat cell membranes to reduce glucose level. Promotes conversion of glucose to its storage form, glycogen; triggers amino acid uptake and conversion to protein in muscle cells and inhibits protein degradation; stimulates triglyceride formation and inhibits release of free fatty acids from adipose tissue; stimulates lipoprotein lipase activity, which converts circulating lipoproteins to fatty acids.
Therapeutic effect: Lowers glucose level.

Available forms

insulin injection
Injection (human): 100 units/ml (Actrapid HM ◊, Humulin R†, Novolin R†, Humalog [lispro], Velosulin Human ◊); 100 units/ml in

1.5-ml cartridge system† (Actrapid HM Penfill ◊, Novolin R PenFill†)
Injection (from pork): 100 units/ml†
Injection (purified beef): 100 units/ml (Hypurin Neutral ◊, Insulin 2 ◊)
Injection (purified pork): 100 units/ml (Actrapid MC ◊, Pork Regular Iletin II†, Regular Purified Pork Insulin†); 100 units/ml in 1.5-ml cartridge system ◊ (Actrapid MC Penfill ◊); 100 units/ml in 2-ml cartridge system ◊ ; 500 units/ml (Regular [Concentrated] Iletin II)
insulin zinc suspension, prompt
Injection (purified pork): 100 units/ml† (Semilente MC ◊)
isophane insulin suspension
Injection (from beef): 100 units/ml† (NPH Insulin†)
Injection (human, recombinant): 100 units/ml (Humulin N†, Humulin NPH ◊, Insulatard Human ♦, Novolin N†, Protaphane HM ◊); 100 units/ml in 1.5-ml cartridge system (Protaphane HM PenFill ◊, Novolin N PenFill†)
Injection (purified beef): 100 units/ml (Hypurin Isophane ◊, Isotard MC ◊)
Injection (purified pork): 100 units/ml (Insulatard ◊, NPH Purified Pork†, Pork NPH Iletin II, Protaphane MC ◊)
isophane insulin suspension 50% with insulin injection 50%
Injection (human): 100 units/ml (Humulin 50/50†)
isophane insulin suspension 70% with insulin injection 30%
Injection (human): 100 units/ml (Actraphane HM ◊, Humulin 70/30†, Novolin 70/30†); 100 units/ml in 1.5-ml cartridge system (Actraphane HM Penfil ◊, Novolin 70/30 PenFill†)
Injection (purified pork): 100 units/ml (Actraphane MC ◊)
insulin zinc suspension
Injection (from beef): 100 units/ml (Lente Insulin†, Lente MC ◊)
Injection (purified beef): 100 units/ml (Lente MC ◊)
Injection (purified pork): 100 units/ml (Lente Iletin II†, Monotard MC ◊, Lente Purified Pork Insulin†)
Injection (human): 100 units/ml† (Humulin L†, Monotard HM ◊,
protamine zinc suspension
Injection (purified pork): Protamine Zinc Insulin MC ◊

insulin zinc suspension, extended
Injection (from beef): 100 units/ml† (Ultralente Insulin†)
Injection (human): 100 units/ml (Ultratard HM ◊, Humulin U†)
Injection (purified pork): 100 units/ml ◊ (Ultratard MC ◊)

NURSING PROCESS

🔬 Assessment
• Assess patient's glucose level before therapy and regularly thereafter. If patient is under stress, unstable, pregnant, recently diagnosed, or taking drugs that can interact with insulin, monitor level more frequently.
• Monitor patient's glycosylated hemoglobin regularly.
• Monitor urine ketone level when glucose level is elevated.
• Be alert for adverse reactions and drug interactions.
• Monitor injection sites for local reactions.
• Evaluate patient's and family's knowledge of drug therapy.

🔲 Nursing diagnoses
• Ineffective health maintenance related to hyperglycemia
• Risk for injury related to drug-induced hypoglycemia
• Deficient knowledge related to drug therapy

▶ Planning and implementation
🔆 **ALERT:** Regular insulin is used in patients with circulatory collapse, diabetic ketoacidosis, or hyperkalemia. Don't use regular insulin concentrated (500 units/ml) I.V. Don't use intermediate- or long-acting insulins for coma or other emergency that needs rapid drug action.
🔆 **ALERT:** Dosage is always expressed in USP units. Use only syringes calibrated for particular concentration of insulin given.
• Insulin resistance may develop and large insulin doses are needed to control symptoms of diabetes in these patients. U-500 insulin is available as Regular (Concentrated) Iletin II for such patients. Although not normally stocked in every pharmacy, it's readily available. Give hospital pharmacy sufficient notice before needing to refill in-house prescription. Never store U-500 insulin in same area with other insulin

preparations because of danger of severe over-dose if given accidentally to other patients.

● To mix insulin suspension, swirl vial gently or rotate between palms or between palm and thigh. Don't shake vigorously because doing so causes bubbling and air in syringe.

● Humalog insulin has a rapid onset of action; give 15 minutes before meals.

● Lente, semilente, and ultralente insulins may be mixed in any proportion.

● Regular insulin may be mixed with NPH or lente insulins in any proportion.

● Switching from separate injections to pre-pared mixture may alter patient response. Whenever NPH or lente is mixed with regular insulin in same syringe, give immediately to avoid loss of potency.

● Don't use insulin that has changed color or become clumped or granular.

● Check expiration date on vial before using.

● Usual route is S.C. Pinch fold of skin with fin-gers starting at least 3 inches apart, and insert needle at 45- to 90-degree angle.

● Press but don't rub site after injection. Rotate and chart injection sites to avoid overuse of one area. Rotate injection sites within same anatom-ic region to help diabetic patients achieve better control.

● Ketosis-prone type 1, severely ill, and newly diagnosed diabetic patients with very high glucose levels may require hospitalization and I.V. treatment with regular fast-acting in-sulin.

● Store drug in cool area. Refrigeration is desir-able but not essential except for concentrated regular insulin.

● Notify prescriber of sudden changes in glu-cose levels, dangerously high or low levels, or ketosis.

● If patient develops diabetic ketoacidosis or hy-perglycemic hyperosmolar nonketotic coma, provide supportive measures.

● Treat hypoglycemic reaction with oral form of rapid-acting glucose if patient can swallow or with glucagon or I.V. glucose if patient can't be roused. Follow with complex carbohydrate snack when patient is awake, and determine cause of reaction.

● Make sure patient is following appropriate diet and exercise programs. Adjust insulin dosage when other aspects of regimen are changed.

● Discuss with prescriber how to deal with non-compliance.

● Treat lipoatrophy or lipohypertrophy accord-ing to prescribed protocol.

● **ALERT:** Spell out units to reduce the risk of er-ror by misreading the "U" as "0" (zero).

Patient teaching

● Tell patient that insulin relieves symptoms but doesn't cure disease.

● Inform patient about nature of disease; impor-tance of following therapeutic regimen; adher-ence to specific diet, weight reduction, exercise, and personal hygiene programs; and ways of avoiding infection. Review timing of injections and eating, and explain that meals must not be skipped.

● Stress that accuracy of measurement is very important, especially with concentrated regular insulin. Aids, such as magnifying sleeve or dose magnifier, may improve accuracy. Instruct pa-tient and family how to measure and give in-sulin.

● Advise patient not to alter order of mixing in-sulins or change model or brand of syringe or needle.

● Tell patient that glucose monitoring and urine ketone tests are essential guides to dosage and success of therapy. Stress the importance of rec-ognizing hypoglycemic symptoms because in-sulin-induced hypoglycemia is hazardous and may cause brain damage if prolonged; most ad-verse effects are self-limiting and temporary.

● Teach patient about proper use of equipment for monitoring glucose level.

● Instruct patient to avoid alcohol consumption during drug therapy.

● Advise patient not to smoke within 30 min-utes after insulin injection. Smoking decreases absorption.

● Tell patient that marijuana use may increase insulin requirements.

● Advise patient to wear or carry medical iden-tification at all times, to carry ample insulin sup-ply and syringes on trips, to have carbohydrates (lump of sugar or candy) on hand for emergen-cies, and to note time-zone changes for dose scheduling when traveling.

☑ Evaluation

● Patient's glucose level is normal.

● Patient sustains no injury from drug-induced hypoglycemia.

• Patient and family state understanding of drug therapy.

interferon alfa-2a, recombinant (rIFN-A)
(in-ter-FEER-on AL-fuh too-ay ree-COM-bih-nent)
Roferon-A

interferon alfa-2b, recombinant (IFN-alpha 2)
Intron-A

Pharmacologic class: biological response modifier
Therapeutic class: antineoplastic
Pregnancy risk category: C

Indications and dosages

▶ **Hairy cell leukemia.** *Adults:* For induction, 3 million IU alfa-2a S.C. or I.M. daily for 16 to 24 weeks. For maintenance, 3 million IU alfa-2a S.C. or I.M. three times weekly. Or, 2 million IU/m² alfa-2b I.M. or S.C. three times weekly for induction and maintenance.
▶ **Condylomata acuminata.** *Adults:* 1 million IU alfa-2b per lesion, intralesionally, three times weekly for 3 weeks.
▶ **Kaposi's sarcoma.** *Adults:* For induction, 36 million IU alfa-2a S.C. or I.M. daily for 10 to 12 weeks; for maintenance, 36 million IU alfa-2a three times weekly. Doses may begin at 3 million IU and escalate every 3 days until patient is given 36 million IU daily, in order to decrease toxicity Or, 30 million IU/m² alfa-2b S.C. or I.M. three times weekly. Maintain dose unless disease progresses rapidly or intolerance occurs.
▶ **Chronic hepatitis C.** *Adults:* 3 million IU alfa-2a three times weekly S.C. or I.M. for 12 months (48 to 52 weeks). Alternatively, induction dose of 6 million IU alfa-2a three times weekly for the first 3 months (12 weeks) followed by 3 million IU alfa-2a three times weekly for 9 months (36 weeks). If no response after 3 months, stop therapy. Re-treatment with either 3 or 6 million IU alfa-2a three times weekly for 6 to 12 months may be considered. Or, 3 million IU alfa-2b S.C. or I.M. three times weekly. In patients tolerating therapy with normalization of ALT at 16 weeks of treatment, ex-

tend therapy to 18 to 24 months. If no normalization of ALT at 16 weeks of treatment, consider discontinuing therapy.
▶ **Chronic hepatitis B.** *Adults:* 30 to 35 million IU alfa-2b S.C. or I.M. weekly either as 5 million IU daily or 10 million IU three times weekly for 16 weeks.
Children ages 1 to 17: 3 million IU/m² alfa-2b S.C. three times weekly for 1 week, then escalate dose to 6 million IU/m² S.C. three times weekly (up to 10 million IU/m² S.C. three times weekly) for 16 to 24 weeks.
▶ **Chronic myelogenous leukemia.** *Adults:* 9 million IU alfa-2a daily I.M or S.C. An escalating dosing regimen in which daily doses of 3 million and 6 million IU are given over 3 days, followed by 9 million IU daily for remainder of therapy, may produce increased short-term tolerance.
Children: 2.5 to 5 million IU/m² alfa-2a I.M. daily.
▶ **Malignant melanoma.** *Adults:* 20 million IU/m² alfa-2b daily given as I.V. infusion 5 days in a row for 4 weeks. For maintenance therapy, 10 million IU/m² S.C. three times weekly for 48 weeks. If adverse effects occur, stop therapy until they subside and then resume therapy at 50% of the previous dose. If intolerance persists, stop therapy.
▶ **Initial treatment of aggressive follicular non-Hodgkin's lymphoma in conjunction with anthracycline-containing combination chemotherapy.** *Adults:* 5 million IU alfa-2b S.C. three times weekly for up to 18 months.
▶ **Metastatic renal cell carcinoma‡.** *Adults:* 5 to 20 million IU alfa-2b S.C. daily or three times weekly.

Contraindications and precautions

• Contraindicated in patients hypersensitive to drug or to mouse protein.
• Use cautiously in patients with severe hepatic or renal function impairment, seizure disorders, compromised CNS function, cardiac disease, or myelosuppression.
• Alpha interferons, cause or aggravate fatal or life-threatening neuropsychiatric, autoimmune, ischemic, and infectious disorders. Monitor patient closely. Stop drug in patients with persistently severe or worsening signs or symptoms of these conditions.
☀ Lifespan: In pregnant women, use cautiously. In breast-feeding women, drug isn't recom-

mended. In children, safety of drug hasn't been established.

Adverse reactions

CNS: *dizziness,* confusion, paresthesia, numbness, lethargy, depression, nervousness, difficulty in thinking or concentrating, insomnia, sedation, apathy, anxiety, irritability, syncope, fatigue, vertigo, gait disturbances, poor coordination.
CV: hypotension, chest pain, *arrhythmias,* palpitations, *heart failure,* hypertension, edema, flushing, *MI.*
EENT: excessive salivation, visual disturbances, dry or inflamed oropharynx, rhinorrhea, sinusitis, conjunctivitis, earache, eye irritation, rhinitis.
GI: *anorexia, nausea, diarrhea,* vomiting, abdominal fullness, abdominal pain, flatulence, constipation, hypermotility, gastric distress, dysgeusia.
GU: transient impotence.
Hematologic: *anemia, leukopenia, neutropenia, mild thrombocytopenia.*
Hepatic: *hepatitis.*
Respiratory: coughing, dyspnea, tachypnea, *cyanosis.*
Skin: *rash,* dryness, *pruritus,* partial alopecia, diaphoresis, urticaria.
Other: flulike syndrome (fever, fatigue, myalgia, headache, chills, arthralgia), hot flushes.

Interactions

Drug-drug. *Aminophylline, theophylline:* May reduce theophylline clearance. Monitor level.
Cardiotoxic, hematotoxic, or neurotoxic drugs: Effects of previously or concurrently administered drugs may be increased by interferons. Monitor patient closely.
CNS depressants: May enhance CNS effects. Avoid using together.
Interleukin-2: May increase risk of renal impairment from interleukin-2. Monitor patient closely.
Live-virus vaccines: May increase risk of adverse reactions and decreased antibody response. Don't use together.
Zidovudine: May have synergistic adverse effects between alfa-2b and zidovudine. Carefully monitor WBC count.
Drug-lifestyle. *Alcohol use:* May increase risk of GI bleeding. Discourage using together.

Sun exposure: May cause photosensitivity reactions. Discourage prolonged or unprotected sun exposure.

Effects on lab test results

- May increase calcium, potassium, AST, ALT, alkaline phosphatase, LDH, and fasting glucose levels and triglycerides.
- May increase PT, INR, and PTT. May decrease hemoglobin, hematocrit, and WBC, neutrophil, and platelet counts.

Pharmacokinetics

Absorption: More than 80% absorbed after I.M. or S.C. injection.
Distribution: Wide and rapid.
Metabolism: Drug appears to be metabolized in liver and kidneys.
Excretion: Reabsorbed from glomerular filtrate with minor biliary elimination.

Route	Onset	Peak	Duration
I.M.	Unknown	3¾ hr	Unknown
S.C.	Unknown	7¼ hr	Unknown
Intralesional	Unknown	Unknown	Unknown

Action

Chemical effect: May involve direct antiproliferative action against tumor cells or viral cells to inhibit replication and change immune response by enhancing phagocytic activity of macrophages and by augmenting specific cytotoxicity of lymphocytes for target cells.
Therapeutic effect: Inhibits growth of certain tumor cells and viral cells.

Available forms

alfa-2a
Powder for injection with diluent: 18 million IU/multidose vial
Prefilled syringes: 3 million IU/0.5 ml. 6 million IU/0.5 ml, 9 million IU/0.5 ml
Solution for injection: 3 million IU/vial, 6 million IU/vial, 9 million IU/vial, 9 million IU/multidose vial, 18 million IU/multidose vial, 36 million IU/multidose vial
alfa-2b
Powder for injection with diluent: 3 million IU/vial; 5 million IU/vial; 10 million IU/vial; 18 million IU/multidose vial; 25 million IU/vial; 50 million IU/vial
Solution for injection: 3 million IU/vial or syringe, 5 million IU/vial or syringe, 10 million

---

IU/vial, 18 million IU/multidose vial, 25 million IU/vial

NURSING PROCESS

◆ Assessment
• Assess patient's condition before therapy and regularly thereafter.
• Obtain allergy history. Drug contains phenol as preservative and albumin as stabilizer.
• At beginning of therapy, assess for flulike symptoms, which tend to diminish with continued therapy.
• Alpha interferons may cause or aggravate fatal or life-threatening neuropsychiatric, autoimmune, ischemic, and infectious disorders. Monitor patients closely. Stop drug in patients with persistently severe or worsening signs or symptoms of these conditions. In many, but not all, cases, these disorders resolve after stopping therapy.
• Monitor blood studies. Any effects are dose-related and reversible. Recovery occurs within several days or weeks after withdrawal.
• Be alert for adverse reactions and drug interactions.
• Evaluate patient's and family's knowledge of drug therapy.

◆ Nursing diagnoses
• Ineffective health maintenance related to underlying condition
• Risk for injury related to drug-induced adverse CNS reactions
• Deficient knowledge related to drug therapy

◆ Planning and implementation
• Premedicate patient with acetaminophen to minimize flulike symptoms.
• Give drug h.s. to minimize daytime drowsiness.
• Make sure patient is well hydrated, especially during initial stages of treatment.
• **ⓢ ALERT:** Different brands of interferon may not be equivalent and may require different dosages.
• Use S.C. administration route in patients whose platelet count is below 50,000/mm³.
• When giving interferon alfa-2b for condylomata acuminata, use only 10 million-IU vial because dilution of other strengths is needed for intralesional use results in hypertonic solution. Don't reconstitute 10-million-IU vial with more

than 1 ml of diluent. Use tuberculin or similar syringe and 25G to 30G needle. Don't inject too deeply beneath lesion or too superficially. As many as five lesions can be treated at one time. To ease discomfort, give drug in evening with acetaminophen.
• Refrigerate drug.
• Notify prescriber of severe adverse reactions, which may require dosage reduction or discontinuation.
• Using drug with blood dyscrasia-causing drugs, bone marrow suppressants, or radiation therapy may increase bone marrow suppression. Dosage reduction may be needed.

Patient teaching
• Advise patient that laboratory tests will be performed before therapy and periodically thereafter. Tests include CBC with differential, platelet count, blood chemistry and electrolyte studies, liver function test results, and, if patient has cardiac disorder or advanced stages of cancer, ECGs.
• Instruct patient in proper oral hygiene because bone marrow-suppressant effects may lead to microbial infection, delayed healing, and gingival bleeding. Drug may decrease salivary flow.
• Emphasize need to follow prescriber's instructions about taking and recording temperature. Explain how and when to take acetaminophen.
• Advise patient to check with prescriber for instructions after missing dose.
• Tell patient that drug may cause temporary hair loss; explain that it will grow back when therapy ends.
• Teach patient how to prepare and give drug and how to dispose of used needles, syringes, containers, and unused drug. Give him a copy of information for patients included with product, and make sure he understands it. Also provide information on drug stability.
• Warn patient not to receive any immunization without prescriber's approval and to avoid contact with people who have taken polio vaccine. Use with live-virus vaccine may increase adverse reactions and decrease patient's antibody response. Patient is at increased risk for infection.
• Instruct patient to avoid alcohol during drug therapy.
• Advise patient to report signs of depression.

☑ Evaluation

• Patient shows improved health.
• Patient sustains no injury from adverse CNS reactions.
• Patient and family state understanding of drug therapy.

---

interferon beta-1b, recombinant

(in-ter-FEER-on BAY-tuh wun bee ree-COM-bih-nent)
Betaseron

Pharmacologic class: biological response modifier
Therapeutic class: antiviral, immunoregulator
Pregnancy risk category: C

Indications and dosages

▶ **To reduce frequency of exacerbations in patients with relapsing forms of multiple sclerosis (MS).** *Adults:* 0.625 mg S.C. q other day for weeks 1 and 2; then 0.125 mg S.C. q other day for weeks 3 and 4; then 0.1875 mg S.C. q other day for weeks 5 and 6; then 0.25 mg S.C. q other day thereafter.

Contraindications and precautions

• Contraindicated in patients hypersensitive to interferon beta or human albumin.
⚠ **Lifespan:** In pregnant and breast-feeding women, drug isn't recommended. It's unknown whether drug appears in breast milk. In women of child-bearing age, use cautiously. In children, safety of drug hasn't been established.

Adverse reactions

CNS: depression, anxiety, emotional lability, depersonalization, *malaise,* **suicidal tendencies,** confusion, somnolence, *seizures,* headache, dizziness.
CV: *hemorrhage.*
EENT: laryngitis.
GI: *nausea, diarrhea, constipation.*
GU: *menstrual disorders (bleeding or spotting, early or delayed menses, decreased days of menstrual flow, menorrhagia).*
Hematologic: *leukopenia, neutropenia.*
Respiratory: dyspnea.
Other: *flulike symptoms (fever, chills, myalgia, diaphoresis);* breast pain; *pelvic pain; lymphadenopathy;* hypersensitivity reaction, *inflammation, pain, and necrosis at injection site.*

Interactions

Drug-lifestyle. *Sun exposure:* May cause photosensitivity reactions. Discourage prolonged or unprotected sun exposure.

Effects on lab test results

• May increase ALT and bilirubin levels.
• May decrease WBC and neutrophil counts.

Pharmacokinetics

Absorption: Bioavailability is 50% after SC injection.
Distribution: Unknown.
Metabolism: Unknown.
Excretion: Unknown. *Half-life:* 8 minutes to 4¼ hours.

Route	Onset	Peak	Duration
S.C.	Unknown	1-8 hr	Unknown

Action

Chemical effect: Attaches to membrane receptors and causes cellular changes, including increased protein synthesis.
Therapeutic effect: Decreases exacerbations in multiple sclerosis.

Available forms

Powder for injection: 0.3 mg

NURSING PROCESS

☞ Assessment

• Assess patient's underlying condition before therapy.
• Monitor frequency of exacerbations after drug therapy begins.
• Monitor WBC counts, platelet counts, and blood chemistries, including liver function test results.
• Be alert for adverse reactions.
• Monitor patient for depression and suicidal ideation.
• Evaluate patient's and family's knowledge of drug therapy.

🔄 Nursing diagnoses

• Ineffective health maintenance related to exacerbations of multiple sclerosis
• Risk for injury related to drug-induced adverse CNS reactions
• Deficient knowledge related to drug therapy

⧉ Planning and implementation
- Premedicate patient with acetaminophen to minimize flulike symptoms.
- To reconstitute, inject 1.2 ml of supplied diluent (0.54% saline solution for injection) into vial and gently swirl to dissolve drug. Don't shake. Reconstituted solution will contain 8 million units (0.25 mg)/ml. Discard vials that contain particles or discolored solution.
- Inject immediately after preparation.
- Store at room temperature. Once reconstituted, may refrigerate for up to 3 hours before use.
- Rotate injection sites to minimize local reactions.

Patient teaching
- Warn woman of childbearing age about dangers to fetus. Tell her to notify prescriber promptly if she becomes pregnant.
- Teach patient how to give S.C. injections, including solution preparation, use of aseptic technique, rotation of injection sites, and equipment disposal. Periodically reevaluate patient's technique.
- Advise patient to take drug h.s. to minimize mild flulike symptoms.
- Advise patient to report thoughts of depression or suicidal ideation.

☑ Evaluation
- Patient exhibits decreased frequency of exacerbations.
- Patient sustains no injury from adverse CNS reactions.
- Patient and family state understanding of drug therapy.

---

interferon gamma-1b
(in-ter-FEER-on GAH-muh wun bee)
Actimmune

Pharmacologic class: biological response modifier
Therapeutic class: immunomodulator; antineoplastic
Pregnancy risk category: C

Indications and dosages
▶ **To delay disease progression in patients with severe, malignant osteopetrosis; chronic granulomatous disease.** *Patients with body surface area greater than 0.5 m²:* 50 mcg/m²

(1 million IU/m²) S.C. three times weekly in the deltoid or anterior thigh.
Patients with body surface area 0.5 m² or less: 1.5 mcg/kg/dose S.C. three times weekly in the deltoid or anterior thigh.

Contraindications and precautions
- Contraindicated in patients hypersensitive to drug or to genetically engineered products derived from *Escherichia coli.*
- Use cautiously in patients with cardiac disease, compromised CNS function, or seizure disorders.
- ☀ **Lifespan:** In pregnant women, use cautiously. In breast-feeding women, drug isn't recommended. In children younger than age 1, safety of drug hasn't been established.

Adverse reactions
CNS: *fatigue, decreased mental status, gait disturbance.*
GI: *nausea, vomiting, diarrhea.*
Hematologic: *neutropenia, thrombocytopenia.*
Skin: *rash.*
Other: flulike syndrome, erythema and tenderness at injection site.

Interactions
Drug-drug. *Myelosuppressive drugs:* May have additive myelosuppression. Monitor patient closely.
Zidovudine: May have additive bone marrow suppression. Consider reducing dosage.

Effects on lab test results
- May increase liver enzyme levels.
- May decrease neutrophil and platelet counts.

Pharmacokinetics
Absorption: About 90% absorbed after S.C. or I.M. administration.
Distribution: Unknown.
Metabolism: Unknown.
Excretion: Unknown. *Half-life:* 6 hours.

Route	Onset	Peak	Duration
S.C.	Unknown	≤ 7 hr	Unknown

Action
Chemical effect: Acts as interleukin-type lymphokine. Drug has potent phagocyte-activating properties and enhances oxidative metabolism of tissue macrophages.

Therapeutic effect: Promotes phagocyte activity.

Available forms

Injection: 100 mcg (2 million IU)/0.5-ml vial

NURSING PROCESS

💀 Assessment
• Assess patient's condition before therapy and regularly thereafter.
• Be alert for adverse reactions and drug interactions. Symptoms of flulike syndrome include headache, fever, chills, myalgia, and arthralgia.
• If adverse GI reactions occur, monitor patient's hydration status.
• Evaluate patient's and family's knowledge of drug therapy.

🔷 Nursing diagnoses
• Ineffective health maintenance related to underlying condition
• Risk for fluid volume deficit related to adverse GI reactions
• Deficient knowledge related to drug therapy

🔷 Planning and implementation
• Premedicate with acetaminophen to minimize symptoms at beginning of therapy. Flulike symptoms tend to diminish with continued therapy.
• Discard unused portion. Each vial is for single-dose use and doesn't contain preservative.
• Give drug h.s. to reduce discomfort from flulike symptoms.
• Refrigerate drug immediately. Vials must be stored at 36° to 46° F (2° to 8° C); don't freeze. Don't shake vial; avoid excessive agitation. Discard vials that have been left at room temperature for more than 12 hours.
Patient teaching
• Teach patient how to give drug and how to dispose of used needles, syringes, containers, and unused drug. Give him a copy of patient information included with product, and make sure he understands it.
• Instruct patient to notify prescriber if adverse reactions occur.

✓ Evaluation
• Patient responds well to drug.
• Patient maintains adequate hydration.

• Patient and family state understanding of drug therapy.

ipratropium bromide
(ip-ruh-TROH-pee-um BROH-mighd)
Atrovent

Pharmacologic class: anticholinergic
Therapeutic class: bronchodilator
Pregnancy risk category: B

Indications and dosages

▶ **Bronchospasm caused by COPD.** *Adults and children age 12 and older:* 1 to 2 inhalations q.i.d. Additional inhalations may be needed. However, don't exceed 12 total inhalations in 24 hours. Or, use inhalation solution, giving up to 500 mcg q 6 to 8 hours via oral nebulizer.
▶ **Rhinorrhea linked to allergic and non-allergic perennial rhinitis.** *Adults and children age 6 and older:* 2 sprays of 0.03% nasal spray in each nostril b.i.d. or t.i.d.
▶ **Rhinorrhea caused by the common cold.** *Adults and children age 12 and older:* 2 sprays of 0.06% nasal spray per nostril t.i.d. or q.i.d. *Children ages 5 to 11:* 2 sprays of 0.06% nasal spray per nostril t.i.d.
▶ **Rhinorrhea linked to seasonal allergic rhinitis.** *Adults and children age 5 and older:* 2 sprays of 0.06% nasal spray per nostril q.i.d.

Contraindications and precautions

• Contraindicated in patients hypersensitive to drug or to atropine or its derivatives and in those hypersensitive to soya lecithin or related food products such as soybeans and peanuts.
• Use cautiously in patients with angle-closure glaucoma, prostatic hyperplasia, or bladder-neck obstruction.
• Safety and effectiveness of use beyond 4 days for rhinorrhea from the common cold haven't been established.
🜲 **Lifespan:** In pregnant and breast-feeding women, use cautiously. In children younger than age 12, safety of oral inhaler or nebulizer hasn't been established.

Adverse reactions

CNS: nervousness, dizziness, headache.
CV: palpitations.
EENT: blurred vision, epistaxis.

Reactions may be *common*, uncommon, *life-threatening*, or COMMON AND LIFE-THREATENING.

GI: nausea, GI distress, dry mouth.
Respiratory: cough, *upper respiratory tract infection, bronchitis, bronchospasm.*
Skin: rash.

Interactions

Drug-drug. *Anticholinergics:* May increase anticholinergic effects. Avoid using together.
Cromolyn sodium: Will form precipitate if mixed in same nebulizer. Don't use together.
Drug-herb. *Jaborandi tree, pill-bearing spurge:* May decrease drug effects. Use cautiously.

Effects on lab test results

None reported.

Pharmacokinetics

Absorption: Not readily absorbed into systemic circulation.
Distribution: Not distributed.
Metabolism: Small amount that is absorbed is metabolized in liver.
Excretion: Absorbed drug excreted in urine and bile; remainder excreted unchanged in feces.
Half-life: About 2 hours.

Route	Onset	Peak	Duration
Inhalation	5-15 min	1-2 hr	3-6 hr

Action

Chemical effect: Inhibits vagally mediated reflexes by antagonizing acetylcholine.
Therapeutic effect: Relieves bronchospasms and symptoms of seasonal allergic rhinitis.

Available forms

Inhaler: Each metered dose supplies 18 mcg
Nasal spray: 0.03% (21 mcg), 0.06% (42 mcg)
Solution for inhalation: 0.02% (500 mcg vial)
Solution for nebulizer: 0.025% (250 mcg/ml) ◊, 0.02% (200 mcg/ml)

NURSING PROCESS

Assessment
• Assess patient's condition before and after drug therapy; monitor peak expiratory flow.
• Be alert for adverse reactions and drug interactions.
• Evaluate patient's and family's knowledge of drug therapy.

Nursing diagnoses
• Ineffective breathing pattern related to patient's underlying condition
• Acute pain related to drug-induced headache
• Deficient knowledge related to drug therapy

Planning and implementation
ALERT: Don't confuse Atrovent with Alupent.
ALERT: Drug isn't effective for treating acute episodes of bronchospasm when rapid response is needed.
• Don't exceed 12 total inhalations in 24 hours, and total nasal sprays shouldn't exceed eight in each nostril in 24 hours.
• If giving more than one inhalation, 2 minutes should elapse between inhalations. If giving more than one type of inhalant, always give bronchodilator first and wait 5 minutes before giving the other.
• Give drug on time to ensure maximal effect.
• If drug fails to relieve bronchospasms, notify prescriber.
Patient teaching
• Warn patient that drug isn't effective for treating acute episodes of bronchospasm where rapid response is needed.
• Give patient these instructions for using metered-dose inhaler: Clear nasal passages and throat. Breathe out, expelling as much air from lungs as possible. Place mouthpiece well into mouth and inhale deeply as you release dose from inhaler. Hold breath for several seconds, remove mouthpiece, and exhale slowly.
• Tell patient to avoid accidentally spraying into eyes. Temporary blurring of vision may result.
• Tell patient to wait at least 2 minutes before repeating when using more than one inhalation.
• If patient also uses a corticosteroid inhaler, tell him to use ipratropium first, and then wait about 5 minutes before using the corticosteroid. This process allows bronchodilator to open air passages for maximum effectiveness of the corticosteroid.
• Tell patient to take a missed dose as soon as remembered, unless it's almost time for next dose. In that case, tell him to skip the missed dose. Advise against doubling the dose.

Evaluation
• Patient's bronchospasms are relieved.
• Patient doesn't suffer from any drug-induced headaches.

• Patient and family state understanding of drug therapy.

irbesartan
(ir-buh-SAR-tun)
Avapro

Pharmacologic class: angiotensin II receptor antagonist
Therapeutic class: antihypertensive
Pregnancy risk category: C (D in second and third trimesters)

Indications and dosages

▶ **Hypertension.** *Adults and children age 13 and older:* Initially, 150 mg P.O. daily; increase to a maximum of 300 mg daily, if needed.
Children ages 6 to 12 years: Initially, 75 mg P.O. daily; increase to a maximum of 150 mg daily, if needed.
▶ **Nephropathy in type 2 diabetic patients.** *Adults:* 300 mg P.O. daily.

Contraindications and precautions

• Contraindicated in patients hypersensitive to drug or its components.
• Use cautiously in volume- or salt-depleted patients and in patients with renal impairment or renal artery stenosis.
⚜ Lifespan: In pregnant women, drug is contraindicated. In children younger than age 6, safety of drug hasn't been established.

Adverse reactions

CNS: fatigue, anxiety, dizziness, headache.
CV: chest pain, edema, tachycardia.
EENT: pharyngitis, rhinitis, sinus abnormality.
GI: diarrhea, dyspepsia, abdominal pain, nausea, vomiting.
GU: UTI.
Metabolic: *hyperkalemia.*
Musculoskeletal: musculoskeletal trauma or pain.
Respiratory: upper respiratory tract infection.
Skin: rash.

Interactions

None reported.

Effects on lab test results

May increase potassium level.

Pharmacokinetics

Absorption: Rapid and complete, with an average absolute bioavailability of 60% to 80%.
Distribution: Wide; 90% bound to proteins.
Metabolism: Primarily by conjugation and oxidation.
Excretion: By biliary and renal routes. About 20% is recovered in urine and the rest in feces.
Half-life: 11 to 15 hours.

Route	Onset	Peak	Duration
P.O.	Unknown	1½-2 hr	24 hr

Action

Chemical effect: Inhibits the vasoconstricting and aldosterone-secreting effects of angiotensin II by selectively blocking binding of angiotensin II to receptor sites in many tissues.
Therapeutic effect: Lowers blood pressure.

Available forms

Tablets: 75 mg, 150 mg, 300 mg

NURSING PROCESS

☰ Assessment
• Monitor patient's blood pressure regularly. Dizziness and orthostatic hypotension may occur more frequently in patients with type 2 diabetes mellitus and renal disease.
• Monitor patient's electrolytes, and assess patient for volume or salt depletion before starting drug therapy.
• Make sure woman of child-bearing age is using effective birth control before starting this drug because of danger to fetus.
• Evaluate patient's and family's knowledge of drug therapy.

⊞ Nursing diagnoses
• Risk for hypotension in volume- or salt-depleted patients
• Risk of injury related to the presence of hypertension
• Deficient knowledge related to drug therapy

▷ Planning and implementation
• If drug is needed to control blood pressure, give with a diuretic or other antihypertensive.

Reactions may be *common*, uncommon, *life-threatening*, or COMMON AND LIFE-THREATENING.

• If patient becomes hypotensive, place in a supine position and give an I.V. infusion of normal saline solution.

Patient teaching

• Warn woman of child-bearing age about consequences of exposing fetus to drug. Tell her to call prescriber immediately if pregnancy is suspected.

• Tell patient that drug may be taken once daily with or without food.

• Instruct patient to avoid driving and hazardous activities until CNS effects of drug are known.

☑ Evaluation

• Patient doesn't experience hypotension as a result of volume or salt depletion.

• Patient's blood pressure remains within normal limits and drug therapy doesn't cause injury.

• Patient and family state understanding of drug therapy.

iron dextran
(IGH-ern DEKS-tran)
DexFerrum, Dexiron ♦ , InFeD

Pharmacologic class: parenteral iron supplement
Therapeutic class: hematinic
Pregnancy risk category: C

Indications and dosages

▶ **Iron-deficiency anemia.** Total dose (in ml) is based on patient's weight and hemoglobin level using the following formula:

$$0.0476 \times weight\ (kg) \times [Hemoglobin_N - Hemoglobin_O] + 1\ ml/5\ kg\ of\ weight\ (max.\ 14\ ml)$$

One ml iron dextran provides 50 mg elemental iron.

Adults and children: For I.M. use, 0.5-ml test dose injected by Z-track method. If no reactions occur, maximum daily doses are 0.5 ml (25 mg) for infants weighing less than 5 kg (11 lb), 1 ml (50 mg) for children weighing less than 10 kg (22 lb), and 2 ml (100 mg) for heavier children and adults. For I.V. use, 0.5-ml test dose injected over 30 seconds. If no reactions occur in 1 hour, remainder of therapeutic dose is given I.V. Therapeutic dose repeated I.V. daily. Maxi-

mum single dose is 100 mg. Give slowly (1 ml/minute).

▽ I.V. administration

• Check facility policy before giving I.V.

• Use I.V. when patient has insufficient muscle mass for deep I.M. injection, impaired absorption from muscle as a result of stasis or edema, possibility of uncontrolled I.M. bleeding from trauma (as may occur in hemophilia), or massive and prolonged parenteral therapy (as may be needed in chronic substantial blood loss).

• When I.V. dose is complete, flush vein with 10 ml of normal saline solution. Have patient rest for 15 to 30 minutes after I.V. administration.

Contraindications and precautions

• Contraindicated in patients hypersensitive to drug and in those with acute infectious renal disease or anemia disorders (except iron-deficiency anemia).

• Use cautiously patients who have serious hepatic impairment, rheumatoid arthritis, or other inflammatory diseases, and in patients with history of significant allergies or asthma.

⚖ **Lifespan:** In pregnant women, use only when the potential benefits to the mother outweigh the potential risks to the fetus. In breastfeeding women, use cautiously. In children younger than age 4 months, drug is contraindicated.

Adverse reactions

CNS: headache, transitory paresthesia, arthralgia, myalgia, dizziness, malaise, syncope.
CV: chest pain, chest tightness, *shock,* hypertension, *arrhythmias, hypotensive reaction, peripheral vascular flushing with overly rapid I.V. administration, tachycardia.*
GI: nausea, vomiting, metallic taste, transient loss of taste, abdominal pain, diarrhea.
Respiratory: *bronchospasm.*
Skin: rash, urticaria, *brown discoloration* at I.M. injection site.
Other: *soreness, inflammation, and local phlebitis* at I.V. injection site; sterile abscess; necrosis; atrophy; fibrosis; *anaphylaxis;* delayed sensitivity reactions.

Interactions

Drug-Drug. *Chloramphenicol:* May increase iron level because of decreased iron clearance and erythropoiesis. Consult prescriber about using together.

Effects on lab test results

• May increase bilirubin levels. May decrease calcium levels.
• May increase hemoglobin and hematocrit.

Pharmacokinetics

Absorption: In two stages: 60% after 3 days and up to 90% by 3 weeks. Remainder is absorbed over several months or longer.
Distribution: During first 3 days, local inflammation facilitates passage of drug into lymphatic system; drug is then ingested by macrophages, which enter lymph and blood.
Metabolism: Cleared from plasma by reticuloendothelial cells of liver, spleen, and bone marrow.
Excretion: Trace amounts in urine, bile, and feces. *Half-life:* 6 hours.

Route	Onset	Peak	Duration
I.V., I.M.	72 hr	Unknown	3-4 wk

Action

Chemical effect: Provides elemental iron, a component of hemoglobin.
Therapeutic effect: Increases level of iron, an essential component of hemoglobin.

Available forms

Injection: 50 mg elemental iron/ml

NURSING PROCESS

⬛ Assessment

• Assess patient's iron deficiency before therapy.
• Monitor effectiveness by evaluating hemoglobin, hematocrit, and reticulocyte count, and monitor patient's health status.
• Be alert for adverse reactions and drug interactions.
• Observe patient for delayed reactions (1 to 2 days), which may include arthralgia, backache, chills, dizziness, headache, malaise, fever, myalgia, nausea, and vomiting.
• Evaluate patient's and family's knowledge of drug therapy.

⬛ Nursing diagnoses

• Ineffective health maintenance related to iron deficiency
• Risk for injury related to potential drug-induced anaphylaxis
• Deficient knowledge related to drug therapy

▷ Planning and implementation

• Don't give iron dextran with oral iron preparations.
• I.M. or I.V. injections of iron are recommended only for patients for whom oral administration is impossible or ineffective.
• **ⓢ ALERT:** I.M. or I.V. test dose is required.
• When giving I.M., use a 19G or 20G needle that is 2 to 3 inches long. Inject drug deep into upper outer quadrant of buttock—never into arm or other exposed area. Use Z-track method to avoid leakage into S.C. tissue and staining of skin.
• Minimize skin staining by using separate needle to withdraw drug from its container.
• Keep epinephrine and resuscitation equipment readily available to treat anaphylaxis.
Patient teaching
• Warn patient to avoid OTC vitamins that contain iron.
• Teach patient to recognize and report symptoms of reaction or toxicity.

☑ Evaluation

• Patient's hemoglobin, hematocrit, and reticulocyte counts are normal.
• Patient doesn't experience anaphylaxis.
• Patient and family state understanding of drug therapy.

iron sucrose injection
(IGH-ern SOO-krohs inn-JECK-shun)
Venofer

Pharmacologic classification: polynuclear iron (III)-hydroxide in sucrose
Therapeutic classification: hematinic
Pregnancy risk category: B

Indications and dosages

▶ **Iron deficiency anemia in patients undergoing long-term hemodialysis who are receiving supplemental erythropoietin therapy.**
Adults: 100 mg (5 ml) of elemental iron I.V. di-

rectly in the dialysis line either by slow injection (1 ml per minute) or by infusion over 15 minutes during the dialysis session, one to three times weekly for a total of 1,000 mg in 10 doses. Repeat, if needed.

▼ I.V. administration

• Don't mix with other drugs or add to parenteral nutrition solutions of I.V. infusion.
• Inspect for particulate matter and discoloration before administration.
• For slow injection, administer at 1 ml (20 mg elemental iron) undiluted solution per minute, not exceeding one vial (100 mg elemental iron) per injection.
• For infusion, dilute to a maximum of 100 ml in normal saline solution immediately before infusion, and infuse 100 mg elemental iron over at least 15 minutes. Administering by infusion may reduce the risk of hypotension.
• Transferrin saturation values increase rapidly after I.V. administration of iron sucrose. Obtain iron level values 48 hours after I.V. dosing.

Contraindications and precautions

• Contraindicated in patients with evidence of iron overload, patients hypersensitive to drug or any of its inactive components, and patients with anemia not caused by iron deficiency.
⚠ Lifespan: In breast-feeding women, use cautiously; it's not known whether drug appears in breast milk. In children, safety and effectiveness of drug haven't been established. In elderly patients, make dose selection conservatively; these patients may have decreased hepatic, renal, and cardiac function and other diseases and drug therapies.

Adverse reactions

CNS: fever, headache, asthenia, malaise, dizziness, pain.
CV: *hypotension,* chest pain, **heart failure,** hypertension, fluid retention.
GI: nausea, vomiting, diarrhea, abdominal pain, taste perversion.
Musculoskeletal: *leg cramps,* bone and muscle pain.
Respiratory: dyspnea, pneumonia, cough.
Skin: pruritus.
Other: accidental injury, hypersensitivity reaction (e.g., wheezing, dyspnea, rash, pruritus), *sepsis,* application site reaction.

Interactions

Drug-drug. *Oral iron preparations:* May reduce absorption of these compounds. Avoid using together.

Effects on lab test results

• May increase liver enzyme levels.

Pharmacokinetics

Absorption: Administered I.V.
Distribution: Mainly in blood and somewhat in extravascular fluid. A significant amount of iron is also distributed in the liver, spleen, and bone marrow.
Metabolism: Dissociated by the reticuloendothelial system into iron and sucrose.
Excretion: About 75% of sucrose and 5% of the iron component are eliminated by urinary excretion in 24 hours. *Half-life:* 6 hours.

Route	Onset	Peak	Duration
I.V.	Unknown	Unknown	Variable

Action

Chemical effect: Dissociated by the reticuloendothelial system into iron and sucrose. The released iron component eventually replenishes depleted body iron stores, resulting in significant increases in iron and ferritin levels and significant decreases in total iron binding capacity.
Therapeutic effect: Increases iron level.

Available forms

Injection: 20 mg/ml of elemental iron

NURSING PROCESS

⬛ Assessment
• Assess underlying condition before therapy and reassess regularly.
• Monitor hemoglobin, hematocrit, ferritin level, and transferrin saturation.
• Monitor patient for adverse reactions or hypersensitivity reactions to the drug.
• Evaluate patient's and family's knowledge of drug therapy.

⊞ Nursing diagnoses
• Acute pain related to adverse drug effects
• Ineffective health maintenance related to iron deficiency
• Deficient knowledge related to iron sucrose therapy

⟩⟩ Planning and implementation

- Monitor patient for symptoms of overdose or too-rapid infusion, which include hypotension, headache, nausea, dizziness, joint aches, paresthesia, abdominal and muscle pain, edema, and CV collapse.
- Observe patient for rare but fatal hypersensitivity reactions characterized by anaphylaxis, loss of consciousness, collapse, hypotension, dyspnea, or seizures.
- Withhold dose in patients with evidence of iron overload.

Patient teaching

- Instruct patient to notify prescriber if symptoms of overdose occur, such as headache, nausea, dizziness, joint aches, paresthesia, or abdominal and muscle pain.
- Warn patient not to take OTC vitamins containing iron.

☑ Evaluation

- Patient does not experience pain.
- Patient's hemoglobin and hematocrit are normal.
- Patient and family state understanding of iron sucrose therapy.

---

isoniazid (isonicotinic acid hydride INH)

(igh-soh-NIGH-uh-sid)

Isotamine ◆, Laniazid, Nydrazid, PMS Isoniazid ◆

Pharmacologic class: isonicotinic acid hydrazine
Therapeutic class: antituberculotic
Pregnancy risk category: C

Indications and dosages

▶ **Actively growing tubercle bacilli.** *Adults:* 5 mg/kg P.O. or I.M. daily in single dose, maximum 300 mg P.O. or I.M. daily, continued for 6 months to 2 years.
Infants and children: 10 mg/kg P.O. or I.M. daily in single dose, maximum 300 mg P.O. or I.M. daily, continued for 18 months to 2 years. Administration with at least one other antituberculotic is recommended.
▶ **Prevention of tubercle bacilli in those closely exposed to tuberculosis or those with** positive skin tests whose chest X-rays and bacteriologic studies are consistent with nonprogressive tuberculosis. *Adults:* 300 mg P.O. daily in single dose, for 6 months to 1 year. *Infants and children:* 10 mg/kg P.O. daily in single dose. Maximum, 300 mg P.O. daily for 1 year.

Contraindications and precautions

- Contraindicated in patients with acute hepatic disease or isoniazid-related liver damage.
- Use cautiously in patients with chronic non–isoniazid-related liver disease, seizure disorders (especially in those taking phenytoin), severe renal impairment, or chronic alcoholism.
- ⚘ **Lifespan:** In pregnant and breast-feeding women and in elderly patients, use cautiously.

Adverse reactions

CNS: *peripheral neuropathy* (especially in patients who are malnourished, alcoholic, diabetic, or slow acetylators), usually preceded by paresthesia of hands and feet; psychosis; *seizures.*
GI: nausea, vomiting, epigastric distress, constipation, dry mouth.
Hematologic: *agranulocytosis,* hemolytic anemia, *aplastic anemia,* eosinophilia, *leukopenia, neutropenia, thrombocytopenia, methemoglobinemia,* pyridoxine-responsive hypochromic anemia.
Hepatic: *hepatitis* (occasionally severe and sometimes fatal, especially in elderly patients).
Metabolic: hyperglycemia, *metabolic acidosis.*
Other: rheumatic syndrome and lupuslike syndrome, hypersensitivity reactions (fever, rash, lymphadenopathy, vasculitis), irritation at I.M. injection site.

Interactions

Drug-drug. *Acetaminophen:* May increase hepatotoxic effects of acetaminophen. Don't give together.
Antacids and laxatives containing aluminum: May decrease rate and amount of isoniazid absorbed. Give isoniazid at least 1 hour before antacid or laxative.
Carbamazepine: May increase risk of isoniazid hepatotoxicity. Use together cautiously.
Carbamazepine, phenytoin: May increase levels of these anticonvulsants. Monitor patient closely.
Corticosteroids: May decrease therapeutic effect of isoniazid. Monitor patient's need for larger isoniazid dose.

Cyclosporine: May increase adverse CNS effects of cyclosporine. Monitor patient closely.
Disulfiram: May cause neurologic symptoms, including changes in behavior and coordination. Avoid using together.
Ketoconazole: May decrease ketoconazole levels. Monitor patient closely.
Oral anticoagulants: May increase anticoagulant activity. Monitor patient for signs of bleeding.
Rifampin: May increase risk of hepatotoxicity. Monitor patient closely.
Theophylline: May increase theophylline level. Monitor level closely, and adjust theophylline dosage.
Drug-food. *Foods containing tyramine:* May cause hypertensive crisis. Tell patients to avoid such foods altogether.
Drug-lifestyle. *Alcohol use:* May increase risk of isoniazid-related hepatitis. Discourage using together.

Effects on lab test results

● May increase transaminase, glucose, and bilirubin levels. May decrease calcium and phosphate levels.
● May increase eosinophil count. May decrease hemoglobin, hematocrit, and WBC, granulocyte, neutrophil, and platelet counts.

Pharmacokinetics

Absorption: Complete and rapid after P.O. administration. Also absorbed readily after I.M. injection.
Distribution: Wide.
Metabolism: Primarily in liver. Rate of metabolism varies individually; fast acetylators metabolize drug five times as rapidly as others. About 50% of blacks and whites are slow acetylators, whereas more than 80% of Chinese, Japanese, and Eskimos are fast acetylators.
Excretion: Primarily in urine; some in saliva, sputum, feces, and breast milk. *Half-life:* 1 to 4 hours.

Route	Onset	Peak	Duration
P.O., I.M.	Unknown	1-2 hr	Unknown

Action

Chemical effect: May inhibit cell wall biosynthesis by interfering with lipid and DNA synthesis.

Therapeutic effect: Kills susceptible bacteria, such as *Mycobacterium tuberculosis, M. bovis,* and some strains of *M. kansasii.*

Available forms

Injection: 100 mg/ml
Oral solution: 50 mg/5 ml
Tablets: 100 mg, 300 mg

NURSING PROCESS

Assessment
● Assess patient's infection before therapy.
● Monitor patient for improvement, and evaluate culture and sensitivity tests.
● Be alert for adverse reactions and drug interactions.
● Monitor hepatic function closely for changes.
● Monitor patient for paresthesia of hands and feet, which usually precedes peripheral neuropathy, especially in patients who are malnourished, alcoholic, diabetic, or slow acetylators.
● Evaluate patient's and family's knowledge of drug therapy.

Nursing diagnoses
● Infection related to presence of susceptible bacteria
● Disturbed sensory perception (tactile) related to drug-induced peripheral neuropathy
● Deficient knowledge related to drug therapy

Planning and implementation
● Give oral form of drug 1 hour before or 2 hours after meals to avoid decreased absorption.
● When giving I.M., switch to P.O. form as soon as possible.
● Always give isoniazid with other antituberculotics to prevent development of resistant organisms.
● Give pyridoxine to prevent peripheral neuropathy, especially in malnourished patients.
Patient teaching
● Tell patient to take drug as prescribed; warn against stopping drug without prescriber's consent.
● Advise patient to take with food if GI irritation occurs.
● Instruct patient to avoid alcohol during drug therapy.
● Instruct patient to avoid certain foods (fish, such as skipjack and tuna, and tyramine-containing products, such as aged cheese, beer,

and chocolate) because drug has some MAO inhibitor activity.
• Tell patient to notify prescriber immediately if symptoms of liver impairment occur (loss of appetite, fatigue, malaise, jaundice, dark urine).
• Urge patient to comply with treatment, which may last for months or years.

☑ Evaluation
• Patient is free from infection.
• Patient maintains normal peripheral nervous system function.
• Patient and family state understanding of drug therapy.

isoproterenol (isoprenaline)
(igh-soh-proh-TEER-uh-nol)
Isuprel

isoproterenol hydrochloride

isoproterenol sulfate
Medihaler-Iso

Pharmacologic class: adrenergic
Therapeutic class: bronchodilator, cardiac stimulant
Pregnancy risk category: C

Indications and dosages
▶ **Bronchospasm.** *Adults and children:* For acute dyspneic episodes, one inhalation of sulfate form initially. Repeat, if needed, after 2 to 5 minutes. Maintenance dosage is one to two inhalations four to six times daily. Repeat once more 10 minutes after second dose. Give no more than three doses for each attack.
▶ **Bronchospasm in COPD.** Give by IPPB or for nebulization by compressed air or oxygen. *Adults:* 2 ml of 0.125% or 2.5 ml of 0.1% solution (prepared by diluting 0.5 ml of 0.5% solution to 2 or 2.5 ml or by diluting 0.25 ml of 1% solution to 2 or 2.5 ml with water or half-normal or normal saline solution) up to five times daily.
Children: 2 ml of 0.125% solution or 2.5 ml of 0.1% solution up to five times daily.
▶ **Heart block and ventricular arrhythmias.** *Adults:* Initially, 0.02 to 0.06 mg hydrochloride I.V. Subsequent doses 0.01 to 0.2 mg I.V. or

5 mcg/minute I.V. Or, 0.2 mg I.M. initially; then 0.02 to 1 mg, p.r.n.
Children: Give half of initial adult dose of hydrochloride.
▶ **Shock.** *Adults and children:* 0.5 to 5 mcg/minute hydrochloride by continuous I.V. infusion. Usual concentration is 1 mg (5 ml) in 500 ml D_5W. Infusion rate adjusted according to heart rate, central venous pressure, blood pressure, and urine flow.
▶ **Postoperative cardiac patients with bradycardia‡.** *Children:* I.V. infusion of 0.029 mcg/kg/minute.
▶ **As an aid in diagnosing the cause of mitral regurgitation‡.** *Adults:* 4 mcg/minute I.V. infusion.
▶ **As an aid in diagnosing coronary artery disease or lesions‡.** *Adults:* 1 to 3 mcg/minute I.V. infusion.

▽ I.V. administration
• If injection solution is discolored or contains precipitate, don't use.
• Give drug by direct injection or I.V. infusion. For infusion, drug may be diluted with most common I.V. solutions. However, don't use with sodium bicarbonate injection; drug decomposes rapidly in alkaline solutions.
ⓢ **ALERT:** If heart rate exceeds 110 beats/min with I.V. infusion, notify prescriber. Doses sufficient to increase heart rate to more than 130 beats/min may induce ventricular arrhythmias.
• When giving I.V. isoproterenol to treat shock, closely monitor blood pressure, central venous pressure, ECG, arterial blood gas measurements, and urine output. Carefully adjust infusion rate according to these measurements. Use continuous infusion pump to regulate flow rate.

Contraindications and precautions
• Contraindicated in patients with tachycardia caused by digitalis intoxication, in those with arrhythmias (other than those that may respond to treatment with isoproterenol), and in those with angina pectoris.
• Use cautiously in patients with renal or CV disease, coronary insufficiency, diabetes, hyperthyroidism, or history of sensitivity to sympathomimetic amines.
⚠ **Lifespan:** In pregnant and breast-feeding women and in children and elderly patients, use cautiously.

Adverse reactions

CNS: *headache,* mild tremor, weakness, dizziness, nervousness, insomnia, ***Stokes-Adams seizures.***
CV: *palpitations, tachycardia, angina,* flushing of face, ***cardiac arrest,*** *blood pressure that rises and then falls,* ***arrhythmias.***
GI: nausea, vomiting.
Metabolic: hyperglycemia.
Respiratory: ***bronchospasm.***
Skin: diaphoresis.

Interactions

Drug-drug. *Epinephrine, other sympathomimetics:* Increases risk of arrhythmias. Avoid using together.
Propranolol, other beta blockers: Blocks bronchodilating effect of isoproterenol. If used together, monitor patient carefully.

Effects on lab test results

• May increase glucose level.

Pharmacokinetics

Absorption: Rapid after P.O. inhalation.
Distribution: Wide.
Metabolism: By conjugation in GI tract and by enzymatic reduction in liver, lungs, and other tissues.
Excretion: Primarily in urine.

Route	Onset	Peak	Duration
I.V.	Immediate	Unknown	< 1 hr
Inhalation	2-5 min	Unknown	½-2 hr

Action

Chemical effect: Relaxes bronchial smooth muscle by acting on beta$_2$-adrenergic receptors. As cardiac stimulant, acts on beta$_1$-adrenergic receptors in heart.
Therapeutic effect: Relieves bronchospasms and heart block and restores normal sinus rhythm after ventricular arrhythmia.

Available forms

isoproterenol
Nebulizer inhaler: 0.25%, 0.5%, 1%
isoproterenol hydrochloride
Aerosol inhaler: 131 mcg/metered spray
Injection: 20 mcg/ml, 200 mcg/ml
Solution for inhalation: 0.5%, 1%
isoproterenol sulfate
Aerosol inhaler: 80 mcg/metered spray

NURSING PROCESS

⚗ Assessment
• Assess patient's underlying condition before therapy.
• Monitor cardiopulmonary status frequently.
• Be alert for adverse reactions and drug interactions.
• This drug may aggravate ventilation and perfusion abnormalities. Even when ease of breathing is improved, arterial oxygen tension may fall paradoxically.
• Evaluate patient's and family's knowledge of drug therapy.

⊞ Nursing diagnoses
• Ineffective health maintenance related to underlying condition
• Risk for injury related to drug-induced adverse reactions
• Deficient knowledge related to drug therapy

▷ Planning and implementation
• Drug doesn't treat blood or fluid volume deficit. Correct volume deficit before giving vasopressors.
⊛ ALERT: Don't confuse Isuprel with Ismelin or Isordil.
• If drug is given by inhalation with oxygen, make sure oxygen concentration won't suppress respiratory drive.
• Follow same instructions for metered powder nebulizer, although deep inhalation isn't needed.
• If adverse reactions occur, notify prescriber; adjust dosage or stop drug if needed.
• If precordial distress or angina occurs, stop drug immediately.
Patient teaching
• Give patient the following instructions for using metered-dose inhaler: Clear nasal passages and throat. Breathe out, expelling as much air from lungs as possible. Place mouthpiece well into mouth and inhale deeply as you release dose from inhaler. Hold breath for several seconds, remove mouthpiece, and exhale slowly.
• Tell patient to wait at least 2 minutes before repeating when using more than one inhalation.
• If patient also uses a corticosteroid inhaler, tell him to use bronchodilator first, and then wait about 5 minutes before using corticosteroid. This process allows bronchodilator to open air passages for maximum effectiveness of the corticosteroid.

• Warn patient using oral inhalant that this drug may turn sputum and saliva pink.
• Tell patient to stop drug and notify prescriber about chest tightness or dyspnea.
• Warn patient against overuse of drug. Tell him that tolerance can develop.
• Tell patient to reduce caffeine intake during therapy.

☑ **Evaluation**
• Patient exhibits improved health.
• Patient doesn't experience injury from adverse reactions.
• Patient and family state understanding of drug therapy.

isosorbide dinitrate
(igh-soh-SOR-bighd digh-NIGH-trayt)
**Apo-ISDN♦ , Cedocard SR♦ , Coronex♦ ,
Dilatrate-SR, Isordil, Isordil Titradose,
Isotrate, Sorbitrate**

isosorbide mononitrate
IMDUR, ISMO, Isotrate ER, Monoket

Pharmacologic class: nitrate
Therapeutic class: antianginal, vasodilator
Pregnancy risk category: C

Indications and dosages

▶ **Acute angina, prophylaxis in situations likely to cause angina.** *Adults:* 2.5 to 10 mg isosorbide dinitrate S.L. for prompt relief of angina pain, repeated q 2 to 3 hours during acute phase, or q 4 to 6 hours for prophylaxis. Or, 2.5 to 10 mg chewable tablets, p.r.n., for acute attack or q 2 to 3 hours for prophylaxis but only after initial test dose of 5 mg to determine risk of severe hypotension. Or, initially, 5 to 20 mg P.O., then maintain on 10 to 40 mg P.O. q 6 hr. Or. initially, 40 mg extended-release tablets P.O., then maintain on 40 to 80 mg P.O. q 8 to 12 hours. Use isosorbide mononitrate for prophylaxis only: 20 mg P.O. b.i.d. with doses 7 hours apart and first dose upon awakening. For sustained-release form, 30 to 60 mg P.O. once daily on arising; after several days, dosage may be increased to 120 mg once daily; rarely, 240 mg may be needed.
▶ **Adjunctive treatment of heart failure‡.** *Adults:* 80 mg isosorbide dinitrate P.O. daily

with hydralazine. Maximum dose is 160 mg isosorbide dinitrate and 300 mg hydralazine.
▶ **Diffuse esophageal spasm without gastroesophageal reflux‡.** *Adults:* 10 to 30 mg isosorbide dinitrate P.O. q.i.d.

Contraindications and precautions

• Contraindicated in patients hypersensitive to nitrates, in those with idiosyncratic reactions to nitrates, and in those with severe hypotension, shock, or acute MI with low–left-ventricular filling pressure.
• Use cautiously in patients with blood volume depletion (such as that resulting from diuretic therapy) or mild hypotension.
☆ **Lifespan:** In pregnant and breast-feeding women, use cautiously. In children, safety of drug hasn't been established.

Adverse reactions

CNS: *headache, sometimes with throbbing; dizziness;* weakness.
CV: orthostatic hypotension, tachycardia, palpitations, ankle edema, fainting, *flushing.*
GI: nausea, vomiting.
Skin: cutaneous vasodilation.
Other: hypersensitivity reactions, S.L. burning.

Interactions

Drug-drug. *Antihypertensives:* Possibly increased hypotensive effects. Monitor patient closely during initial therapy.
Sildenafil, vardenafil: May cause severe hypotension. Avoid using together.
Drug-lifestyle. *Alcohol use:* May increase hypotension. Discourage using together.

Effects on lab test results

None reported.

Pharmacokinetics

Absorption: Dinitrate is well absorbed from GI tract but undergoes first-pass metabolism, resulting in bioavailability of about 50% (depending on dosage form used). Mononitrate is also absorbed well, with almost 100% bioavailability.
Distribution: Distributed widely throughout body.
Metabolism: Metabolized in liver to active metabolites.

Excretion: Excreted in urine. *Half-life:* Dinitrate P.O., 5 to 6 hours; S.L., 2 hours; mononitrate, about 5 hours.

Route	Onset	Peak	Duration
P.O.	2-60 min	2-60 min	1-12 hr
S.L.	2-5 min	2-5 min	1-2 hr

Action

Chemical effect: May reduce cardiac oxygen demand by decreasing left–ventricular-end diastolic pressure (preload) and, to a lesser extent, systemic vascular resistance (afterload). Drug also may increase blood flow through collateral coronary vessels. Most isosorbide dinitrate activity is attributed to its active metabolite, isosorbide mononitrate.

Therapeutic effect: Relieves angina.

Available forms

isosorbide dinitrate
Tablets: 5 mg, 10 mg, 20 mg, 30 mg, 40 mg
Tablets (chewable): 5 mg, 10 mg
Tablets (S.L.): 2.5 mg, 5 mg, 10 mg
Tablets (sustained-release): 40 mg
isosorbide mononitrate
Tablets: 10 mg, 20 mg
Tablets (extended-release): 30 mg, 60 mg, 120 mg

NURSING PROCESS

🜂 Assessment

• Assess patient's angina before therapy and regularly thereafter.
• Monitor blood pressure, heart rate and rhythm, and intensity and duration of drug response.
• Be alert for adverse reactions and drug interactions.
• Evaluate patient's and family's knowledge of drug therapy.

🜂 Nursing diagnoses

• Acute pain related to angina
• Risk for injury related to drug-induced adverse reactions
• Deficient knowledge related to drug therapy

▷ Planning and implementation

🜋 **ALERT:** Don't confuse Isordil with Isuprel or Inderal.

🜋 **ALERT:** Don't confuse Coronex (isosorbide dinitrate) with Coronex (the herbal supplement).
• To prevent development of tolerance, don't give drug during an 8- to 12-hour period daily. The dosage regimen for isosorbide mononitrate (one tablet upon awakening with second dose in 7 hours, or one extended-release tablet daily) is intended to offer nitrate-free period during the day to minimize nitrate tolerance.
• Give drug on empty stomach, either 30 minutes before or 1 to 2 hours after meals, and have patient swallow tablets whole. Have patient chew chewable tablets thoroughly before swallowing.
• Give S.L. form of drug at first sign of angina. Have patient wet tablet with saliva, place it under his tongue until completely absorbed, and sit down and rest. Dose may be repeated every 10 to 15 minutes for maximum of three doses.
🜋 **ALERT:** Don't stop drug abruptly because coronary vasospasm may occur.
• If patient's pain doesn't subside, notify prescriber immediately.

Patient teaching
• Advise patient to take drug regularly, as prescribed, and to keep it accessible at all times.
🜋 **ALERT:** Advise patient that abrupt discontinuation causes coronary vasospasm.
• Tell patient to take S.L. tablet at first sign of attack. Explain that tablet should be wet with saliva and placed under tongue until completely absorbed, and that patient should sit down and rest until pain subsides. Tell patient that dose may be repeated every 10 to 15 minutes for maximum of three doses. If drug doesn't provide relief, tell him to get medical help promptly.
• Tell patient who complains of tingling sensation with drug placed S.L. to try holding tablet in buccal pouch.
🜋 **ALERT:** Warn patient not to confuse S.L. form with P.O. form.
• Instruct patient taking oral form to take tablet on empty stomach, either 30 minutes before or 1 to 2 hours after meals, and to swallow tablet whole or chew chewable tablet thoroughly before swallowing.
• Tell patient to minimize orthostatic hypotension by changing to upright position slowly. Tell him to go up and down stairs carefully and to lie down at first sign of dizziness.
• Instruct patient to avoid alcohol consumption during therapy.

• Tell patient to store drug in cool place, in tightly closed container, away from light.

☑ Evaluation
• Patient is free from pain.
• Patient doesn't experience injury from adverse reactions.
• Patient and family state understanding of drug therapy.

isotretinoin
(igh-soh-TREH-tih-noyn)
Accutane, Accutane Roche ♦, Amnesteem, Claravis, Roaccutane ◇, Sotret

Pharmacologic class: retinoic acid derivative
Therapeutic class: antiacne drug
Pregnancy risk category: X

Indications and dosages

▶ **Severe recalcitrant nodular acne unresponsive to conventional therapy.** *Adults and children ages 12 to 17:* 0.5 to 2 mg/kg P.O. daily in two divided doses for 15 to 20 weeks.
▶ **Keratinization disorders resistant to conventional therapy, prevention of skin cancer‡.** *Adults:* Dosage varies with specific disease and severity of the disorder. Dosages up to 2 to 4 mg/kg P.O. daily have been used. Consult literature for specific recommendations.
▶ **Squamous cell cancer of the head and neck‡.** *Adults:* 50 to 100 mg/m² P.O.

Contraindications and precautions

• Contraindicated in patients hypersensitive to parabens, which are used as preservatives.
• Use cautiously in patients with genetic predisposition or history of osteoporosis, osteomalacia, or other disorders of bone metabolism. Also use cautiously in patients with a history of mental illness or a family history of psychiatric disorders, asthma, liver disease, diabetes, heart disease, osteoporosis, weak bones, or anorexia nervosa.
⚡ Lifespan: In women of child-bearing age, drug is contraindicated unless patient has had negative serum pregnancy test within 2 weeks of beginning therapy, will begin drug therapy on second or third day of next menstrual period, and will comply with stringent contraceptive measures for 1 month before therapy, during

therapy, and at least 1 month after therapy. In pregnant women, drug is contraindicated. In breast-feeding women, drug isn't recommended. In children younger than age 12, safety of drug hasn't been established. In children ages 12 to 17, use cautiously.

Adverse reactions

CNS: headache, fatigue, depression, psychosis, *suicide, depression, psychosis, aggressive and violent behavior,* emotional instability, *pseudotumor cerebri (benign intracranial hypertension).*
CV: *hypertriglyceridemia.*
EENT: *conjunctivitis,* corneal deposits, dry eyes, visual disturbances, hearing impairment, decreased night vision.
GI: nonspecific GI symptoms, gum bleeding and inflammation, nausea, vomiting, *acute pancreatitis,* inflammatory bowel disease.
Hepatic: *hepatitis.*
Hematologic: anemia.
Metabolic: hyperglycemia.
Musculoskeletal: skeletal hyperostosis, calcification of tendons and ligaments, premature epiphyseal closure, decreases in bone mineral density, musculoskeletal symptoms (sometimes severe) including back pain and arthralgia, arthritis, tendonitis, other types of bone abnormalities, *rhabdomyolysis.*
Skin: *cheilosis, rash, dry skin,* peeling of palms and toes, skin infection, thinning of hair, photosensitivity.

Interactions

Drug-drug. *Corticosteroids:* May increase risk of osteoporosis. Use together cautiously.
Medicated soaps and cleansers, medicated cover-ups, topical resorcinol peeling agents (benzoyl peroxide), and preparations containing alcohol: Cumulative drying effect. Use cautiously.
Micro-dosed progesterone birth control pills that don't contain estrogen: May decrease effectiveness of birth control. Advise patient to use alternative contraceptive methods.
Phenytoin: May increase risk of osteomalacia. Use together cautiously.
Tetracyclines: May increase the potential for the development of pseudotumor cerebri. Avoid use together.
Vitamin A products: May have additive toxic effect. Avoid use together.

Drug-food. *Any food:* May enhance absorption of drug. Have patient take drug with food.
Drug-lifestyle. *Alcohol use:* May increase risk of hypertriglyceridemia. Discourage using together.
Sun exposure: May increase photosensitivity reactions. Advise patient to use sunscreen and wear protective clothing.

Effects on lab test results

• May increase CPK, ALT, AST, alkaline phosphatase, glucose, and triglyceride levels.
• May increase platelet count. May decrease hemoglobin and hematocrit.

Pharmacokinetics

Absorption: Rapid.
Distribution: Wide; 99.9% protein-bound, primarily to albumin.
Metabolism: Metabolized in liver and possibly in gut wall.
Excretion: Unknown. *Half-life:* 30 minutes to 39 hours.

Route	Onset	Peak	Duration
P.O.	Unknown	3 hr	Unknown

Action

Chemical effect: May normalize keratinization, reversibly decrease size of sebaceous glands, and alter composition of sebum to less viscous form that is less likely to plug follicles.
Therapeutic effect: Improves skin integrity.

Available forms

Capsules: 10 mg, 20 mg, 30 mg, 40 mg

NURSING PROCESS

Assessment

• Assess patient's skin before therapy and regularly thereafter.
• Obtain baseline lipid studies, liver function test results, and pregnancy test before therapy. Monitor these values at regular intervals until response to drug is established (usually about 4 weeks).
• Monitor glucose and CK levels in patients who engage in vigorous physical activity.
• Be alert for adverse reactions and drug interactions.
• Osteoporosis, osteopenia, bone fractures, and delayed healing of bone fractures have been seen in patients taking isotretinoin. While causality to drug hasn't been established, an effect can't be ruled out. Long-term effects haven't been studied. It's important to not exceed the recommended dose or duration.
• Most adverse reactions appear to be dose-related, occurring at dosages greater than 1 mg/kg daily. They're usually reversible when therapy is stopped or dosage reduced.
• Evaluate patient's and family's knowledge of drug therapy.

Nursing diagnoses

• Impaired skin integrity related to underlying skin condition
• Impaired tissue integrity related to adverse reactions
• Deficient knowledge related to drug therapy

Planning and implementation

• Start second course of therapy at least 8 weeks after completion of first course because improvement may continue after stopping drug.
• Give drug with meals or shortly thereafter to enhance absorption.
• **ALERT:** Screen patient with headache, nausea and vomiting, or visual disturbances for papilledema. Signs and symptoms of pseudotumor cerebri require an immediate stop to therapy and prompt neurologic intervention.
Patient teaching
• Advise patient to take drug with milk, meals, or shortly after meals to ensure adequate absorption.
• Tell patient to immediately report visual disturbances and bone, muscle, or joint pain.
• Warn patient that contact lenses may feel uncomfortable during therapy.
• Warn patient against using abrasives, medicated soaps and cleansers, acne preparations containing peeling agents, and topical alcohol preparations (including cosmetics, after-shave, cologne) because these agents cause cumulative irritation or excessive drying of skin.
• Instruct patient to avoid alcohol during therapy.
• Tell patient to avoid prolonged exposure to sunlight, to use sunblock, and to wear protective clothing.
• **ALERT:** Advise patient not to donate blood during or for 30 days after therapy; severe fetal abnormalities may occur if a pregnant woman receives blood containing isotretinoin.

• Advise women of child-bearing age to use two reliable forms of contraception simultaneously within 1 month of treatment.

☑ **Evaluation**
• Patient has improved skin condition.
• Patient is free from conjunctivitis, corneal deposits, and dry eyes.
• Patient and family state understanding of drug therapy.

itraconazole
(ih-truh-KAHN-uh-zohl)
Sporanox

Pharmacologic class: synthetic triazole
Therapeutic class: antifungal
Pregnancy risk category: C

Indications and dosages

▶ **Pulmonary and extrapulmonary blastomycosis, histoplasmosis.** *Adults:* 200 mg P.O. (capsules) daily. Dosage may be increased as needed and tolerated in 100-mg increments to maximum of 400 mg daily. Divide doses larger than 200 mg daily into two doses. Continue treatment for at least 3 months. In life-threatening illness, loading dose of 200 mg t.i.d. is given for 3 days. Or, give 200 mg by I.V. infusion over 1 hour twice daily for four doses; then 200 mg I.V. once daily.
▶ **Aspergillosis.** *Adults:* 200 to 400 mg P.O. (capsules) daily. Or, give 200 mg by I.V. infusion over 1 hour twice daily for four doses; then decrease to 200 mg I.V. once daily for up to 14 days.
▶ **Onychomycosis for toenails with or without fingernail involvement.** *Adults:* 200 mg P.O. (capsules) once daily for 12 weeks.
▶ **Onychomycosis for fingernails.** *Adults:* Two treatment phases each consisting of 200 mg P.O. (capsules) b.i.d. for 1 week. Phases are separated by a 3-week period without drug.
▶ **Esophageal candidiasis.** *Adults:* 100 to 200 mg P.O. (oral solution) swished in mouth vigorously and swallowed daily for a minimum of 3 weeks.
▶ **Oropharyngeal candidiasis.** *Adults:* 200 mg P.O. (oral solution) swished in mouth vigorously and swallowed daily for 1 to 2 weeks. For patients unresponsive to fluconazole tablets, give 100 mg swished in mouth vigorously and swallowed twice daily for 2 to 4 weeks.

▼ **I.V. administration**
• Dilute in normal saline solution for injection. Add dose to 50-ml I.V. bag of normal saline solution.
• Compatibility with other drugs is unknown.
• Infuse over 60 minutes, using an infusion set with a filter. Flush I.V. line with 15 to 20 ml of normal saline solution after each infusion.

Contraindications and precautions

• Contraindicated in patients hypersensitive to drug and in those receiving oral triazolam or oral midazolam. Also contraindicated in patients with ventricular dysfunction, heart failure, or a history of heart failure. Don't use injection in patients with a creatinine clearance less than 30 ml/minute. Also contraindicated in patients receiving pimozide, dofetilide, or quinidine.
• Use cautiously in patients with hypochlorhydria (they may not absorb drug as readily as patients with normal gastric acidity), in HIV-infected patients (hypochlorhydria can accompany HIV infection), and in those with liver disease.
⚠ Lifespan: In pregnant women, use cautiously. In breast-feeding women, drug is contraindicated because it appears in breast milk. In children, safety of drug hasn't been established.

Adverse reactions

CNS: malaise, fatigue, *headache,* dizziness, somnolence, fever, asthenia, pain, tremor, abnormal dreaming, anxiety, depression.
CV: edema, hypertension, orthostatic hypotension, *heart failure,* hypertriglyceridemia.
EENT: rhinitis, sinusitis, pharyngitis.
GI: *nausea,* vomiting, diarrhea, abdominal pain, anorexia, dyspepsia, flatulence, increased appetite, constipation, gastritis, gastroenteritis, ulcerative stomatitis, gingivitis.
GU: albuminuria, impotence, cystitis, UTI.
Hematologic: *neutropenia.*
Hepatic: *impaired hepatic function, hepatotoxicity, liver failure (fatal).*
Metabolic: hypokalemia.
Musculoskeletal: myalgia.

Reactions may be *common,* uncommon, *life-threatening,* or COMMON AND LIFE-THREATENING.

Respiratory: upper respiratory tract infection, *pulmonary edema.*
Skin: rash, pruritus.
Other: decreased libido, injury, herpes zoster, *hypersensitivity reactions (urticaria, angioedema, Steven-Johnson syndrome).*

Interactions

Drug-drug. *Antacids, H₂-receptor antagonists, phenytoin, rifampin:* May decrease itraconazole level. Avoid using together.
Alprazolam, chlordiazepoxide, clonazepam, clorazepate, diazepam, estazolam, flurazepam, midazolam, quazepam, triazolam: May increase and prolong levels of these drugs, CNS depression, and psychomotor impairment. Don't use together.
Atorvastatin, fluvastatin, lovastatin, pravastatin, simvastatin: May increase levels and adverse effects of these HMG-CoA reductase inhibitors. Avoid this combination. If they must be given together, reduce dose of HMG-CoA reductase inhibitor.
Cyclosporine, digoxin: May increase levels of these drugs. Monitor level closely.
Dofetilide, pimozide, quinidine: May increase levels of these drugs by CYP 3A4 metabolism, causing serious CV events, including torsades de pointes, prolonged QT interval, ventricular tachycardia, cardiac arrest, or sudden death. Avoid using together.
Isoniazid: May decrease itraconazole level. Monitor patient closely.
Oral anticoagulants: May enhance anticoagulant effects. Monitor PT and INR closely.
Oral antidiabetics: May cause hypoglycemia. Monitor glucose level.
Drug-food. *Colas:* May increase drug level and adverse effects. Advise patient to take drug with water.
Grapefruit: May delay absorption of drug. Advise patient to avoid grapefruit products.
Orange juice: May decrease level and therapeutic effects of drug. Advise patient to avoid taking drug with orange juice.

Effects on lab test results

• May increase alkaline phosphatase, ALT, AST, bilirubin, and GGT levels. May decrease potassium level.

Pharmacokinetics

Absorption: Bioavailability is maximal when taken without food. Absolute bioavailability is 55%.
Distribution: Protein binding is 99.8%; that of its metabolite, hydroxyitraconazole, is 99.5%. Extensively distributed in tissues susceptible to infection.
Metabolism: Extensively metabolized by liver into large number of metabolites, including hydroxyitraconazole, the major metabolite.
Excretion: In feces and urine. *Half-life:* 1 to 8½ hours.

Route	Onset	Peak	Duration
P.O.			
fasting	Unknown	2 hr	Unknown
not fasting	Unknown	5 hr	Unknown
I.V.	Unknown	Unknown	Unknown

Action

Chemical effect: Interferes with fungal cell wall synthesis by inhibiting formation of ergosterol and increasing cell wall permeability.
Therapeutic effect: Hinders fungi, including *Aspergillus* sp. and *Blastomyces dermatitidis.*

Available forms

Capsules: 100 mg
Injection: 10 mg/ml
Oral solution: 10 mg/ml

NURSING PROCESS

Assessment
• Assess patient's infection before therapy and regularly thereafter.
• Before starting treatment, obtain nail specimens for KOH preparation, fungal culture, or nail biopsy to confirm diagnosis of onychomycosis.
• Monitor liver and renal function test results.
• Be alert for adverse reactions and drug interactions.
• Evaluate patient's and family's knowledge of drug therapy.

Nursing diagnoses
• Infection related to presence of susceptible fungi
• Risk for deficient fluid volume related to adverse reactions
• Deficient knowledge related to drug therapy

▶ Planning and implementation

• Don't use in patients with baseline liver impairment, unless there is a life-threatening situation where benefit exceeds risk. If signs of liver dysfunction occur, monitor liver function closely and stop therapy; don't restart unless the benefit exceeds risk.

• Give capsules with food. Don't give oral solution with food.

⊛ **ALERT:** Oral solution and capsules aren't interchangeable.

• If signs and symptoms of heart failure occur, stop drug.

• Report signs and symptoms of liver disease and abnormal liver test results.

Patient teaching

• Teach patient to recognize and report signs and symptoms of liver disease (anorexia, dark urine, pale feces, unusual fatigue, or jaundice).

• Tell patient to take capsules with food to ensure maximal absorption.

• Instruct patient to swish oral solution vigorously in the mouth (10 ml at a time) for several seconds and then swallow.

☑ Evaluation

• Patient is free from infection.

• Patient maintains adequate fluid balance.

• Patient and family state understanding of drug therapy.

kaolin and pectin mixtures
(KAY-oh-lin and PEK-tin MIX-cherz)
K-Pek, Kaodene Non-Narcotic†, Kaolin w/Pectin†, Kao-Spen, Kapectolin†

Pharmacologic class: absorbent
Therapeutic class: antidiarrheal
Pregnancy risk category: NR

Indications and dosages

▶ **Mild, nonspecific diarrhea.** *Adults:* With regular-strength suspension, 60 to 120 ml P.O. after each bowel movement. With liquid, 45 ml P.O. one to three times daily or after each loose bowel movement.

Children ages 6 to 12: With regular-strength suspension, 30 to 60 ml P.O. after each bowel movement. With liquid, 22.5 ml P.O. one to three times daily or after each loose bowel movement.

Children ages 3 to 6: With regular-strength suspension, 15 to 30 ml P.O. after each bowel movement. With liquid, 15 ml P.O. one to three times daily or after each loose bowel movement.

Contraindications and precautions

• Do not use in patients with diarrhea linked to pseudomembranous colitis or caused by toxigenic bacteria.

• Use cautiously in patients with bleeding disorders or salicylate sensitivity.

☀ **Lifespan:** In pregnant women and in children, use cautiously.

Adverse reactions

GI: constipation; fecal impaction or ulceration (in infants and elderly or debilitated patients after long-term use).

Interactions

Drug-drug. *Oral drugs:* May decrease drug absorption. Separate administration times by at least 2 to 3 hours.

Effects on lab test results

None reported.

Pharmacokinetics

Absorption: None.
Distribution: None.
Metabolism: None.
Excretion: In stool. *Half-life:* Unknown.

Route	Onset	Peak	Duration
P.O.	Unknown	Unknown	Unknown

Action

Chemical effect: Decreases fluid content of feces, although total water loss seems to remain the same.
Therapeutic effect: Alleviates diarrhea.

Available forms

Liquid: 3.9 g kaolin and 194.4 mg pectin per 30 ml with bismuth subsalicylate (Kaodene)
Oral suspension: 5.2 g kaolin and 260 mg pectin per 30 ml† (Kao-Spen), 90 g kaolin and

2 g pectin per 30 ml† (Kapectolin†, Kaolin w/Pectin†)

NURSING PROCESS

⚡ Assessment
- Assess patient's bowel patterns before and after therapy.
- Be alert for adverse GI reactions and drug interactions.
- Evaluate patient's and family's knowledge of drug therapy.

🔷 Nursing diagnoses
- Diarrhea related to underlying condition
- Constipation related to long-term use of drug
- Deficient knowledge related to drug therapy

❯ Planning and implementation
- Read label carefully. Check dosage and strength.
- Give dose after each loose bowel movement.
- Don't use in place of specific therapy for underlying cause of diarrhea.

Patient teaching
- Warn patient not to use drug to replace therapy for underlying cause.
- Advise patient not to use drug for more than 2 days.

✔ Evaluation
- Patient reports decrease in or absence of loose stools.
- Patient doesn't have constipation.
- Patient and family state understanding of drug therapy.

ketoconazole
(kee-toh-KAHN-uh-zohl)
Nizoral, Nizoral A-D

Pharmacologic class: imidazole derivative
Therapeutic class: antifungal
Pregnancy risk category: C

Indications and dosages

▶ **Systemic candidiasis, chronic mucocandidiasis, oral thrush, candiduria, coccidioidomycosis, histoplasmosis, chromomycosis, paracoccidioidomycosis, severe cutaneous dermatophyte infection resistant to therapy with topical or oral griseofulvin.** *Adults and children weighing more than 40 kg (88 lb):* Initially, 200 mg P.O. daily in single dose. Dosage may be increased to 400 mg once daily in patients who don't respond to lower dosage.
Children age 2 and older: 3.3 to 6.6 mg/kg P.O. daily as single dose.

Contraindications and precautions

- Contraindicated in patients hypersensitive to drug and in those taking oral midazolam or triazolam.
- Use cautiously in patients with hepatic disease and in those taking other hepatotoxic drugs.
⚖ **Lifespan:** In pregnant women, use cautiously. Breast-feeding women shouldn't breast-feed during therapy.

Adverse reactions

CNS: headache, nervousness, dizziness, *suicidal tendencies.*
GI: *nausea, vomiting,* abdominal pain, diarrhea, constipation.
Hematologic: *thrombocytopenia.*
Hepatic: *hepatotoxicity.*
Skin: itching.
Other: gynecomastia with tenderness.

Interactions

Drug-drug. *Alprazolam, chlordiazepoxide, clonazepam, clorazepate, diazepam, estazolam, flurazepam, midazolam, quazepam, triazolam:* May increase and prolong levels, CNS depression, and psychomotor impairment. Don't use together.
Antacids, anticholinergics, H₂-receptor antagonists, proton pump inhibitors, sucralfate: May decrease ketoconazole absorption. Wait at least 2 hours after ketoconazole dose before giving these drugs.
Atorvastatin, fluvastatin, lovastatin, pravastatin, simvastatin: May cause increased level and adverse effects of these HMG-CoA reductase inhibitors. Avoid this combination. If they must be given together, reduce dose of HMG-CoA reductase inhibitor.
Corticosteroids: May increase corticosteroid bioavailability and may decrease clearance, possibly resulting in toxicity. Monitor patient closely.
Cyclosporine, methylprednisolone, tacrolimus: May increase levels of these drugs. Adjust their dosages, and monitor their levels closely.

Isoniazid, rifampin: May increase ketoconazole metabolism. Monitor patient for decreased antifungal effect.

Oral anticoagulants: May enhance anticoagulant response may be enhanced. Monitor PT and INR.

Oral midazolam, triazolam: May elevate levels of these drugs, which may potentiate or prolong sedative or hypnotic effects. Avoid using together.

Effects on lab test results

• May increase lipid, alkaline phosphatase, ALT, and AST levels.
• May decrease hemoglobin, hematocrit, and platelet and WBC counts.

Pharmacokinetics

Absorption: Decreased by raised gastric pH and may be increased in extent and consistency by food.

Distribution: Distributed into bile, saliva, cerumen, synovial fluid, and sebum. Penetration into CSF is erratic and probably minimal. 84% to 99% bound to proteins.

Metabolism: Metabolized in liver.

Excretion: Primarily in feces, with smaller amount excreted in urine. *Half-life:* 8 hours.

Route	Onset	Peak	Duration
P.O.	Unknown	1-2 hr	Unknown

Action

Chemical effect: Inhibits purine transport and DNA, RNA, and protein synthesis; increases cell wall permeability, making fungus more susceptible to osmotic pressure.

Therapeutic effect: Kills or hinders growth of susceptible fungi, including most pathogenic fungi.

Available forms

Tablets: 200 mg
Shampoo: 1%†

NURSING PROCESS

⚡ Assessment

• Assess patient's infection before therapy and regularly thereafter.
• Evaluate laboratory studies for eradication of fungi.

• Be alert for adverse reactions and drug interactions.
• If adverse GI reactions occur, monitor patient's hydration status.
• Evaluate patient's and family's knowledge of drug therapy.

Nursing diagnoses

• Infection related to presence of susceptible fungi
• Risk for deficient fluid volume related to adverse GI reactions
• Deficient knowledge related to drug therapy

Planning and implementation

• Because of risk of serious hepatotoxicity, don't use for less serious conditions, such as fungus infections of skin or nails.
• To minimize nausea, divide daily amount into two doses. Also, giving drug with meals helps to decrease nausea.
• Have patient dissolve each tablet in 4 ml aqueous solution of 0.2*N* hydrochloric acid and sip mixture through a straw to avoid contact with teeth. Have patient drink full glass (8 oz) of water afterward.

Patient teaching

• Instruct patient with achlorhydria to dissolve each tablet in 4 ml aqueous solution of 0.2*N* hydrochloric acid, sip mixture through a straw (to avoid contact with teeth), and drink a glass of water after the dose because ketoconazole requires gastric acidity for dissolution and absorption.
• Make sure patient understands that treatment will continue until all tests indicate that active fungal infection has subsided. If drug is stopped too soon, infection will recur. Minimum treatment for candidiasis is 7 to 14 days; for other systemic fungal infections, 6 months; for resistant dermatophyte infections, at least 4 weeks.
• Reassure patient that nausea will subside.

✓ Evaluation

• Patient is free from infection.
• Patient maintains adequate hydration.
• Patient and family state understanding of drug therapy.

ketoprofen

(kee-toh-PROH-fen)

Actron caplets†, Apo-Keto ♦, Apo-Keto-E ♦, Novo-Keto-EC ♦, Orudis, Orudis-E ♦, Orudis KT†, Orudis SR ♦ ◇, Oruvail, Rhodis ♦, Rhodis-EC ♦

Pharmacologic class: NSAID
Therapeutic class: non-opioid analgesic, antipyretic, anti-inflammatory
Pregnancy risk category: B

Indications and dosages

▶ **Rheumatoid arthritis and osteoarthritis.**
Adults: 75 mg t.i.d., 50 mg q.i.d., or 200 mg as sustained-release tablet once daily. Maximum, 300 mg daily. Or, where suppository is available, 100 mg P.R. b.i.d. or one suppository h.s. (with ketoprofen P.O. during day).
▶ **Mild-to-moderate pain; dysmenorrhea.**
Adults: 25 to 50 mg P.O. q 6 to 8 hours, p.r.n.
▶ **Minor aches and pain or fever.** *Adults:*
12.5 mg with full glass of water q 4 to 6 hours. Don't exceed 25 mg in 4 hours or 75 mg in 24 hours.

Contraindications and precautions

• Contraindicated in patients hypersensitive to drug and in those with a history of aspirin- or NSAID-induced asthma, urticaria, or other allergic reactions.
• Use cautiously in patients with history of peptic ulcer disease, renal dysfunction, hypertension, heart failure, or fluid retention.
⚖ **Lifespan:** In pregnant women, avoid use of drug in third trimester of pregnancy. In breast-feeding women, drug isn't recommended. In children, safety of drug hasn't been established. Children younger than age 16 shouldn't be given drug unless directed by prescriber.

Adverse reactions

CNS: *headache,* dizziness, *CNS excitation* or depression.
EENT: tinnitus, visual disturbances, *laryngeal edema.*
GI: *nausea, abdominal pain, diarrhea, constipation, flatulence,* peptic ulceration, anorexia, vomiting, stomatitis.
GU: *nephrotoxicity.*

Hematologic: prolonged bleeding time, *thrombocytopenia, agranulocytosis.*
Respiratory: dyspnea, *bronchospasm.*
Skin: rash, photosensitivity, exfoliative dermatitis.

Interactions

Drug-drug. *Anticoagulants:* May increase anticoagulant effect. Monitor patient for signs and symptoms of bleeding.
Aspirin: May increase risk of adverse GI reactions and increased ketoprofen levels. Avoid using together.
Corticosteroids: May increase risk of adverse GI reactions. Avoid using together.
Hydrochlorothiazide, other diuretics: May decrease diuretic effectiveness. Monitor patient for lack of effect.
Lithium, methotrexate: May increase levels of these drugs, leading to toxicity. Monitor levels closely.
Other NSAIDS: May increase risk of bleeding. Monitor patient.
Probenecid: May increase ketoprofen level. Avoid using together.
Drug-herb. *Dong quai, feverfew, garlic, ginger, horse chestnut, red clover:* May increase risk of bleeding. Monitor patient closely.
St. John's wort: May increase risk of photosensitivity reactions. Advise patient to avoid unprotected or prolonged exposure to sunlight.
Drug-lifestyle. *Alcohol use:* May increase risk of GI toxicity. Discourage using together.
Sun exposure: May cause photosensitivity reactions. Advise patient to avoid unprotected or prolonged exposure to sunlight.

Effects on lab test results

• May increase BUN level.
• May increase bleeding time. May decrease WBC and platelet counts.

Pharmacokinetics

Absorption: Rapid and complete.
Distribution: Highly protein-bound.
Metabolism: Metabolized extensively in liver.
Excretion: Excreted in urine. *Half-life:* 2 to 5½ hours for extended-release forms.

Route	Onset	Peak	Duration
P.O., P.R.	1-2 hr	½-2 hr	3-4 hr

Action

Chemical effect: May inhibit prostaglandin synthesis.
Therapeutic effect: Relieves pain, fever, and inflammation.

Available forms

Capsules: 25 mg, 50 mg, 75 mg
Capsules (extended-release): 100 mg, 150 mg, 200 mg
Suppositories: 100 mg ♦
Tablets: 12.5 mg†
Tablets (enteric-coated): 50 mg ♦, 100 mg ♦
Tablets (sustained-release): 200 mg ♦

NURSING PROCESS

Assessment

• Assess patient's pain before and after drug administration. Full effect may not occur for 2 to 4 weeks.
• Check renal and hepatic function every 6 months during long-term therapy.
• Be alert for adverse reactions and drug interactions.
• If adverse GI reactions occur, monitor patient's hydration status.
• Evaluate patient's and family's knowledge of drug therapy.

Nursing diagnoses

• Chronic pain related to underlying condition
• Risk for deficient fluid volume related to adverse GI reactions
• Deficient knowledge related to drug therapy

Planning and implementation

• Sustained-release form isn't recommended for patients in acute pain.
• May give drug with antacids, food, or milk to minimize adverse GI effects.
• Inform laboratory personnel that patient is taking ketoprofen. Drug may interfere with some laboratory determinations of glucose and iron levels, depending on testing method used.
Patient teaching
• Patient may take drug with milk or meals if he experiences adverse GI effects.
• Tell patient that full therapeutic effect may be delayed for 2 to 4 weeks.
• Instruct patient to report adverse visual or auditory reactions immediately.

• Teach patient to recognize and immediately report evidence of GI bleeding. Also, explain that serious GI toxicity, including peptic ulceration and bleeding, can occur in patients taking NSAIDs despite an absence of GI symptoms.
• Inform patient that use with aspirin, alcohol, or corticosteroids may increase risk of adverse GI reactions.
• Advise patient to use sunblock, wear protective clothing, and avoid prolonged exposure to sunlight. Explain that drug may cause photosensitivity reactions.

Evaluation

• Patient is free from pain.
• Patient maintains normal hydration status.
• Patient and family state understanding of drug therapy.

ketorolac tromethamine
(KEE-toh-roh-lak troh-METH-uh-meen)
Toradol

Pharmacologic class: NSAID
Therapeutic class: analgesic
Pregnancy risk category: C

Indications and dosages

▶ **Short-term management of pain.** *Adults younger than age 65:* Dosage based on patient response. Initially, 60 mg I.M. or 30 mg I.V. as single dose or doses of 30 mg I.M. or I.V. q 6 hours. Maximum, 120 mg daily. To switch to P.O. dosing, initially give 20 mg P.O., and then 10 mg P.O. q 4 to 6 hours, p.r.n., up to 40 mg daily. Maximum combined use of drug not to exceed 5 days.
Adults age 65 and older, renally impaired patients, and those weighing less than 50 kg (110 lb): Initially, 30 mg I.M. or 15 mg I.V. as single dose or doses of 15 mg I.M. or I.V. q 6 hours. Maximum, 60 mg daily. To switch to P.O. dosing, 10 mg P.O. q 4 to 6 hours, p.r.n., up to 40 mg daily. Maximum combined use of drug not to exceed 5 days.

I.V. administration

• Give I.V. bolus over at least 15 seconds.

Reactions may be *common*, uncommon, *life-threatening*, or COMMON AND LIFE-THREATENING.

Contraindications and precautions

• Contraindicated in patients hypersensitive to drug and in those with a history of syndrome of nasal polyps, angioedema, bronchospastic reactivity, or allergic reactions to aspirin or other NSAIDs; in patients receiving aspirin or other NSAIDs; in those with advanced renal impairment; and in those at risk for renal impairment as a result of volume depletion. Also contraindicated in patients with a high risk of bleeding and in those with suspected or confirmed cerebrovascular bleeding, hemorrhage diathesis, and incomplete hemostasis.

• Not recommended for intrathecal or epidural administration because of its alcohol content.

• Use cautiously in women and patients in the perioperative period, and in patients with hepatic or renal impairment, history of serious GI events or peptic ulcer disease, cardiac decompensation, hypertension, or coagulation disorders.

⚒ **Lifespan:** In women giving birth and in breast-feeding women, use cautiously; trace amounts have been detected in breast milk. In children, safety of drug hasn't been established

Adverse reactions

CNS: drowsiness, insomnia, syncope, dizziness, *headache.*
CV: edema, hypertension, palpitations.
GI: *nausea, dyspepsia, GI pain,* diarrhea.
GU: hematuria, polyuria.
Hematologic: purpura, eosinophilia, anemia.
Skin: sweating.
Other: pain at injection site.

Interactions

Drug-drug. *Antihypertensives, diuretics:* May decrease effectiveness of these drugs. Monitor reactions closely.
Lithium: May increase lithium level. Monitor level closely.
Methotrexate: May decrease methotrexate clearance and increase toxicity. Don't use together.
Salicylates, warfarin: May increase levels of free (unbound) salicylates or warfarin in blood. Significance is unknown.
Drug-herb. *Dong quai, feverfew, garlic, ginger, horse chestnut, red clover:* May increase risk of bleeding. Monitor patient closely.

St. John's wort: May increase risk of photosensitivity reactions. Advise patient to avoid unprotected or prolonged exposure to sunlight.

Effects on lab test results

• May increase eosinophil count. May decrease hemoglobin and hematocrit.

Pharmacokinetics

Absorption: Complete after I.M. use. After P.O. use, food delays absorption but doesn't decrease amount absorbed.
Distribution: More than 99.9% protein-bound.
Metabolism: Mainly in liver.
Excretion: More than 90% in urine, with the remainder in feces. *Half-life:* 4 to 6 hours.

Route	Onset	Peak	Duration
P.O.	30-60 min	30-60 min	6-8 hr
I.V.	Immediate	Immediate	8 hr
I.M.	≤ 10 min	30-60 min	6-8 hr

Action

Chemical effect: May inhibit prostaglandin synthesis.
Therapeutic effect: Relieves pain.

Available forms

Injection: 15 mg/ml, 30 mg/ml
Tablets: 10 mg

NURSING PROCESS

⚖ Assessment
• Assess patient's pain before and after drug therapy.
• Be alert for adverse reactions and drug interactions.
• Evaluate patient's and family's knowledge of drug therapy.

⊞ Nursing diagnoses
• Acute pain related to underlying condition
• Risk for injury related to drug-induced adverse CNS reactions
• Deficient knowledge related to drug therapy

▷ Planning and implementation
• When switching from injectable to P.O. form, don't exceed 120 mg of drug (including maximum of 40 mg P.O.) on day of transition.
• Administration by I.M. route may cause pain at injection site. Apply pressure to site for 15 to

30 seconds after injection to minimize local effects.

• If pain persists or worsens, notify prescriber.

⊛ **ALERT:** Don't confuse Toradol with Foradil.

Patient teaching

• Teach patient to recognize and immediately report signs and symptoms of GI bleeding. Also explain that serious GI toxicity, including peptic ulceration and bleeding, can occur in patient taking oral NSAIDs despite an absence of GI symptoms.

• Advise patient to report persistent or worsening pain.

• Explain that drug is intended only for short-term use.

☑ Evaluation

• Patient is free from pain.

• Patient sustains no injury from adverse reactions.

• Patient and family state understanding of drug therapy.

ketotifen fumarate
(kee-toe-TYE-fen FOO-muh-rayt)
Zaditor

Pharmacologic class: histamine (H_1-receptor) antagonist and mast cell stabilizer
Therapeutic class: ophthalmic antihistamine
Pregnancy risk category: C

Indications and dosages

▶ **Temporary prevention of itching of eye caused by allergic conjunctivitis.** *Adults and children age 3 and older:* Instill 1 drop in affected eye q 8 to 12 hours.

Contraindications and precautions

• Contraindicated in patients hypersensitive to drug or its component.

⚖ **Lifespan:** In breast-feeding women, use cautiously; it's unknown if topical ocular product appears in breast milk. In children younger than age 3, safety and effectiveness of drug haven't been established.

Adverse reactions

CNS: *headaches.*
EENT: *conjunctival infection, rhinitis,* ocular allergic reactions, burning or stinging of eyes,

conjunctivitis, eye discharge, dry eyes, eye pain, eyelid disorder, itching of eyes, keratitis, lacrimation disorder, mydriasis, photophobia, ocular rash, pharyngitis.
Other: flulike syndrome.

Interactions

None reported.

Effects on lab test results

None reported.

Pharmacokinetics

Absorption: Unknown.
Distribution: Unknown.
Metabolism: Unknown.
Excretion: Unknown. *Half-life:* Unknown.

Route	Onset	Peak	Duration
Ophthalmic	Within minutes	Unknown	Unknown

Action

Chemical effect: Inhibits release of mediators from cells involved in hypersensitivity reactions.
Therapeutic effect: Temporary prevention of eye itching.

Available forms

Ophthalmic solution: 0.025%; supplied as 5-ml solution in 7.5-ml bottles

NURSING PROCESS

⚗ Assessment

• Assess underlying condition before therapy and reassess regularly throughout therapy.

• Monitor patient for sensitivity reactions.

• Monitor patient for signs of infection.

• Evaluate patient's and family's knowledge of drug therapy.

⊕ Nursing diagnoses

• Risk for injury related to ocular infection and possible altered vision

• Impaired tissue integrity related to drug-induced adverse EENT reactions

• Deficient knowledge related to ketotifen fumarate therapy

▷ Planning and implementation

• Drug is for ophthalmic use only; not for injection or oral use.

Reactions may be *common,* uncommon, *life-threatening*, or COMMON AND LIFE-THREATENING.

• Drug isn't indicated for use with irritation related to contact lenses.
• Preservative in drug may be absorbed by soft contact lenses. Have patient remove contact lenses before giving drops and tell him not to reinsert for at least 10 minutes.

Patient teaching
• Teach patient proper instillation technique. Tell him to avoid contaminating dropper tip and solution and not to touch eyelids or surrounding areas with dropper tip of bottle.
• Tell patient not to wear contact lenses if eyes are red. Warn patient not to use drug to treat irritation related to contact lenses.
• Instruct patient who wears soft contact lenses and whose eyes aren't red to wait at least 10 minutes after instilling drug before inserting contact lenses.
• Advise patient to report adverse reactions to drug.
• Instruct patient to keep bottle tightly closed when not in use.

☑ Evaluation
• Patient does not sustain any injury.
• Patient demonstrates appropriate management of any adverse EENT reactions.
• Patient and family state understanding of therapy.

labetalol hydrochloride
(lah-BAY-tuh-lol high-droh-KLOR-ighd)
Normodyne, Presolol ◇ , Trandate

Pharmacologic class: alpha-adrenergic and beta blocker
Therapeutic class: antihypertensive
Pregnancy risk category: C

Indications and dosages

▶ **Hypertension.** *Adults:* 100 mg P.O. b.i.d. with or without diuretic. Increase dosage to 200 mg b.i.d. after 2 days. Increase q 2 to 3 days until reaching ideal response. Maintenance dosage, 200 to 400 mg b.i.d.

▶ **Severe hypertension, hypertensive emergency.** *Adults:* 200 mg diluted in 160 ml of D₅W; infuse at 2 mg/minute until obtaining satisfactory response; then stop infusion. Repeat dose may q 6 to 12 hours. Or, give by repeated I.V. injection; initially, 20 mg I.V. slowly over 2 minutes. Then, repeat injections of 40 to 80 mg q 10 minutes, p.r.n., until maximum dose of 300 mg is reached.

▼ I.V. administration

③ **ALERT:** Sodium bicarbonate injection and furosemide are incompatible with I.V. drug.
• Take blood pressure immediately before and 5 to 10 minutes after injection.
• Prepare infusion by diluting with D₅W or normal saline solutions; for example, 200 mg of drug to 160 ml D₅W to yield 1 mg/ml.
• Give diluted infusion with infusion-control device.
• Give by slow, direct I.V. injection over 2 minutes at 10-minute intervals.
• Monitor blood pressure q 5 minutes for 30 minutes, then q 30 minutes for 2 hours, then hourly for 6 hours.
• When given I.V. for hypertensive emergency, drug produces rapid, predictable fall in blood pressure within 5 to 10 minutes.
• Have patient lie down for 3 hours after infusion.

Contraindications and precautions

• Contraindicated in patients hypersensitive to drug and in those with bronchial asthma, overt cardiac failure, greater than first-degree heart block, cardiogenic shock, severe bradycardia, and other conditions linked to severe and prolonged hypotension.
• Use cautiously in patients with heart failure, hepatic impairment, chronic bronchitis, emphysema, peripheral vascular disease, or pheochromocytoma.
⚖ **Lifespan:** In pregnant and breast-feeding women, use cautiously. In children, safety of drug hasn't been established.

Adverse reactions

CNS: vivid dreams, *dizziness,* fatigue, headache, transient scalp tingling.
CV: *orthostatic hypotension,* peripheral vascular disease, **bradycardia, ventricular arrhythmias.**
EENT: nasal stuffiness.

GI: nausea, vomiting, diarrhea.
GU: sexual dysfunction, urine retention.
Respiratory: increased airway resistance.
Skin: rash.

Interactions

Drug-drug. *Beta-adrenergic agonists:* May blunt the bronchodilator effect of these drugs in patients with bronchospasm. Increase dosage of these bronchodilators.
Cimetidine: May enhance labetalol's effect. Give together cautiously; monitor patient for adverse reactions.
Diuretics and other hypotensives: May increase hypotensive effects. Monitor patient and adjust dosage.
Glutethimide: May decrease effects of labetalol. Adjust labetalol dose carefully to reach optimal blood pressure control.
Halothane: May have additive hypotensive effect. Monitor blood pressure.

Effects on lab test results

• May increase transaminase and blood urea levels.

Pharmacokinetics

Absorption: 90% to 100%; however, drug undergoes extensive first-pass metabolism in liver and only about 25% reaches systemic circulation unchanged.
Distribution: Distributed widely throughout body; about 50% protein-bound.
Metabolism: Metabolized extensively in liver and, possibly, GI mucosa.
Excretion: About 5% excreted unchanged in urine; remainder excreted as metabolites in urine and feces. *Half-life:* About 5½ hours after I.V. dose; 6 to 8 hours after P.O. dose.

Route	Onset	Peak	Duration
P.O.	≤ 20 min	2-4 hr	8-12 hr
I.V.	2-5 min	5 min	2-4 hr

Action

Chemical effect: Unknown; may be related to reduced peripheral vascular resistance as result of alpha-adrenergic blockade.
Therapeutic effect: Lowers blood pressure.

Available forms

Injection: 5 mg/ml
Tablets: 100 mg, 200 mg, 300 mg

NURSING PROCESS

Assessment
• Obtain history of patient's hypertension before therapy.
• Monitor blood pressure frequently. Drug masks common signs of shock.
• Be alert for adverse reactions and drug interactions.
• Evaluate patient's and family's knowledge of drug therapy.

Nursing diagnoses
• Ineffective health maintenance related to presence of hypertension
• Risk for trauma related to drug-induced hypotension
• Deficient knowledge related to drug therapy

Planning and implementation
• If dizziness occurs, give h.s. or give smaller doses t.i.d. to help minimize this reaction.
ALERT: Don't confuse Trandate with Tridrate or Trental.
Patient teaching
• Tell patient that abruptly stopping therapy can worsen angina and cause MI.
• Inform patient that rising slowly and avoiding sudden position changes can minimize dizziness.

Evaluation
• Patient's blood pressure is normal.
• Patient doesn't experience trauma caused by drug-induced hypotension.
• Patient and family state understanding of drug therapy.

lactulose
(LAK-tyoo-lohs)
Cephulac, Cholac, Chronulac, Constilac, Constulose, Duphalac, Enulose, Generlac, Kristalose, Lac-Dol ◇

Pharmacologic class: disaccharide
Therapeutic class: laxative
Pregnancy risk category: B

Indications and dosages

▶ **Constipation.** *Adults:* 10 to 20 g (15 to 30 ml) P.O. daily, increase to 60 ml/day, if needed.

▶ **Prevention and treatment of hepatic encephalopathy, including hepatic precoma and coma in patients with severe hepatic disease.** *Adults:* Initially, 20 to 30 g (30 to 45 ml) P.O. t.i.d. or q.i.d. until two to three soft stools are produced daily. Usual dosage, 30 to 50 g t.i.d. Or, 200 g (300 ml) diluted with 700 ml of water or normal saline solution and given as retention enema q 4 to 6 hours, p.r.n.
Adolescents and older children: 40 to 90 ml daily.
Infants: 2.5 to 10 ml daily in divided doses.
For all patients, the desired effect is two to three stools per day. If diarrhea occurs with first dose, reduce dose immediately. If diarrhea persists, stop drug.

▶ **To induce bowel evacuation in geriatric patients with colonic retention of barium and severe constipation after a barium meal examination‡.** *Adults:* 3.3 to 6.7 g P.O. b.i.d. for 1 to 4 weeks.

▶ **To restore bowel movements after hemorrhoidectomy‡.** *Adults:* 10 g P.O. twice during day before surgery and for 5 days postoperatively.

Contraindications and precautions

● Contraindicated in patients on low-galactose diet.
● Use cautiously in patients with diabetes mellitus.
⚖ Lifespan: In breast-feeding women, use cautiously. In children, information is limited for treatment of hepatic encephalopathy. In children, use for chronic constipation is contraindicated. In elderly patients, use cautiously because they may be more susceptible to hyponatremia.

Adverse reactions

GI: *abdominal cramps, belching, diarrhea, distention, flatulence.*

Interactions

Drug-drug. *Antacids, antibiotics, oral neomycin:* May decrease effectiveness of lactulose. Avoid using together.

Effects on lab test results

● May decrease ammonia level.

Pharmacokinetics

Absorption: Minimal.
Distribution: Local, primarily in colon.
Metabolism: Metabolized by colonic bacteria (absorbed portion isn't metabolized).
Excretion: Mostly in feces; absorbed portion excreted in urine.

Route	Onset	Peak	Duration
P.O.	24-48 hr	Varies	Varies
P.R.	Unknown	Unknown	Unknown

Action

Chemical effect: Produces osmotic effect in colon. Resulting distention promotes peristalsis. Also decreases blood ammonia, probably as result of bacterial degradation, which lowers pH of colon contents.
Therapeutic effect: Relieves constipation.

Available forms

Crystals for reconstitution: 10 g/packet, 20 g/packet
Solution: 10 g/15 ml, 3.33 g/5 ml

NURSING PROCESS

🔖 **Assessment**
● Assess patient's condition before therapy and regularly thereafter; if patient has hepatic encephalopathy, also assess mental status.
● Monitor sodium and other electrolyte levels.
● Be alert for adverse reactions and drug interactions.
● Evaluate patient's and family's knowledge of drug therapy.

💠 **Nursing diagnoses**
● Constipation related to underlying condition
● Deficient knowledge related to drug therapy

▶ **Planning and implementation**
⚠ **ALERT:** Don't confuse lactulose with lactose.
● Replace fluid loss.
● Diarrhea may indicate overdose.
● To minimize sweet taste, dilute with water or fruit juice or give with food.
● If enema isn't retained for at least 30 minutes, repeat dose.

⊛ **ALERT:** A hazard may exist for patients undergoing electrocautery procedures during proctoscopy or colonoscopy. The accumulation of hydrogen gas in significant concentration combined with an electrical spark may cause an explosion. For patients undergoing electrocautery procedures, give an enema with a nonfermentable solution.

• Store drug at room temperature, preferably below 86° F (30° C). Don't freeze.

Patient teaching
• Advise patient to dilute drug with juice or water or to take with food to improve taste.
• Inform patient of adverse reactions and tell him to notify prescriber if reactions become bothersome or if diarrhea occurs.

☑ Evaluation
• Patient's constipation is relieved.
• Patient and family state understanding of drug therapy.

lamivudine
(la-MI-vyoo-deen)
Epivir, Epivir-HBV

Pharmacologic class: synthetic nucleoside analogue
Therapeutic class: antiviral
Pregnancy risk category: C

Indications and dosages

▶ **HIV infection (with other antiretrovirals).**
Adults and children age 16 and older: 300 mg Epivir P.O. once daily or 150 mg P.O. b.i.d.
Children ages 3 months to 16 years: 4 mg/kg Epivir P.O. b.i.d. Maximum dosage, 150 mg b.i.d.
Neonates 30 days and younger‡: 2 mg/kg Epivir P.O. b.i.d.
◳ **Adjust-a-dose:** For adult and adolescent patients with renal impairment, if creatinine clearance is 30 to 49 ml/minute, give 150 mg Epivir P.O. daily; if clearance is 15 to 29 ml/minute, give 150 mg P.O. on day 1, then 100 mg daily; if clearance is 5 to 14 ml/minute, give 150 mg on day 1, then 50 mg daily; if clearance is less than 5 ml/minute, give 50 mg on day 1, then 25 mg daily.

▶ **Chronic hepatitis B with evidence of hepatitis B virus (HBV) replication and active liv-** er inflammation. *Adults:* 100 mg Epivir-HBV P.O. once daily.
Children ages 2 to 17: 3 mg/kg Epivir-HBV once daily, up to a maximum dose of 100 mg.
◳ **Adjust-a-dose:** For adult patients with renal impairment, if creatinine clearance is 30 to 49 ml/minute, give 100 mg Epivir-HBV as first dose, then 50 mg P.O. daily; if clearance is 15 to 29 ml/minute, give 100 mg first dose, then 25 mg P.O. daily; if clearance is 5 to 14 ml/minute, give 35 mg first dose, then 15 mg P.O. daily; if clearance is less than 5 ml/minute, give 35 mg first dose, then 10 mg P.O. daily.

Contraindications and precautions

• Contraindicated in patients hypersensitive to drug.
• Epivir-HBV is contraindicated for patients co-infected with HBV and HIV.
• Safety and effectiveness of treatment with Epivir-HBV in all patients beyond 1 year haven't been established; optimum duration of treatment isn't known.
• Use cautiously in patients with liver disease. Use cautiously and at a reduced dosage in patients with renal impairment.
⚥ **Lifespan:** Women shouldn't breast feed. In children younger than age 2, safety and effectiveness for chronic hepatitis B haven't been established. In children with history of pancreatitis or other significant risk factors for development of pancreatitis, use cautiously, if at all.

Adverse reactions

For HIV-infected patients
CNS: *fever, headache, fatigue, neuropathy, malaise, dizziness, insomnia,* sleep disorders, depressive disorders.
EENT: *nasal symptoms.*
GI: *nausea, diarrhea, vomiting, anorexia,* abdominal pain, abdominal cramps, dyspepsia, *pancreatitis, hepatomegaly* (children).
Hematologic: *neutropenia,* anemia, *thrombocytopenia,* lymphadenopathy (in children).
Musculoskeletal: *musculoskeletal pain,* myalgia, arthralgia.
Respiratory: *cough.*
Skin: rash (*rashes* in children).
Other: *chills.*
For hepatitis B patients
CNS: *malaise, fatigue, headache,* fever.

EENT: *ear, nose, and throat infections, sore throat.*
GI: *abdominal pain and discomfort, nausea, vomiting, diarrhea.*
Musculoskeletal: *myalgia,* arthralgia.
Skin: rash.

Interactions

Drug-drug. *Co-trimoxazole:* Increases bioavailability of lamivudine. Dosage modification isn't needed. Avoid giving lamivudine with high doses of co-trimoxazole for *Pneumocystis carinii* pneumonia and toxoplasmosis.
Zalcitabine: May inhibit activation of one another. Avoid using together.

Effects on lab test results

• May increase ALT and bilirubin levels.
• May decrease hemoglobin, hematocrit, and neutrophil and platelet counts.

Pharmacokinetics

Absorption: Rapid, for HIV-infected patients.
Distribution: May distribute into extravascular spaces. Volume of distribution is independent of dose and doesn't correlate with body weight. Less than 36% is bound to proteins.
Metabolism: The only known metabolite is trans-sulfoxide.
Excretion: Primarily, unchanged in urine. *Half-life:* 5 to 7 hours.

Route	Onset	Peak	Duration
P.O.	Unknown	1-3 hr	Unknown

Action

Chemical effect: Inhibits HIV reverse transcription via viral DNA chain termination and RNA- and DNA-dependent DNA polymerase activities.
Therapeutic effect: Reduces the symptoms of HIV infection.

Available forms

Epivir
Oral solution: 5 mg/ml
Tablets: 150 mg, 300 mg
Epivir-HBV
Oral solution: 10 mg/ml
Tablets: 100 mg

NURSING PROCESS

✍ Assessment

• Obtain history of patient's underlying condition before therapy, and reassess regularly thereafter.
• Test patient with HBV for HIV before and during treatment because drug isn't appropriate for those dually infected.
⚠ **ALERT:** Some patients with chronic HBV infection may have recurrent hepatitis upon stopping drug. Patients with liver disease may have more severe consequences; periodically monitor both liver function test results and markers of HBV replication.
• Monitor renal function before and during therapy.
• Monitor patient's CBC, platelet count, and renal and liver function studies. Report any abnormalities to prescriber.
• Evaluate patient's and family's knowledge of drug therapy.

Nursing diagnoses

• Risk for infection related to the presence of HIV
• Risk for injury related to drug-induced CNS adverse reactions
• Deficient knowledge related to drug therapy

Planning and implementation

• Safety and effectiveness of drug hasn't been established for chronic hepatitis B in patients infected with both HIV and HBV. Drug-resistant HBV variations may occur in these patients. However, if using drug in these patients, use higher dosage indicated for HIV therapy as part of an appropriate combination regimen.
⚠ **ALERT:** Lactic acidosis and severe hepatomegaly, including fatal cases, have been reported.
• If signs, symptoms, or laboratory abnormalities suggest pancreatitis, stop treatment immediately and notify prescriber if clinical signs, symptoms, or laboratory abnormalities suggest pancreatitis.
• An Antiretroviral Pregnancy Registry has been established to monitor maternal-fetal outcomes of pregnant women exposed to drug. To register a pregnant woman, call 1-800-258-4263.
⚠ **ALERT:** Don't confuse lamivudine with lamotrigine.

Patient teaching
- Inform patient that long-term effects of drug are unknown.
- Stress importance of taking drug exactly as prescribed.
- Teach parents the signs and symptoms of pancreatitis. Advise them to report signs and symptoms immediately.

☑ **Evaluation**
- Patient responds well to drug therapy.
- Patient sustains no injury as a result of drug-induced CNS adverse reactions.
- Patient and family state understanding of drug therapy.

lamivudine and zidovudine
(la-MI-vyoo-deen and zye-DOE-vyoo-deen)
Combivir

Pharmacologic class: reverse transcriptase inhibitor
Therapeutic class: antiretroviral
Pregnancy risk category: C

Indications and dosages

▶ **HIV infection.** *Adults and children age 12 and older weighing more than 50 kg (110 lb):* One tablet P.O. b.i.d.

Contraindications and precautions

- Contraindicated in patients hypersensitive to drug or its components, in those who need dosage adjustments (such as those weighing less than 50 kg), and in those with creatinine clearance less than 50 ml/minute. Also contraindicated in patients experiencing dose-limiting adverse effects.
- Safety and effectiveness of lamivudine haven't been established for treatment of chronic hepatitis B in patients infected with both HIV and hepatitis B virus (HBV). Drug-resistant HBV variations may occur in these patients who have also received antiretroviral regimens with drug.
- ⚕ Lifespan: Women shouldn't breast feed. In children younger than age 12, drug is contraindicated.

Adverse reactions

CNS: *fever, headache, malaise, fatigue, insomnia, dizziness, neuropathy,* depression.

EENT: *nasal signs and symptoms.*
GI: *nausea, diarrhea, vomiting, anorexia,* abdominal pain, abdominal cramps, dyspepsia.
Hematologic: *neutropenia, severe anemia.*
Musculoskeletal: *musculoskeletal pain,* myalgia, arthralgia.
Respiratory: *cough.*
Skin: rash.
Other: *chills.*

Interactions

Drug-drug. *Atovaquone, fluconazole, methadone, probenecid, and valproic acid co-administered with zidovudine:* Increases bioavailability of zidovudine. Dosage modification isn't needed.
Co-trimoxazole or nelfinavir: Increases bioavailability of lamivudine. Dosage modification isn't needed.
Ganciclovir, interferon-alfa, and other bone marrow suppressive or cytotoxic drugs: May increase hematologic toxicity of zidovudine. Use cautiously as with other reverse transcriptase inhibitors.
Nelfinavir, ritonavir: Decreases bioavailability of zidovudine. Dosage modification isn't needed.
Zalcitabine: Zalcitabine and lamivudine may inhibit intracellular phosphorylation of one another. Avoid using together.

Effects on lab test results

- May increase ALT, AST, and amylase levels.
- May decrease hemoglobin, hematocrit, and neutrophil count.

Pharmacokinetics

Absorption: Rapid for both drugs, with bioavailability of 86% and 64%, respectively.
Distribution: Both drugs are extensively distributed with low protein binding.
Metabolism: Only about 5% of lamivudine is metabolized; zidovudine is primarily metabolized (74%) in the liver.
Excretion: Lamivudine is primarily eliminated unchanged in the urine. Zidovudine and its major metabolite are primarily eliminated in the urine. *Half-lives of lamivudine and zidovudine:* 5 to 7 hours and ½ to 3 hours, respectively. Hemodialysis and peritoneal dialysis have negligible effect on the removal of zidovudine, but removal of its metabolite, GZDV, is enhanced.

The effect of dialysis on lamivudine is unknown.

Route	Onset	Peak	Duration
P.O.	Unknown	Unknown	Unknown

Action

Chemical effect: Inhibits reverse transcriptase via DNA chain termination. Both drugs are also weak inhibitors of DNA polymerase. Together, they have synergistic antiretroviral activity by suppressing or delaying the emergence of resistant strains that can occur with retroviral monotherapy, because dual resistance requires multiple mutations.
Therapeutic effect: Reduces the symptoms of HIV infection.

Available forms

Tablets: 150 mg lamivudine and 300 mg zidovudine

NURSING PROCESS

Assessment

• Obtain history of patient's underlying condition before therapy, and reassess regularly thereafter.
• Watch for hematologic toxicity with frequent blood counts, especially in patients with advanced HIV infection.
• Assess patient's fine motor skills and peripheral sensation for evidence of peripheral neuropathies.
ALERT: Patients with chronic hepatitis B virus (HBV) infection may experience recurrence of hepatitis upon discontinuation of lamivudine. Patients with liver disease may have more severe consequences. Periodically monitor liver function test results and markers of HBV replication in patients with liver disease and HBV.
• Evaluate patient's and family's knowledge of drug therapy.

Nursing diagnoses

• Risk for infection related to the presence of HIV
• Disturbed sensory perception (tactile) related to drug-induced peripheral neuropathy
• Deficient knowledge related to drug therapy

Planning and implementation

ALERT: Lactic acidosis and severe hepatomegaly, including fatal cases, have been reported. Stop treatment in any patient who develops signs or symptoms of lactic acidosis or severe hepatotoxicity.
• Use drug cautiously in patients with bone marrow suppression (granulocyte count below 1,000 cells/mm^3 or hemoglobin below 9.5 g/dl).
• An Antiretroviral Pregnancy Registry has been established to monitor maternal-fetal outcomes of pregnant women exposed to Combivir. To register a pregnant patient, prescriber can call 1-800-258-4263.
Patient teaching
• Advise patient that therapy with lamivudine and zidovudine won't cure HIV infection and that he may continue to experience illness, including opportunistic infections.
• Warn patient that HIV transmission can still occur with drug therapy. Educate patient about using barrier contraception when engaging in sexual activities to prevent disease transmission.
• Teach patient signs and symptoms of neutropenia and anemia (fever, chills, infection, fatigue) and instruct him to report such occurrences immediately to prescriber.
• Tell patient to have blood counts followed closely while on drug, especially if he has advanced disease.
• Advise patient to consult prescriber or pharmacist before taking other drugs.
• Warn patient to report abdominal pain immediately.
• Instruct patient to report signs and symptoms of myopathy or myositis (muscle inflammation, pain, weakness, decrease in muscle size).
• Stress importance of taking combination drug therapy exactly as prescribed to reduce the development of resistance.
• Tell patient he may take combination with or without food.
• Inform women that breast-feeding is contraindicated in HIV infection and during drug therapy.

Evaluation

• Patient responds well to drug.
• Patient doesn't develop peripheral neuropathy.
• Patient and family state understanding of drug therapy.

---

lamotrigine
(lah-MOH-trigh-jeen)
Lamictal

Pharmacologic class: phenyltriazine
Therapeutic class: anticonvulsant
Pregnancy risk category: C

Indications and dosages

▶ **Adjunct therapy for partial seizures caused by epilepsy or generalized seizures of Lennox-Gastaut syndrome.** *Adults and children older than age 12:* For patients taking valproic acid with other enzyme-inducing antiepileptics, 25 mg P.O. q other day for 2 weeks; then 25 mg P.O. daily for 2 weeks. Continue to increase, p.r.n., by 25 to 50 mg/day q 1 to 2 weeks until effective maintenance dosage of 100 to 400 mg daily, given in one or two divided doses, is reached. When added to valproic acid alone, maintenance dose is 100 to 200 mg P.O. daily. For patients receiving enzyme-inducing antiepileptics and not valproic acid, 50 mg P.O. daily for 2 weeks; then 100 mg P.O. daily in two divided doses for 2 weeks. Increase, p.r.n., by 100 mg daily q 1 to 2 weeks. Maintenance dosage, 300 to 500 mg P.O. daily in two divided doses.
Children ages 2 to 12 weighing 6.7 to 40 kg (15 to 88 lb): For patients taking valproic acid with other enzyme-inducing antiepileptics, 0.15 mg/kg P.O. daily in one or two divided doses (round down to nearest whole tablet) for 2 weeks, followed by 0.3 mg/kg daily in one or two divided doses for another 2 weeks. Then, maintenance dosage, 1 to 5 mg/kg daily (maximum, 200 mg daily in one to two divided doses). For patients receiving enzyme-inducing antiepileptics and not valproic acid, 0.6 mg/kg P.O. daily in two divided doses (round down to nearest whole tablet) for 2 weeks, followed by 1.2 mg/kg daily in two divided doses for another 2 weeks. Maintenance dosage, 5 to 15 mg/kg daily (maximum, 400 mg daily in two divided doses).
▶ **To convert patients from monotherapy with a hepatic enzyme-inducing anticonvulsant drug to lamotrigine therapy.** *Adults and children age 16 and older:* Add 50 mg P.O. once daily to current drug regimen for 2 weeks, followed by 100 mg P.O. daily in two divided doses for 2 weeks. Then, increase daily dosage by 100 mg q 1 to 2 weeks until maintenance dose of 500 mg daily in two divided doses is reached. Gradually withdraw hepatic enzyme-inducing anticonvulsant in 20% decrements weekly for 4 weeks.
◩ **Adjust-a-dose:** For patients with severe renal impairment, use lower maintenance dosage.

Contraindications and precautions

• Contraindicated in patients hypersensitive to drug.
• Use cautiously in patients with renal, hepatic, or cardiac impairment.
⚠ **Lifespan:** In pregnant women, use cautiously. In breast-feeding women, drug isn't recommended. In children, drug is only indicated as adjunctive therapy for the generalized seizures of Lennox-Gastaut syndrome. For other uses, safety and effectiveness haven't been established in children younger than age 16.

Adverse reactions

CNS: fever, *dizziness, headache, ataxia, somnolence,* incoordination, insomnia, tremor, depression, anxiety, *seizures,* irritability, speech disorder, decreased memory, aggravated reaction, concentration disturbance, sleep disorder, emotional lability, vertigo, malaise, mind racing, *suicide attempts.*
CV: palpitations.
EENT: *diplopia, blurred vision,* vision abnormality, nystagmus, rhinitis, pharyngitis.
GI: *nausea, vomiting,* diarrhea, dyspepsia, abdominal pain, constipation, anorexia, dry mouth.
GU: dysmenorrhea, vaginitis, amenorrhea.
Musculoskeletal: dysarthria, muscle spasm, neck pain.
Respiratory: cough, dyspnea.
Skin: *Stevens-Johnson syndrome, toxic epidermal necrolysis,* rash, pruritus, alopecia, acne.
Other: hot flushes, flulike syndrome, infection, chills, tooth disorder.

Interactions

Drug-drug. *Acetaminophen:* May reduce lamotrigine level, decreasing therapeutic effects. Monitor patient.
Carbamazepine, phenobarbital, phenytoin, primidone: Decreases steady-state level of lamotrigine. Monitor patient closely for decreased clinical effect.

Reactions may be *common,* uncommon, *life-threatening,* or COMMON AND LIFE-THREATENING.

Folate inhibitors (such as co-trimoxazole, methotrexate): May have additive effect because lamotrigine inhibits dihydrofolate reductase, an enzyme involved in folic acid synthesis. Monitor patient closely for adverse effects and toxicities.

Valproic acid: Decreases lamotrigine clearance, which increases steady-state levels. Monitor patient closely for toxicity.

Drug-herb. *Evening primrose oil:* May lower the seizure threshold. Discourage using together.

Drug-lifestyle. *Sun exposure:* Photosensitivity reactions may occur. Urge patient to avoid unprotected or prolonged exposure to sunlight.

Effects on lab test results

None reported.

Pharmacokinetics

Absorption: Rapid and complete with negligible first-pass metabolism.
Distribution: 55% protein-bound.
Metabolism: Predominantly by glucuronic acid conjugation.
Excretion: Excreted primarily in urine. *Half-life:* 14½ to 70¼ hours, depending on dosage schedule and use of other anticonvulsants.

Route	Onset	Peak	Duration
P.O.	Unknown	1½-4¾ hr	Unknown

Action

Chemical effect: Unknown; may inhibit release of glutamate and aspartate, excitatory neurotransmitters in the brain, through action at sodium channels.
Therapeutic effect: Prevents partial seizure activity.

Available forms

Tablets: 25 mg, 100 mg, 150 mg, 200 mg
Tablets (chewable dispersible): 2 mg, 5 mg, 25 mg

NURSING PROCESS

✍ Assessment
• Obtain history of patient's seizure disorder before therapy.
• Evaluate patient for reduction in frequency and duration of seizures after therapy begins. Check adjunct anticonvulsant level periodically.

• Evaluate patient's and family's knowledge of drug therapy.

🔆 Nursing diagnoses
• Risk for trauma related to seizures
• Risk for impaired skin integrity related to dermatologic reactions
• Deficient knowledge related to drug therapy

▶ Planning and implementation
• If drug is added to multidrug regimen that includes valproic acid, lower dosage.
⑤ **ALERT:** Don't stop drug abruptly because doing so increases the risk of seizures. Instead, taper drug over at least 2 weeks.
⑤ **ALERT:** Rash may be life-threatening. Stop drug and notify prescriber at first sign of rash.
⑤ **ALERT:** Don't confuse Lamictal with Lamisil.
Patient teaching
• Inform patient that drug may cause rash. Combination therapy with valproic acid and lamotrigine is more likely to cause a serious rash. Tell patient to report rash or signs or symptoms of hypersensitivity immediately because they could be life-threatening.
• Instruct patient to avoid prolonged exposure to sunlight, use sunblock, and wear protective clothing.
• Warn patient not to engage in hazardous activity until CNS effects of drug are known.

☑ Evaluation
• Patient is seizure-free.
• Patient doesn't develop drug-induced skin reactions.
• Patient and family state understanding of drug therapy.

lansoprazole
(lan-soh-PRAY-zohl)
Prevacid, Prevacid SoluTab

Pharmacologic class: substituted benzimidazole
Therapeutic class: antiulcer drug
Pregnancy risk category: B

Indications and dosages

▶ **Short-term therapy for active duodenal ulcer.** *Adults:* 15 mg P.O. daily before meals for 4 weeks.

▶ **Maintenance of healed duodenal ulcers.**
Adults: 15 mg P.O. daily.
▶ **Short-term therapy for erosive esophagitis.** *Adults:* 30 mg P.O. daily before meals for up to 8 weeks. If healing doesn't occur, give additional 8 weeks of therapy. Maintenance dosage for healing is 15 mg P.O. daily.
Children ages 1 to 11 weighing 30 kg (66 lb) or less: 15 mg P.O. daily for up to 12 weeks.
Children ages 1 to 11 weighing more than 30 kg: 30 mg P.O. daily for up to 12 weeks.
▶ **Short-term therapy for active benign gastric ulcer.** *Adults:* 30 mg P.O. daily for up to 8 weeks.
▶ *Helicobacter pylori* **eradication to reduce risk of duodenal ulcer recurrence.** *Adults:* For triple therapy, 30 mg P.O. lansoprazole with 500 mg P.O. clarithromycin and 1 g P.O. amoxicillin, each given q 12 hours for 14 days. For dual therapy, 30 mg P.O. lansoprazole with 1 g P.O. amoxicillin, each given q 8 hours for 14 days.
▶ **Long-term therapy for pathologic hypersecretory conditions, including Zollinger-Ellison syndrome.** *Adults:* Initially, 60 mg P.O. daily. Increase dosage, as needed. If more than 120 mg daily, give in divided doses.
▶ **Short-term therapy for symptomatic gastroesophageal reflux disease.** *Adults:* 15 mg P.O. daily for up to 8 weeks.
Children ages 1 to 11 weighing 30 kg (66 lb) or less: 15 mg P.O. daily for up to 12 weeks.
Children ages 1 to 11 weighing more than 30 kg: 30 mg P.O. daily for up to 12 weeks.
▶ **NSAID-related ulcer in patients who are continuing NSAIDs.** *Adults:* 30 mg P.O. daily for 8 weeks.
▶ **To reduce risk of NSAID-related ulcer in patient with a history of gastric ulcer who needs NSAIDs.** *Adults:* 15 mg P.O. daily for up to 12 weeks.

Contraindications and precautions

• Contraindicated in patients hypersensitive to drug.
• Drug isn't recommended as maintenance therapy for patients with active duodenal ulcers or erosive esophagitis.
🕊 Lifespan: In pregnant women, use cautiously. In breast-feeding women, drug isn't recommended. In children younger than age 1 and those ages 12 to 17, safety and effectiveness of drug haven't been established

Adverse reactions

GI: diarrhea, nausea, abdominal pain.

Interactions

Drug-drug. *Ampicillin esters, digoxin, iron salts, ketoconazole:* Lansoprazole may interfere with absorption. Monitor patient closely.
Sucralfate: Delays lansoprazole absorption. Give lansoprazole at least 30 minutes before sucralfate.
Theophylline: Theophylline clearance may increase slightly. Use together cautiously. Adjust dosage, if needed when lansoprazole is started or stopped.
Drug-food. *Food:* Decreases absorption of drug when taken with meals. Take drug on an empty stomach, before meals.
Drug-herb. *Male fern:* Inactivated in alkaline environments. Discourage using together.
St. John's wort: Increases risk of photosensitivity reactions. Advise patient to avoid unprotected or prolonged exposure to sunlight.

Effects on lab test results

None reported.

Pharmacokinetics

Absorption: Rapid.
Distribution: 97% bound to proteins.
Metabolism: Metabolized extensively in liver.
Excretion: Excreted mainly in feces, minimally in urine. *Half-life:* Less than 2 hours.

Route	Onset	Peak	Duration
P.O.	Unknown	2 hr	> 24 hr

Action

Chemical effect: Inhibits activity of proton pump and binds to hydrogen or potassium adenosine triphosphatase, located at secretory surface of gastric parietal cells.
Therapeutic effect: Decreases gastric acid formation.

Available forms

Capsules (delayed-release): 15 mg, 30 mg
Oral suspension (delayed-release): 15 mg/packet, 30 mg/packet
Tablets (orally disintegrating, delayed-release): 15 mg, 30 mg
Orally disintegrating tablets contain 2.5 mg phenylalanine/15 mg tablet and 5.1 mg phenylalanine/30 mg tablet.

NURSING PROCESS

🕮 Assessment
- Assess patient's condition before therapy and regularly thereafter.
- Be alert for adverse reactions and drug interactions.
- Evaluate patient's and family's knowledge of drug therapy.

🕮 Nursing diagnoses
- Impaired tissue integrity related to underlying condition
- Ineffective health maintenance related to drug-induced adverse reactions
- Deficient knowledge related to drug therapy

⟫ Planning and implementation
- Give drug on empty stomach.
- Contents of capsule can be mixed with 40 ml of apple juice in a syringe and given within 3 to 5 minutes via NG tube. Flush with additional apple juice to ensure entire dose is given and to maintain patency of the tube.
- Empty contents of capsule into about 2 oz (60 ml) of apple, cranberry, grape, orange, pineapple, prune, tomato, or vegetable juice, mix briefly, and use within 30 minutes. To ensure complete delivery of the dose, rinse glass with two or more servings of juice and have patient drink immediately. Or, mix contents of capsule with 1 tbs of applesauce, pudding, cottage cheese, yogurt, or strained pears and have patient swallow immediately. Tell him not to chew or crush granules.
- For the oral suspension, empty packet contents into 30 ml of water. Stir well and have patient drink immediately. Tell patient not to chew or crush the contents of the capsules or the suspension. Don't use with other liquids or food. If any material remains after drinking, add more water, stir, and have patient drink immediately.
- Dosage adjustment may be needed for patients with severe liver disease.
- Place orally disintegrating tablets on the patient's tongue and allow to dissolve completely. Water isn't necessary.
- ⊗ **ALERT:** Drug shouldn't be crushed or chewed.
- Notify prescriber if adverse reactions occur and provide supportive care.

Patient teaching
- Inform patient not to crush or chew lansoprazole preparations.

- Explain to patients who have difficulty swallowing how to mix drug with other liquids.
- Tell patient to allow orally disintegrating tablets to dissolve on tongue until the particles can be swallowed.
- Instruct patient to notify prescriber if any adverse reactions occur.

☑ Evaluation
- Patient regains normal GI tissue integrity.
- Patient doesn't experience serious adverse reactions.
- Patient and family state understanding of drug therapy.

leflunomide
(leh-FLOO-noh-mighd)
Arava

Pharmacologic class: pyrimidine synthesis inhibitor
Therapeutic class: immunomodulator
Pregnancy risk category: X

Indications and dosages

▶ **Active rheumatoid arthritis, to reduce signs and symptoms and to retard structural damage based on X-ray evidence of erosions and joint space narrowing, to improve physical function.** *Adults:* 100 mg P.O. q 24 hours for 3 days followed by 20 mg (maximum daily dose) P.O. q 24 hours. Decrease dosage to 10 mg daily if higher dosage isn't tolerated.

Contraindications and precautions

- Contraindicated in patients hypersensitive to drug or its components.
- Drug isn't recommended for patients with hepatic insufficiency, hepatitis B or C, severe immunodeficiency, bone marrow dysplasia, or severe uncontrolled infections. It's also not recommended for men attempting to father children.
- Vaccination with live vaccines isn't recommended. Long half-life of drug should be considered when contemplating giving a live vaccine after stopping drug treatment.
- Use cautiously in patients with renal insufficiency.
- Some immunosuppression drugs, including leflunomide, cause an increased risk of malig-

nancy, particularly lymphoproliferative disorders.

⚶ **Lifespan:** In pregnant and breast-feeding women, drug is contraindicated. In children, drug isn't recommended.

Adverse reactions

CNS: asthenia, dizziness, fever, headache, paresthesia, malaise, migraine, sleep disorder, vertigo, neuritis, anxiety, depression, insomnia, neuralgia.
CV: angina pectoris, *hypertension,* chest pain, peripheral edema, palpitations, tachycardia, vasculitis, vasodilation, varicose veins.
EENT: pharyngitis, rhinitis, sinusitis, epistaxis, enlarged salivary gland, blurred vision, cataracts, conjunctivitis, eye disorders.
GI: mouth ulcer, oral candidiasis, stomatitis, dry mouth, anorexia, *diarrhea,* dyspepsia, gastroenteritis, nausea, abdominal pain, vomiting, cholelithiasis, colitis, constipation, esophagitis, flatulence, gastritis, melena, gingivitis, taste perversion.
GU: UTI, albuminuria, cystitis, dysuria, hematuria, menstrual disorder, pelvic pain, vaginal candidiasis, prostate disorder, urinary frequency.
Hematologic: anemia, hyperlipidemia.
Metabolic: weight loss, *diabetes mellitus,* hyperglycemia, hyperthyroidism, hypokalemia.
Musculoskeletal: arthrosis, back pain, bursitis, muscle cramps, myalgia, bone necrosis, bone pain, arthralgia, leg cramps, joint disorder, neck pain, synovitis, tendon rupture, tenosynovitis.
Respiratory: bronchitis, increased cough, pneumonia, *respiratory infection,* **asthma,** dyspnea, lung disorders.
Skin: *alopecia,* eczema, pruritus, *rash,* dry skin, acne, contact dermatitis, fungal dermatitis, hair discoloration, hematoma, nail disorder, skin nodule, subcutaneous nodule, maculopapular rash, skin disorder, skin discoloration, skin ulcer, increased sweating, ecchymosis.
Other: allergic reaction, flulike syndrome, injury or accident, pain, abscess, cyst, hernia, tooth disorder, herpes simplex, herpes zoster.

Interactions

Drug-drug. *Cholestyramine, charcoal:* Decreases leflunomide level. Sometimes used for this effect in overdose.
Methotrexate, other hepatotoxic drugs: Increases risk of hepatotoxicity. Monitor liver enzyme levels.

NSAIDs (diclofenac, ibuprofen): Increases NSAID levels. Clinical significance is unknown; monitor patient.
Rifampin: Increases active leflunomide metabolite level. Use together cautiously.
Tolbutamide: Increases tolbutamide levels. Clinical significance is unknown; monitor patient.

Effects on lab test results

• May increase AST, ALT, glucose, lipid, T_4, and CK levels. May decrease potassium and TSH levels.
• May decrease hemoglobin and hematocrit.

Pharmacokinetics

Absorption: 80% of dose is absorbed after P.O. administration.
Distribution: Extensively bound to albumin; has low volume of distribution.
Metabolism: Primary route of metabolism hasn't been identified.
Excretion: Excreted renally as well as by direct biliary elimination; 43% excreted in urine, 48% eliminated in feces.

Route	Onset	Peak	Duration
P.O.	Unknown	6-12 hr	Unknown

Action

Chemical effect: Inhibits dihydroorotate dehydrogenase, an enzyme involved in pyrimidine synthesis, and has antiproliferative activity and anti-inflammatory effects.
Therapeutic effect: Reduces pain and inflammation related to rheumatoid arthritis.

Available forms

Tablets: 10 mg, 20 mg, 100 mg

NURSING PROCESS

▓ **Assessment**
• Assess patient's condition before therapy and regularly thereafter.
• Be alert for adverse reactions and drug interactions.
• Monitor ALT, platelet, WBC, and hemoglobin and hematocrit at baseline and at monthly intervals during the first 6 months, then, if stable, q 6 to 8 weeks thereafter. If used with methotrexate or other potential immunosuppressive drugs, monitor patient's AST, ALT, and albumin levels monthly.

Reactions may be *common,* uncommon, **_life-threatening_**, or **COMMON AND LIFE-THREATENING.**

⊛ **ALERT:** Severe liver injury, sometimes fatal, may rarely occur. Most cases of severe liver injury occur within 6 months of therapy in patients with multiple risk factors for hepatotoxicity (liver disease, other hepatotoxins).

• Monitor for overlapping hematologic toxicity when switching to another antirheumatics.
• Because of drug's long half-life, carefully observe patient after reducing dose, since level may take several weeks to decline.
• Evaluate patient's and family's knowledge of drug therapy.

🔳 Nursing diagnoses
• Ineffective health maintenance related to underlying disease
• Deficient knowledge related to drug therapy

▶ Planning and implementation
• If ALT level increases between 2 and 3 times ULN, reducing dose to 10 mg/day may allow continued administration under close monitoring. If increases between 2 and 3 times ULN persist despite dose reduction or if ALT level increases more than 3 times ULN, stop drug and give cholestyramine or charcoal and monitor closely. Give additional doses of cholestyramine or charcoal as indicated.
⊛ **ALERT:** Drug can cause fetal harm when given to pregnant women. Discontinue drug in women planning to become pregnant, and notify prescriber.
• Stop drug in man who plans to father a child. Tell him to take prescribed cholestyramine 8 g P.O. t.i.d. for 11 days to remove drug.
• Stop drug and initiate cholestyramine or charcoal therapy if bone marrow suppression occurs.
Patient teaching
• Explain need for and frequency of required blood test monitoring.
• Instruct patient to use contraceptive measures during drug therapy and until drug is no longer active.
• Advise patient to notify prescriber immediately if pregnancy is suspected.
• Advise breast-feeding woman not to breast-feeding during drug therapy.
• Inform patient that aspirin, other NSAIDs, and low-dose corticosteroids may be continued during treatment; however, combined use of drug with antimalarials, I.M. or P.O. gold, penicillamine, azathioprine, or methotrexate hasn't been adequately studied.

✅ Evaluation
• Patient's symptoms of rheumatoid arthritis improve.
• Patient and family state understanding of drug therapy.

leucovorin calcium (citrovorum factor, folinic acid)
(loo-koh-VOR-in KAL-see-um)

Pharmacologic class: formyl derivative (active reduced form of folic acid)
Therapeutic class: vitamin, antidote
Pregnancy risk category: C

Indications and dosages
▶ **Overdose of folic acid antagonist.** *Adults and children:* P.O., I.M., or I.V. dose equivalent to weight of antagonist given.
▶ **Rescue after high methotrexate dose given as cancer therapy.** *Adults and children:* 10 mg/m² P.O., I.M., or I.V. q 6 hours until methotrexate level falls below 5×10^{-8} M.
▶ **Megaloblastic anemia caused by congenital enzyme deficiency.** *Adults and children:* 3 to 6 mg I.M. daily; then 1 mg P.O. or I.M. daily for life.
▶ **Folate-deficient megaloblastic anemia.** *Adults and children:* Up to 1 mg P.O. or I.M. daily. Duration of treatment depends on hematologic response.
▶ **Hematologic toxicity caused by pyrimethamine or trimethoprim therapy.** *Adults and children:* 5 to 15 mg P.O. or I.M. daily.
▶ **Palliative treatment of advanced colorectal carcinoma.** *Adults:* 20 mg/m² I.V., followed by fluorouracil, for 5 consecutive days. Repeat q 4 weeks for two additional courses; then q 4 to 5 weeks, if tolerated.

▽ I.V. administration
• Give drug I.V. to patients with GI toxicity when doses exceed 25 mg.
• When using powder for injection, reconstitute drug in 50-mg vial with 5 ml, 100-mg vial with 10 ml, or 350-mg vial with 17 ml of sterile water or bacteriostatic water for injection. When doses are greater than 10 mg/m², don't use diluents containing benzyl alcohol, especially in neonates.

Rapid onset   *Liquid form contains alcohol.   ◆Canada   ◇ Australia   †OTC   ‡Off-label use

⊛ **ALERT:** Don't exceed 160 mg/minute when giving by I.V. infusion because of the calcium concentration.

● Protect drug from light and heat, especially reconstituted parenteral forms.

Contraindications and precautions

● Contraindicated in patients with pernicious anemia and other megaloblastic anemias caused by lack of vitamin B$_{12}$.

⚖ **Lifespan:** In breast-feeding women, use cautiously. In children, use cautiously; may increase risk of seizures. In neonates, injection form is contraindicated because it contains benzyl alcohol.

Adverse reactions

Respiratory: *bronchospasm.*
Skin: hypersensitivity reactions (rash, pruritus, erythema).

Interactions

Drug-drug. *Anticonvulsants:* May decrease anticonvulsant effectiveness. Monitor patient closely.
Fluorouracil: May enhance fluorouracil toxicity. Avoid using together.
Methotrexate: May decrease effectiveness of intrathecal methotrexate. Avoid using together.

Effects on lab test results

None reported.

Pharmacokinetics

Absorption: Rapid, after P.O. administration.
Distribution: Throughout body; liver contains about one-half of total body folate stores.
Metabolism: In liver.
Excretion: By kidneys. *Half-life:* 6¼ hours.

Route	Onset	Peak	Duration
P.O.	20-30 min	2-3 hr	3-6 hr
I.V.	5 min	10 min	3-6 hr
I.M.	10-20 min	< 1 hr	3-6 hr

Action

Chemical effect: Readily converts to other folic acid derivatives.
Therapeutic effect: Raises folic acid level.

Available forms

Injection: 1-ml ampule (3 mg/ml with 0.9% benzyl alcohol; 10 mg/ml in 5 ml vial; 50-mg,

100-mg, and 350-mg vials for reconstitution (contain no preservatives)
Tablets: 5 mg, 15 mg, 25 mg

NURSING PROCESS

🜨 Assessment

● Assess patient's condition before therapy and regularly thereafter.
● Monitor creatinine level daily to detect renal dysfunction.
● Be alert for adverse reactions and drug interactions.
● Monitor patient for rash, wheezing, pruritus, and urticaria, which can be signs of drug allergy.
● Evaluate patient's and family's knowledge of drug therapy.

🜨 Nursing diagnoses

● Ineffective health maintenance related to underlying condition
● Deficient knowledge related to drug therapy

▶ Planning and implementation

● Drug may mask diagnosis of pernicious anemia.
● Follow leucovorin rescue schedule and protocol closely to maximize therapeutic response.
● Don't give simultaneously with systemic methotrexate.
⊛ **ALERT:** Don't confuse leucovorin (folinic acid) with folic acid. To avoid confusion, don't refer to leucovorin as folinic acid.
Patient teaching
● Explain to patient reasons for drug therapy.

✓ Evaluation

● Patient's condition improves.
● Patient and family state understanding of drug therapy.

leuprolide acetate

(loo-PROH-lighd AS-ih-tayt)
Eligard, Lucrin ◇, Lupron, Lupron Depot, Lupron Depot-Ped, Lupron Depot-3 Month, Lupron Depot-4 Month, Lupron for Pediatric Use

Pharmacologic class: gonadotropin-releasing hormone

Therapeutic class: antineoplastic, luteinizing hormone-releasing hormone analogue
Pregnancy risk category: X

Indications and dosages

▶ **Advanced prostate cancer.** *Adults:* 1 mg S.C. daily. Or, 7.5 mg I.M. (depot injection) monthly. Or, 7.5 mg Eligard S.C. once monthly. Or, 22.5 mg I.M. q 3 months (84 days). Or, 22.5 mg Eligard S.C. q 3 months. Or, 30 mg I.M. (depot injection) q 4 months (16 weeks). Or, 30 mg Eligard S.C. q 4 months.
▶ **Endometriosis.** *Adults:* 3.75 mg I.M. as single injection once monthly. Or, 11.25 mg I.M. q 3 months (depot injection only) for up to 6 months.
▶ **Central precocious puberty.** *Children:* Initially, 0.3 mg/kg (minimum, 7.5 mg) I.M. (depot injection only) as single injection q 4 weeks. Increase dosage in increments of 3.75 mg q 4 weeks, if needed. This will be considered the maintenance dosage. Or, 50 mcg/kg S.C. (injection form) daily. If total down-regulation isn't achieved, adjust dosage upward by 10 mcg/kg daily. This becomes the maintenance dosage. Stop drug before girl reaches age 11 and before boy reaches age 12.

Contraindications and precautions

• Contraindicated in patients hypersensitive to drug or other gonadotropin-releasing hormone analogues, and in women with undiagnosed vaginal bleeding.
• Use cautiously in patients hypersensitive to benzyl alcohol.
⚖ **Lifespan:** In women, the 30-mg depot formulation is contraindicated. In pregnant and breast-feeding women, drug is contraindicated. In neonates, drug is contraindicated because it contains benzyl alcohol.

Adverse reactions

CNS: dizziness, depression, headache.
CV: *arrhythmias,* angina, *MI,* peripheral edema.
GI: nausea, vomiting.
GU: impotence.
Musculoskeletal: transient bone pain (during first week of treatment).
Respiratory: *pulmonary embolism.*
Skin: skin reactions at injection site.
Other: *hot flushes,* decreased libido, gynecomastia.

Interactions

None significant.

Effects on lab test results

• May increase BUN, creatinine, bilirubin, alkaline phosphatase, LDH, glucose, uric acid, albumin, calcium, and phosphorus levels.
• May decrease hemoglobin and hematocrit.
• May give inaccurate reading of pituitary gonadotropic and gonadal functions during treatment and for up to 12 weeks afterwards.

Pharmacokinetics

Absorption: Rapid and complete after S.C. use; unknown for I.M. use.
Distribution: Unknown; about 7% to 15% bound to proteins at therapeutic level.
Metabolism: Unknown.
Excretion: Unknown. *Half-life:* 3 hours.

Route	Onset	Peak	Duration
I.M., S.C.	Unknown	1-2 mo	1-3 mo

Action

Chemical effect: Initially stimulates but then inhibits release of follicle-stimulating hormone and luteinizing hormone, resulting in testosterone suppression.
Therapeutic effect: Hinders prostatic cancer cell growth and eases signs and symptoms of endometriosis.

Available forms

Micropheres for injection, lyophilized: 3.75 mg, 7.5 mg, 11.25 mg, 15 mg, 22.5 mg, 30 mg
Implant: 72 mg
Injection: 5 mg/ml in 2.8-ml multiple-dose vial
Suspension for depot injection: 7.5 mg, 22.5 mg, 30 mg (single-use kit)

NURSING PROCESS

🔬 Assessment

• Assess patient's condition before therapy and regularly thereafter.
• Be alert for adverse reactions.
• Evaluate patient's and family's knowledge of drug therapy.

Nursing diagnoses
• Ineffective health maintenance related to underlying condition
• Disturbed thought processes related to drug-induced depression
• Deficient knowledge related to drug therapy

Planning and implementation
ALERT: Never give drug by I.V. injection.
• Give once-monthly depot injection under medical supervision. Use supplied diluent to reconstitute drug (extra diluent is provided and should be discarded). Draw 1 ml into syringe with 22G needle. (When preparing Lupron Depot-3 Month 22.5 mg, use a 23G or larger needle.) Withdraw 1.5 ml from ampule for the 3-month formulation. Inject into vial, then shake well. Suspension will appear milky. Although suspension is stable for 24 hours after reconstitution, it contains no bacteriostatic agent. Use immediately.
• When using prefilled dual-chamber syringes, prepare for injection by screwing white plunger into end stopper until stopper begins to turn. Remove and discard tab around base of needle. Hold syringe upright and release diluent by slowly pushing plunger until first stopper is at blue line in middle of barrel. Gently shake syringe to form a uniform milky suspension. If particles adhere to stopper, tap syringe against finger. Remove needle guard and advance plunger to expel air from syringe. Inject entire contents I.M. as for a normal injection.
• Leuprolide is nonsurgical alternative to orchiectomy for prostate cancer.
ALERT: A fractional dose of drug formulated to give q 3 months isn't equivalent to same dose of once-monthly formulation.
Patient teaching
• Before starting therapy in child for central precocious puberty, make sure parents understand importance of continuous therapy.
• Carefully instruct patient who will give S.C. injection about proper administration techniques, and advise him to use only syringes provided by manufacturer.
• Advise patient that if another syringe must be substituted, a low-dose insulin syringe (U-100, 0.5 ml) is acceptable.
• Advise patient to store drug at room temperature, protected from light and heat.
• Reassure patient with history of undesirable effects from other endocrine therapies that this drug is much easier to tolerate. Tell patient that adverse effects are transient and will disappear after about 1 week.
• Warn patient that worsening of prostate cancer symptoms may occur when therapy starts.

Evaluation
• Patient exhibits improvement in underlying condition.
• Patient demonstrates pretreatment thought processes.
• Patient and family state understanding of drug therapy.

levalbuterol hydrochloride
(leev-al-BYOO-teh-rohl high-droh-KLOR-ighd)
Xopenex

Pharmacologic class: beta$_2$ agonist
Therapeutic class: bronchodilator
Pregnancy risk category: C

Indications and dosages

▶ **To prevent or treat bronchospasm in patients with reversible obstructive airway disease.** *Adults and children age 12 and older:* 0.63 mg given t.i.d. q 6 to 8 hours by P.O. inhalation via a nebulizer. Patients with more severe asthma who don't respond adequately to 0.63-mg doses may benefit from 1.25 mg t.i.d. *Children ages 6 to 11:* 0.31 mg given t.i.d. by nebulization. Routine dosing shouldn't exceed 0.63 mg t.i.d.

Contraindications and precautions

• Contraindicated in patients hypersensitive to drug or racemic albuterol, or any of its components.
• Use cautiously in patients with CV disorders, especially coronary insufficiency, hypertension, and arrhythmias. Also use cautiously in patients with seizure disorders, hyperthyroidism, or diabetes mellitus and in patients who are unusually responsive to sympathomimetic amines.
☀ Lifespan: In pregnant women, use only if the potential benefits outweigh the potential harm to the fetus. In breast-feeding women, use cautiously. In children younger than age 6 and in patients age 65 and older, safety of drug has not been established.

Adverse reactions

CNS: dizziness, migraine, nervousness, tremor, anxiety, pain.
CV: tachycardia.
EENT: *rhinitis,* sinusitis, turbinate edema.
GI: dyspepsia.
Musculoskeletal: leg cramps.
Respiratory: increased cough.
Other: flulike syndrome, accidental injury, *viral infection.*

Interactions

Drug-drug. *Beta blockers:* Blocks pulmonary effect of the drug and, possibly, severe bronchospasm. Don't use together, if possible. If drug is needed, a cardioselective beta blocker may be considered but give it with caution.
Digoxin: Decreases digoxin levels up to 22%. Monitor digoxin level and for loss of therapeutic effect.
Epinephrine, short-acting sympathomimetic aerosol bronchodilators: Increases adverse adrenergic effects. To avoid serious CV effects, use additional adrenergics with caution.
Loop and thiazide diuretics: Increases risk of ECG changes and hypokalemia. Use together cautiously; monitor cardiac status and potassium level.
MAO inhibitors, tricyclic antidepressants: May potentiate action of levalbuterol on the vascular system. Use caution when giving these drugs within 2 weeks of each other.

Effects on lab test results

None reported.

Pharmacokinetics

Absorption: Some.
Distribution: Unknown.
Metabolism: Unknown.
Excretion: Unknown. *Half-life:* 3¼ to 4 hours.

Route	Onset	Peak	Duration
Inhalation	10-17 min	90 min	5-8 hr

Action

Chemical effect: Activates beta$_2$ receptors on airway smooth muscle, which causes smooth muscle from trachea to terminal bronchioles to relax, thereby relieving bronchospasm and reducing airway resistance. Also inhibits the release of mediators from mast cells in the airway.
Therapeutic effect: Improves ventilation.

Available forms

Solution for inhalation: 0.31 mg, 0.63 mg, or 1.25 mg in 3-ml vials

NURSING PROCESS

Assessment
• Obtain history of patient's underlying condition before therapy, and reassess regularly thereafter.
• Make sure that patient has a thorough physical examination before starting drug therapy.
• Be alert for adverse reactions and drug interactions.
• Evaluate patient's and family's knowledge of drug therapy.

Nursing diagnoses
• Impaired gas exchange related to underlying respiratory condition
• Risk for injury related to drug-induced adverse reactions
• Deficient knowledge related to drug therapy

Planning and implementation
ALERT: Drug may produce life-threatening paradoxical bronchospasm. If this reaction occurs, stop drug immediately and start alternative therapy.
• Drug may produce significant CV effects in some patients. Although such effects are uncommon at recommended dose, stop drug if they occur.
• Compatibility, effectiveness, and safety of levalbuterol when mixed with other drugs in a nebulizer haven't been established.
Patient teaching
• Warn patient to stop drug and notify prescriber if drug causes breathing to worsen.
• Urge patient not to increase the dosage or frequency without consulting prescriber.
• Tell patient to seek medical attention immediately if levalbuterol becomes less effective, if signs and symptoms worsen, or if drug is needed more often than usual.
• Tell patient that the effects of levalbuterol may last up to 8 hours.
• Urge patient to use other inhalations and antiasthma drugs only as directed while taking levalbuterol.
• Inform patient that common adverse reactions include palpitations, rapid heart rate, headache, dizziness, tremor, and nervousness.

- Tell woman to notify prescriber if she becomes pregnant or intends to breast-feed.
- Tell patient to keep unopened vials in foil pouch. Once the foil pouch is opened, use vials within 2 weeks. Inform patient that vials removed from the pouch, if not used immediately, should be protected from light and heat and used within 1 week.
- Teach patient to correctly use nebulizer.
- Tell patient to breathe as calmly, deeply, and evenly as possible until no more mist is formed in the nebulizer reservoir (5 to 15 minutes). At this point, the treatment is finished.

☑ Evaluation

- Patient's respiratory status improves.
- Patient doesn't experience injury from adverse reactions caused by drug.
- Patient and family state understanding of drug therapy.

---

levetiracetam

(leev-ah-tah-RACE-ah-tam)
Keppra

Pharmacologic class: anticonvulsant
Therapeutic class: anticonvulsant
Pregnancy risk category: C

Indications and dosages

▶ **Adjunctive therapy for partial seizures.**
Adults: Initially, 500 mg b.i.d. Increase dosage 500 mg b.i.d., p.r.n., for seizure control at 2-week intervals to maximum of 1,500 mg b.i.d.
🛇 Adjust-a-dose: For patients with renal impairment, if creatinine clearance is greater than 80 ml/minute, give 500 to 1,500 mg q 12 hours; if clearance is 50 to 80 ml/minute, give 500 to 1,000 mg q 12 hours; if clearance is 30 to 50 ml/minute, give 250 to 750 mg q 12 hours; if clearance is less than 30 ml/minute, give 250 to 500 mg q 12 hours. For dialysis patients, give 500 to 1,000 mg q 24 hours. Give one dose of 250 to 500 mg after dialysis.

Contraindications and precautions

- Contraindicated in patients hypersensitive to drug.
- Use cautiously in immunocompromised patients and in those with poor renal function.

🌡 **Lifespan:** In breast-feeding women, use cautiously because it's not known whether drug appears in breast milk. In children younger than age 16, drug is contraindicated. In elderly patients, use cautiously because they are at an increased risk for falls.

Adverse reactions

CNS: *asthenia, headache, somnolence,* dizziness, depression, vertigo, paresthesia, nervousness, hostility, emotional lability, ataxia, amnesia, anxiety.
EENT: diplopia, pharyngitis, rhinitis, sinusitis.
GI: anorexia.
Hematologic: *leukopenia, neutropenia.*
Musculoskeletal: pain.
Respiratory: cough.
Other: infection.

Interactions

Drug-drug. *Antihistamines, benzodiazepines, opioids, tricyclic antidepressants, other drugs that cause drowsiness:* May lead to severe sedation. Avoid using together.
Carbamazepine, clozapine, and other drugs known to cause leukopenia or neutropenia: May increase the risk of infection. Monitor patient closely; monitor hematologic studies.
Drug-lifestyle. *Alcohol use:* Increases risk of severe sedation. Discourage using together.

Effects on lab test results

- May decrease WBC and neutrophil counts.

Pharmacokinetics

Absorption: Rapid. Level peaks in about 1 hour. When given with food, peak level is delayed by about 1½ hours and level will be slightly lower. Levels reaches steady-state in about 2 days.
Distribution: Protein binding is minimal.
Metabolism: No active metabolites. Drug isn't metabolized through the CYP system.
Excretion: About 66% of drug is eliminated unchanged by glomerular filtration and tubular reabsorption. *Half-life:* About 7 hours in patients with normal renal function.

Route	Onset	Peak	Duration
P.O.	1 hr	1 hr	12 hr

Action

Chemical effect: Unknown. Thought to inhibit kindling activity in hippocampus, thus preventing simultaneous neuronal firing that leads to seizure activity.
Therapeutic effect: Prevents seizure activity.

Available forms

Oral solution: 100 mg/ml
Tablets: 250 mg, 500 mg, 750 mg

NURSING PROCESS

ᴿ Assessment

• Obtain history of patient's underlying condition before therapy, and reassess regularly thereafter.
• Assess renal function before therapy starts.
• Monitor patient closely for dizziness, which may lead to falls.
• Evaluate patient's and family's knowledge of drug therapy.

Nursing diagnoses

• Risk for trauma related to seizures
• Risk for infection related to drug-induced leukopenia and neutropenia
• Deficient knowledge related to drug therapy

Planning and implementation

• Drug can be taken with or without food.
• Use drug only with other anticonvulsants; not recommended for monotherapy.
• Seizures can occur if drug is stopped abruptly. Tapering is recommended.
ⓘ **ALERT:** Don't confuse Keppra with Kaletra.
Patient teaching
• Warn patient to use extra care when rising to a sitting or standing position to avoid dizziness and falling.
• Advise patient to call prescriber and not to stop drug suddenly if adverse reactions occur.
• Tell patient to take with other prescribed seizure drugs.
• Inform patient that drug can be taken with or without food.

✔ Evaluation

• Patient is free from seizure activity.
• Patient doesn't develop infection.
• Patient and family state understanding of drug therapy.

levodopa
(lee-voh-DOH-puh)
Dopar, Larodopa

Pharmacologic class: precursor of dopamine
Therapeutic class: antiparkinsonian
Pregnancy risk category: C

Indications and dosages

▶ **Idiopathic parkinsonism, postencephalitic parkinsonism, and symptomatic parkinsonism after carbon monoxide or manganese intoxication or with cerebral arteriosclerosis.** *Adults and children older than age 12:* Initially, 0.5 to 1 g P.O. daily divided into two or more doses with food; increased by no more than 0.75 g daily q 3 to 7 days until daily dose of 3 to 6 g is reached. Maximum, 8 g daily. Adjust dosage carefully to patient requirements, tolerance, and response. Closely supervise higher dosages.

Contraindications and precautions

• Contraindicated in patients hypersensitive to drug, in those who have taken an MAO inhibitor within 14 days, and in those with acute angle-closure glaucoma, melanoma, or undiagnosed skin lesions.
• Use cautiously in patients with severe CV, renal, hepatic, or pulmonary disorders; peptic ulcer; psychiatric illness; MI with residual arrhythmias; bronchial asthma; emphysema; or endocrine disease.
☀ **Lifespan:** In pregnant women, use cautiously. In breast-feeding women, drug is contraindicated. In children age 12 and younger, safety of drug hasn't been established.

Adverse reactions

CNS: *aggressive behavior, abnormal movements (choreiform, dystonic, dyskinetic), involuntary grimacing and head movements, myoclonic body jerks,* **seizures,** *ataxia, tremor, muscle twitching, bradykinetic episodes, psychiatric disturbance, memory loss, mood changes, nervousness, anxiety, disturbing dreams, euphoria, malaise, fatigue, severe depression,* **suicidal tendencies,** *dementia, delirium, hallucinations.*

CV: *orthostatic hypotension,* cardiac irregularities, flushing, hypertension, phlebitis.
EENT: blepharospasm, blurred vision, diplopia, mydriasis or miosis, widening of palpebral fissures, activation of latent Horner's syndrome, oculogyric crises, nasal discharge.
GI: dry mouth, excessive salivation, bitter taste, *nausea, vomiting, anorexia,* constipation, flatulence, diarrhea, epigastric pain.
GU: urinary frequency, urine retention, incontinence, darkened urine, priapism.
Hematologic: hemolytic anemia, *leukopenia, agranulocytosis.*
Hepatic: *hepatotoxicity.*
Metabolic: weight loss.
Respiratory: hyperventilation, hiccups.
Other: dark perspiration, excessive and inappropriate sexual behavior.

Interactions

Drug-drug. *Antacids:* Increases levodopa absorption. Administer antacids 1 hour after levodopa.
Anticholinergics: Increases gastric deactivation and decreases intestinal absorption of levodopa. Avoid using together.
Benzodiazepine: Levodopa's therapeutic value may be attenuated. Monitor patient closely.
Furazolidone, procarbazine: May increase risk of severe hypertension. Avoid using together.
Inhaled halogen anesthetics, sympathomimetics: May increase risk of arrhythmias. Monitor ECG and vital signs closely.
MAO inhibitors (phenelzine, tranylcypromine): May cause a hypertensive reaction. Don't use together.
Metoclopramide: May accelerate gastric emptying of levodopa. Give metoclopramide 1 hour after levodopa.
Papaverine, phenothiazines and other antipsychotics, phenytoin, rauwolfia alkaloids: May decrease levodopa effect. Use together cautiously.
Pyridoxine (vitamin B₆): May decrease the effectiveness of levodopa. Avoid using together. Pyridoxine has little to no effect on the combination drug levodopa and carbidopa.
Tricyclic antidepressants: Delays absorption and decreases bioavailability of levodopa. Hypertensive episodes have occurred. Monitor patient closely.

Drug-herb. *Kava:* May interfere with drug and with natural dopamine, worsening symptoms of Parkinson's disease. Discourage using together.
Rauwolfia: May decrease effectiveness of levodopa. Discourage using together.
Drug-food. *Foods high in protein:* May decrease levodopa absorption. Don't give with high-protein foods.
Drug-lifestyle. *Cocaine:* Increases risk of arrhythmias. Inform patient of this interaction.

Effects on lab test results

• May increase BUN, ALT, AST, alkaline phosphatase, LDH, bilirubin, and uric acid levels.
• May decrease hemoglobin, hematocrit, and WBC and granulocyte counts.
• May falsely increase urine catecholamine level. May falsely decrease urine vanillylmandelic acid level. May cause false-positive Coombs' test or tests for urine glucose with reagents that use copper sulfate. May cause false-negative results with tests that use glucose enzymatic methods. May cause false-positive or false-negative tests for urine ketones and urine phenylketonuria.

Pharmacokinetics

Absorption: Rapid, by active amino acid transport system, with 30% to 50% reaching general circulation.
Distribution: Wide, to most body tissues but not to CNS, which receives less than 1% of dose because of extensive metabolism in periphery.
Metabolism: 95% of levodopa is converted to dopamine.
Excretion: Primarily in urine. *Half-life:* 1 to 3 hours.

Route	Onset	Peak	Duration
P.O.	Unknown	1-3 hr	About 5 hr but varies greatly

Action

Chemical effect: Unknown; may be decarboxylated to dopamine, countering dopamine depletion in extrapyramidal centers.
Therapeutic effect: Relieves signs and symptoms of parkinsonism.

Available forms

Capsules: 100 mg, 250 mg, 500 mg
Tablets: 100 mg, 250 mg, 500 mg

Reactions may be *common,* uncommon, *life-threatening*, or COMMON AND LIFE-THREATENING.

NURSING PROCESS

🔢 Assessment
- Assess patient's condition before therapy and regularly thereafter.
- Observe and monitor vital signs, especially during dosage adjustments.
- Test patient receiving long-term therapy regularly for diabetes and acromegaly; periodically monitor kidney, liver, and hematopoietic function.
- Be alert for adverse reactions and drug interactions.
- Evaluate patient's and family's knowledge of drug therapy.

🔲 Nursing diagnoses
- Impaired physical mobility related to presence of parkinsonism
- Disturbed thought processes related to drug-induced adverse reactions
- Deficient knowledge related to drug therapy

▶ Planning and implementation
- To minimize GI upset, give drug with food. However, keep in mind that high-protein meals can impair absorption and reduce effectiveness.
- In a patient undergoing surgery, continue drug as long as oral intake is permitted, usually until 6 to 24 hours before surgery. Resume drug as soon as patient can take oral medication.
- Protect drug from heat, light, and moisture. If preparation darkens, discard because it has lost potency.
- ⚠ ALERT: Muscle twitching and eyelid twitching may be early signs of drug overdose; report immediately.
- Reestablish effectiveness of lower dosage regimen with a prescriber-supervised period of withholding drug (called a drug holiday). Because of the risk of this drug holiday causing symptoms that resemble neuroleptic malignant syndrome, observe patient when drug is stopped or reduced abruptly.

Patient teaching
- Advise patient to take drug with food except high-protein meals. If patient has trouble swallowing pills, tell him or family member to crush tablets and mix with applesauce or baby food.
- Warn patient and family not to increase dosage without prescriber's orders.
- Warn patient about possible dizziness and light-headedness, especially at start of therapy.

Tell patient to change positions slowly and dangle legs before getting out of bed. Elastic stockings may help control this reaction.
- Advise patient and family that multivitamin preparations, fortified cereals, and certain OTC drugs may contain pyridoxine (vitamin B_6), which can block effects of levodopa.
- Warn patient about risk of arrhythmias if he uses cocaine, especially when used with drug.

☑ Evaluation
- Patient has improved physical mobility.
- Patient maintains normal thought process.
- Patient and family state understanding of drug therapy.

levofloxacin
(lee-voe-FLOX-a-sin)
Levaquin

Pharmacologic class: fluorinated carboxy-quinolone
Therapeutic class: broad-spectrum antibacterial
Pregnancy risk category: C

Indications and dosages
▶ **Acute maxillary sinusitis caused by susceptible strains of** *Streptococcus pneumoniae,* *Moraxella catarrhalis,* **or** *Haemophilus influenzae. Adults:* 500 mg P.O. or I.V. daily for 10 to 14 days.
▶ **Acute bacterial exacerbation of chronic bronchitis caused by** *Staphylococcus aureus,* *S. pneumoniae, M. catarrhalis,* **or** *H. influenzae* **or** *parainfluenzae. Adults:* 500 mg P.O. or I.V. daily for 7 days.
▶ **Community-acquired pneumonia caused by** *S. aureus, S. pneumoniae, M. catarrhalis,* *H. influenzae, H. parainfluenzae, Klebsiella pneumoniae, Chlamydia pneumoniae, Legionella pneumophila,* **or** *Mycoplasma pneumoniae. Adults:* 500 mg P.O. or I.V. daily for 7 to 14 days.
▶ **Mild to moderate skin and skin-structure infections caused by** *S. aureus* **or** *Streptococcus pyogenes. Adults:* 500 mg P.O. or I.V. daily for 7 to 10 days.
▶ **Mild to moderate uncomplicated UTI caused by** *Escherichia coli, K. pneumoniae,* **or**

Staphylococcus saprophyticus. Adults: 250 mg P.O. daily for 3 days.

▶ **Mild to moderate UTI caused by *Enterococcus faecalis, Enterobacter cloacae, E. coli, K. pneumoniae, Proteus mirabilis,* or *Pseudomonas aeruginosa. Adults:* 250 mg P.O. or I.V. daily for 10 days.

▶ **Mild to moderate acute pyelonephritis caused by *E. coli. Adults:* 250 mg P.O. or I.V. daily for 10 days.

▶ **Community-acquired pneumonia caused by penicillin-resistant *S. pneumoniae. Adults:* 500 mg P.O. or I.V. infusion over 60 minutes once daily for 7 to 14 days.

▤ **Adjust-a-dose:** For patients with renal impairment, if creatinine clearance is 20 to 49 ml/minute, give initial dose of 500 mg, then 250 mg once daily; if clearance is 10 to 19 ml/minute, initial dose is 500 mg, then 250 mg q 48 hours. For patients on hemodialysis or chronic ambulatory peritoneal dialysis, give initial dose of 500 mg, then 250 mg q 48 hours.

▶ **Complicated skin and skin structure infections caused by methicillin-sensitive *S. aureus, E. faecalis, S. pyogenes, P. mirabilis;* nosocomial pneumonia caused by methicillin-susceptible *S. aureus, P. aeruginosa, Serratia marcescens, E. coli, K. pneumoniae, H. influenzae,* or *S. pneumoniae. Adults:* 750 mg P.O or I.V. infusion over 90 minutes daily for 7 to 14 days.

▤ **Adjust-a-dose:** For patients with renal impairment, if creatinine clearance is 20 to 49 ml/min, give 750 mg initially, then 750 mg q 48 hours; if clearance is 10 to 19 ml/minute or patient is on hemodialysis or chronic ambulatory peritoneal dialysis, give 750 mg initially, then 500 mg q 48 hours.

▶ **Chronic bacterial prostatitis caused by *E. coli, E. faecalis,* or *Staphylococcus epidermidis. Adults:* 500 mg P.O. or I.V. daily for 28 days.

▤ **Adjust-a-dose:** For patients with renal impairment, if creatinine clearance is 20 to 49 ml/minute, give initial dose of 500 mg, then 250 mg daily. If clearance is 10 to 19 ml/min, give initial dose of 500 mg, then 250 mg q 48 hours. For patients on dialysis or chronic ambulatory peritoneal dialysis, give initial dose of 500 mg, then 250 mg q 48 hours.

▶ **Traveler's diarrhea‡.** *Adults:* 500 mg P.O. as a single dose with loperamide hydrochloride.

▶ **Prevention of traveler's diarrhea‡.** *Adults:* 500 mg P.O. daily during period of risk, for up to 3 weeks.

▶ **Uncomplicated cervical, urethral, or rectal gonorrhea‡.** *Adults and adolescents :* 250 mg P.O. as a single dose.

▶ **Disseminated gonococcal infection‡.** *Adults and adolescents:* 250 mg I.V. daily and continue for 24 to 48 hours after improvement begins. Switch to 500 mg P.O. daily to complete at least 1 week of therapy.

▶ **Nongonococcal urethritis; urogenital chlamydial infections‡.** *Adults and adolescents:* 500 mg P.O. daily for 7 days.

▶ **Acute pelvic inflammatory disease‡.** *Adults and adolescents:* 500 mg I.V. daily with or without metronidazole 500 mg q 8 hours. Stop parenteral regimen 24 hours after improvement; then begin 100 mg P.O. b.i.d. of doxycycline to complete 14 days of therapy. Or, give 500 mg P.O. levofloxacin daily for 14 days with or without metronidazole 500 mg b.i.d. for 14 days.

▽ I.V. administration

- Give only by I.V. infusion.
- Dilute in single-use vials with D_5W or normal saline solution for injection to a final concentration of 5 mg/ml.
- Reconstituted solution should be clear, slightly yellow, and free of particulates.
- Don't mix with other drugs. Infuse over 60 minutes.
- Diluted solution is stable for 72 hours at room temperature, 14 days when refrigerated in plastic containers, and 6 months when frozen. Thaw at room temperature or in refrigerator.

Contraindications and precautions

- Contraindicated in patients hypersensitive to drug, its components, or other fluoroquinolones.
- ⚘ Lifespan: Breast-feeding women should either stop taking drug or stop breast-feeding. In children, safety of drug hasn't been established. In elderly patients, adjust dose if they have renal impairment.

Adverse reactions

CNS: headache, insomnia, dizziness, encephalopathy, paresthesia, pain, *seizures.*
CV: chest pain, palpitations, vasodilation, abnormal ECG.

GI: nausea, diarrhea, constipation, vomiting, abdominal pain, dyspepsia, flatulence, *pseudomembranous colitis.*
GU: vaginitis.
Hematologic: eosinophilia, hemolytic anemia, *lymphocytopenia.*
Metabolic: *hypoglycemia.*
Musculoskeletal: back pain, tendon rupture.
Respiratory: allergic pneumonitis.
Skin: rash, photosensitivity reactions, pruritus, *erythema multiforme, Stevens-Johnson syndrome.*
Other: hypersensitivity reactions, *anaphylaxis, multisystem organ failure.*

Interactions

Drug-drug. *Aluminum hydroxide, aluminum-magnesium hydroxide, calcium carbonate, magnesium hydroxide:* May decrease effects of levofloxacin. Give antacid at least 6 hours before or 2 hours after levofloxacin.
Antidiabetics: May alter glucose levels. Monitor them closely.
Iron salts: May decrease absorption of levofloxacin reducing anti-infective response. Give at least 2 hours apart.
Products containing zinc, sucralfate: May interfere with GI absorption of levofloxacin. Give at least 2 hours apart.
NSAIDs: May increase CNS stimulation. Monitor patient for seizure activity.
Theophylline: May decrease theophylline clearance with some fluoroquinolones. Monitor theophylline levels.
Warfarin: May enhance anticoagulant effects. Monitor PT and INR closely.
Drug-lifestyle. *Sun exposure:* May cause photosensitivity reactions. Urge patient to avoid unprotected or prolonged exposure to sunlight.

Effects on lab test results

• May decrease glucose level.
• May increase eosinophil count. May decrease hemoglobin, hematocrit, and WBC and lymphocyte counts.
• May cause false-positive opiate assay results.

Pharmacokinetics

Absorption: Level after I.V. administration is comparable to that observed for equivalent P.O. doses (on a mg-per-mg basis). Therefore, P.O. and I.V. routes can be considered interchangeable. Level peaks within 1 to 2 hours after P.O.

dosing. Steady state occurs within 48 hours on a 500 mg/day regimen.
Distribution: Mean volume of distribution ranges from 89 to 112 L after single and multiple 500-mg doses, indicating widespread distribution into body tissues. Drug also penetrates well into lung tissues; levels are generally two to five times higher than plasma levels.
Metabolism: Limited. The only identified metabolites are the desmethyl and *N*-oxide metabolites, which have little relevant pharmacologic activity.
Excretion: Primarily excreted unchanged in the urine. *Half-life:* About 6 to 8 hours.

Route	Onset	Peak	Duration
P.O., I.V.	Unknown	1-2 hr	Unknown

Action

Chemical effect: Inhibits bacterial DNA gyrase and prevents DNA replication, transcription, repair, and recombination in susceptible bacteria.
Therapeutic effect: Kills susceptible bacteria.

Available forms

Infusion (premixed): 250 mg in 50 ml D_5W, 500 mg in 100 ml D_5W, 750 mg in 150 ml D_5W (5 mg/ml)
Single-use vials: 500 mg, 750 mg (25 mg/ml)
Tablets: 250 mg, 500 mg, 750 mg

NURSING PROCESS

Assessment

• Obtain specimen for culture and sensitivity tests before starting therapy and as needed to detect bacterial resistance.
• Obtain history of seizure disorders or other CNS diseases, such as cerebral arteriosclerosis, before therapy starts.
• Monitor glucose level and renal, hepatic, and hematopoietic blood studies.
• Evaluate patient's and family's knowledge of drug therapy.

Nursing diagnoses

• Risk for infection related to presence of bacteria susceptible to drug
• Risk for deficient fluid volume related to drug-induced adverse GI reactions
• Deficient knowledge related to drug therapy

⟩ Planning and implementation
- Give oral drugs with plenty of fluids.
- ⊛ **ALERT:** If *P. aeruginosa* is or is suspected to be the cause, combination therapy with an antipseudomonal beta-lactam is recommended.
- Treat acute hypersensitivity reactions with epinephrine, oxygen, I.V. fluids, antihistamines, corticosteroids, pressor amines, and airway management.
- If patient has symptoms of excessive CNS stimulation (restlessness, tremor, confusion, hallucinations), stop drug and notify prescriber. Take seizure precautions.
- Most antibacterials can cause pseudomembranous colitis. Notify prescriber if diarrhea occurs. Stop drug, if needed.

Patient teaching
- Tell patient to take drug as prescribed, even if symptoms resolve.
- Advise patient to take drug with plenty of fluids and to avoid antacids, sucralfate, and products containing iron or zinc for at least 2 hours before and after each dose.
- Warn patient to avoid hazardous tasks until adverse CNS effects of drug are known.
- Advise patient to avoid excessive sunlight, use sunblock, and wear protective clothing when outdoors.
- Instruct patient to stop drug and notify prescriber if rash or other signs or symptoms of hypersensitivity develop.
- Tell patient to notify prescriber if he experiences pain or inflammation; tendon rupture can occur with drug.
- Instruct diabetic patient to monitor glucose level and notify prescriber if a hypoglycemic reaction occurs.
- Instruct patient to notify prescriber about loose stools or diarrhea.

☑ Evaluation
- Patient is free from infection after drug therapy.
- Patient maintains adequate hydration throughout drug therapy.
- Patient and family state understanding of drug therapy.

levothyroxine sodium (T_4, L-thyroxine sodium)
(lee-voh-thigh-ROKS-een SOH-dee-um)
Eltroxin, Levo-T, Levothroid, Levoxine, Levoxyl, Novothyrox, Oroxine◇, Synthroid, ThyroTabs, Unithroid

Pharmacologic class: thyroid hormone
Therapeutic class: thyroid hormone replacement
Pregnancy risk category: A

Indications and dosages
▶ **Congenital hypothyroidism.** *Neonates:* 0.0375 mg (0.025 to 0.05 mg) P.O. daily.
Infants younger than age 1: Initially, 0.025 to 0.05 mg P.O. daily; increase to 0.05 mg P.O. in 4 to 6 weeks, as needed.
Children age 1 and older: 0.03 to 0.05 mg/kg P.O. daily until adult dose (0.15 mg) is reached in early or mid-adolescence.
▶ **Myxedema coma.** *Adults:* 300 to 500 mcg I.V., followed by parenteral maintenance dosage of 75 to 100 mcg I.V. daily. Switch patient to P.O. maintenance as soon as possible.
▶ **Hypothyroidism and thyroid hormone replacement.** *Adults age 65 and younger:* Initially, 0.025 to 0.05 mg P.O. daily, increased by 0.025 mg P.O. q 2 to 4 weeks until desired response occurs. Maintenance dosage is 0.1 to 0.2 mg P.O. daily. May give I.V. or I.M. when P.O. ingestion is precluded for long periods. Adjust dosage, if needed.
Adults older than age 65: 0.0125 to 0.025 mg P.O. daily. Increase by 0.0125 to 0.025 mg at 3- to 8-week intervals, depending on response.
Children younger than age 1: Initially, 0.025 to 0.075 mg, gradually increased by 0.025 to 0.05 mg q 2 to 4 weeks until desired response occurs.
Children age 1 and older: 3 to 5 mcg/kg P.O. daily, gradually increased by 0.025 to 0.05 mg q 2 to 4 weeks until desired response occurs.

▽ I.V. administration
- Initial I.V. dose is about half the previously established oral dose of Synthroid tablets.
- Prepare I.V. dose immediately before injection. Dilute Synthroid powder for injection with 5 ml of normal saline solution for injection or bacteriostatic saline solution injection with ben-

zyl alcohol to 200- or 500-mcg vial; don't use other diluents. Resulting solutions contain 40 or 100 mcg/ml, respectively.
• Don't mix with other I.V. infusion solutions.
• Inject into vein over 1 to 2 minutes.
• Monitor blood pressure and heart rate closely. High initial I.V. dosage is usually tolerated by patients in myxedema coma. Normal levels of T_4 should occur within 24 hours, followed by a threefold increase in T_3 in 3 days.

Contraindications and precautions

• Contraindicated in patients hypersensitive to drug and in patients with acute MI uncomplicated by hypothyroidism, untreated thyrotoxicosis, or uncorrected adrenal insufficiency.
• Use cautiously in patients with angina pectoris, hypertension, other CV disorders, renal insufficiency, or ischemia. Also use cautiously in patients with diabetes mellitus, diabetes insipidus, or myxedema.
• Rapid replacement in patients with arteriosclerosis may precipitate angina, coronary occlusion, or CVA. Use cautiously in these patients.
⚚ Lifespan: In breast-feeding women and in elderly patients, use cautiously.

Adverse reactions

CNS: fever, headache, *nervousness, insomnia, tremor.*
CV: *tachycardia, palpitations, arrhythmias,* angina pectoris, hypertension, *cardiac arrest.*
GI: appetite change, nausea, diarrhea.
GU: menstrual irregularities.
Metabolic: weight loss.
Musculoskeletal: leg cramps.
Skin: diaphoresis.
Other: heat intolerance.

Interactions

Drug-drug. *Cholestyramine, colestipol:* Impairs levothyroxine absorption. Separate doses by 4 to 5 hours.
Insulin, oral antidiabetics: Alters glucose level. Monitor glucose level. Adjust dosage, if needed.
I.V. phenytoin: Free thyroid released. Monitor patient for tachycardia.
Oral anticoagulants: Alters PT. Monitor PT and INR; monitor patient for bleeding. Adjust dosage, if needed.

Sympathomimetics (such as epinephrine): Increases risk of coronary insufficiency. Monitor patient closely.

Effects on lab test results

None reported.

Pharmacokinetics

Absorption: Well absorbed from GI tract after P.O. administration.
Distribution: Distributed widely; 99% protein-bound.
Metabolism: Metabolized in peripheral tissues, primarily in liver, kidneys, and intestines.
Excretion: 20% to 40% excreted in feces. *Half-life:* 6 to 7 days.

Route	Onset	Peak	Duration
P.O., I.V., I.M.	24 hr	Unknown	Unknown

Action

Chemical effect: Not fully defined; stimulates metabolism by accelerating cellular oxidation.
Therapeutic effect: Raises thyroid hormone levels in body.

Available forms

Injection: 200 mcg/vial, 500 mcg/vial
Tablets: 0.025 mg, 0.05 mg, 0.075 mg, 0.088 mg, 0.1 mg, 0.112 mg, 0.125 mg, 0.137 mg, 0.15 mg, 0.175 mg, 0.2 mg, 0.3 mg

NURSING PROCESS

🔖 Assessment

• Assess patient's condition before therapy and regularly thereafter. Normal levels of T_4 should occur within 24 hours, followed by threefold increase in T_3 level in 3 days.
• Be alert for adverse reactions and drug interactions.
• In patients with coronary artery disease who must receive thyroid hormone, monitor carefully for possible coronary insufficiency.
• Evaluate patient's and family's knowledge of drug therapy.

🔖 Nursing diagnoses

• Ineffective health maintenance related to presence of hypothyroidism

- Risk for injury related to drug-induced adverse reactions
- Deficient knowledge related to drug therapy

> **Planning and implementation**

⊕ **ALERT:** Don't confuse mg with mcg dosage (1 mg = 1,000 mcg).

- Thyroid hormone replacement requirements are about 25% lower in patients older than age 60 than in young adults.
- Patients with adult hypothyroidism are unusually sensitive to thyroid hormone. Start patient at lowest dosage and adjust to higher dosage until reaching a euthyroid state based on symptoms and laboratory data.
- When changing from levothyroxine to liothyronine, stop levothyroxine then begin liothyronine at a low dose. Increase liothyronine dosage in small increments after residual effects of drug disappear. When changing from liothyronine to levothyroxine, start levothyroxine several days before withdrawing liothyronine to avoid relapse.
- Thyroid hormones alter thyroid function test results. Stop drug 4 weeks before test.
- In patients taking a prescribed anticoagulant with thyroid hormones, reduce anticoagulant dosage, if needed.

⊕ **ALERT:** Don't confuse levothyroxine sodium with liothyronine sodium or liotrix.

Patient teaching

- Stress importance of compliance. Tell patient to take thyroid hormones at same time each day, preferably before breakfast, to maintain constant hormone levels. Suggest morning dosage to prevent insomnia.
- Instruct patient (especially elderly patient) to immediately notify prescriber if he experiences chest pain, palpitations, sweating, nervousness, shortness of breath, or other signs of overdose or aggravated CV disease.
- Advise patient who has achieved stable response not to change brands.
- Tell patient to report unusual bleeding and bruising.

☑ **Evaluation**

- Patient's thyroid hormone levels are normal.
- Patient doesn't experience any adverse reactions.
- Patient and family state understanding of drug therapy.

lidocaine hydrochloride (lignocaine hydrochloride)

(LIGH-doh-kayn high-droh-KLOR-ighd)
LidoPen Auto-Injector, Xylocaine, Xylocard ♦ ◇

Pharmacologic class: amide derivative
Therapeutic class: ventricular antiarrhythmic
Pregnancy risk category: B

Indications and dosages

▶ **Ventricular arrhythmias resulting from MI, cardiac manipulation, or digoxin toxicity.** *Adults:* 50 to 100 mg (1 to 1.5 mg/kg) by I.V. bolus at 25 to 50 mg/minute. Repeat bolus dose q 3 to 5 minutes until arrhythmias subside or adverse reactions develop. Don't exceed 300-mg total bolus during 1-hour period. Simultaneously, constant infusion of 20 to 50 mcg/kg/minute (1 to 4 mg/minute) is begun. If single bolus has been given, smaller bolus dose may be repeated 5 to 10 minutes after start of infusion to maintain therapeutic level. After 24 hours of continuous infusion, decrease rate by one-half. Or, 200 to 300 mg I.M., followed by second I.M. dose 60 to 90 minutes later, if needed.
Children: 1 mg/kg by I.V. bolus, followed by infusion of 20 to 50 mcg/kg/minute.

◨ **Adjust-a-dose:** For elderly patients, patients weighing less than 50 kg (110 lb), and patients with heart failure or hepatic disease, give half the normal adult dose.

▶ **Status epilepticus‡.** *Adults:* 1 mg/kg I.V. bolus; then, if seizures continue, give 0.5 mg/kg 2 minutes after first dose. May use an infusion of 30 mcg/kg/minute.

▼ I.V. administration

- Injections (additive syringes and single-use vials) containing 40, 100, or 200 mg/ml are for the preparation of I.V. infusion solutions only and must be diluted before use.
- Add 1 g of drug (using 25 ml of 4% or 5 ml of 20% injection) to 1 L of D_5W injection to provide a solution containing 1 mg/ml.
- A more concentrated solution of up to 8 mg/ml may be used if patient is fluid restricted.
- Patients receiving infusion must be on a cardiac monitor and must be attended at all times. Use infusion-control device to give infusion

precisely. Don't exceed 4 mg/minute; faster rate greatly increases risk of toxicity.
• Don't give injections containing preservatives I.V.

Contraindications and precautions

• Contraindicated in patients hypersensitive to amide-type local anesthetics and in those with Adams-Stokes syndrome, Wolff-Parkinson-White syndrome, or severe degrees of SA, AV, or intraventricular block in absence of artificial pacemaker.
• Use cautiously and reduce dosage in patients with complete or second-degree heart block or sinus bradycardia, in those with heart failure or renal or hepatic disease, and in those weighing less than 50 kg.
⚖ Lifespan: In breast-feeding women and in children, safety of drug hasn't been established. In elderly patients, use cautiously.

Adverse reactions

CNS: *confusion, tremor,* lethargy, somnolence, *stupor, restlessness,* slurred speech, euphoria, depression, *light-headedness,* paresthesia, muscle twitching, *seizures.*
CV: hypotension, *bradycardia, new or worsened arrhythmias, cardiac arrest.*
EENT: *tinnitus, blurred or double vision.*
Respiratory: *respiratory arrest, status asthmaticus.*
Skin: diaphoresis.
Other: *anaphylaxis,* soreness at injection site, cold sensation.

Interactions

Drug-drug. *Atenolol, metoprolol, nadolol, pindolol, propranolol:* May reduce hepatic metabolism of lidocaine, thus increasing risk of lidocaine toxicity. Give bolus doses of lidocaine at a slower rate and monitor lidocaine level closely.
Cimetidine: May decrease clearance of lidocaine, increasing the risk of lidocaine toxicity. Use a different H$_2$-antagonist, if possible. Monitor lidocaine level closely.
Phenytoin, procainamide, propranolol, quinidine: May have additive cardiac depressant effects. Monitor patient.
Succinylcholine: Possible prolonged neuromuscular blockage. Monitor patient for increased effects.
Tocainide: May increase risk of adverse reactions. Avoid using together.

Drug-herb. *Pareira:* May add to or potentiate neuromuscular blockade. Avoid using together.
Drug-lifestyle. *Smoking:* May increase lidocaine metabolism. Monitor patient closely; discourage patient from smoking.

Effects on lab test results

• May increase CK level.

Pharmacokinetics

Absorption: Nearly complete after I.M. administration.
Distribution: Distributed widely, especially to adipose tissue.
Metabolism: Most of drug metabolized in liver to two active metabolites.
Excretion: 90% excreted as metabolites; less than 10% excreted in urine unchanged. *Half-life:* 1½ to 2 hours (may be prolonged in patients with heart failure or hepatic disease).

Route	Onset	Peak	Duration
I.V. bolus	Immediate	30-60 min	10-20 min
I.M.	5-15 min	10 min	2 hr

Action

Chemical effect: Decreases depolarization, automaticity, and excitability in ventricles during diastolic phase by direct action on tissues.
Therapeutic effect: Abolishes ventricular arrhythmias.

Available forms

Infusion (premixed): 0.2% (2 mg/ml), 0.4% (4 mg/ml), 0.8% (8 mg/ml)
Injection for direct I.V. use: 1% (10 mg/ml), 2% (20 mg/ml)
Injection for I.M. use: 300 mg/3 ml automatic injection device
Injection for I.V. admixtures: 4% (40 mg/ml), 10% (100 mg/ml), 20% (200 mg/ml)

NURSING PROCESS

⏚ Assessment

• Assess patient's condition before therapy and regularly thereafter.
⚡ **ALERT:** Patient receiving infusion must be on cardiac monitor and be attended to at all times.
• Monitor patient's response, especially ECG, blood pressure, and electrolytes, BUN, and creatinine levels.
• Check for therapeutic level (2 to 5 mcg/ml).

• Be alert for adverse reactions and drug inter-actions.

⊛ **ALERT:** Monitor patient for toxicity. Seizures may be first clinical sign. Severe reactions usu-ally are preceded by somnolence, confusion, and paresthesia.

• Evaluate patient's and family's knowledge of drug therapy.

⊞ **Nursing diagnoses**

• Decreased cardiac output related to presence of ventricular arrhythmia

• Disturbed thought processes related to adverse CNS reactions

• Deficient knowledge related to drug therapy

▷ **Planning and implementation**

⊛ **ALERT:** If using I.M. drug in patient with sus-pected MI, test isoenzymes before therapy be-cause patients receiving I.M. drug show seven-fold increase in CK level. Such an increase originates in skeletal muscle, not cardiac muscle.

⊛ **ALERT:** Give I.M. injections only in deltoid muscle.

• If signs of toxicity (such as dizziness) occur, stop drug at once and notify prescriber. Contin-ued infusion could lead to seizures and coma. Give oxygen by way of nasal cannula, if not contraindicated. Keep oxygen and cardiopulmo-nary resuscitation equipment available.

• Stop drug and notify prescriber if arrhythmias worsen or if ECG changes, such as with a widening QRS complex or substantially pro-longed PR interval.

Patient teaching

• Explain purpose of drug to patient.

• Tell patient or caregiver to report any adverse reactions.

• Instruct patient to avoid smoking during drug therapy.

☑ **Evaluation**

• Patient's cardiac output returns to normal with abolishment of ventricular arrhythmia.

• Patient maintains normal thought processes throughout therapy.

• Patient and family state understanding of drug therapy.

linezolid
(linn-AYE-zoe-lid)
Zyvox

Pharmacologic class: oxazolidinone
Therapeutic class: antibiotic
Pregnancy risk category: C

Indications and dosages

▶ **Vancomycin-resistant** *Enterococcus faeci-um* **infections, including those with concur-rent bacteremia.** *Adults and children age 12 and older:* 600 mg I.V. or P.O. q 12 hours for 14 to 28 days.
Neonates 7 days or older, infants, and children age 11 and younger: 10 mg/kg I.V. or P.O. q 8 hours for 14 to 28 days.
Neonates less than 7 days old: 10 mg/kg I.V. or P.O. q 12 hours for 14 to 28 days. Increase to 10 mg/kg q 8 hours when patient is 7 days old. Consider this dosage increase if neonate has sub-clinical response.
▶ **Nosocomial pneumonia caused by** *Staphy-lococcus aureus* **(methicillin-susceptible [MSSA] and methicillin-resistant [MRSA] strains) or** *Streptococcus pneumonia* **(penicillin-susceptible strains only); compli-cated skin and skin-structure infections, in-cluding diabetic foot infections without osteo-myelitis, caused by** *S. aureus* **(MSSA and MRSA),** *Streptococcus pyogenes,* **or** *Strepto-coccus agalactiae;* **community-acquired pneumonia caused by** *S. pneumoniae* **(penicillin-susceptible strains only), including those with concurrent bacteremia, or** *S. au-reus* **(MSSA only).** *Adults and children age 12 and older:* 600 mg I.V. or P.O. q 12 hours for 10 to 14 days.
Neonates 7 days or older, infants, and children age 11 and younger: 10 mg/kg I.V. or P.O. q 8 hours for 10 to 14 days.
Neonates less than 7 days old: 10 mg/kg I.V. or P.O. q 12 hours for 14 to 28 days. Increase to 10 mg/kg q 8 hours when patient is 7 days old. Consider this dosage increase if neonate has subclinical response.
▶ **Uncomplicated skin and skin-structure infections caused by** *S. aureus* **(MSSA only) or** *S. pyogenes.* *Adults:* 400 mg P.O. q 12 hours for 10 to 14 days.

Reactions may be *common*, uncommon, *life-threatening*, or **COMMON AND LIFE-THREATENING**.

Children ages 12 to 18: 600 mg P.O. q 12 hours
for 10 to 14 days.
Children ages 5 to 11: 10 mg/kg P.O. q 12 hours
for 10 to 14 days.
*Neonates 7 days or older, infants, and children
younger than age 5:* 10 mg/kg P.O. q 8 hours for
10 to 14 days.
Neonates less than 7 days old: 10 mg/kg I.V. or
P.O. q 12 hours for 14 to 28 days. Increase to
10 mg/kg q 8 hours when patient is 7 days old.
Consider this dosage increase if neonate has
sub-clinical response.

▼ I.V. administration

• Drug is compatible with D₅W, normal saline
solution for injection, and lactated Ringer's injection.
• Drugs is incompatible with linezolid include
amphotericin B, ceftriaxone sodium, chlorpromazine hydrochloride, diazepam, erythromycin
lactobionate, pentamidine isethionate, phenytoin
sodium, and trimethoprim-sulfamethoxazole.
• Don't inject additives into the infusion bag.
Give other I.V. drugs separately or in a separate
I.V. line to avoid physical incompatibilities. If a
single I.V. line is used, flush the line with a
compatible solution before and after linezolid
infusion.
• Infuse over 30 to 120 minutes. Don't infuse
linezolid in a series connection.
• Store drug at room temperature in its protective overwrap. The solution may turn yellow
over time, but this doesn't indicate a change in
potency. Use within 21 days.

Contraindications and precautions

• Contraindicated in patients hypersensitive to
drug or any inactive components of the formulation.
• Safety and effectiveness of therapy for longer
than 28 days haven't been studied.
⚠ Lifespan: In children, safety and effectiveness of drug haven't been established.

Adverse reactions

CNS: *headache,* insomnia, dizziness, fever.
GI: *diarrhea, nausea,* constipation, vomiting,
altered taste, tongue discoloration, oral candidiasis, *pseudomembranous colitis.*
GU: vaginal candidiasis.
Hematologic: anemia, *leukopenia, neutropenia, thrombocytopenia.*

Skin: rash.
Other: fungal infection.

Interactions

Drug-drug. *Adrenergics (such as dopamine, epinephrine, pseudoephedrine):* Increases risk of
hypertension. Monitor blood pressure and heart
rate. Start continuous infusions of dopamine and
epinephrine at lower doses, and adjust to response.
Serotoninergic drugs: Increases risk of serotonin syndrome (confusion, delirium, restlessness, tremor, blushing, diaphoresis, hyperpyrexia). If these symptoms occur, consider stopping
serotoninergic drug as directed.
Drug-food. *Foods and beverages high in tyramine (such as aged cheese, tap beer, red wine,
air-dried meat, soy sauce, sauerkraut):* Increases blood pressure. Advise patient to avoid these
foods, if possible. Tyramine content of meals
shouldn't exceed 100 mg.

Effects on lab test results

• May increase ALT, AST, bilirubin, alkaline
phosphatase, creatinine, BUN, amylase, and lipase levels.
• May decrease hemoglobin, hematocrit, and
WBC, neutrophil, and platelet counts.

Pharmacokinetics

Absorption: Rapid and complete. Bioavailability is about 100%.
Distribution: Distributed readily into well-
perfused tissues. Protein-binding is about 31%.
Metabolism: Undergoes oxidative metabolism
to two inactive metabolites. Linezolid doesn't
appear to be metabolized by the CYP oxidative
system.
Excretion: At steady-state, about 30% of a dose
appears in urine as linezolid and about 50% as
metabolites. Linezolid undergoes significant renal tubular reabsorption, such that renal clearance is low. Non-renal clearance accounts for
about 65% of the total clearance. *Half-life:*
6½ hours.

Route	Onset	Peak	Duration
P.O.			
tablet	Unknown	1 hr	4¾ -5½ hr
suspension	Unknown	1 hr	4½ hr
I.V.	Unknown	½ hr	4¾ hr

Action

Chemical effect: Bacteriostatic against enterococci and staphylococci. Bactericidal against most strains of streptococci. Exerts antimicrobial effects by interfering with bacterial protein synthesis. Binds to the 23S ribosomal DNA on the bacterial 50S ribosomal subunit. This action prevents formation of a functional 70S ribosomal subunit, thereby blocking the translation step of bacterial protein synthesis.
Therapeutic effect: Hinders or kills susceptible bacteria.

Available forms

Injection: 2 mg/ml
Powder for oral suspension: 100 mg/5 ml when reconstituted
Tablets: 400 mg, 600 mg

NURSING PROCESS

✍ Assessment

• Obtain history of patient's underlying condition before therapy, and reassess regularly thereafter.
• Obtain specimen for culture and sensitivity tests before starting therapy. Use sensitivity results to guide subsequent therapy.
• Monitor platelet count in patients with increased risk of bleeding, patients with thrombocytopenia, patients receiving drugs that may cause thrombocytopenia, and patients receiving linezolid for more than 14 days.
• Monitor patient for persistent diarrhea; consider pseudomembranous colitis.
• Evaluate patient's and family's knowledge of drug therapy.

⊕ Nursing diagnoses

• Infection related to susceptible bacteria
• Risk for injury related to drug-induced adverse reactions
• Deficient knowledge related to drug therapy

▷ Planning and implementation

• Because inappropriate use of antibiotics may lead to resistant organisms, carefully consider other drugs before starting therapy, especially in the outpatient setting.
• No dosage adjustment is needed when switching from I.V. to P.O. dosage forms.
• **⚠ ALERT:** Don't confuse Zyvox with Zovirax. They both come in a 400-mg strength.

Patient teaching

• Inform patient that tablets and oral suspension may be taken with or without meals.
• Stress the importance of completing the entire course of therapy, even if the patient feels better.
• Tell patient to alert prescriber if he has hypertension, is taking cough or cold preparations, or is being treated with selective serotonin-reuptake inhibitors or other antidepressants.
• Inform patient with phenylketonuria that each 5 ml of linezolid oral suspension contains 20 mg of phenylalanine. Linezolid tablets and injection don't contain phenylalanine.

☑ Evaluation

• Patient is free from infection.
• Patient doesn't experience injury as a result of drug-induced adverse reactions.
• Patient and family state understanding of drug therapy.

liothyronine sodium (T₃)

(lee-oh-THIGH-roh-neen SOH-dee-um)
Cytomel, Tertroxin ◇ , Triostat

Pharmacologic class: thyroid hormone
Therapeutic class: thyroid hormone replacement
Pregnancy risk category: A

Indications and dosages

▶ **Congenital hypothyroidism.** *Children:* 5 mcg P.O. daily with a 5-mcg increase q 3 to 4 days until desired response is achieved.
▶ **Myxedema.** *Adults:* Initially, 5 mcg P.O. daily; increase by 5 to 10 mcg q 1 to 2 weeks until daily dose reaches 25 mcg. Then, increase by 12.5 to 25 mcg daily q 1 to 2 weeks. Maintenance dosage is 50 to 100 mcg daily.
▶ **Myxedema coma, precoma.** *Adults:* Initially, 10 to 20 mcg I.V. for patients with known or suspected CV disease; 25 to 50 mcg I.V. for those not known to have CV disease. Subsequent dosages are based on patient's condition and response.
▶ **Nontoxic goiter.** *Adults:* Initially, 5 mcg P.O. daily; may increase by 5 to 10 mcg daily q 1 to 2 weeks until daily dose reaches 25 mcg. Then, increase by 12.5 to 25 mcg daily q 1 to 2 weeks. Usual maintenance dosage is 75 mcg daily.

▶ **Thyroid hormone replacement.** *Adults:* Initially, 25 mcg P.O. daily, increased by 12.5 to 25 mcg q 1 to 2 weeks until satisfactory response is achieved. Usual maintenance dosage is 25 to 75 mcg daily.

▶ **T₃ suppression test to differentiate hyperthyroidism from euthyroidism.** *Adults:* 75 to 100 mcg P.O. daily for 7 days.

▼ I.V. administration

• Give repeat doses more than 4 hours but less than 12 hours apart.

Contraindications and precautions

• Contraindicated in patients hypersensitive to drug and in those with untreated thyrotoxicosis, uncorrected adrenal insufficiency, and acute MI uncomplicated by hypothyroidism.
• Use cautiously in patients with angina pectoris, hypertension, other CV disorders, renal insufficiency, or ischemia. Also use cautiously in patients with diabetes mellitus, diabetes insipidus, or myxedema.
• Rapid replacement in patients with arteriosclerosis may precipitate angina, coronary occlusion, or CVA. Use cautiously in these patients.
⚖ **Lifespan:** In breast-feeding women and in elderly patients, use cautiously.

Adverse reactions

CNS: irritability, *nervousness, insomnia, tremor,* headache.
CV: *tachycardia,* **arrhythmias,** angina, hypertension, *cardiac arrest.*
GI: diarrhea, abdominal cramps, vomiting.
GU: menstrual irregularities.
Metabolic: weight loss.
Musculoskeletal: accelerated bone maturation in infants and children.
Skin: diaphoresis.
Other: heat intolerance.

Interactions

Drug-drug. *Cholestyramine, colestipol:* Impairs liothyronine absorption. Separate doses by 4 to 5 hours.
Insulin, oral antidiabetics: Initial thyroid replacement therapy may increase insulin or oral hypoglycemic requirements. Monitor glucose levels. Adjust dosage, if needed.
I.V. phenytoin: Free thyroid released. Monitor patient for tachycardia.

Oral anticoagulants: Alters PT. Monitor PT and INR; monitor patient for bleeding. Adjust dosage, if needed.
Sympathomimetics (such as epinephrine): Increases risk of coronary insufficiency. Monitor patient closely.
Drug-herb. *Kelp:* May interfere with thyroid hormone replacement therapy. Discourage using together.
Lemon balm: Has antithyroid effects; inhibits thyroid-stimulating hormone. Discourage using together.

Effects on lab test results

None reported.

Pharmacokinetics

Absorption: 95%.
Distribution: Highly protein-bound.
Metabolism: Unknown.
Excretion: Unknown. *Half-life:* 1 to 2 days.

Route	Onset	Peak	Duration
P.O.	Unknown	2-3 days	3 days
I.V.	Unknown	Unknown	Unknown

Action

Chemical effect: Not clearly defined; enhances oxygen consumption by most body tissues and increases basal metabolic rate and metabolism of carbohydrates, lipids, and proteins.
Therapeutic effect: Raises thyroid hormone levels in body.

Available forms

Injection: 10 mcg/ml
Tablets: 5 mcg, 25 mcg, 50 mcg

NURSING PROCESS

📖 Assessment

• Assess patient's condition before therapy and regularly thereafter.
• Monitor pulse rate and blood pressure.
• Observe patient with coronary artery disease for coronary insufficiency.
• Be alert for adverse reactions and drug interactions.
• Evaluate patient's and family's knowledge of drug therapy.

⊞ Nursing diagnoses
• Ineffective health maintenance related to underlying thyroid condition
• Disturbed sleep pattern related to drug-induced insomnia
• Deficient knowledge related to drug therapy

▷ Planning and implementation
• Give drug at same time every day, preferably in the morning to prevent insomnia.
• **ALERT:** Don't give I.M. or S.C.
• Use levothyroxine for thyroid hormone replacement therapy. Use liothyronine when rapid onset or rapidly reversible drug is desirable or in patients with impaired peripheral conversion of levothyroxine to liothyronine.
• In most patients, regulation of drug dosage is difficult.
• Thyroid hormone replacement requirements are about 25% lower in patients older than age 60 than in young adults.
• **ALERT:** When changing from levothyroxine to liothyronine, stop levothyroxine and begin liothyronine at low dosage and increase in small increments after residual effects of levothyroxine have disappeared. When changing from liothyronine to levothyroxine, start levothyroxine several days before withdrawing liothyronine to avoid relapse.
• Thyroid hormones alter thyroid function tests. Stop drug 7 to 10 days before test.
• Patient who takes thyroid hormone and anticoagulant usually needs decreased anticoagulant dosage.
• **ALERT:** Don't confuse liothyronine with levothyroxine or liotrix.
• **ALERT:** Don't confuse Cytomel with Cytotec.
Patient teaching
• Stress importance of compliance. Tell patient to take thyroid hormones at same time each day, preferably before breakfast, to maintain constant hormone levels and prevent insomnia.
• Advise patient who has achieved stable response not to change brands to avoid problems with bioequivalence.
• Warn patient (especially elderly patient) to notify prescriber at once if chest pain, palpitations, sweating, nervousness, or other signs of overdose occur or if signs of aggravated CV disease (chest pain, dyspnea, and tachycardia) develop.
• Tell patient to report unusual bleeding and bruising.

☑ Evaluation
• Patient's thyroid hormone levels are normal.
• Patient doesn't have insomnia.
• Patient and family state understanding of drug therapy.

lisinopril
(ligh-SIN-uh-pril)
Prinivil, Zestril

Pharmacologic class: ACE inhibitor
Therapeutic class: antihypertensive
Pregnancy risk category: C (D in second and third trimesters)

Indications and dosages
▷ **Hypertension.** *Adults:* Initially, 10 mg P.O. daily. If patient also takes a diuretic, reduce initial dosage to 5 mg P.O. daily. Most patients are well controlled on 20 to 40 mg daily. Maximum dosage, 80 mg daily.
▷ **Adjunct therapy in heart failure (with diuretics and digoxin).** *Adults:* Initially, 5 mg P.O. daily. Usual effective dosage range is 5 to 20 mg daily. In patients with hyponatremia (sodium level below 130 mEq/L) or creatinine above 3 mg/dl, start with 2.5 mg P.O. once daily.
▷ **Hemodynamically stable patients within 24 hours of acute MI to improve survival.** *Adults:* Initially, 5 mg P.O. Then 5 mg P.O. after 24 hours, 10 mg P.O. after 48 hours, and 10 mg P.O. once daily for 6 weeks. In patients with systolic blood pressure of 120 mm Hg or less at start of therapy or during first 3 days after an infarct, reduce dosage to 2.5 mg.

Contraindications and precautions
• Contraindicated in patients hypersensitive to ACE inhibitors and in those with a history of angioedema from previous treatment with an ACE inhibitor.
• Use cautiously in patients with impaired kidney function; adjust dosage as directed. Also use cautiously in patients at risk for hyperkalemia (those with renal insufficiency or diabetes or who use drugs that raise potassium level).
▲ **Lifespan:** In pregnant women, drug is contraindicated. In breast-feeding women, use cautiously. In children, safety of drug hasn't been established.

Adverse reactions

CNS: *dizziness, headache, fatigue,* depression, somnolence, paresthesia.
CV: hypotension, *orthostatic hypotension,* chest pain.
EENT: *nasal congestion.*
GI: *diarrhea,* nausea, dyspepsia, dysgeusia.
GU: impotence.
Metabolic: *hyperkalemia.*
Musculoskeletal: *muscle cramps.*
Respiratory: *dry, persistent, tickling, nonproductive cough.*
Skin: rash.
Other: *angioedema, anaphylaxis,* decreased libido.

Interactions

Drug-drug. *Capsaicin:* May cause or worsen coughing caused by ACE inhibitors. Monitor patient closely.
Diuretics: May cause excessive hypotension. Discontinue diuretics 2 to 3 days or increase salt intake before lisinopril therapy or reduce lisinopril dosage to 5 mg P.O. once daily. Monitor blood pressure closely until stabilized.
Indomethacin: Attenuated hypotensive effect. Monitor blood pressure.
Insulin, oral antidiabetics: May increase risk of hypoglycemia, especially when starting lisinopril. Monitor blood glucose closely.
Lithium: May increase lithium level. Monitor patient for toxicity.
Potassium-sparing diuretics, potassium supplements: May increase risk of hyperkalemia. Monitor potassium level.
Thiazide diuretics: Attenuation of potassium loss caused by thiazide diuretics. Monitor potassium level.
Drug-herb. *Licorice:* May cause sodium retention and increase blood pressure, thereby interfering with the therapeutic effects of ACE inhibitors. Discourage using together.
Drug-food. *Potassium-containing salt substitutes:* May increase risk of hyperkalemia. Monitor patient closely; discourage patient from using unless directed by prescriber.

Effects on lab test results

• May increase liver function test results and BUN, creatinine, potassium, and bilirubin levels.

Pharmacokinetics

Absorption: Variable.
Distribution: Wide, although minimally to brain. Protein-binding appears insignificant.
Metabolism: Not metabolized.
Excretion: Unchanged in urine. *Half-life:* 12 hours.

Route	Onset	Peak	Duration
P.O.	1 hr	7 hr	24 hr

Action

Chemical effect: Unknown; may result primarily from suppression of renin-angiotensin-aldosterone system.
Therapeutic effect: Lowers blood pressure.

Available forms

Tablets: 2.5 mg, 5 mg, 10 mg, 20 mg, 40 mg

NURSING PROCESS

⚷ Assessment
• Assess patient's condition before therapy and regularly thereafter. Beneficial effects of drug may require several weeks of therapy.
• Monitor WBC with differential counts before therapy, q 2 weeks for first 3 months of therapy, and periodically thereafter.
• Be alert for adverse reactions and drug interactions.
• Evaluate patient's and family's knowledge of drug therapy.

⊞ Nursing diagnoses
• Risk for injury related to presence of hypertension
• Decreased cardiac output related to drug-induced hypotension
• Deficient knowledge related to drug therapy

▶ Planning and implementation
• If drug doesn't control blood pressure, add diuretics.
Ⓢ **ALERT:** Don't confuse lisinopril with fosinopril or Lioresal.
Ⓢ **ALERT:** Don't confuse Prinivil with Proventil or Prilosec.
Ⓢ **ALERT:** Don't confuse Zestril with Zostrix, Zetia, Zebeta, or Zyrtec.
Patient teaching
• Advise patient to report signs or symptoms of angioedema (including laryngeal edema), such

as breathing difficulty or swelling of face, eyes, lips, or tongue.
- Tell patient that light-headedness may occur, especially during first few days of therapy. Tell him to rise slowly to avoid this effect and to report symptoms to prescriber. If syncope occurs, tell patient to stop taking drug and call prescriber immediately.
- Tell patient not to stop drug suddenly but to call prescriber if adverse reactions occur.
- Advise patient to report signs of infection, such as fever and sore throat.
- Tell patient to notify prescriber if she becomes pregnant. Drug will need to be stopped.

☑ **Evaluation**
- Patient's blood pressure is within normal limits.
- Patient maintains adequate cardiac output throughout therapy.
- Patient and family state understanding of drug therapy.

lithium carbonate
(LITH-ee-um KAR-buh-nayt)
Carbolith ◆ , Duralith ◆ , Eskalith, Eskalith CR, Lithane, Lithicarb ◇ , Lithizine ◆ , Lithobid, Lithonate, Lithotabs

lithium citrate
Lithium Citrate Syrup*

Pharmacologic class: alkali metal
Therapeutic class: antimanic
Pregnancy risk category: D

Indications and dosages
▶ **Prevention or control of mania.** *Adults:* 300 to 600 mg P.O. up to q.i.d., increasing on basis of blood levels to achieve optimal dosage, usually 1,800 mg P.O. daily. Recommended therapeutic lithium blood levels: 1 to 1.5 mEq/L for acute mania; 0.6 to 1.2 mEq/L for maintenance therapy; and 2 mEq/L as maximum dosage.
▶ **Major depression, schizoaffective disorder, schizophrenic disorder, alcohol dependence‡.** *Adults:* 300 mg lithium carbonate P.O. t.i.d. or q.i.d.
▶ **Apparent mixed bipolar disorder in children‡.** *Children:* Initially, 15 to 60 mg/kg or

0.5 to 1.5 g/m² lithium carbonate P.O. daily in three divided doses. Don't exceed usual adult dosage. Adjust dosage based upon patient's response and lithium level. Usual range, 150 to 300 mg daily in divided doses to maintain lithium level of 0.5 to 1.2 mEq/L.
▶ **Chemotherapy-induced neutropenia in children and patients with AIDS receiving zidovudine‡.** *Adults and children:* 300 to 1,000 mg P.O. daily.

Contraindications and precautions
- Contraindicated if therapy can't be closely monitored.
- Use cautiously in patients receiving neuroleptics, neuromuscular blockers, or diuretics; in debilitated patients; and in patients with thyroid disease, seizure disorder, renal or CV disease, severe debilitation or dehydration, or sodium depletion.
- ☀ **Lifespan:** In pregnant and breast-feeding women, drug shouldn't be used. In children younger than age 12, drug isn't recommended. In elderly patients, use cautiously.

Adverse reactions
CNS: tremor, drowsiness, headache, confusion, restlessness, dizziness, psychomotor retardation, stupor, lethargy, *coma,* syncope, *epileptiform seizures,* EEG changes, worsened organic mental syndrome, impaired speech, ataxia, weakness, incoordination.
CV: *reversible ECG changes,* **arrhythmias,** hypotension, ankle and wrist edema.
EENT: tinnitus, blurred vision.
GI: dry mouth, metallic taste, nausea, vomiting, anorexia, diarrhea, thirst, abdominal pain, flatulence, indigestion.
GU: polyuria, glycosuria, **renal toxicity** with long-term use, albuminuria.
Hematologic: *leukocytosis with leukocyte count of 14,000 to 18,000/mm³* (reversible).
Metabolic: transient hyperglycemia, goiter, hypothyroidism, hyponatremia.
Skin: pruritus, rash, diminished or absent sensation, drying and thinning of hair, psoriasis, acne, alopecia.

Interactions
Drug-drug. *Aminophylline, sodium bicarbonate, urine alkalizers:* Increases lithium excretion. Avoid salt loads and monitor lithium levels.

Carbamazepine, indomethacin, methyldopa, piroxicam, probenecid: Increases effect of lithium. Monitor patient for lithium toxicity.
Diuretics: Increases reabsorption of lithium by kidneys with possible toxic effect. Use cautiously, and monitor lithium and electrolyte levels (especially sodium).
Fluoxetine: Increases lithium levels. Monitor patient for toxicity.
Neuroleptics: May cause encephalopathy. Watch for signs and symptoms (lethargy, tremor, extrapyramidal symptoms), and stop drug if they occur.
Neuromuscular blockers: May cause prolonged paralysis or weakness. Monitor patient closely.
Thyroid hormones: May induce hypothyroidism. Monitor thyroid function.
Drug-herb. *Parsley:* May promote or produce serotonin syndrome. Discourage using together.

Effects on lab test results

• May increase glucose level. May decrease sodium, T_3, T_4, and protein-bound iodine levels.
• May increase ^{131}I uptake and WBC and neutrophil counts.

Pharmacokinetics

Absorption: Rate and extent vary with dosage form; absorption is complete within 8 hours of P.O. use.
Distribution: Distributed widely; levels in thyroid gland, bone, and brain exceed serum levels.
Metabolism: Not metabolized.
Excretion: 95% excreted unchanged in urine.
Half-life: 18 hours (adolescents) to 36 hours (elderly).

Route	Onset	Peak	Duration
P.O.	1-3 wk	30 min-3 hr	Unknown

Action

Chemical effect: Unknown; probably alters chemical transmitters in CNS, possibly by interfering with ionic pump mechanisms in brain cells, and may compete with sodium ions.
Therapeutic effect: Prevents or controls mania.

Available forms

lithium carbonate
Capsules: 150 mg, 300 mg, 600 mg
Tablets: 300 mg (300 mg = 8.12 mEq lithium)
Tablets (controlled-release): 300 mg, 450 mg

lithium citrate
Syrup (sugarless): 8 mEq (of lithium) per 5 ml (8 mEq lithium = 300 mg of lithium carbonate)

NURSING PROCESS

▚ Assessment
• Assess patient's condition before therapy and regularly thereafter. Expect delay of 1 to 3 weeks before drug's beneficial effects are noticed.
• Monitor baseline ECG, thyroid and kidney studies, and electrolyte levels. Monitor lithium blood levels 8 to 12 hours after first dose, usually before morning dose, two or three times weekly in first month, then weekly to monthly during maintenance therapy.
• With blood levels of lithium below 1.5 mEq/L, adverse reactions usually remain mild.
• Check urine-specific gravity and report level below 1.005, which may indicate diabetes insipidus.
• Lithium may alter glucose tolerance in diabetic patient. Monitor glucose level closely.
• Perform outpatient follow-up of thyroid and kidney function q 6 to 12 months. Palpate thyroid to check for enlargement.
• Be alert for adverse reactions and drug interactions.
• Evaluate patient's and family's knowledge of drug therapy.

▣ Nursing diagnoses
• Disturbed thought processes related to presence of manic disorder
• Ineffective health maintenance related to drug-induced endocrine dysfunction
• Deficient knowledge related to drug therapy

▷ Planning and implementation
Ⓢ **ALERT:** Don't confuse Lithobid with Levbid, Lithonate with Lithostat, or Lithotabs with Lithobid or Lithostat.
• Monitoring lithium blood level is crucial to safe use of drug. Don't use in patient who can't have level checked regularly.
• Give with plenty of water and after meals to minimize GI reactions.
• Before leaving bedside, make sure patient has swallowed drug.
• Notify prescriber if patient's behavior hasn't improved in 3 weeks or if it worsens.

Patient teaching
- Tell patient to take drug with plenty of water and after meals to minimize GI upset.
- Explain that lithium has narrow therapeutic margin of safety. A blood level that is even slightly high can be dangerous.
- Warn patient and family to watch for signs of toxicity (diarrhea, vomiting, tremor, drowsiness, muscle weakness, ataxia) and to expect transient nausea, polyuria, thirst, and discomfort during first few days. Tell patient to withhold one dose and call prescriber if toxic symptoms appear but not to stop drug abruptly.
- Warn patient to avoid activities that require alertness and good psychomotor coordination until CNS effects of drug are known.
- Tell patient not to switch brands or take other prescription or OTC drugs without prescriber's approval.
- Advise patient to wear or carry medical identification.

☑ Evaluation
- Patient exhibits improved behavior and thought processes.
- Patient maintains normal endocrine function throughout therapy.
- Patient and family state understanding of drug therapy.

lomustine (CCNU)
(loh-MUH-steen)
CeeNU

Pharmacologic class: alkylating drug, nitrosourea (cell cycle–phase nonspecific)
Therapeutic class: antineoplastic
Pregnancy risk category: D

Indications and dosages
▶ **Brain tumor, Hodgkin's disease, lymphomas.** *Adults and children:* 100 to 130 mg/m² P.O. as single dose q 6 weeks. Reduce dosage according to degree of bone marrow suppression. Don't repeat doses until WBC count is more than 4,000/mm³ and platelet count is more than 100,000/mm³.

Contraindications and precautions
- Contraindicated in patients hypersensitive to drug.

- Use cautiously in patients with decreased platelet, WBC, or RBC count and in those receiving other myelosuppressant drugs.
- ⚠ Lifespan: In pregnant and breast-feeding women, drug isn't recommended.

Adverse reactions
GI: *nausea, vomiting* (beginning within 4 to 5 hours), stomatitis.
GU: *nephrotoxicity,* progressive azotemia, *renal impairment.*
Hematologic: anemia, *leukopenia* (delayed up to 6 weeks, lasting 1 to 2 weeks), *thrombocytopenia* (delayed up to 4 weeks, lasting 1 to 2 weeks), *bone marrow suppression* (delayed up to 6 weeks).
Hepatic: *hepatotoxicity.*
Respiratory: *pulmonary fibrosis.*
Other: *secondary malignant disease.*

Interactions
Drug-drug. *Anticoagulants, aspirin:* Increases bleeding risk. Avoid using together.

Effects on lab test results
- May increase urine urea, liver enzyme, BUN, and creatinine levels.
- May decrease hemoglobin, hematocrit, and WBC, RBC, and platelet counts.

Pharmacokinetics
Absorption: Absorbed rapidly and well.
Distribution: Distributed widely in body tissues and crosses blood-brain barrier to significant extent.
Metabolism: Rapidly and extensive in liver.
Excretion: Metabolites excreted primarily in urine with smaller amounts excreted in feces and through lungs. *Half-life:* 1 to 2 days.

Route	Onset	Peak	Duration
P.O.	Unknown	Unknown	Unknown

Action
Chemical effect: Cross-links strands of cellular DNA and interferes with RNA transcription.
Therapeutic effect: Kills selected cancer cells.

Available forms
Capsules: 10 mg, 40 mg, 100 mg, dose pack (two 10-mg, two 40-mg, two 100-mg capsules)

NURSING PROCESS

🔖 Assessment

• Assess patient's condition before therapy and regularly thereafter.
• Monitor CBC weekly; bone marrow toxicity is delayed.
• Periodically monitor liver function test results.
• Be alert for adverse reactions and drug interactions.
• Evaluate patient's and family's knowledge of drug therapy.

🌐 Nursing diagnoses

• Ineffective health maintenance related to presence of neoplastic disease
• Ineffective protection related to adverse hematologic reactions
• Deficient knowledge related to drug therapy

⧉ Planning and implementation

• To avoid nausea, give antiemetic before giving drug.
• Give 2 to 4 hours after meals; drug is better absorbed if taken on empty stomach.
• Repeat dose only when CBC results reveal safe blood counts.
• Institute infection control and bleeding precautions.

Patient teaching
• Warn patient to watch for signs of infection (fever, sore throat, fatigue) and bleeding (easy bruising, nosebleeds, bleeding gums, melena) and to take temperature daily.
• Instruct patient to avoid OTC products containing aspirin.
• Advise woman of childbearing age to avoid becoming pregnant during therapy and to consult with prescriber before becoming pregnant.

✅ Evaluation

• Patient responds well to therapy.
• Patient regains normal hematologic function.
• Patient and family state understanding of drug therapy.

loperamide
(loh-PEH-ruh-mighd)
Imodium, Imodium A-D†, Kaopectate II Caplets†, Maalox Anti-Diarrheal Caplets†, Neo-Diaral†, Pepto Diarrhea Control†

Pharmacologic class: piperidine derivative
Therapeutic class: antidiarrheal
Pregnancy risk category: B

Indications and dosages

▶ **Acute diarrhea.** *Adults and children age 12 and older:* Initially, 4 mg P.O.; then 2 mg after each unformed stool. Maximum dosage is 16 mg daily.
Children ages 9 to 11: 10 ml (2 mg) t.i.d. P.O. on first day. Subsequent doses of 5 ml (1 mg)/10 kg (22 lb) of body weight may be given after each unformed stool. Maximum dosage is 6 mg daily.
Children ages 6 to 8: 10 ml (2 mg) P.O. b.i.d. on first day. Report persistent diarrhea.
Children ages 2 to 5: 5 ml (1 mg) P.O. t.i.d. on first day. Report persistent diarrhea.
▶ **Chronic diarrhea.** *Adults:* Initially, 4 mg P.O.; then 2 mg after each unformed stool until diarrhea subsides. Adjust dosage to individual response.
Children‡: 0.08 to 0.24 mg/kg P.O. daily in two to three divided doses.
▶ **Acute diarrhea including traveler's diarrhea†.** *Adults:* 4 mg after first loose bowel movement followed by 2 mg after each subsequent loose bowel movement; maximum, 8 mg P.O. daily for 2 days.

Contraindications and precautions

• Contraindicated in patients hypersensitive to drug, and in patients in whom constipation must be avoided. OTC form is contraindicated in patients with bloody diarrhea and those with temperature over 101° F (38° C).
• Use cautiously in patients with hepatic disease.
⚘ **Lifespan:** In pregnant and breast-feeding women, use cautiously. In children younger than age 2, drug is contraindicated.

Adverse reactions

CNS: drowsiness, fatigue, dizziness.
GI: dry mouth; abdominal pain, distention, or discomfort; *constipation;* nausea; vomiting.

Skin: rash.
Other: hypersensitivity reactions.

Interactions

None significant.

Effects on lab test results

None reported.

Pharmacokinetics

Absorption: Poor.
Distribution: Unknown.
Metabolism: Metabolized in liver.
Excretion: Excreted primarily in feces; less than 2% excreted in urine. *Half-life:* 9 to 14½ hours.

Route	Onset	Peak	Duration
P.O.	Unknown	2½-5 hr	24 hr

Action

Chemical effect: Inhibits peristaltic activity, prolonging transit of intestinal contents.
Therapeutic effect: Relieves diarrhea.

Available forms

Capsules: 2 mg
Oral liquid*: 1 mg/5 ml†, 1 mg/ml†
Tablets: 2 mg†

NURSING PROCESS

◤ Assessment
• Assess patient's diarrhea before therapy and regularly thereafter.
• Be alert for adverse reactions.
⊛ **ALERT:** Monitor children closely for CNS effects because they may be more sensitive than adults to such effects.
• Monitor patient's hydration status if adverse GI reactions occur.
• Evaluate patient's and family's knowledge of drug therapy.

◤ Nursing diagnoses
• Diarrhea related to underlying condition
• Risk for deficient fluid volume related to drug-induced adverse GI reactions
• Deficient knowledge related to drug therapy

◤ Planning and implementation
• Notify prescriber if acute abdominal signs occur or drug is ineffective.

• If drug is given by NG tube, flush tube to clear it and ensure drug's passage to stomach.
⊛ **ALERT:** Oral liquids are available in different concentrations. Check dosage carefully. For children, consider an oral liquid product that doesn't contain alcohol.
⊛ **ALERT:** Don't confuse Imodium with Ionamin.

Patient teaching
• Advise patient not to exceed recommended dosage.
• Tell patient with acute diarrhea to stop drug and seek medical attention if no improvement occurs within 48 hours; for chronic diarrhea, tell him to notify prescriber and stop drug if no improvement occurs after giving 16 mg daily for at least 10 days.
• Advise patient to stop taking drug and to notify prescriber immediately if abdominal distention or other symptoms develop in acute colitis.

☑ Evaluation
• Patient's diarrhea is relieved.
• Patient maintains adequate hydration throughout therapy.
• Patient and family state understanding of drug therapy.

lopinavir and ritonavir
(loe-PIN-a-veer and rih-TOH-nuh-veer)
Kaletra

Pharmacologic class: protease inhibitor
Therapeutic class: antiviral
Pregnancy risk category: C

Indications and dosages

▶ **HIV infection (with other antiretrovirals).**
Adults and children older than age 12: 400 mg lopinavir/100 mg ritonavir (3 capsules or 5 ml) P.O. b.i.d. with food. In treatment-experienced patient also taking efavirenz or nevirapine in whom reduced susceptibility to lopinavir might be suspected, consider a dose of 533/133 mg (4 capsules or 6.5 ml) P.O. b.i.d. with food.
Children ages 6 months to 12 years weighing 15 to 40 kg (33 to 88 lb): 10 mg/kg (lopinavir content) P.O. b.i.d. with food, up to a maximum of 400/100 mg in children weighing more than 40 kg. In treatment-experienced patient also taking efavirenz or nevirapine who weighs 15 to

50 kg (33 to 110 lb) and in whom reduced susceptibility to lopinavir is suspected, consider a dose of 11 mg/kg (lopinavir content) P.O. b.i.d. Children who weigh more than 50 kg can receive the adult dose.

Children ages 6 months to 12 years weighing 7 to 14 kg (15 to 31 lb): 12 mg/kg (lopinavir content) P.O. b.i.d. with food. In treatment-experienced patient also taking efavirenz or nevirapine in whom reduced susceptibility to lopinavir is suspected, consider a dose of 13 mg/kg (lopinavir content) P.O. b.i.d. with food.

Contraindications and precautions

• Contraindicated in patients hypersensitive to any of drug's ingredients.

• Use cautiously in patients with a history of pancreatitis or with hepatic impairment, hepatitis B or C, marked elevations in liver enzyme levels, or hemophilia.

⚑ Lifespan: Women shouldn't breast feed. In infants younger than age 6 months, safety and effectiveness of drug haven't been established. In elderly patients, use cautiously.

Adverse reactions

CNS: pain, asthenia, headache, fever, insomnia, malaise, abnormal dreams, agitation, amnesia, anxiety, ataxia, confusion, depression, dizziness, dyskinesia, emotional lability, *encephalopathy,* hypertonia, nervousness, neuropathy, paresthesia, peripheral neuritis, somnolence, abnormal thinking, tremor.

CV: chest pain, *deep vein thrombosis,* hypertension, palpitations, peripheral edema, thrombophlebitis, vasculitis, facial edema, edema.

EENT: sinusitis, abnormal vision, eye disorder, otitis media, tinnitus.

GI: abdominal pain, abnormal stools, *diarrhea, nausea,* vomiting, anorexia, cholecystitis, constipation, dry mouth, dyspepsia, dysphagia, enterocolitis, eructation, esophagitis, fecal incontinence, flatulence, gastritis, gastroenteritis, GI disorder, *hemorrhagic colitis,* increased appetite, *pancreatitis,* sialadenitis, stomatitis, ulcerative stomatitis.

GU: abnormal ejaculation, taste perversion, hypogonadism, renal calculus, urine abnormality.

Hematologic: anemia, *leukopenia, neutropenia,* lymphadenopathy; *thrombocytopenia* in children.

Hepatic: hyperbilirubinemia in children.

Metabolic: Cushing's syndrome, hypothyroidism, dehydration, decreased glucose tolerance, *lactic acidosis,* weight loss, hyperglycemia, hyperuricemia, *hypercholesterolemia,* hyponatremia in children.

Musculoskeletal: back pain, arthralgia, arthrosis, myalgia.

Respiratory: bronchitis, dyspnea, *lung edema.*

Skin: rash, acne, alopecia, dry skin, exfoliative dermatitis, furunculosis, nail disorder, pruritus, benign skin neoplasm, skin discoloration, sweating.

Other: chills, flulike syndrome, viral infection, gynecomastia, decreased libido.

Interactions

Drug-drug. *Amiodarone, bepridil, lidocaine, quinidine:* Increases levels of antiarrhythmics. Use cautiously. Monitor levels of these drugs, if possible; adjust dosage, if needed.

Amprenavir, indinavir, saquinavir: Increases levels of these drugs. Avoid using together.

Antiarrhythmics (flecainide, propafenone), pimozide: Increases risk of cardiac arrhythmias. Don't use together.

Atovaquone, methadone: Decreases levels of these drugs. Consider increasing doses of these drugs.

Carbamazepine, dexamethasone, phenobarbital, phenytoin: Decreases lopinavir levels. Use cautiously.

Clarithromycin: Increases clarithromycin levels in patients with renal impairment. Adjust clarithromycin dose.

Cyclosporine, rapamycin, tacrolimus: Increases levels of these drugs. Monitor therapeutic levels.

Delavirdine, ritonavir: Increases levels of lopinavir. Avoid using together.

Didanosine: Decreases absorption of didanosine because lopinavir and ritonavir is taken with food. Give didanosine 1 hour before or 2 hours after lopinavir and ritonavir.

Dihydroergotamine, ergonovine, ergotamine, methylergonovine: Increases risk of ergot toxicity characterized by peripheral vasospasm and ischemia. Don't use together.

Disulfiram, metronidazole: May increase risk of disulfiram-like reaction. Avoid using together.

Efavirenz, nevirapine: Decreases lopinavir levels. Consider increasing lopinavir and ritonavir dose.

Felodipine, nicardipine, nifedipine: Increases levels of these drugs. Use cautiously. Monitor patient.

Itraconazole, ketoconazole: Increases levels of these drugs. Don't give more than 200 mg/day of these drugs.

HMG-CoA reductase inhibitors: Increases risk of adverse reactions, such as myopathy, rhabdomyolysis. Atorvastatin, fluvastatin, and pravastatin may be used with careful monitoring; Avoid using lovastatin or simvastatin.

Methadone: Methadone AUC decreased. May need to increase dose. Monitor patient closely.

Midazolam, triazolam: Increases risk of prolonged or increased sedation or respiratory depression. Don't use together.

Hormonal contraceptives (ethinyl estradiol): Decreases effectiveness of contraceptives. Recommend alternative contraception measures.

Rifabutin: Increases rifabutin levels. Decrease rifabutin dose by 75%; monitor patient for adverse effects.

Rifampin: Decreases effectiveness of lopinavir and ritonavir. Avoid using together.

Sildenafil: Increases sildenafil levels. Don't exceed 25 mg of sildenafil in a 48-hour period. Use cautiously, and monitor patient for adverse reactions.

Warfarin: May affect warfarin level. Monitor PT and INR.

Drug-herb. *St. John's wort:* Loss of virologic response and possible resistance to Kaletra. Discourage using together.

Drug-food. *Any food:* Increases absorption of drug. Give drug with food.

Effects on lab test results

- May increase amylase, liver enzyme, glucose, uric acid, cholesterol, and triglyceride levels. In children, may increase bilirubin level and decrease sodium level.
- May decrease hemoglobin, hematocrit, and WBC, neutrophil, and platelet counts.

Pharmacokinetics

Absorption: Peak levels are achieved in 4 hours. Lopinavir and ritonavir is better absorbed when taken with food.

Distribution: Lopinavir is 98 or 99% protein-bound.

Metabolism: Lopinavir is extensively metabolized by the CYP 3A isoenzyme. Ritonavir is a potent inhibitor of the CYP 3A, which inhibits the metabolism of lopinavir, and therefore increases lopinavir level.

Excretion: In urine and feces. Less than 3% of the drug is excreted unchanged. *Half-life:* About 6 hours.

Route	Onset	Peak	Duration
P.O.	Unknown	4 hr	6 hr

Action

Chemical effects: Inhibits the HIV protease. Ritonavir inhibits the metabolism of lopinavir, thereby increasing lopinavir level.

Therapeutic effect: Prevents the cleavage of the Gag-Pol polyprotein, resulting in the production of immature, noninfectious viral particles.

Available forms

Capsules: lopinavir 133.3 mg/ritonavir 33.3 mg
Solution: lopinavir 400 mg/ritonavir 100 mg per 5 ml (80 mg/20 mg per ml)

NURSING PROCESS

Assessment
- Assess underlying condition before therapy and reassess regularly throughout therapy.
- Monitor total cholesterol and triglycerides before starting therapy and periodically thereafter.
- To monitor maternal-fetal outcomes of pregnant women exposed to lopinavir/ritonavir, an antiretroviral registry has been established. Enroll patients by calling 1-800-258-4263.
- **ⓈALERT:** This drug interacts with many other drugs. Review current drugs that patient is taking.
- Evaluate patient's and family's knowledge of drug therapy.

Nursing diagnoses
- Risk for falls related to drug-induced adverse CNS effects
- Risk for powerlessness related to chronic disease and need for aggressive medical management
- Deficient knowledge related to drug therapy

Planning and implementation
- Give drug with food.
- Refrigerated drug remains stable until expiration date on package. If stored at room temperature, use drug within 2 months.

Reactions may be *common,* uncommon, *life-threatening,* or **COMMON AND LIFE-THREATENING.**

- Monitor patient for signs of fat redistribution, including central obesity, buffalo hump, peripheral wasting, breast enlargement, and cushingoid appearance.
- Monitor patient for signs of pancreatitis: nausea, vomiting, abdominal pain, increased lipase and amylase values.
- Monitor patient for signs of bleeding.
- For an overdose, induce emesis or perform gastric lavage. Activated charcoal may be used to aid in the removal of unabsorbed drug. Dialysis is unlikely to help remove drug.
- ⊛ **ALERT:** Don't confuse Kaletra with Keppra.

Patient teaching
- Tell patient to take drug with food.
- Tell patient also taking didanosine to take it 1 hour before or 2 hours after lopinavir and ritonavir.
- Advise patient to report side effects to prescriber.
- Tell patient to immediately report severe nausea, vomiting, or abdominal pain.
- Warn patient to tell prescriber about any other prescription or nonprescription medicine that he is taking, including herbal supplements.
- Tell patient that drug is not a cure for HIV.
- Advise patient taking sildenafil that there is an increased risk of sildenafil-associated adverse events including hypotension, visual changes, and priapism, and he should promptly report any symptoms. Tell him not to exceed 25 mg of sildenafil in a 48-hour period.
- Inform HIV-infected mothers they shouldn't breast-feed to avoid HIV transmission.

☑ Evaluation
- Patient doesn't experience falls.
- Patient has adequate support, personal and professional, to deal with emotional aspects of having HIV disease.
- Patient and family state understanding of drug therapy.

loracarbef
(loh-ruh-KAR-bef)
Lorabid

Pharmacologic class: synthetic beta-lactam antibiotic of carbacephem class
Therapeutic class: antibiotic
Pregnancy risk category: B

Indications and dosages

▶ **Secondary bacterial infections of acute bronchitis.** *Adults:* 200 to 400 g P.O. q 12 hours for 7 days.
▶ **Acute bacterial exacerbations of chronic bronchitis.** *Adults:* 400 mg P.O. q 12 hours for 7 days.
▶ **Pneumonia.** *Adults:* 400 mg P.O. q 12 hours for 14 days.
▶ **Pharyngitis, sinusitis, tonsillitis.** *Adults:* 200 to 400 mg P.O. q 12 hours for 10 days. *Children:* 15 mg/kg P.O. daily in divided doses q 12 hours for 10 days.
▶ **Acute otitis media.** *Children:* 30 mg/kg (oral suspension) P.O. daily in divided doses q 12 hours for 10 days.
▶ **Uncomplicated skin and skin-structure infections.** *Adults:* 200 mg P.O. q 12 hours for 7 days.
▶ **Impetigo.** *Children:* 15 mg/kg P.O. daily in divided doses q 12 hours for 7 days.
▶ **Uncomplicated cystitis.** *Adults:* 200 mg P.O. daily for 7 days.
▶ **Uncomplicated pyelonephritis.** *Adults:* 400 mg P.O. q 12 hours for 14 days.
Ⓢ **Adjust-a-dose:** For patients with renal impairment, if creatinine clearance is 10 to 49 ml/minute, give half of usual dose at same interval. If clearance is below 10 ml/minute, give usual dose q 3 to 5 days. Give hemodialysis patients another dose after dialysis.

Contraindications and precautions

- Contraindicated in patients hypersensitive to drug or other cephalosporins and in patients with diarrhea caused by pseudomembranous colitis.
- ⚕ **Lifespan:** In pregnant and breast-feeding women, use cautiously. In infants younger than age 6 months, safety and effectiveness of drug haven't been established.

Adverse reactions

CNS: headache, somnolence, nervousness, insomnia, dizziness.
CV: vasodilation.
GI: diarrhea, nausea, vomiting, abdominal pain, anorexia, *pseudomembranous colitis.*
GU: vaginal candidiasis.
Hematologic: *transient thrombocytopenia, leukopenia,* eosinophilia.
Skin: rash, urticaria, pruritus, *erythema multiforme.*

Other: hypersensitivity reactions, *anaphylaxis.*

Interactions

Drug-drug. *Probenecid:* Decreases loracarbef excretion, causing increased levels. Monitor patient for toxicity.
Drug-food. *Any food:* Decreases absorption. Give drug 1 hour before or 2 hours after meals.

Effects on lab test results

• May increase BUN, creatinine, ALT, AST, and alkaline phosphatase levels.
• May increase PT, INR, and eosinophil count. May decrease platelet, WBC, RBC, and neutrophil counts.
• May cause false-positive direct Coombs' test.

Pharmacokinetics

Absorption: About 90%. Absorption of suspension is greater than that of capsule.
Distribution: About 25% of circulating drug is bound to proteins.
Metabolism: Doesn't appear to be metabolized.
Excretion: Excreted primarily in urine. *Half-life:* About 1 hour.

Route	Onset	Peak	Duration
P.O.	Unknown	30-60 min	Unknown

Action

Chemical effect: Inhibits cell-wall synthesis, promoting osmotic instability; usually bactericidal.
Therapeutic effect: Kills susceptible bacteria, including gram-positive aerobes, such as *Staphylococcus aureus* and *saprophyticus, Streptococcus pneumoniae* and *pyogenes;* and gram-negative aerobes, such as *Escherichia coli, Haemophilus influenzae,* and *Moraxella catarrhalis.*

Available forms

Powder for oral suspension: 100 mg/5 ml, 200 mg/5 ml in 50-, 75-, and 100-ml bottles
Pulvules: 200 mg, 400 mg

NURSING PROCESS

Assessment

• Assess patient's infection before therapy and regularly thereafter.

• Obtain specimen for culture and sensitivity tests before giving first dose. Therapy may begin pending test results.
• Be alert for adverse reactions and drug interactions.
⚡ ALERT: Watch for seizures. Beta-lactam antibiotics may trigger seizures in susceptible patients, especially when given without dosage modification to those with renal impairment.
• Monitor patient's hydration status if adverse GI reactions occur.
• Evaluate patient's and family's knowledge of drug therapy.

Nursing diagnoses

• Infection related to presence of susceptible bacteria
• Risk for deficient fluid volume related to drug-induced adverse GI reactions
• Deficient knowledge related to drug therapy

Planning and implementation

• To reconstitute powder for oral suspension, add 30 ml of water in two portions to 50-ml bottle or 60 ml of water in two portions to 100-ml bottle. Shake after each addition.
• After reconstitution, store oral suspension for 14 days at constant room temperature (59° to 86° F [15° to 30° C]).
• If seizures occur, stop drug and tell prescriber. Give anticonvulsants.
⚡ ALERT: Don't confuse Lorabid with Lortab.
Patient teaching
• Tell patient to take drug on an empty stomach, at least 1 hour before or 2 hours after meals.
• Tell patient to shake suspension well before measuring dose and to take drug exactly as prescribed.
• Instruct patient to discard unused portion after 14 days.

✓ Evaluation

• Patient is free from infection.
• Patient maintains adequate hydration throughout therapy.
• Patient and family state understanding of drug therapy.

loratadine

(loo-RAH-tuh-deen)
Alavert†, Claratyne ◇, Claritin†, Claritin Reditabs†, Claritin Syrup†, Claritin-D 12-hour†, Claritin-D 24 Hour†, Tavist ND Allergy†

Pharmacologic class: tricyclic antihistamine
Therapeutic class: antihistamine
Pregnancy risk category: B

Indications and dosages

▶ **Allergic rhinitis, chronic idiopathic urticaria.** *Adults and children age 6 and older:* 10 mg P.O. daily.
Children ages 2 to 5: 5 mg P.O. daily.
⊠ Adjust-a-dose: For patients with renal or hepatic impairment, adjust dosage as follows: In adults and children age 6 and older with liver impairment or creatinine clearance less than 30 ml/minute, give 10 mg q other day. In children ages 2 to 5 with liver impairment or renal insufficiency, give 5 mg q other day.

Contraindications and precautions

• Contraindicated in patients hypersensitive to drug.
• Use cautiously in patients with hepatic impairment.
⚕ **Lifespan:** In pregnant women, use only when absolutely necessary. In breast-feeding women, drug isn't recommended. In children younger than age 2, safety of drug hasn't been established.

Adverse reactions

CNS: *headache,* drowsiness, fatigue, insomnia, nervousness.
GI: dry mouth.

Interactions

Drug-drug. *Erythromycin, ketoconazole:* Increases loratadine levels. Monitor patient closely.
Drug-lifestyle. *Alcohol use:* Increases CNS depression. Discourage using together.

Effects on lab test results

None reported.

Pharmacokinetics

Absorption: Readily absorbed. Food may delay peak levels by 1 hour.
Distribution: Doesn't readily cross blood-brain barrier; about 97% bound to protein.
Metabolism: Extensively metabolized, although specific enzyme systems responsible for metabolism haven't been identified.
Excretion: About 80% distributed equally between urine and feces. *Half-life:* 8.4 hours.

Route	Onset	Peak	Duration
P.O.	1 hr	4-6 hr	24 hr

Action

Chemical effect: Blocks effects of histamine at H_1-receptor sites. Drug's chemical structure prevents entry into CNS, preventing sedation.
Therapeutic effect: Relieves allergy symptoms.

Available forms

Syrup: 1 mg/ml†
Tablets: 10 mg†
Tablets (rapidly disintegrating): 10 mg†

NURSING PROCESS

⚕ Assessment

• Assess patient's condition before therapy and regularly thereafter.
• Be alert for adverse reactions and drug interactions.
• Evaluate patient's and family's knowledge of drug therapy.

⚕ Nursing diagnoses

• Ineffective health maintenance related to underlying allergy condition
• Fatigue related to drug's adverse effect
• Deficient knowledge related to drug therapy

▶ Planning and implementation

• Give drug on empty stomach.
• Notify prescriber if drug is ineffective.
Patient teaching
• Tell patient to take drug at least 2 hours after meal, to avoid eating for at least 1 hour after taking drug, and to take drug only once daily.
• Advise patient taking rapidly disintegrating tablets to place tablet on the tongue, where it

disintegrates within a few seconds. It can be swallowed with or without water.
- Tell patient to contact prescriber if symptoms persist or worsen.
- Advise patient to stop taking drug 4 days before allergy skin tests to preserve accuracy of tests.
- Tell patient to avoid alcohol and driving or other activities that require alertness until CNS effects of drug are known.

☑ **Evaluation**
- Patient states that allergy symptoms are relieved.
- Patient describes coping strategies for fatigue.
- Patient and family state understanding of drug therapy.

lorazepam
(loo-RAZ-eh-pam)
Apo-Lorazepam ◆ , Ativan, Lorazepam Intensol, Novo-Lorazem ◆ , Nu-Loraz ◆

Pharmacologic class: benzodiazepine
Therapeutic class: anxiolytic, sedative-hypnotic
Pregnancy risk category: D
Controlled substance schedule: IV

Indications and dosages

▶ **Anxiety.** *Adults:* 2 to 6 mg P.O. daily in divided doses. Maximum, 10 mg daily.
▶ **Insomnia caused by anxiety.** *Adults:* 2 to 4 mg P.O. h.s.
▶ **Premedication before operative procedure.** *Adults:* 0.05 mg/kg I.M. 2 hours before procedure. Maximum dosage, 4 mg. Or, 2 mg total or 0.044 mg/kg I.V., whichever is smaller. Larger doses up to 0.05 mg/kg I.V. (to total of 4 mg) may be needed.
▶ **Nausea and vomiting caused by emetogenic cancer chemotherapy‡.** *Adults:* 2.5 mg P.O. the evening before chemotherapy; repeat just after the initiation of chemotherapy. Or, 1.5 mg/m² (maximum, 3 mg) I.V. over 5 minutes, 45 minutes before chemotherapy. *Elderly patient:* Initially, 1 to 2 mg P.O. daily in divided doses. Adjust as needed and as tolerated.
▶ **Status epilepticus‡.** *Adults and children:* 0.05 to 0.1 mg/kg I.V. Doses may be repeated at 10- to 15-minute intervals p.r.n. for seizure control. Alternatively, adults may be given 4 to 8 mg I.V.

▼ I.V. administration
- Dilute with equal volume of sterile water for injection, normal saline solution for injection, or D₅W injection.
- Preoperative I.V. dose shouldn't exceed 2 mg in patients older than age 50.
- Give drug slowly, at no more than 2 mg/minute.
- ⑤ **ALERT:** Check respirations before each I.V. dose and every 5 to 15 minutes thereafter until respiratory status is stable. Have emergency resuscitation equipment and oxygen available.

Contraindications and precautions
- Contraindicated in patients hypersensitive to drug, other benzodiazepines, or vehicle used in parenteral dosage form; also contraindicated in patients with acute angle-closure glaucoma.
- Use cautiously in patients with pulmonary, renal, or hepatic impairment. Also use cautiously and at a reduced dosage in acutely ill or debilitated patients.
- ⚖ **Lifespan:** In pregnant women, avoid use, especially during first trimester. In breast-feeding women, avoid use. In children, safety of drug hasn't been established. In elderly patients, use cautiously and at a reduced dosage.

Adverse reactions
CNS: *drowsiness, lethargy, hangover,* fainting, anterograde amnesia, restlessness, psychosis.
CV: transient hypotension.
EENT: visual disturbances.
GI: dry mouth, abdominal discomfort.
GU: incontinence, urine retention.
Other: *acute withdrawal syndrome* (after suddenly stopping drug in physically dependent patients).

Interactions
Drug-drug. *CNS depressants:* May increase CNS depression. Avoid using together.
Digoxin: May increase digoxin level, increasing toxicity. Monitor level.
Drug-herb. *Catnip, kava, lady's slipper, lemon balm, passion flower, sassafras, skullcap, valer-*

---

ian: Sedative effects may be enhanced. Discourage using together.
Drug-lifestyle. *Alcohol use:* May cause additive CNS effects. Strongly discourage using together.
Smoking: Decreases benzodiazepine effectiveness. Monitor patient closely; discourage patient from smoking.

Effects on lab test results

• May increase liver function test results.

Pharmacokinetics

Absorption: Well absorbed after P.O. administration; unknown after I.M. administration.
Distribution: Distributed widely throughout body; about 85% protein-bound.
Metabolism: Metabolized in liver.
Excretion: Excreted in urine. *Half-life:* 10 to 20 hours.

Route	Onset	Peak	Duration
P.O.	1 hr	2 hr	12-24 hr
I.V.	1-5 min	1-1½ hr	6-8 hr
I.M.	15-30 min	1-1½ hr	6-8 hr

Action

Chemical effect: Unknown; probably stimulates gamma-aminobutyric receptors in ascending reticular activating system.
Therapeutic effect: Relieves anxiety and promotes calmness and sleep.

Available forms

Injection: 2 mg/ml, 4 mg/ml
Oral solution (concentrated): 2 mg/ml
S.L. tablets: 0.5 mg◆, 1 mg◆, 2 mg◆
Tablets: 0.5 mg, 1 mg, 2 mg

NURSING PROCESS

Assessment

• Assess patient's condition before therapy and regularly thereafter.
• Monitor liver, kidney, and hematopoietic function studies periodically in patient receiving repeated or prolonged therapy.
• Be alert for adverse reactions and drug interactions.
• Evaluate patient's and family's knowledge of drug therapy.

Nursing diagnoses

• Anxiety related to underlying condition
• Risk for injury related to drug-induced adverse CNS effects
• Deficient knowledge related to drug therapy

Planning and implementation

• For I.M. injection, inject drug deep into muscle mass. Don't dilute.
• Refrigerate parenteral form to prolong shelf life.
ALERT: Possibility of abuse and addiction exists. Don't withdraw drug abruptly after long-term use; withdrawal symptoms may occur.
ALERT: Don't confuse lorazepam with alprazolam.
Patient teaching
• Warn patient to avoid hazardous activities until CNS effects of drug are known.
• Tell patient to avoid alcohol and smoking during drug therapy.
• As premedication before surgery, drug provides substantial preoperative amnesia. Teach patient about drug before giving preoperative dose. Provide written materials or inform family member, if possible.

Evaluation

• Patient is less anxious.
• Patient doesn't experience injury as result of adverse CNS reactions.
• Patient and family state understanding of drug therapy.

losartan potassium
(loh-SAR-tan poh-TAH-see-um)
Cozaar

Pharmacologic class: angiotensin II receptor antagonist
Therapeutic class: antihypertensive
Pregnancy risk category: C (D in second and third trimesters)

Indications and dosages

▶ **Nephropathy in type 2 diabetes mellitus.**
Adults: 50 mg P.O. daily. Increase dose to 100 mg daily based on blood pressure response.
▶ **Hypertension.** *Adults:* Initially, 25 to 50 mg P.O. daily. Maximum daily dose is 100 mg in one or two divided doses.

▶ **To reduce risk of CVA in patients with hypertension and left ventricular hypertrophy.**
Adults: Initially, 50 mg P.O. once daily. Adjust dosage based on blood pressure response, adding hydrochlorothiazide 12.5 mg once daily, increasing losartan to 100 mg daily, or both. If further adjustments are required, may increase the daily dosage of hydrochlorothiazide to 25 mg.

Contraindications and precautions

• Contraindicated in patients hypersensitive to drug.
• Use cautiously in patients with impaired kidney or liver function.
⚠ Lifespan: In pregnant women, drug should be used only when absolutely necessary. In breast-feeding women, avoid breast-feeding during drug therapy. In children, safety of drug hasn't been established.

Adverse reactions

For hypertension and left ventricular hypertrophy
CNS: dizziness, asthenia, fatigue, headache, insomnia.
CV: edema, chest pain.
EENT: nasal congestion, sinusitis, pharyngitis, sinus disorder.
GI: abdominal pain, nausea, diarrhea, dyspepsia.
Musculoskeletal: muscle cramps, myalgia, back or leg pain.
Respiratory: cough, upper respiratory tract infection.
Other: *angioedema.*
For nephropathy
CNS: *asthenia, fatigue,* fever, hypesthesia, diabetic neuropathy.
CV: *chest pain,* hypotension, orthostatic hypotension, *diabetic vascular disease.*
EENT: sinusitis, cataract.
GI: *diarrhea,* dyspepsia, gastritis.
GU: *UTI.*
Hematologic: *anemia.*
Metabolic: *hyperkalemia,* **HYPOGLYCEMIA,** weight gain.
Musculoskeletal: *back pain,* leg or knee pain, muscle weakness.
Respiratory: *cough, bronchitis.*
Skin: cellulitis.
Other: infection, *flulike syndrome,* trauma, *angioedema.*

Interactions

Drug-drug. *Potassium-sparing diuretics, potassium supplements:* May cause possible hyperkalemia. Monitor potassium level.
Drug-herb. *Red yeast rice:* Contains components similar to those of statin drugs, increasing the risk of adverse events or toxicity. Discourage using together.
Drug-food. *Salt substitutes containing potassium:* May increase risk of hyperkalemia. Monitor patient closely; advise patient to use only under prescriber's guidance.

Effects on lab test results

None reported.

Pharmacokinetics

Absorption: Absorbed well and undergoes extensive first-pass metabolism; systemic bioavailability of drug is about 33%.
Distribution: Highly bound to proteins.
Metabolism: CYP 2C9 and 3A4 are involved in biotransformation of drug to metabolites.
Excretion: Excreted primarily in feces with smaller amount excreted in urine. *Half-life:* About 2 hours.

Route	Onset	Peak	Duration
P.O.	Unknown	1-4 hr	Unknown

Action

Chemical effect: Inhibits vasoconstricting and aldosterone-secreting effects of angiotensin II by selectively blocking binding of angiotensin II to receptor sites in many tissues, including vascular smooth muscle and adrenal glands.
Therapeutic effect: Lowers blood pressure.

Available forms

Tablets: 25 mg, 50 mg, 100 mg

NURSING PROCESS

▨ **Assessment**

• Assess patient's blood pressure before therapy and regularly thereafter. When drug is used alone, its effect on blood pressure is notably less in black patients than in those of other races.
• Regularly assess creatinine and BUN levels to check kidney function. Patients with severe heart failure whose kidney function depends on angiotensin-aldosterone system may experience acute renal impairment during therapy. Closely

monitor patient, especially during first few weeks of therapy.
- Be alert for adverse reactions.
- Monitor patient for symptomatic hypotension if he is taking a diuretic.
- Evaluate patient's and family's knowledge of drug therapy.

🖭 Nursing diagnoses
- Risk for injury related to presence of hypertension
- Disturbed sleep pattern related to drug-induced insomnia
- Deficient knowledge related to drug therapy

⊠ Planning and implementation
- In patients with impaired liver function and in those with volume depletion (such as those receiving diuretics), use initial dose of 25 mg.
- Black patients with hypertension and left ventricular hypertrophy have a lower risk of CVA on atenolol than on this drug, but the cause is unknown.
- Drug can be used alone or with other antihypertensives.
- Determine trough level to measure effect. If effect of once-daily dosing is inadequate, give a twice-daily regimen using same total daily dose or increase dosage.
- Give once-daily dosing in morning to prevent insomnia.
- If pregnancy is suspected, stop drug and notify prescriber immediately.
- ⊛ **ALERT:** Don't confuse Cozaar with Zocor.

Patient teaching
- Tell patient to avoid sodium substitutes; these products may contain potassium, which can cause hyperkalemia in patients taking losartan.
- Inform woman of childbearing age to notify prescriber immediately if pregnancy occurs or is suspected.

☑ Evaluation
- Patient's blood pressure is normal.
- Patient states that insomnia hasn't occurred.
- Patient and family state understanding of drug therapy.

lovastatin (mevinolin)
(loh-vuh-STAH-tin)
Altocor, Mevacor

Pharmacologic class: HMG-CoA reductase inhibitor
Therapeutic class: cholesterol-lowering drug
Pregnancy risk category: X

Indications and dosages

▶ **Primary prevention of coronary artery disease; coronary artery disease; hyperlipidemia.** *Adults:* Initially, 20 mg immediate-release tablets P.O. once daily with evening meal. Recommended range is 10 to 80 mg in single or two divided doses; maximum recommended dosage is 80 mg daily. Or, 20 to 60 mg extended-release P.O. h.s. Starting dose of 10 mg can be used for patients requiring smaller reductions. Usual dosage range is 10 to 60 mg daily for the extended release tablets.
▶ **Heterozygous familial hypercholesterolemia.** *Children ages 10 to 17:* 10 to 40 mg P.O. (immediate-release) daily with evening meal. In patients requiring reductions in LDL level of 20% or more, start with 20 mg daily.
☒ **Adjust-a-dose:** For patients also taking cyclosporine, give 10 mg P.O. daily, not to exceed 20 mg daily. Use of drug with fibrates or niacin should generally be avoided; if used with either, don't give more than 20 mg of lovastatin daily. For patients with renal impairment, if creatinine clearance is less than 30 ml/minute, exercise caution and careful consideration for dosage increases above 20 mg daily.

Contraindications and precautions

- Contraindicated in patients hypersensitive to drug, and in those with active liver disease or conditions linked to unexplained persistent elevations of transaminase levels.
- Use cautiously in patients who consume substantial quantities of alcohol or have history of liver disease.
- 🜲 **Lifespan:** In pregnant and breast-feeding women, drug is contraindicated. In women of childbearing age, drug is contraindicated unless they have no risk of pregnancy. In children younger than age 10, safety of drug hasn't been established.

Adverse reactions

CNS: headache, dizziness, peripheral neuropathy.
EENT: blurred vision.
GI: constipation, diarrhea, dyspepsia, flatulence, abdominal pain or cramps, heartburn, dysgeusia, nausea.
Musculoskeletal: muscle cramps, myalgia, myositis, *rhabdomyolysis*.
Skin: rash, pruritus.

Interactions

Drug-drug. *Bile acid sequestrants:* Decreases lovastatin bioavailability. Administer separately.
Cyclosporine or other immunosuppressants, erythromycin, gemfibrozil, niacin: Increases risk of polymyositis and rhabdomyolysis. Monitor patient closely.
Digoxin: Slight elevation in digoxin levels is possible. Monitor patient.
Isradipine: Increases clearance of lovastatin and its metabolites via increased hepatic blood flow. Monitor patient for loss of therapeutic effect.
Fluconazole, itraconazole, ketoconazole: May increase level and adverse effects of lovastatin. Avoid this combination. If drugs must be given together, reduce dose of lovastatin.
Oral anticoagulants: Lovastatin may enhance oral anticoagulant effects. Monitor PT and INR.
Drug-herb. *Red yeast rice:* Herb contains components similar to those of drug, increasing the risk of adverse events or toxicity. Discourage using together.
Drug-lifestyle. *Alcohol use:* Increases risk of hepatotoxicity. Discourage using together.
Sun exposure: Photosensitivity reactions may occur. Tell patient to avoid unprotected or prolonged exposure to sunlight.

Effects on lab test results

• May increase ALT, AST, and CK levels.

Pharmacokinetics

Absorption: About 30%. Giving with food improves levels of total inhibitors by about 30%. Extended-release tablets have greater bioavailability than immediate-release tablets.
Distribution: Less than 5% of dose reaches systemic circulation because of extensive first-pass hepatic extraction; liver is principal site of action. Drug and its principal metabolite are more than 95% bound to proteins.

Metabolism: Metabolized in liver. Studies with extended-release tablets have not been conducted.
Excretion: About 80% excreted in feces, about 10% in urine. *Half-life:* 3 hours. Extended-release tablets incur negligible excretion through the kidneys.

Route	Onset	Peak	Duration
P.O.	Unknown	2-6 hr	4-6 wk
extended-release	Unknown	14 hr	Unknown

Action

Chemical effect: Inhibits HMG-CoA reductase. This enzyme is an early and rate-limiting step in synthetic pathway of cholesterol.
Therapeutic effect: Lowers LDL and total cholesterol levels.

Available forms

Tablets: 10 mg, 20 mg, 40 mg
Tablets (extended-release): 10 mg, 20 mg, 40 mg, 60 mg

NURSING PROCESS

Assessment

• Obtain history of patient's lipoprotein and cholesterol levels before therapy, and reassess regularly thereafter.
• Use for heterozygous familial hypercholesterolemia in girls who are at least 1 year postmenarche and boys (ages 10 to 17) who have these findings after an adequate trial of diet therapy: 1) LDL cholesterol level remains > 189 mg/dl; or 2) LDL cholesterol level remains >160 mg/dl and a family history of premature CV disease or two or more other CV disease risk factors.
• Perform liver function tests at start of therapy and periodically thereafter.
• Be alert for adverse reactions and drug interactions.
• Evaluate patient's and family's knowledge of drug therapy.

Nursing diagnoses

• Risk for injury related to underlying condition
• Pain related to drug-induced adverse musculoskeletal reactions
• Deficient knowledge related to drug therapy

⧉ Planning and implementation

• Begin drug therapy only after diet and other nonpharmacologic therapies have proven ineffective. Patient should follow a standard low-cholesterol diet.

• Give drug with evening meal; absorption is enhanced and cholesterol biosynthesis is greater in evening.

ⓢ **ALERT:** Don't confuse lovastatin with Lotensin, Leustatin, or Livostin. Don't confuse Mevacor with Mivacron.

ⓢ **ALERT:** Don't confuse Altocor with Advicor.

Patient teaching

• Instruct patient to take drug with evening meal.

• Advise patient not to crush or chew extended-release tablets.

• Teach patient to restrict total fat and cholesterol intake to manage lipid level and to control other cardiac disease risk factors. If appropriate, recommend weight control, exercise, and smoking cessation programs.

• Advise patient to have periodic eye examinations.

• Tell patient to store drug at room temperature in light-resistant container.

• Instruct patient to avoid alcohol consumption during drug therapy.

ⓢ **ALERT:** Inform woman that drug is contraindicated during pregnancy. Tell her to notify prescriber immediately if she becomes pregnant.

☑ Evaluation

• Patient's LDL and cholesterol levels are within normal limits.

• Patient doesn't experience musculoskeletal pain.

• Patient and family state understanding of drug therapy.

---

lymphocyte immune globulin (antithymocyte globulin [equine], ATG), (LIG)

(LIM-foh-sight ih-MYOON GLOH-byoo-lin)
Atgam

Pharmacologic class: immunoglobulin
Therapeutic class: immunosuppressant
Pregnancy risk category: C

Indications and dosages

▶ **Prevention of acute renal allograft rejection.** *Adults and children:* 15 mg/kg I.V. daily for 14 days, followed by alternate-day dosing for 14 days. Give first dose within 24 hours of transplantation.

▶ **Acute renal allograft rejection.** *Adults and children:* 10 to 15 mg/kg I.V. daily for 14 days, followed by alternate-day dosing for 14 days. Start therapy when rejection is diagnosed.

▶ **Aplastic anemia.** *Adults:* 10 to 20 mg/kg I.V. daily for 8 to 14 days. Additional alternate-day therapy up to total of 21 doses can be given.

▶ **Skin allotransplantation‡.** *Adults:* 10 mg/kg I.V. 24 hours before allograft; then 10 to 15 mg/kg q other day. Maintenance dose ranges from 5 to 40 mg/kg daily based on response. Therapy usually continues until allograft covers less than 20% of total body surface area, usually 40 to 60 days.

▼ I.V. administration

• Dilute dose in 250 to 1,000 ml of half-normal or normal saline solution for injection. Don't exceed final concentration of 1 mg/ml. When adding drug to solution, make sure container is inverted so drug doesn't contact air inside container. Gently rotate or swirl container to mix contents; don't shake because this may cause excessive foaming and may alter drug.

• Don't dilute drug with dextrose solutions or solutions with low salt concentration because precipitate may form. The proteins in drug can be denatured by air. Drug is unstable in acidic solutions.

• Allow diluted drug to reach room temperature before infusion.

• Infuse with in-line filter with pore size of 0.2 to 1 micron over no less than 4 hours (most facilities specify 4 to 8 hours) into a vascular shunt, arterial venous fistula, or high-flow central vein. Drug solutions must be filtered during administration; use filters with pore sizes of 0.2 to 5 microns.

• Don't use solutions that are more than 12 hours old, including actual infusion time.

• Refrigerate drug at 35° to 47° F (2° to 8° C). Don't freeze. Drug is heat-sensitive.

Contraindications and precautions

• Contraindicated in patients hypersensitive to drug.

• Use cautiously in patients receiving additional immunosuppressive therapy (such as corticosteroids and azathioprine) because of increased potential for infection.

🕸 Lifespan: In pregnant women, use cautiously. In breast-feeding women, drug isn't recommended.

Adverse reactions

CNS: malaise, *seizures,* headache.
CV: *hypotension, chest pain,* thrombophlebitis, tachycardia, edema, *iliac vein obstruction,* renal artery stenosis.
EENT: *laryngospasm.*
GI: *nausea, vomiting,* diarrhea, epigastric pain, abdominal distention, stomatitis.
Hematologic: *leukopenia, thrombocytopenia,* hemolysis, *aplastic anemia,* lymphadenopathy.
Metabolic: hyperglycemia.
Musculoskeletal: arthralgia.
Respiratory: *dyspnea,* hiccups, *pulmonary edema.*
Skin: rash.
Other: febrile reactions, serum sickness, *anaphylaxis,* infection, night sweats.

Interactions

Drug-drug. *Muromonab-CD3:* May increase risk of infection. Monitor patient closely.

Effects on lab test results

• May increase liver enzyme and glucose levels.
• May decrease hemoglobin, hematocrit, and WBC and platelet counts.

Pharmacokinetics

Absorption: Administered I.V.
Distribution: Unknown.
Metabolism: Unknown.
Excretion: About 1% excreted in urine, principally as unchanged drug. *Half-life:* About 6 days.

Route	Onset	Peak	Duration
I.V.	Unknown	5 days	Unknown

Action

Chemical effect: Unknown; inhibits cell-mediated immune responses by either altering T-cell function or eliminating antigen-reactive T cells.

Therapeutic effect: Prevents or relieves signs and symptoms of renal allograft rejection; also relieves signs and symptoms of aplastic anemia.

Available forms

Injection: 50 mg of equine immunoglobulin/ml in 5-ml ampules

NURSING PROCESS

🕮 Assessment
• Assess patient's condition before therapy and regularly thereafter.
• Be alert for adverse reactions and drug interactions.
• Evaluate patient's and family's knowledge of drug therapy.

🕮 Nursing diagnoses
• Ineffective health maintenance related to underlying condition
• Ineffective immune protection related to adverse hematologic reactions
• Deficient knowledge related to drug therapy

🕮 Planning and implementation
• An intradermal skin test is recommended at least 1 hour before first dose. Marked local swelling or erythema larger than 10 mm indicates increased risk of severe systemic reaction, such as anaphylaxis. Severe reactions to skin test, such as hypotension, tachycardia, dyspnea, generalized rash, or anaphylaxis, usually preclude further administration. Anaphylaxis has occurred in patients with negative skin tests.
🕮 **ALERT:** Keep airway adjuncts and anaphylaxis drugs at bedside during administration.
Patient teaching
• Warn patient that fever is likely. Instruct him to report adverse drug effects.
• Instruct patient to take infection-control and bleeding precautions.

🕮 Evaluation
• Patient responds well to therapy.
• Patient doesn't experience serious adverse hematologic reactions.
• Patient and family state understanding of drug therapy.

magaldrate (aluminum-magnesium complex)

(muh-GAL-drayt)

Iosopan†, Riopan†

Pharmacologic class: aluminum-magnesium salt
Therapeutic class: antacid
Pregnancy risk category: A

Indications and dosages

▶ **Antacid.** *Adults:* 540 to 1,080 mg (5 to 10 ml) P.O. with water between meals and h.s.

Contraindications and precautions

• Contraindicated in patients with severe renal disease. Drug isn't typically used in patients with renal impairment to help control hypophosphatemia because it contains magnesium, which may accumulate.
• Use cautiously in patients with mild renal impairment.
≈ **Lifespan:** In pregnant and breast-feeding women, use cautiously.

Adverse reactions

GI: mild constipation, diarrhea.

Interactions

Drug-drug. *Allopurinol, antibiotics (including fluoroquinolones and tetracyclines), diflunisal, digoxin, iron, isoniazid, penicillamine, phenothiazines, quinidine:* May decrease pharmacologic effects of these drugs because of impaired absorption. Separate administration times.
Enteric-coated drugs: May release prematurely in stomach. Separate doses by at least 1 hour.

Effects on lab test results

• May increase gastrin level and, in patients with renal impairment, magnesium level.

Pharmacokinetics

Absorption: May be absorbed systemically, posing risk to patient with renal impairment.

Absorption is unrelated to mechanism of action.
Distribution: Primarily local.
Metabolism: None.
Excretion: Excreted in feces. *Half-life:* Unknown.

Route	Onset	Peak	Duration
P.O.			
fasting	≤ 20 min	Unknown	20-60 min
non-fasting	≤ 20 min	3 hr	20-60 min

Action

Chemical effect: Reduces total acid load in GI tract, elevates gastric pH to reduce pepsin activity, strengthens gastric mucosal barrier, and increases esophageal sphincter tone.
Therapeutic effect: Soothes stomach upset.

Available forms

Liquid, oral suspension: 540 mg/5 ml†

NURSING PROCESS

Assessment
• Assess patient's condition before therapy and regularly thereafter.
• Record amount and consistency of stools.
• Monitor magnesium level in patient with mild renal impairment. Symptomatic hypermagnesemia usually occurs only in severe renal impairment.
• Be alert for adverse reactions and drug interactions.
• Evaluate patient's and family's knowledge of drug therapy.

Nursing diagnoses
• Chronic pain related to gastric hyperacidity
• Diarrhea related to drug-induced adverse GI reactions
• Deficient knowledge related to drug therapy

Planning and implementation
• Shake suspension well. Give with water to facilitate passage.
• When giving through NG tube, make sure tube is placed properly and is patent. After instilling drug, flush tube with water to ensure passage to stomach and to clear tube.

• Drug has very low sodium content and is acceptable for patient on restricted sodium intake.

Patient teaching

• Advise patient not to take drug indiscriminately or to switch antacids without prescriber's advice.

☑ **Evaluation**

• Patient states that pain is relieved.
• Patient maintains normal bowel patterns throughout therapy.
• Patient and family state understanding of drug therapy.

---

magnesium chloride
(mag-NEE-see-um KLOR-ighd)
Slow-Mag

magnesium sulfate

Pharmacologic class: magnesium salt
Therapeutic class: anticonvulsant, electrolyte supplement, antiarrhythmic
Pregnancy risk category: A

Indications and dosages

▶ **Mild hypomagnesemia.** *Adults:* 1 g I.M. q 6 hours for four doses, depending on magnesium level.

▶ **Severe hypomagnesemia (magnesium level 0.8 mEq/L or less with symptoms).** *Adults:* 5 g I.V. in 1 L of solution over 3 hours. Subsequent doses depend on magnesium level.

▶ **Magnesium supplementation.** *Adults:* 54 to 483 mg P.O. daily in divided doses.

▶ **Magnesium supplementation in total parenteral nutrition (TPN).** *Adults:* 4 to 24 mEq I.V. daily added to TPN solution. *Infants:* 2 to 10 mEq I.V. daily added to TPN solution. Each 2 ml of 50% solution contains 1 g, or 8.12 mEq, magnesium sulfate.

▶ **Hypomagnesemic seizures.** *Adults:* 1 to 2 g of 10% solution I.V. over 15 minutes; then 1 g I.M. q 4 to 6 hours, based on patient's response and magnesium level.

▶ **Seizures caused by hypomagnesemia in acute nephritis.** *Children:* 0.2 ml/kg of 50% solution I.M. q 4 to 6 hours, p.r.n., or 100 mg/kg of 10% solution I.V. very slowly. Adjust dosage

according to magnesium level and seizure response.

▶ **Paroxysmal atrial tachycardia in patients unresponsive to other treatments.** *Adults:* 3 to 4 g I.V. of 10% solution over 30 seconds with close monitoring of ECG.

▶ **To reduce CV morbidity and mortality from acute MI.** *Adults:* 2 g I.V. over 5 to 15 minutes, followed by infusion of 18 g over 24 hours (12.5 mg/minute). Initiate therapy as soon as possible, but no longer than 6 hours after MI.

▼ I.V. administration

• Drug may form precipitate when mixed with solutions containing arsenates, barium, calcium, clindamycin, ethanol, heavy metals, hydrocortisone sodium succinate, phosphates, polymyxin B sulfate, procaine, salicylates, or tartrates.
• Drug is incompatible with alkalis, including carbonates and bicarbonates.
• Inject I.V. bolus dose slowly, using infusion pump for continuous infusion to avoid respiratory or cardiac arrest. Don't exceed 150 mg/minute; rapid drip causes heat sensation.
• When giving I.V. for severe hypomagnesemia, watch for respiratory depression and signs and symptoms of heart block. Respirations should be more than 16 breaths/minute before dose is given.

Contraindications and precautions

• Contraindicated in patients with myocardial damage or heart block.
• Use parenteral magnesium cautiously in patients with impaired kidney function.
⚞ **Lifespan:** In women who are actively progressing in labor, drug is contraindicated.

Adverse reactions

CNS: *weak or absent deep tendon reflexes,* flaccid paralysis, hypothermia, drowsiness, perioral paresthesia, twitching carpopedal spasm, tetany, *seizures.*
CV: flushing; slow, weak pulse; *arrhythmias; hypotension; circulatory collapse.*
Metabolic: hypocalcemia.
Respiratory: *respiratory paralysis.*
Skin: diaphoresis.

Interactions

Drug-drug. *Digoxin:* May cause serious cardiac conduction changes. Give cautiously.

Neuromuscular blockers: May increase neuromuscular blockage. Use cautiously; monitor patient for increased effects.

Nitrofurantoin, penicillamine, tetracyclines: Decreases bioavailability with oral magnesium supplements. Separate administration times by 2 to 3 hours.

Effects on lab test results

• May increase magnesium level. May decrease calcium level.

Pharmacokinetics

Absorption: 35% to 40% of P.O. dose is absorbed through GI tract. High-fat diets may interfere with absorption.
Distribution: About 30% of magnesium is bound intracellularly to proteins and energy-rich phosphates.
Metabolism: Unknown.
Excretion: Parenteral dose excreted primarily in urine; P.O. dose excreted in urine and feces.
Half-life: Unknown.

Route	Onset	Peak	Duration
P.O.	Unknown	4 hr	4-6 hr
I.V., I.M.	Unknown	Unknown	4-6 hr

Action

Chemical effect: Replaces and maintains magnesium levels; as anticonvulsant, reduces muscle contractions by interfering with release of acetylcholine at myoneural junction.
Therapeutic effect: Raises magnesium levels, alleviates seizure activity, and restores normal sinus rhythm.

Available forms

magnesium chloride
Injectable solutions: 20% in 50-ml vials
Tablets (delayed-release): 64 mg
magnesium sulfate
Injectable solutions: 10%, 12.5%, 50% in 2-ml, 5-ml, 10-ml, 20-ml, and 30-ml ampules, vials, and prefilled syringes

NURSING PROCESS

Assessment

• Assess patient's condition before therapy and regularly thereafter.
• Check magnesium level after repeated doses.

• After giving to toxemic pregnant woman within 24 hours before delivery, watch neonate for signs and symptoms of magnesium toxicity, including neuromuscular and respiratory depression.
• Monitor patient's fluid intake and output. Output should be 100 ml or more during 4-hour period before dose.
• Be alert for adverse reactions and drug interactions.
• Evaluate patient's and family's knowledge of drug therapy.

Nursing diagnoses

• Ineffective health maintenance related to underlying condition
• Risk for injury related to drug-induced adverse reactions
• Deficient knowledge related to drug therapy

Planning and implementation

• Keep I.V. calcium available to reverse magnesium intoxication.
• Undiluted 50% solutions may be given to adults by deep I.M. injection. When giving to children, dilute solutions to 20% or less.
⚡ ALERT: Test knee-jerk and patellar reflexes before each additional dose. If no reflex, notify prescriber and don't give magnesium until reflexes return; otherwise, patient may develop temporary respiratory failure and need cardiopulmonary resuscitation or I.V. administration of calcium.
Patient teaching
• Instruct patient taking parenteral drug to report adverse reactions immediately.
• Review oral administration schedule with patient. Tell him not to take more than prescribed.

Evaluation

• Patient has positive response to drug administration.
• Patient sustains no injury from adverse reactions.
• Patient and family state understanding of drug therapy.

magnesium citrate (citrate of magnesia)

(mag-NEE-see-um SIH-trayt)

Citro-Mag ♦ , Evac-Q-Mag

magnesium hydroxide (milk of magnesia)

Milk of Magnesia†, Milk of Magnesia Concentrate†, Phillips' Milk of Magnesia†, Phillips' Milk of Magnesia Concentrated†

magnesium sulfate (epsom salts)

Pharmacologic class: magnesium salt
Therapeutic class: saline laxative
Pregnancy risk category: NR

Indications and dosages

▶ **Constipation; to evacuate bowel before surgery.** *Adults and children age 12 and older:* 11 to 25 g magnesium citrate P.O. daily as single dose or divided. Or, 2 to 4 tbs magnesium hydroxide h.s. or upon rising, followed by a full glass (8 oz) of liquid. Or, 10 to 30 g magnesium sulfate P.O. daily as single dose or divided.
Children ages 6 to 11: 5.5 to 12.5 g magnesium citrate P.O. daily as single dose or divided. Or, 1 to 2 tbs magnesium hydroxide followed by a full glass (8 oz) of liquid. Don't use dosage cup. Or, 5 to 10 g magnesium sulfate P.O. daily as single dose or divided.
Children ages 2 to 5: 2.7 to 6.25 g magnesium citrate P.O. daily as single dose or divided. Or, 1 to 3 tsp magnesium hydroxide followed by a full glass (8 oz) of liquid. Don't use dosage cup. Or, 2.5 to 5 g P.O. daily as single dose or divided.
▶ **Acid indigestion, gastroesophageal reflux disease, peptic ulcer disease, heartburn.** *Adults and children age 12 and older:* Don't use dosage cup. 1 to 3 tsp magnesium hydroxide with a little water, up to four times a day, or as directed by prescriber. Or, for adults, 5 to 15 ml magnesium citrate P.O. t.i.d. or q.i.d.

Contraindications and precautions

● Contraindicated in patients with abdominal pain, nausea, vomiting, other symptoms of appendicitis or acute surgical abdomen, myocardial damage, heart block, fecal impaction, rectal fissures, intestinal obstruction or perforation, or renal disease.
● Use cautiously in patients with rectal bleeding.
☙ Lifespan: In women during labor and delivery, drug is contraindicated. In pregnant and breast-feeding women, use cautiously.

Adverse reactions

GI: *abdominal cramping, nausea, diarrhea,* laxative dependence with long-term or excessive use.
Metabolic: fluid and electrolyte disturbances.

Interactions

Drug-drug. *Ciprofloxacin, gatifloxacin, levofloxacin, lomefloxacin, moxifloxacin, norfloxacin, ofloxacin:* Magnesium hydroxide may decrease effects of quinolones. Give drug at least 6 hours before or 2 hours after quinolones.
Oral drugs: Impairs absorption. Separate administration times.

Effects on lab test results

● May alter fluid and electrolyte levels with prolonged use.

Pharmacokinetics

Absorption: About 15% to 30% may be absorbed systemically (posing risk to patients with renal impairment).
Distribution: Unknown.
Metabolism: Unknown.
Excretion: Unabsorbed drug excreted in feces; absorbed drug excreted rapidly in urine. *Half-life:* Unknown.

Route	Onset	Peak	Duration
P.O.	30 min-3 hr	Varies	Varies

Action

Chemical effect: Reduces total acid load in GI tract, elevates gastric pH to reduce pepsin activity, strengthens gastric mucosal barrier, and increases esophageal sphincter tone.
Therapeutic effect: Soothes stomach upset, relieves constipation, and raises magnesium level.

Available forms

magnesium citrate
Oral solution: about 168 mEq magnesium/
240 ml†
magnesium hydroxide
Oral suspension: 7% to 8.5% (about 80 mEq
magnesium/30 ml)†
magnesium sulfate
Granules: about 40 mEq magnesium/5 g†

NURSING PROCESS

🔍 Assessment

• Assess patient's condition before therapy and
regularly thereafter.
• Before giving for constipation, determine
whether patient has adequate fluid intake, exercise, and diet.
⚠ **ALERT:** Monitor electrolyte levels during prolonged use. Magnesium may accumulate in patients with renal insufficiency.
• Be alert for adverse reactions and drug interactions.
• Evaluate patient's and family's knowledge of
drug therapy.

🔲 Nursing diagnoses

• Constipation related to underlying condition
• Diarrhea related to therapy
• Deficient knowledge related to drug therapy

▶ Planning and implementation

• Time drug administration so that it doesn't interfere with scheduled activities or sleep.
• Chill magnesium citrate before use to improve
its palatability.
• Shake suspension well. Give with large
amount of water when used as laxative. When
giving through NG tube, make sure tube is
placed properly and is patent. After instilling
drug, flush tube with water to ensure passage to
stomach and to maintain tube patency.
⚠ **ALERT:** Drug is for short-term therapy only.
• Magnesium sulfate is more potent than other
saline laxatives.
Patient teaching
• Teach patient about dietary sources of bulk,
such as bran and other cereals, fresh fruit, and
vegetables.
• Warn patient that frequent or prolonged use
may cause dependence.

☑ Evaluation

• Patient's constipation is relieved.
• Diarrhea doesn't develop.
• Patient and family state understanding of drug
therapy.

magnesium oxide
(mag-NEE-see-um OKS-ighd)
Mag-Ox 400, Maox, Uro-Mag

Pharmacologic class: magnesium salt
Therapeutic class: antacid, laxative
Pregnancy risk category: NR

Indications and dosages

▶ **Antacid use.** *Adults:* 140 mg P.O. with water
or milk after meals and h.s.
▶ **Constipation.** *Adults:* 4 g P.O. with water or
milk, usually h.s.
▶ **Mild hypomagnesemia.** *Adults:* 400 to
840 mg P.O. daily. Monitor magnesium level
response.

Contraindications and precautions

• Contraindicated in patients with severe renal
disease.
• Use cautiously in patients with mild renal impairment.
⚠ **Lifespan:** In pregnant and breast-feeding
women, use cautiously.

Adverse reactions

GI: *diarrhea,* nausea, abdominal pain.
Metabolic: hypermagnesemia.

Interactions

Drug-drug. *Allopurinol, antibiotics (including
fluoroquinolones and tetracyclines), diflunisal,
digoxin, iron, isoniazid, penicillamine, phenothiazines, quinidine:* Decreases pharmacologic effect, possibly because of impaired absorption.
Separate administration times.
Enteric-coated drugs: May release prematurely
in stomach. Separate doses by at least 1 hour.

Effects on lab test results

• May increase magnesium level.

Pharmacokinetics

Absorption: Small amount absorbed from GI
tract.

Distribution: Unknown.
Metabolism: None.
Excretion: Unabsorbed drug excreted in feces; absorbed drug excreted in urine. *Half-life:* Unknown.

Route	Onset	Peak	Duration
P.O.			
fasting	20 min	Unknown	20-60 min
non-fasting	20 min	3 hr	20-60 min

Action

Chemical effect: Reduces total acid load in GI tract, elevates gastric pH to reduce pepsin activity, strengthens gastric mucosal barrier, and increases esophageal sphincter tone.
Therapeutic effect: Soothes stomach upset, relieves constipation, and raises magnesium level.

Available forms

Capsules: 140 mg†
Tablets: 400 mg†, 420 mg†, 500 mg†

NURSING PROCESS

⚗ Assessment
• Assess patient's condition before therapy and regularly thereafter.
• **⊛ ALERT:** Monitor magnesium level. With prolonged use and renal impairment, watch for symptoms of hypermagnesemia (signs and symptoms include hypotension, nausea, vomiting, depressed reflexes, respiratory depression, and coma).
• Be alert for adverse reactions and drug interactions.
• Evaluate patient's and family's knowledge of drug therapy.

⊞ Nursing diagnoses
• Ineffective health maintenance related to underlying condition
• Risk for injury related to potential for hypermagnesemia
• Deficient knowledge related to drug therapy

▶ Planning and implementation
• Don't give other oral drugs 1 to 2 hours before or after treatment.
• If diarrhea occurs, use a different drug.

Patient teaching
• Advise patient not to take drug indiscriminately or to switch antacids without prescriber's advice.

✓ Evaluation
• Patient responds well to therapy.
• Patient maintains normal magnesium level throughout therapy.
• Patient and family state understanding of drug therapy.

magnesium sulfate
(mag-NEE-see-um SUL-fayt)

Pharmacologic class: mineral, electrolyte
Therapeutic class: anticonvulsant
Pregnancy risk category: A

Indications and dosages

▶ **Control of seizures caused by epilepsy, glomerulonephritis, or hypothyroidism.**
Adults: 1 g I.M. or I.V.
▶ **Control of seizures in preeclampsia or eclampsia.** *Women:* For severe cases, total initial dose is 10 to 14 g (81 to 113.4 mEq) I.V. For all others, initially, 4 g I.V. in 250 ml of D_5W or normal saline solution given with 4 to 5 g (of undiluted 50% solution) deep I.M. into each buttock. Or, after the initial 4 g I.V. loading dose, follow by 1 to 3 g hourly as continuous I.V. infusion. Maximum total dosage, 30 to 40 g daily.
▶ **Hypomagnesemia.** *Adults:* 1 g I.M. q 6 hours for four doses for mild deficiency. Or, 3 g P.O. q 6 hours for four doses. For severe hypomagnesemia, up to 2 mEq (0.5 ml of 50% solution)/kg I.M. within a 4- hour period may be given. Or, 5 g (approximately 40 mEq) added to 1 L of D_5W or normal saline solution I.V. over 3 hours.
▶ **Prevention of hypomagnesia as part of TPN.** *Adults:* 5 to 8 mEq daily. *Infants:* 0.25 to 0.6 mEq/kg daily.
▶ **Seizures, hypertension, and encephalopathy linked to acute nephritis in children.**
Children: 0.2 ml/kg of 50% solution I.M. q 4 to 6 hours, p.r.n. For severe symptoms, 100 to 200 mg/kg as a 1% to 3% solution I.V. very slowly over 1 hour with one-half of dose given in first 15 to 20 minutes. Adjust dosage according to magnesium level and seizure response.

▶ **Management of paroxysmal atrial tachycardia‡.** *Adults:* 3 to 4 g (30 to 40 ml of a 10% solution) I.V. over 30 seconds with caution.
▶ **Management of life-threatening ventricular arrhythmias, such as sustained ventricular tachycardia or torsades de pointes‡.** *Adults:* 1 to 6 g I.V. over several minutes, followed by continuous infusion of 3 to 20 mg/minute for 5 to 48 hours. Dosage and duration of therapy based on patient response and magnesium level. Or, loading dose 1 to 2 g (8 to 16 mEq) I.V. diluted in 50 to 100 ml D₅W injection given over 5 to 10 minutes, followed with infusion of 0.5 to 1.0 ml (4 to 8 mEq)/hour.
▶ **Management of preterm labor‡.** *Adults:* 4 to 6 g I.V. over 20 minutes as a loading dose, followed by maintenance infusions of 2 to 4 g/hour for 12 to 24 hours, as tolerated, after contractions subside.
▶ **Asthma‡.** *Children:* 25 to 50 mg/kg (up to 2 g) I.V. over 10 to 20 minutes.

▼ I.V. administration

• Dilute to maximum concentration of 200 mg/ml (20%).
• Drug is compatible with D₅W and normal saline solution.
• Infuse no faster than 150 mg/minute (1.5 ml/minute of 10% solution or 0.75 ml/minute of 20% solution). Rapid drip induces uncomfortable heat sensation.
• Monitor vital signs q 15 minutes when giving drug I.V.
• For preterm labor, monitor I.V. fluids and rates carefully to avoid circulatory overload. Monitor patient for pulmonary edema.

Contraindications and precautions

• Parenteral administration contraindicated in patients with heart block or myocardial damage.
• Use cautiously in patients with impaired kidney function.
🔥 **Lifespan:** In women who are in labor and in breast-feeding women, use cautiously.

Adverse reactions

CNS: drowsiness, *depressed reflexes,* flaccid paralysis, hypothermia.
CV: *hypotension, flushing,* **circulatory collapse,** depressed cardiac function, *heart block.*
Metabolic: hypocalcemia.
Respiratory: *respiratory paralysis.*
Skin: diaphoresis.

Interactions

Drug-drug. *Anesthetics, CNS depressants:* May cause additive CNS depression. Use together cautiously.
Digoxin: May exacerbate arrhythmias. Use together cautiously; monitor ECG.
Neuromuscular blockers: May increase neuromuscular blockade. Use together cautiously; monitor patient for enhanced drug effects.

Effects on lab test results

• May increase magnesium level. May decrease calcium level.

Pharmacokinetics

Absorption: Unknown.
Distribution: Throughout body.
Metabolism: None.
Excretion: Unchanged in urine. *Half-life:* Unknown.

Route	Onset	Peak	Duration
I.V.	1-2 min	Almost immediate	30 min
I.M.	1 hr	Unknown	3-4 hr

Action

Chemical effect: May decrease acetylcholine released by nerve impulses, but anticonvulsant mechanism is unknown.
Therapeutic effect: Prevents or controls seizures, raises magnesium level, stops paroxysmal atrial tachycardia, and alleviates selected symptoms of acute nephritis in children.

Available forms

Injection: 10%, 12.5%, 50%

NURSING PROCESS

📖 Assessment

• Assess patient's condition before therapy and regularly thereafter.
🔔 **ALERT:** Watch for respiratory depression and signs of heart block. Respirations should be about 16 breaths/minute before each dose.
• Monitor fluid intake and output. Output should be 100 ml or more in 4-hour period before each dose.
• Be alert for adverse reactions and drug interactions.
🔔 **ALERT:** Check magnesium level after repeated doses. Disappearance of knee-jerk and patellar

reflexes is sign of early stages of magnesium toxicity. Signs of hypermagnesemia begin to appear at a level of 4 mEq/L.

• Observe neonate for signs of magnesium toxicity, including neuromuscular or respiratory depression, when giving I.V. form to toxemic mother within 24 hours before delivery.
• Evaluate patient's and family's knowledge of drug therapy.

⊞ Nursing diagnoses
• Ineffective health maintenance related to underlying condition
• Risk for injury related to drug-induced adverse reactions
• Deficient knowledge related to drug therapy

⊠ Planning and implementation
• For I.M. use, maximum concentration in adults is 250 mg/ml (25%) or 500 mg/ml (50%). In infants and children, maximum concentration is 200 mg/ml (20%).
• Keep I.V. calcium gluconate available at bedside at all times to reverse magnesium intoxication.
• For cases of severe hypermagnesia, peritoneal dialysis or hemodialysis may be needed.
• If used to treat seizures, institute appropriate seizure precautions.
⊛ **ALERT:** Don't confuse magnesium sulfate with manganese sulfate.
Patient teaching
• Stress importance of reporting adverse reactions immediately.

☑ Evaluation
• Patient responds well to therapy.
• Patient doesn't experience injury.
• Patient and family state understanding of drug therapy.

---

mannitol
(MAN-ih-tol)
Osmitrol

Pharmacologic class: osmotic diuretic
Therapeutic class: diuretic, diagnostic and nephrotic treatment drug, treatment of drug intoxication, reduction of intracranial or intraocular pressure
Pregnancy risk category: C

Indications and dosages

▶ **Test dose for marked oliguria or suspected inadequate kidney function.** *Adults and children older than age 12:* 200 mg/kg or 12.5 g as 15% or 20% I.V. solution over 3 to 5 minutes. Response is adequate if 30 to 50 ml of urine/hour is excreted over 2 to 3 hours. If response is inadequate, give second test dose. If still no response after second dose, stop drug.
Children age 12 and younger‡: 0.2 g/kg or 6 g/m² I.V. over 3 to 5 minutes.
▶ **Oliguria.** *Adults and children older than age 12:* 100 g I.V. as 15% to 20% solution over 90 minutes to several hours.
Children age 12 and younger ‡: 2 g/kg or 60 g/m² I.V.
▶ **Prevention of oliguria or acute renal impairment.** *Adults and children older than age 12:* 50 to 100 g I.V. of concentrated solution, followed by 5% to 10% solution. Exact concentration determined by fluid requirements.
▶ **Edema; ascites caused by renal, hepatic, or cardiac failure.** *Adults and children older than age 12:* 100 g I.V. as 10% to 20% solution over 2 to 6 hours.
Children age 12 and younger‡: 2 g/kg or 60 g/m² I.V. as a 15% to 20% solution over 2 to 6 hours.
▶ **Reduction of intraocular or intracranial pressure.** *Adults and children older than age 12:* 1.5 to 2 g/kg as 15% to 25% I.V. solution over 30 to 60 minutes.
Children age 12 and younger‡: 2 g/kg or 60 g/m² I.V. as a 15% to 20% solution over 30 to 60 minutes.
▶ **Diuresis in drug intoxication.** *Adults and children older than age 12:* 25-g loading dose followed by an infusion maintaining 100- to 500-ml urine output/hour and positive fluid balance.
Children age 12 and younger ‡: 2 g/kg or 60 g/m² I.V. of a 5% to 10% solution, p.r.n.
▶ **Irrigating solution during transurethral resection of prostate.** *Adults:* 2.5% solution, p.r.n.

▼ I.V. administration

• To dissolve crystallized solution (occurs at low temperatures or in concentrations greater than 15%), warm bottle in hot water bath and shake vigorously. Cool to body temperature before giving. Don't use solution with undissolved crystals.

• Give as intermittent or continuous infusion, using in-line filter and infusion pump. Direct injection isn't recommended. Check I.V. line patency at infusion site before and during administration.

• Watch for signs of infiltration, including inflammation, edema, and necrosis.

Contraindications and precautions

• Contraindicated in patients hypersensitive to drug and in those with anuria, severe pulmonary congestion, frank pulmonary edema, severe heart failure, severe dehydration, metabolic edema, progressive renal disease or dysfunction, or active intracranial bleeding except during craniotomy.

⚞ Lifespan: In pregnant women, use cautiously. In breast-feeding women, drug isn't recommended.

Adverse reactions

CNS: headache, confusion, *seizures.*
CV: transient expansion of plasma volume during infusion, causing **circulatory overload** and **heart failure;** tachycardia; chest pains.
EENT: blurred vision, rhinitis.
GI: thirst, nausea, vomiting, *diarrhea.*
GU: urine retention.
Metabolic: *water intoxication,* cellular dehydration.

Interactions

Drug-drug. *Lithium:* Increases urinary excretion of lithium. Monitor patient closely; monitor lithium level.

Effects on lab test results

• May cause electrolyte imbalance.

Pharmacokinetics

Absorption: Administered I.V.
Distribution: Remains in extracellular compartment; doesn't cross blood-brain barrier.
Metabolism: Metabolized minimally to glycogen in liver.
Excretion: Excreted in urine. *Half-life:* About 1½ hours.

Route	Onset	Peak	Duration
I.V.	30-60 min	≤ 1 hr	6-8 hr

Action

Chemical effect: Increases osmotic pressure of glomerular filtrate, inhibiting tubular reabsorption of water and electrolytes. This elevates blood osmolality, enhancing water flow into extracellular fluid.

Therapeutic effect: Increases water excretion, decreases intracranial or intraocular pressure, prevents or treats kidney dysfunction, and alleviates drug intoxication.

Available forms

Injection: 5%, 10%, 15%, 20%, 25%

NURSING PROCESS

▨ **Assessment**
• Assess patient's condition before therapy and regularly thereafter.
• Monitor vital signs, central venous pressure, and fluid intake and output hourly. Insert urethral catheter in comatose or incontinent patient because therapy is based on strict evaluation of fluid intake and output. In patient with urethral catheter, use hourly urometer collection bag to facilitate accurate evaluation.
• Monitor weight, kidney function, and serum and urine sodium and potassium levels daily.
• Be alert for adverse reactions and drug interactions.
• Evaluate patient's and family's knowledge of drug therapy.

✥ **Nursing diagnoses**
• Ineffective health maintenance related to underlying condition
• Risk for deficient fluid volume related to drug-induced adverse GI reactions
• Deficient knowledge related to drug therapy

▷ **Planning and implementation**
• For maximum intraocular pressure reduction before surgery, give 1 to 1½ hours preoperatively.
• When used as irrigating solution for prostate surgery, a concentration of 3.5% or greater is needed to avoid hemolysis.
• Notify prescriber immediately if oliguria increases or adverse reactions occur.
Patient teaching
• Tell patient he may feel thirsty or have a dry mouth, and emphasize the importance of drinking only amount of fluid provided.

• Instruct patient to immediately report pain in chest, back, or legs, or shortness of breath.

☑ **Evaluation**
• Patient responds well to mannitol.
• Patient maintains adequate hydration throughout therapy.
• Patient and family state understanding of drug therapy.

mebendazole
(meh-BEN-duh-zohl)
Vermox

Pharmacologic class: benzimidazole
Therapeutic class: anthelmintic
Pregnancy risk category: C

Indications and dosages

▶ **Pinworm.** *Adults and children older than age 2:* 100 mg P.O. as single dose. If infection persists for 3 weeks, repeat treatment.
▶ **Roundworm, whipworm, hookworm.** *Adults and children older than age 2:* 100 mg P.O. b.i.d. for 3 days. If infection persists for 3 weeks, repeat treatment.
▶ **Trichinosis‡.** *Adults and children older than age 2:* 200 to 400 mg P.O. t.i.d. for 3 days, then 400 to 500 mg t.i.d. for 10 days.
▶ **Capillariasis‡.** *Adults and children older than age 2:* 200 mg P.O. b.i.d. for 20 days.
▶ **Toxocariasis‡.** *Adults and children:* 100 to 200 mg P.O. b.i.d. for 5 days.
▶ **Dracunculiasis‡.** *Adults and children older than age 2:* 400 to 800 mg P.O. daily for 6 days.

Contraindications and precautions

• Contraindicated in patients hypersensitive to drug.
⚘ **Lifespan:** In pregnant women, use cautiously. In breast-feeding women, safety of drug hasn't been established.

Adverse reactions

GI: transient abdominal pain, diarrhea.

Interactions

Drug-drug. *Carbamazepine, hydantoins:* May reduce level of mebendazole, possibly decreasing its therapeutic effect. Monitor patient for effect.

Cimetidine: Increases mebendazole levels. Monitor patient for toxicity.

Effects on lab test results

None reported.

Pharmacokinetics

Absorption: About 5% to 10% of dose is absorbed; varies widely among patients.
Distribution: Highly bound to proteins.
Metabolism: Metabolized to inactive metabolites.
Excretion: Mostly excreted in feces; 2% to 10% excreted in urine. *Half-life:* 3 to 9 hours.

Route	Onset	Peak	Duration
P.O.	Unknown	2-5 hr	Varies

Action

Chemical effect: Selectively and irreversibly inhibits uptake of glucose and other nutrients in susceptible helminths.
Therapeutic effect: Kills helminth infestation.

Available forms

Tablets (chewable): 100 mg

NURSING PROCESS

⚗ Assessment
• Assess patient's condition before therapy and regularly thereafter.
• Be alert for adverse reactions and drug interactions.
• Evaluate patient's and family's knowledge of drug therapy.

⊕ Nursing diagnoses
• Infection related to presence of helminths
• Diarrhea related to drug-induced adverse GI reactions
• Deficient knowledge related to drug therapy

▶ Planning and implementation
• Tablets may be chewed, swallowed whole, or crushed and mixed with food.
• Give drug to all family members to decrease risk of spreading infection.
• No dietary restrictions, laxatives, or enemas are needed.
Patient teaching
• Teach patient about personal hygiene, especially good hand-washing technique. To avoid

reinfection, teach patient to wash perianal area daily, to change undergarments and bedclothes daily, and to wash hands and clean fingernails before meals and after bowel movements.

• Advise patient not to prepare food for others.

✓ Evaluation

• Patient is free from infestation.

• Patient's bowel pattern returns to normal after therapy is stopped.

• Patient and family state understanding of drug therapy.

mechlorethamine hydrochloride (nitrogen mustard)
(meh-klor-ETH-uh-meen high-droh-KLOR-ighd)
Mustargen

Pharmacologic class: alkylating drug (cell cycle–phase nonspecific)
Therapeutic class: antineoplastic
Pregnancy risk category: D

Indications and dosages

▶ **Hodgkin's disease.** *Adults and children:* 6 mg/m² daily on days 1 and 8 of 28-day cycle given with other antineoplastics, such as mechlorethamine-vincristine-procarbazine-prednisone (MOPP) regimen. Dosage repeated for six cycles.

⊠ Adjust-a-dose: Subsequent doses reduced by 50% in MOPP regimen when WBC count is between 3,000 and 3,999/mm³ and by 75% when WBC count is between 1,000 and 2,999/mm³ or platelet count is between 50,000 and 100,000/mm³.

▶ **Polycythemia vera, chronic lymphocytic leukemia, chronic myelocytic leukemia, bronchogenic cancer, lymphosarcoma, mycosis fungoides.** Dosage based on ideal dry body weight, so the presence of edema or ascites must be considered so the dose will be based on actual weight unaugmented by these conditions.

Adults and children: 0.4 mg/kg as single dose or divided into two to four daily doses of 0.2 or 0.1 mg/kg respectively. Subsequent courses can't be given until patient has recovered hematologically, usually within 3 weeks.

▶ **Malignant effusions.** *Adults:* 0.2 to 0.4 mg/ kg intracavitarily.

▼ I.V. administration

• Follow facility policy to reduce risks. Preparation and administration of parenteral form are linked to carcinogenic, mutagenic, and teratogenic risks for personnel.

• Reconstitute drug using 10 ml of sterile water for injection or normal saline solution injection. Resulting solution contains 1 mg/ml of drug. Give by direct injection into vein or into I.V. line containing freeflowing solution.

• Prepare immediately before infusion. Solution is very unstable. Use within 15 minutes, and discard unused solution.

• Don't use solutions that are discolored or contain particulates. Don't use vials that appear to contain droplets of water.

• Dispose of equipment used in drug preparation and administration properly and according to facility policy. Neutralize unused solution with equal volume of 5% sodium bicarbonate and 5% sodium thiosulfate for 45 minutes.

• Make sure I.V. solution doesn't extravasate because mechlorethamine is a potent vesicant. If it does, apply cold compresses and infiltrate area with isotonic sodium thiosulfate.

Contraindications and precautions

• Contraindicated in patients with infectious disease or previous anaphylactic reactions to the drug.

• Routine use in patients with widely disseminated neoplasms is discouraged. In patients with inoperable neoplasms or in the terminal stage of the disease, weigh potential risks and discomfort from use of the drug against limited obtainable gain.

• Use cautiously in patients with chronic lymphatic lymphoma caused by increased drug toxicity.

⚠ Lifespan: In pregnant women, use cautiously because of the risk of harm to the fetus. Women of childbearing potential should avoid becoming pregnant. Breast-feeding women should stop breast-feeding or avoid taking the drug, taking into account the importance of the drug to the mother. In children, safety and effectiveness of drug haven't been established.

Adverse reactions

CNS: headache, weakness, drowsiness, vertigo.
CV: *thrombophlebitis.*
EENT: tinnitus, hearing loss with high doses.
GI: *metallic taste, nausea, vomiting, anorexia.*
Hematologic: *thrombocytopenia, agranulocytosis, lymphocytopenia, myelosuppression* that peaks in 4 to 10 days and lasts 10 to 21 days, mild anemia that begins in 2 to 3 weeks.
Skin: *alopecia,* rash, sloughing, severe irritation if drug extravasates or touches skin.
Other: precipitation of herpes zoster, *anaphylaxis, secondary malignant disease.*

Interactions

Drug-drug. *Anticoagulants, aspirin:* Increases risk of bleeding. Monitor PT and INR and monitor patient for bleeding; adjust dosage, if needed.

Effects on lab test results

• May increase urine urea level.
• May decrease hemoglobin, hematocrit, and platelet, granulocyte, lymphocyte, WBC, and RBC counts.

Pharmacokinetics

Absorption: Incomplete, probably from deactivation by body fluids in cavity.
Distribution: Doesn't cross blood-brain barrier.
Metabolism: Converted rapidly to its active form, which reacts quickly with various cellular components before being deactivated.
Excretion: Metabolites excreted in urine.

Route	Onset	Peak	Duration
I.V., intracavitary	Rapid	Unknown	Unknown

Action

Chemical effect: Cross-links strands of cellular DNA and interferes with RNA transcription, causing imbalance of growth that leads to cell death.
Therapeutic effect: Kills certain cancer cells.

Available forms

Injection: 10-mg vials

NURSING PROCESS

🗚 Assessment

• Assess patient's condition before therapy and regularly thereafter.

• Monitor CBC and platelet counts regularly.
• Monitor uric acid level.
• Be alert for adverse reactions and drug interactions.
• Monitor patient for signs and symptoms of infection caused by immunosuppression.
• Neurotoxicity increases with dose and patient age.
• Evaluate patient's and family's knowledge of drug therapy.

🗱 Nursing diagnoses

• Ineffective health maintenance related to presence of neoplastic disease
• Ineffective immune protection related to adverse hematologic reactions
• Deficient knowledge related to drug therapy

▷ Planning and implementation

🏵 **ALERT:** Mustargen is highly toxic. Inhalation of dust, vapors, and contact with skin or mucous membranes must be avoided.
• When giving by intracavitary route for sclerosing effect, dilute with up to 100 ml of normal saline solution for injection. Turn patient from side to side q 15 minutes to 1 hour to distribute drug.
• To prevent hyperuricemia with resulting uric acid nephropathy, make sure patient is adequately hydrated.
• If patient suffers from the acute phase of herpes zoster, stop drug to avoid progression to generalized herpes zoster.
• If extravasation occurs, quickly infiltrate the area with sterile isotonic sodium thiosulfate (1/6 molar) and apply an ice compress for 6 to 12 hours. Notify prescriber immediately.

Patient teaching
• Warn patient to watch for signs of infection (fever, sore throat, fatigue) and bleeding (easy bruising, nosebleeds, bleeding gums, melena). Have patient take temperature daily.
• Instruct patient to avoid OTC products that contain aspirin.
• Advise woman of childbearing age to avoid becoming pregnant during therapy and to consult with prescriber before becoming pregnant.

☑ Evaluation

• Patient responds positively to drug.
• Patient regains normal hematologic parameters.

Reactions may be *common,* uncommon, *life-threatening*, or **COMMON AND LIFE-THREATENING**.

• Patient and family state understanding of drug therapy.

meclizine hydrochloride (meclozine hydrochloride)

(MEK-lih-zeen high-droh-KLOR-ighd)
Ancolan ◇, Antivert†, Antivert/25, Antivert/50, Antrizine, Bonamine ♦, Bonine†, Dramamine Less Drowsy Formula†, Meni-D, Vergon†

Pharmacologic class: piperazine-derivative antihistamine
Therapeutic class: antiemetic, antivertigo drug
Pregnancy risk category: B

Indications and dosages

▶ **Vertigo, dizziness.** *Adults:* 25 to 100 mg P.O. daily in divided doses. Dosage varies with patient response.
▶ **Motion sickness.** *Adults:* 25 to 50 mg P.O. 1 hour before travel, repeat daily for duration of journey.

Contraindications and precautions

• Contraindicated in patients hypersensitive to drug.
• Use cautiously in patients with asthma, glaucoma, or prostatic hyperplasia.
⚖ **Lifespan:** In pregnant women, safety of drug hasn't been established. In breast-feeding women, use cautiously. In children, safety of drug hasn't been established.

Adverse reactions

CNS: *drowsiness,* fatigue.
EENT: blurred vision.
GI: dry mouth.

Interactions

Drug-drug. *CNS depressants:* May increase drowsiness. Use together cautiously; monitor patient for safety.

Effects on lab test results

None reported.

Pharmacokinetics

Absorption: Unknown.
Distribution: Well distributed throughout body.

Metabolism: Unknown. Thought to be metabolized in liver.
Excretion: Excreted unchanged in feces; metabolites found in urine. *Half-life:* About 6 hours.

Route	Onset	Peak	Duration
P.O.	1 hr	Unknown	8-24 hr

Action

Chemical effect: Unknown; may affect neural pathways originating in labyrinth to inhibit nausea and vomiting.
Therapeutic effect: Relieves vertigo and nausea.

Available forms

Capsules: 25 mg, 30 mg†
Tablets: 12.5 mg, 25 mg†, 50 mg
Tablets (chewable): 25 mg†

NURSING PROCESS

✍ Assessment

• Assess patient's condition before therapy and regularly thereafter.
• Be alert for adverse reactions and drug interactions.
• Evaluate patient's and family's knowledge of drug therapy.

Nursing diagnoses

• Risk for injury related to vertigo
• Risk for deficient fluid volume related to motion sickness
• Deficient knowledge related to drug therapy

⊿ Planning and implementation

• Don't stop drug abruptly after long-term therapy because paradoxical reactions or sudden reversal of improved state may occur.
⚠ **ALERT:** Don't confuse Antivert with Axert.
Patient teaching
• Advise patient to refrain from driving and performing other hazardous activities that require alertness until CNS effects of drug are known.
• If drug is to be used long-term, stress importance of not stopping abruptly.
• Advise patient not to use alcohol while taking this drug and to consult a prescriber before taking drug if already taking sedatives or tranquilizers.

Rapid onset   *Liquid form contains alcohol.   ♦Canada   ◇ Australia   †OTC   ‡Off-label use

☑ **Evaluation**
- Patient states that vertigo is relieved.
- Patient states that motion sickness doesn't occur.
- Patient and family state understanding of drug therapy.

medroxyprogesterone acetate
(med-roks-ee-proh-JES-ter-ohn AS-ih-tayt)
Amen, Cycrin, Depo-Provera, Provera

Pharmacologic class: progestin
Therapeutic class: progestin antineoplastic
Pregnancy risk category: X

Indications and dosages

▶ **Abnormal uterine bleeding caused by hormonal imbalance.** *Women:* 5 to 10 mg P.O. daily for 5 to 10 days beginning on day 16 of menstrual cycle. If patient also has received estrogen, 10 mg P.O. daily for 10 days beginning on day 16 of cycle.
▶ **Secondary amenorrhea.** *Women:* 5 to 10 mg P.O. daily for 5 to 10 days.
▶ **Endometrial or renal carcinoma.** *Women:* 400 to 1,000 mg I.M. weekly.
▶ **Contraception.** *Women:* 150 mg I.M. once q 3 months.
▶ **Paraphilia.** *Men:* Initially, 200 mg I.M. b.i.d. or t.i.d. or 500 mg I.M. weekly. Adjust dosage based on response.

Contraindications and precautions

- Contraindicated in patients hypersensitive to drug and in those with active thromboembolic disorders, breast cancer, undiagnosed abnormal vaginal bleeding, missed abortion, hepatic dysfunction, or a history of thromboembolic disorders, cerebrovascular disease, or apoplexy. Tablets are also contraindicated in patients with liver dysfunction or known or suspected cancer of genital organs.
- Use cautiously in patients with diabetes mellitus, seizure disorder, migraine, cardiac or renal disease, asthma, or depression.
⚠ **Lifespan:** In pregnant women, drug is contraindicated. In breast-feeding women, drug isn't recommended.

Adverse reactions

CNS: dizziness, migraine, lethargy, depression, nervousness, asthenia.
CV: hypertension, thrombophlebitis, *pulmonary embolism,* edema, *thromboembolism, CVA.*
EENT: intolerance to contact lenses.
GI: nausea, vomiting, abdominal cramps.
GU: breakthrough bleeding, dysmenorrhea, amenorrhea, cervical erosion, abnormal secretions, uterine fibromas, vaginal candidiasis.
Hepatic: cholestatic jaundice, *tumors,* gallbladder disease.
Metabolic: hyperglycemia, weight gain.
Skin: melasma, rash, pain, induration, sterile abscesses, acne, alopecia.
Other: breast tenderness, enlargement, or secretion; decreased libido, hypersensitivity reactions.

Interactions

Drug-drug. *Aminoglutethimide, rifampin:* May decrease progestin effects. Monitor patient for diminished therapeutic response. Tell patient to use nonhormonal contraceptive during therapy with these drugs.
Bromocriptine: May cause amenorrhea, interfering with bromocriptine's effects. Avoid using together.
Drug-food. *Caffeine:* May increase caffeine levels. Monitor patient for effect.
Drug-lifestyle. *Smoking:* Increases risk of adverse CV effects. If smoking continues, may need alternative therapy. Discourage patient from smoking.

Effects on lab test results

- May increase thyroxin-binding globulin and T_4 levels.
- May increase liver function test values.

Pharmacokinetics

Absorption: Slow after I.M. use; unknown for P.O. use.
Distribution: Unknown.
Metabolism: Primarily in liver.
Excretion: Primarily in urine. *Half-life:* 2¼ hours.

Route	Onset	Peak	Duration
P.O., I.M.	Unknown	Unknown	Unknown

Reactions may be *common,* uncommon, *life-threatening*, or COMMON AND LIFE-THREATENING.

Action

Chemical effect: Suppresses ovulation, possibly by inhibiting pituitary gonadotropin secretion, and forms thick cervical mucus.
Therapeutic effect: Stops abnormal uterine bleeding, reverses secondary amenorrhea, prevents pregnancy, and hinders cancer cell growth.

Available forms

Injection (suspension): 150 mg/ml, 400 mg/ml
Tablets: 2.5 mg, 5 mg, 10 mg

NURSING PROCESS

Assessment
• Assess patient's condition before therapy and regularly thereafter.
• Be alert for adverse reactions and drug interactions.
• Monitor injection sites for evidence of sterile abscess.
• Evaluate patient's and family's knowledge of drug therapy.

Nursing diagnoses
• Ineffective health maintenance related to underlying condition
• Excessive fluid volume related to drug-induced edema
• Deficient knowledge related to drug therapy

Planning and implementation
• Rotate injection sites to prevent muscle atrophy.
Patient teaching
• Explain to patient adverse effects of progestins before first dose.
• Instruct patient to avoid caffeine and smoking during drug therapy.
• **ALERT:** Tell patient to report unusual symptoms immediately and to stop drug and notify prescriber if visual disturbance or migraine occurs.
• Teach woman how to perform routine monthly breast self-examination.
• Warn patient that I.M. injection may be painful.

Evaluation
• Patient responds well to drug therapy.
• Patient doesn't develop fluid excess throughout drug therapy.

• Patient and family state understanding of drug therapy.

mefloquine hydrochloride
(MEF-loh-kwin high-droh-KLOR-ighd)
Lariam

Pharmacologic class: quinine derivative
Therapeutic class: antimalarial
Pregnancy risk category: C

Indications and dosages

▶ **Acute malaria infections caused by mefloquine-sensitive strains of** *Plasmodium falciparum* **and** *P. vivax. Adults:* 1,250 mg P.O. as single dose. Give patients with *P. vivax* infections primaquine or other 8-aminoquinolones to avoid relapse after treatment of initial infection.
▶ **Malaria prevention.** *Adults:* 250 mg P.O. once weekly. Give 1 week before patient enters endemic area and continue for 4 weeks after return.

Contraindications and precautions

• Contraindicated in patients hypersensitive to drug or related compounds. Drug shouldn't be given for prevention in patients with active depression, a recent history of depression, generalized anxiety disorder, psychosis, or schizophrenia or other major psychiatric disorders, or with a history of convulsions.
• Use cautiously in patients with a previous history of depression and in patients with cardiac disease or seizure disorders.
• **Lifespan:** In pregnant and breast-feeding women, use cautiously. In children, safety of drug hasn't been established.

Adverse reactions

CNS: dizziness, fever, fatigue, syncope, headache, *seizures,* tremor, ataxia, mood changes, panic attacks, *suicide.*
CV: extrasystoles, chest pain, edema.
EENT: tinnitus.
GI: loss of appetite, vomiting, *nausea,* loose stools, diarrhea, GI discomfort, dyspepsia.
Skin: rash.
Other: chills.

Interactions

Drug-drug. *Beta blockers, quinidine, quinine:* ECG abnormalities and cardiac arrest may occur. Avoid using together.
Chloroquine, quinine: May increase risk of seizures. Monitor patient.
Halofantrine: May increase risk of fatal prolongation of QTc interval. Don't use together.
Valproic acid: Decreases valproic acid level and may cause loss of seizure control at start of mefloquine therapy. Check anticonvulsant level.

Effects on lab test results

• May increase transaminase levels.
• May decrease hematocrit, hemoglobin, and WBC and platelet counts.

Pharmacokinetics

Absorption: Well absorbed.
Distribution: Concentrated in RBCs; about 98% protein-bound.
Metabolism: Metabolized by liver.
Excretion: Excreted primarily by liver; small amounts found in urine. *Half-life:* About 21 days.

Route	Onset	Peak	Duration
P.O.	Unknown	7-24 hr	Unknown

Action

Chemical effect: Unknown; may be related to its ability to form complexes with hemin.
Therapeutic effect: Kills malaria-causing organisms. Spectrum of activity includes all human types of malaria, including chloroquine-resistant malaria and strains of *P. falciparum* and *P. vivax.*

Available forms

Tablets: 250 mg

NURSING PROCESS

🔬 Assessment

• Assess patient's condition before therapy and regularly thereafter.
• Monitor liver function test results periodically.
• Be alert for adverse reactions and drug interactions.
• Monitor patient's hydration status if adverse GI reactions occur.
• Evaluate patient's and family's knowledge of drug therapy.

💠 Nursing diagnoses

• Infection related to presence of malaria organisms
• Risk of deficient fluid volume related to drug-induced adverse reactions
• Deficient knowledge related to drug therapy

▶ Planning and implementation

⚠ ALERT: During prophylactic use, if psychiatric symptoms such as acute anxiety, depression, restlessness or confusion occur, these may be considered prodromal to a more serious event. Stop drug and use an alternative.
• Because health risks from simultaneous administration of quinine and mefloquine are great, don't begin therapy within 12 hours of last dose of quinine or quinidine.
• Patients with infections caused by *P. vivax* are at high risk for relapse because drug doesn't eliminate hepatic phase (exoerythrocytic parasites). Follow-up therapy with primaquine is advisable.
• Give drug with food and full glass of water to minimize adverse GI reactions.
Patient teaching
• Advise patient to take drug on same day of week when using it for prevention.
• Advise patient to use caution when performing hazardous activities that require alertness and coordination because dizziness, disturbed sense of balance, and neuropsychiatric reactions may occur.
• Instruct patient taking drug as prevention to stop drug and notify prescriber if he notices signs or symptoms of impending toxicity, such as unexplained anxiety, depression, confusion, or restlessness.
• For patient undergoing long-term therapy, recommend that he have periodic ophthalmologic examinations.

✅ Evaluation

• Patient is free from infection.
• Patient maintains adequate hydration throughout therapy.
• Patient and family state understanding of drug therapy.

Reactions may be *common*, uncommon, *life-threatening*, or COMMON AND LIFE-THREATENING.

megestrol acetate
(meh-JES-trol AS-ih-tayt)
Megace, Megostat ◊

Pharmacologic class: progestin
Therapeutic class: antineoplastic
Pregnancy risk category: D

Indications and dosages

▶ **Breast cancer.** *Adults:* 40 mg P.O. q.i.d.
▶ **Endometrial cancer.** *Adults:* 40 to 320 mg P.O. daily in divided doses.
▶ **Anorexia, cachexia, or unexplained significant weight loss in patients with AIDS.**
Adults: 800 mg P.O. (oral suspension) daily in divided doses; 100 to 400 mg for AIDS-related cachexia.
▶ **Anorexia or cachexia in patients with neoplastic disease.** *Adults:* 480 to 600 mg P.O. daily.

Contraindications and precautions

● Contraindicated in patients hypersensitive to drug.
● Use cautiously in patients with history of thrombophlebitis.
⚖ **Lifespan:** In pregnant women, drug is contraindicated in the first 4 months of pregnancy. In breast-feeding women, drug isn't recommended. In children, safety of drug hasn't been established.

Adverse reactions

CV: hypertension, thrombophlebitis, *heart failure, thromboembolic phenomena.*
GI: nausea, vomiting, abdominal pain.
GU: breakthrough menstrual bleeding.
Metabolic: weight gain, increased appetite.
Musculoskeletal: carpal tunnel syndrome, back pain.
Respiratory: *pulmonary embolism.*
Skin: alopecia, hirsutism.
Other: breast tenderness.

Interactions

None significant.

Effects on lab test results

● May increase glucose level.

Pharmacokinetics

Absorption: Well absorbed across GI tract.
Distribution: Appears to be stored in fatty tissue; highly bound to proteins.
Metabolism: Completely metabolized in liver.
Excretion: Excreted in urine.

Route	Onset	Peak	Duration
P.O.	Unknown	Unknown	Unknown

Action

Chemical effect: Changes tumor's hormonal environment and alters neoplastic process. Mechanism of appetite stimulation is unknown.
Therapeutic effect: Hinders cancer cell growth and increases appetite.

Available forms

Oral suspension: 40 mg/ml
Tablets: 20 mg, 40 mg

NURSING PROCESS

⚕ **Assessment**
● Assess patient's condition before therapy and regularly thereafter.
● Be alert for adverse reactions.
● Monitor patient's hydration status if adverse GI reactions occur.
● Evaluate patient's and family's knowledge of drug therapy.

⊕ **Nursing diagnoses**
● Ineffective health maintenance related to underlying condition
● Risk for deficient fluid volume related to drug-induced adverse GI reactions
● Deficient knowledge related to drug therapy

▷ **Planning and implementation**
● Two months is adequate trial when treating cancer.
● Notify prescriber if patient develops pronounced back pain, abdominal pain, headache, or nausea and vomiting.
Patient teaching
● Inform patient that therapeutic response isn't immediate.
● Advise breast-feeding woman to stop during therapy because of possible infant toxicity.
● Encourage women to use contraceptive measures during therapy.

☑ Evaluation
- Patient responds well to therapy.
- Patient maintains adequate hydration throughout therapy.
- Patient and family state understanding of drug therapy.

meloxicam
(mell-OX-ih-kam)
Mobic

Pharmacologic class: enolic acid NSAID
Therapeutic class: anti-inflammatory, analgesic
Pregnancy risk category: C

Indications and dosages

▶ **To relieve signs and symptoms of osteoarthritis.** *Adults:* 7.5 mg P.O. once daily. May increase to maximum of 15 mg daily, p.r.n.

Contraindications and precautions

- Contraindicated in patients hypersensitive to drug and in those who have experienced asthma, urticaria, or allergic-type reactions after taking aspirin or other NSAIDs.
- Use cautiously in patients with a history of ulcers or GI bleeding and in patients with dehydration, anemia, hepatic disease, renal disease, hypertension, fluid retention, heart failure, or asthma.
- ⚖ **Lifespan:** In late pregnancy, avoid using. In elderly and debilitated patients, use cautiously because of increased risk of fatal GI bleeding.

Adverse reactions

CNS: dizziness, headache, insomnia, fatigue, *seizures,* paresthesia, fever, tremor, vertigo, anxiety, confusion, depression, nervousness, somnolence, malaise, syncope.
CV: *arrhythmias,* palpitations, tachycardia, angina, *heart failure,* hypertension, hypotension, *MI,* edema.
EENT: pharyngitis, abnormal vision, conjunctivitis, tinnitus.
GI: abdominal pain, diarrhea, dyspepsia, flatulence, nausea, constipation, colitis, dry mouth, duodenal ulcer, esophagitis, gastric ulcer, gastritis, GI reflux, *hemorrhage, pancreatitis,* vomiting, increased appetite, taste perversion.
GU: albuminuria, hematuria, urinary frequency, *renal impairment,* UTI.
Hematologic: anemia, *leukopenia, thrombocytopenia, purpura.*
Hepatic: bilirubinemia, *hepatitis.*
Metabolic: dehydration, weight changes.
Musculoskeletal: arthralgia, back pain.
Respiratory: upper respiratory tract infection, *asthma, bronchospasm,* dyspnea, cough.
Skin: rash, pruritus, alopecia, bullous eruption, photosensitivity reactions, sweating, urticaria.
Other: accidental injury, allergic reaction, *angioedema,* flulike symptoms.

Interactions

Drug-drug. *ACE inhibitors:* Diminishes antihypertensive effects. Monitor patient's blood pressure.
Aspirin: Increases risk of adverse effects. Avoid using together.
Furosemide, thiazide diuretics: NSAIDs may reduce sodium excretion linked to diuretics, leading to sodium retention. Monitor patient for edema and increased blood pressure.
Lithium: Increases lithium level. Monitor lithium level closely for toxicity during treatment.
Warfarin: Increases PT or INR and risk of bleeding complications. Monitor PT and INR, and check for signs and symptoms of bleeding.
Drug-herb. *Dong quai, feverfew, garlic, ginger, horse chestnut, red clover:* Possible increased risk of bleeding. Discourage use together.
St. John's wort: Increases risk of photosensitivity reactions. Advise patient to avoid unprotected or prolonged exposure to sunlight.
Drug-lifestyle. *Smoking:* Increases risk of GI irritation and bleeding. Monitor patient for bleeding; discourage patient from smoking.
Alcohol use: Increases risk of GI irritation and bleeding. Monitor patient for bleeding; discourage using together.

Effects on lab test results

- May increase BUN, creatinine, ALT, AST, and bilirubin levels.
- May decrease hemoglobin, hematocrit, and WBC and platelet counts.

Pharmacokinetics

Absorption: Bioavailability is 89% and doesn't appear to be affected by food or antacids. Steady-state conditions are reached after 5 days of daily administration.

Reactions may be *common,* uncommon, *life-threatening,* or COMMON AND LIFE-THREATENING.

Distribution: 99.4% bound to proteins.
Metabolism: Almost completely metabolized to pharmacologically inactive metabolites.
Excretion: Excreted in both urine and feces, primarily as metabolites. *Half-life:* 15 to 20 hours.

Route	Onset	Peak	Duration
P.O.	Unknown	Unknown	Unknown

Action

Chemical effect: Mechanism of action may be related to prostaglandin (cyclooxygenase) synthetase inhibition.
Therapeutic effect: Relief of signs and symptoms of osteoarthritis.

Available forms

Tablets: 7.5 mg

NURSING PROCESS

⚗ Assessment

• Obtain accurate history of drug allergies; drug can produce allergic-like reactions in patients hypersensitive to aspirin and other NSAIDs.
• Assess patient for increased risk of GI bleeding. Risk factors include history of ulcers or GI bleeding, treatment with corticosteroids or anticoagulants, longer duration of NSAID treatment, smoking, alcoholism, older age, and poor overall health.
• Monitor patient for signs and symptoms of overt and occult bleeding.
• Monitor patient for fluid retention; closely monitor patients who have hypertension, edema, or heart failure.
• Monitor liver function.
• Evaluate patient's and family's knowledge of drug therapy.

⊕ Nursing diagnoses

• Chronic pain related to underlying condition
• Risk for injury related to drug-induced adverse reactions
• Deficient knowledge related to drug therapy

▷ Planning and implementation

• Drug may be taken with food to prevent GI upset.
• Rehydrate patient who is dehydrated before starting treatment.

• If patient develops evidence of liver disease (eosinophilia, rash), stop drug.

Patient teaching

• Tell patient to notify prescriber about history of allergic reactions to aspirin or other NSAIDs before starting therapy.
• Tell patient to report signs and symptoms of GI ulcerations and bleeding, such as vomiting blood, blood in stool, and black, tarry stools.
• Instruct patient to report skin rash, weight gain, or edema.
• Advise patient to report warning signs of hepatotoxicity (nausea, fatigue, lethargy, pruritus, jaundice, right upper quadrant tenderness, and flulike symptoms).
• Warn patient with a history of asthma that it may recur during therapy and that he should stop taking the drug and notify prescriber if it does.
• Tell woman to notify prescriber if she becomes pregnant or is planning to become pregnant during therapy.
• Inform patient that it may take several days before consistent pain relief is achieved.

☑ Evaluation

• Patient is free from pain.
• Patient sustains no injury as a result of drug-induced adverse reactions.
• Patient and family state understanding of drug therapy.

melphalan (L-phenylalanine mustard)

(MEL-feh-len)
Alkeran

Pharmacologic class: alkylating drug (cell cycle–phase nonspecific)
Therapeutic class: antineoplastic
Pregnancy risk category: D

Indications and dosages

▶ **Multiple myeloma.** *Adults:* 6 mg P.O. daily for 2 to 3 weeks; then stop drug for up to 4 weeks or until WBC and platelet counts begin to rise again; then give maintenance dosage of 2 mg daily.
Alternative therapy: 0.15 mg/kg P.O. daily for 7 days at 2- to 6-week intervals. Or, 0.25 mg/kg

P.O. daily for 4 days, repeat q 4 to 6 weeks. Or, give I.V. to patients who can't tolerate oral therapy: 16 mg/m² given by infusion over 15 to 20 minutes q 2 weeks for four doses. After patient has recovered from toxicity, drug is given q 4 weeks.

◪ **Adjust-a-dose:** For patients with renal impairment, reduce I.V. dosage by 50% to reduce risk of severe leukopenia and drug-related death.

▶ **Nonresectable advanced ovarian cancer.**
Adults: 0.2 mg/kg P.O. daily for 5 days. Repeat q 4 to 6 weeks, depending on bone marrow recovery.

▼ I.V. administration

● Follow facility policy to reduce risks. Preparation and administration of parenteral form are linked to carcinogenic, mutagenic, and teratogenic risks for personnel.

● Because drug isn't stable in solution, reconstitute immediately before giving with 10 ml of sterile diluent supplied by manufacturer. Shake vigorously until solution is clear. Resulting solution contains 5 mg of melphalan per ml. Immediately dilute required dose in normal saline solution for injection. Don't exceed a final concentration of 0.45 mg/ml.

● Give by I.V. infusion over 15 to 20 minutes.

● Give promptly after diluting; reconstituted product begins to degrade within 30 minutes. After final dilution, nearly 1% of drug degrades q 10 minutes. Administration must be completed within 60 minutes of reconstitution.

● Don't refrigerate reconstituted product because precipitate will form.

Contraindications and precautions

● Contraindicated in patients hypersensitive to drug and in those whose disease is resistant to drug. Patients hypersensitive to chlorambucil may have cross-sensitivity to melphalan.

● Drug isn't recommended for patients with severe leukopenia, thrombocytopenia, anemia, or chronic lymphocytic leukemia.

⚘ **Lifespan:** In pregnant and breast-feeding women, drug isn't recommended. In children, safety of drug hasn't been established.

Adverse reactions

Hematologic: *thrombocytopenia, leukopenia, bone marrow suppression.*
Hepatic: *hepatotoxicity.*

Respiratory: pneumonitis, *pulmonary fibrosis.*
Skin: dermatitis, pruritus, rash, alopecia.
Other: *anaphylaxis,* hypersensitivity reactions.

Interactions

Drug-drug. *Anticoagulants, aspirin:* Increases risk of bleeding. Avoid using together.
Antigout drugs: Decreases effectiveness. Dosage adjustments may be needed.
Bone marrow suppressants: May have additive toxicity. Monitor patient closely.
Carmustine: Carmustine lung toxicity threshold may be reduced. Monitor patient closely for signs of toxicity.
Cisplatin: Cisplatin may affect melphalan kinetics by inducing renal dysfunction and subsequently altering melphalan clearance. Monitor patient for toxicity.
Cyclosporine: Increases toxicity of cyclosporine, particularly nephrotoxicity. Monitor cyclosporine level and renal function tests.
Interferon alfa: May decrease melphalan level. Monitor level closely.
Nalidixic acid: May increase risk of severe hemorrhagic necrotic enterocolitis in children. Monitor patient closely.
Vaccines: Decreases effectiveness of killed-virus vaccines and increases risk of toxicity from live-virus vaccines. Postpone routine immunization for at least 3 months after last dose of melphalan.
Drug-food. *Any food:* Decreases absorption of oral drug. Separate administration times; give drug on an empty stomach.

Effects on lab test results

● May increase urine urea level.
● May decrease hemoglobin, hematocrit, and RBC, WBC, and platelet counts.

Pharmacokinetics

Absorption: Incomplete and variable.
Distribution: Distributed rapidly and widely in total body water; initially 50% to 60% bound to proteins and increases to 80% to 90% over time.
Metabolism: Extensively deactivated by hydrolysis.
Excretion: Excreted primarily in urine. *Half-life:* 2 hours.

Route	Onset	Peak	Duration
P.O., I.V.	Unknown	Unknown	Unknown

Action

Chemical effect: Cross-links strands of cellular DNA and interferes with RNA transcription.
Therapeutic effect: Kills certain cancer cells.

Available forms

Injection: 50 mg
Tablets (scored): 2 mg

NURSING PROCESS

Assessment

- Assess patient's condition before therapy and regularly thereafter.
- Monitor uric acid level and CBC.
- Be alert for adverse reactions and drug interactions.
- Evaluate patient's and family's knowledge of drug therapy.

Nursing diagnoses

- Ineffective health maintenance related to presence of neoplastic disease
- Ineffective immune protection related to adverse hematologic reactions
- Deficient knowledge related to drug therapy

Planning and implementation

- Dosage may need to be reduced in patient with renal impairment.
- Melphalan is drug of choice with prednisone in patients with multiple myeloma.
- Give drug on empty stomach.
- Anaphylaxis may occur. Keep antihistamines and steroids readily available.
- **ALERT:** Don't confuse melphalan with Mephyton.

Patient teaching

- Tell patient to take oral drug on empty stomach.
- Warn patient to watch for signs of infection (fever, sore throat, fatigue) and bleeding (easy bruising, nosebleeds, bleeding gums, melena). Have patient take temperature daily.
- Instruct patient to avoid OTC products that contain aspirin.
- Advise woman of childbearing age to avoid becoming pregnant during therapy and to consult with prescriber before becoming pregnant.

Evaluation

- Patient responds well to therapy.
- Patient regains normal hematologic function when therapy is completed.
- Patient and family state understanding of drug therapy.

memantine hydrochloride

(MEHM-en-tyn high-droh-KLOR-ighd)
Namenda

Pharmacologic class: N-methyl-D-aspartate (NMDA) receptor antagonist
Therapeutic class: Alzheimer's disease drug
Pregnancy risk category: B

Indications and dosages

▶ **Moderate to severe Alzheimer's type dementia.** *Adults:* Initially, 5 mg P.O. once daily. Increase by 5 mg/day each week up to the target dose. Maximum, 10 mg P.O. b.i.d. Doses above 5 mg should be divided b.i.d.
Adjust-a-dose: Consider reducing the dosage if the patient has moderate renal impairment.

Contraindications and precautions

- Contraindicated in patients allergic to drug or its components. Not recommended for patients with severe renal impairment.
- Use cautiously in patients with seizures, hepatic impairment, or moderate renal impairment. Also use cautiously in patients who may have an increased urine pH (from drugs, diet, renal tubular acidosis, or severe UTI).
- **Lifespan:** In pregnant women, use only if potential benefit justifies the risk. In breast-feeding women, use cautiously; it isn't known whether the drug appears in breast milk. In children, safety and efficacy haven't been established. In elderly patients, use cautiously.

Adverse reactions

CNS: abnormal gait, aggressiveness, agitation, anxiety, ataxia, confusion, *CVA,* depression, dizziness, fatigue, hallucinations, headache, hypokinesia, insomnia, pain, somnolence, syncope, TIA, vertigo.
CV: edema, *heart failure,* hypertension.

EENT: cataracts, conjunctivitis.
GI: anorexia, constipation, diarrhea, nausea, vomiting.
GU: incontinence, urinary frequency, UTI.
Hematologic: anemia.
Metabolic: weight loss.
Musculoskeletal: arthralgia, back pain.
Respiratory: bronchitis, coughing, dyspnea, pneumonia, upper respiratory tract infection.
Skin: rash.
Other: falls, flulike symptoms, inflicted injury.

Interactions

Drug-drug. *Cimetidine, hydrochlorothiazide, quinidine, ranitidine, triamterene:* Altered levels of both drugs. Monitor patient.
NMDA antagonists (amantadine, ketamine, dextromethorphan): Combined use not studied. Use together cautiously.
Urine alkalinizers (carbonic anhydrase inhibitors, sodium bicarbonate): Decreased memantine clearance. Monitor patient for adverse effects.
Drug-herb. *Herbs that alkalinize urine:* May increase drug level and adverse effects. Discourage use together.
Drug-food. *Foods that alkalinize urine:* May increase drug level and adverse effects. Discourage use together.
Drug-lifestyle. *Alcohol use:* May decrease drug's effectiveness or increase adverse effects. Discourage use together.
Smoking: Altered levels of drug and nicotine. Discourage use together.

Effects on lab test results

- May increase alkaline phosphatase level.
- May decrease hemoglobin and hematocrit.

Pharmacokinetics

Absorption: Well absorbed. Peak level occurs in 3 to 7 hours.
Distribution: About 45% bound to plasma proteins.
Metabolism: Little.
Excretion: Unchanged, primarily in the urine.
Half-life: 60 to 80 hours.

Route	Onset	Peak	Duration
P.O.	Unknown	3-7 hr	Unknown

Action

Chemical effect: Antagonizes NMDA receptors, the persistent activation of which seems to increase Alzheimer's symptoms.
Therapeutic effect: Decreases dementia related to Alzheimer's disease.

Available forms

Tablets: 5 mg, 10 mg

NURSING PROCESS

Assessment
- Assess underlying condition before therapy and regularly thereafter.
- Evaluate patient's and family's knowledge of drug therapy.

Nursing diagnoses
- Acute or chronic confusion related to underlying disease
- Risk for imbalanced fluid volume related to drug-induced GI effects
- Deficient knowledge related to drug therapy

Planning and implementation
- Drug isn't indicated for mild Alzheimer's disease or other types of dementia.
- Give drug without regard to food.

Patient teaching
- Explain that drug doesn't cure Alzheimer's disease but may improve the symptoms.
- Tell patient to report adverse effects.
- Urge patient to avoid alcohol during treatment.
- To avoid possible interactions, advise patient not to take herbal or OTC products without first asking a health care provider.

Evaluation
- Patient's cognition improves and he experiences less confusion.
- Patient and family state that adverse GI effects haven't occurred or have been managed effectively.
- Patient and family state understanding of drug therapy.

Reactions may be *common*, uncommon, *life-threatening*, or **COMMON AND LIFE-THREATENING**.

menotropins
(meh-noh-TROH-pins)
Humegon, Pergonal, Repronex

Pharmacologic class: gonadotropin
Therapeutic class: ovulation stimulant, spermatogenesis stimulant
Pregnancy risk category: X

Indications and dosages

▶ **Anovulation.** *Women:* 75 IU each of follicle-stimulating hormone (FSH) and luteinizing hormone (LH) I.M. daily for 7 to 12 days; follow by 5,000 to 10,000 USP units of human chorionic gonadotropin (HCG) I.M. 1 day after last dose of menotropins. Repeat for 1 to 3 to three menstrual cycles until ovulation occurs.
▶ **Infertility with ovulation.** *Women:* 75 IU each of FSH and LH I.M. daily for 7 to 12 days; follow by 5,000 to 10,000 USP units of HCG I.M. 1 day after last dose of menotropins. Repeat for 2 menstrual cycles and then increase to 150 IU each of FSH and LH daily for 7 to 12 days; follow by 5,000 to 10,000 USP units of HCG I.M. 1 day after last dose of menotropins. Repeat for 2 menstrual cycles.
▶ **Infertility.** *Men:* Treat with HCG of 5,000 USP units 3 times a week for 4 to 6 months; then 75 IU each of FSH and LH I.M. 3 times weekly (given with 2,000 USP units of HCG twice weekly) for at least 4 months. If spermatogenesis doesn't increase, dosage increased to 150 IU each of FSH and LH 3 times weekly (dosage of HCG remains unchanged).

Contraindications and precautions

• Contraindicated in patients hypersensitive to drug; in women with primary ovarian failure, uncontrolled thyroid or adrenal dysfunction, pituitary tumor, abnormal uterine bleeding, uterine fibromas, or ovarian cysts or enlargement; and in men with normal pituitary function, primary testicular failure, or infertility disorders other than hypogonadotropic hypogonadism.
⚖ **Lifespan:** In pregnant women, drug is contraindicated. In breast-feeding women or children, don't use drug.

Adverse reactions

CV: *CVA,* fever, tachycardia.
GI: nausea, vomiting, diarrhea.

GU: *ovarian enlargement with pain and abdominal distention,* multiple births, ovarian hyperstimulation syndrome (sudden ovarian enlargement, ascites, or pleural effusion).
Hematologic: hemoconcentration with fluid loss into abdomen.
Respiratory: atelectasis, *acute respiratory distress syndrome, pulmonary embolism, pulmonary infarction, arterial occlusion.*
Other: *gynecomastia,* hypersensitivity reactions, *anaphylaxis.*

Interactions

None significant.

Effects on lab test results

None reported.

Pharmacokinetics

Absorption: Unknown.
Distribution: Unknown.
Metabolism: Unknown.
Excretion: Excreted in urine. *Half-life:* S.C., 54 hours; I.M., 60 hours.

Route	Onset	Peak	Duration
I.M.	9-12 days	Unknown	Unknown

Action

Chemical effect: When given to women who haven't had primary ovarian failure, mimics FSH in inducing follicular growth and LH in aiding follicular maturation.
Therapeutic effect: Stimulates ovulation and fertility.

Available forms

Injection: 75 IU of LH and 75 IU of FSH activity/ampule; 150 IU of LH and 150 IU of FSH activity/ampule

NURSING PROCESS

⬛ Assessment
• Assess patient's condition before therapy and regularly thereafter.
• Be alert for adverse reactions.
• Evaluate patient's and family's knowledge of drug therapy.

⬛ Nursing diagnoses
• Sexual dysfunction related to underlying disorder

• Risk for deficient fluid volume related to drug-induced adverse reactions
• Deficient knowledge related to drug therapy

▶ **Planning and implementation**
• Monitor patient closely to ensure adequate ovarian stimulation.
• Reconstitute with 1 to 2 ml of sterile normal saline solution. Use immediately.
• Rotate injection sites.
Patient teaching
• Discuss risk of multiple births.
• In infertility, encourage daily intercourse from day before HCG is given until ovulation occurs.
• Tell patient that pregnancy usually occurs 4 to 6 weeks after therapy.
• Instruct patient to immediately report severe abdominal pain, bloating, swelling of hands or feet, nausea, vomiting, diarrhea, substantial weight gain, or shortness of breath.

☑ **Evaluation**
• Patient or partner becomes pregnant.
• Patient maintains adequate hydration throughout therapy.
• Patient and family state understanding of drug therapy.

meperidine hydrochloride (pethidine hydrochloride)
(meh-PER-uh-deen high-droh-KLOR-ighd)
Demerol

Pharmacologic class: opioid
Therapeutic class: opioid analgesic, adjunct to anesthesia
Pregnancy risk category: C
Controlled substance schedule: II

Indications and dosages

▶ **Moderate to severe pain.** *Adults:* 50 to 150 mg P.O., I.M., or S.C. q 3 to 4 hours, p.r.n. Or, 15 to 35 mg/hour by continuous I.V. infusion.
Children: 1.1 to 1.76 mg/kg P.O., I.M., or S.C. q 3 to 4 hours. Maximum dosage is 100 mg q 4 hours, p.r.n.
▶ **Preoperatively.** *Adults:* 50 to 100 mg I.M., I.V., or S.C. 30 to 90 minutes before surgery.

Children: 1 to 2.2 mg/kg I.M., I.V., or S.C. up to adult dose 30 to 90 minutes before surgery.
▶ **Adjunct to anesthesia.** *Adults:* Repeat slow I.V. injections of fractional doses (i.e., 10 mg/ ml). Or, continuous I.V. infusion of more dilute solution (1 mg/ml) adjusted to needs of patient.
▶ **Obstetric analgesia.** *Adults:* 50 to 100 mg I.M. or S.C. when pain becomes regular, repeat at 1- to 3-hour intervals.

▼ **I.V. administration**

• Keep resuscitation equipment and naloxone available.
• Give slowly by direct I.V. injection or slow continuous I.V. infusion. Drug is compatible with most I.V. solutions, including D_5W, normal saline solution, and Ringer's or lactated Ringer's solutions.

Contraindications and precautions

• Contraindicated in patients hypersensitive to drug and in those who have received MAO inhibitors within 14 days.
• Use cautiously in debilitated patients and in patients with increased intracranial pressure, head injury, asthma, other respiratory conditions, supraventricular tachycardias, seizures, acute abdominal conditions, hepatic or renal disease, hypothyroidism, Addison's disease, urethral stricture, or prostatic hyperplasia.
⚖ Lifespan: In pregnant and breast-feeding women and in elderly patients, use cautiously.

Adverse reactions

CNS: *sedation, somnolence, clouded sensorium, euphoria, paradoxical excitement, tremors, dizziness, seizures.*
CV: *hypotension, **bradycardia**, tachycardia, **cardiac arrest, shock.***
GI: *nausea, vomiting, constipation,* ileus.
GU: *urine retention.*
Musculoskeletal: muscle twitching.
Respiratory: *respiratory depression, respiratory arrest.*
Skin: local tissue irritation and induration (after S.C. injection), phlebitis (after I.V. use).
Other: pain at injection site, physical dependence.

Interactions

Drug-drug. *Chlorpromazine:* May cause excessive sedation and hypotension. Don't use together.

Reactions may be *common,* uncommon, ***life-threatening***, or COMMON AND LIFE-THREATENING.

CNS depressants, general anesthetics, hypnotics, other opioid analgesics, phenothiazines, sedatives, tricyclic antidepressants: Possible respiratory depression, hypotension, profound sedation, or coma. Use together cautiously. Reduce meperidine dosage as directed.

MAO inhibitors: Increases CNS excitation or depression that can be severe or fatal. Don't use together.

Phenytoin: Decreases level of meperidine. Monitor patient for decreased analgesia.

Drug-herb. Parsley: May promote or produce serotonin syndrome. Discourage using together.

Drug-lifestyle. Alcohol use: May have additive CNS effects. Discourage using together.

Effects on lab test results

• May increase amylase and lipase levels.

Pharmacokinetics

Absorption: Unknown.
Distribution: Distributed widely throughout body.
Metabolism: Metabolized primarily by hydrolysis in liver.
Excretion: Excreted primarily in urine. Excretion enhanced by acidifying urine. Half-life: 2½ to 4 hours.

Route	Onset	Peak	Duration
P.O.	15 min	60-90 min	2-4 hr
I.V.	1 min	5-7 min	2-4 hr
I.M., S.C.	10-15 min	30-50 min	2-4 hr

Action

Chemical effect: binds with opioid receptors in CNS, altering both perception of and emotional response to pain through unknown mechanism.
Therapeutic effect: relieves pain.

Available forms

Injection: 25 mg/ml, 50 mg/ml, 75 mg/ml, 100 mg/ml
Injection (for infusion only): 10 mg/ml
Syrup: 50 mg/5 ml
Tablets: 50 mg, 100 mg

NURSING PROCESS

Assessment

• Assess patient's pain before therapy and regularly thereafter.

• Be alert for adverse reactions and drug interactions.
• Meperidine and its active metabolite normeperidine accumulate in the body. Monitor patient for increased toxic effect, especially in patient with renal impairment.
• Monitor respirations of neonate exposed to drug during labor.
• If drug is stopped abruptly after long-term use, monitor patient for withdrawal symptoms.
• Evaluate patient's and family's knowledge of drug therapy.

Nursing diagnoses

• Acute pain related to underlying condition
• Risk for injury related to drug-induced adverse reactions
• Deficient knowledge related to drug therapy

Planning and implementation

• Drug may be used in some patients who are allergic to morphine.
• Because meperidine toxicity often appears after several days of treatment, it isn't recommended for treatment of chronic pain.
• **ALERT:** Don't give drug if respiratory rate is less than 12 breaths/minute, if respiratory rate or depth is decreased, or if change in pupils is noted.
• **ALERT:** Oral dose is less than half as effective as parenteral dose. Give I.M., if possible. When changing from parenteral to oral route, increase dosage.
• Syrup has local anesthetic effect. Give with full glass of water.
• **ALERT:** Drug is incompatible with aminophylline, barbiturates, heparin, morphine sulfate, phenytoin, sodium bicarbonate, or sulfonamides.
• Don't give subcutaneously because it's painful.
• **ALERT:** Don't confuse Demerol with Demulen, Dymelor, or Temaril.

Patient teaching

• Warn outpatient to avoid hazardous activities until CNS effects of drug are known.
• Instruct patient to avoid alcohol consumption during drug therapy.
• Teach patient to manage adverse reactions, such as constipation.
• Tell family members to withhold drug and notify prescriber if patient's respiratory rate decreases.

☑ **Evaluation**

• Patient is free from pain.
• Patient doesn't experience injury.
• Patient and family state understanding of drug therapy.

mercaptopurine
(6-mercaptopurine, 6-MP)
(mer-cap-toh-PYOO-reen)
Purinethol

Pharmacologic class: antimetabolite (cell cycle–phase specific, S phase)
Therapeutic class: antineoplastic
Pregnancy risk category: D

Indications and dosages

▶ **Acute lymphoblastic leukemia in children, chronic myelocytic leukemia.** *Adults:* 2.5 mg/kg P.O. daily as single dose, up to 5 mg/kg P.O. daily. Maintenance dosage is 1.5 to 2.5 mg/kg P.O. daily.
Children age 5 and older: 2.5 mg/kg P.O. daily. Maintenance dosage is 1.5 to 2.5 mg/kg P.O. daily.
▶ **Acute myeloblastic leukemia‡.** *Adults:* 500 mg/m² P.O. daily with other therapies.

Contraindications and precautions

• Contraindicated in patients whose disease has resisted drug.
⚕ Lifespan: In pregnant and breast-feeding women, drug isn't recommended.

Adverse reactions

GI: *nausea, vomiting, anorexia,* painful oral ulcers.
Hematologic: *leukopenia, thrombocytopenia, anemia* (may persist several days after drug is stopped).
Hepatic: biliary stasis, *jaundice, hepatotoxicity.*
Metabolic: hyperuricemia.
Skin: rash, hyperpigmentation.

Interactions

Drug-drug. *Allopurinol:* Slows inactivation of mercaptopurine. Decrease mercaptopurine to one-fourth or one-third normal dose, as directed.

Hepatotoxic drugs: May enhance hepatotoxicity of mercaptopurine. Monitor patient closely; monitor liver function test results.
Nondepolarizing neuromuscular blockers: Antagonized muscle relaxant effect. Notify anesthesiologist that patient is receiving drug.
Warfarin: Antagonizes anticoagulant effect. Monitor PT and INR.

Effects on lab test results

• May increase uric acid level.
• May decrease hemoglobin, hematocrit, and WBC, RBC, and platelet counts.

Pharmacokinetics

Absorption: Incomplete and variable; about 50% of dose is absorbed.
Distribution: Distributed widely in total body water.
Metabolism: Extensively metabolized in liver.
Excretion: Excreted in urine. *Half-life:* Unknown.

Route	Onset	Peak	Duration
P.O.	Unknown	Unknown	Unknown

Action

Chemical effect: Inhibits RNA and DNA synthesis.
Therapeutic effect: Inhibits growth of certain cancer cells.

Available forms

Tablets (scored): 50 mg

NURSING PROCESS

☑ **Assessment**

• Assess patient's condition before therapy and regularly thereafter.
• Monitor blood count and transaminase, alkaline phosphatase, and bilirubin levels weekly during induction and monthly during maintenance.
• Observe for signs of bleeding and infection.
• Monitor fluid intake and output and uric acid level.
• Be alert for adverse reactions and drug interactions. Adverse GI reactions are less common in children.
⚕ ALERT: Watch for jaundice, clay-colored stools, and frothy, dark urine. Hepatic dysfunction is reversible when drug is stopped. If hepat-

Photoguide to tablets and capsules

This photoguide provides full-color photographs of some of the most commonly prescribed tablets and capsules. These drugs, organized by generic name, are shown in actual size and color with page references to corresponding drug information. Each drug is labeled with its trade name and its strength.

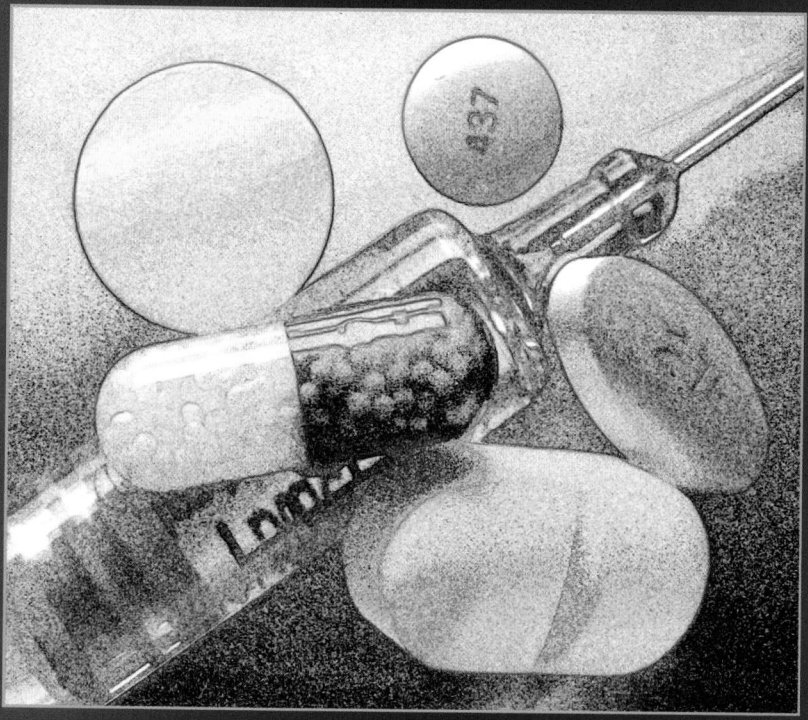

Adapted from Facts and Comparisons, St. Louis, Missouri.
For the list of companies permitting use of these photographs, see pages 1400-1401.

ALENDRONATE SODIUM

Fosamax
(page 115)

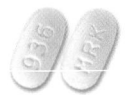 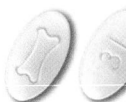

10 mg   40 mg   70 mg

ALPRAZOLAM

Xanax
(page 124)

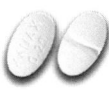 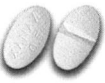 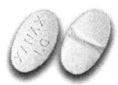

0.25 mg   0.5 mg   1 mg

AMLODIPINE BESYLATE

Norvasc
(page 145)

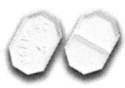 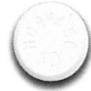

5 mg   10 mg

AMOXICILLIN AND POTASSIUM CLAVULANATE

Augmentin
(page 147)

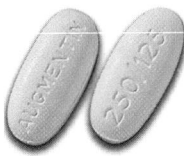 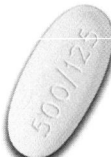

250 mg   500 mg

AMOXICILLIN TRIHYDRATE

Amoxil
(page 149)

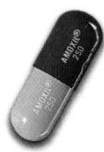 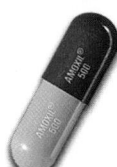

250 mg   500 mg

ANASTROZOLE

Arimidex
(page 164)

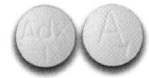

1 mg

ATENOLOL

Tenormin
(page 186)

 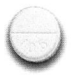 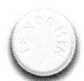

25 mg   50 mg   100 mg

ATORVASTATIN CALCIUM

Lipitor
(page 189)

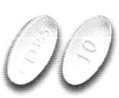 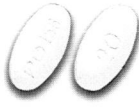 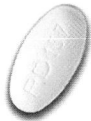

10 mg   20 mg   40 mg

AZITHROMYCIN

Zithromax
(page 204)

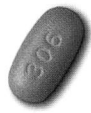

250 mg

BUPROPION HYDROCHLORIDE

Wellbutrin SR
(page 256)

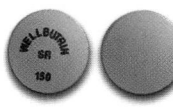

150 mg

CAPTOPRIL

Capoten
(page 276)

12.5 mg   25 mg

CARVEDILOL

Coreg
(page 290)

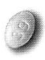

3.125 mg   6.25 mg   12.5 mg

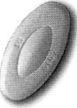

25 mg

CEFADROXIL MONOHYDRATE

Duricef
(page 295)

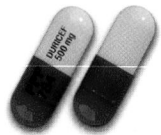

500 mg   1,000 mg

CEFUROXIME AXETIL

Ceftin
(page 318)

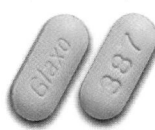 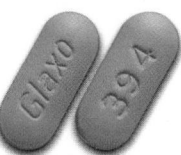

250 mg   500 mg

CELECOXIB

Celebrex
(page 320)

 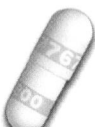

100 mg   200 mg

CIPROFLOXACIN

Cipro
(page 347)

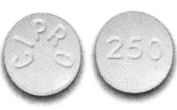 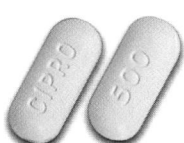 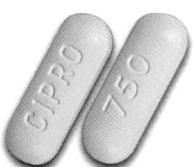

250 mg   500 mg   750 mg

CITALOPRAM HYDROBROMIDE

Celexa
(page 352)

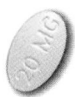

20 mg   40 mg

DESLORATADINE

Clarinex
(page 415)

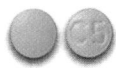

5 mg

DIAZEPAM

Valium
(page 431)

| 2 mg | 5 mg | 10 mg |

DIGOXIN

Lanoxin
(page 442)

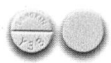 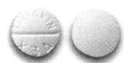

0.125 mg   0.25 mg

DILTIAZEM HYDROCHLORIDE

Cardizem
(page 446)

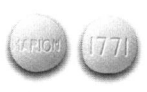 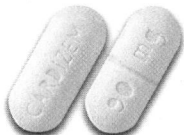

30 mg   90 mg

Cardizem CD
(page 446)

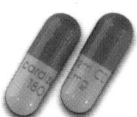 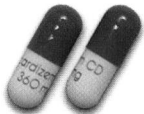

180 mg   360 mg

Cardizem LA
(page 446)

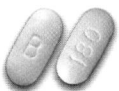 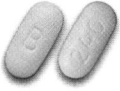 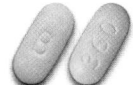

180 mg   240 mg   360 mg

DIVALPROEX SODIUM

Depakote
(page 1292)

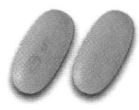 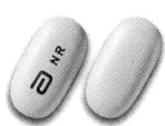 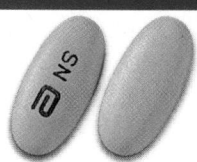

125 mg   250 mg   500 mg

ENALAPRIL MALEATE

Vasotec
(page 503)

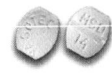

2.5 mg

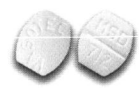

5 mg

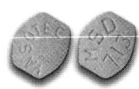

10 mg

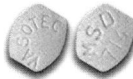

20 mg

ERYTHROMYCIN BASE

ERYC
(page 527)

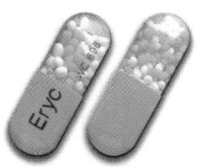

250 mg

ESTRADIOL

Estrace
(page 536)

2 mg

ESTROGENS, CONJUGATED

Premarin
(page 539)

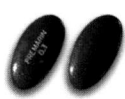

0.3 mg

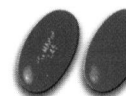

0.45 mg

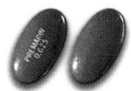

0.625 mg

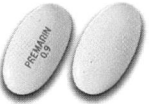

0.9 mg

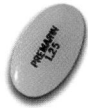

1.25 mg

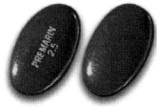

2.5 mg

ETHINYL ESTRADIOL AND NORETHINDRONE

Ovcon-35
(page 550)

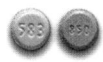

0.4/35-28

FAMOTIDINE

Pepcid
(page 571)

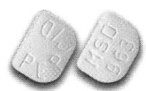

20 mg   40 mg

FLUCONAZOLE

Diflucan
(page 585)

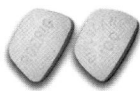 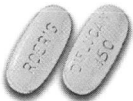 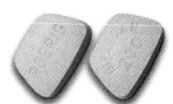

100 mg   150 mg   200 mg

FLUOXETINE HYDROCHLORIDE

Prozac
(page 595)

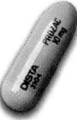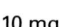 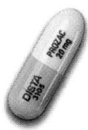 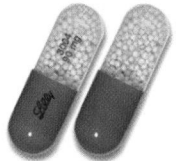

10 mg   20 mg   90 mg

FOSINOPRIL SODIUM

Monopril
(page 620)

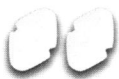 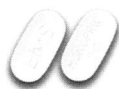 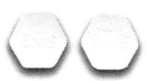

10 mg   20 mg   40 mg

FROVATRIPTAN SUCCINATE

Frova
(page 623)

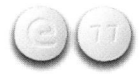

2.5 mg

FUROSEMIDE

Lasix
(page 626)

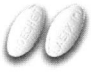 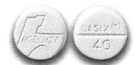

20 mg   40 mg

GABAPENTIN

Neurontin
(page 628)

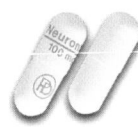 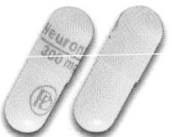 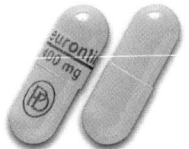

100 mg   300 mg   400 mg

GLIPIZIDE

Glucotrol
(page 647)

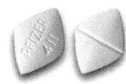 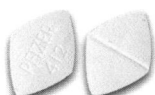

5 mg   10 mg

Glucotrol XL
(page 647)

5 mg   10 mg

GLYBURIDE

DiaBeta
(page 652)

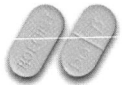 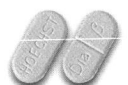 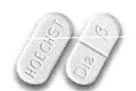

1.25 mg   2.5 mg   5 mg

Micronase
(page 652)

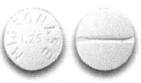 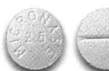 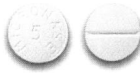

1.25 mg   2.5 mg   5 mg

LANSOPRAZOLE

Prevacid
(page 749)

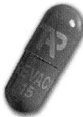 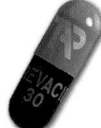

15 mg   30 mg

LEVOFLOXACIN

Levaquin
(page 761)

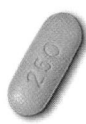   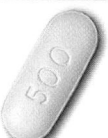

250 mg   500 mg

LEVOTHYROXINE SODIUM

Levoxyl
(page 764)

25 mcg   50 mcg   75 mcg

88 mcg   100 mcg   112 mcg

125 mcg   137 mcg   150 mcg

175 mcg   200 mcg   300 mcg

    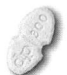

LISINOPRIL

Prinivil
(page 772)

    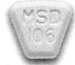

2.5 mg   5 mg   10 mg

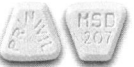

20 mg   40 mg

LOSARTAN POTASSIUM

Cozaar
(page 785)

25 mg 50 mg

LOVASTATIN

Mevacor
(page 787)

  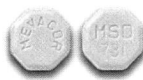

10 mg 20 mg 40 mg

MEDROXYPROGESTERONE ACETATE

Provera
(page 804)

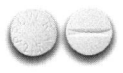 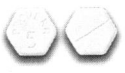 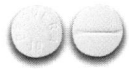

2.5 mg 5 mg 10 mg

METFORMIN HYDROCHLORIDE

Glucophage
(page 825)

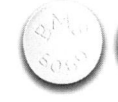 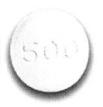 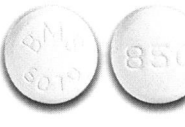 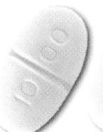

500 mg 850 mg 1000 mg

Glucophage XR
(page 825)

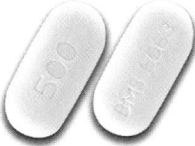

500 mg

METHYLPHENIDATE HYDROCHLORIDE

Ritalin
(page 839)

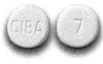 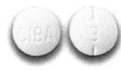 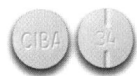

5 mg 10 mg 20 mg

METOPROLOL SUCCINATE

Toprol-XL
(page 848)

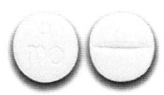 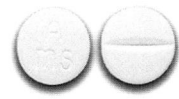 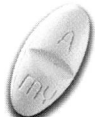

| 50 mg | 100 mg | 200 mg |

MONTELUKAST SODIUM

Singulair
(page 873)

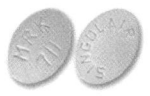

| 4 mg | 5 mg | 10 mg |

NABUMETONE

Relafen
(page 885)

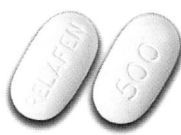 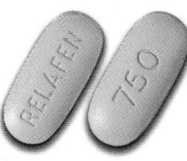

| 500 mg | 750 mg |

NEFAZODONE HYDROCHLORIDE

Serzone
(page 900)

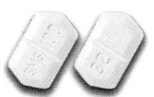 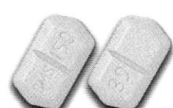 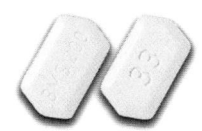

| 100 mg | 150 mg | 200 mg |

NIFEDIPINE

Procardia XL
(page 914)

  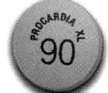

| 30 mg | 60 mg | 90 mg |

NORTRIPTYLINE HYDROCHLORIDE

Pamelor
(page 928)

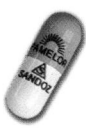 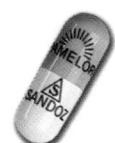 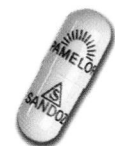

| 10 mg | 25 mg | 50 mg |

OMEPRAZOLE

Prilosec
(page 941)

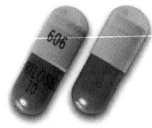

10 mg

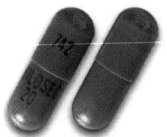

20 mg

OXYCODONE HYDROCHLORIDE

OxyContin
(page 957)

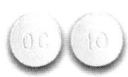

10 mg

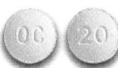

20 mg

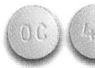

40 mg

80 mg

PAROXETINE HYDROCHLORIDE

Paxil
(page 972)

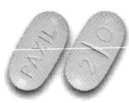

20 mg

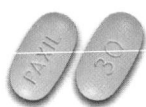

30 mg

PHENYTOIN SODIUM

Dilantin Kapseals
(page 1014)

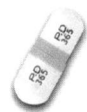

30 mg

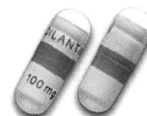

100 mg

POTASSIUM CHLORIDE

K-Dur 20
(page 1037)

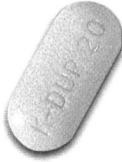

20 mEq

PRAVASTATIN SODIUM

Pravachol
(page 1045)

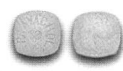 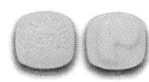 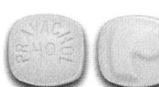

| 10 mg | 20 mg | 40 mg |

PROCHLORPERAZINE

Compazine
(page 1060)

| 5 mg | 10 mg |

PROMETHAZINE HYDROCHLORIDE

Phenergan
(page 1064)

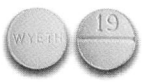 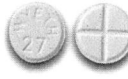 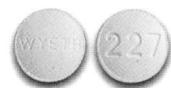

| 12.5 mg | 25 mg | 50 mg |

QUINAPRIL HYDROCHLORIDE

Accupril
(page 1085)

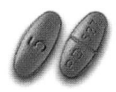

| 5 mg | 10 mg | 20 mg |

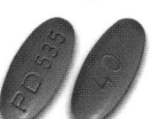

40 mg

RANITIDINE HYDROCHLORIDE

Zantac
(page 1097)

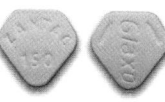 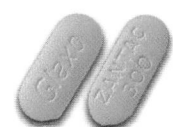

| 150 mg | 300 mg |

RISEDRONATE SODIUM

Actonel
(page 1115)

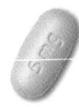

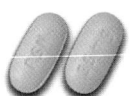

5 mg

35 mg

RISPERIDONE

Risperdal
(page 1117)

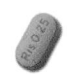

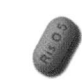

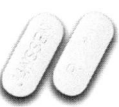

0.25 mg

0.5 mg

1 mg

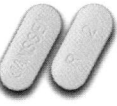

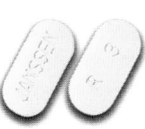

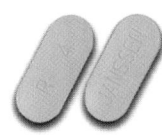

2 mg

3 mg

4 mg

Risperdal M-Tab
(page 1117)

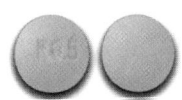

0.5 mg

ROFECOXIB

Vioxx
(page 1125)

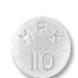

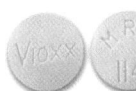

12.5 mg

25 mg

50 mg

ROSIGLITAZONE MALEATE

Avandia
(page 1129)

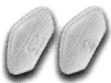

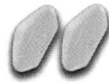

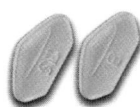

2 mg

4 mg

8 mg

ROSUVASTATIN CALCIUM

Crestor
(page 1133)

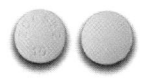 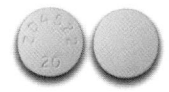

10 mg   20 mg

SERTRALINE HYDROCHLORIDE

Zoloft
(page 1146)

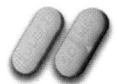 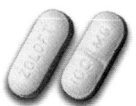

50 mg   100 mg

SILDENAFIL CITRATE

Viagra
(page 1151)

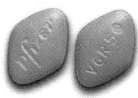 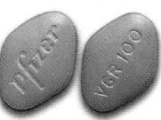

50 mg   100 mg

SIMVASTATIN

Zocor
(page 1153)

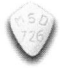 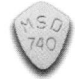

5 mg   10 mg   20 mg

TERAZOSIN HYDROCHLORIDE

Hytrin
(page 1209)

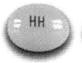

1 mg   5 mg   10 mg

VALDECOXIB

Bextra
(page 1289)

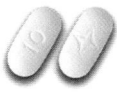 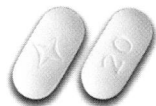

10 mg   20 mg

VARDENAFIL HYDROCHLORIDE

Levitra
(page 1297)

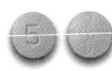   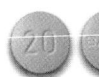

5 mg   10 mg   20 mg

VENLAFAXINE HYDROCHLORIDE

Effexor XR
(page 1302)

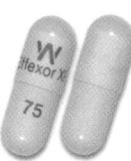 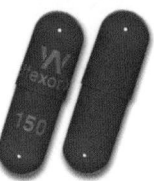

75 mg   150 mg

WARFARIN SODIUM

Coumadin
(page 1319)

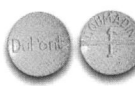 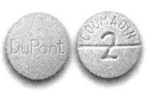 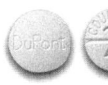

1 mg   2 mg   2.5 mg

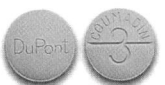 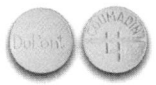 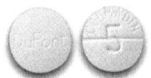

3 mg   4 mg   5 mg

  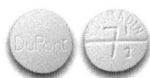 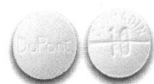

6 mg   7.5 mg   10 mg

ZOLPIDEM TARTRATE

Ambien
(page 1335)

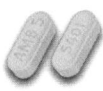 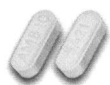

5 mg   10 mg

ic tenderness occurs, stop drug and notify prescriber.
• Evaluate patient's and family's knowledge of
drug therapy.

Nursing diagnoses
• Ineffective health maintenance related to pres-
ence of leukemia
• Ineffective immune protection related to drug-
induced adverse hematologic reactions
• Deficient knowledge related to drug therapy

Planning and implementation
• Dosage modifications may be needed after
chemotherapy or radiation therapy and in patient with depressed neutrophil or platelet count
or impaired liver or kidney function.
ALERT: Sometimes drug is ordered as
6-mercaptopurine or 6-MP. The numeral 6 is
part of drug name and doesn't signify number of
dosage units. To prevent confusion, avoid these
designations.
• Drug regimen must continue despite nausea
and vomiting. Notify prescriber if adverse GI
reactions occur and give an antiemetic.
• Encourage adequate fluid intake (3 L daily).
• Give allopurinol cautiously.
• If hepatic tenderness occurs, stop drug and notify prescriber.
ALERT: Don't confuse Purinethol with propylthiouracil.
Patient teaching
• Tell patient to notify prescriber if vomiting occurs shortly after taking dose because antiemetic will be needed so drug therapy can continue.
• Instruct patient to watch for signs of infection
(fever, sore throat, fatigue) and bleeding (easy
bruising, nosebleeds, bleeding gums, melena).
Have patient take his temperature daily.
• Advise woman of childbearing age to avoid
becoming pregnant during therapy and to consult with prescriber before becoming pregnant.

Evaluation
• Patient responds well to therapy.
• Patient doesn't develop serious ill effects
when hematologic studies are abnormal.
• Patient and family state understanding of drug
therapy.

meropenem
(mer-oh-PEN-em)
Merrem I.V.

Pharmacologic class: synthetic broad-spectrum
carbapenem antibiotic
Therapeutic class: antibiotic
Pregnancy risk category: B

Indications and dosages
▶ **Complicated appendicitis and peritonitis
caused by viridans group streptococci,** *Escherichia coli, Klebsiella pneumoniae, Pseudomonas aeruginosa, Bacteroides fragilis,
Bacteroides thetaiotaomicron,* **and** *Peptostreptococcus* **species; bacterial meningitis
(children only) caused by** *Streptococcus pneumoniae, Haemophilus influenzae,* **and** *Neisseria meningitidis. Adults:* 1 g I.V. q 8 hours over
15 to 30 minutes or over 3 to
5 minutes as I.V. bolus injection (5 to 20 ml).
Children weighing more than 50 kg (110 lb):
1 g I.V. q 8 hours for intra-abdominal infections
and 2 g I.V. q 8 hours for meningitis.
Children age 3 months and older: 20 mg/kg
(intra-abdominal infection) or 40 mg/kg (bacterial meningitis) q 8 hours over 15 to 30 minutes
as I.V. infusion or over 3 to 5 minutes as I.V. bolus injection (5 to 20 ml). Maximum dosage is
2 g I.V. q 8 hours.
Adjust-a-dose: For adults with renal impairment, if creatinine clearance is 26 to 50 ml/
minute, give usual dose q 12 hours; if clearance
is 10 to 25 ml/minute, give ½ usual dose q 12
hours; if clearance is less than 10 ml/minute,
give ½ dose q 24 hours.

I.V. administration
• For I.V. bolus administration, add 10 ml of
sterile water for injection to 500-mg/20-ml vial
or add 20 ml to 1-g/30-ml vial. Shake to dissolve, and let stand until clear.
• For I.V. infusion, infusion vials (500 mg/
100 ml and 1 g/100 ml) may be directly reconstituted with compatible infusion fluid. Or, an
injection vial may be reconstituted, then the resulting solution added to an I.V. container, and
further diluted with appropriate infusion fluid.
Don't use ADD-Vantage vials for this purpose.
• Follow manufacturer's guidelines closely
when using ADD-Vantage vials.

● Don't mix meropenem with solutions containing other drugs.
● Use freshly prepared solutions of drug immediately whenever possible.
● Stability of drug varies with form of drug used (injection vial, infusion vial, or ADD-Vantage container).

Contraindications and precautions

● Contraindicated in patients hypersensitive to drug, its components, or other drugs in same class. Also contraindicated in those who have had anaphylactic reactions to beta-lactams.
● Use cautiously and at a reduced dosage in patients with renal impairment.
❧ **Lifespan:** In pregnant women, use only if clearly needed. In breast-feeding women, use cautiously; it is unknown whether drug appears in breast milk. In infants younger than age 3 months, safety and effectiveness of drug haven't been established.

Adverse reactions

CNS: *seizures,* headache.
CV: thrombophlebitis at injection site.
GI: diarrhea, nausea, vomiting, constipation, oral candidiasis, *pseudomembranous colitis,* glossitis.
Hematologic: anemia, eosinophilia.
Respiratory: *apnea.*
Skin: rash, pruritus, phlebitis.
Other: hypersensitivity reactions, *anaphylaxis,* inflammation.

Interactions

Drug-drug. *Probenecid:* Inhibits renal excretion of meropenem. Don't give together.

Effects on lab test results

● May increase ALT, AST, bilirubin, alkaline phosphatase, LDH, creatinine, and BUN levels.
● May increase eosinophil count. May decrease hemoglobin, hematocrit, and WBC count. May increase or decrease platelet count and PT.

Pharmacokinetics

Absorption: Administered I.V.
Distribution: Protein-binding is 2%. Penetrates into most body fluids and tissues including CSF.
Metabolism: Metabolized in kidneys.
Excretion: Excreted in urine. *Half-life:* 1 hour.

Route	Onset	Peak	Duration
I.V.	Unknown	Within 1 hr	Unknown

Action

Chemical effect: Readily penetrates the cell wall of most gram-positive and gram-negative bacteria to reach penicillin-binding protein targets, where it inhibits cell wall synthesis.
Therapeutic effect: Bactericidal.

Available forms

Powder for injection: 500 mg/15 ml, 500 mg/20 ml, 500 mg/100 ml, 1 g/15 ml, 1 g/30 ml, 1 g/100 ml

NURSING PROCESS

⚕ Assessment

● Obtain specimen for culture and sensitivity tests before giving first dose.
⊛ **ALERT:** Serious and occasionally fatal hypersensitivity reactions have been reported in patients receiving therapy with beta-lactams. Before starting therapy, determine whether previous hypersensitivity reactions have occurred to penicillins, cephalosporins, other beta-lactams, or other allergens.
● Monitor patient for signs and symptoms of superinfection.
● Periodically assess organ system functions during prolonged therapy.
● Evaluate patient's and family's knowledge of drug therapy.

⊞ Nursing diagnoses

● Infection related to bacteria
● Risk for deficient fluid volume related to effect on kidneys
● Deficient knowledge related to drug therapy

⊳ Planning and implementation

● Drug isn't used to treat methicillin-resistant staphylococci.
● If patient develops diarrhea, suspect pseudomembranous colitis. If confirmed, stop drug, begin fluid and electrolyte management, and give an antibacterial effective against *C. difficile.*
● If overdose occurs (usually in patients with renal impairment), stop drug and provide general supportive therapy until renal elimination occurs. Drug and its metabolites are removable by hemodialysis, if needed.

Patient teaching
- Advise breast-feeding patient of risk of drug transmission to infant.
- Instruct patient to report adverse reactions.

☑ Evaluation
- Patient is free from infection.
- Patient maintains adequate hydration.
- Patient and family state understanding of drug therapy.

mesalamine
(mez-AL-uh-meen)
Asacol, Canasa, Pentasa, Rowasa

Pharmacologic class: salicylate
Therapeutic class: anti-inflammatory
Pregnancy risk category: B

Indications and dosages

▶ **Active mild to moderate distal ulcerative colitis, proctitis, proctosigmoiditis.** *Adults:* 800 mg P.O. (tablets) t.i.d. for total dose of 2.4 g daily for 6 weeks, or 1 g P.O. (capsules) q.i.d. for total dose of 4 g up to 8 weeks. Or, 500 mg P.R. (suppository) b.i.d., increased to t.i.d. after 2 weeks; retain for 1 to 3 hours or longer, or 4 g as retention enema once daily (preferably h.s.) retained overnight (for about 8 hours). Usual course of therapy for P.R. form is 3 to 6 weeks.
▶ **Maintenance of remission of ulcerative colitis.** *Adults:* 1.6 g P.O. daily in divided doses for 6 months. Or, 60 ml (4 g) rectal suspension q 2 to 3 nights or 1 to 3 g rectal suspension daily.

Contraindications and precautions

- Contraindicated in patients hypersensitive to drug, its components, or salicylates.
- Use cautiously in patients with renal impairment. Nephrotoxic potential from absorbed mesalamine exists.
⚕ **Lifespan:** In pregnant women, use cautiously. In breast-feeding women, suppository form of drug isn't recommended; oral form may be used with caution. In children, drug is contraindicated. In the elderly, use cautiously.

Adverse reactions

CNS: headache, dizziness, fatigue, fever, malaise.
GI: abdominal pain, cramps, or discomfort; flatulence; diarrhea; rectal pain; bloating; *nausea;* vomiting; *belching; pancolitis; pancreatitis.*
Respiratory: wheezing.
Skin: pruritus, rash, urticaria, hair loss, acne.
Other: *anaphylaxis.*

Interactions

None significant.

Effects on lab test results

- May increase BUN, creatinine, AST, ALT, alkaline phosphatase, LDH, amylase, and lipase levels.

Pharmacokinetics

Absorption: Poorly absorbed with P.R. administration; P.O. tablets and capsules are made to have delayed absorption from GI tract.
Distribution: Not clearly defined.
Metabolism: Undergoes acetylation, but whether this takes place at colonic or systemic sites is unknown.
Excretion: P.O. form primarily excreted in urine; most of P.R. form excreted in feces. *Half-life:* Mesalamine, 30 to 75 minutes; acetylated metabolite, about 5 to 10 hours.

Route	Onset	Peak	Duration
P.O., P.R.	Unknown	3-12 hr	Unknown

Action

Chemical effect: Unknown; probably acts topically by inhibiting prostaglandin production in colon.
Therapeutic effect: Relieves inflammation in lower GI tract.

Available forms

Capsules (controlled-release): 250 mg
Rectal suspension: 4 g/60 ml
Suppositories: 500 mg
Tablets (delayed-release): 400 mg

NURSING PROCESS

☑ Assessment
- Assess patient's condition before therapy and regularly thereafter.
- Monitor periodic kidney function studies in patient on long-term therapy.

• Because it contains potassium metabisulfite, drug may cause hypersensitivity reactions in patient sensitive to sulfites.
• Be alert for adverse reactions.
• Evaluate patient's and family's knowledge of drug therapy.

⊞ Nursing diagnoses
• Impaired tissue integrity related to underlying condition
• Acute pain related to drug-induced adverse GI reactions
• Deficient knowledge related to drug therapy

⊠ Planning and implementation
• Have patient swallow tablets and capsules whole; don't t crush or let him chew them.
• For maximum effectiveness, have patient retain suppository as long as possible (1 to 3 hours). When giving suspension, shake bottle before application.
⊛ ALERT: Don't confuse Asacol with Os-Cal.
Patient teaching
• Teach patient how to take oral and rectal form, and instruct him to carefully follow instructions supplied with drug.
• Instruct patient to stop taking drug if he experiences fever or rash. Patient intolerant of sulfasalazine may also be hypersensitive to this drug.

☑ Evaluation
• Patient reports relief from GI symptoms.
• Patient states that no new pain is experienced during therapy.
• Patient and family state understanding of drug therapy.

---

mesna
(MEZ-nah)
MESNEX

Pharmacologic class: thiol derivative
Therapeutic class: uroprotectant
Pregnancy risk category: B

Indications and dosages

▶ **Prevention of hemorrhagic cystitis in patients receiving ifosfamide.** *Adults:* Dosage varies with amount of ifosfamide given. Usual dose is 240 mg/m² as I.V. bolus with ifosfa-

mide. Repeat dose at 4 hours and 8 hours after ifosfamide is given. Alternatively, calculate daily dose as 100% of the ifosfamide dose. Give as a single bolus injection (20%) followed by two oral administrations (40% each). Protocols that use 1.2 g/m² ifosfamide would employ 240 mg/m² I.V. mesna at 0 hours, then 480 mg/m² P.O. at 2 and 6 hours.
▶ **Prevention of hemorrhagic cystitis in bone marrow recipients receiving cyclophosphamide‡.** *Adults:* 60% to 160% of the cyclophosphamide daily dose given I.V. in three to five divided doses or by continuous infusion. Or, in patients receiving cyclophosphamide (50 to 60 mg/kg I.V. daily for 2 to 4 days), give 10 mg/kg I.V. loading dose followed by 60 mg/kg by continuous infusion over 24 hours. Give with each cyclophosphamide dose and continue for 24 hours after last dose of cyclophosphamide.

▼ I.V. administration

• Dilute drug in commercially available ampules of D₅W, dextrose 5% and normal saline solution for injection, normal saline solution for injection, or lactated Ringer's solution to obtain final solution of 20 mg/ml.
• Although diluted solutions are stable for 24 hours at room temperature, refrigerate after preparation and use them within 6 hours. After opening ampule, discard any unused drug because it decomposes quickly into inactive compound.
• Mesna and ifosfamide are compatible in same I.V. infusion.
⊛ ALERT: Don't mix mesna with cisplatin because they're incompatible.

Contraindications and precautions

• Contraindicated in patients hypersensitive to drug or thiol-containing compounds.
☙ Lifespan: In pregnant women, use cautiously. In breast-feeding women and in children, safety of drug hasn't been established.

Adverse reactions

CNS: *fatigue, fever, asthenia,* dizziness, headache, somnolence, anxiety, confusion, insomnia, pain.
CV: chest pain, edema, hypotension, tachycardia, flushing.
GI: *nausea, vomiting,* diarrhea, *constipation, anorexia, abdominal pain,* dyspepsia.

Reactions may be *common,* uncommon, *life-threatening*, or COMMON AND LIFE-THREATENING.

GU: hematuria.
Hematologic: *leukopenia, thrombocytopenia, anemia, granulocytopenia.*
Metabolic: hypokalemia, dehydration.
Musculoskeletal: back pain.
Respiratory: dyspnea, coughing, pneumonia.
Skin: alopecia, increased sweating, pallor.
Other: allergy, injection site reaction.

Interactions

None significant.

Effects on lab test results

None reported.

Pharmacokinetics

Absorption: Food does not have an effect on oral absorption.
Distribution: Remains in vascular compartment; isn't distributed through tissues.
Metabolism: Rapidly metabolized to mesna disulfide, its only metabolite.
Excretion: Excreted in urine. *Half-life:* Mesna, 1¼ hour; mesna disulfide, 1 hour.

Route	Onset	Peak	Duration
P.O., I.V.	Unknown	Unknown	Unknown

Action

Chemical effect: Prevents ifosfamide-induced hemorrhagic cystitis by reacting with urotoxic ifosfamide metabolites.
Therapeutic effect: Prevents ifosfamide from adversely affecting bladder tissue.

Available forms

Injection: 100 mg/ml in 2- and 10-ml vials
Tablets: 400 mg

NURSING PROCESS

⚡ Assessment
• Assess patient's condition before therapy and regularly thereafter.
• Up to 6% of patients may not respond to drug's protective effects.
• Monitor urine samples daily in patient taking mesna for hematuria.
• Be alert for adverse reactions.
• Monitor patient's hydration status if adverse GI reactions occur.
• Evaluate patient's and family's knowledge of drug therapy.

⬚ Nursing diagnoses
• Risk for deficient fluid volume related to drug-induced adverse GI reactions
• Deficient knowledge related to drug therapy

⬚ Planning and implementation
• For patients who vomit within 2 hours of taking P.O. drug, repeat the dose or give I.V.
• Because drug is used with ifosfamide and other chemotherapeutic drugs, it's difficult to determine adverse reactions attributable solely to this drug.
• Drug isn't effective in preventing hematuria from other causes (such as thrombocytopenia).
• Although formulated to prevent hemorrhagic cystitis from ifosfamide, drug won't protect against other toxicities linked to ifosfamide.
• Drug may interfere with diagnostic tests for urine ketones.
Patient teaching
• Instruct patient to report hematuria immediately and to notify prescriber about adverse GI reactions.

☑ Evaluation
• Patient maintains adequate hydration throughout therapy.
• Patient and family state understanding of drug therapy.

mesoridazine besylate
(mes-oh-RID-eh-zeen BES-eh-layt)
Serentil, Serentil Concentrate*

Pharmacologic class: phenothiazine (piperidine derivative)
Therapeutic class: antipsychotic
Pregnancy risk category: C

Indications and dosages

▶ **Management of psychotic disorders and for schizophrenic patients who don't show an acceptable response to other antipsychotics.**
Adults and children older than age 12: Initially, 50 mg P.O. t.i.d., up to 400 mg P.O. daily. Or, 25 mg I.M. repeated in 30 to 60 minutes, if needed, up to 200 mg I.M. daily.

Contraindications and precautions

• Contraindicated in patients hypersensitive to drug and in those experiencing severe CNS depression or coma.

⚕ Lifespan: In pregnant women, use cautiously. In breast-feeding women, drug isn't recommended. In children younger than age 12, safety of drug hasn't been established.

Adverse reactions

CNS: extrapyramidal reactions, drowsiness, *tardive dyskinesia, sedation,* EEG changes, dizziness, *neuroleptic malignant syndrome.*
CV: *orthostatic hypotension,* tachycardia, ECG changes, *prolonged QT interval, torsades de pointes, sudden death.*
EENT: *ocular changes, blurred vision,* retinitis pigmentosa.
GI: *dry mouth, constipation,* increased appetite.
GU: *urine retention,* dark urine, menstrual irregularities, inhibited ejaculation.
Hematologic: *leukopenia, agranulocytosis, aplastic anemia, thrombocytopenia,* hyperprolactinemia.
Hepatic: cholestatic jaundice.
Metabolic: weight gain.
Skin: *mild photosensitivity reactions,* sterile abscess.
Other: allergic reactions, gynecomastia, pain at I.M. injection site.

Interactions

Drug-drug. *Antacids:* Inhibits absorption of oral phenothiazines. Separate doses by at least 2 hours.
Anticholinergics: May increase anticholinergic effects. Use together cautiously.
Anticonvulsants: Phenothiazines may decrease the seizure threshold. Monitor patient. Dose of anticonvulsant may need to be increased.
Antihypertensives: May increase hypotensive effects. Monitor blood pressure closely.
Barbiturates: May decrease phenothiazine effect. Observe patient.
CNS depressants: Increases CNS depression. Use together cautiously.
Drugs that increase QT interval (disopyramide, procainamide, quinidine): Prolonged QT interval may result in arrhythmias. Don't use together.
Lithium, phenothiazine: May cause possible disorientation, unconsciousness, and extrapyramidal symptoms. Use cautiously.

Drug-herb. *Dong quai, St. John's wort:* Increases risk of photosensitivity reactions. Advise patient to avoid unprotected or prolonged exposure to sunlight.
Evening primrose oil: May decrease the seizure threshold. Discourage using together.
Kava: Increases risk or severity of dystonic reactions. Discourage using together.
Yohimbe: Phenothiazines may increase the risk of toxicity. Discourage using together.
Drug-lifestyle. *Alcohol use:* May increase CNS depression, particularly psychomotor skills. Strongly discourage use together.
Sun exposure: Increases photosensitivity reactions. Urge patient to avoid unprotected or prolonged exposure to sunlight.

Effects on lab test results

• May increase liver function test values and eosinophil count. May decrease hemoglobin, hematocrit, and WBC, granulocyte, and platelet counts.

Pharmacokinetics

Absorption: Erratic and variable with P.O. use; unknown with I.M. use.
Distribution: Wide; 91% to 99% protein-bound.
Metabolism: Extensively by liver.
Excretion: Excreted primarily in urine with some excretion in feces by way of biliary tract.

Route	Onset	Peak	Duration
P.O., I.M.	Up to several wk	Unknown	Unknown

Action

Chemical effect: Unknown. A piperidine phenothiazine and major sulfoxide metabolite of thioridazine, mesoridazine may block postsynaptic dopamine receptors in brain.
Therapeutic effect: Relieves psychotic signs and symptoms.

Available forms

Injection: 25 mg/ml
Oral concentrate: 25 mg/ml*
Tablets: 10 mg, 25 mg, 50 mg, 100 mg

NURSING PROCESS

☑ Assessment

• Assess patient's condition before therapy and regularly thereafter.

Reactions may be *common*, uncommon, *life-threatening*, or COMMON AND LIFE-THREATENING.

• Obtain baseline measures of blood pressure before starting therapy and monitor regularly. Watch for orthostatic hypotension, especially with parenteral administration.

• Monitor therapy with weekly bilirubin tests during first month, periodic blood tests (CBC and liver function), and ophthalmologic tests (long-term use).

⚠ **ALERT:** Because drug is linked to a dose-related prolonged QT interval, which is potentially life threatening, use only in schizophrenic patients who fail to respond to other antipsychotics.

⚠ **ALERT:** Before treatment, obtain baseline ECG and measure potassium level. Normalize potassium level before starting therapy. Don't give drug to patient with a baseline QTc interval longer than 450 msec. Stop drug in patients with a QTc interval longer than 500 msec.

• Monitor patient for tardive dyskinesia. It may occur after prolonged use, although it may not appear until months or years later and may disappear spontaneously or persist for life, despite discontinuation of drug.

⚠ **ALERT:** Watch for symptoms of neuroleptic malignant syndrome (extrapyramidal effects, hyperthermia, autonomic disturbance), which is rare but can be fatal.

• Evaluate patient's and family's knowledge of drug therapy.

🔷 Nursing diagnoses
• Disturbed thought processes related to underlying condition
• Constipation related to drug-induced adverse GI reactions
• Deficient knowledge related to drug therapy

▶ Planning and implementation
• Oral liquid and parenteral forms may cause contact dermatitis. Wear gloves when preparing solutions, and avoid contact with skin and clothing.

• Replace parenteral therapy with P.O. therapy to as soon as possible. When P.O. concentrate solution is used, dilute dose with water, orange juice, or grape juice just before administration.

• Give drug deep in upper outer quadrant of buttocks. Massage slowly afterward to prevent sterile abscess. Injection may sting.

• Protect drug from light. Slight yellowing of injection or concentrate is common; this doesn't

affect potency. Discard markedly discolored solutions.

⚠ **ALERT:** Withhold dose and notify prescriber if jaundice, symptoms of blood dyscrasia (fever, sore throat, infection, cellulitis, weakness), or persistent extrapyramidal reactions (longer than a few hours) develop, especially in pregnant women or in children.

• Acute dystonic reactions may be treated with diphenhydramine.

⚠ **ALERT:** Don't stop drug abruptly unless severe adverse reactions occur. After abrupt withdrawal of long-term therapy, patient may experience gastritis, nausea, vomiting, dizziness, tremors, feeling of warmth or cold, diaphoresis, tachycardia, headache, and insomnia.

⚠ **ALERT:** Don't confuse Serentil with Serevent or Aventyl.

Patient teaching
• Warn patient to avoid activities that require alertness and psychomotor coordination until CNS effects of drug are known.
• Advise patient to change positions slowly.
• Tell patient to avoid alcohol during drug therapy.
• Have patient report urine retention or constipation.
• Tell patient that drug may discolor urine.
• Advise patient to relieve dry mouth with sugarless gum or hard candy.
• Tell patient to avoid prolonged exposure to sunlight, use sunblock, and wear protective clothing to avoid photosensitivity reactions.

☑ Evaluation
• Patient exhibits improved behavior.
• Patient maintains normal bowel pattern.
• Patient and family state understanding of drug therapy.

---

metaproterenol sulfate
(met-uh-proh-TER-eh-nul SUL-fayt)
Alupent

Pharmacologic class: beta-adrenergic agonist
Therapeutic class: bronchodilator
Pregnancy risk category: C

Indications and dosages
▶ **Acute episodes of bronchial asthma.** *Adults and children older than age 12:* 2 to 3 inhala-

tions. Don't repeat inhalations more often than q
3 to 4 hours. Maximum, 12 inhalations daily.
▶ **Bronchial asthma and reversible bronchospasm.** *Adults and children older than age 9 or
weighing more than 27 kg (60 lb):* 20 mg P.O. q
6 to 8 hours.
*Children ages 6 to 9 or weighing less than
27 kg:* 10 mg P.O. q 6 to 8 hours.
Or, by way of IPPB or nebulizer. *Adults and
children age 12 and older:* by IPPB, 0.2 to
0.3 ml of 5% solution diluted in 2.5 ml of normal saline solution or 2.5 ml of commercially
available 0.4% or 0.6% solution q 4 hours, p.r.n.
By hand-bulb nebulizer, 10 inhalations of an
undiluted 5% solution.
Children ages 6 to 12: 0.1 to 0.2 ml of 5% solution diluted in normal saline solution to final
volume of 3 ml q 4 hours, p.r.n.

Contraindications and precautions

• Contraindicated in patients hypersensitive to
drug or its ingredients, in those receiving cyclopropane or halogenated hydrocarbon general
anesthetics, and in those with tachycardia or arrhythmias caused by tachycardia, peripheral or
mesenteric vascular thrombosis, or profound hypoxia or hypercapnia.
• Use cautiously in patients with hypertension,
hyperthyroidism, heart disease, diabetes, or cirrhosis and in those receiving digoxin.
⚖ Lifespan: In pregnant and breast-feeding
women, use cautiously.

Adverse reactions

CNS: nervousness, weakness, drowsiness,
tremors.
CV: tachycardia, hypertension, ECG changes,
palpitations, *cardiac arrest.*
GI: vomiting, nausea, bad taste.
Respiratory: *paradoxical bronchoconstriction.*

Interactions

Drug-drug. *Other sympathomimetics:* May
have additive effects and toxicity. Separate administration times.
Propranolol, other beta blockers: Blocks bronchodilating effect of metaproterenol. Monitor
patient.
Theophylline, aminophylline: May increase risk
of cardiotoxicity. Monitor ECG and vital signs
closely.

Effects on lab test results

None reported.

Pharmacokinetics

Absorption: Well absorbed from the GI tract.
Inhaled doses are minimally absorbed through
the lungs.
Distribution: Widely distributed.
Metabolism: Extensively metabolized on first
pass through liver.
Excretion: Excreted in urine.

Route	Onset	Peak	Duration
P.O.	1 min	≤ 1 hr	1-4 hr
Inhalation	15 min	≤ 1 hr	2-6 hr
Nebulization	5-30 min	≤ 1 hr	2-6 hr

Action

Chemical effect: Relaxes bronchial smooth
muscle by acting on beta$_2$-adrenergic receptors.
Therapeutic effect: Improves breathing.

Available forms

Aerosol inhaler: 0.65 mg/metered spray
Solution for nebulizer inhalation: 0.4%, 0.6%,
5% solution
Syrup: 10 mg/5 ml
Tablets: 10 mg, 20 mg

NURSING PROCESS

⚕ Assessment
• Assess patient's condition before therapy and
regularly thereafter.
• Be alert for adverse reactions and drug inter-
actions.
• Monitor patient's hydration status if adverse
GI reactions occur.
• Evaluate patient's and family's knowledge of
drug therapy.

⬛ Nursing diagnoses
• Impaired gas exchange related to underlying
respiratory condition
• Risk for deficient fluid volume related to
drug-induced adverse GI reactions
• Deficient knowledge related to drug therapy

▶ Planning and implementation
• Patient may use tablets and aerosol together.
Watch for toxicity.

- Aerosol nebulization solution can be given by IPPB with drug diluted in normal saline solution or by hand-bulb nebulizer at full strength.

⊗ **ALERT:** Don't confuse metaproterenol with metoprolol or metipranolol.

⊗ **ALERT:** Don't confuse Alupent with Atrovent.

Patient teaching
- Give patient the following instructions for using metered-dose inhaler: Clear nasal passages and throat. Breathe out, expelling as much air from lungs as possible. Place mouthpiece well into mouth and inhale deeply as you release a dose from inhaler. Hold breath for several seconds, remove mouthpiece, and exhale slowly. Allow 2 minutes between inhalations.
- Instruct patient to store drug in light-resistant container.
- Advise patient that these inhalations should precede corticosteroid inhalations by 10 to 15 minutes to maximize effectiveness of corticosteroid therapy.
- Tell patient using corticosteroid inhaler to use bronchodilator first, and then wait 5 minutes before using corticosteroid. This allows bronchodilator to open air passages for maximum effectiveness of corticosteroid.
- Tell patient who takes multiple inhalations to wait at least 2 minutes between each inhalation.
- Warn patient to stop taking drug immediately and notify prescriber if paradoxical bronchospasm occurs.
- If no response is derived from dosage, tell patient to notify prescriber or request dosage adjustments.

☑ **Evaluation**
- Patient's status improves.
- Patient maintains adequate hydration.
- Patient and family state understanding of drug therapy.

metformin hydrochloride
(met-FOR-min high-droh-KLOR-ighd)
Glucophage, Glucophage XR, Riomet

Pharmacologic class: biguanide
Therapeutic class: antidiabetic
Pregnancy risk category: B

Indications and dosages

▶ **Adjunct to diet and exercise to lower glucose level in patients with type 2 (non–insulin-dependent) diabetes mellitus.** *Adults:* Initially, 500 mg P.O. b.i.d. with morning and evening meals, or 850 mg P.O. once daily with morning meal. When 500-mg dose form is used, increase dosage by 500 mg weekly, up to a maximum of 2,000 mg tablets or oral solution daily. Or, 500 mg P.O. b.i.d.; increase to 850 mg P.O. b.i.d. after 2 weeks. When 850-mg dose form is used, increase dosage by 850 mg q other week, maximum 2,550 mg P.O. daily, p.r.n. Doses greater than 2,000 mg may be better tolerated if divided t.i.d. If using extended-release form, initiate therapy at 500 mg P.O. daily with the evening meal. May increase dose weekly in increments of 500 mg P.O. daily, to a maximum dose of 2,000 mg P.O. once daily. If higher doses are needed, consider using the regular-release form up to its maximum dose.
Children ages 10 to 16: 500 mg P.O. b.i.d. using the regular-release form only. Increase dosage in increments of 500 mg weekly up to a maximum of 2,000 mg daily in divided doses. Don't use extended-release form in children.

Contraindications and precautions

- Contraindicated in patients hypersensitive to drug and in those with hepatic disease, renal disease or renal dysfunction, acute or chronic metabolic acidosis, and heart failure patients who require medication. Temporarily withhold drug in patients undergoing radiologic studies involving parenteral administration of iodinated contrast materials; using such products may result in acute renal dysfunction. If patient enters hypoxic state, stop drug.
- Use cautiously in debilitated or malnourished patients and in those with adrenal or pituitary insufficiency because of increased risk of hypoglycemia.
⚘ **Lifespan:** In pregnant women, safety hasn't been established. In breast-feeding women, drug isn't recommended. In children younger than age 10, safety of regular form of drug hasn't been established. In children younger than age 17, safety of extended-release form hasn't been established. In elderly patients, use cautiously.

Adverse reactions

CNS: headache, dizziness, asthenia.

GI: *diarrhea, nausea, vomiting,* abdominal discomfort, *flatulence,* indigestion, unpleasant or metallic taste.
Hematologic: megaloblastic anemia.
Metabolic: *lactic acidosis.*

Interactions

Drug-drug. *Calcium channel blockers, corticosteroids, estrogens, isoniazid, nicotinic acid, hormonal contraceptives, phenothiazines, phenytoin, sympathomimetics, thiazide and other diuretics, thyroid drugs:* May produce hyperglycemia. Monitor patient's glycemic control. Metformin dosage may need to be increased.
Cationic drugs (such as amiloride, cimetidine, digoxin, morphine, procainamide, quinidine, quinine, ranitidine, triamterene, trimethoprim, vancomycin): May compete for common renal tubular transport systems, which may reduce metformin clearance and increase metformin level. Monitor patient's glucose level. Adjust dosages, if needed.
Furosemide, nifedipine: Increases metformin levels. Monitor patient. Metformin dosage may need to be decreased.
Iodinated contrast material: Parenteral contrast studies with iodinated materials have been linked to lactic acidosis leading to acute renal impairment. Withhold metformin on or before the day of the study, and resume after 48 hours, provided renal function is within normal limits.
Drug-herb. *Aloe, bilberry leaf, bitter melon, burdock, dandelion, fenugreek, garlic, ginseng:* Improved glucose control may allow reduction of antidiabetic. Tell patient to discuss use of herbal remedies with prescriber before therapy.
Drug-lifestyle. *Alcohol use:* May potentiate drug effects. Discourage using together.

Effects on lab test results

• May decrease pH and bicarbonate levels.
• May decrease hemoglobin, hematocrit, and RBC count.

Pharmacokinetics

Absorption: Food decreases rate and extent of absorption of tablets, but increases extent of absorption of oral solution.
Distribution: Negligibly bound to proteins.
Metabolism: Not metabolized.
Excretion: Unchanged in urine. *Half-life:* About 6 hours.

Route	Onset	Peak	Duration
P.O.	Unknown	Unknown	Unknown
P.O. extended-release	Unknown	4-8 hr	Unknown
oral solution	Unknown	2½ hr	Unknown

Action

Chemical effect: Decreases hepatic glucose production and intestinal absorption of glucose and improves insulin sensitivity (increases peripheral glucose uptake and utilization).
Therapeutic effect: Lowers glucose level.

Available forms

Oral solution: 500 mg/5 ml
Tablets: 500 mg, 850 mg, 1,000 mg
Tablets (extended-release): 500 mg, 750 mg

NURSING PROCESS

Assessment
• Assess patient's glucose level before therapy and regularly thereafter.
• Before beginning therapy, assess patient's kidney function, and then reassess at least annually. If renal impairment is detected, expect prescriber to switch to different antidiabetic.
• Monitor patient's hematologic status for megaloblastic anemia. Patients with inadequate vitamin B_{12} or calcium intake or absorption seem predisposed to developing subnormal vitamin B_{12} levels when taking metformin. Check their vitamin B_{12} level determinations every 2 to 3 years.
• Be alert for adverse reactions and drug interactions.
• Monitor patient closely during times of increased stress, such as infection, fever, surgery, or trauma; insulin therapy may be needed.
• Risk of metformin-induced lactic acidosis is very low. Cases have been reported primarily in diabetic patients with significant renal insufficiency; with other medical or surgical problems; and with multiple, concomitant drug regimens. The risk of lactic acidosis increases with the degree of renal impairment and patient's age.
• Evaluate patient's and family's knowledge of drug therapy.

🕀 Nursing diagnoses

- Ineffective health maintenance related to presence of hyperglycemia
- Risk for deficient fluid volume related to drug-induced adverse GI reactions
- Deficient knowledge related to drug therapy

▶ Planning and implementation

- When switching from standard oral antidiabetic (except chlorpropamide) to metformin, no transition period usually is needed. When switching patient from chlorpropamide to metformin, use care during first 2 weeks of metformin therapy because prolonged retention of chlorpropamide increases risk of hypoglycemia during this time.
- Notify prescriber if glucose level rises despite therapy.
- If patient hasn't responded to 4 weeks of therapy using maximum dosage, prescriber may add oral sulfonylurea while continuing metformin at maximum dosage. If patient still doesn't respond after several months, prescriber may stop both drugs and start insulin therapy.
- Ⓢ **ALERT:** If patient develops conditions linked to hypoxemia or dehydration, stop drug immediately and notify prescriber because of risk of lactic acidosis.
- Metformin therapy may be temporarily suspended for surgical procedure (except minor procedures not related to restricted intake of food and fluids) and not restarted until patient's oral intake has resumed and kidney function is normal.

Patient teaching

- Tell patient to take once-daily dose with breakfast and twice-daily dose with breakfast and dinner.
- Tell patient not to crush or chew extended-release tablets (Glucophage XR).
- Instruct patient to stop drug and tell prescriber about unexplained hyperventilation, myalgia, malaise, unusual somnolence, or other symptoms of early lactic acidosis.
- Warn patient to minimize alcohol consumption while taking drug.
- Ⓢ **ALERT:** Teach patient about diabetes and the importance of following therapeutic regimen; adhering to diet, weight reduction, exercise, and hygiene programs; and avoiding infection. Explain how and when to monitor glucose level and how to differentiate between hypoglycemia and hyperglycemia.

- Tell patient not to change dosage without prescriber's consent. Encourage patient to report abnormal glucose test results.
- Advise patient not to take other drugs, including OTC drugs, without checking with prescriber.
- Instruct patient to wear or carry medical identification.

☑ Evaluation

- Patient's glucose level is normal.
- Patient maintains adequate hydration throughout therapy.
- Patient and family state understanding of drug therapy.

methadone hydrochloride
(METH-eh-dohn high-droh-KLOR-ighd)
Dolophine, Methadose, Physeptone ◊

Pharmacologic class: opioid
Therapeutic class: opioid analgesic, opioid detoxification adjunct
Pregnancy risk category: C
Controlled substance schedule: II

Indications and dosages

▶ **Severe pain.** *Adults:* 2.5 to 10 mg P.O., I.M., or S.C. q 3 to 4 hours, p.r.n.
Children‡: 0.7 mg/kg P.O. q 4 to 6 hours.
▶ **Opiate withdrawal syndrome.** *Adults:* 15 to 20 mg P.O. daily (highly individualized). Maintenance dosage is 20 to 120 mg P.O. daily. Adjust dosage, p.r.n. Daily doses greater than 120 mg require state and federal approval.

Contraindications and precautions

- Contraindicated in patients hypersensitive to drug.
- Use cautiously in debilitated patients and in patients with acute abdominal conditions, severe hepatic or renal impairment, hypothyroidism, Addison's disease, prostatic hyperplasia, urethral stricture, head injury, increased intracranial pressure, asthma, or other respiratory conditions.
- 🔥 **Lifespan:** In pregnant and breast-feeding women, use cautiously. In children, safety of drug hasn't been established. In elderly patients, use cautiously.

Rapid onset   *Liquid form contains alcohol.   ♦Canada   ◊ Australia   †OTC   ‡Off-label use

Adverse reactions

CNS: *sedation, somnolence, clouded sensorium, euphoria,* dizziness, chorea, *seizures.*
CV: *hypotension, **bradycardia, shock, cardiac arrest, arrhythmias.***
EENT: visual disturbances.
GI: *nausea, vomiting, constipation,* ileus.
GU: *urine retention.*
Respiratory: *respiratory depression, respiratory arrest.*
Skin: diaphoresis.
Other: decreased libido, physical dependence, pain at injection site, tissue irritation, induration after S.C. injection.

Interactions

Drug-drug. *Ammonium chloride and other urine acidifiers, phenytoin:* May reduce methadone effect. Monitor patient for decreased pain control.
CNS depressants, general anesthetics, hypnotics, MAO inhibitors, sedatives, tranquilizers, tricyclic antidepressants: Possible respiratory depression, hypotension, profound sedation, or coma. Use together cautiously. Monitor patient.
Rifampin: May cause withdrawal symptoms; reduces blood levels of methadone. Use together cautiously.
Drug-lifestyle. *Alcohol use:* May have additive effects. Discourage patient from using together.

Effects on lab test results

• May increase amylase or lipase levels.

Pharmacokinetics

Absorption: Well absorbed from GI tract; unknown for I.M. route.
Distribution: Highly bound to tissue protein.
Metabolism: Metabolized primarily in liver.
Excretion: Excreted primarily in urine; metabolites excreted in feces. *Half-life:* 15 to 25 hours.

Route	Onset	Peak	Duration
P.O.	30-60 min	½-1 hr	4-6 hr
I.M.	10-20 min	1-2 hr	4-5 hr
S.C.	Unknown	Unknown	Unknown

Action

Chemical effect: Binds to opioid receptors at many sites in CNS, altering both perception of and emotional response to pain through unknown mechanism.

Therapeutic effect: Relieves pain and symptoms of opioid withdrawal.

Available forms

Dispersible tablets (for maintenance therapy): 40 mg
Injection: 10 mg/ml
Oral solution: 5 mg/5 ml, 10 mg/5 ml, 10 mg/ml (concentrate)
Tablets: 5 mg, 10 mg

NURSING PROCESS

Assessment

• Assess patient's pain or opioid dependence before and during therapy.
• Monitor patient closely because drug has cumulative effect; marked sedation can occur after repeated doses.
• Be alert for adverse reactions and drug interactions.
• Evaluate patient's and family's knowledge of drug therapy.

Nursing diagnoses

• Chronic pain related to underlying condition
• Ineffective individual coping related to opioid dependence
• Deficient knowledge related to drug therapy

Planning and implementation

• Liquid form is legally required in maintenance programs. Dissolve tablets in 120 ml of orange juice or powdered citrus drink.
• P.O. dose is one-half as potent as injected dose.
• For parenteral use, I.M. injection is preferred. Rotate injection sites.
• Around-the-clock regimen is needed to manage severe, chronic pain.
• **ALERT:** Very high doses of methadone may cause QT interval prolongation and torsades de pointe.

Patient teaching
• Warn patient about getting out of bed or walking. Warn outpatient to avoid hazardous activities until drug's CNS effects are known.
• Instruct patient to avoid alcohol consumption during drug therapy.

Evaluation

• Patient is free from pain.

Reactions may be *common,* uncommon, *life-threatening,* or COMMON AND LIFE-THREATENING.

- Patient doesn't exhibit opioid withdrawal symptoms.
- Patient and family state understanding of drug therapy.

methamphetamine hydrochloride
(meth-am-FET-uh-meen high-droh-KLOR-ighd)
Desoxyn

Pharmacologic class: amphetamine
Therapeutic class: CNS stimulant, short-term adjunct anorexigenic, sympathomimetic amine
Pregnancy risk category: C
Controlled substance schedule: II

Indications and dosages

▶ **Attention deficit hyperactivity disorder.**
Children age 6 and older: Initially, 5 mg P.O. once daily or b.i.d., increase by 5-mg increments weekly, p.r.n. Usual effective dosage is 20 to 25 mg daily.
▶ **Short-term adjunct in exogenous obesity.**
Adults: 2.5 to 5 mg P.O. b.i.d. to t.i.d. 30 minutes before meals.

Contraindications and precautions

- Contraindicated in patients hypersensitive to sympathomimetic amines; patients with idiosyncratic reactions to sympathomimetic amines; patients with moderate to severe hypertension, hyperthyroidism, symptomatic CV disease, advanced arteriosclerosis, glaucoma, or history of drug abuse; patients who have taken an MAO inhibitor within 14 days; and agitated patients.
- Use cautiously in patients who are debilitated, asthenic, or psychopathic or who have history of suicidal or homicidal tendencies.
⚠ **Lifespan:** In pregnant and breast-feeding women, drug is contraindicated. In elderly patients, use cautiously.

Adverse reactions

CNS: *nervousness, insomnia,* irritability, *talkativeness,* dizziness, headache, hyperexcitability, tremors.
CV: hypertension, hypotension, *tachycardia, palpitations, **arrhythmias.***
EENT: blurred vision, mydriasis.
GI: metallic taste, dry mouth, nausea, vomiting, abdominal cramps, diarrhea, constipation, anorexia.
GU: impotence.
Skin: urticaria.
Other: altered libido.

Interactions

Drug-drug. *Acetazolamide, antacids, sodium bicarbonate:* Increases renal reabsorption. Monitor patient for enhanced effects.
Ammonium chloride, ascorbic acid: Decreases level and increases renal excretion of methamphetamine. Monitor patient for decreased methamphetamine effects.
Guanethidine: Amphetamines may decrease the antihypertensive effectiveness of guanethidine. Monitor blood pressure.
Haloperidol, phenothiazines, tricyclic antidepressants: Increases CNS effects. Avoid using together.
Insulin, oral antidiabetics: May decrease antidiabetic requirement. Monitor glucose level.
MAO inhibitors: May cause severe hypertension; possible hypertensive crisis. Don't use within 14 days of MAO inhibitor therapy.
Drug-herb. *Melatonin:* Enhances monoaminergic effects of methamphetamine; may worsen insomnia. Discourage using together.
Drug-food. *Caffeine-containing beverages:* May increase amphetamine and related amine effects. Discourage using together.

Effects on lab test results

- May increase corticosteroid level.

Pharmacokinetics

Absorption: Rapid.
Distribution: Widely distributed.
Metabolism: Metabolized in liver to at least seven metabolites.
Excretion: Excreted in urine. *Half-life:* 4 to 5 hours.

Route	Onset	Peak	Duration
P.O.	Unknown	Unknown	≤ 24 hr

Action

Chemical effect: Unknown; probably promotes nerve impulse transmission by releasing stored norepinephrine from nerve terminals in brain. Main sites of activity appear to be cerebral cortex and reticular activating system. In hyperkinetic children, drug has paradoxical calming effect.

Therapeutic effect: Promotes calmness in children with attention deficit disorder and causes weight loss.

Available forms

Tablets: 5 mg

⚗ Assessment
• Assess patient's condition before therapy and regularly thereafter.
• Be alert for adverse reactions and drug interactions.
• Evaluate patient's and family's knowledge of drug therapy.

🔀 Nursing diagnoses
• Ineffective health maintenance related to underlying condition
• Disturbed sleep pattern related to drug-induced insomnia
• Deficient knowledge related to drug therapy

⟩⟩ Planning and implementation
⊕ **ALERT:** Don't confuse Desoxyn with digitoxin or digoxin.
• Drug isn't the first-line treatment for obesity. Use as anorexigenic is prohibited in some states.
• When used for obesity, make sure patient is on weight-reduction program.
• If tolerance to anorexigenic effect develops, notify prescriber and stop drug.
Patient teaching
• Warn patient of high potential for abuse. Advise him that drug shouldn't be used to prevent fatigue.
• Advise patient to take last dose of drug at least 6 hours before bedtime.
• Warn patient to avoid activities that require alertness or good coordination until CNS effects are known.
• Tell patient to avoid caffeine during drug therapy.
• Instruct patient to report signs of excessive stimulation.
• Instruct patient not to crush long-acting tablets.

☑ Evaluation
• Patient exhibits positive response to drug therapy.
• Patient doesn't experience insomnia.

• Patient and family state understanding of drug therapy.

methimazole
(meth-IH-muh-zohl)
Tapazole

Pharmacologic class: thyroid hormone antagonist
Therapeutic class: antithyroid drug
Pregnancy risk category: D

Indications and dosages
▶ **Hyperthyroidism.** *Adults:* If mild, 15 mg P.O. daily. If moderately severe, 30 to 40 mg daily. If severe, 60 mg daily. Daily dose divided into three doses at 8-hour intervals. Maintenance dosage is 5 to 15 mg daily.
Children: 0.4 mg/kg P.O. daily in divided doses q 8 hours. Maintenance dosage is 0.2 mg/kg P.O. daily in divided doses q 8 hours.

Contraindications and precautions
• Contraindicated in patients hypersensitive to drug.
⚖ **Lifespan:** In pregnant women, use cautiously. In breast-feeding women, drug isn't recommended.

Adverse reactions
CNS: headache, drowsiness, vertigo.
GI: diarrhea, nausea, vomiting, salivary gland enlargement, loss of taste.
Hematologic: *agranulocytosis, leukopenia, thrombocytopenia, aplastic anemia,* lymphadenopathy.
Hepatic: jaundice.
Metabolic: hypothyroidism.
Musculoskeletal: arthralgia, myalgia.
Skin: abnormal hair loss, rash, urticaria, skin discoloration.
Other: drug-induced fever.

Interactions
Drug-drug. *Anticoagulants:* Enhances effects from anti–vitamin K activity attributed to drug. Monitor PT and INR as indicated.
Beta blockers, digoxin, theophylline: May increase levels of these drugs when a hyperthyroid patient becomes euthyroid. Reduce dosage of these drugs, if needed.

Reactions may be *common,* uncommon, *life-threatening*, or COMMON AND LIFE-THREATENING.

Effects on lab test results

• May decrease hemoglobin, hematocrit, and granulocyte, WBC, RBC, and platelet counts.

Pharmacokinetics

Absorption: Rapid.
Distribution: Concentrated in thyroid and isn't protein-bound.
Metabolism: Hepatic.
Excretion: Primarily in urine. *Half-life:* 5 to 13 hours.

Route	Onset	Peak	Duration
P.O.	≤ 5 days	30 min-1 hr	Unknown

Action

Chemical effect: Inhibits oxidation of iodine in thyroid gland, blocking iodine's ability to combine with tyrosine to form T_4. Also may prevent coupling of monoiodotyrosine and diiodotyrosine to form T_4 and T_3.
Therapeutic effect: Reduces thyroid hormone level.

Available forms

Tablets: 5 mg, 10 mg

NURSING PROCESS

🎓 Assessment

• Assess patient's thyroid condition before therapy and regularly thereafter.
• Monitor thyroid function studies.
• Monitor CBC and liver function periodically.
⚛ **ALERT:** Dosages higher than 30 mg daily increase risk of agranulocytosis, especially in patients older than age 40.
• Be alert for adverse reactions.
• Evaluate patient's and family's knowledge of drug therapy.

🔲 Nursing diagnoses

• Ineffective health maintenance related to presence of hyperthyroidism
• Ineffective immune protection related to drug-induced adverse hematologic reactions
• Deficient knowledge related to drug therapy

▶ Planning and implementation

• Pregnant women may need reduced dose as pregnancy progresses. Thyroid hormone may be added. Drug may be stopped during last weeks of pregnancy.
• Notify prescriber about signs and symptoms of hypothyroidism because dosage may need to be adjusted.
⚛ **ALERT:** If severe rash occurs or cervical lymph nodes become enlarged, stop drug and notify prescriber.
⚛ **ALERT:** Don't confuse methimazole with mebendazole or methazolamide.

Patient teaching
• Tell patient to take drug with meals.
• Warn patient to immediately report fever, sore throat, or mouth sores (signs of agranulocytosis); skin eruptions (sign of hypersensitivity); and anorexia, pruritus, right upper quadrant pain, and yellow skin or sclera (signs of hepatic dysfunction).
• Tell patient to ask prescriber about using iodized salt and eating shellfish.
• Warn patient against taking OTC cough medications; many contain iodine.
• Instruct patient to store drug in light-resistant container.

✔ Evaluation

• Patient has normal thyroid hormone level.
• Patient maintains normal hematologic parameters throughout therapy.
• Patient and family state understanding of drug therapy.

methocarbamol

(meth-oh-KAR-buh-mol)
Robaxin, Robaxin-750

Pharmacologic class: carbamate derivative of guaifenesin
Therapeutic class: centrally acting skeletal muscle relaxant
Pregnancy risk category: C

Indications and dosages

▶ **As adjunct in acute, painful musculoskeletal conditions.** *Adults:* 1.5 g P.O. q.i.d. for 2 to 3 days; then 1 g P.O. q.i.d., or not more than 500 mg (5 ml) I.M. into each buttock. Repeat q 8 hours, p.r.n. Or, 1 to 3 g daily (10 to 30 ml) I.V. directly into vein at 3 ml/minute, or 10 ml may be added to no more than 250 ml of

D_5W or normal saline solution. Maximum dosage is 3 g daily I.M. or I.V. for 3 consecutive days.

▶ **Supportive therapy in tetanus management.** *Adults:* 1 to 2 g by direct I.V., or 1 to 3 g as infusion q 6 hours.
Children: 15 mg/kg or 500 mg/m² I.V. q 6 hours.

▽ I.V. administration

● Dilute 10 ml of drug in no more than 250 ml of D_5W or normal saline solution injection.
● Infuse slowly; maximum rate is 300 mg (3 ml)/minute.
● Drug irritates veins. It may cause phlebitis and fainting and aggravate seizures if injected rapidly. Keep patient supine during infusion and for 15 minutes afterward. Drug is an irritant. Watch for irritation and infiltration; extravasation can cause tissue damage and necrosis.

Contraindications and precautions

● Contraindicated in patients hypersensitive to drug and in those with impaired kidney function or seizure disorder (injectable form).
● Use cautiously in patients with myasthenia gravis who are receiving anticholinesterases.
⚠ **Lifespan:** In women who are or may become pregnant, drug is not recommended, unless the benefits outweigh the risk. In breast-feeding women, use cautiously. In children, safety and effectiveness of drug haven't been established except in tetanus.

Adverse reactions

CNS: drowsiness, dizziness, light-headedness, headache, syncope, fever, mild muscle incoordination with I.M. or I.V. use, *seizures* with I.V. use.
CV: hypotension, *bradycardia* with I.M. or I.V. use, thrombophlebitis, flushing.
EENT: blurred vision.
GI: nausea, anorexia, GI upset, metallic taste.
GU: hematuria with I.V. use, discoloration of urine.
Hematologic: hemolysis.
Skin: urticaria, pruritus, rash.
Other: extravasation with I.V. use, *anaphylaxis* with I.M. or I.V. use.

Interactions

Drug-drug. *CNS depressants:* Increases CNS depression. Avoid using together.

Pyridostigmine bromide: Methocarbamol may inhibit the effects of pyridostigmine. Use methocarbamol cautiously in myasthenia gravis patients receiving anticholinesterases.
Drug-lifestyle. *Alcohol use:* Increases CNS depression. Discourage using together.

Effects on lab test results

● May decrease hemoglobin and hematocrit (with I.V. use).
● Drug may interfere with urine tests to determine 5-hydroxyindoleacetic acid and vanillylmandelic acid levels.

Pharmacokinetics

Absorption: Rapid and complete after P.O. administration; unknown after I.M. administration.
Distribution: Widely distributed throughout body.
Metabolism: Extensively metabolized in liver.
Excretion: Excreted primarily in urine. *Half-life:* 1 to 2 hours.

Route	Onset	Peak	Duration
P.O.	≤ 30 min	≤ 2 hr	Unknown
I.V.	Immediate	Immediate	Unknown
I.M.	Unknown	Unknown	Unknown

Action

Chemical effect: Unknown; probably modifies central perception of pain without modifying pain reflexes.
Therapeutic effect: Relieves skeletal muscle pain.

Available forms

Injection: 100 mg/ml
Tablets: 500 mg, 750 mg

NURSING PROCESS

✍ Assessment

● Assess patient's condition before therapy and regularly thereafter.
● Watch for orthostatic hypotension, especially with parenteral route.
● Monitor CBC periodically during prolonged therapy.
● Be alert for adverse reactions and drug interactions.
● If adverse GI reactions occur, monitor patient's hydration status.

Reactions may be *common*, uncommon, *life-threatening*, or COMMON AND LIFE-THREATENING.

- Evaluate patient's and family's knowledge of drug therapy.

⊞ Nursing diagnoses
- Acute pain related to underlying musculoskeletal condition
- Risk for deficient fluid volume related to drug-induced adverse GI reactions
- Deficient knowledge related to drug therapy

▶ Planning and implementation
- Give tablets with meals or milk.
- For patient with NG tube, crush tablets and mix in water or saline solution.
- For I.M. administration, give deep into upper outer quadrant of buttocks, with maximum of 5 ml in each buttock.
- ⑤ **ALERT:** Don't give drug S.C.
- For tetanus, methocarbamol is used with tetanus antitoxin, penicillin, tracheotomy, and aggressive supportive care. Long course of I.V. methocarbamol therapy is needed.
- Have epinephrine, antihistamines, and corticosteroids available.
- ⑤ **ALERT:** Don't confuse methocarbamol with mephobarbital.

Patient teaching
- Advise patient to get up slowly after parenteral administration.
- Tell patient that urine may turn green, black, or brown.
- Instruct patient to follow prescriber's orders regarding physical activity.
- Warn patient to avoid activities that require alertness until drug's CNS effects are known.
- Tell patient not to combine drug with alcohol or other CNS depressants. Instruct patient to avoid alcohol consumption during drug therapy.

✓ Evaluation
- Patient is free from pain.
- Patient maintains adequate hydration throughout therapy.
- Patient and family state understanding of drug therapy.

methotrexate (amethopterin, MTX)
(meth-oh-TREKS-ayt)
Trexall

methotrexate sodium
Methotrexate LPF, Rheumatrex Dose Pack

Pharmacologic class: antimetabolite (cell cycle–phase specific, S phase)
Therapeutic class: antineoplastic, immunosuppressant, antirheumatic
Pregnancy risk category: X

Indications and dosages

▶ **Trophoblastic tumors (choriocarcinoma, hydatidiform mole).** *Adults:* 15 to 30 mg P.O. or I.M. daily for 5 days. May repeat course after 1 or more weeks, based on response or toxicity. Three to five courses usually are used.
▶ **Acute lymphoblastic and lymphatic leukemia.** *Adults and children:* 3.3 mg/m² P.O. or I.M. daily for 4 to 6 weeks or until remission occurs; then 20 to 30 mg/m² P.O. or I.M. twice weekly. Or, 2.5 mg/kg I.V. q 14 days.
▶ **Meningeal leukemia.** *Adults and children older than age 12:* 12 mg/m² intrathecally, or an empirical dose of 15 mg q 2 to 5 days and repeat until cell count of CSF returns to normal, then give one additional dose. Or, 12 mg/m² once weekly for 2 weeks, then once monthly thereafter.
▶ **Burkitt's lymphoma (stage I or stage II).** *Adults:* 10 to 25 mg P.O. daily for 4 to 8 days with 1-week rest intervals.
▶ **Lymphosarcoma (stage III).** *Adults:* 0.625 to 2.5 mg/kg P.O., I.M., or I.V. daily.
▶ **Osteosarcoma.** *Adults:* Initially, 12 g/m² I.V. as 4-hour infusion. Subsequent doses 12 to 15 g/m² I.V. as 4-hour infusion given weeks 4, 5, 6, 7, 11, 12, 15, 16, 29, 30, 44, and 45 after surgery. Give with leucovorin, 15 mg P.O. q 6 hours for 10 doses 24 hours after start of methotrexate infusion.
▶ **Mycosis fungoides.** *Adults:* 2.5 to 10 mg P.O. daily, or 50 mg I.M. weekly, or 25 mg I.M. twice weekly.
▶ **Psoriasis.** *Adults:* 10 to 25 mg P.O., I.M., or I.V. as single weekly dose.
▶ **Rheumatoid arthritis.** *Adults:* Initially, 7.5 mg P.O. once weekly, or divided as 2.5 mg

P.O. q 12 hours for three doses once a week. Dosage may be gradually increased to maximum of 20 mg weekly.

Adults‡: 7.5 to 15 mg I.M. once weekly.

▶ **Head and neck carcinoma‡.** *Adults:* 40 to 60 mg/m^2 I.V. once weekly. Response to therapy is limited to 4 months.

▽ I.V. administration

• Follow facility policy to reduce risks. Preparation and administration of parenteral forms are linked to carcinogenic, mutagenic, and teratogenic risks.

• For reconstitution of lyophilized powders, reconstitute immediately before use, and discard unused drug. Dilute with D$_5$W or normal saline solution. Dilute the 20 mg vial to a concentration no greater than 25 mg/ml. Reconstitute 1 g vial with 19.4 ml of diluent for a maximum concentration of 50 mg/ml. For intrathecal injection, reconstitute to a concentration of 1 mg/ml.

• Liquid methotrexate sodium injection products, with preservatives, may be given undiluted. If further dilution is desired, use normal saline solution. Storage for 24 hours at 70° to 77° F (21° to 25° C) results in a product that is within 90% of label potency.

• Preservative-free liquid methotrexate sodium injection products may be given undiluted or may be further diluted with D$_5$W or normal saline solution.

• Drug may be given daily or weekly, depending on the disease.

• Store at room temperature. Protect from light.

Contraindications and precautions

• Contraindicated in patients hypersensitive to drug; and in those with psoriasis or rheumatoid arthritis who also have alcoholism, alcoholic liver, chronic liver disease, immunodeficiency syndromes, or blood dyscrasias.

• Use cautiously and at modified dosage in patients with impaired liver or kidney function, bone marrow suppression, aplasia, leukopenia, thrombocytopenia, or anemia. Also use cautiously in patients with infection, peptic ulceration, or ulcerative colitis and in debilitated patients.

⚖ **Lifespan:** In pregnant and breast-feeding women, drug is contraindicated. In children younger than age 2, safety hasn't been estab-

lished for uses other than treatment of cancers. In elderly patients, use cautiously.

Adverse reactions

CNS: *arachnoiditis* (within hours of intrathecal use), subacute neurotoxicity (may begin few weeks later), demyelination, *leukoencephalopathy.*

EENT: pharyngitis.

GI: *stomatitis, diarrhea,* enteritis, *intestinal perforation, nausea, vomiting.*

GU: nephropathy, TUBULAR NECROSIS, *renal impairment.*

Hematologic: WBC and platelet count nadirs on day 7, *anemia, leukopenia, thrombocytopenia.*

Hepatic: *acute toxicity, chronic toxicity, cirrhosis, hepatic fibrosis.*

Metabolic: hyperuricemia.

Musculoskeletal: osteoporosis in children with long-term use.

Respiratory: *pulmonary fibrosis, pulmonary interstitial infiltrates,* pneumonitis.

Skin: *urticaria,* pruritus, alopecia, hyperpigmentation, psoriatic lesions, rash, photosensitivity reactions.

Other: *sudden death.*

Interactions

Drug-drug. *Digoxin:* May decrease digoxin level. Monitor digoxin level.

Folic acid derivatives: Antagonizes methotrexate effect. Monitor patient.

NSAIDs, phenylbutazone, salicylates, sulfonamides: Increases methotrexate toxicity. Use together cautiously; monitor methotrexate levels.

Phenytoin: May decrease phenytoin level. Monitor phenytoin level.

Probenecid: May impair excretion of methotrexate causing increased levels, effects, and toxicity. Monitor level closely and decrease dosage accordingly.

Procarbazine: May increase nephrotoxicity of methotrexate. Monitor renal function closely.

Vaccines: Immunizations may be ineffective; may increase risk of disseminated infection with live-virus vaccines. Consult with prescriber about safe time to give vaccine.

Drug-food. *Food:* Delays drug absorption and reduces peak levels of methotrexate. Take on empty stomach.

Drug-lifestyle. *Alcohol use:* May increase hepatotoxicity. Discourage using together.

Reactions may be *common,* uncommon, *life-threatening,* or COMMON AND LIFE-THREATENING.

Sun exposure: Photosensitivity reactions may occur. Urge patient to avoid unprotected or prolonged exposure to sunlight.

Effects on lab test results

- May increase uric acid, BUN, creatinine, and liver enzyme levels.
- May decrease hemoglobin, hematocrit, and WBC, RBC, and platelet counts.

Pharmacokinetics

Absorption: Smaller P.O. doses are almost completely absorbed, but absorption of larger doses is incomplete and variable. I.M. doses are absorbed completely.
Distribution: Distributed widely throughout body with highest levels in kidneys, gallbladder, spleen, liver, and skin; about 50% bound to protein.
Metabolism: Metabolized only slightly in liver.
Excretion: Excreted primarily in urine. *Half-life:* 4 hours. *Terminal half-life for doses below 30 mg/m²:* About 3 to 10 hours. *Terminal half-life for doses of 30 mg/m² and above:* 8 to 15 hours.

Route	Onset	Peak	Duration
P.O.	Unknown	1-2 hr	Unknown
I.V., intrathecal	Unknown	Immediate	Unknown
I.M.	Unknown	30 min-1 hr	Unknown

Action

Chemical effect: Prevents reduction of folic acid to tetrahydrofolate by binding to dihydrofolate reductase.
Therapeutic effect: Kills certain cancer cells and reduces inflammation.

Available forms

Methotrexate
Tablets: 5 mg, 7.5 mg, 10 mg, 15 mg
Methotrexate sodium
Injection (lyophilized powder, preservative free): 20 mg, 1 g vials
Injection (preservative free): 25 mg/ml in 2, 4, 8, 10 ml vials
Injection (with preservatives): 25 mg/ml in 2, 10 ml vials
Tablets: 2.5 mg

NURSING PROCESS

Assessment
- Assess patient's condition before therapy and regularly thereafter.
- Perform baseline pulmonary function tests and repeat periodically.
- Monitor fluid intake and output daily.
- Monitor uric acid level.
- Watch for increases in AST, ALT, and alkaline phosphatase levels—signs of hepatic dysfunction.
- Monitor CBC regularly.
- Be alert for adverse reactions and drug interactions.
- Evaluate patient's and family's knowledge of drug therapy.

Nursing diagnoses
- Ineffective health maintenance related to underlying condition
- Ineffective immune protection related to drug-induced adverse hematologic reactions
- Deficient knowledge related to drug therapy

Planning and implementation
- For intrathecal use, only use 20-, 50-, or 100-mg vials of powder with no preservatives. Reconstitute immediately before using with preservative-free normal saline solution injection. Dilute to maximum of 1 mg/ml. Use only new vials of drug and diluent.
- CSF volume depends on age, not body surface area (BSA). Using BSA for dosing when treating meningeal leukemia has resulted in low CSF methotrexate level in children and high level and neurotoxicity in adults. Instead, a dosing regimen based on age may be used. Elderly patients may require a reduced dosage because CSF volume and turnover may decrease with age.
- Have patient drink 2 to 3 L of fluids daily.
- **ALERT:** Alkalinize urine by giving sodium bicarbonate tablets to prevent precipitation of drug, especially with high doses. Maintain urine pH at more than 6.5. If BUN level reaches 20 to 30 mg/dl or creatinine level reaches 1.2 to 2 mg/dl, reduce dosage. Report BUN level over 30 mg/dl or creatinine level over 2 mg/dl, and stop drug.
- Rash, redness, or ulcerations in mouth or adverse pulmonary reactions may signal serious complications. If ulcerative stomatitis or other

severe adverse GI reaction occurs or if pulmonary toxicity is detected, stop drug.
• Leucovorin rescue is used with high-dose (greater than 100 mg) protocols. This technique works against systemic toxicity but doesn't interfere with tumor cells' absorption of methotrexate.

Patient teaching
• Teach and encourage diligent mouth care to reduce risk of superinfection in mouth.
• Tell patient to take oral form on empty stomach.
• Advise patient to avoid prolonged exposure to sunlight and to wear protective clothing and use highly protective sunblock.
• Tell patient to continue leucovorin rescue despite severe nausea and vomiting and to tell prescriber. Parenteral leucovorin therapy may be needed.
• Warn patient to avoid becoming pregnant during and immediately after therapy because of risk of abortion or congenital anomalies.
• Instruct patient to avoid alcohol consumption during drug therapy.

☑ **Evaluation**
• Patient exhibits positive response to drug therapy.
• Patient doesn't experience serious complications when hematologic parameters are depressed during therapy.
• Patient and family state understanding of drug therapy.

methylcellulose
(meth-il-SEL-yoo-lohs)
Citrucel†, Citrucel Sugar Free†

Pharmacologic class: adsorbent
Therapeutic class: bulk-forming laxative
Pregnancy risk category: NR

Indications and dosages

▶ **Chronic constipation.** *Adults and children age 12 and older:* Usual dosage is up to 6 g daily, given in divided doses of 0.45 to 3 g per dose. Usually given one to three times daily with at least one full glass of liquid with each dose.
Children ages 6 to 11: Usual dosage is up to 3 g daily, given in divided doses of 0.45 to 1.5 g per

dose. Usually given one to three times daily with at least one full glass of liquid with each dose.

Contraindications and precautions

• Contraindicated in patients with abdominal pain, nausea, vomiting, or other symptoms of appendicitis or acute surgical abdomen and in those with intestinal obstruction or ulceration, disabling adhesions, or difficulty swallowing.
⚕ **Lifespan:** In pregnant and breast-feeding women, use cautiously.

Adverse reactions

GI: *nausea,* vomiting, and diarrhea with excessive use; esophageal, gastric, small intestinal, or colonic strictures when drug is chewed or taken in dry form; *abdominal cramps,* especially in severe constipation; laxative dependence with long-term or excessive use.

Interactions

None significant.

Effects on lab test results

None reported.

Pharmacokinetics

Absorption: Not absorbed.
Distribution: Distributed in intestine.
Metabolism: None.
Excretion: Excreted in feces.

Route	Onset	Peak	Duration
P.O.	12-24 hr	≤ 3 days	Varies

Action

Chemical effect: Absorbs water and expands to increase bulk and moisture content of stool, which encourages peristalsis and bowel movement.
Therapeutic effect: Relieves constipation.

Available forms

Powder: 105 mg/g, 196 mg/g

NURSING PROCESS

🔀 **Assessment**
• Assess patient's constipation before therapy and regularly thereafter.

• Before giving drug for constipation, determine whether patient has adequate fluid intake, exercise, and diet.
• Be alert for adverse reactions.
• If adverse GI reactions occur, monitor patient's hydration status.
• Evaluate patient's and family's knowledge of drug therapy.

⊞ Nursing diagnoses
• Constipation related to underlying condition
• Risk for deficient fluid volume related to drug-induced adverse GI reactions
• Deficient knowledge related to drug therapy

�longrightarrow Planning and implementation
• Drug is especially useful in debilitated patients and in those with postpartum constipation, irritable bowel syndrome, diverticulitis, or colostomies. Drug is also used to treat laxative abuse and to empty colon before barium enema.
⊛ ALERT: Don't confuse Citrucel with Citracal.
Patient teaching
• Tell patient to take drug with at least 8 ounces of pleasant-tasting liquid.
• Teach patient about dietary sources of bulk, such as bran and other cereals, fresh fruit, and vegetables.

☑ Evaluation
• Patient's constipation is relieved.
• Patient maintains adequate hydration throughout therapy.
• Patient and family state understanding of drug therapy.

---

methyldopa
(meth-il-DOH-puh)
Aldomet, Apo-Methyldopa ♦, Dopamet ♦, Hydopa ◊, Novomedopa ♦, Nu-Medopa ♦

methyldopate hydrochloride
Aldomet

Pharmacologic class: centrally acting antiadrenergic
Therapeutic class: antihypertensive
Pregnancy risk category: B (P.O.), C (I.V.)

Indications and dosages

▶ **Hypertension, hypertensive crisis.** *Adults:* Initially, 250 mg P.O. b.i.d. to t.i.d. in first 48 hours. Then increase p.r.n. q 2 days. Entire daily dose may be given in evening or h.s. If other antihypertensives are added to or deleted from therapy, adjust dosages, p.r.n. Maintenance dosage is 500 mg to 2 g daily in two to four divided doses. Maximum recommended daily dose is 3 g. Or, 250 to 500 mg I.V. q 6 hours, diluted in D_5W and given over 30 to 60 minutes. Maximum dosage is 1 g q 6 hours. Switch to P.O. antihypertensives as soon as possible. *Children:* Initially, 10 mg/kg P.O. daily in two to four divided doses. Or, 20 to 40 mg/kg I.V. daily in four divided doses. Increase dosage at least q 2 days until desired response occurs. Maximum 65 mg/kg, 2 g/m², or 3 g daily, whichever is least.

▽ I.V. administration

• Dilute appropriate dose in 100 ml D_5W. Alternatively, the required dose may be administered in 5% dextrose injection in a concentration of 10 mg/ml.
• Infuse slowly over 30 to 60 minutes.
• When control has been obtained, substitute oral therapy starting with the same parenteral dosage schedule.

Contraindications and precautions

• Contraindicated in patients hypersensitive to drug or any of its components (including sulfites) and in those with active hepatic disease (such as acute hepatitis) or active cirrhosis. Also contraindicated if previous methyldopa therapy has been linked to liver disorders. Coadministration with MAO inhibitors is contraindicated.
• Use cautiously in patients with renal impairment or a history of impaired liver function.
⚖ **Lifespan:** In breast-feeding women, use cautiously. In elderly patients, use cautiously because they may experience syncope related to increased sensitivity.

Adverse reactions

CNS: *sedation,* headache, asthenia, weakness, dizziness, *decreased mental acuity,* involuntary choreoathetoid movements, psychic disturbances, depression, nightmares.
CV: *bradycardia, heart failure,* orthostatic hypotension, aggravated angina, *myocarditis, edema.*

EENT: *nasal congestion.*
GI: nausea, vomiting, diarrhea, *pancreatitis, dry mouth.*
GU: impotence.
Hematologic: hemolytic anemia, *reversible agranulocytosis, thrombocytopenia.*
Hepatic: *hepatic necrosis.*
Metabolic: *weight gain.*
Skin: rash.
Other: gynecomastia, galactorrhea, *drug-induced fever.*

Interactions

Drug-drug. *Amphetamines, norepinephrine, phenothiazines, tricyclic antidepressants:* Possible decreased hypotensive effects. Monitor blood pressure carefully.
Antihypertensives, diuretics: Increases hypotensive effects. Decreased methyldopa dosage may be needed.
Barbiturates: May increase the potential for orthostatic hypotension. Monitor patient and blood pressure.
Haloperidol: May produce dementia and sedation. Use together cautiously.
Levodopa: May have additive hypotensive effects and may increase adverse CNS reactions. Monitor patient closely.
Lithium: May increase lithium levels. Monitor patient for increased lithium levels and lithium toxicity.
MAO inhibitors: May increase sympathetic stimulation, which may result in hypertensive crisis. Don't use together.
Oral iron therapy: May increase hypotensive effects. Use together cautiously; monitor blood pressure.
Drug-herb. *Capsicum:* May reduce antihypertensive effectiveness. Discourage using together.
Yohimbe: May interfere with blood pressure. Discourage using together.

Effects on lab test results

- May increase creatinine level.
- May decrease hemoglobin, hematocrit, liver function test results, and granulocyte, platelet, RBC, and WBC counts.
- May cause positive direct Coombs' test.

Pharmacokinetics

Absorption: Partial.
Distribution: Distributed throughout body; bound weakly to proteins.

Metabolism: Metabolized extensively in liver and intestinal cells.
Excretion: Absorbed drug excreted in urine; unabsorbed drug excreted in feces. *Half-life:* About 2 hours.

Route	Onset	Peak	Duration
P.O.	Unknown	4-6 hr	12-48 hr
I.V.	Unknown	4-6 hr	10-16 hr

Action

Chemical effect: Unknown; thought to involve inhibition of central vasomotor centers, thereby decreasing sympathetic outflow to heart, kidneys, and peripheral vasculature.
Therapeutic effect: Lowers blood pressure.

Available forms

methyldopa
Oral suspension: 250 mg/5 ml
Tablets: 125 mg, 250 mg, 500 mg
methyldopate hydrochloride
Injection: 50 mg/ml in 5- and 10-mg vials

NURSING PROCESS

✍ Assessment
- Assess patient's blood pressure before therapy and regularly thereafter.
- Monitor CBC with differential counts before therapy, q 2 weeks for first 3 months of therapy, and periodically thereafter.
- Monitor patient's Coombs' test results. In patient who has received this drug for several months, positive reaction to direct Coombs' test indicates hemolytic anemia.
- Be alert for adverse reactions and drug interactions.
- Evaluate patient's and family's knowledge of drug therapy.

⊕ Nursing diagnoses
- Ineffective health maintenance related to presence of hypertension
- Risk for injury related to drug-induced adverse CNS reactions
- Deficient knowledge related to drug therapy

▶ Planning and implementation
- Report involuntary choreoathetoid movements; drug may be stopped.
- Occasionally tolerance may occur, usually between the second and third months of therapy.

The addition of a diuretic or a dosage adjustment may be needed. If patient's response changes significantly, notify prescriber.
• If hypertension occurs after dialysis, notify prescriber; patient may need extra dose of drug.
• In a patient who needs blood transfusions, perform direct and indirect Coombs' tests to prevent crossmatching problems.
⑤ **ALERT:** Don't confuse Aldomet with Aldoril or Anzemet.

Patient teaching
• Advise patient to report signs of infection, such as fever and sore throat.
• Tell patient to report adverse reactions but not to stop taking drug.
• Tell patient to check his weight daily and to report weight gain of more than 5 lb (2.27 kg). Diuretics can relieve sodium and water retention.
• Warn patient that drug may impair mental alertness, particularly at start of therapy. Once-daily dose h.s. minimizes daytime drowsiness.
• Tell patient to rise slowly and avoid sudden position changes.
• Tell patient that dry mouth can be relieved with ice chips, sugarless gum, or hard candy.
• Advise patient that urine may turn dark in bleached toilet bowls.

☑ Evaluation
• Patient's blood pressure is normal.
• Patient doesn't experience injury as result of drug-induced adverse CNS reactions.
• Patient and family state understanding of drug therapy.

methylphenidate hydrochloride
(meth-il-FEN-ih-dayt high-droh-KLOR-ighd)
Concerta, Metadate CD, Metadate ER, Methylin, Methylin ER, Ritalin, Ritalin LA, Ritalin SR

Pharmacologic class: piperidine CNS stimulant
Therapeutic class: CNS stimulant (analeptic)
Pregnancy risk category: NR (Metadate ER, Methylin, Methylin ER, Ritalin, Ritalin SR); C (Concerta, Metadate CD, Ritalin LA)
Controlled substance schedule: II

Indications and dosages

▶ **Attention deficit hyperactivity disorder (ADHD).** *Children age 6 and older:* Initially 5 mg Metadate ER, Methylin, Methylin ER, Ritalin, or Ritalin SR P.O. b.i.d. before breakfast and lunch, increased in 5- to 10-mg increments weekly, p.r.n., until an optimum daily dose of 2 mg/kg is reached, not to exceed 60 mg/day. Ritalin SR, Metadate ER, and Methylin ER tablets may be used in place of tablets by calculating the dose of methylphenidate in intervals of 8 hours. Or, initially, 20 mg Metadate CD P.O. daily before breakfast, increased in 20 mg increments weekly to a maximum of 60 mg daily.
Children age 6 and older not currently on methylphenidate or for patients on stimulants other than methylphenidate: 18 mg P.O. extended-release Concerta once daily in the morning. Adjust dosage by 18 mg at weekly intervals to a maximum of 54 mg P.O. once daily in the morning.
Children age 6 and older currently on methylphenidate: If the previous methylphenidate daily dose is 5 mg b.i.d. or t.i.d. or 20 mg sustained-release, the recommended dose of Concerta is 18 mg P.O. q morning. If the previous methylphenidate daily dose is 10 mg b.i.d. or t.i.d. or 40 mg sustained-release, the recommended dose of Concerta is 36 mg P.O. q morning. If the previous methylphenidate daily dose is 15 mg b.i.d. or t.i.d. or 60 mg sustained-release, the recommended dose of Concerta is 54 mg P.O. q morning. Maximum daily dose is 54 mg.
Or, 20 mg Ritalin LA P.O. once daily. Adjust dosage in weekly 10-mg increments to a maximum of 60 mg daily. If the previous methylphenidate daily dose is 10 mg b.i.d. or 20 mg sustained-release, the recommended dose of Ritalin LA is 20 mg P.O. once daily. If the previous methylphenidate daily dose is 15 mg b.i.d., the recommended dose of Ritalin LA is 30 mg P.O. once daily. If the previous methylphenidate daily dose is 20 mg b.i.d. or 40 mg sustained-release, the recommended dose of Ritalin LA is 40 mg P.O. once daily. If the previous methylphenidate daily dose is 30 mg b.i.d. or 60 mg sustained-release, the recommended dose of Ritalin LA is 60 mg P.O. once daily.
▶ **Narcolepsy.** *Adults:* 10 mg Metadate ER, Methylin, Methylin ER, Ritalin, or Ritalin SR P.O. b.i.d. or t.i.d. 30 to 45 minutes before

meals. Dosage varies with patient needs; average dose is 40 to 60 mg P.O. daily. Ritalin SR, Metadate ER, and Methylin ER tablets may be used in place of methylphenidate tablets by calculating the dose of methylphenidate in intervals of 8 hours.

Contraindications and precautions

• Contraindicated in patients hypersensitive to drug and in those with glaucoma, motor tics, family history or diagnosis of Tourette syndrome, or history of marked anxiety, tension, or agitation. Ritalin, Ritalin SR, and Ritalin LA are contraindicated during treatment with MAO inhibitors and within 14 days of MAO inhibitor therapy.
• Use cautiously in patients with hypertension, history of drug abuse, seizures, or EEG abnormalities.
☀ **Lifespan:** In pregnant and breast-feeding women, use cautiously. In children younger than age 6, drug isn't recommended.

Adverse reactions

CNS: *nervousness, insomnia,* Tourette syndrome, dizziness, headache, akathisia, dyskinesia, *seizures.*
CV: *palpitations,* angina, *tachycardia,* changes in blood pressure and pulse rate.
EENT: dry throat, pharyngitis and sinusitis.
GI: vomiting; nausea, abdominal pain, and anorexia.
Hematologic: *thrombocytopenia, thrombocytopenic purpura, leukopenia.*
Metabolic: weight loss, delayed growth.
Respiratory: upper respiratory tract infection, cough.
Skin: rash, urticaria, exfoliative dermatitis, *erythema multiforme.*

Interactions

Drug-drug. *Anticonvulsants (phenytoin, phenobarbital, primidone):* Increases level of anticonvulsants. Patient may need dosage adjustment.
Centrally acting antihypertensives: Decreases antihypertensive effect. Monitor blood pressure.
Clonidine: May cause serious adverse events. Avoid using together.
Coumadin: May increase levels. Monitor PT and INR and monitor patient for bleeding.
Drugs that increase gastric pH (antacids, proton pump inhibitors, H_2 receptor antagonists): May

alter the release of Ritalin LA extended-release capsules. Separate administration times.
MAO inhibitors: May cause severe hypertension; possible hypertensive crisis. Don't use together or within 14 days of MAO inhibitor therapy.
Tricyclic antidepressants: Increases levels of these drugs. Avoid using together.
Drug-food. *Caffeine:* May increase amphetamine and related amine effects. Discourage using together.

Effects on lab test results

• May decrease hemoglobin, hematocrit, and WBC and platelet counts.

Pharmacokinetics

Absorption: Absorbed rapidly and completely after oral administration. Ritalin LA and Metadate CD have bimodal absorption (two distinct peaks).
Distribution: Unknown. Ritalin LA is 10% to 33% protein bound.
Metabolism: Metabolized by the liver.
Excretion: Excreted in urine.

Route	Onset	Peak	Duration
P.O.			
Concerta	Unknown	6-8 hr	8-12 hr
Metadate CD	Unknown	1st peak 1½ hr; 2nd peak 4½ hr	8-12 hr
Methylin, Ritalin	Unknown	2 hr	3-6 hr
Methylin ER, Ritalin-SR	Unknown	4¾ hr	3-8 hr
Ritalin LA	Unknown	1st peak 1-3 hr; 2nd peak 4-7 hr	8-12 hr

Action

Chemical effect: Unknown; probably promotes nerve impulse transmission by releasing stored norepinephrine from nerve terminals in brain. Main site of activity appears to be cerebral cortex and reticular activating system. In hyperkinetic children, drug has paradoxical calming effect.
Therapeutic effect: Promotes calmness and prevents sleep.

Available forms

Tablets (Ritalin, Methylin): 5 mg, 10 mg, 20 mg

Extended-release
Capsules (Metadate CD): 20 mg
Capsules (Ritalin LA): 20 mg, 30 mg, 40 mg
Tablets (Concerta): 18 mg, 27 mg, 36 mg,
54 mg
Tablets (Metadate ER, Methylin ER): 10 mg,
20 mg
Sustained-release
Oral solution (Methylin): 5 mg/5 ml, 10 mg/
5 ml
Tablets (Ritalin-SR): 20 mg

NURSING PROCESS

🗒 Assessment
• Assess patient's condition before therapy and regularly thereafter.
• Drug may precipitate Tourette syndrome in children. Monitor effects, especially at start of therapy.
• Observe patient for signs of excessive stimulation. Monitor blood pressure.
• Monitor results of periodic CBC, differential, and platelet counts with long-term use.
• Monitor height and weight in child receiving prolonged therapy. Drug may delay growth, but child will attain normal height when drug is stopped.
⊛ **ALERT:** Chronic abuse can lead to marked tolerance and psychic dependence. Careful supervision is needed. Monitor patient for tolerance or psychological dependence.
• Be alert for adverse reactions and drug interactions.
• Evaluate patient's and family's knowledge of drug therapy.

🗹 Nursing diagnoses
• Ineffective health maintenance related to underlying condition
• Disturbed sleep pattern related to drugnduced insomnia
• Deficient knowledge related to drug therapy

▷ Planning and implementation
⊛ **ALERT:** This is drug of choice for ADHD and is usually stopped after puberty.
• Don't use to prevent fatigue.
• Metadate CD may be swallowed whole, or the contents of the capsule may be sprinkled onto a small amount of applesauce and given immediately.

• Give at least 6 hours before bedtime to prevent insomnia. Give after meals to reduce appetite suppression.
• Ritalin SR tablets have a duration of about 8 hours and may be used in place of regular tablets when 8-hour dosage of sustained release tablets corresponds to the adjusted dosage of the regular tablets.
⊛ **ALERT:** Don't confuse Ritalin with Rifadin.
Patient teaching
• Tell patient to swallow Ritalin SR and Concerta tablets whole and not to chew or crush them. Metadate CD may be swallowed whole, or the contents of the capsule may be sprinkled onto a small amount of applesauce and given immediately.
• Warn patient to avoid activities that require alertness until CNS effects of drug are known.
• Tell patient to avoid caffeine.
• Advise patient with seizure disorder to notify prescriber.
• Inform patient that he will need more rest as drug effects wear off.
• Warn patient that the shell of the Concerta tablet may appear in the stool.

🗹 Evaluation
• Patient responds positively to drug therapy.
• Patient doesn't experience insomnia during therapy.
• Patient and family state understanding of drug therapy.

methylprednisolone
(meth-il-pred-NIS-uh-lohn)
Medrol, Meprolone

methylprednisolone acetate
depMedalone 40, depMedalone 80, Depo-Medrol, Depopred-40, Depopred-80

methylprednisolone sodium succinate
A-MethaPred, Solu-Medrol

Pharmacologic class: glucocorticoid
Therapeutic class: anti-inflammatory, immunosuppressant
Pregnancy risk category: NR

Indications and dosages

▶ **Severe inflammation or immunosuppression.** *Adults:* 2 to 60 mg methylprednisolone P.O. daily in four divided doses. Or, 10 to 80 mg methylprednisolone acetate I.M. daily, or 4 to 80 mg into joint or soft tissue, p.r.n. May repeat q 1 to 5 weeks p.r.n. Or, 10 to 250 mg methylprednisolone succinate I.M. or I.V. q 4 hours. *Children:* 0.03 to 0.2 mg/kg or 1 to 6.25 mg/m² methylprednisolone succinate I.M. once or twice daily. Although dosage may be reduced in infants and children, give dose based more on severity of condition and response by age or size. Don't give less than 0.5 mg/kg daily.

▶ **Shock.** *Adults:* 100 to 250 mg methylprednisolone succinate I.V. at 2- to 6-hour intervals. Or, 30 mg/kg I.V. initially, repeat q 4 to 6 hours, p.r.n. Continue therapy for 2 to 3 days or until patient is stable.

▶ **Acute exacerbations of multiple sclerosis.** *Adults:* Give 200 mg I.M. daily for 2 weeks, followed by 800 mg q other day for 1 month.

▶ **Severe lupus nephritis‡.** *Adults:* 1 g methylprednisolone succinate I.V. over 1 hour for 3 days. Continue orally at 0.5 mg/kg daily using prednisone or prednisolone. *Children:* 30 mg/kg methylprednisolone succinate I.V. q other day for 6 doses.

▶ **To minimize motor and sensory defects caused by acute spinal cord injury‡.** *Adults:* Initially, 30 mg/kg I.V. over 15 minutes followed in 45 minutes by 5.4 mg/kg/hour I.V. infusion for 23 hours.

▶ **Adjunct to moderate-to-severe** *Pneumocystis carinii* **pneumonia‡.** *Adults and children older than age 13:* 30 mg I.V. b.i.d. for 5 days; 30 mg I.V. daily for 5 days; 15 mg I.V. daily for 11 days (or until completion of anti-infective regimen).

▼ I.V. administration

● Compatible solutions include D₅W, normal saline solution, and D₅W in normal saline solution.

● Use within 48 hours after mixing.

● Give only methylprednisolone sodium succinate I.V., never the acetate form. Reconstitute according to manufacturer's directions using supplied diluent or bacteriostatic water for injection with benzyl alcohol.

● For direct injection, inject diluted drug into vein or I.V. line containing free-flowing compatible solution over at least 1 minute. For treatment of shock, give massive doses over at least 10 minutes to prevent arrhythmias and circulatory collapse.

● When giving as intermittent or continuous infusion, dilute solution according to manufacturer's instructions and give over prescribed duration. If used for continuous infusion, change solution q 24 hours.

Contraindications and precautions

● Contraindicated in patients allergic to drug or its components and in those with systemic fungal infections.

● Use cautiously in patients with GI ulceration or renal disease, hypertension, osteoporosis, diabetes mellitus, hypothyroidism, cirrhosis, diverticulitis, nonspecific ulcerative colitis, recent intestinal anastomoses, thromboembolic disorders, seizures, myasthenia gravis, heart failure, tuberculosis, ocular herpes simplex, emotional instability, or psychotic tendencies.

⚖ **Lifespan:** In pregnant women, use cautiously. For breast-feeding women, drug isn't recommended. In premature infants, methylprednisolone acetate and methylprednisolone succinate are contraindicated because they contain benzyl alcohol.

Adverse reactions

CNS: *euphoria, insomnia,* psychotic behavior, pseudotumor cerebri.

CV: *heart failure,* hypertension, edema, ***thromboembolism, fatal arrest or circulatory collapse*** after rapid administration of large I.V. doses.

EENT: cataracts, glaucoma.

GI: peptic ulceration, GI irritation, increased appetite, ***pancreatitis.***

Metabolic: hypokalemia, hyperglycemia, carbohydrate intolerance, growth suppression in children.

Musculoskeletal: muscle weakness, osteoporosis.

Skin: hirsutism, delayed wound healing, acne, various skin eruptions.

Other: susceptibility to infections, ***acute adrenal insufficiency*** with increased stress (infection, surgery, or trauma) or abrupt withdrawal after long-term therapy.

Interactions

Drug-drug. *Anticholinesterases:* May cause profound weakness. Use together cautiously.
Aspirin, indomethacin, other NSAIDs: Increases risk of GI distress and bleeding. Give together cautiously.
Cyclosporins: May increase risk of adverse events and convulsions. May need to increase methylprednisolone dose.
CYP 3A4 inducers (barbiturates, phenytoin, rifampin, ephedrine): Decreases corticosteroid effect. Increase corticosteroid dosage.
CYP 3A4 inhibitors (ketoconazole, macrolides): May decrease glucocorticoid clearance. Adjust dosage, if needed.
Hormonal contraceptives: Reduces metabolism of corticosteroids. Dose of steroid may need to be reduced.
Oral anticoagulants: Alters dosage requirements. Monitor PT and INR closely.
Potassium-depleting drugs (such as thiazide and loop diuretics): Enhances potassium-wasting effects. Monitor potassium level.
Skin-test antigens: Decreases response. Defer skin testing until therapy is completed.
Toxoids, live-virus vaccines: Decreases antibody response and increases risk of neurologic complications. Avoid using together.

Effects on lab test results

• May increase glucose and cholesterol levels. May decrease potassium and calcium levels.

Pharmacokinetics

Absorption: Absorbed readily after P.O. administration; sodium succinate is absorbed rapidly while acetate is absorbed much more slowly.
Distribution: Distributed rapidly to muscle, liver, skin, intestines, and kidneys.
Metabolism: Metabolized in liver.
Excretion: Excreted primarily in urine; insignificant amount excreted in feces. *Half-life:* 18 to 36 hours.

Route	Onset	Peak	Duration
P.O.	Rapid	1-2 hr	30-36 hr
I.V.	Immediate	Immediate	Unknown
I.M.	6-48 hr	Unknown	4-8 days

Action

Chemical effect: Not clear; decreases inflammation, mainly by stabilizing leukocyte lysosomal membranes. Drug also suppresses immune response, stimulates bone marrow, and influences protein, fat, and carbohydrate metabolism.
Therapeutic effect: Relieves inflammation and suppresses immune system function.

Available forms

methylprednisolone
Tablets: 2 mg, 4 mg, 8 mg, 16 mg, 24 mg, 32 mg
methylprednisolone acetate
Injection (suspension): 20 mg/ml, 40 mg/ml, 80 mg/ml
methylprednisolone sodium succinate
Injection: 40-, 125-, 500-, 1,000-, and 2,000-mg vials

NURSING PROCESS

🏥 Assessment

• Assess patient's condition before therapy and regularly thereafter.
• Watch for enhanced response in patient with hypothyroidism or cirrhosis.
• Monitor patient's weight, blood pressure, electrolyte levels (especially glucose), and sleep patterns. Euphoria may initially interfere with sleep, but patient typically adjusts to drug after 1 to 3 weeks.
• Be alert for adverse reactions and drug interactions.
• Evaluate patient's and family's knowledge of drug therapy.

💠 Nursing diagnoses

• Ineffective health maintenance related to underlying condition
• Risk for injury related to drug-induced adverse reactions
• Deficient knowledge related to drug therapy

⟩ Planning and implementation

⚘ ALERT: Salt formulations are not interchangeable.
• Drug may be used for alternate-day therapy.
• For better results and less risk of toxicity, give once-daily dose in morning.
• Avoid S.C. injection because atrophy and sterile abscesses may occur.
• Give with food when possible. Critically ill patients may also need antacid or H_2-receptor antagonist therapy.

• Give I.M. injections deep into gluteal muscle.
• Dermal atrophy may occur with large doses of acetate salt. Use multiple small injections rather than single large dose and rotate injection sites.
⊛ **ALERT:** Don't give intrathecally because severe adverse reactions may occur.
• Don't use acetate salt when immediate onset of action is needed.
• Discard reconstituted solutions after 48 hours.
• Always adjust to lowest effective dose.
• Give potassium supplements, p.r.n.
• Gradually reduce drug dosage after long-term therapy. Abrupt withdrawal may cause inflammation, fatigue, weakness, arthralgia, fever, dizziness, lethargy, depression, fainting, orthostatic hypotension, dyspnea, anorexia, and hypoglycemia. After prolonged use, sudden withdrawal may be fatal.
⊛ **ALERT:** Don't confuse Solu-Medrol with Solu-Cortef.
⊛ **ALERT:** Don't confuse methylprednisolone with medroxyprogesterone.

Patient teaching
• Tell patient most adverse reactions are dose- or duration-dependent.
• Tell patient not to stop drug abruptly or without prescriber's consent.
• Teach patient signs of early adrenal insufficiency: fatigue, muscle weakness, joint pain, fever, anorexia, nausea, dyspnea, dizziness, and fainting.
• Instruct patient to wear or carry medical identification.
• Warn patient receiving long-term therapy about cushingoid symptoms, and tell him to report sudden weight gain or swelling. Suggest exercise or physical therapy, and advise him to ask prescriber about vitamin D or calcium supplements.

✓ **Evaluation**
• Patient responds positively to drug therapy.
• Patient sustains no injury from adverse reactions.
• Patient and family state understanding of drug therapy.

metoclopramide hydrochloride
(met-oh-KLOH-preh-mighd high-droh-KLOR-ighd)
Apo-Metoclop ♦ , Clopra, Maxeran ♦ , Maxolon, Octamide, Octamide PFS, Pramin ◇ , Reclomide, Reglan

Pharmacologic class: para-aminobenzoic acid derivative; dopamine-receptor agonist
Therapeutic class: antiemetic, GI stimulant
Pregnancy risk category: B

Indications and dosages

▶ **Prevention or reduction of nausea and vomiting induced by cisplatin alone or with other chemotherapeutics.** *Adults:* 1 to 2 mg/kg I.V. 30 minutes before chemotherapy; then repeat q 2 hours for two doses; then q 3 hours for three doses.
▶ **Prevention or reduction of postoperative nausea and vomiting.** *Adults:* 10 to 20 mg I.M. near end of surgical procedure, repeat q 4 to 6 hours, p.r.n.
▶ **To facilitate small-bowel intubation and aid in radiologic examinations.** *Adults and children older than age 14:* 10 mg (2 ml) I.V. as single dose over 1 to 2 minutes.
Children ages 6 to 14: 2.5 to 5 mg I.V. (0.5 to 1 ml).
Children younger than age 6: 0.1 mg/kg I.V.
▶ **Delayed gastric emptying caused by diabetic gastroparesis.** *Adults:* 10 mg P.O. for mild symptoms; slow I.V. infusion for severe symptoms 30 minutes before meals and h.s. for 2 to 8 weeks, depending on response.
▶ **Gastroesophageal reflux disease.** *Adults:* 10 to 15 mg P.O. q.i.d., p.r.n., 30 minutes before meals and h.s.
⧄ **Adjust-a-dose:** For patients with renal impairment, if creatinine clearance is less than 40 ml/minute, reduce initial dose by 50% and adjust dose, as tolerated.

▽ I.V. administration

• Give doses of 10 mg or less by direct injection over 1 to 2 minutes.
• Dilute doses larger than 10 mg in 50 ml of compatible diluent and infuse over at least 15 minutes.
• Drug is compatible with D_5W, normal saline solution injection, dextrose 5% in half-normal saline solution, Ringer's injection, and lactated

Ringer's injection. Normal saline is the preferred diluent because drug is most stable in this solution.
• If giving infusion mixture within 24 hours, protection from light is unnecessary. If protected from light and refrigerated, it's stable for 48 hours.
• Closely monitor blood pressure.

Contraindications and precautions

• Contraindicated in patients hypersensitive to drug; patients allergic to procainamide may also be allergic to metoclopramide. Also contraindicated in patients taking medications that are likely to cause extrapyramidal reactions (phenothiazines, butyrophenones), in those for whom stimulation of GI motility might be dangerous (such as those with hemorrhage), and in those with pheochromocytoma or seizure disorder.
• Use cautiously in patients with a history of depression, Parkinson's disease, hypertension, or renal impairment.
• Safety and effectiveness haven't been established for therapy that lasts longer than 12 weeks.
⚖ Lifespan: In pregnant and breast-feeding women, use cautiously. In elderly patients, use cautiously and at a reduced dose.

Adverse reactions

CNS: *restlessness, anxiety, drowsiness,* fatigue, fever, *lassitude,* insomnia, **suicide ideation, seizures,** headache, dizziness, extrapyramidal symptoms, tardive dyskinesia, dystonic reactions, sedation.
CV: transient hypertension.
GI: nausea, bowel disturbances.
Hematologic: *agranulocytosis, neutropenia.*
Skin: rash.
Other: prolactin secretion, loss of libido.

Interactions

Drug-drug. *Acetaminophen, aspirin, cyclosporine, diazepam, levodopa, lithium, tetracycline:* Increases absorption of these drugs. Monitor patient for adverse effects.
Anticholinergics, opioid analgesics: Antagonizes GI motility effects of metoclopramide. Use together cautiously.
Butyrophenones, phenothiazines: Increases risk of extrapyramidal effects. Avoid using together.

CNS depressants: May cause additive CNS depression. Avoid using together.
Digoxin: Decreases absorption of digoxin. Monitor digoxin levels.
Insulin: Metoclopramide influences the rate of absorption of food. Adjust insulin dosage, if needed.
Drug-lifestyle. *Alcohol use:* May cause additive CNS depression. Discourage using together.

Effects on lab test results

• May increase aldosterone and prolactin levels.
• May decrease neutrophil and granulocyte counts.

Pharmacokinetics

Absorption: After P.O. dose, rapid and complete. After I.M. dose, about 74% to 96% bioavailable.
Distribution: Distributed to most body tissues and fluids, including brain.
Metabolism: Not metabolized extensively; small amount metabolized in liver.
Excretion: Excreted in urine and feces. *Half-life:* 4 to 6 hours.

Route	Onset	Peak	Duration
P.O.	30-60 min	1-2 hr	1-2 hr
I.V.	1-3 min	Unknown	1-2 hr
I.M.	10-15 min	Unknown	1-2 hr

Action

Chemical effect: Stimulates motility of upper GI tract by increasing lower esophageal sphincter tone and blocks dopamine receptors at chemoreceptor trigger zone.
Therapeutic effect: Prevents or minimizes nausea and vomiting from chemotherapy or surgery. Also reduces gag reflex in small-bowel intubation and radiologic examinations, improves gastric emptying when diabetic gastroparesis is present, and reduces gastric reflux.

Available forms

Injection: 5 mg/ml
Syrup: 5 mg/5 ml (sugar-free), 10 mg/ml
Tablets: 5 mg, 10 mg

NURSING PROCESS

🔖 Assessment

• Assess patient's condition before therapy and regularly thereafter.

- Monitor blood pressure frequently in patient taking I.V. form of drug.
- Be alert for adverse reactions and drug interactions.
- Evaluate patient's and family's knowledge of drug therapy.

⊕ Nursing diagnoses
- Risk for deficient fluid volume related to nausea and vomiting
- Risk for injury related to drug-induced adverse CNS reactions
- Deficient knowledge related to drug therapy

⊇ Planning and implementation
- Dilute oral concentrate just before administration in water, juice, or carbonated beverage. Semisolid food such as applesauce or pudding also may be used.
- Commercially available preparation may be used without further dilution for I.M. use.
- ⊛ **ALERT:** Diphenhydramine 25 mg I.V. counteracts extrapyramidal effects caused by high drug doses.

Patient teaching
- Instruct patient to avoid alcohol consumption during drug therapy.
- Advise patient to avoid activities requiring alertness for 2 hours after taking each dose.

☑ Evaluation
- Patient responds positively to drug and doesn't develop fluid volume deficit.
- Patient doesn't experience injury from adverse reactions.
- Patient and family state understanding of drug therapy.

metolazone
(meh-TOH-luh-zohn)
Mykrox, Zaroxolyn

Pharmacologic class: quinazoline derivative (thiazide-like) diuretic
Therapeutic class: diuretic, antihypertensive
Pregnancy risk category: B

Indications and dosages

▶ **Edema in heart failure or renal disease.**
Adults: 5 to 20 mg Zaroxolyn P.O. daily.

▶ **Mild to moderate essential hypertension.**
Adults: Initially, 2.5 to 5 mg Zaroxolyn P.O. daily until desired therapeutic response has been achieved; then reduce daily dose. Maintenance dosage determined by patient's blood pressure. Or, 0.5 mg Mykrox P.O. once daily in morning; increase to 1 mg P.O. daily, if needed. If response is inadequate, add another antihypertensive.

Contraindications and precautions

- Contraindicated in patients hypersensitive to thiazides or other sulfonamide-derived drugs and in patients with anuria, hepatic coma, or precoma.
- Use cautiously in patients with impaired kidney or liver function.
- ⚖ **Lifespan:** In pregnant women, drug isn't recommended. In breast-feeding women and in children, safety of drug hasn't been established.

Adverse reactions

CNS: dizziness, headache, fatigue.
CV: volume depletion, orthostatic hypotension, palpitations, chest pain.
GI: anorexia, nausea, *pancreatitis.*
GU: nocturia, polyuria, frequent urination.
Hematologic: *aplastic anemia, agranulocytosis, leukopenia, thrombocytopenia,* hyperlipidemia.
Hepatic: *hepatic encephalopathy.*
Metabolic: hyperglycemia and glucose tolerance impairment; hyperuricemia, fluid and electrolyte imbalances, including hypokalemia, *metabolic alkalosis,* hypercalcemia, and dilutional hyponatremia and hypochloremia, dehydration.
Musculoskeletal: acute gouty attacks, muscle cramps, swelling.
Skin: dermatitis, photosensitivity reactions, rash.
Other: hypersensitivity reactions.

Interactions

Drug-drug. *Amphotericin B, corticosteroids:* May potentiate hypokalemia. Monitor potassium level.
Barbiturates, opioids: Increases orthostatic hypotensive effect. Monitor blood pressure closely.
Bumetanide, ethacrynic acid, furosemide, torsemide: May cause excessive diuretic re-

sponse resulting in serious electrolyte abnormalities or dehydration. Adjust doses carefully while monitoring patient closely.

Cholestyramine, colestipol: Decreases intestinal absorption of thiazides. Separate doses by 1 hour.

Diazoxide: Increases antihypertensive, hyperglycemic, and hyperuricemic effects. Use together cautiously.

Digoxin: Increases risk of digitalis toxicity from metolazone-induced hypokalemia. Monitor potassium and digitalis levels.

Insulin, sulfonylureas: Increases requirements in diabetic patients. Dosages may need to be adjusted.

Lithium: Decreases lithium clearance, increasing risk of lithium toxicity. Avoid giving together.

NSAIDs: Increases risk of NSAID-induced renal impairment. Monitor patient for signs of renal impairment.

Drug-lifestyle. *Alcohol use:* Increases orthostatic hypotensive effect. Discourage using together.

Sun exposure: Photosensitivity reactions may occur. Urge patient to avoid unprotected or prolonged exposure to sunlight.

Effects on lab test results

- May increase glucose, calcium, cholesterol, pH, bicarbonate, uric acid, and triglyceride levels. May decrease potassium, sodium, magnesium, and chloride levels.
- May decrease hemoglobin, hematocrit, and granulocyte, platelet, and WBC counts.

Pharmacokinetics

Absorption: About 65% in healthy people; in cardiac patients, falls to 40%. Rate and extent vary among preparations. Mykrox is more rapidly available and completely bioavailable than Zaroxolyn.

Distribution: 50% to 70% erythrocyte-bound; 33% protein-bound.

Metabolism: Insignificant.

Excretion: 70% to 95% excreted unchanged in urine. *Half-life:* About 14 hours.

Route	Onset	Peak	Duration
P.O.	1 hr	2-8 hr	12-24 hr

Action

Chemical effect: Increases sodium and water excretion by inhibiting sodium reabsorption in cortical diluting site of ascending loop of Henle.

Therapeutic effect: Promotes water and sodium elimination and lowers blood pressure.

Available forms

Tablets (Mykrox): 0.5 mg
Tablets (Zaroxolyn): 2.5 mg, 5 mg, 10 mg

NURSING PROCESS

Assessment

- Assess patient's condition before therapy and regularly thereafter. In hypertensive patients, therapeutic response may be delayed several days.
- Unlike thiazide diuretics, drug is effective in patient with decreased kidney function.
- Monitor fluid intake and output, weight, blood pressure, and electrolyte level.
- Monitor uric acid level, especially in patient with history of gout.
- Be alert for adverse reactions and drug interactions.
- Evaluate patient's and family's knowledge of drug therapy.

Nursing diagnoses

- Excessive fluid volume related to presence of edema
- Risk for injury related to presence of hypertension
- Deficient knowledge related to drug therapy

Planning and implementation

⑤ **ALERT:** Zaroxolyn and Mykrox are not therapeutically equivalent or interchangable.
- Drug may be used with potassium-sparing diuretic to prevent potassium loss.
- Give drug in morning to prevent nocturia.
- Drug is used as adjunct in furosemide-resistant edema.

⑤ **ALERT:** Don't confuse Zaroxolyn with Zarontin or Metolazone with Metoprolol.

⑤ **ALERT:** Mykrox tablets are more rapidly and completely absorbed than other brands, mimicking oral solution. Don't interchange Mykrox with Zaroxolyn tablets.

Patient teaching

- Advise patient to avoid sudden posture changes and to rise slowly to avoid orthostatic hypotension.
- Advise patient to wear protective clothing, avoid prolonged exposure to sunlight, and use sunblock to prevent photosensitivity reactions.
- Instruct patient to avoid alcohol consumption during drug therapy.

☑ Evaluation

- Patient doesn't have edema.
- Patient's blood pressure is normal.
- Patient and family state understanding of drug therapy.

metoprolol succinate
(meh-TOH-pruh-lol SUHK-seh-nayt)
Toprol-XL

metoprolol tartrate
(meh-TOH-pruh-lol TAR-trayt)
Apo-Metoprolol ♦ , Apo-Metoprolol (Type L) ♦ , Betaloc ♦ ◇ , Betaloc Durules ♦ , Lopresor ♦ , Lopressor, Minax ◇ , Novometoprol ♦ , Nu-Metop ♦

Pharmacologic class: beta₁ selective blocker
Therapeutic class: antihypertensive, adjunct treatment of acute MI
Pregnancy risk category: C

Indications and dosages

▶ **Hypertension.** *Adults:* Initially, 50 to 100 mg metoprolol succinate P.O. (extended-release tablets) once daily. Adjust dosage as needed and tolerated at intervals of not less than 1 week to maximum of 400 mg daily. For metoprolol tartrate, initially, 50 to 100 mg P.O. daily in single or divided doses; usual maintenance dosage is 100 to 450 mg daily.
▶ **Early intervention in acute MI.** *Adults:* 5 mg metoprolol tartrate I.V. push q 2 to 5 minutes to a total of 15 mg. Then, 15 minutes after last dose, 25 to 50 mg P.O. q 6 hours for 48 hours. Maintenance dosage is 100 mg P.O. b.i.d.
▶ **Angina pectoris.** *Adults:* Initially, 100 mg metoprolol succinate P.O. (extended-release tablets) daily as single dose. Dosage increased at weekly intervals until adequate response or pronounced decrease in heart rate is seen. Daily

dose beyond 400 mg hasn't been studied. Or, 100 mg metoprolol tartrate P.O. in two divided doses. Dosage increased at weekly intervals until adequate response or pronounced decrease in heart rate is seen. Maintenance dosage is 100 to 400 mg P.O. daily.
▶ **Stable, symptomatic heart failure (New York Heart Association class II) resulting from ischemia, hypertension, or cardiomyopathy.** *Adults:* 25 mg metoprolol succinate P.O. (extended-release) once daily for 2 weeks. In patients with more severe heart failure, start with 12.5 mg P.O. (extended-release) once daily for 2 weeks. Double the dose q 2 weeks as tolerated to a maximum of 200 mg daily.
▶ **Atrial tachyarrhythmias after acute MI‡.** *Adults:* 2.5 to 5 mg I.V. q 2 to 5 minutes to control rate up to 15 mg over a 10- to 15-minute period. Once heart rate is controlled or normal sinus rhythm is restored, therapy may continue with 50 mg P.O. b.i.d. for 24 hours starting 15 minutes after the last I.V. dose. Increase dosage to 100 mg P.O. b.i.d. as tolerated. Stop drug when therapeutic response is achieved or if systolic blood pressure is less than 100 mm Hg or heart rate is less than 50 beats/minute.
▶ **Unstable angina or non–ST-segment elevation MI at high risk for ischemic events‡.** *Adults:* 5 mg I.V. bolus q 5 minutes for 3 doses. May continue therapy with P.O. regimen.

▼ I.V. administration

- Give drug undiluted and by direct injection.
- Don't mix this drug with other drugs. Drug is only compatible with meperidine hydrochloride or morphine sulfate, or with alteplase infusions at Y-site connection.
- Store drug at room temperature and protect from light. Discard solution if it is discolored or contains particulates.

Contraindications and precautions

- Contraindicated in patients hypersensitive to drug or other beta blockers and in those with sinus bradycardia, heart block greater than first-degree, cardiogenic shock, or overt cardiac failure when used to treat hypertension or angina. When used to treat MI, drug is also contraindicated in patients with heart rate below 45 beats/minute, second- or third-degree heart block, PR interval of 0.24 second or more with first-degree heart block, systolic blood pressure under

---

100 mm Hg, or moderate-to-severe cardiac failure.

• Use cautiously in patients with heart failure, diabetes, or respiratory or hepatic disease.

🔆 Lifespan: In pregnant women, use cautiously. In breast-feeding women, drug isn't recommended. In children, safety of drug hasn't been established.

Adverse reactions

CNS: fatigue, lethargy, dizziness, fever.
CV: *bradycardia, hypotension, heart failure, AV block,* peripheral vascular disease.
GI: nausea, vomiting, diarrhea.
Musculoskeletal: arthralgia.
Respiratory: dyspnea, *bronchospasm.*
Skin: rash.

Interactions

Drug-drug. *Amobarbital, aprobarbital, butabarbital, butalbital, mephobarbital, pentobarbital, phenobarbital, primidone, secobarbital:* May reduce the effects of metoprolol. Consider an increased beta blocker dose.
Chlorpromazine: Decreases hepatic clearance. Monitor patient for increased beta blocking effect.
Cimetidine: May increase the pharmacologic effects of beta blocker. Consider another H₂ agonist or decrease the dose of beta blocker.
CYP 2D6 inhibitors, such as quinidine, fluoxetine, paroxetine, propafenone, amiodarone: May increase metoprolol levels. Monitor patient for increased adverse effects.
Digoxin, diltiazem: May cause excessive bradycardia and increase depressant effect on myocardium. Use together cautiously.
Hydralazine: May increase levels and effects of both drugs. Monitor patient closely. Adjust dosage of either drug, if needed.
Indomethacin: Decreases antihypertensive effect. Monitor blood pressure and adjust dosage.
Insulin, oral antidiabetics: Alters dosage requirements in previously stabilized diabetic patient. Observe patient carefully.
I.V. lidocaine: May reduce metabolism of lidocaine, increasing the risk of toxicity. Give bolus doses of lidocaine at a slower rate and monitor lidocaine levels closely.
MAO inhibitors: Bradycardia may develop during use with MAO inhibitors. Monitor ECG and patient closely.

Other antihypertensives: May produce additive effects. Monitor blood pressure.
Prazosin: May increase the risk of orthostatic hypotension in the early phases of use together. Assist patient to stand slowly until effects are known.
Rifampin: Increases metabolism of metoprolol. Monitor patient for decreased effect.
Thioamines: Pharmacokinetics of metoprolol may be altered, increasing the effects of metoprolol. Monitor patient.
Thyroid hormones: Actions of metoprolol may be impaired when patient is converted to euthyroid state. Monitor patient.
Verapamil: May increase the effects of both drugs. Monitor cardiac function closely and decrease dosages p.r.n.
Drug-food. *Any food:* May increase absorption. Give together.

Effects on lab test results

• May increase transaminase, alkaline phosphatase, LDH, and uric acid levels.

Pharmacokinetics

Absorption: Rapidly and almost complete; food enhances absorption of metoprolol tartrate.
Distribution: Distributed widely throughout body; about 12% protein-bound.
Metabolism: Metabolized in liver.
Excretion: About 95% excreted in urine. *Half-life:* 3 to 7 hours.

Route	Onset	Peak	Duration
P.O.	≤ 15 min	1-12 hr	6-24 hr
I.V.	≤ 5 min	20 min	5-8 hr

Action

Chemical effect: Unknown for antihypertensive action. Drug decreases myocardial contractility, heart rate, and cardiac output; lowers blood pressure; reduces myocardial oxygen consumption; and depresses renin secretion.
Therapeutic effect: Reduces blood pressure and angina and helps to prevent myocardial tissue damage.

Available forms

metoprolol succinate
Tablets (extended-release): 25 mg, 50 mg, 100 mg, 200 mg
metoprolol tartrate
Injection: 1 mg/ml in 5-ml ampules

Tablets: 50 mg, 100 mg
Tablets (extended-release): 100 mg ◆ ,
200 mg ◆

NURSING PROCESS

▨ Assessment
- Assess patient's condition before therapy and regularly thereafter.
- Monitor blood pressure frequently. Drug masks common signs of shock.
- Be alert for adverse reactions and drug interactions.
- Evaluate patient's and family's knowledge of drug therapy.

⊞ Nursing diagnoses
- Ineffective health maintenance related to underlying disorder
- Risk for injury related to drug-induced adverse CNS reactions
- Deficient knowledge related to drug therapy

▶ Planning and implementation
⊛ **ALERT:** Always check patient's apical pulse rate before giving drug. If it's slower than 60 beats/minute, withhold drug and call prescriber immediately.
- Give drug with meals because food may increase absorption of metoprolol tartrate.
⊛ **ALERT:** Don't confuse metoprolol with metaproterenol or metolazone or Toprol XL with Topamax.

Patient teaching
- Tell patient that abrupt discontinuation of therapy can worsen angina and precipitate MI. Withdraw drug gradually over 1 to 2 weeks.
- Instruct patient to take oral form of drug with meals to enhance absorption.
- Advise patient to report adverse reactions to prescriber.
- Warn patient to avoid performing hazardous activities until CNS effects of drug are known.

☑ Evaluation
- Patient responds well to therapy.
- Patient doesn't experience injury from adverse CNS reactions.
- Patient and family state understanding of drug therapy.

metronidazole
(met-roh-NIGH-duh-zohl)
Apo-Metronidazole ◆ , Flagyl, Flagyl ER,
Flagyl 375, Metric 21, Metrogyl ◇ ,
Metrozine ◇ , Novonidazol ◆ , Protostat,
Trikacide ◆

metronidazole hydrochloride
Flagyl I.V. RTU, Metro I.V., Novonidazol ◆

Pharmacologic class: nitroimidazole
Therapeutic class: antibacterial, antiprotozoal, amebicide
Pregnancy risk category: B

Indications and dosages

▶ **Amebic hepatic abscess.** *Adults:* 500 to 750 mg P.O. t.i.d. for 5 to 10 days.
Children: 35 to 50 mg/kg daily (in three doses) for 10 days.

▶ **Intestinal amebiasis.** *Adults:* 750 mg P.O. t.i.d. for 5 to 10 days.
Children: 35 to 50 mg/kg daily (in three doses) for 10 days. Therapy is followed by P.O. iodoquinol.

▶ **Trichomoniasis.** *Adults:* 500 mg P.O. b.i.d. for 7 days or 2 g P.O. in single dose (may give 2-g dose as two 1-g doses on same day); allow 4 to 6 weeks between courses of therapy.
Children: 5 mg/kg dose P.O. t.i.d. for 7 days. Maximum dose is 2 g daily.

▶ **Refractory trichomoniasis.** *Adults:* 500 mg P.O. b.i.d. for 7 days. For repeated failures, 2 g P.O. daily for 3 to 5 days.

▶ **Bacterial infections caused by anaerobic microorganisms.** *Adults:* Loading dose is 15 mg/kg I.V. infused over 1 hour (about 1 g for 70-kg [154-lb] adult). Maintenance dosage is 7.5 mg/kg I.V. or P.O. q 6 hours (about 500 mg for 70-kg adult). Give first maintenance dose 6 hours after loading dose. Maximum, 4 g daily.

▶ **Prevention of postoperative infection in contaminated or potentially contaminated colorectal surgery.** *Adults:* 15 mg/kg I.V. infused over 30 to 60 minutes and completed about 1 hour before surgery. Then, 7.5 mg/kg I.V. infused over 30 to 60 minutes at 6 and 12 hours after initial dose.

▶ **Pelvic inflammatory disease‡.** *Adults:* 500 mg I.V. q 8 hours with other drugs. Or,

500 mg P.O. b.i.d. for 14 days given with ofloxacin, 400 mg P.O. b.i.d.

▶ **Bacterial vaginosis‡.** *Adults:* 500 mg P.O. b.i.d. for 7 days. Or, 2 g P.O. as a single dose. Or, 250 mg P.O. t.i.d. for 7 days.

▶ **Active Crohn's disease‡.** *Adults:* 400 mg P.O. b.i.d. For refractory perineal disease, 20 mg/kg (1 to 1.5 g) P.O. daily in three to five divided doses.

▶ **Prevention of sexually transmitted disease in sexual assault victims** ‡. *Adults:* 2 g P.O. given with other drugs.

▶ *Helicobacter pylori* **with peptic ulcer disease‡.** *Adults:* 250 to 500 mg P.O. t.i.d. to q.i.d. given with other drugs. Continue for 7 to 14 days depending on the regimen used. *Children:* 15 to 20 mg/kg P.O. daily, divided in two doses for 4 weeks given with other drugs.

▼ I.V. administration

● No preparation is needed for RTU form.
● Add 4.4 ml of sterile water for injection, bacteriostatic water for injection, sterile normal saline solution injection, or bacteriostatic normal saline solution injection. Reconstituted drug contains 100 mg/ml.
● Add contents of vial to 100 ml of D_5W, lactated Ringer's injection, or normal saline solution for final concentration of 5 mg/ml.
● The resulting highly acidic solution must be neutralized before giving. Carefully add 5 mEq of sodium bicarbonate for each 500 mg of metronidazole. Carbon dioxide will form and may need to be vented.
● Don't use equipment (needles, hubs) containing aluminum to reconstitute the drug or to transfer reconstituted medication. Equipment that contains aluminum will turn the solution orange; the potency isn't affected.
● **ALERT:** Infuse drug over at least 1 hour. Don't give I.V. push.
● Don't refrigerate neutralized diluted solution. Precipitation may occur. If Flagyl I.V. RTU is refrigerated, crystals may form. These will disappear after solution is gently warmed to room temperature.

Contraindications and precautions

● Contraindicated in patients hypersensitive to drug or other nitroimidazole derivatives.
● Use cautiously in patients receiving hepatotoxic drugs and in patients with history of blood dyscrasia or CNS disorder, retinal or visual field changes, hepatic disease, or alcoholism.
● **Lifespan:** In pregnant women, don't use in first trimester unless absolutely necessary. In breast-feeding women, drug isn't recommended.

Adverse reactions

CNS: vertigo, headache, ataxia, fever, incoordination, confusion, irritability, depression, restlessness, weakness, fatigue, drowsiness, insomnia, sensory neuropathy, paresthesia of limbs, psychic stimulation, *seizures,* neuropathy.
CV: flattened T wave, edema, flushing, thrombophlebitis after I.V. infusion.
GI: abdominal cramping, stomatitis, *nausea, vomiting, anorexia,* diarrhea, constipation, proctitis, dry mouth, metallic taste.
GU: darkened urine, polyuria, dysuria, pyuria, incontinence, cystitis, dyspareunia, dry vagina and vulva, sense of pelvic pressure.
Hematologic: *transient leukopenia, neutropenia, thrombocytopenia.*
Skin: pruritus, rash.
Other: decreased libido, gynecomastia, overgrowth of nonsusceptible organisms, especially *Candida* (glossitis, furry tongue).

Interactions

Drug-drug. *Barbiturates, phenobarbital, phenytoin:* Decreases metronidazole effectiveness because of increased hepatic clearance. Monitor patient closely for effect.
Cimetidine: Increases risk of metronidazole toxicity because of inhibited hepatic metabolism. Monitor patient.
Disulfiram: May cause acute psychoses and confusional states. Don't use together.
Fluorouracil, azathioprine: May increase risk of transient neutropenia. Use cautiously.
Lithium: Increases lithium level, possibly resulting in toxicity. Monitor lithium level closely.
Oral anticoagulants: Increases anticoagulant effects. Monitor patient for bleeding; monitor PT and INR.
Drug-lifestyle. *Alcohol use:* May cause disulfiram-like reaction (nausea, vomiting, headache, cramps, flushing). Discourage using together.

Effects on lab test results

● May decrease WBC and neutrophil counts.

Rapid onset   *Liquid form contains alcohol.   ◆Canada   ◇ Australia   †OTC   ‡Off-label use

Pharmacokinetics

Absorption: About 80%; food delays peak levels to about 2 hours.
Distribution: Distributed in most body tissues and fluids; less than 20% bound to proteins.
Metabolism: Metabolized to active metabolite and to other metabolites.
Excretion: Excreted primarily in urine; 6% to 15% in feces. *Half-life:* 6 to 8 hours (may be longer in patients with impaired liver function).

Route	Onset	Peak	Duration
P.O.	Unknown	1-2 hr	Unknown
I.V.	Immediate	Immediate	Unknown

Action

Chemical effect: Direct-acting trichomonacide and amebicide that works at both intestinal and extraintestinal sites.
Therapeutic effect: Hinders growth of selected organisms, including most anaerobic bacteria and protozoa.

Available forms

Capsules: 375 mg
Injection: 5 mg/ml
Oral suspension (benzoyl metronidazole): 200 mg/5 ml ◇
Tablets: 200 mg ◇, 250 mg, 400 mg ◇, 500 mg
Tablets (extended release): 750 mg

NURSING PROCESS

⚗ Assessment

• Assess patient's infection before therapy and regularly thereafter.
• Watch carefully for edema, especially in patients also receiving corticosteroids, because Flagyl I.V. RTU may cause sodium retention.
• Record number and character of stools when used in amebiasis.
• Be alert for adverse reactions and drug interactions.
• Evaluate patient's and family's knowledge of drug therapy.

Nursing diagnoses

• Infection related to presence of susceptible organisms
• Risk for deficient fluid volume related to drug-induced adverse GI reactions
• Deficient knowledge related to drug therapy

▶ Planning and implementation

• Give drug (except Flagyl ER) with meals to minimize GI distress. Give Flagyl ER at least 1 hour before or 2 hours after meals.
• Use only after *T. vaginalis* has been confirmed by wet smear or culture or *E. histolytica* has been identified. Also treat asymptomatic sexual partners simultaneously to avoid reinfection.
• During pregnancy, 7-day regimen is preferred over 2-g single-dose regimen for trichomoniasis.

Patient teaching
• Tell patient to avoid alcohol or alcohol-containing drugs during therapy and for at least 48 hours after therapy is completed.
• Tell patient that metallic taste and dark or red-brown urine may occur.
• Instruct patient to take oral form with meals to minimize reactions.
• Urge patient to complete full course of therapy even if he feels better.
• Instruct patient in proper hygiene.

☑ Evaluation

• Patient is free from infection.
• Patient maintains adequate hydration throughout therapy.
• Patient and family state understanding of drug therapy.

mexiletine hydrochloride
(MEKS-il-eh-teen high-droh-KLOR-ighd)
Mexitil

Pharmacologic class: lidocaine analogue, sodium channel antagonist
Therapeutic class: class IB ventricular antiarrhythmic
Pregnancy risk category: C

Indications and dosages

▶ **Refractory life-threatening ventricular arrhythmias, including ventricular tachycardia and PVCs.** *Adults:* 200 to 400 mg P.O., followed by 200 mg q 8 hours. If satisfactory control isn't obtained, increase dose q 2 to 3 days to 400 mg q 8 hours. Patients who respond well to q-12-hour schedule may be given up to 450 mg q 12 hours. Maximum daily dose is 1,200 mg.
▶ **Diabetic neuropathy‡.** *Adults:* 150 mg P.O. daily for 3 days; then give 300 mg P.O. daily for 3 days followed by 10 mg/kg P.O. daily.

Contraindications and precautions

- Contraindicated in patients with cardiogenic shock or second- or third-degree AV block in absence of artificial pacemaker.
- Use cautiously in patients with first-degree heart block, ventricular pacemaker, sinus node dysfunction, intraventricular conduction disturbances, hypotension, severe heart failure, or seizure disorder.

⚘ **Lifespan:** In pregnant women, use cautiously. In breast-feeding women, drug isn't recommended. In children, safety of drug hasn't been established.

Adverse reactions

CNS: *tremor, dizziness,* blurred vision, ataxia, diplopia, confusion, nystagmus, nervousness, headache.
CV: *hypotension, bradycardia, widened QRS complex, arrhythmias,* palpitations, chest pain.
GI: nausea, vomiting.
Skin: rash.

Interactions

Drug-drug. *Antacids, atropine, opioids:* Slows mexiletine absorption. Monitor patient; separate administration times.
Cimetidine: Increases or decreases mexiletine level. Monitor patient for effect or toxicities.
Methylxanthines (such as theophylline): Reduces clearance of methylxanthines, possibly resulting in toxicity. Monitor levels.
Metoclopramide: Mexiletine absorption may be accelerated. Monitor patient for toxicity.
Phenobarbital, phenytoin, rifampin, urine acidifiers: Decreases mexiletine blood levels. Monitor patient.
Urine alkalinizers: Increases mexiletine blood levels. Monitor patient.
Drug-food. *Caffeine:* Reduces clearance of methylxanthines, possibly resulting in toxicity. Monitor patient.

Effects on lab test results

- May increase AST level.

Pharmacokinetics

Absorption: About 90%.
Distribution: Distributed widely throughout body. Distribution volume declines in patients with liver disease, resulting in toxic levels with usual doses. About 50% to 60% of circulating drug is bound to proteins.

Metabolism: Most of drug metabolized in liver.
Excretion: Excreted in urine. *Half-life:* 10 to 12 hours.

Route	Onset	Peak	Duration
P.O.	½-2 hr	2-3 hr	Unknown

Action

Chemical effect: Blocks fast sodium channel in cardiac tissues without involvement of autonomic nervous system. Drug reduces rate of rise and amplitude of action potential and decreases automaticity in Purkinje fibers. It also shortens action potential and, to a lesser extent, decreases effective refractory period in Purkinje fibers.
Therapeutic effect: Abolishes ventricular arrhythmias.

Available forms

Capsules: 100 mg ♦, 150 mg, 200 mg, 250 mg

NURSING PROCESS

🔎 Assessment

- Assess patient's condition until arrhythmia is abolished.
- Monitor drug levels. Therapeutic levels are 0.75 to 2 mcg/ml.
- Be alert for adverse reactions and drug interactions.
- Monitor patient for toxicity. An early sign is tremors, usually fine tremor of hands. This progresses to dizziness and later to ataxia and nystagmus as drug's blood level increases. Ask patient about these symptoms.
- If adverse GI reactions occur, monitor patient's hydration status.
- Evaluate patient's and family's knowledge of drug therapy.

📋 Nursing diagnoses

- Decreased cardiac output related to presence of ventricular arrhythmia
- Risk for deficient fluid volume related to drug-induced adverse GI reactions
- Deficient knowledge related to drug therapy

▶ Planning and implementation

- Give with meals or antacids to lessen GI distress.
- If patient appears to be good candidate for q-12-hour therapy, notify prescriber. Twice-daily dose enhances compliance.

Rapid onset　　*Liquid form contains alcohol.*　　♦ Canada　　◇ Australia　　†OTC　　‡Off-label use

- Notify prescriber of any significant changes in blood pressure, heart rate, and heart rhythm.

Patient teaching
- Instruct patient taking oral form of drug to take it with food.
- Instruct patient to report adverse reactions.

☑ **Evaluation**
- Patient regains normal cardiac output.
- Patient maintains adequate hydration throughout therapy.
- Patient and family state understanding of drug therapy.

midazolam hydrochloride
(MID-ayz-oh-lam high-droh-KLOR-ighd)
Hypnovel ◇ , Versed, Versed Syrup

Pharmacologic class: benzodiazepine
Therapeutic class: preoperative sedative, drug for conscious sedation, adjunct for induction of general anesthesia
Pregnancy risk category: D
Controlled substance schedule: IV

Indications and dosages

▶ **Preoperative sedation (to induce sleepiness or drowsiness and relieve apprehension).** *Adults younger than age 60:* 0.07 mg to 0.08 mg/kg I.M. about 1 hour before surgery.
▶ **Conscious sedation before short diagnostic or endoscopic procedures.** *Adults younger than age 60:* Initially, give slowly a dose no greater than 2.5 mg I.V.; repeat in 2 minutes if needed in small increments of initial dose over at least 2 minutes. Maximum total dose, 5 mg. *Adults age 60 and older:* 1.5 mg or less over at least 2 minutes. If additional adjustment is needed, give at no more than 1 mg over 2 minutes. Total doses exceeding 3.5 mg aren't usually needed.
▶ **Induction of general anesthesia.** *Adults younger than age 55:* 0.3 to 0.35 mg/kg I.V. over 20 to 30 seconds if patient hasn't received preanesthesia drug, or 0.15 to 0.35 mg/kg I.V. over 20 to 30 seconds if patient has received preanesthesia drug. Additional increments of 25% of initial dose may be needed to complete induction. *Adults age 55 and older:* 0.3 mg/kg I.V. over 20 to 30 seconds if patient hasn't received premedication, or 0.2 mg/kg I.V. over 20 to 30 sec-

onds if patient has received sedation or narcotic premedication. Additional increments of 25% of initial dose may be needed to complete induction.
▶ **To induce sleepiness and amnesia and to relieve apprehension before anesthesia or before or during procedures in children.** *Children:* 0.1 to 0.15 mg/kg I.M. Doses up to 0.5 mg/kg can be used for more anxious patients. Total dose usually doesn't exceed 10 mg. I.V. depending on age of child. *Children ages 6 months to 5 years:* Initially, 0.05 to 0.1 mg/kg I.V. over 2 to 3 minutes. Additional doses may be given in small increments after 2 to 3 minutes. Total dose of up to 0.6 mg/kg (not to exceed 6 mg) may be given. *Children ages 6 to 12:* 0.025 to 0.05 mg/kg I.V. over 2 to 3 minutes. Additional doses may be given in small increments after 2 to 3 minutes. Total dose of up to 0.4 mg/kg (not to exceed 10 mg) may be given. *Children ages 12 to 16:* Initially, give dose of 2.5 mg I.V. or less slowly; repeat in 2 minutes, if needed, in small increments of initial dose over at least 2 minutes to achieve desired effect. Slowly titrate additional doses to maintain desired level of sedation in increments of 25% of dose used to first reach the sedative endpoint. Total dose of up to 10 mg may be used.
▶ **Continuous infusion for sedation of intubated patients in the critical care setting.** *Adults:* Initially, 0.01 to 0.05 mg/kg I.V. over several minutes, repeat at 10- to 15-minute intervals, until adequate sedation is achieved. To maintain sedation, infuse initially at 0.02 to 0.1 mg/kg/hour. Some patients may need higher loading doses or infusion rates. Use the lowest effective rate. *Children:* Initially, 0.05 to 0.2 mg/kg I.V. over at least 2 to 3 minutes; then continuous infusion at 0.06 to 0.12 mg/kg/hour. Increase or decrease infusion to maintain desired effect. *Neonates born at 32 weeks' gestation or later:* Initially 0.06 mg/kg/hour. Adjust rate, p.r.n., using lowest possible rate. *Neonates born earlier than 32 weeks' gestation:* Initially 0.03 mg/kg/hour. Adjust rate, p.r.n., using lowest possible rate.

▼ I.V. administration

- When mixing infusion, use 5-mg/ml vial, dilute to 0.5 mg/ml with D_5W or normal saline solution.

• Give slowly over at least 2 minutes, and wait at least 2 minutes when adjusting doses to effect.
• Watch for irritation and infiltration; extravasation can cause tissue damage and necrosis.

Contraindications and precautions

• Contraindicated in patients hypersensitive to drug and in those with acute angle-closure glaucoma, shock, coma, or acute alcohol intoxication.
• Use cautiously in patients with uncompensated acute illness and in debilitated patients.
⚖ Lifespan: In pregnant women, drug isn't recommended. In breast-feeding women and in elderly patients, use cautiously.

Adverse reactions

CNS: headache, oversedation, involuntary movements, combativeness, amnesia.
CV: variations in blood pressure *(hypotension)* and pulse rate, *cardiac arrest.*
GI: *nausea,* vomiting, *hiccups.*
Respiratory: *decreased respiratory rate,* APNEA.
Other: pain, tenderness at injection site.

Interactions

Drug-drug. *Cimetidine, verapamil:* May increase effects of benzodiazepine. Monitor patient closely.
CNS depressants: May increase risk of apnea. Monitor vital signs and respiratory status closely if used together.
CYP 3A4 inducers (rifampin, carbamazepine, phenytoin, phenobarbital): May decrease midazolam concentration. Monitor patient for effect; adjust dosage if needed.
Diltiazem: May increase CNS depression and prolonged effects of midazolam. Use lower dose of midazolam.
Fluconazole, ketoconazole, itraconazole, miconazole: May increase and prolong levels, and may increase CNS depression and psychomotor impairment. Don't use together.
Indinavir, ritonavir: Possible prolonged or severe sedation and respiratory depression. Monitor patient closely.
Opioid analgesics: May increase midazolam's hypnotic effect and increase risk of hypotension. Monitor patient closely; adjust dosage.
Hormonal contraceptives: May prolong benzodiazepine half-life. Monitor patient closely.

Rifamycin: May decrease midazolam levels. Monitor patient for effect.
Drug-food. *Grapefruit juice:* May increase bioavailability of oral midazolam. Discourage use together.
Drug-lifestyle. *Alcohol use:* May cause additive CNS effects. Strongly discourage use together.

Effects on lab test results

None reported.

Pharmacokinetics

Absorption: 80% to 100%.
Distribution: Large volume; about 97% protein-bound.
Metabolism: In liver by CYP 3A4 isoenzyme.
Excretion: In urine. *Half-life:* 2 to 6 hours.

Route	Onset	Peak	Duration
P.O.	10-20 min	45-60 min	2-6 hr
I.V.	1½-5 min	Rapid	2-6 hr
I.M.	≤ 15 min	15-60 min	2-6 hr

Action

Chemical effect: May depress CNS at limbic and subcortical levels of brain by potentiating effects of GABA.
Therapeutic effect: Promotes calmness and sleep.

Available forms

Injection: 1 mg/ml, 5 mg/ml
Syrup: 2 mg/ml

NURSING PROCESS

🔲 Assessment

• Assess patient's condition before therapy and regularly thereafter.
• Monitor blood pressure, heart rate and rhythm, respirations, airway integrity, and arterial oxygen saturation during procedure, especially in patients premedicated with opioids.
• Evaluate patient's and family's knowledge of drug therapy.

🔲 Nursing diagnoses

• Anxiety related to surgery
• Ineffective breathing pattern related to drug's effect on respiratory system
• Deficient knowledge related to drug therapy

⧎ Planning and implementation
• Before giving drug, have oxygen and resuscitation equipment available in case of severe respiratory depression. Excessive dosages or rapid infusions may cause respiratory arrest, particularly in elderly or debilitated patients.
• Drug may be mixed in same syringe with morphine sulfate, meperidine, atropine sulfate, or scopolamine.
• For I.M. dose, give deep into large muscle mass.
ⓈＡＬＥＲＴ: Don't confuse Versed with VePesid.
Patient teaching
• Use extra caution for teaching patients because drug will diminish predrug memory. Provide written information, family member instruction, and follow-up contact to ensure that patient has adequate information.
• Instruct patient not to use alcohol and drug together.

☑ Evaluation
• Patient exhibits calmness.
• Patient maintains adequate breathing pattern throughout therapy.
• Patient and family state understanding of drug therapy.

miglitol
(MIG-lih-tall)
Glyset

Pharmacologic class: alpha-glucosidase inhibitor
Therapeutic class: antidiabetic
Pregnancy risk category: B

Indications and dosages
▶ **Monotherapy as an adjunct to diet to improve glycemic control in patients with type 2 diabetes mellitus whose hyperglycemia can't be managed with diet alone; with a sulfonylurea when diet plus either miglitol or sulfonylurea alone yield inadequate glycemic control.** *Adults:* 25 mg P.O. t.i.d. with the first bite of each main meal; some patients may start at 25 mg P.O. daily to minimize GI side effects. Increase dosage after 4 to 8 weeks to maintenance dosage of 50 mg P.O. t.i.d. Further increase dosage after 3 months, based on glycosy-

lated hemoglobin, to maximum of 100 mg P.O. t.i.d.

Contraindications and precautions
• Contraindicated in patients hypersensitive to drug or its components. Also contraindicated in patients with diabetic ketoacidosis, inflammatory bowel disease, colonic ulceration, or partial intestinal obstruction; patients predisposed to intestinal obstruction or those with chronic intestinal diseases related to disorders of digestion or absorption; and patients with conditions that may deteriorate as a result of increased gas formation in the intestine.
• Drug isn't recommended for patients with creatinine more than 2 mg/dl.
• Use cautiously in patients also receiving insulin or oral sulfonylureas.
⚖ **Lifespan:** In pregnant women, use only if clearly needed. In breast-feeding women, don't use. In children, safety and effectiveness of drug haven't been established.

Adverse reactions
GI: abdominal pain, diarrhea, flatulence.
Skin: rash.

Interactions
Drug-drug. *Digoxin, propranolol, ranitidine:* May decrease the bioavailability of these drugs. Monitor patient for loss of effectiveness and adjust dosages.
Insulin, oral sulfonylureas: May increase the effect of these drugs. Adjust dosage of these drugs if needed. Monitor these patients for hypoglycemia.
Intestinal absorbents (such as charcoal) and digestive enzyme preparations (such as amylase, pancreatin): May reduce the effectiveness of miglitol. Avoid using together.
Drug-herb. *Aloe, bilberry leaf, bitter melon, burdock, dandelion, fenugreek, garlic, ginseng, stinging nettle:* May improve glucose level control, allowing for a reduced antidiabetic dosage. Advise patient to discuss the use of herbal remedies with prescriber before therapy.

Effects on lab test results
• May decrease iron and glucose levels.

Pharmacokinetics
Absorption: Saturable at high doses. A 25-mg dose is completely absorbed, whereas a dose of

100 mg is only 50% to 70% absorbed; levels peak in 2 to 3 hours.

Distribution: Distributed primarily into the extracellular fluid. Protein-binding is less than 4%.

Metabolism: None.

Excretion: Primarily renal. More than 95% of a dose appears in urine as unchanged drug. *Half-life:* About 2 hours.

Route	Onset	Peak	Duration
P.O.	Unknown	2-3 hr	Unknown

Action

Chemical effect: Lowers glucose level through reversible inhibition of alpha glucosidases in the small intestine; they convert oligosaccharides and disaccharides to glucose. Inhibiting these enzymes delays glucose absorption. Drug has no effect on insulin secretion.

Therapeutic effect: Lowers glucose level.

Available forms

Tablets: 25 mg, 50 mg, 100 mg

NURSING PROCESS

Assessment

• Obtain history of patient's underlying condition before therapy, and reassess regularly.

• Monitor glucose level regularly, especially during situations of increased stress, such as infection, fever, surgery, and trauma.

• Check glycosylated hemoglobin q 3 months to monitor long-term glycemic control.

• Evaluate patient's and family's knowledge of drug therapy.

Nursing diagnoses

• Ineffective health maintenance related to hyperglycemia

• Risk for injury related to drug-induced hypoglycemia

• Deficient knowledge related to drug therapy

Planning and implementation

• Give with the first bite of each main meal.

• Manage type 2 diabetes with diet control, exercise program, and regular testing of urine and glucose levels.

• Treat mild to moderate hypoglycemia with dextrose, such as glucose tablets or gel or orange juice with sugar packets. Severe hypoglycemia may require I.V. glucose or glucagon.

Patient teaching

• Tell patient about the importance of adhering to prescriber's diet, weight reduction, and exercise instructions and to have glucose level and glycosylated hemoglobin tested regularly.

• Inform patient that drug therapy relieves symptoms but doesn't cure diabetes.

• Tell patient the signs and symptoms of hyperglycemia and hypoglycemia.

• Instruct patient to treat hypoglycemia with glucose tablets and to have a source of glucose readily available when miglitol is taken with a sulfonylurea or insulin.

• Advise patient to seek medical advice promptly during periods of stress such as fever, trauma, infection, or surgery because drug requirements may change.

• Instruct patient to take drug t.i.d. with the first bite of each main meal.

• Show patient how and when to monitor glucose level.

• Advise patient that adverse GI effects are most common during the first few weeks of therapy and should improve over time.

• Urge patient to always carry medical identification.

Evaluation

• Patient's glucose level is normal.

• Patient sustains no injury from drug-induced hypoglycemia.

• Patient and family state understanding of drug therapy.

milrinone lactate
(MIL-rih-nohn LAK-tayt)
Primacor

Pharmacologic class: bipyridine phosphodiesterase inhibitor
Therapeutic class: inotropic vasodilator
Pregnancy risk category: C

Indications and dosages

▶ **Short-term therapy for acute decompensated heart failure.** *Adults:* Loading dose is 50 mcg/kg I.V., given slowly over 10 minutes, followed by continuous I.V. infusion of 0.375 to 0.75 mcg/kg/minute. Adjust infusion dose based on response.

⧄ Adjust-a-dose: For patients with renal impairment, if creatinine clearance is 50 ml/minute or less, adjust dosage to maximum effect, not to exceed 1.13 mg/kg I.V. daily.

▼ I.V. administration

• Dilute with half-normal or normal saline solution or D₅W. Prepare 100-mcg/ml solution by adding 180 ml of diluent per 20-mg (20-ml) vial, 150-mcg/ml solution by adding 113 ml of diluent per 20-mg (20-ml) vial, and 200-mcg/ml solution by adding 80 ml of diluent per 20-mg (20-ml) vial.

• **⧖ ALERT:** Giving furosemide in an I.V. line containing this drug causes precipitate to form. Don't give in the same line.

• Drop in blood pressure requires stopping or slowing infusion.

• Drug hasn't been shown to be safe or effective for more than 48 hours. Avoid using longer.

Contraindications and precautions

• Contraindicated in patients hypersensitive to drug.

• Drug isn't recommended for patients with severe aortic or pulmonic valvular disease in place of surgical correction of obstruction, or for patients in acute phase of MI.

• Use cautiously in patients with atrial flutter or fibrillation because drug slightly shortens AV node conduction time and may increase ventricular response rate.

⚐ **Lifespan:** In pregnant and breast-feeding women, use cautiously. In children, safety of drug hasn't been established.

Adverse reactions

CNS: headache.
CV: VENTRICULAR ARRHYTHMIAS, *ventricular ectopic activity, nonsustained ventricular tachycardia, sustained ventricular tachycardia, ventricular fibrillation.*

Interactions

Drug-drug. *Natrecor:* May increase hypotensive effect. Avoid using together.

Effects on lab test results

None reported.

Pharmacokinetics

Absorption: Administered I.V.
Distribution: About 70% bound to protein.

Metabolism: About 12% metabolized to glucuronide metabolite.
Excretion: About 83% excreted unchanged in urine. *Half-life:* 2¼ to 2¾ hours.

Route	Onset	Peak	Duration
I.V.	5-15 min	1-2 hr	3-6 hr

Action

Chemical effect: Produces inotropic action by increasing cellular levels of cAMP; produces vasodilation by relaxing vascular smooth muscle.
Therapeutic effect: Relieves acute signs and symptoms of heart failure.

Available forms

Injection: 1 mg/ml
Premixed injection: 200 mcg/ml in 100 ml D₅W injection; 200 mcg/ml in 200 ml D₅W injection.

NURSING PROCESS

⚕ Assessment

• Assess patient's heart failure before therapy and regularly thereafter.

• Monitor fluid and electrolyte status, blood pressure, heart rate, and kidney function during therapy.

• Monitor patient's ECG continuously during therapy.

• Be alert for adverse reactions.

• Evaluate patient's and family's knowledge of drug therapy.

⊕ Nursing diagnoses

• Impaired gas exchange related to presence of heart failure

• Decreased cardiac output related to drug-induced cardiac arrhythmias

• Deficient knowledge related to drug therapy

▷ Planning and implementation

• Drug is typically given with digoxin and diuretics.

• Inotropics may aggravate outflow tract obstruction in hypertrophic subaortic stenosis.

• **⧖ ALERT:** Improvement of cardiac output may result in enhanced urine output. Reduce diuretic dosage as heart failure improves. Potassium loss may predispose patient to digitalis toxicity.

⊕ **ALERT:** Don't confuse milrinone with inamrinone.

Patient teaching
• Tell patient to report headache; mild analgesic can be given for relief.

☑ **Evaluation**
• Patient exhibits adequate gas exchange, as heart failure is resolved.
• Drug-induced arrhythmias don't develop during therapy.
• Patient and family state understanding of drug therapy.

minocycline hydrochloride
(migh-noh-SIGH-kleen high-droh-KLOR-ighd)
Akamin ◇ , **Alti-Minocycline** ♦ , **Apo-Minocycline** ♦ , **Dynacin, Minocin, Minomycin** ◇ , **Novo-Minocycline** ♦ , **PMS-Minocycline** ♦

Pharmacologic class: tetracycline
Therapeutic class: antibiotic
Pregnancy risk category: D

Indications and dosages

▶ **Infections caused by sensitive gram-negative and gram-positive organisms, trachoma, amebiasis.** *Adults:* 200 mg I.V.; then 100 mg I.V. q 12 hours. Maximum 400 mg I.V. daily. Or, 200 mg P.O. initially; then 100 mg P.O. q 12 hours. Some clinicians use 100 or 200 mg P.O. initially, followed by 50 mg q.i.d. *Children older than age 8:* Initially, 4 mg/kg P.O. or I.V., followed by 2 mg/kg P.O. q 12 hours. Give I.V. in 500- to 1,000-ml solution without calcium over 6 hours.
▶ **Gonorrhea in patients sensitive to penicillin.** *Adults:* Initially, 200 mg P.O.; then 100 mg q 12 hours for at least 4 days.
▶ **Syphilis in patients sensitive to penicillin.** *Adults:* Initially, 200 mg P.O.; then 100 mg q 12 hours for 10 to 15 days.
▶ **Meningococcal carrier state.** *Adults:* 100 mg P.O. q 12 hours for 5 days.
▶ **Uncomplicated urethral, endocervical, or rectal infection caused by** *Chlamydia trachomatis* **or** *Ureaplasma urealyticum.* *Adults:* 100 mg P.O. b.i.d. for at least 7 days.
▶ **Uncomplicated gonococcal urethritis in men.** *Adults:* 100 mg P.O. b.i.d. for 5 days.

▶ **Multibacillary leprosy‡.** *Adults:* 100 mg P.O. daily with clofazimine and ofloxacin for 6 months, followed by 100 mg P.O. daily for an additional 18 months in conjunction with clofazimine.
▶ **Nocardiosis‡.** *Adults:* Usual dose for 12 to 18 months.
▶ **Nongonococcal urethritis caused by** *C. trachomatis* **or** *mycoplasma‡.* *Adults:* 100 mg P.O. daily in one or two divided doses for 1 to 3 weeks.

▼ I.V. administration

• Reconstitute 100 mg of powder with 5 ml of sterile water for injection, with further dilution of 500 to 1,000 ml for I.V. infusion.
• Infusions are usually given over 6 hours.
• Solution is stable for 24 hours at room temperature.
• Thrombophlebitis may develop. Watch for irritation and infiltration; extravasation can cause tissue damage and necrosis.
• Switch to P.O. form as soon as possible.

Contraindications and precautions

• Contraindicated in patients hypersensitive to drug or other tetracyclines.
• Use cautiously in patients with impaired kidney or liver function.
⚖ **Lifespan:** During last half of pregnancy and in children younger than age 8, drug may cause permanent discoloration of teeth, enamel defects, and bone growth retardation. In breastfeeding women, drug isn't recommended.

Adverse reactions

CNS: *light-headedness or dizziness from vestibular toxicity,* **intracranial hypertension** *(pseudotumor cerebri).*
CV: pericarditis, *thrombophlebitis.*
EENT: dysphagia, glossitis.
GI: *anorexia,* epigastric distress, oral candidiasis, *nausea,* vomiting, *diarrhea,* enterocolitis, inflammatory lesions in anogenital region.
Hematologic: *neutropenia,* eosinophilia, *thrombocytopenia.*
Musculoskeletal: bone growth retardation if used in children younger than age 8; superinfection.
Skin: *maculopapular and erythematous rashes, photosensitivity reactions, increased pigmentation, urticaria.*

Other: permanent discoloration of teeth, enamel defects, *hypersensitivity reactions (anaphylaxis)*.

Interactions

Drug-drug. *Antacids (including sodium bicarbonate) and laxatives containing aluminum, magnesium, or calcium; antidiarrheals:* May decrease antibiotic absorption. Give antibiotic 1 hour before or 2 hours after these drugs.
Cimetidine: May decrease absorption of minocycline. Monitor patient.
Digoxin: Increases digoxin level. Decrease digoxin dose, if needed.
Ferrous sulfate, other iron products, zinc: Decreases antibiotic absorption. Give drug 3 hours after or 2 hours before iron.
Hormonal contraceptives: Decreases contraceptive effectiveness and increased risk of breakthrough bleeding. Recommend nonhormonal form of birth control.
Methoxyflurane: May cause nephrotoxicity with tetracyclines. Avoid using together; monitor patient carefully.
Oral anticoagulants: May increase anticoagulant effect. Monitor PT and INR. Adjust dosage if needed.
Penicillins: May interfere with bactericidal action of penicillins. Avoid using together.
Drug-herb. *St. John's wort:* May increase photosensitivity reactions. Urge patient to avoid unprotected or prolonged exposure to sunlight.
Drug-lifestyle. *Sun exposure:* Photosensitivity reactions may occur. Urge patient to avoid unprotected or prolonged exposure to sunlight.

Effects on lab test results

- May increase BUN and liver enzyme levels.
- May increase eosinophil count. May decrease hemoglobin and hematocrit and platelet and neutrophil counts.
- Parenteral form may cause false-positive reading of copper sulfate tests (Clinitest). All forms may cause false-negative reading of glucose enzymatic tests (Diastix).

Pharmacokinetics

Absorption: 90% to 100%.
Distribution: Distributed widely in body tissues and fluids, including synovial, pleural, prostatic, and seminal fluids; bronchial secretions; saliva; and aqueous humor. CSF penetration is poor. Drug is 70% to 80% protein-bound.

Metabolism: Partial.
Excretion: Excreted primarily unchanged in liver. *Half-life:* 11 to 26 hours.

Route	Onset	Peak	Duration
P.O.	Unknown	1-4 hr	Unknown
I.V.	Immediate	Immediate	Unknown

Action

Chemical effect: Unknown; may exert bacteriostatic effect by binding to ribosomal subunit of microorganisms, inhibiting protein synthesis.
Therapeutic effect: Hinders bacterial cell growth.

Available forms

Akamin ◇, *Minomycin* ◇
Capsules: 100 mg
Tablets: 50 mg
Alti-Minocycline ◆, *Apo-Minocycline* ◆, *Novo-Minocycline* ◆, *PMS-Minocycline* ◆
Capsules: 50 mg, 100 mg
Dynacin
Capsules: 50 mg, 75 mg, 100 mg
Tablets: 50 mg, 75 mg, 100 mg
Minocin
Capsules (pellet-filled): 50 mg, 100 mg
Injection: 100 mg/vial

NURSING PROCESS

⚕ Assessment

- Assess patient's infection before therapy and regularly thereafter.
- Obtain specimen for culture and sensitivity tests before giving first dose. Therapy may begin pending results.
- Be alert for adverse reactions and drug interactions.
- If adverse GI reactions occur, monitor patient's hydration status.
- Evaluate patient's and family's knowledge of drug therapy.

⚕ Nursing diagnoses

- Infection related to presence of susceptible bacteria
- Risk for deficient fluid volume related to drug-induced adverse reactions
- Deficient knowledge related to drug therapy

Reactions may be *common,* uncommon, *life-threatening,* or **COMMON AND LIFE-THREATENING.**

▶ Planning and implementation

⊛ **ALERT:** Check expiration date. Outdated or deteriorated tetracyclines have been linked to reversible nephrotoxicity (Fanconi's syndrome).

• Don't expose these drugs to light or heat. Keep cap tightly closed.

• Drug may cause tooth discoloration in children and young adults. If it occurs, inform prescriber.

⊛ **ALERT:** Don't confuse Minocin with niacin and Mithracin.

⊛ **ALERT:** Don't confuse Dynacin with Dyna-Circ.

Patient teaching

• Inform patient that drug may be taken with food, and instruct him to take drug exactly as prescribed.

• Instruct patient to take oral form of drug with full glass of water, and to avoid taking it within 1 hour of bedtime to avoid esophagitis.

• Warn patient to avoid hazardous tasks until adverse CNS effects of drug are known.

• Instruct patient to avoid direct sunlight and ultraviolet light, to use sunblock, and to wear protective clothing.

• Advise patient using hormonal contraceptives that another form of birth control should be used. Also inform her that she may experience breakthrough bleeding.

☑ Evaluation

• Patient is free from infection.

• Patient maintains adequate hydration throughout therapy.

• Patient and family state understanding of drug therapy.

---

minoxidil

(migh-NOKS-uh-dil)
Loniten

Pharmacologic class: peripheral vasodilator
Therapeutic class: antihypertensive
Pregnancy risk category: C

Indications and dosages

▶ **Severe hypertension.** *Adults and children age 12 and older:* Initially, 5 mg P.O. as single dose. Effective dosage range, 10 to 40 mg daily. Increase dose q 3 days up to a maximum dosage of 100 mg.

Children younger than age 12: 0.2 mg/kg P.O. (maximum 5 mg) as single daily dose. Effective dosage range, 0.25 to 1 mg/kg daily. Maximum dosage, 50 mg P.O. daily.

Contraindications and precautions

• Contraindicated in patients hypersensitive to drug and in those with pheochromocytoma.

• Use cautiously in patients with impaired kidney function or recent acute MI.

⚖ **Lifespan:** In pregnant women, use cautiously. In breast-feeding women, drug isn't recommended.

Adverse reactions

CV: *edema, tachycardia, pericardial effusion and tamponade,* **heart failure,** ECG changes.
Metabolic: weight gain.
Skin: *hypertrichosis* (elongation, thickening, and enhanced pigmentation of fine body hair), rash, **Stevens-Johnson syndrome.**
Other: breast tenderness.

Interactions

Drug-drug. *Guanethidine:* May cause severe orthostatic hypotension. Advise patient to stand up slowly.
Drug-herb. *Yohimbe:* May interfere with blood pressure control. Monitor blood pressure closely.

Effects on lab test results

• May increase BUN, creatinine, and alkaline phosphatase levels.

• May decrease hemoglobin and hematocrit.

Pharmacokinetics

Absorption: Rapid.
Distribution: Distributed widely in body tissues; not bound to proteins.
Metabolism: About 90%.
Excretion: Excreted primarily in urine. *Half-life:* 4¼ hours.

Route	Onset	Peak	Duration
P.O.	About 30 min	≤ 1 hr	2-5 days

Action

Chemical effect: Unknown; produces direct arteriolar vasodilation.
Therapeutic effect: Lowers blood pressure.

Available forms

Tablets: 2.5 mg, 10 mg, 25 mg ◊

NURSING PROCESS

⚗ Assessment

• Obtain history of patient's blood pressure and pulse rate before therapy and reassess regularly thereafter.
• Be alert for adverse reactions and drug interactions.
• Monitor fluid intake and output and check for weight gain and edema.
• Evaluate patient's and family's knowledge of drug therapy.

🔄 Nursing diagnoses

• Risk for injury related to presence of hypertension
• Excessive fluid volume related to drug-induced edema
• Deficient knowledge related to drug therapy

▶ Planning and implementation

• Drug is removed by hemodialysis. Give dose after dialysis.
• Give with beta blocker to control tachycardia and a diuretic to counteract fluid retention.
• If blood pressure changes significantly or pulse rate rises more than 20 beats/minute from baseline, notify prescriber.
• Titration of drug must be done carefully, and adjustments should be made every 3 days because full effect of a given dose is not obtained until then. If more rapid management is needed, adjustments can be made every 6 hours with careful monitoring.
⊛ **ALERT:** Don't confuse Loniten with Lotensin.

Patient teaching

• Make sure patient reads package insert describing drug's adverse reactions. Provide verbal explanation.
• Teach patient how to take his own pulse and instruct him to report increases over 20 beats/minute to prescriber.
• Tell patient not to suddenly stop taking drug but to call prescriber if unpleasant adverse effects occur.
• Tell patient to weigh himself at least weekly and to report weight gain of more than 5 lb (2.27 kg).
• Inform patient that excessive hair growth commonly occurs within 3 to 6 weeks of beginning treatment. Assure patient that extra hair will disappear within 1 to 6 months of stopping drug. Advise him not to stop drug without prescriber's approval.

☑ Evaluation

• Patient's blood pressure is normal.
• Patient exhibits no evidence of edema throughout therapy.
• Patient and family state understanding of drug therapy.

mirtazapine

(mir-TAH-zuh-peen)
Remeron, Remeron SolTab

Pharmacologic class: piperazinoazepine group of compounds
Therapeutic class: antidepressant
Pregnancy risk category: C

Indications and dosages

▶ **Depression.** *Adults:* Initially, 15 mg P.O. h.s. Maintenance dosage is 15 to 45 mg daily. Adjust dosage at intervals of at least 1 to 2 weeks.

Contraindications and precautions

• Contraindicated in patients hypersensitive to drug and in those taking MAO inhibitors.
• Use cautiously in patients with CV or cerebrovascular disease, seizure disorders, suicidal ideations, impaired hepatic or renal function, or history of mania or hypomania.
🕸 **Lifespan:** In pregnant women, use only if clearly needed. In breast-feeding women, use cautiously. In children, safety and effectiveness haven't been established.

Adverse reactions

CNS: *somnolence,* dizziness, asthenia, abnormal dreams, abnormal thinking, tremor, confusion.
CV: edema, peripheral edema.
GI: nausea, *increased appetite, dry mouth, constipation.*
GU: urinary frequency.
Hematologic: *neutropenia, agranulocytosis.*
Metabolic: *weight gain.*
Musculoskeletal: back pain, myalgia.
Respiratory: dyspnea.
Other: flulike syndrome.

Interactions

Drug-drug. *Diazepam, other CNS depressants:* Possible additive CNS effects. Avoid using together.
MAO inhibitors: May cause potentially serious, sometimes fatal reactions. Don't use drug within 14 days of an MAO inhibitor.
Drug-lifestyle. *Alcohol use:* May have possible additive CNS effects. Discourage using together.

Effects on lab test results

• May increase ALT levels.

Pharmacokinetics

Absorption: Rapid.
Distribution: 85% bound to proteins.
Metabolism: Extensively metabolized in liver.
Excretion: Mainly excreted in urine; some in feces. *Half-life:* About 20 to 40 hours.

Route	Onset	Peak	Duration
P.O.	Unknown	Within 2 hr	Unknown

Action

Chemical effect: Enhances central noradrenergic and serotonergic activity; potent antagonist of histamine receptors.
Therapeutic effect: Relieves depression.

Available forms

Orally disintegrating tablets: 15 mg, 30 mg, 45 mg
Tablets: 15 mg, 30 mg, 45 mg

NURSING PROCESS

Assessment

• If patient develops a sore throat, fever, stomatitis, or other signs of infection together with a low WBC count, stop drug and monitor him closely.
• Evaluate patient's and family's knowledge of drug therapy.

Nursing diagnoses

• Disturbed thought processes related to adverse effects
• Risk for injury related to sedation and orthostatic hypotension
• Deficient knowledge related to drug therapy

Planning and implementation

• Use cautiously when giving drug to breast-feeding women.
• Don't abruptly stop drug. Drug has an increased risk of suicidal behavior. Monitor patient and take suicide precautions.
Patient teaching
• Instruct patient to remove orally disintegrating tablet from blister pack and immediately place on the tongue. Tell him he won't need water to swallow the tablet because drug dissolves rapidly.
• Tell patient not to break or split tablet.
• Warn patient to avoid hazardous activities if somnolence occurs.
• Tell patient to report signs and symptoms of infection or flulike symptoms.
• Advise patient to avoid alcohol or other CNS depressants.
• Stress importance of compliance with therapy.
• Instruct patient not to take other drugs without prescriber's approval.
• Tell woman to notify prescriber if she suspects pregnancy or if she is breast-feeding.

Evaluation

• Patient regains normal thought processes.
• Patient sustains no injury from adverse reactions.
• Patient and family state understanding of drug therapy.

misoprostol
(mee-SOH-pruh-stol)
Cytotec

Pharmacologic class: prostaglandin E₁ analogue
Therapeutic class: gastric mucosal protectant
Pregnancy risk category: X

Indications and dosages

▶ **Prevention of NSAID-induced gastric ulcer in elderly or debilitated patients at high risk for complications from gastric ulcer and in patients with history of NSAID-induced ulcer.**
Adults: 200 mcg P.O. q.i.d. with food. If dosage isn't tolerated, decrease to 100 mcg P.O. q.i.d.
▶ **Duodenal or gastric ulcer‡.** *Adults:* 100 to 200 mcg P.O. q.i.d. with meals and h.s. for 4 to 8 weeks.

Contraindications and precautions

• Contraindicated in those with a known allergy to prostaglandins.

≋ Lifespan: In pregnant women, avoid using drug. In breast-feeding women, avoid using drug because significant diarrhea in infants has been reported.

Adverse reactions

CNS: headache.
GI: *diarrhea, abdominal pain,* nausea, flatulence, dyspepsia, vomiting, constipation.
GU: hypermenorrhea, dysmenorrhea, spotting, cramps, menstrual disorders.

Interactions

Drug-drug. *Antacids:* Reduces misoprostol level insignificantly. Monitor patient.

Effects on lab test results

None reported.

Pharmacokinetics

Absorption: Rapid.
Distribution: Highly bound to proteins.
Metabolism: Rapidly de-esterified to misoprostol acid, the biologically active metabolite.
Excretion: About 15% excreted in feces; balance excreted in urine. *Half-life:* 20 to 40 minutes.

Route	Onset	Peak	Duration
P.O.	30 min	10-15 min	3 hr

Action

Chemical effect: Replaces gastric prostaglandins depleted by NSAID therapy. Decreases basal and stimulated gastric acid secretion and may increase gastric mucus and bicarbonate production.
Therapeutic effect: Protects gastric mucosa from ulcerating.

Available forms

Tablets: 100 mcg, 200 mcg

NURSING PROCESS

⚕ Assessment

• Obtain history of patient's GI condition before therapy.

• In woman of childbearing age, make sure that negative pregnancy test is obtained within 2 weeks before therapy begins.
• Be alert for adverse reactions and drug interactions.
• Evaluate patient's and family's knowledge of drug therapy.

✦ Nursing diagnoses

• Risk for injury related to potential for gastric ulceration
• Acute pain related to headache
• Deficient knowledge related to drug therapy

▶ Planning and implementation

✦ ALERT: Take special precautions not to use drug in pregnant women. Make sure she is fully aware of dangers of drug to fetus and that she receives both verbal and written warnings regarding these dangers. Also make sure she can comply with effective contraceptive use.
• Uterine rupture is linked to certain risk factors, including later trimester pregnancies, higher doses of the drug, prior cesarean delivery or uterine surgery, or five or more previous pregnancies.
✦ ALERT: Don't confuse misoprostol with mifepristone.

Patient teaching

• Instruct patient not to share drug. Remind her that drug may cause miscarriage, usually with life-threatening bleeding.
• Advise her not to begin therapy until second or third day of next normal menstrual period.

✓ Evaluation

• Patient remains free from signs and symptoms of gastric ulceration.
• Patient states that drug-induced headache doesn't occur.
• Patient and family state understanding of drug therapy.

mitomycin (mitomycin-C)

(might-oh-MIGH-sin)
Mitozytrex, Mutamycin

Pharmacologic class: antineoplastic antibiotic (cell cycle–phase nonspecific)
Therapeutic class: antineoplastic
Pregnancy risk category: NR

Indications and dosages

▶ **Disseminated pancreatic and stomach cancers.** *Adults:* 15 mg/m² Mitozytrex or 20 mg/m² Mutamycin I.V. as single dose. Repeat cycle after 6 to 8 weeks; adjust dosage if needed based on lowest WBC and platelet counts.
▶ **Bladder cancer‡.** *Adults:* 20 to 60 mg Mutamycin intravesically once per week for 8 weeks.

▼ I.V. administration

• Follow facility policy to reduce risks. Preparation and administration of parenteral form are related to mutagenic, teratogenic, and carcinogenic risks to personnel.
• To reconstitute 5-mg vial Mitozytrex, use 8.5 ml sterile water for injection; for 5-mg vial of Mutamycin, use 10 ml of sterile water for injection; to reconstitute 20-mg vial, use 40 ml of sterile water for injection; to reconstitute a 40-mg vial, use 80 ml sterile water for injection, to give a concentration of 0.5 mg/ml. Allow to stand at room temperature until complete dissolution occurs.
• When reconstituted with sterile water for injection to a concentration of 0.5 mg/ml, Mitozytrex is stable for 24 hours. When diluted, stable in D₅W for 4 hours, normal saline solution for 48 hours, sodium lactate for 24 hours.
• When reconstituted with sterile water for injection to a concentration of 0.5 mg/ml, Mutamycin is stable for 14 days refrigerated or 7 days at room temperature. When diluted, stable in D₅W for 3 hours, normal saline solution for 12 hours, sodium lactate for 24 hours.
• The combination of this drug (5 mg to 15 mg) and heparin (1,000 units to 10,000 units) in 30 ml of normal saline solution injection is stable at room temperature for 48 hours for Mutamycin and 72 hours for Mitozytrex.
• Give drug into the side arm of a free-flowing I.V.
• Watch for irritation and infiltration; extravasation can cause tissue damage and necrosis. If extravasation occurs, stop infusion immediately and notify prescriber because of potential for severe ulceration and necrosis.

Contraindications and precautions

• Contraindicated in patients hypersensitive to drug and in those with thrombocytopenia, coagulation disorder, or increased bleeding tendency from other causes.

※ **Lifespan:** In pregnant and breast-feeding women, drug isn't recommended. In children, safety of drug hasn't been established.

Adverse reactions

CNS: headache, neurologic abnormalities, confusion, drowsiness, fatigue, *fever.*
GI: *nausea, vomiting,* anorexia, stomatitis.
GU: *renal toxicity, hemolytic uremic syndrome.*
Hematologic: THROMBOCYTOPENIA, LEUKO-PENIA (may be delayed up to 8 weeks and be cumulative with successive doses), *microangiopathic hemolytic anemia.*
Respiratory: *pulmonary edema,* dyspnea, nonproductive cough, *acute respiratory distress syndrome, interstitial pneumonitis.*
Skin: desquamation, induration, pruritus, and *pain* at injection site; *septicemia,* cellulitis, ulceration, and sloughing with extravasation; *reversible alopecia;* purple coloration of nail beds.

Interactions

Drug-drug. *Vinca alkaloids:* May cause acute respiratory distress. Avoid using together.

Effects on lab test results

• May decrease hemoglobin, hematocrit, and platelet and WBC counts.

Pharmacokinetics

Absorption: Administered I.V.
Distribution: Distributed widely in body tissues; doesn't cross blood-brain barrier.
Metabolism: Metabolized by hepatic microsomal enzymes and deactivated in kidneys, spleen, brain, and heart.
Excretion: Excreted primarily in urine; small portion excreted in bile and feces. *Half-life:* About 50 minutes.

Route	Onset	Peak	Duration
I.V.	Unknown	Unknown	Unknown

Action

Chemical effect: Acts like alkylating drug, cross-linking strands of DNA. This causes imbalance of cell growth, leading to cell death.
Therapeutic effect: Kills certain cancer cells.

Available forms

Injection: 5-, 20-, and 40-mg vials

⚕ Assessment
• Assess patient's condition before therapy and regularly thereafter.
• Obtain CBC and blood studies.
• Monitor kidney function tests.
• Be alert for adverse reactions and drug interactions.
• Evaluate patient's and family's knowledge of drug therapy.

⊕ Nursing diagnoses
• Ineffective health maintenance related to presence of neoplastic disease
• Ineffective protection related to adverse hematologic reactions
• Deficient knowledge related to drug therapy

▷ Planning and implementation
• Never give drug I.M. or S.C.
• If WBC count is less than 4,000/mm³ and platelet count is less than 150,000/mm³, stop drug. Restart drug when counts rise above these levels.
• Hemolytic uremic syndrome is characterized by microangiopathic hemolytic anemia, thrombocytopenia, and renal impairment.
⊛ ALERT: Don't confuse mitomycin with mithramycin.
Patient teaching
• Instruct patient to watch for signs of infection and bleeding and to take temperature daily.
• Warn patient that alopecia may occur but assure him that it's reversible.
• Tell patient to report adverse reactions to prescriber promptly.

☑ Evaluation
• Patient responds well to therapy.
• Patient doesn't develop serious complications.
• Patient and family state understanding of drug therapy.

mitoxantrone hydrochloride
(migh-toh-ZAN-trohn high-droh-KLOR-ighd)
Novantrone

Pharmacologic class: antibiotic antineoplastic
Therapeutic class: antineoplastic
Pregnancy risk category: D

Indications and dosages
▷ **Combination initial therapy for acute non-lymphocytic leukemia.** *Adults:* Induction begins with 12 mg/m² I.V. daily on days 1 through 3, given with 100 mg/m² daily of cytarabine on days 1 through 7. If response isn't adequate, give second induction. Maintenance therapy: 12 mg/m² on days 1 and 2, given with cytarabine on days 1 through 5.
▷ **To reduce neurologic disability and frequency of relapse in chronic progressive, progressive relapsing, or worsening relapsing-remitting multiple sclerosis.** *Adults:* 12 mg/m² I.V. over 5 to 15 minutes q 3 months.
▷ **Combination initial therapy for pain from advanced hormone-refractory prostate cancer.** *Adults:* 12 to 14 mg/m² I.V. infusion over 15 to 30 minutes q 21 days.

▼ I.V. administration
• Preparation and administration of parenteral form carries mutagenic, teratogenic, and carcinogenic risks.
• Dilute dose (available as aqueous solution of 2 mg/ml in volumes of 10, 12.5, and 15 ml) in at least 50 ml of normal saline solution injection or D₅W injection. Give drug by direct injection into free-flowing I.V. line of normal saline solution or D₅W injection over at least 3 minutes, usually 15 to 30 minutes.
⊛ ALERT: Don't mix with other drugs, especially heparin because it's physically incompatible.
• Although drug isn't a vesicant, if dose extravasates, stop infusion immediately and notify prescriber.
• Store undiluted solution at room temperature. Once vial is penetrated, undiluted solution may be stored at room temperature for 7 days, or 14 days in refrigerator. Don't freeze.

Contraindications and precautions
• Contraindicated in patients hypersensitive to drug.
• Use cautiously in patients previously exposed to anthracyclines or other cardiotoxic drugs.
⚖ Lifespan: In pregnant and breast-feeding women, drug isn't recommended. In children, safety of drug hasn't been established.

Adverse reactions
CNS: *seizures,* headache.
CV: *heart failure, arrhythmias,* tachycardia.
EENT: conjunctivitis.

GI: BLEEDING, *abdominal pain, diarrhea, nausea, mucositis, vomiting, stomatitis.*
GU: uric acid nephropathy, *renal impairment.*
Hematologic: *myelosuppression.*
Hepatic: jaundice.
Metabolic: hyperuricemia.
Respiratory: dyspnea, cough.
Skin: petechiae, ecchymoses, alopecia.

Interactions

None significant.

Effects on lab test results

• May increase ALT, AST, bilirubin, BUN, creatinine, and uric acid levels.
• May decrease hemoglobin, hematocrit, and WBC, RBC, and platelet counts.

Pharmacokinetics

Absorption: Administered I.V.
Distribution: 78% protein-bound.
Metabolism: Metabolized by liver.
Excretion: Excreted by way of renal and hepatobiliary systems. *Half-life:* 5¾ days.

Route	Onset	Peak	Duration
I.V.	Unknown	Unknown	Unknown

Action

Chemical effect: Not fully understood; probably cell cycle–nonspecific. Drug reacts with DNA, producing cytotoxic effect.
Therapeutic effect: Hinders susceptible cancer cell growth.

Available forms

Injection: 2 mg/ml in 10-, 12.5-, and 15-ml vials

NURSING PROCESS

Assessment

• Assess patient's condition before therapy and regularly thereafter.
• Monitor CBC and other lab test results.
• Monitor left ventricular ejection fraction.
• Be alert for adverse reactions and drug interactions.
• Evaluate patient's and family's knowledge of drug therapy.

Nursing diagnoses

• Ineffective health maintenance related to presence of leukemia
• Ineffective immune protection related to drug-induced myelosuppression
• Deficient knowledge related to drug therapy

Planning and implementation

• Don't give to patient with neutrophil count below 1,500 cells/mm³ unless benefits outweigh risks.
• Give allopurinol, if needed. Uric acid nephropathy can be avoided by adequately hydrating patient before and during therapy.
• If severe nonhematologic toxicity occurs during first course of therapy, delay second course until patient recovers.
Patient teaching
• Inform patient that urine may appear blue-green within 24 hours after administration and that some bluish discoloration of sclera may occur. These effects aren't harmful.
• Teach patient infection control and bleeding precautions. Tell him to watch for and report signs of bleeding and infection.
• Advise woman of childbearing age to avoid pregnancy during therapy and to consult prescriber before becoming pregnant.

Evaluation

• Patient responds well to therapy.
• Patient develops no serious complications from drug-induced myelosuppression.
• Patient and family state understanding of drug therapy.

mivacurium chloride
(migh-vuh-KYOO-ree-um KLOR-ighd)
Mivacron

Pharmacologic class: nondepolarizing neuromuscular blocker
Therapeutic class: skeletal muscle relaxant
Pregnancy risk category: C

Indications and dosages

▶ **Adjunct to general anesthesia, to facilitate endotracheal intubation, and to relax skeletal muscles during surgery or mechanical ventilation.** *Adults:* Dosage is highly individualized. Usually, 0.15 mg/kg I.V. push over 5 to 15 sec-

onds provides adequate muscle relaxation within 135 seconds for endotracheal intubation. Supplemental doses of 0.1 mg/kg I.V. q 15 minutes is usually sufficient to maintain muscle relaxation. Or, maintain neuromuscular blockade with continuous infusion of 4 mcg/kg/minute begun simultaneously with initial dose, or 9 to 10 mcg/kg/minute started after evidence of spontaneous recovery caused by initial dose. When used with isoflurane or enflurane anesthesia, reduce dosage about 35% to 40%.
Children ages 2 to 12: 0.2 mg/kg I.V. push given over 5 to 15 seconds. Neuromuscular blockade is usually evident in less than 2 minutes. Maintenance doses are generally needed more frequently in children. Or, maintain neuromuscular blockade with continuous I.V. infusion adjusted to effect. Most children respond to 5 to 31 mcg/kg/minute.
❚ **Adjust-a-dose:** For patients with end-stage renal or hepatic disease, decrease infusion rates by as much as 50%.

▼ I.V. administration

● Give only under direct medical supervision of clinician skilled in use of neuromuscular blockers and techniques for maintaining airway. Don't use unless emergency equipment for respiratory support and antagonist are within reach.
● To avoid patient distress, don't give until patient is unconscious by general anesthetic because drug has no effect on consciousness or pain threshold.
● Drug may be given by direct injection over 5 to 15 seconds.
● Use with D_5W, normal saline solution injection, D_5W in normal saline solution injection, lactated Ringer's injection, or D_5W in lactated Ringer's injection. Diluted solutions are stable for 24 hours at room temperature.
● For premixed infusion in D_5W, remove protective outer wrap and check container for minor leaks by squeezing bag before giving. Don't add other drugs to container, and don't use container in series connections.
● Drug is compatible with alfentanil, fentanyl, sufentanil, droperidol, and midazolam.
● Alkaline solutions, such as barbiturate solutions, are physically incompatible; precipitate may form. Don't give through same I.V. line.

Contraindications and precautions

● Contraindicated in patients hypersensitive to drug or other drugs containing benzylisoquinolinium or in patients with allergy to benzyl alcohol.
● Use cautiously, if at all, in patients who are homozygous for atypical pseudocholinesterase gene. Drug is metabolized to inactive compounds by pseudocholinesterase.
● Use cautiously in patients with significant CV disease and in those who may be adversely affected by release of histamine (such as asthmatic patients).
● Also use cautiously, possibly at reduced dosage, in debilitated patients; in patients with metastatic cancer, severe electrolyte disturbances, or neuromuscular diseases; and in those in whom potentiation or difficulty in reversal of neuromuscular blockade is anticipated. Patients with myasthenia gravis or myasthenic syndrome (Eaton-Lambert syndrome) are particularly sensitive to effects of nondepolarizing relaxants.
⚞ **Lifespan:** In pregnant and breast-feeding women, use cautiously. In children younger than age 2, safety and effectiveness of drug haven't been established.

Adverse reactions

CNS: dizziness.
CV: *flushing,* hypotension, tachycardia, ***bradycardia, arrhythmias,*** phlebitis.
Musculoskeletal: prolonged muscle weakness, muscle spasms.
Respiratory: ***bronchospasm,*** wheezing, ***respiratory insufficiency, apnea.***
Skin: rash, urticaria, erythema.

Interactions

Drug-drug. *Alkaline solutions (such as barbiturate solutions):* Physically incompatible; precipitate may form. Don't give through same I.V. line.
Amikacin, gentamicin, neomycin, streptomycin, tobramycin: May increase the effects of mivacurium, including prolonged respiratory depression. Use together only when necessary. Reduce mivacurium dose if needed.
Bacitracin, clindamycin, colistimethate, colistin, ketamine, parenteral verapamil, polymyxin B sulfate, tetracycline: May potentiate neuromuscular blockade, leading to increased skeletal

---

muscle relaxation and prolonged effect. Use together cautiously.

Carbamazepine, phenytoin: May decrease the effects of mivacurium. Increase dose, if needed.

Inhaled anesthetics (especially enflurane, isoflurane), magnesium salts, quinidine: May enhance activity or prolong action of nondepolarizing neuromuscular blockers. Monitor patient for excessive weakness.

Effects on lab test results

None reported.

Pharmacokinetics

Absorption: Administered I.V.
Distribution: Not extensively distributed to tissues.
Metabolism: Rapidly hydrolyzed by pseudocholinesterase to inactive components.
Excretion: Metabolites excreted in urine and bile. *Half-life:* cis-trans and trans-trans isomers, less than 2¼ minutes; cis-cis isomer, 55 minutes.

Route	Onset	Peak	Duration
I.V.	1-2 min	2-5 min	20-35 min

Action

Chemical effect: Competes with acetylcholine for receptor sites at motor end plate. Because cholinesterase inhibitors may antagonize this action, drug is considered a competitive antagonist. Drug is mixture of three stereoisomers, each with neuromuscular blocking activity.
Therapeutic effect: Relaxes skeletal muscles.

Available forms

Infusion: 0.5 mg/ml in 50 ml of D₅W
Injection: 2 mg/ml in 5- and 10-ml vials

NURSING PROCESS

🗓 Assessment

• Assess patient's need for drug before therapy and regularly thereafter.
• Monitor respiratory rate closely until patient is fully recovered from neuromuscular blockade, as evidenced by tests of muscle strength (hand grip, head lift, and ability to cough).
• Be alert for adverse reactions and drug interactions.

• Evaluate patient's and family's knowledge of drug therapy.

🗓 Nursing diagnoses

• Ineffective breathing pattern related to drug's effect on respiratory muscle
• Deficient knowledge related to drug therapy

▷ Planning and implementation

Ⓢ **ALERT:** Give test dose to assess patient's sensitivity to drug. Patients with severe burns develop resistance to nondepolarizing neuromuscular blockers; however, they also may have reduced pseudocholinesterase activity.
• Monitor nerve stimulator and train-of-four to document antagonism of neuromuscular blockade and recovery of muscle strength. Before attempting reversal with neostigmine or edrophonium, wait for some signs of spontaneous recovery.
• Experimental evidence suggests that acid-base and electrolyte balances may influence actions of nondepolarizing neuromuscular blockers. Alkalosis may counteract paralysis; acidosis may enhance it.
• In patients 30% or more above their ideal weight, adjust dosage to ideal body weight to avoid prolonged neuromuscular blockade.
• Duration of effect is increased about 150% in patients with end-stage renal disease and 300% in patients with hepatic dysfunction.
• Like other neuromuscular blockers, dosage requirements for children are higher on mg/kg basis than those for adults. Onset and recovery of neuromuscular blockade occur more rapidly in children.
Ⓢ **ALERT:** Don't confuse Mivacron with Mazicon or Mevacor.
Patient teaching
• Describe use of drug to patient and family, and answer their questions.

☑ Evaluation

• Patient maintains adequate ventilation with or without assistance.
• Patient and family state understanding of drug therapy.

---

modafinil

(moh-DAF-ih-nil)

Provigil

Pharmacologic class: nonamphetamine CNS stimulant
Therapeutic class: analeptic
Pregnancy risk category: C
Controlled substance schedule: IV

Indications and dosages

▶ **To improve wakefulness in patients with excessive daytime sleepiness caused by narcolepsy.** *Adults:* 200 mg P.O. daily, given as a single dose in the morning.
◩ **Adjust-a-dose:** For patients with severe hepatic impairment, reduce dosage by 50%.

Contraindications and precautions

• Contraindicated in patients hypersensitive to drug. Don't use in patients with a history of left ventricular hypertrophy or ischemic ECG changes, chest pain, arrhythmias, or other signs or symptoms of mitral valve prolapse caused by CNS stimulant use.
• Use cautiously in patients with recent MI or unstable angina, in those with history of psychosis, and in those receiving treatment with MAO inhibitors.
• Use cautiously and at reduced dosage in patients with severe hepatic impairment, with or without cirrhosis.
⚱ **Lifespan:** In pregnant women, use only when the potential benefits outweigh the potential harm to the fetus. In breast-feeding women, use cautiously. In patients younger than age 16 or older than age 65, safety and effectiveness of drug haven't been established. In elderly patients with renal or hepatic impairment, use cautiously and at a reduced rate.

Adverse reactions

CNS: *headache,* nervousness, dizziness, depression, anxiety, fever, cataplexy, insomnia, paresthesia, dyskinesia, hypertonia, confusion, amnesia, emotional lability, ataxia, syncope, tremor.
CV: hypotension, hypertension, vasodilation, *arrhythmias,* chest pain.
EENT: *rhinitis,* pharyngitis, epistaxis, amblyopia, abnormal vision.

GI: *nausea,* diarrhea, dry mouth, mouth ulcer, gingivitis, thirst, anorexia, vomiting.
GU: abnormal urine, urine retention, abnormal ejaculation.
Hematologic: eosinophilia.
Metabolic: hyperglycemia.
Musculoskeletal: neck pain, rigid neck, joint disorder.
Respiratory: lung disorders, dyspnea, *asthma.*
Skin: herpes simplex, dry skin.
Other: chills.

Interactions

Drug-drug. *Carbamazepine, phenobarbital, rifampin, other inducers of CYP 3A4; itraconazole, ketoconazole, other inhibitors of CYP 3A4:* Alters modafinil levels. Monitor patient closely.
Cyclosporine, theophylline: Reduces levels of these drugs. Use together cautiously.
Diazepam, phenytoin, propranolol, other drugs metabolized by CYP 2C9: May increase levels of these drugs. Use together cautiously. Adjust dosage p.r.n.
Hormonal contraceptives: Reduces levels of these drugs, resulting in reduced contraceptive effectiveness. Recommend additional or alternative contraceptive method during modafinil therapy and for 1 month afterward.
Methylphenidate: Delays modafinil absorption. Separate administration times.
Phenytoin, warfarin: May cause concentration-dependent inhibition of CYP 2C9 activity and increase levels of phenytoin and warfarin. Monitor patient closely for signs of toxicity.
Tricyclic antidepressants (clomipramine, desipramine): May increase tricyclic antidepressant levels. Reduce dosage of these drugs.

Effects on lab test results

• May increase glucose, GGT, and AST levels.
• May increase eosinophil count.

Pharmacokinetics

Absorption: Rapid, with levels peaking in 2 to 4 hours.
Distribution: Well distributed in body tissue. About 60% binds to protein, primarily albumin.
Metabolism: About 90% of drug is metabolized in the liver, with subsequent renal elimination of the metabolites.
Excretion: Less than 10% is excreted from the kidneys as unchanged drug. *Half-life:* Unknown.

Reactions may be *common,* uncommon, *life-threatening,* or **COMMON AND LIFE-THREATENING.**

Route	Onset	Peak	Duration
P.O.	Unknown	2-4 hr	Unknown

Action

Chemical effect: Unknown. It has wake-promoting actions similar to those of sympathomimetics, including amphetamines, but it's structurally distinct from amphetamines and doesn't appear to alter the release of either dopamine or norepinephrine to produce CNS stimulation.

Therapeutic effect: Improves daytime wakefulness.

Available forms

Tablets: 100 mg, 200 mg

NURSING PROCESS

Assessment

• Obtain history of patient's underlying condition before therapy, and reassess regularly thereafter.
• Assess patient's renal function before starting drug therapy.
• Monitor hypertensive patients on modafinil therapy closely.
• Evaluate patient's and family's knowledge of drug therapy.

Nursing diagnoses

• Disturbed sleep pattern related to drug-induced insomnia
• Risk for injury related to drug-induced CNS adverse effects
• Deficient knowledge related to drug therapy

Planning and implementation

• Food has no effect on overall bioavailability, but it may delay modafinil absorption by 1 hour.
• Although single, daily, 400-mg doses have been well tolerated, no consistent evidence exists that this dosage provides additional benefit beyond the 200-mg dose.

Patient teaching

• Drug may impair judgment. Advise patient to be careful while driving or performing other activities that require alertness until full effects of drug are known.
• Instruct patient not to take other prescription or OTC drugs without consulting prescriber because of possible drug interactions.

• Advise patient to avoid alcohol while taking modafinil.
• Tell patient to notify prescriber if he develops a rash, hives, or a related allergic reaction.
• Caution woman that use of hormonal contraceptives (including depot or implantable contraceptives) with modafinil tablets may increase the risk of pregnancy. Recommend an alternative or additional method of contraception during modafinil therapy and for 1 month afterward.
• Advise woman to notify prescriber if she becomes pregnant or intends to become pregnant during therapy.
• Tell woman to notify prescriber if she's breast-feeding.

Evaluation

• Patient develops and maintains normal sleep-wake patterns.
• Patient has no adverse CNS effects.
• Patient and family state understanding of drug therapy.

moexipril hydrochloride
(moh-EKS-eh-pril high-droh-KLOR-ighd)
Univasc

Pharmacologic class: ACE inhibitor
Therapeutic class: antihypertensive
Pregnancy risk category: C (D in second and third trimesters)

Indications and dosages

▶ **Hypertension.** *Adults:* Initially, 7.5 mg P.O. daily 1 hour before meals. If inadequate response, increase or divide dose. Maintenance dosage, 7.5 to 30 mg daily in one or two divided doses 1 hour before meals.

Adjust-a-dose: For patients with renal impairment, if creatinine clearance is 40 ml/minute or less, initiate dosage at 3.75 mg P.O. daily. Maximum is 15 mg P.O. daily. For patients taking diuretics, if diuretic cannot be discontinued initial dose should be 3.75 mg P.O. daily.

Contraindications and precautions

• Contraindicated in patients hypersensitive to drug and in those with history of angioedema with previous treatment with ACE inhibitor.

• Use cautiously in patients with impaired kidney function, heart failure, or renal artery stenosis.

⚖ **Lifespan:** In pregnant women, drug isn't recommended. In breast-feeding women, use cautiously. In children, safety of drug hasn't been established.

Adverse reactions

CNS: *dizziness,* headache, fatigue, pain.
CV: peripheral edema, hypotension, orthostatic hypotension, chest pain, flushing.
EENT: pharyngitis, rhinitis, sinusitis.
GI: diarrhea, dyspepsia, nausea.
GU: urinary frequency.
Hematologic: *neutropenia.*
Metabolic: *hyperkalemia.*
Musculoskeletal: myalgia.
Respiratory: *persistent, nonproductive cough;* upper respiratory tract infection.
Skin: rash.
Other: *anaphylaxis, angioedema,* flulike syndrome.

Interactions

Drug-drug. *Antacids:* Bioavailability of ACE inhibitors may be decreased. Give drug on an empty stomach.
Digoxin: Increases digoxin level. Monitor digoxin level and patient closely.
Diuretics: May increase risk of excessive hypotension. Monitor blood pressure closely.
Indomethacin: May reduce hypotensive effects of ACE inhibitors. Avoid using together; monitor blood pressure.
Lithium: Increases lithium level and lithium toxicity. Use together cautiously. Monitor lithium level frequently.
Potassium-sparing diuretics, potassium supplements: Increases risk of hyperkalemia. Monitor potassium level closely.
Drug-herb. *Capsaicin:* May cause or worsen coughing linked to ACE inhibitor treatment. Discourage using together.
Drug-food. *Salt substitutes that contain potassium:* May increase risk of hyperkalemia. Monitor potassium level closely; urge patient to avoid salt substitutes containing potassium.

Effects on lab test results

• May increase potassium level.
• May decrease neutrophil count.

Pharmacokinetics

Absorption: Incomplete, with bioavailability of about 13%. Food significantly decreases bioavailability.
Distribution: About 50% protein-bound.
Metabolism: Metabolized extensively to the active metabolite moexiprilat.
Excretion: Excreted primarily in feces, with small amount in urine. *Half-life:* 2 to 9 hours.

Route	Onset	Peak	Duration
P.O.	1 hr	3-6 hr	24 hr

Action

Chemical effect: Unknown; may suppress renin-angiotensin-aldosterone system. Inhibits ACE, thereby inhibiting production of angiotensin II (a potent vasoconstrictor and stimulator of aldosterone secretion).
Therapeutic effect: Lowers blood pressure.

Available forms

Tablets: 7.5 mg, 15 mg

NURSING PROCESS

🔍 **Assessment**

• Assess patient's blood pressure before therapy.
• Measure blood pressure at lowest point just before dose to verify adequate control. Drug is less effective in reducing trough blood pressure in blacks than in nonblacks.
• Monitor patient for hypotension.
• Assess kidney function before therapy and periodically thereafter. Monitor potassium level.
• May cause agranulocytosis and neutropenia. Monitor CBC with differential counts before therapy, especially in patient who has collagen-vascular disease with impaired kidney function.
• Be alert for adverse reactions and interactions.
• Evaluate patient's and family's knowledge of drug therapy.

🔲 **Nursing diagnoses**

• Risk for injury related to presence of hypertension
• Disturbed sleep pattern related to cough
• Deficient knowledge related to drug therapy

▷ **Planning and implementation**
⚠ **ALERT:** Excessive hypotension can occur when drug is given with diuretics. If possible, stop di-

---

uretics 2 to 3 days before starting this drug to decrease potential for reaction. If drug doesn't adequately control blood pressure, restart diuretic with care.

• Angioedema involving tongue, glottis, or larynx may be fatal because of airway obstruction. Give epinephrine and use equipment to ensure a patent airway.

• If cough interferes with patient's ability to sleep, notify prescriber.

Patient teaching

• Instruct patient to take drug on an empty stomach; high-fat meals can impair absorption.

• Tell patient to avoid salt substitutes; these products may contain potassium, which can cause hyperkalemia.

• Advise patient to rise slowly to minimize light-headedness. If syncope occurs, tell him to stop drug and call prescriber immediately.

• Urge patient to use caution in hot weather and during exercise. Inadequate fluid intake, vomiting, diarrhea, and excessive perspiration can lead to light-headedness and syncope.

• Advise patient to report signs of infection, such as fever and sore throat; easy bruising or bleeding; swelling of tongue, lips, face, eyes, mucous membranes, or limbs; difficulty swallowing or breathing; and hoarseness.

• Tell woman to notify prescriber if she becomes pregnant.

Evaluation

• Patient's blood pressure is normal.

• Patient states that sleep disturbance doesn't occur.

• Patient and family state understanding of drug therapy.

montelukast sodium
(mon-tih-LOO-kist SOH-dee-um)
Singulair

Pharmacologic class: leukotriene receptor antagonist
Therapeutic class: antiasthmatic
Pregnancy risk category: B

Indications and dosages

▶ **Asthma, seasonal allergic rhinitis.** *Adults and children age 15 and older:* 10 mg P.O. daily in evening.

Children ages 6 to 14: 5 mg chewable tablet P.O. daily in the evening.
Children ages 2 to 5: 4 mg chewable tablet P.O. or one packet of 4-mg oral granules daily in the evening.

▶ **Asthma.** *Children ages 12 to 23 months:* One packet of 4-mg granules P.O. daily in the evening.

▶ **Prevention of exercise-induced bronchoconstriction‡.** *Adults and children age 15 and older:* 10 mg P.O. daily.
Children ages 6 to 14: 5 mg P.O. daily.

Contraindications and precautions

• Contraindicated in patients hypersensitive to drug or its components and in patients with acute asthmatic attacks or status asthmaticus.

• Use cautiously and with appropriate monitoring when systemic corticosteroid dosages are reduced.

⚠ Lifespan: In children younger than age 1, safety and effectiveness of drug haven't been established.

Adverse reactions

CNS: *headache,* dizziness, fatigue, fever, asthenia.
EENT: nasal congestion.
GI: dyspepsia, infectious gastroenteritis, abdominal pain.
GU: pyuria.
Respiratory: cough.
Skin: rash.
Other: trauma, influenza, dental pain.

Interactions

Drug-drug. *Phenobarbital, rifampin:* May decrease bioavailability of montelukast via induction of hepatic metabolism. Monitor patient closely for decreased effects.

Effects on lab test results

• May increase ALT and AST levels.

Pharmacokinetics

Absorption: Rapid with an oral bioavailability of 64%.
Distribution: More than 99% bound to proteins.
Metabolism: Extensively metabolized by CYP isoenzymes.
Excretion: About 86% is recovered in the feces, indicating montelukast and its metabolites

are excreted almost exclusively via the bile.
Half-life: 2¾ to 5½ hours.

Route	Onset	Peak	Duration
P.O.			
coated	Unknown	3-4 hr	Unknown
chewable	Unknown	2-2½ hr	Unknown

Action

Chemical effect: Inhibits action cysteinyl leukotriene$_1$ (CysLT$_1$) receptor by binding with CysLT$_1$. This reduces early- and late-phase bronchoconstriction caused by antigen challenge.
Therapeutic effect: Improves breathing.

Available forms

Granules: 4-mg packets
Tablets (chewable): 4 mg, 5 mg
Tablets (film-coated): 10 mg

NURSING PROCESS

⚖ Assessment
• Assess patient's underlying condition and monitor drug's effectiveness.
• Monitor patient for adverse reactions and drug interactions.
• Evaluate patient's and family's knowledge of drug therapy.

⊞ Nursing diagnoses
• Impaired gas exchange related to asthma
• Activity intolerance related to asthma
• Deficient knowledge related to drug therapy

▷ Planning and implementation
• Don't abruptly substitute drug for inhaled or oral corticosteroids.
• Drug isn't indicated for patients with acute asthmatic attacks or status asthmaticus. Also not indicated as monotherapy for managing exercise-induced bronchospasm. Continue rescue drug for acute exacerbations.
• Give oral granules directly in mouth or mixed with a teaspoonful of cold or room temperature applesauce, carrots, rice, or ice cream. After opening packet, give within 15 minutes. If mixed with food, don't store excess for future use; discard any unused portion.
• Don't dissolve oral granules in liquid before giving. However, patient may take liquids afterwards.

• Don't give oral granules with high-fat meals.
• Give drug daily; don't use on an as-needed basis.

Patient teaching
• Advise patient to take drug daily, even if asymptomatic, and to contact prescriber if asthma isn't well controlled.
• Warn patient not to reduce or stop taking other prescribed antiasthma drugs without prescriber's approval.
• Give patient directions for administration of oral granules mixed in with applesauce, carrots, rice, or ice cream. Tell him to discard any unused portion.
• Warn patient that drug isn't beneficial in acute asthma attacks or in exercise-induced bronchospasm, and advise him to keep appropriate rescue drugs available.
• Advise patient with known aspirin sensitivity to continue to avoid using aspirin and NSAIDs.
• Advise patient with phenylketonuria that chewable tablet contains phenylalanine.

☑ Evaluation
• Patient's respiratory signs and symptoms improve.
• Patient can perform normal activities of daily living.
• Patient and family state understanding of drug therapy.

moricizine hydrochloride
(MOR-ih-sigh-zeen high-droh-KLOR-ighd)
Ethmozine

Pharmacologic class: sodium channel blocker
Therapeutic class: antiarrhythmic
Pregnancy risk category: B

Indications and dosages

▶ **Life-threatening ventricular arrhythmias.**
Adults: Individualized dosage is based on response and patient tolerance. Begin therapy in hospital. Most patients respond to 600 to 900 mg P.O. daily in divided doses q 8 hours. Daily dose is increased within this range q 3 days by 150 mg until desired effect is achieved.
⚠ **Adjust-a-dose:** For patients with hepatic or renal impairment, give 600 mg or less P.O. daily. Monitor ECG before increasing dosage.

Contraindications and precautions

• Contraindicated in patients hypersensitive to drug, in patients with second- or third-degree AV block or right bundle-branch heart block when linked to left hemiblock (bifascicular block) unless artificial pacemaker is present, and in patients with cardiogenic shock.

• Use cautiously in patients with sick-sinus syndrome because drug may cause sinus bradycardia or sinus arrest. Also use cautiously in patients with coronary artery disease and left ventricular dysfunction because these patients may be at risk for sudden death when treated with drug.

• Give cautiously to patients with hepatic or renal impairment.

⚙ **Lifespan:** In pregnant women, use cautiously. In breast-feeding women, drug isn't recommended. In children, safety of drug hasn't been established.

Adverse reactions

CNS: *dizziness, headache, fatigue,* anxiety, hypoesthesia, asthenia, nervousness, paresthesia, sleep disorders.
CV: *proarrhythmic events (ventricular tachycardia, PVCs, supraventricular arrhythmias), ECG abnormalities (including conduction defects, sinus pause, junctional rhythm, or AV block), heart failure,* palpitations, *cardiac death,* chest pain.
EENT: blurred vision.
GI: *nausea, vomiting, abdominal pain, dyspepsia, diarrhea, dry mouth.*
GU: urine retention, urinary frequency, dysuria.
Musculoskeletal: muscle pain.
Respiratory: dyspnea.
Skin: diaphoresis, rash.
Other: drug-induced fever.

Interactions

Drug-drug. *Cimetidine:* Increases levels and decreases clearance of moricizine. Begin moricizine therapy at low dosage (not more than 600 mg daily) and monitor levels and therapeutic effect closely.
Digoxin, propranolol: May cause additive prolongation of PR interval. Monitor patient closely; monitor ECG.
Theophylline: Increases clearance and reduces levels of theophylline. Monitor levels and therapeutic response; adjust theophylline dosage.

Effects on lab test results

• May increase liver function test results.

Pharmacokinetics

Absorption: Administration within 30 minutes of mealtime delays absorption and lowers peak levels but has no effect on extent of absorption.
Distribution: 95% protein-bound.
Metabolism: Undergoes significant first-pass metabolism. At least 26 metabolites have been found; none represent more than 1% of a dose. Drug induces its own metabolism.
Excretion: 50% excreted in feces; 39% excreted in urine; some recycled through enterohepatic circulation. *Half-life:* 1½ to 3½ hours.

Route	Onset	Peak	Duration
P.O.	≤ 2 hr	30 min-2 hr	10-24 hr

Action

Chemical effect: Reduces fast inward current carried by sodium ions across myocardial cell membranes. Has potent local anesthetic activity and membrane-stabilizing effect.
Therapeutic effect: Alleviates ventricular arrhythmias.

Available forms

Tablets: 200 mg, 250 mg, 300 mg

NURSING PROCESS

🖉 **Assessment**
• Assess patient's condition before therapy and regularly thereafter.
• Be alert for adverse reactions and drug interactions.
• Evaluate patient's and family's knowledge of drug therapy.

🔷 **Nursing diagnoses**
• Decreased cardiac output related to presence of ventricular arrhythmia
• Risk for injury related to drug-induced adverse reactions
• Deficient knowledge related to drug therapy

▶ **Planning and implementation**
• When substituting this drug for another antiarrhythmic, withdraw previous drug for one or two of drug's half-lives before starting this drug. When withdrawing or adjusting drug, hospitalize patient with tendency to develop life-

threatening arrhythmias after drug withdrawal. Start this drug as follows: 6 to 12 hours after last dose of disopyramide; 8 to 12 hours after last dose of mexiletine; 3 to 6 hours after last dose of procainamide; 8 to 12 hours after last dose of propafenone; 6 to 12 hours after last dose of quinidine; 8 to 12 hours after last dose of tocainide.

• Determine electrolyte status and correct imbalances before therapy. Hypokalemia, hyperkalemia, and hypomagnesemia may alter effects of drug.

⊛ **ALERT:** Don't confuse Ethmozine with Erythrocin.

Patient teaching

• Tell patient to report adverse reactions promptly.

☑ **Evaluation**

• Patient regains normal cardiac output with alleviation of ventricular arrhythmia.
• Patient sustains no injury from adverse reactions.
• Patient and family state understanding of drug therapy.

---

morphine hydrochloride
(MOR-feen high-droh-KLOR-ighd)
M.O.S. ♦, M.O.S.-SR ♦

morphine sulfate
Astramorph PF, Avinza, DMS Concentrate, Duramorph PF, Infumorph 200, Infumorph 500, Kadian, Morphine H.P. ♦, MS Contin, MSIR, MS/L, MS/L concentrate, OMS concentrate, Oramorph SR, RMS Uniserts, Roxanol, Roxanol 100, Roxanol T, Statex ♦

morphine tartrate ◇

Pharmacologic class: opioid
Therapeutic class: opioid analgesic
Pregnancy risk category: C
Controlled substance schedule: II

Indications and dosages

▶ **Severe pain.** *Adults:* 5 to 20 mg/70 kg S.C. or I.M. q 4 hours, p.r.n. Or, 2 to 10 mg/70 kg I.V. q 4 hours, p.r.n. Or, 10 to 30 mg P.O. Or, 10 to 20 mg P.R. q 4 hours, p.r.n. Or, 30 mg controlled-release tablets P.O. q 8 to 12 hours.

Or, 5 mg epidural injection by epidural catheter. If adequate pain relief not obtained within 1 hour, give additional doses of 1 to 2 mg at intervals sufficient to assess effectiveness. Maximum total epidural dose, 10 mg.

▶ **Severe pain associated with terminal cancer.** *Adults:* Give loading dose of 15 mg or more I.V. by continuous I.V. infusion; then continuous infusion of 0.8 to 80 mg/hour. *Children:* 0.1 to 0.2 mg/kg S.C. q 4 hours. Maximum single dose is 15 mg.

▼ I.V. administration

• For direct injection, dilute 2.5 to 15 mg in 4 or 5 ml of sterile water for injection and give over 4 to 5 minutes.
• For continuous infusion, mix with D_5W to yield 0.1 to 1 mg/ml.
• In adults with severe, chronic pain, maintenance I.V. infusions may last 0.8 to 80 mg/hour. Higher doses may be needed.
• Drug is compatible with most common I.V. solutions.

Contraindications and precautions

• Contraindicated in patients hypersensitive to drug and in those with conditions that preclude I.V. administration of opioids (acute bronchial asthma or upper airway obstruction).
• Use cautiously in debilitated patients and in patients with head injury, increased intracranial pressure, seizures, chronic pulmonary disease, prostatic hyperplasia, severe hepatic or renal disease, acute abdominal conditions, hypothyroidism, Addison's disease, or urethral stricture.

⚘ **Lifespan:** In pregnant women, use cautiously. In breast-feeding women, wait 2 to 3 hours after last dose before breast-feeding to avoid sedation in infant. In elderly patients, use cautiously.

Adverse reactions

CNS: *sedation, somnolence, clouded sensorium, euphoria, **seizures*** (with large doses), *dizziness, nightmares* (with long-acting oral forms).
CV: *hypotension, flushing, **bradycardia, shock, cardiac arrest.***
GI: *nausea, vomiting, constipation, ileus.*
GU: *urine retention.*
Hematologic: ***thrombocytopenia.***
Respiratory: ***respiratory depression, respiratory arrest.***

Reactions may be *common*, uncommon, *life-threatening*, or COMMON AND LIFE-THREATENING.

Skin: pruritus and flushing with epidural administration.
Other: *physical dependence.*

Interactions

Drug-drug. *Antihistamines, chloral hydrate, CNS depressants, general anesthetics, glutethimide, hypnotics, MAO inhibitors, methocarbamol, other opioid analgesics, sedatives, tranquilizers, tricyclic antidepressants:* May cause possible respiratory depression, hypotension, profound sedation, or coma. Use together cautiously. Reduce morphine dosage and monitor patient response.
Drug-lifestyle. *Alcohol use:* May have additive CNS effects. Urge patient to avoid using alcohol during drug therapy.

Effects on lab test results

• May increase amylase level.
• May decrease platelet count.

Pharmacokinetics

Absorption: Variable when given P.O.; unknown for other routes.
Distribution: Distributed widely throughout body.
Metabolism: Metabolized primarily in liver.
Excretion: Excreted in urine and bile. *Half-life:* 2 to 3 hours.

Route	Onset	Peak	Duration
P.O.	1 hr	1-2 hr	4-12 hr
I.V.	< 5 min	20 min	4-5 hr
I.M.	10-30 min	30-60 min	4-5 hr
S.C.	10-30 min	50-90 min	4-5 hr
P.R.	20-60 min	20-60 min	4-5 hr
Epidural	15-60 min	15-60 min	24 hr
Intrathecal	15-60 min	Unknown	24 hr

Action

Chemical effect: Binds with opioid receptors in CNS, altering both perception of and emotional response to pain through unknown mechanism.
Therapeutic effect: Relieves pain.

Available forms

morphine hydrochloride
Oral solution ◆: 1 mg/ml, 5 mg/ml, 10 mg/ml, 20 mg/ml, 50 mg/ml
Suppositories: 10 mg ◆, 20 mg ◆, 30 mg ◆

Syrup: 1 mg/ml ◆, 5 mg/ml ◆, 10 mg/ml ◆, 20 mg/ml ◆, 50 mg/ml ◆
Tablets: 10 mg ◆, 20 mg ◆, 40 mg ◆, 60 mg ◆
Tablets (extended-release): 30 mg ◆, 60 mg ◆
morphine sulfate
Capsules: 15 mg, 30 mg
Capsules (extended-release) (Avinza): 30 mg, 60 mg, 90 mg, 120 mg
Capsules (sustained-release): 20 mg, 50 mg, 100 mg
Injection (with preservative): 500 mcg/ml, 1 mg/ml, 2 mg/ml, 3 mg/ml, 4 mg/ml, 5 mg/ml, 8 mg/ml, 10 mg/ml, 15 mg/ml, 25 mg/ml, 50 mg/ml
Injection (without preservative): 500 mcg/ml, 1 mg/ml, 10 mg/ml, 15 mg/ml, 25 mg/ml
Oral solution: 10 mg/5 ml, 20 mg/5 ml, 20 mg/ml
Oral solution (concentrated): 20 mg/ml, 30 mg/1.5 ml, 100 mg/5 ml
Soluble tablets: 10 mg, 15 mg, 30 mg
Suppositories: 5 mg, 10 mg, 20 mg, 30 mg
Syrup: 1 mg/ml, 5 mg/ml
Tablets: 15 mg, 30 mg
Tablets (controlled-release): 15 mg, 30 mg, 60 mg, 100 mg, 200 mg
Tablets (extended-release): 15 mg, 30 mg, 60 mg, 100 mg, 200 mg
morphine tartrate
Injection: 80 mg/ml ◇

NURSING PROCESS

⚕ Assessment

• Assess patient's pain before therapy and regularly thereafter.
• Drug may worsen or mask gallbladder pain.
• Monitor patient for respiratory depression after administration. When given epidurally, monitor patient for up to 24 hours after injection. Check respiratory rate and depth q 30 to 60 minutes for 24 hours.
• Be alert for adverse reactions and drug interactions.
• Evaluate patient's and family's knowledge of drug therapy.

🔲 Nursing diagnoses

• Acute pain related to underlying condition
• Ineffective breathing pattern related to drug's depressive effect on respiratory system
• Deficient knowledge related to drug therapy

▷ Planning and implementation

• Preservative-free preparations are available for epidural or intrathecal administration.

❸ ALERT: Highly concentrated injections containing 10 or 25 mg/ml are meant for continuous, controlled microinfusion devices. Don't use for I.M., S.C., I.V epidural, or intrathecal individual doses because of the risk of substantial overdose.

• Solutions of various concentrations are available as well as intensified P.O. solution (20 mg/ml). Carefully note the strength you are giving.

• Don't crush or break extended-release tablets.

• If using S.L., measure solution with tuberculin syringe. Give dose a few drops at a time to allow maximal S.L. absorption and minimize swallowing.

• Refrigeration of rectal suppository isn't needed.

• In some patients, P.R. and P.O. absorption may not be equivalent.

• Morphine is drug of choice in relieving pain of MI. It may cause transient decrease in blood pressure.

• Keep opioid antagonist and resuscitation equipment available.

• An around-the-clock regimen best manages severe, chronic pain.

❸ ALERT: If respiratory rate is below 12 breaths/minute, withhold dose and notify prescriber.

• Because constipation is often severe with maintenance dosage, give stool softener or other laxative.

❸ ALERT: Don't confuse morphine with hydromorphone.

❸ ALERT: Don't confuse Avinza with Invanz.

Patient teaching

• Warn patient about getting out of bed or walking. Warn outpatient not to drive or perform other potentially hazardous activities until full CNS effects of drug are known.

• Tell patient to report continued pain.

• Instruct patient to avoid alcohol consumption during drug therapy.

☑ Evaluation

• Patient states that pain is relieved.

• Patient maintains adequate breathing patterns throughout therapy.

• Patient and family state understanding of drug therapy.

moxifloxacin hydrochloride
(mox-ih-FLOX-uh-sin high-droh-CLOR-ighd)
Avelox, Avelox I.V.

Pharmacologic class: fluoroquinolone
Therapeutic class: antibiotic
Pregnancy risk category: C

Indications and dosages

▶ **Acute bacterial sinusitis caused by** *Streptococcus pneumoniae, Haemophilus influenzae,* **or** *Moraxella catarrhalis. Adults:* 400 mg P.O. or I.V. once daily for 10 days.

▶ **Acute bacterial exacerbation of chronic bronchitis caused by** *S. pneumoniae, H. influenzae, H. parainfluenzae, Klebsiella pneumoniae, Staphylococcus aureus,* **or** *M. catarrhalis. Adults:* 400 mg P.O. or I.V. once daily for 5 days.

Community-acquired pneumonia caused by *S. pneumoniae* **(including penicillin-resistant strains, minimal inhibitory concentration (MIC) value for penicillin is 2 mcg/ml or greater),** *H. influenzae, Mycoplasma pneumoniae, Chlamydia pneumoniae, M. catarrhalis, S. aureus,* **or** *K. pneumoniae. Adults:* 400 mg P.O. or I.V. once daily for 7 to 14 days.

▶ **Uncomplicated skin and skin-structure infections caused by** *S. aureus* **and** *Streptococcus pyogenes. Adults:* 400 mg P.O daily for 7 days.

▽ I.V. administration

• Flush I.V. line with a compatible solution such as D_5W, normal saline solution, or Ringer's lactate solution before and after use.

• If particulate matter is visible, don't use.

• Infuse I.V. over 60 minutes by direct infusion or through a Y-type IV infusion set. Avoid rapid or bolus infusion.

❸ ALERT: Don't mix or infuse drug simultaneously with other substances because of limited compatibility data.

• Switch from I.V. to P.O. form when warranted.

Contraindications and precautions

• Contraindicated in patients hypersensitive to drug, its components, or other fluoroquinolones.

• Use cautiously in patients with known or suspected CNS disorders and in patients with risk

---

Reactions may be *common,* uncommon, *life-threatening,* or **COMMON AND LIFE-THREATENING.**

factors that may predispose them to seizures or lower the seizure threshold. Use cautiously in patients with prolonged QT interval or uncorrected hypokalemia.

☀ **Lifespan:** In pregnant and breast-feeding women and in children, safety and effectiveness of drug haven't been established. In elderly patients, monitor cardiac function carefully, especially with I.V. form of drug.

Adverse reactions

CNS: dizziness, headache, asthenia, pain, malaise, insomnia, nervousness, anxiety, confusion, somnolence, tremor, vertigo, paresthesia.

CV: *prolonged QT interval,* chest pain, palpitations, tachycardia, hypertension, peripheral edema.

GI: *pseudomembranous colitis,* nausea, diarrhea, abdominal pain, vomiting, dyspepsia, dry mouth, constipation, oral candidiasis, anorexia, stomatitis, glossitis, flatulence, gastrointestinal disorder, taste perversion.

GU: vaginitis, vaginal candidiasis.

Hematologic: *thrombocytosis, thrombocytopenia, leukopenia,* eosinophilia.

Hepatic: liver dysfunction, cholestatic jaundice.

Musculoskeletal: leg pain, back pain, arthralgia, myalgia, tendon rupture.

Respiratory: dyspnea.

Skin: rash (maculopapular, purpuric, pustular), pruritus, sweating.

Other: candidiasis, *allergic reaction,* injection site reaction.

Interactions

Drug-drug. *Aluminum hydroxide, aluminum-magnesium hydroxide, calcium carbonate, magnesium hydroxide:* May decrease effects of moxifloxacin. Give antacid at least 6 hours before or 2 hours after.

Didanosine, metal cations (such as aluminum, magnesium, iron, zinc), multivitamins: May decrease absorption and lower levels. Give moxifloxacin at least 4 hours before or 8 hours after these drugs.

Class IA (quinidine, procainamide) or Class III (amiodarone, sotalol) antiarrhythmics: May have possible enhanced adverse CV effects. Avoid using together.

Drugs known to prolong the QT interval (e.g., erythromycin, antipsychotics, tricyclic antidepressants): May have an additive effect when combined with these drugs. Avoid using together.

NSAIDs: May increase risk of CNS stimulation and seizures. Don't use together.

Sucralfate: May decrease absorption of moxifloxacin reducing anti-infective effect. If use together can't be avoided, give at least 6 hours apart.

Warfarin: Enhances anticoagulant effects. Monitor PT and INR closely.

Drug-lifestyle. *Sun exposure:* Although photosensitivity reactions haven't occurred with moxifloxacin, it has been reported with other fluoroquinolones. Discourage prolonged or unprotected exposure to sunlight.

Effects on lab test results

• May increase GGT, amylase, and LDH levels.
• May increase eosinophil count. May decrease PT and WBC count. May increase or decrease platelet count.

Pharmacokinetics

Absorption: Well absorbed, with an absolute bioavailability of about 90%. Level peaks in 1 to 3 hours. Steady-state is reached after 3 days on a 400 mg once-daily dose.

Distribution: Widely distributed with a distribution volume of 1.7 to 2.7 L/kg. Protein-binding is about 50%. Penetrates well into nasal and bronchial secretions, sinus mucosa, and saliva.

Metabolism: Drug is metabolized to inactive glucuronide and sulfate conjugates. About 14% of dose is converted to the glucuronide metabolite. Sulfate metabolite accounts for about 38% of the dose.

Excretion: About 45% of dose is excreted unchanged, about 20% in urine and 25% in feces. Sulfate metabolite is eliminated mainly in feces; glucuronide metabolite undergoes renal excretion. *Half-life:* About 12 hours.

Route	Onset	Peak	Duration
P.O., I.V.	Unknown	1-3 hr	Unknown

Action

Chemical effect: Inhibits the activity of topoisomerase I (DNA gyrase) and topoisomerase IV in susceptible bacteria. These enzymes are needed for bacterial DNA replication, transcription, repair, and recombination.

Rapid onset   *Liquid form contains alcohol.   ◆Canada   ◇ Australia   †OTC   ‡Off-label use

Therapeutic effect: Kills susceptible bacteria, including *S. pneumoniae, H. influenzae, H. parainfluenzae, K. pneumoniae, S. aureus, M. pneumoniae, C. pneumoniae,* and *M. catarrhalis.*

Available forms

Injection (premixed solution): 400 mg
Tablets (film-coated): 400 mg

NURSING PROCESS

Assessment

● Obtain history of patient's underlying condition before therapy, and reassess regularly thereafter.
● Obtain specimen for culture and sensitivity tests before first dose. Therapy may begin pending culture results.
● Monitor patient for hypersensitivity reactions, CNS toxicities including seizures, prolonged QT interval, pseudomembranous colitis, phototoxicity, and tendon rupture.
● Evaluate patient's and family's knowledge of drug therapy.

Nursing diagnoses

● Infection related to presence of bacteria susceptible to drug
● Risk for injury related to drug-induced adverse reactions
● Deficient knowledge related to drug therapy

Planning and implementation

● Correct hypokalemia before starting therapy.
● Give without regard to meals. Give at same time to provide consistent absorption.
● Provide liberal fluid intake.
● Give drug 4 hours before or 8 hours after antacids, sucralfate, and products containing iron or zinc.
● The most common adverse reactions are nausea, vomiting, stomach pain, diarrhea, dizziness, and headache.
● Store drug at controlled room temperature.
Patient teaching
● Instruct patient to take drug once daily, at the same time each day.
● Tell patient to finish the entire course of therapy, even if symptoms resolve.
● Advise the patient to drink plenty of fluids and to take moxifloxacin 4 hours before or 8

hours after antacids, sucralfate, and products containing iron and zinc.
● Most common adverse reactions are nausea, vomiting, stomach pain, diarrhea, dizziness, and headache.
● Tell patient to avoid hazardous activities, such as driving or operating machinery, until effects of drug are known.
● Instruct patient to contact prescriber if he experiences allergic reaction, palpitations, fainting, persistent diarrhea, severe sunburn, injury to a muscle tendon, or seizures.

Evaluation

● Patient is free from infection after drug therapy.
● Patient sustains no injury as a result of drug-induced adverse reactions.
● Patient and family state understanding of drug therapy.

moxifloxacin hydrochloride ophthalmic solution

(mocks-ih-FLOCKS-ah-sin high-droe-KLOR-ighd off-THAL-mick suh-LOO-shun)
Vigamox

Pharmacologic class: fluoroquinolone antibiotic
Therapeutic class: antibiotic
Pregnancy risk category: C

Indications and dosages

▶ **Bacterial conjunctivitis.** *Adults and children age 1 and older:* 1 drop into affected eye t.i.d. for 7 days.

Contraindications and precautions

● Contraindicated in patients hypersensitive to drug, fluoroquinolones, or their components.
⚖ Lifespan: In pregnant women, use only if benefits justify potential risk to fetus. In breastfeeding women, use cautiously. In children younger than age 1, don't use drug.

Adverse reactions

EENT: conjunctivitis; dry eyes; increased lacrimation; keratitis; ocular hyperemia; ocular discomfort, pain, and pruritus; otitis media;

pharyngitis; reduced visual acuity; rhinitis; subconjunctival hemorrhage.
Respiratory: increased cough.
Skin: rash.
Other: infection, fever.

Interactions

None reported.

Effects on lab test results

None reported.

Pharmacokinetics

Absorption: Unknown.
Distribution: Unknown.
Metabolism: Unknown.
Excretiont: Unknown.

Route	Onset	Peak	Duration
Ocular	Unknown	Unknown	Unknown

Action

Chemical effect: Inhibits DNA gyrase and topoisomerase IV, preventing cell replication, transcription, repair of bacterial DNA, and cell division.
Therapeutic effect: Kills susceptible bacteria causing infection.

Available forms

Solution: 0.5%

NURSING PROCESS

Assessment
• Assess patient's allergy history before initiating therapy.
• Monitor patient for superinfection.
• Monitor patient for adverse reactions.
• Evaluate patient's and family's knowledge of drug therapy.

Nursing diagnoses
• Infection related to presence of bacteria susceptible to drug
• Disturbed visual sensory perception related to adverse effects of the drug.
• Deficient knowledge related to drug therapy

Planning and implementation
• Don't inject solution subconjunctivally or into anterior chamber of the eye.

• Drug has caused serious hypersensitivity reactions. If allergic reaction occurs, stop drug and treat symptoms.

Patient teaching
• Tell patient to stop drug and seek medical treatment immediately if evidence of hypersensitivity reaction (itching, rash, swelling of the face or throat, or difficulty breathing) develops.
• Tell patient not to wear contact lenses during treatment.
• Instruct patient not to touch dropper tip to anything, including eyes and fingers.

Evaluation
• Patient is free from infection after drug therapy.
• Patient does not experience adverse drug effects.
• Patient and family state understanding of drug therapy.

muromonab-CD3
(myoo-roh-MOH-nab see dee three)
Orthoclone OKT3

Pharmacologic class: monoclonal antibody
Therapeutic class: immunosuppressive
Pregnancy risk category: C

Indications and dosages

▶ **Acute allograft rejection in heart, liver, or kidney transplant.** *Adults:* 5 mg I.V. daily for 10 to 14 days.
Children: Initially, 2.5 mg/day (if 30 kg or less) or 5 mg/day (if more than 30 kg) I.V. as a single bolus over less than 1 minute for 10 to 14 days. Increase daily dose in 2.5 mg increments to decrease CD3-positive cells.

I.V. administration

• Draw solution into syringe through low–protein-binding 0.2- or 0.22-micron filter. Discard filter and attach needle for I.V. bolus injection.
• Give bolus over less than 1 minute.
ALERT: Don't give by I.V. infusion or with other drug solutions.

Contraindications and precautions

• Contraindicated in patients hypersensitive to drug or to other products of murine origin. Also contraindicated in patients who have antimouse antibody titers of 1:1,000 or more, who have fluid overload, as evidenced by chest X-ray or weight gain greater than 3% within week before treatment, and who have history of or predisposition to seizures.

⚖ Lifespan: In pregnant and breast-feeding women, drug is contraindicated. In children, safety of drug hasn't been established.

Adverse reactions

CNS: *asthenia*, fatigue, lethargy, malaise, *fever, seizures,* dizziness, *headache, meningitis, tremor,* confusion, depression, nervousness, somnolence.
CV: vasodilation, *arrhythmia, bradycardia,* hypertension, hypotension, chest pain, *tachycardia,* vascular occlusion, *edema, cardiac arrest, shock, heart failure.*
EENT: photophobia, tinnitus.
GI: anorexia, *diarrhea, nausea,* abdominal pain, GI pain, *vomiting,*
GU: *renal dysfunction.*
Hematologic: anemia, *leukocytosis, leukopenia, thrombocytopenia.*
Musculoskeletal: arthralgia, myalgia.
Respiratory: *dyspnea,* hyperventilation, *hypoxia,* pneumonia, *pulmonary edema,* respiratory congestion, wheezing, *acute respiratory distress syndrome.*
Skin: diaphoresis, pruritus, *rash.*
Other: *chills,* pain in trunk area, *cytokine release syndrome, hypersensitivity reactions.*

Interactions

Drug-drug. *Immunosuppressants:* Increases risk of infection. Monitor patient closely.
Indomethacin: Increases muromonab-CD3 levels with CNS effects. Encephalopathy may occur. Monitor patient closely.
Live-virus vaccines: May increase replication and effects of vaccine. Postpone vaccination when possible and consult prescriber.

Effects on lab test results

• May increase BUN and creatinine levels.

Pharmacokinetics

Absorption: Administered I.V.
Distribution: Unknown.

Metabolism: Unknown.
Excretion: Unknown.

Route	Onset	Peak	Duration
I.V.	Almost immediately	Unknown	1 wk after therapy stops

Action

Chemical effect: Reacts in T-lymphocyte membrane with CD3 needed for antigen recognition and depletes blood of CD3-positive T cells.
Therapeutic effect: Halts acute allograft rejection in kidney transplantation.

Available forms

Injection: 1 mg/ml in 5-ml ampules

NURSING PROCESS

☑ Assessment
• Assess patient's condition before therapy and regularly thereafter.
• Obtain chest X-ray within 24 hours before drug treatment.
• Assess patient for signs of fluid overload before treatment.
• Be alert for adverse reactions and drug interactions.
• If adverse GI reactions occur, monitor patient's hydration status.
• Evaluate patient's and family's knowledge of drug therapy.

⊕ Nursing diagnoses
• Risk for injury related to presence of acute allograft rejection
• Risk for deficient fluid volume related to drug-induced adverse GI reactions
• Deficient knowledge related to drug therapy

▶ Planning and implementation
• Begin treatment in facility equipped and staffed for cardiopulmonary resuscitation where patient can be monitored closely.
• Most adverse reactions develop within 30 minutes to 6 hours after first dose.
• **ALERT:** Give antipyretic before giving drug to help lower risk of expected pyrexia and chills. It is recommended that methylprednisolone sodium succinate 8 mg/kg be administered I.V. 1 to 4 hours before initial dose of muromonab-CD3 to reduce the risk for and severity of cytokine release syndrome.

• If second course of therapy is attempted, patient may develop antibodies to drug that can lead to loss of effectiveness and more severe adverse reactions; use for one course of treatment only.

Patient teaching
• Inform patient of expected adverse reactions, and reassure him that they will lessen as treatment progresses.

☑ **Evaluation**
• Patient shows no signs of organ rejection.
• Patient maintains adequate hydration.
• Patient and family state understanding of drug therapy.

mycophenolate mofetil
(migh-koh-FEN-oh-layt MOH-feh-til)
CellCept

mycophenolate mofetil hydrochloride
CellCept Intravenous

Pharmacologic class: mycophenolic acid derivative
Therapeutic class: immunosuppressant
Pregnancy risk category: C

Indications and dosages

▶ **Prevention of organ rejection in patients receiving allogeneic renal transplant.** *Adults:* 1 g I.V. infused over 2 hours b.i.d. with cyclosporine and corticosteroids. Begin I.V. infusion within 24 hours after transplantation. For oral dosing, give 1 g P.O. b.i.d. as soon as possible after surgery.
Children age 1 and older: 600 mg/m² oral suspension P.O. b.i.d. up to a maximum daily dose of 2 g/10 ml. Or, give child with 1.25 m² to 1.5 m² body surface area 750 mg capsules P.O. b.i.d. Give child with a greater than 1.5 m² body surface area 1 g P.O. tablets or capsules b.i.d. For oral dosing, give as soon as possible after surgery.
◩ **Adjust-a-dose:** For patients with renal impairment, if GFR is less than 25 ml/minute outside the immediate posttransplant period, avoid doses above 1 g b.i.d. If neutropenia develops, interrupt or reduce dosing.

▶ **Prevention of organ rejection in patients receiving allogeneic cardiac transplant.**
Adults: 1.5 g P.O. or I.V. b.i.d. with cyclosporine and corticosteroids.
▶ **Prevention of organ rejection in patients receiving allogenic hepatic transplants.**
Adults: 1 g I.V. b.i.d. over no less than 2 hours or 1.5 g P.O. b.i.d., with cyclosporine and corticosteroids.
◩ **Adjust-a-dose:** If neutropenia develops, interrupt or reduce dosing.

▼ **I.V. administration**
• Avoid direct contact with solution.
• Reconstitute under aseptic conditions.
• Reconstitute the contents of each CellCept Intravenous vial with 14 ml of D₅W. Use two vials to prepare a 1-g dose and 3 vials for a 1.5-g dose. Gently shake the vial to dissolve drug.
• For a 1 g dose, 2 vials are further diluted into 140 ml of D₅W; for a 1.5-g dose, 3 vials are further diluted into 210 ml of 5% dextrose injection. The final concentration of both solutions is 6 mg/ml.
• Use within 4 hours of reconstitution and dilution.
⊛ **ALERT:** Never give drug by rapid or bolus I.V. injection. Give infusion over at least 2 hours.
• Drug is incompatible with other I.V. solutions.

Contraindications and precautions

• Contraindicated in patients hypersensitive to drug, mycophenolic acid, or other components of product.
• Use cautiously in patients with GI disorders.
☀ **Lifespan:** In pregnant and breast-feeding women, drug is contraindicated unless benefits outweigh risks. In children, safety of drug for cardiac and hepatic transplantation hasn't been established.

Adverse reactions

CNS: *tremor,* insomnia, dizziness, *headache, pain, fever, asthenia.*
CV: *chest pain, hypertension, edema,* peripheral edema.
EENT: pharyngitis.
GI: *diarrhea, constipation, nausea, dyspepsia, vomiting, oral candidiasis, abdominal pain,* HEMORRHAGE.
GU: UTI, hematuria, **kidney tubular necrosis.**

Hematologic: anemia, *leukopenia*, THROMBO-CYTOPENIA, hypochromic anemia, leukocytosis. **Metabolic:** *hypercholesteremia, hypophosphatemia, hypokalemia, hyperkalemia,* hyperglycemia. **Musculoskeletal:** *back pain.* **Respiratory:** *dyspnea, cough,* infection, bronchitis, pneumonia. **Skin:** *acne,* rash. **Other:** *infection, sepsis.*

Interactions

Drug-drug. *Acyclovir, ganciclovir, other drugs known to undergo tubular secretion:* Increases risk of toxicity for both drugs. Monitor patient closely.
Antacids with magnesium and aluminum hydroxides: Decreases absorption of mycophenolate mofetil. Separate administration times.
Azathioprine: Hasn't been studied. Avoid using together.
Cholestyramine: May interfere with enterohepatic recirculation, reducing mycophenolate bioavailability. Don't give together.
Hormonal contraceptives: May affect effectiveness of hormonal contraceptives. Advise patient to use barrier birth control methods.

Effects on lab test results

• May increase cholesterol and glucose levels. May decrease phosphorous level. May increase or decrease potassium level.
• May decrease hemoglobin, hematocrit, and platelet counts. May increase or decrease WBC count.

Pharmacokinetics

Absorption: Absorbed from GI tract.
Distribution: 97% bound to proteins.
Metabolism: Undergoes complete presystemic metabolism to mycophenolic acid.
Excretion: Excreted primarily in urine, with small amount in feces. *Half-life:* About 18 hours.

Route	Onset	Peak	Duration
P.O.	Unknown	Unknown	Unknown
I.V.	Unknown	Unknown	10-17 hr

Action

Chemical effect: Inhibits proliferative responses of T- and B-lymphocytes, suppresses antibody formation by B-lymphocytes, and may inhibit recruitment of leukocytes into sites of inflammation and graft rejection.
Therapeutic effect: Prevents organ rejection.

Available forms

mycophenolate mofetil
Capsules: 250 mg
Powder for oral suspension: 200 mg/ml
Tablets: 500 mg
mycophenolate mofetil hydrochloride
Injection: 500 mg/vial

NURSING PROCESS

⚗ Assessment
• Obtain history of patient's kidney transplant.
• Monitor CBC regularly.
• Be alert for adverse reactions and drug interactions.
• Evaluate patient's and family's knowledge of drug therapy.

⊕ Nursing diagnoses
• Ineffective health maintenance related to need for kidney transplant
• Ineffective immune protection related to drug-induced immunosuppression
• Deficient knowledge related to drug therapy

▷ Planning and implementation
• Give drug on an empty stomach.
• **ALERT:** Because of potential teratogenic effects, don't open or crush capsules. Avoid inhaling powder in capsules or letting it contact skin or mucous membranes. If contact occurs, wash skin thoroughly with soap and water and rinse eyes with plain water.
• If neutropenia occurs, notify prescriber.
Patient teaching
• Warn patient not to open or crush capsule but to swallow it whole on an empty stomach.
• Stress importance of not interrupting therapy without consulting prescriber.
• Inform woman that a pregnancy test should be done 1 week before therapy. Advise her to use effective contraception until at least 6 weeks after therapy stops, even if she has a history of infertility (unless she has had a hysterectomy). Tell her to use two forms of contraception simultaneously unless abstinence is the chosen method. If pregnancy occurs despite these measures, have patient contact prescriber immediately.

Reactions may be *common,* uncommon, *life-threatening*, or COMMON AND LIFE-THREATENING.

☑ Evaluation

- Patient shows no signs and symptoms of organ rejection.
- Neutropenia doesn't develop.
- Patient and family state understanding of drug therapy.

N

nabumetone
(nuh-BYOO-meh-tohn)
Apo-Nabumetone ♦ , Relafen

Pharmacologic class: NSAID
Therapeutic class: anti-inflammatory, analgesic, antipyretic
Pregnancy risk category: C

Indications and dosages

▶ **Rheumatoid arthritis, osteoarthritis.**
Adults: Initially, 1,000 mg P.O. daily as single dose or in divided doses b.i.d. Maximum dose, 2,000 mg daily.

Contraindications and precautions

- Contraindicated in patients hypersensitive to drug and in patients with history of aspirin- or NSAID-induced asthma, urticaria, or other allergic reactions.
- Use cautiously in patients with renal or hepatic impairment, peptic ulcer disease, heart failure, hypertension, or other conditions that may predispose patient to fluid retention.
⚖ **Lifespan:** In women in the third trimester of pregnancy and breast-feeding women, drug isn't recommended. Use during pregnancy only if clearly needed. In children, safety of drug hasn't been established. In geriatric patients, use cautiously.

Adverse reactions

CNS: *dizziness, headache,* fatigue, insomnia, nervousness, somnolence.
CV: vasculitis, *edema.*
EENT: *tinnitus.*
GI: *diarrhea, dyspepsia, abdominal pain, constipation, flatulence, nausea,* dry mouth,

gastritis, stomatitis, vomiting, *bleeding,* ulceration.
Respiratory: dyspnea, pneumonitis.
Skin: *pruritus, rash,* increased sweating.

Interactions

Drug-drug. *Diuretics:* NSAIDs may decrease diuretic effectiveness. Monitor patient for effect.
Drugs highly bound to proteins (such as warfarin): Increases risk of adverse effects from displacement of drug by nabumetone. Use together cautiously; monitor patient for adverse effects.
Drug-herb. *Dong quai, feverfew, garlic, ginger, horse chestnut, red clover:* Increases risk of bleeding. Discourage using together.
St. John's wort: Increases risk of photosensitivity. Advise patient to avoid unprotected or prolonged exposure to sunlight.
Drug-food. *Any food:* Increases the rate of absorption. Give together.
Drug-lifestyle. *Alcohol use:* Increases risk of additive GI toxicity. Discourage using together.

Effects on lab test results

None reported.

Pharmacokinetics

Absorption: Well absorbed from GI tract. Administration with food increases absorption rate and peak levels of principal metabolite but doesn't change total drug absorbed.
Distribution: Over 99% of metabolite is bound to proteins.
Metabolism: Metabolized to inactive metabolites in liver.
Excretion: Metabolites excreted primarily in urine; about 9% appears in feces. *Half-life:* About 24 hours.

Route	Onset	Peak	Duration
P.O.	Unknown	2-4 hr	Unknown

Action

Chemical effect: Unknown; may inhibit prostaglandin synthesis.
Therapeutic effect: Relieves pain.

Available forms

Tablets: 500 mg, 750 mg

NURSING PROCESS

🔀 Assessment
• Assess patient's arthritis before therapy and regularly thereafter.
• During long-term therapy, periodically monitor renal and liver function, CBC, and hematocrit; assess these patients for evidence of GI bleeding.
• Watch for fluid retention, especially among patients with heart failure and hypertension.
• Be alert for adverse reactions and drug interactions.
• Evaluate patient's and family's knowledge of drug therapy.

🔁 Nursing diagnoses
• Chronic pain related to arthritic condition
• Impaired tissue integrity related to adverse drug effect on GI mucosa
• Deficient knowledge related to drug therapy

▷ Planning and implementation
• Give drug with food to increase absorption rate.
• Notify prescriber about adverse reactions.
• ⚫ ALERT: Don't confuse Relafen with Rifadin.
Patient teaching
• Instruct patient to take drug with food, milk, or antacids for best absorption.
• Advise patient to limit alcohol intake because of additive GI toxicity.
• Teach patient to recognize and report signs and symptoms of GI bleeding.

☑ Evaluation
• Patient is free from pain.
• Patient's GI tissue integrity is maintained throughout drug therapy.
• Patient and family state understanding of drug therapy.

nadolol
(nay-DOH-lol)
Apo-Nadol ♦ , Corgard

Pharmacologic class: nonselective beta blocker
Therapeutic class: antihypertensive, antianginal
Pregnancy risk category: C

Indications and dosages
▶ **Angina pectoris.** *Adults:* Initially, 40 mg P.O. once daily. Increase in 40- to 80-mg increments q 3 to 7 days until optimum response occurs. Usual maintenance dosage is 40 to 240 mg daily.
▶ **Hypertension.** *Adults:* Initially, 20 to 40 mg P.O. once daily. Increase by 40- to 80-mg increments q 2 to 14 days until optimum response occurs. Usual maintenance dosage is 40 to 320 mg daily (rarely, 640 mg).
🔲 **Adjust-a-dose:** In patients with renal impairment, if creatinine clearance is 31 to 50 ml/minute, give q 24 to 36 hours; if 10 to 30 ml/minute, give q 24 to 48 hours; if less than 10 ml/minute, give q 40 to 60 hours.
▶ **Arrhythmias‡.** *Adults:* 60 to 160 mg P.O. daily.
▶ **Prevention of vascular headaches‡.** *Adults:* 20 to 40 mg P.O. daily; gradually increase to 120 mg daily, if needed.

Contraindications and precautions
• Contraindicated in patients with bronchial asthma, sinus bradycardia, greater than first-degree heart block, and cardiogenic shock.
• Use cautiously in patients undergoing major surgery involving general anesthesia and in those with heart failure, chronic bronchitis, emphysema, renal or hepatic impairment, or diabetes.
🔥 **Lifespan:** In pregnant women, use only if the benefits justify the risks. In breast-feeding women, drug isn't recommended. In children, safety of drug hasn't been established.

Adverse reactions
CNS: fatigue, lethargy, dizziness, fever.
CV: *bradycardia,* hypotension, **heart failure,** peripheral vascular disease.
GI: nausea, vomiting, diarrhea, constipation.
Respiratory: *increased airway resistance.*
Skin: rash.

Interactions
Drug-drug. *Antihypertensives:* Enhances antihypertensive effect. Monitor patient's blood pressure closely.
Digoxin, diltiazem: May cause excessive bradycardia and affect AV conduction. Use together cautiously; monitor ECG.
Epinephrine: May cause an initial hypertensive episode followed by bradycardia. Stop beta

blocker 3 days before anticipated epinephrine use. Monitor patient closely.

Insulin: May mask symptoms of hypoglycemia as a result of beta blockade (such as tachycardia). Use cautiously in patients with diabetes.

I.V. lidocaine: May reduce hepatic metabolism of lidocaine increasing the risk of toxicity. Give bolus doses of lidocaine at a slower rate and monitor lidocaine level closely.

NSAIDs: Decreases antihypertensive effect. Monitor blood pressure and adjust dosage.

Oral antidiabetics: Can alter dosage requirements in diabetic patients. Monitor glucose level.

Prazosin: May increase the risk of orthostatic hypotension in the early phases of use together. Help patient to stand slowly until effects are known.

Verapamil: May increase the effects of both drugs. Monitor cardiac function closely for excessive bradycardia and decrease dosages as necessary.

Effects on lab test results

None reported.

Pharmacokinetics

Absorption: 30% to 40%.
Distribution: Distributed throughout body; about 30% protein-bound.
Metabolism: None.
Excretion: Most excreted unchanged in urine; remainder in feces. *Half-life:* About 20 hours.

Route	Onset	Peak	Duration
P.O.	Unknown	2-4 hr	Unknown

Action

Chemical effect: Reduces cardiac oxygen demand by blocking catecholamine-induced increases in heart rate, blood pressure, and myocardial contraction. Depresses renin secretion.
Therapeutic effect: Lowers blood pressure and relieves angina.

Available forms

Tablets: 20 mg, 40 mg, 80 mg, 120 mg, 160 mg

NURSING PROCESS

Assessment

● Assess patient's condition before therapy and regularly thereafter.

● Drug masks common signs of shock and hyperthyroidism.
● Be alert for adverse reactions and drug interactions.
● Evaluate patient's and family's knowledge of drug therapy.

Nursing diagnoses

● Risk for injury related to presence of hypertension
● Acute pain related to angina
● Deficient knowledge related to drug therapy

Planning and implementation

● **ALERT:** Always check apical pulse before giving drug. If slower than 60 beats/minute, withhold drug and notify prescriber.
● If patient develops severe hypotension, give vasopressor.
● **ALERT:** Reduce dosage gradually over 1 to 2 weeks. Stopping abruptly can worsen angina and MI.
● **ALERT:** Don't confuse Corgard with Coreg.
Patient teaching
● Explain importance of taking drug as prescribed, even when feeling well. Warn patient not to stop drug suddenly.

Evaluation

● Patient's blood pressure is normal.
● Patient reports reduced angina.
● Patient and family state understanding of drug therapy.

nafcillin sodium
(naf-SIL-in SOH-dee-um)

Pharmacologic class: penicillinase-resistant penicillin
Therapeutic class: antibiotic
Pregnancy risk category: B

Indications and dosages

▶ **Systemic infections caused by susceptible organisms (methicillin-sensitive *Staphylococcus aureus*).** *Adults:* 500 mg to 1 g I.V. q 4 hours depending on severity of the infection.
Infants and children older than age 1 month: 50 to 200 mg/kg I.V. daily in divided doses q 4 to 6 hours depending on the severity of the infection.

Neonates age 7 days or younger weighing less than 2 kg (4.4 lb): 25 mg/kg I.V. q 12 hours.
Neonates age 7 days or younger weighing more than 2 kg: 25 mg/kg I.V. q 8 hours.
Neonates older than 7 days weighing less than 2 kg: 25 mg/kg I.V. q 8 hours.
Neonates older than 7 days weighing more than 2 kg: 25 mg/kg I.V. q 6 hours.

▶ **Meningitis.** *Adults:* 100 to 200 mg/kg I.V. daily in divided doses q 4 to 6 hours.
Neonates age 7 days or younger weighing less than 2 kg: 50 mg/kg I.V. q 12 hours.
Neonates age 7 days or younger weighing more than 2 kg: 50 mg/kg I.V. q 8 hours.
Neonates older than 7 days weighing less than 2 kg: 50 mg/kg I.V. q 8 hours.
Neonates older than 7 days weighing more than 2 kg: 50 mg/kg I.V. q 6 hours.

▶ **Acute or chronic osteomyelitis caused by susceptible organism.** *Adults:* 1 to 2 g I.V. q 4 hours for 4 to 8 weeks.
Children older than age 1 month: 100 to 200 mg/kg daily in equally divided doses q 4 to 6 hours for 4 to 8 weeks.

▶ **Native valve endocarditis caused by susceptible organisms.** *Adults:* 2 g I.V. q 4 hours for 4 to 6 weeks with gentamicin.
Children older than age 1 month: 100 to 200 mg/kg daily in equally divided doses q 4 to 6 hours for 4 to 8 weeks with gentamicin.

▼ I.V. administration

• After thawing at room temperature or under refrigeration, check and discard container with leaks, cloudiness, or precipitate.
• Give by intermittent I.V. infusion over 30 to 60 minutes.
• Change I.V. site q 48 hours to reduce the risk of vein irritation.
• Avoid continuous I.V. infusion to avoid vein irritation.
⊛ **ALERT:** Aminoglycosides are chemically and physically incompatible with drug. Don't mix together in same I.V. solution.

Contraindications and precautions

• Contraindicated in patients hypersensitive to drug or other penicillins.
• Use cautiously in patients with GI distress and those with other drug allergies, especially to cephalosporins.
⚖ **Lifespan:** In pregnant and breast-feeding women, use cautiously.

Adverse reactions

GI: *nausea,* vomiting, diarrhea.
Hematologic: *transient leukopenia, neutropenia, granulocytopenia, thrombocytopenia* (with high doses).
Other: hypersensitivity reactions (chills, fever, rash, pruritus, urticaria, *anaphylaxis*), vein irritation, thrombophlebitis.

Interactions

Drug-drug. *Aminoglycosides:* May have synergistic effect; may use together for this effect. Monitor patient closely.
Cyclosporine: May cause subtherapeutic cyclosporine level. Monitor level.
Probenecid: Increases level of nafcillin. Probenecid may be used for this purpose.
Rifampin: Dose-dependent antagonism. Monitor patient closely.
Warfarin: Increases risk of bleeding when used with I.V. nafcillin. Monitor patient for bleeding.

Effects on lab test results

• May decrease neutrophil, granulocyte, WBC, and platelet counts.
• May falsely elevate urine or serum proteins or cause false-positive results in certain tests for them.

Pharmacokinetics

Absorption: Administered I.V.
Distribution: Distributed widely. CSF penetration is poor but enhanced by meningeal inflammation. Drug is 70% to 90% protein-bound.
Metabolism: Metabolized primarily in liver; undergoes enterohepatic circulation.
Excretion: Excreted primarily in bile; 25% to 30% is excreted in urine unchanged. *Half-life:* 30 to 90 minutes.

Route	Onset	Peak	Duration
I.V.	Immediate	Immediate	Unknown

Action

Chemical effect: Inhibits cell wall synthesis during microorganism multiplication; bacteria resist penicillins by producing penicillinases—enzymes that hydrolyze penicillins. Drug resists these enzymes.
Therapeutic effect: Kills susceptible bacteria, such as penicillinase-producing staphylococci, and some gram-positive aerobic and anaerobic bacilli.

Available forms

Injection (for I.V. infusion): 1 g, 2 g

🏶 Assessment

• Assess patient's infection before therapy and regularly thereafter.
• Before giving drug, ask patient about allergic reactions to penicillin. Remember that allergic reactions may occur even in patients with no history of penicillin allergy.
• Obtain specimen for culture and sensitivity tests before giving first dose. Therapy may begin pending results.
⊛ **ALERT:** Monitor WBC counts twice weekly in patients receiving nafcillin for longer than 2 weeks. Neutropenia commonly occurs in the third week.
• Be alert for adverse reactions and drug interactions.
• If adverse GI reactions occur, monitor patient's hydration status.
• Evaluate patient's and family's knowledge of drug therapy.

🔲 Nursing diagnoses

• Infection related to susceptible bacteria
• Risk for deficient fluid volume related to drug-induced adverse GI reactions
• Deficient knowledge related to drug therapy

🔁 Planning and implementation

• Give drug at least 1 hour before bacteriostatic antibiotics.
• If urinalysis is abnormal; notify prescriber; this may indicate drug-induced interstitial nephritis.
Patient teaching
• Tell patient to call prescriber if rash, fever, or chills develop.

🗹 Evaluation

• Patient is free from infection.
• Patient maintains adequate hydration throughout drug therapy.
• Patient and family state understanding of drug therapy.

nalbuphine hydrochloride

(NAL-byoo-feen high-droh-KLOR-ighd)
Nubain

Pharmacologic class: opioid agonist-antagonist, opioid partial agonist
Therapeutic class: opioid analgesic, adjunct to anesthesia
Pregnancy risk category: B

Indications and dosages

▶ **Moderate to severe pain.** *Adults:* For patient weighing about 70 kg (154 lb), give 10 to 20 mg I.V., I.M., or S.C., q 3 to 6 hours, p.r.n. Maximum daily dosage is 160 mg.
▶ **Adjunct in balanced anesthesia.** *Adults:* 0.3 mg/kg to 3 mg/kg I.V. over 10 to 15 minutes, followed by maintenance doses of 0.25 to 0.5 mg/kg in single I.V. doses p.r.n.

▼ I.V. administration

• Inject slowly over at least 2 minutes into vein or into I.V. line containing compatible, free-flowing I.V. solution, such as D_5W, normal saline solution, or lactated Ringer's solution.
⊛ **ALERT:** Respiratory depression can be reversed with naloxone. Keep resuscitation equipment available.

Contraindications and precautions

• Contraindicated in patients hypersensitive to drug.
• Use cautiously in substance abusers and in those with emotional instability, head injury, increased intracranial pressure, impaired ventilation, MI accompanied by nausea and vomiting, upcoming biliary surgery, and hepatic or renal disease.
🜲 **Lifespan:** In pregnant and breast-feeding women, use cautiously. In children, safety of drug hasn't been established.

Adverse reactions

CNS: *headache, sedation, dizziness, vertigo,* nervousness, depression, restlessness, crying, euphoria, hostility, unusual dreams, confusion, hallucinations, speech difficulty, delusions.
CV: hypertension, hypotension, tachycardia, *bradycardia.*
EENT: blurred vision.

Rapid onset   *Liquid form contains alcohol.*   ♦ Canada   ◇ Australia   †OTC   ‡Off-label use

GI: cramps, dyspepsia, bitter taste, *dry mouth, nausea, vomiting,* constipation.
GU: urinary urgency.
Respiratory: *respiratory depression, pulmonary edema.*
Skin: itching; burning; urticaria; *sweaty, clammy feeling.*

Interactions

Drug-drug. *CNS depressants, general anesthetics, hypnotics, MAO inhibitors, sedatives, tranquilizers, tricyclic antidepressants:* May cause respiratory depression, hypertension, profound sedation, or coma. Don't use together.
Opioid analgesics: May cause decrease in analgesic effect and increase withdrawal symptoms. Avoid using together.
Drug-lifestyle. *Alcohol use:* May cause respiratory depression, hypertension, profound sedation, or coma. Discourage using together.

Effects on lab test results

None reported.

Pharmacokinetics

Absorption: Unknown.
Distribution: Not measurably bound to proteins.
Metabolism: Metabolized in liver.
Excretion: Excreted in urine and bile. *Half-life:* 5 hours.

Route	Onset	Peak	Duration
I.V.	2-3 min	≤ 30 min	3-4 hr
I.M.	≤ 15 min	≤ 60 min	3-6 hr
S.C.	≤ 15 min	Unknown	3-6 hr

Action

Chemical effect: Binds with opioid receptors in CNS, altering pain perception and response to pain by unknown mechanism.
Therapeutic effect: Relieves pain and enhances anesthesia.

Available forms

Injection: 10 mg/ml, 20 mg/ml
I.V. PCA infusion: 1.5 mg/ml

NURSING PROCESS

Assessment
● Assess patient's pain or anesthetic requirement before therapy and regularly thereafter.

● Observe for signs of withdrawal in patient receiving long-term opioid therapy.
● Monitor patient closely for respiratory depression.
● Monitor patient for signs and symptoms of constipation.
● Be alert for adverse reactions and drug interactions.
● Evaluate patient's and family's knowledge of drug therapy.

Nursing diagnoses
● Acute pain related to condition
● Disturbed thought processes related to drug's effect on CNS
● Deficient knowledge related to drug therapy

Planning and implementation
● Psychological and physical dependence may occur with prolonged use.
● Drug acts as an opioid antagonist and may precipitate withdrawal syndrome. For patients receiving long-term opioid therapy, start with 25% of usual dose.
● Give a stool softener or other laxative to prevent constipation. Encourage patient to drink fluids and eat fiber.
⊛ **ALERT:** If patient's respirations are shallow or rate is below 12 breaths/minute, withhold dose and notify prescriber.
⊛ **ALERT:** Don't confuse Nubain with Navane.
Patient teaching
● Warn ambulatory patient about getting out of bed or walking.
● Instruct outpatient to avoid hazardous activities until CNS effects of drug are known.

Evaluation
● Patient is free from pain.
● Patient maintains normal thought processes throughout therapy.
● Patient and family state understanding of drug therapy.

naloxone hydrochloride
(nal-OKS-ohn high-droh-KLOR-ighd)
Narcan

Pharmacologic class: opioid antagonist
Therapeutic class: adjunct to opiate cessation
Pregnancy risk category: B

Indications and dosages

▶ **Known or suspected opioid-induced respiratory depression, including that caused by pentazocine and propoxyphene.** *Adults:* 0.4 to 2 mg I.V., I.M., or S.C. Repeat q 2 to 3 minutes, p.r.n. If no response is observed after 10 mg has been given, re-evaluate diagnosis.

▶ **Postoperative opioid depression.** *Adults:* 0.1 to 0.2 mg I.V. q 2 to 3 minutes, p.r.n. *Children:* 0.005 to 0.01 mg/kg dose I.V. Repeat q 2 to 3 minutes, p.r.n. *Neonates (asphyxia neonatorum):* 0.01 mg/kg I.V. into umbilical vein. May repeat q 2 to 3 minutes for three doses.

▶ **Naloxone challenge for diagnosing opiate dependence‡.** *Adults:* 0.16 mg I.M. naloxone; if no signs of withdrawal after 20 to 30 minutes, give second dose of 0.24 mg

▽ I.V. administration

• Give continuous I.V. infusion to control adverse effects of epidural morphine.
• For neonatal concentration, if 0.02 mg/ml isn't available, adult concentration (0.4 mg) may be diluted by mixing 0.5 ml with 9.5 ml of sterile water or saline solution for injection to make neonatal concentration (0.02 mg/ml).
⊛ **ALERT:** Don't mix with drugs containing bisulfite, metabisulfite, long-chain, or high molecular weight anions or any solution with an alkaline pH.

Contraindications and precautions

• Contraindicated in patients hypersensitive to drug.
• Use cautiously in patients with cardiac irritability and opioid addiction. Abrupt reversal of opioid-induced CNS depression may cause nausea, vomiting, diaphoresis, tachycardia, CNS excitement, and increased blood pressure.
⚖ **Lifespan:** In pregnant women, use cautiously. In breast-feeding women, safety of drug hasn't been established.

Adverse reactions

CNS: tremors, *seizures.*
CV: tachycardia and hypertension with high doses, *ventricular fibrillation.*
GI: nausea and vomiting with high doses.
Respiratory: *pulmonary edema.*
Other: *withdrawal symptoms* in opioid-dependent patients with higher-than-recommended doses.

Interactions

None significant.

Effects on lab test results

None reported.

Pharmacokinetics

Absorption: Unknown.
Distribution: Rapidly distributed into body tissues and fluids.
Metabolism: Rapidly metabolized in liver.
Excretion: Excreted in urine. *Half-life:* 60 to 90 minutes in adults, 3 hours in neonates.

Route	Onset	Peak	Duration
I.V.	1-2 min	Unknown	Varies
I.M., S.C.	2-5 min	Unknown	Varies

Action

Chemical effect: Unknown; may displace opioid analgesics from their receptors (competitive antagonism). Has no pharmacologic activity.
Therapeutic effect: Reverses opioid effects.

Available forms

Injection: 0.02 mg/ml, 0.4 mg/ml, 1 mg/ml

NURSING PROCESS

🗒 Assessment

• Assess patient's opioid use before therapy.
• Assess effectiveness of drug regularly throughout therapy.
• Duration of narcotic may exceed that of naloxone, causing relapse into respiratory depression. Monitor patient's respiratory depth and rate.
• Patients who receive naloxone to reverse opioid-induced respiratory depression may develop tachypnea.
• If adverse GI reactions occur, monitor patient's hydration status.
• Evaluate patient's and family's knowledge of drug therapy.

🔲 Nursing diagnoses

• Ineffective health maintenance related to opioid use
• Risk for deficient fluid volume related to drug-induced adverse GI reactions
• Deficient knowledge related to drug therapy

▷ Planning and implementation

⊛ **ALERT:** Drug is effective only in reversing respiratory depression caused by opioids. Use flumazenil to treat respiratory depression caused by diazepam or other benzodiazepines.

⊛ **ALERT:** Provide oxygen, ventilation, and other resuscitation measures to patient with severe respiratory depression from acute opioid overdose.

⊛ **ALERT:** Don't confuse naloxone with naltrexone.

Patient teaching
• Instruct patient and family to report adverse reactions.

☑ Evaluation
• Patient responds well to drug.
• Patient maintains adequate hydration.
• Patient and family state understanding of drug therapy.

---

naltrexone hydrochloride
(nal-TREKS-ohn high-droh-KLOR-ighd)
Depade, ReVia

Pharmacologic class: opioid antagonist
Therapeutic class: adjunct in opioid detoxification
Pregnancy risk category: C

Indications and dosages

▶ **Adjunct in maintaining opioid-free state in detoxified patients.** *Adults:* Initially, 25 mg P.O. If no withdrawal signs occur within 1 hour, additional 25 mg is given. Once patient receives 50 mg q 24 hours, flexible maintenance schedule may be used.
▶ **Alcohol dependence.** *Adults:* 50 mg P.O. once daily for up to 12 weeks.

Contraindications and precautions

• Contraindicated in patients hypersensitive to drug; in those who are receiving opioid analgesics, have a positive urine screen for opioids, or are opioid dependent; in those who have acute opioid withdrawal; and in those with acute hepatitis or liver failure.
• Use cautiously in patients with mild hepatic disease or history of recent hepatic disease.

※ **Lifespan:** In pregnant women, use cautiously. In breast-feeding women and in children, safety of drug hasn't been established.

Adverse reactions

CNS: *insomnia, anxiety, nervousness, headache,* depression, **suicidal ideation.**
GI: *nausea, vomiting,* anorexia, *abdominal pain.*
Hematologic: lymphocytosis.
Hepatic: *hepatotoxicity.*
Musculoskeletal: *muscle and joint pain.*

Interactions

Drug-drug. *Products containing opioids (such as cough and cold and antidiarrheal products):* Decreases response to these products. Recommend using a nonopioid product.
Thioridazine: Increases somnolence and lethargy. Monitor patient closely.

Effects on lab test results
• May increase AST, ALT, and LDH levels.
• May increase lymphocyte count.

Pharmacokinetics

Absorption: Well absorbed from GI tract.
Distribution: Widely distributed throughout body but varies considerably. Drug is about 21% to 28% protein-bound.
Metabolism: Undergoes extensive first-pass hepatic metabolism. Its major metabolite may be pure antagonist and contribute to its effectiveness. Drug and metabolites may undergo enterohepatic recirculation.
Excretion: Excreted mainly by kidneys. *Half-life:* About 4 hours.

Route	Onset	Peak	Duration
P.O.	15-30 min	> 12 hr	24 hr

Action

Chemical effect: Unknown; may reversibly block subjective effects of I.V. opioids by occupying opioid receptors in brain.
Therapeutic effect: Helps prevent opioid dependence and treats alcohol dependence.

Available forms

Tablets: 25 mg, 50 mg

Reactions may be *common,* uncommon, *life-threatening,* or COMMON AND LIFE-THREATENING.

NURSING PROCESS

⚡ Assessment

• Assess patient's opioid or alcohol dependence before therapy.
• Monitor effectiveness of drug.
• Evaluate patient's and family's knowledge of drug therapy.

🔷 Nursing diagnoses

• Health-seeking behavior related to desire to remain free from opioid dependence
• Disturbed sleep pattern related to drug-induced insomnia
• Deficient knowledge related to drug therapy

➤ Planning and implementation

🔹 **ALERT:** Begin treatment for opioid dependency after giving naloxone challenge, a provocative test of opioid dependency. If signs of opioid withdrawal persist after challenge, withhold drug.

🔹 **ALERT:** Patient must be completely free from opioids before using drug or severe withdrawal symptoms may occur. Wait at least 7 days in patient addicted to short-acting opioids, such as heroin and meperidine. Wait at least 10 days in patient addicted to longer-acting opioids, such as methadone.

• Generally, if analgesia is necessary, a non-opiate analgesic should be used. If an opioid analgesic is necessary in an emergency, give an opioid analgesic in a higher dose than usual to surmount naltrexone's effect. Respiratory depression caused by opioid analgesic may be longer and deeper.

• For patient with opioid dependence who isn't expected to comply, use flexible maintenance regimen: 100 mg on Monday and Wednesday, 150 mg on Friday.

• Use naltrexone only as part of comprehensive rehabilitation program.

🔹 **ALERT:** Don't confuse naloxone and naltrexone.

Patient teaching

• Advise patient to wear or carry medical identification. Warn him to tell medical personnel that he takes naltrexone.
• Give patient names of nonopioid drugs he can take for pain, diarrhea, or cough.

☑ Evaluation

• Patient maintains opioid-free state.
• Patient reports no insomnia.
• Patient and family state understanding of drug therapy.

nandrolone decanoate

(NAN-druh-lohn deh-kuh-NOH-ayt)
Androlone-D, Deca-Durabolin, Hybolin Decanoate, Kabolin, Neo-Durabolic

nandrolone phenpropionate

Durabolin, Hybolin Improved

Pharmacologic class: anabolic steroid
Therapeutic class: erythropoietic and anabolic (nandrolone decanoate), antineoplastic (nandrolone phenpropionate)
Pregnancy risk category: X
Controlled substance schedule: III

Indications and dosages

➤ **Severe debility or disease states, refractory anemias.** *Adults:* 50 to 100 mg nandrolone decanoate I.M. weekly for women; 100 to 200 mg I.M. weekly for men. Therapy should be intermittent.
Children ages 2 to 13: 25 to 50 mg nandrolone decanoate I.M. q 3 to 4 weeks.
➤ **Metastatic breast cancer.** *Adults:* 50 to 100 mg nandrolone phenpropionate I.M. weekly.

Contraindications and precautions

• Contraindicated in patients hypersensitive to anabolic steroids, in men with breast or prostate cancer, in patients with nephrosis, in patients experiencing the nephrotic phase of nephritis, in women with breast cancer and hypercalcemia.

• Use cautiously in patients with diabetes; cardiac, renal, or hepatic disease; epilepsy; or migraine or other conditions that may be aggravated by fluid retention.

⚘ **Lifespan:** In pregnant and breast-feeding women, drug is contraindicated. In children, use cautiously. In elderly patients, use cautiously because older men may be at increased risk for prostatic hypertrophy and prostatic carcinoma.

Adverse reactions

CV: edema.
GI: gastroenteritis, nausea, vomiting, diarrhea, change in appetite.
GU: bladder irritability.
Hematologic: *thrombocytopenia.*
Hepatic: reversible jaundice, *peliosis hepatis, liver cell tumors.*
Metabolic: hypercalcemia.
Musculoskeletal: muscle cramps or spasms.
Other: androgenic effects in women (acne, edema, *weight gain, hirsutism,* hoarseness, clitoral enlargement, *decreased breast size,* altered libido, male-pattern baldness, *oily skin or hair*), hypoestrogenic effects in women (flushing, diaphoresis, vaginitis, vaginal bleeding, nervousness, emotional lability, menstrual irregularities), excessive hormonal effects in prepubertal men (premature epiphyseal closure, *acne,* priapism, *growth of body and facial hair,* phallic enlargement), excessive hormonal effects in postpubertal men (testicular atrophy, oligospermia, decreased ejaculatory volume, impotence, gynecomastia, epididymitis), pain, induration at injection site.

Interactions

Drug-drug. *Hepatotoxic drugs:* Increases risk of hepatotoxicity. Monitor liver function test results.
Insulin, oral antidiabetics: Alters antidiabetic dosage requirements. Monitor glucose levels in diabetic patients.
Oral anticoagulants: Alters anticoagulant dosage requirements. Monitor PT and INR.

Effects on lab test results

• May increase creatinine, lipid, sodium, potassium, calcium, phosphate, cholesterol, and liver enzyme levels.
• May decrease platelet count and thyroid function test values.

Pharmacokinetics

Absorption: Nandrolone decanoate is slowly released from I.M. depot. Nandrolone phenpropionate's absorption is unknown.
Distribution: Unknown.
Metabolism: Nandrolone decanoate is hydrolyzed to free nandrolone by esterase and metabolized in liver. Nandrolone phenpropionate is metabolized in liver.

Excretion: Excreted in urine. *Half-life:* 6 to 8 days for nandrolone decanoate; unknown for nandrolone phenpropionate.

Route	Onset	Peak	Duration
I.M.			
decanoate	Unknown	3-6 days	Unknown
phenpro-pionate	Unknown	1-2 days	Unknown

Action

Chemical effect: Promotes tissue building, reverses catabolism, and stimulates erythropoiesis.
Therapeutic effect: Promotes tissue building and RBC growth (decanoate); hinders growth of breast cancer cells (phenpropionate).

Available forms

nandrolone decanoate
Injection (in oil): 50 mg/ml, 100 mg/ml, 200 mg/ml
nandrolone phenpropionate
Injection (in oil): 25 mg/ml, 50 mg/ml

NURSING PROCESS

☑ Assessment

• Assess patient's condition before therapy and regularly thereafter.
• Make sure that pregnancy test is negative for woman of childbearing age before therapy starts.
• In child, obtain X-ray of wrist bones before treatment to assess bone maturation. During treatment, bone maturation may proceed rapidly; periodically review X-ray results to monitor it.
• Closely observe boy younger than age 7 for precocious development of male sexual characteristics.
• Semen evaluation is routinely performed q 3 to 4 months, especially in adolescent male.
• Evaluate hepatic function.
• Watch for symptoms of hypoglycemia in diabetic patient. Check glucose level regularly because antidiabetic dosage may need to be adjusted.
• Check quantitative urine and serum calcium levels.
• Check weight regularly and assess for fluid retention.

- Be alert for adverse reactions and drug interactions.
- Evaluate patient's and family's knowledge of drug therapy.

✚ Nursing diagnoses
- Ineffective health maintenance related to underlying condition
- Disturbed body image related to adverse androgenic reactions
- Deficient knowledge related to drug therapy

▶ Planning and implementation
- Inject I.M. drug deeply, preferably into upper outer quadrant of gluteal muscle in adults. Rotate injection sites to prevent muscle atrophy.
- Duration of treatment depends on response of condition and adverse reactions.

⊛ **ALERT:** Notify prescriber immediately about signs of virilization; they may be irreversible despite stopping therapy promptly.
- Adjust dosage to try to reverse jaundice. If liver function test results are abnormal, stop therapy.
- Drug-induced edema usually can be controlled with sodium restrictions or diuretics.
- When used to promote erythropoiesis, make sure patient has adequate daily iron intake.
- Duration of treatment depends on response and adverse reactions.
- Anabolic steroids may alter results of laboratory studies performed during therapy and for 2 to 3 weeks after therapy ends.

Patient teaching
- Make sure patient understands importance of using effective nonhormonal contraceptive during therapy.
- Advise women to shower or bathe after intercourse to decrease risk of vaginitis. Instruct her to wear only cotton underwear.
- Tell woman to report menstrual irregularities and to stop drug until the cause of irregularity has been determined.
- Instruct patient to report sudden weight gain.

☑ Evaluation
- Patient responds well to therapy.
- Patient states acceptance of body image changes.
- Patient and family state understanding of drug therapy.

naproxen
(nuh-PROK-sin)
Apo-Naproxen♦ , EC-Naprosyn, Naprosyn, Naprosyn SR♦ ◇ , Naxen♦ ◇ , Novo-Naprox♦ , Nu-Naprox♦

naproxen sodium
Aleve†, Anaprox, Anaprox DS, Apo-Napro-Na♦ , Apo-Napro-Na DS♦ , Naprelan, Novo-Naprox Sodium♦ , Synflex♦ , Synflex DS♦

Pharmacologic class: NSAID
Therapeutic class: nonopioid analgesic, antipyretic, anti-inflammatory
Pregnancy risk category: B

Indications and dosages

▶ **Rheumatoid arthritis, osteoarthritis, ankylosing spondylitis.** *Adults:* 250 to 500 mg naproxen P.O. b.i.d. Or, 375 mg to 500 mg EC-Naprosyn P.O. b.i.d, 275 to 550 mg naproxen sodium P.O. b.i.d. Or, 750 mg or 1,000 mg Naprelan P.O. daily. Or, where suppository is available, 500 mg P.R. h.s. with naproxen P.O. during day.
▶ **Juvenile arthritis.** *Children:* 10 mg/kg naproxen P.O. in two divided doses.
▶ **Acute gout.** *Adults:* 750 mg naproxen P.O., followed by 250 mg q 8 hours until attack subsides. Or, 825 mg naproxen sodium initially; then 275 mg q 8 hours until attack subsides. Or, 1,000 mg to 1,500 mg Naprelan P.O. on the first day, then 1,000 mg daily until attack subsides.
▶ **Mild to moderate pain, primary dysmenorrhea, acute tendinitis and bursitis.** *Adults:* 500 mg naproxen P.O., followed by 250 mg q 6 to 8 hours p.r.n. Or, 550 mg naproxen sodium P.O. initially; then 275 mg P.O. q 6 to 8 hours p.r.n. Or, 1,000 mg Naprelan P.O. daily; use 1,500 mg P.O. daily for limited period.

Contraindications and precautions

- Contraindicated in patients hypersensitive to drug and patients with asthma, rhinitis, or nasal polyps.
- Use cautiously in those with renal disease, CV disease, GI disorders, hepatic disease, or peptic ulcer disease.

≛ **Lifespan:** In women in the last trimester of pregnancy and in breast-feeding women, drug is contraindicated. In elderly patients, use cautiously.

Adverse reactions

CNS: *headache, drowsiness, dizziness,* tinnitus, cognitive dysfunction, aseptic meningitis.
CV: *peripheral edema,* palpitations, digital vasculitis.
EENT: visual disturbances, *tinnitus.*
GI: *epigastric distress, occult blood loss,* nausea, peptic ulceration.
GU: *nephrotoxicity.*
Hematologic: *agranulocytosis, thrombocytopenia, neutropenia.*
Metabolic: *hyperkalemia.*
Respiratory: dyspnea.
Skin: *pruritus, rash,* urticaria.

Interactions

Drug-drug. *Antihypertensives, diuretics:* Decreases effect of these drugs. Monitor patient.
Aspirin, corticosteroids: Increases risk of adverse GI reactions. Use cautiously and monitor patient for abdominal pain, bleeding.
Cyclosporine: Increases nephrotoxicity of both drugs. Monitor renal function tests.
Methotrexate: Increases risk of toxicity. Monitor levels.
Oral anticoagulants, sulfonylureas, drugs that are highly protein-bound: Increases risk of toxicity. Monitor patient closely.
Probenecid: Decreases elimination of naproxen. Monitor patient for toxicity.
Drug-herb. *Dong quai, feverfew, garlic, ginger, horse chestnut, red clover:* Increases risk of bleeding. Discourage using together.
St. John's wort: Increases risk of photosensitivity. Advise patient to avoid unprotected or prolonged exposure to sunlight.
Drug-lifestyle. *Alcohol use:* Increases risk of adverse GI reactions. Discourage using together.

Effects on lab test results

• May increase BUN, creatinine, ALT, AST, and potassium levels.
• May increase bleeding time. May decrease granulocyte, platelet, and neutrophil counts.
• May interfere with urinary assays of 5-hydroxyindoleacetic acid and may falsely elevate urine 17-ketosteroid concentrations.

Pharmacokinetics

Absorption: Rapid and complete.
Distribution: Highly protein-bound.
Metabolism: Metabolized in liver.
Excretion: Excreted in urine. *Half-life:* 1¼ hours.

Route	Onset	Peak	Duration
P.O.	≤ 1 hr	1-6 hr	7-12 hr
P.R.	Unknown	Unknown	Unknown

Action

Chemical effect: Unknown; produces anti-inflammatory, analgesic, and antipyretic effects, possibly by inhibiting prostaglandin synthesis.
Therapeutic effect: Relieves pain, fever, and inflammation.

Available forms

naproxen
Oral suspension: 125 mg/5 ml
Suppositories: 500 mg ◇
Tablets: 250 mg, 375 mg, 500 mg
Tablets (delayed-release, enteric coated): 375 mg, 500 mg
Tablets (extended-release) ♦ **:** 750 mg, 1,000 mg
naproxen sodium
275 mg naproxen sodium = 250 mg naproxen
Tablets (controlled-release): 375 mg, 500 mg (equivalent to 412.5 mg or 550 mg naproxen sodium, respectively)
Tablets (film-coated): 220 mg, 275 mg, 550 mg

NURSING PROCESS

ᴧᴱ Assessment

• Assess patient's condition before therapy and regularly thereafter.
• Monitor CBC and renal and hepatic function q 4 to 6 months during long-term therapy.
• NSAIDs may mask signs and symptoms of infection.
• If adverse GI reactions occur, monitor patient's hydration status.
• Evaluate patient's and family's knowledge of drug therapy.

⊕ Nursing diagnoses

• Acute pain related to condition

Reactions may be *common,* uncommon, ***life-threatening,*** or COMMON AND LIFE-THREATENING.

• Risk for deficient fluid volume related to drug-induced adverse GI reactions
• Deficient knowledge related to drug therapy

⊠ Planning and implementation

⊛ **ALERT:** Don't exceed 1.25 g of naproxen or 1.375 of naproxen sodium daily.
• Give drug with food or milk to minimize GI upset.
• Tell patient to take a full glass of water or other liquid with each dose.
• Don't break, crush or chew delayed-release tablets.
• Suppository isn't available in the United States.
• Don't use in patients with inflammatory lesion of the rectum or anus.

Patient teaching
• Tell patient taking prescription doses of naproxen for arthritis that full therapeutic effect may take 2 to 4 weeks.
⊛ **ALERT:** Warn patient against taking naproxen and naproxen sodium at the same time.
• Teach patient to recognize and report evidence of GI bleeding. Serious GI toxicity, including peptic ulceration and bleeding, can occur in patients taking NSAIDs, despite absence of GI symptoms.
• Warn patient that use with aspirin, alcohol, or corticosteroids may increase risk of adverse GI reactions.
• Advise patient to have periodic eye examinations.

☑ Evaluation
• Patient is free from pain.
• Patient maintains adequate hydration.
• Patient and family state understanding of drug therapy.

naratriptan hydrochloride
(nah-rah-TRIP-tin high-droh-KLOR-ighd)
Amerge, Naramig ◊

Pharmacologic class: selective 5-hydroxy-tryptamine 1 (5-HT$_1$) receptor subtype agonist
Therapeutic class: antimigraine drug
Pregnancy risk category: C

Indications and dosages

▶ **Acute migraine headaches with or without aura.** *Adults:* 1 or 2.5 mg P.O. as a single dose. If headache returns or responds only partially, dose may be repeated after 4 hours, for maximum dose of 5 mg in 24 hours.
⊠ **Adjust-a-dose:** For patients with mild renal or hepatic impairment, don't use more than 2.5 mg P.O. in 24 hours. If creatinine clearance is less than 15 ml/minute or if patient has severe hepatic impairment, don't use drug.

Contraindications and precautions

• Contraindicated in patients hypersensitive to drug or its components and in those who have received ergot-containing, ergot-type, or other 5-HT$_1$ agonists in the previous 24 hours. Also contraindicated in patients with a history, symptoms, or signs of cardiac ischemia, cerebrovascular disease, peripheral vascular disease, significant underlying CV disease, uncontrolled hypertension, creatinine clearance below 15 ml/minute, or Child-Pugh grade C.
• Unless a CV evaluation determines that patient is free from cardiac disease, use cautiously in patient with risk factors for coronary artery disease, such as hypertension, hypercholesterolemia, obesity, diabetes, a strong family history of coronary artery disease, surgical or physiologic menopause (women), age older than 40 (men), and smoking. For patients with cardiac risk factors but a satisfactory CV evaluation, give first dose in a medical facility and consider ECG monitoring.
• Safety and effectiveness haven't been established for cluster headaches or for treating more than four migraine headaches in a 30-day period.
⚖ **Lifespan:** In pregnant women and elderly patients, drug is contraindicated.

Adverse reactions

CNS: paresthesias, dizziness, drowsiness, malaise, fatigue, vertigo, syncope.
CV: palpitations, increased blood pressure, *tachyarrhythmias, abnormal ECG changes (PR and QT interval prolongation, ST/T wave abnormalities,* PVCs, atrial flutter or fibrillation), *coronary vasospasm, coronary artery vasospasm, transient myocardial ischemia, MI, ventricular tachycardia, ventricular fibrillation.*

EENT: ear, nose, and throat infections; photophobia.
GI: nausea, hyposalivation, vomiting.
Other: warm or cold temperature sensations; pressure, tightness, and heaviness sensations.

Interactions

Drug-drug. *Ergot-containing or ergot-type drugs (methysergide, dihydroergotamine), other 5-HT$_1$ agonists:* Prolong vasospastic reactions. Don't give within 24 hours of naratriptan.
Hormonal contraceptives: Slightly higher naratriptan levels. Monitor patient.
SSRIs, such as fluoxetine, fluvoxamine, paroxetine, sertraline: May cause weakness, hyperreflexia, and incoordination. Monitor patient.
Sibutramine: Signs of serotonin syndrome including CNS irritability, motor weakness, shivering, myoclonus may occur. Use together cautiously.
Drug-lifestyle. *Smoking:* Increases naratriptan clearance. Discourage using together; urge patient to stop smoking.

Effects on lab test results

None reported.

Pharmacokinetics

Absorption: Well absorbed with a bioavailability of 70%.
Distribution: About 28% to 31% protein-bound.
Metabolism: Metabolized to a number of inactive metabolites by wide range of CYP isoenzymes.
Excretion: Primarily excreted in urine with 50% of dose recovered unchanged and 30% as metabolites. *Half-life:* 6 hours.

Route	Onset	Peak	Duration
P.O.	Unknown	2-3 hr	Unknown

Action

Chemical effect: May activate receptors in intracranial blood vessels leading to vasoconstriction and relief of migraine headache; activation of receptors on sensory nerve endings in trigeminal system may inhibit proinflammatory neuropeptide release.
Therapeutic effect: Relieves migraine pain.

Available forms

Tablets: 1 mg, 2.5 mg

NURSING PROCESS

▧ Assessment
• Assess baseline cardiac function before starting therapy. Perform periodic cardiac reevaluation in patients who develop risk factors for coronary artery disease.
• Monitor renal and liver function test results before starting drug therapy, and report abnormalities.
• Evaluate patient's and family's knowledge of drug therapy.

⊕ Nursing diagnoses
• Acute pain related to presence of migraine headache
• Risk for injury related to drug-induced adverse CV reactions
• Deficient knowledge related to drug therapy

▶ Planning and implementation
• Give drug only for a definite diagnosis of migraine. Drug isn't intended for preventing migraine headaches or treating hemiplegic headaches, basilar migraines, or cluster headaches.
• If patient has pain or tightness in chest or throat, arrhythmias, or increased blood pressure, withhold drug and notify prescriber.
• Don't give drug to patients with history of coronary artery disease, hypertension, arrhythmias, or risk factors for coronary artery disease because drug may cause coronary vasospasm and hypertension.
• For patients with cardiac risk factors who have had a satisfactory cardiac evaluation, give first dose while monitoring ECG. Keep emergency equipment readily available.
Patient teaching
• Instruct patient to take drug only as prescribed.
• Tell patient that drug is intended to relieve migraine headaches, not prevent them.
• Instruct patient to take dose soon after headache starts. If no response occurs to first tablet, tell patient to seek prescriber approval before taking second tablet. If prescriber approves a second dose, patient may take a second tablet, but no sooner than 4 hours after first tablet. Warn patient not to exceed two tablets in 24 hours.

- Teach patient to alert prescriber about bothersome adverse effects or risk factors for coronary artery disease.

☑ Evaluation

- Patient has relief of migraine headache.
- Patient has no pain or tightness in chest or throat, arrhythmias, or increase in blood pressure.
- Patient and family state understanding of drug therapy.

nateglinide
(na-TEG-li-nide)
Starlix

Pharmacologic class: amino acid derivative
Therapeutic class: antidiabetic
Pregnancy risk category: C

Indications and dosages

▶ **Alone or with metformin or a thiazolidinedione to lower glucose levels in patients with type 2 diabetes whose hyperglycemia isn't adequately controlled by diet and exercise and who haven't received long-term therapy with other antidiabetics.** *Adults:* 120 mg P.O. t.i.d., taken 1 to 30 minutes before meals. If patient's glycosylated hemoglobin (HbA_{1c}) is near goal when treatment starts, he may receive 60 mg P.O. t.i.d.

Contraindications and precautions

- Contraindicated in patients hypersensitive to drug and in patients with type 1 diabetes or diabetic ketoacidosis.
- Use cautiously in malnourished patients and patients with moderate-to-severe liver dysfunction or adrenal or pituitary insufficiency.
- ⚖ **Lifespan:** In breast-feeding women, avoid drug because it isn't known whether drug appears in breast milk. In children, safety and effectiveness of drug haven't been established. In elderly patients, use cautiously; some elderly patients may have greater sensitivity to the glucose-lowering effects than others.

Adverse reactions

CNS: dizziness.
GI: diarrhea.
Metabolic: *hypoglycemia.*

Musculoskeletal: back pain, arthropathy.
Respiratory: *upper respiratory tract infection,* bronchitis, coughing.
Other: flulike symptoms, accidental trauma.

Interactions

Drug-drug. *MAO inhibitors, nonselective beta blockers, NSAIDs, salicylates:* May increase the hypoglycemic action of nateglinide. Monitor patient for hypoglycemia and monitor glucose levels closely.
Corticosteroids, sympathomimetics, thiazides, thyroid drugs: May reduce the hypoglycemic action of nateglinide. Monitor patient for hyperglycemia and monitor glucose levels closely.

Effects on lab test results

- May decrease glucose level.

Pharmacokinetics

Absorption: Rapidly absorbed when taken immediately before a meal. Levels peak within 1 hour. The rate of absorption is slower when nateglinide is taken with or after a meal, but the extent of absorption is unaffected.
Distribution: 98% bound to proteins, primarily albumin.
Metabolism: Metabolized in the liver by hydroxylation followed by glucuronide conjugation. Drug is metabolized by CYP 2C9 (70%) and CYP 3A4 (30%).
Excretion: Drug and its metabolites are rapidly and completely eliminated in urine and feces after oral use. *Half-life:* About 1½ hours.

Route	Onset	Peak	Duration
P.O.	20 min	1 hr	4 hr

Action

Chemical effect: Stimulates insulin secretion from the pancreas. This action is dependent on the presence of functioning beta cells in the pancreas.
Therapeutic effect: Lowers glucose level.

Available forms

Tablets: 60 mg, 120 mg

NURSING PROCESS

� Assessment

- Assess underlying condition before therapy and reassess regularly throughout therapy.

- Monitor glucose level regularly to evaluate drug effectiveness.
- When other drugs are started or stopped, monitor glucose level closely to detect possible drug interactions.
- Periodically monitor HbA_{1c} levels.
- Evaluate patient's and family's knowledge of drug therapy.

🔷 Nursing diagnoses
- Ineffective health maintenance related to hyperglycemia
- Risk for injury related to adverse drug effect of hypoglycemia
- Deficient knowledge related to nateglinide therapy

▶ Planning and implementation
- Don't use with or instead of glyburide or other oral antidiabetics. Drug may be used with metformin.
- Give drug 1 to 30 minutes before a meal. If patient misses a meal, skip the scheduled dose.
- ⚡ **ALERT:** Risk of hypoglycemia rises with strenuous exercise, alcohol ingestion, insufficient caloric intake, and use with other oral antidiabetics.
- Symptoms of hypoglycemia may be masked in patients with autonomic neuropathy and in those who use beta blockers.
- Insulin may be needed for glycemic control in patients with fever, infection, trauma, or impending surgery.
- Effectiveness may decline over time.
- ⚡ **ALERT:** Observe patient for evidence of hypoglycemia, including sweating, rapid pulse, trembling, confusion, headache, irritability, and nausea. To minimize the risk of hypoglycemia, follow dose immediately by a meal. If hypoglycemia occurs and the patient remains conscious, give an oral form of glucose. If unconscious, give I.V. glucose.

Patient teaching
- Tell patient to take nateglinide 1 to 30 minutes before a meal.
- To reduce the risk of hypoglycemia, advise patient to skip the scheduled dose if he misses a meal.
- Educate patient about the risk of hypoglycemia and its signs and symptoms (sweating, rapid pulse, trembling, confusion, headache, irritability, and nausea). Advise patient to treat

these symptoms by eating or drinking something containing sugar.
- Teach patient how to monitor and log glucose levels to evaluate diabetes control.
- Instruct patient to adhere to the prescribed diet and exercise regimen.
- Explain the possible long-term complications of diabetes and the importance of regular preventive therapy.
- Encourage patient to wear or carry medical identification that shows he has diabetes.

☑ Evaluation
- Patient's glucose level is normal.
- Patient does not become hypoglycemic and therefore sustains no injury.
- Patient and family state understanding of drug therapy.

---

nefazodone hydrochloride
(nef-AZ-oh-dohn high-droh-KLOR-ighd)
Serzone

Pharmacologic class: synthetically derived phenylpiperazine
Therapeutic class: antidepressant
Pregnancy risk category: C

Indications and dosages
▶ **Depression.** *Adults:* Initially, 200 mg P.O. daily in two divided doses. Dosage increased in increments of 100 to 200 mg daily at intervals of no less than 1 week, as indicated. Usual daily dosage range is 300 to 600 mg.

Contraindications and precautions
- Contraindicated in patients hypersensitive to drug or other phenylpiperazine antidepressants and within 14 days of MAO inhibitor therapy. Also contraindicated in patients who are withdrawn from drug because of liver injury.
- Use cautiously in patients with CV or cerebrovascular disease that could be worsened by hypotension (such as history of MI, angina, or CVA) and conditions that predispose to hypotension (such as dehydration, hypovolemia, and treatment with antihypertensives).
- Also use cautiously in patients with history of mania.

♨ **Lifespan:** In pregnant and breast-feeding women, use cautiously. In children, safety of drug hasn't been established.

Adverse reactions

CNS: headache, fever, *somnolence, dizziness, asthenia,* insomnia, *light-headedness, confusion,* memory impairment, paresthesia, abnormal dreams, decreased concentration, ataxia, incoordination, psychomotor retardation, tremor, hypertonia.
CV: vasodilation, orthostatic hypotension, hypotension, peripheral edema.
EENT: *blurred vision, abnormal vision,* pharyngitis, tinnitus, visual field defect.
GI: *dry mouth, nausea, constipation,* dyspepsia, diarrhea, increased appetite, vomiting, taste perversion.
GU: urinary frequency, UTI, urine retention, vaginitis.
Metabolic: hyponatremia.
Musculoskeletal: neck rigidity, arthralgia.
Respiratory: cough.
Skin: pruritus, rash.
Other: infection, flulike syndrome, chills, thirst, breast pain.

Interactions

Drug-drug. *Alprazolam, triazolam:* Increases effects of these drugs. Either avoid using together or reduce dosage of alprazolam and triazolam greatly.
Calcium channel blockers, HMG-CoA reductase inhibitors: May increase levels of these drugs. Adjust dosage if needed.
CNS-active drugs: May alter CNS activity. Use together cautiously.
Digoxin: May increase digoxin level. Use together cautiously, and monitor digoxin levels.
MAO inhibitors (phenelzine, selegiline, tranylcypromine): May cause serotonin syndrome (CNS irritability, shivering, and altered consciousness). Don't give together. Wait at least 2 weeks after stopping an MAO inhibitor before giving any SSRIs.
Other drugs highly bound to proteins: May increase adverse reactions. Monitor patient closely.
Sibutramine, sumatriptan: May cause severe excitation, hyperpyrexia, seizures, delirium, coma, or a fatal reaction. Avoid using together.
Drug-herb. *St. John's wort:* May cause additive effects and serotonin syndrome (CNS irritabili-

ty, shivering, and altered consciousness}. Discourage using together.
Drug-lifestyle. *Alcohol use:* Enhances CNS depression. Discourage using together.

Effects on lab test results

• May decrease sodium level.

Pharmacokinetics

Absorption: Rapid and complete with low, variable absolute bioavailability (about 20%).
Distribution: Widely distributed in body tissues, including CNS. Drug is extensively bound to proteins.
Metabolism: Extensively metabolized.
Excretion: Excreted in urine. *Half-life:* 2 to 4 hours.

Route	Onset	Peak	Duration
P.O.	Unknown	1 hr	Unknown

Action

Chemical effect: Not precisely defined. Drug inhibits neuronal uptake of serotonin (5-HT$_2$) and norepinephrine; it also occupies serotonin and alpha$_1$-adrenergic receptors in CNS.
Therapeutic effect: Relieves depression.

Available forms

Tablets: 50 mg, 100 mg, 150 mg, 200 mg, 250 mg

NURSING PROCESS

☜ Assessment

• Assess patient's depression before therapy and regularly thereafter.
• Record mood changes. Monitor patient for suicidal tendencies.
• Be alert for adverse reactions and drug interactions.
• Evaluate patient's and family's knowledge of drug therapy.

🖫 Nursing diagnoses

• Disturbed thought processes related to depression
• Risk for injury related to drug-induced adverse CNS reactions
• Deficient knowledge related to drug therapy

▶ Planning and implementation

⊛ **ALERT:** Allow at least 1 week after stopping drug before patient starts an MAO inhibitor. Allow at least 14 days after stopping an MAO inhibitor before patient starts drug.

⊛ **ALERT:** Don't initiate therapy in patients with active liver disease or with elevated baseline transaminases levels. Preexisting liver disease doesn't appear to increase the likelihood of developing liver failure; however, baseline abnormalities can complicate patient monitoring.

⊛ **ALERT:** If signs and symptoms of liver dysfunction occur, such as increased AST or ALT levels greater than or equal to 3 times upper limit of normal, stop drug and don't restart.

⊛ **ALERT:** Don't confuse Serzone with Seroquel.

Patient teaching

• Warn patient not to engage in hazardous activity until CNS effects of drug are known.

⊛ **ALERT:** Instruct man with prolonged or inappropriate erections to stop drug at once and call prescriber.

• Instruct woman to call prescriber if she becomes pregnant or intends to become pregnant during therapy.

• Teach patient the signs and symptoms of liver dysfunction (jaundice, anorexia, gastrointestinal complaints, and malaise), and tell him to report them to prescriber immediately.

• Instruct patient not to drink alcoholic beverages during drug therapy.

• Tell patient who develops rash, hives, or related allergic reaction to notify prescriber.

• Inform patient that several weeks of therapy may be needed to obtain full antidepressant effect. Once improvement occurs, tell patient not to stop drug until directed by prescriber.

• Urge patient to notify prescriber before taking any OTC medications.

☑ Evaluation

• Patient exhibits improved behavior.

• Patient sustains no injuries from drug-induced adverse CNS reactions.

• Patient and family state understanding of drug therapy.

nelfinavir mesylate
(nel-FIN-uh-veer MES-ih-layt)
Viracept

Pharmacologic class: HIV protease inhibitor
Therapeutic class: antiviral
Pregnancy risk category: B

Indications and dosages

▶ **HIV infection when antiretroviral therapy is warranted.** *Adults:* 750 mg P.O. t.i.d., or 1,250 mg P.O. b.i.d. with meal.
Children ages 2 to 13: 20 to 30 mg/kg/dose P.O. t.i.d. with meal. Give dose t.i.d. as shown in table.

Body weight (kg)	Level 1-g scoops	Level teaspoons	Tablets
7 to < 8.5	4	1	-
8.5 to < 10.5	5	1.25	-
10.5 to < 12	6	1.5	-
12 to < 14	7	1.75	-
14 to < 16	8	2	-
16 to < 18	9	2.25	-
18 to < 23	10	2.5	2
> 23	15	3.75	3

▶ **Post-exposure prophylaxis following occupational exposure to HIV‡.** *Adults:* 750 mg P.O. t.i.d. with two other antiretrovirals for 4 weeks.

Contraindications and precautions

• Contraindicated in patients hypersensitive to drug or its components and in patients receiving amiodarone, ergot derivatives, lovastatin, midazolam, pimozide, quinidine, simvastatin, or triazolam.

• Use cautiously in patients with hepatic dysfunction or hemophilia type A and B.

⚕ **Lifespan:** In breast-feeding women, stop breast-feeding to avoid transmitting HIV virus to infant.

Adverse reactions

CNS: *seizures, suicidal ideation.*
GI: nausea, *diarrhea*, flatulence, *pancreatitis.*
Hematologic: *leukopenia, thrombocytopenia.*
Hepatic: *hepatitis.*

Metabolic: dehydration, *diabetes mellitus,* hyperlipidemia, hyperuricemia, *hypoglycemia.*
Skin: rash.
Other: redistribution or accumulation of body fat.

Interactions

Drug-drug. *Amiodarone, ergot derivatives, lovastatin, midazolam, pimozide, quinidine, simvastatin or triazolam:* May increase levels of these drugs, causing increased risk of serious or life-threatening adverse reactions. Avoid use together.
Atorvastatin: May increase level of atorvastatin. Use lowest possible dose or consider using pravastatin or fluvastatin instead.
Azithromycin: May increase azithromycin levels. Monitor patient for liver impairment.
Carbamazepine, phenobarbital: May reduce the effectiveness of nelfinavir. Use together cautiously.
Cyclosporine, sirolimus, tacrolimus: May increase levels of these immunosuppressants. Use together cautiously.
Delavirdine, HIV protease inhibitors (indinavir or saquinavir), nevirapine: May increase levels of protease inhibitors. Use together cautiously.
Didanosine: May decrease didanosine absorption. Take nelfinavir with food at least 2 hours before or 1 hour after didanosine.
Ethinyl estradiol: May decrease level of contraceptive. Advise patient to use alternative contraceptive measures during therapy.
Methadone, phenytoin: May decrease levels of these drugs. Adjust dosage of these drugs accordingly.
Rifabutin: Increases rifabutin level, and decreases level of nelfinavir. Reduce dose of rifabutin to one-half the usual dose, and increase nelfinavir to 1,250 mg b.i.d.
Sildenafil: May increase adverse effects of sildenafil. Use together cautiously. Don't exceed 25 mg of sildenafil in a 48-hour period.
Drug-herb. *St. John's wort:* Decreases nelfinavir level. Discourage using together.

Effects on lab test results

• May increase ALT, AST, alkaline phosphatase, bilirubin, GGT, amylase, CPK, and uric acid levels. May increase or decrease glucose level.
• May decrease hemoglobin, hematocrit, and WBC and platelet counts.

Pharmacokinetics

Absorption: Level peaks higher when drug is taken with food.
Distribution: More than 98% bound to protein.
Metabolism: Metabolized primarily by CYP 3A.
Excretion: Excreted mainly in feces. *Half-life:* 3½ to 5 hours.

Route	Onset	Peak	Duration
P.O.	Unknown	2-4 hr	Unknown

Action

Chemical effect: Inhibits protease enzyme and prevents splitting of the viral polyprotein.
Therapeutic effect: Produces immature, noninfectious virus.

Available forms

Powder: 50 mg/g powder
Tablets: 250 mg, 625 mg

NURSING PROCESS

Assessment
• Obtain baseline assessment of patient's condition, and reassess regularly thereafter to monitor drug effectiveness.
• Monitor liver function test results.
• Assess patient for increased bleeding tendencies, especially if he has hemophilia type A or B.
• Monitor patient for excessive diarrhea, and treat as directed.
• Evaluate patient's and family's knowledge of drug therapy.

Nursing diagnoses
• Risk for injury related to adverse GI effects of drug
• Risk for impaired skin integrity secondary to drug adverse effects
• Deficient knowledge related to drug therapy

Planning and implementation
• Give oral powder to children unable to take tablets. May mix oral powder with small amount of water, milk, formula, soy formula, soy milk, or dietary supplements. Tell patient to consume entire contents.
• Don't reconstitute drug with water in its original container.
• Use reconstituted powder within 6 hours.

- Mixing with acidic foods or juice isn't recommended because of the bitter taste.
- **⊛ ALERT:** Don't confuse nelfinavir with nevirapine.

Patient teaching
- Advise patient to take drug with food.
- Inform patient that drug doesn't cure HIV infection and it doesn't reduce the risk of transmitting HIV to others.
- Tell patient that long-term effects of drug are unknown.
- Instruct patient to take drug daily as prescribed and not to alter dose or stop drug without medical approval.
- Tell patient that diarrhea is most common adverse effect and it can be controlled with loperamide.
- If patient misses a dose, tell him to take it as soon as possible and then return to his normal schedule. If a dose is skipped, advise patient not to double the dose.
- Instruct patient taking hormonal contraceptives to use an additional (or different) contraceptive measure while taking nelfinavir.
- **⊛ ALERT:** Warn patient with phenylketonuria that powder contains 11.2 mg phenylalanine per gram.
- Instruct patient to report use of other prescribed or OTC drugs because of possible drug interactions.
- Advise patient taking sildenafil of an increased risk of sildenafil-associated adverse events, including hypotension, visual changes, and priapism; tell him to promptly report any symptoms to prescriber. Tell him not to exceed 25 mg of sildenafil in a 48-hour period.

☑ Evaluation
- Patient has no adverse GI reactions.
- Patient and family state understanding of drug therapy.
- Skin integrity remains intact.

---

neomycin sulfate
(nee-oh-MIGH-sin SUL-fayt)
Mycifradin, Neo-fradin, Neo-Tabs

Pharmacologic class: aminoglycoside
Therapeutic class: antibiotic
Pregnancy risk category: D

Indications and dosages

▶ **Infectious diarrhea caused by entero-pathogenic** *Escherichia coli. Adults:* 50 mg/kg daily P.O. in four divided doses for 2 to 3 days. *Children:* 50 to 100 mg/kg daily P.O. divided q 4 to 6 hours for 2 to 3 days.

▶ **Preoperative suppression of intestinal bacteria.** *Adults:* 1 g P.O. q hour for four doses; then, 1 g q 4 hours for balance of 24 hours. Give a saline cathartic before first dose. *Children:* 40 to 100 mg/kg daily P.O. divided q 4 to 6 hours. Give a saline cathartic before first dose.

▶ **Adjunct in hepatic coma.** *Adults:* 1 to 3 g P.O. q.i.d. for 5 to 6 days. Or, 200 ml of 1% solution or 100 ml of 2% solution as enema retained for 20 to 60 minutes q 6 hours.

Contraindications and precautions

- Contraindicated in patients hypersensitive to other aminoglycosides and in those with intestinal obstruction.
- Use cautiously in patients with renal impairment, neuromuscular disorders, or ulcerative bowel lesions.
- ☀ **Lifespan:** In breast-feeding women, safety of drug hasn't been established. In elderly patients, use cautiously.

Adverse reactions

CNS: headache, lethargy.
EENT: *ototoxicity.*
GI: nausea, vomiting.
GU: *nephrotoxicity* (cells or casts in urine, oliguria, proteinuria).
Skin: rash, urticaria.
Other: *hypersensitivity reactions.*

Interactions

Drug-drug. *Acyclovir, amphotericin B, cisplatin, methoxyflurane, other aminoglycosides, vancomycin:* Increases risk of nephrotoxicity. Use together cautiously.
Atracurium, doxacurium, mivacurium, pancuronium, rocuronium, tubocurarine, vecuronium: May increase the effects of nondepolarizing muscle relaxant, such as prolonged respiratory depression. Use together only when necessary. Reduce dose.
Cephalothin: Increases risk of nephrotoxicity. Use together cautiously; monitor renal function.
Digoxin: Decreases digoxin absorption. Monitor patient for loss of therapeutic effect.

Reactions may be *common,* uncommon, *life-threatening,* or **COMMON AND LIFE-THREATENING.**

Dimenhydrinate: May mask symptoms of oto-toxicity. Use cautiously.

I.V. loop diuretics (such as furosemide): Increases risk of ototoxicity. Use cautiously; monitor hearing function.

Methotrexate: Decreases effects of methotrexate. Monitor patient for decreased effect.

Oral anticoagulants: Inhibits vitamin K–producing bacteria; may increase anticoagulant effect. Monitor patient for bleeding; monitor PT and INR.

Effects on lab test results

• May increase BUN, creatinine, and nonprotein nitrogen levels.

Pharmacokinetics

Absorption: About 3%. Enhanced in patients with impaired GI motility or mucosal intestinal ulcerations.
Distribution: Distributed locally in GI tract.
Metabolism: Not metabolized.
Excretion: Excreted primarily unchanged in feces. *Half-life:* 2 to 3 hours.

Route	Onset	Peak	Duration
P.O.	Unknown	1-4 hr	8 hr

Action

Chemical effect: Inhibits protein synthesis by binding directly to 30S ribosomal subunit.
Therapeutic effect: Kills susceptible bacteria, such as many aerobic gram-negative organisms and some aerobic gram-positive organisms. Inhibits ammonia-forming bacteria in GI tract, reducing ammonia and improving neurologic status of patients with hepatic encephalopathy.

Available forms

Oral solution: 125 mg/5 ml
Tablets: 500 mg

NURSING PROCESS

⚙ Assessment

• Assess patient's condition before therapy and regularly thereafter.
• Evaluate patient's hearing before therapy and regularly thereafter.
• Monitor renal function (output, specific gravity, urinalysis, BUN and creatinine levels, and creatinine clearance).

• Be alert for adverse reactions and drug interactions.
• If adverse GI reactions occur, monitor patient's hydration status.
• Evaluate patient's and family's knowledge of drug therapy.

⚙ Nursing diagnoses

• Infection related to organisms
• Risk for deficient fluid volume related to drug-induced adverse GI reactions
• Deficient knowledge related to drug therapy

⟩ Planning and implementation

⚠ **ALERT:** Never give drug parenterally.
• Drug is nonabsorbable at recommended dosage. More than 4 g daily may be systemically absorbed and lead to nephrotoxicity.
• Make sure patient is well hydrated while taking drug to minimize chemical irritation of renal tubules.
• For preoperative disinfection, provide low-residue diet and cathartic immediately before oral administration of drug.
• In adjunct treatment of hepatic coma, decrease patient's dietary protein and assess neurologic status frequently during therapy.
• The ototoxic and nephrotoxic properties of neomycin limit its usefulness.
• Drug is available with polymyxin B as urinary bladder irrigant.
• Notify prescriber about signs of decreasing renal function or complaints of tinnitus, vertigo, or hearing loss. Deafness may begin several weeks after drug is stopped.
Patient teaching
• Instruct patient to report adverse reactions, especially hearing loss or change in urinary elimination.
• Emphasize the need to drink 2 L of fluid each day.
• Tell patient to alert prescriber if infection worsens or doesn't improve.

✓ Evaluation

• Patient is free from infection.
• Patient maintains adequate hydration throughout drug therapy.
• Patient and family state understanding of drug therapy.

neostigmine bromide
(nee-oh-STIG-meen BROH-mighd)
Prostigmin

neostigmine methylsulfate
Prostigmin

Pharmacologic class: cholinesterase inhibitor
Therapeutic class: muscle stimulant
Pregnancy risk category: C

Indications and dosages

▶ **Myasthenia gravis.** *Adults:* 15 to 30 mg P.O.
t.i.d. (range, 15 to 375 mg daily). Or, 0.5 mg
S.C. or I.M.
Children: 7.5 to 15 mg P.O. t.i.d. or q.i.d. Sub-
sequent dosages must be highly individualized,
depending on response and tolerance of adverse
effects. Therapy may be required day and night.
▶ **To diagnose myasthenia gravis.** *Adults:*
0.022 mg/kg I.M. 30 minutes after 0.011 mg/kg
I.M. of atropine sulfate.
Children: 0.025 to 0.04 mg/kg. I.M. after
0.011 mg/kg atropine sulfate S.C.
▶ **Postoperative abdominal distention and
bladder atony.** *Adults:* 0.25 to 0.5 mg I.M. or
S.C. q 4 to 6 hours for 2 to 3 days.
▶ **Antidote for nondepolarizing neuromuscular blockers.** *Adults:* 0.5 to 2 mg I.V. slowly.
Repeat p.r.n. to total of 5 mg. Before antidote
dose, give 0.6 to 1.2 mg I.V. atropine sulfate.
▶ **Supraventricular tachycardia from tricyclic antidepressant overdose‡.** *Children:*
0.5 to 1 mg I.V., followed by 0.25 to 0.5 mg I.V.
q 1 to 3 hours, p.r.n.
▶ **Decrease small bowel transit time during
radiography‡.** *Adults:* 0.5 to 0.75 mg S.C.

▼ I.V. administration

• 1:1,000 solution of injectable solution contains 1 mg/ml; 1:2,000 solution contains
0.5 mg/ml.
• Give drug at slow, controlled rate of no more
than 1 mg/minute in adults and 0.5 mg/minute
in children.

Contraindications and precautions

• Contraindicated in patients hypersensitive to
cholinergics or bromide and in those with peri-

tonitis or mechanical obstruction of intestine or
urinary tract.
• Use cautiously in patients with bronchial asthma, bradycardia, seizure disorders, recent coronary occlusion, vagotonia, hyperthyroidism,
arrhythmias, or peptic ulcer.
❧ Lifespan: In pregnant women, safety of
drug has not been established.

Adverse reactions

CNS: dizziness, headache, mental confusion,
jitters.
CV: *bradycardia,* hypotension, *cardiac arrest.*
EENT: blurred vision, lacrimation, miosis.
GI: *nausea, vomiting, diarrhea, abdominal
cramps,* excessive salivation.
GU: urinary frequency.
Musculoskeletal: *muscle cramps,* muscle
weakness, muscle fasciculations.
Respiratory: *depressed respiratory drive,
bronchospasm, bronchoconstriction, respirato-
ry arrest.*
Skin: rash (with bromide), diaphoresis.
Other: *hypersensitivity reactions (anaphy-
laxis).*

Interactions

Drug-drug. *Aminoglycosides, anticholinergics,
atropine, corticosteroids, magnesium sulfate,
procainamide, quinidine:* May reverse cholinergic effects. Observe patient for lack of drug effect.

Effects on lab test results

None reported.

Pharmacokinetics

Absorption: 1% to 2% after P.O. administration. Unknown after S.C. or I.M. administration.
Distribution: About 15% to 25% of dose binds
to proteins.
Metabolism: Hydrolyzed by cholinesterases
and metabolized by microsomal liver enzymes.
Excretion: About 80% of drug excreted in
urine. *Half-life:* 52 to 53 minutes.

Route	Onset	Peak	Duration
P.O.	45-75 min	1-2 hr	2-4 hr
I.V.	4-8 min	1-2 hr	2-4 hr
I.M.	20-30 min	1-2 hr	2-4 hr
S.C.	Unknown	1-2 hr	2-4 hr

Reactions may be *common*, uncommon, *life-threatening*, or COMMON AND LIFE-THREATENING.

Action

Chemical effect: Inhibits destruction of acetylcholine released from parasympathetic and somatic efferent nerves. Acetylcholine accumulates, promoting increased stimulation of receptor.
Therapeutic effect: Stimulates muscle contraction.

Available forms

neostigmine bromide
Tablets: 15 mg
neostigmine methylsulfate
Injection: 0.25 mg/ml, 0.5 mg/ml, 1 mg/ml

NURSING PROCESS

✏ Assessment

• Assess patient's condition before therapy.
• Monitor patient's response after each dose. Watch closely for improvement in strength, vision, and ptosis 45 to 60 minutes after each dose. Show patient how to record variations in muscle strength.
• Monitor vital signs frequently.
• Evaluate patient's and family's knowledge of drug therapy.

⚏ Nursing diagnoses

• Impaired physical mobility related to condition
• Diarrhea related to drug's adverse effect on GI tract
• Deficient knowledge related to drug therapy

⟫ Planning and implementation

🟉 **ALERT:** For diagnosis of myasthenia gravis, stop any anticholinesterases for at least 8 hours before giving drug.
• In myasthenia gravis, schedule doses before fatigue. For example, if patient has dysphagia, schedule dose 30 minutes before each meal.
• Give atropine injection; provide respiratory support p.r.n.
• When drug is used to prevent abdominal distention and GI distress, use a rectal tube to help passage of gas.
🟉 **ALERT:** Although drug is commonly used to reverse effects of nondepolarizing neuromuscular blockers in patients who have undergone surgery, it may worsen blockade produced by succinylcholine.
• Patient may develop resistance to drug.

• Give oral drug with food or milk.
• Give hospitalized patient a bedside supply of tablets. A patient with long-standing disease may insist on self-administration.
🟉 **ALERT:** Use I.M. drug instead of edrophonium to diagnose myasthenia gravis. May be preferable to use edrophonium when lengthy procedures involving testing of limb strength are used.
🟉 **ALERT:** Don't confuse neostigmine with etomidate (Amidate) vials; they may look alike.
Patient teaching
• Tell patient to take drug with food or milk to reduce GI distress.
• When using for myasthenia gravis, explain that drug will relieve ptosis, double vision, difficulty chewing and swallowing, and trunk and limb weakness. Stress need to take drug exactly as ordered. Explain that it may have to be taken for life.
• Advise patient to wear or carry medical identification indicating that he has myasthenia gravis.

✓ Evaluation

• Patient performs activities of daily living without assistance.
• Patient has normal bowel patterns.
• Patient and family state understanding of drug therapy.

nesiritide
(ne-SIR-I-tide)
Natrecor

Pharmacologic class: human B-type natriuretic peptide
Therapeutic class: inotropic vasodilator
Pregnancy risk category: C

Indications and dosages

▶ **Acutely decompensated heart failure in patients with dyspnea at rest or with minimal activity.** *Adults:* 2 mcg/kg by I.V. bolus over 60 seconds followed by continuous infusion of 0.01 mcg/kg/minute.

▼ I.V. administration

• Reconstitute one 1.5-mg vial with 5 ml of diluent (such as D₅W, normal saline solution, 5% dextrose and 0.2% saline solution injection,

or 5% dextrose and half-normal saline solution) from a prefilled 250-ml I.V. bag.
• Don't shake vial. Gently rock vial until a clear, colorless solution results.
• Withdraw contents of vial and add back to the 250-ml I.V. bag to yield 6 mcg/ml. Invert the bag several times to ensure complete mixing, and use the solution within 24 hours.
• Use these formulas to calculate bolus volume (2 mcg/kg) and infusion flow rate (0.01 mcg/kg/minute):

$$\frac{\text{Bolus volume}}{(\text{ml})} = 0.33 \times \frac{\text{patient weight}}{(\text{kg})}$$

$$\frac{\text{Infusion flow rate}}{(\text{ml/hr})} = 0.1 \times \frac{\text{patient weight}}{(\text{kg})}$$

• Before starting bolus dose, prime the I.V. tubing. Withdraw the bolus and giveover 60 seconds through an I.V. port in the tubing.
• Immediately after giving bolus, infuse drug at 0.1 ml/kg/hour to deliver 0.01 mcg/kg/minute.
⚡ **ALERT:** Drug is incompatible with injectable forms of bumetanide, enalaprilat, ethacrynate sodium, furosemide, heparin, hydralazine, and insulin.
⚡ **ALERT:** Nesiritide binds heparin and could bind the heparin lining of a heparin-coated catheter, decreasing the amount of nesiritide delivered. Don't give nesiritide through a central heparin-coated catheter.
⚡ **ALERT:** The preservative sodium metabisulfite is incompatible with drug. Don't give injectable drugs with this preservative in the same line as this drug.
• Store drug at a controlled room temperature.

Contraindications and precautions

• Contraindicated in patients hypersensitive to drug or its components.
• Avoid using drug as primary therapy in patients with cardiogenic shock or patients with systolic blood pressure below 90 mm Hg, low cardiac filling pressures, conditions in which cardiac output is dependent on venous return, or conditions that make vasodilators inappropriate, such as valvular stenosis, restrictive or obstructive cardiomyopathy, constrictive pericarditis, or pericardial tamponade.
🍼 **Lifespan:** In breast-feeding women, use cautiously because it isn't known whether drug appears in breast milk. In children, safety and effectiveness haven't been established. Some

older patients may be more sensitive to drug effects than younger patients, but no overall difference in effectiveness has been noted.

Adverse reactions

CNS: headache, confusion, somnolence, insomnia, dizziness, anxiety, paresthesia, tremor, fever.
CV: *hypotension, ventricular tachycardia,* ventricular extrasystoles, angina, *bradycardia,* atrial fibrillation, AV node conduction abnormalities.
GI: nausea, vomiting, abdominal pain.
Hematologic: anemia.
Musculoskeletal: back pain, leg cramps.
Respiratory: *apnea,* cough.
Skin: rash, sweating, pruritus.
Other: injection site reactions, pain at the site.

Interactions

Drug-drug. *ACE inhibitors:* Increases hypotension symptoms. Monitor blood pressure closely.

Effects on lab test results

• May increase creatinine level more than 0.5 mg/dl above baseline.
• May decrease hemoglobin and hematocrit.

Pharmacokinetics

Absorption: Administered I.V.
Distribution: Unknown.
Metabolism: Unknown.
Excretion: Three independent paths clear drug: lysosomal proteolysis after drug binds to cell surface receptors, proteolytic cleavage by endopeptidases in the vascular lumen, and renal filtration. *Mean terminal half-life:* 18 minutes.

Route	Onset	Peak	Duration
I.V.	15 min	1 hr	3 hr

Action

Chemical effect: Binds to receptors on vascular smooth muscle and endothelial cells, which leads to an increase in guanosine 3′5′-cyclic monophosphate level, relaxation of smooth muscles, and dilation of veins and arteries.
Therapeutic effect: Produces a dose-dependent reduction in pulmonary capillary wedge pressure and systemic arterial pressure in patients with heart failure.

Available forms

Injection: Single-dose vials of 1.5 mg sterile, lyophilized powder

NURSING PROCESS

Assessment
• Assess underlying condition before therapy and reassess regularly throughout therapy.
• **ALERT:** Drug may cause hypotension. Monitor patient's blood pressure closely, particularly if patient also takes an ACE inhibitor.
• Evaluate patient's renal function. Nesiritide may affect renal function in some people. In patients with severe heart failure whose renal function depends on the renin-angiotensin-aldosterone system, treatment may lead to azotemia.
• Monitor patient's cardiac status before, during, and after drug administration.
• Evaluate patient's and family's knowledge of drug therapy.

Nursing diagnoses
• Ineffective tissue perfusion (cardiopulmonary) related to drug-induced hypotension
• Excess fluid volume related to heart failure
• Deficient knowledge related to nesiritide therapy

Planning and implementation
• Because of possible hypotension, don't start drug at dosage higher than recommended. If hypotension develops during administration, reduce dosage or stop drug. Restart dosage; reduce by 30% with no bolus doses.
• Limited experience exists giving this drug for longer than 48 hours.
Patient teaching
• Tell patient to report discomfort at I.V. site.
• Urge patient to report symptoms of hypotension, such as dizziness, light-headedness, blurred vision, or sweating.
• Tell patient to report other adverse effects promptly.

Evaluation
• Patient's blood pressure remains normal during therapy.
• Patient's volume status improves.
• Patient and family state understanding of drug therapy.

nevirapine
(neh-VEER-uh-peen)
Viramune

Pharmacologic class: nonnucleoside reverse transcriptase inhibitor
Therapeutic class: antiviral
Pregnancy risk category: C

Indications and dosages

▶ **Adjunct for deteriorating patients with HIV-1 infection .** *Adults:* 200 mg P.O. daily for first 14 days, followed by 200 mg P.O. b.i.d. with nucleoside analogue antiretroviral drugs.
▶ **Adjunct therapy in children infected with HIV-1.** *Children age 8 and older:* 4 mg/kg P.O. once daily for first 14 days, followed by 4 mg/kg P.O. b.i.d. thereafter. Maximum 400 mg daily.
Children ages 2 months to 7 years: 4 mg/kg P.O. once daily for first 14 days, followed by 7 mg/kg P.O. b.i.d. thereafter. Maximum dose is 400 mg daily.
▶ **Prevention of maternal-fetal transmission of HIV‡.** *Mother:* Give 200 mg P.O. as a single dose at the onset of labor.
Neonate: Give 2 mg/kg P.O. as a single dose 48 to 72 hours after birth. Usually given with a three-part zidovudine regimen.

Contraindications and precautions

• Contraindicated in patients hypersensitive to drug and in those with severe hepatic impairment.
• Use cautiously in patients with impaired renal and hepatic function.
• **Lifespan:** Women of childbearing age should avoid hormonal contraceptives during therapy. Drug appears in breast milk; breast-feeding women should stop nursing during therapy to reduce risk of giving HIV to infant.

Adverse reactions

CNS: *headache,* paresthesia, *fever.*
GI: *nausea,* diarrhea, abdominal pain, ulcerative stomatitis.
Hepatic: *hepatitis, hepatotoxicity.*
Musculoskeletal: myalgia.
Skin: rash, blistering, ***Stevens-Johnson syndrome.***

Interactions

Drug-drug. *CYP 3A4 inhibitors (cimetidine, macrolides):* May increase nevirapine levels. Monitor patient for adverse effects.
Drugs extensively metabolized by CYP 3A (rifabutin, rifampin): May decrease nevirapine levels of these drugs. Adjust dosages of these drugs if needed.
Ketoconazole: Decreases ketoconazole levels and increase nevirapine levels. Avoid using together.
Protease inhibitors, hormonal contraceptives: Decreases levels of these drugs. Monitor patient for effect; advise patient to use nonhormonal contraception.
Drug-herb. *St. John's wort:* Decreases nevirapine levels. Discourage using together.

Effects on lab test results

- May increase ALT, AST, GGT, and bilirubin levels.
- May decrease hemoglobin, hematocrit, and neutrophil count.

Pharmacokinetics

Absorption: Readily absorbed.
Distribution: Widely distributed.
Metabolism: Metabolized by liver.
Excretion: Excreted in urine and feces. *Terminal phase half-life:* 45 hours (single dose); 25 to 30 hours (multiple dosing).

Route	Onset	Peak	Duration
P.O.	Unknown	4 hr	Unknown

Action

Chemical effect: Binds to reverse transcriptase and blocks RNA-dependent and DNA-dependent DNA polymerase activities.
Therapeutic effect: May inhibit replication of HIV-1.

Available forms

Oral suspension: 50 mg/5 ml
Tablets: 200 mg

NURSING PROCESS

Assessment

- Obtain lab tests, including liver and renal function tests, before and during therapy.
- Monitor patient for blistering, oral lesions, conjunctivitis, muscle or joint aches, or general malaise. Be especially alert for severe rash or rash accompanied by fever. Report such signs and symptoms immediately to prescriber.

Nursing diagnoses

- Infection related to presence of virus
- Deficient knowledge related to drug therapy

Planning and implementation

- Use drug with at least one other antiretroviral.
- **ALERT:** Don't confuse nelfinavir with nevirapine.

Patient teaching

- Inform patient that drug doesn't cure HIV infection and that he can still develop illnesses linked to advanced HIV infection. Explain that drug doesn't reduce the risk of HIV transmission.
- Instruct patient to report rash at once and to stop drug if rash develops.
- Tell patient not to use other drugs unless approved by prescriber.
- If therapy is interrupted for more than 7 days, instruct patient to resume it as if for the first time.

Evaluation

- Patient shows no signs of worsening condition.
- Patient and family state understanding of drug therapy.

---

niacin (vitamin B₃, nicotinic acid)
(NIGH-uh-sin)
Niacin TR Tablets, Niacor, Niaspan, Nico-400, Nicobid , Nicolar, Nicotinex*, Slo-Niacin

niacinamide (nicotinamide)†

Pharmacologic class: B-complex vitamin
Therapeutic class: vitamin B₃, antilipemic, peripheral vasodilator
Pregnancy risk category: A (C in dosages that exceed the RDA)

Indications and dosages

▶ **RDA.** *Neonates and infants younger than 6 months:* 5 mg.
Infants ages 6 months to 1 year: 6 mg.
Children ages 1 to 3: 9 mg.

Children ages 4 to 6: 12 mg.
Children ages 7 to 10: 13 mg.
Men ages 11 to 14: 17 mg.
Men ages 15 to 18: 20 mg.
Men ages 19 to 50: 19 mg.
Men age 51 and older: 15 mg.
Women ages 11 to 50: 15 mg.
Women age 51 and older: 13 mg.
Pregnant women: 17 mg.
Breast-feeding women: 20 mg.

▶ **Pellagra.** Adults: 300 to 500 mg P.O., S.C., I.M., or I.V. infusion daily in divided doses, depending on severity of niacin deficiency.
Children: Up to 300 mg P.O. or 100 mg I.V. daily, depending on severity of niacin deficiency.
After symptoms subside, advise adequate nutrition and RDA supplements to prevent recurrence.

▶ **Hartnup disease.** Adults: 50 to 200 mg P.O. daily.

▶ **Niacin deficiency.** Adults: up to 100 mg P.O. daily.

▶ **Hyperlipidemias, especially with hypercholesterolemia.** Adults: Initially, 250 mg P.O. as a single dose following evening meal. Then increase q 4 to 7 days to 1 to 2 g P.O. b.i.d or t.i.d. with meals until desired LDL level is achieved. Maximum, 6 g daily. Or, for extended-release tablets, initially start at 500 mg P.O. daily h.s. for 1 to 4 weeks; then increase to 1,000 mg h.s. during weeks 5 to 8. After week 8, increase dose by 500 mg q 4 weeks. Maximum, 2 g daily.

▼ I.V. administration

• Give drug by slow I.V. (no more than 2 mg/minute).

Contraindications and precautions

• Contraindicated in patients hypersensitive to drug and in those with hepatic dysfunction, active peptic ulcers, severe hypotension, or arterial hemorrhage.
• Use cautiously in patients with gallbladder disease, diabetes mellitus, or coronary artery disease and in patients with history of liver disease, peptic ulcer, allergy, or gout.
⚖ Lifespan: In pregnant women, assess benefits and risks of therapy. In breast-feeding women, avoid breast-feeding because drug appears in breast milk. In children, safety of doses that exceed the RDA hasn't been established.

Adverse reactions

CNS: dizziness, transient headache.
CV: *flushing, excessive peripheral vasodilation, arrhythmias.*
GI: *nausea, vomiting, diarrhea,* possible activation of peptic ulceration, epigastric or substernal pain.
Hepatic: *hepatic dysfunction.*
Metabolic: hyperglycemia, hyperuricemia.
Skin: pruritus, dryness, tingling.

Interactions

Drug-drug. *Antihypertensives:* May increase risk of orthostatic hypotension. Use together cautiously; also warn patient about orthostatic hypotension.
HMG-CoA reductase inhibitors, such as lovastatin: Co-administration may result in myopathy and rhabdomyolysis. Avoid using together. Monitor patient for muscle pain and weakness.

Effects on lab test results

• May increase glucose, AST, ALT, and uric acid levels.

Pharmacokinetics

Absorption: Rapid after P.O. use. Unknown after S.C. or I.M. use.
Distribution: Coenzymes are distributed widely in body tissues.
Metabolism: Metabolized by liver to active metabolites.
Excretion: Excreted in urine. *Half-life:* About 45 minutes.

Route	Onset	Peak	Duration
P.O.	Unknown	45 min	Unknown
I.V., I.M., S.C.	Unknown	Unknown	Unknown

Action

Chemical effect: Niacin and niacinamide stimulate lipid metabolism, tissue respiration, and glycogenolysis; niacin decreases synthesis of low-density lipoproteins and inhibits lipolysis in adipose tissue.
Therapeutic effect: Restores normal level of vitamin B_3, lowers triglyceride and cholesterol levels, and dilates peripheral blood vessels.

Available forms

niacin
Capsules (timed-release): 125 mg†, 250 mg†, 300 mg†, 400 mg†, 500 mg
Elixir: 50 mg/5 ml†
Injection: 100 mg/ml in 30-ml vials
Tablets: 50 mg†, 100 mg†, 250 mg†, 500 mg
Tablets (extended-release): 500 mg, 750 mg, 1 g
Tablets (timed-release): 250 mg†, 500 mg†, 750 mg†
niacinamide
Tablets: 50 mg†, 100 mg†, 500 mg†

NURSING PROCESS

⚗ Assessment
• Assess patient's condition before therapy and regularly thereafter.
• Monitor hepatic function and glucose levels.
• Be alert for adverse reactions and drug interactions.
• If adverse GI reactions occur, monitor patient's hydration status.
• Evaluate patient's and family's knowledge of drug therapy.

⊕ Nursing diagnoses
• Imbalanced nutrition: less than body requirements related to decreased intake of vitamin B₃
• Risk for deficient fluid volume related to drug-induced adverse GI reactions
• Deficient knowledge related to drug therapy

▶ Planning and implementation
⊛ **ALERT:** Give aspirin (325 mg P.O. 30 minutes before niacin dose) to help reduce persistent or distressing flushing.
• Timed-release niacin or niacinamide may prevent excessive flushing that occurs with large doses. However, timed-release niacin has been linked to hepatic dysfunction, even at doses as low as 1 g daily.
• Give drug with meals to minimize GI adverse effects.
⊛ **ALERT:** Don't confuse Nicobid and Nicotinex with Nicoderm, Nicotrol, or Nicorette.
Patient teaching
• Explain that skin flushing or warm sensation is usually harmless and will usually subside with continued use.
• To decrease flushing, advise patient to take drug with a low-fat snack and to avoid taking it

after alcohol, hot beverages, hot or spicy foods, a hot shower, or exercise.
• Stress that drug is a potent medication that may cause serious adverse effects. Explain importance of adhering to therapeutic regimen.
• Advise patient against self-medicating for hyperlipidemia.

☑ Evaluation
• Patient's vitamin B₃ levels are normal.
• Patient maintains adequate hydration throughout drug therapy.
• Patient and family state understanding of drug therapy.

---

nicardipine hydrochloride
(nigh-KAR-dih-peen high-droh-KLOR-ighd)
Cardene, Cardene I.V., Cardene SR

Pharmacologic class: calcium channel blocker
Therapeutic class: antianginal, antihypertensive
Pregnancy risk category: C

Indications and dosages
▶ **Chronic stable angina (alone or with other antianginals).** *Adults:* Initially, 20 mg P.O. t.i.d. (immediate-release only). Dosage titrated based on response q 3 days. Usual dosage range is 20 to 40 mg t.i.d.
▶ **Hypertension.** *Adults:* Initially, 20 to 40 mg P.O. t.i.d. (immediate-release) or 30 to 60 mg b.i.d. (sustained-release). Dosage increase based on response. Or, for patients unable to take oral nicardipine, initially, 50 ml/hour (5 mg/hour) I.V. infusion, increased by 25 ml/hour (2.5 mg/hour) q 15 minutes up to 150 ml/hour (15 mg/hour).

▽ I.V. administration
• Dilute with compatible solution before administration. The drug is compatible with D₅W, dextrose 5% in normal saline solution or half-normal saline solution, and normal saline solution or half-normal saline solution for 24 hours at room temperature.
⊛ **ALERT:** The drug is incompatible with sodium bicarbonate and lactated Ringer's solution.
• Give by slow I.V. infusion at 0.1 mg/ml.
• Closely monitor blood pressure during infusion and after completion of infusion.

• If hypotension or tachycardia occurs, titrate infusion rate.
• Change peripheral infusion site every 12 hours to minimize risk of venous irritation.

Contraindications and precautions

• Contraindicated in patients hypersensitive to drug and in those with advanced aortic stenosis.
• Use cautiously in patients with cardiac conduction disturbances, hypotension, heart failure, and impaired hepatic or renal function.
⚜ **Lifespan:** In pregnant women, use cautiously. In breast-feeding women, drug isn't recommended. In children, safety of drug hasn't been established.

Adverse reactions

CNS: dizziness, light-headedness, *headache* (I.V. form), paresthesia, drowsiness, asthenia.
CV: peripheral edema, palpitations, angina, tachycardia, flushing.
GI: nausea, abdominal discomfort, dry mouth.
Skin: rash.

Interactions

Drug-drug. *Antihypertensives:* Enhances antihypertensive effect. Monitor patient's blood pressure closely.
Beta blockers: May increase cardiac depressant effects. Monitor patient.
Cimetidine: May decrease metabolism of calcium channel blockers. Monitor patient for toxicity.
Cyclosporine: May increase cyclosporine level. Monitor level closely.
Theophylline: Effects of theophylline may be enhanced. Monitor patient.
Drug-food. *Grapefruit juice:* May increase bioavailability of drug. Give drug with another liquid.
High-fat meal: Decreases bioavailability of drug by 20% to 30%. Don't give drug with a high fat meal.

Effects on lab test results

None reported.

Pharmacokinetics

Absorption: Complete; may decrease if taken with food.
Distribution: Over 95% bound to proteins.
Metabolism: Absolute bioavailability of about 35%; extensively metabolized in liver.

Excretion: About 60% excreted in urine, 35% in bile. *Half-life:* 2 to 4 hours.

Route	Onset	Peak	Duration
P.O.	< 20 min	30 min-4 hr	6-12 hr
I.V.	Immediate	Within min	Soon after therapy stops

Action

Chemical effect: Inhibits calcium ion influx across cardiac and smooth-muscle cells, decreasing myocardial contractility and oxygen demand. Also dilates coronary arteries and arterioles.
Therapeutic effect: Lowers blood pressure and relieves angina.

Available forms

Capsules (immediate-release): 20 mg, 30 mg
Capsules (sustained-release): 30 mg, 45 mg, 60 mg
Injection: 2.5 mg/ml

NURSING PROCESS

Assessment

• Assess patient's condition before therapy and regularly thereafter.
• Measure blood pressure frequently during initial therapy. Maximum blood pressure response occurs about 1 hour after immediate-release form and 2 to 4 hours after sustained-release form. Check for orthostatic hypotension. Because blood pressure may vary widely based on blood level of drug, assess adequacy of antihypertensive effect 8 hours after dosing.
• Be alert for adverse reactions and drug interactions.
• Evaluate patient's and family's knowledge of drug therapy.

Nursing diagnoses

• Risk for injury related to hypertension
• Acute pain related to angina
• Deficient knowledge related to drug therapy

Planning and implementation

• When switching to oral nicardipine, give first dose of t.i.d. regimen 1 hour before stopping infusion. If switching to an oral antihypertensive other than nicardipine, start therapy after stopping infusion.

Rapid onset   *Liquid form contains alcohol.   ◆Canada   ◇ Australia   †OTC   ‡Off-label use

Ⓢ **ALERT:** Use extended-release form because of improved medication adherence and fewer fluctuations in blood pressure, and because the short-acting form has an increased risk for mortality

Ⓢ **ALERT:** Don't confuse nicardipine with nifedipine or nimodipine.

ⓈALERT: Don't confuse Cardene with Cardura or codeine. Don't confuse Cardene SR with Cardizem SR.

Patient teaching
● Advise patient to report chest pain immediately. Some patients may experience increased frequency, severity, or duration of chest pain at start of therapy or during dosage adjustments.
● Stress need to take drug exactly as prescribed even when feeling well.
● Instruct patient how to minimize orthostatic hypotension.

✓ **Evaluation**
● Patient's blood pressure is normal.
● Patient's anginal attacks are less frequent and less severe.
● Patient and family state understanding of drug therapy.

nifedipine
(nigh-FEH-duh-peen)
**Adalat, Adalat CC, Adalat P.A. ◆,
Adalat XL ◆, Nifedical XL, Nu-Nifed ◆,
Procardia, Procardia XL**

Pharmacologic class: calcium channel blocker
Therapeutic class: antianginal
Pregnancy risk category: C

Indications and dosages
▶ **Vasospastic angina (also called Prinzmetal's [variant] angina) and classic chronic stable angina pectoris.** *Adults:* Initially, 10 mg P.O. (capsules) t.i.d. Usual effective dosage range is 10 to 20 mg t.i.d. Some patients may need up to 30 mg q.i.d. Maximum daily dose is 180 mg.
▶ **Hypertension.** *Adults:* 30 or 60 mg P.O. (extended-release) once daily. Adjust over 7- to 14-day period. Maximum, 120 mg daily.

Contraindications and precautions
● Contraindicated in patients hypersensitive to drug.
● Use cautiously in those with heart failure or hypotension.
● Use extended-release tablets cautiously in patients with severe GI narrowing because obstructive symptoms may occur.
⚠ Lifespan: In pregnant and breast-feeding women, drug is contraindicated. In children, safety of drug hasn't been established. In geriatric patients, use cautiously.

Adverse reactions
CNS: *dizziness, light-headedness, headache,* weakness, syncope.
CV: *flushing,* peripheral edema, hypotension, palpitations, **heart failure, MI.**
EENT: nasal congestion.
GI: nausea, heartburn, diarrhea.
Metabolic: hypokalemia.
Musculoskeletal: muscle cramps.
Respiratory: dyspnea, **pulmonary edema.**
Skin: rash, pruritus.

Interactions
Drug-drug. *Cimetidine, ranitidine:* Decreases nifedipine metabolism. Monitor patient closely for increased adverse effects.
I.V. magnesium sulfate: May cause neuromuscular blockade and hypotension. Don't use together. Monitor patient.
Propranolol, other beta blockers: May cause hypotension and heart failure. Use together cautiously; monitor vital signs.
Quinidine: May cause hypotension, bradycardia, ventricular tachycardia, AV block, and pulmonary edema. Reduce quinidine dosage and monitor level. Monitor ECG and vital signs.
Drug-food. *Grapefruit juice:* Increases drug bioavailability. Discourage using together because effects vary.

Effects on lab test results
● May increase ALT, AST, alkaline phosphatase, and LDH levels. May decrease potassium level.

Pharmacokinetics
Absorption: About 90% of drug is absorbed rapidly from GI tract; however, only about 65% to 70% of drug reaches systemic circulation because of significant first-pass effect in liver.

Reactions may be *common,* uncommon, ***life-threatening***, or COMMON AND LIFE-THREATENING.

Distribution: About 92% to 98% of circulating drug is bound to proteins.
Metabolism: Metabolized in liver.
Excretion: Excreted in urine and feces as inactive metabolites. *Half-life:* 2 to 5 hours.

Route	Onset	Peak	Duration
P.O.	20 min	30 min-2 hr	4-24 hr

Action

Chemical effect: Unknown; may inhibit calcium ion influx across cardiac and smooth-muscle cells, decreasing myocardial contractility and oxygen demand. Also may dilate coronary arteries and arterioles.
Therapeutic effect: Reduces blood pressure and prevents angina.

Available forms

Capsules: 10 mg, 20 mg
Tablets (extended-release): 30 mg, 60 mg, 90 mg

NURSING PROCESS

⚕ Assessment
• Assess patient's condition before therapy and regularly thereafter.
• Monitor blood pressure regularly, especially if patient also takes a beta blocker or an antihypertensive.
• Monitor potassium level regularly.
• Be alert for adverse reactions and drug interactions.
• Evaluate patient's and family's knowledge of drug therapy.

🔲 Nursing diagnoses
• Risk for injury related to presence of hypertension
• Pain related to angina
• Deficient knowledge related to drug therapy

▷ Planning and implementation
🔹 **ALERT:** When rapid response to drug is desired, instruct patient to bite and swallow capsule. If he can't chew capsules, liquid can be withdrawn by puncturing capsule with needle and squeezing contents into mouth. When using these methods, continuous blood pressure and ECG monitoring is recommended.
🔹 **ALERT:** Despite widespread S.L. use of nifedipine capsules, avoid this route of adminis-

tration. Peak level will be lower and it will take longer for level to peak than when capsule is bitten and swallowed.
🔹 **ALERT:** Procardia XL and Adalat CC aren't equivalent.
• S.L. nitroglycerin may be prescribed for acute angina.
• Although rebound effect hasn't been observed when drug is stopped, reduce dosage slowly.
🔹 **ALERT:** Don't confuse nifedipine with nicardipine or nisoldipine.
Patient teaching
• If patient is kept on nitrate therapy while nifedipine dosage is being adjusted, urge continued compliance.
• Warn patient that angina may worsen when therapy starts or dosage increases. Reassure him that this is temporary.
• Instruct patient to swallow extended-release tablets without breaking, crushing, or chewing them.
• Advise patient who takes extended-release form of drug that he may pass wax-matrix "ghost" of tablet in stool.
🔹 **ALERT:** Warn patient not to switch brands. Procardia XL and Adalat CC aren't equivalent because of their differing pharmacokinetics.
• Tell patient to protect capsules from direct light and moisture and to store them at room temperature.

🔲 Evaluation
• Patient's blood pressure is normal.
• Patient's angina is less frequent and severe.
• Patient and family state understanding of drug therapy.

nisoldipine
(nigh-SOHL-dih-peen)
Sular

Pharmacologic class: calcium channel blocker
Therapeutic class: antihypertensive
Pregnancy risk category: C

Indications and dosages

▶ **Hypertension.** *Adults:* Initially, 20 mg P.O. once daily; then increase by 10 mg weekly or at longer intervals, as indicated. Usual maintenance dosage is 20 to 40 mg once daily. Dosages above 60 mg daily aren't recommended.

⊠ **Adjust-a-dose:** For patients older than age 65 and those who have liver dysfunction, initial dosage is 10 mg P.O. daily.

Contraindications and precautions

• Contraindicated in patients hypersensitive to dihydropyridine calcium channel blockers.
• Use cautiously in patients with severe hepatic impairment, heart failure, or compromised ventricular function, and particularly in those taking beta blockers.
⚘ **Lifespan:** In pregnant women, use cautiously. In breast-feeding women, avoid using drug.

Adverse reactions

CNS: *headache,* dizziness.
CV: vasodilation, palpitations, chest pain, *peripheral edema.*
EENT: sinusitis, pharyngitis.
GI: nausea.
Skin: rash.

Interactions

Drug-drug. *Cimetidine:* Increases bioavailability and peak levels of nisoldipine. Monitor patient for increased adverse effects.
Quinidine: Decreases bioavailability, but not peak levels, of nisoldipine. Monitor patient.
Drug-food. *Grapefruit juice:* May increase drug level, increasing therapeutic and adverse effects. Discourage patients from taking drug with grapefruit products.
High-fat meal: Increases peak drug level. Discourage high-fat meals during drug therapy.

Effects on lab test results

None reported.

Pharmacokinetics

Absorption: Well absorbed from GI tract; high-fat foods significantly affect release of drug from coat-core form.
Distribution: About 99% protein-bound.
Metabolism: Extensively metabolized, with five major metabolites identified.
Excretion: Excreted in urine. *Half-life:* 7 to 12 hours.

Route	Onset	Peak	Duration
P.O.	Unknown	6-12 hr	Unknown

Action

Chemical effect: Prevents entry of calcium ions into vascular smooth-muscle cells, causing dilation of arterioles, which decreases peripheral vascular resistance.
Therapeutic effect: Lowers blood pressure.

Available forms

Extended-release tablets: 10 mg, 20 mg, 30 mg, 40 mg

NURSING PROCESS

🗚 Assessment
• Assess patient's blood pressure before therapy and monitor regularly thereafter, especially during dosage adjustment.
• Monitor patient carefully. Some patients, especially those with severe obstructive coronary artery disease, have developed increased frequency, duration, or severity of angina or acute MI when starting calcium channel blocker therapy or increasing dosage.
• Be alert for adverse reactions and interactions.
• Evaluate patient's and family's knowledge of drug therapy.

⊞ Nursing diagnoses
• Risk for injury related to hypertension
• Excessive fluid volume related to edema
• Deficient knowledge related to drug therapy

▷ Planning and implementation
• Don't give drug with a high-fat meal or grapefruit products.
⚠ ALERT: Don't confuse nisoldipine with nifedipine or nicardipine.
Patient teaching
• Tell patient to take drug as prescribed.
• Instruct patient to swallow tablet whole and not to chew, divide, or crush.

☑ Evaluation
• Patient's blood pressure is normal.
• Patient doesn't exhibit signs of edema.
• Patient and family state understanding of drug therapy.

nitrofurantoin macrocrystals
(nigh-troh-fyoo-RAN-toyn MAH-kroh-kris-tuls)
Macrobid, Macrodantin

nitrofurantoin microcrystals
Apo-Nitrofurantoin ♦, Furadantin, Furalan,
Macrodantin

Pharmacologic class: nitrofuran
Therapeutic class: urinary tract anti-infective
Pregnancy risk category: B

Indications and dosages

▶ **UTI caused by susceptible** *Escherichia coli, Staphylococcus aureus,* **enterococci, and certain strains of** *Klebsiella, Proteus,* **and** *Enterobacter. Adults and children older than age 12:* 50 to 100 mg P.O. q.i.d. with milk or meals. Or, 100 mg Macrobid PO q 12 hours for 7 days. *Children ages 1 month to 12 years:* 5 to 7 mg/kg P.O. daily, divided q.i.d.
▶ **Long-term suppression therapy.** *Adults:* 50 to 100 mg P.O. q h.s. *Children:* 1 to 2 mg/kg P.O. q h.s.

Contraindications and precautions

● Contraindicated in patients with moderate-to-severe renal impairment (creatinine clearance less than 60 ml/minute), anuria, or oliguria.
● Use cautiously in patients with renal impairment, anemia, diabetes mellitus, electrolyte abnormalities, vitamin B deficiency, debilitating disease, or G6PD deficiency.
⚖ Lifespan: In pregnant and breast-feeding women, use cautiously. In infants age 1 month and younger, drug is contraindicated.

Adverse reactions

CNS: *peripheral neuropathy,* headache, dizziness, drowsiness, *ascending polyneuropathy with high doses or renal impairment.*
GI: anorexia, nausea, vomiting, abdominal pain, diarrhea.
Hematologic: *hemolysis in patients with G6PD deficiency (reversed after stopping drug), agranulocytosis, thrombocytopenia.*
Hepatic: *hepatitis, hepatic necrosis.*
Respiratory: *asthmatic attacks in patients with history of asthma,* pulmonary sensitivity (cough, chest pains, fever, chills, dyspnea).

Skin: maculopapular, erythematous, or eczematous eruption; pruritus; urticaria; exfoliative dermatitis; *Stevens-Johnson syndrome.*
Other: hypersensitivity reactions, *anaphylaxis,* transient alopecia, drug fever, overgrowth of nonsusceptible organisms in urinary tract.

Interactions

Drug-drug. *Magnesium-containing antacids:* Decreases nitrofurantoin absorption. Separate ingestion by 1 hour.
Quinolones (like nalidixic acid, norfloxacin): Possible decreased effectiveness of quinolone derivatives. Avoid using together.
Probenecid, sulfinpyrazone: Increases blood level and decreases urine level. May result in increased toxicity and lack of therapeutic effect. Don't use together.
Drug-food. *Any food:* Increases drug absorption. Give drug with food.

Effects on lab test results

● May increase bilirubin and alkaline phosphatase levels. May decrease glucose level.
● May decrease granulocyte and platelet counts.
● May cause false-positive results with urine glucose test using copper sulfate reduction method (Clinitest).

Pharmacokinetics

Absorption: Well absorbed from GI tract. Food aids drug's dissolution and speeds absorption. Macrocrystal form has slower dissolution and absorption.
Distribution: Drug crosses into bile; 60% binds to proteins.
Metabolism: Metabolized partially in liver.
Excretion: About 30% to 50% of dose is eliminated in urine. *Half-life:* 15 minutes to 1 hour.

Route	Onset	Peak	Duration
P.O.	Unknown	Unknown	Unknown

Action

Chemical effect: Unknown; may interfere with bacterial enzyme systems and cell wall formation.
Therapeutic effect: Hinders growth of many common gram-positive and gram-negative urinary pathogens including *E. coli, S. aureus,* enterococci, and certain strains of *Klebsiella* and *Enterobacter.*

Available forms

nitrofurantoin macrocrystals
Capsules: 25 mg, 50 mg, 100 mg
Capsules (dual-release): 100 mg
nitrofurantoin microcrystals
Capsules: 50 mg, 100 mg
Oral suspension: 25 mg/5 ml
Tablets: 50 mg, 100 mg

NURSING PROCESS

⚚ Assessment
• Assess patient's infection before therapy and regularly thereafter.
• Obtain urine specimen for culture and sensitivity tests before starting therapy, and repeat p.r.n. Therapy may begin pending results.
• Monitor fluid intake and output. May turn urine brown or darker.
• Monitor CBC and pulmonary status regularly.
• Be alert for adverse reactions and drug interactions.
• If adverse GI reactions occur, monitor patient's hydration status.
• Evaluate patient's and family's knowledge of drug therapy.

⚙ Nursing diagnoses
• Infection related to susceptible bacteria
• Risk for deficient fluid volume related to drug-induced adverse GI reactions
• Deficient knowledge related to drug therapy

⬘ Planning and implementation
• Drug has no effect on blood or tissue outside urinary tract.
⚕ ALERT: Hypersensitivity may develop during long-term therapy.
• Dual-release capsules (25 mg nitrofurantoin macrocrystals combined with 75 mg nitrofurantoin monohydrate) enable twice-daily dosing.
• Continue treatment for 3 days after urine specimens become sterile.
• Some patients may experience fewer adverse GI effects with nitrofurantoin macrocrystals.
• Store drug in amber container. Avoid metals other than stainless steel or aluminum to avoid precipitate formation.
Patient teaching
• Tell patient to take drug with food or milk to minimize GI distress.

• Teach patient how to measure intake and output. Warn him that drug will turn urine brown or darker.
• Instruct patient how to store drug.

☑ Evaluation
• Patient is free from infection.
• Patient maintains adequate hydration throughout drug therapy.
• Patient and family state understanding of drug therapy.

nitroglycerin (glyceryl trinitrate)
(nigh-troh-GLIH-suh-rin)
Anginine◇, Deponit, GTN-Poh◇, Minitran, Nitradisc◇, Nitro-Bid, Nitro-Bid IV, Nitrodisc, Nitro-Dur, Nitrogard, Nitroglyn, Nitroject, Nitrolingual, Nitrong, NitroQuick, Nitrostat, Nitro-Time, Transderm-Nitro, Transiderm-Nitro◇, Tridil

Pharmacologic class: nitrate
Therapeutic class: antianginal, vasodilator
Pregnancy risk category: C

Indications and dosages

▶ **Prevention of chronic anginal attacks.**
Adults: 2.5 mg or 2.6 mg sustained-release capsule q 8 to 12 hours. Or, 2% ointment: Start with ½ inch of ointment and increase by ½ inch increments until headache occurs; then decrease to previous dose. Range of dosage with ointment is ½ to 5 inches. Usual dose is 1 to 2 inches. Or, Nitrodisc, Nitro-Dur, or Transderm-Nitro transdermal disk or pad, 0.2 to 0.4 mg/hour once daily.
▶ **Acute angina pectoris; to prevent or minimize anginal attacks when taken immediately before stressful events.** *Adults:* 1 S.L. tablet (grain [gr] ¼₀₀, ½₀₀, ⅟₁₅₀, ⅟₁₀₀) dissolved under tongue or in buccal pouch as soon as angina begins. Repeat q 5 minutes for up to 15 minutes if symptoms persist. Or, using Nitrolingual spray, 1 or 2 sprays into mouth, preferably onto or under tongue. Repeat q 3 to 5 minutes if symptoms persist, to maximum of three doses in 15-minute period. Or, 1 to 3 mg transmucosally q 3 to 5 hours during waking hours.
▶ **Hypertension related to surgery; heart failure linked to MI; angina pectoris in acute situations; to produce controlled hypotension**

during surgery (**by I.V. infusion**). *Adults:* Initial infusion rate is 5 mcg/minute. Increase p.r.n. by 5 mcg/minute q 3 to 5 minutes until response occurs. If 20-mcg/minute rate doesn't produce response, dosage is increased by as much as 20 mcg/minute q 3 to 5 minutes. Up to 100 mcg/minute may be needed.

▶ **Hypertensive crisis‡.** *Adults:* Infuse at 5 to 100 mcg/minute I.V.

▼ I.V. administration

• Dilute drug with D₅W or normal saline solution for injection. Concentration should not exceed 400 mcg/ml.
• Give with infusion control device and titrate to desired response.
• ⊛ **ALERT:** Mix in glass bottles and avoid I.V. filters because drug binds to plastic. Regular polyvinyl chloride tubing can bind up to 80% of drug, making it necessary to infuse higher dosages. A special nonabsorbent, nonpolyvinyl chloride tubing is available from manufacturer.
• Always use same type of infusion set when changing I.V. lines.
• When changing concentration of nitroglycerin infusion, flush I.V. administration set with 15 to 20 ml of new concentration before use. This will clear line of old drug solution.

Contraindications and precautions

• Contraindicated in patients hypersensitive to nitrates and in those with early MI (S.L. form), severe anemia, increased intracranial pressure, angle-closure glaucoma, orthostatic hypotension, and allergy to adhesives (transdermal form). I.V. nitroglycerin is contraindicated in patients with cardiac tamponade, restrictive cardiomyopathy, constrictive pericarditis, or hypersensitivity to I.V. form.
• Use cautiously in patients with hypotension or volume depletion.
• ⚘ **Lifespan:** In pregnant and breast-feeding women, use cautiously. In children, safety of drug hasn't been established.

Adverse reactions

CNS: *headache, sometimes with throbbing; dizziness;* weakness.
CV: *orthostatic hypotension, tachycardia, flushing, palpitations,* fainting.
EENT: sublingual burning.
GI: nausea, vomiting.

Skin: cutaneous vasodilation, contact dermatitis (patch), rash.
Other: hypersensitivity reactions.

Interactions

Drug-drug. *Alteplase:* Decreases t-PA antigen concentrations. Avoid using together. If use together is unavoidable, use the lowest effective dose of nitroglycerin.
Antihypertensives: May enhance hypotensive effect. Monitor patient closely.
Dihydroergotamine: May decrease antianginal effect. Avoid use together.
Sildenafil: May cause severe hypotension. Use of nitrates in any form with sildenafil is contraindicated.
Drug-lifestyle. *Alcohol use:* May increase hypotension. Urge patient to avoid alcohol during therapy.

Effects on lab test results

None reported.

Pharmacokinetics

Absorption: Well absorbed from GI tract. However, because it undergoes first-pass metabolism in liver, drug is incompletely absorbed into systemic circulation. For S.L. form, absorption from oral mucosa is relatively complete. For topical or transdermal form, well absorbed. Data not reported for other forms.
Distribution: Distributed widely; about 60% of circulating drug is bound to proteins.
Metabolism: Metabolized in liver.
Excretion: Metabolites excreted in urine. *Half-life:* About 1 to 4 minutes.

Route	Onset	Peak	Duration
P.O.	20-45 min	Unknown	8-12 hr
I.V.	Immediate	Immediate	3-5 min
Topical	30 min	Unknown	4-8 hr
Transdermal	30 min	Unknown	≤ 24 hr
S.L.	1-3 min	Unknown	30-60 min
Buccal	3 min	Unknown	5 hr
Translingual	2-4 min	Unknown	30-60 min

Action

Chemical effect: Reduces cardiac oxygen demand by decreasing left ventricular end-diastolic pressure (preload) and, to a lesser extent, systemic vascular resistance (afterload).

Also increases blood flow through collateral coronary vessels.

Therapeutic effect: Prevents or relieves acute angina, lowers blood pressure, and helps minimize heart failure caused by MI.

Available forms

Aerosol (translingual): 0.4 mg metered spray
Capsules (sustained-release): 2.5 mg, 6.5 mg, 9 mg, 13 mg
I.V.: 0.5 mg/ml, 0.8 mg/ml, 5 mg/ml
I.V. premixed solutions in dextrose: 100 mcg/ml, 200 mcg/ml, 400 mcg/ml
Tablets (buccal): 1 mg, 2 mg, 3 mg
Tablets (S.L.): 0.3 mg (gr ½₀₀) 4 mg (gr ½₅₀), 0.6 mg (gr ½₀₀)
Tablets (sustained-release): 2.6 mg, 6.5 mg, 9 mg
Topical: 2% ointment
Transdermal: 2.5 mg/24 hours, 5 mg/24 hours, 7.5 mg/24 hours, 10 mg/24 hours, 15 mg/24 hours

NURSING PROCESS

Assessment
● Assess patient's condition before therapy and regularly thereafter.
● Monitor vital signs and drug response. Be particularly aware of blood pressure. Excessive hypotension may worsen MI.
● Be alert for adverse reactions and drug interactions.
● Evaluate patient's and family's knowledge of drug therapy.

Nursing diagnoses
● Pain related to angina
● Risk for injury related to drug-induced adverse reactions
● Deficient knowledge related to drug therapy

Planning and implementation
● Give P.O. tablets on empty stomach, either 30 minutes before or 1 to 2 hours after meals.
● Don't allow patient to swallow or chew S.L. tablets.
● Give S.L. tablet at first sign of attack. Wet tablet with patient's saliva, then place under patient's tongue until completely absorbed. Have patient sit down and rest until pain subsides.

● Repeat dose q 10 to 15 minutes for up to three doses. If drug doesn't provide relief, notify prescriber promptly.
● If patient complains of tingling sensation with S.L. form, place tablet in buccal pouch.
● When giving translingual aerosol form, make sure patient doesn't inhale spray. Release it onto or under tongue, and have patient wait about 10 seconds or so before swallowing.
● To apply ointment, measure prescribed amount on application paper, then place paper on any nonhairy area. Don't rub in. Cover with plastic film to aid absorption and protect clothing.
● If using Tape-Surrounded Appli-Ruler (TSAR) system, keep TSAR on skin to protect patient's clothing and to make sure that ointment remains in place.
● Remove excess ointment from previous site before applying next dose. Avoid getting ointment on fingers.
● Apply transdermal forms to any nonhairy area, except lower parts of arms or legs, to promote maximum absorption.
● **ALERT:** Remove transdermal patch before defibrillation. Because of aluminum backing on patch, electric current may cause patch to explode.
● When stopping transdermal treatment of angina, gradually reduce dose and frequency of application over 4 to 6 weeks.
● If drug is ineffective, notify prescriber immediately; keep patient at rest.
● Drug may cause headache, especially at start of therapy. Reduce dosage temporarily; tolerance may develop. Treat headache with aspirin or acetaminophen.
● Minimize drug tolerance with 10- to 12-hour daily nitrate-free interval. For example, remove transdermal system in early evening and apply a new system the next morning. Or omit last daily dose of buccal, sustained-release, or ointment form. If tolerance is suspected, alter dosage.
● **ALERT:** Don't confuse Nitro-Bid with Nicobid.
● **ALERT:** Don't confuse nitroglycerin with nitroprusside.

Patient teaching
● Teach patient how to use form of drug prescribed.
● Tell patient to place transmucosal tablet between lip and gum above incisors, or between cheek and gum.

- Tell patient to swallow oral tablets whole and not to chew them.
- Instruct patient to take drug regularly, as prescribed, and to have it accessible at all times.
- Tell patient that stopping drug abruptly causes coronary vasospasm.
- Inform patient that an additional dose may be taken before anticipated stress or h.s. if angina is nocturnal.
- Instruct patient to use caution when wearing transdermal patch near microwave oven. Leaking radiation may heat metallic backing of patch and cause burns.
- Advise patient to avoid alcohol during drug therapy.
- Tell patient to change to upright position slowly. Advise him to go up and down stairs carefully and to lie down at first sign of dizziness.
- Urge patient to store drug in cool, dark place in tightly closed container. To ensure freshness, tell him to replace S.L. tablets q 3 months and to remove cotton because it absorbs drug.
- Tell patient to store S.L. tablets in original container or other container specifically approved for this use and to carry container in jacket pocket or purse, not in a pocket close to body.

☑ **Evaluation**
- Patient reports pain relief.
- Patient doesn't experience injury from adverse reactions.
- Patient and family state understanding of drug therapy.

nitroprusside sodium
(nigh-troh-PRUS-ighd SOH-dee-um)
Nipride ♦ , Nitropress

Pharmacologic class: vasodilator
Therapeutic class: antihypertensive
Pregnancy risk category: C

Indications and dosages

▶ **To lower blood pressure quickly in hypertensive emergencies; to produce controlled hypotension during anesthesia; to reduce preload and afterload in cardiac pump failure or cardiogenic shock (may be used with or without dopamine).** *Adults:* Begin infusion

at 0.25 to 0.3 mcg/kg/minute I.V. and gradually titrate q few minutes to a maximum infusion rate of 10 mcg/kg/minute. Average dose is 3 mcg/kg/minute. Patients taking other antihypertensives are extremely sensitive to nitroprusside. Dosage is adjusted accordingly.

▼ I.V. administration
- Don't use bacteriostatic water for injection or sterile saline solution for reconstitution.
- Prepare solution by dissolving 50 mg in 2 to 3 ml of D_5W injection or according to manufacturer's instructions. Further dilute concentration in 250, 500, or 1,000 ml of D_5W to provide solutions with 200, 100, or 50 mcg/ml, respectively. Reconstitute ADD-Vantage vials labeled as containing 50 mg of drug according to manufacturer's directions.
- Because drug is sensitive to light, wrap I.V. solution in foil; it isn't necessary to wrap tubing. Fresh solution should have faint brownish tint. Discard drug after 24 hours.
- Infuse with infusion pump. Drug is best given by piggyback through peripheral line with no other medication. Don't adjust rate of main I.V. line while drug is being infused. Even small bolus of nitroprusside can cause severe hypotension.
- Check blood pressure q 5 minutes at start of infusion and q 15 minutes thereafter.
- ⓢ **ALERT:** If severe hypotension occurs, stop infusion. Effects of drug quickly reverse. Notify prescriber.
- If possible, start arterial pressure line. Adjust flow to specified level.
- If cyanide toxicity occurs, stop drug immediately and notify prescriber.

Contraindications and precautions
- Contraindicated in patients hypersensitive to drug and in those with compensatory hypertension (as in arteriovenous shunt or coarctation of aorta), inadequate cerebral circulation, congenital optic atrophy, or tobacco-induced amblyopia.
- Use cautiously in patients with increased intracranial pressure and in those with hypothyroidism, hepatic or renal disease, hyponatremia, or low vitamin B_{12} level.
- ❄ **Lifespan:** In pregnant women, use cautiously. In breast-feeding women and in children, safety of drug hasn't been established.

Adverse reactions

CNS: *headache, dizziness,* ataxia, loss of consciousness, *coma, increased intracranial pressure,* weak pulse, absent reflexes, dilated pupils, *restlessness, muscle twitching.*
CV: distant heart sounds, palpitations, *bradycardia,* tachycardia, hypotension.
GI: vomiting, nausea, abdominal pain.
Hematologic: *methemoglobinemia.*
Metabolic: *acidosis.*
Respiratory: dyspnea, shallow breathing.
Skin: pink color, *diaphoresis.*
Other: *thiocyanate toxicity, cyanide toxicity.*

Interactions

Drug-drug. *Antihypertensives:* May cause sensitivity to nitroprusside. Adjust dosage.
Ganglionic blockers, general anesthetics, negative inotropics, other antihypertensives: May have additive effects. Monitor blood pressure closely.
Sildenafil: Increases hypotensive effects. Don't use together.
Tricyclic antidepressants: May potentiate the pressor response and cause arrhythmias. Use with caution.

Effects on lab test results

• May increase creatinine and methemoglobin levels.

Pharmacokinetics

Absorption: Administered I.V.
Distribution: Unknown.
Metabolism: Metabolized rapidly in erythrocytes and tissues to cyanide radical and then converted to thiocyanate in liver.
Excretion: Excreted primarily as metabolites in urine. *Half-life:* 2 minutes.

Route	Onset	Peak	Duration
I.V.	Almost immediate	1-2 min	10 min

Action

Chemical effect: Relaxes arteriolar and venous smooth muscle.
Therapeutic effect: Lowers blood pressure and reduces preload and afterload.

Available forms

Injection: 50 mg/vial in 2-ml, 5-ml vials

NURSING PROCESS

⚖ Assessment
• Assess patient's condition before therapy.
• Obtain baseline vital signs before giving drug, and find out what parameters prescriber wants to achieve.
⚠ **ALERT:** Excessive doses or rapid infusion (more than 15 mcg/kg/minute) can cause cyanide toxicity; therefore, check thiocyanate levels q 72 hours. Levels above 100 mcg/ml may cause toxicity. Watch for profound hypotension, metabolic acidosis, dyspnea, headache, loss of consciousness, ataxia, and vomiting.
• Be alert for adverse reactions and drug interactions.
• Evaluate patient's (if appropriate) and family's knowledge of drug therapy.

⊕ Nursing diagnoses
• Risk for injury related to hypertension
• Decreased cardiac output related to heart failure
• Deficient knowledge related to drug therapy

▶ Planning and implementation
• Keep patient in supine position when starting therapy or adjusting dosage.
⚠ **ALERT:** Don't confuse nitroprusside with nitroglycerin.
Patient teaching
• Advise patient, if alert, to report adverse reactions or discomfort at the I.V. site immediately.

☑ Evaluation
• Patient's blood pressure is normal.
• Patient has normal cardiac output.
• Patient and family state understanding of drug therapy.

nizatidine
(nigh-ZAT-ih-deen)
Axid, Axid AR†, Tazac ◆

Pharmacologic class: histamine$_2$ (H$_2$)-receptor antagonist
Therapeutic class: antiulcer drug
Pregnancy risk category: B

Indications and dosages

▶ **Active duodenal ulcer.** *Adults:* 300 mg P.O. daily h.s. Or, 150 mg P.O. b.i.d.
▶ **Maintenance therapy for duodenal ulcer.** *Adults:* 150 mg P.O. daily h.s.
▶ **Benign gastric ulcer.** *Adults:* 150 mg P.O. b.i.d. or 300 mg P.O. h.s. for 8 weeks.
▶ **Gastroesophageal reflux disease.** *Adults:* 150 mg P.O. b.i.d.
◩ **Adjust-a-dose:** For patients with renal impairment, if creatinine clearance is 20 to 50 ml/minute, give 150 mg P.O. daily for treatment of active duodenal ulcer or 150 mg q other day for maintenance therapy. If creatinine clearance is less than 20 ml/minute, give 150 mg P.O. q other day for treatment or 150 mg q third day for maintenance.

Contraindications and precautions

• Contraindicated in patients hypersensitive to H_2-receptor antagonists.
• Use cautiously in patients with renal impairment.
⚞ **Lifespan:** In pregnant and breast-feeding women, use cautiously. In children, safety of drug hasn't been established.

Adverse reactions

CNS: *somnolence,* fever.
CV: *arrhythmias.* ⬤
Hematologic: *thrombocytopenia.*
Hepatic: *liver damage.*
Metabolic: hyperuricemia.
Skin: *diaphoresis,* rash, urticaria, exfoliative dermatitis.

Interactions

Drug-drug. *Aspirin:* May elevate salicylate levels (with high doses). Monitor patient for salicylate toxicity.
Drug-food. *Tomato-based, mixed-vegetable juices:* May decrease drug potency. Monitor diet.
Drug-lifestyle. *Alcohol:* May increase alcohol level. Discourage using together.

Effects on lab test results

• May increase liver enzyme and uric acid levels.
• May decrease platelet count.
• May cause false-positive test results for urobilinogen.

Pharmacokinetics

Absorption: Greater than 90%. May be slightly enhanced by food and slightly impaired by antacids.
Distribution: About 35% of drug is bound to proteins.
Metabolism: Unknown, but may undergo hepatic metabolism.
Excretion: More than 90% excreted in urine; less than 6% in feces. *Half-life:* 1 to 2 hours.

Route	Onset	Peak	Duration
P.O.	≤ 30 min	30 min-3 hr	≤ 12 hr

Action

Chemical effect: Competitively inhibits action of H_2 at receptor sites of parietal cells.
Therapeutic effect: Decreases gastric acid secretion.

Available forms

Capsules: 75 mg†, 150 mg, 300 mg

NURSING PROCESS

▨ **Assessment**
• Assess patient's condition before therapy and regularly thereafter.
• Be alert for adverse reactions and drug interactions.
• Assess patient for abdominal pain. Note presence of blood in emesis, stool, or gastric aspirate.
• Evaluate patient's and family's knowledge of drug therapy.

▨ **Nursing diagnoses**
• Impaired tissue integrity related to ulceration of GI mucosa
• Decreased cardiac output related to drug-induced arrhythmias
• Deficient knowledge related to drug therapy

▷ **Planning and implementation**
• If necessary, open capsules and mix contents with apple juice. However, drug loses some potency when combined with tomato-based, mixed-vegetable juices.
Patient teaching
• Urge patient to avoid cigarette smoking because it may increase gastric acid secretion and worsen disease.
• Have patient report blood in stool or emesis.

• Warn patient to take drug as directed, even after pain subsides, to allow for adequate healing.

☑ **Evaluation**

• Patient reports pain relief.
• Patient maintains normal cardiac output throughout drug therapy.
• Patient and family state understanding of drug therapy.

norepinephrine bitartrate (levarterenol bitartrate, noradrenaline acid tartrate)

(nor-ep-ih-NEF-rin bigh-TAR-trayt)
Levophed

Pharmacologic class: adrenergic (direct acting)
Therapeutic class: vasopressor
Pregnancy risk category: C

Indications and dosages

▶ **To restore blood pressure in acute hypotensive states.** *Adults:* Initially, 8 to 12 mcg/minute by I.V. infusion, adjusted to maintain normal blood pressure. Average maintenance dosage is 2 to 4 mcg/minute.
Children: 2 mcg/m²/minute by I.V. infusion; dosage adjusted based on patient response.
▶ **Severe hypotension during cardiac arrest.** *Children:* Initial I.V. infusion rate is 0.1 mcg/kg/minute. Rate adjusted based on response.
▶ **GI bleeding‡.** *Adults:* Give 8 mg in 250 ml normal saline solution intraperitoneally. Or give 8 mg in 100 ml of normal saline solution via NG tube q 1 hour for 6 to 8 hours and then q 2 hours for 4 to 6 hours.

▼ I.V. administration

• Use central venous catheter or large vein, such as in antecubital fossa, to minimize risk of extravasation. Dilute in dextrose 5% in normal saline solution for injection; normal saline solution for injection alone isn't recommended. Use continuous infusion pump to regulate flow rate and piggyback setup so I.V. line remains open if drug is stopped.
• The infusion is usually prepared by adding 4 mg of norepinephrine to 1 L of 5% dextrose injection to equal a concentration of 4 mcg/ml.

• Titrate infusion rate according to assessment findings and prescriber's guidelines. In previously hypertensive patients, blood pressure should be raised no higher than 40 mm Hg below previous systolic pressure.
⊛ **ALERT:** Never leave patient unattended during infusion.
• Check site frequently for extravasation. If it occurs, stop infusion immediately and call prescriber. Counteract effect by infiltrating area with 5 to 10 mg phentolamine and 10 to 15 ml of normal saline solution. Also check for blanching along course of infused vein; may progress to superficial sloughing.
• Drug solutions deteriorate after 24 hours.
• Protect drug from light. Discard discolored solutions or solutions that contain precipitate. Drug solutions deteriorate after 24 hours.
⊛ **ALERT:** Avoid mixing with alkaline solutions, oxidizing drugs, or iron salts.
• If prolonged I.V. therapy is needed, change injection site frequently.

Contraindications and precautions

• Contraindicated in patients receiving cyclopropane or halothane anesthesia and in patients with mesenteric or peripheral vascular thrombosis, profound hypoxia, hypercapnia, or hypotension caused by blood volume deficits.
• Use cautiously in patients receiving MAO inhibitors, tricyclic antidepressants, or certain antihistamines and in patients with sulfite sensitivity.
⚖ **Lifespan:** In pregnant and breast-feeding women, drug is contraindicated.

Adverse reactions

CNS: *headache,* anxiety, fever, weakness, dizziness, tremor, restlessness, insomnia.
CV: *bradycardia, severe hypertension,* marked increase in peripheral resistance, decreased cardiac output, *arrhythmias.*
GU: decreased urine output.
Metabolic: *metabolic acidosis,* hyperglycemia, increased glycogenolysis.
Respiratory: *respiratory difficulties, asthmatic episodes.*
Other: irritation with extravasation, swelling and enlargement of thyroid, *anaphylaxis.*

Interactions

Drug-drug. *Alpha-adrenergic blockers:* May antagonize drug effects. Monitor patient.

Reactions may be *common,* uncommon, *life-threatening,* or **COMMON AND LIFE-THREATENING.**

Antihistamines, ergot alkaloids, guanethidine, methyldopa: Use with sympathomimetics may cause severe hypertension. Don't give together.
Bretylium: May cause arrhythmias. Monitor ECG closely.
Inhaled anesthetics: Increases risk of arrhythmias. Monitor ECG closely.
MAO inhibitors: Increases risk of hypertensive crisis. Monitor patient closely.
Tricyclic antidepressants: May potentiate the pressor response and cause arrhythmias. Use with caution.

Effects on lab test results

• May increase glucose level.

Pharmacokinetics

Absorption: Administered I.V.
Distribution: Drug localizes in sympathetic nerve tissues.
Metabolism: Metabolized in liver and other tissues to inactive compounds.
Excretion: Excreted in urine. *Half-life:* About 1 minute.

Route	Onset	Peak	Duration
I.V.	Immediate	Immediate	1-2 min

Action

Chemical effect: Stimulates alpha- and beta$_1$-adrenergic receptors in sympathetic nervous system.
Therapeutic effect: Raises blood pressure.

Available forms

Injection: 1 mg/ml

NURSING PROCESS

⏳ Assessment

• Assess patient's condition before therapy.
• During infusion, frequently monitor ECG, cardiac output, central venous pressure, pulmonary capillary wedge pressure, pulse rate, urine output, and color and temperature of limbs. Also, check blood pressure q 2 minutes until stabilized; then check q 5 minutes.
• Be alert for adverse reactions and drug interactions.
• Monitor vital signs closely when therapy ends. Watch for sudden drop in blood pressure.
• Evaluate patient's and family's knowledge of drug therapy.

🩺 Nursing diagnoses

• Decreased cardiac output related to hypotension
• Risk for injury related to drug-induced adverse reactions
• Deficient knowledge related to drug therapy

▶ Planning and implementation

• Drug isn't a substitute for blood or fluid volume deficit. If deficit exists, replace fluid before giving vasopressors.
• Keep emergency drugs on hand to reverse effects of norepinephrine: atropine for reflex bradycardia, phentolamine for vasopressor effects, and propranolol for arrhythmias.
• Report decreased urine output to prescriber immediately.
• When stopping drug, gradually slow infusion rate and report sudden drop in blood pressure.
Patient teaching
• Tell patient to immediately report discomfort at infusion site or difficulty breathing.

☑ Evaluation

• Patient has normal cardiac output.
• Patient sustains no injuries from drug-induced adverse reactions.
• Patient and family state understanding of drug therapy.

norethindrone

(nor-ETH-in-drohn)
Camila, Errin, Jolivette, Micronor, Nora-BE, Nor-Q.D.

norethindrone acetate

Aygestin, Norlutate ♦

Pharmacologic class: progestin
Therapeutic class: contraceptive
Pregnancy risk category: X

Indications and dosages

▶ **Amenorrhea, abnormal uterine bleeding.**
Women: 2.5 to 10 mg norethindrone acetate P.O. daily on days 5 to 25 of menstrual cycle.
▶ **Endometriosis.** *Women:* 5 mg norethindrone acetate P.O. daily for 14 days; then increase by 2.5 mg daily q 2 weeks up to 15 mg daily.

▶ **To prevent pregnancy.** *Women:* Initially, 0.35 mg norethindrone P.O. on first day of menstruation; then 0.35 mg daily.

Contraindications and precautions

• Contraindicated in patients hypersensitive to drug; patients with thromboembolic disorders, cerebral apoplexy, or a history of these conditions; and patients with breast cancer, undiagnosed abnormal vaginal bleeding, severe hepatic disease, or missed abortion.
• Use cautiously in patients with diabetes mellitus, seizure disorder, migraine, cardiac or renal disease, asthma, and depression.
⚖ Lifespan: In pregnant women, drug is contraindicated. In breast-feeding women, drug isn't recommended. In children, safety of drug hasn't been established.

Adverse reactions

CNS: dizziness, migraine, lethargy, depression.
CV: hypertension, thrombophlebitis, *pulmonary embolism, thromboembolism, CVA,* edema.
GI: nausea, vomiting, abdominal cramps.
GU: breakthrough bleeding, dysmenorrhea, amenorrhea, cervical erosion, abnormal secretions, uterine fibromas, vaginal candidiasis.
Hepatic: cholestatic jaundice.
Metabolic: hyperglycemia.
Skin: melasma, rash.
Other: decreased libido; breast tenderness, enlargement, or secretion.

Interactions

Drug-drug. *Barbiturates, carbamazepine, rifampin:* Decreases progestin effects. Monitor patient for lack of effect.
Bromocriptine: May cause amenorrhea, thus interfering with bromocriptine effects. Avoid using together.
Drug-food. *Caffeine:* May increase caffeine level. Monitor patient for caffeine effects.
Drug-lifestyle. *Smoking:* Increases risk of CV effects. If smoking continues, may need alternative therapy.

Effects on lab test results

• May increase glucose level.
• May increase liver function test results.

Pharmacokinetics

Absorption: Well absorbed from GI tract.

Distribution: Distributed widely; about 80% protein-bound.
Metabolism: Metabolized primarily in liver; it undergoes extensive first-pass metabolism.
Excretion: Excreted primarily in feces. *Half-life:* 5 to 14 hours.

Route	Onset	Peak	Duration
P.O.	Unknown	Unknown	Unknown

Action

Chemical effect: Suppresses ovulation, possibly by inhibiting pituitary gonadotropin secretion, and forms thick cervical mucus.
Therapeutic effect: Prevents pregnancy and relieves symptoms of endometriosis, amenorrhea, and abnormal uterine bleeding.

Available forms

norethindrone
Tablets: 0.35 mg, 0.5 mg
norethindrone acetate
Tablets: 5 mg

NURSING PROCESS

🔆 Assessment
• Assess patient's condition before therapy and regularly thereafter.
• Be alert for adverse reactions and drug interactions.
• Evaluate patient's and family's knowledge of drug therapy.
• Monitor blood pressure and edema.

🔆 Nursing diagnoses
• Ineffective health maintenance related to underlying condition
• Excessive fluid volume related to drug-induced edema
• Deficient knowledge related to drug therapy

▶ Planning and implementation
⊛ **ALERT:** Norethindrone acetate is twice as potent as norethindrone. Don't use as contraception.
• Preliminary estrogen treatment is usually needed by patients with menstrual disorders.
⊛ **ALERT:** If visual disturbance, migraine, or headache occurs or if pulmonary emboli are suspected, withhold drug, notify prescriber, and provide supportive care.

🅢 **ALERT:** Don't confuse Micronor with Micro-K or Micronase.

Patient teaching
• If switching from combined hormonal contraceptives to progestin-only pills (POPs), tell patient to take the first POPs the day after the last active combined pill.
• If switching from POPs to combined pills, tell patient to take the first active combined pill on the first day of menstruation, even if the POPs pack isn't finished.
• Explain adverse effects of progestin and have patient read package insert before taking first dose.
• Tell patient to take drug at same time each day when used as a contraceptive. If she is more than 3 hours late or has missed a pill, she should take pill as soon as she remembers, then continue normal schedule. A backup method of contraception should be used for the next 48 hours.
• Instruct patient to report unusual symptoms immediately. Tell her to stop drug and call prescriber if visual disturbance or migraine occurs.
• Teach patient how to perform routine monthly breast self-examination.
• Warn patient that edema and weight gain are likely. Advise her to restrict sodium intake.

☑ **Evaluation**
• Patient responds well to therapy.
• Patient's drug-induced edema is minimized with sodium restriction.
• Patient and family state understanding of drug therapy.

norfloxacin
(nor-FLOKS-uh-sin)
Noroxin

Pharmacologic class: fluoroquinolone
Therapeutic class: broad-spectrum antibiotic
Pregnancy risk category: C

Indications and dosages

▶ **UTI caused by susceptible strains of *Escherichia coli*, *Klebsiella*, *Enterobacter*, *Proteus*, *Pseudomonas aeruginosa*, *Citrobacter*, *Staphylococcus aureus*, *Staphylococcus epidermidis*, and group D streptococci.** *Adults:* For uncomplicated infections, 400 mg P.O. b.i.d. for 7 to 10 days. For complicated infections, 400 mg b.i.d. for 10 to 21 days.
▶ **Cystitis caused by *E. coli*, *K. pneumoniae*, or *Proteus mirabilis*.** *Adults:* 400 mg P.O. b.i.d. for 3 days.
▶ **Acute, uncomplicated gonorrhea.** *Adults:* 800 mg P.O. as single dose, followed by doxycycline therapy to treat coexisting chlamydial infection.
▶ **Gastroenteritis‡.** *Adults:* 400 mg P.O. b.i.d. for 5 days.
▶ **Traveler's diarrhea‡.** *Adults:* 400 mg P.O. b.i.d. for 3 days.
🅢 **Adjust-a-dose:** For patients with renal impairment, if creatinine clearance is less than 30 ml/minute, give 400 mg once daily.

Contraindications and precautions

• Contraindicated in patients hypersensitive to fluoroquinolones.
• Use cautiously in patients with conditions that may predispose them to seizure disorders, such as cerebral arteriosclerosis.
⚖ Lifespan: In pregnant women, use cautiously. In breast-feeding women and in children, safety of drug hasn't been established.

Adverse reactions

CNS: fatigue, somnolence, headache, fever, dizziness, *seizures*.
GI: nausea, constipation, flatulence, heartburn, dry mouth.
GU: crystalluria.
Hematologic: eosinophilia.
Musculoskeletal: arthralgia, arthritis, myalgia, joint swelling.
Skin: rash, photosensitivity reaction.
Other: hypersensitivity reactions (rash, *anaphylactoid reactions*).

Interactions

Drug-drug. *Aluminum hydroxide, aluminum-magnesium hydroxide, calcium carbonate, magnesium hydroxide:* May decrease effects of norfloxacin. Give antacid at least 6 hours before or 2 hours after norfloxacin.
Cyclosporine: Increases cyclosporine level. Monitor level.
Iron salts: May decrease absorption of norfloxacin reducing anti-infective response. Give at least 2 hours apart.
Nitrofurantoin: Decreases norfloxacin's effectiveness. Don't use together.

Oral anticoagulants: Increases anticoagulant effect. Monitor patient closely for bleeding; monitor PT and INR.

Probenecid: May increase levels of norfloxacin by decreasing its excretion. Monitor patient for toxicity.

Sucralfate: May decrease absorption of the norfloxacin reducing anti-infective response. If use together can't be avoided, give at least 6 hours apart.

Theophylline: May impair theophylline metabolism, resulting in increased level and risk of toxicity. Monitor theophylline level closely.

Warfarin: May increase anticoagulant effect. Monitor patient and INR closely.

Drug-food. *Any food:* Decreases absorption of drug. Give drug 1 hour before or 2 hours after meals.

Drug-lifestyle. *Sunlight:* May cause photosensitivity reaction. Urge patient to avoid unprotected or prolonged sun exposure.

Effects on lab test results

• May increase BUN, creatinine, ALT, AST, and alkaline phosphatase levels.
• May increase eosinophil count. May decrease hemoglobin, hematocrit, and neutrophil count.

Pharmacokinetics

Absorption: About 30% to 40%. As dose increases, percentage absorbed decreases. Food may reduce absorption.

Distribution: Into renal tissue, liver, gallbladder, prostatic fluid, testicles, seminal fluid, bile, and sputum. 10% to 15% binds to proteins.

Metabolism: Unknown.

Excretion: Mostly excreted by kidneys with about 30% appearing in bile. *Half-life:* 3 to 4 hours.

Route	Onset	Peak	Duration
P.O.	Unknown	1-2 hr	Unknown

Action

Chemical effect: Inhibits bacterial DNA synthesis, mainly by blocking DNA gyrase.

Therapeutic effect: Kills certain bacteria.

Available forms

Tablets: 400 mg

NURSING PROCESS

Assessment

• Assess patient's infection before therapy and regularly thereafter.
• Obtain culture and sensitivity tests before starting therapy, and repeat p.r.n. throughout therapy.
• Be alert for adverse reactions and drug interactions.
• Evaluate patient's and family's knowledge of drug therapy.

Nursing diagnoses

• Infection related to bacteria
• Risk for injury related to drug-induced adverse CNS reactions
• Deficient knowledge related to drug therapy

Planning and implementation

• Give drug on empty stomach.
• Make sure patient is well hydrated before and during therapy to avoid crystalluria.
⚠ ALERT: Don't confuse Noroxin with Neurontin or Floxin.

Patient teaching

• Urge patient to take drug 1 hour before or 2 hours after meals to promote absorption.
• Warn patient not to exceed recommended dosage.
• Encourage patient to drink several glasses of water throughout day to maintain hydration and adequate urine output.
• Warn patient to avoid hazardous activities until CNS effects of drug are known.

Evaluation

• Patient is free from infection.
• Patient has no injuries from drug-induced adverse CNS reactions.
• Patient and family state understanding of drug therapy.

---

nortriptyline hydrochloride
(nor-TRIP-teh-leen high-droh-KLOR-ighd)
Allegron◇, Aventyl*, Pamelor*

Pharmacologic class: tricyclic antidepressant
Therapeutic class: antidepressant
Pregnancy risk category: NR

Indications and dosages

▶ **Depression, panic disorder‡.** *Adults:* 25 mg P.O. t.i.d. or q.i.d., gradually increased to maximum of 150 mg daily. Or, entire dosage may be given h.s.

▧ **Adjust-a-dose:** For elderly and debilitated patients, give 30 mg to 50 mg P.O. once daily or in divided doses.

Contraindications and precautions

• Contraindicated in patients hypersensitive to drug, patients in acute recovery phase after MI, and patients who have taken an MAO inhibitor within 14 days.
• Use cautiously in patients taking thyroid drugs and in patients with glaucoma, suicidal tendency, history of urine retention or seizures, CV disease, or hyperthyroidism.
⚘ **Lifespan:** In pregnant and breast-feeding women and in children, drug isn't recommended. In elderly patients, use cautiously and at a reduced dosage.

Adverse reactions

CNS: *drowsiness, dizziness,* excitation, *seizures,* tremor, weakness, confusion, headache, nervousness, EEG changes, extrapyramidal reactions.
CV: *tachycardia,* ECG changes, hypertension, *heart block, CVA, MI.*
EENT: *blurred vision,* tinnitus, mydriasis.
GI: dry mouth, *constipation,* nausea, vomiting, anorexia, paralytic ileus.
GU: urine retention.
Hematologic: *bone marrow depression,* eosinophilia, *agranulocytosis, thrombocytopenia.*
Skin: diaphoresis, rash, urticaria, photosensitivity.
Other: hypersensitivity reaction.

Interactions

Drug-drug. *Anticholinergics:* Increases anticholinergic effect. Paralytic ileus may occur. Monitor patient.
Barbiturates, CNS depressants: Enhances CNS depression. Avoid using together.
Bupropion, cimetidine, methylphenidate, SSRIs, valproic acid: May increase nortriptyline levels. Monitor patient for adverse reactions.
Clonidine: May cause loss of blood pressure control with potentially life threatening elevations in blood pressure. Don't use together.

Epinephrine, norepinephrine: Increases hypertensive effect. Use together cautiously; monitor blood pressure.
MAO inhibitors: May cause severe excitation, hyperpyrexia, or seizures. Use together cautiously.
Quinolones: Increases risk of life-threatening arrhythmias, including torsade de pointes. Don't use together.
Rifamycin: Decreases nortriptyline levels. Monitor levels for decreased effect.
Drug-herb. *SAMe, St. John's wort, yohimbe:* Use with some tricyclic antidepressants may increase serotonin levels. Discourage using together.
Drug-lifestyle. *Alcohol use:* Enhances CNS depression. Discourage using together.
Smoking: May lower nortriptyline level. Monitor patient for lack of drug effect.
Sun exposure: Increases risk of photosensitivity reaction. Urge patient to avoid unprotected or prolonged exposure to sunlight.

Effects on lab test results

• May increase or decrease glucose level.
• May increase liver function test values and eosinophil count. May decrease RBC, WBC, granulocyte, and platelet counts.

Pharmacokinetics

Absorption: Rapid.
Distribution: Distributed widely into body, including CNS. Drug is 95% protein-bound.
Metabolism: Metabolized by liver; significant first-pass effect may account for variability of levels in different patients taking same dosage.
Excretion: Most excreted in urine; some in feces. *Half-life:* 18 to 24 hours.

Route	Onset	Peak	Duration
P.O.	Unknown	7-8½ hr	Unknown

Action

Chemical effect: Unknown; increases amount of norepinephrine, serotonin, or both in CNS by blocking their reuptake by presynaptic neurons.
Therapeutic effect: Relieves depression.

Available forms

Capsules: 10 mg, 25 mg, 50 mg, 75 mg
Oral solution: 10 mg/5 ml*
Tablets: 10 mg ◊ , 25 mg ◊

⚡ Assessment
- Assess patient's depression before therapy and regularly thereafter.
- Be alert for adverse reactions and drug interactions.
- Evaluate patient's and family's knowledge of drug therapy.

⊕ Nursing diagnoses
- Disturbed thought processes related to depression
- Risk for injury related to drug-induced adverse CNS reactions
- Deficient knowledge related to drug therapy

▶ Planning and implementation
- Reduce dosage in geriatric or debilitated patient.
- ⊛ **ALERT:** Don't withdraw drug abruptly. After abrupt withdrawal of long-term therapy, patient may experience nausea, headache, and malaise.
- ⊛ **ALERT:** Because hypertensive episodes have occurred during surgery in patients receiving tricyclic antidepressants, stop drug gradually several days before surgery.
- If signs of psychosis occur or increase, reduce dosage.
- ⊛ **ALERT:** Don't confuse nortriptyline with amitriptyline.

Patient teaching
- Whenever possible, advise patient to take full dose h.s. to reduce risk of orthostatic hypotension.
- Warn patient to avoid hazardous activities until CNS effects of drug are known. Drowsiness and dizziness usually subside after a few weeks.
- Tell patient to avoid alcohol during drug therapy.
- Warn patient not to stop drug suddenly.
- Advise patient to consult prescriber before taking other prescription or OTC drugs.
- Advise patient to use sunblock, wear protective clothing, and avoid prolonged exposure to sunlight.

☑ Evaluation
- Patient's depression improves.
- Patient experiences no injuries from drug-induced adverse CNS reactions.
- Patient and family state understanding of drug therapy.

nystatin
(nigh-STAT-in)
Mycostatin*, Nilstat, Nystex*

Pharmacologic class: polyene macrolide
Therapeutic class: antifungal
Pregnancy risk category: C

Indications and dosages
▶ **GI tract infections.** *Adults:* 500,000 to 1 million units as oral tablets P.O. t.i.d.
▶ **Oral, vaginal, and intestinal infections caused by** *Candida albicans* **and other** *Candida* **sp.** *Adults:* 500,000 to 1 million units suspension P.O. t.i.d. for oral candidiasis.
Children and infants older than age 3 months: 250,000 to 500,000 units suspension P.O. q.i.d. *Neonates and premature infants:* 100,000 units suspension P.O. q.i.d.
▶ **Vaginal infections.** *Adults:* 100,000 units, as vaginal tablets, inserted high into vagina, daily or b.i.d. for 14 days.

Contraindications and precautions
- Contraindicated in patients hypersensitive to drug.
- ≋ **Lifespan:** In breast-feeding women, safety of drug hasn't been established.

Adverse reactions
GI: transient nausea, vomiting, diarrhea (with large oral dosage).

Interactions
None significant.

Effects on lab test results
None reported.

Pharmacokinetics
Absorption: Not absorbed from GI tract, intact skin, or mucous membranes.
Distribution: None.
Metabolism: None.
Excretion: Oral form excreted almost entirely unchanged in feces. *Half-life:* Unknown.

Route	Onset	Peak	Duration
P.O., topical, vaginal	Unknown	Unknown	Unknown

Reactions may be *common,* uncommon, *life-threatening,* or COMMON AND LIFE-THREATENING.

Action

Chemical effect: Unknown; probably acts by binding to sterols in fungal cell membrane, altering cell permeability and allowing leakage of intracellular components.
Therapeutic effect: Kills susceptible yeasts and fungi.

Available forms

Oral suspension: 100,000 units/ml
Tablets: 500,000 units
Vaginal suppositories: 100,000 units

NURSING PROCESS

◪ Assessment
• Assess patient's infection before therapy and regularly thereafter.
• Be alert for adverse reactions.
• If adverse GI reactions occur, monitor patient's hydration status.
• Evaluate patient's and family's knowledge of drug therapy.

🔁 Nursing diagnoses
• Infection related to organisms
• Risk for deficient fluid volume related to drug-induced adverse GI reactions
• Deficient knowledge related to drug therapy

▶ Planning and implementation
• Drug isn't effective against systemic infections.
• When treating oral candidiasis (thrush), clean food debris from patient's mouth and have patient hold suspension in mouth for several minutes before swallowing.
• When treating an infant, swab medication on oral mucosa.
• Immunosuppressed patients with oral candidiasis are sometimes instructed by prescriber to suck on vaginal tablets (100,000 units) because doing so provides prolonged contact with oral mucosa.
• Pregnant patients can use vaginal tablets up to 6 weeks before term to treat infection that may cause thrush in neonates.
Patient teaching
• Advise patient to take drug for at least 2 days after symptoms disappear to prevent reinfection. Consult prescriber for duration of therapy.
• Instruct patient to continue therapy during menstruation.

• Instruct patient in oral hygiene techniques. Poorly fitting dentures and overuse of mouthwash may alter oral flora and promote infection.
• Explain that predisposing factors for vaginal infection include use of antibiotics, hormonal contraceptives, and corticosteroids; diabetes; reinfection by sexual partner; and tight-fitting undergarments. Encourage patient to wear cotton (not synthetic) underpants.
• Teach patient about hygiene for affected areas, including wiping perineal area from front to back.
• Advise patient to report redness, swelling, or irritation.

☑ Evaluation
• Patient is free from infection.
• Patient maintains adequate hydration throughout drug therapy.
• Patient and family state understanding of drug therapy.

octreotide acetate
(ok-TREE-oh-tighd AS-ih-tayt)
Sandostatin, Sandostatin LAR Depot

Pharmacologic class: synthetic octapeptide
Therapeutic class: somatotropic hormone
Pregnancy risk category: B

Indications and dosages

▶ **Flushing and diarrhea caused by carcinoid tumors.** *Adults:* 0.1 to 0.6 mg daily S.C. in two to four divided doses for first 2 weeks (usual daily dosage is 0.3 mg). Subsequent dosage based on patient's response. Patients currently on Sandostatin can switch to Sandostatin LAR Depot 20 mg I.M. to gluteal area q 4 weeks for 2 months.
▶ **Watery diarrhea caused by vasoactive intestinal polypeptide secreting tumors (vipomas).** *Adults:* 0.2 to 0.3 mg daily S.C. in two to four divided doses for first 2 weeks of therapy. Subsequent dosage based on individual response; typically doesn't exceed 0.45 mg daily. Patients currently on Sandostatin can switch

to Sandostatin LAR Depot 20 mg I.M. to gluteal area q 4 weeks for 2 months.

▶ **Acromegaly.** *Adults:* Initially, 0.05 mg S.C. t.i.d.; then adjusted according to somatomedin C levels q 2 weeks. Usual effective dosage is 0.1 mg S.C. t.i.d. Some patients may require up to 0.5 mg S.C. t.i.d. for maximum effectiveness. Patients on Sandostatin can switch to Sandostatin LAR Depot 20 mg I.M. to gluteal area q 4 weeks for 3 months.

▶ **GI fistula‡.** *Adults:* 0.05 to 0.2 mg S.C. q 8 hours.

▶ **Variceal bleeding‡.** *Adults:* 0.025 to 0.05 mg/hour continuous I.V. infusion. Duration is from 18 hours to 5 days.

▶ **AIDS-related diarrhea‡.** *Adults:* 0.1 to 0.5 mg S.C. t.i.d.

▶ **Short bowel (ileostomy) syndrome‡.** *Adults:* 0.025 mg/hour continuous I.V. infusion or 0.05 mg S.C. b.i.d.

▶ **Chemotherapy- and radiation-induced diarrhea‡.** *Adults:* 0.05 to 0.1 mg S.C. t.i.d. for 1 to 3 days.

▶ **Pancreatic fistula‡.** *Adults:* 0.05 to 0.2 mg S.C. q 8 hours.

▶ **Irritable bowel syndrome‡.** *Adults:* 0.1 mg single dose to 0.125 mg S.C. b.i.d.

▶ **Dumping syndrome‡.** *Adults:* 0.05 to 0.15 mg S.C. daily.

Contraindications and precautions

• Contraindicated in patients hypersensitive to drug or its components.

☀ **Lifespan:** In pregnant women, use cautiously. In breast-feeding women and in children, safety of drug hasn't been established.

Adverse reactions

CNS: pain, dizziness, headache, lightheadedness, fatigue.
CV: flushing, *arrhythmias, bradycardia.*
GI: *nausea, diarrhea, abdominal pain or discomfort,* loose stools, vomiting, fat malabsorption, gallbladder abnormalities.
Metabolic: hyperglycemia, *hypoglycemia,* hypothyroidism.
Skin: edema, wheal, erythema and pain at injection site.
Other: burning at S.C. injection site.

Interactions

Drug-drug. *Cyclosporine:* May decrease cyclosporine level. Monitor patient.

Drug-food. *Dietary fats:* Drug may alter the absorption of dietary fats. Also may decrease vitamin B_{12} level; monitor level.

Effects on lab test results

• May decrease T_4 and thyroid-stimulating hormone levels. May increase or decrease glucose level.

Pharmacokinetics

Absorption: Rapid and complete after S.C. injection.
Distribution: Distributed to plasma, where it binds to lipoprotein and albumin.
Metabolism: Not clearly defined.
Excretion: About 35% of drug is unchanged in urine. *Half-life:* About 1½ hours.

Route	Onset	Peak	Duration
I.M., S.C.	≤ 30 min	30-60 min	12 hr-6 wk

Action

Chemical effect: Mimics action of naturally occurring somatostatin.
Therapeutic effect: Relieves flushing and diarrhea caused by certain tumors and treats acromegaly.

Available forms

Depot: 10 mg/5 ml, 20 mg/5 ml, 30 mg/5 ml
Injection: 0.05-mg, 0.1-mg, 0.5-mg ampules; 0.2-mg/ml, 1-mg/ml multidose vials

NURSING PROCESS

☑ Assessment

• Assess patient's condition before therapy and regularly thereafter.
• Monitor somatomedin C levels q 2 weeks. Dosage is adjusted based on this level.
• Monitor laboratory tests at baseline and then periodically, such as thyroid function tests, urine 5-hydroxyindoleacetic acid, plasma serotonin, plasma substance P (for carcinoid tumors), and plasma vasoactive intestinal peptide (for vipomas).
• Monitor fluid and electrolyte status.
• Be alert for adverse reactions and drug interactions.
• Evaluate patient's and family's knowledge of drug therapy.

🔄 Nursing diagnoses
• Diarrhea related to condition
• Fatigue related to drug-induced adverse CNS reaction
• Deficient knowledge related to drug therapy

▣ Planning and implementation
• Give drug in divided doses for first 2 weeks of therapy; subsequent daily dosage depends on patient's response.
• Read drug labels carefully, and check dosage and strength.
⚠ **ALERT:** For LAR Depot injection, give drug I.M. only. Avoid deltoid muscle because of possible discomfort at site.
• Drug therapy may alter fluid and electrolyte balance and may require adjustment of other drugs.

Patient teaching
• Tell patient to report signs of gallbladder disease such as abdominal discomfort. Drug may be linked to development of cholelithiasis.
• Inform patient that laboratory tests are needed during therapy.
• Advise diabetic patient to monitor glucose level closely. Antidiabetics may need dosage adjustment.

☑ Evaluation
• Patient's bowel pattern is normal.
• Patient uses energy-saving measures to combat fatigue.
• Patient and family state understanding of drug therapy.

---

ofloxacin
(oh-FLOKS-eh-sin)
Apo-Oflox ♦ , Floxin

Pharmacologic class: fluoroquinolone
Therapeutic class: antibiotic
Pregnancy risk category: C

Indications and dosages

▶ **Lower respiratory tract infections caused by susceptible strains of *Haemophilus influenzae* or *Streptococcus pneumoniae*.** *Adults:* 400 mg P.O. q 12 hours for 10 days.
▶ **Cervicitis or urethritis caused by *Chlamydia trachomatis* or *Neisseria gonorrhoeae*.** *Adults:* 300 mg P.O. q 12 hours for 7 days.

▶ **Acute, uncomplicated gonorrhea.** *Adults:* 400 mg P.O. as single dose.
▶ **Mild to moderate skin and skin-structure infections caused by susceptible strains of *Staphylococcus aureus*, *Staphylococcus epidermidis*, *Streptococcus pyogenes*, or *Proteus mirabilis*.** *Adults:* 400 mg P.O. q 12 hours for 10 days.
▶ **Cystitis caused by *Escherichia coli* or *Klebsiella pneumoniae*.** *Adults:* 200 mg P.O. q 12 hours for 3 days.
▶ **UTIs caused by susceptible strains of *Citrobacter diversus*, *Enterobacter aerogenes*, *E. coli*, *P. mirabilis*, or *Pseudomonas aeruginosa*.** *Adults:* 200 mg P.O. q 12 hours for 7 days. Complicated infections may need 10 days of therapy.
▶ **Prostatitis caused by *E. coli*.** *Adults:* 300 mg P.O. q 12 hours for 6 weeks.
▶ **Adjunct to *Brucella* infections‡.** *Adults:* 400 mg P.O. daily for 6 weeks.
▶ **Typhoid fever‡.** *Adults:* 200 to 400 mg P.O. q 12 hours for 7 to 14 days.
▶ **Antituberculosis drug (adjunct) ‡.** *Adults:* 300 mg P.O. daily.
▶ **Postoperative sternotomy or soft tissue wounds caused by *Mycobacterium fortuitum*‡.** *Adults:* 300 to 600 mg P.O. daily for 3 to 6 months.
▶ **Acute Q fever pneumonia‡.** *Adults:* 600 mg P.O. daily for up to 16 days.
▶ **Mediterranean spotted fever‡.** *Adults:* 200 mg P.O. q 12 hours for 7 days.
▶ **Traveler's diarrhea‡.** *Adults:* 300 mg P.O. b.i.d. for 3 days.
▣ **Adjust-a-dose:** For patients with renal impairment, if creatinine clearance is 20 to 50 ml/minute, give usual recommended dose q 24 hours; if creatinine clearance is less than 20 ml/minute, give one-half of recommended dose q 24 hours.
For patients with hepatic impairment, maximum daily dose is 400 mg.

Contraindications and precautions

• Contraindicated in patients hypersensitive to drug or other fluoroquinolones.
• Use cautiously in patients with renal impairment, history of seizures, or other CNS diseases such as cerebral arteriosclerosis.
🔥 **Lifespan:** In pregnant women, use cautiously. In children and breast-feeding women, safety of drug hasn't been established.

Adverse reactions

CNS: headache, dizziness, fever, fatigue, lethargy, malaise, drowsiness, sleep disorders, nervousness, light-headedness, insomnia, *seizures*.
CV: chest pain.
EENT: visual disturbances.
GI: nausea, anorexia, abdominal pain or discomfort, diarrhea, vomiting, dry mouth, flatulence, dysgeusia.
GU: vaginitis, vaginal discharge, genital pruritus.
Hematologic: eosinophilia, anemia, leukocytosis, *neutropenia, lymphocytopenia, leukopenia*.
Metabolic: *hypoglycemia,* hyperglycemia.
Musculoskeletal: trunk pain, transient arthralgia, myalgia.
Skin: rash, pruritus, photosensitivity reaction.
Other: hypersensitivity reactions, *anaphylaxis*.

Interactions

Drug-drug. *Aluminum hydroxide, aluminum-magnesium hydroxide, calcium carbonate, magnesium hydroxide:* May decrease effects of ofloxacin. Give antacid at least 6 hours before or 2 hours after ofloxacin.
Divalent or trivalent cations (such as zinc), or didanosine (chewable/buffered tablets or pediatric powder for oral solution): Interferes with GI absorption of ofloxacin. Give these drugs at least 2 hours before or 2 hours after taking ofloxacin.
Cimetidine: May interfere with the elimination of ofloxacin. Monitor patient for toxicity.
Iron salts: May decrease absorption of ofloxacin, reducing anti-infective response. Give at least 2 hours apart.
NSAIDs: Increases risk of CNS stimulation and convulsive seizures. Avoid using together; however, monitor patient for tremors and seizures if used together.
Oral anticoagulants: Increases anticoagulant effect. Monitor patient for bleeding and altered PT and INR.
Procainamide: May increase procainamide concentration. Monitor procainamide concentration; adjust dose accordingly.
Sucralfate: May decrease absorption of the ofloxacin, reducing anti-infective response. If use together can't be avoided, give at least 6 hours apart.
Theophylline: Decreases theophylline clearance with some fluoroquinolones. Monitor theophylline level.

Warfarin: May enhance anticoagulant effects. Monitor PT and INR closely.
Drug-food. *Any food:* May decrease drug absorption. Give drug on an empty stomach.
Drug-lifestyle. *Sun exposure:* Photosensitivity reactions may occur. Urge patient to avoid unprotected or prolonged sun exposure.

Effects on lab test results

• May increase ALT, AST, and alkaline phosphatase levels. May increase or decrease glucose level.
• May increase eosinophil count. May decrease hemoglobin, hematocrit, and neutrophil and lymphocyte counts. May increase or decrease WBC count.
• May produce false-positive opiate assay results.

Pharmacokinetics

Absorption: Well absorbed.
Distribution: Widely distributed to body tissues and fluids.
Metabolism: Pyridobenzoxazine ring decreases extent of metabolism in liver.
Excretion: 70% to 80% of drug is excreted unchanged in urine; less than 5% in feces. half-life: 4 to 7½ hours.

Route	Onset	Peak	Duration
P.O.	Unknown	1-2 hr	Unknown

Action

Chemical effect: Unknown; may inhibit bacterial DNA gyrase and prevent DNA replication in susceptible bacteria.
Therapeutic effect: Kills susceptible aerobic gram-positive and gram-negative organisms.

Available forms

Tablets: 200 mg, 300 mg, 400 mg

NURSING PROCESS

☑ Assessment

• Assess patient's infection before therapy and regularly thereafter.
• Monitor regular blood studies and hepatic and renal function tests during prolonged therapy.
• Give serologic test for syphilis to patient treated for gonorrhea. Drug isn't effective against syphilis, and treatment of gonorrhea may mask or delay symptoms of syphilis.

Reactions may be *common,* uncommon, *life-threatening,* or COMMON AND LIFE-THREATENING.

- Be alert for adverse reactions and drug interactions.
- If adverse GI reactions occur, monitor patient's hydration status.
- Evaluate patient's and family's knowledge of drug therapy.

🔄 Nursing diagnoses
- Infection related to presence of bacteria
- Risk for deficient fluid volume related to drug-induced adverse GI reactions
- Deficient knowledge related to drug therapy

⟫ Planning and implementation
- Give oral drug on empty stomach.
- ⓢ ALERT: If patient experiences restlessness, tremor, confusion, or hallucinations, stop medication and notify prescriber. Take seizure precautions.

Patient teaching
- Advise patient to take drug with plenty of fluids but not with meals. Also, tell patient to avoid antacids, sucralfate, and products containing iron or zinc for at least 2 hours before and after each dose.
- Advise patient to complete full course of antibiotics, as directed.
- Warn patient to avoid hazardous tasks until CNS effects of drug are known.
- Advise patient to use sunblock and protective clothing to avoid photosensitivity reactions.
- Tell patient to stop drug and notify prescriber if rash or other signs of hypersensitivity reactions develop.

☑ Evaluation
- Patient is free from infection.
- Patient maintains adequate hydration throughout drug therapy.
- Patient and family state understanding of drug therapy.

---

olanzapine
(oh-LAN-za-peen)
Zyprexa, Zyprexa Zydis

Pharmacologic class: thienobenzodiazepine derivative
Therapeutic class: antipsychotic
Pregnancy risk category: C

Indications and dosages

▶ **Short-term therapy for acute manic episodes related to bipolar I disorder.** *Adults:* Initially, 10 to 15 mg P.O. daily. Adjust dosage p.r.n. by increments of 5 mg daily at intervals of 24 hours or more. Maximum dose is 20 mg P.O. daily. Duration of treatment is 3 to 4 weeks.
▶ **Long-term therapy for schizophrenia.** *Adults:* Initially, 5 to 10 mg P.O. daily. Goal is 10 mg P.O. daily within several days of starting therapy. Dosage may be increased weekly in increments of 5 mg daily to a maximum of 20 mg daily. Clinical assessment is recommended for dosages that exceed 10 mg daily.
▶ **Short-term therapy for acute manic episodes of bipolar I disorder, given with lithium or valproate.** *Adults:* 10 mg P.O. once daily. Dosage range is 5 to 20 mg daily. Duration of treatment is 6 weeks.
▶ **Long-term therapy for bipolar I disorder.** *Adults:* 5 to 20 mg P.O. daily.
▧ **Adjust-a-dose:** For patients who are debilitated, have a predisposition to hypotensive reactions, have risk factors for slower metabolism of olanzapine (nonsmoking women older than age 65), or may be more pharmacodynamically sensitive to olanzapine, the recommended starting dosage is 5 mg P.O. daily. In these patients, increase dose with caution.

Contraindications and precautions
- Contraindicated in patients hypersensitive to drug.
- Use cautiously in patients with heart disease, cerebrovascular disease, conditions that predispose patient to hypotension, history of seizures or conditions that might lower the seizure threshold, or hepatic impairment. Also use cautiously in patients with a history of paralytic ileus and in those at risk for aspiration pneumonia, prostatic hyperplasia, or angle-closure glaucoma.
⚕ Lifespan: In pregnant women, drug should be given only if potential benefits justify risks to fetus. Breast-feeding women should avoid breast-feeding. In elderly patients, use cautiously.

Adverse reactions

CNS: *dizziness, somnolence, asthenia, insomnia,* personality disorder, akathisia, tremor, fever, abnormal gait, speech impairment, tardive

---

dyskinesia, *parkinsonism, **neuroleptic malig-
nant syndrome, suicide attempt.***
CV: orthostatic hypotension, chest pain, tachy-
cardia, hypertension, peripheral edema.
EENT: rhinitis, pharyngitis, amblyopia, con-
junctivitis.
GI: *constipation, dry mouth, dyspepsia,* in-
creased appetite, vomiting, increased salivation
and thirst.
GU: urinary incontinence, UTI, amenorrhea,
hematuria, metrorrhagia, vaginitis.
Hematologic: *leukopenia.*
Metabolic: weight gain, hyperglycemia.
Musculoskeletal: joint pain, joint stiffness and
twitching, extremity pain, back pain, hypertonia.
Respiratory: increased cough, dyspnea.
Skin: ecchymosis, sweating.
Other: dental pain, flu syndrome, injury.

Interactions

Drug-drug. *Antihypertensives:* May increase
hypotensive effects. Monitor blood pressure
closely.
Carbamazepine, omeprazole, rifampin: Increases olanzapine clearance. Monitor patient.
Diazepam: Increases CNS effects. Monitor patient closely.
Dopamine agonists, levodopa: Antagonizes activity of these drugs. Monitor patient.
Fluvoxamine: Decreases the clearance of olanzapine. Consider lower doses of olanzapine.
Drug-herb. *Nutmeg:* May reduce effectiveness
of or interfere with drug therapy. Discourage using together.
Drug-lifestyle. *Alcohol use:* Increases CNS effects. Discourage using together.

Effects on lab test results

• May increase AST, ALT, GGT, CK, and prolactin levels.

Pharmacokinetics

Absorption: Level peaks in about 6 hours.
Food doesn't affect rate or extent of absorption.
About 40% of dose is limited by first-pass metabolism.
Distribution: Distributes extensively throughout the body, with a volume of distribution of
about 1,000 L. About 93% protein-bound, primarily to albumin and alpha$_1$-acid glycoprotein.
Metabolism: Metabolized by direct glucuronidation and CYP-mediated oxidation.

Excretion: About 57% of drug appears in urine
and 30% in feces as metabolites. Only 7% of
dose is recovered in urine unchanged. *Half-life:*
21 to 54 hours.

Route	Onset	Peak	Duration
P.O.	Unknown	6 hr	Unknown

Action

Chemical effect: Unknown. Binds to dopamine
and serotonin receptors; may antagonize adrenergic, cholinergic, and histaminergic receptors.
Therapeutic effect: Relieves signs and symptoms of psychosis.

Available forms

Zyprexa
Tablets: 2.5 mg, 5 mg, 7.5 mg, 10 mg, 15 mg,
20 mg
Zyprexa Zydis
Tablets (orally disintegrating): 5 mg, 10 mg,
15 mg, 20 mg

NURSING PROCESS

Assessment
• Obtain history of patient's underlying condition before therapy, and reassess regularly thereafter.
• Obtain baseline and periodic glucose levels
and liver function tests.
• Monitor patient for signs of neuroleptic malignant syndrome (hyperpyrexia, muscle rigidity,
altered mental status, autonomic instability),
which is rare but commonly fatal. Stop drug immediately, monitor patient, and treat p.r.n.
• Monitor patient for tardive dyskinesia, which
may occur after prolonged use. It may not appear until months or years later, and it may disappear spontaneously or persist for life despite
stopping therapy.
• Monitor patient for abnormal body temperature regulation, especially if patient is exercising
strenuously, exposed to extreme heat, receiving
anticholinergics, or at risk for dehydration.
• Evaluate patient's and family's knowledge of
drug therapy.

Nursing diagnoses
• Disturbed thought processes related to underlying condition

---

• Risk for injury related to drug-induced adverse CNS reactions
• Deficient knowledge related to drug therapy

⟫ **Planning and implementation**

• Therapy starts at 5-mg dose in patients who are debilitated, predisposed to hypotension, pharmacologically sensitive to drug, or affected by altered metabolism caused by smoking status, sex, or age.
• Orally disintegrating tablets contain phenylalanine.
Ⓢ **ALERT:** Don't confuse olanzapine with olsalazine.
Ⓢ **ALERT:** Don't confuse Zyprexa with Zyrtec or Celexa.

Patient teaching
• Drug can be taken without regard to food.
• Tell patient to avoid hazardous tasks until adverse CNS effects of drug are known.
• Warn patient against exposure to extreme heat; drug may impair body's ability to reduce core temperature.
• Tell patient to avoid alcohol during therapy.
• Tell patient to rise slowly to avoid effects of orthostatic hypotension.
• Instruct patient to relieve dry mouth with ice chips or sugarless candy or gum.
• Advise woman to notify prescriber if she becomes pregnant or intends to become pregnant during drug therapy. Advise her not to breast-feed during therapy.

✔ **Evaluation**
• Patient's behavior and communication show improved thought processes.
• Patient sustains no injury from adverse CNS reactions.
• Patient and family state understanding of drug therapy.

---

olmesartan medoxomil
(ol-meh-SAHR-tan me-DOKS-oh-mil)
Benicar

Pharmacologic class: angiotensin II receptor antagonist
Therapeutic class: antihypertensive
Pregnancy risk category: C (first trimester) and D (second and third trimesters)

Indications and dosages

▶ **Hypertension.** *Adults:* 20 mg P.O. daily in patients who aren't volume-contracted. If blood pressure isn't reduced after 2 weeks of therapy, increase dosage to 40 mg P.O. once daily.
Ⓢ **Adjust-a-dose:** In patients whose intravascular volume may be depleted, consider lower starting dose.

Contraindications and precautions

• Contraindicated in patients hypersensitive to drug or any of its components.
• Use cautiously in patients who are volume- or salt-depleted, in those whose renal function depends on the renin-angiotensin-aldosterone system (such as patients with severe heart failure), and in those with renal artery stenosis.
⚛ **Lifespan:** In pregnant women, drug is contraindicated. If woman becomes pregnant, stop drug immediately. Breast-feeding women should either stop breast-feeding or stop taking the drug. It's unknown whether drug appears in breast milk. In children, safety and effectiveness of drug haven't been established. In elderly patients, use cautiously because they may have greater sensitivity to drug.

Adverse reactions

CNS: headache.
EENT: pharyngitis, rhinitis, sinusitis.
GI: diarrhea.
GU: hematuria.
Metabolic: hyperglycemia, hypertriglyceridemia.
Musculoskeletal: back pain.
Respiratory: bronchitis, upper respiratory tract infection.
Other: flulike symptoms, accidental injury.

Interactions

None reported.

Effects on lab test results

• May increase glucose, triglyceride, uric acid, liver enzyme, bilirubin, and CK levels.
• May decrease hemoglobin and hematocrit.

Pharmacokinetics

Absorption: Rapid and complete. Steady-state concentrations are achieved within 3 to 5 days.
Distribution: 99% bound to proteins.
Metabolism: After absorption, virtually no further drug metabolism occurs.

Rapid onset   *Liquid form contains alcohol.   ♦Canada   ◊ Australia   †OTC   ‡Off-label use

Excretion: In the urine and feces. *Half-life:* 13 hours.

Route	Onset	Peak	Duration
P.O.	Rapid	1-2 hr	24 hr

Action

Chemical effect: Blocks the vasoconstrictor and aldosterone-secreting effects of angiotensin II by selectively blocking the binding of angiotensin II to the AT_1 receptor in the vascular smooth muscle.
Therapeutic effect: Lowers blood pressure

Available forms

Tablets: 5 mg, 20 mg, 40 mg

NURSING PROCESS

⚕ Assessment
• Monitor patients with heart failure closely for oliguria, azotemia, and acute renal impairment.
• Monitor BUN and creatinine levels in patients with renal artery stenosis.
• Be alert for adverse reactions.
• Evaluate patient's and family's knowledge of drug therapy.

⚕ Nursing diagnoses
• Risk for injury related to presence of hypertension
• Disturbed sleep pattern related to drug-induced cough
• Deficient knowledge related to drug therapy

⚕ Planning and implementation
• Symptomatic hypotension may occur in patients who are volume- or salt-depleted, especially those being treated with high doses of a diuretic. If hypotension occurs, place patient supine and treat supportively. Treatment may continue when blood pressure is stabilized.
• If blood pressure isn't adequately controlled, a diuretic or other antihypertensive may be added.
Patient teaching
• Tell patient to take drug exactly as prescribed and not to stop even if he feels better.
• Tell patient that drug may be taken without regard to meals.
• Tell patient to report adverse reactions to prescriber promptly, especially lightheadedness and syncope.

• Advise women of childbearing age to immediately report pregnancy to prescriber.
• Inform diabetic patients that glucose readings may become higher, and the dosage of their antidiabetics may need adjustment.
• Warn patient that reduced fluid volume from inadequate fluid intake, excessive perspiration, diarrhea, or vomiting may cause a drop in blood pressure, leading to lightheadedness and fainting.
• Inform patient that other antihypertensives can have additive or synergistic effects. Patient should inform prescriber of all drugs (including OTC) that he's taking.

☑ Evaluation
• Patient's blood pressure is normal.
• Patient's sleep patterns are undisturbed throughout therapy.
• Patient and family state understanding of drug therapy.

olsalazine sodium
(olh-SAL-uh-zeen SOH-dee-um)
Dipentum

Pharmacologic class: salicylate
Therapeutic class: anti-inflammatory
Pregnancy risk category: C

Indications and dosages

▶ **Maintenance of remission of ulcerative colitis in patients intolerant of sulfasalazine.**
Adults: 500 mg P.O. b.i.d. with meals.

Contraindications and precautions

• Contraindicated in patients hypersensitive to salicylates.
• Use cautiously in patients with renal disease. Renal tubular damage may result from absorbed drug or its metabolites.
⚖ **Lifespan:** In pregnant and breast-feeding women, use cautiously. In children, safety of drug hasn't been established.

Adverse reactions

CNS: headache, depression, vertigo, dizziness.
GI: *diarrhea,* nausea, abdominal pain, heartburn.
Musculoskeletal: arthralgia.
Skin: rash, itching.

Reactions may be *common*, uncommon, *life-threatening*, or COMMON AND LIFE-THREATENING.

Interactions

Drug-drug. *Anticoagulants, coumarin derivatives:* Prolongs PT and INR. Monitor patient closely for bleeding.

Effects on lab test results

None reported.

Pharmacokinetics

Absorption: About 2% of single dose is absorbed.
Distribution: Liberated mesalamine is absorbed slowly from colon, resulting in very high local levels.
Metabolism: 0.1% is metabolized in liver; remainder reaches colon, where it's rapidly converted to mesalamine by colonic bacteria.
Excretion: About 80% excreted in feces; less than 1% in urine. *Half-life:* About 1 hour.

Route	Onset	Peak	Duration
P.O.	Unknown	1 hr	Unknown

Action

Chemical effect: Unknown; converts to 5-aminosalicylic acid (5-ASA or mesalamine) in colon, where it has local anti-inflammatory effect.
Therapeutic effect: Prevents flare-up of ulcerative colitis.

Available forms

Capsules: 250 mg

NURSING PROCESS

Assessment

• Assess patient's condition before therapy and regularly thereafter.
• Monitor BUN and creatinine levels and urinalysis in patient with renal disease.
• Be alert for adverse reactions.
• Evaluate patient's and family's knowledge of drug therapy.

Nursing diagnoses

• Impaired tissue integrity related to ulcerative colitis
• Diarrhea related to drug's adverse effect on GI tract
• Deficient knowledge related to drug therapy

Planning and implementation

• Give drug in evenly divided doses with food to decrease GI irritation.
• Report diarrhea to prescriber. Although diarrhea appears dose-related, it's difficult to distinguish from worsening of disease symptoms. Worsening of disease has been noted with similar drugs.
ALERT: Don't confuse olsalazine with olanzapine.

Patient teaching

• Tell patient to take drug in evenly divided doses and with food to minimize adverse GI reactions.
• Urge patient to notify prescriber about adverse reactions, especially diarrhea or increased pain.

Evaluation

• Patient has no evidence of ulcerative colitis.
• Patient is free from diarrhea.
• Patient and family state understanding of drug therapy.

omalizumab

(oh-mah-LIZZ-uh-mahb)
Xolair

Pharmacologic class: DNA-derived humanized Ig (immunoglobulin) G1k monoclonal antibody
Therapeutic class: antiasthmatic
Pregnancy risk category: B

Indications and dosages

▶ **Moderate to severe persistent asthma in patients who have positive skin test or in vitro reactivity to a seasonal allergen and whose symptoms are inadequately controlled with inhaled corticosteroids.** *Adults and children age 12 and older:* Dosage is determined by total IgE level (IU/ml) measured before the start of treatment and by body weight (kg). See table on next page. Divide doses greater than 150 mg and use more than one injection site. Inject S.C.q 2 to 4 weeks.

Contraindications and precautions

• Contraindicated in patients hypersensitive to drug.
Lifespan: In pregnant women, use only if clearly needed. In breast-feeding women, use cautiously. In children younger than age 12,

DOSE EVERY 4 WEEKS

Pretreatment IgE (IU/ml)	Body weight (kg)			
	30-60	> 60-70	> 70-90	> 90-150
≥ 30-100	150 mg	150 mg	150 mg	300 mg
> 100-200	300 mg	300 mg	300 mg	Don't give
> 200-300	300 mg	Don't give	Don't give	Don't give

DOSE EVERY 2 WEEKS

Pretreatment IgE (IU/ml)	Body weight (kg)			
	30-60	> 60-70	> 70-90	> 90-150
≥ 30-100	Don't give	Don't give	Don't give	Don't give
> 100-200	Don't give	Don't give	Don't give	225
> 200-300	Don't give	225	225	300
> 300-400	225	225	300	Don't give
> 400-500	300	300	375	Don't give
> 500-600	300	375	Don't give	Don't give
> 600-700	375	Don't give	Don't give	Don't give

safety and effectiveness of drug haven't been established.

Route	Onset	Peak	Duration
S.C.	Unknown	7-8 days	Unknown

Adverse reactions

CNS: *headache,* pain, fatigue, dizziness.
EENT: sinusitis, pharyngitis, earache.
Musculoskeletal: arthralgia, fracture, leg pain, arm pain.
Respiratory: *upper respiratory tract infection.*
Skin: pruritus, dermatitis.
Other: *injection site reaction, viral infections.*

Interactions

None reported.

Effects on lab test results

• May increase IgE levels for up to 1 year after therapy.

Pharmacokinetics

Absorption: Slowly absorbed with a bioavailability of about 62%.
Distribution: Tissues distribution studies show no specific uptake by any organ or tissue.
Metabolism: Unknown.
Excretion: Liver elimination of IgG includes degradation in the reticuloendothelial system and endothelial cells. Intact IgG is also excreted in bile. *Half-life:* About 26 days.

Action

Chemical effect: Inhibits binding of IgE to the high-affinity receptor FceRI on the surface of mast cells and basophils. Reducing IgE limits the release of mediators of the allergic response and reduces the number of FceRI receptors on basophils.
Therapeutic effect: Treats asthma symptoms.

Available forms

Powder for injection: 150 mg in 5-ml vial

NURSING PROCESS

Assessment

• Assess patient's respiratory condition before therapy and regularly thereafter.
• Be alert for adverse reactions.
ALERT: Observe patient after injection and have medications available to treat severe hypersensitivity reactions. If a severe hypersensitivity reaction occurs, stop therapy.
• Evaluate patient's and family's knowledge of drug therapy.

🔆 Nursing diagnoses

- Impaired gas exchange related to presence of bronchospasms
- Acute pain related to drug-induced headache
- Deficient knowledge related to drug therapy

▷ Planning and implementation

💲 **ALERT:** Drug shouldn't be used for acute bronchospasm or status asthmaticus.

- Don't abruptly stop systemic or inhaled corticosteroids when starting this drug. Decreases in corticosteroids should be gradual and medically supervised.
- Because the solution is slightly viscous, it may take 5 to 10 seconds to inject.
- Injection site reactions, including bruising, redness, warmth, burning, stinging, itching, hives, pain, induration, and inflammation, may occur. Most reactions occur within 1 hour of injection, last less than 8 days, and decrease in frequency with subsequent injections.
- Total IgE levels are elevated during treatment and remain elevated for up to 1 year after treatment has stopped. Therefore, testing IgE levels during therapy can't be used as a guide to determine dose. If treatment has been stopped for less than 1 year, use IgE levels from the original dose determination. If treatment has been stopped for 1 year or more, retest total IgE levels.

Patient teaching

- Tell patient not to decrease the dose or stop taking his other antiasthmatics unless directed by prescriber.
- Tell patient not to expect immediate improvement in his asthma after starting therapy.

☑ Evaluation

- Patient exhibits normal breathing pattern.
- Patient states that drug-induced headache is relieved by analgesic.
- Patient and family state understanding of drug therapy.

---

omeprazole
(oh-MEH-pruh-zohl)
Losec ◆ ◇ , Prilosec, Prilosec OTC†

Pharmacologic class: substituted benzimidazole
Therapeutic class: gastric acid suppressant.
Pregnancy risk category: C

Indications and dosages

▶ **Erosive esophagitis; symptomatic, poorly responsive gastroesophageal reflux disease (GERD).** *Adults:* 20 mg P.O. daily for 4 to 8 weeks. (Patients with GERD should have been unresponsive to H_2-receptor antagonist.)
▶ **Pathologic hypersecretory conditions (such as Zollinger-Ellison syndrome).** *Adults:* Initially, 60 mg P.O. daily, adjusted according to patient response. If daily amount exceeds 80 mg, give in divided doses. Dosages up to 120 mg t.i.d. have been given. Continue therapy as long as indicated.
▶ **Duodenal ulcer (short-term therapy).** *Adults:* 20 mg P.O. daily for 4 to 8 weeks.
▶ **Gastric ulcer.** *Adults:* 40 mg P.O. daily for 4 to 8 weeks.
▶ *Helicobacter pylori* **eradication to reduce risk of duodenal ulcer recurrence as part of triple therapy with clarithromycin and amoxicillin.** *Adults:* 20 mg P.O. with 500 mg clarithromycin P.O. and 1,000 mg amoxicillin P.O., each given b.i.d. for 10 days. For patients with ulcers when therapy starts, another 18 days of 20 mg omeprazole P.O. once daily is recommended.
▶ **Posterior laryngitis‡.** *Adults:* 40 mg q h.s. for 6 to 24 weeks.
▶ **Heartburn on 2 or more days per week.** *Adults:* 20 mg P.O. (Prilosec OTC) daily before breakfast for 14 days. May repeat the 14-day course q 4 months.

Contraindications and precautions

- Contraindicated in patients hypersensitive to drug or its components.

☀ **Lifespan:** In pregnant and breast-feeding women, use cautiously. In children, safety of drug hasn't been established.

Adverse reactions

CNS: headache, dizziness.
GI: diarrhea, abdominal pain, nausea, vomiting, constipation, flatulence.
Musculoskeletal: back pain.
Respiratory: cough.
Skin: rash.

Interactions

Drug-drug. *Ampicillin esters, iron derivatives, ketoconazole:* These drugs may have poor bioavailability because optimal absorption requires low gastric pH. Give separately.

Clarithromycin: Increases levels of either drug. Monitor patient for drug toxicity.

Diazepam, phenytoin, warfarin: Decreases hepatic clearance of these drugs, possibly leading to increased levels. Monitor patient closely.

Sucralfate: Delays absorption and reduces omeprazole bioavailability. Separate administration times by 30 minutes or more.

Drug-herb. *Male fern:* Herb is inactivated in alkaline environments. Discourage using together.

Pennyroyal: May change the rate at which toxic metabolites of herb form. Discourage using together.

Effects on lab test results

None reported.

Pharmacokinetics

Absorption: Absorbed rapidly after drug leaves stomach. However, bioavailability is about 40% because of instability in gastric acid as well as substantial first-pass effect. Bioavailability increases slightly with repeated dosing.
Distribution: Protein-binding is about 95%.
Metabolism: Metabolized primarily in liver.
Excretion: Excreted primarily in urine. *Half-life:* 30 to 60 minutes.

Route	Onset	Peak	Duration
P.O.	≤ 1 hr	2 hr	< 3 days

Action

Chemical effect: Inhibits activity of acid (proton) pump and binds to hydrogen-potassium adenosine triphosphatase on secretory surface of gastric parietal cells to block formation of gastric acid.
Therapeutic effect: Relieves symptoms caused by excessive gastric acid.

Available forms

Capsules (delayed-release): 10 mg, 20 mg, 40 mg
Tablets (delayed-release): 20 mg

NURSING PROCESS

🔲 Assessment
● Assess patient's condition before therapy and regularly thereafter.
● Be alert for adverse reactions and drug interactions.

● If adverse GI reactions occur, monitor patient's hydration status.
● Evaluate patient's and family's knowledge of drug therapy.

🔲 Nursing diagnoses
● Impaired tissue integrity related to upper gastric disorder
● Risk for deficient fluid volume related to drug-induced adverse GI reactions
● Deficient knowledge related to drug therapy

▶ Planning and implementation
● Give drug 30 minutes before meals.
● Dosage adjustments aren't needed for patients with renal or hepatic impairment.
🖲 **ALERT:** Don't confuse Prilosec with Prozac, prilocaine, or Prinivil.
🖲 **ALERT:** Don't confuse Losec with Lasix.
Patient teaching
● Explain importance of taking drug exactly as prescribed.
● Warn patient not to crush or chew tablets or capsules.
● Advise patient that Prilosec OTC isn't intended for immediate relief of heartburn or to treat infrequent heartburn (one episode of heartburn a week or less).
● Inform patient that Prilosec OTC may take 1 to 4 days for full effect, although some patients may get complete relief of symptoms within 24 hours.

☑ Evaluation
● Patient responds well to therapy.
● Patient maintains adequate hydration throughout drug therapy.
● Patient and family state understanding of drug therapy.

ondansetron hydrochloride
(on-DAN-seh-tron high-droh-KLOR-ighd)
Zofran, Zofran ODT

Pharmacologic class: serotonin (5-HT₃) receptor antagonist
Therapeutic class: antiemetic
Pregnancy risk category: B

Indications and dosages

▶ **Prevention of nausea and vomiting caused by moderately emetogenic chemotherapy.**
Adults and children age 12 and older: 8 mg P.O. 30 minutes before start of chemotherapy. Follow with 8 mg P.O. 8 hours after first dose. Then follow with 8 mg q 12 hours for 1 to 2 days. Or, give single dose of 32 mg by I.V. infusion over 15 minutes beginning 30 minutes before chemotherapy; or three divided doses of 0.15 mg/kg I.V. Give first dose 30 minutes before chemotherapy; give subsequent doses 4 and 8 hours after first dose. Infuse drug over 15 minutes.
Children ages 4 to 11: 4 mg P.O. 30 minutes before start of chemotherapy. Follow with 4 mg P.O. 4 and 8 hours after first dose. Then follow with 4 mg q 8 hours for 1 to 2 days. Or, three doses of 0.15 mg/kg I.V. Give first dose 30 minutes before chemotherapy; give subsequent doses 4 and 8 hours after first dose. Infuse drug over 15 minutes.

▶ **Prevention of nausea and vomiting caused by highly emetogenic chemotherapy.** *Adults:* 24 mg P.O. 30 minutes before start of chemotherapy.

▶ **Prevention of postoperative nausea and vomiting.** *Adults:* 4 mg I.V. (undiluted) over 2 to 5 minutes immediately before induction of anesthesia or postoperatively. Or, 4 mg I.M. as a single injection immediately before induction of anesthesia or postoperatively. Or, 16 mg P.O. 1 hour before induction of anesthesia.
Children ages 2 to 12 weighing 40 kg (88 lb) or less: 0.1 mg/kg I.V. Give dose over 2 to 5 minutes as a single dose.
Children ages 2 to 12 weighing more than 40 kg: Give 4 mg I.V. over 2 to 5 minutes as a single dose.

▶ **Prevention of nausea and vomiting related to radiotherapy, either total body irradiation or single high-dose fraction or daily fractions to the abdomen.** *Adults:* 8 mg P.O. t.i.d.
⊠ Adjust-a-dose: For patients with severe liver impairment, don't exceed total daily dose of 8 mg P.O. daily or a single maximum dose of 8 mg I.V. over 15 minutes.

▽ I.V. administration

- Dilute drug in 50 ml of D₅W injection or normal saline solution for injection before giving.
- Infuse drug over 15 minutes.

- Drug is stable for up to 48 hours after dilution in 5% dextrose in normal saline solution for injection, 5% dextrose in half-normal saline solution for injection, and 3% saline solution for injection.

Contraindications and precautions

- Contraindicated in patients hypersensitive to drug.
- Use cautiously and at a reduced dosage in patients with liver failure.
⚘ Lifespan: In pregnant and breast-feeding women, use cautiously. In children, safety and effectiveness of the 24-mg tablet or the use of oral forms of drug for postoperative nausea and vomiting or radiation-induced nausea and vomiting haven't been established. In children younger than age 2, information on safety and effectiveness of injection forms of drug is limited.

Adverse reactions

CNS: headache.
GI: diarrhea, constipation.
Skin: rash.

Interactions

Drug-drug. *Drugs that alter hepatic drug-metabolizing enzymes (such as cimetidine, phenobarbital):* May alter pharmacokinetics of ondansetron. No dosage adjustment appears necessary.
Rifampin: Ondansetron levels may be reduced, thereby decreasing antiemetic effect. Monitor patient for adequate antiemetic effect; adjust dosage as necessary.

Effects on lab test results

- May increase ALT and AST levels.

Pharmacokinetics

Absorption: Variable; bioavailability is 50% to 60%.
Distribution: 70% to 76% is protein-bound.
Metabolism: Extensively metabolized.
Excretion: Primarily excreted in urine. *Half-life:* 4 hours.

Route	Onset	Peak	Duration
P.O., I.V.	Unknown	Unknown	Unknown

Rapid onset   *Liquid form contains alcohol.   ◆ Canada   ◇ Australia   †OTC   ‡Off-label use

Action

Chemical effect: Blocking action may take place in CNS at area postrema (chemoreceptor trigger zone) and in peripheral nervous system on terminals of vagus nerve.
Therapeutic effect: Prevents nausea and vomiting from emetogenic chemotherapy or surgery.

Available forms

Injection: 2 mg/ml, 4 mg/ml
Oral solution: 4 mg/5 ml
Tablets: 4 mg, 8 mg, 24 mg
Tablets (orally disintegrating): 4 mg, 8 mg

NURSING PROCESS

⚖ Assessment
● Assess patient's condition before therapy and regularly thereafter.
● Be alert for adverse reactions and drug interactions.
● Evaluate patient's and family's knowledge of drug therapy.

⚕ Nursing diagnoses
● Risk for deficient fluid volume related to nausea and vomiting
● Pain related to drug-induced headache
● Deficient knowledge related to drug therapy

▶ Planning and implementation
⊛ ALERT: Don't confuse Zofran with Zantac or Zosyn.
⊛ ALERT: Don't confuse Zofran with Precedex. These vials appear very similar.
Patient teaching
● Instruct patient when to take drug.
● Tell patient to report adverse reactions.
● Advise patient to report any discomfort at I.V. site.

☑ Evaluation
● Patient maintains adequate hydration.
● Patient does not experience any drug-induced headaches.
● Patient and family state understanding of drug therapy.

opium tincture*
(OH-pee-um TINK-shur)

opium tincture, camphorated* (paregoric)

Pharmacologic class: opiate
Therapeutic class: antidiarrheal
Pregnancy risk category: C
Controlled substance schedule: II (III for opium tincture, camphorated)

Indications and dosages

▶ **Acute, nonspecific diarrhea.** *Adults:* 0.6 ml (range 0.3 to 1 ml) opium tincture P.O. q.i.d. Maximum dosage is 6 ml daily. Or, 5 to 10 ml camphorated opium tincture once daily, b.i.d., t.i.d., or q.i.d. until diarrhea subsides.
Children: 0.25 to 0.5 ml/kg camphorated opium tincture P.O. once daily, b.i.d., t.i.d., or q.i.d. until diarrhea subsides.
▶ **Severe opiate withdrawal symptoms in neonates born to women addicted to opiates‡.**
Neonates: Camphorated opium tincture (paregoric) or a 1:25 dilution of opium tincture in water given as 3 to 6 drops or 0.2 ml q 3 hours. Adjust dose to control symptoms. May be increased by 0.05 ml q 3 hours until symptoms are controlled. Don't exceed 0.7 ml per dose. Once symptoms are stabilized for 3 to 5 days, gradually decrease dose over a 2- to 4-week period.

Contraindications and precautions

● Contraindicated in patients with acute diarrhea resulting from poisoning, until toxic material is removed from GI tract. Also contraindicated in patients with diarrhea caused by organisms that penetrate intestinal mucosa.
● Use cautiously in patients with asthma, prostatic hyperplasia, hepatic disease, or opioid dependence.
⚖ **Lifespan:** In pregnant and breast-feeding women, safety of drug hasn't been established.

Adverse reactions

CNS: dizziness, light-headedness.
GI: nausea, vomiting.
Other: physical dependence after long-term use.

Reactions may be *common*, uncommon, *life-threatening*, or **COMMON AND LIFE-THREATENING**.

Interactions

None significant.

Effects on lab test results

• May increase amylase and lipase levels.

Pharmacokinetics

Absorption: Variable.
Distribution: Distributed widely in body.
Metabolism: Metabolized in liver.
Excretion: Excreted in urine. *Half-life:* Unknown.

Route	Onset	Peak	Duration
P.O.	Unknown	Unknown	Unknown

Action

Chemical effect: Increases smooth-muscle tone in GI tract, inhibits motility and propulsion, and diminishes secretions.
Therapeutic effect: Relieves diarrhea.

Available forms

opium tincture
Oral solution: 50 mg/5 ml (equivalent to morphine 10 mg/ml*)
opium tincture, camphorated
Oral solution: Each 5 ml contains morphine, 2 mg; anise oil, 0.2 ml; benzoic acid, 20 mg; camphor, 20 mg; glycerin, 0.2 ml; and ethanol to make 5 ml*

NURSING PROCESS

Assessment
• Assess patient's condition before therapy and regularly thereafter.
• Be alert for adverse reactions.
• Monitor patient's hydration status throughout drug therapy.
• Evaluate patient's and family's knowledge of drug therapy.

Nursing diagnoses
• Diarrhea related to GI disorder
• Risk for deficient fluid volume related to diarrhea and drug-induced adverse GI reactions
• Deficient knowledge related to drug therapy

Planning and implementation
ⓘ ALERT: Read label carefully. Opium content of opium tincture is 25 times greater than that of camphorated opium tincture (paregoric). Don't

confuse the two. Also, camphorated opium tincture (paregoric) is more dilute, and teaspoonful doses are easier to measure than dropper quantities of opium tincture.
• Mix drug with water to form a milky fluid.
• Store drug in tightly capped, light-resistant container.
• For overdose, use opioid antagonist naloxone to reverse respiratory depression.

Patient teaching
• Advise patient against using drug for more than 2 days; risk of dependence increases with long-term use.
• Encourage proper storage to keep drug out of children's hands.

☑ Evaluation
• Patient's diarrhea ceases.
• Patient maintains adequate hydration.
• Patient and family state understanding of drug.

orlistat

(OR-lih-stat)
Xenical

Pharmacologic class: lipase inhibitor
Therapeutic class: antiobesity drug
Pregnancy risk category: B

Indications and dosages

▶ **Management of obesity, including weight loss and weight maintenance, given with a reduced-calorie diet; reduction of risk of weight regain after weight loss.** *Adults:*
120 mg P.O. t.i.d. with each main meal containing fat (during or up to 1 hour after the meal).

Contraindications and precautions

• Contraindicated in patients hypersensitive to drug or any of its components and in patients with chronic malabsorption syndrome or cholestasis.
• Use cautiously in patients with a history of hyperoxaluria or calcium oxalate nephrolithiasis and in patients who are at risk for anorexia nervosa or bulimia, or who are receiving cyclosporine therapy because of possible changes in cyclosporine absorption related to variations in diet.

☆ Lifespan: In pregnant and breast-feeding women, drug isn't recommended. In children, safety of drug hasn't been established.

Adverse reactions

CNS: *headache,* dizziness, fatigue, sleep disorder, anxiety, depression.
CV: pedal edema.
EENT: otitis.
GI: *oily spotting, flatus with discharge, fecal urgency, fatty or oily stool, oily evacuation, increased defecation, abdominal pain,* fecal incontinence, nausea, infectious diarrhea, rectal pain, vomiting.
GU: menstrual irregularity, vaginitis, UTI.
Musculoskeletal: *back pain,* leg pain, arthritis, myalgia, joint disorder, tendinitis.
Respiratory: *influenza, upper respiratory tract infection,* lower respiratory tract infection.
Skin: rash, dry skin.
Other: tooth and gingival disorders.

Interactions

Drug-drug. *Fat-soluble vitamins such as vitamin E, beta-carotene:* Decreases vitamin absorption. Separate administration times by 2 hours.
Pravastatin: Slightly increases pravastatin levels and increases lipid-lowering effects of drug. Monitor patient.
Warfarin: Possible change in coagulation parameters. Monitor INR.

Effects on lab test results

• May decrease vitamin D, beta-carotene, LDL, and total cholesterol levels.

Pharmacokinetics

Absorption: Systemic exposure is minimal because only a small amount of drug is absorbed.
Distribution: More than 99% binds to proteins. Lipoproteins and albumin are major binding proteins.
Metabolism: Primarily in GI wall.
Excretion: Most unabsorbed drug is excreted in feces. *Half-life:* Unknown.

Route	Onset	Peak	Duration
P.O.	Unknown	Unknown	Unknown

Action

Chemical effect: Bonds with the active site of gastric and pancreatic lipases. These inactivated enzymes are thus unavailable to hydrolyze dietary fat, in the form of triglycerides, into absorbable free fatty acids and monoglycerides. Because the undigested triglycerides aren't absorbed, the resulting caloric deficit may help with weight control. The recommended dosage of 120 mg t.i.d. inhibits dietary fat absorption by about 30%.
Therapeutic effect: Weight loss and weight maintenance.

Available forms

Capsules: 120 mg

NURSING PROCESS

🗹 Assessment
• Obtain history of patient's underlying condition before therapy, and reassess regularly thereafter.
• Screen patient for anorexia nervosa or bulimia; as with any weight-loss drug, drug can be misused.
• Organic causes of obesity, such as hypothyroidism, must be ruled out before patient starts orlistat therapy.
• In diabetic patients, monitor glucose frequently during weight loss. Dosage of oral antidiabetic or insulin may need to be reduced.
• Evaluate patient's and family's knowledge of drug therapy.

🖭 Nursing diagnoses
• Imbalanced nutrition: More than body requirements related to obesity
• Disturbed body image related to obesity
• Deficient knowledge related to drug therapy

➤ Planning and implementation
• Drug is recommended for patients with an initial body mass index of 30 kg/m² or more (27 kg/m² or more if patient has other risk factors, such as hypertension, diabetes, or dyslipidemia).
• It's unknown whether drug is safe and effective to use longer than 2 years.
• Tell patient to follow dietary guidelines. GI effects may increase when patient takes drug with high-fat foods—specifically, when more than 30% of total daily calories come from fat.
• Drug reduces absorption of some fat-soluble vitamins and beta-carotene.
⚠ ALERT: Don't confuse Xenical with Xeloda.

Reactions may be *common,* uncommon, *life-threatening,* or COMMON AND LIFE-THREATENING.

Patient teaching
• Advise patient to follow a nutritionally balanced, reduced-calorie diet that derives only 30% of its calories from fat. Daily intake of fat, carbohydrate, and protein should be distributed over three main meals. If a meal is occasionally missed or contains no fat, tell patient that dose can be skipped.
• To ensure adequate nutrition, advise patient to take a daily multivitamin supplement that contains fat-soluble vitamins within at least 2 hours of taking drug, such as h.s.
• Tell patient with diabetes that weight loss may improve glycemic control, so the dosage of his oral antidiabetic or insulin may need to be reduced.
• Tell woman to inform prescriber if she is pregnant, plans to become pregnant, or is breast-feeding.

☑ Evaluation
• Patient's nutritional intake is adequate according to proper dietary guidelines.
• Patient reaches and maintains a stable weight.
• Patient and family state understanding of drug therapy.

---

oseltamivir phosphate
(ah-sul-TAM-ih-veer FOS-fayt)
Tamiflu

Pharmacologic class: neuraminidase inhibitor
Therapeutic class: antiviral
Pregnancy risk category: C

Indications and dosages
▶ **Uncomplicated, acute illness from influenza in patients who have been symptomatic for 2 days or less.** *Adults and children age 13 and older:* 75 mg P.O. b.i.d. for 5 days.
Children age 1 and older who weigh 15 kg (33 lb) or less: 30 mg oral suspension P.O. b.i.d.
Children age 1 and older who weigh more than 15 to 23 kg (33 to 51 lb): 45 mg oral suspension P.O. b.i.d.
Children age 1 and older who weigh more than 23 to 40 kg (51 to 88 lb): 60 mg oral suspension P.O. b.i.d.
Children who weigh more than 40 kg (88 lb): 75 mg oral suspension P.O. b.i.d.

◩ **Adjust-a-dose:** For patients with renal impairment, if creatinine clearance is 10 to 30 ml/minute, give 75 mg once daily for 5 days.
▶ **Prevention of influenza after close contact with infected person.** *Adults and children age 13 and older:* 75 mg P.O. once daily beginning within 2 days of exposure and lasting at least 7 days.
◩ **Adjust-a-dose:** For patients with renal impairment, if creatinine clearance is 10 to 30 ml/minute, give 75 mg once q other day or 30 mg of oral suspension daily.
▶ **Prevention of influenza during a community outbreak.** *Adults and children age 13 and older:* 75 mg P.O. daily for up to 6 weeks.
◩ **Adjust-a-dose:** For patients with renal impairment, if creatinine clearance is 10 to 30 ml/minute, give 75 mg once q other day or 30 mg of oral suspension daily.

Contraindications and precautions
• Contraindicated in patients hypersensitive to drug or its components.
⚖ **Lifespan:** In breast-feeding women, use drug only if potential benefits outweigh risks to the infant. In children younger than age 1, use for treatment of influenza hasn't been established. In children younger than age 13, use for prevention of influenza hasn't been established.

Adverse reactions
CNS: dizziness, insomnia, headache, vertigo, fatigue.
GI: abdominal pain, diarrhea, nausea, vomiting.
Respiratory: bronchitis, cough.

Interactions
None significant.

Effects on lab test results
None reported.

Pharmacokinetics
Absorption: Well absorbed. More than 75% reaches systemic circulation as oseltamivir carboxylate.
Distribution: Protein-binding for oseltamivir is 42%; 3% for oseltamivir carboxylate.
Metabolism: Extensively metabolized by hepatic esterases to its active component, oseltamivir carboxylate.
Excretion: Oseltamivir carboxylate is almost entirely eliminated in urine via glomerular fil-

tration and tubular secretion. Less than 20% is eliminated in feces.

Route	Onset	Peak	Duration
P.O.	Unknown	Unknown	Unknown

Action

Chemical effect: Oseltamivir carboxylate, the active form of oseltamivir, inhibits the enzyme neuraminidase in influenza virus particles. This action is thought to inhibit viral replication, possibly by interfering with viral particle aggregation and release from the host cell.
Therapeutic effect: Lessens the symptoms of influenza.

Available forms

Capsules: 75 mg
Oral suspension: 12 mg/ml after reconstitution

NURSING PROCESS

Assessment
• Obtain complete medical history before treatment.
• Evaluate renal function before giving drug, as directed.
• Evaluate patient's and family's knowledge of drug therapy.

Nursing diagnoses
• Infection related to influenza virus
• Imbalanced nutrition: Less than body requirements related to drug's adverse GI effects
• Deficient knowledge related to drug therapy

Planning and implementation
• Drug is used primarily to treat symptoms; it is not a replacement for an annual influenza vaccination.
• No evidence supports use in treating other viral infections.
• Drug may be given with meals to decrease adverse GI effects.
• Safety and effectiveness of repeated treatment courses haven't been established.
• Store at controlled room temperature (59° to 86° F [15° to 30° C]).
Patient teaching
• Tell patient to take drug within 2 days of start of symptoms.
• Inform patient that receiving this drug isn't a substitute for receiving the flu vaccination. Urge

patient to continue receiving an annual vaccination.

Evaluation
• Patient recovers from influenza.
• Patient has no adverse GI effects and maintains adequate hydration.
• Patient and family state understanding of drug therapy.

oxaliplatin
(ox-ah-leh-PLA-tin)
Eloxatin

Pharmacologic class: alkylating drug
Therapeutic class: antineoplastic
Pregnancy risk category: D

Indications and dosages

▶ **Metastatic colon or rectal cancer that has recurred or progressed during or within 6 months of completion of first-line therapy with 5-fluorouracil (5-FU) or leucovorin and irinotecan.** *Adults:* On day one, 85 mg/m² oxaliplatin I.V. in 250 to 500 ml D_5W and 200 mg/m² leucovorin I.V. in D_5W, given simultaneously over 2 hours in separate bags using a Y-line. Then, 400 mg/m² 5-FU I.V. bolus given over 2 to 4 minutes, followed by 600 mg/m² 5-FU I.V. infusion in 500 ml D_5W over 22 hours. On day two, 200 mg/m² leucovorin I.V. infusion over 2 hours. Then, 400 mg/m² 5-FU I.V. bolus given over 2 to 4 minutes, followed by 600 mg/m² 5-FU I.V. infusion in 500 ml D_5W over 22 hours. Repeat cycle q 2 weeks.
Adjust-a-dose: In patients with unresolved and persistent grade 2 neurosensory events (events that interfere with function, but not daily activities), reduce dose to 65 mg/m². In patients with persistent grade 3 neurosensory events (pain and functional impairment that affect daily activity), consider stopping drug. In patients recovering from grade 3 or 4 GI (severe or life-threatening altered function) or hematologic (neutrophil count less than $1.5 \times 10^9/L$ and platelet count less than $100 \times 10^9/L$) events, reduce dose to 65 mg/m². Also reduce dose of 5-FU by 20%.

▼ I.V. administration

• Preparing and giving drug may have carcinogenic, mutagenic, and teratogenic risks. Follow facility policy to reduce risks.
• Reconstitute powder using sterile water for injection or D_5W. Add 10 ml to a 50-mg vial or 20 ml to a 100-mg vial for a final concentration of 5 mg/ml. Never reconstitute with sodium chloride solution or other solution containing chloride.
• Further dilute reconstituted solutions in an infusion solution of 250 to 500 ml of D_5W.
• Inspect bag for particulate matter and discoloration before giving and discard if present.
• Don't use needles or I.V. administration sets that contain aluminum because they will react with platinum in drug, causing loss of potency and formation of a black precipitate.
• Drug doesn't require prehydration.
• Premedicate with antiemetics with or without dexamethasone.
• Give oxaliplatin and leucovorin over 2 hours at the same time in separate bags, using a Y-line. Extend the infusion time to 6 hours to decrease acute toxicities.
• Avoid ice and cold exposure during infusion of drug because cold temperatures can exacerbate acute neurologic symptoms. Cover patient with a blanket during infusion.
⊛ **ALERT:** Don't give this drug in the same line as 5-FU or other alkaline solutions. Flush infusion line with D_5W before giving any other drugs simultaneously.
• Store unopened vials at room temperature. Reconstituted solutions are stable if refrigerated (36° to 46° F [2° to 8° C]) for up to 24 hours. After final dilution, solutions are stable for 6 hours at room temperature and up to 24 hours under refrigeration.

Contraindications and precautions

• Contraindicated in patients allergic to drug or other platinum-containing compounds.
• Use cautiously in patients with preexisting renal impairment or peripheral sensory neuropathy.
⚠ **Lifespan:** In pregnant women, drug is contraindicated. In breast-feeding women and in children, safety and effectiveness of drug haven't been established. In elderly patients, use cautiously because diarrhea, dehydration, hypokalemia, and fatigue may occur more frequently in these patients.

Adverse reactions

CNS: *pain, peripheral neuropathy, fatigue, headache, dizziness, insomnia, fever.*
CV: chest pain, **thromboembolism**, edema, *flushing, peripheral edema.*
EENT: *rhinitis*, pharyngitis, epistaxis, abnormal lacrimation.
GI: *nausea, vomiting, diarrhea, stomatitis, abdominal pain, anorexia, constipation, dyspepsia, taste perversion,* gastroesophageal reflux, flatulence, mucositis.
GU: dysuria, hematuria.
Hematologic: FEBRILE NEUTROPENIA, *anemia,* LEUKOPENIA, THROMBOCYTOPENIA.
Metabolic: hypokalemia, dehydration.
Musculoskeletal: *back pain, arthralgia.*
Respiratory: *dyspnea, cough, upper respiratory tract infection,* hiccups, **pulmonary toxicity.**
Skin: rash, alopecia.
Other: *injection site reaction,* **anaphylaxis,** *hand-foot syndrome, allergic reaction,* rigors.

Interactions

Drug-drug. *Nephrotoxic drugs (such as gentamicin):* May decrease elimination of drug and increase levels. Monitor patient for signs and symptoms of toxicity.

Effects on lab test results

• May increase creatinine, bilirubin, AST, and ALT levels. May decrease potassium level.
• May decrease hemoglobin and neutrophil, WBC, and platelet counts.

Pharmacokinetics

Absorption: Administered I.V.
Distribution: Wide tissue distribution. More than 90% protein-bound.
Metabolism: Undergoes non-enzymatic biotransformation. No evidence of CYP-mediated metabolism.
Excretion: Primarily renal. *Half-life:* Unknown.

Route	Onset	Peak	Duration
I.V.	Unknown	Unknown	Unknown

Action

Chemical effect: May inhibit cell replication and transcription by forming platinum complexes that cross-link with DNA molecules.
Therapeutic effect: Inhibits cancer cell formation

Available forms

Injection: 50- or 100-mg vials

NURSING PROCESS

⚗ Assessment
• Monitor CBC, platelet count, and liver and kidney function before each chemotherapy cycle.
• Monitor patient for hypersensitivity reactions, which may occur within minutes of giving drug.
• Monitor patient for injection site reaction. Extravasation may occur.
• Monitor patient for neuropathy and pulmonary toxicity. Peripheral neuropathy may be acute or persistent. Acute neuropathy is reversible; it occurs within 2 days of therapy and resolves within 14 days. Persistent peripheral neuropathy occurs more than 14 days after therapy and causes paresthesias, dysesthesias, hypoesthesias, and decrease in sensation that can interfere with daily activities (such as walking or swallowing).
• Evaluate patient's and family's knowledge of drug therapy.

🔲 Nursing diagnoses
• Ineffective health maintenance related to cancer
• Ineffective protection related to drug-induced adverse hematologic reactions
• Deficient knowledge related to drug therapy

▷ Planning and implementation
• Drug clearance is reduced in patients with renal impairment. Dosage adjustment for patients with renal impairment hasn't been established.
Patient teaching
• Inform patient of potential adverse reactions.
• Tell patient to avoid exposure to cold or cold objects (such as cold drinks or ice cubes), which can bring on or worsen acute symptoms of peripheral neuropathy. Advise patient to have warm drinks, wear warm clothing, and cover any exposed skin, such as on hands, face, and head. Have patient warm the air going into his lungs by wearing a scarf or ski mask. Have him wear gloves when touching cold objects (such as foods in the freezer, outside door handles, and mailbox).
• Tell patient to contact prescriber immediately if he has trouble breathing or experiences signs

and symptoms of an allergic reaction (rash, hives, swelling of lips or tongue, sudden cough).
• Tell patient to contact prescriber if fever, signs and symptoms of an infection, persistent vomiting, diarrhea, or signs and symptoms of dehydration (thirst, dry mouth, lightheadedness, and decreased urination) occur.

✓ Evaluation
• Patient responds well to therapy.
• Patient develops no serious complications from drug-induced adverse hematologic reactions.
• Patient and family state understanding of drug therapy.

oxaprozin potassium
(oks-uh-PROH-zin)
Apo-Oxaprozin ◆, Daypro, Daypro ALTA, Rhoxal-Oxaprozin ◆

Pharmacologic class: NSAID
Therapeutic class: non-opioid analgesic, antipyretic, anti-inflammatory
Pregnancy risk category: C

Indications and dosages

▶ **Osteoarthritis, rheumatoid arthritis.**
Adults: 1,200 mg P.O. once daily. Divided doses may be used in patients unable to tolerate single doses. For osteoarthritis patients with low body weight and milder disease, an initial dose of 600 mg once daily may be appropriate. Maximum daily dose, 1,200 mg.
◻ Adjust-a-dose: For patients with renal impairment or those undergoing hemodialysis, initial dose is 600 mg P.O. daily.

Contraindications and precautions

• Contraindicated in patients hypersensitive to drug and in those with syndrome of nasal polyps, angioedema, and bronchospastic reactivity to aspirin or other NSAIDs.
• Use cautiously in patients with history of peptic ulcer disease, hepatic or renal dysfunction, hypertension, CV disease, or conditions that predispose to fluid retention.
🕭 **Lifespan:** In pregnant and breast-feeding women, use cautiously. In children, safety of drug hasn't been established.

Adverse reactions

CNS: depression, sedation, somnolence, confusion, sleep disturbances.
EENT: tinnitus, visual disturbances.
GI: *nausea, dyspepsia, diarrhea, constipation,* abdominal pain or distress, anorexia, flatulence, vomiting, *GI hemorrhage.*
GU: dysuria, renal insufficiency, urinary frequency.
Skin: *rash,* photosensitivity.

Interactions

Drug-drug. *Antihypertensives, diuretics:* Decreases effect. Monitor patient closely and adjust dosage.
Aspirin: Oxaprozin displaces salicylates from protein-binding sites, increasing risk of salicylate toxicity. Avoid using together.
Aspirin, corticosteroids: Increases risk of adverse GI reactions. Avoid using together.
Cyclosporine: Risk of nephrotoxicity by both drugs may increase. Monitor renal function tests.
Methotrexate: Increases risk of methotrexate toxicity. Avoid using together.
Oral anticoagulants: Increases risk of bleeding. Use together cautiously; monitor patient for bleeding.
Drug-herb. *Dong quai, feverfew, garlic, ginger, horse chestnut, red clover:* May increase risk of bleeding. Discourage using together.
St. John's wort: Increases risk of photosensitivity. Advise patient to avoid unprotected or prolonged exposure to sunlight.
Drug-lifestyle. *Alcohol use:* Increases risk of adverse GI reactions. Discourage using together.
Sun exposure: Photosensitivity reactions may occur. Urge patient to avoid unprotected or prolonged exposure to sunlight.

Effects on lab test results

• May increase ALT, AST, BUN, and creatinine levels.
• May increase bleeding time. May decrease hemoglobin and hematocrit.

Pharmacokinetics

Absorption: Oral bioavailability is 95%; food may reduce rate but not extent of absorption.
Distribution: About 99.9% protein-bound.
Metabolism: Metabolized in liver.
Excretion: Metabolites are excreted in urine (65%) and feces (35%). *Half-life:* 5 hours.

Route	Onset	Peak	Duration
P.O.	Unknown	2 hr	Unknown

Action

Chemical effect: Unknown; may inhibit prostaglandin synthesis.
Therapeutic effect: Relieves pain, fever, and inflammation.

Available forms

Caplets: 600 mg
Tablets: 600 mg

NURSING PROCESS

⚕ Assessment

• Assess patient's condition before therapy and regularly thereafter.
• Monitor liver function test results periodically during long-term therapy, and closely monitor patient with abnormal test results. Liver function values may be elevated. These abnormal findings may persist, worsen, or resolve with continued therapy. Rarely, patient may progress to severe hepatic dysfunction.
• Be alert for adverse reactions and drug interactions.
• Evaluate patient's and family's knowledge of drug therapy.

🔲 Nursing diagnoses

• Chronic pain related to condition
• Impaired tissue integrity related to adverse GI effects of drug
• Deficient knowledge related to drug therapy

▶ Planning and implementation

• Give drug on empty stomach unless adverse GI reactions occur.
• Notify prescriber immediately about adverse reactions, especially GI symptoms.
⑤ ALERT: Don't confuse oxaprozin with oxazepam.
Patient teaching
• To minimize adverse GI effects, tell patient to take drug with milk or meals.
• Explain that full therapeutic effects may be delayed for 2 to 4 weeks.
• Tell patient to report adverse visual or auditory reactions immediately.
• Teach patient to recognize and promptly report signs and symptoms of GI bleeding.

- Advise patient to use sunscreen, wear protective clothing, and avoid prolonged exposure to sunlight.
- Warn patient to avoid hazardous activities until CNS effects of drug are known.

☑ Evaluation
- Patient is free from pain.
- Patient maintains GI tissue integrity.
- Patient and family state understanding of drug therapy.

oxazepam
(oks-AZ-ih-pam)
Alepam◇, Apo-Oxazepam◆, Murelax◇, Novoxapam◆, Serax, Serepax◇

Pharmacologic class: benzodiazepine
Therapeutic class: antianxiety, sedative-hypnotic
Pregnancy risk category: D
Controlled substance schedule: IV

Indications and dosages
▶ **Alcohol withdrawal.** *Adults:* 15 to 30 mg P.O. t.i.d. or q.i.d.
▶ **Severe anxiety.** *Adults:* 15 to 30 mg P.O. t.i.d. or q.i.d.
▶ **Mild-to-moderate anxiety.** *Adults:* 10 to 15 mg P.O. t.i.d. or q.i.d.
▶ **Older patients with anxiety, tension, irritability, and agitation.** *Adults:* 10 mg P.O. t.i.d. May increase cautiously to 15 mg P.O. t.i.d. to q.i.d.

Contraindications and precautions
- Contraindicated in patients hypersensitive to drug.
- Use cautiously in patients with history of drug abuse and in those for whom a drop in blood pressure could lead to cardiac problems.
- ☀ **Lifespan:** In pregnant and breast-feeding women, avoid using drug. In children, safety of drug hasn't been established. In geriatric patients, use cautiously.

Adverse reactions
CNS: drowsiness, lethargy, hangover, fainting, *mental status changes.*
CV: transient hypotension.
GI: nausea, vomiting, abdominal discomfort.

Hepatic: *hepatic dysfunction.*
Other: increased risk for falls.

Interactions
Drug-drug. *Cimetidine, CNS depressants:* Increases CNS depression. Avoid using together.
Digoxin: May increase digoxin levels, increasing toxicity. Monitor levels closely.
Hormonal contraceptives: Increases clearance of oxazepam. Monitor patient for decreased effect.
Phenytoin: May increase oxazepam clearance and increase phenytoin concentration. Monitor patient closely for phenytoin toxicity.
Drug-herb. *Catnip, kava, lady's slipper, lemon balm, passionflower, sassafras, skullcap, valerian:* Sedative effects may be enhanced. Discourage using together.
Drug-lifestyle. *Alcohol use:* Increases CNS depression. Discourage using together.
Smoking: Increases benzodiazepine clearance. Monitor patient for lack of drug effect.

Effects on lab test results
- May increase liver enzyme function values.

Pharmacokinetics
Absorption: Well absorbed.
Distribution: Distributed widely throughout body. Drug is 85% to 95% protein-bound.
Metabolism: Metabolized in liver.
Excretion: Metabolites are excreted in urine.
Half-life: 5 to 13 hours.

Route	Onset	Peak	Duration
P.O.	Unknown	3 hr	Unknown

Action
Chemical effect: Unknown; believed to stimulate gamma-aminobutyric receptors in ascending reticular activating system.
Therapeutic effect: Relieves anxiety and promotes calmness.

Available forms
Capsules: 10 mg, 15 mg, 30 mg
Tablets: 10 mg, 15 mg, 30 mg

NURSING PROCESS

☑ Assessment
- Assess patient's condition before therapy and regularly thereafter.

- Monitor liver, renal, and hematopoietic function studies periodically in patient receiving repeated or prolonged therapy.
- Be alert for adverse reactions and drug interactions.
- Evaluate patient's and family's knowledge of drug therapy.

⊕ **Nursing diagnoses**
- Disturbed thought processes related to condition
- Risk for injury related to drug-induced adverse CNS reactions
- Deficient knowledge related to drug therapy

▷ **Planning and implementation**
- Reduce dosage in geriatric or debilitated patient.
- Possibility of abuse and addiction exists. Don't stop drug abruptly; withdrawal symptoms may occur.
- ⊛ **ALERT:** Don't confuse oxazepam with oxaprozin.

Patient teaching
- Warn patient to avoid hazardous activities until CNS effects of drug are known.
- Tell patient to avoid alcohol during drug therapy.
- Warn patient not to stop drug abruptly; withdrawal signs may occur.

☑ **Evaluation**
- Patient has less anxiety.
- Patient sustains no injury as result of drug therapy.
- Patient and family state understanding of drug therapy.

oxcarbazepine
(ox-car-bay-zah-peen)
Trileptal

Pharmacologic class: carboxamide derivative
Therapeutic class: antiepileptic
Pregnancy risk category: C

Indications and dosages

▶ **Adjunctive therapy for partial seizures in patients with epilepsy.** *Adults:* Initially, 300 mg P.O. b.i.d. Increase by maximum of 600 mg daily (300 mg P.O. b.i.d.) at weekly intervals. Recommended daily dosage is 600 mg P.O. b.i.d.
Children ages 4 to 16: Initially, 4 to 5 mg/kg P.O. b.i.d., not to exceed 600 mg P.O. daily. Target maintenance dosage depends on patient weight. If patient weighs 20 to 29 kg (44 to 64 lb), target maintenance dosage is 900 mg daily. If 29.1 to 39 kg (64 to 86 lb), target maintenance dosage is 1,200 mg daily. If more than 39 kg (86 lb), target maintenance dosage is 1,800 mg daily. Achieve target dosage over 2 weeks.
▶ **Conversion to monotherapy for partial seizures in patients with epilepsy.** *Adults:* Initially, 300 mg P.O. b.i.d. with simultaneous reduction in dosage of other antiepileptics. Increase by a maximum of 600 mg daily at weekly intervals over 2 to 4 weeks. Recommended daily dose is 2,400 mg P.O., divided b.i.d. Withdraw other antiepileptics completely over 3 to 6 weeks.
Children ages 4 to 16: Initially 8 to 10 mg/kg P.O. daily divided b.i.d., with simultaneous reduction in dose of other antiepileptics. Increase by a maximum of 10 mg/kg daily at weekly intervals. Withdraw other antiepileptics completely over 3 to 6 weeks.
▶ **Initial monotherapy for partial seizures in patients with epilepsy.** *Adults:* Initially, 300 mg P.O. b.i.d. Increase by 300 mg daily q third day to a total daily dose of 1,200 mg.
Children ages 4 to 16: Initially, 8 to 10 mg/kg P.O. daily divided b.i.d., increasing the dosage by 5 mg/kg daily q third day to the recommended daily dosage: 20 to 24 kg (44 to 54 lb), 600 to 900 mg; 25 to 34 kg (55 to 76 lb), 900 to 1,200 mg; 35 to 44 kg (77 to 98 lb), 900 to 1,500 mg; 45 to 49 kg (99 to 109 lb), 1,200 to 1,500 mg; 50 to 59 kg (110 to 131 lb), 1,200 to 1,800 mg; 60 to 69 kg (132 to 153 lb), 1,200 to 2,100 mg; 70 kg (154 lb), 1,500 to 2,100 mg.
⊠ **Adjust-a-dose:** For patients with renal impairment, if creatinine clearance is less than 30 ml/minute, therapy starts at 150 mg P.O. b.i.d. (one-half the usual starting dose) and increases slowly to achieve desired clinical response.

Contraindications and precautions

- Contraindicated in patients hypersensitive to drug or its components.
- Use cautiously in patients who have had hypersensitivity reactions to carbamazepine.

≜ Lifespan: Breast-feeding women should either stop breast-feeding or stop the drug, taking into account the importance of drug to her.

Adverse reactions

CNS: *fatigue,* fever, asthenia, feeling abnormal, *headache, dizziness, somnolence, ataxia, abnormal gait,* insomnia, *tremor,* nervousness, agitation, abnormal coordination, speech disorder, confusion, anxiety, amnesia, **aggravated seizures,** hypoesthesia, emotional lability, impaired concentration, *vertigo.*
CV: hypotension, edema, chest pain.
EENT: *nystagmus, diplopia, abnormal vision,* abnormal accommodation, rhinitis, sinusitis, pharyngitis, epistaxis.
GI: *nausea, vomiting, abdominal pain,* diarrhea, dyspepsia, constipation, gastritis, anorexia, dry mouth, rectal hemorrhage, taste perversion, thirst.
GU: UTI, urinary frequency, vaginitis.
Metabolic: hyponatremia, weight gain.
Musculoskeletal: muscle weakness, back pain.
Respiratory: *upper respiratory tract infection,* coughing, bronchitis, chest infection.
Skin: acne, purpura, rash, bruising, increased sweating.
Other: allergic reaction, hot flushes, toothache.

Interactions

Drug-drug. *Carbamazepine, valproic acid, verapamil:* Decreases levels of the active metabolite of oxcarbazepine. Monitor patient and levels closely.
Felodipine: Decreases felodipine level. Monitor patient closely.
Hormonal contraceptives: Decreases levels of ethinyl estradiol and levonorgestrel, which reduces contraceptive effect. Women of childbearing age should use other forms of contraception.
Phenobarbital: Decreases levels of the active metabolite of oxcarbazepine and increases phenobarbital level. Monitor patient closely.
Phenytoin: Decreases levels of the active metabolite of oxcarbazepine. May increase phenytoin level in adults receiving high doses of oxcarbazepine. Monitor phenytoin levels closely when starting therapy in these patients.
Drug-lifestyle. *Alcohol use:* Increases CNS depression. Discourage using together.

Effects on lab test results

• May decrease sodium and T_4 levels.

Pharmacokinetics

Absorption: Complete.
Distribution: About 40% of active metabolite is bound to proteins, mostly to albumin.
Metabolism: Rapidly metabolized in the liver to active metabolite. 4% of dose is oxidized to inactive metabolite.
Excretion: Drug and its metabolites are mainly excreted by the kidneys. More than 95% of dose appears in urine, with less than 1% as unchanged drug. Fecal excretion accounts for less than 4% of dose. *Half-life:* About 2 hours for drug, about 9 hours for active metabolite. Children younger than age 8 have about 30% to 40% increased clearance of drug.

Route	Onset	Peak	Duration
P.O.	Unknown	Variable	Unknown

Action

Chemical effect: Effect may result from blockade of voltage-sensitive sodium channels, which causes stabilized hyperexcited neural membranes, inhibited repetitive neuronal firing, and reduced synaptic impulses. Also may stem from increased potassium conductance and modulation of high-voltage activated calcium channels.
Therapeutic effect: Controls partial seizures.

Available forms

Oral suspension: 60 mg/ml, 300 mg/5 ml*
Tablets (film-coated): 150 mg, 300 mg, 600 mg

NURSING PROCESS

⚗ Assessment
⊛ ALERT: Ask patient about history of hypersensitivity reaction to carbamazepine because 25% to 30% of affected patients may develop hypersensitivity to this drug. If signs or symptoms of hypersensitivity occur, stop drug immediately.
• Obtain history of patient's underlying condition before therapy, and reassess regularly thereafter.
⊛ ALERT: Drug is linked to several adverse neurologic events, including psychomotor slowing, difficulty with concentration, speech or language problems, somnolence, fatigue, and abnormal coordination (including ataxia and gait disturbances). Monitor patient closely.

Reactions may be *common,* uncommon, *life-threatening,* or **COMMON AND LIFE-THREATENING.**

• Monitor patient for evidence of hyponatremia, including nausea, malaise, headache, lethargy, confusion, and decreased sensation.
• Evaluate patient's and family's knowledge of drug therapy.

🔄 Nursing diagnoses
• Risk for trauma related to seizures
• Risk for injury related to drug-induced adverse reactions
• Deficient knowledge related to drug therapy

▶ Planning and implementation
🔆 **ALERT:** Withdraw drug gradually to minimize risk of increased seizure frequency.
• Correct hyponatremia p.r.n.
• Shake oral suspension well before giving. Suspension can be mixed with water or may be swallowed directly from the syringe. Oral suspension and tablets may be interchanged at equal doses. Suspension can be taken without regard to food.
Patient teaching
• Advise patient to tell prescriber if he has ever had a hypersensitivity reaction to carbamazepine.
• Tell patient that drug may be taken with or without food.
• Warn patient to avoid hazardous activities until effects of drug are known.
• Tell patient to avoid alcohol while taking drug.
• Advise patient not to interrupt therapy without consulting prescriber.
• Advise patient to report signs and symptoms of hyponatremia, such as nausea, malaise, headache, lethargy, or confusion.
• Advise women using hormonal contraceptives for birth control to use another form of birth control while taking drug.

☑ Evaluation
• Patient experiences no or fewer seizures during drug therapy.
• Patient sustains no injury from drug-induced adverse reactions.
• Patient and family state understanding of drug therapy.

oxybutynin chloride
(oks-ee-BYOO-tih-nin KLOR-ighd)
Apo-Oxybutynin ◆ , Ditropan, Ditropan XL, Oxytrol

Pharmacologic class: synthetic tertiary amine
Therapeutic class: antispasmodic
Pregnancy risk category: B

Indications and dosages
▶ **Antispasmodic for uninhibited or reflex neurogenic bladder.** *Adults:* 5 mg P.O. b.i.d. to t.i.d., up to 5 mg q.i.d.
Children older than age 5: 5 mg P.O. b.i.d., up to 5 mg t.i.d.
▶ **Overactive bladder.** *Adults:* Initially, 5 mg Ditropan XL P.O. once daily. Adjust dosage weekly in 5-mg increments, p.r.n., to a maximum of 30 mg P.O. daily. Or, 1 transdermal patch (Oxytrol) twice weekly applied to dry, intact skin on abdomen, hip, or buttocks.

Contraindications and precautions
• Contraindicated in patients hypersensitive to drug and in debilitated patients with intestinal atony, in hemorrhaging patients with unstable CV status, and in patients with myasthenia gravis, GI obstruction, glaucoma, adynamic ileus, megacolon, severe colitis, ulcerative colitis with megacolon, or obstructive uropathy.
• Use cautiously in patients with autonomic neuropathy, reflux esophagitis, or hepatic or renal disease. Use transdermal patch cautiously in patients with bladder outflow obstruction, gastroesophageal reflux, intestinal atony, and in those taking bisphosphonates.
⚖ Lifespan: In pregnant and breast-feeding women and in geriatric patients, use cautiously. In geriatric patients with intestinal atony, drug is contraindicated.

Adverse reactions
Oral form
CNS: *drowsiness,* fever, dizziness, insomnia, restlessness, impaired alertness.
CV: flushing, palpitations, tachycardia.
EENT: *transient blurred vision,* mydriasis, cycloplegia.
GI: nausea, vomiting, *constipation,* bloated feeling, *dry mouth.*

GU: impotence, urinary hesitancy, urine retention.
Skin: decreased diaphoresis, rash, urticaria.
Other: suppressed lactation, allergic reactions.
Transdermal form
CNS: fatigue, somnolence, headache.
CV: flushing.
EENT: abnormal vision.
GI: *dry mouth,* diarrhea, abdominal pain, flatulence, nausea.
GU: dysuria.
Musculoskeletal: back pain.
Skin: *pruritus,* erythema, vesicles, macules, rash, burns.

Interactions

Drug-drug. *Anticholinergics:* Increases anticholinergic effects. Use together cautiously.
Atenolol, digoxin: Increases levels of these drugs. Monitor patient closely.
CNS depressants: Increases CNS effects. Use cautiously.
Drug-lifestyle. *Alcohol use:* Increases CNS effects. Discourage using together.
Exercise, hot weather: May precipitate heatstroke. Urge patient to avoid exercise or any increased activity during hot and humid weather and maintain adequate hydration.

Effects on lab test results

None reported.

Pharmacokinetics

Absorption: Rapid.
Distribution: Unknown. Transdermal system is widely distributed.
Metabolism: By liver. Transdermal system is metabolized by liver and gut wall via CYP 3A4; bypasses first-pass metabolism.
Excretion: Excreted primarily in urine. *Transdermal half-life:* 2 hours.

Route	Onset	Peak	Duration
P.O.	30-60 min	3-4 hr	6-10 hr
Transdermal	24-48 hr	Varies	96 hr

Action

Chemical effect: Produces direct spasmolytic effect and antimuscarinic (atropine-like) effect on smooth muscles of urinary tract, increasing bladder capacity and providing some local anesthesia and mild analgesia.
Therapeutic effect: Relieves bladder spasms.

Available forms

Syrup: 5 mg/5 ml
Tablets: 5 mg
Tablets (extended-release): 5 mg, 10 mg, 15 mg
Transdermal patch: 36 mg patch (delivers 3.9 mg/day)

NURSING PROCESS

Assessment
• Assess patient's bladder condition before therapy.
• Before giving drug, confirm neurogenic bladder by cystometry and rule out partial intestinal obstruction in patients with diarrhea, especially those with colostomy or ileostomy.
• Prepare patient for periodic cystometry to evaluate response to therapy.
• Watch geriatric patients for confusion and mental status changes.
• Be alert for adverse reactions.
• Drug may aggravate symptoms of hyperthyroidism, coronary artery disease, heart failure, arrhythmias, tachycardia, hypertension, or prostatic hyperplasia.
• Evaluate patient's and family's knowledge of drug therapy.

Nursing diagnoses
• Acute pain related to bladder spasms
• Risk for injury related to drug-induced adverse CNS reactions
• Deficient knowledge related to drug therapy

Planning and implementation
• If patient has a UTI, give antibiotics.
• To minimize tendency toward tolerance, stop therapy periodically to determine whether patient can be weaned off medication.
 ALERT: Don't confuse Ditropan with diazepam or Dithranol.
Patient teaching
• Warn patient to avoid hazardous activities until CNS effects of drug are known.
• Tell patient to avoid alcohol during drug therapy.
• Advise patient that taking drug in hot weather raises the risk of fever or heatstroke and urge patient to take precautions to avoid excessive heat and maintain adequate hydration.
• Instruct patient to change transdermal patch two times per week and avoid using the same

site within 7 days. Also warn patient to wear only one patch at a time and to properly dispose of old patches to prevent accidental application or ingestion.
• Advise patient to store drug in tightly closed containers at room temperature.

☑ **Evaluation**
• Patient is free from bladder pain.
• Patient sustains no injuries from drug-induced adverse CNS reactions.
• Patient and family state understanding of drug therapy.

oxycodone hydrochloride
(oks-ee-KOH-dohn high-droh-KLOR-ighd)
Endocodone, Endone◇, M-Oxy, OxyContin, Oxydose, OxyFAST, OxyIR, OxyNorm◇, Percolone, Roxicodone*, Roxicodone Intensol, Supeudol◆

oxycodone pectinate
Proladone◇

Pharmacologic class: opioid
Therapeutic class: analgesic
Pregnancy risk category: B
Controlled substance schedule: II

Indications and dosages

▶ **Moderate to severe pain.** *Adults:* 5 mg P.O. q 6 hours, p.r.n. Or, 1 to 3 suppositories P.R. daily, p.r.n.
Adults not currently receiving opioids who need a continuous around-the-clock analgesic for an extended period of time: 10 mg extended-release tablets P.O. q 12 hours. May increase dose q 1 to 2 days, p.r.n. 80-mg formulation is for opioid-tolerant patients only.
🔲 **Adjust-a-dose:** For patients with impaired hepatic function, start extended-release tablets at ⅓ to ½ of usual dosage and adjust carefully. In patients with impaired renal function, if creatinine clearance is less than 60 ml/minute, reduce initial extended-release dose and adjust carefully.

Contraindications and precautions

• Contraindicated in patients hypersensitive to drug.
• Use cautiously in debilitated patients and in those with head injury, increased intracranial

pressure, seizures, asthma, COPD, prostatic hyperplasia, severe hepatic or renal disease, acute abdominal conditions, urethral stricture, hypothyroidism, Addison's disease, or arrhythmias.
▒ **Lifespan:** In pregnant and breast-feeding women, use cautiously. In children, drug isn't recommended. In geriatric patients, use cautiously.

Adverse reactions

CNS: *sedation, somnolence, clouded sensorium, euphoria,* dizziness.
CV: *hypotension, **bradycardia**.*
GI: nausea, vomiting, constipation, ileus.
GU: urine retention.
Respiratory: *respiratory depression.*
Other: physical dependence.

Interactions

Drug-drug. *Anticoagulants:* Oxycodone products containing aspirin may increase anticoagulant effect. Monitor PT and INR. Use together cautiously; monitor patient for bleeding.
CNS depressants, general anesthetics, hypnotics, MAO inhibitors, other opioid analgesics, protease inhibitors, sedatives, tranquilizers, tricyclic antidepressants: May have additive effects. Use together cautiously. Reduce oxycodone dose as directed, and monitor patient response.
Drug-lifestyle. *Alcohol use:* Increases CNS depression. Discourage using together.

Effects on lab test results

• May increase amylase and lipase levels.

Pharmacokinetics

Absorption: Unknown.
Distribution: Unknown.
Metabolism: Metabolized in liver.
Excretion: Excreted primarily in urine. *Half-life:* 2 to 3 hours.

Route	Onset	Peak	Duration
P.O.	10-15 min	≤1 hr	3-6 hr
P.R.	Unknown	Unknown	Unknown

Action

Chemical effect: Binds with opioid receptors in CNS, altering response to pain via unknown mechanism.
Therapeutic effect: Relieves pain.

Available forms

oxycodone hydrochloride
Capsules: 5 mg
Oral solution: 5 mg/ml, 20 mg/ml
Tablets: 5 mg, 15 mg, 30 mg
Tablets (sustained-release): 10 mg, 20 mg, 40 mg, 80 mg
oxycodone pectinate
Suppositories: 10 mg ♦ , 30 mg ◊

NURSING PROCESS

⚗ Assessment
• Assess patient's pain before and after giving drug.
• Monitor circulatory and respiratory status.
• Be alert for adverse reactions and drug interactions.
• Evaluate patient's and family's knowledge of drug therapy.

⚕ Nursing diagnoses
• Acute pain related to condition
• Ineffective breathing pattern related to drug-induced respiratory depression
• Deficient knowledge related to drug therapy

▷ Planning and implementation
• Give drug with food or milk to avoid GI upset.
• **⚡ ALERT:** OxyContin isn't intended for p.r.n. use or for immediate postoperative pain. Drug is only indicated for postoperative use if patient was receiving it prior to surgery or if pain is expected to persist for an extended period of time.
• For best results, give drug before patient has intense pain.
• Single-agent oxycodone solution or tablet is especially useful for patient who shouldn't take aspirin or acetaminophen.
• **⚡ ALERT:** If respirations are shallow or rate falls below 12 breaths/minute, withhold dose and notify prescriber.
• **⚡ ALERT:** Don't confuse oxycodone immediate-release tablets with OxyContin extended-release tablets.
• **⚡ ALERT:** OxyContin is potentially addictive and abused as much as morphine. Chewing, crushing, snorting, or injecting it can lead to overdose and death.
Patient teaching
• Instruct patient to take drug with food or milk to minimize GI upset.

• Tell patient to ask for drug before pain becomes intense.
• Tell patient not to chew or crush OxyIR or extended-release forms.
• Warn ambulatory patient about getting out of bed or walking. Warn outpatient to avoid hazardous activities until CNS effects of drug are known.

☑ Evaluation
• Patient is free from pain.
• Patient's respiratory rate and pattern remain within normal limits.
• Patient and family state understanding of drug therapy.

oxymorphone hydrochloride
(oks-ee-MOR-fohn high-droh-KLOR-ighd)
Numorphan

Pharmacologic class: opioid
Therapeutic class: analgesic
Pregnancy risk category: C
Controlled substance schedule: II

Indications and dosages

▶ **Moderate to severe pain.** *Adults:* 1 to 1.5 mg I.M. or S.C. q 4 to 6 hours, p.r.n. Or, 0.5 mg I.V. q 4 to 6 hours, p.r.n. Or, 5 mg P.R. q 4 to 6 hours, p.r.n.

▽ I.V. administration
• Give drug by direct I.V. injection. If needed, dilute in normal saline solution.
• Keep patient supine while giving to minimize hypotension.

Contraindications and precautions
• Contraindicated in patients hypersensitive to drug.
• Use cautiously in debilitated patients and in those with head injury, increased intracranial pressure, seizures, asthma, COPD, acute abdominal conditions, prostatic hyperplasia, severe hepatic or renal disease, urethral stricture, respiratory depression, hypothyroidism, Addison's disease, or arrhythmias.
⚖ Lifespan: In pregnant and breast-feeding women and in elderly patients, use cautiously. In children, drug is contraindicated.

Adverse reactions

CNS: *sedation, somnolence, clouded sensorium, euphoria,* dizziness, *seizures* with large doses.
CV: *hypotension,* **bradycardia.**
GI: *nausea, vomiting, constipation,* ileus.
GU: urine retention.
Respiratory: *respiratory depression.*
Other: physical dependence.

Interactions

Drug-drug. *CNS depressants, general anesthetics, MAO inhibitors, tricyclic antidepressants:* May have additive effects. Use together cautiously.
Drug-lifestyle. *Alcohol use:* May have additive effects. Discourage using together.

Effects on lab test results

• May increase amylase level.

Pharmacokinetics

Absorption: Well absorbed.
Distribution: Widely distributed.
Metabolism: Metabolized primarily in liver.
Excretion: Excreted primarily in urine. *Half-life:* Unknown.

Route	Onset	Peak	Duration
I.V.	5-10 min	15-30 min	3-4 hr
I.M.	10-15 min	30-90 min	3-6 hr
S.C.	10-20 min	60-90 min	3-6 hr
P.R.	15-30 min	2 hr	3-6 hr

Action

Chemical effect: Binds with opioid receptors in CNS, altering response to pain via unknown mechanism.
Therapeutic effect: Relieves pain.

Available forms

Injection: 1 mg/ml, 1.5 mg/ml
Suppositories: 5 mg

NURSING PROCESS

Assessment

• Assess patient's pain before and after giving drug.
• Be alert for adverse reactions and drug interactions.
• Evaluate patient's and family's knowledge of drug therapy.

Nursing diagnoses

• Acute pain related to condition
• Ineffective breathing pattern related to drug-induced respiratory depression
• Deficient knowledge related to drug therapy

Planning and implementation

• Keep opioid antagonist (naloxone) and resuscitation equipment available.
• Don't give drug for mild to moderate pain.
• Drug may worsen gallbladder pain.
• Give drug before patient's pain becomes too intense.
ALERT: If respirations decrease or rate is below 12 breaths/minute, withhold dose and notify prescriber.
• Dependence can develop with long-term use.
• Giving laxatives or stool softeners may help prevent or relieve constipation.
ALERT: Don't confuse oxymorphone with oxymetholone.
Patient teaching
• Instruct patient to take drug before pain becomes intense.
• Warn ambulatory patient about getting out of bed or walking. Warn outpatient to avoid hazardous activities until CNS effects of drug are known.
• Tell patient to refrigerate suppositories.
• Advise patient or family to report a decreased respiratory rate.
• Teach patient about increasing fluid and fiber intake to prevent constipation.

Evaluation

• Patient is free from pain.
• Patient's respiratory status is within normal limits.
• Patient and family state understanding of drug therapy.

---

oxytocin, synthetic injection
(oks-ih-TOH-sin, sin-THET-ik in-JEK-shun)
Pitocin

Pharmacologic class: exogenous hormone
Therapeutic class: oxytocic, lactation stimulant
Pregnancy risk category: NR

Indications and dosages

▶ **Induction or stimulation of labor.** *Adults:* Initially, 1 ml ampule (10 units) I.V. in 1,000 ml of D₅W, dextrose 5% in normal saline, or normal saline solution infused at 1 to 2 milliunits/minute. Increase rate in increments of no more than 1 to 2 milliunits/minute at 15- to 30-minute intervals until normal contraction pattern is established. Decrease rate when labor is firmly established. Maximum dose, 20 milliunits/minute.

▶ **Reduction of postpartum bleeding after expulsion of placenta.** *Adults:* 10 to 40 units I.V. in 1,000 ml of D₅W or normal saline solution infused at rate necessary to control bleeding, usually 20 to 40 milliunits/minute. Also, 10 units can be given I.M. after delivery of placenta.

▶ **Incomplete or inevitable abortion.** *Adults:* 10 units I.V. in 500 ml of normal saline solution or dextrose 5% in normal saline solution or D₅W. Infuse at 20 to 40 gtt/minute.

▶ **Oxytocin challenge test to assess fetal distress in high-risk pregnancies greater than 31 weeks' gestation‡.** *Adults:* 5 to 10 units I.V. in 1 L of D₅W injection, yielding a solution of 5 to 10 milliunits per ml. Infuse 0.5 milliunits/minute, gradually increasing at 15-minute intervals to a maximum infusion of 20 milliunits/minute. Stop infusion when three moderate uterine contractions occur within a 10-minute period. Response of fetal heart rate may be used to evaluate prognosis.

▼ I.V. administration

• Give only by infusion.
• Give by piggyback infusion so drug can be stopped without interrupting I.V. line.
• Use an infusion pump.

Contraindications and precautions

• Contraindicated in patients hypersensitive to drug. Also contraindicated in cephalopelvic disproportion or delivery that requires conversion, as in transverse lie; in fetal distress when delivery isn't imminent; in prematurity; in other obstetric emergencies; and in severe toxemia, hypertonic uterine patterns, total placenta previa, or vasa previa.
• During first and second stages of labor, use cautiously because cervical laceration, uterine rupture, and maternal and fetal death may occur. In patients with grand multiparity, uterine sep-

sis, traumatic delivery, or overdistended uterus, use cautiously, if at all.
• Also use cautiously, if at all, in patients with invasive cervical carcinoma and in patients with history of cervical or uterine surgery.
 Lifespan: Drug is only indicated for pregnant and postpartum women.

Adverse reactions

Maternal
CNS: *subarachnoid hemorrhage from hypertension, seizures, coma from water intoxication.*
CV: *hypertension;* increased heart rate, systemic venous return, and cardiac output; *arrhythmias.*
GI: nausea, vomiting.
GU: *tetanic uterine contractions, abruptio placentae, impaired uterine blood flow, pelvic hematoma, increased uterine motility.*
Hematologic: afibrinogenemia (may be related to postpartum bleeding).
Other: hypersensitivity reactions, *anaphylaxis.*
Fetal
CV: *bradycardia,* tachycardia, *PVCs.*
Hematologic: hyperbilirubinemia.
Respiratory: *anoxia, asphyxia.*

Interactions

Drug-drug. *Cyclopropane anesthetics:* May cause less pronounced tachycardia but more severe hypotension. Also may cause maternal sinus bradycardia with abnormal atrioventricular arrhythmias. Use together cautiously.
Thiopental anesthetics: Possible delayed induction. Use together cautiously.
Vasoconstrictors: May cause severe hypertension if oxytocin given within 3 or 4 hours of vasoconstrictor in patients receiving caudal block anesthetic. Avoid using together.

Effects on lab test results

None reported.

Pharmacokinetics

Absorption: Unknown.
Distribution: Distributed through extracellular fluid.
Metabolism: Metabolized rapidly in kidneys and liver. In early pregnancy, a circulating enzyme, oxytocinase, can inactivate drug.

Excretion: Small amounts excreted in urine.
Half-life: 3 to 5 minutes.

Route	Onset	Peak	Duration
I.V.	Immediate	Unknown	1 hr
I.M.	3-5 min	Unknown	2-3 hr

Action

Chemical effect: Causes potent and selective stimulation of uterine and mammary gland smooth muscle.
Therapeutic effect: Induces labor and milk ejection and reduces postpartum bleeding.

Available forms

Injection: 10 units/ml in ampule, vial or syringe

NURSING PROCESS

⚖ Assessment
• Assess patient's condition before therapy and regularly thereafter.
• Monitor and record uterine contractions, heart rate, blood pressure, intrauterine pressure, fetal heart rate, and blood loss q 15 minutes.
• Be alert for adverse reactions and drug interactions.
• Monitor fluid intake and output. Antidiuretic effect may lead to fluid overload, seizures, and coma.
• Evaluate patient's and family's knowledge of drug therapy.

🔁 Nursing diagnoses
• Risk for deficient fluid volume related to postpartum bleeding
• Excessive fluid volume related to drug-induced antidiuretic effect
• Deficient knowledge related to drug therapy

⟫ Planning and implementation
• Drug is used to induce or reinforce labor only when pelvis is known to be adequate, vaginal delivery is indicated, fetal maturity is ensured, and fetal position is favorable. Use only in hospital where critical care facilities and experienced clinician are immediately available.
• Drug isn't recommended for routine I.M. use. However, 10 units may be given I.M. after delivery of placenta to control postpartum uterine bleeding.
• Never give oxytocin simultaneously by more than one route.

• Have 20% solution magnesium sulfate available for relaxation of myometrium.
• ⚠ **ALERT:** If contractions are less than 2 minutes apart, if they're above 50 mm Hg, or if they last 90 seconds or longer, stop infusion, turn patient on her side, and notify prescriber.
• ⚠ **ALERT:** Don't confuse Pitocin with Pitressin.
• ⚠ **ALERT:** Don't confuse oxytocin with OxyContin.

Patient teaching
• Instruct patient to report unusual feelings or adverse effects at once.
• Instruct patient to remain lying down during administration.

☑ Evaluation
• Patient maintains adequate fluid balance with drug therapy.
• Patient doesn't develop edema.
• Patient and family state understanding of drug therapy.

paclitaxel
(pak-lih-TAK-sil)
Onxol, Taxol

Pharmacologic class: novel antimicrotubule
Therapeutic class: antineoplastic
Pregnancy risk category: D

Indications and dosages

▶ **First-line and subsequent treatment of advanced ovarian cancer.** *Previously untreated adults:* 175 mg/m² I.V. over 3 hours q 3 weeks followed by cisplatin 75 mg/m²; or, 135 mg/m² I.V. over 24 hours with cisplatin 75 mg/m² q 3 weeks.
Previously treated adults: 135 or 175 mg/m² I.V. over 3 hours q 3 weeks.
▶ **Breast cancer that doesn't respond to combination chemotherapy for metastatic disease or relapse within 6 months of chemotherapy that included an anthracycline; after combination chemotherapy that includes doxorubicin for node-positive breast cancer.** *Adults:* 175 mg/m² I.V. over 3 hours q 3 weeks.

▶ **Initial treatment of advanced non–small-cell lung cancer for patients who aren't candidates for curative surgery or radiation.**
Adults: 135 mg/m^2 I.V. infusion over 24 hours, follow with cisplatin 75 mg/m^2. Repeat cycle q 3 weeks.

For all indications, subsequent courses shouldn't be given until neutrophil count is at least 1,500/mm^3 and platelet count is at least 100,000/mm^3.

▶ **AIDS-related Kaposi's sarcoma.** *Adults:* 135 mg/m^2 I.V. over 3 hours q 3 weeks, or 100 mg/m^2 I.V. over 3 hours q 2 weeks. Don't give if baseline or subsequent neutrophil counts are less than 1,000/mm^3.

▽ I.V. administration

- Preparing and giving drug are linked to carcinogenic, mutagenic, and teratogenic risks. Follow facility policy for safe handling. Mark all waste materials with chemotherapy hazard labels.
- Dilute concentrate to 0.3 to 1.2 mg/ml before infusion. Compatible solutions include normal saline solution for injection, D$_5$W, dextrose 5% in normal saline for injection, and dextrose 5% in lactated Ringer's injection. Diluted solutions are stable for 27 hours at room temperature.
- Prepare and store infusion solutions in glass containers. Don't allow undiluted concentrate to come in contact with polyvinyl chloride I.V. bags or tubing. Store diluted solution in glass or polypropylene bottles, or use polypropylene or polyolefin bags. Administer through polyethylene-lined administration sets, and use in-line 0.22-micron filter.
- Take care to avoid extravasation.

Contraindications and precautions

- Contraindicated in patients hypersensitive to drug or polyoxyethylated castor oil, a vehicle used in drug solution, and in patients with solid tumors with baseline neutrophil counts below 1,500/mm^3. When used to treat AIDS-related Kaposi's sarcoma, contraindicated in patients with baseline neutrophil counts below 1,000/mm^3.
- Use cautiously in patients who have received radiation therapy; they may have more frequent or severe myelosuppression.
- ☀ **Lifespan:** In pregnant and breast-feeding women, drug isn't recommended. In children, safety of drug hasn't been established.

Adverse reactions

CNS: peripheral neuropathy.
CV: *bradycardia*, hypotension, abnormal ECG.
GI: *nausea, vomiting, diarrhea, mucositis.*
Hematologic: NEUTROPENIA, LEUKOPENIA, THROMBOCYTOPENIA, anemia, bleeding.
Musculoskeletal: *myalgia, arthralgia.*
Skin: alopecia, phlebitis, cellulitis at injection site.
Other: *hypersensitivity reactions (anaphylaxis).*

Interactions

Drug-drug. *Cisplatin:* May have additive myelosuppressive effects. Use together cautiously.
Cyclosporine, dexamethasone, diazepam, estradiol, etoposide, ketoconazole, quinidine, retinoic acid, teniposide, testosterone, verapamil, vincristine: Inhibits paclitaxel metabolism. Use together cautiously.
Doxorubicin: May increase levels of doxorubicin and its metabolites. Dose adjustments may be needed.

Effects on lab test results

- May increase alkaline phosphatase, AST, and triglyceride levels.
- May decrease hemoglobin, hematocrit, and neutrophil, WBC, and platelet counts.

Pharmacokinetics

Absorption: Administered I.V.
Distribution: About 89% to 98% of drug is bound to proteins.
Metabolism: May be metabolized in liver.
Excretion: Unknown. *Half-life:* 2¼ to 5¾ hours.

Route	Onset	Peak	Duration
I.V.	Unknown	Unknown	Unknown

Action

Chemical effect: Inhibits normal reorganization of microtubule network necessary for mitosis and other vital cellular functions.
Therapeutic effect: Stops ovarian and breast cancer cell activity.

Available forms

Injection: 6 mg/ml

NURSING PROCESS

⏳ Assessment

- Assess patient's condition before therapy and regularly thereafter.
- Continuously monitor patient for first 30 minutes of infusion. Monitor patient closely throughout infusion.
- Monitor blood counts and liver function test results frequently during therapy.
- Be alert for adverse reactions and drug interactions.
- Evaluate patient's and family's knowledge of drug therapy.

🔲 Nursing diagnoses

- Ineffective health maintenance related to cancer
- Ineffective protection related to drug-induced adverse hematologic reactions
- Deficient knowledge related to drug therapy

▷ Planning and implementation

- To reduce severe hypersensitivity, pretreat patient with corticosteroids, such as dexamethasone, and antihistamines. H_1-receptor antagonists, such as diphenhydramine, and H_2-receptor antagonists, such as cimetidine or ranitidine, may be used.
- ⚕ ALERT: Don't confuse paclitaxel with paroxetine.
- ⚕ ALERT: Don't confuse Taxol with Paxil or Taxotere.

Patient teaching

- Warn patient to watch for signs of bleeding and infection.
- Teach patient symptoms of peripheral neuropathy, such as tingling, burning, or numbness in limbs, and urge her to report them immediately to prescriber. Dosage reduction may be necessary.
- Warn patient that alopecia occurs in up to 82% of patients.
- Advise woman of childbearing age to avoid pregnancy during therapy. Also recommend consulting with prescriber before becoming pregnant.

✅ Evaluation

- Patient responds well to therapy.
- Patient develops no serious complications from drug-induced adverse hematologic reactions.

- Patient and family state understanding of drug therapy.

palivizumab
(pal-ih-VYE-zoo-mab)
Synagis

Pharmacologic class: recombinant monoclonal antibody immunoglobulin $(Ig)G1_k$
Therapeutic class: RSV prophylactic
Pregnancy risk category: C

Indications and dosages

▶ **Prevention of serious lower respiratory tract disease caused by RSV in children at high risk.** *Infants and children:* 15 mg/kg I.M. monthly throughout RSV season, with first dose before RSV season.

Contraindications and precautions

- Contraindicated in children hypersensitive to drug or its components.
- Use cautiously in children with thrombocytopenia or other coagulation disorders.
- 🔁 Lifespan: Drug is only indicated in children.

Adverse reactions

CNS: nervousness, pain.
EENT: *otitis media, rhinitis,* pharyngitis, sinusitis, conjunctivitis.
GI: diarrhea, vomiting, gastroenteritis, oral candidiasis.
Hematologic: anemia.
Respiratory: *upper respiratory tract infection,* cough, wheeze, bronchiolitis, ***apnea***, pneumonia, bronchitis, ***asthma***, croup, dyspnea.
Skin: *rash,* fungal dermatitis, eczema, seborrhea.
Other: hernia, failure to thrive, injection site reaction, viral infection, flulike syndrome.

Interactions

None significant.

Effects on lab test results

- May increase ALT and AST levels.
- May decrease hemoglobin and hematocrit.

Rapid onset   *Liquid form contains alcohol.   ◆ Canada   ◇ Australia   †OTC   ‡Off-label use

Pharmacokinetics

Absorption: Unknown.
Distribution: Unknown.
Metabolism: Unknown.
Excretion: Unknown. *Half-life:* About 18 days.

Route	Onset	Peak	Duration
I.M.	Unknown	Unknown	Unknown

Action

Chemical effect: Inhibits RSV replication.
Therapeutic effect: Prevents RSV infection in high-risk children.

Available forms

Injection (single use vial): 50 mg, 100 mg

NURSING PROCESS

⚗ Assessment
• Obtain accurate medical history before giving drug; ask if child has any coagulation disorders or liver dysfunction.
• Be alert for adverse reactions.
• Evaluate patient's and family's knowledge of drug therapy.

⊕ Nursing diagnoses
• Risk for infection related to RSV infection
• Risk for injury related to drug-induced adverse reactions
• Deficient knowledge related to drug therapy

▷ Planning and implementation
• Very rare non-fatal cases of anaphylaxis have been reported following re-exposure to drug. Rare severe acute hypersensitivity reactions have also been reported on initial exposure or re-exposure to palivizumab. If a severe hypersensitivity reaction occurs, permanently stop drug. If milder hypersensitivity reactions occur, readminister drug cautiously. If anaphylaxis or severe allergic reactions occur, give drug such as epinephrine and provide supportive care as required.
• To reconstitute, slowly add 1 ml of sterile water for injection into a 100-mg vial. Gently swirl vial for 30 seconds to avoid foaming; don't shake. Let reconstituted solution stand at room temperature for 20 minutes. Give within 6 hours of reconstitution.
• Give drug in front thigh muscle, off to one side. Don't use gluteal muscle routinely as an injection site because of risk of damage to sciatic nerve. Divide injections over 1 ml.
• Patient should receive monthly doses throughout RSV season, even if RSV infection develops. In the northern hemisphere, RSV season typically lasts from November to April.

Patient teaching
• Explain to parent or caregiver that drug is used to prevent RSV and not to treat it.
• Advise parent that monthly injections are recommended throughout RSV season.
• Tell parent to immediately report adverse reactions or unusual bruising, bleeding, or weakness.

☑ Evaluation
• Patient doesn't develop RSV infection.
• Patient sustains no injury from drug-induced adverse reactions.
• Patient and family state understanding of drug therapy.

palonosetron hydrochloride
(pa-LOW-no-suh-tron high-droh-KLOHR-ighd)
Aloxi

Pharmacologic class: selective serotonin subtype 3 receptor antagonist (5-HT$_3$ antagonist)
Therapeutic class: antiemetic
Pregnancy risk category: B

Indications and dosages

▶ **Prevention of acute and delayed nausea and vomiting caused by moderately or highly emetogenic chemotherapy.** *Adults:* 0.25 mg I.V. over 30 seconds; give 30 minutes before the start of chemotherapy. Give once per cycle, not more than q 7 days.

▽ I.V. administration

• Don't mix with other drugs.
• Give by rapid I.V. injection over 30 seconds. Flush I.V. line before and after with normal saline.
• Give by either peripheral or central I.V. access.
• Store vials at room temperature. Protect vials from light, and don't freeze the solution.

Contraindications and precautions

• Contraindicated in patents hypersensitive to drug or its components.

• Use cautiously in patients hypersensitive to other 5-HT$_3$ antagonists; cross-sensitivity may occur. Also use cautiously in patients with cardiac conduction abnormalities, hypokalemia, or hypomagnesemia and in patients taking drugs that affect cardiac conduction.

☀ Lifespan: In pregnant women, use drug only if the potential benefits outweigh the risks. Breast-feeding women should consider stopping breast-feeding or using a different antiemetic; it's unknown if drug appears in breast milk. In children, safety and effectiveness of drug haven't been established.

Adverse reactions

CNS: anxiety, dizziness, headache, weakness.
CV: *bradycardia,* hypotension, *nonsustained ventricular tachycardia.*
GI: constipation, diarrhea.
Metabolic: *hyperkalemia.*

Interactions

Drug-drug. *Diuretics with potential for inducing electrolyte abnormalities, antiarrhythmics or other drugs that may prolong the QT interval, high doses of anthracycline:* May increase risk of prolonged QT interval. Use together cautiously.

Effects on lab test results

• May increase potassium level.

Pharmacokinetics

Absorption: Administered I.V.
Distribution: Distributes well into tissues. Drug is 60% bound to proteins.
Metabolism: 50% is metabolized to inactive metabolites via CYP 2D6 and, to a lesser extent, CYP 3A4 and 1A2.
Excretion: 40% of drug and inactive metabolites are eliminated unchanged in the urine. *Half-life:* 40 hours.

Route	Onset	Peak	Duration
I.V.	30 min	Unknown	5 days

Action

Chemical effect: Binds to the 5-HT$_3$ receptor, which inhibits emesis caused by cytotoxic chemotherapy.

Therapeutic effect: Prevents vomiting because of chemotherapy.

Available forms

Injection: 0.25 mg/5 ml (single-use vial).

NURSING PROCESS

🔖 Assessment
• Assess patient's condition before therapy and regularly thereafter.
• Obtain baseline potassium level.
• In patients with known cardiac conduction abnormalities, obtain baseline ECG.
• Be alert for adverse reactions and drug interactions.
• Evaluate patient's and family's knowledge of drug therapy.

🔲 Nursing diagnoses
• Risk for deficient fluid volume related to nausea and vomiting
• Pain related to drug-induced headache
• Deficient knowledge related to drug therapy

▶ Planning and implementation
• Give 30 minutes before chemotherapy on day one of each cycle.
• Consider giving with corticosteroids as part of the antiemetic therapy, particularly for patients receiving highly emetogenic chemotherapy.
• Give additional antiemetics for breakthrough nausea and vomiting.
Patient teaching
• Advise patients to take a different antiemetic for breakthrough nausea and vomiting, and tell patient to take it at the first sign of nausea and not to wait until symptoms are severe.
• Tell patients with a history of cardiac conduction abnormalities to report any changes in their drug regimen, such as the adding or stopping of antiarrhythmics.

✅ Evaluation
• Patient maintains adequate hydration.
• Patient doesn't experience drug-induced headaches.
• Patient and family state understanding of drug therapy.

---

pamidronate disodium
(pam-ih-DROH-nayt digh-SOH-dee-um)
Aredia

Pharmacologic class: bisphosphonate, pyrophosphate analogue
Therapeutic class: antihypercalcemic
Pregnancy risk category: D

Indications and dosages

▶ **Moderate to severe hypercalcemia related to malignancy (with or without metastases).**
Adults: Dosage depends on severity of hypercalcemia. Calcium levels are corrected for serum albumin as follows:

$$\text{Corrected serum calcium (CCa)} = \text{serum calcium} + 0.8 (4 - \text{serum albumin})$$
(in mg/dl)   (in mg/dl)   (in g/dl)

Patients with moderate hypercalcemia (CCa levels of 12 to 13.5 mg/dl) may receive 60 to 90 mg I.V. infusion as a single dose over 2 to 24 hours. Patients with severe hypercalcemia (CCa levels higher than 13.5 mg/dl) may receive 90 mg over 2 to 24 hours. Wait at least 7 days to give repeat dose to allow for full response to initial dose.
▶ **Osteolytic bone lesions of multiple myeloma.** *Adults:* 90 mg I.V. daily over 4 hours once monthly.
▶ **Osteolytic bone lesions of breast cancer.**
Adults: 90 mg I.V. daily over 2 hours q 3 to 4 weeks.
▶ **Moderate to severe Paget's disease.** *Adults:* 30 mg I.V. as 4-hour infusion on 3 consecutive days for total dose of 90 mg. Cycle repeated, p.r.n.

▼ I.V. administration

● Reconstitute vial with 10 ml sterile water for injection. Once drug is completely dissolved, add to 250-ml (2-hour infusion), 500-ml (4-hour infusion), or 1,000-ml (up to 24-hour infusion) bag of half-normal or normal saline solution injection or D₅W.
● Don't mix with infusion solutions that contain calcium, such as Ringer's injection or lactated Ringer's injection. Inspect for precipitate before administering.
● Give drug only by I.V. infusion. Nephropathy may occur with rapid bolus injections.
● Infusions of more than 2 hours may reduce the risk for renal toxicity, particularly in patients with preexisting renal insufficiency.
● Solution is stable for 24 hours at room temperature.

Contraindications and precautions

● Contraindicated in patients hypersensitive to drug or to other bisphosphonates, such as etidronate.
● Use cautiously in patients with renal impairment.
🔺 **Lifespan:** In pregnant women, drug may cause fetal harm. In breast-feeding women, use cautiously. In children, safety of drug hasn't been established.

Adverse reactions

CNS: *pain, fever, fatigue, headache, insomnia, anxiety, seizures.*
CV: hypertension, atrial fibrillation.
GI: *abdominal pain, anorexia, constipation, nausea, vomiting, diahrrhea, dyspepsia, GI hemorrhage.*
GU: *UTI, renal failure.*
Hematologic: *leukopenia,* THROMBOCYTOPE-
NIA, GRANULOCYTOPENIA, *anemia.*
Metabolism: hypophosphatemia, *hypokalemia,* hypomagnesemia, hypocalcemia.
Musculoskeletal: *bone pain, arthralgia, myalgia.*
Other: METASTASES.

Interactions

None significant.

Effects on lab test results

● May increase creatinine levels. May decrease phosphate, potassium, magnesium, and calcium levels.
● May decrease hemoglobin, hematocrit, and WBC and platelet counts.

Pharmacokinetics

Absorption: Administered I.V.
Distribution: About 50% to 60% of dose is rapidly taken up by bone; drug is also taken up by kidneys, liver, spleen, teeth, and tracheal cartilage.
Metabolism: None.

Reactions may be *common,* uncommon, *life-threatening,* or COMMON AND LIFE-THREATENING.

Excretion: Excreted by kidneys. *Half-life:* Alpha, 1½ hours; beta, 27¼ hours.

Route	Onset	Peak	Duration
I.V.	Unknown	Unknown	Unknown

Action

Chemical effect: Inhibits bone resorption. Adsorbs to hydroxyapatite crystals in bone and may directly block calcium phosphate dissolution.
Therapeutic effect: Lowers calcium levels.

Available forms

Powder for injection: 30 mg/vial, 90 mg/vial
Solution for injection: 3 mg/ml, 6 mg/ml, 9 mg/ml in 10-ml vials

NURSING PROCESS

Assessment
• Assess patient's condition before therapy and regularly thereafter.
• Assess hydration before therapy.
• Closely monitor electrolytes, and creatinine levels, CBC counts and differential, hematocrit, and hemoglobin.
• Carefully monitor patient with anemia, leukopenia, or thrombocytopenia during first 2 weeks of therapy.
• Monitor patient's temperature. Fever is most likely 24 to 48 hours after therapy.
• Be alert for adverse reactions and drug interactions. Patients with renal impairment are at a greater risk for adverse reactions.
• Evaluate patient's and family's knowledge of drug therapy.

Nursing diagnoses
• Ineffective health maintenance related to hypercalcemia
• Risk for injury related to drug-induced hypocalcemia
• Deficient knowledge related to drug therapy

Planning and implementation
• Use drug only after patient has been vigorously hydrated with saline solution. In patients with mild to moderate hypercalcemia, hydration alone may be sufficient.
• If patient has severe hypocalcemia, short-term administration of calcium may be needed.

• For patients with multiple myeloma, there is limited information on use in patients with creatinine greater than 3 mg/dl. Before infusion, adequately hydrate patients with marked Bence-Jones proteinuria and dehydration. Optimal duration of therapy is unknown; in studies, 21 months demonstrated overall benefits.
 ALERT: Because of the risk of renal dysfunction leading to renal failure, single doses shouldn't exceed 90 mg.
• In patients treated for bone metastases who have renal dysfunction, withhold dose until renal function returns to baseline. Use in patients with severe renal impairment isn't recommended.
• For breast cancer patients, optimal duration of therapy is unknown; in studies, 24 months demonstrated overall benefits.
 ALERT: Don't confuse Aredia with Meridia.
Patient teaching
• Instruct patient to report unusual signs or symptoms at once.
• Inform patient of need for frequent tests to monitor effectiveness of drug and detect adverse reactions.

Evaluation
• Patient's calcium level returns to normal.
• Patient doesn't develop hypocalcemia during drug therapy.
• Patient and family state understanding of drug therapy.

pancuronium bromide
(pan-kyoo-ROH-nee-um BROH-mighd)

Pharmacologic class: nondepolarizing neuromuscular blocker
Therapeutic class: skeletal muscle relaxant
Pregnancy risk category: C

Indications and dosages

▶ **Adjunct to anesthesia to induce skeletal muscle relaxation; to facilitate intubation; to lessen muscle contractions in pharmacologically or electrically induced seizures; to assist with mechanical ventilation.** Dosage depends on anesthetic used, individual needs, and response. Dosages are representative and must be adjusted.

Adults and children age 1 month and older: Initially, 0.04 to 0.1 mg/kg I.V.; then 0.01 mg/kg q 25 to 60 minutes.

Neonates younger than age 1 month: Dosages are individualized.

▼ I.V. administration

• Mix drug only with fresh solutions; precipitates will form if alkaline solutions such as barbiturate solutions are used.

• Store drug in refrigerator. Don't store in plastic containers or syringes, although plastic syringes may be used for administration.

Contraindications and precautions

• Contraindicated in patients hypersensitive to bromides, in those with tachycardia, and in those for whom even a minor increase in heart rate is undesirable.

• Use cautiously in debilitated patients and in those with respiratory depression, myasthenia gravis, myasthenic syndrome of lung cancer, bronchogenic carcinoma, dehydration, thyroid disorders, collagen diseases, porphyria, electrolyte disturbances, hyperthermia, toxemic states, or renal, hepatic, or pulmonary impairment.

⚖ Lifespan: In pregnant women undergoing cesarean section and in breast-feeding women, use large doses cautiously. In elderly patients, use cautiously.

Adverse reactions

CV: tachycardia, increased blood pressure.
EENT: excessive salivation.
Musculoskeletal: residual muscle weakness.
Respiratory: *prolonged, dose-related respiratory insufficiency or apnea;* wheezing.
Skin: transient rashes, excessive diaphoresis.
Other: burning sensation, *allergic or idiosyncratic hypersensitivity reactions.*

Interactions

Drug-drug. *Amikacin, gentamicin, neomycin, streptomycin, tobramycin:* May increase the effects of nondepolarizing muscle relaxant including prolonged respiratory depression. Use together only when necessary. Dose of nondepolarizing muscle relaxant may need to be reduced.

Carbamazepine, phenytoin: May decrease the effects of pancuronium causing it to be less ef-

fective. May need to increase the dose of the pancuronium.

Kanamycin; clindamycin; general anesthetics; polymyxin antibiotics, such as polymyxin B sulfate and colistin; quinidine: Potentiates neuromuscular blockade, leading to increased skeletal muscle relaxation and prolonged effect. Use cautiously during surgical and postoperative periods.

Lithium, opioid analgesics: Potentiates neuromuscular blockade, leading to increased skeletal muscle relaxation and respiratory paralysis. Use cautiously and reduce pancuronium dosage, as directed.

Succinylcholine: Increases intensity and duration of blockade. Allow succinylcholine effects to subside before giving pancuronium.

Effects on lab test results

None reported.

Pharmacokinetics

Absorption: Administered I.V.
Distribution: Little protein-binding regardless of dose.
Metabolism: Unknown.
Excretion: Excreted mainly in urine; some biliary excretion. *Half-life:* About 2 hours.

Route	Onset	Peak	Duration
I.V.	30-45 sec	3-4½ min	35-45 min

Action

Chemical effect: Prevents acetylcholine from binding to receptors on muscle end plate, thus blocking depolarization.
Therapeutic effect: Relaxes skeletal muscles.

Available forms

Injection: 1 mg/ml, 2 mg/ml

NURSING PROCESS

⚕ Assessment

• Assess patient's condition before therapy and regularly thereafter.

• Monitor baseline electrolyte determinations (electrolyte imbalance can increase neuromuscular effects) and vital signs.

• Measure fluid intake and output; renal dysfunction may prolong duration of action because 25% of drug is unchanged before excretion.

• Nerve stimulator and train-of-four monitoring are recommended to confirm antagonism of neuromuscular blockade and recovery of muscle strength. Before attempting reversal with neostigmine, some evidence of spontaneous recovery should be observed.

• Monitor respirations closely until patient fully recovers from neuromuscular blockade, as evidenced by tests of muscle strength (hand grip, head lift, and ability to cough).

• Be alert for adverse reactions and drug interactions.

• Evaluate patient's and family's knowledge of drug therapy.

🔷 Nursing diagnoses
• Ineffective health maintenance related to condition
• Ineffective breathing pattern related to drug's effect on respiratory muscles
• Deficient knowledge related to drug therapy

⧛ Planning and implementation
• Administer sedatives or general anesthetics before neuromuscular blockers. Neuromuscular blockers don't reduce consciousness or alter pain threshold. Give analgesics for pain.

• Drug should be used only by personnel skilled in airway management.

• If giving with succinylcholine, allow succinylcholine effects to subside before giving this drug.

• Have emergency respiratory support equipment (endotracheal equipment, ventilator, oxygen, atropine, edrophonium, epinephrine, and neostigmine) immediately available.

• Once spontaneous recovery starts, drug-induced neuromuscular blockade may be reversed with anticholinesterase drug (such as neostigmine or edrophonium). Usually given with an anticholinergic such as atropine.

⚠ **ALERT:** Don't confuse pancuronium with pipecuronium.

Patient teaching
• Explain all events to patient because he can still hear.

• Reassure patient that he'll be monitored at all times and that pain medication will be provided, if appropriate.

• Tell patient that he may feel burning sensation at injection site.

☑ Evaluation
• Patient's condition improves.
• Patient maintains adequate ventilation with mechanical assistance.
• Patient and family state understanding of drug therapy.

pantoprazole sodium
(pan-TOE-pra-zole SOH-dee-um)
Protonix, Protonix I.V.

Pharmacologic class: substituted benzimidazole
Therapeutic class: proton pump inhibitor
Pregnancy risk category: B

Indications and dosages

▶ **Short-term treatment of erosive esophagitis related to gastroesophageal reflux disease (GERD).** *Adults:* 40 mg P.O. once daily for up to 8 weeks. For those patients who haven't healed after 8 weeks of therapy, an additional 8-week course may be considered.

▶ **Short-term treatment of GERD related to history of erosive esophagitis.** *Adults:* 40 mg I.V. daily for 7 to 10 days. Switch to oral form as soon as patient is able to take oral medications.

▶ **Long-term maintenance of healing erosive esophagitis and reduction in relapse rates of daytime and nighttime heartburn symptoms in patients with GERD.** *Adults:* 40 mg P.O. once daily.

▶ **Short-term treatment of pathological hypersecretion conditions related to Zollinger-Ellison syndrome or other neoplastic conditions.** *Adults:* Individualize dosage. Usual dose is 80 mg I.V. q 12 hours for no more than 6 days. For those needing a higher dose, 80 mg q 8 hours is expected to maintain acid output below 10 mEq/h. Maximum daily dose, 240 mg.

▶ **Long-term treatment of pathological hypersecretory conditions, including with Zollinger-Ellison syndrome.** *Adults:* Individualize dosage. Usual starting dose is 40 mg P.O. b.i.d. Adjust dose to a maximum of 240 mg daily.

▽ I.V. administration
• Reconstitute each vial with 10 ml of normal saline solution.

• Compatible diluents for infusion include 5% dextrose, normal saline solution, or lactated Ringer's injection.

• For GERD, further dilute with 100 ml of diluent to a final concentration of 0.4 mg/ml.

• For hypersecretion conditions, combine 2 reconstituted vials and further dilute with 80 ml of diluent to a total volume of 100 ml, with a final concentration of 0.8 mg/ml.

• Infuse diluted solutions I.V. over 15 minutes at a rate not greater than 3 mg/min (7 ml/min) for GERD and 6 mg/min (7 ml/min) for pathological hypersecretory conditions.

• Don't give another infusion simultaneously through the same line.

• The reconstituted solution may be stored for up to 2 hours at room temperature, and the diluted solutions may be stored for up to 12 hours at room temperature.

• Stop I.V. drug as soon as P.O. use is possible.

Contraindications and precautions

• Contraindicated in patients hypersensitive to any component of the drug.

⚕ **Lifespan:** In breast-feeding women, use cautiously. In children, safety and effectiveness of drug haven't been established.

Adverse reactions

CNS: headache, insomnia, asthenia, migraine, anxiety, dizziness, pain.
CV: chest pain.
EENT: pharyngitis, rhinitis, sinusitis.
GI: diarrhea, flatulence, abdominal pain, eructation, constipation, dyspepsia, gastroenteritis, gastrointestinal disorder, nausea, vomiting.
GU: rectal disorder, urinary frequency, UTI.
Metabolic: hyperglycemia, hyperlipidemia.
Musculoskeletal: back pain, neck pain, arthralgia, hypertonia.
Respiratory: bronchitis, increased cough, dyspnea, upper respiratory tract infection.
Skin: rash.
Other: flulike syndrome, infection.

Interactions

Drug-drug. *Ampicillin esters, iron salts, ketoconazole:* May decrease absorption of these drugs. Monitor patient closely and try to space out the time intervals of administration.
Drug-herb. *St. John's wort:* May increase risk of sunburn. Discorage use together.

Drug-food. *Food:* Delays absorption of pantoprazole for up to 2 hours, however the extent of absorption isn't affected. Can be given without regard to meals.

Effects on lab test results

• May increase glucose and lipid levels. May increase or decrease liver function levels.

Pharmacokinetics

Absorption: Well absorbed with an absolute bioavailability of 77%. Peak level occurs at 2.5 hours. Food may delay its absorption up to 2 hours; however, the extent of absorption isn't affected.
Distribution: Distributes mainly in the extracellular fluid. Protein binding is approximately 98%, mainly to albumin.
Metabolism: Extensively metabolized in the liver through the CYP system.
Excretion: About 71% of a dose is excreted in the urine with 18% excreted in the feces by biliary excretion. *Half-life:* 1 hour.

Route	Onset	Peak	Duration
P.O.	Unknown	2½ hr	Unknown
I.V.	15-30 min	Unknown	24 hr

Action

Chemical effect: Inhibits the activity of the proton pump by binding to hydrogen-potassium adenosine triphosphatase, located at secretory surface of the gastric parietal cells.
Therapeutic effect: Suppresses gastric acid secretion.

Available forms

Injection: 40-mg vial.
Tablet (delayed-release): 20 mg, 40 mg

NURSING PROCESS

⚗ Assessment

• Assess underlying condition before therapy and reassess regularly throughout therapy.

• Assess patient for complaints of epigastric or abdominal pain and for bleeding (such as blood in stool or emesis).

• Be alert for adverse reactions and interactions.

• Evaluate patient's and family's knowledge of drug therapy.

Reactions may be *common,* uncommon, *life-threatening*, or COMMON AND LIFE-THREATENING.

🔄 Nursing diagnoses

• Risk for imbalanced fluid volume related to drug-induced adverse reactions
• Risk for aspiration related to underlying gastrointestinal disorder
• Deficient knowledge deficit related to pantoprazole therapy

▶ Planning and implementation

• Symptomatic response to therapy doesn't mean there isn't gastric malignancy.
Ⓢ **ALERT:** Don't confuse Protonix with Lotronex, Prilosec, Prozac, or Prevacid.
Patient teaching
• Instruct patient to take exactly as prescribed and at approximately the same time every day.
• Tell patient that drug can be taken without regard to meals.
• Inform patient that tablet is to be swallowed whole and not crushed, split, or chewed.
• Tell patient that antacids don't affect the absorption of pantoprazole.
• Instruct patient to report abdominal pain or signs of bleeding, such as tarry stool.
• Advise patient to avoid alcohol, food, or other medications (aspirin, NSAIDs) that could cause gastric irritation.

☑ Evaluation

• Patient maintains adequate hydration throughout therapy.
• Patient responds well to therapy and doesn't aspirate.
• Patient and family state understanding of pantoprazole therapy.

papaverine hydrochloride

(puh-PAV-eh-reen high-droh-KLOR-ighd)
Pavabid Plateau Caps, Pavagen TD

Pharmacologic class: benzylisoquinoline derivative, opioid alkaloid
Therapeutic class: peripheral vasodilator
Pregnancy risk category: C

Indications and dosages

▶ **Relief of cerebral and peripheral ischemia from arterial spasm and myocardial ischemia; coronary occlusion and certain cerebral angiospastic states.** *Adults:* 150 to 300 mg P.O. q 8 to 12 hours. Or, 30 to 120 mg I.M. or

I.V. q 3 hours, as indicated. For extrasystoles, give two doses 10 minutes apart.
Children: 6 mg/kg I.M. or I.V. divided q.i.d.
▶ **Impotence‡.** *Adults:* 2.5 to 37.5 mg by intracavernous injection.

▽ I.V. administration

• Give drug by direct injection over 1 to 2 minutes to minimize risk of serious adverse reactions. Don't add to lactated Ringer's injection because precipitate forms.

Contraindications and precautions

• I.V. use is contraindicated in patients with Parkinson's disease or complete AV block.
• Use cautiously in patients with glaucoma or acute coronary thrombosis. Use cautiously in large doses.
🌿 **Lifespan:** In pregnant women, use cautiously. In breast-feeding women and in children, safety of drug hasn't been established.

Adverse reactions

CNS: *headache,* depression, malaise.
CV: *flushing, increased heart rate, increased blood pressure* (parenteral use), depressed AV and intraventricular conduction, hypotension, *arrhythmias.*
GI: constipation, dry mouth, *nausea.*
Hepatic: *hepatitis, cirrhosis.*
Respiratory: increased depth of respiration, *apnea.*
Skin: *diaphoresis.*

Interactions

Drug-drug. *Levodopa:* Papaverine may interfere with therapeutic effects of levodopa in patients with Parkinson's disease. Monitor patient closely for lack of effect.
Drug-herb. *Hawthorne:* May have additive vasodilatory effects. Discourage using together.

Effects on lab test results

• May increase liver function test values.

Pharmacokinetics

Absorption: 54% of oral drug is bioavailable; sustained-release forms are sometimes absorbed poorly and erratically. Unknown after I.M. administration.
Distribution: Drug tends to localize in adipose tissue and in liver; remainder is distributed

---

Rapid onset   *Liquid form contains alcohol.   ◆ Canada   ◇ Australia   †OTC   ‡Off-label use

throughout body. About 90% of drug is protein-bound.

Metabolism: Metabolized by the liver.
Excretion: Excreted in urine as metabolites.
Half-life: Varies widely.

Route	Onset	Peak	Duration
P.O.	Rapid	1-2 hr	12 hr
I.V., I.M.	Unknown	Unknown	Unknown

Action

Chemical effect: Has direct, nonspecific relaxant effect on vascular, cardiac, and other smooth muscle.
Therapeutic effect: Relieves vascular spasms.

Available forms

Capsules (sustained-release): 150 mg
Injection: 30 mg/ml in 2- and 10-ml ampules

NURSING PROCESS

℞ Assessment

• Assess patient's condition before therapy and regularly thereafter.
• Monitor blood pressure and heart rate and rhythm, especially in patient with cardiac disease.
• Be alert for adverse reactions and drug interactions.
• Monitor patient for adverse hepatic reactions during long-term therapy.
• Evaluate patient's and family's knowledge of drug therapy.

Nursing diagnoses

• Ineffective tissue perfusion (cerebral, cardiopulmonary, peripheral, GI) related to vascular spasms
• Constipation related to drug's effect on GI tract
• Deficient knowledge related to drug therapy

Planning and implementation

• Drug is most effective when given early in course of disorder.
• If vital signs change, hold dose and notify prescriber at once.
Patient teaching
• Tell patient that long-term therapy is required.
• Advise patient to avoid hazardous activities until CNS effects of drug are known.

• Instruct patient to avoid sudden position changes.

☑ Evaluation

• Patient maintains adequate tissue perfusion.
• Patient states measures used to prevent constipation.
• Patient and family state understanding of drug therapy.

---

paroxetine hydrochloride
(par-OKS-eh-teen high-droh-KLOR-ighd)
Paxil, Paxil CR

Pharmacologic class: SSRI
Therapeutic class: antidepressant
Pregnancy risk category: C

Indications and dosages

▶ **Major depressive disorder.** *Adults:* Initially, 20 mg P.O. daily, preferably in morning, as directed. Increase by 10 mg daily at weekly intervals, to maximum of 50 mg daily, if necessary. Or, initially, 25 mg Paxil CR P.O. as a single daily dose, usually in the morning, with or without food. May increase dose at intervals of at least 1 week by 12.5 mg daily increments, up to a maximum of 62.5 mg daily.
▶ **Obsessive-compulsive disorder.** *Adults:* Initially, 20 mg P.O. daily, preferably in morning, as directed. Increase by 10 mg daily at weekly intervals to target of 40 mg daily. Maximum daily dose, 60 mg.
▶ **Panic disorder.** *Adults:* Initially, 10 mg P.O. daily. Increase by 10-mg increments at no less than weekly intervals to target dose of 40 mg daily. Maximum daily dose is 60 mg. Or, initially, 12.5 mg Paxil CR P.O. as a single daily dose, usually in the morning, with or without food. May increase dose at intervals of at least 1 week by 12.5 mg daily increments, up to a maximum daily dose of 75 mg.
▶ **Social anxiety disorder.** *Adults:* Initially, 20 mg P.O. daily, usually in the morning. Maintain lowest effective dosage, and periodically assess patient to determine need for continued therapy. Maximum daily dose, 60 mg.
▶ **Generalized anxiety disorder.** *Adults:* Initially, 20 mg P.O. daily. Increase dose by 10 mg daily at increments of at least 1 week. Maximum daily dose, 50 mg.

▶ **Posttraumatic stress disorder.** *Adults:* Initially, 20 mg P.O. daily. Increase dose by 10 mg daily at increments of at least 1 week. Maximum daily dose, 50 mg.

◩ **Adjust-a-dose:** For geriatric or debilitated patients and patients with severe hepatic or renal disease, initially, give 10 mg P.O. (immediate-release) daily, preferably in morning. If patient doesn't respond, increase by 10-mg increments at weekly intervals to maximum daily dose of 40 mg. The recommended initial dosage of Paxil CR is 12.5 mg daily. Dosage shouldn't exceed 50 mg daily.

▶ **Premenstrual dysphoric disorder.** *Adults:* Initially, 12.5 mg Paxil CR P.O. daily, usually in the morning, with or without food. Maximum, 25 mg daily.

▶ **Diabetic neuropathy‡.** *Adults:* 10 to 60 mg P.O. daily.

▶ **Headache‡.** *Adults:* 10 to 50 mg P.O daily.

▶ **Premature ejaculation‡.** *Adults:* 20 mg P.O. daily.

Contraindications and precautions

• Contraindicated in patients taking MAO inhibitors or thioridazine.

• Use cautiously in patients with a history of seizures or mania; patients with severe, concomitant systemic illness; and patients at risk for volume depletion.

⚜ **Lifespan:** In pregnant and breast-feeding women, use cautiously. In children, safety of drug hasn't been established.

Adverse reactions

CNS: *asthenia,* blurred vision, *somnolence, dizziness, insomnia, tremor, headache,* nervousness, anxiety, paresthesia, confusion.
CV: palpitations, vasodilation, orthostatic hypotension.
EENT: lump or tightness in throat, dysgeusia.
GI: *dry mouth, nausea, constipation, diarrhea,* taste perversion, increased or decreased appetite, flatulence, vomiting, dyspepsia.
GU: *abnormal ejaculation, male genital disorders (including anorgasmy, erectile difficulties, delayed ejaculation or orgasm, impotence, and sexual dysfunction),* urinary frequency, other urinary disorder, *female genital disorder (including anorgasmy, difficulty with orgasm).*
Metabolic: hyponatremia.
Musculoskeletal: myopathy, myalgia, myasthenia.

Skin: *excessive sweating,* rash.
Other: decreased libido, yawning.

Interactions

Drug-drug. *Cimetidine:* Decreases hepatic metabolism of paroxetine, leading to risk of toxicity. Dosage adjustments may be necessary.
Digoxin: May decrease digoxin level. Monitor level closely.
Phenelzine, selegiline, tranylcypromine: May cause serotonin syndrome, including CNS irritability, shivering, and altered consciousness. Don't give together. Wait at least 2 weeks after stopping an MAO inhibitor before giving any SSRI.
Phenobarbital, phenytoin: May alter pharmacokinetics of both drugs. Dosage adjustments may be needed.
Procyclidine: May increase procyclidine levels. Monitor patient for excessive anticholinergic effects.
Sumatriptan: Weakness, hyperreflexia, and incoordination may occur. Monitor patient.
Theophylline: Theophylline clearance may decrease threefold. Dosage reduction may be necessary.
Thioridazine: Prolongation of QT interval and increased risk of serious ventricular arrhythmias, such as torsades de pointes and sudden death. Avoid use together.
Tricyclic antidepressants: May inhibit tricyclic antidepressant metabolism. Dose of tricyclic antidepressant may need to be reduced. Monitor patient closely.
Tryptophan: May increase risk of adverse reactions, such as nausea and dizziness. Avoid using together.
Warfarin: Increases risk of bleeding. Use with caution; monitor patient closely for bleeding.
Drug-herb. *St. John's wort:* May result in sedative-hypnotic intoxication. Discourage using together.
Drug-lifestyle. *Alcohol use:* May alter psychomotor function. Discourage using together.

Effects on lab test results

• May decrease sodium level.

Pharmacokinetics

Absorption: Completely absorbed.
Distribution: Distributed throughout body, including CNS; only 1% remains in plasma. About 93% to 95% bound to protein.

Metabolism: About 36% metabolized in liver.
Excretion: About 64% excreted in urine. *Half-life:* About 24 hours.

Route	Onset	Peak	Duration
P.O.			
immediate-release	1-4 wk	2-8 hr	Unknown
controlled-release	Unknown	6-10 hr	Unknown

Action

Chemical effect: Unknown; presumed to be linked to inhibition of CNS neuronal uptake of serotonin.
Therapeutic effect: Relieves depression.

Available forms

Suspension: 10 mg/5ml
Tablets: 10 mg, 20 mg, 30 mg, 40 mg
Tablets (controlled-release): 12.5 mg, 25 mg, 37.5 mg

NURSING PROCESS

🗒 Assessment
• Assess patient's depression before therapy and regularly thereafter.
• Be alert for adverse reactions and drug interactions.
• Evaluate patient's and family's knowledge of drug therapy.

🔲 Nursing diagnoses
• Disturbed thought processes related to depression
• Risk for injury related to drug-induced adverse CNS reactions
• Deficient knowledge related to drug therapy

🔷 Planning and implementation
• Don't give drug within 14 days of MAO inhibitor therapy.
• Don't crush CR tablet. If patient can't swallow a CR tablet whole, consider giving regular-release paroxetine hydrochloride.
• If signs of psychosis occur or increase, reduce dosage.
• **ALERT:** Don't confuse paroxetine with paclitaxel.
• **ALERT:** Don't confuse Paxil with Doxil, Taxol, or Plavix.

Patient teaching
• Warn patient to avoid hazardous activities until CNS effects of drug are known.
• Warn patient that the Paxil CR tablet shouldn't be chewed or crushed, and should be swallowed whole.
• Tell patient that he may notice improvement in 1 to 4 weeks but that he must continue with prescribed regimen to obtain continued benefits.
• Tell patient to abstain from alcohol during drug therapy.
• **ALERT:** If patient wishes to switch from an SSRI to St. John's wort, tell him to wait a few weeks for the SSRI to fully leave his system before starting the herb. The exact time required will depend on which SSRI he takes.

☑ Evaluation
• Patient's depression improves.
• Patient sustains no injuries because of drug-induced adverse CNS reactions.
• Patient and family state understanding of drug therapy.

pegaspargase (PEG-L-asparaginase)
(peg-AHS-per-jays)
Oncaspar

Pharmacologic class: modified version of enzyme L-asparaginase
Therapeutic class: antineoplastic
Pregnancy risk category: C

Indications and dosages

▶ **Acute lymphoblastic leukemia (ALL) in patients who need L-asparaginase but have developed hypersensitivity to native forms of L-asparaginase.** *Adults and children with body surface area of at least 0.6 m²:* 2,500 IU/m² I.M. or I.V. q 14 days.
Children with body surface area less than 0.6 m²: 82.5 IU/kg I.M. or I.V. q 14 days.

▽ I.V. administration

• Handle and give solution with care; wear gloves. Avoid inhaling vapors and contact with skin or mucous membranes, especially in eyes. If contact occurs, wash with copious amounts of water for at least 15 minutes.

• Avoid excessive agitation; don't shake. Keep refrigerated at 36° to 46° F (2° to 8° C). Don't use if cloudy, precipitated, or stored at room temperature for more than 48 hours.
• Give drug over 1 to 2 hours in 100 ml of normal saline solution or D_5W through infusion that is already running.
• Keep patient under observation for 1 hour after use and keep resuscitation equipment (such as epinephrine, oxygen, and I.V. steroids) within reach to treat anaphylaxis. If moderate to life-threatening hypersensitivity reactions occur, stop drug.
• Discard unused portions. Use only one dose per vial; don't reenter vial. Don't save unused drug for later use.

Contraindications and precautions

• Contraindicated in patients with pancreatitis or history of pancreatitis; in those who have had significant hemorrhagic events with previous L-asparaginase therapy; and in those with previous serious allergic reactions, such as generalized urticaria, bronchospasm, laryngeal edema, hypotension, or other unacceptable adverse reactions to pegaspargase.
• Use cautiously in patients with liver dysfunction.
Lifespan: In pregnant and breast-feeding women, drug isn't recommended.

Adverse reactions

CNS: ***seizures,*** headache, paresthesia, ***status epilepticus,*** somnolence, ***coma,*** mental status changes, dizziness, emotional lability, mood changes, parkinsonism, confusion, disorientation, fatigue, malaise.
CV: hypotension, tachycardia, chest pain, subacute bacterial endocarditis, hypertension, edema.
EENT: epistaxis.
GI: nausea, vomiting, abdominal pain, anorexia, diarrhea, constipation, indigestion, flatulence, GI pain, mucositis, ***pancreatitis (sometimes fulminant and fatal),*** colitis, mouth tenderness.
GU: increased urinary frequency, hematuria, severe hemorrhagic cystitis, renal dysfunction, ***renal failure.***
Hematologic: ***thrombosis, leukopenia, pancytopenia, agranulocytosis, thrombocytopenia, disseminated intravascular coagulation,*** hemolytic anemia, easy bruising, ***hemorrhage.***
Hepatic: jaundice, bilirubinemia, ascites, hypoalbuminemia, fatty changes in liver, ***liver failure.***
Metabolic: hyperuricemia, hyponatremia, uric acid nephropathy, hypoproteinemia, proteinuria, weight loss, ***metabolic acidosis,*** hyperglycemia, ***hypoglycemia.***
Musculoskeletal: arthralgia, myalgia, musculoskeletal pain, joint stiffness, cramps.
Respiratory: cough, ***severe bronchospasm,*** upper respiratory tract infection.
Skin: ecchymosis, itching, alopecia, fever blister, purpura, white hands, urticaria, fungal changes, nail whiteness and ridging, erythema simplex, petechial rash, nighttime sweating.
Other: ***hypersensitivity reactions (including anaphylaxis,*** pain, fever, chills, peripheral edema; infection); ***sepsis; septic shock;*** injection pain or reaction; localized edema.

Interactions

Drug-drug. *Aspirin, dipyridamole, heparin, NSAIDs, warfarin:* Imbalances in coagulation factors may occur, predisposing patient to bleeding or thrombosis. Use together cautiously.
Methotrexate: May interfere with action of methotrexate, which requires cell replication for its lethal effect. Monitor patient for decreased effectiveness.
Protein-bound drugs: Protein depletion may increase toxicity of other drugs that bind to proteins. Monitor patient for toxicity. May interfere with enzymatic detoxification of other drugs, particularly in liver. Give together cautiously.

Effects on lab test results

• May increase BUN, creatinine, amylase, lipase, bilirubin, ALT, AST, uric acid, and ammonia levels. May decrease sodium and protein levels. May increase or decrease glucose level.
• May increase PT, INR, PTT, and thromboplastin. May decrease antithrombin III, fibrinogen, hemoglobin, hematocrit, and WBC, RBC, platelet, and granulocyte counts.

Pharmacokinetics

Absorption: Unknown.
Distribution: Unknown.
Metabolism: Unknown.
Excretion: Unknown. *Half-life:* 2 to 6 days.

Route	Onset	Peak	Duration
I.V., I.M.	Unknown	Unknown	Unknown

Action

Chemical effect: Destroys cancer cells by inactivating the amino acid asparagine. Asparagine is required by tumor cells to synthesize proteins. Because tumor cells can't synthesize their own asparagine, protein synthesis and, eventually, synthesis of DNA and RNA are inhibited.
Therapeutic effect: Kills selected leukemic cells.

Available forms

Injection: 750 IU/ml

NURSING PROCESS

🔏 Assessment

• Assess patient's condition before therapy and regularly thereafter.
• Monitor patient closely for hypersensitivity reactions, including life-threatening anaphylaxis, which may occur during therapy, especially in patient hypersensitive to other forms of L-asparaginase.
• Monitor patient's peripheral blood count and bone marrow. A drop in circulating lymphoblasts is often noted after therapy begins. This may be accompanied by marked rise in uric acid levels.
• Monitor amylase levels to detect early evidence of pancreatitis. Monitor patient's glucose levels during therapy because hyperglycemia may occur.
• Monitor patient for liver dysfunction when used with hepatotoxic chemotherapeutics.
• Drug may affect a number of plasma proteins; therefore, monitor fibrinogen, PT, and PTT.
• Be alert for adverse reactions and drug interactions.
• Evaluate patient's and family's knowledge of drug therapy.

🔁 Nursing diagnoses

• Ineffective health maintenance related to leukemia
• Ineffective protection related to drug-induced adverse hematologic reactions
• Deficient knowledge related to drug therapy

▶ Planning and implementation

• Use as monotherapy only in unusual situation when combined regimen that uses other chemotherapeutic drugs is inappropriate because of toxicity, because patient is refractory to other

therapy, or because of other specific patient-related factors.
• Don't use drug that has been frozen. Although drug may not look different, freezing destroys its activity. Obtain new dose from pharmacist.
• Hydrate patient before therapy. Hyperuricemia may result from rapid lysis of leukemic cells. Allopurinol may be ordered.
• I.M. route is preferred over I.V. route because of its lower risk of hepatotoxicity, coagulopathy, and GI and renal disorders.
• Limit volume administered at single injection site to 2 ml. If volume is larger than 2 ml, use multiple injection sites.
Patient teaching
• Inform patient about hypersensitivity reactions and importance of alerting staff at once if they occur.
• Instruct patient to ask prescriber before taking other drugs, including OTC preparations. Using together may increase risk of bleeding or may increase toxicity of other drugs.
• Instruct patient to report signs and symptoms of infection (fever, chills, and malaise) to prescriber because drug may suppress immune system.

☑ Evaluation

• Patient responds well to therapy.
• Patient develops no serious complications caused by drug-induced adverse hematologic reactions.
• Patient and family state understanding of drug therapy.

---

pegfilgrastim
(peg-FILL-grass-tihm)
Neulasta

Pharmacologic class: colony-stimulating factor
Therapeutic class: neutrophil-growth stimulator
Pregnancy risk category: C

Indications and dosages

▶ **To reduce frequency of infection in patients with nonmyeloid malignancies receiving myelosuppressive anticancer drugs that may cause febrile neutropenia.** *Adults:* 6 mg S.C. once per chemotherapy cycle. Don't give in

---

the period between 14 days before and 24 hours after administration of cytotoxic chemotherapy.

Contraindications and precautions

• Contraindicated in patients hypersensitive to *Escherichia coli*–derived proteins, filgrastim, or any component of the drug.
• Don't give from 14 days before to 24 hours after cytotoxic chemotherapy.
• Don't use for peripheral blood progenitor cell (PBPC) mobilization.
• Use cautiously in patients with sickle cell disease, those receiving chemotherapy causing delayed myelosuppression, or those receiving radiation therapy.

⚠ Lifespan: In pregnant women, use drug only if potential benefit to mother justifies potential risk to fetus. In breast-feeding women, use cautiously. Infants, children, and adolescents weighing less than 45 kg (99 lb) shouldn't use the 6-mg single-use syringe dose. In children, safety and effectiveness of drug haven't been established.

Adverse reactions

CNS: *dizziness, headache, fatigue, insomnia, fever.*
CV: *peripheral edema.*
GI: *nausea, diarrhea, vomiting, constipation, anorexia, taste perversion, dyspepsia, abdominal pain, stomatitis, mucositis.*
Hematologic: GRANULOCYTOPENIA, NEUTROPENIC FEVER.
Musculoskeletal: *skeletal pain, generalized weakness, arthralgia, myalgia, bone pain.*
Respiratory: *acute respiratory distress syndrome (ARDS).*
Skin: *alopecia.*

Interactions

Drug-drug. *Lithium:* May increase the release of neutrophils. Monitor neutrophil counts closely.

Effects on lab test results

• May increase LDH, alkaline phosphatase, and uric acid levels.
• May increase WBC, granulocyte, and neutrophil counts.

Pharmacokinetics

Absorption: Unknown.
Distribution: Unknown.

Metabolism: Unknown.
Excretion: Unknown. *Half-life:* 15 to 80 hours.

Route	Onset	Peak	Duration
S.C.	Unknown	Unknown	Unknown

Action

Chemical effect: Binds cell receptors to stimulate proliferation, differentiation, commitment, and end-cell function of neutrophils. Pegfilgrastim and filgrastim have the same mechanism of action. Pegfilgrastim has a reduced renal clearance and therefore a longer half-life than filgrastim.
Therapeutic effect: Increases WBC count.

Available forms

Injection: 6 mg/0.6 ml single-use, preservative-free, prefilled syringes.

NURSING PROCESS

✍ Assessment

• Assess underlying condition before therapy and reassess regularly throughout therapy.
• Obtain CBC and platelet count before therapy.
• Monitor patient's hemoglobin, hematocrit, and CBC and platelet counts; and LDH, alkaline phosphatase, and uric acid levels during therapy.
• Evaluate patient's and family's knowledge of drug therapy.

⊕ Nursing diagnoses

• Acute pain related to adverse musculoskeletal effects of drug
• Risk for infection related to underlying condition and treatment
• Deficient knowledge related to pegfilgrastim therapy

▶ Planning and implementation

• The maximum amount of filgrastim that can be given is unknown. Treat patients having symptomatic leukocytosis with leukapheresis.
⚠ **ALERT:** Splenic rupture may occur rarely with filgrastim use. Evaluate patient who experiences signs or symptoms of left upper abdominal or shoulder pain for an enlarged spleen or splenic rupture.
• Monitor patient for allergic-type reactions, including anaphylaxis, skin rash, and urticaria.

• Evaluate patient who develops fever, lung infiltrates, or respiratory distress for ARDS. If ARDS occurs, stop drug.
• Keep patient with sickle cell disease well hydrated, and monitor patient for symptoms of sickle cell crisis.
• Pegfilgrastim may act as a growth factor for tumors.

Patient teaching
• Inform patient of the potential side effects of the drug.
• Tell patient to report signs and symptoms of allergic reactions, left upper abdominal or shoulder pain, fever, or breathing problems.
• Tell patient with sickle cell disease to maintain hydration and report signs or symptoms of sickle cell crisis.
• Instruct patient or caregiver how to give drug if it is to be given at home.
• Instruct patient or caregiver that the drug shouldn't be frozen. If accidentally frozen, thaw in refrigerator before administration. Drug should be discarded if frozen twice.

☑ **Evaluation**
• Patient states that pain management is adequate.
• Patient's WBC count is normal.
• Patient and family state understanding of drug therapy.

peginterferon alfa-2a
(peg-inter-FEAR-on AL-fah TOO AY)
Pegasys

Pharmacologic class: biological response modifier
Therapeutic class: antiviral
Pregnancy risk category: C

Indications and dosages

▶ **Chronic hepatitis C in patients not previously treated with interferon alfa.** *Adults:* 180 mcg S.C. in abdomen or thigh, once weekly for 48 weeks.
🔲 **Adjust-a-dose:** For patients who experience moderate to severe adverse reactions, decrease dose to 135 mcg S.C. once a week; in some cases, decrease to 90 mcg S.C. once a week. For patients who experience hematologic reactions, if neutrophil count is less than

750/mm³, reduce dose to 135 mcg S.C. once a week; if absolute neutrophil count (ANC) is less than 500/mm³, stop drug until ANC exceeds 1,000/mm³ and restart at 90 mcg S.C. once a week. If platelet count is less than 50,000/mm³, reduce dose to 90 mcg S.C. once a week; stop drug if platelet count drops below 25,000/mm³. In patients on hemodialysis, decrease dose to 135 mcg S.C. once a week. In patients with ALT level increases above baseline, decrease dose to 90 mcg S.C. once a week; if hepatic impairment worsens or bilirubin level increases, stop therapy.

Contraindications and precautions

• Contraindicated in patients hypersensitive to interferon alfa-2a or its components and in patients with autoimmune hepatitis or decompensated liver disease before or during therapy.
• Use cautiously in patients with a history of depression, suicidal ideation, or suicide attempts. Also use cautiously in patients with baseline neutrophil counts less than 1,500/mm³, baseline platelet counts less than 90,000/mm³, or baseline hemoglobin less than 10 g/dl. Use cautiously in patients with cardiac disease or hypertension, thyroid disease, autoimmune disorders, pulmonary disorders, colitis, pancreatitis, or ophthalmologic disorders. Also use cautiously in patients with creatinine clearance less than 50 ml/minute.
• Safety and effectiveness of drug haven't been established for hepatitis C in liver- or other organ-transplant recipients, for patients with hepatitis C co-infected with HIV or hepatitis B, or in patients who haven't responded to other alpha interferon therapy.
🔺 **Lifespan:** In pregnant women, use only if benefit outweighs risk. Women of childbearing potential must use effective contraception. Breast-feeding women should stop during therapy. It's unknown whether drug appears in breast milk. In neonates and premature infants, avoid using drug because it contains benzyl alcohol. In children, safety and effectiveness of drug haven't been established. In elderly patients, use cautiously because they may be at increased risk for adverse reactions.

Adverse reactions

CNS: *fever, pain, fatigue,* asthenia, *headache, insomnia, dizziness,* concentration and memory

---

impairment, *depression, irritability,* anxiety, *suicide, cerebral hemorrhage, coma.*
CV: *pulmonary embolism.*
GI: *nausea, diarrhea, abdominal pain,* vomiting, dry mouth, *anorexia, pancreatitis.*
Hematologic: NEUTROPENIA, *thrombocytopenia.*
Musculoskeletal: *myalgia, arthralgia,* back pain.
Skin: *alopecia, pruritus,* increased sweating, dermatitis, rash.
Other: *rigors, injection site reaction.*

Interactions

Drug-drug. *Theophylline:* May increase theophylline level. Monitor theophylline level and adjust dosage, p.r.n.

Effects on lab test results

• May increase ALT level.
• May decrease hemoglobin, hematocrit, and ANC, WBC, and platelet counts. May increase or decrease thyroid function test values.

Pharmacokinetics

Absorption: Unknown.
Distribution: Unknown.
Metabolism: Possibly in liver and kidney.
Excretion: Probably renal because patients on hemodialysis have decreased clearance of drug. *Half-life:* 80 hours.

Route	Onset	Peak	Duration
S.C.	Unknown	72-96 hr	Up to 1 wk

Action

Chemical effect: Binds to specific receptors on the cell surface, which inhibits viral replication in infected cells, inhibits cell proliferation, and causes immunomodulation. Partially stimulates production of effector proteins in vitro.
Therapeutic effect: Increases effector proteins and body temperature, and decreases leukocyte and platelet counts.

Available forms

Injection: 180 mcg/ml single-dose vials, 180 mcg/0.5 ml prefilled syringes

NURSING PROCESS

Assessment

• Monitor patient for psychiatric reactions, including depression and suicidal ideation. These symptoms may occur in patients without prior psychiatric illness. If severe depression occurs, stop drug and start psychiatric therapy.
• Obtain CBC before therapy and monitor routinely thereafter. Stop drug for large decrease in neutrophil or platelet counts.
• Obtain baseline eye examination and periodically monitor eye exams during therapy. If new or worsening eye disorders occur, stop drug.
• Monitor lab values for kidney or liver impairment.

Nursing diagnoses

• Ineffective health maintenance related to underlying condition
• Risk for suicide related to adverse CNS effects of drug
• Deficient knowledge related to peginterferon alfa-2a therapy

Planning and implementation

• If uncontrollable thyroid disease, hyperglycemia, hypoglycemia, or diabetes mellitus occur, stop drug.
• If persistent or unexplained pulmonary infiltrates or pulmonary dysfunction occur, stop drug.
• If signs and symptoms of colitis (abdominal pain, bloody diarrhea, and fever) occur, stop drug. Symptoms should resolve within 1 to 3 weeks.
• If signs and symptoms of pancreatitis occur, stop drug.
Patient teaching
• Teach patient proper technique for giving drug and disposing of needles and syringes.
• Tell patient to immediately report depression or suicidal ideation.
• Tell patient to report signs and symptoms of pancreatitis, colitis, eye disorders, or respiratory disorders.
• Advise patient to avoid driving or operating machinery if dizziness, fatigue, confusion, or somnolence occur.

Evaluation

• Patient has improved health.
• Patient denies suicidal ideation.
• Patient and family state understanding of drug therapy.

peginterferon alfa-2b
(pehg-in-ter-FEAR-ahn AL-fah TOO BEE)
PEG-Intron

Pharmacologic class: biological response modifier
Therapeutic class: antiviral
Pregnancy risk category: C

Indications and dosages

▶ **Chronic hepatitis C.** *Adults:* Recommended regimen is approximately 1 mcg/kg S.C. once weekly for 48 weeks on the same day each week. Recommended doses are as follows:
37 to 45 kg (81 to 99 lb): 40 mcg (0.4 ml) of 100-mcg/ml strength
46 to 56 kg (100 to 123 lb): 50 mcg (0.5 ml) of 100-mcg/ml strength
57 to 72 kg (124 to 158 lb): 64 mcg (0.4 ml) of 160-mcg/ml strength
73 to 88 kg (159 to 194 lb): 80 mcg (0.5 ml) of 160-mcg/ml strength
89 to 106 kg (195 to 233 lb): 96 mcg (0.4 ml) of 240-mcg/ml strength
107 to 136 kg (234 to 299 lb): 120 mcg (0.5 ml) of 240-mcg/ml strength
137 to 160 kg (300 to 352 lb): 150 mcg (0.5 ml) of 300-mcg/ml strength

▶ **Chronic hepatitis C in patients not previously treated with interferon alpha, given with ribavirin.** *Adults:* Recommended regimen is approximately 1.5 mcg/kg S.C. once weekly for 48 weeks on same day each week. Specific doses are as follows:
Less than 40 kg (<88 lb): 50 mcg (0.5 ml) of 100-mcg/ml strength
40 to 50 kg (88 to 110 lb): 64 mcg (0.4 ml) of 160-mcg/ml strength
51 to 60 kg (111 to 132 lb): 80 mcg (0.5 ml) of 160-mcg/ml strength
61 to 75 kg (133 to 165 lb): 96 mcg (0.4 ml) of 240 mcg-mcg/ml strength
76 to 85 kg (166 to 187 lb): 120 mcg (0.5 ml) of 240 mcg-mcg/ml strength
More than 85 kg (187 lb): 150 mcg (0.5 ml) of 300-mcg/ml strength

⬛ **Adjust-a-dose:** In patients with WBC counts less than 1,500/mm³, neutrophil counts less than 750/mm³, or platelet counts less than 80,000/mm³, decrease dose by one-half. Oral ribavirin dose can be continued. If hemoglobin is less than 10 g/dl, reduce oral ribavirin dose by 200 mg daily. If hemoglobin is less than 8.5 g/dl, WBC counts less than 1000/mm³, neutrophil counts less than 500/mm³, or platelet counts less than 50,000/mm³, stop both drugs.

If patient develops mild depression, drug can be continued, but he should be evaluated weekly. For moderate depression, reduce dose by one-half for 4 to 8 weeks and evaluate patient q week. If symptoms improve and remain stable for 4 weeks, continue at present dose or resume previous dose. If severe depression occurs, stop drug.

For patients with stable CV disease whose hemoglobin decreases more than 2 g/dl in any 4-week period, decrease peginterferon alfa-2b dosage by one-half and ribavirin dosage by 200 mg daily. If hemoglobin is less than 12 g/dl after 4 weeks of reduced dosages, stop both drugs.

Contraindications and precautions

● Contraindicated in patients hypersensitive to drug or its components and in patients with renal impairment (creatinine clearance below 50 ml/minute), pulmonary infiltrates, autoimmune hepatitis, or decompensated liver disease (Child-Pugh class B and C).
● Don't use drug in organ transplant recipients, patients who haven't responded to other alpha interferon therapy, or those with HIV or hepatitis B virus.
● Use cautiously in patients with psychiatric disorders; diabetes mellitus; cardiovascular disease; pulmonary function impairment; or autoimmune, ischemic, and infectious disorders.
🔥 **Lifespan:** In pregnant women and men whose sexual partners are pregnant, drug is contraindicated. Breast-feeding women should either stop breast-feeding or drug; it isn't known whether drug appears in breast milk. In neonates and infants, drug is contraindicated because it contains benzyl alcohol. In children, safety and effectiveness of drug haven't been established.

Adverse reactions

CNS: dizziness, hypertonia, fever, depression, insomnia, anxiety, emotional lability, irritability, headache, fatigue, malaise, *suicidal behavior.*
CV: flushing.
EENT: pharyngitis, sinusitis.

Reactions may be *common*, uncommon, *life-threatening*, or COMMON AND LIFE-THREATENING.

GI: nausea, anorexia, diarrhea, abdominal pain, vomiting, dyspepsia, right upper quadrant pain.
Hematologic: *neutropenia, thrombocytopenia.*
Hepatic: hepatomegaly.
Metabolic: hypothyroidism, hyperthyroidism, weight decrease.
Musculoskeletal: musculoskeletal pain.
Respiratory: cough.
Skin: alopecia, pruritus, dry skin, rash, increased sweating.
Other: injection site reaction (inflammation), injection site pain, viral infection, flulike symptoms, rigors.

Interactions

None reported.

Effects on lab test results

• May increase ALT levels. May increase or decrease TSH levels.
• May decrease neutrophil and platelet counts.

Pharmacokinetics

Absorption: Levels peak 15 to 44 hours after a dose and persist for 48 to 72 hours.
Distribution: Unknown.
Metabolism: Unknown.
Excretion: About 30% is excreted by the kidneys. *Half-life:* 40 hours.

Route	Onset	Peak	Duration
S.C.	Unknown	15-44 hr	Unknown

Action

Chemical effect: Binds to certain receptors on the cell surface, which induces enzymes to suppress cell proliferation. This modifies immune function and inhibits virus replication in infected cells.
Therapeutic effect: Increases effector proteins and body temperature, and it decreases leukocyte and platelet counts.

Available forms

Injection: 100 mcg/ml, 160 mcg/ml, 240 mcg/ml, 300 mcg/ml

NURSING PROCESS

Assessment
• Assess underlying condition before therapy and regularly thereafter.

• Assess patients for preexisting uncontrolled diabetes or thyroid disorders. Peginterferon alfa-2b may cause or aggravate hypothyroidism, hyperthyroidism, or diabetes.
• If patient has cardiac history, obtain ECG before starting drug.
• Evaluate patient's volume status and make sure patient is well hydrated before starting drug.
• Obtain eye examination in patients with diabetes or hypertension before starting drug. Retinal hemorrhages, cotton wool spots, and retinal artery or vein obstruction may occur.
• Monitor CBC, platelet count, and AST, ALT, bilirubin, and TSH levels before starting drug and periodically during therapy.
• Evaluate patient's and family's knowledge of drug therapy.

Nursing diagnoses
• Ineffective health maintenance related to underlying condition
• Risk for suicide related to adverse CNS effects of drug
• Deficient knowledge related to peginterferon alfa-2b therapy

Planning and implementation
• Drug may be used alone or with Copegus for chronic hepatitis B.
• If patient has history of MI or arrhythmias, watch closely for hypotension, arrhythmias, tachycardia, cardiomyopathy, and MI.
• **ALERT:** Alpha interferons may cause or aggravate fatal or life-threatening neuropsychiatric, autoimmune, ischemic, and infectious disorders. Monitor patients closely with periodic evaluations of these disorders. Stop therapy in patients with persistently severe or worsening signs or symptoms of these conditions. In many, but not all, cases these disorders resolve after stopping therapy.
• Monitor patient for depression and other psychiatric illness. If symptoms are severe, stop drug and refer patient for psychiatric care.
• Monitor patient for signs and symptoms of colitis, such as abdominal pain, bloody diarrhea, and fever. If colitis occurs, stop drug. Symptoms should resolve 1 to 3 weeks after stopping drug.
• Monitor patient for signs and symptoms of pancreatitis or hypersensitivity reactions. If these occur, stop drug.

- Monitor patient with pulmonary disease for dyspnea, pulmonary infiltrates, pneumonitis, and pneumonia.
- If patient has renal disease, watch for signs and symptoms of toxicity.
- If patient has severe neutropenia or thrombocytopenia, stop drug.

Patient teaching
- Explain appropriate use of the drug and its benefits and risks. Tell patient that adverse reactions may continue for several months after therapy stops.
- Advise patient that laboratory tests are required before therapy starts and periodically thereafter.
- Tell patient to take drug h.s. and to use antipyretics to decrease the effect of flulike symptoms.
- Emphasize the importance of properly disposing of needles and syringes, and warn against reusing old needles and syringes.
- Tell patient that drug isn't known to prevent transmission of hepatitis C. It also isn't known whether drug cures hepatitis C or prevents cirrhosis, liver failure, or liver cancer that may result from hepatitis C.
- Advise patient to immediately report symptoms of depression or thoughts of suicide.

☑ **Evaluation**
- Patient has improved health.
- Patient reports no suicidal ideation.
- Patient and family state understanding of drug therapy.

pemoline
(PEH-moh-leen)
Cylert, Cylert Chewable, PemADD, PemADD CT

Pharmacologic class: oxazolidinedione derivative
Therapeutic class: CNS stimulant
Pregnancy risk category: B
Controlled substance schedule: IV

Indications and dosages

▶ **Attention deficit hyperactivity disorder (ADHD).** *Children age 6 and older:* Initially, 37.5 mg P.O. in morning. Increase by 18.75 mg daily q week, as necessary. Effective dosage

range is 56.25 to 75 mg daily. Maximum dosage, 112.5 mg daily.
▶ **Narcolepsy‡.** *Adults:* 50 to 200 mg P.O. daily in divided doses after breakfast and after lunch.

Contraindications and precautions

- Contraindicated in patients hypersensitive to drug, in those who have idiosyncratic reactions to drug, and in those with hepatic dysfunction.
- Because of risk of hepatic failure, don't use drug as first-line therapy.
- Use cautiously in patients with impaired renal function.
- ⚘ **Lifespan:** In children, drug may precipitate Tourette syndrome.

Adverse reactions

CNS: *insomnia,* malaise, dyskinetic movements, irritability, fatigue, mild depression, dizziness, headache, drowsiness, hallucinations, nervousness, *seizures, Tourette syndrome,* psychosis.
GI: anorexia, abdominal pain, nausea, diarrhea.
Hematologic: *aplastic anemia.*
Hepatic: *hepatitis,* jaundice, *hepatic failure.*
Metabolic: growth suppression.
Skin: rash.

Interactions

Drug-drug. *Anticonvulsants:* May decrease seizure threshold. Monitor patient closely; take seizure precautions.
Drugs with CNS activity: May have additive side effects. Monitor patient closely.

Effects on lab test results

- May increase liver enzyme levels.
- May decrease hemoglobin and hematocrit.
- May increase prostate-specific antigen (PSA) levels.

Pharmacokinetics

Absorption: Well absorbed.
Distribution: Distribution is unknown. Drug is 50% protein-bound.
Metabolism: Metabolized in liver.
Excretion: Excreted in urine. *Half-life:* 12 hours.

Route	Onset	Peak	Duration
P.O.	Unknown	2-4 hr	Unknown

Action

Chemical effect: Releases stored norepinephrine from nerve terminals in brain (mainly in the cerebral cortex and reticular activating system), which may promote transmission of nerve impulses.
Therapeutic effect: Promotes calmness in children with ADHD.

Available forms

Tablets: 18.75 mg, 37.5 mg, 75 mg
Tablets (chewable and containing povidone): 37.5 mg

NURSING PROCESS

⚖ Assessment

• Assess patient's condition, including liver function test results, before and during therapy.
• May precipitate Tourette syndrome in children. Monitor patient closely, especially at start of therapy.
• Monitor patient for blood or hepatic function changes and growth suppression.
• If significant hepatic dysfunction occurs, stop drug.
• Drug may produce adverse reactions similar to those from amphetamines or methylphenidate, including lowered seizure threshold. Has potential for abuse and dependence.
• Evaluate patient's and family's knowledge of drug therapy.

🔄 Nursing diagnoses

• Risk for injury related to ADHD
• Disturbed sleep pattern related to drug-induced insomnia
• Deficient knowledge related to drug therapy

▶ Planning and implementation

• Give drug at least 6 hours before bedtime.
• **⚠ ALERT:** Don't use drug as first-line therapy for ADHD because of risk of life-threatening hepatic failure.
• Discuss therapy with patient and patient's family, and obtain a signed consent form before starting therapy.
Patient teaching
• Warn patient and parent to avoid hazardous activities until effects of drug are known.
• Tell patient to report insomnia and other adverse effects.

☑ Evaluation

• Patient shows less hyperactivity.
• Patient can sleep without difficulty throughout drug therapy.
• Patient and family state understanding of drug therapy.

penicillamine
(pen-ih-SIL-uh-meen)
Cuprimine, Depen

Pharmacologic class: chelate
Therapeutic class: heavy metal antagonist, antirheumatic
Pregnancy risk category: NR

Indications and dosages

▶ **Wilson's disease.** *Adults and children:* 250 mg P.O. q.i.d. 30 to 60 minutes before meals. Adjust dosage to achieve urinary copper excretion of 0.5 to 1 mg daily.
▶ **Cystinuria.** *Adults:* 250 mg to 1 g P.O. q.i.d. before meals. Adjust dosage to achieve urinary cystine excretion of less than 100 mg daily when renal calculi are present or 100 to 200 mg daily when no calculi are present. Maximum, 4 g daily.
Children: 30 mg/kg P.O. daily divided q.i.d. before meals. Adjust dosage to achieve urinary cystine excretion of less than 100 mg daily when renal calculi are present or 100 to 200 mg daily when no calculi are present.
▶ **Rheumatoid arthritis.** *Adults:* Initially, 125 to 250 mg P.O. daily, with increases of 125 to 250 mg q 1 to 3 months, if necessary. Maximum, 1.5 g daily.
▶ **Adjunct in heavy metal poisoning‡.** *Adults:* 500 to 1,500 mg P.O. daily for 1 to 2 months.
▶ **Primary biliary cirrhosis‡.** *Adults:* Initially, 250 mg P.O. daily with increases of 250 mg P.O. q 2 weeks. Maximum, 1 g daily in divided doses.

Contraindications and precautions

• Contraindicated in patients with previous penicillamine-related aplastic anemia or granulocytosis, patients with rheumatoid arthritis and renal insufficiency.
• Use cautiously, if at all, in patients hypersensitive to penicillin.

≉ **Lifespan:** In pregnant women, except those with Wilson's disease, drug is contraindicated. In breast-feeding women, safety of drug hasn't been established.

Adverse reactions

EENT: tinnitus, *optic neuritis.*
GI: *anorexia, epigastric pain, nausea, vomiting, diarrhea, loss of taste or altered taste perception, stomatitis,* oral ulcerations.
GU: nephrotic syndrome, glomerulonephritis, proteinuria, hematuria.
Hematologic: *leukopenia, eosinophilia, thrombocytopenia,* monocytosis, *agranulocytopenia, aplastic anemia,* lymphadenopathy.
Hepatic: *hepatotoxicity.*
Musculoskeletal: *arthralgia.*
Respiratory: *pneumonitis.*
Skin: alopecia; friability, especially at pressure spots; wrinkling; erythema; urticaria; ecchymoses.
Other: lupus-like syndrome, myasthenia gravis syndrome with long-term use, allergic reactions.

Interactions

Drug-drug. *Antacids, oral iron:* Decreases effectiveness of penicillamine. Give at least 2 hours apart.
Antimalaria drugs, cytotoxic drugs, gold therapy, oxyphenbutazone, phenylbutazone: Increases risk of toxicity. Avoid giving together.
Digoxin: May decrease digoxin effect. Dosage adjustment may be required.
Drug-food. *Any food:* Delays absorption of drug. Give drug 1 hour before or 3 hours after meals.

Effects on lab test results

• May increase liver enzyme levels.
• May increase eosinophil count and sedimentation rate. May decrease hemoglobin, hematocrit, and platelet, WBC, and granulocyte counts.

Pharmacokinetics

Absorption: Well absorbed from GI tract.
Distribution: Limited data available.
Metabolism: Uncomplexed penicillamine is metabolized in liver to inactive disulfides.
Excretion: Only small amount of penicillamine excreted unchanged; after 24 hours, 50% of drug excreted in urine, 20% in feces, and 30% is unaccounted for.

Route	Onset	Peak	Duration
P.O.	Unknown	1 hr	Unknown

Action

Chemical effect: Chelates heavy metals and may inhibit collagen formation; unknown for rheumatoid arthritis.
Therapeutic effect: Chelates copper in Wilson's disease, combines with cystine to form complex more soluble than cystine alone, and relieves symptoms of rheumatoid arthritis.

Available forms

Capsules: 125 mg, 250 mg
Tablets (scored): 250 mg

NURSING PROCESS

☑ Assessment
• Obtain history of patient's underlying condition before therapy.
• Monitor effectiveness by evaluating patient's urinary copper or cysteine excretion or improvement in rheumatoid arthritis.
• Monitor CBC and kidney and liver function q 2 weeks for first 6 months, and then monthly.
• Monitor urinalysis regularly for protein loss.
• Check patient's range of motion and joint mobility.
• Be alert for adverse reactions and drug interactions.
• Evaluate patient's and family's knowledge of drug therapy.

⊕ Nursing diagnoses
• Impaired physical mobility related to Wilson's disease
• Impaired urinary elimination related to drug-induced renal dysfunction
• Deficient knowledge related to drug therapy

⊳ Planning and implementation
• Give dose on empty stomach to facilitate absorption, preferably 1 hour before or 3 hours after meals.
• Give supplemental pyridoxine daily.
• If patient has a skin reaction, give antihistamines. Handle patient carefully to avoid skin damage.
⊛ **ALERT:** Report rash and fever (important signs of toxicity) to prescriber immediately.
• If WBC count falls below 3,500/mm³ or platelet count falls below 100,000/mm³, with-

hold drug and notify prescriber. A progressive decline in platelet or WBC count in three successive blood tests may necessitate temporary cessation of therapy, even if such counts are within normal limits.

⊕ **ALERT:** Don't confuse penicillamine with penicillin.

Patient teaching
• Tell patient with rheumatoid arthritis that drug may not take effect for up to 3 months.
• Tell patient to maintain adequate fluid intake, especially at night.
• Advise patient to report early signs of granulocytopenia: fever, sore throat, chills, bruising, and prolonged bleeding time.
• Reassure patient that taste impairment usually resolves in 6 weeks without change in dosage.

☑ **Evaluation**
• Patient reports increase in physical mobility.
• Patient maintains normal urinary elimination pattern.
• Patient and family state understanding of drug therapy.

penicillin G benzathine (benzylpenicillin benzathine)
(pen-ih-SIL-in gee BENZ-uh-theen)
Bicillin L-A, Permapen

Pharmacologic class: natural penicillin
Therapeutic class: antibiotic
Pregnancy risk category: B

Indications and dosages
▶ **Congenital syphilis.** *Children younger than age 2:* 50,000 units/kg I.M. as single dose.
▶ **Group A streptococcal upper respiratory tract infections.** *Adults:* 1.2 million units I.M. as single injection.
Children weighing more than 27 kg (59 lb): 900,000 units I.M. as single injection.
Children weighing less than 27 kg (59 lb): 300,000 to 600,000 units I.M. as single injection.
▶ **Prophylaxis of poststreptococcal rheumatic fever.** *Adults and children:* 1.2 million units I.M. once monthly or 600,000 units twice monthly.

▶ **Syphilis of less than 1 year's duration.** *Adults:* 2.4 million units I.M. as single dose.
▶ **Syphilis of more than 1 year's duration.** *Adults:* 2.4 million units I.M. weekly for 3 successive weeks.

Contraindications and precautions
• Contraindicated in patients hypersensitive to drug or other penicillins.
• Use cautiously in patients with other drug allergies, especially to cephalosporins.
⚠ **Lifespan:** In pregnant women, use cautiously. Drug appears in breast milk. In breastfeeding women, use of drug may sensitize infant to penicillin and cause some adverse effects.

Adverse reactions
CNS: pain, neuropathy, *seizures.*
Hematologic: eosinophilia, hemolytic anemia, *thrombocytopenia, leukopenia.*
Other: hypersensitivity reactions (maculopapular and exfoliative dermatitis, chills, fever, edema, *anaphylaxis*), sterile abscess at injection site.

Interactions
Drug-drug. *Colestipol:* Decreases levels of penicillin G benzathine. Give penicillin 1 hour before or 4 hours after colestipol.
Heparin, oral anticoagulants: Increases risk of bleeding. Monitor PT, PTT, and INR and patient for bleeding.
Hormonal contraceptives: Decreases effectiveness of hormonal contraceptives, and increased breakthrough bleeding may occur. Advise patient to use alternate method during therapy.
Probenecid: Increases levels of penicillin. Probenecid may be used for this purpose.

Effects on lab test results
• May increase eosinophil count. May decrease hemoglobin, hematocrit, and platelet, WBC, and granulocyte counts.

Pharmacokinetics
Absorption: Absorbed slowly from I.M. injection site.
Distribution: Distributed widely into synovial, pleural, pericardial, and ascitic fluids; bile; and liver, skin, lungs, kidneys, muscle, intestines, tonsils, maxillary sinuses, saliva, and erythrocytes. CSF penetration is poor but enhanced in

patients with inflamed meninges. Drug is 45% to 68% protein-bound.

Metabolism: Between 16% and 30% of drug is metabolized to inactive compounds.

Excretion: Excreted primarily in urine. *Half-life:* 30 to 60 minutes.

Route	Onset	Peak	Duration
I.M.	Unknown	13-24 hr	1-4 wk

Action

Chemical effect: Inhibits cell wall synthesis during microorganism multiplication; bacteria resist penicillins by producing penicillinases, enzymes that convert penicillins to inactive penicilloic acid. Penicillin G benzathine resists these enzymes.

Therapeutic effect: Kills susceptible bacteria, such as most non–penicillinase-producing strains of gram-positive and gram-negative aerobic cocci; spirochetes; and some gram-positive aerobic and anaerobic bacilli.

Available forms

Injection: 600,000 units/ml, 1,200,000 units/dose, 2,400,000 units/dose

NURSING PROCESS

Assessment

● Assess patient's infection before therapy and regularly thereafter.
● Before giving drug, ask patient about allergic reactions to penicillin. However, negative history of penicillin allergy is no guarantee against future allergic reaction.
● Obtain specimen for culture and sensitivity tests before giving first dose. Therapy may begin pending results.
● Be alert for adverse reactions and drug interactions.
● Observe patient closely. Large doses and prolonged therapy raise the risk of bacterial or fungal superinfection, especially in geriatric, debilitated, or immunosuppressed patients.
● Evaluate patient's and family's knowledge of drug therapy.

Nursing diagnoses

● Infection related to presence of bacteria
● Ineffective protection related to risk of hypersensitivity reactions to drug
● Deficient knowledge related to drug therapy

Planning and implementation

● Shake drug well before injection.
● **ALERT:** Never give drug I.V.; doing so has caused cardiac arrest and death.
● Inject deep into upper outer quadrant of buttocks in adult; in midlateral thigh in infant and young child. Avoid injection into or near major nerves or blood vessels to prevent neurovascular damage.
● Give drug at least 1 hour before bacteriostatic antibiotics.
● Drug's extremely slow absorption makes allergic reactions difficult to treat. If patient develops signs of anaphylactic shock, such as rapidly developing dyspnea and hypotension, stop drug immediately. Notify prescriber and immediately give epinephrine, corticosteroids, antihistamines, or other resuscitative measures.
● **ALERT:** Be aware of the various preparations of penicillin. They aren't interchangable.
● **ALERT:** Don't confuse penicillin with penicillamine.

Patient teaching

● Tell patient to call prescriber if rash, fever, or chills develop.
● Warn patient that injection may be painful but that ice applied to site may ease discomfort.

Evaluation

● Patient is free from infection.
● Patient shows no signs of allergy.
● Patient and family state understanding of drug therapy.

penicillin G potassium (benzylpenicillin potassium)
(pen-ih-SIL-in gee poh-TAH-see-um)
Pfizerpen

Pharmacologic class: natural penicillin
Therapeutic class: antibiotic
Pregnancy risk category: B

Indications and dosages

▶ **Moderate to severe systemic infections.**
Adults: 12 to 24 million units I.M. or I.V. daily in divided doses q 4 hours.
Children: 25,000 to 300,000 units/kg I.M. or I.V. daily in divided doses q 4 hours.

Reactions may be *common*, uncommon, *life-threatening*, or COMMON AND LIFE-THREATENING.

▶ **Anthrax.** *Adults:* 5 to 20 million units I.V. daily given in divided doses q 4 to 6 hours for at least 14 days after symptoms abate. Alternatively, may give 80,000 units/kg body weight in the first hour followed by a maintenance dose of 320,000 units/kg body weight daily. The average adult dose is 4 million units q 4 hours; can also be given as 2 million units q 2 hours. *Children:* 100,000 to 150,000 units/kg I.V. daily in divided doses q 4 to 6 hours for at least 14 days after symptoms abate.

🔲 **Adjust-a-dose:** For patients with renal impairment, if creatinine clearance is less than 10 ml/min, give one-half of usual dose q 8 to 10 hours or usual dose q 12 to 18 hours. If patient is uremic and creatinine clearance is less than 10 ml/minute, give full loading dose, then give one-quarter dose q 4 to 5 hours for additional doses.

▼ I.V. administration

• Use continuous I.V. infusion when large doses are required (10 million units or more). Otherwise, give via intermittent I.V. infusion over 1 to 2 hours.
• Aminoglycosides are physically and chemically incompatible with drug. Administer separately.

Contraindications and precautions

• Contraindicated in patients hypersensitive to drug or other penicillins.
• Use cautiously in patients with other drug allergies, especially to cephalosporins.
⚕ Lifespan: In pregnant women, use cautiously. Drug appears in breast milk. In breastfeeding women, use of drug may sensitize infant to penicillin and cause some adverse effects.

Adverse reactions

CNS: neuropathy, *seizures.*
CV: thrombophlebitis.
Hematologic: hemolytic anemia, *thrombocytopenia, leukopenia.*
Metabolic: *severe potassium poisoning with high doses (hyperreflexia, seizures, coma).*
Other: hypersensitivity reactions (rash, urticaria, maculopapular eruptions, exfoliative dermatitis, chills, fever, edema, *anaphylaxis*), overgrowth of nonsusceptible organisms, pain at injection site.

Interactions

Drug-drug. *Heparin, oral anticoagulants:* Increases risk of bleeding. Monitor PT, PTT, and INR and patient for bleeding.
Hormonal contraceptives: Decreases effectiveness of hormonal contraceptives, and increased breakthrough bleeding may occur. Advise patient to use alternate method during therapy.
Potassium-sparing diuretics: May increase risk of hyperkalemia. Don't use together.
Probenecid: Increases levels of penicillin. Probenecid may be used for this purpose.

Effects on lab test results

• May increase potassium level.
• May increase eosinophil count. May decrease hemoglobin and hematocrit and platelet, WBC, and granulocyte counts.

Pharmacokinetics

Absorption: Absorbed rapidly from I.M. injection site.
Distribution: Distributed widely into synovial, pleural, pericardial, and ascitic fluids; bile; and liver, skin, lungs, kidneys, muscle, intestines, tonsils, maxillary sinuses, saliva, and erythrocytes. CSF penetration is poor but is enhanced in patients with inflamed meninges. Drug is 45% to 68% protein-bound.
Metabolism: Hepatic metabolism accounts for less than 30% of biotransformation of penicillin.
Excretion: Excreted primarily in urine. *Half-life:* 30 to 60 minutes.

Route	Onset	Peak	Duration
I.V.	Immediate	Immediate	Unknown
I.M.	Unknown	15-30 min	Unknown

Action

Chemical effect: Inhibits cell wall synthesis during microorganism multiplication; bacteria resist penicillins by producing penicillinases, enzymes that convert penicillins to inactive penicilloic acid. Drug resists these enzymes.
Therapeutic effect: Kills susceptible bacteria.

Available forms

Injection (powder): 1 million units, 5 million units, 10 million units, 20 million units
Injection (premixed in dextrose): 20,000 units, 40,000 units, 60,000 units

---

NURSING PROCESS

⚞ Assessment
● Assess patient's infection before therapy and regularly thereafter.
● Before giving, ask patient about any allergic reactions to penicillin. However, negative history of penicillin allergy is no guarantee against future allergic reaction.
● Obtain specimen for culture and sensitivity tests before first dose. Therapy may begin pending results.
● Be alert for adverse reactions and drug interactions.
● Observe patient closely. Large doses and prolonged therapy raise the risk of bacterial or fungal superinfection, especially in geriatric, debilitated, or immunosuppressed patients.
● Evaluate patient's and family's knowledge of drug therapy.

⊕ Nursing diagnoses
● Infection related to presence of bacteria
● Ineffective protection related to risk of hypersensitivity reactions to drug
● Deficient knowledge related to drug therapy

▶ Planning and implementation
● Reconstitute vials with sterile water for injection, D_5W, or normal saline solution for injection. Volume of diluent varies with manufacturer.
● Give drug at least 1 hour before bacteriostatic antibiotics.
● **⚠ ALERT:** Be aware of the various preparations of penicillin. They aren't interchangable.
● Monitor level in patients taking large doses. A high level may lead to seizures. Take precautions.
● Give drug I.M. deep into large muscle; warn patient that injection may be painful.
● **⚠ ALERT:** Don't confuse penicillamine with penicillin.

Patient teaching
● Tell patient to take drug exactly as prescribed, even after he feels better.
● Warn patient never to use leftover penicillin for a new illness or to share penicillin with family and friends.
● Tell patient to call prescriber if rash, fever, or chills develop.
● Warn patient that I.M. injection may be painful but that ice applied to site may ease discomfort.

☑ Evaluation
● Patient is free from infection.
● Patient shows no signs of allergy.
● Patient and family state understanding of drug therapy.

penicillin G procaine
(benzylpenicillin procaine)
(pen-ih-SIL-in gee PROH-kayn)

Pharmacologic class: natural penicillin
Therapeutic class: antibiotic
Pregnancy risk category: B

Indications and dosages
▶ **Moderate to severe systemic infections.**
Adults: 600,000 to 1.2 million units I.M. daily in single dose.
Children older than age 1 month: 25,000 to 50,000 units/kg I.M. daily in single dose.
▶ **Uncomplicated gonorrhea.** *Adults and children older than age 12:* 1 g probenecid; after 30 minutes, 4.8 million units of penicillin G procaine I.M., divided between two injection sites.
▶ **Pneumococcal pneumonia.** *Adults and children older than age 12:* 600,000 units to 1.2 million units I.M. daily for 7 to 10 days.
▶ **Anthrax caused by** *Bacillus anthracis,* **including inhalational anthrax (postexposure).**
Adults: 1.2 million units I.M. q 12 hours.
Children: 25,000 units/kg I.M. (maximum, 1.2 million units) q 12 hours.
▶ **Cutaneous anthrax.** *Adults:* 600,000 to 1 million units I.M. daily.

Contraindications and precautions
● Contraindicated in patients hypersensitive to drug or other penicillins.
● Use cautiously in patients with other drug allergies, especially to cephalosporins.
⚖ Lifespan: In pregnant women, use cautiously. Drug appears in breast milk. In breast-feeding women, use of drug may sensitize infant to penicillin and cause some adverse effects.

Adverse reactions
CNS: *seizures.*
Hematologic: *thrombocytopenia,* hemolytic anemia, *leukopenia.*

Reactions may be *common,* uncommon, *life-threatening,* or COMMON AND LIFE-THREATENING.

Musculoskeletal: arthralgia.
Other: hypersensitivity reactions (rash, urticaria, chills, fever, edema, prostration, *anaphylaxis*), overgrowth of nonsusceptible organisms.

Interactions

Drug-drug. *Colestipol:* Decreases levels of penicillin G procaine. Give penicillin 1 hour before or 4 hours after colestipol.
Heparin, oral anticoagulants: Increases risk of bleeding. Monitor PT, PTT, and INR and patient for bleeding.
Hormonal contraceptives: Decreases effectiveness of hormonal contraceptives, and increased breakthrough bleeding may occur. Advise patient to use alternate method during therapy.
Probenecid: Increases blood levels of penicillin. Probenecid may be used for this purpose.

Effects on lab test results

• May increase eosinophil count. May decrease hemoglobin, hematocrit, and platelet, WBC, and granulocyte counts.

Pharmacokinetics

Absorption: Slow.
Distribution: Distributed widely into synovial, pleural, pericardial, and ascitic fluids; bile; and liver, skin, lungs, kidneys, muscle, intestines, tonsils, maxillary sinuses, saliva, and erythrocytes. CSF penetration usually poor, but enhanced in patients with inflamed meninges. Drug is 45% to 68% protein-bound.
Metabolism: From 16% to 30% metabolized to inactive compounds.
Excretion: Excreted primarily in urine. *Half-life:* 30 to 60 minutes.

Route	Onset	Peak	Duration
I.M.	Unknown	1-4 hr	1-2 days

Action

Chemical effect: Inhibits cell wall synthesis during microorganism multiplication; bacteria resist penicillins by producing penicillinases, enzymes that convert penicillins to inactive penicilloic acid. Penicillin G procaine resists these enzymes.
Therapeutic effect: Kills susceptible bacteria, such as most non–penicillinase-producing strains of gram-positive and gram-negative aerobic cocci, spirochetes, and some gram-positive aerobic and anaerobic bacilli.

Available forms

Injection: 600,000 units/ml, 1.2 million units/ml, 2.4 million units/ml

NURSING PROCESS

Assessment
• Assess patient's infection before therapy and regularly thereafter.
• Before giving, ask patient about allergic reactions to penicillin. However, negative history of penicillin allergy is no guarantee against future allergic reaction.
• Obtain specimen for culture and sensitivity tests before giving first dose. Therapy may begin pending results.
• Be alert for adverse reactions and drug interactions.
• Observe patient closely. Large doses and prolonged therapy raise the risk of bacterial or fungal superinfection, especially in geriatric, debilitated, or immunosuppressed patients.
• Evaluate patient's and family's knowledge of drug therapy.

Nursing diagnoses
• Infection related to presence of bacteria
• Ineffective protection related to risk of hypersensitivity reactions to drug
• Deficient knowledge related to drug therapy

Planning and implementation
• Shake drug well before injection.
• Never give I.V.; doing so has caused cardiac arrest and death.
• Inject deep into upper outer quadrant of buttocks in adults; in midlateral thigh in infants and small children. Avoid injection into or near major nerves or blood vessels to prevent neurovascular damage.
• Give penicillin G procaine at least 1 hour before bacteriostatic antibiotics.
• Drug's extremely slow absorption makes allergic reactions difficult to treat. If patient develops signs of anaphylactic shock, such as rapidly developing dyspnea and hypotension, stop drug immediately. Notify prescriber and immediately give epinephrine, corticosteroids, antihistamines, or other resuscitative measures.

⊛ ALERT: Be aware of the various preparations of penicillin. They aren't interchangable.

Patient teaching
• Tell patient to call prescriber if rash, fever, or chills develop.
• Warn patient that injection may be painful but that ice applied to site may ease discomfort.

☑ Evaluation
• Patient is free from infection.
• Patient shows no signs of allergy.
• Patient and family state understanding of drug therapy.

penicillin G sodium (benzylpenicillin sodium)
(pen-ih-SIL-in gee SOH-dee-um)
Crystapen ◆

Pharmacologic class: natural penicillin
Therapeutic class: antibiotic
Pregnancy risk category: B

Indications and dosages

▶ **Moderate to severe systemic infections.**
Adults: 12 to 24 million units daily I.M. or I.V. in divided doses q 4 to 6 hours.
Children: 25,000 to 300,000 units/kg daily I.M. or I.V. in divided doses q 4 to 6 hours.
▶ **Endocarditis prophylaxis for dental surgery.** *Adults and children weighing more than 27 kg (59 lb):* 2 million units I.V. or I.M. 30 to 60 minutes before procedure; then 1 million units 6 hours later.
🔲 **Adjust-a-dose:** For patients with renal impairment, if creatinine clearance is less than 10 ml/min, give one-half of usual dose q 8 to 10 hours or usual dose q 12 to 18 hours. If patient is uremic and creatinine clearance is greater than 10 ml/minute, give full loading dose, then give one-half dose q 4 to 5 hours.

▼ I.V. administration

• Reconstitute vials with sterile water for injection, normal saline solution for injection, or D$_5$W. Volume of diluent varies with manufacturer and concentration needed.
• For patient receiving 10 million units of drug or more daily, dilute in 1 to 2 liters of compatible solution and administer over 24 hours. Oth-

erwise, give by intermittent I.V. infusion: Dilute drug in 50 to 100 ml and give over 1 to 2 hours q 4 to 6 hours.
• In neonate or child, give divided doses usually over 15 to 30 minutes.
• Aminoglycosides are physically and chemically incompatible with drug. Administer separately.

Contraindications and precautions

• Contraindicated in patients hypersensitive to drug or other penicillins.
• Use cautiously in patients with other drug allergies, especially to cephalosporins.
🔆 **Lifespan:** In pregnant women, use cautiously. Drug appears in breast milk. In breastfeeding women, use of drug may sensitize infant to penicillin and cause some adverse effects.

Adverse reactions

CNS: neuropathy, *seizures.*
CV: thrombophlebitis.
Hematologic: hemolytic anemia, *leukopenia, thrombocytopenia.*
Musculoskeletal: arthralgia.
Other: hypersensitivity reactions (exfoliative dermatitis, urticaria, *anaphylaxis*), overgrowth of nonsusceptible organisms, vein irritation, pain at injection site.

Interactions

Drug-drug. *Colestipol:* Decreases levels of penicillin G sodium. Give penicillin 1 hour before or 4 hours after colestipol.
Heparin, oral anticoagulants: Increases risk of bleeding. Monitor PT, PTT, and INR and patient for bleeding.
Hormonal contraceptives: Decreases effectiveness of hormonal contraceptives and increased breakthrough bleeding may occur. Advise patient to use alternate method during therapy.
Probenecid: Increases blood levels of penicillin. Probenecid may be used for this purpose.

Effects on lab test results

• May increase eosinophil count. May decrease hemoglobin, hematocrit, and platelet, WBC, and granulocyte counts.

Pharmacokinetics

Absorption: Rapid.
Distribution: Distributed widely into synovial, pleural, pericardial, and ascitic fluids; bile; and

---

Reactions may be *common,* uncommon, *life-threatening*, or COMMON AND LIFE-THREATENING.

liver, skin, lungs, kidneys, muscle, intestines, tonsils, maxillary sinuses, saliva, and erythrocytes. CSF penetration is poor but is enhanced in patients with inflamed meninges. Drug is 45% to 68% protein-bound.

Metabolism: 16% to 30% of drug is metabolized to inactive compounds.

Excretion: Excreted primarily in urine. *Half-life:* 30 to 60 minutes.

Route	Onset	Peak	Duration
I.V.	Immediate	Immediate	Unknown
I.M.	Unknown	15-30 min	Unknown

Action

Chemical effect: Inhibits cell wall synthesis during microorganism multiplication; bacteria resist penicillins by producing penicillinases, enzymes that convert penicillins to inactive penicilloic acid. Penicillin G sodium resists these enzymes.

Therapeutic effect: Kills susceptible bacteria, such as most non–penicillinase-producing strains of gram-positive and gram-negative aerobic cocci, spirochetes, and some gram-positive aerobic and anaerobic bacilli.

Available forms

Injection: 5-million-unit vial

NURSING PROCESS

Assessment
• Assess patient's infection before therapy and regularly thereafter.
• Before giving, ask patient about allergic reactions to penicillin. However, negative history of penicillin allergy is no guarantee against future allergic reaction.
• Obtain specimen for culture and sensitivity tests before first dose. Therapy may begin pending results.
• Be alert for adverse reactions and drug interactions.
• Observe patient closely. Large doses and prolonged therapy raise the risk of bacterial or fungal superinfection, especially in geriatric, debilitated, or immunosuppressed patients.
• Evaluate patient's and family's knowledge of drug therapy.

Nursing diagnoses
• Infection related to presence of bacteria

• Ineffective protection related to risk of hypersensitivity reactions to drug
• Deficient knowledge related to drug therapy

Planning and implementation
• Give drug I.M. deep in upper outer quadrant of buttocks in adult; in midlateral thigh in young child. Don't massage injection site. Avoid injection near major nerves or blood vessels to prevent neurovascular damage.
⊛ **ALERT:** Don't give by S.C. route.
• Give penicillin G sodium at least 1 hour before bacteriostatic antibiotics.
⊛ **ALERT:** Be aware of the various preparations of penicillin. They aren't interchangable.
• Monitor level in patient taking large doses. A high level may lead to seizures. Take precautions.
⊛ **ALERT:** Don't confuse penicillamine with penicillin.
Patient teaching
• Tell patient to report discomfort at I.V. site
• Warn patient that I.M. injection may be painful but that ice applied to site may ease discomfort.

Evaluation
• Patient is free from infection.
• Patient shows no signs of allergy.
• Patient and family state understanding of drug therapy.

penicillin V
(phenoxymethylpenicillin)
(pen-ih-SIL-in VEE)

penicillin V potassium
(phenoxymethylpenicillin potassium)
Abbocillin VK ◇ , Apo-Pen-VK ◇ , Beepen-VK, Cilicaine VK ◇ , Nadopen-V ♦ , Nadopen-V-200 ♦ , Nadopen-V 400 ♦ , Novo-Pen-VK ♦ , Nu-Pen-VK ♦ , Pen-Vee K, PVF K ♦ , PVK ◇ , V-Cillin K, Veetids

Pharmacologic class: natural penicillin
Therapeutic class: antibiotic
Pregnancy risk category: B

Indications and dosages

▶ **Mild to moderate systemic infections.**
Adults: 125 to 500 mg (200,000 to 800,000 units) P.O. q 6 hours.
Children: 15 to 50 mg/kg (25,000 to 90,000 units/kg) P.O. daily, in divided doses q 6 to 8 hours.
▶ **Endocarditis prophylaxis for dental surgery.** *Adults:* 2 g P.O. 30 to 60 minutes before procedure; then 500 mg P.O. q 6 hours for eight doses.
Children weighing less than 30 kg (66 lb): Give half of adult dose.
▶ **Necrotizing ulcerative gingivitis.** *Adults and children older than age 12:* 250 mg to 500 mg P.O. q 6 to 8 hours.
▶ **Prophylaxis for rheumatic fever.** *Adults and children:* 250 mg P.O. b.i.d.
▶ **Prophylaxis for pneumococcal infections‡.**
Children age 5 and older: 250 mg P.O. b.i.d.
Children younger than age 5: 125 mg P.O. b.i.d.
▶ **Lyme disease‡.** *Adults:* 250 to 500 mg P.O. q.i.d. for 10 to 20 days.

Contraindications and precautions

• Contraindicated in patients hypersensitive to drug or other penicillins.
• Use cautiously in patients with other drug allergies, especially to cephalosporins.
⚖ Lifespan: In pregnant women, use cautiously. Drug appears in breast milk. In breastfeeding women, use of drug may sensitize infant to penicillin and cause some adverse effects.

Adverse reactions

CNS: neuropathy, *seizures.*
GI: *epigastric distress,* vomiting, diarrhea, *nausea.*
Hematologic: eosinophilia, hemolytic anemia, *leukopenia, thrombocytopenia.*
Other: hypersensitivity reactions (rash, urticaria, chills, fever, edema, *anaphylaxis*), overgrowth of nonsusceptible organisms.

Interactions

Drug-drug. *Heparin, oral anticoagulants:* Increases risk of bleeding. Monitor PT, PTT, and INR and patient for bleeding.
Hormonal contraceptives containing estrogen: Decreases effectiveness of hormonal contraceptive. Monitor patient for breakthrough bleeding. Advise patient to use alternative forms of birth control.

Probenecid: Increases level of penicillin. Probenecid may be used for this purpose.

Effects on lab test results

• May increase eosinophil count. May decrease hemoglobin, hematocrit, and platelet, WBC, and granulocyte counts.

Pharmacokinetics

Absorption: About 60% to 75%.
Distribution: Distributed widely into synovial, pleural, pericardial, and ascitic fluids; bile; and liver, skin, lungs, kidneys, muscle, intestines, tonsils, maxillary sinuses, saliva, and erythrocytes. CSF penetration is poor but is enhanced in patients with inflamed meninges. Drug is 75% to 89% protein-bound.
Metabolism: Between 35% and 70% metabolized to inactive compounds.
Excretion: Excreted primarily in urine. *Half-life:* 30 minutes.

Route	Onset	Peak	Duration
P.O.	Unknown	30-60 min	Unknown

Action

Chemical effect: Inhibits cell wall synthesis during microorganism multiplication; bacteria resist penicillins by producing penicillinases. Penicillin V resists those enzymes.
Therapeutic effect: Kills susceptible bacteria, such as most non–penicillinase-producing strains of gram-positive and gram-negative aerobic cocci, spirochetes, and some gram-positive aerobic and anaerobic bacilli.

Available forms

penicillin V
Oral suspension: 125 mg/5 ml, 250 mg/5 ml (after reconstitution)
Tablets: 250 mg, 500 mg
penicillin V potassium
Capsules: 250 mg ◊
Oral suspension: 125 mg/5 ml, 250 mg/5 ml (after reconstitution)
Tablets: 125 mg, 250 mg, 500 mg
Tablets (film-coated): 250 mg, 500 mg

NURSING PROCESS

☞ Assessment

• Assess patient's infection before therapy and regularly thereafter.

Reactions may be *common,* uncommon, *life-threatening,* or COMMON AND LIFE-THREATENING.

• Before giving drug, ask patient about any allergic reactions to penicillin. However, negative history of penicillin allergy is no guarantee against future allergic reaction.

• Obtain specimen for culture and sensitivity tests before giving first dose. Therapy may begin pending results.

• Periodically assess renal and hematopoietic function in patient receiving long-term therapy.

• Be alert for adverse reactions and drug interactions.

• Observe patient closely. Large doses and prolonged therapy raise the risk of bacterial or fungal superinfection, especially in geriatric, debilitated, or immunosuppressed patients.

• Evaluate patient's and family's knowledge of drug therapy.

▦ Nursing diagnoses
• Infection related to presence of bacteria
• Ineffective protection related to risk of hypersensitivity reactions to drug
• Deficient knowledge related to drug therapy

▧ Planning and implementation
• Give drug at least 1 hour before bacteriostatic antibiotics.

• American Heart Association considers amoxicillin the preferred drug for endocarditis prophylaxis because GI absorption is better and levels are sustained longer. Penicillin V is considered an alternative choice.

⊛ **ALERT:** Be aware of the various preparations of penicillin. They aren't interchangable.

⊛ **ALERT:** Don't confuse penicillamine with penicillin.

Patient teaching
• Tell patient to take drug exactly as prescribed, even after he feels better.

• Tell patient that drug may be taken without regard to meals. However, if GI disturbances occur, drug may be taken with meals.

• Warn patient never to use leftover penicillin V for new illness or to share penicillin with family and friends.

• Tell patient to call prescriber if rash, fever, or chills develop.

☑ Evaluation
• Patient is free from infection.
• Patient shows no signs of allergy.
• Patient and family state understanding of drug therapy.

pentamidine isethionate
(pen-TAM-eh-deen ighs-eh-THIGH-oh-nayt)
NebuPent, Pentacarinat, Pentam 300

Pharmacologic class: diamidine derivative
Therapeutic class: antiprotozoal
Pregnancy risk category: C

Indications and dosages

▶ **Pneumocystis carinii pneumonia.** *Adults and children:* 4 mg/kg I.V. or I.M. once daily for 14 to 21 days.

▶ **Prevention of** *P. carinii* **pneumonia in high-risk patients.** *Adults:* 300 mg by inhalation (using Respirgard II nebulizer) once q 4 weeks.

▼ I.V. administration

• Reconstitute drug with 3 ml of sterile water for injection; then dilute in 50 to 250 ml of D_5W. Inject over at least 1 hour.

• To minimize hypotension, infuse drug slowly with patient lying down.

Contraindications and precautions

• Contraindicated in patients with history of anaphylactic reaction to drug.

• Use cautiously in patients with hypertension, hypotension, hypoglycemia, hypocalcemia, leukopenia, thrombocytopenia, anemia, or hepatic or renal dysfunction.

⚖ **Lifespan:** In pregnant women, use cautiously. In breast-feeding women, drug isn't recommended.

Adverse reactions

Parenteral form
CNS: confusion, fever, hallucinations.
CV: *severe hypotension,* hypotension, facial flushing, tachycardia.
GI: *pancreatitis.*
GU: *renal toxicity, acute renal failure.*
Hematologic: *leukopenia, thrombocytopenia, anemia.*
Hepatic: hepatic dysfunction, *hepatitis,* hepatomegaly.
Metabolic: *hypoglycemia,* hyperglycemia, hypocalcemia.
Respiratory: cough, *bronchospasm.*
Skin: pruritus, *Stevens-Johnson syndrome.*
Other: *sterile abscess, pain and induration* at injection site.

Aerosol form
CNS: *fatigue, dizziness.*
CV: *chest pain.*
GI: *nausea, pharyngitis, vomiting, metallic taste.*
Metabolic: *decreased appetite.*
Respiratory: *shortness of breath, chest congestion, cough,* BRONCOSPASM.
Skin: *rash.*
Other: *night sweats, chills.*

Interactions

Drug-drug. *Aminoglycosides, amphotericin B, capreomycin, cisplatin, colistin, methoxyflurane, polymyxin B, vancomycin:* Increases risk of nephrotoxicity. Monitor patient closely.

Effects on lab test results

• May increase BUN, creatinine, potassium, and liver enzyme levels. May decrease calcium level. May increase or decrease glucose levels.
• May decrease hemoglobin, hematocrit, and WBC and platelet counts.

Pharmacokinetics

Absorption: Limited after aerosol administration. Unknown after I.M. administration.
Distribution: Drug appears to be extensively tissue-bound. CNS penetration is poor. Extent of protein-binding is unknown.
Metabolism: Unknown.
Excretion: Excreted unchanged in urine. *Half-life:* Varies according to route of administration: 9 to 13¼ hours for I.M., about 6½ hours for I.V., and unknown for aerosol.

Route	Onset	Peak	Duration
I.V.	Unknown	Immediate	Unknown
I.M.	Unknown	30 min-1 hr	Unknown
Aerosol	Unknown	Unknown	Unknown

Action

Chemical effect: Interferes with infectious organism's biosynthesis of DNA, RNA, phospholipids, and proteins.
Therapeutic effect: Hinders growth of susceptible organisms.

Available forms

Aerosol: 300-mg vial
Injection: 300-mg vial

NURSING PROCESS

⚖ Assessment

• Assess patient's infection before therapy and regularly thereafter.
• Monitor glucose, calcium, creatinine, and BUN levels daily. After parenteral administration, glucose level may decrease initially; hypoglycemia may be severe in 5% to 10% of patients. This may be followed by hyperglycemia and insulin-dependent diabetes mellitus, which may be permanent.
• Monitor CBC, platelet count, liver function tests, and renal function periodically during therapy.
• Closely monitor blood pressure during I.V. administration.
• Be alert for adverse reactions and drug interactions.
• Evaluate patient's and family's knowledge of drug therapy.

⊕ Nursing diagnoses

• Infection related to presence of organisms
• Risk for injury related to drug-induced adverse CNS reactions
• Deficient knowledge related to drug therapy

▷ Planning and implementation

• For I.M. use, reconstitute drug with 3 ml of sterile water for solution containing 100 mg/ml; administer deeply. Expect pain and induration.
• In patient with AIDS, this drug may produce less severe adverse reactions than co-trimoxazole and may be drug of choice.
• Administer aerosol form only by Respirgard II nebulizer manufactured by Marquest. Dosage recommendations are based on particle size and delivery rate of this device.
• To use aerosol, mix contents of one vial in 6 ml of sterile water for injection. Don't use normal saline solution; it will cause precipitation.
• Don't mix with other drugs.
• Don't use low-pressure (below 20 pounds per square inch [psi]) compressors. The flow rate should be 5 to 7 liters/minute from 40- to 50-psi air or oxygen source.
• Inhalation of pentamidine may induce bronchospasm or cough, especially in patients with a history of smoking or asthma.

Patient teaching

• Instruct patient to use aerosol device until chamber is empty, which may take up to 45 minutes.
• Warn patient that I.M. injection is painful. However, application of warm soaks is helpful.
• Tell patient to report lightheadedness or signs and symptoms of hypoglycemia immediately.

☑ Evaluation

• Patient is free from infection.
• Patient sustains no injuries because of drug-induced adverse CNS reactions.
• Patient and family state understanding of drug therapy.

---

pentazocine hydrochloride
(pen-TAZ-oh-seen high-droh-KLOR-ighd)
Fortral ◊

pentazocine hydrochloride and acetaminophen
Talacen

pentazocine hydrochloride and aspirin
Talwin Compound

pentazocine hydrochloride and naloxone hydrochloride
Talwin NX

pentazocine lactate
Fortral ◊ , Talwin

Pharmacologic class: opioid agonist-antagonist, opioid partial agonist
Therapeutic class: opioid analgesic, adjunct to anesthesia
Pregnancy risk category: C
Controlled substance schedule: IV

Indications and dosages

▶ **Moderate to severe pain.** *Adults:* 50 to 100 mg Talwin NX P.O. q 3 to 4 hours, p.r.n. Maximum oral dosage, 600 mg daily. Or, 2 tablets Talwin Compound P.O. t.i.d. or q.i.d. Or, 1 tablet Talacen P.O. q 4 hours, up to 6 tablets dai-

ly. Or, 30 mg I.M., I.V., or S.C. q 3 to 4 hours, p.r.n. Maximum total parenteral dosage is 360 mg in 24 hours. Single doses above 30 mg I.V. or 60 mg I.M. or S.C. aren't recommended.
▶ **Labor.** *Women:* 30 mg I.M. or 20 mg I.V. q 2 to 3 hours when contractions become regular.

▽ I.V. administration

• Don't mix in same syringe with aminophylline, barbiturates, or other alkaline substances.
• Give drug by direct I.V. injection.
• Administer slowly.

Contraindications and precautions

• Contraindicated in patients hypersensitive to drug or its components.
• Use cautiously in patients with hepatic or renal disease, acute MI, head injury, increased intracranial pressure, or respiratory depression.
⚞ Lifespan: In pregnant and breast-feeding women, use cautiously. In children younger than age 12, drug isn't recommended. In elderly patients, use cautiously because they may be more sensitive to adverse CNS effects of drug.

Adverse reactions

CNS: *sedation,* visual disturbances, hallucinations, drowsiness, *dizziness, light-headedness,* confusion, *euphoria,* headache, psychotomimetic effects.
CV: hypotension, *shock.*
EENT: dry mouth, dysgeusia.
GI: *nausea, vomiting,* constipation.
GU: urine retention.
Respiratory: *respiratory depression.*
Skin: induration, nodules, sloughing, and sclerosis of injection site.
Other: *hypersensitivity reactions (anaphylaxis),* physical and psychological dependence.

Interactions

Drug-drug. *CNS depressants:* May have additive effects. Use together cautiously.
Fluoxetine: May cause diaphoresis, ataxia, flushing, and tremor. Use together cautiously.
Opioid analgesics: May decrease analgesic effect. Avoid using together.
Drug-lifestyle. *Alcohol use:* May have additive effects. Discourage using together.

Smoking: May increase requirements for pentazocine. Monitor drug's effectiveness; urge patient to stop smoking.

Effects on lab test results

• May interfere with laboratory tests for urinary 17-hydroxycorticosteroids.

Pharmacokinetics

Absorption: Well absorbed after P.O. or parenteral administration, although P.O. form undergoes first-pass metabolism in liver and less than 20% of dose reaches systemic circulation unchanged. Bioavailability is increased in patients with hepatic dysfunction; patients with cirrhosis absorb 60% to 70% of drug.
Distribution: Appears to be widely distributed throughout body.
Metabolism: Metabolized in liver. Metabolism may be prolonged in patients with impaired hepatic function.
Excretion: Excreted primarily in urine, with very small amounts excreted in feces. *Half-life:* 2 to 3 hours.

Route	Onset	Peak	Duration
P.O.	15-30 min	60-90 min	2-3 hr
I.V.	2-3 min	15-30 min	2-3 hr
I.M., S.C.	15-20 min	15-60 min	4-6 hr

Action

Chemical effect: Binds with opioid receptors at many sites in CNS, altering pain response by unknown mechanism.
Therapeutic effect: Relieves pain.

Available forms

pentazocine hydrochloride
Tablets: 25 mg ◇, 50 mg ◇
pentazocine hydrochloride and acetaminophen
Tablets: 25 mg pentazocine hydrochloride and 650 mg acetaminophen
pentazocine hydrochloride and aspirin
Tablets: 12.5 mg pentazocine hydrochloride and 325 mg aspirin
pentazocine hydrochloride and naloxone hydrochloride
Tablets: 50 mg pentazocine hydrochloride and 500 mcg naloxone hydrochloride
pentazocine lactate
Injection: 30 mg/ml

NURSING PROCESS

Assessment
• Assess patient's pain before and after drug administration.
• Monitor vital signs closely, especially respirations.
• Be alert for adverse reactions and drug interactions.
• Evaluate patient's and family's knowledge of drug therapy.

Nursing diagnoses
• Acute pain related to condition
• Ineffective breathing pattern related to drug-induced respiratory depression
• Deficient knowledge related to drug therapy

Planning and implementation
• Talwin NX, the oral pentazocine available in the U.S., contains the opioid antagonist naloxone, which prevents illicit I.V. use.
ALERT: Talwin NX is for P.O. use only. Severe, potentially fatal reaction may occur if given by injection.
• When using I.M. or S.C, rotate injection sites to minimize tissue irritation. If possible, avoid giving by S.C. route.
• Drug has opioid antagonist properties. May precipitate withdrawal syndrome in opioid-dependent patient.
• Dependence may occur with prolonged use.
ALERT: If respiratory rate drops significantly, hold drug and notify prescriber. Have naloxone readily available to reverse respiratory depression.

Patient teaching
• Warn ambulatory patient about getting out of bed or walking. Warn outpatient to avoid hazardous activities until CNS effects of drug are known.
• Inform patient about the risk of dependence.

Evaluation
• Patient is free from pain.
• Patient maintains respiratory rate and pattern within normal limits.
• Patient and family state understanding of drug therapy.

---

pentobarbital (pentobarbitone)
(pen-toh-BAR-beh-tol)
Nembutal*

pentobarbital sodium
Carbrital◇, Nembutal Sodium*

Pharmacologic class: barbiturate
Therapeutic class: anticonvulsant, sedative-hypnotic
Pregnancy risk category: D
Controlled substance schedule: II, III (suppositories)

Indications and dosages

▶ **Sedation.** *Adults:* 20 to 40 mg P.O. b.i.d., t.i.d., or q.i.d.
Children: 2 to 6 mg/kg daily P.O. or P.R. in three divided doses. Maximum daily dosage, 100 mg.
▶ **Short-term therapy for insomnia.** *Adults:* 100 to 200 mg P.O. h.s. or 150 to 200 mg I.M. Or, initially, 100 mg I.V. with additional small doses, to a total of 500 mg. Or, 120 or 200 mg P.R.
Children: 2 to 6 mg/kg I.M. Maximum dose is 100 mg. P.R. doses are 30 mg for children ages 2 months to 1 year, 30 or 60 mg for children ages 1 to 4, 60 mg for children ages 5 to 12, and 60 or 120 mg for children ages 12 to 14.
▶ **Preoperative sedation.** *Adults:* 150 to 200 mg I.M.
Children age 10 or older: 5 mg/kg P.O. or I.M.
Children younger than age 10: 5 mg/kg P.R.

▽▼ I.V. administration

• I.V. use of barbiturates may cause severe respiratory depression, laryngospasm, or hypotension. Have emergency resuscitation equipment available.
• To minimize deterioration, use I.V injection solution within 30 minutes after opening container. Don't use cloudy solution.
• Reserve I.V. injection for emergencies and give under close supervision. Give slowly (50 mg/minute or less).
• Parenteral solution is alkaline. Local tissue reactions and injection site pain may result. Monitor for irritation and infiltration; extravasation can lead to tissue damage and necrosis. Assess patency of I.V. site before and during administration.

• Don't mix with other drugs in syringe or in I.V. solutions or lines.

Contraindications and precautions

• Contraindicated in patients with porphyria or hypersensitivity to barbiturates.
• Use cautiously in debilitated patients and in those with acute or chronic pain, depression, suicidal tendencies, history of drug abuse, or hepatic impairment.
⚖ Lifespan: In pregnant and breast-feeding women, drug isn't recommended. In elderly patients, use cautiously.

Adverse reactions

CNS: *drowsiness, lethargy, hangover,* paradoxical excitement in elderly patients.
GI: nausea, vomiting.
Hematologic: worsening of porphyria.
Respiratory: *respiratory depression.*
Skin: rash, urticaria, *Stevens-Johnson syndrome.*
Other: *angioedema.*

Interactions

Drug-drug. *CNS depressants, including opioid analgesics:* Excessive CNS and respiratory depression may occur. Use together cautiously.
Corticosteroids, doxycycline, estrogens and hormonal contraceptives, oral anticoagulants: Pentobarbital may enhance metabolism of these drugs. Monitor patient for decreased effect.
Griseofulvin: Decreases absorption of griseofulvin. Separate administration times.
MAO inhibitors: Inhibits barbiturate metabolism and prolongs CNS depression. Reduce barbiturate dosage.
Metoprolol, propranolol: May reduce the effects of these drugs. Consider an increased beta blocker dose.
Rifampin: May decrease barbiturate levels. Monitor patient for decreased effect.
Drug-lifestyle. *Alcohol use:* May impair coordination, increase CNS effects, and cause death. Strongly discourage use together.

Effects on lab test results

None reported.

Pharmacokinetics

Absorption: Rapid after P.O. or P.R. administration. Unknown after I.M. administration.

Distribution: Distributed widely throughout body. About 35% to 45% of drug is protein-bound.
Metabolism: In liver.
Excretion: 99% of drug is excreted in urine.
Half-life: 35 to 50 hours.

Route	Onset	Peak	Duration
P.O.	≤ 15 min	30-60 min	1-4 hr
I.V.	Immediate	Immediate	15 min
I.M.	10-25 min	Unknown	Unknown
P.R.	≤ 15 min	Unknown	1-4 hr

Action

Chemical effect: Unknown; may interfere with transmission of impulses from thalamus to cortex of brain.
Therapeutic effect: Promotes sleep and calmness.

Available forms

pentobarbital
Elixir: 20 mg/5 ml
pentobarbital sodium
Capsules: 50 mg, 100 mg
Injection: 50 mg/ml
Suppositories: 30 mg, 60 mg, 120 mg, 200 mg

NURSING PROCESS

Assessment
• Assess patient's condition before therapy and regularly thereafter.
• Geriatric patients are more sensitive to adverse CNS effects of drug.
• Inspect patient's skin. Skin eruptions may precede life-threatening reactions to barbiturate therapy.
• Be alert for adverse reactions and drug interactions.
• Evaluate patient's and family's knowledge of drug therapy.

Nursing diagnoses
• Disturbed sleep pattern related to condition
• Risk for injury related to drug-induced adverse CNS reactions
• Deficient knowledge related to drug therapy

Planning and implementation
• Give I.M. injection deeply. Superficial injection may cause pain, sterile abscess, and sloughing.

• To ensure accurate dosage, don't divide suppositories.
⊛ **ALERT:** If skin reactions occur, stop drug and notify prescriber. In some patients, high fever, stomatitis, headache, or rhinitis may precede skin reactions.
• Pentobarbital has no analgesic effect and may cause restlessness or delirium in patients with pain.
⊛ **ALERT:** Long-term use isn't recommended; drug loses its effectiveness in promoting sleep after 14 days of continued use. Long-term high doses may cause dependence and may lead to withdrawal symptoms if drug is suddenly stopped. Withdraw barbiturates gradually.
⊛ **ALERT:** Don't confuse pentobarbital with phenobarbital.
Patient teaching
• Warn patient about performing activities that require alertness or physical coordination. For inpatient, particularly geriatric patient, supervise walking and raise bed rails.
• Inform patient that morning hangover is common after hypnotic dose, which suppresses REM sleep. Patient may experience increased dreaming after therapy stops.
• Tell patient who uses hormonal contraceptives to use a different birth control method because drug may decrease contraceptive effect.

Evaluation
• Patient reports satisfactory sleep.
• Patient sustains no injuries from drug-induced adverse CNS reactions.
• Patient and family state understanding of drug therapy.

pentostatin (2'-deoxycoformycin)
(pen-toh-STAH-tin)
Nipent

Pharmacologic class: antimetabolite (adenosine deaminase [ADA] inhibitor)
Therapeutic class: antineoplastic
Pregnancy risk category: D

Indications and dosages

▶ **Alpha-interferon–refractory hairy-cell leukemia.** *Adults:* 4 mg/m^2 I.V. q other week.

▼ I.V. administration

• Preparing and giving drug may have mutagenic, teratogenic, and carcinogenic risks. Follow facility policy to reduce risks.
• Treat all spills and waste products with 5% sodium hypochlorite (household bleach).
• Add 5 ml of sterile water for injection to vial containing pentostatin powder for injection. Mix thoroughly to make solution of 5 mg/ml. Drug may be administered by I.V. bolus injection or diluted further in 25 or 50 ml of D_5W or normal saline solution for injection and infused over 20 to 30 minutes.
• Use reconstituted solution within 8 hours; it contains no preservatives.

Contraindications and precautions

• Contraindicated in patients hypersensitive to drug and in patients with renal impairment (creatinine clearance of 60 ml/minute or less).
⚖ Lifespan: In pregnant and breast-feeding women, drug isn't recommended. In children, safety of drug hasn't been established.

Adverse reactions

CNS: pain, asthenia, malaise, fever, *headache, neurologic symptoms, anxiety, confusion, depression, dizziness, insomnia, nervousness, paresthesia, somnolence, abnormal thinking, fatigue.*
CV: chest pain, *arrhythmias,* abnormal ECG, thrombophlebitis, peripheral edema, *hemorrhage.*
EENT: abnormal vision, conjunctivitis, ear pain, eye pain, epistaxis, pharyngitis, rhinitis, sinusitis.
GI: abdominal pain, nausea, vomiting, anorexia, diarrhea, constipation, flatulence, stomatitis.
GU: *hematuria, dysuria.*
Hematologic: *myelosuppression,* LEUKOPENIA, anemia, THROMBOCYTOPENIA, *lymphocytopenia,* lymphadenopathy.
Metabolic: weight loss.
Musculoskeletal: back pain, myalgia, arthralgia.
Respiratory: *cough, bronchitis, dyspnea, pulmonary edema,* pneumonia.
Skin: diaphoresis, photosensitivity reaction, contact dermatitis, ecchymosis, petechiae, rash, eczema, dry skin, herpes simplex or zoster, maculopapular rash, vesiculobullous rash, pruritus, seborrhea, discoloration.

Other: INFECTION, HYPERSENSITIVITY REACTIONS, *neoplasm,* chills, *sepsis,* flulike syndrome.

Interactions

Drug-drug. *Cytarabine, vidarabine:* May increase adverse reactions. Avoid use together. *Fludarabine:* May increase risk of fatal pulmonary toxicity. Don't use together.

Effects on lab test results

• May increase BUN, creatinine, liver enzyme, and uric acid levels.
• May decrease hemoglobin, hematocrit, and platelet, WBC, lymphocyte, and granulocyte counts.

Pharmacokinetics

Absorption: Administered I.V.
Distribution: Protein–binding is about 4%.
Metabolism: Unknown.
Excretion: More than 90% excreted in urine.
Half-life: About 6 hours.

Route	Onset	Peak	Duration
I.V.	Unknown	Unknown	Unknown

Action

Chemical effect: Inhibits the enzyme ADA, which causes an increase in intracellular levels of deoxyadenosine triphosphate. This leads to cell damage and death. ADA has the greatest activity in cells of the lymphoid system, especially malignant T cells.
Therapeutic effect: Kills certain leukemic cells.

Available forms

Powder for injection: 10 mg/vial

NURSING PROCESS

▨ Assessment

• Assess patient's condition before therapy and regularly thereafter.
• Be alert for adverse reactions and drug interactions.
• Evaluate patient's and family's knowledge of drug therapy.

⊞ Nursing diagnoses

• Ineffective health maintenance related to leukemia

- Ineffective protection related to drug-induced adverse hematologic reactions
- Deficient knowledge related to drug therapy

> **Planning and implementation**
- Use drug only in patients with hairy-cell leukemia that progresses after minimum of 3 months of treatment with alpha-interferon or disease that doesn't respond to alpha-interferon after 6 months.
- Use drug only under supervision of prescriber qualified and experienced in use of chemotherapy drugs. Adverse reactions after therapy are common.
- Make sure patient is well hydrated before therapy; administer 500 to 1,000 ml of dextrose 5% in half-normal saline solution for injection.
- Give additional 500 ml of D₅W for hydration after drug is administered.
- Optimal duration of therapy is unknown. Current recommendations suggest two additional courses of therapy after complete response. If partial response isn't evident after 6 months, stop drug. If partial response is evident, continue drug for another 6 months or for two courses of therapy after complete response.
- Withhold drug in patients with CNS toxicity, severe rash, or active infection and notify prescriber. Drug may be resumed when infection clears.
- **⊛ ALERT:** If absolute neutrophil count falls below 200/mm³ and pretreatment level was over 500/mm³, temporarily withhold drug and notify prescriber. No recommendations exist for dosage adjustments in patients with anemia, neutropenia, or thrombocytopenia.
- **⊛ ALERT:** Don't confuse pentostatin with pentosan.

Patient teaching
- Teach patient how to take infection-control and bleeding precautions.
- Tell patient to notify prescriber of adverse reactions.

✓ Evaluation
- Patient responds well to therapy.
- Patient doesn't develop serious complications from adverse reactions.
- Patient and family state understanding of drug therapy.

pentoxifylline
(pen-tok-SIH-fi-lin)
Trental

Pharmacologic class: xanthine derivative
Therapeutic class: hemorrheologic
Pregnancy risk category: C

Indications and dosages

▶ **Intermittent claudication caused by chronic occlusive vascular disease.** *Adults:* 400 mg P.O. t.i.d. with meals for at least 8 weeks.

Contraindications and precautions

- Contraindicated in patients who are intolerant of methylxanthines, such as caffeine and theophylline, and in those with recent cerebral or retinal hemorrhage.
- **⚖ Lifespan:** In pregnant women, use cautiously. In breast-feeding women, drug isn't recommended. In children, safety of drug hasn't been established.

Adverse reactions

CNS: headache, dizziness.
GI: dyspepsia, nausea, vomiting.

Interactions

Drug-drug. *Anticoagulants:* Increases anticoagulant effect. Adjust anticoagulant dosage; monitor patient for bleeding.
Antihypertensives: Increases hypotensive effect. Dosage adjustments may be necessary; monitor patient's blood pressure closely.
Theophylline: Increases theophylline level. Monitor level; adjust theophylline dosage.
Drug-lifestyle. *Smoking:* Vasoconstriction may result. Advise patient to avoid smoking because it may worsen his condition.

Effects on lab test results

None reported.

Pharmacokinetics

Absorption: Almost complete but slowed by food. Undergoes first-pass hepatic metabolism.
Distribution: Bound by erythrocyte membrane.
Metabolism: Metabolized extensively by erythrocytes and liver.

Excretion: Excreted primarily in urine; less than 4% of drug is excreted in feces. *Half-life:* About 30 to 45 minutes.

Route	Onset	Peak	Duration
P.O.	Unknown	2-4 hr	Unknown

Action

Chemical effect: Unknown; thought to increase RBC flexibility and lower blood viscosity.
Therapeutic effect: Improves capillary blood flow.

Available forms

Tablets (controlled-release): 400 mg
Tablets (extended-release): 400 mg

NURSING PROCESS

Assessment
• Assess patient's condition before therapy and regularly thereafter.
• Be alert for adverse reactions and drug interactions.
• Be aware that geriatric patients may be more sensitive to drug's effects.
• If adverse GI reactions occur, monitor patient's hydration.
• Evaluate patient's and family's knowledge of drug therapy.

Nursing diagnoses
• Ineffective peripheral tissue perfusion related to condition
• Risk for deficient fluid volume related to drug-induced adverse GI reactions
• Deficient knowledge related to drug therapy

Planning and implementation
• Drug is useful in patients who aren't good surgical candidates.
• Report adverse reactions to prescriber; dosage may need to be reduced.
• **ALERT:** Don't confuse Trental with Trendar or Trandate.
Patient teaching
• Advise patient to take drug with meals to minimize GI upset.
• Instruct patient to swallow drug whole, without breaking, crushing, or chewing.
• Tell patient to report adverse GI or CNS reactions.

• Advise patient to avoid smoking because nicotine causes vasoconstriction that can worsen his condition.
• Advise patient that effects of drug may not be seen for 2 to 4 weeks.
• Tell patient not to stop drug during first 8 weeks of therapy unless directed by prescriber.

Evaluation
• Patient has adequate peripheral tissue perfusion.
• Patient maintains adequate hydration throughout therapy.
• Patient and family state understanding of drug therapy.

pergolide mesylate
(PER-goh-lighd MES-ih-layt)
Permax

Pharmacologic class: dopaminergic agonist
Therapeutic class: antiparkinsonian
Pregnancy risk category: B

Indications and dosages

▶ **Adjunct treatment with levodopa-carbidopa in management of symptoms caused by Parkinson's disease.** *Adults:* Initially, 0.05 mg P.O. daily for first 2 days followed by increased dosage of 0.1 to 0.15 mg q third day over 12 days. Subsequent dosage increased by 0.25 mg q third day until optimum response is seen, if needed. Drug usually is given in divided doses t.i.d. Gradual reductions in levodopa-carbidopa dosage may be made during dosage adjustment.

Contraindications and precautions

• Contraindicated in patients hypersensitive to drug or ergot alkaloids.
• Use cautiously in patients prone to arrhythmias and in patients with a history of pleuritis, pleural effusion, pleural fibrosis, pericarditis, pericardial effusion, cardiac valvulopathy or retroperitoneal fibrosis.
• **Lifespan:** In pregnant women, use cautiously. In breast-feeding women and in children, safety of drug hasn't been established.

Adverse reactions

CNS: headache, asthenia, *dyskinesia, dizziness, hallucinations,* dystonia, confusion, *somnolence,* syncope, insomnia, anxiety, depression, tremor, abnormal dreams, personality disorder, psychosis, abnormal gait, akathisia, extrapyramidal syndrome, incoordination, akinesia, hypertonia, neuralgia, speech disorder, twitching paresthesia.
CV: chest pain; *orthostatic hypotension;* vasodilation; palpitations; hypotension; hypertension; *arrhythmias; MI;* facial, peripheral, or generalized edema.
EENT: *rhinitis,* epistaxis, abnormal vision, diplopia, eye disorder.
GI: dry mouth, dysgeusia, abdominal pain, *nausea, constipation,* diarrhea, dyspepsia, anorexia, vomiting.
GU: urinary frequency, UTI, hematuria.
Metabolic: weight gain.
Musculoskeletal: neck and back pain, arthralgia, bursitis, myalgia.
Skin: diaphoresis, rash.
Other: flulike syndrome, chills, infection.

Interactions

Drug-drug. *Butyrophenones, metoclopramide, other dopamine antagonists, phenothiazines, thioxanthenes:* May antagonize effects of pergolide. Avoid using together.
CNS depressants: May cause additive CNS effects. Monitor patient closely.
Levodopa: May cause additive neurologic effects, such as hallucinations. Monitor patient closely.

Effects on lab test results

None reported.

Pharmacokinetics

Absorption: Well absorbed.
Distribution: About 90% protein-bound.
Metabolism: Metabolized to at least 10 different compounds, some of which retain pharmacologic activity.
Excretion: Excreted mainly by kidneys. *Half-life:* Unknown.

Route	Onset	Peak	Duration
P.O.	Unknown	Unknown	Unknown

Action

Chemical effect: Directly stimulates dopamine receptors in nigrostriatal system.
Therapeutic effect: Helps to relieve signs and symptoms of Parkinson's disease.

Available forms

Tablets: 0.05 mg, 0.25 mg, 1 mg

NURSING PROCESS

Assessment
● Assess patient's condition before therapy. Monitor drug effectiveness by regularly checking patient's body movements for improvement.
● Monitor blood pressure and heart rate and rhythm. Symptomatic orthostatic or sustained hypotension may occur in some patients, especially at start of therapy. Drug also may induce arrhythmias.
● Be alert for adverse reactions and drug interactions.
● Evaluate patient's and family's knowledge of drug therapy.

Nursing diagnoses
● Impaired physical mobility related to Parkinson's disease
● Decreased cardiac output related to drug-induced adverse CV reactions
● Deficient knowledge related to drug therapy

Planning and implementation
● Dosage is gradually increased according to patient's response and tolerance.
● If patient has significant changes in vital signs or mental status, notify prescriber.
Patient teaching
● Inform patient of potential adverse reactions, especially hallucinations and confusion.
● Warn patient to avoid activities that could result in injury from orthostatic hypotension and syncope.

Evaluation
● Patient has improved mobility.
● Patient maintains cardiac output.
● Patient and family state understanding of drug therapy.

perindopril erbumine
(PER-in-doh-pril ER-buh-mighn)
Aceon

Pharmacologic class: ACE inhibitor
Therapeutic class: antihypertensive
Pregnancy risk category: C (first trimester), D (second and third trimesters)

Indications and dosages

▶ **Essential hypertension.** *Adults:* Initially, 4 mg P.O. once daily. Increase until blood pressure is controlled or a maximum of 16 mg daily is reached. Usual maintenance dosage, 4 to 8 mg daily; may be divided into two doses. *Adults older than age 65:* Initially, 4 mg P.O. daily as one dose or two divided doses. Daily dosage increases exceeding 8 mg should occur only under close medical supervision.
☒ **Adjust-a-dose:** For patients with renal impairment, if creatinine clearance is above 30 ml/minute, initially give 2 mg P.O. daily with a maximum maintenance dosage of 8 mg daily. For patients taking diuretics, initially give 2 to 4 mg P.O. daily as one dose or divided into two doses with close medical supervision for several hours and until blood pressure is stable. Adjust dosage based on patient's response.

Contraindications and precautions

• Contraindicated in patients hypersensitive to drug or any other ACE inhibitor. Also contraindicated in patients with a history of angioedema secondary to ACE inhibitors.
• Use cautiously in patients with a history of angioedema unrelated to ACE inhibitor therapy. Also use cautiously in patients with impaired renal function, heart failure, ischemic heart disease, cerebrovascular disease, renal artery stenosis, or collagen vascular disease, such as systemic lupus erythematosus or scleroderma.
⚖ **Lifespan:** In pregnant women, drug is contraindicated.

Adverse reactions

CNS: dizziness, asthenia, fever, sleep disorder, paresthesia, depression, somnolence, nervousness, *headache.*
CV: palpitations, edema, chest pain, abnormal ECG.
EENT: rhinitis, sinusitis, ear infection, pharyngitis, tinnitus.
GI: dyspepsia, diarrhea, abdominal pain, nausea, vomiting, flatulence.
GU: proteinuria, UTI, sexual dysfunction in men, menstrual disorder.
Metabolic: *hyperkalemia.*
Musculoskeletal: back pain, hypertonia, neck pain, joint pain, myalgia, arthritis, leg or arm pain.
Respiratory: *cough,* upper respiratory tract infection.
Skin: rash.
Other: viral infection, injury, seasonal allergy.

Interactions

Drug-drug. *Antacids:* Decreases drug bioavailability. Separate administration times by at least 2 hours.
Diuretics: May have additive hypotensive effect. Monitor patient closely.
Lithium: Increases lithium level and may cause lithium toxicity. Use together cautiously, and monitor lithium levels. Use of a diuretic may further increase the risk of lithium toxicity.
Potassium supplements, potassium-sparing diuretics, other drugs capable of increasing potassium (such as indomethacin, heparin, cyclosporine): May have additive hyperkalemic effect. Use together cautiously, and monitor potassium levels frequently.
Drug-herb. *Capsaicin:* Increases risk of cough. Discourage using together.
Licorice: May cause sodium retention and increase blood pressure, interfering with therapeutic effects of ACE inhibitors. Discourage using together.
Drug-food. *Salt substitutes containing potassium:* May increase risk of hyperkalemia. Use together cautiously.

Effects on lab test results

• May increase ALT, triglyceride, and potassium levels.

Pharmacokinetics

Absorption: Rapid; level peaks at about 1 hour. Absolute P.O. bioavailability of perindopril is around 75%. Perindopril and perindoprilat levels are about doubled in geriatric patients.

Rapid onset   *Liquid form contains alcohol.*   ♦Canada   ◊ Australia   †OTC   ‡Off-label use

Distribution: Perindopril and perindoprilat are about 60% and 10% to 20% bound to proteins, respectively.

Metabolism: Extensively metabolized by the liver to the active ACE inhibitor, perindoprilat.

Excretion: About 4% to 12% of drug is excreted in the urine as unchanged drug. Clearance is reduced in geriatric patients and patients with heart failure or renal insufficiency. *Half-life:* 1 hour.

Route	Onset	Peak	Duration
P.O.	Unknown	1 hr	Unknown

Action

Chemical effect: This is a prodrug converted by the liver to the active metabolite perindoprilat. Perindoprilat probably inhibits ACE activity, thereby preventing conversion of angiotensin I to angiotensin II, a potent vasoconstrictor. ACE inhibition results in decreased vasoconstriction and decreased aldosterone, thus reducing sodium and water retention.

Therapeutic effect: Lowers blood pressure.

Available forms

Tablets: 2 mg, 4 mg, 8 mg

NURSING PROCESS

Assessment

• Obtain complete medical history before therapy.

• Monitor CBC with differential before therapy, especially in renally impaired patients with systemic lupus erythematosus or scleroderma. Other ACE inhibitors have been linked to agranulocytosis and neutropenia.

• Monitor renal function before and periodically throughout therapy. If creatinine clearance is less than 30 ml/minute, don't use drug.

• Assess patient for volume or sodium depletion as a result of prolonged diuretic therapy, dietary salt restriction, dialysis, diarrhea, or vomiting.

• Monitor potassium level closely.

• If patient is at risk for hypotension, watch closely during first dose, for the first 2 weeks, and whenever increasing the dose of this drug or a diuretic. If severe hypotension occurs, place patient in supine position and treat symptomatically.

• Evaluate patient's and family's knowledge of drug therapy.

Nursing diagnoses

• Risk for injury related to presence of hypertension

• Risk for activity intolerance related to drug-induced adverse effects

• Deficient knowledge related to drug therapy

Planning and implementation

• Correct volume and salt depletion before starting drug.

ALERT: Angioedema of the face, limbs, lips, tongue, glottis, and larynx has been reported in patients treated with perindopril. Angioedema involving the tongue, glottis, or larynx may cause fatal airway obstruction. Give appropriate therapy, such as S.C. epinephrine solution, promptly. Stop drug, notify prescriber, and observe patient until the swelling resolves.

• Swelling confined to the face and lips will probably resolve without treatment, but antihistamines may help relieve symptoms.

• Patients with a history of angioedema unrelated to ACE inhibitor therapy may be at increased risk of angioedema while receiving an ACE inhibitor.

• Excessive hypotension can occur when drug is given with diuretics. If possible, stop diuretics 2 to 3 days before starting this drug. If diuretic can't be stopped, prescriber may consider starting this drug at a reduced dosage, decreasing the diuretic dosage, or both.

• ACE inhibitors rarely are linked to a fatal syndrome of cholestatic jaundice and fulminant hepatic necrosis. If patient develops jaundice or marked elevation of hepatic enzyme levels during therapy, notify prescriber and stop drug.

Patient teaching

• Inform patient that angioedema, including laryngeal edema, can occur during therapy, especially with the first dose. Advise patient to stop taking the drug and immediately report any signs or symptoms that suggest angioedema (swelling of face, limbs, eyes, lips, tongue; hoarseness or difficulty in swallowing or breathing).

• Advise patient to report promptly any sign of infection (sore throat, fever) or jaundice (yellowing of eyes or skin).

• Tell patient to avoid salt substitutes containing potassium unless instructed otherwise by prescriber.

• Warn patient that light-headedness may occur, especially during the first few days of therapy. Advise patient to report light-headedness and, if fainting occurs, to stop taking drug and consult prescriber promptly.

• Warn patient that inadequate fluid intake or excessive perspiration, diarrhea, or vomiting can lead to an excessive drop in blood pressure.

• Advise patient to notify prescriber immediately if she suspects pregnancy.

☑ **Evaluation**

• Patient's blood pressure is controlled and he remains free of injury.

• Patient has no adverse effects that limit mobility.

• Patient and family state understanding of drug therapy.

perphenazine
(per-FEN-uh-zeen)
Apo-Perphenazine ♦ , Trilafon, Trilafon Concentrate

Pharmacologic class: phenothiazine (piperazine derivative)
Therapeutic class: antipsychotic, antiemetic
Pregnancy risk category: NR

Indications and dosages

▶ **Psychosis in nonhospitalized patients.**
Adults: Initially, 4 to 8 mg P.O. t.i.d., reduced as soon as possible to minimum effective dosage.
Children older than age 12: Lowest adult dose.
▶ **Psychosis in hospitalized patients.** *Adults:* Initially, 8 to 16 mg P.O. b.i.d., t.i.d., or q.i.d.; increase to 64 mg daily, p.r.n. Or, 5 to 10 mg I.M. q 6 hours, p.r.n. Maximum daily I.M. dose shouldn't exceed 30 mg.
Children older than age 12: Lowest limit of adult dosage.
▶ **Severe nausea and vomiting.** *Adults:* 5 to 10 mg I.M., p.r.n.

Contraindications and precautions

• Contraindicated in patients hypersensitive to drug, in comatose patients, in patients with CNS depression, blood dyscrasia, bone marrow depression, liver damage, or subcortical damage, and in those receiving large doses of CNS depressants.

• Use cautiously with other CNS depressants or anticholinergics. Also use cautiously in debilitated patients and patients with alcohol withdrawal, depression, suicidal tendency, severe adverse reactions to other phenothiazines, impaired renal function, or respiratory disorders.

⚠ Lifespan: In pregnant and breast-feeding women and in elderly patients, use cautiously. In children age 12 and younger, safety of drug hasn't been established.

Adverse reactions

CNS: *extrapyramidal reaction, tardive dyskinesia,* sedation, pseudoparkinsonism, EEG changes, dizziness, *seizures, neuroleptic malignant syndrome.*
CV: *orthostatic hypotension,* tachycardia, ECG changes, *cardiac arrest.*
EENT: ocular changes, blurred vision.
GI: dry mouth, constipation.
GU: *urine retention,* dark urine, menstrual irregularities, inhibited ejaculation.
Hematologic: transient *leukopenia,* hyperprolactinemia, *agranulocytosis,* hemolytic anemia, *thrombocytopenia.*
Hepatic: cholestatic jaundice.
Metabolic: weight gain, increased appetite.
Skin: *mild photosensitivity reaction,* sterile abscess.
Other: allergic reactions, pain at I.M. injection site, gynecomastia.

Interactions

Drug-drug. *Antacids:* Inhibits oral phenothiazine absorption. Administer drugs separately.
Anticonvulsants: Phenothiazines may lower the seizure threshold. Monitor patient.
Barbiturates: May decrease phenothiazine effect. Observe patient closely.
Bromocriptine: Decreases bromocriptine effectiveness. Monitor patient for effect.
CNS depressants: Increases CNS depression. Avoid using together.
Lithium: Causes severe neurological toxicity with encephalitis-like syndrome; decreased therapeutic response to perphenazine. Don't use together.

Rapid onset   *Liquid form contains alcohol.   ♦Canada   ◊ Australia   †OTC   ‡Off-label use

Drug-herb. *Dong quai, St. John's wort:* Increases photosensitivity reactions. Discourage using together.
Evening primrose oil: May increase risk of seizures. Discourage using together.
Kava: Increases risk of dystonic reactions. Discourage using together.
Milk thistle: Decreases liver toxicity caused by phenothiazines. Monitor liver enzyme levels.
Yohimbe: Increases risk of yohimbe toxicity. Discourage using together.
Drug-lifestyle. *Alcohol use:* Increases CNS depression, particularly psychomotor skills. Strongly discourage use together.
Sun exposure: Increases photosensitivity reaction. Urge patient to avoid unprotected or prolonged exposure to sunlight.

Effects on lab test results

• May increase prolactin levels.
• May increase liver function test values and eosinophil count. May decrease hemoglobin, hematocrit, and WBC, granulocyte, and platelet counts.

Pharmacokinetics

Absorption: Rate and extent vary. Erratic and variable for P.O. tablet; much more predictable for P.O. concentrate. Rapid from I.M. injection.
Distribution: Distributed widely; 91% to 99% of drug is protein-bound.
Metabolism: Metabolized extensively by liver.
Excretion: Most of drug excreted in urine; some in feces. *Half-life:* Unknown.

Route	Onset	Peak	Duration
P.O., I.M.	Varies	Unknown	Unknown

Action

Chemical effect: Unknown; probably blocks postsynaptic dopamine receptors in brain and inhibits medullary chemoreceptor trigger zone.
Therapeutic effect: Relieves signs and symptoms of psychosis; also relieves nausea and vomiting.

Available forms

Injection: 5 mg/ml
Oral concentrate: 16 mg/5 ml*
Syrup: 2 mg/5 ml ♦
Tablets: 2 mg, 4 mg, 8 mg, 16 mg

NURSING PROCESS

✒ Assessment

• Assess patient's condition before therapy and regularly thereafter.
• Obtain baseline blood pressure before therapy, and monitor regularly. Watch for orthostatic hypotension, especially with I.M. administration.
• Monitor weekly bilirubin tests during first month, and obtain periodic blood tests (CBC and liver function) and ophthalmic tests (long-term use).
• Be alert for adverse reactions and drug interactions.
• Monitor patient for tardive dyskinesia, which may occur after prolonged use. It may not appear until months or years later and may disappear spontaneously or persist for life despite stopping drug.
• If drug is used for nausea and vomiting, monitor patient's hydration.
• Evaluate patient's and family's knowledge of drug therapy.

⊞ Nursing diagnoses

• Disturbed thought processes related to psychosis
• Risk for deficient fluid volume related to nausea or vomiting
• Deficient knowledge related to drug therapy

▷ Planning and implementation

• When giving liquid form, dilute with fruit juice, milk, carbonated beverage, or semisolid food just before giving.
• Concentrate causes turbidity or precipitation in colas, black coffee, grape or apple juice, or tea. Don't mix with them.
• When given I.M., inject drug deep in upper outer quadrant of buttocks. Injection may sting.
• Massage slowly after injection to prevent sterile abscess.
• Keep patient supine for 1 hour after injection because of risk of hypotension.
• Prevent contact dermatitis by keeping drug away from skin and clothes. Wear gloves when preparing liquid forms.
• Protect drug from light. Slight yellowing of injection or concentrate doesn't affect potency. Discard markedly discolored solutions.
• Don't stop drug abruptly unless severe adverse reactions demand it. After abrupt withdrawal of long-term therapy, patient may experi-

ence gastritis, nausea, vomiting, dizziness, tremors, feeling of warmth or cold, diaphoresis, tachycardia, headache, or insomnia.

• If patient develops jaundice, symptoms of blood dyscrasia (fever, sore throat, infection, cellulitis, weakness), or extrapyramidal reactions that last longer than a few hours, withhold dose and notify prescriber.

• Acute dystonic reactions may be treated with diphenhydramine.

⊛ **ALERT:** Don't confuse perphenazine with prochlorperazine.

Patient teaching

• Advise patient to change positions slowly to minimize effects of orthostatic hypotension.

• Teach patient which fluids are appropriate for dilution of concentrate.

• Warn patient to avoid hazardous activities until CNS effects of drug are known. Drowsiness and dizziness usually subside after a few weeks.

• Tell patient to avoid alcohol during drug therapy.

• Advise patient to report urine retention or constipation.

• Tell patient to use sunblock and to wear protective clothing to avoid photosensitivity reactions.

• Tell patient to relieve dry mouth with sugarless gum or hard candy.

☑ Evaluation

• Patient's thought processes are normal.

• Patient maintains adequate hydration throughout drug therapy.

• Patient and family state understanding of drug therapy.

---

phenazopyridine hydrochloride (phenylazo diamino pyridine hydrochloride)

(fen-eh-soh-PEER-eh-deen high-droh-KLOR-ighd)
Azo-Dine, Azo-Gesic, Azo-Standard†, Baridium†, Geridium, Phenazol, Prodium†, Pyridiate, Pyridium, Pyridium Plus, Re-Azo, Urodine†, Urogesic, UTI Relief

Pharmacologic class: azo dye
Therapeutic class: urinary analgesic
Pregnancy risk category: B

Indications and dosages

▶ **Urinary tract irritation or infection.**
Adults: 200 mg P.O. t.i.d.
Children: 12 mg/kg P.O. daily divided into three equal doses.

Contraindications and precautions

• Contraindicated in patients with glomerulonephritis, severe hepatitis, uremia, or renal insufficiency.

⚖ **Lifespan:** In pyelonephritis during pregnancy, drug is contraindicated. In breast-feeding women, safety of drug hasn't been established. In children, use cautiously.

Adverse reactions

CNS: headache, vertigo.
EENT: staining of contact lenses.
GI: nausea, mild GI disturbance.
Skin: rash, pruritus.

Interactions

None significant.

Effects on lab test results

• May alter urine glucose results when Diastix is used. May interfere with urinalysis based on spectrometry or color reactions.

Pharmacokinetics

Absorption: Unknown.
Distribution: Unknown.
Metabolism: In liver.
Excretion: 65% excreted in urine unchanged.
Half-life: Unknown.

Route	Onset	Peak	Duration
P.O.	Unknown	Unknown	Unknown

Action

Chemical effect: Unknown; has local anesthetic effect on urinary mucosa.
Therapeutic effect: Relieves urinary tract pain.

Available forms

Tablets: 95 mg†, 97 mg, 97.2 mg, 100 mg†, 150 mg, 200 mg

NURSING PROCESS

🕮 Assessment

• Assess patient's pain before and after giving drug.

• Be alert for adverse reactions.
• If nausea occurs, monitor patient's hydration.
• Evaluate patient's and family's knowledge of drug therapy.

⊕ **Nursing diagnoses**
• Acute pain related to underlying urinary tract condition
• Risk for deficient fluid volume related to drug-induced nausea
• Deficient knowledge related to drug therapy

▷ **Planning and implementation**
• Administer drug with food to minimize nausea.
⊛ **ALERT:** Don't confuse Pyridium with pyridoxine or pyridine.
Patient teaching
• Advise patient that taking drug with meals may minimize nausea.
• Tell patient to stop taking drug and to notify prescriber if skin or sclera becomes yellow-tinged.
• Warn patient that drug colors urine red or orange. It may stain fabrics and contact lenses.
• Tell patient to notify prescriber if urinary tract pain persists. Drug isn't for long-term therapy.

☑ **Evaluation**
• Patient is free from pain.
• Patient maintains adequate hydration.
• Patient and family state understanding of drug therapy.

---

phenobarbital (phenobarbitone)
(feen-oh-BAR-bih-tol)
Solfoton

phenobarbital sodium (phenobarbitone sodium)
Luminal Sodium

Pharmacologic class: barbiturate
Therapeutic class: anticonvulsant, sedative-hypnotic
Pregnancy risk category: D
Controlled substance schedule: IV

Indications and dosages

▶ **All forms of epilepsy except absence seizures; febrile seizures in children.** *Adults:* 60 to 250 mg P.O. daily, in divided doses t.i.d. or as single dose h.s.
Children: 1 to 6 mg/kg P.O. daily, divided q 12 hours for total of 100 mg; can be given once daily, usually h.s.
▶ **Status epilepticus.** *Adults:* 10 to 20 mg/kg I.V.; may repeat, if necessary.
Children: 15 to 20 mg/kg I.V. Don't exceed 50 mg/minute.
▶ **Sedation.** *Adults:* 30 to 120 mg P.O. daily in two or three divided doses.
Children: 3 to 5 mg/kg P.O. daily in divided doses t.i.d.
▶ **Insomnia.** *Adults:* 100 to 200 mg P.O. or I.M. h.s.
▶ **Preoperative sedation.** *Adults:* 100 to 200 mg I.M. 60 to 90 minutes before surgery.
Children: 1 to 3 mg/kg I.V. or I.M. 60 to 90 minutes before surgery.

▽ I.V. administration

• Don't mix parenteral form with acidic solutions.
• If injectable solution contains precipitate, don't use.
⊛ **ALERT:** I.V. injection is reserved for emergencies. Monitor respirations closely.
⊛ **ALERT:** Don't give more than 60 mg/minute.
• Have resuscitation equipment available.

Contraindications and precautions

• Contraindicated in patients hypersensitive to barbiturates and in those with hepatic dysfunction, respiratory disease with dyspnea or obstruction, nephritis, or a history of manifest or latent porphyria.
• Use cautiously in debilitated patients and in patients with acute or chronic pain, depression, suicidal tendencies, history of drug abuse, altered blood pressure, CV disease, shock, or uremia.
⚕ **Lifespan:** In pregnant and breast-feeding women, drug isn't recommended. In elderly patients, use cautiously; drug causes paradoxical excitement in these patients.

Adverse reactions

CNS: drowsiness, lethargy, hangover.
CV: *bradycardia,* hypotension.
GI: nausea, vomiting.

Hematologic: exacerbation of porphyria.
Respiratory: *respiratory depression, apnea.*
Skin: rash; *erythema multiforme, Stevens-Johnson syndrome,* urticaria.
Other: *angioedema;* pain, swelling, thrombophlebitis, necrosis, nerve injury at injection site.

Interactions

Drug-drug. *Chloramphenicol, MAO inhibitors, valproic acid:* Increases barbiturate effect. Monitor patient for increased CNS and respiratory depression.
CNS depressants, including opioid analgesics: Excessive CNS depression. Use together cautiously.
Corticosteroids, digitoxin, doxycycline, estrogens and hormonal contraceptives, oral anticoagulants, tricyclic antidepressants: Phenobarbital may enhance metabolism of these drugs. Monitor patient for decreased effect.
Diazepam: Increases effects of both drugs. Use together cautiously.
Griseofulvin: Decreases griseofulvin absorption. Administer drug separately.
Mephobarbital, primidone: Excessive phenobarbital levels. Monitor patient closely.
Metoprolol, propranolol: May reduce the effects of these drugs. Consider an increased beta blocker dose.
Rifampin: May decrease barbiturate levels. Monitor patient for decreased effect.
Valproic acid: Increases phenobarbital levels. Monitor patient for toxicity.
Drug-lifestyle. *Alcohol use:* May impair coordination, increase CNS effects, and cause death. Strongly discourage use together.

Effects on lab test results

• May decrease bilirubin level.

Pharmacokinetics

Absorption: Absorbed well after P.O. administration. 100% from I.M. injection.
Distribution: Distributed widely throughout body. Drug is about 25% to 30% protein-bound.
Metabolism: Metabolized in liver.
Excretion: Excreted in urine. *Half-life:* 5 to 7 days.

Route	Onset	Peak	Duration
P.O.	20-60 min	Unknown	10-12 hr
I.V.	5 min	≥ 15 min	10-12 hr
I.M.	> 60 min	Unknown	10-12 hr

Action

Chemical effect: Unknown; may depress CNS synaptic transmission and increase seizure activity threshold in motor cortex. As sedative, may interfere with transmission of impulses from thalamus to brain cortex.
Therapeutic effect: Prevents and stops seizure activity; promotes calmness and sleep.

Available forms

Capsules: 16 mg
Elixir*: 15 mg/5 ml, 20 mg/5 ml
Injection: 30 mg/ml, 60 mg/ml, 65 mg/ml, 130 mg/ml
Tablets: 15 mg, 16 mg, 30 mg, 32 mg, 60 mg, 65 mg, 100 mg

NURSING PROCESS

Assessment
• Assess patient's condition before therapy and regularly thereafter.
• Monitor blood level closely. Therapeutic level is 15 to 40 mcg/ml.
• Be alert for adverse reactions and drug interactions.
• Evaluate patient's and family's knowledge of drug therapy.

Nursing diagnoses
• Risk for trauma related to seizures
• Risk for injury related to drug-induced adverse CNS reactions
• Deficient knowledge related to drug therapy

Planning and implementation
• Don't stop drug abruptly; seizures may worsen. If adverse reactions occur, notify prescriber immediately.
• Give drug by deep I.M. injection. Superficial injection may cause pain, sterile abscess, and tissue sloughing.
⚕ ALERT: Don't confuse pentobarbital with phenobarbital.
Patient teaching
• Tell patient that phenobarbital is available in different strengths and sizes. Advise him to check prescription and refills closely.
• Inform patient that full effects don't occur for 2 to 3 weeks except when loading dose is used.
• Advise patient to avoid hazardous activities until CNS effects of drug are known.

- Warn patient and parents not to stop drug abruptly.
- Tell patient using hormonal contraceptives to use a different birth control method.

☑ Evaluation

- Patient is free from seizure activity.
- Patient has no injury from drug-induced adverse CNS reactions.
- Patient and family state understanding of drug therapy.

phentermine hydrochloride
(FEN-ter-meen high-droh-KLOR-ighd)
Adipex-P, Duromine ◇ , Ionamin, Pro-Fast HS, Pro-Fast SA, Pro-Fast SR

Pharmacologic class: indirect-acting sympathomimetic amine
Therapeutic class: short-term adjunct anorexigenic
Pregnancy risk category: C
Controlled substance schedule: IV

Indications and dosages

▶ **Short-term adjunct in exogenous obesity.**
Adults: 8 mg P.O. t.i.d. 30 minutes before meals. Or, 15 to 37.5 mg daily before breakfast. Give Pro-fast HS or Pro-fast SR capsules 2 hours after breakfast. Give Adipex-P before breakfast or 1 to 2 hours after breakfast.

Contraindications and precautions

- Contraindicated in agitated patients, patients hypersensitive to sympathomimetic amines, patients who have idiosyncratic reactions to them, patients who have taken an MAO inhibitor within 14 days, and patients with hyperthyroidism, moderate-to-severe hypertension, advanced arteriosclerosis, symptomatic CV disease, or glaucoma.
- Use cautiously in patients with mild hypertension.
- ☀ Lifespan: In pregnant and breast-feeding women, drug isn't recommended. In children, safety of drug hasn't been established.

Adverse reactions

CNS: overstimulation, headache, euphoria, dysphoria, dizziness, *insomnia.*

CV: palpitations, tachycardia, increased blood pressure.
EENT: mydriasis, eye irritation, blurred vision.
GI: dry mouth, dysgeusia, constipation, diarrhea, other GI disturbances.
GU: impotence.
Skin: urticaria.
Other: altered libido.

Interactions

Drug-drug. *Acetazolamide, antacids, sodium bicarbonate:* Increases renal reabsorption. Monitor patient.
Ammonium chloride, ascorbic acid: Decreases levels and increases renal excretion of phentermine. Monitor patient for decreased effects.
Guanethidine: May decrease hypotensive effect. Monitor blood pressure closely.
Haloperidol, phenothiazines, tricyclic antidepressants: Increases CNS effects. Avoid using together.
Insulin, oral antidiabetics: May alter antidiabetic requirements. Monitor glucose levels.
MAO inhibitors: May cause severe hypertension and hypertensive crisis. Don't use together or within 14 days of MAO inhibitor.
Drug-food. *Caffeine:* May increase CNS stimulation. Discourage using together.

Effects on lab test results

None reported.

Pharmacokinetics

Absorption: Absorbed readily from GI tract.
Distribution: Distributed throughout body.
Metabolism: Unknown.
Excretion: Excreted in urine. *Half-life:* 19 to 24 hours.

Route	Onset	Peak	Duration
P.O.	Unknown	Unknown	12-14 hr

Action

Chemical effect: Unknown; probably works by releasing stored norepinephrine from nerve terminals in the brain (primarily in the cerebral cortex and reticular activating system), thus promoting nerve impulse transmission
Therapeutic effect: Depresses appetite.

Available forms

Capsules: 18.75 mg (15 mg base), 30 mg (24 mg base), 37.5 mg (30 mg base)

Reactions may be *common,* uncommon, *life-threatening*, or COMMON AND LIFE-THREATENING.

Capsules (resin complex): 15 mg, 30 mg
Tablets: 8 mg, 37.5 mg (30-mg base)

NURSING PROCESS

⚕ Assessment
• Weigh patient before therapy and regularly thereafter.
• Be alert for adverse reactions and drug interactions.
• Monitor patient for habituation and tolerance.
• Evaluate patient's and family's knowledge of drug therapy.

⚕ Nursing diagnoses
• Imbalanced nutrition: more than body requirements related to food intake
• Disturbed sleep pattern related to drug-induced insomnia
• Deficient knowledge related to drug therapy

⟩ Planning and implementation
• Give drug at least 6 hours before bedtime to avoid insomnia.
• Make sure patient is following a weight-reduction program.
⚙ **ALERT:** Don't confuse phentermine with phentolamine.
Patient teaching
• Instruct patient to take drug at least 6 hours before bedtime to avoid sleep interference.
• Warn patient to avoid hazardous activities until CNS effects of drug are known.
• Tell patient to avoid caffeine because it increases the effects of amphetamines and related amines.
• Tell patient to report signs of excessive stimulation.
• Inform patient that fatigue may result as drug effects wear off.

⚕ Evaluation
• Patient loses weight.
• Patient doesn't have insomnia.
• Patient and family state understanding of drug therapy.

phenylephrine hydrochloride
(fen-il-EF-rin high-droh-KLOR-ighd)
Neo-Synephrine

Pharmacologic class: adrenergic
Therapeutic class: vasoconstrictor
Pregnancy risk category: C

Indications and dosages
▶ **Hypotensive emergencies during spinal anesthesia.** *Adults:* Initially, 0.1 to 0.2 mg I.V., followed by 0.1 to 0.2 mg, p.r.n.
▶ **Maintenance of blood pressure during spinal or inhalation anesthesia.** *Adults:* 2 to 3 mg S.C. or I.M. 3 or 4 minutes before anesthesia.
Children: 0.044 to 0.088 mg/kg S.C. or I.M.
▶ **Prolongation of spinal anesthesia.** *Adults:* 2 to 5 mg added to anesthetic solution.
▶ **Vasoconstrictor for regional anesthesia.** *Adults:* 1 mg phenylephrine added to 20 ml local anesthetic.
▶ **Mild to moderate hypotension.** *Adults:* 2 to 5 mg S.C. or I.M.; repeated in 1 to 2 hours as needed and tolerated. Initial dose shouldn't exceed 5 mg. Or, 0.1 to 0.5 mg slow I.V., no more than q 10 to 15 minutes.
Children: 0.1 mg/kg I.M. or S.C.; repeated in 1 to 2 hours as needed and tolerated.
▶ **Severe hypotension and shock (including drug-induced).** *Adults:* 0.1 to 0.18 mg/minute I.V. infusion. After blood pressure stabilizes, maintain at 0.04 to 0.06 mg/minute, adjusted to patient response.
▶ **Paroxysmal supraventricular tachycardia.** *Adults:* Initially, 0.5 mg rapid I.V. Subsequent doses may be increased by 0.1 to 0.2 mg. Maximum dose shouldn't exceed 1 mg.

▼ I.V. administration
• For direct injection, dilute 10 mg (1 ml) with 9 ml sterile water for injection to provide solution containing 1 mg/ml.
• Prepare I.V. infusions by adding 10 mg of drug to 500 ml of D_5W or normal saline solution for injection.
• Initial infusion rate is usually 100 to 180 mcg/minute; maintenance rate is usually 40 to 60 mcg/minute.
• Use continuous infusion pump to regulate flow rate.

• During infusion, frequently monitor ECG, blood pressure, cardiac output, central venous pressure, pulmonary capillary wedge pressure, pulse rate, urine output, and color and temperature of limbs. Titrate infusion rate according to findings and prescriber's guidelines.

• Use central venous catheter or large vein, as in antecubital fossa, to minimize risk of extravasation.

• To treat extravasation, infiltrate site promptly with 10 to 15 ml of normal saline solution for injection that contains 5 to 10 mg phentolamine. Use a fine needle.

• After prolonged I.V. infusion, avoid abrupt withdrawal.

Contraindications and precautions

• Contraindicated in patients hypersensitive to drug and in patients with severe hypertension or ventricular tachycardia.

• Use cautiously in patients with heart disease, hyperthyroidism, severe atherosclerosis, bradycardia, partial heart block, myocardial disease, or sulfite sensitivity.

⚠ Lifespan: In pregnant and breast-feeding women and in elderly patients, use cautiously.

Adverse reactions

CNS: *headache, restlessness, light-headedness, weakness.*
CV: palpitations, *bradycardia, arrhythmias,* hypertension, angina, decreased cardiac output.
EENT: blurred vision.
GI: vomiting.
Respiratory: *asthma attacks.*
Skin: pilomotor response, feeling of coolness.
Other: tachyphylaxis, *decreased organ perfusion with prolonged use,* tissue sloughing with extravasation, *anaphylaxis.*

Interactions

Drug-drug. *Alpha-adrenergic blockers, phenothiazines:* Decreases vasopressor response. Monitor patient closely.
Beta blockers: Blocks cardiostimulatory effects. Monitor patient closely.
Bretylium: Increases risk of arrhythmias. Monitor ECG.
Oxytocics, guanethidine: Increases pressor response and causes severe, persistent hypertension. Monitor patient and blood pressure closely.

Phenelzine, tranylcypromine: May cause severe headache, hypertension, fever, and hypertensive crisis. Avoid using together.
Tricyclic antidepressants: May potentiate the pressor response and cause arrhythmias. Use cautiously.

Effects on lab test results

None reported.

Pharmacokinetics

Absorption: Unknown after I.M. and S.C. administration.
Distribution: Unknown.
Metabolism: Metabolized in liver and intestine.
Excretion: Unknown. *Half-life:* Unknown.

Route	Onset	Peak	Duration
I.V.	Immediate	Unknown	15-20 min
I.M.	10-15 min	Unknown	½-2 hr
S.C.	10-15 min	Unknown	50-60 min

Action

Chemical effect: Mainly stimulates alpha-adrenergic receptors in sympathetic nervous system.
Therapeutic effect: Raises blood pressure and stops paroxysmal supraventricular tachycardia.

Available forms

Injection: 10 mg/ml

NURSING PROCESS

🔏 **Assessment**
• Assess patient's condition before therapy and regularly thereafter.
• Monitor blood pressure frequently; avoid severe increase. Maintain blood pressure slightly below patient's normal level. In previously normotensive patient, maintain systolic pressure at 80 to 100 mm Hg; in previously hypertensive patient, maintain systolic pressure at 30 to 40 mm Hg below usual level.
• Monitor ECG throughout therapy.
• Be alert for adverse reactions and drug interactions.
• Evaluate patient's and family's knowledge of drug therapy.

⊕ Nursing diagnoses
- Ineffective tissue perfusion (cerebral, cardiopulmonary, peripheral, GI, renal) related to underlying condition
- Decreased cardiac output related to drug-induced adverse reaction
- Deficient knowledge related to drug therapy

▶ Planning and implementation
- Drug is incompatible with butacaine sulfate, alkalis, ferric salts, and oxidizing drugs.

Patient teaching
- Tell patient to report discomfort at infusion site immediately.

✓ Evaluation
- Patient maintains tissue perfusion and cellular oxygenation.
- Patient maintains adequate cardiac output.
- Patient and family state understanding of drug therapy.

phenylephrine hydrochloride (intranasal)

(fen-il-EF-rin high-droh-KLOR-ighd)
Afrin Children's Pump Mist†, Alconefrin 12†, Alconefrin 25†, Alconefrin 50†, Duration†, Little Colds for Infants and Children†, Little Noses Gentle Formula†, Neo-Synephrine 4 Hour†, Nostril†, Rhinall†, Vicks Sinex†

Pharmacologic class: adrenergic
Therapeutic class: vasoconstrictor
Pregnancy risk category: C

Indications and dosages

▶ **Nasal congestion.** *Adults and children age 12 and older:* 2 to 3 drops (gtt) or 1 to 2 sprays in each nostril, p.r.n.
Children ages 6 to 11: 2 to 3 gtt or 1 to 2 sprays of 0.25% solution in each nostril q 3 to 4 hours, p.r.n.
Children younger than age 6: 2 to 3 gtt of 0.125% solution q 4 hours, p.r.n.

Contraindications and precautions

- Contraindicated in patients hypersensitive to drug.
- Use cautiously in patients with hyperthyroidism, marked hypertension, type 1 diabetes mellitus, cardiac disease, or advanced arteriosclerotic changes.
- ♨ **Lifespan:** In pregnant and breast-feeding women, children with low body weight, and elderly patients, use cautiously.

Adverse reactions

CNS: headache, tremor, dizziness, nervousness.
CV: *palpitations, tachycardia, PVCs,* hypertension, pallor.
EENT: transient burning or stinging, dry nasal mucosa, rebound nasal congestion with chronic use.
GI: nausea.

Interactions

Drug-drug. *Guanethidine:* May potentiate phenylephrine hydrochloride and decrease pressor response (hypotension). Monitor patient's blood pressure closely.
Methyldopa: Increases pressor response and increases risk of arrhythmias. Don't use together.
Phenelzine, tranylcypromine: May cause severe headache, hypertension, fever, and hypertensive crisis. Avoid use together.
Tricyclic antidepressants: May potentiate the pressor response and cause arrhythmias. Use cautiously.

Effects on lab test results

None reported.

Pharmacokinetics

Absorption: Minimal.
Distribution: Locally to nasal tissue.
Metabolism: In liver.
Excretion: In urine. *Half-life:* Unknown.

Route	Onset	Peak	Duration
Intranasal	Rapid	Unknown	½-4 hr

Action

Chemical effect: Causes local vasoconstriction of dilated arterioles, reducing blood flow.
Therapeutic effect: Relieves nasal congestion.

Available forms

Nasal solution: 0.125%, 0.16%, 0.25%, 0.5%, 1%

NURSING PROCESS

✍ Assessment
- Assess patient's condition before therapy and regularly thereafter.
- Be alert for adverse reactions.
- Evaluate patient's and family's knowledge of drug therapy.

⊕ Nursing diagnoses
- Ineffective health maintenance related to nasal congestion
- Impaired tissue integrity related to adverse effect on nasal tissue
- Deficient knowledge related to drug therapy

▶ Planning and implementation
- Have patient hold head upright; insert nozzle and have patient sniff spray briskly.

Patient teaching
- Teach patient how to give drug.
- Tell patient not to share drug to prevent spread of infection.
- Warn patient not to exceed recommended dosage.
- Advise patient to contact prescriber if symptoms persist beyond 3 days.

☑ Evaluation
- Patient's nasal congestion is relieved.
- Patient maintains normal nasal tissue integrity.
- Patient and family state understanding of drug therapy.

phenytoin (diphenylhydantoin)
(FEN-uh-toyn)
Dilantin-125, Dilantin Infatabs

phenytoin sodium (extended)
Dilantin Kapseals, Phenytek

phenytoin sodium (prompt)
Dilantin

Pharmacologic class: hydantoin derivative
Therapeutic class: anticonvulsant
Pregnancy risk category: D

Indications and dosages

▶ **Control of tonic-clonic (grand mal) and complex partial (temporal lobe) seizures.**

Adults: Highly individualized. Initially, 100 mg P.O. (extended-release) t.i.d., increased in increments of 100 mg P.O. q 2 to 4 weeks until desired response is obtained. Usual range is 300 to 600 mg daily. If patient is stabilized with extended-release capsules, once-daily dosing with 300-mg extended-release capsules is possible as an alternative.
Children: 5 mg/kg or 250 mg/m^2 P.O. (extended-release) divided b.i.d. or t.i.d. Maximum daily dose is 300 mg.

▶ **For patient requiring a loading dose.**
Adults: Initially, 1 g P.O. daily divided into three doses and administered at 2-hour intervals. Or, 10 to 15 mg/kg I.V. at a rate not exceeding 50 mg/minute. Normal maintenance dose is started 24 hours later with frequent level determinations.
Children: Initially, 5 mg/kg P.O. daily in two or three equally divided doses with subsequent dose individualized to maximum of 300 mg daily. Usual dosage is 4 to 8 mg/kg P.O. daily. Children older than age 6 may require the minimum adult dosage (300 mg daily).

▶ **Prevention and treatment of seizures occurring during neurosurgery.** *Adults:* 100 to 200 mg I.M or I.V. q 4 hours during surgery and continued in the immediate postoperative period.

▶ **Status epilepticus.** *Adults:* Loading dose of 10 to 15 mg/kg I.V. (1 to 1.5 g may be needed) at a rate not exceeding 50 mg/minute; then maintenance dosages of 100 mg P.O. or I.V. q 6 to 8 hours.
Children: Loading dose of 15 to 20 mg/kg I.V., at a rate not exceeding 1 to 3 mg/kg/minute; then highly individualized maintenance doses.

▪ **Adjust-a-dose:** Elderly patients may need lower dosages.

▽ I.V. administration
- Check patency of I.V. catheter before administering. Extravasation may cause severe local tissue damage.
- Never use cloudy solution.
- ⑤ **ALERT:** If giving as infusion, don't mix drug with D$_5$W because it will precipitate. Clear I.V. tubing first with normal saline solution. May mix with normal saline solution if necessary and infuse over 30 to 60 minutes when possible.
- Infusion must begin within 1 hour after preparation and run through in-line filter.

Reactions may be *common*, uncommon, *life-threatening*, or COMMON AND LIFE-THREATENING.

- Administer drug slowly (50 mg/minute) as I.V. bolus.
- Avoid giving phenytoin by I.V. push into veins on back of hand to avoid discoloration known as purple glove syndrome. Inject into larger veins or central venous catheter.
- Discard 4 hours after preparation.

Contraindications and precautions

- Contraindicated in patients hypersensitive to hydantoin and in patients with sinus bradycardia, SA block, second- or third-degree AV block, or Adams-Stokes syndrome.
- Use cautiously in debilitated patients, in patients receiving other hydantoin derivatives, and in patients with hepatic dysfunction, hypotension, myocardial insufficiency, diabetes, or respiratory depression.

⚖ **Lifespan:** In pregnant and breast-feeding women, drug isn't recommended. In geriatric patients, use cautiously; geriatric patients tend to metabolize phenytoin slowly and may need lower dosages.

Adverse reactions

CNS: *ataxia, slurred speech, confusion,* dizziness, insomnia, nervousness, twitching, headache.
CV: hypotension.
EENT: nystagmus, diplopia, blurred vision, gingival hyperplasia.
GI: nausea, vomiting.
Hematologic: *thrombocytopenia, leukopenia, agranulocytosis, pancytopenia,* macrocythemia, megaloblastic anemia, lymphadenopathy.
Hepatic: *toxic hepatitis.*
Metabolic: hyperglycemia.
Musculoskeletal: osteomalacia.
Skin: scarlatiniform or morbilliform rash; bullous, exfoliative, or purpuric dermatitis; *Stevens-Johnson syndrome; hirsutism; toxic epidermal necrolysis;* photosensitivity reaction, hypertrichosis.
Other: periarteritis nodosa; lupus erythematosus; pain, necrosis, or inflammation at injection site; discoloration (purple glove syndrome) if given by I.V. push in back of hand.

Interactions

Drug-drug. *Amiodarone, antihistamines, chloramphenicol, cimetidine, clonazepam, cycloserine, diazepam, disulfiram, influenza vaccine, isoniazid, phenylbutazone, salicylates, sulfame-*thizole, valproate: Increases therapeutic effects of phenytoin. Monitor patient for toxicity.
Atracurium, cisatracurium, doxacurium, mivacurium, pancuronium, rocuronium, tubocurarine, vecuronium: May decrease the effects of nondepolarizing muscle relaxant causing it to be less effective. May need to increase the dose of the nondepolarizing muscle relaxant.
Carbamazepine, dexamethasone, diazoxide, folic acid, phenobarbital: Decreases phenytoin activity. Monitor patient closely.
Disulfiram: May increase toxic effects of phenytoin. Monitor phenytoin level closely and adjust dose as necessary.
Lithium: Increases toxicity. Monitor lithium levels.
Meperidine: Toxic effects of meperidine may be increased while decreasing analgesic effects. Monitor patient for decreased effects and toxicity.
Warfarin: Displacement of warfarin can occur. Monitor patient for bleeding complications.
Drug-herb. *Milk thistle:* May decrease risk of liver toxicity. Monitor patient.
Drug-food. *Enteral nutrition therapy:* May reduce orally administered phenytoin concentrations. Consider giving phenytoin 2 hours before starting enteral feeding, or wait 2 hours after stopping enteral feeding to administer phenytoin.
Drug-lifestyle. *Alcohol use:* Decreases phenytoin activity. Discourage using together.

Effects on lab test results

- May increase alkaline phosphatase, GGT, and glucose levels. May reduce protein–bound iodine, free thyroxine, urinary 17-hydroxysteroid, and 17-ketosteroid levels.
- May increase urine 6-hydroxycortisol excretion. May decrease hemoglobin, hematocrit, and platelet, WBC, RBC, and granulocyte counts.
- May decrease dexamethasone suppression and metyrapone test values.

Pharmacokinetics

Absorption: Slow after P.O. administration. Formulation-dependent; bioavailability may differ among products. Erratic from I.M. site.
Distribution: Distributed widely throughout body. Drug is about 90% protein-bound.
Metabolism: Metabolized by liver.
Excretion: Excreted in urine; exhibits dose-dependent (zero-order) elimination kinetics.

Above certain dosage level, small increases in dosage disproportionately increase levels. *Half-life:* Varies with dose and concentration changes.

Route	Onset	Peak	Duration
P.O.	Unknown	½-2 hr	Unknown
P.O. extended	Unknown	4-12 hr	Unknown
I.V.	Immediate	1-2 hr	Unknown
I.M.	Unknown	Unknown	Unknown

Action

Chemical effect: Unknown; probably limits seizure activity by either increasing efflux or decreasing influx of sodium ions across cell membranes in motor cortex during generation of nerve impulses.
Therapeutic effect: Prevents and stops seizure activity.

Available forms

phenytoin
Oral suspension: 125 mg/5 ml
Tablets (chewable): 50 mg
phenytoin sodium (prompt)
Capsules: 100 mg (92-mg base)
Injection: 50 mg/ml (46-mg base)
phenytoin sodium (extended)
Capsules: 30 mg (27.6-mg base), 100 mg (92-mg base), 200 mg (184-mg base), 300 mg (276-mg base)

NURSING PROCESS

⚗ Assessment
• Assess patient's condition before therapy and regularly thereafter.
• Monitor blood levels; therapeutic level is 10 to 20 mcg/ml.
• Monitor CBC and calcium level q 6 months, and periodically monitor hepatic function.
• Check vital signs, blood pressure, and ECG during I.V. administration.
• Be alert for adverse reactions and drug interactions.
• Mononucleosis may decrease phenytoin level. Monitor patient for increased seizure activity.
• Evaluate patient's and family's knowledge of drug therapy.

🔃 Nursing diagnoses
• Risk for trauma related to seizures
• Impaired oral mucous membrane related to gingival hyperplasia
• Deficient knowledge related to drug therapy

⊳ Planning and implementation
• Use only clear or slightly yellow solution for injection. Don't refrigerate.
• Divided doses given with or after meals may decrease adverse GI reactions.
• Dilantin capsule is only P.O. form that can be given once daily. If any other brand or form is given once daily, toxic levels may result.
• Don't give drug I.M. unless dosage adjustments are made. Drug may precipitate at site, cause pain, and be erratically absorbed.
• If rash appears, stop drug. If rash is scarlatiniform or morbilliform, drug may be resumed after rash clears. If rash reappears, stop drug. If rash is exfoliative, purpuric, or bullous, don't resume.
• Don't withdraw drug suddenly; seizures may worsen. If adverse reactions develop, notify prescriber immediately.
• If patient has megaloblastic anemia, prescriber may order folic acid and vitamin B_{12}.
ⓈＡＬＥＲＴ: Don't confuse phenytoin with Mephyton or fosphenytoin.
ⓈＡＬＥＲＴ: Don't confuse Dilantin with Dilaudid.
Patient teaching
• Advise patient to avoid hazardous activities until CNS effects of drug are known.
• Advise patient not to change brands or dosage forms.
• Warn patient and parents not to stop drug abruptly.
• Promote oral hygiene and regular dental examinations. Gingivectomy may be necessary periodically if dental hygiene is poor.
• Inform patient that drug may color urine pink, red, or red-brown.
• Tell patient that heavy alcohol use may diminish drug's benefits.

☑ Evaluation
• Patient is free from seizure activity.
• Patient expresses importance of good oral hygiene and regular dental examinations.
• Patient and family state understanding of drug therapy.

Reactions may be *common*, uncommon, *life-threatening*, or COMMON AND LIFE-THREATENING.

physostigmine salicylate (eserine salicylate)

(fiz-oh-STIG-meen sa-LIS-il-ayt)
Antilirium

Pharmacologic class: cholinesterase inhibitor
Therapeutic class: antimuscarinic antidote
Pregnancy risk category: C

Indications and dosages

▶ **To reverse CNS toxicity caused by anti-cholinergic drugs.** *Adults:* 0.5 to 2 mg I.M. or I.V. (1 mg/minute I.V.) repeated q 10 minutes as necessary if life-threatening signs (coma, seizures, arrhythmias) recur.
Children: 0.02 mg/kg I.M. or slow I.V. repeated q 5 to 10 minutes until response is obtained. Maximum dosage, 2 mg. Drug is reserved for life-threatening situations.

▼ I.V. administration

• Use only clear solution. Darkening of solution may indicate loss of potency.
• Give drug I.V. at controlled rate; use direct injection at no more than 1 mg/minute. Rapid administration may cause bradycardia and hypersalivation, leading to respiratory difficulties and seizures.

Contraindications and precautions

• Contraindicated in patients receiving choline esters or depolarizing neuromuscular blockers and in patients with mechanical obstruction of intestine or urogenital tract, asthma, gangrene, diabetes, CV disease, or vagotonia.
• Use cautiously in patients with sensitivity or allergy to sulfites.
※ **Lifespan:** In pregnant women, use cautiously. In breast-feeding women, safety of drug hasn't been established. In children, reserve use for life-threatening situations only.

Adverse reactions

CNS: *seizures,* hallucinations, muscle twitching, muscle weakness, ataxia, *restlessness, excitability, sweating.*
CV: irregular pulse, palpitations, **bradycardia,** hypotension.
EENT: miosis.
GI: nausea, vomiting, epigastric pain, *diarrhea, excessive salivation.*

GU: urinary urgency.
Respiratory: *bronchospasm,* bronchial constriction, dyspnea.

Interactions

Drug-drug. *Anticholinergics, atropine, procainamide, quinidine:* May reverse cholinergic effects. Observe patient for lack of drug effect. *Ganglionic blockers:* May decrease blood pressure. Avoid using together.
Drug-herb. *Jaborandi tree, pill-bearing spurge:* May have additive effects and increase risk of toxicity. Discourage using together.

Effects on lab test results

None reported.

Pharmacokinetics

Absorption: Absorbed well from injection site.
Distribution: Distributed widely and crosses blood-brain barrier.
Metabolism: Cholinesterase hydrolyzes physostigmine relatively quickly.
Excretion: Primary mode of excretion unknown; small amount excreted in urine. *Half-life:* 1 to 2 hours.

Route	Onset	Peak	Duration
I.V.	3-5 min	≤ 5 min	30-60 min
I.M.	3-5 min	20-30 min	30-60 min

Action

Chemical effect: Inhibits destruction of acetylcholine released from parasympathetic and somatic efferent nerves. Acetylcholine accumulates, promoting increased stimulation of receptor.
Therapeutic effect: Reverses anticholinergic signs and symptoms.

Available forms

Injection: 1 mg/ml

NURSING PROCESS

⚡ Assessment

• Assess patient's condition before therapy and regularly thereafter. Effect is often immediate and dramatic, but may be transient and require repeated doses.
• Monitor vital signs frequently, especially respirations.

Rapid onset   *Liquid form contains alcohol.   ◆ Canada   ◇ Australia   †OTC   ‡Off-label use

- Be alert for adverse reactions and drug interactions.
- Evaluate patient's and family's knowledge of drug therapy.

🔲 **Nursing diagnoses**
- Ineffective health maintenance related to underlying condition
- Risk for injury related to drug-induced adverse CNS reactions
- Deficient knowledge related to drug therapy

▶ **Planning and implementation**
- Position patient to ease breathing. If hypersensitivity or cholinergic crisis occurs, have atropine injection readily available and give 0.5 mg S.C. or slow I.V. push. Provide respiratory support p.r.n. Best administered in presence of prescriber.
- If patient becomes restless or hallucinates, raise side rails of bed. Adverse reactions may indicate drug toxicity. Notify prescriber.
- If excessive salivation or emesis, frequent urination, or diarrhea occur, stop drug.
- If excessive sweating or nausea occurs, give lower dose.

Patient teaching
- Tell patient to report adverse reactions, especially pain at the I.V. site.

☑ **Evaluation**
- Patient responds well to therapy.
- Patient doesn't experience injury from adverse CNS reactions.
- Patient and family state understanding of drug therapy.

phytonadione (vitamin K₁)
(figh-toh-neh-DIGH-ohn)
Mephyton

Pharmacologic class: vitamin K
Therapeutic class: blood coagulation modifier
Pregnancy risk category: C

Indications and dosages

▶ **RDA.** *Infants age 6 months and younger:* 5 mcg.
Infants ages 6 months to 1 year: 10 mcg.
Children ages 1 to 3: 15 mcg.
Children ages 4 to 6: 20 mcg.

Children ages 7 to 10: 30 mcg.
Children ages 11 to 14: 45 mcg.
Men ages 15 to 18: 65 mcg.
Men ages 19 to 24: 70 mcg.
Men age 25 and older: 80 mcg.
Women ages 15 to 18: 55 mcg.
Women ages 19 to 24: 60 mcg.
Women age 25 and older, pregnant or breast-feeding women: 65 mcg.
▶ **Hypoprothrombinemia secondary to vitamin K malabsorption, drug therapy, or excessive vitamin A.** *Adults:* Depending on severity, 2 to 25 mg P.O., S.C., or I.M.; repeat and increase up to 50 mg, if necessary.
Children: 5 to 10 mg P.O. or parenterally. I.V. injection rate for infants and children shouldn't exceed 3 mg/m²/minute or total of 5 mg.
Infants: 2 mg P.O. or parenterally.
▶ **Hypoprothrombinemia secondary to effect of oral anticoagulants.** *Adults:* 2.5 to 10 mg P.O., S.C., or I.M. based on PT; repeat if necessary within 12 to 48 hours after P.O. dose or within 6 to 8 hours after parenteral dose. In emergency, 10 to 50 mg slow I.V., maximum rate 1 mg/minute; repeat q 4 hours, p.r.n.
▶ **Prevention of hemorrhagic disease of newborn.** *Neonates:* 0.5 to 1 mg I.M. or S.C. within 1 hour after birth.
▶ **Hemorrhagic disease of newborn.** *Neonates:* 1 mg S.C. or I.M. based on laboratory tests. Higher doses may be necessary if mother has been receiving anticoagulants P.O.
▶ **To differentiate between hepatocellular disease or biliary obstruction as source of hypoprothrombinemia.** *Adults and children:* 10 mg I.M. or S.C.
▶ **Prevention of hypoprothrombinemia related to vitamin K deficiency in long-term parenteral nutrition.** *Adults:* 5 to 10 mg I.M. weekly.
Children: 2 to 5 mg I.M. weekly.
▶ **Prevention of hypoprothrombinemia in infants receiving less than 0.1 mg/L vitamin K in breast milk or milk substitutes.** *Infants:* 1 mg I.M. monthly.

▽ I.V. administration

- Dilute drug with normal saline solution for injection, D₅W, or 5% dextrose in normal saline solution for injection.
- Give I.V. by slow infusion over 2 to 3 hours. Maximum infusion rate 1 mg/minute in adult or 3 mg/m²/minute in child.

• Protect parenteral products from light. Wrap infusion container with aluminum foil.

Contraindications and precautions

• Contraindicated in patients hypersensitive to drug.

⚠ **Lifespan:** In pregnant and breast-feeding women, use cautiously.

Adverse reactions

CNS: dizziness, *seizurelike movements.*
CV: flushing, transient hypotension after I.V. administration, rapid and weak pulse, cardiac irregularities.
Skin: diaphoresis, erythema.
Other: cramplike pain; *anaphylaxis and anaphylactoid reactions* (usually after rapid I.V. administration); pain, swelling, and hematoma at injection site.

Interactions

Drug-drug. *Anticoagulants:* Temporary resistance to prothrombin-depressing anticoagulants may result, especially when larger doses of phytonadione are used. Monitor patient closely.
Cholestyramine resin, mineral oil: Inhibits GI absorption of oral vitamin K. Administer separately.

Effects on lab test results

None reported.

Pharmacokinetics

Absorption: Drug requires presence of bile salts for GI tract absorption after P.O. administration. Unknown after I.M. or S.C. administration.
Distribution: Concentrates in liver for short time.
Metabolism: Metabolized rapidly by liver.
Excretion: Not clearly defined. *Half-life:* Unknown.

Route	Onset	Peak	Duration
P.O.	6-12 hr	Unknown	12-14 hr
I.V., I.M., S.C.	1-2 hr	Unknown	12-14 hr

Action

Chemical effect: An antihemorrhagic factor that promotes hepatic formation of active prothrombin.

Therapeutic effect: Controls abnormal bleeding.

Available forms

Injection (aqueous colloidal solution): 2 mg/ml, 10 mg/ml
Injection (aqueous dispersion): 2 mg/ml, 10 mg/ml
Tablets: 5 mg

NURSING PROCESS

⚕ Assessment
• Assess patient's condition before therapy and regularly thereafter.
• Monitor PT to determine dosage effectiveness
• Failure to respond to vitamin K may indicate coagulation defects.
• Be alert for adverse reactions and drug interactions.
• If adverse GI reactions occur, monitor patient's hydration.
• Evaluate patient's and family's knowledge of drug therapy.

🔲 Nursing diagnoses
• Ineffective protection related to underlying vitamin K deficiency
• Risk for deficient fluid volume related to adverse GI reactions
• Deficient knowledge related to drug therapy

▷ Planning and implementation
• Check brand name labels for administration route restrictions.
• Anticipate order for weekly addition of 5 to 10 mg of phytonadione to total parenteral nutrition solutions.
• S.C. is the preferred route of administration.
• Give drug I.M. in upper outer quadrant of buttocks in adult or older child; inject in anterolateral aspect of thigh or deltoid region in infant.
• If severe bleeding occurs, don't delay other treatment, such as fresh frozen plasma or whole blood.
Patient teaching
• Explain drug's purpose.
• Instruct patient to report adverse reactions.

✓ Evaluation
• Patient achieves normal PT levels with drug therapy.

- Patient maintains adequate hydration throughout drug therapy.
- Patient and family state understanding of drug therapy.

pimecrolimus
(py-meck-roh-LY-muhs)
Elidel

Pharmacologic class: topical immunomodulator
Therapeutic class: topical skin product
Pregnancy risk category: C

Indications and dosages

▶ **Short-term and intermittent long-term therapy for mild to moderate atopic dermatitis in non-immunocompromised patients, in whom the use of alternative, conventional therapies is deemed inadvisable or for patients who aren't adequately responding to or are intolerant of conventional therapies.**
Adults and children age 2 and older: Apply a thin layer to the affected skin twice daily and rub in gently and completely.

Contraindications and precautions

- Contraindicated in patients hypersensitive to drug or the components of the cream.
- Don't use on areas of active cutaneous viral infections or infected atopic dermatitis.
- Not recommended for use in patients with Netherton's syndrome or in immunocompromised patients.
- Use cautiously in patients with varicella zoster virus infection, herpes simplex virus infection, or eczema herpeticum.
- ⚠ Lifespan: In pregnant women, safety of drug hasn't been established. In breast-feeding women, a decision should be made to stop nursing or drug. In children younger than age 2, drug isn't recommended. In patients age 65 and older, safety of drug hasn't been established.

Adverse reactions

CNS: *headache.*
EENT: *nasopharyngitis,* otitis media, sinusitis, pharyngitis, eye infection, nasal congestion, rhinorrhea, sinus congestion, rhinitis, epistaxis, conjunctivitis, earache.

GI: gastroenteritis, abdominal pain, sore throat, tonsillitis, vomiting, diarrhea, nausea, toothache, constipation, loose stools.
GU: dysmenorrhea.
Musculoskeletal: back pain, arthralgias.
Respiratory: *upper respiratory tract infections,* pneumonia, *bronchitis, cough, asthma,* wheezing, dyspnea.
Skin: skin infections, impetigo, folliculitis, molluscum contagiosum, varicella, skin papilloma, urticaria, acne.
Other: herpes simplex, *application site reaction* (burning, irritation, erythema, pruritus), *influenza, pyrexia,* influenzalike illness, hypersensitivity reaction, bacterial infection, staphylococcal infection, viral infection.

Interactions

Drug-drug. *CYP 3A family of inhibitors (erythromycin, itraconazole, ketoconazole, fluconazole, calcium channel blockers):* May have an effect on metabolism of pimecrolimus. Use together cautiously.
Drug-lifestyle. *Natural or artificial sunlight:* Pimecrolimus may shorten the time to skin tumor formation. Avoid or minimize exposure to sunlight.

Effects on lab test results

None reported.

Pharmacokinetics

Absorption: Low systemic absorption.
Distribution: 74% to 87% bound to proteins.
Metabolism: No evidence of skin mediated drug metabolism exists.
Excretion: Following the administration of a single oral radiolabeled dose of pimecrolimus, about 81% of the administered radioactivity was recovered, primarily in the feces (78.4%) as metabolites. Less than 1% of the radioactivity found in the feces was because of unchanged drug. *Half-life:* Unknown.

Route	Onset	Peak	Duration
Topical	Unknown	Unknown	Unknown

Action

Chemical effect: Unknown. May inhibit T cell activation by blocking the transcription of early cytokines. May also prevent the release of inflammatory cytokines and mediators from mast

---

cells in vitro after stimulation by antigen/immunoglobulin E.

Therapeutic effect: Improves skin integrity.

Available forms

Cream: 1% in tubes of 15 grams, 30 grams, and 100 grams. Base contains the following alcohols: benzyl alcohol, cetyl alcohol, oleyl alcohol, and stearyl alcohol.

NURSING PROCESS

Assessment

• Assess underlying skin condition before therapy and reassess regularly throughout therapy. Infections at treatment sites should be cleared before use.

• Evaluate patient's and family's knowledge of drug therapy.

Nursing diagnoses

• Risk for situational low self-esteem related to skin disorder

• Impaired skin integrity related to underlying skin condition

• Deficient knowledge related to pimecrolimus therapy

▶ Planning and implementation

• May be used on all skin surfaces, including the head, neck, and intertriginous areas.

• If disease resolves, stop drug.

• If symptoms persist beyond 6 weeks, reevaluate patient.

⊛ **ALERT:** Don't use with occlusive dressing; this may promote systemic exposure.

• May cause local symptoms such as skin burning. Most local reactions start within 1 to 5 days, are mild to moderately severe, and last no more than 5 days.

• Monitor patient for lymphadenopathy. In the absence of a clear etiology for the lymphadenopathy, or in the presence of acute infectious mononucleosis, consider stopping drug.

• Papillomas or warts may occur with use. If skin papillomas worsen or don't respond to conventional treatment, consider stopping drug.

Patient teaching

• Instruct patient to use as directed; this medication is for external use on the skin only. Tell patient to report any signs or symptoms of adverse reactions.

• Tell patient not to use medication with an occlusive dressing.

• Instruct patient to wash hands after application if hands aren't being treated.

• Tell patient to stop drug after signs and symptoms of atopic dermatitis have resolved. Tell patient to contact prescriber if symptoms persist beyond 6 weeks.

• Advise patient to resume therapy at the first signs or symptoms of recurrence.

• Instruct patient to minimize or avoid exposure to natural or artificial sunlight (including tanning beds and ultraviolet A/B treatment) while using this medication.

• Tell patient that application site reactions are expected, but to notify prescriber if reaction is severe or persists for more than 1 week.

✓ Evaluation

• Patient has improved self-esteem as skin condition clears.

• Patient has improved skin condition.

• Patient and family state understanding of drug therapy.

pimozide
(PIH-mih-zighd)
Orap

Pharmacologic class: diphenylbutylpiperidine
Therapeutic class: antipsychotic
Pregnancy risk category: C

Indications and dosages

▶ **Suppression of motor and phonic tics in patients with Tourette syndrome refractory to first-line therapy.** *Adults and children older than age 12:* Initially, 1 to 2 mg P.O. daily in divided doses. Increase q other day, p.r.n. Maximum dosage is 20 mg daily.

Contraindications and precautions

• Contraindicated in patients hypersensitive to drug, patients with simple tics or tics other than those caused by Tourette syndrome, patients receiving concurrent therapy with drugs known to cause motor and phonic tics, and patients with congenital long–QT interval syndrome, history of arrhythmias, severe toxic CNS depression, or coma.

- Use cautiously in patients with hepatic or renal dysfunction, glaucoma, prostatic hyperplasia, seizure disorder, or EEG abnormalities.
- **Lifespan:** In breast-feeding women, safety of drug hasn't been established.

Adverse reactions

CNS: *parkinsonian-like symptoms,* other extrapyramidal symptoms (dystonia, akathisia, hyperreflexia, opisthotonos, oculogyric crisis), *tardive dyskinesia, sedation,* **neuroleptic malignant syndrome.**
CV: *ECG changes (prolonged QT interval),* hypotension.
EENT: visual disturbances.
GI: dry mouth, constipation.
GU: impotence.
Musculoskeletal: muscle rigidity.

Interactions

Drug-drug. *Antiarrhythmics, phenothiazines, tricyclic antidepressants:* Increases risk of ECG abnormalities. Monitor patient closely.
CNS depressants: Increases CNS depression. Avoid using together.
Drug-lifestyle. *Alcohol use:* Increases CNS depression. Discourage using together.

Effects on lab test results

None reported.

Pharmacokinetics

Absorption: Slow and incomplete.
Distribution: Distributed widely into body.
Metabolism: Metabolized by liver; significant first-pass effect.
Excretion: About 40% of drug is excreted in urine as parent drug and metabolites; about 15% is excreted in feces. *Half-life:* About 29 hours.

Route	Onset	Peak	Duration
P.O.	Unknown	4-12 hr	Unknown

Action

Chemical effect: May block dopamine nonselectively at presynaptic and postsynaptic receptors on neurons in CNS.
Therapeutic effect: Stops tics linked to Tourette syndrome.

Available forms

Tablets: 1 mg, 2 mg, 4 mg ♦, 10 mg ♦

NURSING PROCESS

Assessment
- Assess patient's tics before therapy and regularly thereafter.
- Perform ECG before therapy and periodically thereafter. Check for prolonged QT interval.
- Monitor patient for tardive dyskinesia, which may occur after prolonged use. It may not appear until months or years later and may disappear spontaneously or persist for life despite stopping drug.
- Monitor patient who also is taking anticonvulsants for increased seizure activity. Pimozide may lower seizure threshold.
- Be alert for adverse reactions and drug interactions.
- Evaluate patient's and family's knowledge of drug therapy.

Nursing diagnoses
- Disturbed body image related to presence of tics
- Impaired physical mobility related to adverse reactions
- Deficient knowledge related to drug therapy

Planning and implementation
- Acute dystonic reactions may be treated with diphenhydramine.
- **ALERT:** Avoid giving other drugs that prolong QT interval, such as antiarrhythmics.

Patient teaching
- Warn patient not to stop taking drug abruptly and not to exceed prescribed dosage.
- Tell patient to avoid alcohol during drug therapy.
- Tell patient to use sugarless hard candy, gum, and liquids to relieve dry mouth.

Evaluation
- Patient states positive feelings about self with absence of tics.
- Patient is able to perform activities of daily living.
- Patient and family state understanding of drug therapy.

---

pindolol
(PIN-duh-lol)
Novo-Pindol ♦ , Visken

Pharmacologic class: beta blocker
Therapeutic class: antihypertensive
Pregnancy risk category: B

Indications and dosages

▶ **Hypertension.** *Adults:* Initially, 5 mg P.O.
b.i.d. Increase as needed and tolerated to maximum of 60 mg daily.
▶ **Angina‡.** *Adults:* 15 to 40 mg P.O. daily in four divided doses.

Contraindications and precautions

• Contraindicated in patients hypersensitive to drug and in those with bronchial asthma, severe bradycardia, heart block greater than first degree, cardiogenic shock, or cardiac failure. Contraindicated for use with thioridazine.
• Use cautiously in patients with heart failure, nonallergic bronchospastic disease, diabetes, hyperthyroidism, or impaired renal or hepatic function.
⚖ **Lifespan:** In pregnant women, use cautiously. In breast-feeding women, drug isn't recommended. In children, safety of drug hasn't been established.

Adverse reactions

CNS: insomnia, fatigue, dizziness, nervousness, vivid dreams, hallucinations, lethargy.
CV: *edema, bradycardia, heart failure,* peripheral vascular disease, hypotension.
EENT: visual disturbances.
GI: *nausea,* vomiting, diarrhea.
Metabolic: *hypoglycemia without tachycardia.*
Musculoskeletal: *muscle pain, joint pain.*
Respiratory: increased airway resistance.
Skin: rash.

Interactions

Drug-drug. *Aminophylline, theophylline:* May act antagonistically, reducing the effects of one or both drugs. The elimination of theophylline may also be reduced. Monitor theophylline level and patient closely.
Digoxin, diltiazem: May cause excessive bradycardia and additive depression of AV node. Use together cautiously.

Epinephrine: May cause an initial hypertensive episode followed by bradycardia. Stop the beta blocker 3 days before anticipated epinephrine use. Monitor patient closely.
Indomethacin: Decreases antihypertensive effect. Monitor blood pressure and adjust dosage, as directed.
Insulin: May mask symptoms of hypoglycemia as a result of beta blockade (such as tachycardia). Use cautiously in patients with diabetes.
I.V. lidocaine: May reduce hepatic metabolism of lidocaine, increasing the risk of toxicity. Give bolus doses of lidocaine at a slower rate and monitor lidocaine levels closely.
Prazosin: May increase the risk of orthostatic hypotension in the early phases of use together. Assist patient to stand slowly until effects are known.
Thioridazine: May prolong QT interval and increase the risk of potentially fatal cardiac arrhythmias. Pindolol level may increase. Avoid using together.
Verapamil: May increase the effects of both drugs. Monitor cardiac function closely and decrease dosages as necessary.

Effects on lab test results

• May increase transaminase, alkaline phosphatase, LDH, and uric acid levels. May decrease glucose level.

Pharmacokinetics

Absorption: Rapid. Food doesn't reduce bioavailability but may increase rate of GI absorption.
Distribution: Distributed widely throughout body and is 40% to 60% protein-bound.
Metabolism: About 60% to 65% of drug is metabolized in liver.
Excretion: 35% to 50% of dose excreted unchanged in urine. *Half-life:* About 3 to 4 hours.

Route	Onset	Peak	Duration
P.O.	Unknown	1-2 hr	24 hr

Action

Chemical effect: Unknown; may include reduced cardiac output, decreased sympathetic outflow to peripheral vasculature, and inhibition of renin release by kidneys.
Therapeutic effect: Lowers blood pressure.

Available forms

Tablets: 5 mg, 10 mg, 15 mg ◆

NURSING PROCESS

🗚 Assessment

• Assess patient's blood pressure before therapy and regularly thereafter.
• Always check patient's apical pulse rate before giving drug.
• Be alert for adverse reactions and drug interactions.
• Evaluate patient's and family's knowledge of drug therapy.

🆔 Nursing diagnoses

• Risk for injury related to presence of hypertension
• Fatigue related to drug's adverse effect
• Deficient knowledge related to drug therapy

⯮ Planning and implementation

• If you detect extreme pulse rates, withhold medication and call prescriber immediately.
• If severe hypotension occurs, notify prescriber.
• Stopping drug abruptly can worsen angina and precipitate MI. Withdraw over 1 to 2 weeks after long-term administration.
⊛ **ALERT:** Don't confuse pindolol with Parlodel, perindopril, Panadol, or Plendil.
Patient teaching
• Teach patient how to take his pulse, and tell him to do so before taking each dose. Tell him to notify prescriber before taking any more doses if his pulse rate varies significantly from its usual level.
• Tell patient not to stop drug suddenly even if he has unpleasant adverse reactions; urge him to discuss them with prescriber. Explain that stopping drug abruptly can worsen angina and increase the risk of MI.
• Instruct patient to check with prescriber before taking OTC medications.
• Teach patient and family caregiver how to take blood pressure measurements. Tell them to notify prescriber of any significant change.
• Advise patient to monitor glucose levels closely. Drug may mask signs of hypoglycemia.

☑ Evaluation

• Patient's blood pressure is normal.

• Patient states energy-conserving measures to combat fatigue.
• Patient and family state understanding of drug therapy.

pioglitazone hydrochloride
(pigh-oh-GLIH-tah-zohn high-droh-KLOR-ighd)
Actos

Pharmacologic class: thiazolidinedione
Therapeutic class: antidiabetic
Pregnancy risk category: C

Indications and dosages

▶ **Monotherapy adjunct to diet and exercise to improve glycemic control in patients with type 2 diabetes mellitus, or combination therapy with a sulfonylurea, metformin, or insulin when diet and exercise plus the single drug doesn't yield adequate glycemic control.** *Adults:* Initially, 15 or 30 mg P.O. once daily. For patients who respond inadequately to initial dose, it may be increased in increments; maximum daily dose is 45 mg. If used in combination therapy, daily dosage shouldn't exceed 30 mg.

Contraindications and precautions

• Contraindicated in patients hypersensitive to drug or its components. Not recommended for New York Heart Association Class III and IV cardiac status patients.
• Also contraindicated in patients with type 1 diabetes mellitus or diabetic ketoacidosis, patients with evidence of active liver disease, patients with ALT levels more than two and one-half times the upper limit of normal, and patients who experience jaundice while taking troglitazone.
⚖ **Lifespan:** In pregnant women, drug should be used only if benefit justifies risk to fetus. Insulin is the preferred antidiabetic for use during pregnancy.

Adverse reactions

CNS: headache.
CV: *edema, **heart failure.***
EENT: sinusitis, pharyngitis.
Hematologic: anemia.

Metabolic: *hypoglycemia with combination therapy, aggravated diabetes mellitus,* weight gain.
Musculoskeletal: myalgia.
Respiratory: upper respiratory tract infection.
Other: tooth disorder.

Interactions

Drug-drug. *Ketoconazole:* May inhibit pioglitazone metabolism. Monitor patient's glucose levels more frequently.
Hormonal contraceptives: May reduce levels of hormonal contraceptives, resulting in less effective contraception. Advise patients taking pioglitazone and hormonal contraceptives to consider additional birth control measures.
Drug-herb. *Aloe, bitter melon, bilberry leaf, burdock, dandelion, fenugreek, garlic, ginseng:* May improve blood glucose control and allow reduction of antidiabetic dosage. Advise patient to discuss herbal remedies with prescriber before using them.

Effects on lab test results

• May increase liver function test results and high-density lipoprotein levels. May decrease glucose and triglyceride levels.
• May decrease hemoglobin and hematocrit.

Pharmacokinetics

Absorption: When taken on an empty stomach, rapidly absorbed and measurable in serum within 30 minutes; level peaks within 2 hours. Food slightly delays time to peak levels (to 3 to 4 hours), but doesn't affect the overall extent of absorption.
Distribution: Drug and its metabolites are extensively protein-bound (more than 98%), primarily to albumin.
Metabolism: Extensively metabolized by the liver. Three metabolites, M-II, M-III, and M-IV, are pharmacologically active.
Excretion: About 15% to 30% of dose is recovered in urine, primarily as metabolites and their conjugates. Most of P.O. dose is excreted in bile and eliminated in feces. *Half-life:* 3 to 7 hours.

Route	Onset	Peak	Duration
P.O.	Unknown	Within 2 hr	Unknown

Action

Chemical effect: Decreases insulin resistance in the periphery and in the liver, resulting in decreased glucose output by the liver.
Therapeutic effect: Lowers glucose level.

Available forms

Tablets: 15 mg, 30 mg, 45 mg

NURSING PROCESS

⚕ Assessment

• Obtain history of patient's underlying condition before therapy, and reassess regularly thereafter.
• Assess patient for excessive fluid volume. Monitor patient with heart failure for increased edema.
• Measure liver enzymes at start of therapy, q 2 months for the first year of therapy, and periodically thereafter. Obtain liver function test results in patients who develop evidence of liver dysfunction, such as nausea, vomiting, abdominal pain, fatigue, anorexia, or dark urine.
• Monitor hemoglobin and hematocrit, especially during the first 4 to 12 weeks of therapy.
• Monitor glucose level regularly, especially during situations of increased stress, such as infection, fever, surgery, and trauma.
• Check glycosylated hemoglobin periodically to evaluate therapeutic response to drug.
• Evaluate patient's and family's knowledge of drug therapy.

⚕ Nursing diagnoses

• Ineffective health maintenance related to hyperglycemia
• Risk for injury related to drug-induced hyperglycemia
• Deficient knowledge related to drug therapy

⚕ Planning and implementation

• If patient develops jaundice or if results of liver function tests show ALT elevations greater than three times the upper limit of normal, notify prescriber and stop drug.
• Drug alone or with insulin can cause fluid retention that may lead to or exacerbate heart failure. Observe patients for these signs or symptoms of heart failure. If cardiac status deteriorates, stop drug.
• Management of type 2 diabetes should include diet control. Because calorie restrictions,

weight loss, and exercise help improve insulin sensitivity and help make drug therapy more effective, these measures are essential for proper diabetes management.

• Watch for hypoglycemia in patients receiving pioglitazone with insulin or a sulfonylurea. Dosage adjustments of these drugs may be needed.

• Because ovulation may resume in premenopausal, anovulatory women with insulin resistance, contraceptive measures may need to be considered.

Patient teaching
• Instruct patient to adhere to dietary instructions and to have glucose level and glycosylated hemoglobin tested regularly.

• Inform patient taking pioglitazone with insulin or an oral antidiabetic about the signs and symptoms of hypoglycemia.

• Tell patient to notify prescriber about periods of stress, such as fever, trauma, infection, or surgery, because medication requirements may change.

• Inform patient that blood tests for liver function will be performed before the start of therapy, q 2 months for the first year, and periodically thereafter.

• Tell patient to report unexplained nausea, vomiting, abdominal pain, fatigue, anorexia, or dark urine immediately because these signs and symptoms may indicate liver problems.

• Advise patient to contact prescriber if he has signs or symptoms of heart failure (unusually rapid increase in weight or edema, shortness of breath).

• Inform patient that pioglitazone can be taken with or without meals.

• If patient misses a dose, warn against doubling the dose the following day.

• Advise premenopausal, anovulatory woman with insulin resistance that drug may restore ovulation; recommend that she consider contraception as needed.

☑ Evaluation
• Patient's glucose level is normal with drug therapy.
• Patient doesn't experience hypoglycemia.
• Patient and family state understanding of drug therapy.

piperacillin sodium and tazobactam sodium
(pigh-PER-uh-sil-in SOH-dee-um and taz-oh-BAK-tem SOH-dee-um)
Zosyn

Pharmacologic class: extended-spectrum penicillin, beta-lactamase inhibitor
Therapeutic class: antibiotic
Pregnancy risk category: B

Indications and dosages

▶ **Moderate to severe infections caused by piperacillin-resistant, piperacillin and tazobactam-susceptible, beta-lactamase-producing strains of microorganisms in the following conditions: appendicitis (complicated by rupture or abscess) and peritonitis caused by** *Escherichia coli, Bacteroides fragilis, B. ovatus, B. thetaiotaomicron, B. vulgatus;* **skin and skin-structure infections caused by** *Staphylococcus aureus;* **postpartum endometritis or pelvic inflammatory disease caused by** *E. coli;* **moderately severe community-acquired pneumonia caused by** *Haemophilus influenzae. Adults:* 3.375 g (3 g piperacillin/0.375 g tazobactam) q 6 hours as a 30-minute I.V. infusion for 7 to 10 days.
❑ **Adjust-a-dose:** For patients with renal impairment, if creatinine clearance is 20 to 40 ml/minute, give 2.25 g (2 g piperacillin/0.25 g tazobactam) q 6 hours; if clearance is less than 20 ml/minute, give same dose q 8 hours. In continuous ambulatory peritoneal dialysis (CAPD) patients, give same dose q 12 hours. In hemodialysis patients, give same dose q 12 hours with a supplemental dose of 0.75 g (0.67 g piperacillin/0.08 g tazobactam) after each dialysis period.
▶ **Moderate to severe nosocomial pneumonia caused by piperacillin-resistant, beta-lactamase-producing strains** *S. aureus* **and by piperacillin/tazobactam-susceptible** *Acinetobacter baumannii, H. influenzae, Klebsiella pneumoniae,* **and** *Pseudomonas aeruginosa. Adults:* 4.5 g (4 g piperacillin/0.5 g tazobactam) q 6 hours given with an aminoglycoside for 7 to 14 days. Patients with *P. aeruginosa* should continue aminoglycoside therapy; if *P. aeruginosa* isn't isolated, aminoglycoside therapy may be stopped.

⬛ **Adjust-a-dose:** For patients with renal impairment, if creatinine clearance is 20 to 40 ml/minute, give 3.375 g (3 g piperacillin and 0.375 g tazobactam) q 6 hours; if clearance is less than 20 ml/minute, give 2.25 g (2 g piperacillin and 0.25 g tazobactam) q 6 hours. In CAPD patients, give 2.25 g (2 g piperacillin and 0.25 g tazobactam) q 8 hours.

▼ I.V. administration

• Reconstitute each gram of piperacillin with 5 ml of diluent, such as sterile or bacteriostatic water for injection, normal saline solution for injection, bacteriostatic normal saline solution for injection, D_5W, 5% dextrose in normal saline solution for injection, or dextran 6% in normal saline solution for injection. Don't use lactated Ringer's injection. Shake until dissolved. Further dilute to final volume of 50 ml before infusion.

• Don't mix with other drugs.

⚠ **ALERT:** Infuse drug over at least 30 minutes. Stop other primary infusions during administration if possible. Aminoglycoside antibiotics (such as gentamicin and tobramycin) are chemically incompatible with drug. Don't mix in same I.V. container.

• Use drug immediately after reconstitution. Discard unused drug in single-dose vials after 24 hours if held at room temperature; after 48 hours if refrigerated. Diluted drug is stable in I.V. bags for 24 hours at room temperature or 1 week if refrigerated.

• Change I.V. site every 48 hours.

Contraindications and precautions

• Contraindicated in patients hypersensitive to drug or other penicillins.

• Use cautiously in patients with other drug allergies, especially to cephalosporins (possible cross-sensitivity), and in those with bleeding tendencies, uremia, or hypokalemia.

⚠ **Lifespan:** In pregnant and breast-feeding women, use cautiously. In children younger than age 12, safety of drug hasn't been established.

Adverse reactions

CNS: pain, *headache, insomnia,* agitation, fever, dizziness, anxiety.
CV: hypertension, tachycardia, chest pain, edema.
EENT: rhinitis.

GI: *diarrhea, nausea, constipation,* vomiting, dyspepsia, stool changes, abdominal pain.
Hematologic: *thrombocytopenia.*
Respiratory: dyspnea.
Skin: rash (including maculopapular, bullous, urticarial, and eczematoid), pruritus.
Other: *anaphylaxis,* candidiasis, inflammation and phlebitis at I.V. site.

Interactions

Drug-drug. *Anticoagulants:* Increases risk of bleeding. Monitor PT, PTT, and INR, and monitor patient for bleeding.
Hormonal contraceptives: Potential for decreased effectiveness of hormonal contraceptives. Advise alternative barrier method while on drug therapy.
Probenecid: Increases blood levels of piperacillin. Probenecid may be used for this purpose.
Vecuronium: Prolongs neuromuscular blockage. Monitor patient closely.

Effects on lab test results

• May increase eosinophil count. May decrease hemoglobin, hematocrit, and WBC and platelet counts.

Pharmacokinetics

Absorption: Administered I.V.
Distribution: Both drugs are about 30% protein-bound.
Metabolism: Piperacillin is metabolized to a minor, microbiologically active desethyl metabolite. Tazobactam is metabolized to a single metabolite that lacks pharmacologic and antibacterial activities.
Excretion: Excreted in urine and bile. *Half-life:* piperacillin, 40 minutes; tazobactam, 70 minutes.

Route	Onset	Peak	Duration
I.V.	Immediate	Immediate	Unknown

Action

Chemical effect: Piperacillin inhibits cell wall synthesis during microorganism multiplication; tazobactam increases piperacillin effectiveness by inactivating beta-lactamases, which destroy penicillins.
Therapeutic effect: Kills susceptible bacteria.

Available forms

Powder for injection: 2 g piperacillin and 0.25 g tazobactam per vial, 3 g piperacillin and 0.375 g tazobactam per vial, 4 g piperacillin and 0.5 g tazobactam per vial

NURSING PROCESS

⚕ Assessment

• Before giving drug, ask patient about previous allergic reactions to this drug or other penicillins. However, negative history of penicillin allergy doesn't guarantee future safety.
• Assess patient's infection before therapy and regularly thereafter.
• Obtain specimen for culture and sensitivity tests before first dose. Therapy may begin pending results.
• Be alert for adverse reactions and drug interactions.
• If adverse GI reactions occur, monitor patient's hydration.
• Evaluate patient's and family's knowledge of drug therapy.

⊕ Nursing diagnoses

• Infection related to presence of bacteria
• Risk of deficient fluid volume related to adverse GI reactions
• Deficient knowledge related to drug therapy

⊠ Planning and implementation

• Because hemodialysis removes 6% of piperacillin dose and 21% of tazobactam dose, supplemental doses may be needed after hemodialysis.
Patient teaching
• Tell patient to report pain or discomfort at I.V. site.
• Advise patient to limit salt intake while taking drug because piperacillin contains 1.98 mEq of sodium per gram.
• Tell patient to report adverse reactions.

☑ Evaluation

• Patient is free from infection.
• Patient maintains adequate hydration.
• Patient and family state understanding of drug therapy.

pirbuterol acetate

(pir-BYOO-teh-rol AS-ih-tayt)
Maxair

Pharmacologic class: beta-adrenergic agonist
Therapeutic class: bronchodilator
Pregnancy risk category: C

Indications and dosages

▶ **Prevention and reversal of bronchospasm, asthma.** *Adults and children age 12 and older:* 1 or 2 inhalations (0.2 to 0.4 mg) repeated q 4 to 6 hours. Maximum, 12 inhalations daily.

Contraindications and precautions

• Contraindicated in patients hypersensitive to drug.
• Use cautiously in patients who are unusually responsive to sympathomimetic amines, and in patients with CV disorders, hyperthyroidism, diabetes, or seizure disorders.
⚖ **Lifespan:** In pregnant and breast-feeding women, use cautiously. In children younger than age 12, safety of drug hasn't been established.

Adverse reactions

CNS: tremor, nervousness, dizziness, insomnia, headache.
CV: tachycardia, palpitations, increased blood pressure.
EENT: dry or irritated throat.

Interactions

Drug-drug. *MAO inhibitors, tricyclic antidepressants:* May potentiate action of beta-adrenergic agonist on vascular system. Use together cautiously.
Propranolol, other beta blockers: Decreases bronchodilating effects. Avoid using together.

Effects on lab test results

None reported.

Pharmacokinetics

Absorption: Negligible level after inhalation.
Distribution: Distributed locally.
Metabolism: Metabolized in liver.
Excretion: About 50% of inhaled dose is excreted in urine as parent drug and metabolites. *Half-life:* Unknown.

Reactions may be *common*, uncommon, *life-threatening*, or COMMON AND LIFE-THREATENING.

Route	Onset	Peak	Duration
Inhalation	≤ 5 min	30-60 min	5-8 hr

Action

Chemical effect: Relaxes bronchial smooth muscle by acting on beta$_2$-adrenergic receptors. **Therapeutic effect:** Improves breathing ability. *Half-life:* Unknown.

Available forms

Inhaler: 0.2 mg/metered dose

NURSING PROCESS

Assessment

• Assess patient's condition before therapy.
• Monitor effectiveness by checking respiratory rate, auscultating lung fields frequently, and following laboratory studies (such as arterial blood gases).
• Be alert for adverse reactions and drug interactions.
• Evaluate patient's and family's knowledge of drug therapy.

Nursing diagnoses

• Impaired gas exchange related to presence of bronchospasms
• Disturbed sleep pattern related to drug-induced insomnia
• Deficient knowledge related to drug therapy

Planning and implementation

• Shake canister well before each use.
• Store drug away from heat and direct sunlight.
• If patient also uses a corticosteroid inhaler, always give pirbuterol first, and then wait about 5 minutes before giving the corticosteroid inhaler.
• If patient's condition doesn't improve or worsens, notify prescriber.
Patient teaching
• Give these instructions for using metered-dose inhaler: Clear nasal passages and throat. Breathe out, expelling as much air from lungs as possible. Place mouthpiece well into mouth and inhale deeply as you release a dose from inhaler. Hold breath for several seconds, remove mouthpiece, and exhale slowly.
• If more than one inhalation is ordered, tell patient to wait at least 2 minutes before repeating procedure.

• If patient also uses a corticosteroid inhaler, tell him to use the bronchodilator first and then wait about 5 minutes before using the corticosteroid. This allows the bronchodilator to open air passages for maximum effectiveness.
• Tell patient to notify prescriber if bronchospasm increases after drug use.
• Advise patient to seek medical attention if previously effective dosage no longer controls symptoms; this change may signify worsening of disease.

Evaluation

• Patient has improved gas exchange, as demonstrated by improved lung sounds and arterial blood gas measurements.
• Patient doesn't have insomnia.
• Patient and family state understanding of drug therapy.

piroxicam
(peer-OK-sih-cam)
Apo-Piroxicam ♦ , Feldene, Novo-Pirocam ♦

Pharmacologic class: NSAID
Therapeutic class: nonopioid analgesic, antipyretic, anti-inflammatory
Pregnancy risk category: C

Indications and dosages

▶ **Osteoarthritis, rheumatoid arthritis.**
Adults: 20 mg P.O. daily. If desired, dosage may be divided b.i.d.
▶ **Juvenile rheumatoid arthritis‡.** *Children weighing 15 to 30 kg (33 to 67 lb):* 5 mg P.O. daily.
Children weighing 31 to 45 kg (68 to100 lb): 10 mg P.O. daily.
Children weighing 46 to 55 kg (101 to 121 lb): 15 mg P.O. daily.

Contraindications and precautions

• Contraindicated in patients hypersensitive to drug and in patients with bronchospasm or angioedema caused by aspirin or NSAIDs.
• Use cautiously in patients with GI disorders, history of renal or peptic ulcer disease, cardiac disease, hypertension, or conditions predisposing to fluid retention.

⚖ **Lifespan:** In pregnant and breast-feeding women, drug is contraindicated. In children, long-term use of drug hasn't been established. In elderly patients, use cautiously.

Adverse reactions

CNS: headache, drowsiness, dizziness, paresthesia, somnolence.
CV: peripheral edema.
EENT: auditory disturbances.
GI: *epigastric distress, nausea, occult blood loss,* peptic ulceration, *severe GI bleeding.*
GU: *nephrotoxicity.*
Hematologic: anemia, *leukopenia, aplastic anemia, agranulocytosis, thrombocytopenia.*
Metabolism: *hyperkalemia, acidosis,* dilutional hypernatremia.
Respiratory: *bronchospasm.*
Skin: pruritus, rash, urticaria, *photosensitivity reaction.*

Interactions

Drug-drug. *Aspirin, corticosteroids:* Increases risk of GI toxicity. Decreases piroxicam levels. Monitor patient closely.
Lithium: Increased lithium levels. Monitor patient for toxicity.
Oral anticoagulants: Increases risk of bleeding. Monitor patient closely for bleeding.
Oral antidiabetics: Increases antidiabetic effects. Monitor patient and glucose levels closely.
Probenecid, ritonavir: Increases toxicity of piroxicam. Don't use together.
Drug-herb. *Dong quai, feverfew, garlic, ginger, horse chestnut, red clover:* May increase risk of bleeding. Monitor patient closely.
St. John's wort: May increase risk of photosensitivity. Advise patient to avoid unprotected or prolonged exposure to sunlight.
Drug-lifestyle. *Alcohol use:* Increases risk of GI toxicity. Decreases drug levels. Discourage using together.
Sun exposure: Increases risk of photosensitivity reaction. Advise patient to avoid unprotected or prolonged exposure to sunlight.

Effects on lab test results

• May increase BUN, creatinine, liver enzyme, sodium, and potassium levels. May decrease glucose level.

• May decrease hemoglobin, hematocrit, and WBC, granulocyte, platelet, and eosinophil counts. May prolong bleeding time.

Pharmacokinetics

Absorption: Rapid. Food delays absorption.
Distribution: Drug is highly protein-bound.
Metabolism: Metabolized in liver.
Excretion: Excreted in urine. *Half-life:* About 50 hours.

Route	Onset	Peak	Duration
P.O.	15-30 min	3-5 hr	24 hr

Action

Chemical effect: Unknown; produces antiinflammatory, analgesic, and antipyretic effects, possibly by inhibiting prostaglandin synthesis.
Therapeutic effect: Relieves pain, fever, and inflammation.

Available forms

Capsules: 10 mg, 20 mg

NURSING PROCESS

🔲 **Assessment**

• Assess patient's condition before therapy and regularly thereafter. Effects don't occur for at least 2 weeks after therapy begins. Evaluate response to drug by assessing for reduced symptoms.
• Check CBC and renal, hepatic, and auditory function periodically during prolonged therapy.
• Be alert for adverse reactions and drug interactions.
• Evaluate patient's and family's knowledge of drug therapy.

⊞ **Nursing diagnoses**

• Chronic pain related to arthritis
• Impaired tissue integrity related to adverse effect on GI mucosa
• Deficient knowledge related to drug therapy

▷ **Planning and implementation**

• If adverse GI reactions occur, give drug with milk, antacids, or food.
• If laboratory abnormalities occur, stop drug and notify prescriber.

Reactions may be *common,* uncommon, *life-threatening,* or COMMON AND LIFE-THREATENING.

Patient teaching
• Tell patient that full effects may be delayed for 2 to 4 weeks.
• Teach patient to recognize and report signs and symptoms of GI bleeding.
• Advise patient to use sunblock, wear protective clothing, and avoid prolonged exposure to sunlight.
• Warn patient to not take any NSAIDs during therapy.

☑ **Evaluation**
• Patient is free from pain.
• Patient maintains normal GI tissue integrity.
• Patient and family state understanding of drug therapy.

plasma protein fraction
(PLAZ-muh PROH-teen FRAK-shun)
Plasmanate, Plasma-Plex, Plasmatein, Protenate

Pharmacologic class: blood derivative
Therapeutic class: plasma volume expander
Pregnancy risk category: C

Indications and dosages

▶ **Hypovolemic shock.** *Adults:* Varies with patient's condition and response, but initial dose may be 250 to 500 ml I.V. (12.5 to 25 g protein), usually no faster than 10 ml/minute. *Infants and young children:* 20 to 30 ml/kg (10 to 15 ml/lb) I.V., infused no faster than 10 ml/minute.
▶ **Hypoproteinemia.** *Adults:* 1,000 to 1,500 ml (50 to 75 g of protein) I.V. daily. Maximum infusion rate is 5 to 8 ml/minute.

▽ I.V. administration

• Maximum rate is 10 ml/minute. Infusion rates greater than 10 ml/minute may cause hypotension.
⑤ **ALERT:** Avoid rapid I.V. infusion. Rate is individualized according to patient's age, condition, and diagnosis.
• If hypotension occurs, slow or stop infusion. Vital signs should return to normal gradually.
• Check expiration date before using. Don't use solutions that are cloudy, contain sediment, or have been frozen. Discard container that has been open for more than 4 hours because solution contains no preservatives.

Contraindications and precautions

• Contraindicated in patients with severe anemia or heart failure and in those having undergone cardiac bypass surgery.
• Use cautiously in patients with hepatic or renal impairment, low cardiac reserve, or restricted sodium intake. Rapid infusion may cause severe, persistent hypotension.
⚖ **Lifespan:** In pregnant and breast-feeding women, use cautiously.

Adverse reactions

CNS: headache, fever.
CV: various effects on blood pressure after rapid infusion or intra-arterial administration, *vascular overload* after rapid infusion, flushing.
GI: nausea, vomiting, hypersalivation.
Musculoskeletal: back pain.
Respiratory: dyspnea, *pulmonary edema.*
Skin: erythema, urticaria.
Other: chills.

Interactions

None significant.

Effects on lab test results

None reported.

Pharmacokinetics

Absorption: Administered I.V.
Distribution: Distributed into intravascular space and extravascular sites, including skin, muscle, and lungs.
Metabolism: Unknown.
Excretion: Unknown. *Half-life:* Unknown.

Route	Onset	Peak	Duration
I.V.	Immediate	Immediate	Unknown

Action

Chemical effect: Supplies colloid to blood and expands plasma volume.
Therapeutic effect: Raises protein levels and expands plasma volume.

Available forms

Injection: 5% solution in 50-ml, 250-ml, 500-ml vials

NURSING PROCESS

⚕ Assessment
- Assess patient's condition before therapy and regularly thereafter.
- Monitor vital signs at least hourly.
- Be alert for adverse reactions, such as hypovolemia (dyspnea, pulmonary edema, and increased blood pressure).
- Drug contains 130 to 160 mEq sodium/L. Monitor patients who are on sodium restriction or who have heart failure carefully for signs and symptoms of hypervolemia.
- Evaluate patient's and family's knowledge of drug therapy.

🔢 Nursing diagnoses
- Decreased cardiac output related to underlying condition
- Acute pain related to headache
- Deficient knowledge related to drug therapy

▶ Planning and implementation
- If patient is dehydrated, give additional fluids P.O. or I.V.
- **🔔 ALERT:** Don't administer drug near area of trauma, injury, or infection.
- Administer mild analgesic for drug-induced headache.
- Drug may be given without regard to patient's blood type or group.
- **Patient teaching**
- Tell patient and family the purpose of drug, and keep them informed of drug effectiveness.
- Instruct patient to report adverse reactions.

✅ Evaluation
- Patient regains normal cardiac output.
- Patient is free from pain.
- Patient and family state understanding of drug therapy.

polyethylene glycol and electrolyte solution
(pol-ee-ETH-ih-leen GLIGH-kohl and ee-LEK-troh-light soh-LOO-shun)
CoLyte, GoLYTELY, NuLYTELY, OCL

Pharmacologic class: polyethylene glycol (PEG) 3350 nonabsorbable solution

Therapeutic class: laxative and bowel evacuant
Pregnancy risk category: C

Indications and dosages
▶ **Bowel preparation before GI examination.**
Adults: 240 ml P.O. q 10 minutes until 4 L are consumed. Typically, give 4 hours before examination, allowing 3 hours for drinking and 1 hour for bowel evacuation.
▶ **Management of acute iron overdose‡.**
Children older than age 3: 2,953 ml/kg over 5 days.

Contraindications and precautions
- Contraindicated in patients with GI obstruction or perforation, gastric retention, toxic colitis, or megacolon.
- 🧬 **Lifespan:** In pregnant and breast-feeding women, use cautiously.

Adverse reactions
GI: nausea, bloating, cramps, vomiting.

Interactions
Drug-drug. *Oral drugs:* Decreases absorption if given within 1 hour of starting therapy. Don't give with other oral drugs.

Effects on lab test results
None reported.

Pharmacokinetics
Absorption: Not absorbed.
Distribution: Not applicable because drug isn't absorbed.
Metabolism: Not applicable because drug isn't absorbed.
Excretion: Excreted via GI tract. *Half-life:* None.

Route	Onset	Peak	Duration
P.O.	≤ 1 hr	Varies	Varies

Action
Chemical effect: Acts as an osmotic agent. Sodium sulfate greatly reduces sodium absorption. The electrolyte concentration causes virtually no net absorption or secretion of ions.
Therapeutic effect: Cleanses bowel.

Available forms
Oral solution: PEG 3350 (6 g), sodium sulfate decahydrate (1.29 g), sodium chloride (146 mg),

potassium chloride (75 mg) sodium bicarbonate (168 mg), polysorbate-80 (30 mg) per 100 ml (OCL)

Powder for oral solution: PEG 3350 (240 g), sodium sulfate (22.72 g), sodium chloride (5.84 g), potassium chloride (2.98 g), sodium bicarbonate (6.72 g) per 4 L (CoLyte); PEG 3350 (236 g), sodium sulfate (22.74 g), sodium bicarbonate (6.74 g), sodium chloride (5.86 g), potassium chloride (2.97 g) per 4 L (GoLYTE-LY); PEG 3350 (420 g), sodium bicarbonate (5.72 g), sodium chloride (11.2 g), potassium chloride (1.48 g) per 4 L (NuLYTELY)

NURSING PROCESS

🕮 Assessment
• Assess patient's condition before therapy and regularly thereafter.
• Be alert for adverse reactions and drug interactions.
• Evaluate patient's and family's knowledge of drug therapy.

⊕ Nursing diagnoses
• Health-seeking behavior (testing) related to need to determine cause of underlying GI problem
• Risk for deficient fluid volume related to adverse GI reactions
• Deficient knowledge related to drug therapy

▷ Planning and implementation
• Use tap water to reconstitute powder. Shake vigorously to make sure all powder is dissolved. Refrigerate solution but use within 48 hours.
• **⊛ ALERT:** Don't add flavoring or additional ingredients to solution or administer chilled solution. Hypothermia has developed after ingestion of large amounts of chilled solution.
• If patient is scheduled for midmorning examination, give solution early in morning. Oral solution induces diarrhea in 30 to 60 minutes that rapidly cleans bowel, usually within 4 hours.
• When used as preparation for barium enema, give solution the evening before examination, to avoid interfering with barium coating of colonic mucosa.
• If given to semiconscious patient or to patient with impaired gag reflex, take care to prevent aspiration.

• No major shifts in fluid or electrolyte balance have been reported.

Patient teaching
• Tell patient to fast for 4 hours before taking solution and to ingest only clear fluids until examination is complete.
• Warn patient about adverse GI reactions to drug.

☑ Evaluation
• Patient is able to have examination.
• Patient maintains adequate fluid volume.
• Patient and family state understanding of drug therapy.

polysaccharide iron complex
(pol-ee-SAK-uh-righd IGH-ern KOM-pleks)
Hytinic, Ferrex 150, Niferex, Niferex-150, Nu-Iron, Nu-Iron 150

Pharmacologic class: oral iron supplement
Therapeutic class: hematinic
Pregnancy risk category: NR

Indications and dosages

▶ **Uncomplicated iron deficiency anemia.**
Adults and children age 12 and older: 100 to 300 mg P.O. daily.
Children ages 6 to 12: 50 to 100 mg P.O. daily as tablets or 1 tsp of elixir P.O. daily.
Children younger than age 6: 3 to 6 mg/kg P.O. daily in three divided doses, as directed by prescriber.
Infants: 10 to 25 mg P.O. daily in three divided doses, as directed by prescriber.

Contraindications and precautions

• Contraindicated in patients hypersensitive to drug or its components and in those with hemochromatosis or hemosiderosis.
⚖ Lifespan: In children, iron overdose may be fatal; treat patient immediately. In children younger than age 6, remind parent or caregiver to give only as directed by prescriber.

Adverse reactions

GI: nausea, constipation, black stools, epigastric pain.

Interactions

Drug-drug. *Antacids, cholestyramine resin, cimetidine, tetracycline, vitamin E:* Decreases iron absorption. Separate doses by 2 to 4 hours.
Chloramphenicol: Delays response to iron therapy. Monitor patient.
Fluoroquinolones, levodopa, methyldopa, penicillamine, tetracycline: Decreases GI absorption of these drugs, possibly resulting in decreased level or effectiveness. Give separately.
Levothyroxine sodium: Decreases levothyroxine effectiveness, leading to hypothyroidism. Avoid using together, or separate administration times by 2 to 4 hours.
Vitamin C: May increase iron absorption. Can be used for this effect.
Drug-food. *Cereals, coffee, dairy products, eggs, teas, whole-grain breads:* Decreases iron absorption. Separate use by 2 to 4 hours.

Effects on lab test results

• May increase hemoglobin, hematocrit, and reticulocyte count.

Pharmacokinetics

Absorption: Iron is absorbed from entire length of GI tract, but primary absorption sites are duodenum and proximal jejunum. Up to 10% of iron is absorbed by healthy people; people with iron-deficiency anemia may absorb up to 60%.
Distribution: Iron is transported through GI mucosal cells directly into blood, where it's immediately bound to carrier protein, transferrin, and transported to bone marrow for incorporation into hemoglobin. Iron is highly protein-bound.
Metabolism: Iron is liberated by destruction of hemoglobin, but is conserved and reused by body.
Excretion: Men and postmenopausal women lose about 1 mg/day; premenopausal women, about 1.5 mg/day. Loss usually occurs in nails, hair, feces, and urine; trace amounts lost in bile and sweat. *Half-life:* Unknown.

Route	Onset	Peak	Duration
P.O.	≤ 3 days	5-30 days	2 mo

Action

Chemical effect: Provides elemental iron, an essential component in formation of hemoglobin.

Therapeutic effect: Restores normal iron levels in body.

Available forms

Capsules†: 150 mg
Solution†: 100 mg/5 ml
Tablets†: 50 mg

NURSING PROCESS

Assessment
• Assess patient's condition before therapy and regularly thereafter.
• Be alert for adverse reactions and drug interactions.
• Evaluate patient's and family's knowledge of drug therapy.

Nursing diagnoses
• Fatigue related to anemia
• Deficient knowledge related to drug therapy

Planning and implementation
• Give drug with juice (preferably orange juice) or water but not with milk or antacids.
Patient teaching
• Inform patient that drug may turn stools black.
• Advise patient to avoid foods that may impair absorption, including yogurt, cheese, eggs, milk, whole-grain breads and cereals, tea, and coffee. Tell him to take drug with juice or water.
• Inform parents that as few as three tablets can cause iron poisoning, which may be fatal in children. Warn them to store drug out of reach of children.
• If patient misses a dose, tell him to take it as soon as he remembers but not to double the dose.

Evaluation
• Patient states that fatigue is relieved as hemoglobin and reticulocyte count return to normal.
• Patient and family state understanding of drug therapy.

Reactions may be *common*, uncommon, *life-threatening*, or COMMON AND LIFE-THREATENING.

potassium acetate
(puh-TAS-ee-um AS-ih-tayt)

Pharmacologic class: potassium supplement
Therapeutic class: electrolyte
Pregnancy risk category: C

Indications and dosages

▶ **Hypokalemia.** *Adults:* No more than 20 mEq
I.V. hourly at concentration of 40 mEq/L or less.
Total 24-hour dose shouldn't exceed 150 mEq.
Potassium replacement should be done with
ECG monitoring and frequent potassium tests.
Use I.v. route only for life-threatening hypokalemia or when oral replacement isn't feasible.
▶ **Prevention of hypokalemia.** *Adults:* Dosage
is individualized to patient's needs, not to exceed 150 mEq daily. Give as an additive to I.V
infusions. Usual dosage is 20 mEq/L infused at
no more than 20 mEq/hour.
Children: Individualized dosage not to exceed
3 mEq/kg daily. Give as an additive to I.V infusions.

▼ I.V. administration

• Give drug only by I.V. infusion, never by I.V.
push or I.M. route.
• Give drug slowly as diluted solution; life-
threatening hyperkalemia may result from too-
rapid infusion.
• Watch for pain and redness at infusion site.
Large-bore needle reduces local irritation.

Contraindications and precautions

• Contraindicated in patients with severe renal
impairment with oliguria, anuria, or azotemia;
those with untreated Addison's disease or
adrenocortical insufficiency; and those with
acute dehydration, heat cramps, hyperkalemia,
hyperkalemic form of familial periodic paralysis, and conditions related to extensive tissue
breakdown.
• Use cautiously in patients with cardiac disease
or renal impairment.
⚠ **Lifespan:** In pregnant and breast-feeding
women, use cautiously.

Adverse reactions

CNS: paresthesia of limbs, listlessness, mental
confusion, weakness or heaviness of legs, flaccid paralysis.

CV: *arrhythmias, cardiac arrest, heart block,*
ECG changes.
GI: nausea, vomiting, abdominal pain, diarrhea,
bowel ulceration.
GU: oliguria.
Respiratory: *respiratory paralysis.*
Skin: cold skin, gray pallor.
Other: pain, redness at infusion site.

Interactions

Drug-drug. *ACE inhibitors, potassium-sparing
diuretics:* Increases risk of hyperkalemia. Use
cautiously.
Drug-herb. *Cascara, licorice:* May antagonize
effects of potassium supplements. Discourage
using together.
Drug-food. *Salt substitutes:* Increases risk of
hyperkalemia. Don't use together.

Effects on lab test results

• May increase potassium level.

Pharmacokinetics

Absorption: Administered I.V.
Distribution: Distributed throughout body.
Metabolism: None significant.
Excretion: Excreted largely by kidneys; small
amounts may be excreted via skin and intestinal
tract, but intestinal potassium is usually reabsorbed. *Half-life:* Unknown.

Route	Onset	Peak	Duration
I.V.	Immediate	Immediate	Unknown

Action

Chemical effect: Aids in transmitting nerve impulses, contracting cardiac and skeletal muscle,
and maintaining intracellular tonicity, cellular
metabolism, acid-base balance, and normal renal function.
Therapeutic effect: Replaces and maintains
potassium level.

Available forms

Injection: 2 mEq/ml in 20-ml, 50-ml, 100-ml
vials; 4 mEq/ml in 50-ml vial

NURSING PROCESS

⚖ Assessment
• Assess patient's condition before therapy and
regularly thereafter.

- During therapy, monitor ECG, renal function, fluid intake and output, and potassium, creatinine, and BUN levels.
- Be alert for adverse reactions and drug interactions.
- Evaluate patient's and family's knowledge of drug therapy.

Nursing diagnoses
- Ineffective health maintenance related to presence of hypokalemia
- Risk for injury related to drug-induced hyperkalemia
- Deficient knowledge related to drug therapy

Planning and implementation
- Don't give potassium postoperatively until urine flow is established.

ALERT: Potassium preparations aren't interchangeable. Verify preparation before giving.

Patient teaching
- Inform patient of need for potassium supplementation.
- Tell patient that drug will be given through an I.V. line.
- Instruct patient to report adverse reactions.

Evaluation
- Patient's potassium level returns to normal with drug therapy.
- Patient doesn't develop hyperkalemia as result of drug therapy.
- Patient and family state understanding of drug therapy.

potassium bicarbonate
(puh-TAS-ee-um bigh-KAR-buh-nayt)
K+ Care ET

Pharmacologic class: potassium supplement
Therapeutic class: mineral
Pregnancy risk category: C

Indications and dosages

▶ **Hypokalemia.** *Adults:* 25 to 50 mEq dissolved in 4 to 8 oz (120 to 240 ml) of water and given once daily to b.i.d.

Contraindications and precautions

- Contraindicated in patients with untreated Addison's disease, acute dehydration, heat cramps, hyperkalemia, hyperkalemic form of familial periodic paralysis, other conditions linked to extensive tissue breakdown, and severe renal impairment with oliguria, anuria, or azotemia.
- Use cautiously in patients with cardiac disease or renal impairment.

Lifespan: In pregnant and breast-feeding women, use cautiously. In children, safety of drug hasn't been established.

Adverse reactions

CNS: paresthesia of limbs, listlessness, mental confusion, weakness or heaviness of legs, flaccid paralysis.
CV: *arrhythmias, cardiac arrest, heart block, ECG changes (prolonged PR interval, widened QRS complex, ST-segment depression, and tall, tented T waves).*
GI: *nausea, vomiting, abdominal pain,* diarrhea, ulcerations, *hemorrhage, obstruction, perforation.*

Interactions

Drug-drug. *ACE inhibitors, potassium-sparing diuretics:* Increases risk of hyperkalemia. Use cautiously.
Drug-food. *Salt substitutes:* Increases risk of hyperkalemia. Don't use together.

Effects on lab test results

- May increase potassium level.

Pharmacokinetics

Absorption: Well absorbed from GI tract.
Distribution: Distributed throughout body.
Metabolism: None significant.
Excretion: Excreted largely by kidneys; small amounts may be excreted via skin and intestinal tract, but intestinal potassium is usually reabsorbed. *Half-life:* Unknown.

Route	Onset	Peak	Duration
P.O.	Unknown	≤ 4 hr	Unknown

Action

Chemical effect: Aids in transmitting nerve impulses, contracting cardiac and skeletal muscle, and maintaining intracellular tonicity, cellular metabolism, acid-base balance, and normal renal function.
Therapeutic effect: Replaces and maintains potassium level.

Available forms

Effervescent tablets: 25 mEq

Assessment
• Assess patient's condition before therapy and regularly thereafter.
• During therapy, monitor ECG, renal function, fluid intake and output, and potassium, creatinine, and BUN levels.
• Be alert for adverse reactions and drug interactions.
• Evaluate patient's and family's knowledge of drug therapy.

Nursing diagnoses
• Ineffective health maintenance related to presence of hypokalemia
• Risk for injury related to potassium-induced hyperkalemia
• Deficient knowledge related to drug therapy

Planning and implementation
• Dissolve potassium bicarbonate tablets completely in 6 to 8 ounces of cold water to minimize GI irritation.
• Ask patient's flavor preference. Available in lime, fruit punch, and orange flavors.
• Have patient take with meals and sip slowly over 5 to 10 minutes.
• Don't give potassium supplements postoperatively until urine flow has been established.
ⓢ ALERT: Potassium preparations aren't interchangeable. Verify preparation before giving.
Patient teaching
• Inform patient about need for potassium supplementation.
• Teach patient how to prepare and take drug.
• Instruct patient to report adverse reactions.

Evaluation
• Patient's potassium level returns to normal.
• Patient doesn't develop hyperkalemia as result of drug therapy.
• Patient and family state understanding of drug therapy.

potassium chloride
(puh-TAS-ee-um KLOR-ighd)
Apo-K*, Cena-K, Gen-K, K-8, K-10*, K+10, Kaochlor, Kaochlor S-F*, Kaon-Cl, Kaon-Cl-10, Kaon-Cl 20%*, Kay Ciel*, K+ Care, K-Dur 10, K-Dur 20, K-Lease, K-Lor, Klor-Con, Klor-Con 8, Klor-Con 10, Klor-Con/25, Klorvess, Klotrix, K·Lyte/Cl, K-Norm, K-Tab, K-vescent Potassium Chloride, Micro-K Extencaps, Micro-K 10 Extencaps, Micro-K LS, Potasalan, Slow-K, Ten-K

Pharmacologic class: potassium supplement
Therapeutic class: mineral
Pregnancy risk category: C

Indications and dosages

▶ **Prevention of hypokalemia.** *Adults and children:* Initially, 20 mEq P.O. daily in divided doses. Adjust dosage, p.r.n., based on potassium level.

▶ **Hypokalemia.** *Adults and children:* 40 to 100 mEq P.O. daily divided into two to four doses. Use I.V. potassium chloride when oral replacement isn't feasible. Maximum dose of diluted I.V. potassium chloride is 20 mEq/hour at 40 mEq/L. Further dose based on potassium level. Don't exceed 150 mEq P.O. daily in adults and 3 mEq/kg P.O. daily in children. Further doses are based on potassium level and blood pH. Monitor ECG and take potassium level frequently when giving I.V. potassium replacement.

▶ **Severe hypokalemia.** *Adults and children:* Potassium chloride should be diluted in a suitable I.V. solution of less than 80 mEq/L and given at no more than 40 mEq/hour. Further dose based on potassium level. Don't exceed 150 mEq I.V. daily in adults and 3 mEq/kg I.V. daily or 40 mEq/m² daily for children. Monitor ECG and take potassium level frequently when giving I.V. potassium replacement.

▶ **Acute MI‡.** *Adults:* High dose—80 mEq/L at 1.5 ml/kg/hour for 24 hours with an I.V. infusion of 25% dextrose and 50 units/L regular insulin. Low dose—40 mEq/L at 1 ml/kg/hour for 24 hours, with an I.V. infusion of 10% dextrose and 20 units/L regular insulin.

▼ I.V. administration

• Give drug only by infusion, never by I.V. push or I.M. route.
• Give slowly as dilute solution; life-threatening hyperkalemia may result from too-rapid infusion.

Contraindications and precautions

• Contraindicated in patients with untreated Addison's disease, adrenocortical insufficiency, acute dehydration, heat cramps, hyperkalemia, hyperkalemic form of familial periodic paralysis, other conditions linked to extensive tissue breakdown, or severe renal impairment with oliguria, anuria, or azotemia.
• Use cautiously in patients with cardiac disease or renal impairment.
⚠ Lifespan: In pregnant and breast-feeding women, use cautiously.

Adverse reactions

CNS: paresthesia of limbs, listlessness, mental confusion, weakness or heaviness of limbs, flaccid paralysis.
CV: *arrhythmias, heart block, cardiac arrest, ECG changes (prolonged PR interval, widened QRS complex, ST-segment depression, and tall, tented T waves).*
GI: *nausea, vomiting, abdominal pain,* diarrhea, *GI ulcerations* (stenosis, *hemorrhage, obstruction, perforation*).
GU: oliguria.
Respiratory: *respiratory paralysis.*
Skin: cold skin, gray pallor, phlebitis.

Interactions

Drug-drug. *ACE inhibitors, potassium-sparing diuretics:* Increases risk of hyperkalemia. Use cautiously.
Drug-herb. *Cascara, licorice:* May antagonize effects of potassium supplements. Discourage using together.
Drug-food. *Salt substitutes:* Increases risk of hyperkalemia. Don't use together.

Effects on lab test results

• May increase potassium level.

Pharmacokinetics

Absorption: Well absorbed.
Distribution: Distributed throughout body.
Metabolism: None significant.

Excretion: Excreted largely by kidneys; small amounts may be excreted via skin and intestinal tract, but intestinal potassium is usually reabsorbed. *Half-life:* Unknown.

Route	Onset	Peak	Duration
P.O.	Unknown	≤ 4 hr	Unknown
I.V.	Immediate	Immediate	Unknown

Action

Chemical effect: Aids in transmitting nerve impulses, contracting cardiac and skeletal muscle, and maintaining intracellular tonicity, cellular metabolism, acid-base balance, and normal renal function.
Therapeutic effect: Replaces and maintains potassium level.

Available forms

Capsules (controlled-release): 8 mEq, 10 mEq
Injection concentrate: 1.5 mEq/ml, 2 mEq/ml
Injection for I.V. infusion: 0.1mEq/ml, 0.2 mEq/ml, 0.3 mEq/ml, 0.4 mEq/ml
Oral liquid: 20 mEq/15 ml, 30 mEq/15 ml, 40 mEq/15 ml
Powder for oral administration: 15 mEq/packet, 20 mEq/packet, 25 mEq/packet
Tablets (controlled-release): 6.7 mEq, 8 mEq, 10 mEq, 20 mEq
Tablets (extended-release): 8 mEq, 10 mEq

NURSING PROCESS

▨ Assessment

• Assess patient's condition before therapy and regularly thereafter.
• During therapy, monitor ECG, renal function, fluid intake and output, and potassium, creatinine, and BUN levels.
• Be alert for adverse reactions and drug interactions.
• Evaluate patient's and family's knowledge of drug therapy.

▦ Nursing diagnoses

• Ineffective health maintenance related to presence of hypokalemia
• Risk for injury related to drug-induced hyperkalemia
• Deficient knowledge related to drug therapy

▶ Planning and implementation

• Give cautiously because different potassium supplements deliver varying amounts of potassium. Never switch products without prescriber's order.

• Make sure powders are completely dissolved before giving.

• Don't crush sustained-release potassium products.

• Give potassium with or after meals with full glass of water or fruit juice to lessen GI distress.

• If tablet or capsule passage is likely to be delayed, as in GI obstruction, use sugar-free liquid (Kaochlor S-F 10%). Have patient sip slowly to minimize GI irritation.

• Enteric-coated tablets aren't recommended because of increased risk of GI bleeding and small-bowel ulcerations.

• Tablets in wax matrix sometimes lodge in esophagus and cause ulceration in cardiac patients who have esophageal compression from enlarged left atrium. Use liquid form in such patients and in those with esophageal stasis or obstruction.

• Drug is commonly given with potassium-wasting diuretics to maintain potassium levels.

⊛ **ALERT:** Potassium preparations aren't interchangeable. Verify preparation before giving.

⊛ **ALERT:** Don't give potassium postoperatively until urine flow is established.

Patient teaching

• Tell patient that controlled-release tablets may appear in stool but that the drug has already been absorbed.

• Instruct patient to report adverse reactions and pain at the I.V. site.

☑ Evaluation

• Patient's potassium level returns to normal.

• Patient doesn't develop hyperkalemia.

• Patient and family state understanding of drug therapy.

---

potassium gluconate
(puh-TAS-ee-um GLOO-kuh-nayt)
Kaon, Kaylixir*, K-G Elixir*

Pharmacologic class: potassium supplement
Therapeutic class: mineral
Pregnancy risk category: C

Indications and dosages

▶ **Hypokalemia.** *Adults:* 40 to 100 mEq P.O. daily in three or four divided doses; 20 mEq P.O. daily for prevention. Further dosage based on potassium level determinations.

Contraindications and precautions

• Contraindicated in patients with untreated Addison's disease, acute dehydration, heat cramps, hyperkalemia, hyperkalemic form of familial periodic paralysis, other conditions related to extensive tissue breakdown, or severe renal impairment with oliguria, anuria, or azotemia.

• Use cautiously in patients with cardiac disease or renal impairment.

⚘ **Lifespan:** In pregnant and breast-feeding women, use cautiously. In children, safety of drug hasn't been established.

Adverse reactions

CNS: paresthesia of limbs, listlessness, mental confusion, weakness or heaviness of legs, flaccid paralysis.

CV: *arrhythmias,* ECG changes (prolonged PR interval, widened QRS complex, ST-segment depression, and tall, tented T waves).

GI: *nausea and vomiting; abdominal pain;* diarrhea; *GI ulcerations* that may be accompanied by stenosis, **hemorrhage, obstruction or perforation** (with oral products, especially enteric-coated tablets).

Interactions

Drug-drug. *ACE inhibitors, potassium-sparing diuretics:* Increases risk of hyperkalemia. Use cautiously.

Drug-food. *Salt substitutes:* Increases risk of hyperkalemia. Don't use together.

Effects on lab test results

• May increase potassium level.

Pharmacokinetics

Absorption: Well absorbed from GI tract.
Distribution: Distributed throughout body.
Metabolism: None significant.
Excretion: Excreted largely by kidneys; small amounts may be excreted via skin and intestinal tract, but intestinal potassium is usually reabsorbed. *Half-life:* Unknown.

Route	Onset	Peak	Duration
P.O.	Unknown	≤ 4 hr	Unknown

Action

Chemical effect: Aids in transmitting nerve impulses, contracting cardiac and skeletal muscle, and maintaining intracellular tonicity, cellular metabolism, acid-base balance, and normal renal function.
Therapeutic effect: Replaces and maintains potassium level.

Available forms

Liquid: 20 mEq/15 ml*
Tablets: 500mg†, 595 mg† (83.45 mg and 99 mg potassium, respectively)

NURSING PROCESS

🏥 Assessment

• Assess patient's condition before therapy and regularly thereafter.
• During therapy, monitor ECG, renal function, fluid intake and output, and potassium, creatinine, and BUN levels.
• Be alert for adverse reactions and drug interactions.
• Evaluate patient's and family's knowledge of drug therapy.

📋 Nursing diagnoses

• Ineffective health maintenance related to presence of hypokalemia
• Risk for injury related to potassium-induced hyperkalemia
• Deficient knowledge related to drug therapy

📊 Planning and implementation

• Give cautiously because different potassium supplements deliver varying amounts of potassium. Never switch products without prescriber's order.
• Give drug with or after meals with glass of water or fruit juice.
• Have patient sip liquid potassium slowly to minimize GI irritation.
• Enteric-coated tablets aren't recommended because of increased risk of GI bleeding and small-bowel ulcerations.
⑤ **ALERT:** Potassium preparations aren't interchangeable. Verify preparation before giving.
⑤ **ALERT:** Don't give potassium supplements postoperatively until urine flow is established.
Patient teaching
• Inform patient of need for potassium supplementation.

• Teach patient how to take drug.
• Instruct patient to report adverse reactions.

☑ Evaluation

• Patient's potassium level returns to normal.
• Patient doesn't develop hyperkalemia as result of drug therapy.
• Patient and family state understanding of drug therapy.

potassium iodide
(puh-TAS-ee-um IGH-uh-dighd)
Iosat, Pima, Thyro-Block

potassium iodide, saturated solution (SSKI)

strong iodine solution (Lugol's Solution)

Pharmacologic class: antithyroid
Therapeutic class: radiation protectant
Pregnancy risk category: D

Indications and dosages

▶ **Preparation for thyroidectomy.** *Adults and children:* 0.1 to 0.3 ml (2 to 6 gtt) strong iodine solution P.O. t.i.d. for 10 days before surgery.
▶ **Thyrotoxic crisis.** *Adults and children:* 500 mg P.O. q 4 hours (about 10 gtt of 1 g/ml solution).
▶ **Radiation protectant for thyroid gland.** *Adults:* 130 mg P.O. daily for 10 days after radiation exposure. Start no later than 3 to 4 hours after acute exposure. Or, 3 ml Pima P.O. daily 24 hours before and for 10 days after exposure.
Children older than age 3: 65 mg P.O. daily for 10 days after exposure. Initiate no later than 3 to 4 hours after acute exposure.
Children older than age 1: 2 ml Pima P.O. once daily 24 hours before and for 10 days after exposure.
Infants and children younger than age 1: 1 ml Pima P.O. daily 24 hours before and for 10 days after exposure to radioactive isotopes of iodine.
▶ **Hyperthyroidism.** *Adults and children:* 50 to 250 mg (1 to 5 gtt of 1g/ml solution) potassium iodide t.i.d. for 10 to 14 days before surgery. Or, 0.1 to 0.3 strong iodine solution (3 to 5 gtt) t.i.d.

Contraindications and precautions

• Contraindicated in patients with tuberculosis, acute bronchitis, iodide hypersensitivity, impaired renal function, or hyperkalemia. Some forms contain sulfites, which may precipitate allergic reactions in hypersensitive people.
• Use cautiously in patients with hypocomplementemic vasculitis, goiter, or autoimmune thyroid disease.
☙ Lifespan: In pregnant and breast-feeding women, drug isn't recommended.

Adverse reactions

CNS: fever, frontal headache.
EENT: acute rhinitis, inflammation of salivary glands, periorbital edema, conjunctivitis, hyperemia.
GI: burning, irritation, *nausea,* vomiting, diarrhea (sometimes bloody), *metallic taste.*
Metabolic: *potassium toxicity* (confusion, irregular heart beat, numbness, tingling, pain or weakness in hands and feet, tiredness).
Skin: acneform rash, mucous membrane ulceration.
Other: hypersensitivity reactions, tooth discoloration.

Interactions

Drug-drug. *ACE inhibitors, potassium-sparing diuretics:* Increases risk of hyperkalemia. Avoid using together.
Antithyroid medications: Potassium iodide may potentiate hypothyroid or goitrogenic effects. Monitor effects closely.
Lithium carbonate: May cause hypothyroidism. Use together cautiously.
Drug-food. *Salt substitutes:* Increases risk of hyperkalemia. Don't use together.

Effects on lab test results

• May increase potassium level.
• May increase or decrease thyroid function test results.

Pharmacokinetics

Absorption: Unknown.
Distribution: Unknown.
Metabolism: Unknown.
Excretion: Unknown. *Half-life:* Unknown.

Route	Onset	Peak	Duration
P.O.	≤ 24 hr	10-15 days	Unknown

Action

Chemical effect: Inhibits thyroid hormone formation by blocking iodotyrosine and iodothyronine synthesis, limits iodide transport into thyroid gland, and blocks thyroid hormone release.
Therapeutic effect: Lowers thyroid hormone levels.

Available forms

potassium iodide
Oral solution: 500 mg/15 ml
Scored tablets: 130 mg
Syrup: 325 mg/5 ml
potassium iodide, saturated solution
Oral solution: 1 g/ml
strong iodine solution
Oral solution: iodine 50 mg/ml and potassium iodide 100 mg/ml

NURSING PROCESS

▧ Assessment

• Assess patient's condition before therapy and regularly thereafter.
• Be alert for adverse reactions and drug interactions.
• Earliest signs of delayed hypersensitivity reactions caused by iodides are irritation and swelling of eyelids.
• Evaluate patient's and family's knowledge of drug therapy.

⊕ Nursing diagnoses

• Ineffective health maintenance related to underlying thyroid condition
• Ineffective protection related to hypersensitivity reactions
• Deficient knowledge related to drug therapy

▶ Planning and implementation

• Potassium iodide is usually given with other antithyroid drugs.
• Dilute oral doses in water, milk, or fruit juice to hydrate patient and mask salty taste; give drug after meals to prevent gastric irritation.
• Give iodide through straw to prevent tooth discoloration.
• Store drug in light-resistant container.
Patient teaching
• Teach patient how to take drug.
• Warn patient that sudden withdrawal may cause thyroid crisis.

Rapid onset   *Liquid form contains alcohol.   ♦Canada   ◊ Australia   †OTC   ‡Off-label use

• Tell patient to ask prescriber whether he can use iodized salt or eat shellfish.
• Tell patient to report adverse reactions.

☑ **Evaluation**
• Patient's thyroid hormone level is lower with potassium iodide therapy.
• Patient doesn't experience hypersensitivity reactions.
• Patient and family state understanding of drug therapy.

pralidoxime chloride (pyridine-2-aldoxime methochloride; 2-PAM chloride)
(pral-ih-DOKS-eem KLOR-ighd)
Protopam Chloride

Pharmacologic class: quaternary ammonium oxime
Therapeutic class: antidote
Pregnancy risk category: C

Indications and dosages

▶ **Antidote for organophosphate poisoning.**
Adults: 1 to 2 g in 100 ml of saline solution by I.V. infusion over 15 to 30 minutes. If patient has pulmonary edema, give by slow I.V. push over at least 5 minutes. Repeat in 1 hour if muscle weakness persists; may give further doses cautiously. Use I.M. or S.C. injection if I.V. route isn't feasible.
▶ **Anticholinesterase overdose.** *Adults:* 1 to 2 g I.V., followed by 250 mg I.V. q 5 minutes.

▼ I.V. administration

• Give I.V. preparation slowly as diluted solution. Dilute with unpreserved sterile water.
• To lessen muscarinic effects and block accumulation of acetylcholine from organophosphate poisoning, give atropine 2 to 6 mg I.V. along with pralidoxime unless patient has cyanosis. (If he is cyanotic, give atropine I.M.) Give atropine q 5 to 60 minutes in adults until muscarinic signs and symptoms disappear; if they reappear, repeat the dose. Maintain atropinization for at least 48 hours.
⏴ **ALERT:** Infuse slowly since tachycardia, laryngospasm, muscle rigidity, and worsening of cholinergic symptoms may occur with rapid

administration. Maximum injection rate is 200 mg/minute.

Contraindications and precautions

• Use cautiously in patients with myasthenia gravis (overdose may cause myasthenic crisis).
⚖ **Lifespan:** In pregnant women, use cautiously. In breast-feeding women and in children, safety of drug hasn't been established.

Adverse reactions

CNS: dizziness, headache, drowsiness, excitement, manic behavior after recovery of consciousness.
CV: tachycardia, increased blood pressure.
EENT: blurred vision, diplopia, impaired accommodation.
GI: nausea.
Musculoskeletal: muscle weakness, muscle rigidity.
Respiratory: hyperventilation.
Other: pain at injection site.

Interactions

Drug-drug. *Atropine:* May cause flushing, tachycardia, dry mouth. Monitor patient.
Barbiturates: Potentiates effects of barbiturates. Use together cautiously.

Effects on lab test results

• May increase AST, ALT, and CPK levels.

Pharmacokinetics

Absorption: Unknown after I.M. or S.C. use.
Distribution: Distributed throughout extracellular fluid; it isn't appreciably bound to protein. It doesn't readily pass into CNS.
Metabolism: Unknown but hepatic metabolism is considered likely.
Excretion: Excreted rapidly in urine. *Half-life:* 1½ hours.

Route	Onset	Peak	Duration
I.V.	Unknown	5-15 min	Unknown
I.M.	Unknown	10-20 min	Unknown
S.C.	Unknown	Unknown	Unknown

Action

Chemical effect: Reactivates cholinesterase that has been inactivated by organophosphorous pesticides and related compounds, permitting degradation of accumulated acetylcholine and facilitating normal functioning of neuromuscular junctions.

Therapeutic effect: Alleviates signs and symptoms of organophosphate poisoning and cholinergic crisis in myasthenia gravis.

Available forms

Injection: 1 g/20 ml in 20-ml vial without diluent or syringe; 1 g/20 ml in 20-ml vial with diluent, syringe, needle, and alcohol swab (emergency kit); 600 mg/2 ml auto-injector (may contain benzyl alcohol), parenteral

NURSING PROCESS

☑ Assessment

• Assess patient's condition before therapy and regularly thereafter. Drug relieves paralysis of respiratory muscles but is less effective in relieving depression of respiratory center.

• Drug isn't effective against poisoning caused by phosphorus, inorganic phosphates, or organophosphates that have no anticholinesterase activity.

• If poison was ingested, observe patient for 48 to 72 hours. Absorption from lower bowel may be delayed. It's difficult to distinguish between toxic effects produced by atropine or organophosphate compounds and those resulting from this drug.

• Watch for signs of rapid weakening in patient with myasthenia gravis who was treated for overdose of cholinergic drugs. Patient can pass quickly from cholinergic crisis to myasthenic crisis and may need more cholinergic drugs to treat myasthenia. Keep edrophonium (Tensilon) available in such situations for establishing differential diagnosis.

• Be alert for adverse reactions.

• Evaluate patient's and family's knowledge of drug therapy.

☷ Nursing diagnoses

• Ineffective health maintenance related to underlying condition

• Risk for injury related to adverse CNS reactions

• Deficient knowledge related to drug therapy

▷ Planning and implementation

• Remove secretions, maintain patent airway, and start artificial ventilation if needed. After dermal exposure to organophosphate, remove patient's clothing and wash his skin and hair with sodium bicarbonate, soap, water, and alcohol as soon as possible. A second washing may be necessary. When washing patient, wear protective gloves and clothes to avoid exposure.

• Draw blood for cholinesterase levels before giving drug.

• Use drug only in hospitalized patients; have respiratory and other supportive measures available. If possible, obtain accurate medical history and chronology of poisoning. Give drug as soon as possible; it's most effective when started within 24 hours.

⊛ **ALERT:** Don't confuse pralidoxime with pramoxine or pyridoxine.

Patient teaching

• Tell patient to report adverse reactions immediately.

• Advise patient treated for organophosphate poisoning to avoid contact with insecticides for several weeks.

☑ Evaluation

• Patient responds well to therapy.

• Patient sustains no injury from adverse CNS reactions.

• Patient and family state understanding of drug therapy.

pramipexole dihydrochloride
(pram-ih-PEKS-ohl digh-high-droh-KLOR-ighd)
Mirapex

Pharmacologic class: dopamine agonist
Therapeutic class: antiparkinsonian
Pregnancy risk category: C

Indications and dosages

▶ **Signs and symptoms of idiopathic Parkinson's disease.** *Adults:* Initially, 0.375 mg P.O. daily in three divided doses; don't increase more often than q 5 to 7 days. Maintenance daily dosage range is 1.5 to 4.5 mg in three divided doses.

☒ **Adjust-a-dose:** For patients with renal impairment, if creatinine clearance is greater than 60 ml/minute, initial dose is 0.125 mg P.O. t.i.d., up to 1.5 mg t.i.d. If creatinine clearance is 35 to 59 ml/minute, initial dose is 0.125 mg P.O. b.i.d. up to 1.5 mg b.i.d. If creatinine clearance is 15 to 34 ml/minute, initial dose is 0.125 mg P.O. daily, up to 1.5 mg daily.

Contraindications and precautions

- Contraindicated in patients hypersensitive to drug or its components.
- Use cautiously in patients with renal impairment; dosage may need adjustment.
- ⚠ Lifespan: In breast-feeding women and geriatric patients, use cautiously.

Adverse reactions

CNS: malaise, akathisia, amnesia, *asthenia, confusion,* delusions, *dizziness, dream abnormalities, dyskinesia,* dystonia, *extrapyramidal syndrome,* gait abnormalities, *hallucinations,* hypoesthesia, hypertonia, *insomnia,* myoclonus, paranoid reaction, *somnolence,* sleep disorders, thought abnormalities, fever.
CV: chest pain, peripheral edema, general edema, *orthostatic hypotension.*
EENT: accommodation abnormalities, diplopia, rhinitis, vision abnormalities.
GI: dry mouth, anorexia, *constipation,* dysphagia, *nausea.*
GU: impotence, urinary frequency, UTI, urinary incontinence.
Metabolic: weight loss.
Musculoskeletal: arthritis, bursitis, twitching, myasthenia.
Respiratory: dyspnea, pneumonia.
Skin: skin disorders.
Other: decreased libido, *accidental injury.*

Interactions

Drug-drug. *Butyrophenones, metoclopramide, phenothiazines, thiothixenes:* May diminish pramipexole effectiveness. Monitor patient closely.
Cimetidine, diltiazem, quinidine, quinine, ranitidine, triamterene, verapamil: Decreases pramipexole clearance. Adjust dosage, as directed.
Levodopa: Increases adverse effects of levodopa. Adjust levodopa dosage, as directed.
Drug-herb. *Black horehound:* May have additive dopaminergic effects. Discourage using together.

Effects on lab test results

None reported.

Pharmacokinetics

Absorption: Rapid. Absolute bioavailability exceeds 90%.
Distribution: Extensively distributed throughout body.
Metabolism: 90% of dose is excreted unchanged in urine.
Excretion: Primary route of elimination is urinary. *Half-life:* 8 to 12 hours.

Route	Onset	Peak	Duration
P.O.	Rapid	2 hr	8-12 hr

Action

Chemical effect: Precise mechanism is unknown, but drug probably stimulates dopamine receptors in striatum.
Therapeutic effect: Relieves symptoms of idiopathic Parkinson's disease.

Available forms

Tablets: 0.125 mg, 0.25 mg, 1 mg, 1.5 mg

NURSING PROCESS

☑ Assessment
- Monitor vital signs carefully because drug may cause orthostatic hypotension, especially during dose escalation.
- Assess patient's risk for physical injury from adverse CNS effects of drug (dyskinesia, dizziness, hallucinations, and somnolence).
- Assess patient's response to drug therapy and adjust dose.
- Evaluate patient's and family's knowledge of drug therapy.

☑ Nursing diagnoses
- Impaired physical mobility related to underlying Parkinson's disease
- Disturbed thought processes related to drug-induced CNS adverse reactions
- Deficient knowledge related to drug therapy

☑ Planning and implementation
- Institute safety precautions.
- ⚠ ALERT: Don't withdraw drug abruptly. Adjust dosage gradually according to patient's response and tolerance.
- Provide ice chips, drinks, or hard, sugarless candy to relieve dry mouth. Increase fluid and fiber intake to prevent constipation.

Reactions may be *common,* uncommon, *life-threatening*, or COMMON AND LIFE-THREATENING.

Patient teaching

- Instruct patient not to rise rapidly after sitting or lying down because of risk of orthostatic hypotension.
- Warn patient to avoid hazardous activities until CNS effects of drug are known.
- Tell patient to contact prescriber before taking this drug with other drugs.
- Tell patient—especially geriatric patient—that hallucinations may occur.
- If nausea develops, advise patient to take drug with food.
- If woman is breast-feeding or intends to do so, tell her to notify prescriber.

☑ Evaluation

- Patient has improved mobility and reduced muscle rigidity and tremor.
- Patient remains mentally alert.
- Patient and family state understanding of drug therapy.

pravastatin sodium (eptastatin)

(PRAH-vuh-stat-in SOH-dee-um)
Pravachol

Pharmacologic class: HMG-CoA reductase inhibitor
Therapeutic class: antilipemic
Pregnancy risk category: X

Indications and dosages

▶ **Primary hypercholesterolemia and mixed dyslipidemia; primary and secondary prevention of coronary events; hyperlipidemia; homozygous familial hypercholesterolemia.**
Adults: Initially, 40 mg P.O. once daily at the same time each day, with or without food. Adjust dosage q 4 weeks based on patient tolerance and response; maximum daily dose, 80 mg.
▶ **Heterozygous familial hypercholesterolemia.** *Children ages 14 to 18:* 40 mg P.O. once daily.
Children ages 8 to 13: 20 mg P.O. once daily.
◨ Adjust-a-dose: For patients with renal or hepatic impairment, start with 10 mg P.O. daily. For patients also taking immunosuppressive drugs, begin therapy with 10 mg P.O. h.s. and adjust to higher doses cautiously. Most patients given combination will receive maximum daily dose of 20 mg.

Contraindications and precautions

- Contraindicated in patients hypersensitive to drug and in patients with active liver disease or unexplained persistent elevations of transaminase levels.
- Use cautiously in patients who consume large quantities of alcohol or have history of liver disease.
- **Lifespan:** In pregnant and breast-feeding women and in women of childbearing age (unless they have no risk of pregnancy), drug is contraindicated. In children younger than age 8, safety of drug hasn't been established.

Adverse reactions

CNS: headache, fatigue, dizziness.
CV: chest pain.
EENT: rhinitis.
GI: vomiting, diarrhea, heartburn, nausea.
GU: *renal failure* secondary to myoglobinuria.
Musculoskeletal: myositis, myopathy, localized muscle pain, myalgia, *rhabdomyolysis.*
Respiratory: cough.
Skin: rash.
Other: flulike symptoms.

Interactions

Drug-drug. *Cholestyramine, colestipol:* Decreases pravastatin levels. Give pravastatin 1 hour before or 4 hours after these drugs.
Drugs that decrease levels or activity of endogenous steroids (such as cimetidine, spironolactone): May increase risk of endocrine dysfunction. No intervention appears necessary. Take complete drug history in patients who develop endocrine dysfunction.
Erythromycin, fibric acid derivatives (such as clofibrate, gemfibrozil), high doses of niacin, immunosuppressants: May increase risk of rhabdomyolysis. Don't use together.
Fluconazole, itraconazole, ketoconazole: May increase level and adverse effects of pravastatin. Avoid this combination. If they must be given together, reduce dose of pravastatin.
Gemfibrozil: Decreases protein-binding and urinary clearance of pravastatin. Avoid using together.
Hepatotoxic drugs: Increases risk of hepatotoxicity. Avoid using together.
Drug-herb. *Kava:* Increases risk of hepatotoxicity. Discourage using together.
Red yeast rice: Herb contains components similar to those of statin drugs. May increase the

risk of adverse events or toxicity. Discourage
using together.
Drug-lifestyle. *Alcohol use:* Increases risk of
hepatotoxicity. Discourage using together.

Effects on lab test results

• May increase ALT, AST, CK, alkaline phosphatase, and bilirubin levels.
• May alter thyroid function test values.

Pharmacokinetics

Absorption: Rapidly absorbed. Although food
reduces bioavailability, drug effects are same if
drug is taken with or 1 hour before meals.
Distribution: About 50% bound to proteins.
Drug undergoes extensive first-pass extraction,
possibly because of active transport system into
hepatocytes.
Metabolism: Metabolized in liver; at least six
metabolites have been identified. Some are active.
Excretion: Excreted by liver and kidneys. *Half-
life:* 1¼ to 2¼ hours

Route	Onset	Peak	Duration
P.O.	Unknown	1 hr	Unknown

Action

Chemical effect: Inhibits HMG-CoA reductase,
which is an early and rate-limiting step in the
synthesis of cholesterol.
Therapeutic effect: Lowers LDL and total cholesterol levels in some patients.

Available forms

Tablets: 10 mg, 20 mg, 40 mg, 80 mg

NURSING PROCESS

🧮 Assessment

• Assess patient's condition before therapy and
regularly thereafter.
• Obtain liver function tests at start of therapy
and periodically thereafter. If elevations persist,
patient should have a liver biopsy.
• Be alert for adverse reactions and drug interactions.
• If adverse GI reactions occur, monitor patient's hydration.
• Evaluate patient's and family's knowledge of
drug therapy.

🔲 Nursing diagnoses

• Risk for injury related to elevated cholesterol
levels
• Risk for deficient fluid volume related to adverse GI reactions
• Deficient knowledge related to drug therapy

▷ Planning and implementation

• Begin only after diet and other nondrug therapies have proved ineffective. Patient should follow a standard low-cholesterol diet.
Patient teaching
• Instruct patient to take recommended dosage
in evening, preferably h.s.
• Teach patient about proper dietary management of lipids (restricting total fat and cholesterol intake), as well as measures to control other cardiac disease risk factors. When
appropriate, recommend weight control, exercise, and smoking cessation programs.
• Inform woman that drug is contraindicated
during pregnancy. Advise her to notify prescriber immediately if she becomes pregnant.

✓ Evaluation

• Patient's LDL and total cholesterol levels are
within normal range.
• Patient maintains adequate hydration.
• Patient and family state understanding of drug
therapy.

prazosin hydrochloride
(PRAH-zoh-sin high-droh-KLOR-ighd)
Minipress

Pharmacologic class: alpha-adrenergic blocker
Therapeutic class: antihypertensive
Pregnancy risk category: C

Indications and dosages

▶ **Mild to moderate hypertension, alone or
with diuretic or other antihypertensive.**
Adults: Initial dosage is 1 mg P.O. b.i.d. to t.i.d.
Increase slowly; maximum daily dosage is
20 mg. Maintenance dosage is 6 to 15 mg daily
in three divided doses. Some patients need larger dosages (up to 40 mg daily). If other antihypertensives or diuretics are added, decrease to
1 to 2 mg t.i.d. and readjust.
Children: 0.5 to 7 mg P.O. t.i.d.

▶ **BPH‡.** *Adults:* Initially, 2 mg P.O. b.i.d. Dose may range from 1 to 9 mg P.O. daily.

Contraindications and precautions

• Use cautiously in patients taking other antihypertensives.

⚕ **Lifespan:** In pregnant women, use cautiously. In breast-feeding women, drug isn't recommended. In children, safety of drug hasn't been established.

Adverse reactions

CNS: *dizziness,* headache, drowsiness, weakness, *first-dose syncope,* depression.
CV: orthostatic hypotension, *palpitations.*
EENT: blurred vision.
GI: vomiting, diarrhea, abdominal cramps, constipation, *nausea,* dry mouth.
GU: priapism, impotence.

Interactions

Drug-drug. *Acebutolol, atenolol, betaxolol, carteolol, esmolol, metoprolol, nadolol, pindolol, propranolol, sotalol, timolol:* May increase risk of orthostatic hypotension in the early phases of use together. Assist patient to stand slowly until effects of drug are known.
Clonidine: May decrease antihypertensive effect of clonidine. Monitor blood pressure.
Diuretics: May increase frequency of syncope with loss of consciousness.
Indomethacin: May decrease antihypertensive action of prazosin. Monitor blood pressure.
Verapamil: May increase prazosin level and increase risk of postural hypotension. Advise patient to sit or lie down if dizziness occurs.
Drug-herb. *Yohimbine:* May antagonize antihypertensive effects. Discourage using together.

Effects on lab test results

• May increase BUN and uric acid levels.
• May increase liver function test values.

Pharmacokinetics

Absorption: Variable.
Distribution: Distributed throughout body; highly protein-bound (about 97%).
Metabolism: Extensive in liver.
Excretion: More than 90% excreted in feces via bile; remainder excreted in urine. *Half-life:* 2 to 4 hours.

Route	Onset	Peak	Duration
P.O.	30-90 min	2-4 hr	7-10 hr

Action

Chemical effect: Unknown; effects probably stem from alpha-adrenergic blocking activity.
Therapeutic effect: Lowers blood pressure.

Available forms

Capsules: 1 mg, 2 mg, 5 mg

NURSING PROCESS

▨ Assessment

• Assess patient's condition before therapy and regularly thereafter.
• Monitor patient's blood pressure and pulse rate frequently.
• Geriatric patients may be more sensitive to hypotensive effects of drug.
• Be alert for adverse reactions and drug interactions.
• Evaluate patient's and family's knowledge of drug therapy.

▨ Nursing diagnoses

• Risk for injury related to presence of hypertension
• Sexual dysfunction related to drug-induced impotence
• Deficient knowledge related to drug therapy

▨ Planning and implementation

• If first dose is larger than 1 mg, severe syncope with loss of consciousness may occur (first-dose syncope).
⚠ **ALERT:** Don't stop therapy abruptly.
• If you suspect compliance problems, discuss twice-daily dosing with prescriber because it may help.
Patient teaching
• Tell patient not to stop taking drug abruptly, but to call prescriber if unpleasant adverse reactions occur.
• Advise patient to minimize effects of orthostatic hypotension by rising slowly and avoiding sudden position changes.
• Dry mouth can be relieved with sugarless chewing gum, sour hard candy, or ice chips.
• Inform male patient of the possibility of impotence, and advise him to seek counseling to learn how to cope with this adverse effect.

☑ **Evaluation**

• Patient's blood pressure is normal.
• Patient seeks counseling for alternative methods of sexual gratification because of drug-induced impotence.
• Patient and family state understanding of drug therapy.

prednisolone (systemic)
(pred-NIS-uh-lohn)
Delta-Cortef, Prelone

prednisolone acetate
Cotolone, Key-Pred-25, Predalone 50, Predcor-50

prednisolone sodium phosphate
Hydeltrasol, Key-Pred SP, Orapred, Pediapred

prednisolone tebutate
Nor-Pred TBA, Predate TBA, Predcor-TBA, Prednisol TBA

Pharmacologic class: glucocorticoid, mineralocorticoid
Therapeutic class: anti-inflammatory, immunosuppressant
Pregnancy risk category: C

Indications and dosages

▶ **Severe inflammation, modification of body's immune response to disease.** *Adults:* 2.5 to 15 mg prednisolone P.O. b.i.d., t.i.d., or q.i.d. Or, 2 to 30 mg prednisolone acetate I.M. q 12 hours. Or, 5 to 60 mg prednisolone sodium phosphate I.M., I.V., or P.O. daily. Or, 4 to 40 mg prednisolone tebutate injected into joints and lesions, p.r.n.
Children: Initially, 0.14 to 2 mg/kg prednisolone P.O. or 4 to 60 mg/m² prednisolone P.O. daily in four divided doses. Or, 0.04 to 0.25 mg/kg prednisolone acetate or 1.5 to 7.5 mg/m² prednisolone acetate I.M. once or twice daily. Or, initially, 0.14 to 2 mg/kg prednisolone sodium phosphate or 4 to 60 mg/m² prednisolone sodium phosphate I.M., I.V., or P.O. daily in three or four divided doses.
▶ **Acute exacerbations of multiple sclerosis.** *Children:* 200 mg prednisolone sodium phosphate P.O. daily for 1 week, followed by 80 mg q other day.

▶ **Nephrotic syndrome.** *Children:* 60 mg/m² prednisolone sodium phosphate P.O. daily in three divided doses for 4 weeks, followed by 4 weeks of single dose alternate-day therapy at 40 mg/m².
▶ **Uncontrolled asthma in patients taking by inhaled corticosteroids and long-acting bronchodilators.** *Children:* 1 to 2 mg/kg prednisolone sodium phosphate P.O. daily in single or divided doses. It is further recommended that short course, or "burst" therapy, be continued until a child achieves a peak expiratory flow rate of 80% of his personal best or symptoms resolve. This usually requires 3 to 10 days of therapy, although it can take longer. No evidence shows that tapering the dose after improvement will prevent a relapse.

▼ **I.V. administration**

⑤ **ALERT:** Never give acetate or tebutate form by I.V. route.
• Give only prednisolone sodium phosphate by I.V. route.
• When giving drug as direct injection, inject undiluted over at least 1 minute.
• When giving drug as intermittent or continuous infusion, dilute solution according to manufacturer's instructions and give over prescribed duration.
• D₅W and normal saline solution are recommended as diluents for I.V. infusions.

Contraindications and precautions

• Contraindicated in patients hypersensitive to drug or its ingredients and in those with fungal infections.
• Use cautiously in patients with recent MI, GI ulcer, renal disease, hypertension, osteoporosis, diabetes mellitus, hypothyroidism, cirrhosis, diverticulitis, nonspecific ulcerative colitis, recent intestinal anastomoses, thromboembolic disorders, seizures, myasthenia gravis, heart failure, tuberculosis, ocular herpes simplex, emotional instability, and psychotic tendencies.
⚘ **Lifespan:** In pregnant women, use cautiously. In breast-feeding women, high doses aren't recommended.

Adverse reactions

Most reactions to corticosteroids are dose- or duration-dependent.

CNS: *euphoria, insomnia,* psychotic behavior, *pseudotumor cerebri, seizures.*
CV: *heart failure, thromboembolism,* hypertension, edema.
EENT: cataracts, glaucoma.
GI: *peptic ulceration,* GI irritation, increased appetite, *pancreatitis.*
Metabolic: hypokalemia, hyperglycemia, carbohydrate intolerance, growth suppression in children.
Musculoskeletal: muscle weakness, osteoporosis.
Skin: hirsutism, delayed wound healing, acne, various skin eruptions.
Other: susceptibility to infections, *acute adrenal insufficiency with increased stress (infection, surgery, or trauma) or abrupt withdrawal after long-term therapy.*

Interactions

Drug-drug. *Aspirin, indomethacin, other NSAIDs:* Increases risk of GI distress and bleeding. Avoid using together.
Barbiturates, phenytoin, rifampin: Decreases corticosteroid effect. Increase corticosteroid dosage.
Oral anticoagulants: Alters dosage requirements. Monitor PT and INR closely.
Potassium-depleting drugs (such as thiazide diuretics): Enhances potassium-wasting effects of prednisolone. Monitor potassium levels.
Skin-test antigens: Decreases skin test response. Defer skin testing until therapy is completed.
Toxoids, vaccines: Decreases antibody response and increases risk of neurologic complications. Check with prescriber about when to reschedule vaccine, if possible.

Effects on lab test results

• May increase glucose and cholesterol levels. May decrease potassium and calcium levels.

Pharmacokinetics

Absorption: Absorbed readily after P.O. use; variable with other routes.
Distribution: Distributed to muscle, liver, skin, intestine, and kidneys. Drug is extensively bound to proteins. Only unbound portion is active.
Metabolism: Metabolized in liver.
Excretion: Inactive metabolites and small amounts of unmetabolized drug are excreted in

urine; insignificant amount excreted in feces. *Half-life:* 18 to 36 hours.

Route	Onset	Peak	Duration
P.O.	Rapid	1-2 hr	30-36 hr
I.V.	Rapid	< 1 hr	Unknown
I.M.	Rapid	< 1 hr	< 4 wk
P.R.	Unknown	Unknown	Unknown
Intra-articular, intralesional	1-2 days	Unknown	3 days-4 wk

Action

Chemical effect: Not clearly defined; decreases inflammation, mainly by stabilizing leukocyte lysosomal membranes; suppresses immune response; stimulates bone marrow; and influences protein, fat, and carbohydrate metabolism.
Therapeutic effect: Relieves inflammation and induces immunosuppression.

Available forms

prednisolone
Syrup: 5 mg/ml, 15 mg/5 ml
Tablets: 5 mg
prednisolone acetate
Injection: 25 mg/ml, 50 mg/ml suspension
prednisolone sodium phosphate
Injection: 20 mg/ml solution
Oral liquid: 5 mg/5 ml, 15 mg/5 ml
prednisolone tebutate
Injection: 20 mg/ml suspension

NURSING PROCESS

⚗ Assessment

• Assess patient's condition before therapy and regularly thereafter.
• Monitor patient's weight, blood pressure, and electrolyte levels.
• Watch for depression or psychotic episodes, especially at high doses.
• Diabetic patient may need increased insulin; monitor glucose levels.
• Monitor patient's stress level; dosage adjustment may be needed.
• Be alert for adverse reactions and drug interactions.
• Evaluate patient's and family's knowledge of drug therapy.

⊕ Nursing diagnoses

• Ineffective health maintenance related to underlying condition

---

• Ineffective protection related to drug-induced adverse reactions
• Deficient knowledge related to drug therapy

▶ Planning and implementation
• Always adjust to lowest effective dosage. However, dosage may need to be increased during times of physiologic stress (such as surgery, trauma, or infection).
• Prednisolone salts (acetate, sodium phosphate, and tebutate) are used parenterally less often than other corticosteroids that have more potent anti-inflammatory action.
• Drug may be used for alternate-day therapy.
• Give dose with food when possible to reduce GI irritation.
• Refrigerate Orapred at 36° to 46° F (2° to 8° C).
• Inject drug I.M. deep into gluteal muscle.
• Alternate injection sites to prevent muscle atrophy.
• Avoid S.C. injection because atrophy and sterile abscesses may occur.
• Unless contraindicated, give low-sodium diet high in potassium and protein. Give potassium supplements, p.r.n.
• Notify prescriber immediately if serious adverse reactions occur, and give supportive care.
• After long-term therapy, reduce dosage gradually. Abrupt withdrawal may cause rebound inflammation, fatigue, weakness, arthralgia, fever, dizziness, lethargy, depression, fainting, orthostatic hypotension, dyspnea, anorexia, or hypoglycemia. Sudden withdrawal after prolonged use may be fatal.
• **⑤ ALERT:** Don't confuse prednisolone with prednisone.

Patient teaching
• Tell patient not to stop drug without prescriber's knowledge.
• Tell patient to take drug as ordered, and tell him what to do if he misses a dose.
• Advise patient to take oral form with meals to minimize GI reactions.
• Warn patient receiving long-term therapy about cushingoid symptoms.
• Teach signs of early adrenal insufficiency: fatigue, muscle weakness, joint pain, fever, anorexia, nausea, dyspnea, dizziness, and fainting.
• Instruct patient to wear or carry medical identification that indicates his need for systemic glucocorticoids during stress.

• Tell patient to report sudden weight gain, swelling, or slow healing.
• Advise patient receiving long-term therapy to exercise or have physical therapy and to ask prescriber about vitamin D or calcium supplements.

✓ Evaluation
• Patient responds well to therapy.
• Patient has no serious adverse reactions.
• Patient and family state understanding of drug therapy.

prednisone
(PRED-nih-sohn)
Apo-Prednisone ♦ , Deltasone, Liquid Pred*, Meticorten, Novo-Prednisone ♦ , Orasone, Panafcort ♦ , Panasol-S, Prednicen-M, Prednisone Intensol*, Sone ♦ , Sterapred, Winpred ♦

Pharmacologic class: adrenocorticoid
Therapeutic class: anti-inflammatory, immunosuppressant
Pregnancy risk category: NR

Indications and dosages
▶ **Severe inflammation or immunosuppression.** *Adults:* 5 to 60 mg P.O. daily in single or divided doses. Maximum, 250 mg daily. Maintenance dosage given once daily or q other day. Dosage must be individualized.
▶ **Acute exacerbations of multiple sclerosis.** *Adults:* 200 mg P.O. daily for 1 week; then 80 mg P.O. q other day for 1 month.

Contraindications and precautions
• Contraindicated in patients hypersensitive to drug and in those with systemic fungal infections.
• Use cautiously in patients with GI ulcer, renal disease, hypertension, osteoporosis, diabetes mellitus, hypothyroidism, cirrhosis, diverticulitis, nonspecific ulcerative colitis, recent intestinal anastomoses, thromboembolic disorders, seizures, myasthenia gravis, heart failure, tuberculosis, ocular herpes simplex, emotional instability, and psychotic tendencies.
• ⚘ Lifespan: In pregnant women, use cautiously. In breast-feeding women, high doses aren't recommended.

Reactions may be *common*, uncommon, *life-threatening*, or COMMON AND LIFE-THREATENING.

Adverse reactions

Most reactions are dose- or duration-dependent.
CNS: *euphoria, insomnia,* psychotic behavior, *pseudotumor cerebri, seizures.*
CV: *heart failure, thromboembolism,* hypertension, edema.
EENT: cataracts, glaucoma.
GI: *peptic ulceration,* GI irritation, increased appetite, *pancreatitis.*
Metabolic: hypokalemia, hyperglycemia, carbohydrate intolerance, growth suppression in children.
Musculoskeletal: muscle weakness, osteoporosis.
Skin: hirsutism, delayed wound healing, acne, various skin eruptions.
Other: susceptibility to infections.

Interactions

Drug-drug. *Aspirin, indomethacin, other NSAIDs:* Increases risk of GI distress and bleeding. Give together cautiously.
Barbiturates, phenytoin, rifampin: Decreases corticosteroid effect. Increase corticosteroid dosage.
Oral anticoagulants: Alters dosage requirements. Monitor PT and INR closely.
Potassium-depleting drugs (such as thiazide diuretics): Enhances potassium-wasting effects of prednisone. Monitor potassium levels.
Skin-test antigens: Decreases skin test response. Defer skin testing until therapy is completed.
Toxoids, vaccines: Decreases antibody response and increases risk of neurologic complications. Don't give together.

Effects on lab test results

• May increase glucose and cholesterol levels. May decrease potassium and calcium levels.

Pharmacokinetics

Absorption: Absorbed readily after P.O. use.
Distribution: Distributed to muscle, liver, skin, intestine, and kidneys. Drug is extensively bound to proteins. Only unbound portion is active.
Metabolism: Metabolized in liver.
Excretion: Inactive metabolites and small amounts of unmetabolized drug are excreted in urine; insignificant amounts excreted in feces.
Half-life: 18 to 36 hours.

Route	Onset	Peak	Duration
P.O.	Varies	Varies	Varies

Action

Chemical effect: Not clearly defined; decreases inflammation; suppresses immune response; stimulates bone marrow; and influences protein, fat, and carbohydrate metabolism.
Therapeutic effect: Relieves inflammation and induces immunosuppression.

Available forms

Oral solution: 5 mg/5 ml*, 5 mg/ml (concentrate)*
Syrup: 5 mg/5 ml*
Tablets: 1 mg, 2.5 mg, 5 mg, 10 mg, 20 mg, 25 mg, 50 mg

NURSING PROCESS

Assessment

• Assess patient's condition before therapy and regularly thereafter.
• Monitor patient's weight, blood pressure, and electrolyte levels.
• Watch for depression or psychotic episodes, especially at high doses.
• Diabetic patient may need increased insulin; monitor glucose level.
• Monitor patient's stress level; dosage adjustment may be needed.
• Be alert for adverse reactions and drug interactions.
• Evaluate patient's and family's knowledge of drug therapy.

Nursing diagnoses

• Ineffective health maintenance related to underlying condition
• Ineffective protection related to drug-induced adverse reactions
• Deficient knowledge related to drug therapy

Planning and implementation

• Always adjust to lowest effective dosage. However, dosage may need to be increased during times of physiologic stress (such as surgery, trauma, or infection).
• Drug may be used for alternate-day therapy.
• For better results and less toxicity, give once-daily dose in morning.
• Give oral dose with food when possible to reduce GI irritation.

Rapid onset   *Liquid form contains alcohol.   ◆Canada   ◇ Australia   †OTC   ‡Off-label use

• After long-term therapy, reduce dosage gradually. Abrupt withdrawal may cause rebound inflammation, fatigue, weakness, arthralgia, fever, dizziness, lethargy, depression, fainting, orthostatic hypotension, dyspnea, anorexia, or hypoglycemia. After long-term therapy, increased stress or abrupt withdrawal may cause acute adrenal insufficiency. Sudden withdrawal after prolonged use may be fatal.

• Unless contraindicated, give low-sodium diet high in potassium and protein. Give potassium supplements, p.r.n.

• If serious adverse reactions occur, notify prescriber immediately and give supportive care.

⊕ **ALERT:** Don't confuse prednisone with prednisolone.

Patient teaching

• Tell patient not to stop drug without prescriber's knowledge.

• Advise patient to take oral form with meals to minimize GI reactions.

• Tell patient to report sudden weight gain, swelling, or slow healing.

• Advise patient receiving long-term therapy to exercise or have physical therapy, to ask prescriber about vitamin D or calcium supplements, and to have periodic eye examinations.

• Instruct patient to wear or carry medical identification that indicates his need for systemic glucocorticoids during stress.

• Warn patient receiving long-term therapy about cushingoid symptoms.

• Teach signs of early adrenal insufficiency: fatigue, muscular weakness, joint pain, fever, anorexia, nausea, dyspnea, dizziness, and fainting.

☑ **Evaluation**

• Patient responds well to therapy.

• Patient doesn't experience serious adverse reactions.

• Patient and family state understanding of drug therapy.

---

primaquine phosphate
(PRIH-muh-kwin FOS-fayt)

Pharmacologic class: 8-aminoquinoline
Therapeutic class: antimalarial
Pregnancy risk category: NR

Indications and dosages

▶ **Radical cure of relapsing *Plasmodium vivax* malaria, eliminating symptoms and infection completely; prevention of relapse.** *Adults:* 15 mg (base) P.O. daily for 14 days. (26.3-mg tablet = 15 mg of base.)
Children: 0.5 mg/kg (base = 0.3 mg/kg daily) P.O. daily for 14 days.

▶ ***Pneumocystis carinii* pneumonia‡.** *Adults:* 15 to 30 mg (base) P.O. daily.

Contraindications and precautions

• Contraindicated in patients with systemic diseases in which granulocytopenia may develop (such as lupus erythematosus or rheumatoid arthritis) and in those taking bone marrow suppressants and potentially hemolytic drugs.

• Use cautiously in patients with previous idiosyncratic reaction (hemolytic anemia, methemoglobinemia, or leukopenia), in those with family or personal history of favism, and in those with erythrocytic G6PD deficiency or nicotinamide adenine dinucleotide (NADH) methemoglobin reductase deficiency.

☙ Lifespan: In pregnant women, use cautiously. In children and breast-feeding women, safety of drug hasn't been established.

Adverse reactions

GI: nausea, vomiting, epigastric distress, abdominal cramps.
Hematologic: *leukopenia,* hemolytic anemia in G6PD deficiency, *methemoglobinemia* in NADH methemoglobin reductase deficiency.

Interactions

Drug-drug. *Quinacrine:* Enhances primaquine toxicity. Don't use together.

Effects on lab test results

• May increase or decrease WBC count.
• May decrease RBC count, hemoglobin, and hematocrit.

Pharmacokinetics

Absorption: Well absorbed.
Distribution: Distributed widely into liver, lungs, heart, brain, skeletal muscle, and other tissues.
Metabolism: Metabolized in liver.
Excretion: Small amount excreted unchanged in urine. *Half-life:* 4 to 10 hours.

Route	Onset	Peak	Duration
P.O.	Unknown	2-3 hr	Unknown

Action

Chemical effect: Unknown; it may be effective because it can bind to and alter properties of DNA.
Therapeutic effect: Prevents or treats relapsing *P. vivax* malaria.

Available forms

Tablets: 15 mg (base)

NURSING PROCESS

Assessment
• Assess patient's condition before therapy and regularly thereafter.
• Obtain frequent blood studies and urine examinations in light-skinned patients taking more than 30 mg (base) daily, dark-skinned patients taking more than 15 mg (base) daily, and patients with severe anemia or suspected sensitivity.
• Monitor patient for sudden drop in hemoglobin level, decreased erythrocyte or leukocyte count, or marked darkening of urine, each of which suggests impending hemolytic reactions.
• Be alert for adverse reactions and drug interactions.
• Evaluate patient's and family's knowledge of drug therapy.

Nursing diagnoses
• Infection related to malaria
• Ineffective protection related to adverse hematologic reactions
• Deficient knowledge related to drug therapy

Planning and implementation
• Give drug with meals.
• A fast-acting antimalarial (such as chloroquine) is usually given with primaquine to reduce possibility of drug-resistant strains.
• Stop drug immediately and notify prescriber about abnormal CBC results or pronounced darkening of urine.
Patient teaching
• Instruct patient to take drug with meals.
• Tell patient to notify prescriber if adverse reactions occur, especially a marked darkening of urine.

• Tell patient to avoid hazardous activities if visual disturbances occur.

Evaluation
• Patient is free from malaria.
• Patient doesn't develop serious adverse hematologic reactions.
• Patient and family state understanding of drug therapy.

primidone
(PRIH-mih-dohn)
Apo-Primidone ♦ , Mysoline, PMS Primidone, Sertan ♦

Pharmacologic class: barbiturate analogue
Therapeutic class: anticonvulsant
Pregnancy risk category: NR

Indications and dosages

▶ **Generalized tonic-clonic, focal, and complex-partial (psychomotor) seizures.**
Adults and children age 8 and older: Initially, 100 to 125 mg P.O. h.s. on days 1 to 3; then 100 to 125 mg P.O. b.i.d. on days 4 to 6; then 100 to 125 mg P.O. t.i.d. on days 7 to 9; followed by maintenance dosage of 250 mg P.O. t.i.d. to q.i.d.; maximum dosage, 2 g daily.
Children younger than age 8: Initially, 50 mg P.O. h.s. for 3 days; then 50 mg P.O. b.i.d. for 4 to 6 days; then 100 mg P.O. b.i.d. for 7 to 9 days; followed by maintenance dosage of 125 to 250 mg P.O. t.i.d., or 10 to 25 mg/kg daily in divided doses.
▶ **Benign familial tremor (essential tremor).**
Adults: 750 mg P.O. daily.

Contraindications and precautions

• Contraindicated in patients with phenobarbital hypersensitivity or porphyria.
⚠ Lifespan: In pregnant and breast-feeding women, drug is contraindicated.

Adverse reactions

CNS: *drowsiness, ataxia,* emotional disturbances, vertigo, hyperirritability, fatigue.
CV: edema.
EENT: *diplopia,* nystagmus, edema of eyelids.
GI: anorexia, nausea, vomiting, thirst.
GU: impotence, polyuria.

Hematologic: ***leukopenia,*** eosinophilia, ***thrombocytopenia.***
Skin: morbilliform rash, alopecia.

Interactions

Drug-drug. *Acetazolamide:* May decrease primidone level. Monitor patient for effect.
Carbamazepine: May decrease primidone level and increase carbamazepine level. Observe patient for lack of effect or carbamazepine toxicity.
Isoniazid, nicotinamide: May increase primidone level. Monitor patient for toxicity.
Metoprolol, propranolol: May reduce the effects of these drugs. Consider an increased beta blocker dose.
Phenytoin: May increase conversion of primidone to phenobarbital. Observe patient for increased phenobarbital effect.
Drug-herb. *Glutamate:* May antagonize anticonvulsant effects of drug. Discourage using together.
Drug-lifestyle. *Alcohol use:* May impair coordination, increase CNS effects, and cause death. Strongly discourage use together.

Effects on lab test results

- May increase eosinophil count. May decrease hemoglobin, hematocrit, and WBC and platelet counts.

Pharmacokinetics

Absorption: Absorbed readily.
Distribution: Wide.
Metabolism: Metabolized slowly by liver to phenylethylmalonamide (PEMA) and phenobarbital; PEMA is the major metabolite.
Excretion: Excreted in urine. *Half-life:* 5 to 15 hours.

Route	Onset	Peak	Duration
P.O.	Unknown	3-4 hr	Unknown

Action

Chemical effect: Unknown; some activity may be caused by PEMA and phenobarbital.
Therapeutic effect: Prevents seizures.

Available forms

Oral suspension: 250 mg/5 ml
Tablets: 50 mg, 250 mg

NURSING PROCESS

Assessment

- Assess patient's condition before therapy and regularly thereafter.
- Monitor blood levels. Therapeutic primidone level is 5 to 12 mcg/ml. Therapeutic phenobarbital level is 15 to 40 mcg/ml.
- Monitor CBC and routine blood chemistry q 6 months.
- Monitor patient's hydration throughout drug therapy.
- Evaluate patient's and family's knowledge of drug therapy.

Nursing diagnoses

- Risk for trauma related to seizures
- Risk for deficient fluid volume related to adverse reactions
- Deficient knowledge related to drug therapy

Planning and implementation

- Shake liquid suspension well.
- Don't withdraw drug suddenly because seizures may worsen.
- Call prescriber immediately if adverse reactions develop.

ALERT: Don't confuse primidone with prednisone.

Patient teaching

- Advise patient to avoid hazardous activities until CNS effects of drug are known.
- Warn patient and parents not to stop drug suddenly.
- Tell patient that full therapeutic response may take 2 weeks or more.

Evaluation

- Patient is free from seizure activity.
- Patient maintains adequate hydration throughout drug therapy.
- Patient and family state understanding of drug therapy.

probenecid

(proh-BEN-uh-sid)
Benemid, Benuryl ♦, Probalan

Pharmacologic class: sulfonamide derivative
Therapeutic class: uricosuric
Pregnancy risk category: B

Indications and dosages

▶ **Adjunct to penicillin therapy.** *Adults and children older than age 14 or weighing more than 50 kg (110 lb):* 500 mg P.O. q.i.d.
Children ages 2 to 14 weighing 50 kg or less: Initially, 25 mg/kg P.O.; then 40 mg/kg in divided doses q.i.d.

▶ **Gonorrhea.** *Adults:* 3.5 g ampicillin P.O. with 1 g probenecid P.O. given together. Or, 1 g probenecid P.O. 30 minutes before 4.8 million units of aqueous penicillin G procaine I.M., injected at two different sites.

▶ **Hyperuricemia of gout, gouty arthritis.** *Adults:* 250 mg P.O. b.i.d. for first week; then 500 mg b.i.d., to maximum of 3 g daily. Maintenance dosage should be reviewed q 6 months and reduced by increments of 500 mg, if indicated.

▶ **To diagnose parkinsonian syndrome or mental depression‡.** *Adults:* 500 mg P.O. q 12 hours for 5 doses.

◻ **Adjust-a-dose:** For patients with renal impairment with a GFR of 30 ml/minute or greater, dose may need to be increased. Increases can be made in 0.5 g increments q 4 weeks. Usual dose is 2 g daily or less.

Contraindications and precautions

• Contraindicated in patients hypersensitive to drug and in patients with uric acid kidney stones, blood dyscrasias, or acute gout attack.
• Use cautiously in patients with peptic ulcer or renal impairment.
▒ Lifespan: In pregnant and breast-feeding women, use cautiously. In children younger than age 2, drug is contraindicated.

Adverse reactions

CNS: *headache,* fever, dizziness.
CV: flushing, hypotension.
GI: anorexia, nausea, vomiting, sore gums, *gastric distress.*
GU: urinary frequency, renal colic.
Hematologic: hemolytic anemia, *aplastic anemia.*
Hepatic: *hepatic necrosis.*
Skin: alopecia, dermatitis, pruritus.
Other: hypersensitivity reaction, *anaphylaxis.*

Interactions

Drug-drug. *Methotrexate:* May impair excretion of methotrexate, causing increased level,

effects, and toxicity. Monitor level closely and adjust dosage accordingly.
NSAIDs: May increase NSAID levels and increase risk of toxicity. Adjust dosage, p.r.n.
Oral antidiabetics: Enhances hypoglycemic effect. Monitor glucose levels closely. Dosage adjustment may be needed.
Rifampin: May decrease rifampin levels. Monitor patient for lack of effect.
Salicylates: Inhibits uricosuric effect of probenecid, causing urate retention. Don't use together.
Sulfonamides: May decrease sulfonamide excretion. Monitor patient for signs of toxicity.
Sulfonylureas: Half-life of these drugs may be increased. Monitor blood glucose.
Zidovudine: May increase absorption of zidovudine. Monitor patient for cutaneous drug eruption, malaise, myalgia, and fever.
Drug-lifestyle. *Alcohol use:* Increases urate levels. Discourage using together.

Effects on lab test results

• May decrease hemoglobin and hematocrit.
• May cause false-positive glucose test results with Benedict's solution or Clinitest.

Pharmacokinetics

Absorption: Complete.
Distribution: Distributed throughout body; about 75% protein-bound.
Metabolism: Metabolized in liver to active metabolites, with some uricosuric effect.
Excretion: Drug and metabolites excreted in urine; probenecid is actively reabsorbed but metabolites aren't. *Half-life:* 3 to 8 hours after 500-mg dose, 6 to 12 hours after larger doses.

Route	Onset	Peak	Duration
P.O.	Unknown	2-4 hr	8 hr

Action

Chemical effect: Blocks renal tubular reabsorption of uric acid, increasing excretion, and inhibits active renal tubular secretion of many weak organic acids, such as penicillins and cephalosporins.
Therapeutic effect: Lowers uric acid and prolongs penicillin action.

Available forms

Tablets: 500 mg

NURSING PROCESS

⚕ Assessment
• Assess patient's condition before therapy and regularly thereafter.
• Monitor periodic BUN and renal function tests in long-term therapy.
• Be alert for adverse reactions and drug interactions.
• If adverse GI reactions occur, monitor patient's hydration.
• Evaluate patient's and family's knowledge of drug therapy.

⊞ Nursing diagnoses
• Ineffective health maintenance related to underlying condition
• Risk for deficient fluid volume related to adverse GI reactions
• Deficient knowledge related to drug therapy

≫ Planning and implementation
• Drug is ineffective in patients with chronic renal insufficiency and a GFR less than 30 ml/ minute.
• Give drug with milk, food, or antacids to minimize GI distress. Continued disturbances may indicate need to lower dosage.
• Encourage patient to drink to maintain minimum daily output of 2 L of water a day. Alkalinize urine with sodium bicarbonate or potassium citrate. These measures will prevent hematuria, renal colic, urate stone development, and costovertebral pain.
• Keep in mind that therapy doesn't start until acute attack subsides. Drug contains no analgesic or anti-inflammatory drug and isn't useful during acute gout attacks.
• Drug may increase frequency, severity, and duration of acute gout attacks during first 6 to 12 months of therapy. Prophylactic colchicine or another anti-inflammatory is given during first 3 to 6 months.
• **ALERT:** Don't confuse probenecid with Procanbid or Benemid with Beminal.

Patient teaching
• Instruct patient to take drug with food or milk to minimize GI distress.
• Advise patient with gout to avoid all drugs that contain aspirin, which may precipitate gout. Acetaminophen may be used for pain.
• Tell patient with gout to avoid alcohol during drug therapy; it increases urate level.

• Tell patient with gout to limit intake of foods high in purine, such as anchovies, liver, sardines, kidneys, sweetbreads, peas, and lentils.
• Instruct patient and family that drug must be taken regularly as ordered or gout attacks may result. Tell patient to visit prescriber regularly so uric acid can be monitored and dosage adjusted, if necessary. Lifelong therapy may be required in patients with hyperuricemia.

☑ Evaluation
• Patient responds positively to therapy.
• Patient maintains adequate hydration.
• Patient and family state understanding of drug therapy.

---

procainamide hydrochloride
(proh-KAYN-uh-mighd high-droh-KLOR-ighd)
Procainamide Durules ♦ , Procan SR, Procanbid, Promine, Pronestyl, Pronestyl-SR

Pharmacologic class: procaine derivative
Therapeutic class: ventricular antiarrhythmic, supraventricular antiarrhythmic
Pregnancy risk category: C

Indications and dosages
▶ **Symptomatic PVCs; life-threatening ventricular tachycardia.** *Adults:* 100 mg q 5 minutes by slow I.V. push, no faster than 25 to 50 mg/minute, until arrhythmias disappear, adverse effects develop, or 500 mg has been given. Usual effective loading dose is 500 to 600 mg. Alternatively, give a loading dose of 500 to 600 mg I.V. infusion over 25 to 30 minutes. Maximum total dose is 1 g. When arrhythmias disappear, give continuous infusion of 2 to 6 mg/minute. If arrhythmias recur, repeat bolus as above and increase infusion rate. For I.M. administration, give 50 mg/kg/day divided q 3 to 6 hours; for arrhythmias during surgery, 100 to 500 mg I.M. For oral therapy, initiate dosage at 50 mg/kg P.O. in divided doses q 3 hours until therapeutic levels are reached. For the maintenance dose, substitute sustained-release form q 6 hours or extended-release form (Procanbid) at dosage of 50 mg/kg P.O. in two divided doses q 12 hours.
Children‡: Dosage not established. Recommendations include 2 to 5 mg/kg not exceeding

---

100 mg repeated, p.r.n., at 5 to 10-minute intervals not exceeding 15 mg/kg in 24 hours or 500 mg in a 30 minute period; or 15 mg/kg infused over 30 to 60 minutes, followed by maintenance infusion of 0.02 to 0.08 mg/kg/minute.

◎ **Adjust-a-dose:** For patients with renal or hepatic dysfunction, decreased dosages or longer dosing intervals may be needed.

▶ **Maintenance of NSR after conversion of atrial flutter‡.** *Adults:* 0.5 to 1 g P.O. q 4 to 6 hours.

▶ **Loading dose to prevent atrial fibrillation or paroxysmal atrial tachycardia‡.** *Adults:* 1.25 g P.O. If arrhythmias persist after 1 hour, give additional 750 mg. If no change occurs, give 500 mg to 1 g P.O. q 2 hours until arrhythmias disappear or adverse effects occur. Maintenance dose is 1 g q 6 hours.

▶ **Malignant hyperthermia‡.** *Adults:* 200 to 900 mg I.V., followed by an infusion.

▼ I.V. administration

• Vials for I.V. injection contain 1 g of drug: 100 mg/ml (10 ml) or 500 mg/ml (2 ml).
• Use infusion control device to give infusion precisely.
• Keep patient in supine position during I.V. use. If drug is given too rapidly, hypotension can occur. Watch closely for adverse reactions during infusion, and notify prescriber if they occur.
• Patient receiving infusions must be monitored at all times.
• If solution becomes discolored, check with pharmacy and expect to discard.

Contraindications and precautions

• Contraindicated in patients hypersensitive to procaine and related drugs; in those with complete, second-, or third-degree heart block in absence of artificial pacemaker; and in those with myasthenia gravis or systemic lupus erythematosus. Also contraindicated in patients with atypical ventricular tachycardia (torsades de pointes) because procainamide may aggravate this condition.
• Use cautiously when giving drug to treat ventricular tachycardia during coronary occlusion.
• Use cautiously in patients with hepatic or renal insufficiency, blood dyscrasias, bone marrow suppression, heart failure, or other conduction disturbances, such as bundle-branch heart block, sinus bradycardia, or digoxin intoxication.

☙ **Lifespan:** In pregnant women, use cautiously. In breast-feeding women, drug isn't recommended. In children, safety of drug hasn't been established.

Adverse reactions

CNS: hallucinations, *fever,* confusion, depression, dizziness.
CV: hypotension, *ventricular asystole, bradycardia, AV block, ventricular fibrillation* after parenteral use, *heart failure.*
GI: nausea, vomiting, anorexia, diarrhea, bitter taste with large doses.
Hematologic: *thrombocytopenia, neutropenia* (especially with sustained-release forms), *agranulocytosis,* hemolytic anemia.
Musculoskeletal: *myalgia.*
Skin: maculopapular rash.
Other: *lupuslike syndrome* (especially after prolonged use).

Interactions

Drug-drug. *Amiodarone:* Increases procainamide levels and toxicity; additive effects on QT interval and QRS complex. Avoid using together.
Anticholinergics: May have additive anticholinergic effects. Monitor patient closely.
Anticholinesterases: Decreases anticholinesterase effect. Anticholinesterase dosage may need to be increased.
Cimetidine: May increase procainamide level. Avoid this combination if possible. Monitor procainamide level closely and adjust the dose as necessary.
Lidocaine: additive cardiodepressant effects. Monitor ECG.
Neuromuscular skeletal muscle relaxants: Increases skeletal muscle relaxant effects. Monitor patient.
Propranolol, ranitidine: May increase procainamide level. Monitor patient for toxicity.
Quinidine, trimethoprim: May elevate procainamide and *N*-acetylprocainamide (NAPA) levels. Monitor patient for toxicity.
Drug-herb. *Jimson weed:* May adversely affect CV function. Discourage using together.
Licorice: May prolong QT interval and be additive. Discourage using together.

Effects on lab test results

- May increase ALT, AST, alkaline phosphatase, LDH, and bilirubin levels.
- May increase antinuclear antibody titer. May decrease hemoglobin, hematocrit, and neutrophil, granulocyte, and platelet counts.

Pharmacokinetics

Absorption: Usually 75% to 95% of P.O. dose. Unknown after I.M. use.
Distribution: Distributed widely in most body tissues, including CSF, liver, spleen, kidneys, lungs, muscles, brain, and heart. About 15% binds to proteins.
Metabolism: Metabolized in liver.
Excretion: Excreted in urine. *Half-life:* About 2½ to 4¾ hours.

Route	Onset	Peak	Duration
P.O.	2 hr	1-1½ hr	Unknown
I.V.	Immediate	Immediate	Unknown
I.M.	10-30 min	15-60 min	Unknown

Action

Chemical effect: Class Ia antiarrhythmic that decreases excitability, conduction velocity, automaticity, and membrane responsiveness with prolonged refractory period. Larger doses may induce AV block.
Therapeutic effect: Restores normal sinus rhythm.

Available forms

Capsules: 250 mg, 375 mg, 500 mg
Injection: 100 mg/ml, 500 mg/ml
Tablets: 250 mg, 375 mg, 500 mg
Tablets (extended-release): 500 mg, 1000 mg
Tablets (sustained-release): 250 mg, 500 mg, 750 mg

NURSING PROCESS

Assessment

- Assess patient's condition before therapy and regularly thereafter.
- Monitor levels of procainamide and its active metabolite, NAPA. To suppress ventricular arrhythmias, therapeutic level of procainamide is 4 to 8 mcg/ml; therapeutic level of NAPA is 10 to 30 mcg/ml.
- Monitor QT interval closely in patient with renal impairment.

- Hypokalemia predisposes patient to arrhythmias; monitor electrolytes, especially potassium level.
- Monitor blood pressure and ECG continuously during I.V. use. Watch for prolonged QT intervals and QRS complexes, heart block, or increased arrhythmias.
- Monitor CBC frequently during first 3 months, particularly in patient taking sustained-release form.
- Be alert for adverse reactions and drug interactions.
- Evaluate patient's and family's knowledge of drug therapy.

Nursing diagnoses

- Decreased cardiac output related to presence of arrhythmia
- Ineffective protection related to adverse hematologic reactions
- Deficient knowledge related to drug therapy

Planning and implementation

ALERT: Some drug products contain tartrazine and sulfites. Ask if patient is allergic to these agents.
ALERT: If blood pressure changes significantly or ECG changes occur, withhold drug, obtain rhythm strip, and notify prescriber immediately.
ALERT: Don't confuse procainamide with probenecid.

- Positive antinuclear antibody titer occurs in about 60% of patients without lupuslike symptoms. This response seems to be related to prolonged use, not to dosage. May progress to systemic lupus erythematosus if drug isn't stopped.

Patient teaching
- Instruct patient to report fever, rash, muscle pain, diarrhea, bleeding, bruises, or pleuritic chest pain.
- Stress importance of taking drug exactly as prescribed. This may require use of alarm clock for nighttime doses.
- Inform patient taking extended-release form that wax-matrix "ghost" from tablet may be passed in stool. Assure patient that drug is completely absorbed before this occurs.
- Tell patient not to crush or break sustained-release or extended-release tablets.

Evaluation

- Patient regains normal cardiac output after drug stops abnormal heart rhythm.

- Patient maintains normal CBC.
- Patient and family state understanding of drug therapy.

procarbazine hydrochloride
(proh-KAR-buh-zeen high-droh-KLOR-ighd)
Matulane, Natulan

Pharmacologic class: antibiotic antineoplastic (specific to S phase of cell cycle)
Therapeutic class: antineoplastic
Pregnancy risk category: D

Indications and dosages

▶ **Hodgkin's disease, lymphoma, brain and lung cancer.** *Adults:* 2 to 4 mg/kg P.O. daily in single dose or divided doses for first week. Then, 4 to 6 mg/kg daily until WBC count decreases to below 4,000/mm³ or platelet count decreases to below 100,000/mm³. If hematologic toxicity occurs, resume at 1 to 2 mg/kg daily. *Children:* 50 mg/m² P.O. daily for first week; then 100 mg/m² until response or toxicity occurs. Maintenance dosage is 50 mg/m² P.O. daily after bone marrow recovery.

Contraindications and precautions

- Contraindicated in patients hypersensitive to drug and those with inadequate bone marrow reserve as shown by bone marrow aspiration.
- Use cautiously in patients with impaired hepatic or renal function.
- ⚕ **Lifespan:** In pregnant and breast-feeding women, drug isn't recommended.

Adverse reactions

CNS: nervousness, depression, insomnia, nightmares, paresthesia, neuropathy, *hallucinations,* confusion, *seizures, coma.*
EENT: retinal hemorrhage, nystagmus, photophobia.
GI: *nausea, vomiting,* anorexia, stomatitis, dry mouth, dysphagia, diarrhea, constipation.
Hematologic: *bleeding tendency, thrombocytopenia, leukopenia,* anemia.
Hepatic: *hepatotoxicity.*
Respiratory: *pleural effusion,* pneumonitis.
Skin: dermatitis, reversible alopecia.

Interactions

Drug-drug. *CNS depressants:* May have additive depressant effects. Avoid using together.
Digoxin: May decrease digoxin level. Monitor level closely.
Levodopa: May cause flushing and a significant rise in blood pressure within 1 hour of levodopa use. Separate administration times; monitor patient's blood pressure closely.
Local anesthetics, sympathomimetics, tricyclic antidepressants: May cause tremors, palpitations, increased blood pressure. Monitor patient closely.
Opioids: May cause severe hypotension and death. Don't give together.
Drug-food. *Caffeine:* May result in arrhythmias, severe hypertension. Discourage caffeine intake.
Foods high in tyramine (cheese, red wine): May cause tremors, palpitations, and increased blood pressure. Monitor patient closely.
Drug-lifestyle. *Alcohol use:* May cause mild disulfiram-like reaction. Warn patient to avoid alcohol.

Effects on lab test results

- May increase liver enzyme levels.
- May increase eosinophil count. May decrease hemoglobin, hematocrit, and platelet, WBC, and RBC counts.

Pharmacokinetics

Absorption: Rapid and complete.
Distribution: Distributes widely into body tissues, with highest levels in liver, kidneys, intestinal wall, and skin. Drug crosses blood-brain barrier.
Metabolism: Extensively metabolized in liver; some metabolites have cytotoxic activity.
Excretion: Drug and metabolites excreted primarily in urine. *Half-life:* About 10 minutes.

Route	Onset	Peak	Duration
P.O.	Unknown	Unknown	Unknown

Action

Chemical effect: Unknown; thought to inhibit DNA, RNA, and protein synthesis.
Therapeutic effect: Kills selected cancer cells.

Available forms

Capsules: 50 mg

NURSING PROCESS

⚡ Assessment
- Assess patient's condition before therapy and regularly thereafter.
- Monitor CBC and platelet counts.
- Be alert for adverse reactions and drug interactions.
- Evaluate patient's and family's knowledge of drug therapy.

⊞ Nursing diagnoses
- Ineffective health maintenance related to presence of neoplastic disease
- Ineffective protection related to adverse hematologic reactions
- Deficient knowledge related to drug therapy

▶ Planning and implementation
- Give drug h.s. to lessen nausea.
- ⊛ ALERT: If patient becomes confused or if paresthesia or other neuropathies develop, stop drug and notify prescriber.

Patient teaching
- Advise patient to take drug h.s. and in divided doses.
- Warn patient to watch for signs of infection (fever, sore throat, fatigue) and bleeding (easy bruising, nosebleeds, bleeding gums, melena). Tell him to take his temperature daily.
- Warn patient to avoid alcohol during drug therapy.
- Tell patient to stop drug and check with prescriber immediately if disulfiram-like reaction occurs (chest pains, rapid or irregular heartbeat, severe headache, stiff neck).
- Warn patient to avoid hazardous activities until CNS effects of drug are known.
- Advise woman of childbearing age not to become pregnant during therapy and to consult with prescriber before becoming pregnant.

✓ Evaluation
- Patient responds well to therapy.
- Patient develops no serious adverse hematologic reactions.
- Patient and family state understanding of drug therapy.

prochlorperazine
(proh-klor-PER-ah-zeen)
**Compazine, PMS Prochlorperazine ♦,
Prorazin ♦, Stemetil ♦**

prochlorperazine edisylate
**Compa-Z, Compazine Syrup, Cotranzine,
Ultrazine-10**

prochlorperazine maleate
**Anti-Naus ♦, Compazine Spansule, PMS
Prochlorperazine ♦, Prorazin, Stemetil**

Pharmacologic class: phenothiazine (piperazine derivative)
Therapeutic class: antipsychotic, antiemetic, anxiolytic
Pregnancy risk category: NR

Indications and dosages

▶ **Preoperative nausea control.** *Adults:* 5 to 10 mg I.M. 1 to 2 hours before induction of anesthesia; repeat once in 30 minutes, if necessary. Or, 5 to 10 mg I.V. 15 to 30 minutes before induction of anesthesia; repeat once if necessary. Or, 20 mg/L D_5W or normal saline solution by I.V. infusion. Begin infusion 15 to 30 minutes before induction of anesthesia.
▶ **Severe nausea and vomiting.** *Adults:* 5 to 10 mg P.O., t.i.d., or q.i.d. Or, 15 mg P.O. (sustained-release) on arising. Or, 10-mg sustained-release form P.O. q 12 hours. Or, 25 mg P.R., b.i.d. Or, 5 to 10 mg I.M. repeated q 3 to 4 hours, p.r.n. Or, 5 to 10 mg may be given I.V. Maximum parenteral dosage is 40 mg daily.
Children weighing 18 to 39 kg (39 to 86 lb): 2.5 mg P.O. or P.R., t.i.d. Or, 5 mg P.O. or P.R., b.i.d. Maximum dosage is 15 mg daily. Or, give 0.132 mg/kg by deep I.M. injection. Control usually is obtained with one dose.
Children weighing 14 to 17 kg (31 to 38 lb): 2.5 mg P.O. or P.R., b.i.d. or t.i.d. Maximum dosage, 10 mg daily. Or give 0.132 mg/kg by deep I.M. injection. Control usually is obtained with one dose.
Children weighing 9 to 14 kg (20 to 30 lb): 2.5 mg P.O. or P.R. once daily or b.i.d. Maximum dosage is 7.5 mg daily. Or give 0.132 mg/kg by deep I.M. injection. Control usually is obtained with one dose.

▶ **To manage symptoms of psychotic disorders.** *Adults:* 5 to 10 mg P.O., t.i.d. or q.i.d. *Children ages 2 to 12:* 2.5 mg P.O. or P.R., b.i.d. or t.i.d. Don't exceed 10 mg on day 1. Increase dosage gradually to recommended maximum, if necessary. In children ages 2 to 5, maximum daily dosage is 20 mg. In children ages 6 to 12, maximum daily dosage is 25 mg.

▶ **To manage symptoms of severe psychoses.** *Adults:* 10 to 20 mg I.M. repeated in 1 to 4 hours, if needed. Rarely, patients may require 10 to 20 mg q 4 to 6 hours. Institute P.O. therapy after symptoms are controlled.

▶ **Nonpsychotic anxiety.** *Adults:* 5 to 10 mg by deep I.M. injection q 3 to 4 hours, not to exceed 40 mg daily; or 5 to 10 mg P.O., t.i.d., or q.i.d. Or, give 15-mg extended-release capsule once daily or 10-mg extended-release capsule q 12 hours.

▼ I.V. administration

• Drug may be given undiluted or diluted in an isotonic solution.
• Don't give faster than 5 mg/minute. Don't give by bolus injection.

Contraindications and precautions

• Contraindicated in patients hypersensitive to phenothiazines, patients with CNS depression (including coma), patients undergoing pediatric surgery, patients taking adrenergic blockers, and patients under the influence of alcohol.
• Use cautiously in patients who have been exposed to extreme heat and patients with impaired CV function, glaucoma, or seizure disorders.
⚠ Lifespan: In pregnant women, safety of drug hasn't been established. In breast-feeding women and acutely ill children, use cautiously. In children younger than age 2 and weighing less than 9 kg (20 lb), drug is contraindicated. In geriatric patients, use cautiously with gradual increases in dosage.

Adverse reactions

CNS: *extrapyramidal reactions,* sedation, pseudoparkinsonism, EEG changes, dizziness.
CV: *orthostatic hypotension,* tachycardia, ECG changes.
EENT: *ocular changes, blurred vision.*
GI: *dry mouth, constipation.*

GU: *urine retention,* dark urine, menstrual irregularities, inhibited ejaculation.
Hematologic: hyperprolactinemia, *transient leukopenia, agranulocytosis.*
Hepatic: cholestatic jaundice.
Metabolic: weight gain, increased appetite.
Skin: *mild photosensitivity,* exfoliative dermatitis.
Other: allergic reactions, gynecomastia.

Interactions

Drug-drug. *Antacids:* Inhibits absorption of oral phenothiazines. Separate antacid doses by at least 2 hours.
Anticholinergics, including antidepressants and antiparkinsonian drugs: Increases anticholinergic activity and aggravated parkinsonian symptoms. Use together cautiously.
Barbiturates: May decrease phenothiazine effect. Monitor patient for decreased effect.
Lithium: May cause disorientation, unconsciousness, and extrapyramidal symptoms. Monitor patient closely.
Drug-herb. *Dong quai, St. John's wort:* Increases photosensitivity reactions. Discourage using together.
Ginkgo: May decrease effects of phenothiazines. Monitor patient.
Kava: Increases risk of dystonic reactions. Discourage using together.
Milk thistle: Decreases liver toxicity caused by phenothiazines. Monitor liver enzyme levels if used together.
Yohimbe: Increases risk for yohimbe toxicity when used together. Discourage using together.
Drug-lifestyle. *Alcohol use:* May increase CNS depression, particularly psychomotor skills. Strongly discourage alcohol use.
Sun exposure: Potential photosensitivity reaction. Urge patient to avoid unprotected or prolonged sun exposure.

Effects on lab test results

• May decrease WBC and granulocyte counts. May alter liver function test results.

Pharmacokinetics

Absorption: Erratic and variable with P.O. tablet; more predictable with P.O. concentrate. Unknown for P.R. use. Rapid for I.M. use.
Distribution: Distributed widely into body; 91% to 99% protein-bound.

Metabolism: Metabolized extensively by liver, but no active metabolites are formed.
Excretion: Excreted primarily in urine; some excreted in feces. *Half-life:* Unknown.

Route	Onset	Peak	Duration
P.O.	30-40 min	Unknown	3-12 hr
I.V.	Immediate	Immediate	Unknown
I.M.	10-20 min	Unknown	3-4 hr
P.R.	60 min	Unknown	3-4 hr

Action

Chemical effect: Acts on chemoreceptor trigger zone to inhibit nausea and vomiting; in larger doses, partially depresses vomiting center.
Therapeutic effect: Relieves nausea and vomiting, signs and symptoms of psychosis, and anxiety.

Available forms

prochlorperazine
Injection: 5 mg/ml
Suppositories: 2.5 mg, 5 mg, 25 mg
Tablets: 5 mg, 10 mg
prochlorperazine edisylate
Syrup: 1 mg/ml
prochlorperazine maleate
Capsules (sustained-release): 10 mg, 15 mg, 30 mg
Tablets: 5 mg, 10 mg, 25 mg

NURSING PROCESS

Assessment
• Assess patient's condition before therapy and regularly thereafter.
• Watch for orthostatic hypotension, especially when giving drug I.V.
• Monitor CBC and liver function test results during prolonged therapy.
• Be alert for adverse reactions and drug interactions.
• Evaluate patient's and family's knowledge of drug therapy.

Nursing diagnoses
• Risk for deficient fluid volume related to nausea and vomiting
• Disturbed thought processes related to presence of psychosis
• Deficient knowledge related to drug therapy

Planning and implementation
• Dilute solution with tomato or fruit juice, milk, coffee, carbonated beverage, tea, water, or soup; or mix with pudding.
• Inject I.M. deep into upper outer quadrant of gluteal region.
• Don't give S.C. or mix in syringe with another drug.
• Avoid getting concentrate or injection solution on hands or clothing.
• Drug is used only if vomiting can't be otherwise controlled or if only a few doses are needed. If more than four doses are needed in 24 hours, notify prescriber.
• Store drug in light-resistant container. Slight yellowing doesn't affect potency; discard extremely discolored solutions.
Patient teaching
• Tell patient to mix oral solution with flavored liquid to mask taste.
• Advise patient to wear protective clothing when exposed to sunlight.
• Tell patient to notify prescriber about adverse reactions.

Evaluation
• Patient's nausea and vomiting are relieved.
• Patient's behavior and communication show better thought processes.
• Patient and family state understanding of drug therapy.

progesterone
(proh-JES-teh-rohn)
Crinone 4%, Crinone 8%, Gesterol 50, PMS-Progesterone ◆, Progestasert, Prometrium

Pharmacologic class: progestin
Therapeutic class: hormone
Pregnancy risk category: D (injection); B (capsules); NR (gel)

Indications and dosages
▶ **Amenorrhea.** *Adults:* 5 to 10 mg I.M. daily for 6 to 8 days usually beginning 8 to 10 days before anticipated start of menstruation.
▶ **Secondary amenorrhea.** *Adults:* 400 mg P.O. in the evening for 10 days. Or, Crinone 4% gel given intravaginally q other day up to 6 doses. Those who fail may try Crinone 8% gel given intravaginally q other day up to 6 doses.

▶ **Prevention of endometrial hyperplasia.**
Adult women with intact uterus: 200 mg P.O. in the evening for 12 contiguous days per 28-day cycle, given with conjugated estrogen tablets.
▶ **Dysfunctional uterine bleeding.** *Adults:* 5 to 10 mg I.M. daily for six doses.
▶ **Contraception (with an intrauterine device).** *Adults:* Progestasert system inserted into uterine cavity; replaced annually.
▶ **Infertility.** *Adults:* 90 mg gel given intravaginally daily to b.i.d. May use up to 10 to 12 weeks after pregnancy to maintain placental autonomy.

Contraindications and precautions

• Contraindicated in patients hypersensitive to drug; in patients with thromboembolic disorders, cerebral apoplexy, or a history of these conditions; and in patients with breast cancer, undiagnosed abnormal vaginal bleeding, severe hepatic disease, or missed abortion.
• Use cautiously in patients with diabetes mellitus, seizure disorder, migraine, cardiac or renal disease, asthma, and depression.
⚕ Lifespan: In pregnant women, drug is contraindicated. In breast-feeding women, use cautiously. Drug appears in breast milk. In children, safety of drug hasn't been established.

Adverse reactions

CNS: dizziness, migraine, lethargy, depression.
CV: hypertension, thrombophlebitis, *thromboembolism, pulmonary embolism, CVA,* edema.
GI: nausea, vomiting, abdominal cramps.
GU: breakthrough bleeding, dysmenorrhea, amenorrhea, cervical erosion, abnormal secretions, uterine fibromas, vaginal candidiasis.
Hepatic: cholestatic jaundice.
Metabolic: hyperglycemia.
Skin: melasma, rash.
Other: breast tenderness, enlargement, or secretion; decreased libido; pain at injection site.

Interactions

Drug-drug. *Barbiturates, carbamazepine, rifampin:* Decreases progestin effects. Avoid using together.
Bromocriptine: May cause amenorrhea. Monitor patient.

Effects on lab test results

• May increase glucose level.

• May increase liver function test values. May decrease pregnanediol excretion. May alter thyroid function test results.

Pharmacokinetics

Absorption: Rapidly absorbed orally and intramuscularly; absorption is prolonged for gel form.
Distribution: Gel form is extensively (96 to 99%) protein bound.
Metabolism: Metabolized in liver.
Excretion: Excreted in mostly in urine. *Half-life:* Few minutes for I.M., 2 to 9 hours for P.O., and 5 to 20 hours for intravaginal gel.

Route	Onset	Peak	Duration
P.O.	Unknown	1-2 hr	Unknown
I.M.	Unknown	24 hr	Unknown
Intra-vaginal	Unknown	3-6 hr	Unknown

Action

Chemical effect: Suppresses ovulation and forms thick cervical mucus.
Therapeutic effect: Alleviates amenorrhea and dysfunctional uterine bleeding.

Available forms

Capsules: 100 mg
Gel: 4%, 8%
Injection (in oil): 50 mg/ml
IUD: 38 mg (with barium sulfate, dispersed in silicone fluid)

NURSING PROCESS

⚕ Assessment
• Assess patient's condition before therapy and regularly thereafter.
• Be alert for adverse reactions and drug interactions.
• Evaluate patient's and family's knowledge of drug therapy.

⚕ Nursing diagnoses
• Risk for deficient fluid volume related to excessive uterine bleeding
• Risk for injury related to dizziness
• Deficient knowledge related to drug therapy

▶ Planning and implementation
• Preliminary estrogen treatment is usually needed in menstrual disorders.

• Give peanut or sesame oil solutions by deep I.M. injection. Check sites frequently for irritation. Rotate injection sites.

Patient teaching
• Tell patient not to perform hazardous activities if dizziness occurs.
• Tell patient to report any unusual symptoms immediately and to stop drug and call prescriber if visual disturbances or migraine occurs.
• Teach patient how to perform routine breast self-examination.

☑ Evaluation
• Patient's uterine bleeding ceases.
• Patient doesn't experience injury from drug-induced dizziness.
• Patient and family state understanding of drug therapy.

promethazine hydrochloride
(proh-METH-uh-zeen high-droh-KLOR-ighd)
Anergan 50, Phenergan*

promethazine theoclate
Avomine ◇

Pharmacologic class: phenothiazine derivative
Therapeutic class: antiemetic, antivertigo drug, antihistamine (H_1-receptor antagonist), sedative
Pregnancy risk category: C

Indications and dosages

▶ **Motion sickness.** *Adults:* 25 mg P.O. or P.R. b.i.d. Take initial dose 30 to 60 minutes before anticipated travel and repeat in 8 to 12 hours, if needed.
Children older than age 2: 12.5 to 25 mg P.O. or P.R. b.i.d.
▶ **Nausea and vomiting.** *Adults:* 12.5 to 25 mg P.O., I.M., or P.R. q 4 to 6 hours, p.r.n.
Children older than age 2: 12.5 to 25 mg P.O. or P.R. q 4 to 6 hours, p.r.n. Or, 6.25 to 12.5 mg I.M. q 4 to 6 hours, p.r.n.
▶ **Rhinitis, allergy symptoms.** *Adults:* 12.5 mg P.O. or P.R. q.i.d. (before meals and h.s.). Or, 25 mg P.O. or P.R. h.s.
Children older than age 2: 6.25 to 12.5 mg P.O. or P.R. t.i.d. Or, 25 mg P.O. or P.R. h.s.
▶ **Sedation.** *Adults:* 25 to 50 mg P.O., P.R., or I.M. h.s. or p.r.n.

Children older than age 2: 12.5 to 25 mg P.O., I.M., or P.R. h.s.
▶ **Routine preoperative or postoperative sedation or adjunct to analgesics.** *Adults:* 25 to 50 mg I.M., I.V., P.R., or P.O.
Children older than age 2: 0.5 to 1.1 mg/kg I.M., P.R., or P.O.

▼ I.V. administration
• Don't give in concentration greater than 25 mg/ml or at rate exceeding 25 mg/minute.
• Shield I.V. infusion from direct light.

Contraindications and precautions
• Contraindicated in patients hypersensitive to drug and in those with intestinal obstruction, prostatic hyperplasia, bladder-neck obstruction, seizure disorders, coma, CNS depression, or stenosing peptic ulcerations.
• Use cautiously in patients with pulmonary, hepatic, or CV disease or asthma.
⚜ **Lifespan:** In pregnant women, safety of drug hasn't been established. In breast-feeding women, neonates, premature neonates, and acutely ill or dehydrated children, drug is contraindicated. Don't use in children for nausea and vomiting when the etiology of the vomiting is unknown. In children younger than age 2, tablets and suppositories aren't recommended. In elderly patients, use cautiously.

Adverse reactions
CNS: *sedation,* confusion, restlessness, tremors, *drowsiness* (especially geriatric patients).
CV: hypotension, EKG changes.
EENT: transient myopia, nasal congestion.
GI: anorexia, nausea, vomiting, constipation, *dry mouth.*
GU: urine retention.
Hematologic: *leukopenia, agranulocytosis, thrombocytopenia.*
Skin: photosensitivity, venous thrombosis at injection site.

Interactions
Drug-drug. *CNS depressants:* Increases sedation. Use together cautiously.
Epinephrine: Promethazine may block or reverse effects of epinephrine. Use another vasopressor.
Levodopa: Promethazine may decrease antiparkinsonian action of levodopa. Avoid using together.

Lithium: Promethazine may reduce GI absorption or enhance renal elimination of lithium. Avoid using together.
MAO inhibitors: Increases extrapyramidal effects. Don't use together.
Protease inhibitors, SSRIs: Increases levels of these drugs and causes serious adverse cardiac effects. Don't use together.
Drug-herb. *Dong quai, St. John's wort:* Increases photosensitivity reactions. Discourage using together.
Kava: Increases risk of dystonic reactions. Discourage using together.
Yohimbe: Increases risk for yohimbe toxicity when used together. Discourage using together.
Drug-lifestyle. *Alcohol use:* Increases sedation. Discourage using together.
Sun exposure: May cause photosensitivity reaction. Urge patient to avoid unprotected or prolonged sun exposure.

Effects on lab test results

• May increase glucose levels.
• May increase hemoglobin and hematocrit. May decrease WBC, platelet, and granulocyte counts.
• May cause false-positive immunologic urine pregnancy test using Gravindex and false-negative results using Prepurex or Dap tests. May interfere with blood typing of ABO group.

Pharmacokinetics

Absorption: Well absorbed after P.O. use; fairly rapid after P.R. or I.M. use.
Distribution: Distributed widely throughout body.
Metabolism: Metabolized in liver.
Excretion: Excreted in urine and feces. *Half-life:* Unknown.

Route	Onset	Peak	Duration
P.O.	15-60 min	Unknown	≤ 12 hr
I.V.	3-5 min	Unknown	≤ 12 hr
I.M., P.R.	20 min	Unknown	≤ 12 hr

Action

Chemical effect: Competes with histamine for H_1-receptor sites on effector cells. Prevents, but doesn't reverse, histamine-mediated responses.
Therapeutic effect: Prevents motion sickness and relieves nausea, nasal congestion, and allergy symptoms. Also promotes calmness.

Available forms

promethazine hydrochloride
Injection: 25 mg/ml, 50 mg/ml (I.M. use only)
Suppositories: 12.5 mg, 25 mg, 50 mg
Syrup: 6.25 mg/5 ml*
Tablets: 12.5 mg, 25 mg, 50 mg
promethazine theoclate
Tablets: 25 mg†

NURSING PROCESS

⚕ Assessment

• Assess patient's condition before therapy and regularly thereafter.
• Be alert for adverse reactions and drug interactions.
• Evaluate patient's and family's knowledge of drug therapy.

⊞ Nursing diagnoses

• Ineffective health maintenance related to underlying condition
• Risk for injury related to drug's sedating effects
• Deficient knowledge related to drug therapy

❱ Planning and implementation

• Pronounced sedative effect limits use in many ambulatory patients.
• Drug is used as adjunct to analgesics (usually to increase sedation); it has no analgesic activity.
• Give drug with food or milk to reduce GI distress.
• **ALERT:** Phenergan ampules contain sulfite.
• Inject I.M. deep into large muscle mass. Rotate injection sites.
• Don't give S.C.
• Drug may be safely mixed with meperidine (Demerol) in same syringe.
• In patient scheduled for myelogram, stop drug 48 hours before procedure and don't resume drug until 24 hours after procedure because of risk of seizures.
Patient teaching
• When treating for motion sickness, tell patient to take first dose 30 to 60 minutes before travel. On succeeding days of travel, he should take dose after rising and with evening meal.
• Warn patient to avoid alcohol and hazardous activities until drug's CNS effects are known.
• Tell patient that coffee or tea may reduce drowsiness. Sugarless gum, sugarless sour hard candy, or ice chips may relieve dry mouth.

- Warn patient about photosensitivity and precautions to avoid it.
- Advise patient to stop drug 4 days before allergy skin tests.

☑ **Evaluation**
- Patient responds well to therapy.
- Patient doesn't experience injury from adverse reactions.
- Patient and family state understanding of drug therapy.

propafenone hydrochloride
(proh-puh-FEE-nohn high-droh-KLOR-ighd)
Rythmol

Pharmacologic class: sodium channel antagonist
Therapeutic class: antiarrhythmic (class IC)
Pregnancy risk category: C

Indications and dosages

▶ **Suppression of life-threatening ventricular arrhythmias, such as sustained ventricular tachycardia.** *Adults:* Initially, 150 mg P.O. q 8 hours. Dosage may be increased at 3- to 4-day intervals to 225 mg q 8 hours. If necessary, increase dosage to 300 mg q 8 hours. Maximum daily dosage is 900 mg.

⃠ **Adjust-a-dose:** For patients with hepatic failure, manufacturer recommends dosage reduction of 20% to 30%.

Contraindications and precautions

- Contraindicated in patients hypersensitive to drug and in those with severe or uncontrolled heart failure, cardiogenic shock, bradycardia, marked hypotension, bronchospastic disorders, electrolyte imbalance, or SA, AV, or intraventricular disorders of impulse conduction in absence of pacemaker.
- Use cautiously in patients with heart failure because propafenone can have negative inotropic effect. Also use cautiously in patients taking other cardiac depressant drugs and in those with hepatic or renal impairment.
- ⚘ **Lifespan:** In pregnant women, safety of drug hasn't been established. In breast-feeding women, drug isn't recommended. In children, safety of drug hasn't been established.

Adverse reactions

CNS: anxiety, ataxia, dizziness, drowsiness, fatigue, headache, insomnia, syncope, tremor, weakness.
CV: atrial fibrillation, *bradycardia,* bundle branch block, *heart failure,* chest pain, edema, first-degree AV block, hypotension, increased QRS duration, intraventricular conduction delay, palpitations, *proarrhythmic events (ventricular tachycardia, PVCs).*
EENT: blurred vision.
GI: abdominal pain or cramps, constipation, diarrhea, dyspepsia, flatulence, nausea, vomiting, dry mouth, unusual taste, anorexia.
Musculoskeletal: joint pain.
Respiratory: dyspnea.
Skin: rash, diaphoresis.

Interactions

Drug-drug. *Antiarrhythmics:* Increases risk of heart failure. Monitor patient closely.
Cimetidine: Decreases metabolism of propafenone. Monitor patient for toxicity.
Digoxin, oral anticoagulants: Propafenone may increase levels of these drugs by about 35% to 85%, resulting in toxicity. Monitor patient closely.
Local anesthetics: Increases risk of CNS toxicity. Monitor patient closely.
Metoprolol, propranolol: Propafenone slows metabolism of these drugs. Monitor patient for toxicity.
Quinidine: Slows propafenone metabolism. Avoid using together.
Rifampin: Increases propafenone clearance. Monitor patient for lack of effect.

Effects on lab test results

None reported.

Pharmacokinetics

Absorption: Well absorbed from GI tract. Because of significant first-pass effect, bioavailability is limited; however, it increases with dosage.
Distribution: 97% protein-bound.
Metabolism: Metabolized in liver.
Excretion: Excreted mainly in feces; some in urine. *Half-life:* 2 to 32 hours.

Route	Onset	Peak	Duration
P.O.	Unknown	≤ 3½ hr	Unknown

Reactions may be *common*, uncommon, *life-threatening*, or COMMON AND LIFE-THREATENING.

Action

Chemical effect: Reduces inward sodium current in Purkinje and myocardial cells. Decreases excitability, conduction velocity, and automaticity in AV nodal, His-Purkinje, and intraventricular tissue; causes slight but significant prolongation of refractory period in AV nodal tissue.
Therapeutic effect: Restores normal sinus rhythm.

Available forms

Tablets: 150 mg, 225 mg, 300 mg

NURSING PROCESS

▩ Assessment

• Assess patient's condition before therapy and regularly thereafter.
• Continuous cardiac monitoring is recommended at start of therapy and during dosage adjustments.
• Be alert for adverse reactions and drug interactions.
• Evaluate patient's and family's knowledge of drug therapy.

▩ Nursing diagnoses

• Decreased cardiac output related to presence of arrhythmia
• Ineffective protection related to drug-induced proarrhythmias
• Deficient knowledge related to drug therapy

▶ Planning and implementation

• Give drug with food to minimize adverse GI reactions.
⊛ ALERT: If PR interval or QRS complex increases by more than 25%, notify prescriber because reduction in dosage may be necessary.
• During use with digoxin, monitor ECG and digoxin level frequently.
Patient teaching
• Tell patient to take drug with food.
• Stress importance of taking drug exactly as ordered.
• Warn patient to avoid hazardous activities if adverse CNS disturbances occur.

▨ Evaluation

• Patient regains adequate cardiac output when arrhythmia is corrected.
• Patient doesn't develop any proarrhythmic events.

• Patient and family state understanding of drug therapy.

propoxyphene hydrochloride (dextropropoxyphene hydrochloride)
(proh-POK-sih-feen high-droh-KLOR-ighd)
Darvon, 642 ♦

propoxyphene napsylate (dextropropoxyphene napsylate)
Darvon-N

Pharmacologic class: opioid
Therapeutic class: analgesic
Pregnancy risk category: C
Controlled substance schedule: IV

Indications and dosages

▶ **Mild to moderate pain.** *Adults:* 65 mg propoxyphene hydrochloride P.O. q 4 hours p.r.n. Maximum, 390 mg P.O. daily. Or, 100 mg propoxyphene napsylate P.O. q 4 hours p.r.n. Maximum, 600 mg P.O. daily.

Contraindications and precautions

• Contraindicated in patients hypersensitive to drug and in patients who are suicidal or addiction-prone.
• Use cautiously in patients with hepatic or renal disease, emotional instability, or history of drug or alcohol abuse.
⚖ **Lifespan:** In pregnant and breast-feeding women, use cautiously. In children, safety of drug hasn't been established.

Adverse reactions

CNS: *dizziness,* headache, *sedation,* euphoria, paradoxical excitement, insomnia.
GI: nausea, vomiting, constipation.
Respiratory: *respiratory depression.*
Other: psychological and physical dependence.

Interactions

Drug-drug. *Barbiturate anesthetics:* May increase respiratory and CNS depression. Use together cautiously.
Carbamazepine: May increase carbamazepine levels. Monitor levels closely.

CNS depressants: May have additive effects. Use together cautiously.
Protease inhibitors: May increase CNS and respiratory depression. Monitor patient.
Warfarin: Increases anticoagulant effect. Monitor PT and INR and patient for bleeding.
Drug-lifestyle. *Alcohol use:* May have additive effects. Discourage using together.

Effects on lab test results

• May increase or decrease liver function test values.

Pharmacokinetics

Absorption: Absorbed primarily in upper small intestine.
Distribution: Drug enters CSF.
Metabolism: Metabolized in liver; about one-quarter of dose is metabolized to norpropoxyphene, an active metabolite.
Excretion: Excreted in urine. *Half-life:* 6 to 12 hours.

Route	Onset	Peak	Duration
P.O.	15-60 min	2-2½ hr	4-6 hr

Action

Chemical effect: Binds with opioid receptors in CNS, altering both perception of and emotional response to pain through unknown mechanism.
Therapeutic effect: Relieves pain.

Available forms

propoxyphene hydrochloride
Capsules: 65 mg
propoxyphene napsylate
Tablets: 50 mg, 100 mg

NURSING PROCESS

⚕ Assessment

• Assess patient's pain before and after giving drug.
• Be alert for adverse reactions and drug interactions.
• If adverse GI reactions occur, monitor patient's hydration.
• Evaluate patient's and family's knowledge of drug therapy.

🔷 Nursing diagnoses

• Acute pain related to underlying condition

• Risk for deficient fluid volume related to GI reactions
• Deficient knowledge related to drug therapy

▶ Planning and implementation

• Give with food to minimize adverse GI reactions.
• Drug can be considered a mild opioid analgesic, but pain relief is equivalent to that provided by aspirin. Tolerance and physical dependence have been observed. Typically used with aspirin or acetaminophen to maximize analgesia.
⚠ **ALERT:** A dose of 65 mg of propoxyphene hydrochloride equals 100 mg of propoxyphene napsylate.
• Drug may cause false decreases in urinary steroid excretion tests.
Patient teaching
• Advise patient to take drug with food or milk to minimize GI upset.
• Warn patient not to exceed recommended dosage. Respiratory depression, hypotension, profound sedation, and coma may result if used in excessive amounts or with other CNS depressants. Propoxyphene-containing products alone or with other drugs are major cause of drug-related overdose and death.
• Advise patient to avoid alcohol during drug therapy.
• Warn ambulatory patient about getting out of bed or walking. Warn outpatient to avoid driving and other hazardous activities until drug's CNS effects are known.

☑ Evaluation

• Patient is free from pain.
• Patient maintains adequate hydration.
• Patient and family state understanding of drug therapy.

propranolol hydrochloride
(proh-PRAH-nuh-lohl high-droh-KLOR-ighd)
Apo-Propranolol ◆, Detensol ◆, Inderal, Inderal LA, InnoPran XL, Novopranol ◆, PMS Propranolol ◆

Pharmacologic class: beta blocker
Therapeutic class: antihypertensive, antianginal, antiarrhythmic, adjunct therapy for migraine, adjunct therapy for MI
Pregnancy risk category: C

Indications and dosages

▶ **Angina pectoris.** *Adults:* Total daily doses of 80 to 320 mg P.O. when given b.i.d., t.i.d., or q.i.d. Or one 80-mg extended-release capsule daily. Dosage increased at 7- to 10-day intervals.

▶ **Mortality reduction after MI.** *Adults:* 180 to 240 mg P.O. daily in divided doses beginning 5 to 21 days after MI. Usually given t.i.d. or q.i.d.

▶ **Supraventricular, ventricular, and atrial arrhythmias; tachyarrhythmias caused by excessive catecholamine action during anesthesia.** *Adults:* 0.5 to 3 mg by slow I.V. push, not to exceed 1 mg/minute. After 3 mg have been given, another dose may be given in 2 minutes; subsequent doses, no sooner than q 4 hours. May be diluted and infused slowly. Usual maintenance dosage is 10 to 30 mg P.O. t.i.d. to q.i.d.
Children‡: 0.01 to 0.1 mg/kg I.V. to a maximum of 1 mg/dose by slow infusion over 5 minutes.

▶ **Hypertension.** *Adults:* Initially, 80 mg P.O. daily in two to four divided doses or extended-release form once daily. Increase at 3- to 7-day intervals to maximum daily dosage of 640 mg. Usual maintenance dosage is 120 to 240 mg daily in two or three divided doses or 120 to 160 mg sustained-release once daily. Or, 80 mg InnoPran XL P.O. once daily h.s. Take consistently with or without food. Adjust to maximum of 120 mg daily if needed.
Children‡: 1 mg/kg P.O. daily, up to a maximum daily dose of 16 mg/kg.

▶ **Prevention of frequent, severe, uncontrollable, or disabling migraine or vascular headache.** *Adults:* Initially, 80 mg P.O. daily in divided doses or one extended-release capsule daily. Usual maintenance dosage is 160 to 240 mg daily.

▶ **Essential tremor.** *Adults:* 40 mg (tablets, solution) P.O. b.i.d. Usual maintenance dosage is 120 to 320 mg daily in three divided doses.

▶ **Hypertrophic subaortic stenosis.** *Adults:* 10 to 20 mg P.O. t.i.d. or q.i.d. before meals and h.s or 80 to 160 mg extended-release capsule daily.

▶ **Adjunct therapy in pheochromocytoma.** *Adults:* 60 mg P.O. daily in divided doses with alpha-adrenergic blocker 3 days before surgery.

▶ **Adjunctive treatment to anxiety‡.** *Adults:* 10 to 80 mg P.O. 1 hour before anxiety-provoking activity.

▼ I.V. administration

● Give drug by direct injection into large vessel or I.V. line containing free-flowing, compatible solution; continuous I.V. infusion generally isn't recommended.

● Or, dilute drug with normal saline solution and give by intermittent infusion over 10 to 15 minutes in 0.1- to 0.2-mg increments.

● Drug is compatible with D_5W, half-normal and normal saline solutions, and lactated Ringer's solution.

Contraindications and precautions

● Contraindicated in patients with bronchial asthma, sinus bradycardia, heart block greater than first-degree, cardiogenic shock, or overt cardiac failure (unless failure is secondary to tachyarrhythmia that can be treated with propranolol).

● Use cautiously in patients taking other antihypertensives and in those with renal impairment, nonallergic bronchospastic diseases, Wolff-Parkinson-White syndrome, hepatic disease, diabetes mellitus (drug blocks some symptoms of hypoglycemia), or thyrotoxicosis (drug may mask some signs of that disorder).

 Lifespan: In pregnant women, use cautiously. In breast-feeding women, drug isn't recommended. In children, safety of drug hasn't been established.

Adverse reactions

CNS: *fatigue, lethargy,* vivid dreams, fever, hallucinations, mental depression, dizziness (InnoPran XL).
CV: *bradycardia, hypotension, heart failure,* intermittent claudication.
GI: nausea, vomiting, diarrhea, constipation (InnoPran XL).
Hematologic: *agranulocytosis.*
Musculoskeletal: arthralgia.
Respiratory: increased airway resistance.
Skin: rash.

Interactions

Drug-drug. *Aminophylline, theophylline:* May act antagonistically reducing the effects of one or both drugs. The elimination of theophylline may also be reduced. Monitor theophylline levels and patient closely.
Amobarbital, aprobarbital, butabarbital, butalbital, mephobarbital, pentobarbital, phenobarbital, primidone, secobarbital: May reduce the

---

Rapid onset   *Liquid form contains alcohol.   ◆Canada   ◇Australia   †OTC   ‡Off-label use

effects of propranolol. Consider an increased beta blocker dose.

Cimetidine: May increase the pharmacologic effects of beta blocker. Consider a different H$_2$-agonist or decrease the dose of beta blocker.

Digoxin, diltiazem, verapamil: May cause hypotension, bradycardia, and increased depressant effect on myocardium. Use together cautiously.

Epinephrine: May cause an initial hypertensive episode followed by bradycardia. Stop the beta blocker 3 days before anticipated epinephrine use. Monitor patient closely.

Glucagon, isoproterenol: Antagonizes propranolol effect. May be used therapeutically and in emergencies.

Hydralazine: May increase levels and pharmacologic effects of both drugs. Monitor patient closely. Dosage adjustment of either drug may be necessary.

Oral antidiabetics: Can alter requirements for these drugs in previously stabilized diabetic patients. Monitor patient for hypoglycemia.

Insulin: May mask symptoms of hypoglycemia as a result of beta blockade (such as tachycardia). Use cautiously in patients with diabetes.

Lidocaine I.V.: May reduce hepatic metabolism of lidocaine, increasing the risk of toxicity. Give bolus doses of lidocaine at a slower rate and monitor lidocaine levels closely.

Prazosin: May increase the risk of orthostatic hypotension in the early phases of use together. Assist patient to stand slowly until effects are known.

Verapamil: May increase the effects of both drugs. Monitor cardiac function closely and decrease dosages as necessary.

Drug-herb. *Ginkgo:* May alter drug level. Discourage use of herb.

Melatonin: Can reverse the negative effects of drug on nocturnal sleep. Advise patient to discuss use with prescriber.

Drug-lifestyle. *Cocaine use:* Increases angina-inducing potential of cocaine. Inform patient of this potentially dangerous combination.

Effects on lab test results

• May increase BUN, transaminase, alkaline phosphatase, and LDH levels.
• May decrease granulocyte count.

Pharmacokinetics

Absorption: Almost complete. Absorption is enhanced when given with food. Food increases the lag time and the time to maximum concentration of InnoPran XL.

Distribution: Distributed widely throughout body. Drug is more than 90% protein-bound.

Metabolism: Metabolized almost totally in liver. P.O. form undergoes extensive first-pass metabolism.

Excretion: About 96% to 99% excreted in urine as metabolites; remainder excreted in feces as unchanged drug and metabolites. *Half-life:* About 4 hours; 8 hours for InnoPran XL.

Route	Onset	Peak	Duration
P.O.	30 min	60-90 min	12 hr
P.O.			
InnoPran XL	Unknown	12-14 hr	24 hr
I.V.	≤ 1 min	≤ 1 min	< 5 min

Action

Chemical effect: Reduces cardiac oxygen demand by blocking catecholamine-induced increases in heart rate, blood pressure, and force of myocardial contraction. Depresses renin secretion and prevents vasodilation of cerebral arteries.

Therapeutic effect: Relieves anginal and migraine pain, lowers blood pressure, restores normal sinus rhythm, and helps limit MI damage.

Available forms

Capsules (extended-release): 60 mg, 80 mg, 120 mg, 160 mg
Injection: 1 mg/ml
Oral solution: 4 mg/ml, 8 mg/ml, 80 mg/ml (concentrate)
Tablets: 10 mg, 20 mg, 40 mg, 60 mg, 80 mg, 90 mg

NURSING PROCESS

▨ Assessment

• Assess patient's condition before therapy and regularly thereafter.
• Monitor blood pressure, ECG, and heart rate and rhythm frequently, especially during I.V. administration.
• Be alert for adverse reactions and drug interactions.

• Evaluate patient's and family's knowledge of drug therapy.

⚙ Nursing diagnoses
• Ineffective health maintenance related to underlying condition
• Impaired gas exchange related to airway resistance
• Deficient knowledge related to drug therapy

⟩ Planning and implementation
• Check patient's apical pulse before giving drug. If extremes in pulse rate are detected, withhold drug and call prescriber immediately.
• **ALERT:** Don't confuse Inderal with Inderide or Isordil.
• Double-check dose and route. I.V. doses are much smaller than oral doses.
• Give oral drug with meals. Food may increase absorption of propranolol.
• Don't stop drug before surgery for pheochromocytoma. Before any surgical procedure, notify anesthesiologist that patient is receiving propranolol.
• If patient develops severe hypotension, notify prescriber; vasopressor may be prescribed.
• Geriatric patient may have increased adverse reactions and may need dosage adjustment.
• Don't stop drug abruptly.
• For overdose, give I.V. isoproterenol, I.V. atropine, or glucagon; refractory cases may require pacemaker.
Patient teaching
• Teach patient how to check pulse rate, and tell him to do so before each dose. Tell him to notify prescriber if rate changes significantly.
• Tell patient that taking drug twice daily or as extended-release capsule may improve compliance. Advise him to check with prescriber.
• Advise patient to continue taking drug as prescribed, even when he's feeling well. Tell him not to stop drug suddenly because doing so can worsen angina and MI.

✓ Evaluation
• Patient responds well to therapy.
• Patient maintains adequate gas exchange.
• Patient and family state understanding of drug therapy.

propylthiouracil (PTU)
(proh-pil-thigh-oh-YOOR-uh-sil)
Propyl-Thyracil ◆

Pharmacologic class: thyroid hormone antagonist
Therapeutic class: antihyperthyroid drug
Pregnancy risk category: D

Indications and dosages
▶ **Hyperthyroidism.** *Adults:* 300 to 450 mg P.O. daily in divided doses. Continue until patient is euthyroid, then start maintenance dose of 100 mg P.O. daily to t.i.d.
Children age 10 and older: Initially, 150 to 300 mg P.O. daily in divided doses q 8 hours. Continue until patient is euthyroid. Individualize maintenance dose.
Children ages 6 to 10: 50 to 150 mg P.O. daily in divided doses q 8 hours. Continue until patient is euthyroid. Individualize maintenance dose.
Neonates and children: 5 to 7 mg/kg P.O. daily in divided doses q 8 hours, or give according to age.
▶ **Thyrotoxic crisis.** *Adults and children:* 200 to 400 mg P.O. q 4 to 6 hours on first day; after symptoms are under control, gradually reduce dosage to usual maintenance levels.

Contraindications and precautions
• Contraindicated in patients hypersensitive to drug.
• ⚖ **Lifespan:** In pregnant women, use cautiously. Pregnant women may need reduced dosage as pregnancy progresses. Monitor thyroid function studies closely. In breast-feeding women, drug is contraindicated.

Adverse reactions
CNS: headache, drowsiness, vertigo.
CV: vasculitis.
EENT: visual disturbances.
GI: diarrhea, *nausea, vomiting* (may be dose-related), salivary gland enlargement, loss of taste.
Hematologic: *agranulocytosis, thrombocytopenia, aplastic anemia, leukopenia,* lymphadenopathy.
Hepatic: jaundice, *hepatotoxicity.*
Metabolic: dose-related hypothyroidism (mental depression; cold intolerance; hard, nonpitting edema).

Musculoskeletal: arthralgia, myalgia.
Skin: rash, urticaria, skin discoloration, pruritus.
Other: drug-induced fever.

Interactions

Drug-drug. *Aminophylline, oxtriphylline, theophylline:* Decreases drug clearance. Dosage may need adjustment.
Anticoagulants: Anticoagulant effects may be increased. Monitor PT, PTT, or INR and patient for bleeding.
Digoxin: Increases glycoside levels. May need to decrease dose.
Potassium iodide: May decrease response to drug. May need to increase dose of antithyroid drug.

Effects on lab test results

● May increase liver enzyme levels.
● May decrease hemoglobin, hematocrit, and granulocyte, WBC, and platelet counts.

Pharmacokinetics

Absorption: About 80% of drug is absorbed rapidly and readily from GI tract.
Distribution: Drug appears to be concentrated in thyroid gland. About 75% to 80% of drug is protein-bound.
Metabolism: Metabolized rapidly in the liver.
Excretion: About 35% excreted in urine. *Half-life:* 1 to 2 hours.

Route	Onset	Peak	Duration
P.O.	Unknown	1-1½ hr	Unknown

Action

Chemical effect: Inhibits oxidation of iodine in thyroid gland, blocking iodine's ability to combine with tyrosine to form T_4, and may prevent coupling of monoiodotyrosine and diiodotyrosine to form T_4 and T_3.
Therapeutic effect: Lowers thyroid hormone level.

Available forms

Tablets: 50 mg, 100 mg ♦

NURSING PROCESS

⬛ Assessment

● Assess patient's condition before therapy and regularly thereafter.

● Watch for signs of hypothyroidism (depression; cold intolerance; hard, nonpitting edema); adjust dosage as directed.
● Monitor CBC to detect impending leukopenia, thrombocytopenia, and agranulocytosis.
● Be alert for adverse reactions.
● If adverse GI reactions occur, monitor patient's hydration.
● Evaluate patient's and family's knowledge of drug therapy.

🔲 Nursing diagnoses

● Ineffective health maintenance related to thyroid condition
● Risk for deficient fluid volume related to adverse GI reactions
● Deficient knowledge related to drug therapy

⬛ Planning and implementation

● Give drug with meals to reduce adverse GI reactions.
● If patient develops severe rash or enlarged cervical lymph nodes, stop drug and notify prescriber.
● Store drug in light-resistant container.
⚡ **ALERT:** Don't confuse propylthiouracil with Purinethol.
Patient teaching
● Tell patient to report skin eruptions (sign of hypersensitivity), fever, sore throat, or mouth sores (early signs of agranulocytosis).
● Instruct patient to ask prescriber whether he can use iodized salt and eat shellfish.
● Warn patient against OTC cough medicines because many contain iodine.

☑ Evaluation

● Patient's thyroid hormone level is normal.
● Patient maintains adequate hydration.
● Patient and family state understanding of drug therapy.

protamine sulfate
(PROH-tuh-meen SUL-fayt)

Pharmacologic class: antidote
Therapeutic class: heparin antagonist
Pregnancy risk category: C

Indications and dosages

▶ **Heparin overdose.** *Adults:* Dosage based on venous blood coagulation studies, usually 1 mg for each 90 to 115 units of heparin. Give by slow I.V. injection over 10 minutes, not to exceed 50 mg.

▼ I.V. administration

• Incompatible with many antibiotics, including cephalosporins and penicillins.
• May be given without further dilution or diluted in D_5W or normal saline solution.
• Give by slow injection over 10 minutes.
• Refrigerate at 36° to 46° F (2° to 8° C).
• Don't store diluted solutions; they contain no preservatives.

Contraindications and precautions

• Contraindicated in patients hypersensitive to drug.
• Use cautiously after cardiac surgery.
✿ **Lifespan:** In pregnant and breast-feeding women, use cautiously. In children, safety of drug hasn't been established.

Adverse reactions

CV: transitory flushing, *drop in blood pressure, bradycardia, circulatory collapse.*
Respiratory: dyspnea, *pulmonary edema, acute pulmonary hypertension.*
Other: feeling of warmth, *anaphylaxis, anaphylactoid reactions.*

Interactions

None significant.

Effects on lab test results

None reported.

Pharmacokinetics

Absorption: Administered I.V.
Distribution: Unknown.
Metabolism: Unknown, although it appears to be partially degraded, with release of some heparin.
Excretion: Unknown. *Half-life:* Shorter than heparin.

Route	Onset	Peak	Duration
I.V.	30-60 sec	Unknown	2 hr

Action

Chemical effect: Forms inert complex with heparin sodium.
Therapeutic effect: Blocks heparin's effects.

Available forms

Injection: 10 mg/ml

NURSING PROCESS

⚕ Assessment
• Assess patient's heparin overdose before therapy.
• Monitor patient continually. Check vital signs frequently.
• Watch for spontaneous bleeding (heparin rebound), especially in patients undergoing dialysis and in those who have undergone cardiac surgery. Protamine sulfate may act as anticoagulant in very high doses.
• Evaluate patient's and family's knowledge of drug therapy.

✛ Nursing diagnoses
• Ineffective protection related to heparin overdose
• Risk for injury related to anaphylaxis
• Deficient knowledge related to drug therapy

▷ Planning and implementation
• Calculate dosage carefully. One mg of protamine neutralizes 90 to 115 units of heparin depending on salt (heparin calcium or heparin sodium) and source of heparin (beef or pork).
• Give drug slowly by direct injection. Treat shock.
⚠ ALERT: Don't confuse protamine with Protopam.
Patient teaching
• Instruct patient to report adverse reactions immediately.

☑ Evaluation
• Patient doesn't experience injury.
• Patient and family state understanding of drug therapy.

Rapid onset   *Liquid form contains alcohol.   ◆Canada   ◇ Australia   †OTC   ‡Off-label use

pseudoephedrine hydrochloride
(soo-doh-eh-FED-rin high-droh-KLOR-ighd)
Cenafed, Children's Sudafed Liquid†,
Decofed†, DeFed-60†, Dimetapp†, Dorcol
Children's Decongestant†, Drixoral Non-
Drowsy Formula†, Eltor 120♦†,
Genaphed†, Halofed†, Halofed Adult
Strength†, Maxenal♦†, Myfedrine†,
Novafed†, PediaCare Infants' Oral
Decongestant Drops†, Pseudo†,
Pseudofrin♦, Pseudogest†, Robidrine♦†,
Sudafed†, Sudafed 12 Hour†, Sudafed 60†,
Sufedrin†, Triaminic†

pseudoephedrine sulfate
Afrin†, Drixoral†, Drixoral 12 Hour Non-
Drowsy Formula†

Pharmacologic class: adrenergic
Therapeutic class: decongestant
Pregnancy risk category: C

Indications and dosages

▶ **Nasal and eustachian tube decongestion.**
Adults and children age 12 and older: 60 mg
P.O. q 4 to 6 hours; or 120 mg P.O. extended-
release tablet q 12 hours; or 240 mg P.O.
controlled-release tablet daily. Maximum
dosage is 240 mg daily.
Children ages 6 to 11: 30 mg P.O. q 4 to 6
hours. Maximum dosage, 120 mg daily.
Children ages 2 to 5: 15 mg P.O. q 4 to 6 hours.
Maximum dosage is 60 mg daily, or 4 mg/kg or
125 mg/m^2 P.O. divided q.i.d.
Children younger than age 2: Consult a prescriber for specific dosage.

Contraindications and precautions

● Contraindicated in patients taking MAO inhibitors and in patients with severe hypertension
or severe coronary artery disease.
● Use cautiously in patients with hypertension,
cardiac disease, diabetes, glaucoma, hyperthyroidism, or prostatic hyperplasia.
⚠ Lifespan: In breast-feeding women, drug is
contraindicated. In children younger than age
12, extended-release forms are contraindicated.

Adverse reactions

CNS: *anxiety,* transient stimulation, tremor,
dizziness, headache, insomnia, *nervousness.*

CV: *arrhythmias, palpitations,* tachycardia, hy-
pertension.
GI: anorexia, nausea, vomiting, dry mouth.
GU: difficulty urinating.
Respiratory: *respiratory difficulty.*
Skin: pallor.

Interactions

Drug-drug. *Antihypertensives:* May attenuate
hypotensive effect. Monitor blood pressure.
Phenelzine, tranylcypromine: May cause severe
headache, hypertension, fever, and hypertensive
crisis. Avoid using together.
Drug-herb. *Bitter orange:* May increase risk of
hypertension and increased adverse CV effects.
Discourage using together.

Effects on lab test results

None reported.

Pharmacokinetics

Absorption: Unknown.
Distribution: Widely distributed throughout
body.
Metabolism: Incompletely metabolized in liver
to inactive compounds.
Excretion: Excreted in urine; rate is accelerated
with acidic urine. *Half-life:* 3 to 16 hours, depending on urine PH.

Route	Onset	Peak	Duration
P.O.	15-30 min	30-60 min	3-12 hr

Action

Chemical effect: Stimulates alpha-adrenergic
receptors in respiratory tract, resulting in vasoconstriction.
Therapeutic effect: Acts to relieve congestion
of nasal and eustachian tube.

Available forms

pseudoephedrine hydrochloride
Capsules†: 60 mg
Capsules (Liquid gel): 30 mg
Liquid: 7.5 mg/0.8 ml, 15 mg/5 ml, 30 mg/5 ml
Tablets: 30 mg, 60 mg
Tablets (chewable): 15 mg
Tablets (extended-release): 120 mg
pseudoephedrine sulfate
Tablets (extended-release): 120 mg (60 mg
immediate-release, 60 mg delayed-release)

Reactions may be *common,* uncommon, *life-threatening*, or COMMON AND LIFE-THREATENING.

Assessment
- Assess patient's condition before therapy and regularly thereafter.
- Be alert for adverse reactions and drug interactions.
- Geriatric patients are more sensitive to drug's effects.
- Evaluate patient's and family's knowledge of drug therapy.

Nursing diagnoses
- Ineffective health maintenance related to congestion
- Disturbed sleep pattern related to drug-induced insomnia
- Deficient knowledge related to drug therapy

Planning and implementation
- Don't crush or break extended-release forms.
- Give last dose at least 2 hours before bedtime to minimize insomnia.

Patient teaching
- Warn patient against using OTC products containing other sympathomimetics.
- Tell patient not to take drug within 2 hours of bedtime because it can cause insomnia.
- Tell patient to relieve dry mouth with sugarless gum or hard candy.
- Instruct patient to stop drug if he becomes unusually restless and to notify prescriber promptly.

Evaluation
- Patient's congestion is relieved.
- Patient and family state understanding of drug therapy.

psyllium
(SIL-ee-um)
Fiberall†, Genfiber†, Hydrocil Instant†, Konsyl†, Konsyl-D†, Metamucil†, Modane Bulk†, Perdiem Fiber Therapy†, Reguloid†, Serutan†, Syllact†

Pharmacologic class: adsorbent
Therapeutic class: bulk laxative
Pregnancy risk category: NR

Indications and dosages
▶ **Constipation, bowel management, irritable bowel syndrome.** *Adults and children age 12 and older:* 1 to 2 rounded tsp P.O. in 8 oz of liquid once daily, b.i.d., or t.i.d., followed by second glass of liquid. Or, 1 packet dissolved in water once daily, b.i.d., or t.i.d. Or, 2 wafers b.i.d. or t.i.d. with at least 8 oz of water.
Children ages 6 to 11: ½ to 1 level tsp P.O. in 4 oz of liquid once daily, b.i.d., or t.i.d. Or, 1 wafer up to t.i.d. with at least 8 oz of water.

Contraindications and precautions
- Contraindicated in patients hypersensitive to drug and in those with intestinal obstruction or ulceration, disabling adhesions, difficulty swallowing, or symptoms of appendicitis, such as abdominal pain, nausea, and vomiting.
- ≉ Lifespan: In pregnant and breast-feeding women, use cautiously.

Adverse reactions
GI: nausea, vomiting, and diarrhea with excessive use; esophageal, gastric, small intestinal, or colonic strictures with dry form; abdominal cramps in severe constipation.

Interactions
None significant.

Effects on lab test results
None reported.

Pharmacokinetics
Absorption: None.
Distribution: Distributed locally in GI tract.
Metabolism: None.
Excretion: Excreted in feces. *Half-life:* Unknown.

Route	Onset	Peak	Duration
P.O.	12-24 hr	≤ 3 days	Varies

Action
Chemical effect: Absorbs water and expands to increase bulk and moisture content of stool, thus encouraging peristalsis and bowel movement.
Therapeutic effect: Relieves constipation.

Available forms
Granules: 2.5 g/tsp, 4 g/tsp

Powder: 3.3 g/tsp, 3.4 g/packet, 3.4 g/tsp, 3.4 g/tbs, 3.5 g/tsp, 3.5 g/scoopful, 6 g/packet, 6 g/tsp
Wafers: 3.4 g/wafer

NURSING PROCESS

🝥 Assessment
● Assess patient's condition before therapy and regularly thereafter.
● Before giving drug for constipation, determine if patient has adequate fluid intake, exercise, and diet.
● Be alert for adverse reactions.
● Evaluate patient's and family's knowledge of drug therapy.

🝚 Nursing diagnoses
● Constipation related to underlying condition
● Acute pain related to abdominal cramps
● Deficient knowledge related to drug therapy

⟩ Planning and implementation
● Mix drug with at least 8 oz (240 ml) of cold, pleasant-tasting liquid, such as orange juice, to mask grittiness. Stir only a few seconds. Have patient drink mixture immediately, before it congeals. Follow with another glass of liquid.
● For dosages in children younger than age 6, consult prescriber.
● If taken before meals, drug may reduce appetite.
● Drug isn't absorbed systemically and is non-toxic. It's especially useful in debilitated patients and those with postpartum constipation, irritable bowel syndrome, and diverticular disease. Also useful to treat chronic laxative abuse and with other laxatives to empty colon before barium enema examinations.
Patient teaching
● Teach patient how to properly mix drug. To enhance effect and prevent intestinal obstruction, tell him to take drug with plenty of water. Advise him that inhaling powder may cause allergic reactions.
● Tell patient that laxative effect usually occurs in 12 to 24 hours but may be delayed up to 3 days.
● Advise diabetic patient to check label and use brand of drug that doesn't contain sugar.
● Teach patient about dietary sources of bulk, including bran and other cereals, fresh fruit, and vegetables.

☑ Evaluation
● Patient's constipation is relieved.

● Patient's abdominal cramping is minimal and tolerable.
● Patient and family state understanding of drug therapy.

pyrantel embonate
(peer-AN-tul EM-boh-nayt)
Anthel ◆, Combantrin ◆, Early Bird ◆

pyrantel pamoate
Antiminth, Combantrin ◆, Pin-Rid†, Pin-X, Reese's Pinworm Medicine

Pharmacologic class: pyrimidine derivative
Therapeutic class: anthelmintic
Pregnancy risk category: C

Indications and dosages
▶ **Roundworm and pinworm.** *Adults and children older than age 2:* 11 mg/kg P.O. given as single dose. Maximum total dose is 1 g. For pinworm, repeat dosage in 2 weeks.

Contraindications and precautions
● Contraindicated in patients hypersensitive to drug.
● Use cautiously in patients with hepatic dysfunction or severe malnutrition or anemia.
⚘ Lifespan: In pregnant women, use cautiously. In children younger than age 2 and breast-feeding women, safety of drug hasn't been established.

Adverse reactions
CNS: headache, dizziness, fever, drowsiness, insomnia, weakness.
GI: anorexia, nausea, vomiting, gastralgia, cramps, diarrhea, tenesmus.
Skin: rash.

Interactions
Drug-drug. *Piperazine salts:* May cause antagonism. Don't give together.
Theophylline: Increases theophylline levels. Monitor level.

Effects on lab test results
● May increase AST level.

Pharmacokinetics
Absorption: Poor.
Distribution: Unknown.

Reactions may be *common*, uncommon, *life-threatening*, or COMMON AND LIFE-THREATENING.

Metabolism: Small amount partially metabolized in liver.
Excretion: More than 50% excreted in feces; about 7% excreted in urine. *Half-life:* Unknown.

Route	Onset	Peak	Duration
P.O.	Varies	1-3 hr	Varies

Action

Chemical effect: Blocks neuromuscular action, paralyzing worm and causing its expulsion by normal peristalsis.
Therapeutic effect: Relieves roundworm and pinworm infestation, including *Ancylostoma duodenale, Ascaris lumbricoides, Enterobius vermicularis, Necator americanus,* and *Trichostrongylus orientalis.*

Available forms

pyrantel embonate
Granules: 100 mg/g ◆
Oral suspension: 50 mg/ml ◆
Squares (chocolate-flavored): 100 mg ◆
Tablets: 125 mg ◆, 250 mg ◆
pyrantel pamoate
Capsules: 180 mg†
Liquid: 50 mg/ml
Oral suspension: 50 mg/ml
Tablets: 125 mg ◆

NURSING PROCESS

⚗ Assessment
• Assess patient's condition before therapy and regularly thereafter.
• Be alert for adverse reactions and drug interactions.
• If adverse GI reactions occur, monitor patient's hydration.
• Evaluate patient's and family's knowledge of drug therapy.

⊕ Nursing diagnoses
• Infection related to worm infestation
• Risk for deficient fluid volume related to adverse GI reactions
• Deficient knowledge related to drug therapy

▷ Planning and implementation
• No dietary restrictions, laxatives, or enemas are needed.
• Give drug to all family members to prevent risk of spreading infection.

• Drug may be taken with food, milk, or fruit juices. Shake suspension well.
Patient teaching
• Tell patient to shake suspension well before taking it. Inform patient that drug may be taken with food or beverages.
• Teach patient about personal hygiene, especially good hand-washing technique. To avoid reinfection, teach him to wash perianal area daily, to change undergarments and bedclothes daily, and to wash hands and clean fingernails before meals and after bowel movements. Advise patient to refrain from preparing food for others during infestation.

☑ Evaluation
• Patient is free from infestation.
• Patient maintains adequate hydration.
• Patient and family state understanding of drug therapy.

pyrazinamide
(peer-uh-ZIN-uh-mighd)
PMS-Pyrazinamide ◆, Tebrazid ◆, Zinamide ◆

Pharmacologic class: synthetic pyrazine analogue of nicotinamide
Therapeutic class: antituberculotic
Pregnancy risk category: C

Indications and dosages

▶ **Adjunct for tuberculosis when primary and secondary antituberculotics can't be used or have failed.** *Adults:* 15 to 30 mg/kg P.O. once daily, not to exceed 2 g daily. Or, twice-weekly dose of 50 to 70 mg/kg (based on lean body weight) to promote compliance.
⊠ Adjust-a-dose: For patients with renal impairment and geriatric patients, start at the low end of the dosing range.

Contraindications and precautions

• Contraindicated in patients hypersensitive to drug and patients with severe hepatic disease or hyperuricemia with acute gout.
• Use cautiously in patients with diabetes mellitus or renal impairment.
⚘ Lifespan: In pregnant women, use cautiously. In children and breast-feeding women, safety of drug hasn't been established.

Adverse reactions

CNS: malaise, fever.
GI: anorexia, nausea, vomiting, diarrhea.
GU: dysuria.
Hematologic: sideroblastic anemia, ***thrombocytopenia.***
Hepatic: *hepatitis, hepatotoxicity.*
Metabolic: *hyperuricemia.*
Musculoskeletal: arthralgia.

Interactions

Drug-herb. *Kava:* May increase risk of liver damage. Discourage using together.

Effects on lab test results

• May increase uric acid level.
• May decrease platelet count, hemoglobin, and hematocrit.

Pharmacokinetics

Absorption: Well absorbed.
Distribution: Distributed widely into body tissues and fluids, including lungs, liver, and CSF. Drug is 50% protein-bound.
Metabolism: Hydrolyzed in liver and in stomach.
Excretion: Excreted almost completely in urine. *Half-life:* 9 to 10 hours.

Route	Onset	Peak	Duration
P.O.	Unknown	1-2 hr	Unknown

Action

Chemical effect: Unknown.
Therapeutic effect: Helps eradicate tuberculosis. Only active against *Mycobacterium tuberculosis.*

Available forms

Tablets: 500 mg

NURSING PROCESS

🔠 Assessment
• Assess patient's condition before therapy and regularly thereafter.
• Monitor hematopoietic studies and uric acid level.
• Monitor liver function test results; examine patient for jaundice and liver tenderness or enlargement before and frequently during therapy.
• Watch closely for signs of gout and liver impairment.

• If adverse GI reactions occur, monitor patient's hydration.
• Evaluate patient's and family's knowledge of drug therapy.

🔠 Nursing diagnoses
• Infection related to tuberculosis
• Risk for deficient fluid volume related to adverse GI reactions
• Deficient knowledge related to drug therapy

▶ Planning and implementation
• Always give drug with other antituberculotics to prevent development of resistant organisms.
• Reduce dosage in patients with renal impairment because nearly all of drug is excreted in urine.
• Question doses that exceed 35 mg/kg; they may cause liver damage.
• Notify prescriber at once if you suspect liver dysfunction.
• When drug is used with surgical management of tuberculosis, it's started 1 to 2 weeks before surgery and continued for 4 to 6 weeks after.
• HIV-infected patients may need longer course.
• Pyrazinamide may interfere with Acetest and Ketostix urine tests to produce pink-brown color.
Patient teaching
• Instruct patient to take drug exactly as prescribed, and tell him not to stop drug without prescriber's approval.
• Teach patient to watch for and immediately report signs of gout and hepatic impairment.

☑ Evaluation
• Patient is free from infection.
• Patient maintains adequate hydration.
• Patient and family state understanding of drug therapy.

pyridostigmine bromide
(peer-ih-doh-STIG-meen BROH-mighd)
Mestinon*, Mestinon SRI, Mestinon Timespans, Regonol

Pharmacologic class: cholinesterase inhibitor
Therapeutic class: muscle stimulant
Pregnancy risk category: NR

Indications and dosages

▶ **Antidote for nondepolarizing neuromuscu-lar blockers.** *Adults:* 10 to 20 mg I.V. preceded by atropine sulfate 0.6 to 1.2 mg I.V.

▶ **Myasthenia gravis.** *Adults:* 60 to 120 mg P.O. t.i.d. Usual dosage is 600 mg daily but higher dosage may be needed (up to 1,500 mg daily). For I.M. or I.V. use, give ⅟₃₀ of oral dosage. Dosage must be adjusted for each pa-tient, depending on response and tolerance. Or, 180 to 540 mg sustained-release tablets (1 to 3 tablets) P.O. daily to b.i.d., with at least 6 hours between doses.

Children: 7 mg/kg or 200 mg/m² P.O. daily in five or six divided doses. Or, 0.05 to 0.15 mg/kg/dose I.V. or I.M.

▶ **To increase survival after exposure to the nerve agent Soman.** *Adults in the military:* 30 mg P.O. q 8 hours starting about 8 hours be-fore Soman exposure.

▼ I.V. administration

• Give I.V. injection no faster than 1 mg/minute. If I.V. administration is too rapid, bradycardia and seizures may result.

Contraindications and precautions

• Contraindicated in patients hypersensitive to anticholinesterases, in those with mechanical obstruction of intestine or urinary tract, and in those with history of a reaction to bromides.
• Use cautiously in patients with bronchial asth-ma, bradycardia, or arrhythmias.
⚘ **Lifespan:** In pregnant and breast-feeding women, safety of drug hasn't been established. In neonates, Regonol is contraindicated because it contains benzyl alcohol.

Adverse reactions

CNS: headache with large doses, weakness, sweating, *seizures.*
CV: *bradycardia,* hypotension, thrombophle-bitis.
EENT: miosis.
GI: abdominal cramps, nausea, vomiting, diar-rhea, excessive salivation.
Musculoskeletal: muscle cramps, muscle fasci-culations.
Respiratory: *bronchospasm, bronchoconstric-tion,* increased bronchial secretions.
Skin: rash.

Interactions

Drug-drug. *Aminoglycosides:* May increase re-sponse to drug. Use together cautiously.
Anesthetics, anticholinergics, atropine, cortico-steroids, magnesium, procainamide, quinidine: May antagonize cholinergic effects. Observe pa-tient for lack of drug effect.
Ganglionic blockers: Increases risk of hypoten-sion. Monitor patient closely.

Effects on lab test results

None reported.

Pharmacokinetics

Absorption: Poor.
Distribution: Unknown.
Metabolism: Unknown.
Excretion: Excreted in urine. *Half-life:* 1 to 3 hours, depending on route.

Route	Onset	Peak	Duration
P.O.	20-60 min	1-2 hr	3-12 hr
I.V.	2-5 min	Unknown	2-3 hr
I.M.	15 min	Unknown	2-3 hr

Action

Chemical effect: Inhibits destruction of acetyl-choline released from parasympathetic and so-matic efferent nerves. This allows acetylcholine to accumulate.
Therapeutic effect: Reverses effect of nonde-polarizing neuromuscular blockers and myas-thenia gravis.

Available forms

Injection: 5 mg/ml in 2-ml ampules or 5-ml vials
Syrup: 60 mg/5 ml
Tablets: 60 mg
Tablets (military use only): 30 mg
Tablets (sustained-release): 180 mg

NURSING PROCESS

📋 Assessment

• Assess patient's condition before therapy and regularly thereafter.
• Monitor and document patient's response after each dose; optimum dosage is difficult to judge.
• Monitor patient's vital signs, especially respi-rations.
• Be alert for adverse reactions and drug inter-actions.

• Evaluate patient's and family's knowledge of drug therapy.

⊞ **Nursing diagnoses**
• Impaired physical mobility related to underlying condition
• Ineffective breathing pattern related to adverse respiratory reactions
• Deficient knowledge related to drug therapy

⧉ **Planning and implementation**
• Stop all other cholinergics before giving drug.
• Don't crush extended-release tablets.
• When using sweet syrup for patient who has difficulty swallowing, pour over ice chips if he can't tolerate flavor.
• Position patient to ease breathing. Have atropine injection readily available, and provide respiratory support as needed.
• If patient's muscle weakness is severe, prescriber will determine if it's caused by drug-induced toxicity or worsening of myasthenia gravis. Test dose of edrophonium I.V. will aggravate drug-induced weakness but will temporarily relieve weakness caused by disease.
• The U.S. formulation of Regonol contains benzyl alcohol preservative that may cause toxicity in neonates if given in large doses. The Canadian formulation of this drug doesn't contain benzyl ethanol.
• If appropriate, obtain prescriber's order for hospitalized patient to have bedside supply of tablets. Patients with long-standing disease often insist on self-administration.
⊛ **ALERT:** If drug is taken immediately before or during Soman exposure, drug may be ineffective against Soman, and may worsen the effects of Soman.
⊛ **ALERT:** Don't confuse Mestinon with Mesantoin or Metatensin.
Patient teaching
• When giving drug for myasthenia gravis, stress the importance of taking it exactly as ordered, on time, in evenly spaced doses. If prescriber has ordered extended-release tablets, tell patient to take tablets at same time each day, at least 6 hours apart. Tell him that he may have to take drug for life.
• Advise patient to wear or carry medical identification at all times.

☑ **Evaluation**
• Patient has improved physical mobility.

• Patient maintains adequate respiratory pattern.
• Patient and family state understanding of drug therapy.

pyridoxine hydrochloride (vitamin B₆)

(peer-ih-DOKS-een high-droh-KLOR-ighd)
Aminoxin, Beesix, Nestrex†, Rodex

Pharmacologic class: water-soluble vitamin
Therapeutic class: nutritional supplement
Pregnancy risk category: A

Indications and dosages

▶ **RDA.** *Men age 15 and older:* 2 mg.
Men ages 11 to 14: 1.7 mg.
Women age 19 and older: 1.6 mg.
Women ages 15 to 18: 1.5 mg.
Women ages 11 to 14: 1.4 mg.
Pregnant women: 2.2 mg.
Breast-feeding women: 2.1 mg.
Children ages 7 to 10: 1.4 mg.
Children ages 4 to 6: 1.1 mg.
Children ages 1 to 3: 1 mg.
Infants ages 6 months to 1 year: 0.6 mg.
Neonates and infants up to age 6 months: 0.3 mg.
▶ **Dietary vitamin B₆ deficiency.** *Adults:* 2.5 to 10 mg P.O. daily for 3 weeks; then 2 to 5 mg daily as supplement to proper diet.
▶ **Seizures related to vitamin B₆ deficiency or dependency.** *Adults and children:* 10 to 100 mg I.M. or I.V. in single dose.
▶ **Vitamin B₆-responsive anemias or dependency syndrome (inborn errors of metabolism).** *Adults:* up to 600 mg I.M., P.O., or I.V. daily until symptoms subside; then 30 mg daily for life.
▶ **Prevention of vitamin B₆ deficiency during drug therapy.** *Adults:* 6 to 100 mg P.O. daily for isoniazid therapy.
▶ **Drug-induced vitamin B₆ deficiency.** *Adults:* 100 to 200 mg P.O. daily for 3 weeks, followed by 25 to 100 mg P.O. daily to prevent relapse.
▶ **Antidote for isoniazid poisoning.** *Adults:* 1 to 4 g I.V., followed by 1 g I.M. q 30 minutes until amount of pyridoxine given equals amount of isoniazid ingested.

Reactions may be *common*, uncommon, *life-threatening*, or COMMON AND LIFE-THREATENING.

▶ **Premenstrual syndrome‡.** *Adults:* 40 to 500 mg P.O., I.M., or I.V. daily.

▶ **Carpal tunnel syndrome‡.** *Adults:* 100 to 200 mg P.O. daily for 12 weeks or longer.

▶ **Hyperoxaluria type I‡.** *Adults:* 25 to 300 mg P.O. daily.

▼ I.V. administration

• Protect drug from light. Don't use solution if it contains precipitate, although slight darkening is acceptable.

• Inject undiluted drug into I.V. line containing free-flowing compatible solution. Or, infuse diluted drug over prescribed duration for intermittent infusions. Don't use for continuous infusion.

Contraindications and precautions

• Contraindicated in patients hypersensitive to drug and in patients with heart disease.

⚘ Lifespan: No considerations reported.

Adverse reactions

CNS: drowsiness, paresthesia, unstable gait.

Interactions

Drug-drug. *Levodopa:* May decrease the effectiveness of levodopa. Avoid using pyridoxine with levodopa. Pyridoxine has little to no effect on the combination drug levodopa and carbidopa.
Phenobarbital, phenytoin: Decreases anticonvulsant level, increasing risk of seizures. Monitor level closely; institute seizure precautions.
Drug-lifestyle. *Alcohol use:* Increases risk of delirium and lactic acidosis. Discourage using together.

Effects on lab test results

• May increase AST level. May decrease folic acid level.

Pharmacokinetics

Absorption: Drug and its substituents are absorbed readily from GI tract. May be diminished in patients with malabsorption syndromes or following gastric resection.
Distribution: Drug is stored mainly in liver.
Metabolism: Metabolized in liver.
Excretion: In erythrocytes, pyridoxine is converted to pyridoxal phosphate and pyridoxamine is converted to pyridoxamine phosphate. The phosphorylated form of pyridoxine is transami-

nated to pyridoxal and pyridoxamine, which is phosphorylated rapidly. Conversion of pyridoxine phosphate to pyridoxal phosphate requires riboflavin. *Half-life:* 15 to 20 days.

Route	Onset	Peak	Duration
P.O., I.V., I.M.	Unknown	Unknown	Unknown

Action

Chemical effect: Vitamin B_6 stimulates various metabolic functions, including amino acid metabolism.
Therapeutic effect: Raises pyridoxine levels, prevents and relieves seizure activity related to pyridoxine deficiency or dependency, and blocks effects of isoniazid poisoning.

Available forms

Injection: 100 mg/ml
Tablets: 10 mg†, 25 mg†, 50 mg†, 100 mg†, 200 mg†, 250 mg†, 500 mg†
Tablets (enteric-coated): 20 mg†
Tablets (extended-release): 200 mg

NURSING PROCESS

✍ Assessment

• Assess patient before therapy and regularly thereafter.

• Be alert for adverse CNS reactions and drug interactions. Patient taking high doses (2 to 6 g daily) may have difficulty walking because of reduced proprioceptive and sensory function.

• Monitor patient's diet. Excessive protein intake increases daily drug requirements.

• Evaluate patient's and family's knowledge of drug therapy.

✛ Nursing diagnoses

• Ineffective health maintenance related to underlying condition

• Risk for injury related to drug-induced adverse CNS reactions

• Deficient knowledge related to drug therapy

▷ Planning and implementation

• When using drug to treat isoniazid toxicity, give anticonvulsants.

• If sodium bicarbonate is required to control acidosis in isoniazid toxicity, don't mix in same syringe with pyridoxine.

⊛ **ALERT:** Don't confuse pyridoxine with pralidoxime, pyrimethamine, or Pyridium.
Patient teaching
• Advise patient taking levodopa alone to avoid
multivitamins containing pyridoxine because of
decreased levodopa effect.
• If prescribed for maintenance therapy to prevent recurrence of deficiency, stress importance
of compliance and good nutrition. Explain that
pyridoxine with isoniazid has specific therapeutic purpose and isn't just a vitamin.

☑ **Evaluation**
• Patient responds well to therapy.
• Patient doesn't experience injury from adverse
CNS reactions.
• Patient and family state understanding of drug
therapy.

pyrimethamine
(peer-ih-METH-uh-meen)
Daraprim

pyrimethamine with sulfadoxine
Fansidar

Pharmacologic class: aminopyrimidine deriva-
tive (folic acid antagonist)
Therapeutic class: antimalarial
Pregnancy risk category: C

Indications and dosages

▶ **Malaria prophylaxis and transmission
control.** *Adults and children older than age 10:*
25 mg pyrimethamine P.O. weekly.
Children ages 4 to 10: 12.5 mg pyrimethamine
P.O. weekly.
Children younger than age 4: 6.25 mg pyri-
methamine P.O. weekly.
Continued in all age groups at least 10 weeks
after leaving endemic area.
▶ **Acute attacks of malaria.** *Adults and chil-
dren older than age 10:* 25 mg pyrimethamine
P.O. daily for 2 days when used with faster-
acting antimalarials; when used alone, 50 mg
P.O. daily for 2 days.
Children ages 4 to 10: 25 mg pyrimethamine
P.O. daily for 2 days.
▶ **Acute attacks of malaria.** *Adults:* 2 to
3 tablets pyrimethamine with sulfadoxine as

single dose, either alone or in sequence with
quinine.
Children ages 9 to 14: 2 tablets pyrimethamine
with sulfadoxine.
Children ages 4 to 8: 1 tablet pyrimethamine
with sulfadoxine.
Children younger than age 4: ½ tablet pyrimethamine with sulfadoxine.
▶ **Malaria prophylaxis.** *Adults:* 1 tablet
pyrimethamine with sulfadoxine weekly, or
2 tablets q 2 weeks.
Children ages 9 to 14: ¾ tablet pyrimethamine
with sulfadoxine weekly, or 1½ tablets q 2
weeks.
Children ages 4 to 8: ½ tablet pyrimethamine
with sulfadoxine weekly, or 1 tablet q 2 weeks.
Children younger than age 4: ¼ tablet pyrimethamine with sulfadoxine weekly, or ½ tablet
q 2 weeks.
▶ **Toxoplasmosis.** *Adults:* Initially, 50 to 75 mg
pyrimethamine P.O. daily for 1 to 3 weeks; then
25 mg P.O. daily for 4 to 5 weeks along with 1 g
sulfadiazine P.O. q 6 hours.
Children: Initially, 1 mg/kg pyrimethamine P.O.
(not to exceed 100 mg) in two equally divided
doses for 2 to 4 days; then 0.5 mg/kg daily for
4 weeks along with 100 mg sulfadiazine/kg P.O.
daily, divided q 6 hours.
▶ **Isosporiasis‡.** *Adults:* 50 to 75 mg pyrimethamine P.O. daily.

Contraindications and precautions

• Contraindicated in patients hypersensitive to
drug and in those with megaloblastic anemia
caused by folic acid deficiency. Pyrimethamine
with sulfadoxine is contraindicated in patients
with porphyria because it contains sulfadoxine,
a sulfonamide.
• Repeated use of pyrimethamine with sulfadoxine is contraindicated in patients hypersensitive to pyrimethamine or sulfonamides, and in
patients with severe renal insufficiency, marked
liver parenchymal damage or blood dyscrasias,
or megaloblastic anemia caused by folate deficiency.
• Use cautiously in patients with impaired hepatic or renal function, severe allergy or bronchial asthma, or G6PD deficiency; in those with
seizure disorders (smaller doses may be needed); and in those treated with chloroquine.
⚖ **Lifespan:** In infants younger than age 2
months, breast-feeding women, and pregnant

---

women at term, repeated use of pyrimethamine with sulfadoxine is contraindicated.

Adverse reactions

CNS: stimulation, *seizures.*
GI: anorexia, vomiting, diarrhea, atrophic glossitis.
Hematologic: *agranulocytosis, aplastic anemia,* megaloblastic anemia, *bone marrow suppression, leukopenia, thrombocytopenia, pancytopenia.*
Skin: rash, *erythema multiforme, Stevens-Johnson syndrome, toxic epidermal necrolysis.*

Interactions

Drug-drug. *Co-trimoxazole, methotrexate, sulfonamides:* Increases risk of bone marrow suppression. Don't use together.
Folic acid, PABA: Decreases antitoxoplasmic effects. May require dosage adjustment.
Lorazepam: May cause mild hepatotoxicity. Monitor liver enzymes.

Effects on lab test results

• May decrease hemoglobin, hematocrit, and granulocyte, WBC, platelet, and RBC counts.

Pharmacokinetics

Absorption: Well absorbed from intestinal tract.
Distribution: Distributed to kidneys, liver, spleen, and lungs. About 80% bound to proteins.
Metabolism: Metabolized to several unidentified compounds.
Excretion: Excreted in urine. *Half-life:* 4 days.

Route	Onset	Peak	Duration
P.O.	Unknown	1½-8 hr	Unknown

Action

Chemical effect: Inhibits enzyme dihydrofolate reductase, thereby impeding reduction of this enzyme to tetrahydrofolic acid. Sulfadoxine competitively inhibits use of PABA.
Therapeutic effect: Prevents malaria and treats malaria and toxoplasmosis infections. Spectrum of activity includes asexual erythrocytic forms of susceptible plasmodia and *Toxoplasma gondii.*

Available forms

pyrimethamine
Tablets: 25 mg
pyrimethamine with sulfadoxine
Tablets: pyrimethamine 25 mg, sulfadoxine 500 mg

NURSING PROCESS

🔏 Assessment
• Assess patient's condition before therapy and regularly thereafter.
• Obtain twice-weekly blood counts, including platelets, for patients with toxoplasmosis because dosages used approach toxic levels.
• Be alert for adverse reactions and drug interactions.
• Evaluate patient's and family's knowledge of drug therapy.

🔁 Nursing diagnoses
• Infection related to presence of susceptible organism
• Ineffective protection related to adverse hematologic reactions
• Deficient knowledge related to drug therapy

▶ Planning and implementation
• Give drug with meals to minimize GI distress.
• If signs of folic acid or folinic acid deficiency develop, reduce dosage or stop drug while patient receives parenteral folinic acid (leucovorin) until blood counts become normal.
• When used to treat toxoplasmosis in patients with AIDS, therapy may be lifelong. Long-term suppressive therapy for patient's lifetime may also be necessary.
🔆 **ALERT:** Because of possibly severe skin reactions, use pyrimethamine with sulfadoxine only in regions where chloroquine-resistant malaria is prevalent and only when traveler plans to stay in region longer than 3 weeks.
Patient teaching
• Advise patient to take drug with food.
• Teach patient to watch for and immediately report signs of folic or folinic acid deficiency and acute toxicity.
• Warn patient taking pyrimethamine with sulfadoxine to stop drug and notify prescriber at first sign of rash.
• Instruct patient to take first prophylactic dose of pyrimethamine with sulfadoxine 1 to 2 days before traveling to endemic area.

☑ Evaluation

- Patient is free from infection.
- Patient maintains normal hematologic parameters.
- Patient and family state understanding of drug therapy.

quetiapine fumarate
(KWET-ee-uh-peen FYOO-muh-rayt)
Seroquel

Pharmacologic class: dibenzothiazepine derivative
Therapeutic class: antipsychotic
Pregnancy risk category: C

Indications and dosages

▶**Schizophrenia.** *Adults:* Initially, 25 mg P.O. b.i.d.; increase in increments of 25 to 50 mg b.i.d. or t.i.d. on days 2 and 3, as tolerated. Target dosage range is 300 to 400 mg daily, divided into two or three daily doses by day 4. Further dosage adjustments usually occur at intervals of not less than 2 days. Dosages can be increased or decreased by 25 to 50 mg b.i.d. Antipsychotic effectiveness typically occurs at 150 to 750 mg daily. Safety of doses above 800 mg daily hasn't been evaluated.

◻**Adjust-a-dose:** For patients with hepatic impairment, initially give 25 mg P.O. daily. Increase in increments of 25 to 50 mg daily to an effective dose, depending on the patient's response and tolerance.

Contraindications and precautions

- Contraindicated in patients hypersensitive to drug or its ingredients.
- Use cautiously in patients with CV or cerebrovascular disease or conditions that predispose them to hypotension; in those with history of seizures or conditions that lower seizure threshold; in those at risk for aspiration pneumonia; and in those who could experience conditions in which core body temperature may be elevated. Also use cautiously in patients who are debilitated.

☀ Lifespan: In pregnant women, use only if the potential benefits outweigh the potential risks to the fetus. Breast-feeding women should avoid breast-feeding during drug therapy. In children, safety of drug hasn't been established. In elderly patients, use cautiously and at a reduced dose.

Adverse reactions

CNS: fever, asthenia, *dizziness, headache, seizures, somnolence,* hypertonia, dysarthria, *neuroleptic malignant syndrome,* tardive dyskinesia.
CV: orthostatic hypotension, tachycardia, palpitations, peripheral edema.
EENT: pharyngitis, rhinitis, ear pain, cataracts, sinusitis, nasal congestion.
GI: dry mouth, dyspepsia, abdominal pain, constipation, anorexia.
GU: urine retention.
Hematologic: *leukopenia.*
Metabolic: *weight gain,* hypothyroidism, hyperglycemia.
Musculoskeletal: back pain.
Respiratory: increased cough, dyspnea.
Skin: rash, sweating.
Other: flulike syndrome.

Interactions

Drug-drug. *Antihypertensives:* May increase drug effects. Monitor blood pressure.
Carbamazepine, glucocorticoids, phenobarbital, phenytoin, rifampin, thioridazine: Increases quetiapine clearance. Increase quetiapine dose, p.r.n.
CNS depressants: Increases CNS effects. Use together cautiously.
Erythromycin, fluconazole, itraconazole, ketoconazole: Decreases quetiapine clearance. Use together cautiously.
Dopamine agonists, levodopa: Effects of these drugs may be antagonized. Monitor patient for effects.
Lorazepam: Reduces lorazepam clearance. Monitor patient.
Drug-lifestyle. *Alcohol use:* Increases CNS effects. Discourage using together.

Effects on lab test results

- May increase liver enzyme, cholesterol, and triglyceride levels. May decrease T_4 and thyroid-stimulating hormone levels.
- May decrease WBC count.

Reactions may be *common,* uncommon, *life-threatening,* or COMMON AND LIFE-THREATENING.

Pharmacokinetics

Absorption: Rapid; 100% bioavailability.
Distribution: Wide; 83% bound to protein.
Metabolism: Extensive.
Excretion: About 73% in urine, 20% in feces.
Half-life: 6 hours.

Route	Onset	Peak	Duration
P.O.	Unknown	1½ hr	Unknown

Action

Chemical effect: Unknown. May block dopamine D-2 receptors and serotonin 5-HT$_2$ receptors in the brain. It also may act at histamine H$_1$ receptors and alpha$_1$-adrenergic receptors.
Therapeutic effect: Reduces symptoms of psychotic disorders.

Available forms

Tablets: 25 mg, 100 mg, 200 mg, 300 mg

NURSING PROCESS

🔯 Assessment

• Monitor patient for tardive dyskinesia. Condition may not appear until months or years after starting drug and may disappear spontaneously or persist for life, despite stopping drug.
• Monitor patient's vital signs carefully, especially during the 3- to 5-day period of initial dosage adjustment and when restarting or increasing dosage.
• Assess patient's risk of physical injury from adverse CNS effects.
• Be alert for adverse reactions and drug interactions.
• Evaluate patient's and family's knowledge of drug therapy.

🔲 Nursing diagnoses

• Risk for imbalanced body temperature related to drug-induced hyperpyrexia
• Impaired physical mobility related to drug-induced adverse CNS effects
• Deficient knowledge related to drug therapy

▷ Planning and implementation

• Geriatric and debilitated patients and patients with hepatic impairment or predisposition to hypotensive reactions usually require lower initial doses and more gradual dosage adjustment.
⑱ **ALERT:** If symptoms of neuroleptic malignant syndrome (hyperpyrexia, muscle rigidity, al-

tered mental status, and autonomic instability) occur, withhold drug and notify prescriber.
• Provide ice chips, drinks, or sugarless hard candy to help relieve dry mouth.
⑱ **ALERT:** Don't confuse Serzone with Seroquel.
Patient teaching
• Warn patient about risk of orthostatic hypotension. Risk is greatest during 3- to 5-day period of initial dosage adjustment and when restarting or increasing dosage.
• Tell patient to avoid becoming overheated or dehydrated during therapy.
• Advise patient to avoid activities that require mental alertness until CNS effects of drug are known.
• Remind patient to have eye examination before starting drug therapy and every 6 months during therapy to check for cataract formation.
• Tell patient to notify prescriber of other medications (prescription or OTC) he is taking or plans to take.
• Tell woman to notify prescriber if she becomes pregnant or intends to become pregnant during drug therapy. Advise her not to breastfeed during drug therapy.
• Advise patient to avoid alcohol during therapy.
• Tell patient that drug may be taken without regard to food.

☑ Evaluation

• Patient maintains normal body temperature.
• Patient maintains physical mobility and doesn't experience extrapyramidal effects of drug.
• Patient and family state understanding of drug therapy.

quinapril hydrochloride
(KWIN-eh-pril high-droh-KLOR-ighd)
Accupril, Asig ◊

Pharmacologic class: ACE inhibitor
Therapeutic class: antihypertensive
Pregnancy risk category: C (D in second and third trimesters)

Indications and dosages

▶ **Hypertension.** *Adults:* Initially, 10 to 20 mg P.O. daily. Adjust dosage based on patient response at intervals of about 2 weeks. Most patients are controlled at 20, 40, or 80 mg daily as a single dose or in two divided doses.

🚫 **Adjust-a-dose:** For patients with renal impairment, if creatinine clearance exceeds 60 ml/minute, maximum initial dose is 10 mg P.O.; if clearance is 30 to 60 ml/minute, 5 mg; and if clearance is 10 to 30 ml/minute, 2.5 mg. No dose recommendations are available for creatinine clearance less than 10 ml/minute.

▶ **Heart failure.** *Adults:* Initially, 5 mg P.O. b.i.d. if patient is taking a diuretic and 10 mg P.O. b.i.d. if patient isn't taking a diuretic. Increase dosage at weekly intervals. Usual effective dosage is 20 to 40 mg daily in equally divided doses.

🚫 **Adjust-a-dose:** For patients with renal impairment, if creatinine clearance exceeds 30 ml/minute, the recommended initial dose is 5 mg P.O.; if clearance is 10 to 30 ml/minute, 2.5 mg. No dose recommendations are available for creatinine clearance less than 10 ml/minute.

Contraindications and precautions

• Contraindicated in patients hypersensitive to ACE inhibitors, in those with a history of angioedema during previous ACE inhibitor therapy, and in those with renal artery stenosis.
• Use cautiously in patients with impaired kidney function and increased potassium levels.
⚠ **Lifespan:** In pregnant women in the second or third trimester, drug isn't recommended. In breast-feeding women, use cautiously. In children, safety of drug hasn't been established.

Adverse reactions

CNS: somnolence, vertigo, light-headedness, syncope, malaise, nervousness, depression.
CV: palpitations, vasodilation, tachycardia, *hypertensive crisis,* angina, orthostatic hypotension, *arrhythmias.*
EENT: dry throat.
GI: dry mouth, abdominal pain, constipation, *GI hemorrhage.*
Metabolic: *hyperkalemia.*
Musculoskeletal: back pain.
Respiratory: dry, persistent, tickling, nonproductive cough.
Skin: pruritus, exfoliative dermatitis, *photosensitivity reaction,* diaphoresis.
Other: *angioedema.*

Interactions

Drug-drug. *Diuretics, other antihypertensives:* May increase the risk of excessive hypotension. Expect to stop diuretic or lower dosage.
Lithium: May increase lithium levels and lithium toxicity. Avoid using together.
Potassium-sparing diuretics: May increase risk of hyperkalemia. Monitor patient, ECG, and potassium levels closely.
Drug-herb. *Licorice:* May cause sodium retention and increase blood pressure, interfering with the therapeutic effects of ACE inhibitors. Discourage using together.
Drug-food. *High-fat foods:* May impair absorption. Discourage using together.
Sodium substitutes containing potassium: May increase risk of hyperkalemia. Discourage using together; monitor patient closely.

Effects on lab test results

• May increase potassium level.
• May decrease liver function test values.

Pharmacokinetics

Absorption: At least 60%; rate and extent drop by 25% to 30% when given with high-fat meal.
Distribution: About 97% of drug and active metabolite are bound to proteins.
Metabolism: 38% of dose de-esterified in liver to active metabolite.
Excretion: Primarily in urine. *Elimination half-life:* 2 hours; *terminal half-life:* 25 hours.

Route	Onset	Peak	Duration
P.O.	≤ 1 hr	1-2 hr	2 hr

Action

Chemical effect: Unknown; may inhibit conversion of angiotensin I to angiotensin II, which lowers peripheral arterial resistance and decreases aldosterone secretion.
Therapeutic effect: Lowers blood pressure.

Available forms

Tablets: 5 mg, 10 mg, 20 mg, 40 mg

NURSING PROCESS

☑ Assessment

• Assess patient's blood pressure before therapy and regularly thereafter. Take blood pressure 2 to 6 hours after dose and just before dose to verify adequate blood pressure control.

Reactions may be *common,* uncommon, *life-threatening,* or COMMON AND LIFE-THREATENING.

• Assess kidney and liver function before and throughout therapy.
• Monitor potassium levels.
• Other ACE inhibitors have been linked to agranulocytosis and neutropenia. Monitor CBC with differential before therapy, q 2 weeks for first 3 months of therapy, and periodically thereafter.
• Be alert for adverse reactions and drug interactions.
• Evaluate patient's and family's knowledge of drug therapy.

Nursing diagnoses
• Risk for injury related to presence of hypertension
• Disturbed sleep pattern related to drug-induced cough
• Deficient knowledge related to drug therapy

Planning and implementation
• If patient has renal impairment, adjust dosage.
• Give drug on empty stomach; high-fat meals can impair absorption.
Patient teaching
• Advise patient to report signs of infection, such as fever and sore throat.
• Tell patient to immediately report signs of angioedema (breathing difficulty and swelling of face, eyes, lips, or tongue), especially after first dose.
• Warn patient that light-headedness can occur, especially at start of drug therapy. Tell him to rise slowly and to stop drug and notify prescriber if he experiences blackouts.
• Inadequate fluid intake, vomiting, diarrhea, and excessive perspiration can lead to light-headedness and syncope. Tell patient to maintain adequate hydration/fluid intake and to use caution in hot weather and during exercise.
• Warn patient to avoid potassium supplements and sodium substitutes that contain potassium during therapy.
• Tell women to notify prescriber about suspected or confirmed pregnancy. Drug will need to be stopped.

Evaluation
• Patient's blood pressure is normal.
• Patient's sleep patterns are undisturbed throughout therapy.
• Patient and family state understanding of drug therapy.

quinidine bisulfate
(KWIN-eh-deen bigh-SUL-fayt)
(66.4% quinidine base)
Biquin Durules ♦ , Kinidin Durules ◇

quinidine gluconate
(62% quinidine base)
Quinaglute Dura-Tabs, Quinalan, Quinate ♦

quinidine sulfate
(83% quinidine base)
Apo-Quinidine ♦ , Cin-Quin, Quinidex Extentabs, Quinora

Pharmacologic class: cinchona alkaloid
Therapeutic class: antiarrhythmic
Pregnancy risk category: C

Indications and dosages

▶ **Atrial flutter or fibrillation.** *Adults:* 200 mg quinidine sulfate or equivalent base P.O. q 2 to 3 hours for five to eight doses, with subsequent daily increases until sinus rhythm is restored or toxic effects develop. Drug is given only after digitalization to avoid increasing AV conduction. Maximum dosage, 3 to 4 g daily. Or, 300 mg Quinidex Extentabs P.O. (extended-release) q 8 to 12 hours.
▶ **Paroxysmal supraventricular tachycardia.** *Adults:* 400 to 600 mg quinidine sulfate P.O. q 2 to 3 hours until toxic adverse reactions develop or arrhythmia subsides.
▶ **Premature atrial and ventricular contractions; paroxysmal AV junctional rhythm; paroxysmal atrial tachycardia; paroxysmal ventricular tachycardia; maintenance after cardioversion of atrial fibrillation or flutter.** *Adults:* Test dose: 200 mg quinidine sulfate or equivalent base P.O., then 200 to 300 mg P.O. q 4 to 6 hours. Or, test dose with 200 mg quinidine gluconate I.M., then give initial dose of 600 mg I.M., followed by 400 mg I.M. q 2 hours, p.r.n., adjusting each dose by the effect of the previous. Or, 300 to 600 mg quinidine sulfate or gluconate sustained-release tablets P.O. q 8 or 12 hours. Or, 800 mg quinidine gluconate I.V. diluted in 40 ml of D_5W and infused at 1 ml/minute.
Children: Test dose is 2 mg/kg; then 30 mg/kg P.O. daily or 900 mg/m[2] P.O. daily in five divided doses.

▶ **Severe** *Plasmodium falciparum* **malaria.**
Adults: 10 mg/kg quinidine gluconate I.V. diluted in 250 ml of normal saline solution and infused over 1 to 2 hours; then continuous maintenance infusion of 0.02 mg/kg/minute for 72 hours or until parasitemia is reduced to less than 1%. Or, 15 mg/kg quinidine gluconate I.V. diluted in 250 ml of normal saline solution infused over 4 hours; begin maintenance therapy 24 hours after the start of the loading dose, 7.5 mg/kg infused over 4 hours, q 8 hours for 7 days, or until oral therapy can be instituted.

▼ I.V. administration

• Use drug I.V. only for acute arrhythmias.
• Mix 10 ml (800 mg) of quinidine gluconate with 40 ml of D₅W and infuse at a slow rate of 1ml/minute for maximum safety.
• Never use discolored (brownish) quinidine solution.

Contraindications and precautions

• Contraindicated in patients hypersensitive to quinidine or related cinchona derivatives; in patients with idiosyncratic reactions to them; and in patients with intraventricular conduction defects, complete heart block, left bundle branch block, history of drug-induced torsade de pointes or prolonged QT interval, digitalis toxicity with grossly impaired AV conduction, or abnormal rhythms caused by escape mechanisms.
• Use cautiously in patients with asthma, muscle weakness, or infection with fever (hypersensitivity reactions to drug may be masked). Also use cautiously in patients with hepatic, renal, or cardiac impairment.
⚞ **Lifespan:** In pregnant women, use cautiously. In breast-feeding women, drug isn't recommended. In children, safety of drug hasn't been established.

Adverse reactions

CNS: *vertigo, headache, light-headedness,* confusion, restlessness, cold sweats, pallor, fainting, fever, dementia.
CV: *PVCs, ventricular tachycardia, atypical ventricular tachycardia (torsades de pointes), severe hypotension, SA and AV block, ventricular fibrillation, cardiotoxicity,* tachycardia, *aggravated heart failure, ECG changes (widening of QRS complex, notched P waves, widened QT interval, ST-segment depression).*

EENT: *tinnitus, blurred vision.*
GI: *diarrhea, nausea, vomiting,* excessive salivation, anorexia, petechial hemorrhage of buccal mucosa, abdominal pain.
Hematologic: hemolytic anemia, *thrombocytopenia, agranulocytosis.*
Hepatic: *hepatotoxicity.*
Respiratory: *acute asthma attack, respiratory arrest.*
Skin: rash, pruritus.
Other: *angioedema,* cinchonism, hypersensitivity reaction, lupus erythematosus.

Interactions

Drug-drug. *Acetazolamide, antacids, sodium bicarbonate, thiazide diuretics:* May increase quinidine levels because of alkaline urine. Monitor patient for increased effect.
Amiodarone: May increase quinidine level producing potentially fatal cardiac arrhythmias. If use together can't be avoided, monitor quinidine level closely. Adjust quinidine p.r.n.
Anticoagulants: Increases anticoagulant effect. Monitor patient closely for bleeding.
Barbiturates, nifedipine, phenytoin, rifampin: May decrease level of quinidine. Monitor patient for decreased quinidine effect.
Cimetidine: Increases quinidine levels. Monitor patient for increased effect.
Digoxin: Increases digoxin level after quinidine therapy starts. Monitor patient closely for digitalis toxicity.
Other antiarrhythmics (such as lidocaine, procainamide, propranolol): Increases risk of toxicity. Use together cautiously.
Propafenone: May increase propafenone levels and its effects. Use together cautiously.
Succinylcholine and nondepolarizing neuromuscular blockades: May increase neuromuscular blockade. Avoid using together.
Sucralfate: May decrease quinidine levels. Adjust dose, p.r.n.
Verapamil: May result in hypotension, bradycardia, or AV block. Monitor blood pressure and heart rate.
Drug-herb. *Jimson weed:* May adversely affect CV function. Discourage using together.
Licorice: May prolong the QT interval. Discourage using together.
Drug-food. *Grapefruit:* May delay absorption and onset of action of drug. Advise patient to avoid eating or drinking grapefruit.

Effects on lab test results
- May increase liver enzyme levels.
- May decrease hemoglobin, hematocrit, and platelet and granulocyte counts.

Pharmacokinetics
Absorption: Although all salts are well absorbed, levels vary greatly among individuals.
Distribution: Well distributed in all tissues except brain; about 80% bound to proteins.
Metabolism: About 60% to 80% metabolized in liver to two metabolites.
Excretion: 10% to 30% excreted in urine. Urine acidification increases excretion; alkalinization decreases it. *Half-life:* 5 to 12 hours.

Route	Onset	Peak	Duration
P.O.	1-3 hr	1-2 hr	6-8 hr
I.V.	Immediate	Immediate	Unknown
I.M.	Unknown	Unknown	Unknown

Action
Chemical effect: Has direct and indirect (anticholinergic) effects on cardiac tissue. Automaticity, conduction velocity, and membrane responsiveness are decreased. The effective refractory period is prolonged. Anticholinergic action reduces vagal tone.
Therapeutic effect: Restores normal sinus rhythm and relieves signs and symptoms of malaria infection.

Available forms
quinidine bisulfate
Tablets (sustained-release): 250 mg ♦ ◊
quinidine gluconate
Injection: 80 mg/ml
Tablets (sustained-release): 324 mg, 325 mg ♦, 330 mg
quinidine sulfate
Tablets: 200 mg, 300 mg
Tablets (sustained-release): 300 mg

NURSING PROCESS

☑ Assessment
- Assess patient's arrhythmia before therapy and regularly thereafter.
- Monitor quinidine level. Therapeutic level for antiarrhythmic effects is 2 to 5 mcg/ml.
- Check apical pulse rate and blood pressure before starting therapy. Hypotension may occur, usually with parenteral use.

- Monitor liver function test results during first 4 to 8 weeks of therapy.
- Be alert for adverse reactions and drug interactions.
- Evaluate patient's and family's knowledge of drug therapy.

✦ Nursing diagnoses
- Decreased cardiac output related to presence of arrhythmia
- Risk for deficient fluid volume related to drug-induced adverse GI reactions
- Deficient knowledge related to drug therapy

▶ Planning and implementation
- Give anticoagulant before therapy in long-standing atrial fibrillation because restoration of normal sinus rhythm may dislodge thrombi from atrial wall, causing thromboembolism.
- If patient develops unexplained fever or elevated hepatic enzyme level, monitor for hepatotoxicity.
- If patient develops symptoms of cardiotoxicity, such as increased PR and QT intervals, 50% widening of the QRS complex, ventricular tachyarrhythmias, frequent ventricular ectopic beats or tachycardia, stop drug immediately.
- Don't crush sustained-release tablets.
- **⚠ ALERT:** Sustained-release preparations aren't interchangeable.
- **⚠ ALERT:** Don't confuse quinidine with clonidine.

Patient teaching
- Tell patient to take drug with meals.
- Tell patient to report signs of toxicity, including ringing in ears, visual disturbances, dizziness, headache, nausea, rash, or shortness of breath.
- Stress importance of follow-up care.

☑ Evaluation
- Patient regains normal cardiac output with resolution of arrhythmia.
- Patient maintains adequate hydration throughout therapy.
- Patient and family state understanding of drug therapy.

---

quinupristin and dalfopristin
(QUIN-uh-pris-tin and DALF-oh-pris-tin)
Synercid

Pharmacologic class: streptogramin
Therapeutic class: antibiotic
Pregnancy risk category: B

Indications and dosages

▶ Serious or life-threatening infections
linked to vancomycin-resistant *Enterococcus
faecium* bacteremia. *Adults and children age
16 and older:* 7.5 mg/kg I.V. infusion over 1
hour q 8 hours. Length of therapy determined
by site and severity of infection.
▶ Complicated skin and skin-structure
infections caused by *Staphylococcus aureus*
(methicillin susceptible) or *Streptococcus pyogenes. Adults and children age 16 and older:*
7.5 mg/kg by I.V. infusion over 1 hour q 12
hours for at least 7 days.

▼ I.V. administration

• Reconstitute powder for injection by adding
5 ml of sterile water for injection or D_5W. Gently swirl vial to dissolve powder completely;
avoid shaking to limit foaming. Reconstituted
solutions must be further diluted within 30 minutes.
• Add dose of reconstituted solution to 250 ml
of D_5W; maximum concentration, 2 mg/ml. Diluted solution is stable for 5 hours at room temperature or 54 hours when refrigerated.
⊛ ALERT: Drug is incompatible with saline and
heparin solutions. Don't dilute with saline-
containing solutions or infuse into lines that
contain saline or heparin. Flush line with D_5W
before and after each dose.
• Fluid-restricted patient with a central venous
catheter may receive dose in 100 ml of D_5W.
This concentration isn't recommended for peripheral venous administration.
• Give all doses by I.V. infusion over 1 hour.
Use an infusion pump or device to control rate
of infusion.
• If moderate-to-severe peripheral venous irritation occurs, consider increasing infusion volume
to 500 or 750 ml, changing injection site, or infusing by central venous catheter.

Contraindications and precautions

• Contraindicated in patients hypersensitive to
drug or other streptogramin antibiotics.
⚖ Lifespan: In pregnant women, use only if
clearly needed. In breast-feeding women, use
cautiously. In children younger than age 16,
safety and effectiveness of drug haven't been established.

Adverse reactions

CNS: headache, pain.
CV: thrombophlebitis.
GI: nausea, diarrhea, vomiting.
Musculoskeletal: arthralgia, myalgia.
Skin: *inflammation, pain, and edema at infu-
sion site;* rash; pruritus.

Interactions

Drug-drug. *Cyclosporine:* Metabolism of cyclosporine is reduced and levels may be increased. Monitor cyclosporine levels.
*Drugs metabolized by CYP 3A4 (carbamaze-
pine, delavirdine, diazepam, diltiazem, disopyramide, docetaxel, indinavir, lidocaine, lovastatin, methylprednisolone, midazolam,
nevirapine, nifedipine, paclitaxel, ritonavir,
tacrolimus, verapamil, vinblastine, and others):*
Increases levels and increases therapeutic effects and adverse reactions of these drugs. Use
together cautiously.
*Drugs metabolized by CYP 3A4 that may pro-
long the QT interval (such as quinidine):* Decreases metabolism of these drugs, resulting in
prolongation of QT interval. Avoid using together.

Effects on lab test results

• May increase AST, ALT, and bilirubin levels.

Pharmacokinetics

Absorption: Administered I.V.
Distribution: Protein-binding is moderate.
Metabolism: Quinupristin and dalfopristin are
converted to several active major metabolites by
nonenzymatic reactions.
Excretion: About 75% of both drugs and their
metabolites excreted in feces. About 15% of
quinupristin and 19% of dalfopristin excreted in
urine. *Half-life:* About 1 hour for quinupristin;
About ¾ hours for dalfopristin.

Route	Onset	Peak	Duration
I.V.	Unknown	Unknown	Unknown

Reactions may be *common,* uncommon, *life-threatening,* or COMMON AND LIFE-THREATENING.

Action

Chemical effect: Inhibit or destroy susceptible bacteria through combined inhibition of protein synthesis in bacterial cells. Dalfopristin inhibits the early phase of protein synthesis in the bacterial ribosome, and quinupristin inhibits the late phase of protein synthesis.
Therapeutic effect: Inactivation or death of bacterial cells.

Available forms

Injection: 500 mg/10 ml (150 mg quinupristin and 350 mg dalfopristin)

NURSING PROCESS

⏳ Assessment

• Obtain history of patient's underlying condition before therapy, and reassess regularly thereafter.
• Overgrowth of nonsusceptible organisms may occur; monitor patient closely for signs and symptoms of superinfection.
• Monitor liver function during therapy.
• Evaluate patient's and family's knowledge of drug therapy.

🔀 Nursing diagnoses

• Risk for infection related to presence of bacteria
• Diarrhea related to drug-induced adverse effect
• Deficient knowledge related to drug therapy

⮞ Planning and implementation

⚡ **ALERT:** Drug isn't active against *Enterococcus faecalis*. Appropriate blood cultures are needed to avoid misidentifying *E. faecalis* as *E. faecium*.
• To reduce adverse reactions, such as arthralgia and myalgia, decrease dose interval to q 12 hours.
• If patient develops diarrhea during or following therapy, notify prescriber because mild to life-threatening pseudomembranous colitis may occur.
Patient teaching
• Advise patient to immediately report irritation at I.V. site, pain in joints or muscles, and diarrhea.
• Tell patient to report persistent or worsening signs and symptoms of infection, such as pain and erythema.

✅ Evaluation

• Patient is free from infection.
• Patient doesn't experience diarrhea.
• Patient and family state understanding of drug therapy.

rabeprazole sodium
(rah-BEH-pruh-zohl SOH-dee-um)
Aciphex

Pharmacologic class: proton pump inhibitor
Therapeutic class: antiulcerative
Pregnancy risk category: B

Indications and dosages

▶ **Healing of erosive or ulcerative gastroesophageal reflux disease (GERD).** *Adults:* 20 mg P.O. daily for 4 to 8 weeks. Additional 8-week course may be considered, if needed.
▶ **Maintenance of healing of erosive or ulcerative GERD.** *Adults:* 20 mg P.O. daily.
▶ **Healing of duodenal ulcers.** *Adults:* 20 mg P.O. daily after morning meal for up to 4 weeks.
▶ **Pathological hypersecretory conditions including Zollinger-Ellison syndrome.** *Adults:* 60 mg P.O. daily; increase p.r.n. to 100 mg P.O. daily or 60 mg P.O. twice daily.
▶ **Symptomatic GERD, including daytime and nighttime heartburn.** *Adults:* 20 mg P.O. daily for 4 weeks. Additional 4-week course may be considered, if needed.
▶ *Helicobacter pylori* **eradication to reduce the risk of duodenal ulcer recurrence.** *Adults:* Three drug regimen: rabeprazole 20 mg P.O. b.i.d. given with amoxicillin 1,000 mg P.O. b.i.d. and clarithromycin 500 mg P.O. b.i.d. for a total of 7 days.

Contraindications and precautions

• Contraindicated in patients hypersensitive to drug, other benzimidazoles (such as lansoprazole or omeprazole), or components in these formulations. For *H. pylori* eradication, clarithromycin is contraindicated in patients hypersensitive to any macrolide antibiotic and in those taking pimozide. Amoxicillin is contraindicated in patients hypersensitive to any penicillin.

• Use cautiously in patients with severe hepatic impairment.

※ **Lifespan:** In pregnant women, clarithromycin is contraindicated for *H. pylori* eradication. In children, safety of drug hasn't been established.

Adverse reactions

CNS: headache.

Interactions

Drug-drug. *Clarithromycin:* Increases levels of rabeprazole. Monitor patient closely.
Cyclosporine: May inhibit cyclosporine metabolism. Use together cautiously.
Digoxin, ketoconazole, other gastric pH-dependent drugs: Decreases or increases drug absorption at increased pH values. Monitor patient closely.
Drug-herb. *St. John's wort:* May increase risk of sunburn. Discourage using together; urge patient to avoid unprotected or prolonged sun exposure.

Effects on lab test results

None reported.

Pharmacokinetics

Absorption: Acid labile; enteric coating allows drug to pass through the stomach relatively intact. Level peaks over a period of 2 to 5 hours.
Distribution: 96.3% protein-bound.
Metabolism: Extensively metabolized by the liver to inactive compounds.
Excretion: 90% eliminated in urine as metabolites. Remaining 10% of metabolites eliminated in feces. *Half-life:* 1 to 2 hours.

Route	Onset	Peak	Duration
P.O.	< 1 hr	2-5 hr	> 24 hr

Action

Chemical effect: Blocks activity of the acid (proton) pump by inhibiting gastric hydrogen-potassium adenosine triphosphatase at the secretory surface of gastric parietal cells, thereby blocking gastric acid secretion.
Therapeutic effect: Promotes healing of gastric erosion or ulceration by stopping gastric acid secretion.

Available forms

Tablets (delayed-release): 20 mg

NURSING PROCESS

⚗ Assessment

• Obtain history of patient's underlying condition before therapy, and reassess regularly thereafter.
• Determine if patient is hypersensitive to penicillin because anaphylaxis may occur.
• Be alert for adverse reactions and drug interactions.
• Evaluate patient's and family's knowledge of drug therapy.

⊕ Nursing diagnoses

• Acute pain related to underlying condition
• Risk for injury related to drug-induced adverse reactions
• Deficient knowledge related to drug therapy

▷ Planning and implementation

• Don't crush, split, or allow patient to chew tablets.
• If duodenal ulcer or GERD isn't healed after first course of therapy, additional courses of therapy may be needed.
• **ALERT:** Symptomatic response to therapy doesn't rule out presence of gastric malignancy.
• In patients who don't respond to therapy for *H. pylori,* test for susceptibility. If resistance to clarithromycin occurs or susceptibility testing isn't possible, give a different antimicrobial.
• **ALERT:** For *H. pylori* eradication, pseudomembranous colitis may occur with nearly all antibacterials, including clarithromycin and amoxicillin. Monitor patient closely.
Patient teaching
• Explain importance of taking drug exactly as prescribed.
• Advise patient that delayed-release tablets should be swallowed whole and not crushed, chewed, or split.
• Tell patient that drug may be taken without regard to meals.

✓ Evaluation

• Patient experiences decreased pain with drug therapy.
• Patient sustains no injury as a result of drug-induced adverse reactions.

• Patient and family state understanding of drug therapy.

rabies immune globulin, human

(RAY-bees ih-MYOON GLOH-byoo-lin, HYOO-mun)

BayRab, Imogam Rabies-HT

Pharmacologic class: immune serum
Therapeutic class: rabies prophylaxis drug
Pregnancy risk category: C

Indications and dosages

▶ **Rabies exposure.** *Adults and children:*
20 IU/kg at time of first dose of rabies vaccine. If feasible, infiltrate the full dose in the area around and in the wounds. Give remainder, if any, I.M. separate from rabies vaccine injection site.

Contraindications and precautions

• Give only one dose to prevent interference with effectiveness of vaccine.
• Use cautiously in patients hypersensitive to thimerosal, in patients with a history of systemic allergic reactions after administration of human immunoglobulin preparations, and in patients with immunoglobulin A deficiency.
⚘ **Lifespan:** In pregnant women, use cautiously. In breast-feeding women, safety of drug hasn't been established.

Adverse reactions

CV: slight fever, slight headache, malaise.
GU: nephrotic syndrome.
Skin: *rash,* pain, redness, induration at injection site.
Other: *anaphylaxis, angioedema.*

Interactions

Drug-drug. *Corticosteroids, immunosuppressive drugs:* May interfere with the active antibody response, predisposing patient to rabies. Avoid these drugs during postexposure immunization period.
Live-virus vaccines: May interfere with response to vaccine. Delay immunization.
Rabies vaccine: May partially suppress the antibody response to rabies immune globulin. Give full dose of immune globulin into wound.

Effects on lab test results

None reported.

Pharmacokinetics

Absorption: Slow.
Distribution: Unknown.
Metabolism: Unknown.
Excretion: Unknown. *Half-life:* About 24 days.

Route	Onset	Peak	Duration
I.M.	Unknown	2-13 days	Unknown

Action

Chemical effect: Provides passive immunity to rabies.
Therapeutic effect: Prevents rabies.

Available forms

Injection: 150 IU/ml in 2-ml, 10-ml vials

NURSING PROCESS

⚖ Assessment
• Obtain history of animal bites, allergies, and immunization reactions.
• Ask patient when he last received a tetanus immunization; prescriber may order booster.
• Be alert for adverse reactions and drug interactions.
• Evaluate patient's and family's knowledge of drug therapy.

⊕ Nursing diagnoses
• Risk for injury related to rabies exposure
• Ineffective protection related to drug-induced hypersensitivity reaction
• Deficient knowledge related to drug therapy

▷ Planning and implementation
• Use only with rabies vaccine and immediate local treatment of wound. Don't give in same syringe or at same site as rabies vaccine. Give drug regardless of interval between exposure and start of therapy.
• Don't administer live-virus vaccines within 3 months of rabies immune globulin.
⑤ ALERT: Drug provides passive immunity. Don't confuse with rabies vaccine, which is suspension of attenuated or killed microorganisms used to give active immunity. The two drugs usually are given together for prophylaxis after exposure to known or suspected rabid animals.

⊛ **ALERT:** Have epinephrine 1:1,000 immediately available to treat any acute anaphylactic reactions.

⊛ **ALERT:** Don't give more than 5 ml at one I.M. injection site; divide I.M. doses larger than 5 ml, and give at different sites. Use a large muscle, such as the gluteus.

Patient teaching
• Tell patient he may develop a slight fever and pain and redness at injection site.
• Advise patient that tetanus booster may be needed.
• Instruct patient to report signs of hypersensitivity immediately.

☑ **Evaluation**
• Patient has passive immunity to rabies.
• Patient shows no signs of hypersensitivity after receiving drug.
• Patient and family state understanding of drug therapy.

raloxifene hydrochloride
(rah-LOKS-ih-feen high-droh-KLOR-ighd)
Evista

Pharmacologic class: selective estrogen receptor modulator of the benzothiophene class
Therapeutic class: antiosteoporotic
Pregnancy risk category: X

Indications and dosages
▶ **Prevention and treatment of osteoporosis.**
Postmenopausal women: 60 mg P.O. daily.

Contraindications and precautions
• Contraindicated in women hypersensitive to drug or its constituents and in those with current or past venous thromboembolic events, including deep vein thrombosis (DVT), pulmonary embolism, or retinal vein thrombosis.
• Use cautiously in women with severe hepatic impairment.
• Use with hormone replacement therapy or systemic estrogen isn't recommended.
⚕ **Lifespan:** In women who are pregnant or planning to become pregnant, in breast-feeding women, and in children, drug is contraindicated. In men, safety and effectiveness haven't been evaluated.

Adverse reactions
CNS: depression, insomnia, migraine, fever.
CV: chest pain, peripheral edema.
EENT: *sinusitis,* pharyngitis, laryngitis.
GI: nausea, dyspepsia, vomiting, flatulence, GI disorder, gastroenteritis, abdominal pain.
GU: vaginitis, UTI, cystitis, leukorrhea, endometrial disorder, vaginal bleeding.
Metabolic: weight gain.
Musculoskeletal: *arthralgia,* myalgia, arthritis, leg cramps.
Respiratory: increased cough, pneumonia.
Skin: rash, sweating.
Other: *hot flushes, infection, flulike syndrome,* breast pain.

Interactions
Drug-drug. *Cholestyramine:* Significantly reduces raloxifene absorption. Don't give these drugs together.
Highly protein-bound drugs (such as clofibrate, diazepam, diazoxide, ibuprofen, indomethacin, naproxen): May interfere with binding sites. Use together cautiously.
Warfarin: May decrease PT. Monitor PT and INR closely.

Effects on lab test results
• May increase calcium, inorganic phosphate, total protein, albumin, hormone-binding globulin, and apolipoprotein A levels. May decrease total and low-density lipoprotein cholesterol levels and apolipoprotein B levels.

Pharmacokinetics
Absorption: Rapid, with about 60% of dose absorbed after P.O. administration.
Distribution: Widely distributed and highly bound to proteins.
Metabolism: Extensive first-pass metabolism to glucuronide conjugates.
Excretion: Primarily excreted in feces, with less than 0.2% excreted unchanged in urine.
Half-life: 27½ hours.

Route	Onset	Peak	Duration
P.O.	Unknown	Unknown	24 hr

Action
Chemical effect: Reduces resorption of bone and decreases overall bone turnover, resulting in increased bone mineral density.

Therapeutic effect: Prevents bone breakdown in postmenopausal women.

Available forms

Tablets: 60 mg

NURSING PROCESS

Assessment

• Obtain history of patient's condition, and reassess during therapy.
• Monitor patient for signs of blood clots. The greatest risk of thromboembolic events occurs during first 4 months.
• Monitor patient for breast abnormalities.
• Monitor lipid levels, blood pressure, body weight, and liver function.
• Evaluate patient's and family's knowledge of drug therapy.

Nursing diagnoses

• Ineffective peripheral tissue perfusion related to potential DVT formation
• Imbalanced nutrition: less than body requirements related to drug-induced adverse GI reactions
• Deficient knowledge related to drug therapy

Planning and implementation

⊕ ALERT: Stop drug at least 72 hours before prolonged immobilization, and resume only after patient is fully mobile.
• If you suspect thromboembolic event, withhold drug and notify prescriber.
• Report unexplained uterine bleeding immediately to prescriber.
• Effect on bone mineral density with more than 2 years of drug therapy isn't known.
Patient teaching
• Advise patient to avoid long periods of restricted movement (such as during traveling) because it increases the risk of venous thromboembolic events.
• Inform patient that hot flashes or flushing may occur and that drug doesn't aid in reducing them.
• Instruct patient to take other bone-loss prevention measures, including taking supplemental calcium and vitamin D if dietary intake is inadequate, performing weight-bearing exercises, and stopping alcohol consumption and smoking.
• Tell patient that drug may be taken without regard to food.

• Advise patient to report any unexplained uterine bleeding or breast abnormalities.
• Explain adverse effects of drug. Instruct patient to read package insert before starting therapy and to read it again each time prescription is renewed.

Evaluation

• Patient doesn't develop pain, redness, or swelling in legs.
• Patient maintains normal dietary intake.
• Patient and family state understanding of drug therapy.

ramipril
(reh-MIH-pril)
Altace, Ramace ◊ , Tritace ◊

Pharmacologic class: ACE inhibitor
Therapeutic class: antihypertensive
Pregnancy risk category: C (D in second and third trimesters)

Indications and dosages

▶ **Hypertension (either alone or with thiazide diuretics).** *Adults:* Initially, 2.5 mg P.O. daily in patients not receiving diuretic therapy. Adjust dose based on blood pressure response. Usual maintenance dosage is 2.5 to 20 mg daily as a single dose or in two equal doses.
◫ Adjust-a-dose: For patients with renal impairment, if creatinine clearance is less than 40 ml/minute (creatinine above 2.5 mg/dl), recommended initial dose is 1.25 mg daily, adjusted upward to maximum dose of 5 mg based on blood pressure response.
In patients receiving diuretic therapy, symptomatic hypotension may occur. To minimize this, stop diuretic, if possible, 2 to 3 days before starting this drug. When this isn't possible, initial dose of this drug should be 1.25 mg.
▶ **Heart failure post-MI.** *Adults:* Initially, 2.5 mg P.O. b.i.d. Adjust to target dose of 5 mg P.O. b.i.d.
◫ Adjust-a-dose: For patients with renal impairment, start therapy with 1.25 mg P.O. once daily, and increase to 1.25 mg b.i.d. Maximum dosage is 2.5 mg b.i.d.
▶ **Reduction in risk of MI, CVA, and death from CV causes.** *Adults age 55 and older:* 2.5 mg P.O. once daily for 1 week, then 5 mg

P.O. once daily for 3 weeks. Increase as tolerated to a maintenance dosage of 10 mg P.O. once daily.

◩ **Adjust-a-dose:** For patients with renal impairment, if creatinine clearance is less than 40 ml/minute, give one-quarter of recommended dose.

Contraindications and precautions

• Contraindicated in patients hypersensitive to ACE inhibitors, in those with history of angioedema during previous therapy with ACE inhibitor, and in those with renal artery stenosis.
• Use cautiously in patients with renal impairment.
⚕ Lifespan: In pregnant and breast-feeding women, drug isn't recommended. In children, safety of drug hasn't been established.

Adverse reactions

CNS: headache, dizziness, fatigue, syncope, asthenia, malaise, light-headedness, anxiety, amnesia, *seizures,* depression, insomnia, nervousness, neuralgia, neuropathy, paresthesia, somnolence, tremors, vertigo.
CV: orthostatic hypotension, angina, *arrhythmias,* chest pain, palpitations, *MI,* edema.
EENT: epistaxis, tinnitus.
GI: nausea, vomiting, abdominal pain, anorexia, constipation, diarrhea, dyspepsia, dry mouth, gastroenteritis.
GU: impotence.
Metabolic: *hyperkalemia,* weight gain.
Musculoskeletal: arthralgia, arthritis, myalgia.
Respiratory: *dry, persistent, tickling, nonproductive cough;* dyspnea.
Skin: rash, dermatitis, pruritus, photosensitivity reaction, increased diaphoresis.
Other: hypersensitivity reactions, *angioedema.*

Interactions

Drug-drug. *Diuretics:* Excessive hypotension, especially at start of therapy. Stop diuretic at least 3 days before starting ramipril, increase sodium intake, or reduce starting dose of ramipril.
Insulin, oral antidiabetics: May increase risk of hypoglycemia, especially at start of ramipril therapy. Monitor patient closely.
Lithium: May increase lithium levels. Use together cautiously, and monitor lithium levels for toxicity.
Potassium-sparing diuretics, potassium supplements: Increases risk of hyperkalemia because

ramipril attenuates potassium loss. Monitor potassium level closely.
Drug-herb. *Capsaicin:* Increases risk of cough. Discourage using together.
Licorice: May cause sodium retention and increase blood pressure, interfering with therapeutic effects of ACE inhibitors. Discourage using together.
Drug-food. *Salt substitutes containing potassium:* Increases risk of hyperkalemia because ramipril attenuates potassium loss. Monitor potassium level closely.

Effects on lab test results

• May increase BUN, creatinine, bilirubin, liver enzyme, glucose, and potassium levels.
• May decrease hemoglobin and hematocrit.

Pharmacokinetics

Absorption: 50% to 60%.
Distribution: 73% protein-bound; ramiprilat (metabolite), 58%.
Metabolism: Almost completely converted to ramiprilat, which is six times more potent than parent drug.
Excretion: 60% in urine; 40% in feces. *Half-life:* 13 to 17 hours.

Route	Onset	Peak	Duration
P.O.	1-2 hr	< 1 hr	About 24 hr

Action

Chemical effect: Unknown; may inhibit conversion from angiotensin I to angiotensin II, a potent vasoconstrictor. This decreases peripheral arterial resistance, thus decreasing aldosterone secretion.
Therapeutic effect: Lowers blood pressure.

Available forms

Capsules: 1.25 mg, 2.5 mg, 5 mg, 10 mg

NURSING PROCESS

🔎 **Assessment**

• Assess patient's blood pressure before therapy and regularly thereafter.
• Closely assess kidney function during first few weeks of therapy. Regularly assess creatinine and BUN levels. Patient with severe heart failure whose kidney function depends on angiotensin-aldosterone system may experience acute renal impairment during therapy. Hyper-

---

tensive patient with renal artery stenosis also may show signs of worsening kidney function at start of therapy.
• Monitor CBC before therapy, q 2 weeks for first 3 months of therapy, and periodically thereafter.
• Monitor potassium level. Risk factors for hyperkalemia include renal insufficiency, diabetes, and use of drugs that raise potassium levels.
• Be alert for adverse reactions and drug interactions.
• Evaluate patient's and family's knowledge of drug therapy.

🔁 Nursing diagnoses
• Risk for injury related to presence of hypertension
• Disturbed sleep pattern related to drug-induced cough
• Deficient knowledge related to drug therapy

⧁ Planning and implementation
• Stop diuretic 2 to 3 days before starting therapy, if possible.
• If patient has trouble swallowing pills whole, capsule may be opened and the contents sprinkled onto 4 ounces of applesauce or mixed in 4 ounces (118 ml) of water or apple juice. These mixtures may be stored at room temperature for up to 24 hours, or refrigerated for up to 48 hours.

Patient teaching
• Instruct patient to avoid sodium substitutes during therapy.
• If patient has trouble swallowing, tell him to open capsules and sprinkle contents on food.
• Tell patient to rise slowly to avoid initial lightheadedness. If syncope occurs, he should stop drug and call prescriber.
• Tell patient not to stop therapy abruptly.
• Advise patient to report signs of angioedema and laryngeal edema, which may occur after first dose.
• Tell patient to report signs of infection.
• Tell woman to report pregnancy. Drug will need to be stopped.

☑ Evaluation
• Patient's blood pressure is normal.
• Patient's sleep patterns are undisturbed throughout therapy.
• Patient and family state understanding of drug therapy.

ranitidine hydrochloride
(ruh-NIH-tuh-deen high-droh-KLOR-ighd)
Zantac*, Zantac-C♦ , Zantac EFFERdose, Zantac GELdose, Zantac 75†

Pharmacologic class: H₂-receptor antagonist
Therapeutic class: antiulcerative
Pregnancy risk category: B

Indications and dosages
▶ **Intractable duodenal ulcer; pathologic hypersecretory conditions, such as Zollinger-Ellison syndrome; or for short-term use in patients unable to tolerate oral forms (I.V. only).** *Adults:* 150 mg P.O. b.i.d. or 300 mg q h.s. Or, 50 mg I.V. or I.M. q 6 to 8 hours. Patients with Zollinger-Ellison syndrome may need up to 6 g P.O. daily. Or, for Zollinger-Ellison syndrome, 1 mg/kg/hour for 4 hours, then increase in increments of 0.5 mg/kg/hr if needed, to a maximum of 2.5 mg/kg/hour.
▶ **Duodenal and gastric ulcer.** *Children ages 1 month to 16 years:* 2 to 4 mg/kg P.O. twice daily to a maximum of 300 mg/day. Maintenance dosage is 2 to 4 mg/kg P.O. once daily to a maximum of 150 mg daily.
▶ **Maintenance therapy for healing duodenal ulcer.** *Adults:* 150 mg P.O. h.s.
▶ **Gastroesophageal reflux disease.** *Adults:* 150 mg P.O. b.i.d.
Children: 5 to 10 mg/kg P.O. daily in divided doses.
▶ **Erosive esophagitis.** *Adults:* 150 mg P.O. q.i.d.; maintenance dosage, 150 mg P.O. b.i.d.
▶ **Relief of occasional heartburn, acid indigestion, and sour stomach.** *Adults and children age 12 and older:* 75 mg once or twice daily; maximum daily dosage, 150 mg.

▽ I.V. administration
• To prepare I.V. injection, dilute 2 ml (50 mg) with compatible I.V. solution to a total volume of 20 ml, and inject over at least 5 minutes. Compatible solutions include sterile water for injection, normal saline solution for injection, D₅W, and lactated Ringer's injection.
• To give drug by intermittent I.V. infusion, dilute 50 mg (2 ml) in 100 ml compatible solution and infuse at a rate of 5 to 7 ml/minute. The premixed solution is 50 ml and doesn't need further dilution. Infuse over 15 to 20 minutes. After di-

lution, solution is stable for 48 hours at room temperature.
- For premixed I.V. infusion, give by slow I.V. drip (over 15 to 20 minutes). Don't add other drugs to solution. If used with primary I.V. fluid system, stop primary solution during infusion.
- Store I.V. vial at 39° to 86° F (4° to 30° C). Store premixed containers at 36° F to 77° F (2° C to 25° C).

Contraindications and precautions

- Contraindicated in patients hypersensitive to drug.
- Use cautiously in patients with hepatic dysfunction. Adjust dosage in patients with impaired kidney function.
- ⚖ Lifespan: In pregnant and breast-feeding women, use cautiously. In children, safety of drug hasn't been established for pathological hypersecretory conditions or the maintenance of healing duodenal ulcer. In neonates younger than 1 month, safety of drug hasn't been established. In elderly patients, use cautiously.

Adverse reactions

CNS: vertigo, malaise.
EENT: blurred vision.
Hematologic: *reversible leukopenia, pancytopenia, thrombocytopenia.*
Hepatic: jaundice.
Other: burning and itching at injection site, *anaphylaxis, angioedema.*

Interactions

Drug-drug. *Antacids:* May interfere with ranitidine absorption. Stagger doses.
Diazepam: Decreases diazepam absorption. Monitor patient for decreased effectiveness; adjust dose.
Glipizide: May increase hypoglycemic effect. Adjust glipizide dosage.
Procainamide: May decrease renal clearance of procainamide. Monitor patient for procainamide toxicity.
Warfarin: May interfere with warfarin clearance. Monitor patient closely for bleeding.
Drug-lifestyle. *Smoking:* May increase gastric acid secretion and worsen disease. Discourage using together.

Effects on lab test results

- May increase creatinine and ALT levels.
- May decrease RBC, WBC, and platelet counts.

Pharmacokinetics

Absorption: About 50% to 60% of P.O. dose; rapid from parenteral sites after I.M. dose.
Distribution: Distributed to many body tissues and appears in CSF; about 10% to 19% protein-bound.
Metabolism: Metabolized in liver.
Excretion: Excreted in urine and feces. *Half-life:* 2 to 3 hours.

Route	Onset	Peak	Duration
P.O.	≤1 hr	1-3 hr	≤13 hr
I.V., I.M.	Unknown	Unknown	≤13 hr

Action

Chemical effect: Competitively inhibits action of H_2 at receptor sites of parietal cells, decreasing gastric acid secretion.
Therapeutic effect: Relieves GI discomfort.

Available forms

Capsules: 150 mg, 300 mg
Granules (effervescent): 150 mg
Infusion: 0.5 mg/ml in 100-ml containers
Injection: 25 mg/ml
Syrup: 15 mg/ml*
Tablets: 75 mg†, 150 mg, 300 mg
Tablets (dispersible): 150 mg†
Tablets (effervescent): 150 mg

NURSING PROCESS

🔲 Assessment

- Assess patient's GI condition before therapy and regularly thereafter.
- Be alert for adverse reactions and drug interactions.
- Evaluate patient's and family's knowledge of drug therapy.

🔲 Nursing diagnoses

- Impaired tissue integrity related to underlying GI condition
- Risk for injury related to drug-induced adverse CNS reactions
- Deficient knowledge related to drug therapy

🔲 Planning and implementation

- Don't use aluminum-based needles or equipment when mixing or giving drug parenterally because drug is incompatible with aluminum.
- No dilution is needed when giving drug I.M.

ⓢ **ALERT:** Don't confuse ranitidine with rimantadine.

ⓢ **ALERT:** Don't confuse Zantac with Xanax or Zyrtec.

Patient teaching

• Remind patient taking drug once daily to take it h.s.

• Instruct patient to take drug without regard to meals.

• Urge patient to avoid cigarette smoking because it may increase gastric acid secretion and worsen disease.

☑ **Evaluation**

• Patient states that GI discomfort is relieved.

• Patient sustains no injury as result of drug-induced adverse CNS reactions.

• Patient and family state understanding of drug therapy.

repaglinide
(reh-PAG-lih-nighd)
Prandin

Pharmacologic class: meglitinide
Therapeutic class: antidiabetic
Pregnancy risk category: C

Indications and dosages

▶ **Adjunct to diet and exercise to lower glucose levels in patients with type 2 diabetes mellitus (non-insulin-dependent diabetes mellitus) whose hyperglycemia can't be controlled satisfactorily by diet and exercise alone; adjunct to diet, exercise, and metformin, rosiglitazone, or pioglitazone.** *Adults:* For patients not previously treated or whose HbA_{1c} is below 8%, start dose at 0.5 mg P.O. given 15 minutes before meal; however, time may vary from immediately before to as long as 30 minutes before meal. For patients previously treated with glucose-lowering drugs and whose HbA_{1c} is 8% or more, initial dose is 1 to 2 mg P.O. with each meal. Recommended dosage range is 0.5 to 4 mg with meals b.i.d., t.i.d., or q.i.d. Maximum, 16 mg daily. Dosage should be determined by glucose level response. May double dosage up to 4 mg with each meal until satisfactory glucose response is achieved. Allow at least 1 week between dosage adjustments to assess response to each dose.

◹ **Adjust-a-dose:** For patients with severe renal impairment, starting dose is 0.5 mg P.O. with meals.

Contraindications and precautions

• Contraindicated in patients hypersensitive to drug or its inactive ingredients and in those with insulin-dependent diabetes mellitus or diabetic ketoacidosis with or without coma.

• Use cautiously in patients with hepatic insufficiency in whom reduced metabolism could increase repaglinide levels and cause hypoglycemia. Also use cautiously in debilitated and malnourished patients and in those with adrenal or pituitary insufficiency because they're more susceptible to the hypoglycemic effect of glucose-lowering drugs.

⚖ **Lifespan:** In pregnant or breast-feeding women, avoid using. In children, safety hasn't been established. In elderly patients, use cautiously.

Adverse reactions

CNS: *headache,* paresthesia.
CV: angina, chest pain.
EENT: rhinitis, sinusitis.
GI: constipation, diarrhea, dyspepsia, nausea, vomiting.
GU: UTI.
Metabolic: HYPOGLYCEMIA, hyperglycemia.
Musculoskeletal: arthralgia, back pain.
Respiratory: bronchitis, *upper respiratory infection.*
Other: tooth disorder.

Interactions

Drug-drug. *Barbiturates, carbamazepine, rifampin:* May increase repaglinide metabolism. Monitor glucose level.
Beta blockers, chloramphenicol, coumarins, MAO inhibitors, NSAIDs, other drugs that are highly protein-bound, probenecid, salicylates, sulfonamides: May potentiate hypoglycemic action of repaglinide. Monitor glucose level.
Calcium channel blockers, corticosteroids, estrogens, hormonal contraceptives, isoniazid, nicotinic acid, phenothiazines, phenytoin, sympathomimetics, thiazides and other diuretics, thyroid products: May produce hyperglycemia and loss of glycemic control. Monitor glucose level.

Erythromycin, inhibitors of CYP 3A4, gemfi-brozil, ketoconazole, miconazole: May inhibit repaglinide metabolism. Monitor glucose levels and avoid using gemfibrozil and repaglinide together.
Levonorgestrel and ethinyl estradiol, simvastatin: May increase repaglinide levels. Monitor glucose level.
Drug-herb. Aloe, bitter melon, bilberry leaf, burdock, dandelion, fenugreek, garlic, ginseng: May improve glucose control so that antidiabetic dosage needs to be reduced. Advise patient to discuss the use of herbal remedies before taking drug.

Effects on lab test results

● May increase or decrease glucose level.

Pharmacokinetics

Absorption: Rapid and complete. Absolute bioavailability is 56%.
Distribution: More than 98% bound to proteins.
Metabolism: Completely metabolized by oxidative biotransformation and direct conjugation with glucuronic acid.
Excretion: About 90% is recovered in feces and 8% in urine. Half-life: 1 hour.

Route	Onset	Peak	Duration
P.O.	Unknown	1 hr	Unknown

Action

Chemical effect: Stimulates the release of insulin from beta cells in the pancreas.
Therapeutic effect: Lowers glucose level.

Available forms

Tablets: 0.5 mg, 1 mg, 2 mg

NURSING PROCESS

◪ Assessment
● Monitor glucose level before therapy and regularly thereafter.
● Be alert for adverse reactions and drug interactions.
● Monitor geriatric patients and patients taking beta blockers carefully because hypoglycemia may be difficult to recognize in these patients.
● Evaluate patient's and family's knowledge of drug therapy.

⊕ Nursing diagnoses
● Imbalanced nutrition: more than body requirements related to patient's underlying condition
● Risk for injury related to drug-induced hypoglycemic episode
● Deficient knowledge related to drug therapy

❯ Planning and implementation
● Increase dosage carefully in patients with renal impairment who need dialysis.
● If repaglinide alone is inadequate, metformin may be added.
● Loss of glycemic control can occur during stress, such as fever, trauma, infection, or surgery. Stop drug and give insulin.
● Oral antidiabetics have been linked to increased CV mortality compared to changing diet alone.
● Give drug immediately or up to 30 minutes before meals.
Patient teaching
● Teach patient about importance of diet and exercise along with drug therapy.
● Discuss symptoms of hypoglycemia with patient and family.
● Advise patient to monitor glucose level periodically to determine minimum effective dose.
● Encourage patient to keep regular medical appointments and have glucose level checked to monitor long-term glucose control.
● Tell patient to take drug before meals, usually 15 minutes before start of meal; however, time can vary from immediately to up to 30 minutes before meal.
● Tell patient to skip dose if he skips a meal and to add dose if he adds a meal.
● Teach patient how to monitor glucose levels carefully and what to do when he is ill, undergoing surgery, or under added stress.

☑ Evaluation
● Patient's glucose level is controlled and an adequate nutritional balance is maintained.
● Patient doesn't experience severe decreases in glucose level.
● Patient and family state understanding of drug therapy.

reteplase, recombinant
(REE-teh-plays, ree-KUHM-buh-nent)
Retavase

Pharmacologic class: recombinant plasminogen activator, enzyme
Therapeutic class: thrombolytic enzyme
Pregnancy risk category: C

Indications and dosages

▶ **Acute MI.** *Adults:* Double-bolus injection of 10 + 10 units. Give each bolus I.V. over 2 minutes. If complications don't occur after first bolus, give second bolus 30 minutes after start of first.

▼ I.V. administration

• Reconstitute drug according to manufacturer's instructions.
• **ALERT:** Don't give drug with other I.V. drugs through the same line. Heparin and reteplase are incompatible in solution.

Contraindications and precautions

• Contraindicated in patients with active internal bleeding, bleeding diathesis, history of CVA, recent intracranial or intraspinal surgery or trauma, severe uncontrolled hypertension, intracranial neoplasm, arteriovenous malformation, or aneurysm.
• Use cautiously in patients who've had major surgery, obstetric delivery, organ biopsy, or trauma within 10 days and in those with previous puncture of noncompressible vessel, cerebrovascular disease, recent GI or GU bleeding, or heart disease.
• **Lifespan:** In breast-feeding women, use cautiously. In children, safety of drug hasn't been established.

Adverse reactions

CNS: *intracranial hemorrhage.*
CV: *arrhythmias, cholesterol embolization, hemorrhage.*
GI: *hemorrhage.*
GU: hematuria.
Hematologic: anemia, *bleeding tendency.*
Other: bleeding at puncture sites.

Interactions

Drug-drug. *Heparin, oral anticoagulants, platelet inhibitors (abciximab, aspirin, dipyridamole):* May increase risk of bleeding. Use together cautiously.

Effects on lab test results

• May decrease plasminogen and fibrinogen levels.
• May decrease hemoglobin and hematocrit.
• May cause unreliable results of coagulation tests or measurements of fibrinolytic activity.

Pharmacokinetics

Absorption: Administered I.V.
Distribution: Rapid distribution.
Metabolism: Unknown.
Excretion: In urine and feces. *Half-life:* 13 to 16 minutes.

Route	Onset	Peak	Duration
I.V.	Unknown	Unknown	Unknown

Action

Chemical effect: Enhances cleavage of plasminogen to generate plasmin.
Therapeutic effect: Dissolves and breaks up clots.

Available forms

Injection: 10.8 IU (18.8 mg)/vial. Supplied in kit with components for reconstitution for 2 single-use vials.

NURSING PROCESS

Assessment
• Monitor ECG.
• Monitor patient for bleeding. Avoid I.M. injections, invasive procedures, and unneeded handling of patient.
• Evaluate patient's and family's knowledge of drug therapy.

Nursing diagnoses
• Ineffective cardiopulmonary tissue perfusion related to underlying condition
• Risk for injury related to adverse effects of drug
• Deficient knowledge related to drug therapy

≥ Planning and implementation

• Reteplase is administered I.V. as double-bolus injection. If bleeding or anaphylactoid reaction occurs after first bolus, notify prescriber.

• Avoid non-compressible pressure sites during therapy. If an arterial puncture is needed, use a vessel in the arm that can be compressed manually. Apply pressure for at least 30 minutes; then apply a pressure dressing. Check site often for bleeding.

Patient teaching

• Teach patient and family about drug.

• Tell patient to report adverse reactions immediately.

☑ Evaluation

• Patient's cardiopulmonary assessment findings show improved perfusion.

• Patient is free from serious adverse reactions caused by therapy.

• Patient and family state understanding of drug therapy.

Rh₀(D) immune globulin, human
(ARR AITCH OH DEE ih-MYOON GLOH-byoo-lin, HYOO-mun)

Rh₀(D) immune globulin, human (Rho[D] IGIM)
BayRho-D Full Dose, RhoGAM

Rh₀(D) immune globulin, human (Rho[D] IGIV)
WinRho SDF

Rh₀(D) immune globulin, human, microdose (Rho[D] IG microdose)
BayRho-D Mini-Dose, MICRhoGAM

Pharmacologic class: immune serum
Therapeutic class: anti-Rh₀(D)-positive prophylaxis drug
Pregnancy risk category: C

Indications and dosages

▶ **Rh exposure (postabortion, postmiscarriage, ectopic pregnancy, postpartum, or threatened abortion 13 weeks or later).**
Women: Transfusion unit or blood bank deter-

mines fetal packed RBC volume entering patient's blood; then give one vial I.M. if fetal packed RBC volume is below 15 ml. More than one vial I.M. may be required if large fetomaternal hemorrhage occurs. Must be given within 72 hours after delivery or miscarriage.

▶ **Transfusion accident.** *Adults and children:* Usually, 600 mcg I.V. q 8 hours or 1,200 mcg I.M. q 12 hours until total dose given. Total dose depends on volume of packed RBCs or whole blood infused. Consult blood bank or transfusion unit at once. Must be given within 72 hours.

▶ **Postabortion or postmiscarriage to prevent Rh antibody formation up to and including 12 weeks' gestation.** *Women:* Consult transfusion unit or blood bank. One microdose vial suppresses immune reaction to 2.5 ml Rh₀(D)-positive RBCs. Should be given within 3 hours but may be given up to 72 hours after abortion or miscarriage.

▶ **Amniocentesis or abdominal trauma during pregnancy.** *Women:* Dose based on extent of fetomaternal hemorrhage.

▶ **Idiopathic thrombocytopenia purpura.** *Adults and children:* 250 units/kg (50 mcg/kg) I.V. as single dose or in two divided doses given on separate days. If patient responded to initial dose, maintenance dose is 125 to 300 units/kg (25 to 60 mcg/kg) based on platelet count and hemoglobin. If patient had inadequate response to initial dose and hemoglobin is more than 10 g/dl, maintenance dose is 250 to 300 units/kg (50 to 60 mcg/kg); for those with hemoglobin of 8 to 10 g/dl maintenance dose is 125 to 200 units/kg (25 to 40 mcg/kg).

▼ I.V. administration

• Reconstitute only with normal saline solution; 2.5 ml for the 120 mcg and 300 mcg vials and 8.5 ml for the 1,000 mcg vial. Slowly inject diluent into vial and gently swirl vial until dissolved. Don't shake vial.

• Give injection over 3 to 5 minutes.

• Don't give in the same line as other drugs.

• Refrigerate drug at 36° to 46° F (2° to 8° C).

Contraindications and precautions

• Contraindicated in Rh₀(D)-positive or Dᵘ-positive patients, those previously immunized to Rh₀(D) blood factor, those with anaphylactic or severe systemic reaction to human globulin, and those with immunoglobulin A deficiency.

• Use cautiously in patients with thrombocytopenia or bleeding disorders.

≛ **Lifespan:** In pregnant and breast-feeding women, use cautiously. Microdose must not be used for any indication with continuation of pregnancy.

Adverse reactions

CNS: slight fever.
Other: *anaphylaxis,* discomfort at injection site.

Interactions

Drug-drug. *Live-virus vaccines:* May interfere with response to $Rh_o(D)$ immune globulin. Delay immunization for 3 months.

Effects on lab test results

None reported.

Pharmacokinetics

Absorption: Unknown.
Distribution: Unknown.
Metabolism: Unknown.
Excretion: Unknown. *Half-life:* 24 to 30 days.

Route	Onset	Peak	Duration
I.V., I.M.	Unknown	Unknown	Unknown

Action

Chemical effect: Suppresses active antibody response and formation of anti-$Rh_o(D)$ in $Rh_o(D)$-negative, D^u-negative people exposed to Rh-positive blood.
Therapeutic effect: Blocks adverse effects of Rh-positive exposure.

Available forms

I.M. injection: 300 mcg of $Rh_o(D)$ immune globulin/vial (standard dose); 50 mcg of $Rh_o(D)$ immune globulin/vial (microdose)
I.V. infusion: 120 mcg, 300 mcg, 1,000 mcg

NURSING PROCESS

✍ Assessment
• Obtain history of Rh-negative patient's Rh-positive exposure, allergies, and reactions to immunizations.
• Evaluate patient's and family's knowledge of drug therapy.

⊞ Nursing diagnoses
• Risk for injury related to Rh-positive exposure
• Ineffective protection related to drug-induced anaphylaxis
• Deficient knowledge related to drug therapy

▶ Planning and implementation
• Inject I.M. into the anterolateral aspect of the upper thigh or deltoid muscle.
• If administering 1,000 mcg, don't give entire dose in one muscle; divide dose between several different sites.
• Make sure epinephrine 1:1,000 is available in case of anaphylaxis.
• After delivery, have neonate's cord blood typed and crossmatched; confirm if mother is $Rh_o(D)$-negative and Du-negative. Give to mother only if infant is $Rh_o(D)$-positive or Du-positive.
• Drug gives passive immunity to woman exposed to $Rh_o(D)$-positive fetal blood during pregnancy and prevents formation of maternal antibodies, which would endanger future $Rh_o(D)$-positive pregnancies.
• Defer vaccination with live-virus vaccines for 3 months after giving drug.
• MICRhoGAM is recommended for every woman having an abortion or miscarriage up to 12 weeks' gestation unless she is $Rh_o(D)$-positive or Du-positive, she has Rh antibodies, or father or fetus is Rh-negative.
Patient teaching
• Explain how drug protects future $Rh_o(D)$-positive fetuses.

☑ Evaluation
• Patient shows evidence of passive immunity to exposure to $Rh_o(D)$-positive blood.
• Patient doesn't develop anaphylaxis after drug administration.
• Patient and family state understanding of drug therapy.

ribavirin
(righ-beh-VIGH-rin)
Copegus, Rebetol, Virazole

Pharmacologic class: synthetic nucleoside
Therapeutic class: antiviral
Pregnancy risk category: X

Indications and dosages

▶ **Hospitalized infants and young children infected by RSV.** *Infants and young children:* 20-mg/ml solution delivered by small particle aerosol generator (SPAG-2) and mechanical ventilator or oxygen hood, face mask, or oxygen tent at about 12.5 L of mist per minute. Therapy lasts 12 to 18 hours daily for 3 to 7 days.
▶ **Chronic hepatitis C.** *Adults weighing 75 kg (165 lb) or less:* 1,000 mg Rebetol P.O. daily in divided doses (400 mg in morning, 600 mg in evening) with interferon alfa-2b 3 million units S.C. three times weekly. Or, 1,000 mg Copegus with 180 mcg of Pegasys (peginterferon alfa-2a).
Adults weighing over 75 kg: 1,200 mg Rebetol P.O. divided b.i.d. (600 mg in morning, 600 mg in evening) with interferon alfa-2b, 3 million units S.C. three times weekly. Or, 1,200 mg Copegus with 180 mcg of Pegasys.

Contraindications and precautions

• Contraindicated in patients hypersensitive to drug and in those with creatinine clearance less than 50 ml/minute, history of significant or unstable cardiac disease, Child-Pugh class B or C, or hemoglobinopathies, such as sickle cell anemia and thalassemia.
• Use cautiously in patients with renal impairment.
⚠ Lifespan: In women who are or may become pregnant and in men whose sexual partners are pregnant, drug is contraindicated. Breast-feeding women should avoid breast-feeding or the drug taking into consideration the importance of the drug. In children, capsules and tablets are contraindicated. In elderly patients, use cautiously.

Adverse reactions

CNS: *headache,* dizziness, *seizures,* asthenia.
CV: *cardiac arrest,* hypotension, chest pains.
EENT: *conjunctivitis, rhinitis, pharyngitis, lacrimation,* rash or erythema of eyelids.
GI: *nausea.*
Hematologic: reticulocytosis, *severe anemia,* hemolytic anemia.
Respiratory: *worsening of respiratory state, bronchospasms, apnea,* bacterial pneumonia, *pneumothorax.*
Skin: *rash.*

Interactions

Drug-drug. *Acetaminophen, antacids containing magnesium, aluminum and simethicone, aspirin, cimetidine:* May affect drug level. Monitor patient.
Didanosine: May increase toxicity. Avoid using together.
Stavudine, zidovudine: May decrease antiretroviral activity. Use together cautiously.

Effects on lab test results

• May increase bilirubin, AST, and ALT levels.
• May increase reticulocytes. May decrease hemoglobin and hematocrit.

Pharmacokinetics

Absorption: Some ribavirin is absorbed systemically.
Distribution: Concentrates in bronchial secretions.
Metabolism: Metabolized to 1,2,4-triazole-3-carboxamide (deribosylated ribavirin).
Excretion: Most of drug excreted in urine.
Half-life: First phase, 9¼ hours; second phase, 40 hours.

Route	Onset	Peak	Duration
Inhalation	Immediate	Immediate	Unknown

Action

Chemical effect: Inhibits viral activity by unknown mechanism, possibly by inhibiting RNA and DNA synthesis by depleting intracellular nucleotide pools.
Therapeutic effect: Inhibits RSV activity.

Available forms

Capsules: 200 mg
Powder to be reconstituted for inhalation: 6 g in 100-ml glass vial
Tablets: 200 mg

NURSING PROCESS

🔖 Assessment

• Assess patient's respiratory infection before therapy and regularly thereafter.
• Monitor ventilator function. Drug may precipitate in ventilator apparatus, causing equipment malfunction with serious consequences.
• Watch for anemia in patient receiving drug longer than 1 to 2 weeks.
• Be alert for adverse reactions.

- Evaluate patient's and family's knowledge of drug therapy.

🔄 Nursing diagnoses
- Infection related to presence of RSV
- Risk for injury related to drug-induced adverse CV reactions
- Deficient knowledge related to drug therapy

▶ Planning and implementation
- Aerosol form is indicated only for severe lower respiratory tract infection caused by RSV. Start therapy pending test results, but existence of RSV infection must be documented.
- Most infants and children with RSV infection don't need treatment. Infants with underlying conditions, such as prematurity or cardiopulmonary disease, benefit most from using aerosol form of drug.
- Give drug by SPAG-2 only. Don't use any other aerosol generator.
- For reconstitution, use sterile USP water for injection, not bacteriostatic water. Water used to reconstitute this drug must not contain an antimicrobial.
- Discard solutions placed in SPAG-2 unit at least every 24 hours before adding newly reconstituted solution.
- Avoid unneeded occupational exposure to drug. Adverse effects reported in health care personnel exposed to aerosolized drug include eye irritation and headache.
- Capsules and tablets aren't effective as monotherapy for chronic hepatitis C.
- Store reconstituted solutions at room temperature for 24 hours.
- Stop drug at first sign of pancreatitis.
- ⊛ ALERT: Don't confuse ribavirin with riboflavin.

Patient teaching
- Inform parents of children with RSV infection of need for drug therapy, and answer their questions.
- Advise patient to use correct device.
- Explain to women of childbearing age and men with sexual partners of childbearing age the effects of drug on a fetus and the need to inform the prescriber immediately if pregnancy occurs.

☑ Evaluation
- Patient is free from infection.

- Patient doesn't develop adverse CV reactions after drug administration.
- Parents state understanding of drug therapy.

riboflavin (vitamin B$_2$)†
(righ-boh-FLAY-vin)

Pharmacologic class: water-soluble vitamin
Therapeutic class: vitamin B complex vitamin
Pregnancy risk category: A (C in doses that exceed RDA)

Indications and dosages
▶ **RDA.** *Men age 51 and older:* 1.4 mg.
Men ages 19 to 50: 1.7 mg.
Men ages 15 to 18: 1.8 mg.
Men ages 11 to 14: 1.5 mg.
Women age 51 and older: 1.2 mg.
Women ages 11 to 50: 1.3 mg.
Pregnant women: 1.6 mg.
Breast-feeding women (first 6 months): 1.8 mg.
Breast-feeding women (second 6 months): 1.7 mg.
Children ages 7 to 10: 1.2 mg.
Children ages 4 to 6: 1.1 mg.
Children ages 1 to 3: 0.8 mg.
Infants ages 6 months to 1 year: 0.5 mg.
Neonates and infants to age 6 months: 0.4 mg.
▶ **Riboflavin deficiency or adjunct to thiamine therapy for polyneuritis or cheilosis caused by pellagra.** *Adults and children age 12 and older:* 5 to 30 mg P.O. daily, depending on severity.
Children younger than age 12: 3 to 10 mg P.O. daily, depending on severity. For maintenance, increase nutritional intake and supplement with vitamin B complex.
▶ **Microcytic anemia linked to splenomegaly and glutathione reductase deficiency.** *Adults:* 10 mg P.O. daily for 10 days.

Contraindications and precautions
※ Lifespan: In pregnant women, don't exceed RDA. Drug is found in breast milk.

Adverse reactions
GU: bright yellow urine.

Interactions

Drug-drug. *Probenecid:* Reduces urinary excretion of riboflavin. Use together cautiously.
Propantheline, other anticholinergics: Decreases rate and extent of absorption. Avoid using together.

Effects on lab test results

None reported.

Pharmacokinetics

Absorption: Absorbed readily from GI tract, although extent is limited. Occurs at specialized segment of mucosa and is limited by duration of drug's contact with this area. Before being absorbed, riboflavin 5-phosphate is rapidly dephosphorylated in GI lumen. GI absorption increases when drug is given with food and decreases when hepatitis, cirrhosis, biliary obstruction, or probenecid administration is present.
Distribution: Riboflavin, a coenzyme, functions in forms of flavin adenine dinucleotide (FAD) and flavin mononucleotide (FMN). FAD and FMN are distributed widely to body tissues. Riboflavin is stored in limited amounts in liver, spleen, kidneys, and heart, mainly in the form of FAD. FAD and FMN are about 60% protein-bound in blood.
Metabolism: Riboflavin is metabolized to FMN in erythrocytes, GI mucosal cells, and liver. FMN is converted to FAD in liver.
Excretion: Excreted in urine. *Half-life:* 66 to 84 minutes.

Route	Onset	Peak	Duration
P.O.	Unknown	Unknown	Unknown

Action

Chemical effect: Converts to two coenzymes needed for normal tissue respiration.
Therapeutic effect: Relieves riboflavin deficiency.

Available forms

Tablets: 10 mg†, 25 mg†, 50 mg†, 100 mg†
Tablets (sugar-free): 50 mg†, 100 mg†

NURSING PROCESS

🗓 Assessment
• Assess patient's riboflavin deficiency before and during therapy.

• Be alert for change in urine color.
• Evaluate patient's and family's knowledge of drug therapy.

🗓 Nursing diagnoses
• Imbalanced nutrition: less than body's needs, related to drug deficiency
• Deficient knowledge related to drug therapy

🗓 Planning and implementation
• Drug may be given I.M. or I.V. as component of multiple vitamins.
• Riboflavin deficiency usually accompanies other vitamin B–complex deficiencies and may require multivitamin therapy.
• Protect drug from air and light.
⑤ **ALERT:** Don't confuse riboflavin (vitamin B_2) with ribavirin (Virazole).
Patient teaching
• Encourage patient to take with meals to increase absorption.
• Stress proper nutritional habits to prevent return of deficiency.
• Inform patient that urine will likely turn bright yellow or orange.

🗹 Evaluation
• Patient's drug deficiency is resolved.
• Patient and family state understanding of drug therapy.

rifabutin
(rif-uh-BYOO-tin)
Mycobutin

Pharmacologic class: semisynthetic ansamycin
Therapeutic class: antibiotic
Pregnancy risk category: B

Indications and dosages

▶ **Prevention of disseminated *Mycobacterium avium* complex (MAC) in patients with advanced HIV infection.** *Adults:* 300 mg P.O. daily as single dose or divided b.i.d.

Contraindications and precautions

• Contraindicated in patients hypersensitive to drug or other rifamycin derivatives (such as rifampin) and in those with active tuberculosis.
• Use cautiously in patients with neutropenia and thrombocytopenia.

⚱ **Lifespan:** In breast-feeding women, drug isn't recommended. In children, safety of drug hasn't been established.

Adverse reactions

CNS: fever, headache.
CV: ECG changes.
GI: dyspepsia, eructation, flatulence, diarrhea, nausea, vomiting, abdominal pain.
GU: *discolored urine.*
Hematologic: anemia, eosinophilia, LEUKOPENIA, NEUTROPENIA, *thrombocytopenia.*
Musculoskeletal: myalgia.
Skin: *rash.*

Interactions

Drug-drug. *Corticosteroids:* Rifabutin decreases effect of drug. Double dose of corticosteroids, if needed.
Cyclosporine: Reduces immunosuppressive effects. Don't use together.
Drugs metabolized by the liver, benzodiazepines, beta blockers, buspirone, doxycycline, hydantoins, indinavir, losartan, macrolides, methadone, morphine, nelfinavir, quinidine, theophylline, tricyclic antidepressants, zidovudine: Decreases zidovudine level. Because rifabutin, like rifampin, induces liver enzymes, it may lower levels of many other drugs as well. Monitor for effect.
Hormonal contraceptives: Decreases effectiveness. Instruct patient to use non-hormonal forms of birth control.
Warfarin: Decreases anticoagulation effect. Increase dose of anticoagulant.
Drug-food. *High-fat foods:* Slows absorption of drug. Avoid taking drug with high-fat meals.

Effects on lab test results

• May increase alkaline phosphatase, AST, and ALT levels.
• May increase eosinophil count. May decrease hemoglobin, hematocrit, and neutrophil, WBC, and platelet counts.

Pharmacokinetics

Absorption: Readily absorbed from GI tract.
Distribution: Because of its high lipophilicity, rifabutin demonstrates high propensity for distribution and intracellular tissue uptake. About 85% of drug is bound to proteins.
Metabolism: Metabolized in liver.

Excretion: Excreted primarily in urine; about 30% excreted in feces. *Half-life:* 45 hours.

Route	Onset	Peak	Duration
P.O.	Unknown	1½-4 hr	Unknown

Action

Chemical effect: Blocks bacterial protein synthesis by inhibiting DNA-dependent RNA polymerase in susceptible bacteria.
Therapeutic effect: Prevents disseminated MAC in patients with advanced HIV infection.

Available forms

Capsules: 150 mg

NURSING PROCESS

⚖ Assessment

• Assess patient's condition before therapy and regularly thereafter.
• Perform baseline hematologic studies and repeat periodically.
• Be alert for adverse reactions and drug interactions.
• Evaluate patient's and family's knowledge of drug therapy.

⊞ Nursing diagnoses

• Infection related to advanced HIV infection and decreased immune system
• Ineffective protection related to drug-induced adverse hematologic reactions
• Deficient knowledge related to drug therapy

▷ Planning and implementation

• High-fat meals slow rate but not extent of absorption.
• Give drug with food. Mix with soft foods for patient who has difficulty swallowing.
• No evidence exists that drug will provide effective prophylaxis against *Mycobacterium tuberculosis.* Patients requiring prophylaxis against both *M. tuberculosis* and MAC may require rifampin and rifabutin.
⚕ ALERT: Don't confuse rifampin, rifapentine, and rifabutin.
Patient teaching
• Tell patient that drug may turn urine, feces, sputum, saliva, tears, and skin brownish-orange. Tell him not to wear soft contacts because they may be permanently stained.

- Instruct patient to report photophobia, excessive lacrimation, or eye pain. Drug may rarely cause uveitis.

☑ **Evaluation**
- Patient doesn't develop disseminated MAC.
- Patient maintains normal hematologic values throughout therapy.
- Patient and family state understanding of drug therapy.

rifampin (rifampicin)

(rih-FAM-pin)
Rifadin, Rifadin IV, Rimactane, Rimycin ◇ , Rofact ◆

Pharmacologic class: semisynthetic rifamycin B derivative (macrocytic antibiotic)
Therapeutic class: antituberculotic
Pregnancy risk category: C

Indications and dosages

▶ **Pulmonary tuberculosis.** *Adults:* 10 mg/kg P.O. or I.V. daily in single dose. Maximum, 600 mg daily.
Children older than age 5: 10 to 20 mg/kg P.O. or I.V. daily in single dose. Maximum, 600 mg daily. Use with other antituberculotics is recommended.
▶ **Meningococcal carriers.** *Adults:* 600 mg P.O. or I.V. b.i.d. for 2 days or once daily for 4 days.
Children ages 1 month to 12 years: 10 mg/kg P.O. or I.V. b.i.d. for 2 days or once daily for 4 days. Maximum, 600 mg daily.
Neonates: 5 mg/kg P.O. or I.V. b.i.d. for 2 days.
⊠ **Adjust-a-dose:** For patients with liver dysfunction, reduce dosage.
▶ **Prophylaxis of** *Haemophilus influenzae* **type B.** *Adults and children:* 20 mg/kg P.O. daily for 4 days. Maximum, 600 mg daily.
▶ **Leprosy‡.** *Adults:* 600 mg P.O. once monthly, usually with other drugs.

▽ I.V. administration

- Reconstitute vial with 10 ml of sterile water for injection to make solution containing 60 mg/ml.
- Add to 100 ml of D₅W and infuse over 30 minutes, or add to 500 ml of D₅W and infuse over 3 hours.

- When dextrose is contraindicated, drug may be diluted with normal saline solution for injection. Don't use other I.V. solutions.

Contraindications and precautions

- Contraindicated in patients hypersensitive to drug.
- Use cautiously in patients with liver disease.
☆ **Lifespan:** In breast-feeding women, use cautiously. In neonates of rifampin-treated mothers, drug may cause hemorrhage.

Adverse reactions

CNS: ataxia, behavioral changes, confusion, dizziness, fatigue, headache, drowsiness, generalized numbness.
CV: *shock.*
EENT: visual disturbances, exudative conjunctivitis.
GI: epigastric distress, anorexia, nausea, vomiting, abdominal pain, diarrhea, flatulence, sore mouth and tongue, *pseudomembranous colitis, pancreatitis.*
GU: hemoglobinuria, hematuria, *acute renal failure,* menstrual disturbances.
Hematologic: eosinophilia, *transient leukopenia, thrombocytopenia,* hemolytic anemia.
Hepatic: *hepatotoxicity,* worsening of porphyria.
Metabolic: hyperuricemia.
Musculoskeletal: osteomalacia.
Respiratory: shortness of breath, wheezing.
Skin: pruritus, urticaria, rash.
Other: flulike syndrome, discoloration of body fluids.

Interactions

Drug-drug. *Analgesics, anticoagulants, anticonvulsants, barbiturates, beta blockers, chloramphenicol, clofibrate, corticosteroids, cyclosporine, dapsone, diazepam, digoxin, disopyramide, doxycycline, hormonal contraceptives, macrolides, methadone, mexiletine, opioids, progestins, protease inhibitors, quinidine, sulfonylureas, theophylline, verapamil:* Reduces effectiveness of these drugs. Avoid using together.
Halothane: May increase risk of hepatotoxicity in both drugs. Monitor liver function closely.
Ketoconazole, para-aminosalicylate sodium: May interfere with absorption of rifampin. Give these drugs 8 to 12 hours apart.

Probenecid: May increase rifampin levels. Use cautiously.

Drug-herb. *Kava:* May increase the risk of hepatotoxicity. Discourage use.

Drug-lifestyle. *Alcohol use:* May increase risk of hepatotoxicity. Discourage using together.

Effects on lab test results

• May increase ALT, AST, alkaline phosphatase, bilirubin, BUN, creatinine, and uric acid levels.
• May increase eosinophil count. May decrease hemoglobin, hematocrit, and platelet and WBC counts.

Pharmacokinetics

Absorption: Complete. Food delays absorption.
Distribution: Wide. 84% to 91% protein-bound.
Metabolism: Extensive.
Excretion: Primarily in bile; drug, but not metabolite, is reabsorbed. Some in urine. *Half-life:* 1¼ to 5 hours.

Route	Onset	Peak	Duration
P.O.	Unknown	2-4 hr	Unknown
I.V.	Unknown	Unknown	Unknown

Action

Chemical effect: Kills bacteria by inhibiting DNA-dependent RNA polymerase, thus impairing RNA synthesis.
Therapeutic effect: Kills susceptible bacteria.

Available forms

Capsules: 150 mg, 300 mg
Injection: 600 mg

NURSING PROCESS

⚕ Assessment

• Assess patient's infection before therapy and regularly thereafter.
• Monitor liver function, hematopoiesis, and uric acid levels.
• Be alert for adverse reactions and drug interactions.
• Watch closely for signs of hepatic impairment.
• If adverse GI reactions occur, monitor hydration.
• Evaluate patient's and family's knowledge of drug therapy.

⊕ Nursing diagnoses

• Infection related to presence of susceptible bacteria
• Risk for deficient fluid volume related to drug-induced adverse reactions
• Deficient knowledge related to drug therapy

⊠ Planning and implementation

• Give drug 1 hour before or 2 hours after meals for optimal absorption; if GI irritation occurs, patient may take with meals. Drug may inhibit standard assays for folate and vitamin B₁₂. Consider alternative assay method.
• Giving at least one additional antituberculotic is recommended.
⑤ ALERT: Don't confuse rifampin, rifapentine, and rifabutin.

Patient teaching
• Warn patient about drowsiness and red-orange discoloration of urine, feces, saliva, sweat, sputum, and tears. Soft contact lenses may be permanently stained.
• Advise patient to avoid alcoholic beverages while taking drug.

☑ Evaluation

• Patient is free from infection.
• Patient maintains adequate hydration throughout therapy.
• Patient and family state understanding of drug therapy.

rifapentine
(rif-ah-PEN-tin)
Priftin

Pharmacologic class: rifamycin-derivative antibiotic
Therapeutic class: antituberculotic
Pregnancy risk category: C

Indications and dosages

▶ **Pulmonary tuberculosis, with at least one other antituberculotic to which the isolate is susceptible.** *Adults:* During intensive phase of short-course therapy, 600 mg P.O. twice weekly for 2 months, with an interval between doses of not less than 3 days (72 hours). During the continuation phase of short-course therapy, 600 mg P.O. once weekly for 4 months with isoniazid or another drug to which the isolate is susceptible.

Contraindications and precautions

• Contraindicated in patients hypersensitive to rifamycin (rifapentine, rifampin, or rifabutin).
• Use drug cautiously and with frequent monitoring in patients with liver disease.
⚘ Lifespan: During last 2 weeks of pregnancy, drug may lead to postnatal hemorrhage in mother or infant. Monitor clotting parameters closely.

Adverse reactions

CNS: pain, headache, dizziness.
CV: hypertension.
GI: anorexia, nausea, vomiting, dyspepsia, diarrhea, *pseudomembranous colitis.*
GU: pyuria, proteinuria, hematuria, urinary casts.
Hematologic: *neutropenia, lymphopenia,* anemia, *leukopenia,* thrombocytosis.
Metabolic: *hyperuricemia.*
Musculoskeletal: arthralgia.
Respiratory: hemoptysis.
Skin: rash, pruritus, acne, maculopapular rash.

Interactions

Drug-drug. *Antiarrhythmics, antibiotics, anticonvulsants, antifungals, barbiturates, benzodiazepines, beta blockers, calcium channel blockers, clofibrate, corticosteroids, digoxin, haloperidol, HIV protease inhibitors, immunosuppressants, levothyroxine, opioid analgesics (methadone), oral anticoagulants, oral hypoglycemics, hormonal contraceptives, progestins, quinine, reverse transcriptase inhibitors, sildenafil, theophylline, tricyclic antidepressants:* Induces metabolism of CYP, decreasing the activity of these drugs. Dosage adjustments may be needed.

Effects on lab test results

• May increase uric acid, ALT, and AST levels.
• May increase platelet count. May decrease hemoglobin, hematocrit, and neutrophil and WBC counts.

Pharmacokinetics

Absorption: Relative bioavailability is 70%.
Distribution: About 98% bound to proteins.
Metabolism: Hydrolyzed by an esterase enzyme to the microbiologically active 25-desacetyl rifapentine. Rifapentine contributes 62% to drug's activity and 25-desacetyl contributes 38%.

Excretion: About 17% is excreted in urine and 70% in feces. *Half-life:* 13 hours.

Route	Onset	Peak	Duration
P.O.	Unknown	5-6 hr	Unknown

Action

Chemical effect: Kills susceptible strains of *Mycobacterium tuberculosis,* both inside and outside cells, by inhibiting DNA-dependent RNA polymerase. Rifapentine and rifampin share similar antimicrobial action.
Therapeutic effect: Kills susceptible bacteria.

Available forms

Tablets (film-coated): 150 mg

NURSING PROCESS

Assessment

• Assess patient's condition before therapy and regularly thereafter.
• Assess patient's understanding of disease and stress importance of strict compliance with drug and daily companion medications, as well as needed follow-up visits and laboratory tests.
• Monitor liver function, CBC, and uric acid levels.
• Monitor patient for persistent or severe diarrhea and notify prescriber if it occurs.
• Evaluate patient's and family's knowledge of drug therapy.

Nursing diagnoses

• Infection related to patient's underlying condition
• Noncompliance related to long-term therapeutic regimen
• Deficient knowledge related to drug therapy

Planning and implementation

• Administration of pyridoxine (vitamin B_6) during rifapentine therapy is recommended in malnourished patients, those predisposed to neuropathy (alcoholics, diabetics), and adolescents.
• Drug must be given with appropriate daily companion drugs. Compliance with all drugs, especially with daily companion drugs on the days when rifapentine isn't given, is crucial for early sputum conversion and protection from tuberculosis relapse.

⊕ **ALERT:** Don't confuse rifampin, rifapentine, and rifabutin.

Patient teaching

• Stress importance of strict compliance with drug and daily companion drugs, as well as needed follow-up visits and laboratory tests.

• Advise patient to use non-hormonal methods of birth control.

• Tell patient to take drug with food if nausea, vomiting, or GI upset occurs.

• Instruct patient to notify prescriber if any of the following occur: fever, loss of appetite, malaise, nausea, vomiting, darkened urine, yellowish discoloration of skin and eyes, pain or swelling of joints, and excessive loose stools or diarrhea.

• Instruct patient to protect pills from excessive heat.

• Tell patient that drug can turn body fluids red-orange. Contact lenses can become permanently stained.

☑ **Evaluation**

• Patient experiences sputum conversion and recovers from tuberculosis.

• Patient is compliant with therapeutic regimen.

• Patient and family state understanding of drug therapy.

riluzole
(RIGH-loo-zohl)
Rilutek

Pharmacologic class: benzothiazole
Therapeutic class: neuroprotector
Pregnancy risk category: C

Indications and dosages

▶ **Amyotrophic lateral sclerosis (ALS).**
Adults: 50 mg P.O. q 12 hours on empty stomach.

Contraindications and precautions

• Contraindicated in patients severely hypersensitive to drug or components of the tablets.

• Use cautiously in patients with hepatic or renal dysfunction. Also use cautiously in women and Japanese patients (who may have a lower metabolic capacity to eliminate riluzole compared with men and white patients, respectively).

☀ **Lifespan:** In breast-feeding women, drug isn't recommended. In children, safety of drug hasn't been established. In elderly patients, use cautiously.

Adverse reactions

CNS: headache, aggravation reaction, *asthenia,* hypertonia, depression, dizziness, insomnia, malaise, somnolence, vertigo, circumoral paresthesia.

CV: hypertension, tachycardia, palpitations, orthostatic hypotension, peripheral edema.

EENT: *rhinitis, sinusitis.*

GI: abdominal pain, *nausea,* vomiting, dyspepsia, anorexia, diarrhea, flatulence, stomatitis, dry mouth, oral candidiasis.

GU: UTI, dysuria.

Hematologic: *neutropenia.*

Metabolic: weight loss.

Musculoskeletal: back pain, arthralgia.

Respiratory: *decreased lung function,* increased cough.

Skin: pruritus, eczema, alopecia, exfoliative dermatitis.

Other: tooth disorder, phlebitis.

Interactions

Drug-drug. *Allopurinol, methyldopa, sulfasalazine:* Increases risk of hepatotoxicity. Monitor patient closely.

Inducers of CYP 1A2 (omeprazole, rifampicin): May increase riluzole elimination. Monitor patient for loss of therapeutic effect.

Potential inhibitors of CYP 1A2 (amitriptyline, phenacetin, quinolones, theophylline): May decrease riluzole elimination. Monitor patient closely for toxicity.

Drug-food. *Any food:* Decreases drug bioavailability. Give 1 hour before or 2 hours after meals.

Caffeine: May decrease riluzole elimination. Monitor patient for adverse reactions.

Charbroiled foods: May increase riluzole elimination. Discourage patient from eating while on drug therapy.

Drug-lifestyle. *Alcohol use:* May increase risk of hepatotoxicity. Discourage using together.

Smoking: May increase riluzole elimination. Urge patient to stop smoking.

Effects on lab test results

• May increase AST, ALT, bilirubin, and GGT levels.

• May decrease neutrophil count.

Pharmacokinetics

Absorption: Well absorbed from GI tract, with average absolute oral bioavailability of about 60%. High-fat meal decreases absorption.
Distribution: 96% protein-bound.
Metabolism: Extensively metabolized in liver.
Excretion: Excreted primarily in urine, with small amount in feces. *Half-life:* 12 hours with repeated doses.

Route	Onset	Peak	Duration
P.O.	Unknown	Unknown	Unknown

Action

Chemical effect: Unknown.
Therapeutic effect: Improves signs and symptoms of ALS.

Available forms

Tablets: 50 mg

NURSING PROCESS

Assessment
- Obtain history of patient's ALS.
- Obtain liver and renal function studies and CBC before and during therapy.
- Evaluate patient's and family's knowledge of drug therapy.

Nursing diagnoses
- Impaired physical mobility related to ALS.
- Risk for deficient fluid volume related to adverse GI reactions
- Deficient knowledge related to drug therapy

Planning and implementation
- If baseline elevations in liver function test results (especially elevated bilirubin level) occur, don't use drug. Drug may increase aminotransferase level. If level exceeds 10 times upper limit of normal or if jaundice develops, notify prescriber.
- Give drug at least 1 hour before or 2 hours after a meal.
  Patient teaching
- Tell patient to take drug at same time each day. If he misses a dose, instruct him not to double the dose but to take the next dose as scheduled.
- Instruct patient to report febrile illness; his WBC count should be checked.

- Warn patient to avoid hazardous activities until drug's CNS effects are known.
- Advise patient to limit alcohol intake during therapy.
- Tell patient to store drug at room temperature, protected from bright light and out of children's reach.

Evaluation
- Patient responds well to therapy.
- Patient maintains adequate hydration.
- Patient and family state understanding of drug therapy.

rimantadine hydrochloride
(righ-MAN-tuh-deen high-droh-KLOR-ighd)
Flumadine

Pharmacologic class: adamantine
Therapeutic class: antiviral
Pregnancy risk category: C

Indications and dosages

▶ **Prevention of influenza A virus.** *Adults and children age 10 and older:* 100 mg P.O. b.i.d. *Children younger than age 10:* 5 mg/kg P.O. once daily, not to exceed 150 mg daily.
▶ **Influenza A virus infection.** *Adults:* 100 mg P.O. b.i.d. for 7 days from onset of symptoms.
Adjust-a-dose: For elderly patients and patients with severe hepatic or renal dysfunction, give 100 mg P.O. daily.

Contraindications and precautions

- Contraindicated in patients hypersensitive to drug or amantadine.
- Use cautiously in patients with renal or hepatic impairment and in patients with a history of seizures.
  Lifespan: In pregnant women, use cautiously. In breast-feeding women, drug is contraindicated.

Adverse reactions

CNS: insomnia, headache, dizziness, nervousness, fatigue, asthenia.
GI: nausea, vomiting, anorexia, dry mouth, abdominal pain.

Interactions

Drug-drug. *Acetaminophen, aspirin:* Reduces rimantadine level. Monitor patient for decreased rimantadine effectiveness.
Cimetidine: May decrease rimantadine clearance. Monitor patient for adverse reactions.

Effects on lab test results

None reported.

Pharmacokinetics

Absorption: Well absorbed from GI tract.
Distribution: Protein-binding is about 40%.
Metabolism: Metabolized extensively in liver.
Excretion: Excreted in urine. *Half-life:* 25½ to 32 hours.

Route	Onset	Peak	Duration
P.O.	Unknown	1-4 hr	Unknown

Action

Chemical effect: Unknown; appears to prevent viral uncoating, an early step in viral reproductive cycle.
Therapeutic effect: Inhibits viral reproduction of influenza A virus.

Available forms

Syrup: 50 mg/5 ml
Tablets: 100 mg

NURSING PROCESS

Assessment
• Obtain history of patient's exposure to influenza A virus before therapy, and reassess regularly thereafter.
• Monitor patient's hydration throughout therapy.
• Evaluate patient's and family's knowledge of drug therapy.

Nursing diagnoses
• Infection related to exposure to influenza A virus
• Risk for deficient fluid volume related to drug-induced adverse GI reactions
• Deficient knowledge related to drug therapy

Planning and implementation
• Give within 48 hours of onset of influenza symptoms and continue for 7 days after signs and symptoms appeared.

• Consider risk to contacts of treated patients, who may be subject to morbidity from influenza A. Influenza A–resistant strains can emerge during therapy. Patients taking drug may still be able to spread disease.
⑤ ALERT: Don't confuse rimantadine with amantadine.
Patient teaching
• Instruct patient to take drug several hours before bedtime to prevent insomnia.

Evaluation
• Patient is free from infection.
• Patient maintains adequate hydration throughout therapy.
• Patient and family state understanding of drug therapy.

Ringer's injection
(RING-erz in-JEK-shun)

Pharmacologic class: electrolyte solution
Therapeutic class: electrolyte and fluid replenishment
Pregnancy risk category: NR

Indications and dosages

▶ **Fluid and electrolyte replacement.** *Adults and children:* Dosage highly individualized; usually based on the patient's weight, age, and condition.

I.V. administration

• Tear outer wrap and remove solution container.
• The plastic may be opaque. This is normal and doesn't affect the solution.
• If drug is added to solution, use additive port using aseptic technique.
• Discard unused portion.

Contraindications and precautions

• Contraindicated in patients with renal impairment, except as emergency volume expander.
• Use cautiously in patients with heart failure, circulatory insufficiency, renal dysfunction, hypoproteinemia, or pulmonary edema.
⚘ Lifespan: In pregnant women, use cautiously.

Adverse reactions

CV: fluid overload.
Metabolic: electrolyte imbalance.

Interactions

None significant.

Effects on lab test results

• May cause electrolyte imbalances.

Pharmacokinetics

Absorption: Administered I.V.
Distribution: Widely distributed.
Metabolism: Not significant.
Excretion: Excreted primarily in urine and minimally in feces. *Half-life:* Unknown.

Route	Onset	Peak	Duration
I.V.	Immediate	Immediate	Unknown

Action

Chemical effect: Replaces fluids and electrolytes.
Therapeutic effect: Restores normal fluid and electrolyte balance.

Available forms

Injection: 500 ml, 1,000 ml

NURSING PROCESS

⚡ Assessment

• Obtain history of patient's fluid and electrolyte levels before therapy, and reassess regularly thereafter.
• Be alert for fluid overload.
• Evaluate patient's and family's knowledge of drug therapy.

⊞ Nursing diagnoses

• Deficient fluid volume related to underlying condition
• Deficient knowledge related to drug therapy

▷ Planning and implementation

• Drug contains sodium (147 mEq/L), potassium (4 mEq/L), calcium (4.5 mEq/L), and chloride (155.5 mEq/L).
• Electrolyte content isn't enough to treat severe electrolyte deficiencies, but it provides electrolytes in levels approximating those of blood.
• ⚠ ALERT: Don't confuse Ringer's injection with lactated Ringer's solutions.

Patient teaching

• Inform patient of need for drug.
• Instruct patient to report signs of fluid overload, such as difficulty breathing.

☑ Evaluation

• Patient regains normal fluid and electrolyte balance.
• Patient and family state understanding of drug therapy.

Ringer's injection, lactated (Hartmann's solution, lactated Ringer's solution)
(RING-erz in-JEK-shun, LAK-tayt-ed)

Pharmacologic class: electrolyte and carbohydrate solution
Therapeutic class: electrolyte and fluid replenishment
Pregnancy risk category: NR

Indications and dosages

▶ **Fluid and electrolyte replacement.** *Adults and children:* Dosage highly individualized according to patient's age, weight, and condition.

▽ I.V. administration

• Tear outer wrap and remove solution container.
• The plastic may be opaque. This is normal and doesn't affect the solution.
• If drug is added to solution, use additive port using aseptic technique.
• Discard unused portion.

Contraindications and precautions

• Contraindicated in patients with lactic acidosis or renal impairment, except as emergency volume expander.
• Use cautiously in patients with heart failure, circulatory insufficiency, renal dysfunction, hypoproteinemia, or pulmonary edema.
• ⚖ Lifespan: In pregnant women, use cautiously.

Adverse reactions

CV: fluid overload.
Metabolic: electrolyte imbalance.

Interactions

None significant.

Effects on lab test results

• May cause electrolyte imbalance.

Pharmacokinetics

Absorption: Administered I.V.
Distribution: Widely distributed.
Metabolism: Not significant for electrolytes. Lactate is oxidized to bicarbonate.
Excretion: Excreted primarily in urine and minimally in feces. *Half-life:* Unknown.

Route	Onset	Peak	Duration
I.V.	Immediate	Immediate	Unknown

Action

Chemical effect: Replaces fluids and electrolytes.
Therapeutic effect: Restores normal fluid and electrolyte balance.

Available forms

Injection: 250 ml, 500 ml, 1,000 ml

NURSING CONSIDERATIONS

⚗ Assessment

• Obtain history of patient's fluid and electrolyte levels before therapy, and reassess regularly thereafter.
• Be alert for fluid overload.
• Evaluate patient's and family's knowledge of drug therapy.

🔲 Nursing diagnoses

• Deficient fluid volume related to underlying condition
• Deficient knowledge related to drug therapy

⟩ Planning and implementation

• Drug contains sodium (130 mEq/L), potassium (4 mEq/L), calcium (3 mEq/L), chloride (109.7 mEq/L), and lactate (28 mEq/L).
• Lactated Ringer's injection approximates electrolyte concentration in blood.
• **ALERT:** Don't confuse lactated Ringer's solutions with Ringer's injection.
Patient teaching
• Inform patient of need for drug.
• Instruct patient to report signs of fluid overload, such as difficulty breathing.

☑ Evaluation

• Patient regains normal fluid and electrolyte balance.
• Patient and family state understanding of drug therapy.

---

risedronate sodium

(ri-SEH-droe-nate SOE-dee-um)
Actonel

Pharmacologic class: bisphosphonate
Therapeutic class: antiresorptive drug
Pregnancy risk category: C

Indications and dosages

▶ **Prevention and treatment of postmenopausal osteoporosis.** *Adults:* 5-mg tablet P.O. once daily, or 35-mg tablet once weekly. Give at least 30 minutes before first food or drink (except water) of the day.
▶ **Glucocorticoid-induced osteoporosis in patients who are either starting or continuing glucocorticoid therapy at 7.5 mg or more of prednisone or equivalent daily.** *Adults:* 5 mg P.O. daily.
▶ **Paget's disease.** *Adults:* 30 mg P.O. daily for 2 months. If relapse occurs or alkaline phosphatase level doesn't normalize, give same dose for 2 months or longer after first course.

Contraindications and precautions

• Contraindicated in patients hypersensitive to any component of the product and in patients who are hypocalcemic or unable to stand or sit upright for 30 minutes after administration.
• Drug isn't recommended for patients with severe renal impairment (creatinine clearance below 30 ml/minute).
• Use cautiously in patients with upper GI disorders such as dysphagia, esophagitis, and esophageal or gastric ulcers.
🔥 **Lifespan:** In breast-feeding women, consider stopping either drug or breast-feeding, taking into account importance of drug to the mother. In children, safety and effectiveness of drug haven't been established.

Adverse reactions

CNS: asthenia, *headache,* depression, dizziness, insomnia, anxiety, neuralgia, vertigo, hypertonia, paresthesia, *pain.*

CV: *hypertension,* CV disorder, chest pain, peripheral edema.
EENT: pharyngitis, rhinitis, sinusitis, cataract, conjunctivitis, otitis media, amblyopia, tinnitus.
GI: *nausea, diarrhea, abdominal pain,* flatulence, gastritis, rectal disorder, constipation.
GU: *UTI,* cystitis.
Hematologic: anemia.
Musculoskeletal: *arthralgia,* neck pain, *back pain,* myalgia, bone pain, leg cramps, bursitis, tendon disorder.
Respiratory: dyspnea, pneumonia, bronchitis.
Skin: ecchymosis, *rash,* pruritus, *skin carcinoma.*
Other: tooth disorder, *infection.*

Interactions

Drug-drug. *Calcium supplements, antacids that contain calcium, magnesium, or aluminum:* May interfere with risedronate absorption. Advise patient to separate administration times.
Drug-food. *Any food:* May interfere with risedronate absorption. Advise patient to take drug at least 30 minutes before first food or drink of the day (other than water).

Effects on lab test results

• May decrease calcium and phosphorus levels.
• May decrease hemoglobin and hematocrit.

Pharmacokinetics

Absorption: Absorbed via the GI tract. Steady state occurs in 57 days. Mean absolute oral bioavailability of the 30-mg tablet is 0.63%. Food alters absorption; give drug at least 30 minutes before breakfast.
Distribution: The mean steady-state volume of distribution is 6.3 L/kg. Protein-binding is about 24%.
Metabolism: No evidence of systemic metabolism.
Excretion: About 50% of a dose is excreted in urine within 24 hours. Unabsorbed drug is eliminated unchanged in feces. *Half-life:* 1½ hours to 20 days. *Half-life:* Unknown.

Route	Onset	Peak	Duration
P.O.	1 hr	Unknown	Unknown

Action

Chemical effect: Reverses the loss of bone mineral density by reducing bone turnover and bone resorption by inhibiting osteoclasts. In patients with Paget's disease, drug causes bone turnover to return to normal.
Therapeutic effect: Reverses the loss of bone mineral density.

Available forms

Tablets: 5 mg, 30 mg, 35 mg

NURSING PROCESS

⚕ Assessment

• Assess underlying condition before therapy and regularly thereafter.
• Evaluate renal function before beginning therapy. Drug isn't recommended for patients with creatinine clearance below 30 ml/minute.
• Assess for the following risk factors for the development of osteoporosis: family history, previous fracture, smoking, a decrease in bone mineral density below the premenopausal mean, a thin body frame, white or Asian race, and early menopause.
• Evaluate patient's and family's knowledge of drug therapy.

⊕ Nursing diagnoses

• Risk for injury related to decreased bone mass
• Ineffective health maintenance related to underlying disease
• Deficient knowledge related to risedronate sodium therapy

▶ Planning and implementation

⚡ ALERT: Follow dosing instructions carefully because benefits of the drug may be compromised by failure to take it according to instructions. Give drug at least 30 minutes before patient's first food or drink (other than water) of the day.
• Give drug with 6 to 8 oz plain water to facilitate delivery to the stomach. Don't allow patient to lie down for 30 minutes after taking drug.
⚡ ALERT: Bisphosphonates have been linked to such GI disorders as dysphagia, esophagitis, and esophageal or gastric ulcers. Monitor patient for symptoms of esophageal disease (such as dysphagia, retrosternal pain, or severe persistent or worsening heartburn).
• If patient's dietary intake of calcium and vitamin D is inadequate, give supplements. However, because calcium supplements and drugs containing calcium, aluminum, or magnesium may interfere with absorption, separate doses.

Reactions may be *common,* uncommon, *life-threatening,* or COMMON AND LIFE-THREATENING.

- Store drug at 68° to 77° F (20° to 25° C).
- Bisphosphonates can interfere with bone-imaging agents.

Patient teaching
- Explain that risedronate is used to replace bone lost as a result of certain disease processes.
- Instruct patient to adhere to dosing instructions.
- Tell patient to take drug at least 30 minutes before the first food or drink (other than water) of the day. Tell patient to take drug with 6 to 8 oz of water while sitting or standing. Warn against lying down for 30 minutes after taking drug.
- Advise patient not to chew or suck the tablet because doing so could cause mouth irritation.
- Advise patient to contact prescriber immediately if symptoms of esophageal disease (difficulty or pain when swallowing, retrosternal pain, or severe heartburn) develop.
- Advise patient to take calcium and vitamin D if dietary intake is inadequate, but to take them at a different time than risedronate.
- Advise patient to stop smoking and drinking alcohol, as appropriate. Also, instruct patient to perform weight-bearing exercise.
- Tell patient to store drug in a cool (room temperature), dry place and away from children.
- Urge patient to read the Patient Information Guide before starting therapy.
- Tell patient if he misses a dose of the 35-mg tablet, he should take 1 tablet on the morning after he remembers and return to taking 1 tablet once a week, as originally scheduled on his chosen day. Patients shouldn't take 2 tablets on the same day.

✓ Evaluation
- Patient doesn't suffer any injury related to decreased bone mass.
- Patient shows improvement in underlying condition.
- Patient and family state understanding of drug therapy.

risperidone
(ris-PER-ih-dohn)
Risperdal, Risperdal M-Tab

Pharmacologic class: benzisoxazole derivative
Therapeutic class: antipsychotic
Pregnancy risk category: C

Indications and dosages

▶ **Short-term therapy for schizophrenia.**
Adults: Initially, 1 mg P.O. b.i.d. Increase in increments of 1 mg b.i.d. on days 2 and 3 to a target dosage of 3 mg b.i.d. Alternatively, 1 mg P.O. on day 1, increase to 2 mg once daily on day 2, and 4 mg once daily on day 3. Wait at least 1 week before adjusting dosage further. Adjust doses by 1 to 2 mg. Doses above 6 mg daily aren't more effective than lower doses and are linked to more extrapyramidal reactions. Doses up to 8 mg daily are safe and effective. Safety of doses above 16 mg daily hasn't been evaluated.

▶ **Delaying relapse in long-term therapy for schizophrenia.** *Adults:* Initially, 1 mg P.O. on day 1, increase to 2 mg once daily on day 2, and 4 mg once daily on day 3. Dosage range is 2 to 8 mg daily.

🔄 **Adjust-a-dose:** For elderly or debilitated patients, hypotensive patients, or patients with severe renal or hepatic impairment, initially give 0.5 mg P.O. b.i.d. Increase dosage in increments of 0.5 mg b.i.d. Increases in dosages more than 1.5 mg b.i.d. should occur at intervals of at least 1 week. Subsequent switches to once-daily dosing may be made after patient has received a twice-daily regimen for 2 to 3 days at the target dose.

Contraindications and precautions

- Contraindicated in patients hypersensitive to drug or any of its components.
- Use cautiously in patients with prolonged QT interval, CV disease, cerebrovascular disease, dehydration, hypovolemia, history of seizures, exposure to extreme heat, or conditions that could affect metabolism or hemodynamic responses. Also use cautiously in patients at risk for aspiration pneumonia.
- ☀ **Lifespan:** In pregnant women, use cautiously. In breast-feeding women, drug is contraindicated. In children, safety of drug hasn't been established. In elderly patients with dementia, drug is contraindicated.

Adverse reactions

CNS: *somnolence, extrapyramidal symptoms, headache, **suicide attempt**, insomnia, agitation, anxiety,* tardive dyskinesia, aggressiveness, fever, sedation, **neuroleptic malignant syndrome, CVA or TIA in elderly patients with dementia.**

CV: tachycardia, chest pain, orthostatic hypotension, *prolonged QT interval.*
EENT: *rhinitis,* sinusitis, pharyngitis, abnormal vision.
GI: *constipation, nausea, vomiting, dyspepsia.*
Metabolic: weight gain.
Musculoskeletal: arthralgia, back pain.
Respiratory: coughing, upper respiratory tract infection.
Skin: rash, dry skin, photosensitivity reaction.
Other: priapism.

Interactions

Drug-drug. *Antihypertensives:* May enhance hypotensive effects. Monitor blood pressure.
Carbamazepine: Increases risperidone clearance, leading to decreased effectiveness. Monitor patient closely.
Clozapine: Decreases risperidone clearance, increasing toxicity. Monitor patient closely.
CNS depressants: Additive CNS depression. Avoid using together.
Dopamine agonists, levodopa: May antagonize the effects of these drugs. Monitor patient closely.
Drug-lifestyle. *Alcohol use:* Additive CNS depression. Discourage using together.
Sun exposure: Increases photosensitivity reactions. Discourage prolonged or unprotected sun exposure.

Effects on lab test results

• May increase prolactin levels.

Pharmacokinetics

Absorption: Well absorbed; absolute oral bioavailability is 70%.
Distribution: Protein-binding is about 90% for risperidone and 77% for its major active metabolite.
Metabolism: Extensively metabolized in liver.
Excretion: Metabolite excreted in urine. *Half-life:* 3 to 20 hours.

Route	Onset	Peak	Duration
P.O.	Unknown	1 hr	Unknown

Action

Chemical effect: Blocks dopamine and serotonin receptors as well as alpha$_1$, alpha$_2$, and H$_1$ receptors in the CNS.
Therapeutic effect: Relieves signs and symptoms of psychosis.

Available forms

Oral solution: 1 mg/ml
Orally disintegrating tablets: 0.5 mg, 1 mg, 2 mg
Phenylalanine contents of orally disintegrating tablets are as follows: 0.5-mg tablet contains 0.14 mg phenylalanine; 1-mg tablet contains 0.28 mg phenylalanine; 2-mg tablet contains 0.56 mg phenylalanine.
Tablets: 0.25 mg, 0.5 mg, 1 mg, 2 mg, 3 mg, 4 mg

NURSING PROCESS

Assessment
• Assess patient's psychosis before therapy and regularly thereafter.
• Assess blood pressure before therapy, and monitor regularly. Watch for orthostatic hypotension, especially during dosage adjustment.
• Be alert for adverse reactions and drug interactions.
⚠ ALERT: Watch for tardive dyskinesia. It may occur after prolonged use; it may not appear until months or years later and may disappear spontaneously or persist for life despite stopping drug.
• Evaluate patient's and family's knowledge of drug therapy.

Nursing diagnoses
• Disturbed thought processes related to presence of psychosis
• Risk for injury related to drug-induced adverse CNS reactions
• Deficient knowledge related to drug therapy

Planning and implementation
• When restarting therapy for patient who has been off drug, follow 3-day dose initiation schedule.
• When switching patient to drug from another antipsychotic, stop other drug immediately when risperidone therapy starts.
⚠ ALERT: Fatal cerebrovascular adverse events, such as CVA or transient ischemic attacks, may occur in elderly patients with dementia.
Patient teaching
• Warn patient to rise slowly, avoid hot showers, and use extra caution during first few days of therapy to avoid fainting.
• Warn patient to avoid activities that require alertness until CNS effects of drug are known.

Drowsiness and dizziness usually subside after a few days.
- Tell patient to avoid alcohol and prolonged sunlight during therapy.
- Advise patient to use caution in hot weather to prevent heatstroke; drug may affect thermoregulation.
- Tell patient to use sunblock and to wear protective clothing in sunlight.
- Tell woman to notify prescriber if she is or plans to become pregnant.
- Inform patient that drug may be taken without regard to food.
- Tell patient to dissolve orally disintegrating tablets on tongue. Instruct him not to release tablets from blister pack until just prior to administration.
- Tell patient not to split or chew orally disintegrating tablets.

☑ **Evaluation**
- Patient behavior and communication indicate improved thought processes.
- Patient doesn't experience injury as result of drug-induced adverse CNS reactions.
- Patient and family state understanding of drug therapy.

ritonavir
(rih-TOH-nuh-veer)
Norvir

Pharmacologic class: protease inhibitor
Therapeutic class: antiviral
Pregnancy risk category: B

Indications and dosages

▶ **HIV infection.** *Adults:* 600 mg P.O. b.i.d. with meals. If adverse events occur, may give 300 mg b.i.d., then increase at 2-to 3-day intervals by 100 mg b.i.d. If given with saquinavir, reduce saquinavir to 400 mg P.O. b.i.d. and ritonavir to 400 or 600 mg P.O. b.i.d.
Children age 2 and older: Initially, 250 mg/m² P.O. b.i.d. Increase by 50 mg/m² at 2- to 3-day intervals to target dose of 400 mg/m² b.i.d.

Contraindications and precautions

- Contraindicated in patients hypersensitive to drug and in those who are taking dihydroergotamine or ergotamine drugs. Also contraindicated with amiodarone, bepridil, flecainide, propafenone, quinidine, ergot derivatives, pimozide, lovastatin, simvastatin, midazolam, and triazolam.

☀ **Lifespan:** Breast-feeding women shouldn't breast-feed. It isn't known whether drug appears in breast milk. In children younger than age 2, safety of drug hasn't been established.

Adverse reactions

CNS: *asthenia,* headache, circumoral paresthesia, dizziness, insomnia, paresthesia, peripheral paresthesia, somnolence, thinking abnormality, *generalized tonic-clonic seizure,* depression, anxiety, pain, malaise, confusion, fever, syncope.
CV: vasodilation.
EENT: pharyngitis.
GI: abdominal pain, anorexia, constipation, *diarrhea, nausea, vomiting, taste perversion,* dyspepsia, flatulence, *pancreatitis, pseudomembranous colitis.*
Hematologic: *thrombocytopenia, leukopenia.*
Hepatic: *hepatitis.*
Metabolic: *diabetes mellitus,* weight loss.
Musculoskeletal: myalgia, arthralgia.
Skin: sweating, rash.
Other: fat redistribution/accumulation, *hypersensitivity reactions.*

Interactions

Drug-drug. *Amiodarone, ergot derivatives, flecainide, midazolam, pimozide, propafenone, quinidine, triazolam:* Potential for serious and life-threatening adverse reactions. Avoid use with lovastatin and simvastatin. Use cautiously with atorvastatin. Consider using fluvastatin or pravastatin.
Atovaquone, divalproex, lamotrigine, phenytoin, warfarin: Decreases levels of these drugs. Use together cautiously and monitor drug levels closely, if appropriate.
Beta blockers, disopyramide, fluoxetine, mexiletine, nefazodone: May increase levels of these drugs, causing cardiac and neurologic events. Use together with caution.
Bupropion, carbamazepine, calcium channel blockers, clonazepam, clorazepate, cyclosporine, dexamethasone, diazepam, dronabinol, estazolam, ethosuximide, flurazepam, lidocaine, methamphetamine, metoprolol, perphenazine, prednisone, propoxyphene, quinine, risperidone, SSRIs, tacrolimus, tricyclic antidepressants,

thioridazine, timolol, tramadol, zolpidem: May
increase levels of these drugs. Use cautiously
together and consider decreasing the dosage of
these drugs by almost 50%.
Clarithromycin: Increases clarithromycin concentration. Patients with impaired renal function
require 50% reduction in clarithromycin if creatinine clearance is 30 to 60 ml/minute, and a
75% reduction if it's below 30 ml/minute.
Didanosine: Decreases didanosine absorption.
Separate doses by 2.5 hours.
Disulfiram, metronidazole: Increases risk of
disulfiram-like reactions since ritonavir formulations contain alcohol. Monitor patient.
Ethinyl estradiol: Decreases ethinyl estradiol
level. Use an alternative or additional method of
birth control.
HMG CoA reductase inhibitors: Large increase
in statin levels, causing myopathy. Avoid using
together.
Indinavir: Increases indinavir levels. Use together cautiously.
Meperidine: Decreases levels of meperidine and
its metabolite. Dosage adjustment isn't recommended because of CNS effects. Use cautiously
together.
Methadone: Decreases methadone levels. Consider increasing methadone dosage.
Rifabutin: Increases rifabutin levels. Monitor
patient and reduce rifabutin daily dosage by at
least 75% of usual dose.
Rifampin: Decreases ritonavir level. Consider
using rifabutin.
Saquinavir: Increases saquinavir level. Adjust
dose by giving 400 mg saquinavir b.i.d. and
400 mg or 600 mg ritonavir b.i.d.
Sildenafil: Increases level of sildenafil. Use together cautiously. Don't exceed 25 mg of sildenafil in a 48-hour period.
Theophylline: Decreased theophylline levels. Increase dose based on blood levels.
Drug-herb. *St. John's wort:* Substantially reduces ritonavir levels. Discourage using together.
Drug-food. *Any food:* Increased absorption.
Give drug with food.

Effects on lab test results

- May increase ALT, AST, GGT, glucose,
triglycerides, lipids, CPK, and uric acid levels.
- May decrease hemoglobin, hematocrit, and
WBC, RBC, platelet, and neutrophil counts.

Pharmacokinetics

Absorption: Enhanced by food.
Distribution: Absolute bioavailability un-
known; 98% to 100% bound to albumin.
Metabolism: Metabolized in the liver and kid-
neys.
Excretion: Excreted in the urine and feces.
Half-life: Unknown.

Route	Onset	Peak	Duration
P.O.	Unknown	2-4 hr	Unknown

Action

Chemical effect: HIV protease inhibitor with
activity against HIV-1 and HIV-2 proteases;
binds to protease-active site and inhibits enzyme
activity.
Therapeutic effect: Prevents cleavage of viral
polyproteins, resulting in formation of immature
noninfectious viral particles.

Available forms

Capsules: 100 mg
Oral solution: 80 mg/ml

NURSING PROCESS

⚕ Assessment

- Use cautiously in patients with hepatic insufficiency.
- Evaluate patient's and family's knowledge of
drug therapy.

⊕ Nursing diagnoses

- Infection related to presence of virus
- Deficient knowledge related to drug therapy

▷ Planning and implementation

⚠ ALERT: Don't confuse Norvir with Norvasc.
Patient teaching
- Inform patient that drug isn't a cure for HIV
infection and that illnesses caused by HIV infection may occur. Drug doesn't reduce risk of
HIV transmission.
- Tell patient that the taste of oral solution may
be improved by mixing with flavored milk within 1 hour of dose.
- Tell patient to take drug with meal.
- If a dose is missed, instruct patient to take
next dose at once; he shouldn't take double
doses.
- Advise patient to report use of other drugs, including OTC drugs.

• Advise patient taking sildenafil that there is an increased risk of sildenafil-associated adverse events, including hypotension, visual changes, and priapism. He should promptly report any symptoms to his prescriber. Tell patient not to exceed 25 mg of sildenafil in a 48-hour period.
• HIV-positive women shouldn't breast-feed to prevent transmission of HIV.

☑ **Evaluation**
• Patient's infection is eradicated.
• Patient and family state understanding of drug therapy.

rivastigmine tartrate
(ri-va-STIG-meen TAR-trayt)
Exelon

Pharmacologic class: cholinesterase inhibitor
Therapeutic class: Alzheimer's disease drug
Pregnancy risk category: B

Indications and dosages

▶ **Symptoms of mild to moderate Alzheimer's disease.** *Adults:* Initially, 1.5 mg P.O. b.i.d. with food. If tolerated, may be increased to 3 mg b.i.d. after 2 weeks. Further increases to 4.5 mg b.i.d. and 6 mg b.i.d. may be given as tolerated after 2 weeks on the previous dose. Effective dosage range is 6 to 12 mg daily, with maximum recommended dosage of 12 mg daily.

Contraindications and precautions

• Contraindicated in patients hypersensitive to drug, its components, or other carbamate derivatives.
• Use cautiously in patients who take NSAIDs and who have a history of ulcers or GI bleeding and in patients with sick sinus syndrome or other supraventricular cardiac conditions, asthma or obstructive pulmonary disease, or seizures.
⚠ **Lifespan:** In breast-feeding women, drug isn't indicated; it isn't known whether drug appears in breast milk.

Adverse reactions

CNS: syncope, fatigue, asthenia, malaise, *dizziness, headache,* somnolence, tremor, insomnia, confusion, depression, anxiety, hallucination,

aggressive reaction, vertigo, agitation, nervousness, delusion, paranoid reaction, pain.
CV: hypertension, chest pain, peripheral edema.
EENT: rhinitis, pharyngitis.
GI: *nausea, vomiting, diarrhea, anorexia, abdominal pain,* dyspepsia, constipation, flatulence, eructation.
GU: UTI, urinary incontinence.
Metabolic: weight loss.
Musculoskeletal: back pain, arthralgia, bone fracture.
Respiratory: upper respiratory tract infection, cough, bronchitis.
Skin: increased sweating, rash.
Other: *accidental trauma,* flulike symptoms.

Interactions

Drug-drug. *Anticholinergics:* May interfere with anticholinergic activity. Monitor patient closely.
Bethanechol, succinylcholine, and other neuromuscular blockers or cholinergic antagonists: May have synergistic effect. Monitor patient closely.
Drug-lifestyle. *Nicotine:* Increases rivastigmine clearance. Monitor patient closely.

Effects on lab test results

None reported.

Pharmacokinetics

Absorption: Rapid, with levels peaking in about 1 hour. Although drug should be given with food, it delays peak levels by about 1.5 hours. Absolute bioavailability is 36%.
Distribution: Widely distributed throughout body; drug crosses the blood-brain barrier. Protein-binding is about 40%.
Metabolism: Rapid and extensive.
Excretion: Elimination is primarily through the kidneys. *Half-life:* About 1½ hours in patients with normal renal function.

Route	Onset	Peak	Duration
P.O.	Unknown	1 hr	12 hr

Action

Chemical effect: Thought to increase acetylcholine levels by reversibly inhibiting its hydrolysis by cholinesterase. Acetylcholine is probably the primary neurotransmitter that is depleted in Alzheimer's disease.

Therapeutic effect: Improves cognitive function.

Available forms

Capsules: 1.5 mg, 3 mg, 4.5 mg, 6 mg
Solution: 2 mg/ml

NURSING PROCESS

Assessment
• Assess underlying condition before therapy and regularly thereafter.
• Perform complete health history, and carefully monitor patient with a history of GI bleeding, NSAID use, arrhythmias, seizures, or pulmonary conditions for adverse effects.
• Evaluate patient's and family's knowledge of drug therapy.

Nursing diagnoses
• Acute or chronic confusion related to underlying disease
• Risk for imbalanced fluid volume related to drug-induced GI effects
• Deficient knowledge related to rivastigmine tartrate therapy

Planning and implementation
• Expect significant GI adverse effects, such as nausea, vomiting, anorexia, and weight loss. They're less common during maintenance doses.
• **ALERT:** Severe vomiting may occur in patients who resume therapy after an interruption. If therapy is interrupted for more than several days, resume therapy at 1.5 mg b.i.d. Adjust dosage upward to maintenance levels.
• Dramatic memory improvement is unlikely. As disease progresses, the benefits of rivastigmine may decline.
• Monitor patient for symptoms of active or occult GI bleeding.
• Monitor patient for severe nausea, vomiting, and diarrhea, which may lead to dehydration and weight loss.
Patient teaching
• Advise patient to report any episodes of nausea, vomiting, or diarrhea.
• Inform patient and caregiver that memory improvement may be subtle and that a more likely result of therapy is a slower decline in memory loss.

• Tell patient to take rivastigmine with food in the morning and evening.
• Instruct patient to consult prescriber before taking OTC medications.

Evaluation
• Patient's cognition improves and he experiences less confusion.
• Patient and family state that adverse GI effects haven't occurred or have been managed effectively.
• Patient and family state understanding of drug therapy.

rizatriptan benzoate
(rih-zah-TRIP-tin BEN-zoh-ayt)
Maxalt, Maxalt-MLT

Pharmacologic class: selective 5-hydroxytryptamine (5-HT$_1$) receptor agonist
Therapeutic class: antimigraine drug
Pregnancy risk category: C

Indications and dosages

▶ **Acute migraine headaches with or without aura.** *Adults:* Initially, 5 to 10 mg P.O. If first dose is ineffective, another dose can be given at least 2 hours after first dose. Maximum, 30 mg daily. For patients taking propranolol, 5 mg P.O., up to maximum of three doses (15 mg total) in 24 hours.

Contraindications and precautions

• Contraindicated in patients hypersensitive to drug or its inactive ingredients and in the management of hemiplegic or basilar migraines. Also contraindicated in patients with ischemic heart disease (angina pectoris, history of MI, or documented silent ischemia) or those with evidence of ischemic heart disease, coronary artery vasospasm (Prinzmetal's variant angina), or other significant underlying CV disease. Also contraindicated in patients with uncontrolled hypertension and within 24 hours of another 5-HT$_1$ agonist or with ergotamine-containing or ergot-type drugs, such as dihydroergotamine or methysergide.
• Don't use within 2 weeks of an MAO inhibitor.
• Use cautiously in patients with hepatic or renal impairment. Also use cautiously in patients

with risk factors for coronary artery disease (hypertension, hypercholesterolemia, smoking, obesity, diabetes, strong family history of coronary artery disease, women with surgical or physiologic menopause, or men older than age 40), unless a cardiac evaluation provides evidence that patient is free from cardiac disease.

⚕ **Lifespan:** In breast-feeding women, don't use drug because the effects on infants are unknown. In children, safety and effectiveness of drug haven't been established.

Adverse reactions

CNS: dizziness, headache, somnolence, paresthesia, asthenia, fatigue, hypesthesia, decreased mental acuity, euphoria, tremor.
CV: flushing, chest pain, pressure or heaviness, palpitations, *coronary artery vasospasm. transient myocardial ischemia, MI, ventricular tachycardia, ventricular fibrillation.*
EENT: neck, throat, and jaw pain, pressure, or heaviness.
GI: dry mouth, nausea, diarrhea, vomiting.
Respiratory: dyspnea.
Other: pain, warm or cold sensations, hot flushes.

Interactions

Drug-drug. *Ergot-containing or ergot-type drugs (dihydroergotamine, methysergide), other 5-HT₁ agonists:* Prolongs vasospastic reactions. Don't use within 24 hours of rizatriptan.
MAO inhibitors: Increases rizatriptan level. Don't use together. Allow at least 14 days between stopping an MAO inhibitor and giving rizatriptan.
Propranolol: Increases rizatriptan levels. Reduce rizatriptan dose to 5 mg.
SSRIs: Weakness, hyperreflexia, incoordination may occur. Monitor patient.

Effects on lab test results

None reported.

Pharmacokinetics

Absorption: Complete with an absolute bioavailability of 45%.
Distribution: Widely distributed, 14% bound to proteins.
Metabolism: Metabolized primarily by oxidative deamination by MAO-A.
Excretion: 82% in urine. *Half-life:* 2 to 3 hours.

Route	Onset	Peak	Duration
P.O.	Unknown	1-1½ hr	Unknown

Action

Chemical effect: Believed to exert its effect by acting as an agonist at serotonin receptors on extracerebral intracranial blood vessels, which results in vasoconstriction of the affected vessels, inhibition of neuropeptide release, and reduction of pain transmission in the trigeminal pathways.
Therapeutic effect: Relieves migraine pain.

Available forms

Tablets: 5 mg, 10 mg
Tablets (disintegrating): 5 mg, 10 mg

NURSING PROCESS

⚖ Assessment

• Use drug only after a definite diagnosis of migraine is established.
• Assess patient for history of coronary artery disease, hypertension, arrhythmias, or presence of risk factors for coronary artery disease.
• Perform baseline and periodic CV evaluation in patients who develop risk factors for coronary artery disease.
• Monitor renal and liver function tests before starting drug therapy, and report abnormalities.
• Evaluate patient's and family's knowledge of drug therapy.

⊞ Nursing diagnoses

• Acute pain related to presence of migraine headache
• Risk for activity intolerance related to adverse drug reactions
• Deficient knowledge related to drug therapy

▷ Planning and implementation

• Don't give to patients with hemiplegic migraine, basilar migraine, or cluster headaches.
⊗ **ALERT:** Don't give drug within 24 hours of an ergot-containing drug or 5-HT₁ agonist or within 2 weeks of an MAO inhibitor.
• For patients with cardiac risk factors who have had a satisfactory cardiac evaluation, give first dose while monitoring ECG and have emergency equipment readily available.
• If patient develops palpitations or neck, throat, or jaw pain, pressure, or heaviness, withhold drug and notify prescriber.

• Safety of treating more than four headaches in a 30-day period, on average, hasn't been established.

• Drug contains phenylalanine.

Patient teaching

• Inform patient that drug doesn't prevent headache.

• For Maxalt-MLT, tell patient to remove blister pack from sachet and to remove drug from blister pack immediately before use. Tell him not to pop tablet out of blister pack but to carefully peel pack away with dry hands, place tablet on tongue, and let it dissolve. Tablet is then swallowed with saliva. No water is needed or recommended. Tell patient that dissolving tablet doesn't provide more rapid headache relief.

• Advise patient that if headache returns after first dose, a second dose may be taken with medical approval at least 2 hours after the first dose. Don't take more than 30 mg in a 24-hour period.

• Tell patient that food may delay onset of drug action.

• Advise patient to notify prescriber if pregnancy occurs or is suspected.

✓ Evaluation

• Patient has relief from migraine headache.

• Patient maintains baseline activity level.

• Patient and family state understanding of drug therapy.

---

rocuronium bromide
(roh-kyoo-ROH-nee-um BROH-mighd)
Zemuron

Pharmacologic class: nondepolarizing neuromuscular blocker
Therapeutic class: skeletal muscle relaxant
Pregnancy risk category: C

Indications and dosages

▶ **Adjunct to general anesthesia, to facilitate endotracheal intubation, and to provide skeletal muscle relaxation during surgery or mechanical ventilation.** Dosage depends on anesthetic used, individual needs, and response. Dosages are representative and must be adjusted.
Adults and children age 3 months or older: Initially, 0.6 mg/kg (adults, up to 1.2 mg/kg) I.V.

bolus. In most patients, perform tracheal intubation within 2 minutes; muscle paralysis should last about 31 minutes. A maintenance dosage of 0.1 mg/kg should provide additional 12 minutes of muscle relaxation, 0.15 mg/kg will add 17 minutes, and 0.2 mg/kg will add 24 minutes to duration of effect.

▼ I.V. administration

• Compatible solutions include D$_5$W, normal saline solution for injection, dextrose 5% in normal saline solution for injection, sterile water for injection, and lactated Ringer's injection.

• Give drug by rapid I.V. injection or continuous I.V. infusion. Infusion rates are highly individualized but range from 0.004 to 0.16 mg/kg/minute.

• Store reconstituted solution in refrigerator. Discard after 24 hours.

Contraindications and precautions

• Contraindicated in patients hypersensitive to drug.

• Use cautiously in patients with hepatic disease, severe obesity, bronchogenic carcinoma, electrolyte disturbances, neuromuscular disease, or altered circulation time caused by CV disease or edema.

⚖ Lifespan: In pregnant women, use cautiously. In breast-feeding women, safety of drug hasn't been established. In elderly patients, use cautiously because of slower circulation.

Adverse reactions

CV: tachycardia, abnormal ECG, *arrhythmias,* transient hypotension, hypertension.
GI: nausea, vomiting.
Respiratory: hiccups, *asthma.*
Skin: rash, pruritus.
Other: injection site edema.

Interactions

Drug-drug. *Amikacin, gentamicin, neomycin, streptomycin, tobramycin:* May increase the effects, including prolonged respiratory depression, of nondepolarizing muscle relaxants. Use together only when needed. Dose of nondepolarizing muscle relaxant may need to be reduced.
Aminoglycoside antibiotics (kanamycin), anticonvulsants, clindamycin, general anesthetics (such as enflurane, halothane, isoflurane), opioid analgesics, polymyxin antibiotics (colistin,

---

polymyxin B sulfate), quinidine, succinyl-choline, tetracyclines: Potentiates neuromuscular blockade, leading to increased skeletal muscle relaxation and potentiation of effect. Use cautiously during surgical and postoperative periods.

Carbamazepine, phenytoin: May decrease the effects of rocuronium. May need to increase the dose of the rocuronium.

Effects on lab test results

None reported.

Pharmacokinetics

Absorption: Administered I.V.
Distribution: About 30% bound to proteins.
Metabolism: Unknown, although hepatic clearance may be significant.
Excretion: About 33% excreted in urine. *Half-life:* 14 to 18 minutes in adults; ¾ to 1¼ hours in children.

Route	Onset	Peak	Duration
I.V.	≤ 1 min	≤ 2 min	Varies

Action

Chemical effect: Prevents acetylcholine from binding to receptors on motor end plate, thus blocking depolarization.
Therapeutic effect: Relaxes skeletal muscles.

Available forms

Injection: 10 mg/ml

NURSING PROCESS

⚖ Assessment

• Assess patient's condition before therapy and regularly thereafter.
• Be alert for adverse reactions and drug interactions.
• Monitor patients with liver disease; they may need higher doses to achieve adequate muscle relaxation and may exhibit prolonged effects from drug.
• Monitor respirations closely until patient is fully recovered from neuromuscular blockade, as evidenced by tests of muscle strength (hand grip, head lift, and ability to cough).
• Evaluate patient's and family's knowledge of drug therapy.

⊞ Nursing diagnoses

• Ineffective health maintenance related to underlying condition
• Ineffective breathing pattern related to drug's effect on respiratory muscles
• Deficient knowledge related to drug therapy

❯ Planning and implementation

• Drug should be used only by personnel skilled in airway management.
• Give sedatives or general anesthetics before neuromuscular blockers because neuromuscular blockers don't affect consciousness or pain perception.
• Give analgesics for pain.
• Keep airway clear. Have emergency respiratory support equipment (endotracheal equipment, ventilator, oxygen, atropine, edrophonium, epinephrine, and neostigmine) on hand.
• Nerve stimulator and train-of-four monitoring are recommended to confirm antagonism of neuromuscular blockade and recovery of muscle strength. Before attempting reversal with neostigmine, note signs of spontaneous recovery.
• Prior administration of succinylcholine may enhance neuromuscular blocking effect and duration of action.
Patient teaching
• Explain all events and happenings to patient because he can still hear.
• Reassure patient that he is being monitored and that muscle use will return when drug has worn off.

☑ Evaluation

• Patient has positive response to drug therapy.
• Patient maintains adequate breathing pattern with mechanical assistance throughout therapy.
• Patient and family state understanding of drug therapy.

rofecoxib
(roh-feh-COKS-ib)
Vioxx

Pharmacologic class: cyclooxygenase-2 (COX-2) inhibitor
Therapeutic class: nonopioid analgesic, anti-inflammatory
Pregnancy risk category: C

Indications and dosages

▶ **Relief of signs and symptoms of osteo-arthritis.** *Adults:* Initially, 12.5 mg P.O. once daily, increase p.r.n. to maximum of 25 mg P.O. once daily.

▶ **Rheumatoid arthritis.** *Adults:* 25 mg P.O. once daily. Maximum daily dose, 25 mg.

▶ **Management of acute pain; primary dysmenorrhea.** *Adults:* 50 mg P.O. once daily p.r.n. for up to 5 days. Chronic use of 50 mg daily isn't recommended.

Contraindications and precautions

• Contraindicated in patients hypersensitive to drug or any of its components and in patients who have experienced asthma, urticaria, or allergic-type reactions after taking aspirin or other NSAIDs.

• Drug should be avoided in patients with advanced kidney disease or moderate or severe hepatic insufficiency.

• Use cautiously in patients with asthma, renal disease, liver dysfunction, or abnormal liver function tests, and in patients with a history of ulcer disease, GI bleeding, or ischemic heart disease. Also use cautiously in patients being treated with oral corticosteroids or anticoagulants, patients with a history of smoking or alcoholism, and debilitated patients because of the increased risk of GI bleeding. Use cautiously in patients with considerable dehydration. Rehydration is recommended before therapy begins. Use cautiously and start therapy at the lowest recommended dosage in patients with fluid retention, hypertension, or heart failure.

• Because of its lack of platelet effects, drug isn't a substitute for aspirin for CV prophylaxis. Patients shouldn't stop antiplatelet therapy. Patients taking rofecoxib may have more than twice as many MIs, other cardiac events, and CVAs as patients taking naproxen.

☼ Lifespan: In pregnant women, drug should be avoided because it may cause the ductus arteriosus to close prematurely. Report prenatal exposure to the Pregnancy Registry at 1-800-986-8999. In elderly patients older than age 65, use cautiously and start at lowest recommended dosage, because of the increased risk of GI bleeding.

Adverse reactions

CNS: headache, asthenia, fatigue, dizziness, *aseptic meningitis.*

CV: hypertension, leg edema, *thromboembolic events,* fluid retention.

EENT: sinusitis.

GI: diarrhea, dyspepsia, epigastric discomfort, heartburn, nausea, abdominal pain.

GU: UTI.

Metabolic: hyponatremia.

Musculoskeletal: back pain.

Respiratory: bronchitis, upper respiratory tract infection, *pulmonary edema.*

Other: flulike syndrome.

Interactions

Drug-drug. *ACE inhibitors:* Decreases antihypertensive effects of ACE inhibitors. Monitor patient's blood pressure closely.

Aspirin: Increases rate of GI ulceration and other complications. Avoid using together. If used together, monitor patient closely for GI bleeding.

Furosemide, thiazide diuretics: May reduce effectiveness of these drugs. Monitor patient closely.

Lithium: Increases lithium level and decreases lithium clearance. Monitor patient closely for lithium toxicity.

Methotrexate: Increases methotrexate level. Monitor patient closely for toxic reaction to methotrexate.

Rifampin: Decreases rofecoxib levels by about 50%. Start therapy with a higher dosage of rofecoxib.

Theophylline: Increases theophylline concentrations. Monitor levels closely.

Warfarin: Increases effects of warfarin. Monitor INR frequently for a few days after therapy starts or dosage changes.

Drug-lifestyle. *Chronic alcohol use, smoking:* Increases risk of GI bleeding. Discourage drinking and smoking, especially during drug therapy; assess patient for bleeding.

Effects on lab test results

• May decrease sodium level.

Pharmacokinetics

Absorption: Well absorbed, with a mean bioavailability of 93%. Levels peak in 2 to 3 hours (median); range is 2 to 9 hours.

Distribution: About 87% of drug binds to proteins.

Metabolism: Metabolized in liver to inactive metabolites.

Reactions may be *common,* uncommon, *life-threatening,* or **COMMON AND LIFE-THREATENING.**

Excretion: Eliminated mainly through hepatic metabolism. Less than 1% of drug is eliminated via the kidneys as unchanged drug. *Half-life:* About 17 hours.

Route	Onset	Peak	Duration
P.O.	Unknown	2-3 hr	Unknown

Action

Chemical effect: Unknown; anti-inflammatory, analgesic, and antipyretic effects may stem from inhibited prostaglandin synthesis caused by inhibited COX-2 isoenzyme. At therapeutic levels, rofecoxib doesn't inhibit cyclooxygenase-1 (COX-1) isoenzyme.
Therapeutic effect: Relieves inflammation and pain.

Available forms

Oral suspension: 12.5 mg/5 ml, 25 mg/5 ml
Tablets: 12.5 mg, 25 mg, 50 mg

NURSING PROCESS

Assessment
• Obtain history of patient's underlying condition before therapy, and reassess regularly thereafter.
Ⓢ **ALERT:** Ask patient if he has asthma or allergies to aspirin or other NSAIDs. If patient has had severe, potentially fatal bronchospasm after taking aspirin or other NSAIDs, don't give drug.
• Assess patient for dehydration.
• Monitor kidney function closely in patients with renal disease. Drug isn't recommended for patients with advanced kidney disease.
• Monitor patient closely for GI bleeding, which can occur any time without warning.
• Monitor patient for signs and symptoms of liver toxicity. If signs and symptoms of liver disease develop, stop drug.
• If patient receiving long-term therapy experiences signs or symptoms of anemia or blood loss, check hemoglobin and hematocrit.
• Evaluate patient's and family's knowledge of drug therapy.

Nursing diagnoses
• Acute pain related to underlying condition
• Risk for injury related to drug-induced adverse reactions
• Deficient knowledge related to drug therapy

Planning and implementation
• Shake oral suspension well before giving it. Patient may take drug with food to decrease GI upset.
Ⓢ **ALERT:** If patient has fluid retention, hypertension, or heart failure, use cautiously and start therapy at lowest recommended dosage. Monitor blood pressure and check patient for fluid retention or worsening heart failure.
• NSAIDs may cause serious GI toxicity. To minimize the risk of an adverse GI event, use lowest effective dosage for shortest possible time. The risk of GI toxicity with rofecoxib 50 mg once daily is significantly less than with naproxen 500 mg twice daily.
• If patient is dehydrated, rehydrate him before therapy begins.
Patient teaching
• Tell patient that drug may be taken without regard to food, although taking it with food may decrease GI upset.
• Tell patient that the most common adverse effects are dyspepsia, epigastric discomfort, heartburn, and nausea. Taking drug with food may help minimize these effects.
• Tell patient to avoid aspirin, products that contain aspirin, and OTC anti-inflammatory drugs such as ibuprofen (Advil) unless prescriber has instructed him otherwise.
• Warn patient that he may experience GI bleeding. Signs and symptoms include bloody vomitus, blood in urine and stool, and black, tarry stools. Advise patient to seek medical advice if he experiences any of these signs or symptoms.
• Instruct patient to report rash, unexplained weight gain, or edema to prescriber.
• Tell patient that all NSAIDs, including rofecoxib, may adversely affect the liver. Explain that signs and symptoms of liver toxicity include nausea, fatigue, lethargy, itching, jaundice, right upper quadrant tenderness, and flu-like symptoms. Advise patient to stop therapy and seek immediate medical advice if he experiences any of these signs or symptoms.
• Instruct patient to inform her prescriber if she becomes pregnant or plans to become pregnant while taking drug.

Evaluation
• Patient is free from pain.
• Patient sustains no injury from drug-induced adverse reactions.

● Patient and family state understanding of drug therapy.

ropinirole hydrochloride
(roh-PIN-er-ohl high-droh-KLOR-ighd)
Requip

Pharmacologic class: nongoline dopamine agonist
Therapeutic class: antiparkinsonian
Pregnancy risk category: C

Indications and dosages

▶ **Idiopathic Parkinson's disease.** *Adults:* Initially, 0.25 mg P.O. t.i.d. Dosages can be adjusted weekly. After week 4, dosage may be increased by 1.5 mg daily on a weekly basis up to dosage of 9 mg daily, and then increased weekly by up to 3 mg daily to maximum daily dose of 24 mg.

Contraindications and precautions

● Contraindicated in patients hypersensitive to drug.
● Use cautiously in patients with severe hepatic or renal impairment.

⚥ **Lifespan:** In patients older than age 65, clearance is reduced; dosage is individually adjusted to response.

Adverse reactions

Early Parkinson's disease (without levodopa)
CNS: pain, asthenia, fatigue, malaise, hallucinations, dizziness, aggravated Parkinson's disease, syncope, somnolence, headache, confusion, hyperkinesia, hypesthesia, vertigo, amnesia, impaired concentration.
CV: hypotension, orthostatic symptoms, flushing, hypertension, edema, chest pain, extrasystoles, atrial fibrillation, palpitations, tachycardia, peripheral ischemia.
EENT: pharyngitis, abnormal vision, eye abnormality, xerophthalmia, rhinitis, sinusitis.
GI: dry mouth, *nausea, vomiting, dyspepsia,* flatulence, abdominal pain, anorexia, constipation, abdominal pain.
GU: UTI, impotence (male).
Respiratory: bronchitis, dyspnea.
Skin: increased sweating.
Other: *viral infection,* yawning.

Advanced Parkinson's disease (with levodopa)
CNS: dizziness, aggravated parkinsonism, somnolence, headache, insomnia, hallucinations, abnormal dreaming, confusion, tremor, anxiety, nervousness, amnesia, paresthesia, syncope, pain.
CV: hypotension.
EENT: diplopia, increased saliva.
GI: *nausea,* abdominal pain, dry mouth, vomiting, constipation, diarrhea, dysphagia, flatulence.
GU: UTI, pyuria, urinary incontinence.
Hematologic: anemia.
Metabolic: weight loss.
Musculoskeletal: *dyskinesia,* hypokinesia, paresis, arthralgia, arthritis.
Respiratory: upper respiratory infection, dyspnea.
Skin: increased sweating.
Other: injury, *falls,* viral infection.

Interactions

Drug-drug. *CNS depressants:* Increases CNS effects. Use together cautiously.
Dopamine antagonists (butyrophenones, metoclopramide, phenothiazines, thioxanthenes): May decrease ropinirole effectiveness. Monitor patient closely.
Estrogens: Decreases ropinirole clearance. If estrogens are started or stopped during therapy, adjust ropinirole dosage.
Inhibitors or substrates of CYP 1A2 (cimetidine, ciprofloxacin, erythromycin, fluvoxamine, diltiazem, tacrine): Decreases ropinirole clearance. If these drugs are started or stopped during therapy, adjust ropinirole dosage.
Drug-lifestyle. *Alcohol use:* Increases sedative effects. Discourage using together.
Smoking: May increase drug clearance. Urge patient to stop smoking, especially during drug therapy.

Effects on lab test results

● May increase BUN and alkaline phosphatase levels.
● May decrease hemoglobin and hematocrit.

Pharmacokinetics

Absorption: Rapid, with an absolute bioavailability of 55%.
Distribution: Widely distributed, with about 40% bound to protein.
Metabolism: Extensively metabolized by the liver to inactive metabolites.

Excretion: Less than 10% excreted unchanged in urine. *Half-life:* 6 hours.

Route	Onset	Peak	Duration
P.O.	Unknown	1-2 hr	6 hr

Action

Chemical effect: Unknown. A dopamine agonist thought to stimulate postsynaptic dopamine D_2 receptors in the brain.
Therapeutic effect: Improves physical mobility in patients with parkinsonism.

Available forms

Tablets: 0.25 mg, 0.5 mg, 1 mg, 2 mg, 5 mg

NURSING PROCESS

⚕ Assessment
• Assess patient before and during therapy to evaluate effectiveness.
• Monitor patient carefully for orthostatic hypotension, especially during dose escalation.
• Assess patient for adequate nutritional intake.
• Evaluate patient's and family's knowledge of drug therapy.

⚕ Nursing diagnoses
• Impaired physical mobility related to underlying Parkinson's disease
• Disturbed thought processes related to drug-induced CNS adverse reactions
• Deficient knowledge related to drug therapy

⚕ Planing and implementation
• Give drug with food to decrease nausea.
• Drug can potentiate dopaminergic adverse effects of levodopa and may cause or worsen dyskinesia. Levodopa dosage may need to be decreased.
• Don't abruptly stop drug. Withdraw gradually over 7 days to avoid hyperpyrexia and confusion.
Patient teaching
• Tell patient to take drug with food if nausea occurs.
• Explain that hallucinations may occur, particularly in geriatric patients.
• To minimize effects of orthostatic hypotension, instruct patient not to rise rapidly after sitting or lying down, especially when therapy starts or dosage changes.

• Advise patient to avoid hazardous activities until CNS effects of drug are known.
• Tell patient to avoid alcohol during drug therapy.
• Tell woman to notify prescriber if pregnancy is suspected or is planned; also tell her to inform prescriber if she is breast-feeding.

⚕ Evaluation
• Patient has improved mobility and reduced muscle rigidity and tremor.
• Patient remains mentally alert.
• Patient and family state understanding of drug therapy.

rosiglitazone maleate
(roh-sih-GLIH-tah-zohn MAL-ee-ayt)
Avandia

Pharmacologic class: thiazolidinedione
Therapeutic class: antidiabetic
Pregnancy risk category: C

Indications and dosages

▶ **Adjunct to diet and exercise (as monotherapy) to improve glycemic control in patients with type 2 diabetes mellitus, or (as combination therapy) with sulfonylurea, metformin, or insulin when diet, exercise, and a single drug don't result in adequate glycemic control.** *Adults:* Initially, 4 mg P.O. daily in the morning or in divided doses b.i.d. in the morning and evening. If fasting glucose level doesn't improve after 12 weeks, increase to 8 mg P.O. daily or in divided doses b.i.d. Maximum dose is 8 mg daily, except in patients taking insulin. For patients stabilized on insulin, the insulin dose should be continued upon initiation of therapy with rosiglitazone. Doses of rosiglitazone greater than 4 mg daily with insulin aren't indicated.
☒ **Adjust-a-dose:** If patient reports hypoglycemia or if fasting glucose levels decrease to less than 100 mg/dL, decrease insulin dose by 10% to 25%. Base further adjustments on response.

Contraindications and precautions

• Contraindicated in patients hypersensitive to drug or any of its components and in patients with New York Heart Association Class III and IV cardiac status unless expected benefits out-

---

weigh risks. Also contraindicated in patients who developed jaundice while taking troglitazone and in patients with active liver disease, increased baseline liver enzyme levels (ALT level is greater than 3 times the upper limit of normal), type 1 diabetes, or diabetic ketoacidosis.

• Combination therapy with metformin and rosiglitazone is contraindicated in patients with renal impairment. Rosiglitazone can be used as monotherapy in patients with renal impairment.

• Use cautiously in patients with edema or heart failure.

⚖ Lifespan: No considerations reported.

Adverse reactions

CNS: headache, fatigue.
CV: edema, *heart failure,* peripheral edema.
EENT: sinusitis.
GI: diarrhea.
Hematologic: anemia.
Metabolic: hyperglycemia.
Musculoskeletal: back pain.
Respiratory: upper respiratory tract infection.
Other: injury.

Interactions

Drug-herb. *Aloe, bitter melon, bilberry leaf, burdock, dandelion, fenugreek, garlic, ginseng:* May improve glucose control. Patient may need reduced antidiabetic dosage. Discourage using together.

Effects on lab test results

• May increase liver enzyme, lipid, and glucose levels.
• May decrease hemoglobin and hematocrit.

Pharmacokinetics

Absorption: Level peaks about 1 hour after a dose. Absolute bioavailability is 99%.
Distribution: About 99.8% of rosiglitazone binds to proteins, primarily albumin.
Metabolism: Extensively metabolized, with no unchanged drug excreted in the urine. Primarily metabolized through N-demethylation and hydroxylation.
Excretion: About 64% and 23% of the dose is eliminated in urine and feces, respectively. *Half-life:* 3 to 4 hours.

Route	Onset	Peak	Duration
P.O.	Unknown	1 hr	Unknown

Action

Chemical effect: Lowers glucose level by improving insulin sensitivity. Highly selective and potent agonist for receptors in key target areas for insulin action, such as adipose tissue, skeletal muscle, and liver.
Therapeutic effect: Lowers glucose level.

Available forms

Tablets: 2 mg, 4 mg, 8 mg

NURSING PROCESS

℞ Assessment

• Obtain history of patient's underlying condition before therapy, and reassess regularly thereafter.
• Check liver enzyme levels before therapy starts. Don't use drug in patients with increased baseline liver enzyme levels. In patients with normal baseline liver enzyme levels, monitor levels q 2 months for the first 12 months and periodically afterward. If ALT level is elevated, recheck levels as soon as possible. If level remains elevated, notify prescriber because drug should be stopped.
• Monitor glucose level regularly and glycosylated hemoglobin periodically to determine therapeutic response to drug.
• If patient has heart failure, watch for increased edema during rosiglitazone therapy.
• Evaluate patient's and family's knowledge of drug therapy.

⊕ Nursing diagnoses

• Ineffective health maintenance related to hyperglycemia
• Risk for injury related to drug-induced hypoglycemia
• Deficient knowledge related to drug therapy

⊵ Planning and implementation

• Before starting drug, treat patient for other causes of poor glycemic control, such as infection.
• Because calorie restriction, weight loss, and exercise help improve insulin sensitivity and help make drug therapy effective, these measures are essential.
• For patients inadequately controlled with a maximum dose of a sulfonylurea or metformin, this drug should be added to, rather than substituted for, those drugs.

Reactions may be *common,* uncommon, *life-threatening,* or **COMMON AND LIFE-THREATENING.**

• This drug alone or with insulin can cause fluid retention that may lead to or exacerbate heart failure. Observe patient for these signs or symptoms of heart failure. If cardiac health deteriorates, stop drug.

• Because ovulation may resume in premenopausal, anovulatory woman with insulin resistance, contraceptive measures may need to be considered.

Patient teaching

• Advise patient that rosiglitazone can be taken with or without food.

• Inform patient that blood will be tested to check liver function before therapy starts, every 2 months for the first 12 months, and periodically thereafter.

• Tell patient to immediately report unexplained signs and symptoms—such as nausea, vomiting, abdominal pain, fatigue, anorexia, or dark urine—because they may indicate liver problems.

• Instruct patient to contact prescriber if he has signs or symptoms of heart failure, such as unusually rapid increase in weight, edema, or shortness of breath.

• Inform premenopausal, anovulatory woman with insulin resistance that ovulation may resume and that she may want to consider contraceptive measures.

• Advise patient that diabetes management should include diet control. Because calorie restriction, weight loss, and exercise help improve insulin sensitivity and help make drug therapy effective, these measures are essential.

☑ Evaluation

• Patient's glucose level is normal with drug therapy.

• Patient doesn't experience hypoglycemia.

• Patient and family state understanding of drug therapy.

---

rosiglitazone maleate and metformin hydrochloride
roh-si-GLI-ta-zone and met-FOR-min
Avandamet

Pharmacologic class: thiazolidinedione and biguanide
Therapeutic class: antidiabetic
Pregnancy risk category: C

Indications and dosages

▶ **Adjunct to diet and exercise to improve glycemic control in patients with type 2 diabetes mellitus who are already treated with rosiglitazone and metformin or who are inadequately controlled on metformin or rosiglitazone alone.** *Adults:* Dosage is based on patient's current doses of rosiglitazone, metformin, or both. Base dose on effectiveness and tolerance and give in two divided doses with meals. For patients inadequately controlled on metformin alone, 2 mg rosiglitazone P.O. b.i.d., plus the dose of metformin already being taken (500 mg or 1,000 mg P.O. b.i.d.). Dosage may be increased after 8 to 12 weeks. For patients inadequately controlled on rosiglitazone alone, 500 mg metformin P.O. b.i.d., plus the dose of rosiglitazone already being taken (2 mg or 4 mg b.i.d.). Dosage may be increased after 1 to 2 weeks. The total daily dose of this drug may be increased in increments of 4 mg rosiglitazone or 500 mg metformin, or both, up to the maximum daily dose of 8 mg rosiglitazone and 2,000 mg metformin in two divided doses.

⧉ Adjust-a-dose: In elderly patients, initial and maintenance doses should be conservative because these patients' kidney function may be reduced. Don't give elderly, malnourished, and debilitated patients the maximum dose.

Contraindications and precautions

• Contraindicated in patients hypersensitive to rosiglitazone or metformin and in patients with abnormal creatinine clearance or creatinine levels 1.5 mg/dl or higher in men or 1.4 mg/dl or higher in women; heart failure requiring drug therapy; acute or chronic metabolic acidosis, including diabetic ketoacidosis, with or without coma; or evidence of active liver disease or ALT more than 2.5 times the upper limit of normal.

• Don't use with insulin or in patients with type 1 diabetes.

• Use cautiously in patients with edema or at high risk of heart failure.

✱ Lifespan: In pregnant and breast-feeding women, drug isn't recommended. In children, safety and effectiveness of drug haven't been established. In elderly patients, use cautiously because aging often causes reduced renal function. Dose selection should be made carefully and renal function monitored regularly. Don't give elderly patients the maximum daily dose. Don't

---

start drug in patients older than age 80 unless renal function is normal.

Adverse reactions

CNS: headache, fatigue.
CV: edema.
EENT: sinusitis.
GI: *diarrhea.*
Hematologic: anemia.
Metabolic: hyperglycemia, *hypoglycemia.*
Musculoskeletal: back pain, arthralgia.
Respiratory: *upper respiratory tract infection.*
Other: injury, viral infection.

Interactions

Drug-drug. *Calcium channel blockers, corticosteroids, diuretics, estrogens, hormonal contraceptives, isoniazid, nicotinic acid, phenothiazines, phenytoin, sympathomimetics, thyroid products:* May cause hyperglycemia. Monitor glucose level; may need to adjust dosage.
Cationic drugs (amiloride, digoxin, morphine, procainamide, quinidine, quinine, ranitidine, triamterene, trimethoprim, vancomycin): May decrease metformin excretion. Monitor glucose level; may need to adjust cationic drugs or metformin.
Furosemide: May increase metformin level and decrease furosemide level. Monitor patient closely.
Nifedipine: May increase absorption of metformin. Monitor patient closely.
Drug-herb. *Guar gum:* Decreases hypoglycemic effect. Monitor glucose level.
Drug-lifestyle. *Alcohol use:* Potentiates effect of metformin on lactate metabolism and increases risk of lactic acidosis. Discourage using together.

Effects on lab test results

• May decrease vitamin B_{12} level. May increase or decrease glucose level.
• May decrease hemoglobin and hematocrit.

Pharmacokinetics

Absorption: Absolute bioavailability of rosiglitazone and metformin is 99% and 50% to 60%, respectively.
Distribution: Rosiglitazone is 99.8% bound to proteins, primarily albumin; metformin is negligibly bound to proteins.
Metabolism: Rosiglitazone is extensively metabolized, primarily by N-demethylation and

hydroxylation. Rosiglitazone may be predominantly metabolized by CYP 2C8, with CYP 2C9 contributing as a minor pathway. Metformin doesn't undergo hepatic metabolism.
Excretion: 64% and 23% of rosiglitazone is eliminated in the urine and feces, respectively. *Rosiglitazone half-life:* 3 to 4 hours. Metformin is excreted unchanged in the urine. *Metformin half-life:* 6¼ hours to 17½ hours.

Route	Onset	Peak	Duration
P.O.			
rosiglitazone	Unknown	1 hr	Unknown
metformin	Unknown	2½-3 hr	Unknown

Action

Chemical effect: Rosiglitazone improves insulin sensitivity. It's a highly selective and potent agonist for receptors in key target areas for insulin action, such as adipose tissue, skeletal muscle, and the liver. Metformin decreases hepatic glucose production and intestinal absorption of glucose and increases insulin sensitivity.
Therapeutic effect: Lowers glucose level.

Available forms

Tablets: 1 mg rosiglitazone maleate/500 mg metformin hydrochloride, 2 mg rosiglitazone maleate/500 mg metformin hydrochloride, 4 mg rosiglitazone maleate/500 mg metformin hydrochloride

NURSING PROCESS

⛑ Assessment

• Obtain history of patient's underlying condition before therapy, and reassess regularly thereafter.
• Monitor transaminase levels at baseline, q 2 months for the first 12 months, and periodically thereafter. If ALT levels increase to more than three times the upper limit of normal, recheck liver enzymes as soon as possible. If ALT remains more than three times the upper limit of normal, stop drug.
• Monitor CBC and vitamin B_{12} levels.
• Monitor for signs and symptoms of heart failure and hepatic dysfunction. If jaundice occurs, stop drug.
• Monitor renal function at baseline and at least annually during therapy.
• Monitor glycosylated hemoglobin (HbA$_{1C}$) q 3 months.

Reactions may be *common,* uncommon, *life-threatening*, or COMMON AND LIFE-THREATENING.

• Evaluate patient's and family's knowledge of drug therapy.

Nursing diagnoses
• Ineffective health maintenance related to hyperglycemia
• Risk for injury related to drug-induced hypoglycemia
• Deficient knowledge related to drug therapy

Planning and implementation
ALERT: Evaluate patient for ketoacidosis or lactic acidosis. Nonspecific symptoms of lactic acidosis include malaise, myalgias, respiratory distress, abdominal distress, hypotension, and bradyarrhythmias.
• In patients undergoing radiologic studies involving iodinated contrast materials, stop drug before or during the procedure, and withhold for 48 hours after the procedure. Resume drug only after renal function has been re-evaluated and documented to be normal.
• Stop drug temporarily in patients having surgery. Don't restart until oral intake resumes and renal function is normal.
• If shock, acute heart failure, acute MI, or other conditions linked to hypoxemia occur, stop drug.
ALERT: Don't confuse Avandamet with Anzemet.

Patient teaching
• Stress the importance of dietary instructions, weight loss, and a regular exercise program.
• Tell patient to immediately report unexplained hyperventilation, myalgia, malaise, or unusual somnolence.
• Instruct patient to report a rapid increase in weight, swelling, shortness of breath, or other symptoms of heart failure.
• Tell patient to report unexplained nausea, vomiting, abdominal pain, fatigue, anorexia, or dark urine.
• Explain that it may take 1 to 2 weeks for drug to take effect and up to 2 to 3 months for the full effect to occur.
• Stress the importance of avoiding excessive alcohol intake.
• Discuss the need for contraception with premenopausal women as ovulation may resume.
• Advise patient to take the medication in divided doses with meals to reduce GI side effects.

Evaluation
• Patient's glucose level is normal with drug therapy.
• Patient doesn't experience hypoglycemia.
• Patient and family state understanding of drug therapy.

rosuvastatin calcium
(ro-SOO-va-stat-in KAL-see-uhm)
Crestor

Pharmacologic class: HMG-CoA reductase inhibitor
Therapeutic class: antihyperlipidemic
Pregnancy risk category: X

Indications and dosages

▶ **Adjunct to diet to reduce total cholesterol, LDL, apolipoprotein B (ApoB), non-HDL, and triglyceride levels, as well as to increase HDL level in primary hypercholesterolemia (heterozygous familial and nonfamilial), mixed dyslipidemia (Fredrickson Type IIa and IIb); adjunct to diet to treat elevated triglyceride levels (Fredrickson Type IV).**
Adults: Initially, 10 mg P.O. daily. Increase dosage, p.r.n., to a maximum of 40 mg daily. Increase q 2 to 4 weeks based on lipid levels. If aggressive lipid lowering is needed, dose may be initiated at 20 mg once daily.
▶ **Adjunct to other lipid-lowering therapies to reduce LDL, ApoB, and total cholesterol levels in homozygous familial hypercholesterolemia.** *Adults:* Initially, 20 mg once daily. Maximum, 40 mg daily.
Adjust-a-dose: For patients with renal impairment, if creatinine clearance is less than 30 ml/minute, initiate dosage at 5 mg once daily; don't exceed 10 mg once daily. In patients taking 40 mg who develop unexplained persistent proteinuria, reduce dosage. For patients taking gemfibrozil with rosuvastatin, don't exceed 10 mg once daily. In patients taking cyclosporine, limit dose of rosuvastatin to 5 mg once daily.

Contraindications and precautions

• Contraindicated in patients hypersensitive to drug or any of its components and in patients with active liver disease or unexplained persistent elevations in transaminases.

• Use cautiously in patients who drink substantial amounts of alcohol and in patients with a history of liver disease. Also use cautiously in patients at increased risk for developing myopathies, such as those with renal impairment, advanced age, or hypothyroidism.

• Use with gemfibrozil only when the benefit clearly outweighs the risk. Don't exceed recommended dosage.

⚠ **Lifespan:** In pregnant women, drug is contraindicated. In breast-feeding women, a decision should be made to either stop breast-feeding or the drug, taking into account the importance of the drug to the mother. It's unknown whether drug appears breast milk. In children, safety of drug hasn't been established

Adverse reactions

CNS: headache, asthenia, dizziness, insomnia, paresthesia, depression, anxiety, vertigo, pain, neuralgia, hypertonia.
CV: chest pain, hypertension, palpitation, vasodilation
EENT: pharyngitis, rhinitis, sinusitis
GI: diarrhea, dyspepsia, nausea, abdominal pain, vomiting, gastritis, constipation, gastroenteritis, flatulence, periodontal abscess.
GU: UTI.
Hematologic: anemia.
Metabolic: *diabetes mellitus.*
Musculoskeletal: myalgia, back pain, pelvic pain, neck pain, pathological fracture, arthritis.
Respiratory: *asthma*, pneumonia, bronchitis, increased cough, dyspnea.
Skin: rash, pruritus, ecchymosis.
Other: flulike syndrome, accidental injury.

Interactions

Drug-drug. *Antacids.* May decrease level of rosuvastatin. Give antacids 2 hours after rosuvastatin.
Cyclosporine. May increase rosuvastatin level and increase risk of myopathy or rhabdomyolysis. Rosuvastatin dose shouldn't exceed 10 mg daily. Monitor patient for signs and symptoms of toxicity.
Gemfibrozil. May increase rosuvastatin level and increase risk of myopathy or rhabdomyolysis. Rosuvastatin dose shouldn't exceed 5 mg daily. Monitor patient for signs and symptoms of toxicity.

Warfarin. May increase warfarin level and increase risk of bleeding. Monitor INR and look for signs of increased bleeding.
Drug-lifestyle. *Alcohol use.* May increase risk of hepatotoxicity. Avoid using together.

Effects on lab test results

• May increase CK, transaminases, glucose, glutamyl transpeptidase, alkaline phosphatase, bilirubin, and thyroid function levels.
• May cause dipstick-positive proteinuria and microscopic hematuria tests.

Pharmacokinetics

Absorption: About 20%; peak level occurs within 3 to 5 hours. Rate of absorption is decreased by food, but the extent of absorption is unaffected. The drug may be given at anytime of day without any change in level.
Distribution: About 88% bound to proteins, primarily albumin
Metabolism: About 10%.
Excretion: 90% in feces. *Half-life:* About 19 hours.

Route	Onset	Peak	Duration
P.O.	2 wk	Unknown	Unknown

Action

Chemical effect: Inhibits HMG-CoA reductase that is an early and rate-limiting step in the synthetic pathway of cholesterol.
Therapeutic effect: Lowers total cholesterol, LDL, ApoB, non-HDL, and triglyceride levels.

Available forms

Tablets: 5 mg, 10 mg, 20 mg, 40 mg

NURSING PROCESS

⚕ Assessment

• Assess patient's condition before therapy and regularly thereafter.
• Perform liver function tests before therapy and again at 12 weeks. Repeat liver function tests 12 weeks following any dosage increase and then twice a year thereafter. If CK levels increase to greater than 10 times the upper limit of normal, stop drug.
• Be alert for adverse reactions and drug interactions.
• If adverse GI reactions occur, monitor hydration.

• Evaluate patient's and family's knowledge of drug therapy.

✦ Nursing diagnoses
• Risk for injury related to elevated cholesterol levels
• Risk for deficient fluid volume related to adverse GI reactions
• Deficient knowledge related to drug therapy

▷ Planning and implementation
• Begin drug only after diet and other nondrug therapies have proved ineffective. Give standard low-cholesterol diet during therapy.
• Withhold drug temporarily in any condition, such as sepsis, hypotension, major surgery, trauma, uncontrolled seizures, and severe metabolic, endocrine, and electrolyte disorders, that may predispose patient to the development of myopathy or rhabdomyolysis.

Patient teaching
• Instruct patient to take drug exactly as prescribed.
• Teach patient about proper dietary management of lipids (restricting total fat and cholesterol intake), as well as measures to control other cardiac disease risk factors. When appropriate, recommend weight control, exercise, and smoking cessation programs.
• Tell patient to immediately report any signs of unexplained muscle pain, tenderness, or weakness, especially if accompanied by malaise or fever.
• Instruct patient to take antacids containing aluminum or magnesium at least 2 hours after this drug.
• Inform woman that drug is contraindicated during pregnancy. Advise her to notify prescriber immediately if she becomes pregnant.

☑ Evaluation
• Patient's LDL and total cholesterol levels are within normal range.
• Patient maintains adequate hydration.
• Patient and family state understanding of drug therapy.

salmeterol xinafoate
(sal-MEE-ter-ohl zee-neh-FOH-ayt)
Serevent Diskus

Pharmacologic class: selective beta$_2$-adrenergic agonist
Therapeutic class: bronchodilator
Pregnancy risk category: C

Indications and dosages

▶ **Long-term maintenance treatment of asthma; prevention of bronchospasm in patients with nocturnal asthma or reversible obstructive airway disease who need regular treatment with short-acting beta agonists.** *Adults and children older than age 4:* 1 inhalation (50 mcg) q 12 hours, in the morning and in the evening.
▶ **Prevention of exercise-induced bronchospasm.** *Adults and children age 4 and older:* 1 inhalation (50 mcg) at least 30 minutes before exercise.
▶ **Maintenance treatment of bronchospasm with COPD (including emphysema and chronic bronchitis).** *Adults:* 1 inhalation (50 mcg) q 12 hours, in the morning and in the evening.

Contraindications and precautions

• Contraindicated in patients hypersensitive to drug or its components.
• Use cautiously in patients who are unusually responsive to sympathomimetics and patients with coronary insufficiency, arrhythmias, hypertension or other CV disorders, thyrotoxicosis, or seizure disorders.
• ⚖ Lifespan: In pregnant women, use cautiously. In children younger than age 4, safety hasn't been established.

Adverse reactions

CNS: *headache,* sinus headache, tremor, nervousness, dizziness.
CV: tachycardia, palpitations, *ventricular arrhythmias.*

EENT: *nasopharyngitis,* nasal cavity or sinus disorder.
GI: nausea, vomiting, diarrhea, heartburn.
Musculoskeletal: joint and back pain, myalgia.
Respiratory: *upper respiratory tract infection,* cough, lower respiratory tract infection, ***bronchospasm.***
Other: *hypersensitivity reactions, anaphylaxis.*

Interactions

Drug-drug. *Beta agonists, methylxanthines, theophylline:* May cause adverse cardiac effects with excessive use. Monitor patient closely.
MAO inhibitors: Risk of severe adverse CV effects. Don't use within 14 days of MAO therapy.
Tricyclic antidepressants: Risk of moderate to severe adverse CV effects. Use cautiously.

Effects on lab test results

None reported.

Pharmacokinetics

Absorption: Low or undetectable because of low therapeutic dose.
Distribution: Local to lungs; 94% to 99% bound to proteins.
Metabolism: Extensively metabolized by hydroxylation.
Excretion: Excreted primarily in feces.

Route	Onset	Peak	Duration
Inhalation	10-20 min	3 hr	12 hr

Action

Chemical effect: Unclear; selectively activates beta$_2$-adrenergic receptors, which results in bronchodilation. Also blocks release of allergic mediators from mast cells in respiratory tract.
Therapeutic effect: Improves breathing ability.

Available forms

Inhalation powder: 50 mcg/blister

NURSING PROCESS

Assessment
- Assess patient's respiratory condition before therapy and regularly thereafter.
- Assess peak flow readings before starting treatment and periodically thereafter.
- Be alert for adverse reactions and drug interactions.

- Evaluate patient's and family's knowledge of drug therapy.

Nursing diagnoses
- Ineffective breathing pattern related to respiratory condition
- Acute pain related to drug-induced headache
- Deficient knowledge related to drug therapy

Planning and implementation
- Don't give drug for acute bronchospasm.
- Report insufficient relief or worsening condition.
- If headache occurs, give mild analgesic.
- **ALERT:** Rare serious asthma episodes or asthma-related deaths may occur, with Blacks at greatest risk.
- **ALERT:** Don't confuse Serevent with Serentil.
Patient teaching
- Tell patient to take drug at about 12-hour intervals and to take even if he is feeling better.
- Tell patient to prevent exercise-induced bronchospasm by taking drug 30 to 60 minutes before exercise.
- **ALERT:** Instruct patient not to use for acute bronchospasm, but to use short-acting beta agonist (such as albuterol) instead.
- Tell patient to contact prescriber if short-acting beta agonist no longer provides sufficient relief or if taking more than 4 inhalations daily. Tell patient not to increase dosage of drug.
- If patient is taking inhaled corticosteroid, he should continue to use it. Warn him not to take other drugs without prescriber's consent.

Evaluation
- Patient exhibits normal breathing pattern.
- Patient states that drug-induced headache is relieved after analgesic administration.
- Patient and family state understanding of drug therapy.

saquinavir
(sah-KWIN-ah-veer)
Fortovase

saquinavir mesylate
Invirase

Pharmacologic class: HIV-1 and HIV-2 protease inhibitor

Therapeutic class: antiviral
Pregnancy risk category: B

Indications and dosages

▶ **Adjunct treatment for advanced HIV infection in selected patients.** *Adults:* 1,000 mg P.O. b.i.d. with 100 mg ritonavir P.O. b.i.d.

Contraindications and precautions

• Contraindicated in patients hypersensitive to drug or components of capsule and in patients taking triazolam, midazolam, ergot derivatives, or cisapride.
⚖ **Lifespan:** In pregnant and breast-feeding women and in children younger than age 16, safety of drug hasn't been established.

Adverse reactions

CNS: asthenia, paresthesia, headache, dizziness.
CV: chest pain.
GI: diarrhea, ulcerated buccal mucosa, abdominal pain, nausea, *pancreatitis.*
Hematologic: *pancytopenia, thrombocytopenia.*
Musculoskeletal: musculoskeletal pain.
Respiratory: bronchitis, cough.
Skin: rash.

Interactions

Drug-drug. *Amprenavir:* Decreases levels of amprenavir. Use together cautiously.
Carbamazepine, phenobarbital, phenytoin: May decrease saquinavir levels. Avoid using together.
Delavirdine: Increases saquinavir concentration. Use cautiously and monitor hepatic enzymes. Decrease dose when used together.
Dexamethasone: Decreases saquinavir levels. Avoid using together.
Efavirenz: Decreases levels of both drugs. Don't use together.
HMG-CoA reductase inhibitors: Increases levels of these drugs, which increases risk of myopathy, including rhabdomyolysis. Avoid using together.
Indinavir, lopinavir/ritonavir combination, nelfinavir, ritonavir: Increases levels of saquinavir. Use together cautiously.
Ketoconazole: May increase saquinavir levels. No dosage adjustment necessary.
Macrolide antibiotics such as clarithromycin: Increases levels of both drugs. Use together cautiously.

Nevirapine: Decreases saquinavir concentrations. Monitor patient.
Rifabutin, rifampin: Reduces the steady-state concentration of saquinavir. Use rifabutin and saquinavir together cautiously. Don't use with rifampin.
Sildenafil: Increases peak levels and exposure of sildenafil. Reduce initial dose of sildenafil to 25 mg when given with saquinavir.
Drug-herb. *St. John's wort:* May substantially reduce blood levels of the drug that could cause loss of therapeutic effects. Discourage using together.
Garlic supplements: May decrease saquinavir concentrations by half. Discourage using together.
Drug-food. *Any food:* Increases drug absorption. Advise patient to take drug with food.
Grapefruit juice: Increases drug levels. Take with liquid other than grapefruit juice.

Effects on lab test results

• May increase liver enzyme levels.
• May decrease WBC, RBC, and platelet counts.

Pharmacokinetics

Absorption: Poor.
Distribution: More than 98% bound to proteins.
Metabolism: Rapid.
Excretion: Excreted mainly in feces. *Half-life:* 1 to 2 hours.

Route	Onset	Peak	Duration
P.O.	Unknown	Unknown	Unknown

Action

Chemical effect: Inhibits activity of HIV protease and prevents cleavage of HIV polyproteins, which are essential for HIV maturation.
Therapeutic effect: Hinders HIV activity.

Available forms

saquinavir
Capsules (soft gelatin): 200 mg
saquinavir mesylate
Capsules (hard gelatin): 200 mg

NURSING PROCESS

📋 **Assessment**
• Obtain history of patient's HIV infection.

• Monitor CBC and platelet counts and electrolyte, uric acid, liver enzyme, and bilirubin levels before therapy and at appropriate intervals during therapy.
• Be alert for adverse reactions and interactions, including those caused by adjunct therapy (zidovudine or zalcitabine).
• If adverse GI reactions occur, monitor patient's hydration.
• Evaluate patient's and family's knowledge of drug therapy.

Nursing diagnoses
• Infection related to presence of HIV
• Risk for deficient fluid volume related to adverse GI reactions
• Deficient knowledge related to drug therapy

Planning and implementation
⊕ **ALERT:** Don't confuse the two forms of this drug because dosages are different.
• If severe toxicity occurs during treatment, stop drug until cause is identified or toxicity resolves. Therapy may resume with no dosage modifications.
• Notify prescriber of adverse reactions, and obtain an order for a mild analgesic, antiemetic, or antidiarrheal, if needed.
Patient teaching
• Tell patient to take drug within 2 hours after a full meal.
• Instruct patient to notify prescriber of adverse reactions.
• Inform patient that drug is usually given with other AIDS-related antiviral drugs.
• Tell patient that a change from Invirase to Fortovase capsules should be made only under a prescriber's supervision.
⊕ **ALERT:** Advise patient taking sildenafil that there is an increased risk of sildenafil-associated adverse events including hypotension, visual changes, and priapism; any symptoms should be promptly reported. Tell patient not to exceed 25 mg of sildenafil in a 48-hour period.

✔ Evaluation
• Patient responds well to therapy.
• Patient maintains adequate hydration.
• Patient and family state understanding of drug therapy.

sargramostim (granulocyte macrophage colony-stimulating factor, GM-CSF)
(sar-GRAH-moh-stim)
Leukine

Pharmacologic class: biological response modifier
Therapeutic class: colony-stimulating factor; hematopoietic growth factor
Pregnancy risk category: C

Indications and dosages
▶ **Acceleration of hematopoietic reconstitution after autologous bone marrow transplantation in patients with malignant lymphoma or acute lymphoblastic leukemia, or during autologous bone marrow transplantation in patients with Hodgkin's disease.**
Adults: 250 mcg/m^2 daily given as 2-hour I.V. infusion beginning 2 to 4 hours after bone marrow transplantation and not less than 24 hours after last dose of chemotherapy or radiation. Patient's post marrow infusion absolute neutrophil count must be at least 500/mm^3. Continue until patient's ANC is greater than 1,500/mm^3 for 3 consecutive days.
▶ **Bone marrow transplantation failure or engraftment delay.** *Adults:* 250 mcg/m^2 as 2-hour I.V. infusion daily for 14 days. Dose may be repeated after 7 days off therapy. If engraftment still hasn't occurred, a third course of 500 mcg/m^2 I.V. daily for 14 days may be tried after another 7 days off therapy.
▶ **Neutrophil recovery following chemotherapy in acute myelogenous leukemia.** *Adults:* 250 mcg/m^2 I.V. infusion over 4 hours daily. Start therapy about day 11 or 4 days after end of induction therapy.

▼ I.V. administration
• Reconstitute drug with 1 ml of sterile water for injection. Direct stream of sterile water against side of vial and gently swirl contents to minimize foaming. Avoid excessive or vigorous agitation or shaking.
• Dilute in normal saline solution. If final level is less than 10 mcg/ml, add human albumin at final level of 0.1% to saline solution before adding drug to prevent adsorption to compo-

---

nents of delivery system. For final level of 0.1% human albumin, add 1 mg human albumin per 1 ml saline solution.

• Give as soon as possible and no later than 6 hours after reconstituting.

• Discard unused portion. Vials are for single-dose use and contain no preservatives. Don't reenter vial.

⊛ **ALERT:** Don't add other drugs to infusion solution because no data exist on solution compatibility and stability.

• Refrigerate sterile powder, reconstituted solution, and diluted solution for injection. Don't freeze or shake.

Contraindications and precautions

• Contraindicated in patients hypersensitive to drug or its components or to yeast-derived products. Also contraindicated in patients with excessive leukemic myeloid blasts in bone marrow or peripheral blood.

• Use cautiously in patients with cardiac disease, hypoxia, fluid retention, pulmonary infiltrates, heart failure, or impaired kidney or liver function.

⚖ **Lifespan:** In pregnant and breast-feeding women, use cautiously. In children, safety of drug hasn't been established.

Adverse reactions

CNS: *malaise, CNS disorders, asthenia, fever.*
CV: *edema,* **supraventricular arrhythmia,** pericardial effusion.
EENT: *mucous membrane disorder.*
GI: *nausea, vomiting, diarrhea, anorexia,* **hemorrhage,** *GI disorder, stomatitis.*
GU: *urinary tract disorder,* abnormal kidney function.
Hematologic: *blood dyscrasias, hemorrhage.*
Hepatic: *liver damage.*
Respiratory: *dyspnea, lung disorders,* pleural effusion.
Skin: *alopecia, rash.*
Other: SEPSIS.

Interactions

Drug-drug. *Corticosteroids, lithium:* May potentiate myeloproliferative effects of sargramostim. Use together cautiously.

Effects on lab test results

• May increase BUN, creatinine, AST, ALT, and bilirubin levels.

Pharmacokinetics

Absorption: Administered I.V.
Distribution: Bound to specific receptors on target cells.
Metabolism: Unknown.
Excretion: Unknown. *Half-life:* About 2 hours.

Route	Onset	Peak	Duration
I.V.	≤ 30 min	2 hr	Unknown

Action

Chemical effect: Differs from natural human GM-CSF. Induces cellular responses by binding to specific receptors on surfaces of target cells.
Therapeutic effect: Stimulates formation of granulocytes (neutrophils, eosinophils) and macrophages.

Available forms

Liquid: 500 mcg*
Powder for injection: 250 mcg

NURSING PROCESS

Assessment

• Assess patient's condition before therapy and regularly thereafter.

• Drug effect may be limited in patient who has received extensive radiotherapy to hematopoietic sites for treatment of primary disease in abdomen or chest or who has been exposed to multiple drugs (alkylating, anthracycline antibiotics, antimetabolites) before autologous bone marrow transplantation.

• Drug is effective in accelerating myeloid recovery in patients receiving bone marrow purged from monoclonal antibodies.

• Drug can act as growth factor for tumors, particularly myeloid cancers.

• Blood counts return to normal or baseline levels within 3 to 7 days after stopping treatment.

• Monitor CBC with differential, including examination for presence of blast cells, biweekly.

• Be alert for adverse reactions and drug interactions.

• Monitor patient's hydration throughout drug therapy.

• Evaluate patient's and family's knowledge of drug therapy.

Nursing diagnoses

• Ineffective health maintenance related to underlying condition

- Risk for deficient fluid volume related to drug-induced adverse effects
- Deficient knowledge related to drug therapy

▷ Planning and implementation
- If severe adverse reactions occur, notify prescriber; dose may be reduced by half or stopped temporarily. Therapy may be resumed when reactions decrease. Transient rashes and local reactions at injection site may occur; serious allergic or anaphylactic reactions aren't common.
- Stimulation of marrow precursors may result in rapid rise of WBC count. If blast cells appear or increase to 10% or more of WBC count or if underlying disease progresses, stop drug. If absolute neutrophil count is more than 20,000/mm³ or if platelet count is more than 50,000/mm³, temporarily stop drug or reduce dose by half.

Patient teaching
- Inform patient and family about need for therapy.
- Advise patient to report adverse reactions immediately.

☑ Evaluation
- Patient exhibits positive response to drug therapy.
- Patient maintains adequate hydration throughout therapy.
- Patient and family state understanding of drug therapy.

---

scopolamine (hyoscine)
(skoh-POL-uh-meen)
Scop ◇ , Transderm Scōp, Scopace

scopolamine butylbromide (hyoscine butylbromide)
Buscopan ♦ ◇

scopolamine hydrobromide (hyoscine hydrobromide)

Pharmacologic class: anticholinergic
Therapeutic class: antimuscarinic, antiemetic, antivertigo drug, antiparkinsonian
Pregnancy risk category: C

Indications and dosages
▶ **Spastic states.** *Adults:* 0.4 to 0.8 mg Scopace P.O. daily. Or, 10 to 20 mg scopolamine butylbromide S.C., I.M., or I.V. t.i.d. or q.i.d.
▶ **Preoperatively to reduce secretions.** *Adults:* 0.2 to 0.6 mg scopolamine hydrobromide I.M. 30 to 60 minutes before induction of anesthesia.
Children ages 8 to 12: 0.3 mg scopolamine hydrobromide I.M. 45 minutes before induction of anesthesia.
Children ages 3 to 8: 0.2 mg scopolamine hydrobromide I.M. 45 minutes before induction of anesthesia.
Children ages 7 months to 3 years: 0.15 mg scopolamine hydrobromide I.M. 45 minutes before induction of anesthesia.
Infants ages 4 to 7 months: 0.1 mcg scopolamine hydrobromide I.M. 45 minutes before induction of anesthesia.
▶ **Prevention of nausea and vomiting from motion sickness.** *Adults:* 1 Transderm Scōp patch (a circular flat unit), formulated to deliver 1 mg over 3 days (72 hours), applied to skin behind ear at least 4 hours before antiemetic is needed. Or, 0.3 to 0.6 mg scopolamine hydrobromide S.C., I.M., or I.V. Or, 0.4 to 0.8 mg P.O.
Children: 0.006 mg/kg or 0.2 mg/m² scopolamine hydrobromide S.C., I.M., or I.V.

▽ I.V. administration
- Intermittent and continuous infusions aren't recommended.
- For direct injection, dilute with sterile water and inject diluted drug at ordered rate through patent I.V. line.
- Protect I.V. solutions from freezing and light, and store at room temperature.

Contraindications and precautions
- Contraindicated in patients with angle-closure glaucoma, obstructive uropathy, obstructive disease of GI tract, asthma, chronic pulmonary disease, myasthenia gravis, paralytic ileus, intestinal atony, unstable CV status in acute hemorrhage, or toxic megacolon.
- Transderm Scōp is contraindicated in patients allergic to scopolamine and other belladonna alkaloids.
- Use cautiously in patients with autonomic neuropathy, hyperthyroidism, coronary artery disease, arrhythmias, heart failure, hypertension,

---

hiatal hernia with reflux esophagitis, hepatic or renal disease, or ulcerative colitis. Also use cautiously in patients in hot or humid environments because of drug-induced heatstroke.

• Use Transderm Scōp cautiously in patients with liver or renal impairment, pyloric obstruction, or urinary bladder and neck obstruction.

⚖ Lifespan: In pregnant women and children younger than age 6, use cautiously. In breastfeeding women, avoid using drug. In children, Transderm Scōp is contraindicated. In elderly patients, use Transderm Scōp cautiously.

Adverse reactions

CNS: disorientation, restlessness, irritability, dizziness, drowsiness, headache, confusion, hallucinations, delirium, fever.
CV: palpitations, tachycardia, flushing, *paradoxical bradycardia.*
EENT: dilated pupils, blurred vision, photophobia, increased intraocular pressure, difficulty swallowing.
GI: *constipation, dry mouth, nausea, vomiting, epigastric distress.*
GU: urinary hesitancy, urine retention.
Respiratory: bronchial plugging, *depressed respirations.*
Skin: rash, dryness, contact dermatitis with transdermal patch.

Interactions

Drug-drug. *Centrally acting anticholinergics (antihistamines, phenothiazines, tricyclic antidepressants):* Increases risk of adverse CNS reactions. Monitor patient closely.
CNS depressants: Increases risk of CNS depression. Monitor patient closely.
Digoxin: Increases digoxin levels. Monitor patient for cardiac toxicity.
Drug-herb. *Jaborandi tree:* Effects of these drugs may be decreased. Discourage using together.
Pill-bearing spurge: Choline may decrease effect of scopolamine. Discourage using together.
Squaw vine: Tannic acid may decrease metabolic breakdown. Discourage using together.
Drug-lifestyle. *Alcohol use:* Increases risk of CNS depression. Discourage using together.

Effects on lab test results

None reported.

Pharmacokinetics

Absorption: Well absorbed percutaneously from behind ear with transdermal patch application. Well absorbed from GI tract when given P.O. or P.R. Absorbed rapidly when given I.M. or S.C.
Distribution: Distributed widely throughout body tissues; probably crosses blood-brain barrier.
Metabolism: Thought to be metabolized completely in liver.
Excretion: May be excreted in urine as metabolites. *Half-life:* 8 hours.

Route	Onset	Peak	Duration
P.O.	30-60 min	Unknown	4-6 hr
I.V., I.M., S.C.	30 min	Unknown	4 hr
P.R.	Unknown	Unknown	Unknown
Transdermal	Unknown	Unknown	≤ 72 hr

Action

Chemical effect: Inhibits muscarinic actions of acetylcholine in the autonomic nervous system. It also may affect neural pathways originating in the labyrinth (inner ear) to inhibit nausea and vomiting.
Therapeutic effect: Relieves spasticity, nausea, and vomiting; reduces secretions; and blocks cardiac vagal reflexes.

Available forms

scopolamine
Transdermal patch: 1.5 mg
scopolamine butylbromide
Capsules: 0.25 mg
Suppositories: 10 mg ◆
Tablets: 10 mg ◆
scopolamine hydrobromide
Injection: 0.3, 0.4, 0.5, 0.6, and 1 mg/ml in 1-ml vials and ampules; 0.86 mg/ml in 0.5-ml ampules

NURSING PROCESS

📋 **Assessment**
• Assess patient's condition before therapy and regularly thereafter.
• Be alert for adverse reactions and drug interactions.
• Evaluate patient's and family's knowledge of drug therapy.

⊞ Nursing diagnoses
- Risk for deficient fluid volume related to nausea and vomiting
- Risk for injury related to drug-induced adverse CNS reactions
- Deficient knowledge related to drug therapy

⟩⟩ Planning and implementation
- Apply patch the night before patient's expected travel.
- Raise side rails of bed as precaution because some patients become temporarily excited or disoriented. Symptoms disappear when sedative effect is complete.
- In therapeutic doses, scopolamine may produce amnesia, drowsiness, and euphoria; patient may need to be reoriented.
- Tolerance may develop when scopolamine is given over a long time.
- **⚠ ALERT:** Overdose may cause curare-like effects such as respiratory paralysis.

Patient teaching
- Advise patient to apply patch the night before planned trip. Transdermal method releases controlled therapeutic amount of drug. Transderm Scōp is effective if applied 2 to 3 hours before experiencing motion but is more effective if applied 12 hours before.
- Advise patient to wash and dry hands thoroughly before and after applying transdermal patch on dry skin behind ear and before touching eye because pupil may dilate. After removing system, he should discard it and wash hands and application site thoroughly.
- Tell patient that if patch becomes displaced, he should remove it and replace it with another patch on fresh skin site behind ear.
- Alert patient to risk of withdrawal symptoms (nausea, vomiting, headache, dizziness) if transdermal system is used longer than 72 hours.
- Tell patient to ask pharmacist for brochure that comes with transdermal product.
- Inform patient about P.O. or P.R. administration, if applicable.
- Advise patient to refrain from activities that require alertness until drug's CNS effects are known.
- Instruct patient to report signs of urinary hesitancy or urine retention.
- Recommend use of sugarless gum or hard candy to help minimize dry mouth.

☑ Evaluation
- Patient responds well to therapy.
- Patient doesn't experience injury from adverse CNS reactions.
- Patient and family state understanding of drug therapy.

secobarbital sodium
(sek-oh-BAR-bih-tohl SOH-dee-um)
Novosecobarb ◆ , Seconal Sodium

Pharmacologic class: barbiturate
Therapeutic class: sedative-hypnotic, anticonvulsant
Pregnancy risk category: D
Controlled substance schedule: II

Indications and dosages
▶ **Preoperative sedation.** *Adults:* 200 to 300 mg P.O. 1 to 2 hours before surgery. *Children:* 2 to 6 mg/kg P.O. 1 to 2 hours before surgery. Maximum single dose is 100 mg.
▶ **Insomnia.** *Adults:* 100 mg P.O. h.s.

Contraindications and precautions
- Contraindicated in patients hypersensitive to barbiturates and in patients with marked liver impairment, porphyria, or respiratory disease in which dyspnea or obstruction is evident.
- Use cautiously in patients with acute or chronic pain, depression, suicidal tendencies, history of drug abuse, or hepatic impairment.
- ⚖ **Lifespan:** In pregnant or breast-feeding women, drug isn't recommended.

Adverse reactions
CNS: *drowsiness, lethargy, hangover,* paradoxical excitement in geriatric patients, somnolence.
GI: nausea, vomiting.
Hematologic: exacerbation of porphyria.
Respiratory: *respiratory depression.*
Skin: rash, urticaria, *Stevens-Johnson syndrome.*
Other: *angioedema,* physical or psychological dependence.

Interactions
Drug-drug. *Chloramphenicol, MAO inhibitors, valproic acid:* Inhibits metabolism of barbiturates; may cause prolonged CNS depression. Reduce barbiturate dosage.

CNS depressants, including opioid analgesics: May cause excessive CNS and respiratory depression. Use together cautiously.

Corticosteroids, digitoxin, doxycycline, estrogens and hormonal contraceptives, oral anticoagulants, theophylline, tricyclic antidepressants, verapamil: Secobarbital may enhance metabolism of these drugs. Monitor patient for decreased effect.

Griseofulvin: Decreases absorption of griseofulvin. Monitor patient for decreased griseofulvin effectiveness.

Metoprolol, propranolol: May reduce the effects of these drugs. Consider an increased beta blocker dose

Rifampin: May decrease barbiturate levels. Monitor patient for decreased effect.

Drug-lifestyle. *Alcohol use:* May impair coordination, increase CNS effects, and cause death. Strongly discourage alcohol use with this drug.

Effects on lab test results

None reported.

Pharmacokinetics

Absorption: Rapid with 90% of drug absorbed.
Distribution: Rapid; about 30% to 45% protein-bound.
Metabolism: Oxidized in liver to inactive metabolites.
Excretion: Excreted in urine. *Half-life:* About 30 hours.

Route	Onset	Peak	Duration
P.O.	15 min	5-30 min	1-4 hr

Action

Chemical effect: Unknown; probably interferes with transmission of impulses from thalamus to cortex of brain.
Therapeutic effect: Promotes pain relief and calmness and relieves acute seizures.

Available forms

Capsules: 50 mg, 100 mg

NURSING PROCESS

Assessment

• Assess patient's condition before therapy and regularly thereafter.

• Assess mental status before therapy. Geriatric patients are more sensitive to adverse CNS effects of drug.
• Be alert for adverse reactions and drug interactions.
• Evaluate patient's and family's knowledge of drug therapy.

Nursing diagnoses

• Disturbed sleep pattern related to underlying condition
• Risk for injury related to drug-induced adverse CNS reactions
• Deficient knowledge related to drug therapy

Planning and implementation

• Prevent hoarding or intentional overdosing by patient who is depressed, suicidal, or drug-dependent or who has history of drug abuse.
• Skin eruptions may precede potentially fatal reactions to barbiturate therapy. If skin reactions occur, stop drug and notify prescriber. In some patients, high fever, stomatitis, headache, or rhinitis may precede skin reactions.
• Long-term use isn't recommended; drug loses its effectiveness in promoting sleep after 14 days of continued use.

Patient teaching
• Warn patient to avoid activities that require mental alertness or physical coordination. For inpatient, supervise walking and raise bed rails, particularly for the geriatric patient.
• Inform patient that morning hangover is common after hypnotic dose, which suppresses REM sleep. Patient may experience increased dreaming after drug is stopped.
• Advise patient who uses hormonal contraceptives to use a different birth control method, such as a barrier method; drug may enhance contraceptive hormone metabolism and decrease its effect.

Evaluation

• Patient states that drug effectively induces sleep.
• Patient doesn't experience injury from adverse CNS reactions.
• Patient and family state understanding of drug therapy.

---

selegiline hydrochloride (L-deprenyl hydrochloride)

(see-LEJ-eh-leen high-droh-KLOR-ighd)
Atapryl, Carbex, Eldepryl, Selpak

Pharmacologic class: MAO inhibitor
Therapeutic class: antiparkinsonian
Pregnancy risk category: C

Indications and dosages

▶ **Adjunct treatment with levodopa-carbidopa in managing symptoms of Parkinson's disease.** *Adults:* 10 mg P.O. daily, taken as 5 mg at breakfast and 5 mg at lunch. After 2 or 3 days of therapy, gradual decrease of levodopa-carbidopa dosage is attempted.

Contraindications and precautions

• Contraindicated in patients hypersensitive to drug and in those receiving meperidine.
⚠ **Lifespan:** In pregnant women, use cautiously. In breast-feeding women and in children, safety of drug hasn't been established.

Adverse reactions

CNS: *dizziness,* increased tremors, chorea, loss of balance, restlessness, increased bradykinesia, facial grimacing, stiff neck, dyskinesia, involuntary movements, twitching, increased apraxia, behavioral changes, fatigue, headache, confusion, hallucinations, vivid dreams, malaise, syncope.
CV: orthostatic hypotension, hypertension, hypotension, *arrhythmias,* palpitations, angina, tachycardia, peripheral edema.
EENT: blepharospasm.
GI: dry mouth, *nausea,* vomiting, constipation, abdominal pain, anorexia or poor appetite, dysphagia, diarrhea, heartburn.
GU: slow urination, transient nocturia, prostatic hyperplasia, urinary hesitancy, urinary frequency, urine retention, sexual dysfunction.
Skin: rash, hair loss, diaphoresis.
Metabolic: weight loss.

Interactions

Drug-drug. *Adrenergics:* May increase pressor response, particularly in patients who have taken overdose of selegiline. Use together cautiously.

Citalopram, fluoxetine, fluvoxamine, nefazodone, paroxetine, sertraline, venlafaxine: May cause serotonin syndrome involving CNS irritability, shivering, and altered consciousness. Don't give together. Wait at least 2 weeks after stopping an MAO inhibitor before giving any SSRI.
Meperidine: May cause stupor, muscle rigidity, severe agitation, and elevated temperature. Avoid using together.
Drug-herb. *Cacao tree:* Potential vasopressor effects. Discourage using together.
Ginseng: May increase risk of adverse reactions, including headache, tremor, and mania. Discourage using together.
Drug-food. *Foods high in tyramine:* May cause hypertensive crisis. Monitor patient's blood pressure; instruct patient to avoid these foods.

Effects on lab test results

None reported.

Pharmacokinetics

Absorption: Unknown.
Distribution: Unknown.
Metabolism: Three metabolites have been detected in serum and urine: *N*-desmethyldeprenyl, L-amphetamine, and L-methamphetamine.
Excretion: 45% excreted in urine as metabolite. *Half-life:* Selegiline, 2 to 10 hours; *N*-desmethyldeprenyl, 2 hours; L-amphetamine, 17¾ hours; L-methamphetamine, 20½ hours.

Route	Onset	Peak	Duration
P.O.	Unknown	30 min-2 hr	Unknown

Action

Chemical effect: Unknown; probably acts by selectively inhibiting MAO type B (found mostly in brain). It also may directly increase dopaminergic activity by decreasing reuptake of dopamine into nerve cells. Its active metabolites, amphetamine and methamphetamine, may contribute to this effect.
Therapeutic effect: Improves physical mobility.

Available forms

Tablets: 5 mg

NURSING PROCESS

☞ Assessment
• Assess patient's condition before therapy and regularly thereafter.
• Be alert for adverse reactions and drug interactions.
• Evaluate patient's and family's knowledge of drug therapy.

⊕ Nursing diagnoses
• Impaired physical mobility related to underlying condition
• Risk for injury related to drug-induced adverse CNS reactions
• Deficient knowledge related to drug therapy

▶ Planning and implementation
• Some patients experience increased adverse reactions related to levodopa and need a 10% to 30% reduction of levodopa-carbidopa dosage.
⊛ **ALERT:** Don't confuse selegiline with Stelazine or Eldepryl with enalapril.
Patient teaching
• Warn patient to move cautiously at start of therapy because he may experience dizziness.
• Advise patient not to take more than 10 mg daily because greater amount of drug won't improve effectiveness and may increase adverse reactions.

☑ Evaluation
• Patient exhibits improved physical mobility.
• Patient doesn't experience injury from adverse CNS reactions.
• Patient and family state understanding of drug therapy.

senna
(SEN-uh)
Black-Draught†, Fletcher's Castoria†
Senexon†, Senokot†, Senolax†, X-Prep*†

Pharmacologic class: anthraquinone derivative
Therapeutic class: stimulant laxative
Pregnancy risk category: C

Indications and dosages

▶ **Acute constipation; preparation for bowel examination.** *Adults:* 2 tablets or ¼ to ½ tsp of Black-Draught granules mixed with water.

Adults and children age 12 and older: For other preparations, usual dose is 2 tablets, 1 tsp of granules dissolved in water, 1 suppository, or 10 to 15 ml syrup h.s. Maximum dosage varies with preparation used.
Children ages 6 to 11: 1 tablet, ½ tsp of granules dissolved in water, ½ suppository h.s. or 5 to 10 ml syrup. Maximum dosage is 2 tablets b.i.d. or 1 tsp of granules b.i.d.
Children ages 2 to 5: ½ tablet or ¼ tsp of granules dissolved in water. Maximum, 1 tablet b.i.d. or ½ tsp of granules b.i.d.
Children ages 1 to 5: 2.5 to 5 ml syrup h.s.
Children ages 1 month to 12 months: Consult prescriber.

Contraindications and precautions
• Contraindicated in patients with ulcerative bowel lesions; nausea, vomiting, abdominal pain, or other symptoms of appendicitis or acute surgical abdomen; fecal impaction; or intestinal obstruction or perforation.
⚖ **Lifespan:** In pregnant and breast-feeding women, use cautiously.

Adverse reactions
GI: *nausea;* vomiting; diarrhea; malabsorption of nutrients; yellow or yellow-green cast to feces; *abdominal cramps,* especially in severe constipation; "cathartic colon" (syndrome resembling ulcerative colitis radiologically) with long-term misuse; constipation after catharsis; diarrhea in breast-feeding infants of mothers receiving senna; darkened pigmentation of rectal mucosa with long-term use (usually reversible within 4 to 12 months after stopping drug); laxative dependence; loss of normal bowel function with excessive use.
GU: red-pink discoloration in alkaline urine; yellow-brown color to acidic urine.
Metabolic: protein-losing enteropathy, electrolyte imbalance.

Interactions
None significant.

Effects on lab test results
• May alter fluid and electrolyte levels with prolonged use.

Pharmacokinetics
Absorption: Minimal.
Distribution: In bile, saliva, colonic mucosa.

Metabolism: Absorbed portion metabolized in liver.
Excretion: Unabsorbed senna excreted mainly in feces; absorbed drug excreted in urine and feces. *Half-life:* Unknown.

Route	Onset	Peak	Duration
P.O.	6-10 hr	Varies	Varies
P.R.	30 min-2 hr	Varies	Varies

Action

Chemical effect: Unknown; increases peristalsis, probably by direct effect on smooth muscle of intestine. It also promotes fluid accumulation in colon and small intestine.
Therapeutic effect: Relieves constipation and cleanses bowel.

Available forms

Dosages expressed as sennosides (active principle)
Granules†: 15 mg/teaspoon, 20 mg/teaspoon
Liquid†: 3 mg/ml
Suppositories†: 30 mg
Syrup†: 8.8 mg/5 ml
Tablets†: 6 mg, 8.6 mg, 17 mg

NURSING PROCESS

Assessment
- Assess patient's condition before therapy and regularly thereafter.
- Before giving drug for constipation, determine if patient's fluid intake, exercise, and diet are adequate.
- Be alert for adverse reactions.
- Evaluate patient's and family's knowledge of drug therapy.

Nursing diagnoses
- Constipation related to underlying condition
- Diarrhea related to drug-induced adverse GI reactions
- Deficient knowledge related to drug therapy

Planning and implementation
- Limit diet to clear liquids after patient takes X-Prep Liquid.
- Avoid exposing drug to excessive heat or light.
- Drug is used for short-term treatment.

- Senna is one of the most effective laxatives for counteracting constipation caused by opioid analgesics.
Patient teaching
- Teach patient about dietary sources of bulk, which include bran and other cereals, fresh fruit, and vegetables.
- Tell patient to maintain adequate fluid intake of at least 6 to 8 glasses of water or juices daily unless contraindicated.

Evaluation
- Patient's constipation is relieved.
- Patient states that diarrhea doesn't occur.
- Patient and family state understanding of drug therapy.

sertraline hydrochloride
(SER-truh-leen high-droh-KLOR-ighd)
Zoloft

Pharmacologic class: serotonin uptake inhibitor
Therapeutic class: antidepressant
Pregnancy risk category: C

Indications and dosages

▶ **Depression.** *Adults:* 50 mg P.O. daily. Adjust dosage as tolerated and needed. Adjust dosage at intervals of no less than 1 week.
▶ **Posttraumatic stress disorder, social anxiety disorder.** *Adults:* Initially, 25 mg P.O. once daily. Increase dosage to 50 mg P.O. once daily after 1 week of therapy. Dosage may be increased at weekly intervals to a maximum of 200 mg daily. Maintain patient on lowest effective dosage.
▶ **Premenstrual dysphoric disorder.** *Women:* Initially, 50 mg daily P.O. continuously, or limited to the luteal phase of the menstrual cycle. Patients not responding may benefit from dose increases at 50-mg increments per menstrual cycle up to 150 mg daily when dosing daily throughout the menstrual cycle, or 100 mg daily when dosing during the luteal phase of the menstrual cycle. If a 100-mg daily dose has been established with luteal phase dosing, a 50-mg daily adjustment step for 3 days should be used at the beginning of each luteal phase dosing period.

▶ **Premature ejaculation‡.** *Adults:* 25 to 50 mg P.O. daily or p.r.n.

Contraindications and precautions

• Contraindicated in patients hypersensitive to drug or any of the inactive ingredients and in patients receiving pimozide.

• Use cautiously in patients at risk for suicide and in those with seizure disorder, major affective disorder, or diseases or conditions that affect metabolism or hemodynamic responses.

※ Lifespan: In pregnant and breast-feeding women, use cautiously. In children, safety of drug hasn't been established.

Adverse reactions

CNS: *headache, tremor, dizziness, insomnia, somnolence,* paresthesia, hypesthesia, hyperesthesia, *fatigue,* twitching, hypertonia, nervousness, anxiety, confusion.

CV: palpitations, chest pain, hot flushes, flushing.

GI: *dry mouth, nausea, diarrhea, loose stools, dyspepsia,* vomiting, constipation, thirst, flatulence, anorexia, abdominal pain, increased appetite.

GU: *male sexual dysfunction.*

Musculoskeletal: myalgia.

Skin: *diaphoresis,* rash, pruritus.

Other: decreased libido.

Interactions

Drug-drug. *Benzodiazepines (except lorazepam and oxazepam), tolbutamide:* Decreases clearance of these drugs. Significance is unknown; monitor patient for increased drug effects.

Cimetidine: Decreases sertraline clearance. Monitor patient for toxicity.

Disulfiram: Oral concentrate contains alcohol that could cause a reaction. Avoid using together.

Phenelzine, selegiline, tranylcypromine: May cause serotonin syndrome including CNS irritability, shivering, and altered consciousness. Don't give together. Wait at least 2 weeks after stopping an MAO inhibitor before giving any SSRI.

Pimozide: May increase pimozide level and cause bradycardia. Avoid using together.

Sumatriptan: May cause weakness, hyperreflexia, and incoordination. Monitor patient closely.

Tricyclic antidepressants (TCA): May inhibit TCA metabolism. Dose of TCA may need to be reduced. Monitor patient closely.

Warfarin, other highly protein-bound drugs: May increase levels of sertraline or other highly bound drug. Increases of 8% in PT and INR have been noted with use of warfarin. Monitor patient closely.

Drug-herb. *Ginkgo:* Herb may decrease adverse sexual effects of drug. Advise patient to speak to prescriber before taking any herbal remedy.

St. John's wort: May cause additive effects and serotonin syndrome including CNS irritability, shivering, and altered consciousness. Discourage use together.

Drug-lifestyle. *Alcohol use:* May enhance CNS effects. Advise patient to avoid alcohol use.

Effects on lab test results

• May increase ALT, AST, cholesterol, and triglyceride levels. May decrease uric acid level.

Pharmacokinetics

Absorption: Well absorbed from GI tract. Rate and extent enhanced when taken with food.

Distribution: Highly protein-bound (greater than 98%).

Metabolism: Metabolism is probably hepatic.

Excretion: Excreted mostly as metabolites in urine and feces. *Half-life:* 26 hours.

Route	Onset	Peak	Duration
P.O.	2-4 wk	4½-8½ hr	Unknown

Action

Chemical effect: Unknown; may be linked to inhibited neuronal uptake of serotonin in CNS.

Therapeutic effect: Relieves depression.

Available forms

Oral concentrate: 20 mg/ml

Tablets: 25 mg, 50 mg, 100 mg

NURSING PROCESS

🔆 **Assessment**

• Assess patient's condition before therapy, and reassess regularly thereafter.

• Assess patient for risk factors for suicide.

• Be alert for adverse reactions and drug interactions.

• Evaluate patient's and family's knowledge of drug therapy.

Nursing diagnoses
• Disturbed thought processes related to presence of depression
• Risk for injury related to drug-induced adverse CNS reactions
• Deficient knowledge related to drug therapy

Planning and implementation
• Give drug once daily, either in morning or evening. Drug may be given with or without food.
• Don't give within 14 days of MAO inhibitor therapy.
• Avoid using the oral concentrate dropper, which is made of rubber, in a patient with a latex allergy.

Patient teaching
• Advise patient to use caution when performing hazardous tasks that require alertness and to avoid alcohol while taking drug. Drugs that influence CNS may impair judgment.
• Instruct patient to check with prescriber or pharmacist before taking OTC drugs.
• Advise patient to mix the oral concentrate with 4 oz of water, ginger ale, or lemon-lime soda only, and to take the dose right away.

Evaluation
• Patient behavior and communication indicate improved thought processes.
• Patient doesn't experience injury from adverse CNS reactions.
• Patient and family state understanding of drug therapy.

---

sevelamer hydrochloride
(seh-VEL-ah-mer high-droh-KLOR-ighd)
Renagel

Pharmacologic class: polymeric phosphate binder
Therapeutic class: hyperphosphatemia drug
Pregnancy risk category: C

Indications and dosages
▶ **Reduction of phosphorus in patients with end-stage renal disease.** *Adults:* Depends on severity of hyperphosphatemia. Gradually adjust dosage based on phosphorus level with goal of lowering phosphorus to 6 mg/dl or less. If phosphorus level is 9 mg/dl or more, start with 1.6 g P.O. t.i.d. with meals; if phosphorus level is between 7.5 and 9 mg/dl, 1.2 g P.O. t.i.d. with meals; if phosphorus level is between 6 and 7.5 mg/dl, 800 mg P.O. t.i.d. with meals.

Contraindications and precautions
• Contraindicated in patients hypersensitive to drug or its components and in those with hypophosphatemia or bowel obstruction.
• Use cautiously in patients with dysphagia, swallowing disorders, severe GI motility disorders, or major GI tract surgery.
⚶ **Lifespan:** In breast-feeding women, use cautiously. In children, safety and effectiveness of drug haven't been established.

Adverse reactions
CNS: *headache, pain.*
CV: hypertension, *hypotension, **thrombosis**.*
GI: *vomiting,* nausea, constipation, *diarrhea,* flatulence, *dyspepsia.*
Respiratory: cough.
Other: *infection.*

Interactions
Drug-drug. *Antiarrhythmics, anticonvulsants:* May have potential pharmacokinetic interaction. Give drug at least 1 hour before or 3 hours after giving these drugs and monitor blood levels of these drugs.

Effects on lab test results
• May increase alkaline phosphatase level.

Pharmacokinetics
Absorption: None.
Distribution: Unknown.
Metabolism: Unknown.
Excretion: Unknown. *Half-life:* Unknown.

Route	Onset	Peak	Duration
P.O.	Unknown	Unknown	Unknown

Action
Chemical effect: Inhibits intestinal phosphate absorption.
Therapeutic effect: Decreases phosphorus level.

Available forms

Capsules: 403 mg
Tablets: 400 mg, 800 mg

NURSING PROCESS

Assessment
• Obtain history of patient's underlying condition before therapy, and reassess regularly thereafter.
• Monitor calcium, bicarbonate, and chloride levels.
• Watch for symptoms of thrombosis (numbness or tingling of limbs, chest pain, shortness of breath), and notify prescriber if they occur.
• Evaluate patient's and family's knowledge of drug therapy.

Nursing diagnoses
• Ineffective tissue perfusion (cardiopulmonary or peripheral) related to potential drug-induced thrombosis
• Imbalanced nutrition: less than body requirements related to drug-induced adverse GI effects
• Deficient knowledge related to drug therapy

Planning and implementation
• Don't crush or break capsules or tablets, and give only with meals.
• Drug may bind to other drugs given at the same time and decrease their bioavailability. Give other drugs 1 hour before or 3 hours after sevelamer.
ALERT: Drug may reduce vitamins D, E, and K and folic acid; give a multivitamin supplement.
Patient teaching
• Instruct patient to take with meals and adhere to prescribed diet.
• Inform patient that drug must be taken whole because contents expand in water; tell him not to open or chew capsules.
• Tell patient to take other drugs as directed, but they must be taken either 1 hour before or 3 hours after sevelamer.
• Inform patient about common adverse reactions and instruct him to report them immediately. Teach patient signs and symptoms of thrombosis (numbness, tingling limbs, chest pain, changes in level of consciousness).

Evaluation
• Patient doesn't develop a thrombus.
• Patient maintains adequate nutrition.
• Patient and family state understanding of drug therapy.

sibutramine hydrochloride monohydrate
(sigh-BYOO-truh-meen high-droh-KLOR-ighd mah-noh-HIGH-drayt)
Meridia

Pharmacologic class: serotonin, norepinephrine, and dopamine reuptake inhibitor
Therapeutic class: antiobesity drug
Pregnancy risk category: C
Controlled substance schedule: IV

Indications and dosages
▶ **Management of obesity.** *Adults:* 10 mg P.O. once daily with or without food. If weight loss is inadequate after 4 weeks, increase dosage to 15 mg P.O. daily. Patients who don't tolerate the 10-mg dose may receive 5 mg P.O. daily. Doses above 15 mg daily aren't recommended.

Contraindications and precautions
• Contraindicated in patients hypersensitive to drug or its active ingredients, those taking MAO inhibitors or other centrally acting appetite suppressants, and those with anorexia nervosa. Don't use drug in patients with severe renal or hepatic dysfunction, history of hypertension, seizures, coronary artery disease, heart failure, arrhythmias, or CVA.
• Use cautiously in patients with angle-closure glaucoma.
Lifespan: In children younger than age 16, safety and effectiveness of drug haven't been established.

Adverse reactions
CNS: asthenia, *headache, insomnia,* dizziness, nervousness, anxiety, depression, paresthesia, somnolence, CNS stimulation, emotional lability, migraine.
CV: tachycardia, vasodilation, hypertension, palpitations, chest pain, generalized edema.
EENT: thirst, *rhinitis, pharyngitis,* sinusitis, ear disorder, ear pain, laryngitis.

GI: *dry mouth,* taste perversion, *anorexia, constipation,* increased appetite, nausea, dyspepsia, gastritis, vomiting, abdominal pain, rectal disorder.
GU: dysmenorrhea, UTI, vaginal candidiasis, metrorrhagia.
Musculoskeletal: arthralgia, myalgia, tenosynovitis, joint disorder, neck or back pain.
Respiratory: cough.
Skin: rash, sweating, acne.
Other: flulike syndrome, injury, herpes simplex, accident, allergic reaction.

Interactions

Drug-drug. *CNS depressants:* May enhance CNS depression. Use cautiously.
Dextromethorphan, dihydroergotamine, fentanyl, fluoxetine, fluvoxamine, lithium, MAO inhibitors, meperidine, paroxetine, pentazocine, sertraline, sumatriptan, tryptophan, venlafaxine: May cause hyperthermia, tachycardia, and loss of consciousness. Don't use together.
Ephedrine, pseudoephedrine: May increase blood pressure or heart rate. Use cautiously.
Drug-lifestyle. *Alcohol use:* Enhances CNS depression. Discourage using together.

Effects on lab test results

• May increase ALT, AST, GGT, LDH, alkaline phosphatase, and bilirubin levels.

Pharmacokinetics

Absorption: Rapid; about 77% of dose is absorbed.
Distribution: Rapid and extensive. Active metabolites are extensively bound to proteins.
Metabolism: Extensive first-pass metabolism by the liver to two active metabolites, M_1 and M_2.
Excretion: About 77% is excreted in urine.
Half-life: M_1 is 14 hours and M_2 is 16 hours.

Route	Onset	Peak	Duration
P.O.	Unknown	3-4 hr	Unknown

Action

Chemical effect: Inhibits reuptake of norepinephrine, serotonin, and dopamine.
Therapeutic effect: Facilitates weight loss.

Available forms

Capsules: 5 mg, 10 mg, 15 mg

NURSING PROCESS

Assessment
• Monitor patient for adverse reactions and drug interactions.
• Assess patient for organic causes of obesity before starting therapy.
• Assess patient's dietary intake.
• Measure blood pressure and pulse before starting therapy, with dosage changes, and at regular intervals during therapy.
• Evaluate patient's and family's knowledge of drug therapy.

Nursing diagnoses
• Imbalanced nutrition: more than body requirements related to increased caloric intake
• Disturbed sleep pattern related to drug-induced insomnia
• Deficient knowledge related to drug therapy

Planning and implementation
• Don't give drug within 2 weeks of MAO inhibitor therapy.
• Give patient ice chips or sugarless hard candy to relieve dry mouth.
• Make sure patient follows appropriate diet regimen.
Patient teaching
• Advise patient to report rash, hives, or other allergic reactions immediately.
• Instruct patient to inform prescriber if he is taking or plans to take other prescription or OTC drugs.
• Advise patient to have blood pressure and pulse monitored at regular intervals. Stress importance of regular follow-up visits with prescriber.
• Advise patient to use drug with reduced calorie diet.
• Tell patient that weight loss can precipitate gallstone formation. Teach patient about signs and symptoms and the need to report them to prescriber promptly.

Evaluation
• Patient achieves nutritional balance with the use of drugs and a reduced-calorie diet.
• Patient experiences normal sleep patterns.
• Patient and family state understanding of drug therapy.

sildenafil citrate
(sil-DEN-ah-fil SIGH-trayt)
Viagra

Pharmacologic class: selective inhibitor of cyclic guanosine monophosphate-specific phosphodiesterase type 5
Therapeutic class: therapy for erectile dysfunction
Pregnancy risk category: B

Indications and dosages

▶ **Erectile dysfunction.** *Men younger than age 65:* 50 mg P.O., p.r.n., about 1 hour before sexual activity. Dosage range is 25 to 100 mg based on effectiveness and tolerance. Maximum is 1 dose daily.
Men age 65 and older: 25 mg P.O., p.r.n., about 1 hour before sexual activity. Dose may be adjusted based on patient response. Maximum is 1 dose daily.
◩ **Adjust-a-dose:** Men with hepatic or severe renal impairment should take 25 mg P.O. about 1 hour before sexual activity. Dose may be adjusted based on patient response. Maximum is 1 dose daily.

Contraindications and precautions

• Contraindicated in patients hypersensitive to drug or its components, those with underlying CV disease, and those using organic nitrates at any frequency and in any form.
• Use cautiously in patients with hepatic or severe renal impairment; those with anatomic deformation of the penis; those with conditions that may predispose them to priapism (such as sickle-cell anemia, multiple myeloma, leukemia), retinitis pigmentosa, bleeding disorders, or active peptic ulcer disease; those who have had an MI, CVA, or life-threatening arrhythmia during previous 6 months; and those with history of cardiac failure, coronary artery disease, or uncontrolled high or low blood pressure.
⚖ **Lifespan:** In men age 65 and older, use cautiously.

Adverse reactions

CNS: anxiety, *headache,* dizziness, **seizures,** somnolence, vertigo.

CV: *MI, sudden cardiac death, ventricular arrhythmia, cerebrovascular hemorrhage, transient ischemic attack,* hypotension, *flushing.*
EENT: diplopia, temporary vision loss, decreased vision, ocular redness or bloodshot appearance, increased intraocular pressure, retinal vascular disease, retinal bleeding, vitreous detachment or traction, perimacular edema, abnormal vision (photophobia, color tinged vision, blurred vision), ocular burning, ocular swelling or pressure.
GI: dyspepsia, diarrhea.
GU: hematuria, prolonged erection, priapism, UTI.
Musculoskeletal: arthralgia, back pain.
Respiratory: respiratory tract infection.
Skin: rash.
Other: flulike syndrome.

Interactions

Drug-drug. *Beta blockers, loop and potassium-sparing diuretics:* Increases level of major metabolite of sildenafil. Significance of this interaction isn't known.
CYP 3A4 inducers, rifampin: Reduces sildenafil level. Monitor drug effect.
Hepatic isoenzyme inhibitors (such as cimetidine, erythromycin, itraconazole, ketoconazole): May reduce clearance of sildenafil. Avoid using together.
Isosorbide, nitroglycerin, other nitrates: May cause severe hypotension. Use of nitrates in any form with sildenafil is contraindicated.
Protease inhibitors, delavirdine: Increases sildenafil level and may result in an increase in sildenafil-associated adverse events, including hypotension, visual changes, and priapism. Don't exceed 25 mg in a 48-hour period.
Drug-food. *High-fat meals:* Reduces rate of absorption and decreases peak levels. Separate administration time from meals.
Grapefruit: May increase levels and delay absorption. Advise patient to avoid the use of grapefruit products.

Effects on lab test results

None reported.

Pharmacokinetics

Absorption: Rapid. Absolute bioavailability is 40%.
Distribution: Extensively into body tissues. About 96% bound to proteins.

Metabolism: Primarily metabolized in the liver to an active metabolite with properties similar to those of parent drug.
Excretion: About 80% is excreted in feces and 13% in urine. *Half-life:* 4 hours.

Route	Onset	Peak	Duration
P.O.	Unknown	30 min-2 hr	4 hr

Action

Chemical effect: Enhances the effect of nitric oxide (NO) by inhibiting phosphodiesterase type 5 (PDE5). When sexual stimulation causes local release of NO, inhibition of PDE5 by sildenafil causes increased levels of cGMP in the corpus cavernosum, resulting in smooth muscle relaxation and inflow of blood to the corpus cavernosum.
Therapeutic effect: Patient achieves an erection.

Available forms

Tablets: 25 mg, 50 mg, 100 mg

NURSING PROCESS

☝ Assessment
• Discuss patient's history of erectile dysfunction to establish need for drug versus other therapies.
• Assess patient for CV risk factors because serious events have been reported with drug use, and report risk factors to prescriber.
• Evaluate patient's and family's knowledge of drug therapy.

⊞ Nursing diagnoses
• Sexual dysfunction related to patient's underlying condition
• Ineffective tissue perfusion (cardiopulmonary) related to drug-induced effects on blood pressure and cardiac output
• Deficient knowledge related to drug therapy

▶ Planning and implementation
⊛ **ALERT:** Drug's systemic vasodilatory properties cause transient decreases in supine blood pressure and cardiac output (about 2 hours after ingestion). Together with the potential cardiac risk of sexual activity, the risk for patients with underlying CV disease is increased.
⊛ **ALERT:** Serious CV events, including MI, sudden cardiac death, ventricular arrhythmia,

cerebrovascular hemorrhage, transient ischemic attack, and hypertension, have occurred in patients during or shortly after sexual activity.
Patient teaching
• Advise patient that drug is contraindicated with regular or intermittent use of nitrates.
• Warn patient about cardiac risk with sexual activity, especially if he has CV risk factors. If patient has symptoms such as angina pectoris, dizziness, or nausea at the start of sexual activity, instruct him to notify prescriber and refrain from further sexual activity.
• Warn patient that erections lasting more than 4 hours and priapism (painful erections more than 6 hours) can occur and should be reported immediately. If priapism isn't treated immediately, penile tissue damage and permanent loss of potency may result.
• Inform patient that drug doesn't protect against sexually transmitted diseases and that protective measures, such as condoms, should be used.
• Instruct patient to take drug 30 minutes to 4 hours before sexual activity; maximum benefit can be expected less than 2 hours after ingesting drug.
• Advise patient that drug is most rapidly absorbed if taken on an empty stomach.
• Inform patient to avoid potentially hazardous activities that rely on color discrimination because blue/green discrimination may be impaired.
• Instruct patient to notify prescriber if visual changes occur.
• Advise patient that drug is effective only in the presence of sexual stimulation.
• Tell patient to take drug only as prescribed.
• Advise patient taking HIV drugs that there is an increased risk of sildenafil-associated adverse events, including hypotension, visual changes, and priapism, and he should promptly report any symptoms to his prescriber. Tell him not to exceed 25 mg of sildenafil in a 48-hour period.

☑ Evaluation
• Sexual activity improves with drug therapy.
• Patient doesn't experience adverse CV events.
• Patient and family state understanding of drug therapy.

Reactions may be *common*, uncommon, *life-threatening*, or COMMON AND LIFE-THREATENING.

simethicone

(sigh-METH-ih-kohn)

Extra Strength Gas-X†, Gas Relief†, Gas-X†, Maximum Strength Gas Relief†, Maximum Strength Phazyme†, Mylanta Gas†, Mylanta Gas Maximum Strength†, Mylanta Gas Regular Strength†, Mylicon-80†, Mylicon-125†, Ovol ♦, Ovol-40 ♦, Ovol-80 ♦, Phazyme†, Phazyme 95†, Phazyme 125†

Pharmacologic class: dispersant
Therapeutic class: antiflatulent
Pregnancy risk category: C

Indications and dosages

▶ **Flatulence, functional gastric bloating.**
Tablets. Adults and children older than age 12:
40 to 125 mg P.O. (tablets) q.i.d. after each meal and h.s. Or, 125 mg P.O. (capsules) q.i.d. after each meal and h.s. Or, 40 to 80 mg P.O. (drops) q.i.d. after each meal and h.s., up to maximum of 500 mg daily.
Children ages 2 to 12: 40 mg P.O. (drops) q.i.d. after each meal and h.s., up to maximum of 240 mg daily.
Children younger than age 2: 20 mg P.O. (drops) q.i.d. after each meal and h.s.

Contraindications and precautions

• Contraindicated in patients hypersensitive to drug.
⚞ **Lifespan:** In pregnant and breast-feeding women, use cautiously.

Adverse reactions

GI: excessive belching or flatus.

Interactions

None significant.

Effects on lab test results

None reported.

Pharmacokinetics

Absorption: None.
Distribution: None.
Metabolism: None.
Excretion: In feces. *Half-life:* Unknown.

Route	Onset	Peak	Duration
P.O.	Immediate	Immediate	Unknown

Action

Chemical effect: By its defoaming action, disperses or prevents formation of mucus-surrounded gas pockets in GI tract.
Therapeutic effect: Relieves gas.

Available forms

Capsules: 125 mg
Drops: 40 mg/0.6 ml†
Tablets: 40 mg†, 50 mg†, 60 mg†, 80 mg†, 95 mg†, 125 mg†

NURSING PROCESS

⚚ Assessment
• Assess patient's condition before therapy and regularly thereafter.
• Be alert for adverse GI reactions.
• Evaluate patient's and family's knowledge of drug therapy.

⊕ Nursing diagnoses
• Acute pain related to gas in GI tract
• Deficient knowledge related to drug therapy

▶ Planning and implementation
• Make sure patient chews tablet before swallowing.
⚑ **ALERT:** Don't confuse simethicone with cimetidine.
Patient teaching
• Advise patient that drug doesn't prevent formation of gas.
• Encourage patient to change position frequently and ambulate to aid in passing flatus.

☑ Evaluation
• Patient's gas pain is relieved.
• Patient and family state understanding of drug therapy.

simvastatin (synvinolin)

(sim-vuh-STAT-in)
Lipex ◇, Zocor

Pharmacologic class: HMG-CoA reductase inhibitor
Therapeutic class: antilipemic, cholesterol-lowering drug
Pregnancy risk category: X

Indications and dosages

▶ **Reductions in risk of coronary artery disease mortality and CV events in patients at high risk of coronary events.** *Adults:* Initially, 20 mg P.O. daily in evening. Dosage adjusted q 4 weeks based on patient tolerance and response. Maximum, 80 mg daily.

▶ **To reduce total and LDL cholesterol in patients with homozygous familial hypercholesterolemia.** *Adults:* 40 mg daily in evening; or 80 mg daily given in three divided doses of 20 mg in morning, 20 mg in afternoon, and 40 mg in evening.

▶ **Heterozygous familial hypercholesterolemia.** *Children ages 10 to 17:* 10 mg P.O. once daily in the evening. Maximum, 40 mg daily.

▧ **Adjust-a-dose:** For patients taking cyclosporine, initially give 5 mg P.O. daily; don't exceed 10 mg daily. For patients taking fibrates or niacin, maximum is 10 mg P.O. daily. For patients taking amiodarone or verapamil, maximum is 20 mg P.O. daily. For patients with severe renal insufficiency, initially give 5 mg P.O. daily.

Contraindications and precautions

• Contraindicated in patients hypersensitive to drug and in those with active liver disease or conditions that have unexplained persistent elevations of transaminase levels.

• Use cautiously in patients who consume substantial quantities of alcohol or have history of liver disease.

⚹ **Lifespan:** In pregnant and breast-feeding women and in women of childbearing potential, drug is contraindicated. In children, safety of drug hasn't been established.

Adverse reactions

CNS: headache, asthenia.
GI: abdominal pain, constipation, diarrhea, dyspepsia, flatulence, nausea.
Respiratory: upper respiratory tract infection.

Interactions

Drug-drug. *Amiodarone, verapamil:* Increases risk of myopathy and rhabdomyolysis. Don't exceed 20 mg simvastatin daily.
Clarithromycin, erythromycin, HIV protease inhibitors, nefazodone: Increases risk of myopathy and rhabdomyolysis. Avoid using together or suspend therapy during treatment with clar-

ithromycin, erythromycin, itraconazole, and ketoconazole.
Cyclosporine, fibrates, niacin: Increases risk of myopathy and rhabdomyolysis. Monitor patient closely if use together can't be avoided. Don't exceed 10 mg simvastatin daily.
Digoxin: Digoxin level may elevate slightly. Closely monitor digoxin level at the start of simvastatin therapy.
Fluconazole, itraconazole, ketoconazole: May increase levels and adverse effects of simvastatin. Avoid this combination. If they must be given together, reduce dose of simvastatin.
Hepatotoxic drugs: Increases risk for hepatotoxicity. Avoid using together.
Warfarin: Enhanced anticoagulant effect. Monitor PT and INR at the start of therapy and during dose adjustment.
Drug-herb. *Red yeast rice:* Contains similar components to those of statin drugs, increasing the risk of adverse events or toxicity. Discourage using together.
Drug-food. *Grapefruit juice:* Increases drug level, increasing risk of adverse effects, including myopathy and rhabdomyolysis. Give with liquids other than grapefruit juice.
Drug-lifestyle. *Alcohol use:* May increase the risk of hepatotoxicity. Discourage using together.

Effects on lab test results

• May increase liver enzyme and CK levels.

Pharmacokinetics

Absorption: Readily absorbed; however, extensive hepatic extraction limits availability of active inhibitors to 5% of dose or less. Individual absorption varies considerably.
Distribution: Parent drug and active metabolites are more than 95% bound to proteins.
Metabolism: Hydrolysis occurs in plasma; at least three major metabolites have been identified.
Excretion: Excreted primarily in bile. *Half-life:* 3 hours.

Route	Onset	Peak	Duration
P.O.	Unknown	1½-2½ hr	Unknown

Action

Chemical effect: Inhibits HMG-CoA reductase. This enzyme is early (and rate-limiting) step in synthetic pathway of cholesterol.

Therapeutic effect: Lowers LDL and total cholesterol levels.

Available forms

Tablets: 5 mg, 10 mg, 20 mg, 40 mg, 80 mg

NURSING PROCESS

☞ Assessment

• Obtain history of patient's LDL and total cholesterol levels before therapy, and reassess regularly thereafter.
• Obtain liver function test results at start of therapy and periodically thereafter. If enzyme level elevations persist, a liver biopsy may be performed.
• Be alert for adverse reactions and drug interactions.
• Assess patient's dietary fat intake.
• Evaluate patient's and family's knowledge of drug therapy.

⊕ Nursing diagnoses

• Risk for injury related to presence of elevated cholesterol levels
• Constipation related to drug-induced adverse GI reactions
• Deficient knowledge related to drug therapy

▶ Planning and implementation

• Drug therapy starts only after diet and other nondrug therapies have proven ineffective. Make sure patient follows a standard low-cholesterol diet during therapy.
• Give drug with evening meal for enhanced effectiveness.
• If cholesterol level falls below target range, dosage may be reduced.
• Make sure patient follows an appropriate diet.
⊛ **ALERT:** Don't confuse Zocor with Cozaar.
Patient teaching
• Tell patient to take drug with evening meal because absorption and cholesterol biosynthesis are enhanced.
• Teach patient dietary management of lipids (restricting total fat and cholesterol intake) and measures to control other cardiac disease risk factors. If appropriate, suggest weight control, exercise, and smoking cessation programs.
• Tell patient to inform prescriber about adverse reactions, particularly muscle aches and pains.

⊛ **ALERT:** Inform woman that drug is contraindicated during pregnancy. Advise her to notify prescriber immediately if pregnancy occurs.

☑ Evaluation

• Patient's LDL and total cholesterol levels are within normal limits.
• Patient regains and maintains normal bowel pattern throughout therapy.
• Patient and family state understanding of drug therapy.

sirolimus
(sir-AH-lih-mus)
Rapamune

Pharmacologic class: macrocyclic lactone
Therapeutic class: immunosuppressant
Pregnancy risk category: C

Indications and dosages

▶ **Prophylaxis of organ rejection in patients receiving renal transplants.** *Adults and children age 13 and older who weigh 40 kg (88 lb) or more:* Initially, 6 mg P.O. as a one-time loading dose as soon as possible after transplantation; then maintenance dose of 2 mg P.O. once daily. Give 4 hours after cyclosporine and corticosteroids.
Children age 13 and older who weigh less than 40 kg: Initially, 3 mg/m² P.O. as a one-time loading dose after transplantation; then maintenance dose of 1 mg/m² P.O. once daily. Maximum daily dose is 40 mg. If a daily dose exceeds 40 mg because of loading dose, give the loading dose over 2 days. Monitor trough levels at least 3 to 4 days after loading dose.
Ⓢ **Adjust-a-dose:** For patients with hepatic impairment, reduce maintenance dose by 33%. Adjusting loading dose isn't needed.

Contraindications and precautions

• Contraindicated in patients hypersensitive to drug or its derivatives or components.
• Use cautiously in patients with hyperlipidemia or impaired liver or renal function.
• The safety and effectiveness of sirolimus haven't been established in liver and lung transplant patients; therefore, such use isn't recommended.

⚕ **Lifespan:** In breast-feeding women, drug is contraindicated.

Adverse reactions

CNS: *headache, insomnia, tremor, anxiety, depression, asthenia,* malaise, syncope, confusion, dizziness, emotional lability, hypertonia, hypesthesia, hypotonia, neuropathy, paresthesia, somnolence, *fever, pain.*

CV: facial edema, *hypertension,* **heart failure,** atrial fibrillation, tachycardia, hypotension, *peripheral edema, chest pain, edema,* **hemorrhage,** palpitations, peripheral vascular disorder, thrombophlebitis, **thrombosis,** vasodilation.

EENT: *pharyngitis,* epistaxis, rhinitis, sinusitis, abnormal vision, cataracts, conjunctivitis, deafness, ear pain, otitis media, tinnitus.

GI: *diarrhea, nausea, vomiting, constipation, abdominal pain, dyspepsia,* enlarged abdomen, hernia, ascites, **peritonitis,** anorexia, dysphagia, eructation, esophagitis, flatulence, gastritis, gastroenteritis, gingivitis, gum hyperplasia, ileus, mouth ulcerations, oral candidiasis, stomatitis.

GU: dysuria, hematuria, albuminuria, **kidney tubular necrosis, UTI,** pelvic pain, glycosuria, bladder pain, hydronephrosis, impotence, kidney pain, nocturia, oliguria, pyuria, scrotal edema, testis disorder, **toxic nephropathy,** urinary frequency, urinary incontinence, urine retention.

Hematologic: *anemia,* THROMBOCYTOPENIA, **leukopenia, thrombotic thrombocytopenic purpura,** leukocytosis, polycythemia, lymphadenopathy.

Hepatic: *hepatic artery thrombosis.*

Metabolic: *hypercholesteremia, hyperlipidemia, hypokalemia, weight gain, hypophosphatemia,* HYPERKALEMIA, hypervolemia, Cushing's syndrome, **diabetes mellitus, acidosis,** dehydration, hypercalcemia, hyperglycemia, hyperphosphatemia, hypocalcemia, **hypoglycemia,** hypomagnesemia, hyponatremia, weight loss.

Musculoskeletal: *back pain, arthralgia,* myalgia, arthrosis, bone necrosis, leg cramps, osteoporosis, tetany.

Respiratory: *dyspnea, cough, atelectasis, upper respiratory tract infection,* **asthma,** bronchitis, **hypoxia, lung edema,** pleural effusion, pneumonia.

Skin: *rash, acne,* hirsutism, fungal dermatitis, pruritus, skin hypertrophy, skin ulcer, ecchymoses, sweating.

Other: abscess; cellulitis; chills; flulike syndrome; infection; **sepsis;** abnormal healing.

Interactions

Drug-drug. *Aminoglycosides, amphotericin, other nephrotoxic drugs:* Increases risk of nephrotoxicity. Use cautiously.

Bromocriptine, cimetidine, clarithromycin, clotrimazole, danazol, erythromycin, fluconazole, indinavir, itraconazole, metoclopramide, nicardipine, ritonavir, verapamil, other drugs that inhibit CYP 3A4: May decrease sirolimus metabolism, thereby increasing sirolimus level. Monitor patient for loss of therapeutic effect.

Carbamazepine, phenobarbital, phenytoin, rifabutin, rifapentine, other drugs that induce CYP 3A4: May increase sirolimus metabolism, thereby decreasing sirolimus level. Monitor patient closely.

Cyclosporine: Inhibits sirolimus metabolism. Sirolimus levels will decrease when cyclosporine is stopped. Carefully increase sirolimus dose during cyclosporine taper to eventually be about 4-fold higher.

Diltiazem: Increases sirolimus level. Monitor and reduce dosage of sirolimus as needed.

HMG-CoA reductase inhibitors or fibrates: Increases risk of rhabdomyolysis with the combination of sirolimus and cyclosporine. Monitor patient closely.

Ketoconazole: Increases rate and extent of sirolimus absorption. Avoid using together.

Live virus vaccines: Reduces effectiveness of vaccines. Avoid using together.

Rifampin: Decreases sirolimus level. Consider alternatives to rifampin.

Tacrolimus: May increase risk of hepatic artery thrombosis. Don't use together.

Drug-food. *Grapefruit juice:* Decreases metabolism of sirolimus. Avoid using together.

Drug-lifestyle. *Sun exposure:* Increases risk of skin cancer. Take precautions.

Effects on lab test results

• May increase BUN, creatinine, liver enzyme, cholesterol, and lipid levels. May decrease sodium and magnesium levels. May increase or decrease phosphate, potassium, glucose, and calcium levels.

• May increase RBC count. May decrease hemoglobin, hematocrit, and platelet count. May increase or decrease WBC count.

Pharmacokinetics

Absorption: Rapid, with mean peak levels occurring in about 1 to 3 hours. Oral bioavailability is about 14%. Food decreases peak levels and increases time to peak level.

Distribution: Extensively partitioned into formed blood elements. Drug is extensively bound to proteins (about 92%).

Metabolism: Extensively metabolized by the mixed function oxidase system, primarily CYP 3A4. Seven major metabolites have been identified in whole blood.

Excretion: 91% in feces and in 2.2% urine.

Half-life: About 62 hours.

Route	Onset	Peak	Duration
P.O.	Unknown	1-3 hr	Unknown

Action

Chemical effect: An immunosuppressant that inhibits T-lymphocyte activation and proliferation that occur in response to antigenic and cytokine stimulation. Also inhibits antibody formation.

Therapeutic effect: Immunosuppression in patients receiving renal transplants.

Available forms

Oral solution: 1 mg/ml
Tablets: 1 mg

NURSING PROCESS

⏣ Assessment

• Obtain history of patient's organ transplantation before therapy.

• Monitor patient's liver and renal function and triglycerides before therapy.

• Monitor sirolimus levels in children who weigh less than 40 kg (88 lb), patients with hepatic impairment, patients taking drugs that induce or inhibit CYP 3A4, and patients whose cyclosporine dosage is markedly reduced or stopped.

• Monitor patient for infection and development of lymphoma, which may result from immunosuppression.

• Watch for development of rhabdomyolysis if patient is receiving sirolimus and cyclosporine is started as an HMG-CoA reductase inhibitor.

• Evaluate patient's and family's knowledge of drug therapy.

⊞ Nursing diagnoses

• Risk for injury related to potential for organ rejection

• Ineffective protection related to drug-induced immunosuppression

• Deficient knowledge related to drug therapy

⊵ Planning and implementation

• Give drug consistently with or without food.

⚕ **ALERT:** In patients with mild-to-moderate hepatic impairment, reduce maintenance dose by about one-third. Loading dose doesn't need to be reduced.

• Dilute oral solution before giving. After dilution, use it immediately.

• When diluting drug, empty correct amount into glass or plastic container filled with at least 2 ounces (60 ml) of water or orange juice. Don't use grapefruit juice or any other liquid. Stir vigorously and have patient drink immediately. Refill container with at least 4 ounces (120 ml) of water or orange juice, stir again, and have patient drink all contents.

• After opening bottle, use contents within 1 month. If needed, bottles and pouches may be stored at room temperature (up to 77° F [25° C]) for several days. Drug can be kept in oral dosing syringe for 24 hours at room temperature or refrigerated at 36° to 46° F (2° to 8° C).

• A slight haze may develop during refrigeration, but this won't affect quality of drug. If haze develops, bring drug to room temperature and shake gently until haze disappears.

• Use drug in a regimen with cyclosporine and corticosteroids. This drug should be taken 4 hours after cyclosporine dose.

• Two to four months following transplantation, patients with low to moderate risk of graft rejection should be tapered off cyclosporine over 4 to 8 weeks. During the taper, adjust sirolimus dose q 1 to 2 weeks to obtain level between 12 to 24 ng/ml. Dosage adjustments should also be based on condition, tissue biopsies, and laboratory findings.

• After transplantation, give antimicrobials for 1 year as directed to prevent *Pneumocystis carinii* pneumonia and for 3 months as directed to prevent CMV infection.

• If patient has hyperlipidemia, start additional interventions, such as diet, exercise, and lipid-lowering drugs. Use with lipid-lowering drugs is common.

• Cyclosporine withdrawal in patients with high-risk of graft rejection isn't recommended. This includes patients with Banff grade III acute rejection or vascular rejection before cyclosporine withdrawal, those who are dialysis-dependent, or with creatinine greater than 4.5 mg/dl, black patients, re-transplants, multi-organ transplants, patients with high panel of reactive antibodies.

Patient teaching
* Show patient how to properly store, dilute, and take drug.
* Tell patient to take drug consistently with or without food to minimize absorption variability.
* Advise patient to take drug 4 hours after taking cyclosporine.
* Tell patient to wash area with soap and water if solution touches skin or mucous membranes; tell him to rinse eyes with plain water if solution gets in eyes.
* Inform woman of childbearing age of risks during pregnancy. Tell her to use effective contraception before, during, and for 12 weeks after stopping drug.
* Advise patient to take precautions against sun exposure.

☑ Evaluation
* Patient doesn't experience organ rejection.
* Patient is free from infection and serious bleeding episodes throughout drug therapy.
* Patient and family state understanding of drug therapy.

sodium bicarbonate
(SOH-dee-um bigh-KAR-buh-nayt)
Arm and Hammer Pure Baking Soda, Bell/ans, Citrocarbonate, Soda Mint

Pharmacologic class: alkalinizer
Therapeutic class: systemic and urine alkalinizer, systemic hydrogen ion buffer, oral antacid
Pregnancy risk category: C

Indications and dosages

▶ **Adjunct to advanced cardiovascular life support during cardiopulmonary resuscitation.** *Adults:* Although no longer routinely recommended, inject either 300 to 500 ml of a 5% solution or 200 to 300 mEq of a 7.5% or 8.4% solution as rapidly as possible. Base further doses on subsequent blood gas values. Alternatively, 1 mEq/kg dose, then repeat 0.5 mEq/kg q 10 minutes.
Children age 2 and younger: 1 mEq/kg I.V. or intraosseous injection of a 4.2 % to 8.4% solu-

tion. Give slowly. Don't exceed daily dose of 8 Eq/kg.
▶ **Severe metabolic acidosis.** *Adults:* Dose depends on blood carbon dioxide content, pH, and patient's condition. Generally, give 90 to 180 mEq/L I.V. during first hour, then adjust, p.r.n.
▶ **Less urgent metabolic acidosis.** *Adults and children age 12 and older:* 2 to 5 mEq/kg as a 4- to 8-hour I.V. infusion.
▶ **Urine alkalization.** *Adults:* 48 mEq (4 g) P.O. initially, then 12 to 24 mEq (1 to 2 g) q 4 hours. May need doses of 30 to 48 mEq (2.5 to 4 g) q 4 hours, up to 192 mEq (16g) daily.
Children: 1 to 10 mEq (84 to 840 mg)/kg P.O. daily.
▶ **Antacid.** *Adults:* 300 mg to 2 g P.O. one to four times daily.

▼ I.V. administration
* Drug is usually given by I.V. infusion. When immediate treatment is needed, drug may be given by direct, rapid I.V. injection. However, in neonates and children younger than age 2, slow I.V. administration is preferred to avoid hypernatremia, decreased CSF pressure, and intracranial hemorrhage.
* **⑤ ALERT:** Sodium bicarbonate inactivates such catecholamines as norepinephrine and dopamine and forms precipitate with calcium. Don't mix sodium bicarbonate with I.V. solutions of these drugs, and flush I.V. line adequately.

Contraindications and precautions
* Contraindicated in patients with metabolic or respiratory alkalosis; in patients who are losing chlorides from vomiting or continuous GI suction; in patients receiving diuretics known to produce hypochloremic alkalosis; and in patients with hypocalcemia in which alkalosis may produce tetany, hypertension, seizures, or heart failure. Oral sodium bicarbonate is contraindicated in patients with acute ingestion of strong mineral acids.
* Use cautiously in patients with heart failure or other edematous or sodium-retaining conditions or renal insufficiency.
* ⚘ **Lifespan:** In pregnant and breast-feeding women, use cautiously.

Adverse reactions
GI: gastric distention, belching, flatulence.

Metabolic: *metabolic alkalosis,* hypernatremia, hypokalemia, hyperosmolarity (with overdose).
Other: pain and irritation at injection site.

Interactions

Drug-drug. *Anorexigenics, flecainide, mecamylamine, quinidine, sympathomimetics:* Increased urine alkalinization causes decreased renal clearance and increased pharmacologic or toxic effects. Monitor for toxicity.
Chlorpropamide, lithium, methotrexate, salicylates, tetracycline: Urine alkalinization causes increased renal clearance of these drugs, possibly resulting in decreased pharmacologic effects. Monitor for lack of effect.

Effects on lab test results

• May increase sodium and lactate levels. May decrease potassium level.

Pharmacokinetics

Absorption: Well absorbed.
Distribution: Bicarbonate is confined to systemic circulation.
Metabolism: None.
Excretion: Bicarbonate is filtered and reabsorbed by kidneys; less than 1% of filtered bicarbonate is excreted. *Half-life:* Unknown.

Route	Onset	Peak	Duration
P.O.	Unknown	Unknown	Unknown
I.V.	Immediate	Immediate	Unknown

Action

Chemical effect: Restores body's buffering capacity and neutralizes excess acid.
Therapeutic effect: Restores normal acid-base balance and relieves acid indigestion.

Available forms

Injection: 4% (2.4 mEq/5 ml), 4.2% (5 mEq/10 ml), 5% (297.5 mEq/500 ml), 7.5% (8.92 mEq/10 ml and 44.6 mEq/50 ml), 8.4% (10 mEq/10 ml and 50 mEq/50 ml)
Tablets†: 300 mg, 325 mg, 520 mg, 600 mg, 650 mg

NURSING PROCESS

⏰ Assessment

• Assess patient's condition before therapy and regularly thereafter.

• To avoid risk of alkalosis, obtain blood pH, Pao_2, $Paco_2$, and electrolyte levels.
• If sodium bicarbonate is being used to produce alkaline urine, monitor urine pH (should be greater than 7) q 4 to 6 hours.
• Be alert for adverse reactions and drug interactions.
• Evaluate patient's and family's knowledge of drug therapy.

🔄 Nursing diagnoses
• Ineffective health maintenance related to underlying condition
• Risk for injury related to drug-induced adverse reactions
• Deficient knowledge related to drug therapy

⟫ Planning and implementation
• Drug isn't routinely recommended for use in cardiac arrest because it may produce paradoxical acidosis from CO_2 production. It shouldn't be routinely given during early stages of resuscitation unless acidosis is clearly present.
• Drug may be used after such interventions as defibrillation, cardiac compression, or administration of first-line drugs.
• Give drug with water, not milk. Drug may cause hypercalcemia, alkalosis, or possibly renal calculi.
• Inform prescriber of laboratory results.
Patient teaching
• Tell patient not to take with milk.
• Discourage use as antacid. Offer nonabsorbable alternate antacid if it is to be used repeatedly.

✓ Evaluation
• Patient regains normal acid-base balance.
• Patient doesn't experience injury from drug-induced adverse reactions.
• Patient and family state understanding of drug therapy.

sodium chloride
(SOH-dee-um KLOR-ighd)

Pharmacologic class: electrolyte
Therapeutic class: sodium and chloride replacement
Pregnancy risk category: C

Indications and dosages

▶ **Fluid and electrolyte replacement in hyponatremia caused by severe electrolyte loss, severe salt depletion.** *Adults:* Dosage is highly individualized. The 3% and 5% solutions are used only with frequent electrolyte determination and given only by slow I.V. With half-normal saline solution: 3% to 8% of body weight, according to deficiencies, over 18 to 24 hours. With normal saline solution: 2% to 6% of body weight, according to deficiencies, over 18 to 24 hours.

▼ I.V. administration

• Infuse 3% and 5% solutions very slowly and cautiously to avoid pulmonary edema. Use only for critical situations, and observe patient continually.

Contraindications and precautions

• Contraindicated in patients with conditions in which giving sodium and chloride is detrimental. The 3% and 5% saline solution injections are contraindicated in patients with increased, normal, or only slightly decreased electrolyte levels.
• Use cautiously in postoperative patients and patients with heart failure, circulatory insufficiency, renal dysfunction, or hypoproteinemia.
※ **Lifespan:** In pregnant and breast-feeding women and in geriatric patients, use cautiously.

Adverse reactions

CV: *aggravation of heart failure,* edema if given too rapidly or in excess, thrombophlebitis.
Metabolic: hypernatremia, *aggravation of existing metabolic acidosis* with excessive infusion, electrolyte disturbances, hypokalemia.
Respiratory: *pulmonary edema* if given too rapidly or in excess.
Skin: local tenderness, abscess, tissue necrosis at injection site.

Interactions

None significant.

Effects on lab test results

• May increase sodium level. May decrease potassium level.

Pharmacokinetics

Absorption: Absorbed readily.
Distribution: Distributed widely in body.

Metabolism: None significant.
Excretion: Primarily in urine; some excreted in sweat, tears, and saliva. *Half-life:* Unknown.

Route	Onset	Peak	Duration
P.O.	Unknown	Unknown	Unknown
I.V.	Immediate	Immediate	Unknown

Action

Chemical effect: Replaces and maintains sodium and chloride levels.
Therapeutic effect: Restores normal sodium and chloride levels.

Available forms

Injection: *Half-normal saline solution:* 500 ml, 1,000 ml
Normal saline solution: 50 ml, 100 ml, 150 ml, 250 ml, 500 ml, 1,000 ml
3% saline solution: 500 ml
5% saline solution: 500 ml
14.6% saline solution: 20 ml, 40 ml, 200 ml
23.4% saline solution: 30 ml, 50 ml, 200 ml
Tablets (enteric-coated): 650 mg, 1 g, 2.25 g
Tablets (slow-release): 600 mg

NURSING PROCESS

🔍 Assessment
• Obtain history of patient's sodium and chloride levels before therapy, and reassess regularly thereafter.
• Monitor other electrolyte levels.
• Assess patient's fluid status.
• Be alert for adverse reactions.
• Evaluate patient's and family's knowledge of drug therapy.

🔲 Nursing diagnoses
• Imbalanced nutrition: less than body requirements related to subnormal levels of sodium and chloride
• Excess fluid volume related to saline solution's water-drawing power
• Deficient knowledge related to drug therapy

▶ Planning and implementation
• Give tablet with glass of water.
⊛ **ALERT:** Don't confuse concentrates (14.6% and 23.4%) available to add to parenteral nutrient solutions with normal saline solution injection, and never give without diluting. Read label carefully.

Patient teaching
- Tell patient to report adverse reactions promptly.

☑ Evaluation
- Patient's sodium and chloride levels are normal.
- Patient doesn't exhibit signs and symptoms of fluid retention.
- Patient and family state understanding of drug therapy.

sodium ferric gluconate complex
(SOH-dee-um FEH-rik GLOO-kuh-nayt KOM-pleks)
Ferrlecit

Pharmacologic class: macromolecular iron complex
Therapeutic class: hematinic
Pregnancy risk category: B

Indications and dosages
▶ **Treatment of iron deficiency anemia in patients undergoing long-term hemodialysis and receiving supplemental erythropoietin therapy.** *Adults:* Before starting therapeutic doses, give a test dose of 2 ml sodium ferric gluconate complex (25 mg elemental iron) diluted in 50 ml normal saline solution I.V. over 1 hour. If test dose is tolerated, give therapeutic dose of 10 ml (125 mg elemental iron) diluted in 100 ml normal saline solution I.V. over 1 hour. Most patients need a minimum cumulative dose of 1 g elemental iron given at more than eight sequential dialysis treatments to achieve a favorable hemoglobin or hematocrit response.

▼ I.V. administration
- Dilute test dose of sodium ferric gluconate complex in 50 ml normal saline solution and give over 1 hour. Dilute therapeutic doses of drug in 100 ml normal saline solution and give over 1 hour.
- Don't mix sodium ferric gluconate complex with other drugs or add to parenteral nutrition solutions for I.V. infusion. Use immediately after dilution in normal saline solution.
- ⑤ **ALERT:** Patient may develop profound hypotension with flushing, light-headedness, malaise, fatigue, weakness, or severe chest, back, flank, or groin pain after rapid I.V. administra-

tion of iron. These reactions don't indicate hypersensitivity and may result from too-rapid administration of drug. Don't exceed 2.1 mg/minute. Monitor patient closely during infusion.

Contraindications and precautions
- Contraindicated in patients hypersensitive to drug or its components (such as benzyl alcohol) and in patients with anemias not linked to iron deficiency. Don't give to patients with iron overload.
- ⚖ **Lifespan:** In breast-feeding women and geriatric patients, use cautiously. In children, safety of drug hasn't been established.

Adverse reactions
CNS: asthenia, headache, fatigue, malaise, dizziness, paresthesia, agitation, insomnia, somnolence, syncope, pain, fever.
CV: hypotension, hypertension, tachycardia, *bradycardia,* angina, chest pain, *MI,* edema, flushing.
EENT: conjunctivitis, abnormal vision, rhinitis.
GI: nausea, vomiting, diarrhea, rectal disorder, dyspepsia, eructation, flatulence, melena, abdominal pain.
GU: UTI.
Hematologic: abnormal erythrocytes, anemia, lymphadenopathy.
Metabolic: *hyperkalemia, hypoglycemia,* hypokalemia, hypervolemia.
Musculoskeletal: myalgia, arthralgia, back pain, arm pain, cramps.
Respiratory: dyspnea, coughing, upper respiratory tract infections, pneumonia, *pulmonary edema.*
Skin: pruritus, increased sweating, rash.
Other: infection, injection site reaction, rigors, chills, flulike syndrome, *sepsis, carcinoma, hypersensitivity reactions.*

Interactions
None reported.

Effects on lab test results
- May decrease glucose level. May increase or decrease potassium level.
- May decrease hemoglobin and hematocrit.

Pharmacokinetics
Absorption: Administered I.V.
Distribution: Unknown.

Metabolism: Unknown.
Excretion: Unknown. *Half-life:* Unknown.

Route	Onset	Peak	Duration
I.V.	Unknown	Unknown	Unknown

Action

Chemical effect: Drug restores total body iron content, which is critical for normal hemoglobin synthesis and oxygen transport.
Therapeutic effect: Restores total body iron content.

Available forms

Injection: 62.5 mg elemental iron (12.5 mg/ml) in 5-ml ampules

NURSING PROCESS

⚖ Assessment
• Obtain history of patient's underlying condition before therapy, and reassess regularly thereafter.
• Find out about other sources of iron patient may be taking, such as nonprescription iron preparations and iron-containing multiple vitamins with minerals.
• Monitor hematocrit and hemoglobin, ferritin, and iron saturation levels during therapy.
• Evaluate patient's and family's knowledge of drug therapy.

🔄 Nursing diagnoses
• Risk for injury related to drug-induced adverse reactions
• Activity intolerance related to underlying condition
• Deficient knowledge related to drug therapy

🔲 Planning and implementation
• Dose is expressed in mg of elemental iron.
• Don't give drug to patients with iron overload, which commonly occurs in hemoglobinopathies and other refractory anemias.
• **ALERT:** Potentially life-threatening hypersensitivity reactions may occur during infusion (characterized by CV collapse, cardiac arrest, bronchospasm, oral or pharyngeal edema, dyspnea, angioedema, urticaria, or pruritus sometimes linked with pain and muscle spasm of chest or back). Have adequate supportive measures readily available. Monitor patient closely during infusion.

• Some adverse reactions in hemodialysis patients may be related to dialysis itself or to chronic renal impairment.
Patient teaching
• Abdominal pain, diarrhea, vomiting, drowsiness, or hyperventilation may indicate iron poisoning. Advise patient to report any of these symptoms immediately.

☑ Evaluation
• Patient doesn't experience injury as a result of drug-induced adverse reactions.
• Patient experiences improved activity tolerance.
• Patient and family state understanding of drug therapy.

sodium lactate
(SOH-dee-um LAK-tayt)

Pharmacologic class: alkalinizer
Therapeutic class: systemic alkalizer
Pregnancy risk category: NR

Indications and dosages

▶ **Urine alkalinization.** *Adults:* 30 ml of 1/6 molar solution per kg of body weight P.O. given in divided doses over 24 hours.
▶ **Metabolic acidosis.** *Adults:* 1/6 molar injection (167 mEq lactate/L) I.V.; dose depends on degree of bicarbonate deficit.

▽ I.V. administration

• Add drug to other I.V. solutions or give as isotonic 1/6 molar solution. Drug is compatible with most common I.V. solutions.
• Don't mix with sodium bicarbonate because drugs are physically incompatible.

Contraindications and precautions

• Contraindicated in patients with hypernatremia, lactic acidosis, or conditions in which sodium administration is detrimental.
• Use cautiously in patients with metabolic or respiratory alkalosis, severe hepatic or renal disease, shock, hypoxia, or beriberi.
• **Lifespan:** In pregnant and breast-feeding women, use cautiously.

Adverse reactions

CNS: fever.
Metabolic: *metabolic alkalosis,* hypernatremia, hyperosmolarity with overdose.
Other: infection, thrombophlebitis at injection site.

Interactions

None significant.

Effects on lab test results

• May increase sodium level.

Pharmacokinetics

Absorption: Administered I.V.
Distribution: Lactate ion occurs naturally throughout body.
Metabolism: Metabolized in liver.
Excretion: None. *Half-life:* Unknown.

Route	Onset	Peak	Duration
I.V.	Immediate	Immediate	Unknown

Action

Chemical effect: Metabolized to sodium bicarbonate, producing buffering effect.
Therapeutic effect: Restores normal acid-base balance.

Available forms

Injection: 1/6 molar solution (167 mEq/L), 5 mEq/ml

NURSING PROCESS

Assessment
• Obtain history of patient's underlying acid-base imbalance before therapy, and reassess regularly thereafter.
• Monitor electrolyte levels.
• Evaluate patient's and family's knowledge of drug therapy.

Nursing diagnoses
• Ineffective health maintenance related to underlying condition
• Ineffective protection related to drug-induced adverse reactions
• Deficient knowledge related to drug therapy

Planning and implementation
• Consider giving sodium bicarbonate instead of sodium lactate in patients with severe acido-

sis who require immediate restoration of plasma bicarbonate.
• Don't use in patients with lactic acidosis.
Patient teaching
• Instruct patient to report discomfort at I.V. site immediately.

Evaluation
• Patient regains normal acid-base balance.
• Patient doesn't experience serious adverse reactions.
• Patient and family state understanding of drug therapy.

sodium phosphate monohydrate
(SOE-dee-um FOS-fate maw-no-HIGH-drate)

sodium phosphate dibasic anhydrous
(SOE-dee-um FOS-fate die-BAY-sick an-HIGH-drus)
Visicol

Pharmacologic class: osmotic laxative
Therapeutic class: bowel evacuant
Pregnancy risk category: C

Indications and dosages

▶ **Cleansing of the bowel before colonoscopy.**
Adults: 40 tablets taken in the following manner: The evening before the procedure, 3 tablets P.O. with at least 8 oz of clear liquid q 15 minutes for a total of 20 tablets. The last dose will be only 2 tablets. The day of the procedure, 3 tablets P.O. with at least 8 oz of clear liquid q 15 minutes for a total of 20 tablets, starting 3 to 5 hours before the procedure. The last dose will be only 2 tablets.

Contraindications and precautions

• Contraindicated in patients hypersensitive to drug or any of its ingredients. Avoid giving drug to patients with heart failure, ascites, unstable angina, gastric retention, ileus, acute intestinal obstruction, pseudo-obstruction, severe chronic constipation, bowel perforation, acute colitis, toxic megacolon, or hypomotility syndrome (hypothyroidism, scleroderma).
• Use cautiously in patients with a history of electrolyte abnormalities, current electrolyte abnormalities, or impaired renal function. Also,

use cautiously in patients who take drugs that can induce electrolyte abnormalities or prolong the QT interval.

⚠ **Lifespan:** In children, safety and effectiveness of drug haven't been established. In elderly patients, use cautiously because of greater sensitivity to drug.

Adverse reactions

CNS: headache, dizziness.
GI: nausea, vomiting, abdominal bloating, abdominal pain.

Interactions

Drug-drug. *Oral drugs:* Reduces absorption of these drugs because of rapid peristalsis and diarrhea induced by sodium phosphate monohydrate and sodium phosphate dibasic anhydrous. Separate administration times.

Effects on lab test results

• May increase phosphorus level. May decrease potassium and calcium levels.

Pharmacokinetics

Absorption: Quick. Duration of action is 1 to 3 hours after administration.
Distribution: Unknown.
Metabolism: Not expected to be metabolized by the liver.
Excretion: Eliminated almost entirely via the kidneys. *Half-life:* Unknown.

Route	Onset	Peak	Duration
P.O.	Unknown	3 hr	1-3 hr

Action

Chemical effect: The primary mechanism is thought to be the osmotic action of sodium, which causes large amounts of water to be drawn into the colon.
Therapeutic effect: Cleanses the colon.

Available forms

Tablets: 1.5 g sodium phosphate (1.102 g sodium phosphate monohydrate and 0.398 g sodium phosphate dibasic anhydrous)

NURSING PROCESS

📝 Assessment

• Assess underlying condition before therapy and reassess regularly throughout therapy.

• Obtain laboratory studies before beginning therapy and correct electrolyte imbalances before giving drug.
• Evaluate patient's and family's knowledge of drug therapy.

🔲 Nursing diagnoses

• Acute pain related to abdominal discomfort
• Risk for deficient fluid volume related to adverse GI effects
• Deficient knowledge related to drug therapy

▷ Planning and implementation

• Undigested or partially digested tablets and other drugs may be seen in the stool or during colonoscopy.
• As with other sodium phosphate cathartic preparations, this drug may induce colonic mucosal ulceration.
• Monitor patient for signs of dehydration.
• Don't repeat administration within 7 days.
• No enema or laxative is needed with drug.
⊛ **ALERT:** Administration of other sodium phosphate products may result in death from significant fluid shifts, electrolyte abnormalities, and cardiac arrhythmias. Patients with electrolyte disturbances have an increased risk of prolonged QT interval. Use drug cautiously in patients who are taking other drugs known to prolong the QT interval.
Patient teaching
• Instruct patient to drink at least 8 oz of clear liquid with each dose. Inadequate fluid intake may lead to excessive fluid loss and hypovolemia.
• Tell patient to drink only clear liquids for at least 12 hours before starting the purgative regimen.
• Warn patient against taking an additional enema or laxative, particularly one that contains sodium phosphate.
• Tell patient that undigested or partially digested tablets and other drugs may appear in the stool.

☑ Evaluation

• Patient states that pain management methods are effective.
• Patient maintains adequate hydration.
• Patient and family state understanding of therapy.

---

sodium polystyrene sulfonate

(SOH-dee-um pol-ee-STIGH-reen SUL-fuh-nayt)
Kayexalate, SPS

Pharmacologic class: cation-exchange resin
Therapeutic class: potassium-removing resin
Pregnancy risk category: C

Indications and dosages

▶**Hyperkalemia.** *Adults:* 15 g P.O. daily to
q.i.d. in water or sorbitol (3 to 4 ml/g of resin).
Or, mix powder with appropriate medium—
aqueous suspension or diet appropriate for renal
impairment—and instill into NG tube. Or, 30 to
50 g q 6 hours as warm emulsion deep into sigmoid colon (20 cm). In persistent vomiting or
paralytic ileus, high-retention enema of sodium
polystyrene sulfonate (30 g) suspended in
200 ml of 10% methylcellulose, 10% dextrose,
or 25% sorbitol solution may be given.
Children: 1 g of resin P.O. or P.R. for each mEq
of potassium to be removed. P.O. route preferred because drug should stay in intestine for
at least 6 hours.

Contraindications and precautions

• Contraindicated in patients hypersensitive to
drug and in those with hypokalemia.
• Use cautiously in patients with severe heart
failure, severe hypertension, or marked edema.
⚡ **Lifespan:** In pregnant and breast-feeding
women, use cautiously.

Adverse reactions

GI: *constipation, fecal impaction* in geriatric
patients, anorexia, gastric irritation, nausea,
vomiting, *diarrhea* with sorbitol emulsions.
Metabolic: hypokalemia, hypocalcemia, sodium retention.

Interactions

Drug-drug. *Antacids and laxatives (nonabsorbable cation-donating types, including magnesium hydroxide):* May cause systemic alkalosis and reduced potassium exchange capability.
Don't use together.

Effects on lab test results

• May increase sodium level. May decrease
potassium, calcium, and magnesium levels.

Pharmacokinetics

Absorption: None.
Distribution: None.
Metabolism: None.
Excretion: Unchanged in feces. *Half-life:* Un-
known.

Route	Onset	Peak	Duration
P.O., P.R.	Unknown	Unknown	Unknown

Action

Chemical effect: Exchanges sodium ions for
potassium ions in intestine. Much of exchange
capacity is used for cations other than potassium
(calcium and magnesium) and, possibly, fats
and proteins.
Therapeutic effect: Lowers potassium level.

Available forms

Powder: 1-lb jar (3.5 g/teaspoon)
Suspension: 60 ml*, 120 ml*, 200 ml*,
480 ml*, 500 ml*

NURSING PROCESS

⚕ Assessment

• Obtain history of patient's potassium level before therapy.
• Monitor potassium level at least once daily.
Treatment may result in potassium deficiency.
Treatment usually stops when potassium level
declines to 4 or 5 mEq/L.
⊛ **ALERT:** Watch for other signs of hypokalemia,
such as irritability, confusion, arrhythmias, ECG
changes, severe muscle weakness and paralysis,
and cardiac toxicity in digitalized patients.
• Monitor patient for symptoms of other electrolyte deficiencies (magnesium, calcium) because drug is nonselective. Monitor calcium
level in patient receiving sodium polystyrene
therapy for more than 3 days. Supplementary
calcium may be needed.
• Watch for sodium overload. Drug contains
about 100 mg of sodium/g. About one-third of
sodium in resin is retained.
• Be alert for adverse reactions and drug interactions.
• Watch for constipation with P.O. or NG administration.
• Evaluate patient's and family's knowledge of
drug therapy.

Nursing diagnoses

- Ineffective health maintenance related to presence of hyperkalemia
- Constipation related to drug-induced adverse GI reactions
- Deficient knowledge related to drug therapy

Planning and implementation

- Don't heat resin; doing so will impair drug's effectiveness.
- Mix resin only with water or sorbitol for P.O. administration. Never mix with orange juice (high potassium content) to disguise taste.
- Chill oral suspension for greater palatability.
- If sorbitol is given, mix with resin suspension.
- Consider solid form. Resin cookie and candy recipes are available; ask pharmacist or dietitian to supply.
- To prevent constipation, use sorbitol (10 to 20 ml of 70% syrup q 2 hours, p.r.n.) to produce one or two watery stools daily.
- Premixed forms are available (SPS and others) for P.R. use.
- If preparing manually, mix polystyrene resin only with water and sorbitol for P.R. use. Don't use mineral oil for P.R. administration to prevent impaction; ion exchange requires aqueous medium. Sorbitol content prevents impaction.
- Prepare P.R. dose at room temperature. Stir emulsion gently during administration.
- Use #28 French rubber tube. Insert tube 20 cm into sigmoid colon and tape in place. Or, consider indwelling urinary catheter with 30-ml balloon inflated distal to anal sphincter to aid in retention. This is especially helpful for patients with poor sphincter control (for example, after CVA). Use gravity flow. Drain returns constantly through Y-tube connection. Place patient in knee-chest position or with hips on pillow for a while if back leakage occurs.
- After P.R. administration, flush tubing with 50 to 100 ml of nonsodium fluid to ensure delivery of all drug. Flush rectum to remove resin.
- Prevent fecal impaction in geriatric patient by giving resin P.R. Give cleansing enema before P.R. administration. Explain to patient the need to retain enema; 6 to 10 hours is ideal, but 30 to 60 minutes is acceptable.
- If hyperkalemia is severe, prescriber won't depend solely on polystyrene resin to lower potassium level. Dextrose 50% with regular insulin may be given by I.V. push.

Patient teaching

- Explain importance of following prescribed low-potassium diet.
- Explain need to retain enema; 6 to 10 hours is ideal, but 30 to 60 minutes is acceptable.
- Tell patient to report adverse reactions.

Evaluation

- Patient's potassium level is normal.
- Patient doesn't develop constipation.
- Patient and family state understanding of drug therapy.

sodium phosphate

(SOH-dee-um FOS-fayts)
Fleet Enema, Fleet Pediatric Enema, Fleet Phospho-soda†

Pharmacologic class: acid salt
Therapeutic class: saline laxative, mineral
Pregnancy risk category: C (I.V.), NR (P.R.)

Indications and dosages

▶ **Constipation.** *Adults and children age 12 and older:* 20 to 45 ml of solution mixed with 120 ml of cold water P.O. Or, 120 ml P.R. (as enema).
Children ages 10 to 11: 10 to 20 ml of solution mixed with 120 ml of cold water P.O.
Children ages 5 to 9: 5 to 10 ml of solution mixed with 120 ml of cold water P.O.
Children older than age 2: 60 ml P.R.
▶ **TPN.** *Adults and children:* Doses are highly individualized. 10 to 15 millimoles (mM) per liter of TPN solution.
Infants receiving TPN: 1.5 to 2 mM/kg daily.

I.V. administration

- To avoid medication errors, drug should be prescribed in terms of millimoles (mM) of phosphorous.
- Dilute and mix with larger volume of fluid.
- To avoid toxicity, infuse slowly.
- Infusions with high concentrations of phosphate may cause hypocalcemia. Monitor calcium levels.

Contraindications and precautions

- Contraindicated in patients on sodium-restricted diets and in patients with intestinal

obstruction or perforation, edema, heart failure, megacolon, impaired renal function, or symptoms of appendicitis or acute surgical abdomen, such as abdominal pain, nausea, and vomiting.
• I.V. sodium phosphate contraindicated in patients with hypernatremia, high phosphate levels, or low calcium levels.
• Use cautiously in patients with large hemorrhoids or anal abrasions.
• Use I.V. sodium phosphate in patients with cardiac disease, renal impairment, adrenal insufficiency, and cirrhosis.
Lifespan: In pregnant and breast-feeding women, use cautiously. In children younger than age 4, use only as directed by prescriber.

Adverse reactions

GI: *abdominal cramps.*
Metabolic: fluid and electrolyte disturbances (such as hypernatremia or hyperphosphatemia) with daily use.
Other: laxative dependence with long-term or excessive use.

Interactions

None significant.

Effects on lab test results

• May increase sodium and phosphate levels. May decrease electrolyte levels with prolonged use.

Pharmacokinetics

Absorption: About 1% to 20% of P.O. dose absorbed; unknown after P.R. administration.
Distribution: Unknown.
Metabolism: Unknown.
Excretion: Unknown. *Half-life:* Unknown.

Route	Onset	Peak	Duration
P.O.	30 min-3 hr	Varies	Varies
P.R.	5-10 min	Varies	Ends with evacuation
I.V.	Unknown	Unknown	Unknown

Action

Chemical effect: Produces osmotic effect in small intestine by drawing water into intestinal lumen.
Therapeutic effect: Relieves constipation.

Available forms

Enema: 160 mg/ml sodium phosphate and 60 mg/ml sodium biphosphate
Liquid: 2.4 g/5 ml sodium phosphate and 900 mg/5 ml sodium biphosphate
I.V. Infusion: 3 mM phosphate and 4 mEq sodium/L in 10-, 15-, 30-, 50-ml vials

NURSING PROCESS

Assessment

• Assess patient's condition before therapy and regularly thereafter.
• Before giving drug for constipation, determine whether patient has adequate fluid intake, exercise, and diet.
• Be alert for adverse reactions.
ALERT: Up to 10% of sodium content of drug may be absorbed.
• Evaluate patient's and family's knowledge of drug therapy.

Nursing diagnoses

• Constipation related to underlying condition
• Acute pain related to drug-induced abdominal cramping
• Deficient knowledge related to drug therapy

Planning and implementation

• Dilute drug with water before giving. Follow administration with full glass of water.
• Make sure that patient has easy access to bathroom facilities, commode, or bedpan.
ALERT: Severe electrolyte imbalances may occur if recommended dosage is exceeded.

Patient teaching

• Teach patient about dietary sources of bulk, which include bran and other cereals, fresh fruit, and vegetables.
• Tell patient to maintain adequate fluid intake of at least 6 to 8 glasses of water or juices daily unless contraindicated.

Evaluation

• Patient's constipation is relieved.
• Patient's abdominal cramping ceases.
• Patient and family state understanding of drug therapy.

somatrem
(SOH-muh-trem)
Protropin

Pharmacologic class: anterior pituitary hormone
Therapeutic class: human growth hormone (GH)
Pregnancy risk category: C

Indications and dosages

▶ **Long-term treatment of children who have growth failure because of lack of adequate endogenous GH secretion.** *Children (prepuberty):* Highly individualized; up to 0.3 mg/kg of body weight (about 0.9 IU/kg) I.M. or S.C. weekly.

Contraindications and precautions

• Contraindicated in patients hypersensitive to benzyl alcohol and in those with epiphyseal closure or active neoplasia.
• Use cautiously in patients with hypothyroidism and in those whose GH deficiency results from an intracranial lesion.
⚖ Lifespan: Drug is suitable for prepubescent children only.

Adverse reactions

Hematologic: *leukemia.*
Metabolic: hypothyroidism, hyperglycemia.
Other: *antibodies to GH.*

Interactions

Drug-drug. *Glucocorticoids:* May inhibit growth-promoting action of somatrem. Adjust glucocorticoid dosage, p.r.n.

Effects on lab test results

• May increase glucose level. May decrease T_4 level.

Pharmacokinetics

Absorption: Unknown.
Distribution: Unknown.
Metabolism: About 90% metabolized in liver.
Excretion: About 0.1% excreted unchanged in urine. *Half-life:* 20 to 30 minutes.

Route	Onset	Peak	Duration
I.M., S.C.	Unknown	Unknown	12-48 hr

Action

Chemical effect: Purified GH of recombinant DNA origin that stimulates linear, skeletal muscle, and organ growth.
Therapeutic effect: Stimulates growth in children.

Available forms

Injectable lyophilized powder: 5 mg (about 15 IU)/vial; 10 mg (30 about IU)/vial

NURSING PROCESS

✍ Assessment
• Assess child's growth before therapy and regularly thereafter.
• Be alert for adverse reactions and drug interactions.
⊛ **ALERT:** Toxicity in neonates may occur from exposure to benzyl alcohol used in drug as preservative.
• Monitor patient's height and blood with regular checkups; radiologic studies are also needed.
• Observe patient for signs of glucose intolerance and hyperglycemia.
• Monitor patient's periodic thyroid function tests for hypothyroidism, which may require treatment with thyroid hormone.
• Evaluate patient's and family's knowledge of drug therapy.

🏥 Nursing diagnoses
• Delayed growth and development related to lack of adequate endogenous GH
• Ineffective health maintenance related to adverse metabolic reactions
• Deficient knowledge related to drug therapy

▷ Planning and implementation
• Check drug's expiration date.
• To prepare solution, inject supplied bacteriostatic water for injection into vial containing drug. Then swirl vial with gentle rotary motion until contents are dissolved. Don't shake vial.
• After reconstitution, vial solution should be clear. Don't inject if solution is cloudy or contains particles.
• If drug is given to neonate, reconstitute immediately before use with sterile water for injection (without bacteriostat). Use vial once, then discard.
• Store reconstituted drug in refrigerator; use within 7 days.

⊛ **ALERT:** Don't confuse somatrem with somatropin.

Patient teaching
• Reassure patient and family members that somatrem is pure and safe. Drug replaces pituitary-derived human GH, which was removed from market in 1985 because of an association with rare but fatal viral infection (Creutzfeldt-Jakob disease).

☑ **Evaluation**
• Patient exhibits growth.
• Patient's thyroid function studies and glucose level are normal.
• Patient and family state understanding of drug therapy.

---

somatropin
(soh-muh-TROH-pin)
Genotropin, Genotropin Miniquick, Humatrope, Norditropin, Nutropin, Nutropin AQ, Nutropin Depot, Saizen, Serostim

Pharmacologic class: anterior pituitary hormone
Therapeutic class: human growth hormone (GH)
Pregnancy risk category: C

Indications and dosages

▶ **Long-term treatment of growth failure in children with inadequate secretion of endogenous GH.** *Children:* 0.18 mg/kg Humatrope S.C. or I.M. weekly, divided equally and given on 3 alternate days, six times weekly or daily. Or, 0.3 mg/kg Nutropin or Nutropin AQ S.C. weekly in daily divided doses. Or, 0.06 mg/kg Saizen I.M. or S.C. three times weekly. Or, 0.024 to 0.034 mg/kg Norditropin S.C., six to seven times weekly. Or, 0.16 to 0.24 mg/kg Genotropin S.C. weekly, divided into five to seven doses. Or 1.5 mg/kg Nutropin Depot S.C. once monthly or 0.75 mg/kg S.C. twice monthly on the same days of each month.

▶ **Growth failure from chronic renal insufficiency up to time of kidney transplant.** *Children:* Weekly dosage of up to 0.35 mg/kg Nutropin or Nutropin AQ S.C. divided into daily doses.

▶ **Long-term treatment of short stature related to Turner's syndrome.** *Children:* Up to

0.375 mg/kg Humatrope, Nutropin, or Nutropin AQ S.C. weekly, divided into equal doses given three to seven times weekly.

▶ **Long-term treatment of growth failure in children with Prader-Willi syndrome (PWS) diagnosed by genetic testing.** *Children:* 0.24 mg/kg Genotropin S.C. weekly, divided into six to seven doses.

▶ **Replacement of endogenous GH in adult patients with GH deficiency.** *Adults:* Initially, not more than 0.006 mg/kg Humatrope, Nutropin, or Nutropin AQ S.C. daily. Humatrope may be increased to maximum of 0.0125 mg/kg daily. Nutropin and Nutropin AQ may be increased to maximum of 0.025 mg/kg daily in patients younger than age 35 or 0.0125 mg/kg daily in patients older than age 35. With Genotropin, starting dose isn't more than 0.04 mg/kg S.C. weekly, divided into six to seven doses. Dose may be increased at 4- to 8-week intervals to a maximum dose of 0.08 mg/kg S.C. weekly, divided into six to seven doses.

▶ **AIDS wasting or cachexia.** *Adults and children weighing more than 55 kg (121 lb):* 6 mg Serostim S.C. h.s.
Adults and children weighing 45 to 55 kg (99 to 121 lb): 5 mg Serostim S.C. h.s.
Adults and children weighing 35 to 45 kg (77 to 99 lb): 4 mg Serostim S.C. h.s.
Adults and children weighing less than 35 kg: 0.1 mg/kg Serostim S.C. daily h.s.

▶ **Long-term treatment of growth failure in children born small for gestational age who don't achieve catch-up growth by 2 years of age.** *Children:* 0.48 mg/kg Genotropin S.C. weekly, divided into five to seven doses.

Contraindications and precautions

• Contraindicated in patients with closed epiphyses or an active underlying intracranial lesion.
• Don't reconstitute Humatrope with supplied diluent for patients with known sensitivity to either m-cresol or glycerin.
• Genotropin is contraindicated in patients with PWS who are severely obese or have severe respiratory impairment.
⚜ **Lifespan:** In pregnant and breast-feeding women, drug isn't indicated. In children with hypothyroidism and in those whose GH deficiency is caused by an intracranial lesion, use cautiously. These children should be examined

frequently for progression or recurrence of underlying disease.

Adverse reactions

CNS: headache, weakness.
CV: mild, transient edema.
Hematologic: *leukemia.*
Metabolic: mild hyperglycemia, hypothyroidism.
Musculoskeletal: localized muscle pain.
Other: injection site pain, *antibodies to GH.*

Interactions

Drug-drug. *Corticosteroids, corticotropin:*
Long-term use inhibits growth response to GH.
Monitor patient.

Effects on lab test results

• May increase glucose, inorganic phosphorus, alkaline phosphatase, and parathyroid hormone levels.

Pharmacokinetics

Absorption: Unknown.
Distribution: Unknown.
Metabolism: About 90% metabolized in liver.
Excretion: About 0.1% excreted unchanged in urine. *Half-life:* 20 to 30 minutes.

Route	Onset	Peak	Duration
I.M, S.C.	Unknown	7½ hr	12-48 hr

Action

Chemical effect: Purified GH of recombinant DNA origin that stimulates linear, skeletal muscle, and organ growth.
Therapeutic effect: Stimulates growth.

Available forms

Genotropin injection: 1.5 mg (about 4.5 IU/vial), 5.8 mg (about 17.4 IU/vial), 13.8 mg (about 41.4 IU/vial)
Genotropin Mini quick injection: 0.2 mg/vial, 0.4 mg/vial, 0.6 mg/vial, 0.8 mg/vial, 1 mg/vial, 1.2 mg/vial, 1.4 mg/vial, 1.6 mg/vial, 1.8 mg/vial, 2 mg/vial
Humatrope injection: 2 mg (about 6 IU/vial ◆), 5 mg (about 15 IU/vial, 6 mg (18 IU/cartridge), 12 mg (36 IU/cartridge), 24 mg (72 IU/cartridge)
Norditropin injection: 4 mg (about 12 IU/ml), 8 mg (about 24 IU/ml), 5 mg/1.5 ml cartridges, 10 mg/1.5 ml cartridges, 15 mg/1.5 ml cartridges
Nutropin injection: 5 mg (about 15 IU/vial), 10 mg (about 30 IU/vial)
Nutropin AQ injection: 10 mg (about 30 IU/vial)
Nutropin Depot injection: 13.5 mg/vial, 18 mg/vial, 22.5 mg/vial
Saizen injection: 5 mg (about 15 IU/vial)
Serostim injection: 4 mg (about 12 IU/vial), 5 mg (about 15 IU/vial), 6 mg (about 18 IU/vial)

NURSING PROCESS

Assessment

• Assess child's growth before therapy and regularly thereafter.
• Be alert for adverse reactions.
• Toxicity in neonates may occur from exposure to benzyl alcohol used in drug as preservative.
• Regular checkups with monitoring of height and of blood and radiologic studies are needed.
• Observe patient for signs of glucose intolerance and hyperglycemia.
• Monitor patient's periodic thyroid function tests for hypothyroidism, which may require treatment with thyroid hormone.
• Evaluate patient's and family's knowledge of drug therapy.

Nursing diagnoses

• Delayed growth and development related to lack of adequate endogenous GH
• Ineffective health maintenance related to adverse metabolic reactions
• Deficient knowledge related to drug therapy

Planning and implementation

• To prepare solution, inject supplied diluent into vial containing drug by aiming stream of liquid against glass wall of vial. Then swirl vial with gentle rotary motion until contents are completely dissolved. Don't shake vial.
• After reconstitution, solution should be clear. Don't inject solution if it's cloudy or contains particles.
• Store reconstituted drug in refrigerator; use within 14 days.
• If sensitivity to diluent develops, drugs may be reconstituted with sterile water for injection. When drug is reconstituted in this manner, use only one reconstituted dose per vial, refrigerate

solution if it isn't used immediately after reconstitution, use reconstituted dose within 24 hours, and discard unused portion.

• Excessive glucocorticoid therapy inhibits growth-promoting effect of somatropin. In patient with coexisting corticotropin deficiency adjust glucocorticoid-replacement dosage carefully to avoid growth inhibition.

Ⓧ **ALERT:** Don't confuse somatropin with somatrem or sumatriptan.

Patient teaching

• Inform parents that child with endocrine disorders (including GH deficiency) may develop slipped capital epiphyses more frequently. Tell them to notify prescriber if child begins limping.

☑ **Evaluation**

• Patient exhibits growth.

• Patient's thyroid function studies and glucose level are normal.

• Patient and family state understanding of drug therapy.

---

sotalol hydrochloride

(SOH-tuh-lol high-droh-KLOR-ighd)
Betapace, Betapace AF, Sotacor♦ ◇

Pharmacologic class: non-selective beta blocker
Therapeutic class: antiarrhythmic, antihypertensive, antianginal
Pregnancy risk category: B

Indications and dosages

▶ **Documented, life-threatening ventricular arrhythmias.** *Adults:* Initially, 80 mg P.O. b.i.d. Dosage is increased q 2 to 3 days as needed and tolerated; most patients respond to 160 to 320 mg daily. A few patients with refractory arrhythmias have received as much as 640 mg daily.

◻ **Adjust-a-dose:** For patients with renal impairment, if creatinine clearance is greater than 60 ml/minute, dosage adjustment isn't needed. If creatinine clearance is 30 to 60 ml/minute, interval is increased to q 24 hours; if clearance is 10 to 30 ml/minute, give q 36 to 48 hours; if clearance is less than 10 ml/minute, individualize dosage.

▶ **Maintenance of normal sinus rhythm (delay in time to recurrence of atrial fibrillation/atrial flutter) in patients with symptomatic atrial fibrillation/atrial flutter who are** currently in sinus rhythm. *Adults:* Initially, 80 mg Betapace AF P.O. twice daily. If initial dose doesn't reduce the frequency of relapses of atrial fibrillation/atrial flutter and is tolerated without excessive QTc interval prolongation (≥ 520 msec), the dose level may be increased after 3 days to 120 mg P.O. bid. Maximum, 160 mg P.O. bid.

◻ **Adjust-a-dose:** For patients with renal impairment, if creatinine clearance is 40 to 60 ml/minute, give once daily.

Contraindications and precautions

• Contraindicated in patients hypersensitive to drug and patients with severe sinus node dysfunction, sinus bradycardia, second- or third-degree AV block in absence of an artificial pacemaker, congenital or acquired long-QT interval syndrome, cardiogenic shock, uncontrolled heart failure, or bronchial asthma. Don't give to patients with a creatinine clearance less than 40 ml/minute.

• Use cautiously in patients with renal impairment or diabetes mellitus.

⚖ **Lifespan:** In pregnant women, use cautiously. In breast-feeding women and in children, safety of drug hasn't been established.

Adverse reactions

CNS: *asthenia, headache, dizziness, weakness, fatigue,* sleep problems, *light-headedness.*
CV: *bradycardia, arrhythmias, heart failure, AV block, proarrhythmic events (ventricular tachycardia, PVCs, ventricular fibrillation),* edema, *palpitations, chest pain,* ECG abnormalities, hypotension.
GI: *nausea,* vomiting, diarrhea, dyspepsia.
Respiratory: *dyspnea, bronchospasm.*

Interactions

Drug-drug. *Antiarrhythmics:* May have additive effects. Avoid using together.
Antihypertensives, catecholamine-depleting drugs (such as guanethidine, haloperidol, and reserpine): Enhances hypotensive effects. Monitor patient closely.
Calcium channel blockers: Enhances myocardial depression. Monitor patient carefully.
Clonidine: Beta blockers may enhance rebound effect seen after withdrawal of clonidine. Discontinue sotalol several days before withdrawing clonidine.

General anesthetics: May cause additional myocardial depression. Monitor patient closely.
Insulin, oral antidiabetics: May cause hyperglycemia and may mask symptoms of hyperglycemia. Adjust dosage.
Prazosin: May increase the risk of orthostatic hypotension in the early phases of use together. Assist patient to stand slowly until effects are known.
Drug-food. *Any food:* Increases drug absorption. Give drug on an empty stomach.

Effects on lab test results

• May increase glucose level.

Pharmacokinetics

Absorption: Well absorbed with bioavailability of 90% to 100%. Food may interfere with absorption.
Distribution: Unknown; doesn't bind to proteins and crosses blood-brain barrier poorly.
Metabolism: Not metabolized.
Excretion: Excreted primarily in urine in unchanged form. *Half-life:* 12 hours.

Route	Onset	Peak	Duration
P.O.	Unknown	2½-4 hr	Unknown

Action

Chemical effect: Depresses sinus heart rate, slows AV conduction, decreases cardiac output, and lowers systolic and diastolic blood pressure.
Therapeutic effect: Restores normal sinus rhythm, lowers blood pressure, and relieves angina.

Available forms

Tablets: 80 mg, 120 mg, 160 mg, 240 mg

NURSING PROCESS

▨ Assessment

• Assess patient's condition before therapy and regularly thereafter.
• Monitor patient's electrolyte levels and ECG regularly, especially if patient is receiving diuretics. Electrolyte imbalances, such as hypokalemia and hypomagnesemia, may enhance QT-interval prolongation and increase risk of serious arrhythmias such as torsades de pointes.
• Be alert for adverse reactions and drug interactions.

• Evaluate patient's and family's knowledge of drug therapy.

▨ Nursing diagnoses

• Ineffective health maintenance related to underlying condition
• Fatigue related to adverse reactions
• Deficient knowledge related to drug therapy

▸ Planning and implementation

• Because pro-arrhythmic events may occur at start of therapy and during dosage adjustments, patient should be hospitalized. Facilities and personnel should be available to monitor cardiac rhythm and interpret ECG.
• Although patients receiving I.V. lidocaine can start therapy with this drug without ill effect, other antiarrhythmics should be withdrawn before therapy with this drug. Therapy typically is delayed until two or three half-lives of withdrawn drug have elapsed. After withdrawal of amiodarone, this drug shouldn't be given until QT interval normalizes.
• Adjust dosage slowly, allowing 2 to 3 days between dosage increments for adequate monitoring of QT intervals and for drug levels to reach steady-state level.
❧ **ALERT:** The baseline QTc interval must be ≤ 450 msec in order to start a patient on Betapace AF. During initiation and adjustment, monitor QT interval 2 to 4 hours after each dose. If the QTc interval is 500 msec or longer, the dose must be reduced or stopped.
❧ **ALERT:** Don't confuse sotalol with Statural or Stadol. Don't substitute Betapace AF for Betapace.
Patient teaching
• Explain importance of taking drug as prescribed, even when feeling well. Instruct patient not to stop drug suddenly.
• Tell patient to take drug 1 hour before or 2 hours after meals.
• Teach patient how to check his pulse rate.

☑ Evaluation

• Patient responds well to therapy.
• Patient states energy-conserving measures to combat fatigue.
• Patient and family state understanding of drug therapy.

---

spironolactone

(spih-ron-uh-LAK-tohn)

Aldactone, Novospiroton ♦ , Spiractin ◇

Pharmacologic class: potassium-sparing diuretic
Therapeutic class: management of edema, antihypertensive, diagnosis of primary hyperaldosteronism, treatment of diuretic-induced hypokalemia
Pregnancy risk category: NR

Indications and dosages

▶ **Edema.** *Adults:* 25 to 200 mg P.O. daily or in divided doses.
Children: 3.3 mg/kg P.O. daily or in divided doses.
▶ **Essential hypertension.** *Adults:* 50 to 100 mg P.O. daily or in divided doses.
Children: 1 to 2 mg/kg P.O. b.i.d.
▶ **Diuretic-induced hypokalemia.** *Adults:* 25 to 100 mg P.O. daily when P.O. potassium supplements are contraindicated.
▶ **Diagnosis of primary hyperaldosteronism.** *Adults:* 400 mg P.O. daily for 4 days (short test) or 3 to 4 weeks (long test). If hypokalemia and hypertension are corrected, presumptive diagnosis of primary hyperaldosteronism is made.
▶ **Management of primary hyperaldosteronism.** *Adults:* 100 to 400 mg P.O. daily. In patients unwilling or unable to undergo surgery, initiate dose at 400 mg daily and then maintain at lowest possible dose.
▶ **Hirsutism‡.** *Adults:* 50 to 200 mg P.O. daily.
▶ **Premenstrual syndrome‡.** *Adults:* 25 mg P.O. q.i.d. on day 14 of menstrual cycle.
▶ **Heart failure in patients receiving an ACE inhibitor and a loop diuretic with or without digoxin‡.** *Adults:* Initially, 12.5 to 25 mg P.O. daily.
▶ **Decrease risk of metrorrhagia‡.** *Adults:* 50 mg P.O. b.i.d. on days 4 through 21 of menstrual cycle.
▶ **Acne vulgaris‡.** *Adults:* 100 mg P.O. daily.

Contraindications and precautions

• Contraindicated in patients with anuria, acute or progressive renal insufficiency, rapidly deteriorating renal function, or hyperkalemia.

• Use cautiously in patients with fluid or electrolyte imbalances, impaired kidney function, or hepatic disease.
⚹ **Lifespan:** In pregnant women, use cautiously. In breast-feeding women, safety of drug hasn't been established.

Adverse reactions

CNS: headache, drowsiness, lethargy, confusion, ataxia.
GI: diarrhea, gastric bleeding, ulceration, cramping, gastritis, vomiting.
GU: impotence, menstrual disturbances.
Hematologic: *agranulocytosis.*
Metabolic: *hyperkalemia,* hyponatremia, mild acidosis, dehydration.
Skin: urticaria, hirsutism, maculopapular eruptions, erythematous rash.
Other: drug fever, gynecomastia, breast soreness, *anaphylaxis, angioedema.*

Interactions

Drug-drug. *ACE inhibitors, indomethacin, other potassium-sparing diuretics, potassium supplements:* Increases risk of hyperkalemia. Don't use together, especially in patients with renal impairment.
Aspirin: May block diuretic effect of spironolactone. Watch for diminished spironolactone response.
Digoxin: May alter digoxin clearance, increasing risk of digoxin toxicity. Monitor digoxin level.
Drug-food. *Potassium-containing salt substitutes, potassium-rich foods (such as citrus fruits, tomatoes):* Increases risk of hyperkalemia. Tell patient to use low-potassium salt substitutes and to eat high-potassium foods cautiously.

Effects on lab test results

• May increase BUN, creatinine, and potassium levels. May decrease sodium level.
• May decrease granulocyte count.

Pharmacokinetics

Absorption: About 90%.
Distribution: More than 90% protein bound.
Metabolism: Metabolized rapidly and extensively.

Excretion: Canrenone and other metabolites excreted primarily in urine, minimally in feces.
Half-life: 1¼ to 2 hours.

Route	Onset	Peak	Duration
P.O.	Unknown	1-2 hours	Unknown

Action

Chemical effect: Antagonizes aldosterone in distal tubule.
Therapeutic effect: Promotes water and sodium excretion and hinders potassium excretion, lowers blood pressure, and helps to diagnose primary hyperaldosteronism.

Available forms

Tablets: 25 mg, 50 mg, 100 mg

NURSING PROCESS

🔋 Assessment
• Assess patient's condition before therapy and regularly thereafter. Maximum antihypertensive response may be delayed up to 2 weeks.
• Monitor electrolyte levels, fluid intake and output, weight, and blood pressure.
• Be alert for adverse reactions and drug interactions.
• Evaluate patient's and family's knowledge of drug therapy.

🔁 Nursing diagnoses
• Excess fluid volume related to presence of edema
• Impaired urinary elimination related to diuretic therapy
• Deficient knowledge related to drug therapy

➡ Planning and implementation
• Give drug with meals to enhance absorption.
• Protect drug from light.
• Inform laboratory that patient is taking spironolactone because it may interfere with some laboratory tests that measure digoxin levels.
• **ALERT:** Don't confuse Aldactone with Aldactazide.
Patient teaching
• **ALERT:** Warn patient to avoid excessive ingestion of potassium-rich foods, potassium-containing salt substitutes, and potassium supplements to prevent serious hyperkalemia.

• Tell patient to take drug with meals and, if possible, early in day to avoid interruption of sleep by nocturia.

☑ Evaluation
• Patient shows no signs of edema.
• Patient demonstrates adjustment of lifestyle to deal with altered patterns of urinary elimination.
• Patient and family state understanding of drug therapy.

---

stavudine (2,3-didehydro-3-deoxythymidine, d4T)
(stay-VYOO-deen)
Zerit, Zerit XR

Pharmacologic class: synthetic thymidine nucleoside analogue
Therapeutic class: antiviral
Pregnancy risk category: C

Indications and dosages

▶ **Patients with advanced HIV infection who are intolerant of or unresponsive to other antivirals.** *Adults and children who weigh 60 kg (132 lb) or more:* 40 mg P.O. q 12 hours, or 100 mg P.O. extended-release daily.
Adults and children who weigh more than 30 kg (66 lb) but less than 60 kg: 30 mg P.O. q 12 hours, or 75 mg P.O. extended-release daily.
Children who weigh less than 30 kg: 1 mg/kg q 12 hours.
⬛ Adjust-a-dose: For patients with renal impairment undergoing hemodialysis, adjust dosage.

Contraindications and precautions

• Contraindicated in patients hypersensitive to drug.
• Don't use Zerit XR in patients with creatinine clearance of 50 ml/minute or less.
• Use cautiously in patients with renal impairment or a history of peripheral neuropathy.
• **Lifespan:** In pregnant women, use cautiously. In breast-feeding women, safety of drug hasn't been established.

Adverse reactions

CNS: *asthenia, peripheral neuropathy, headache, malaise, insomnia, anxiety, depression, nervousness,* dizziness, *fever.*

CV: chest pain.
EENT: conjunctivitis.
GI: *abdominal pain, diarrhea, nausea, vomiting, anorexia,* dyspepsia, constipation, weight loss, *pancreatitis.*
Hematologic: *neutropenia, thrombocytopenia,* anemia, *leukopenia.*
Hepatic: *hepatotoxicity, severe hepatomegaly with steatosis.*
Metabolic: *lactic acidosis.*
Musculoskeletal: myalgia, *back pain, arthralgia.*
Respiratory: *dyspnea.*
Skin: *rash, diaphoresis, pruritus,* maculopapular rash.
Other: *chills,* breast enlargement, redistribution or accumulation of body fat.

Interactions

Drug-drug. *Ketoconazole, ritonavir:* Increases stavudine level. Monitor patient closely.
Methadone: Decreases stavudine absorption. Avoid using together.
Myelosuppressants: Additive myelosuppression. Avoid using together.
Zidovudine: Inhibits stavudine phosphorylation. Don't use together.

Effects on lab test results

- May increase liver enzyme levels.
- May decrease hemoglobin, hematocrit, and neutrophil and platelet counts.

Pharmacokinetics

Absorption: Rapid with mean absolute bioavailability of 86.4%.
Distribution: Equally between RBCs and plasma; binds poorly to proteins.
Metabolism: Not extensive.
Excretion: About 40% renal. *Half-life:* 1 to 2 hours.

Route	Onset	Peak	Duration
P.O.	Unknown	≤ 1 hr	Unknown

Action

Chemical effect: Prevents replication of HIV by interfering with enzyme reverse transcriptase.
Therapeutic effect: Inhibits HIV replication.

Available forms

Capsules: 15 mg, 20 mg, 30 mg, 40 mg

Capsules (extended-release): 37.5 mg, 50 mg, 75 mg, 100 mg.
Powder for oral solution: 1 mg/ml

NURSING PROCESS

☑ Assessment

- Assess patient's condition before therapy and regularly thereafter.
- Periodically monitor CBC and levels of creatinine, AST, ALT, and alkaline phosphatase.
- Be alert for adverse reactions and drug interactions.
- Evaluate patient's and family's knowledge of drug therapy.

⊞ Nursing diagnoses

- Infection related to presence of HIV
- Disturbed sensory perception (peripheral) related to drug-induced peripheral neuropathy
- Deficient knowledge related to drug therapy

▶ Planning and implementation

⊛ ALERT: Peripheral neuropathy appears to be major dose-limiting adverse effect; withdraw drug temporarily and resume at 50% of recommended dose.
- Dosage is calculated based on patient's weight.
⊛ ALERT: Don't confuse drug with other antivirals that may use initials for identification.
- Motor weakness that mimics Guillain-Barré syndrome (including respiratory failure) may occur in HIV-positive patients taking this drug with other antiretrovirals, usually in those with lactic acidosis. Monitor patient for factors of lactic acidosis, including generalized fatigue, GI problems, tachypnea, or dyspnea. Symptoms may continue or worsen upon stopping of drug. In patients with these symptoms, promptly stop antiretroviral therapy and perform a full medical workup immediately. Permanently stopping drug should be considered.
- Monitor patient for pancreatitis, especially when this drug is used with didanosine or hydroxyurea. Use caution when restarting drug after confirmed diagnosis of pancreatitis.
- If patient has trouble swallowing capsule, mix contents of the capsule in applesauce or yogurt. Instruct patient not to chew or crush the beads while swallowing.

Patient teaching
• Tell patient that drug may be taken without regard to meals.
• Advise patient that he can't take drug if he experienced peripheral neuropathy while taking other nucleoside analogues or if his treatment plan includes cytotoxic antineoplastics.
• Warn patient not to take any other drugs for HIV or AIDS (especially street drugs) unless prescriber has approved them.
• Teach patient signs and symptoms of peripheral neuropathy—pain, burning, aching, weakness, or pins and needles in limbs—and tell him to report these immediately.
• Tell patient to report symptoms of lactic acidosis, including fatigue, GI problems, dyspnea or tachypnea.
• Tell patient to report symptoms of pancreatitis, including abdominal pain, nausea, vomiting, weight loss or fatty stools.

☑ Evaluation
• Patient's infection is controlled.
• Patient maintains normal peripheral neurologic function.
• Patient and family state understanding of drug therapy.

streptokinase
(strep-toh-KIGH-nayz)
Kabikinase, Streptase

Pharmacologic class: plasminogen activator
Therapeutic class: thrombolytic enzyme
Pregnancy risk category: C

Indications and dosages

▶ **Arteriovenous cannula occlusion.** *Adults:*
250,000 IU in 2 ml I.V. solution by I.V. pump infusion into each occluded limb of cannula over 25 to 35 minutes. Clamp cannula for 2 hours. Then aspirate contents of cannula; flush with saline solution and reconnect.
▶ **Venous thrombosis, pulmonary embolism, arterial thrombosis and embolism.** *Adults:*
Loading dose is 250,000 IU by I.V. infusion over 30 minutes. Sustaining dose is 100,000 IU/ hour by I.V. infusion for 72 hours for deep vein thrombosis and 100,000 IU/hour over 24 hours by I.V. infusion pump for pulmonary embolism.

▶ **Lysis of coronary artery thrombi after acute MI.** *Adults:* I.V. infusion preferred using 1,500,000 IU infused over 60 minutes. Or, if using intracoronary infusion, the total dose for intracoronary infusion is 140,000 IU. Loading dose is 15,000 to 20,000 IU by coronary catheter over 15 seconds to 2 minutes, followed by infusion of maintenance dose of 2,000 IU/ minute for 60 minutes.

▼ I.V. administration
• Reconstitute each drug vial with 5 ml of normal saline solution for injection. Further dilute to 45 ml.
• Don't shake; roll gently to mix. Some flocculation may be present; discard if large amounts appear. Filter solution with 0.8-micron or larger filter. Use within 24 hours.
• Store powder at room temperature and refrigerate after reconstitution.

Contraindications and precautions
• Contraindicated in patients with ulcerative wounds, active internal bleeding, uncontrolled hypercoagulation, chronic pulmonary disease with cavitation, subacute bacterial endocarditis or rheumatic valvular disease, visceral or intracranial malignant neoplasms, ulcerative colitis, diverticulitis, severe hypertension, acute or chronic hepatic or renal insufficiency, recent CVA, recent trauma with possible internal injuries, or recent cerebral embolism, thrombosis, or hemorrhage.
• Also contraindicated within 10 days after intra-arterial diagnostic procedure or any surgery, including liver or kidney biopsy, lumbar puncture, thoracentesis, paracentesis, or extensive or multiple cutdowns.
• I.M. injections and other invasive procedures are contraindicated during streptokinase therapy.
• Use cautiously when treating arterial embolism that originates from left side of heart because of danger of cerebral infarction.
▲ Lifespan: In pregnant women, use cautiously. In breast-feeding women and in children, safety of drug hasn't been established.

Adverse reactions
CNS: polyradiculoneuropathy, headache, fever.
CV: *hypotension,* vasculitis, ***reperfusion arrhythmias,*** flushing.
EENT: periorbital edema.

GI: nausea.
Hematologic: *bleeding.*
Musculoskeletal: musculoskeletal pain.
Respiratory: minor breathing difficulty, *bronchospasm, pulmonary edema.*
Skin: urticaria, pruritus.
Other: phlebitis at injection site, *hypersensitivity reactions (anaphylaxis), delayed hypersensitivity reactions* (interstitial nephritis, vasculitis, serum-sickness–like reactions), *angioedema.*

Interactions

Drug-drug. *Anticoagulants:* Increases risk of bleeding. Monitor patient closely.
Antifibrinolytic drugs: Streptokinase activity is inhibited and reversed by antifibrinolytic drugs such as aminocaproic acid. Use only when indicated during streptokinase therapy.
Aspirin, dipyridamole, drugs that affect platelet activity, indomethacin, phenylbutazone: Increases risk of bleeding. Monitor patient closely.
Combined therapy with low-dose aspirin (162.5 mg) or dipyridamole has improved acute and long-term results.

Effects on lab test results

• May increase PT, PTT, and INR. May decrease hemoglobin and hematocrit.

Pharmacokinetics

Absorption: Administered I.V.
Distribution: Unknown.
Metabolism: Insignificant.
Excretion: Removed from circulation by antibodies and reticuloendothelial system. *Half-life:* First phase, 18 minutes; second phase, 83 minutes.

Route	Onset	Peak	Duration
I.V.	Immediate	20 min-2 hr	4 hr

Action

Chemical effect: Activates plasminogen in two steps. Plasminogen and streptokinase form a complex that exposes plasminogen-activating site. Plasminogen is then converted to plasmin by cleavage of peptide bond.
Therapeutic effect: Dissolves blood clots.

Available forms

Injection: 250,000 IU, 750,000 IU, and 1.5 million IU in vials for reconstitution

NURSING PROCESS

Assessment

• Assess patient's condition before therapy and regularly thereafter.
• Assess patient for increased risk of bleeding (such as from recent surgery, CVA, trauma, or hypertension) before starting therapy.
• Before starting therapy, draw blood to determine APTT and PT. Rate of I.V. infusion depends on thrombin time and streptokinase resistance. Then repeat studies often and keep laboratory flow sheet on patient's chart to monitor APTT, PT, hemoglobin, and hematocrit.
• Monitor patient for excessive bleeding q 15 minutes for first hour, q 30 minutes for second through eighth hours, then once q shift.
• Monitor pulse rates, color, and sensation of limbs q hour.
• Be alert for adverse reactions and drug interactions.
• Evaluate patient's and family's knowledge of drug therapy.

Nursing diagnoses

• Ineffective cardiopulmonary tissue perfusion related to condition
• Risk for deficient fluid volume related to potential for bleeding
• Deficient knowledge related to drug therapy

Planning and implementation

• Drug should be used only by prescriber with experience in thrombotic disease management and in a setting where close monitoring can be performed.
• Before using streptokinase to clear an occluded arteriovenous cannula, try flushing with heparinized saline solution.
• **ALERT:** To check for hypersensitivity reactions, give 100 IU I.D.; wheal and flare response within 20 minutes means patient is probably allergic. Monitor vital signs frequently.
• If patient has had either recent streptococcal infection or recent treatment with streptokinase, higher loading dose may be needed.
• If bleeding occurs, stop therapy and notify prescriber. Pretreatment with heparin or drugs affecting platelets causes high risk of bleeding but may improve long-term results.
• Have aminocaproic acid available to treat bleeding, and corticosteroids to treat allergic reactions.

- Have typed and crossmatched packed RBCs and whole blood ready to treat hemorrhage.
- Keep involved limb in straight alignment to prevent bleeding from infusion site.
- Avoid unnecessary handling of patient, and pad side rails. Bruising is more likely during therapy.
- Keep venipuncture sites to minimum; use pressure dressing on puncture sites for at least 15 minutes.

⊛ **ALERT:** Notify prescriber immediately if hypersensitivity occurs. Antihistamines or corticosteroids may be used to treat mild reactions. If severe reaction occurs, stop infusion and notify prescriber.

- Heparin by continuous infusion is usually started within 1 hour after stopping streptokinase. Use infusion pump to give heparin.
- In patient with acute MI, thrombolytic therapy may decrease infarct size, improve ventricular function, and decrease risk of heart failure. Drug must be given within 6 hours of onset of symptoms for optimal effect.

Patient teaching
- Tell patient to report oozing, bleeding, or signs of hypersensitivity immediately.

☑ Evaluation
- Patient responds well to therapy.
- Patient maintains adequate fluid balance.
- Patient and family state understanding of drug therapy.

streptomycin sulfate
(strep-toh-MIGH-sin SUL-fayt)

Pharmacologic class: aminoglycoside
Therapeutic class: antibiotic
Pregnancy risk category: D

Indications and dosages

▶ **Streptococcal endocarditis.** *Adults:* 1 g I.M. q 12 hours for 1 week, and then 500 mg q 12 hours for 1 week, given with penicillin. *Adults older than age 60:* 500 mg I.M. q 12 hours for 14 days.
▶ **Primary and adjunct treatment in tuberculosis.** *Adults:* 1 g or 15 mg/kg I.M. daily for 2 to 3 months, and then 1 g two or three times weekly.

Children: 20 to 40 mg/kg I.M. daily in divided doses injected deep into large muscle mass. Given with other antituberculars but not with capreomycin. Continue until sputum specimen becomes negative.
▶ **Enterococcal endocarditis.** *Adults:* 1 g I.M. q 12 hours for 2 weeks, and then 500 mg q 12 hours for 4 weeks, given with penicillin.
▶ **Tularemia.** *Adults:* 1 to 2 g I.M. daily in divided doses injected deep into upper outer quadrant of buttocks. Continue for 7 to 14 days until patient is afebrile for 5 to 7 days.

⊠ Adjust-a-dose: For patients with renal impairment, initial dose is the same as for normal renal function. Subsequent doses and frequency determined by renal function study results and blood levels. For creatinine clearance of 50 to 80 ml/minute, give 7.5 mg/kg q 24 hours; if 10 to 50 ml/minute, give 7.5 mg/kg q 24 to 72 hours; if less than 10 ml/minute, give 7.5 mg/kg q 72 to 96 hours.

Contraindications and precautions

- Contraindicated in patients hypersensitive to drug or other aminoglycosides and patients with labyrinthine disease.
- Use cautiously in patients with impaired kidney function or neuromuscular disorders.

⚘ **Lifespan:** In pregnant women, drug is contraindicated. In breast-feeding women and geriatric patients, use cautiously.

Adverse reactions

CNS: *neuromuscular blockade.*
EENT: *ototoxicity (tinnitus, vertigo, hearing loss).*
GI: vomiting, nausea.
GU: some *nephrotoxicity* (not as much as other aminoglycosides).
Hematologic: eosinophilia, *leukopenia, thrombocytopenia.*
Respiratory: *apnea.*
Skin: exfoliative dermatitis.
Other: hypersensitivity reactions, *angioedema, anaphylaxis.*

Interactions

Drug-drug. *Atracurium, doxacurium, mivacurium, pancuronium, rocuronium, tubocurarine, vecuronium:* May increase the effects of nondepolarizing muscle relaxant including prolonged respiratory depression. Use together only when

---
Reactions may be *common,* uncommon, *life-threatening,* or **COMMON AND LIFE-THREATENING.**

necessary. Dose of nondepolarizing muscle relaxant may need to be reduced.
Cephalosporins: Increases risk of nephrotoxicity. Use together cautiously.
Dimenhydrinate: May mask symptoms of streptomycin-induced ototoxicity. Use together cautiously.
I.V. loop diuretics (such as furosemide): Increases ototoxicity. Use together cautiously.
Other aminoglycosides, acyclovir, amphotericin B, cisplatin, methoxyflurane, vancomycin: Increases risk of nephrotoxicity. Monitor patient.

Effects on lab test results

• May increase BUN, creatinine, and nonprotein nitrogen levels.
• May increase eosinophil count. May decrease hemoglobin, hematocrit, and WBC and platelet counts.

Pharmacokinetics

Absorption: Unknown after I.M. administration.
Distribution: Wide distribution although CSF penetration is low; 36% protein-bound.
Metabolism: None.
Excretion: Mainly in urine; less so in bile.
Half-life: 2 to 3 hours.

Route	Onset	Peak	Duration
I.M.	Unknown	1-2 hr	Unknown

Action

Chemical effect: Inhibits protein synthesis by binding directly to 30S ribosomal subunit.
Therapeutic effect: Kills bacteria.

Available forms

Injection: 400 mg/ml, 1 g/2.5 ml ampules

NURSING PROCESS

⚗ Assessment
• Assess patient's infection before therapy and regularly thereafter.
• Obtain specimen for culture and sensitivity tests before first dose except when treating tuberculosis. Therapy may begin pending results.
• **ALERT:** Obtain blood for peak streptomycin level 1 to 2 hours after I.M. injection; for trough levels, draw blood just before next dose. Don't

use heparinized tube because heparin is incompatible with aminoglycosides.
• Evaluate patient's hearing before therapy, during therapy, and 6 months after therapy.
• Be alert for adverse reactions and drug interactions.
• Evaluate patient's and family's knowledge of drug therapy.

✛ Nursing diagnoses
• Infection related to presence of susceptible bacteria
• Disturbed sensory perception (auditory) related to drug-induced adverse reactions
• Deficient knowledge related to drug therapy

▶ Planning and implementation
• Protect hands when preparing because drug is irritating.
• Inject drug deep into upper outer quadrant of buttocks. Rotate injection sites.
• **⚗ ALERT:** Never give streptomycin I.V.
• Encourage adequate fluid intake; patient should be well hydrated while taking drug to minimize chemical irritation of renal tubules.
• In primary treatment of tuberculosis, stop drug when sputum becomes negative.
Patient teaching
• Warn patient that injection may be painful.
• Emphasize the need to drink at least 2,000 ml daily (if not contraindicated) during therapy.
• Instruct patient to report hearing loss, roaring noises, or fullness in ears immediately.

☑ Evaluation
• Patient is free from infection.
• Patient's auditory function remains normal.
• Patient and family state understanding of drug therapy.

succimer
(SUK-sih-mer)
Chemet

Pharmacologic class: heavy metal antagonist
Therapeutic class: chelate
Pregnancy risk category: C

Indications and dosages

▶ **Lead poisoning in children with blood lead levels above 45 mcg/dl.** *Children:* 10 mg/kg or 350 mg/m² q 8 hours for 5 days. Round dose to nearest 100 mg (see table). For next 2 weeks, decrease interval to q 12 hours.

Weight (kg)	Dose (mg)
8-15	100
16-23	200
24-34	300
35-44	400
≥ 45	500

Contraindications and precautions

• Contraindicated in patients hypersensitive to drug.
• Use cautiously in patients with compromised kidney function.
⚘ Lifespan: No considerations reported.

Adverse reactions

CNS: *drowsiness, dizziness, sensory motor neuropathy, sleepiness, paresthesia, headache.*
CV: *arrhythmias.*
EENT: plugged ears, cloudy film in eyes, otitis media, watery eyes, sore throat, rhinorrhea, nasal congestion.
GI: *nausea, vomiting, diarrhea, loss of appetite, abdominal cramps, hemorrhoidal symptoms, metallic taste, loose stools.*
GU: decreased urination, difficult urination, proteinuria.
Hematologic: intermittent eosinophilia.
Musculoskeletal: *leg, kneecap, back, stomach, rib, or flank pain.*
Respiratory: cough, head cold.
Skin: papular rash, herpetic rash, mucocutaneous eruptions, pruritus.
Other: *flulike syndrome,* candidiasis.

Interactions

None reported.

Effects on lab test results

• May increase AST, ALT, alkaline phosphatase, and cholesterol levels.
• May increase eosinophil and platelet counts.
• False-positive results for ketones in urine using nitroprusside reagents (Ketostix) and falsely decreased levels of uric acid and CK have been reported.

Pharmacokinetics

Absorption: Rapid but variable.
Distribution: Unknown.
Metabolism: Rapid and extensive.
Excretion: 39% excreted in feces unchanged; remainder excreted mainly in urine. *Half-life:* 48 hours.

Route	Onset	Peak	Duration
P.O.	Unknown	1-2 hr	Unknown

Action

Chemical effect: Forms water-soluble complexes with lead and increases its excretion in urine.
Therapeutic effect: Relieves signs and symptoms of lead poisoning.

Available forms

Capsules: 100 mg

NURSING PROCESS

▨ Assessment

• Assess child's condition before therapy and regularly thereafter.
• Measure severity by initial blood lead level and by rate and degree of rebound of blood lead level. Use severity as guide for more frequent blood lead monitoring.
• Monitor transaminase level before and at least weekly during therapy. Transient, mild elevations of transaminase level may occur. Monitor patient with history of hepatic disease more closely.
• Monitor patient at least once weekly for rebound blood lead levels. Elevated blood lead levels and associated symptoms may return rapidly after drug is stopped because of redistribution of lead from bone to soft tissues and blood.
• Be alert for adverse reactions.
• If adverse GI reactions occur, monitor patient's hydration.
• Evaluate parents' knowledge of drug therapy.

⊞ Nursing diagnoses

• Ineffective health maintenance related to presence of lead poisoning
• Risk for deficient fluid volume related to drug-induced adverse GI reactions
• Deficient knowledge related to drug therapy

⊠ Planning and implementation

- Course of treatment lasts 19 days. Repeated courses may be needed if indicated by weekly monitoring of blood lead levels.
- A minimum of 2 weeks between courses is recommended unless high blood lead level indicates need for immediate therapy.

⚠ **ALERT:** Administration of succimer with other chelates isn't recommended. Patient who has received edetate calcium disodium with or without dimercaprol may use succimer as subsequent therapy after 4-week interval.

Patient teaching

- Tell parents of child who can't swallow capsule to open it and sprinkle contents on small amount of soft food. Or, medicated beads from capsule may be poured on spoon and followed with flavored beverage such as a fruit drink.
- Help parents identify and remove sources of lead in child's environment. Chelation therapy isn't a substitute for preventing further exposure.
- Tell parents to consult prescriber if rash occurs. Consider possibility of allergic or other mucocutaneous reactions each time drug is used.

☑ Evaluation

- Patient responds well to therapy.
- Patient maintains adequate hydration.
- Parents state understanding of drug therapy.

succinylcholine chloride (suxamethonium chloride)
(SUK-seh-nil-KOH-leen KLOR-ighd)
Anectine, Anectine Flo-Pack, Quelicin, Scoline ◇ , Sucostrin

Pharmacologic class: depolarizing neuromuscular blocker
Therapeutic class: skeletal muscle relaxant
Pregnancy risk category: C

Indications and dosages

▶ **Adjunct to anesthesia to induce skeletal muscle relaxation; to facilitate intubation and assist with mechanical ventilation or orthopedic manipulations (drug of choice); to lessen muscle contractions in pharmacologically or electrically induced seizures.**
Dosage depends on anesthetic used, individual needs, and response.
Adults: 0.6 mg/kg I.V. over 10 to 30 seconds; then 2.5 mg/minute, p.r.n. Or, 2.5 to 4 mg/kg I.M. up to maximum of 150 mg I.M. in deltoid muscle.
Children: 1 to 2 mg/kg I.M. or I.V. Maximum I.M. dose is 150 mg.

▼ I.V. administration

- Store injectable form in refrigerator. Store powder form at room temperature in tightly closed container.
- Use immediately after reconstitution.
- Don't mix with alkaline solutions (thiopental sodium, sodium bicarbonate, or barbiturates).

Contraindications and precautions

- Contraindicated in patients hypersensitive to drug and patients with abnormally low pseudocholinesterase level, angle-closure glaucoma, malignant hyperthermia, or penetrating eye injury.
- Use cautiously in debilitated patients, those receiving quinidine or digoxin therapy, and those with severe burns or trauma, electrolyte imbalances, hyperkalemia, paraplegia, spinal neuraxis injury, CVA, degenerative or dystrophic neuromuscular disease, myasthenia gravis, myasthenic syndrome of lung cancer, bronchogenic carcinoma, dehydration, thyroid disorders, collagen diseases, porphyria, fractures, muscle spasms, eye surgery, pheochromocytoma, respiratory depression, or hepatic, renal, or pulmonary impairment.

☀ **Lifespan:** In women undergoing cesarean section and in breast-feeding women, use large doses cautiously. In elderly patients, use cautiously.

Adverse reactions

CV: *bradycardia,* tachycardia, hypertension, hypotension, *arrhythmias,* flushing, *cardiac arrest.*
EENT: increased intraocular pressure.
Musculoskeletal: muscle fasciculation, *postoperative muscle pain,* myoglobinemia.
Respiratory: *prolonged respiratory depression, apnea, bronchoconstriction.*
Other: *malignant hyperthermia,* excessive salivation, allergic or idiosyncratic hypersensitivity reactions *(anaphylaxis).*

Interactions

Drug-drug. *Aminoglycoside antibiotics, including amikacin, gentamicin, kanamycin, neomycin, streptomycin; anticholinesterase, such as echothiophate, edrophonium, neostigmine, physostigmine, or pyridostigmine; general anesthetics, such as enflurane, halothane, isoflurane; polymyxin antibiotics, such as colistin and polymyxin B sulfate:* Potentiates neuromuscular blockade, leading to increased skeletal muscle relaxation and potentiation of effect. Use cautiously during surgical and postoperative periods.
Cyclophosphamide, lithium, MAO inhibitors: May cause prolonged apnea. Avoid using together; monitor patient closely.
Digoxin: May cause arrhythmias. Use together cautiously.
Methotrimeprazine, opioid analgesics: Potentiates neuromuscular blockade, leading to increased skeletal muscle relaxation and, possibly, respiratory paralysis. Use cautiously.
Parenteral magnesium sulfate: Potentiates neuromuscular blockade, leading to increased skeletal muscle relaxation and, possibly, respiratory paralysis. Use cautiously, preferably with reduced doses.
Drug-herb. *Melatonin:* Potentiates blocking properties of succinylcholine. Discourage using together.

Effects on lab test results

• May increase myoglobin and potassium levels.

Pharmacokinetics

Absorption: Unknown.
Distribution: Distributed in extracellular fluid and rapidly reaches its site of action.
Metabolism: Occurs rapidly by plasma pseudocholinesterase.
Excretion: About 10% excreted unchanged in urine. *Half-life:* Unknown.

Route	Onset	Peak	Duration
I.V.	30 sec-1 min	1-2 min	4-10 min
I.M.	2-3 min	Unknown	10-30 min

Action

Chemical effect: Prolongs depolarization of muscle end plate.
Therapeutic effect: Relaxes skeletal muscles.

Available forms

Injection: 20 mg/ml, 50 mg/ml, 100 mg/ml; 100-mg, 500-mg, and 1-g vials

NURSING PROCESS

🔁 Assessment

• Assess patient's condition before therapy and regularly thereafter.
• Monitor baseline electrolyte determinations and vital signs (check respiratory rate q 5 to 10 minutes during infusion).
• Monitor respiratory rate and pulse oximetry closely until patient is fully recovered from neuromuscular blockade, as evidenced by tests of muscle strength (hand grip, head lift, and ability to cough).
• Be alert for adverse reactions and drug interactions.
• Evaluate patient's and family's knowledge of drug therapy.

🔁 Nursing diagnoses

• Ineffective health maintenance related to underlying condition
• Ineffective breathing pattern related to drug's effect on respiratory muscles
• Deficient knowledge related to drug therapy

⬥ Planning and implementation

⚠ **ALERT:** Only personnel skilled in airway management should give drug.
• Succinylcholine is drug of choice for short procedures (less than 3 minutes) and for orthopedic manipulations; use caution in fractures or dislocations.
• Give sedatives or general anesthetics before neuromuscular blockers. Neuromuscular blockers don't obtund consciousness or alter pain threshold.
• Keep airway clear. Have emergency respiratory support equipment immediately available.
⚠ **ALERT:** Careful drug calculation is essential. Always verify with another professional.
• To evaluate patient's ability to metabolize succinylcholine, give test dose (10 mg I.M. or I.V.) after patient has been anesthetized. Normal response (no respiratory depression or transient depression for up to 5 minutes) indicates drug may be given. Don't give subsequent doses if patient develops respiratory paralysis sufficient to permit endotracheal intubation. (Recovery within 30 to 60 minutes.)

• Give deep I.M., preferably high into deltoid muscle.

• Give analgesics.

⚕ **ALERT:** Reversing drugs shouldn't be used. Unlike what happens with nondepolarizing drugs, giving neostigmine or edrophonium with this depolarizing drug may worsen neuromuscular blockade.

• Repeated or continuous infusions of succinylcholine aren't advised; this may reduce response or prolong muscle relaxation and apnea.

Patient teaching

• Explain all events and happenings to patient because he can still hear.

• Reassure patient that he is being monitored at all times.

• Inform patient that postoperative stiffness is normal and will soon subside.

☑ Evaluation

• Patient responds well to therapy.

• Patient maintains adequate respiratory patterns with mechanical assistance.

• Patient and family state understanding of drug therapy.

sucralfate
(SOO-krahl-fayt)
Carafate, SCF ◇

Pharmacologic class: pepsin inhibitor
Therapeutic class: antiulcerative
Pregnancy risk category: B

Indications and dosages

▶ **Maintenance therapy for duodenal ulcer.**
Adults: 1 g P.O. b.i.d.

▶ **Short-term (up to 8 weeks) treatment of duodenal ulcer; gastric ulcer‡.** *Adults:* 1 g P.O. q.i.d. 1 hour before meals and h.s.

Contraindications and precautions

• Use cautiously in patients with chronic renal impairment.

⚕ **Lifespan:** In pregnant and breast-feeding women, use cautiously. In children, safety of drug hasn't been established.

Adverse reactions

CNS: dizziness, sleepiness, headache, vertigo.

GI: constipation, nausea, gastric discomfort, diarrhea, bezoar formation, vomiting, flatulence, dry mouth, indigestion.
Musculoskeletal: back pain.
Skin: rash, pruritus.

Interactions

Drug-drug. *Antacids:* May decrease binding of drug to gastroduodenal mucosa, impairing effectiveness. Don't give within 30 minutes of each other.
Cimetidine, digoxin, phenytoin, ranitidine, tetracycline, theophylline: Decreases absorption. Separate administration times by at least 2 hours.
Ciprofloxacin, lomefloxacin, moxifloxacin, norfloxacin, ofloxacin: May decrease absorption of the quinolone, reducing anti-infective response. If use together can't be avoided, give at least 6 hours apart.

Effects on lab test results

None reported.

Pharmacokinetics

Absorption: About 3% to 5%. Acts locally
Distribution: Distributed to GI tract and small amount to tissues.
Metabolism: None.
Excretion: About 90% excreted in feces; absorbed drug excreted unchanged in urine. *Half-life:* 6 to 20 hours.

Route	Onset	Peak	Duration
P.O.	Unknown	≤ 6 hr	Unknown

Action

Chemical effect: May adhere to and protect ulcer's surface by forming barrier.
Therapeutic effect: Aids in duodenal ulcer healing.

Available forms

Suspension: 500 mg/5 ml
Tablets: 1 g

NURSING PROCESS

☑ Assessment

• Assess patient's GI symptoms before therapy and regularly thereafter.

• Be alert for adverse reactions and drug interactions.

• Monitor patient for severe, persistent constipation.
• Evaluate patient's and family's knowledge of drug therapy.

⊞ Nursing diagnoses
• Impaired tissue integrity related to presence of duodenal ulcer
• Constipation related to drug-induced adverse GI reactions
• Deficient knowledge related to drug therapy

⟩⟩ Planning and implementation
• Give drug on an empty stomach for best results.
Patient teaching
• Instruct patient to take drug 1 hour before each meal and h.s.
• Tell patient to continue on prescribed regimen to ensure complete healing. Pain and ulcerative symptoms may subside within first few weeks of therapy.
• Urge patient to avoid cigarette smoking because it may increase gastric acid secretion and worsen disease. Also tell patient to avoid alcohol, chocolate, and spicy foods.
• Tell patient to sleep with head of bed elevated.
• Tell patient to avoid large meals within 2 hours before bedtime.

☑ Evaluation
• Patient's ulcer pain is gone.
• Patient maintains normal bowel elimination patterns.
• Patient and family state understanding of drug therapy.

sufentanil citrate
(soo-FEN-tih-nil SIGH-trayt)
Sufenta

Pharmacologic class: opioid agonist analgesic
Therapeutic class: analgesic, adjunct to anesthesia, anesthetic
Pregnancy risk category: C
Controlled substance schedule: II

Indications and dosages

▶ **Adjunct to general anesthetic.** *Adults:* 1 to 8 mcg/kg I.V. with nitrous oxide and oxygen.

▶ **As primary anesthetic.** *Adults:* 8 to 30 mcg/kg I.V. with 100% oxygen and muscle relaxant.
◨ **Adjust-a-dose:** In geriatric and debilitated patients, reduce dosage.

▼ I.V. administration

• Give drug by direct I.V. injection. May be given by intermittent I.V. infusion, but compatibility and stability in I.V. solutions aren't fully known.

Contraindications and precautions

• Contraindicated in patients hypersensitive to drug.
• Drug isn't recommended for prolonged use.
• Use cautiously in debilitated patients and in patients with head injury, decreased respiratory reserve, or pulmonary, hepatic, or renal disease.
⚠ **Lifespan:** In pregnant women, drug isn't recommended in high doses at term. In breast-feeding women and in children, safety of drug hasn't been established. In geriatric patients, use cautiously and at reduced dosage.

Adverse reactions

CNS: chills, somnolence.
CV: *hypotension,* hypertension, **bradycardia,** tachycardia, **arrhythmias.**
GI: nausea, vomiting.
Musculoskeletal: intraoperative muscle movement.
Respiratory: *chest wall rigidity, apnea, bronchospasm.*
Skin: *pruritus,* erythema.

Interactions

Drug-drug. *CNS depressants:* May have additive effects. Use together cautiously.
Drug-lifestyle. *Alcohol use:* May have additive effects. Discourage using together.

Effects on lab test results

None reported.

Pharmacokinetics

Absorption: Administered I.V.
Distribution: Highly protein-bound and redistributed rapidly.
Metabolism: Probably in liver and small intestine.
Excretion: Primarily in urine. *Half-life:* About 2½ hours.

Route	Onset	Peak	Duration
I.V.	1-2 min	1-2 min	45 sec-5 min

Action

Chemical effect: Binds with opioid receptors in CNS, altering perception of and emotional response to pain through unknown mechanism.
Therapeutic effect: Relieves pain and promotes loss of consciousness.

Available forms

Injection: 50 mcg/ml in 1-ml, 2-ml, and 5-ml ampules

NURSING PROCESS

⚖ Assessment
• Assess patient's condition before therapy and regularly thereafter.
• Because drug decreases rate and depth of respirations, monitor patient's arterial oxygen saturation to help assess respiratory depression.
• Monitor respiratory rate of neonates exposed to drug during labor.
• Monitor postoperative vital signs.
• Be alert for adverse reactions and drug interactions.
• Evaluate patient's and family's knowledge of drug therapy.

🔲 Nursing diagnoses
• Ineffective health maintenance related to underlying condition
• Ineffective breathing pattern related to respiratory depression
• Deficient knowledge related to drug therapy

⟩ Planning and implementation
• Only personnel specifically trained in use of I.V. anesthetics should give drug.
• For obese patient weighing more than 20% of ideal body weight, base dosage calculations on an estimate of ideal weight.
• When used at doses over 8 mcg/kg, postoperative mechanical ventilation and observation are essential because of prolonged respiratory depression.
• Keep opioid antagonist (naloxone) and resuscitation equipment available.
• If respiratory rate falls below 12 breaths/minute, notify prescriber.

⚠ **ALERT:** High doses can produce muscle rigidity reversible by neuromuscular blockers; however, patient must be artificially ventilated.
⚠ **ALERT:** Don't confuse sufentanil with alfentanil or fentanyl, or Sufenta with Survanta.
Patient teaching
• Inform patient and family that drug will be used as part of patient's anesthesia.

✓ Evaluation
• Patient responds well to therapy.
• Patient maintains adequate ventilation with mechanical support, if needed.
• Patient and family state understanding of drug therapy.

sulfasalazine (salazosulfapyridine, sulphasalazine)
(sul-fuh-SAL-uh-zeen)
Azulfidine, Azulfidine EN-Tabs, PMS-Sulfasalazine E.C. ♦, Salazopyrin ♦, Salazopyrin EN-Tabs ♦ ◇, S.A.S.-500 ♦, S.A.S. Enteric-500 ♦

Pharmacologic class: sulfonamide
Therapeutic class: anti-inflammatory
Pregnancy risk category: B

Indications and dosages

▶ **Mild to moderate ulcerative colitis, adjunct therapy in severe ulcerative colitis, Crohn's disease.** *Adults:* Initially, 3 to 4 g P.O. daily in evenly divided doses; usual maintenance dosage is 2 g P.O. daily in divided doses q 6 hours. Dosage may be started with 1 to 2 g, with gradual increase to minimize adverse effects.
Children older than age 2: Initially, 40 to 60 mg/kg P.O. daily, divided into three to six doses; then 30 mg/kg daily in four doses. If GI intolerance occurs, reduce dosage.
▶ **Rheumatoid arthritis in patients who have responded inadequately to salicylates or NSAIDs.** *Adults:* 2 g P.O. daily b.i.d. in evenly divided doses. Dosage may be started at 0.5 to 1 g daily and be gradually increased over 3 weeks to reduce GI intolerance.
▶ **Patients with polyarticular-course juvenile rheumatoid arthritis who have responded inadequately to salicylates or other NSAIDs.**

Children age 6 and older: 30 to 50 mg/kg P.O. daily in two divided doses (as delayed release tablet). Maximum dose is 2 g daily. To reduce GI intolerance, start with one-fourth to one-third of planned maintenance dose and increase weekly until reaching maintenance dose at 1 month.

Contraindications and precautions

• Contraindicated in patients hypersensitive to drug or its metabolites, and patients with porphyria or intestinal or urinary obstruction.

• Use cautiously and in reduced dosages in patients with impaired liver or kidney function, severe allergy, bronchial asthma, or G6PD deficiency.

⚖ **Lifespan:** In pregnant and breast-feeding women, use cautiously. In infants younger than age 2, drug is contraindicated.

Adverse reactions

CNS: headache, depression, *seizures,* hallucinations.

GI: *nausea, vomiting, diarrhea,* abdominal pain, anorexia, stomatitis.

GU: *toxic nephrosis with oliguria and anuria,* crystalluria, hematuria, oligospermia, infertility.

Hematologic: *agranulocytosis, aplastic anemia,* megaloblastic anemia, *thrombocytopenia, leukopenia,* hemolytic anemia.

Hepatic: jaundice, *hepatotoxicity.*

Skin: *erythema multiforme, Stevens-Johnson syndrome, generalized skin eruption, epidermal necrolysis,* exfoliative dermatitis, photosensitivity reactions, urticaria, pruritus.

Other: *hypersensitivity reactions (serum sickness, drug fever, anaphylaxis).*

Interactions

Drug-drug. *Antibiotics:* May alter action of sulfasalazine by altering internal flora. Monitor patient closely.

Digoxin: May reduce digoxin absorption. Monitor patient closely.

Folic acid: Absorption may be decreased. No intervention needed.

Hormonal contraceptives: Decreases contraceptive effectiveness and increased risk of breakthrough bleeding. Suggest non-hormonal contraceptive.

Iron: Lowers sulfasalazine level caused by iron chelation. Monitor patient closely.

Oral anticoagulants: Increases anticoagulant effect. Monitor patient for bleeding.

Oral antidiabetics: Increases hypoglycemic effect. Monitor glucose level.

Drug-herb. *Dong quai, St. John's wort:* Increases risk of photosensitivity. Discourage using together.

Effects on lab test results

• May increase AST and ALT levels.
• May decrease hemoglobin, hematocrit, and granulocyte, platelet, RBC, and WBC counts.

Pharmacokinetics

Absorption: Poor; 70% to 90% transported to colon, where intestinal flora metabolize drug to its active ingredients, which exert their effects locally. One metabolite, sulfapyridine, is absorbed from colon, but only small portion of metabolite 5-aminosalicylic acid is absorbed.
Distribution: Distributed locally in colon. Distribution of absorbed metabolites is unknown.
Metabolism: Divided by intestinal flora in colon.
Excretion: Systemically absorbed sulfasalazine is excreted chiefly in urine. *Half-life:* 6 to 8 hours.

Route	Onset	Peak	Duration
P.O.			
parent drug	Unknown	1½-6 hr	Unknown
metabolites	Unknown	12-24 hr	Unknown

Action

Chemical effect: Unknown.
Therapeutic effect: Relieves inflammation in GI tract.

Available forms

Oral suspension: 250 mg/5 ml
Tablets (with or without enteric coating): 500 mg

NURSING PROCESS

⏧ Assessment

• Assess patient's condition before therapy and regularly thereafter.
• Be alert for adverse reactions and drug interactions.
• Monitor patient's hydration throughout drug therapy.
• Evaluate patient's and family's knowledge of drug therapy.

Reactions may be *common,* uncommon, *life-threatening,* or **COMMON AND LIFE-THREATENING.**

Nursing diagnoses
- Acute pain related to inflammation of GI tract
- Risk for deficient fluid volume related to drug-induced adverse GI reactions
- Deficient knowledge related to drug therapy

Planning and implementation
- Minimize adverse GI symptoms by spacing doses evenly and giving after food intake.
- Drug colors alkaline urine orange-yellow.
- **ALERT:** If patient shows evidence of hypersensitivity, stop immediately and notify prescriber.
- **ALERT:** Don't confuse sulfasalazine with sulfisoxazole, salsalate, or sulfadiazine.

Patient teaching
- Instruct patient to take drug after meals and to space doses evenly.
- Warn patient that drug may cause skin and urine to turn orange-yellow and may permanently stain soft contact lenses yellow.
- Warn patient to avoid direct sunlight and ultraviolet light to prevent photosensitivity reaction.

Evaluation
- Patient is free from pain.
- Patient maintains adequate hydration.
- Patient and family state understanding of drug therapy.

sulfinpyrazone
(sul-fin-PEER-uh-zohn)
Anturan ◆ , Anturane

Pharmacologic class: uricosuric
Therapeutic class: renal tubular blocker, platelet aggregation inhibitor
Pregnancy risk category: NR

Indications and dosages
▶ **Intermittent or chronic gouty arthritis.**
Adults: Initially, 100 mg to 200 mg P.O. b.i.d. during the first week; then 200 mg to 400 mg P.O. b.i.d. Maximum dosage is 800 mg daily. After urate level is controlled, dosage can sometimes be reduced to 200 mg daily in divided doses.
▶ **Prophylaxis of thromboembolic disorders, including angina, MI, transient (cerebral) ischemic attacks, and presence of prosthetic heart valves‡.** *Adults:* 600 to 800 mg P.O. daily

in divided doses to decrease platelet aggregation.

Contraindications and precautions
- Contraindicated in patients hypersensitive to pyrazole derivatives (including oxyphenbutazone and phenylbutazone) and patients with active peptic ulcer, symptoms of GI inflammation or ulceration, or blood dyscrasias.
- Use cautiously in patients with healed peptic ulcer.
- **Lifespan:** In pregnant women, use cautiously. In breast-feeding women and in children, safety of drug hasn't been established.

Adverse reactions
GI: *nausea, dyspepsia,* epigastric pain, reactivation of peptic ulcerations.
Hematologic: *blood dyscrasias* (such as anemia, *leukopenia, agranulocytosis, thrombocytopenia, aplastic anemia*).
Respiratory: *bronchoconstriction* in patients with aspirin-induced asthma.
Skin: rash.

Interactions
Drug-drug. *Aspirin, niacin, salicylates:* Inhibits uricosuric effect of sulfinpyrazone. Don't use together.
Oral anticoagulants: Increases anticoagulant effect and risk of bleeding. Use together cautiously.
Oral antidiabetics: Increases effects. Monitor glucose level closely.
Probenecid: Inhibits renal excretion of sulfinpyrazone. Use together cautiously.
Drug-lifestyle. *Alcohol use:* Decreases drug effectiveness. Discourage use together.

Effects on lab test results
- May increase BUN and creatinine levels.
- May decrease hemoglobin, hematocrit, and RBC, WBC, granulocyte, and platelet counts.

Pharmacokinetics
Absorption: Complete.
Distribution: 98% to 99% protein-bound.
Metabolism: Rapid.
Excretion: Excreted in urine; about 50% excreted unchanged. *Half-life:* 4 to 6 hours.

Route	Onset	Peak	Duration
P.O.	Unknown	1-2 hr	4-6 hr

Action

Chemical effect: Blocks renal tubular reabsorption of uric acid, increasing excretion, and inhibits platelet aggregation.
Therapeutic effect: Relieves signs and symptoms of gouty arthritis.

Available forms

Capsules: 200 mg
Tablets: 100 mg

NURSING PROCESS

▧ Assessment
• Assess patient's condition before therapy and regularly thereafter.
• Monitor BUN level, CBC, and kidney function studies periodically during long-term use.
• Monitor fluid intake and output. Therapy may lead to renal colic and formation of uric acid stones until acid levels are normal (about 6 mg/dl).
• Be alert for adverse reactions and drug interactions.
• Evaluate patient's and family's knowledge of drug therapy.

⊞ Nursing diagnoses
• Ineffective health maintenance related to presence of gouty arthritis
• Risk for injury related to drug-induced adverse CNS reactions
• Deficient knowledge related to drug therapy

▷ Planning and implementation
• Give drug with milk, food, or antacids to minimize GI disturbances.
• Encourage patient to drink fluids to maintain minimum daily output of 2 to 3 L. Alkalinize urine with sodium bicarbonate or other agent. Keep in mind that alkalinizers are used therapeutically to increase drug activity, preventing urolithiasis.
• Drug is recommended for patients unresponsive to probenecid. Suitable for long-term use; neither cumulative effects nor tolerance develops.
• Drug contains no analgesic or anti-inflammatory and is of no value during acute gout attacks.
• Drug may increase frequency, severity, and length of acute gout attacks during first 6 to 12 months of therapy. Prophylactic colchicine

or another anti-inflammatory is given during first 3 to 6 months.
• Lifelong therapy may be needed in patient with hyperuricemia.
• Drug decreases urinary excretion of aminohippuric acid, interfering with laboratory test results.
⑤ **ALERT:** Don't confuse Anturane with Artane or Antabuse.
Patient teaching
• Warn patient with gout not to take aspirin-containing drugs because they may precipitate gout. Acetaminophen may be used for pain.
• Tell patient to take drug with food, milk, or antacid. Also instruct him to drink plenty of water.
• Instruct patient with gout to avoid foods high in purine, such as anchovies, liver, sardines, kidneys, sweetbreads, peas, and lentils.
• Inform patient and family that drug must be taken regularly or gout attacks may result. Tell patient to visit prescriber regularly so blood levels can be monitored and dosage adjusted if needed.

☑ Evaluation
• Patient regains and maintains normal uric acid level.
• Patient doesn't experience injury from adverse CNS reactions.
• Patient and family state understanding of drug therapy.

sulindac
(SUL-in-dak)
Aclin ◇, Apo-Sulin ♦, Clinoril, Novo-Sundac ♦

Pharmacologic class: NSAID
Therapeutic class: non-opioid analgesic, antipyretic, anti-inflammatory
Pregnancy risk category: NR

Indications and dosages

▶ **Osteoarthritis, rheumatoid arthritis, ankylosing spondylitis.** *Adults:* Initially, 150 mg P.O. b.i.d.; increase to 200 mg b.i.d., p.r.n.
▶ **Acute subacromial bursitis or supraspinatus tendinitis, acute gouty arthritis.** *Adults:* 200 mg P.O. b.i.d. for 7 to 14 days. Reduce dose as symptoms subside.

Contraindications and precautions

• Contraindicated in patients hypersensitive to drug and in patients for whom aspirin or NSAIDs precipitate.
• Use cautiously in patients with history of ulcers and GI bleeding, renal dysfunction, compromised cardiac function or hypertension, or conditions predisposing to fluid retention.
⚖ Lifespan: In pregnant women, drug isn't recommended. In breast-feeding women and in children, safety of drug hasn't been established.

Adverse reactions

CNS: dizziness, headache, nervousness, psychosis.
CV: hypertension, *heart failure,* palpitations, edema.
EENT: tinnitus, transient visual disturbances.
GI: *epigastric distress,* peptic ulceration, *pancreatitis, GI bleeding,* occult blood loss, nausea, constipation, dyspepsia, flatulence, anorexia.
GU: interstitial nephritis, *nephrotic syndrome, renal failure.*
Hematologic: *aplastic anemia, thrombocytopenia, neutropenia, agranulocytosis,* hemolytic anemia.
Skin: *rash,* pruritus.
Other: drug fever, *anaphylaxis,* hypersensitivity syndrome, *angioedema.*

Interactions

Drug-drug. *Anticoagulants:* Increases risk of bleeding. Monitor PT closely.
Aspirin: Decreases sulindac level and increases risk of adverse GI reactions. Avoid using together.
Cyclosporine: Increases nephrotoxicity of cyclosporine. Monitor renal function.
Diflunisal, dimethyl sulfoxide: Decreases metabolism of sulindac to its active metabolite, reducing its effectiveness. Don't use together.
Methotrexate: Increases methotrexate toxicity. Avoid using together.
Probenecid: Increases levels of sulindac and its active metabolite. Monitor patient for toxicity.
Sulfonamides, sulfonylureas, other highly protein-bound drugs: May displace these drugs from protein-binding sites, leading to increased toxicity. Monitor patient closely for toxicity.

Effects on lab test results

• May increase BUN, creatinine, liver enzyme, and potassium levels.
• May increase bleeding time. May decrease hemoglobin, hematocrit, and platelet, neutrophil, and granulocyte counts.

Pharmacokinetics

Absorption: Rapid and complete.
Distribution: Highly protein-bound.
Metabolism: Drug is inactive and metabolized in liver to an active sulfide metabolite.
Excretion: Excreted in urine. *Half-life:* Parent drug, 8 hours; active metabolite, about 16 hours.

Route	Onset	Peak	Duration
P.O.	Unknown	2-4 hr	Unknown

Action

Chemical effect: Unknown; produces anti-inflammatory, analgesic, and antipyretic effects, possibly by inhibiting prostaglandin synthesis.
Therapeutic effect: Relieves pain, fever, and inflammation.

Available forms

Tablets: 100 mg ◊, 150 mg, 200 mg

NURSING PROCESS

Assessment
• Assess patient's condition before therapy and regularly thereafter.
• Periodically monitor liver and kidney function and CBC in patient receiving long-term therapy.
• Be alert for adverse reactions and drug interactions.
• Evaluate patient's and family's knowledge of drug therapy.

Nursing diagnoses
• Acute pain related to presence of arthritis
• Impaired tissue integrity related to drug's adverse effect on GI mucosa
• Deficient knowledge related to drug therapy

Planning and implementation
• Notify prescriber of adverse reactions.
Patient teaching
• Tell patient to take drug with food, milk, or antacids to reduce adverse GI reactions.

• Advise patient to refrain from driving or performing other hazardous activities that require mental alertness until CNS effects are known.

• Teach patient signs and symptoms of GI bleeding, and tell him to contact prescriber immediately if they occur. Serious GI toxicity, including peptic ulceration and bleeding, can occur in patient taking NSAIDs despite absence of GI symptoms.

⊛ **ALERT:** Tell patient to notify prescriber immediately if easy bruising or prolonged bleeding occurs.

• Instruct patient to report edema and have blood pressure checked monthly. Drug causes sodium retention but may not affect kidneys as much as other NSAIDs.

• Instruct patient not to take aspirin or aspirin-containing products with sulindac.

• Tell patient to notify prescriber and undergo complete eye examination if visual disturbances occur.

☑ Evaluation

• Patient is free from pain.

• Patient doesn't experience adverse GI reactions.

• Patient and family state understanding of drug therapy.

---

sumatriptan succinate
(soo-muh-TRIP-ten SEK-seh-nayt)
Imitrex

Pharmacologic class: selective 5-hydroxytryptamine (5-HT$_1$) receptor agonist
Therapeutic class: antimigraine drug
Pregnancy risk category: C

Indications and dosages

▶ **Acute migraine attacks (with or without aura).** *Adults:* 6 mg S.C. Maximum recommended dose is two 6-mg injections in 24 hours, separated by at least 1 hour. Or, 25 to 100 mg P.O. initially. If response isn't achieved in 2 hours, may give second dose of 25 to 100 mg. Additional doses may be used in at least 2-hour intervals. Maximum daily oral dose, 200 mg. Or, 5 mg, 10 mg, or 20 mg administered once in one nostril. May repeat once after 2 hours for maximum daily inhalation dose of 40 mg. A

10-mg dose may be achieved by the administration of a single 5-mg dose in each nostril.

▶ **Acute treatment of cluster headache episodes.** *Adults:* 6 mg S.C. Maximum recommended dose is two 6-mg injections in 24 hours, separated by at least 1 hour.

⩟ **Adjust-a-dose:** For patients with hepatic impairment, don't exceed maximum single oral dose of 50 mg.

Contraindications and precautions

• Contraindicated in patients hypersensitive to drug or its components and in patients with history, symptoms, or signs of ischemic cardiac, cerebrovascular (CVA, transient ischemic attack), or peripheral vascular (ischemic bowel disease) syndromes. Also contraindicated in patients with uncontrolled hypertension, severe hepatic impairment, or significant underlying CV diseases, including angina pectoris, MI, or silent myocardial ischemia. Also contraindicated within 24 hours of another 5-HT agonist or ergotamine-containing medication and within 14 days of MAO inhibitor therapy.

• Use cautiously in patients who may have unrecognized coronary artery disease (CAD), such as postmenopausal women, men older than age 40, and patients with risk factors for CAD, such as hypertension, hypercholesterolemia, obesity, diabetes, smoking, or family history of CAD.

⚖ **Lifespan:** In pregnant women and women who intend to become pregnant, use cautiously. In breast-feeding women and in children, safety of drug hasn't been established.

Adverse reactions

CNS: *dizziness, vertigo,* drowsiness, headache, anxiety, malaise, fatigue.
CV: **atrial fibrillation, ventricular fibrillation, ventricular tachycardia, coronary artery vasospasm, transient myocardial ischemia, MI,** pressure or tightness in chest.
EENT: discomfort of throat, nasal cavity or sinus, mouth, jaw, or tongue; altered vision.
GI: abdominal discomfort, dysphagia, diarrhea; nausea, vomiting, unusual or bad taste (nasal spray).
Musculoskeletal: myalgia, muscle cramps, neck pain.
Respiratory: upper respiratory inflammation and dyspnea (P.O.).
Skin: diaphoresis.

Other: *warm or hot sensation; burning sensation;* heaviness, pressure or tightness; tight feeling in head; cold sensation; numbness; flushing, *tingling, injection site reaction* (S.C.).

Interactions

Drug-drug. *Ergot and ergot derivatives; other Serotonin $_{1B/1D}$ agonists:* Prolongs vasospastic effects. Don't use within 24 hours of sumatriptan therapy.
MAO inhibitors: Reduces sumatriptan clearance. Avoid using sumatriptan tablets or nasal spray within 2 weeks of stopping MAO inhibitor. Use injection cautiously in patients and decrease sumatriptan dose.
SSRIs: May cause weakness, hyperreflexia and incoordination. Monitor patient closely if use together is warranted.
Drug-herb. *Horehound:* May enhance serotonergic effects. Discourage using together.

Effects on lab test results

None reported.

Pharmacokinetics

Absorption: Rapid after P.O. administration but with low absolute bioavailability (about 15%); absorbed well from injection site after S.C. administration.
Distribution: Drug has low protein-binding of about 14% to 21%.
Metabolism: About 80%, in liver.
Excretion: Excreted primarily in urine. *Half-life:* About 2 hours.

Route	Onset	Peak	Duration
P.O.	30 min	2-4 hr	Unknown
S.C.	10-20 min	1-2 hr	Unknown
Intranasal	Rapid	1-2 hr	Unknown

Action

Chemical effect: Unknown; thought to selectively activate vascular serotonin (5-HT) receptors. Stimulation of specific receptor subtype 5-HT$_1$, present on cranial arteries and the dura mater, causes vasoconstriction of cerebral vessels but has minimal effects on systemic vessels, tissue perfusion, and blood pressure.
Therapeutic effect: Relieves acute migraine pain.

Available forms

Injection: 6 mg/0.5 ml (12 mg/ml) in 0.5-ml prefilled syringes and vials
Nasal spray: 5 mg/spray; 20 mg/spray
Tablets: 25 mg, 50 mg, 100 mg (base) ◆

NURSING PROCESS

Assessment
• Assess patient's condition before therapy and regularly thereafter.
• Be alert for adverse reactions and drug interactions.
• Evaluate patient's and family's knowledge of drug therapy.

Nursing diagnoses
• Acute pain related to presence of acute migraine attack
• Risk for injury related to drug-induced adverse reactions
• Deficient knowledge related to drug therapy

Planning and implementation
• If patient has risk of unrecognized CAD, give first dose with prescriber present.
• Give single tablet whole with fluids as soon as patient complains of migraine symptoms. Give second tablet if symptoms come back, but no sooner than 2 hours after first tablet.
• Maximum recommended S.C. dosage in 24-hour period is two 6-mg injections separated by at least 1 hour. If patient doesn't experience relief, notify prescriber.
• Patient will most likely experience relief within 1 to 2 hours.
• Redness or pain at injection site should subside within 1 hour after injection.
⚠ **ALERT:** Serious adverse cardiac effects can follow S.C. administration of this drug, but such events are rare.
• If patient doesn't experience relief, notify prescriber.
⚠ **ALERT:** Don't confuse sumatriptan with somatropin.

Patient teaching
• Make sure patient understands that drug is intended only to treat migraine attack, not to prevent or reduce number of attacks.
• Tell patient that drug may be given at any time during migraine attack but should be given as soon as symptoms appear.

• Drug is available in spring-loaded injector system that makes it easy for the patient to give injection to himself. Review detailed information with patient. Make sure patient understands how to load injector, give injection, and dispose of used syringes.

• Instruct patient taking P.O. form when and how often to take drug. Warn patient not to take more than 300 mg within 24 hours.

• Instruct patient to use intranasal spray in one nostril (if 10 mg dose is ordered, 1 spray into each nostril). A second spray may be used if headache returns, but not before 2 hours has elapsed from the first use.

• Tell patient who experiences persistent or severe chest pain to call prescriber immediately. Patient who experiences pain or tightness in throat, wheezing, heart throbbing, rash, lumps, hives, or swollen eyelids, face, or lips should stop using drug and call prescriber.

• Tell woman who is pregnant or intends to become pregnant not to take this drug.

☑ Evaluation
• Patient is free from pain.
• Patient doesn't experience injury from adverse CV reactions.
• Patient and family state understanding of drug therapy.

tacrine hydrochloride
(TAK-reen high-droh-KLOR-ighd)
Cognex

Pharmacologic class: centrally acting reversible anticholinesterase
Therapeutic class: psychotherapeutic for Alzheimer's disease
Pregnancy risk category: C

Indications and dosages

▶ **Mild to moderate dementia of Alzheimer's type.** *Adults:* Initially, 10 mg P.O. q.i.d. After 6 weeks, if patient tolerates drug and transaminase levels aren't elevated, increase dosage to 20 mg q.i.d. After another 6 weeks, increase

dosage to 30 mg q.i.d. If still tolerated, increase to 40 mg q.i.d. after another 6 weeks.

Contraindications and precautions

• Contraindicated in patients hypersensitive to drug or acridine derivatives and in those who have previously developed drug-related jaundice and been confirmed with elevated total bilirubin level of more than 3 mg/dl.

• Use cautiously in patients with sick sinus syndrome or bradycardia; those at risk for peptic ulceration (including patients taking NSAIDs or those with history of peptic ulcer); those with history of hepatic disease; and those with renal disease, asthma, prostatic hyperplasia, or other urinary outflow impairment.

⚕ Lifespan: In pregnant and breast-feeding women, drug isn't recommended. In children, drug isn't indicated.

Adverse reactions

CNS: agitation, ataxia, insomnia, abnormal thinking, somnolence, depression, anxiety, *headache,* fatigue, *dizziness,* confusion.
CV: chest pain, facial flushing.
EENT: rhinitis.
GI: *nausea, vomiting,* anorexia, *diarrhea,* dyspepsia, loose stools, changes in stool color, constipation.
Hepatic: jaundice.
Metabolic: weight loss.
Musculoskeletal: myalgia.
Respiratory: upper respiratory tract infection, cough.
Skin: rash.

Interactions

Drug-drug. *Anticholinergics:* Drug may decrease effectiveness of anticholinergics. Monitor patient closely.
Anticholinesterases, cholinergics (such as bethanechol): May have additive effects. Monitor patient for toxicity.
Cimetidine: May increase tacrine levels. Monitor patient for toxicity.
Fluvoxamine: May increase tacrine levels. Monitor patient.
Succinylcholine: Enhances neuromuscular blockade and prolongs duration of action. Monitor patient.
Theophylline: Increases theophylline level and prolongs theophylline half-life. Carefully monitor theophylline level and adjust dosage.

Reactions may be *common,* uncommon, *life-threatening,* or COMMON AND LIFE-THREATENING.

Drug-food. *Any food:* Decreases drug absorption. Tell patient to take drug on empty stomach.
Drug-lifestyle. *Smoking:* Decreases levels of drug. Monitor response.

Effects on lab test results

• May increase ALT and AST levels.

Pharmacokinetics

Absorption: Rapid with absolute bioavailability of about 17%. Food reduces bioavailability by 30% to 40%.
Distribution: About 55% bound to plasma proteins.
Metabolism: Undergoes first-pass metabolism, which is dose-dependent; extensively metabolized.
Excretion: Excreted in urine. *Half-life:* 2 to 4 hours.

Route	Onset	Peak	Duration
P.O.	Unknown	30 min-3 hr	Unknown

Action

Chemical effect: Reversibly inhibits enzyme cholinesterase in CNS, allowing buildup of acetylcholine.
Therapeutic effect: Improves thinking in patients with Alzheimer's disease.

Available forms

Capsules: 10 mg, 20 mg, 30 mg, 40 mg

NURSING PROCESS

℞ Assessment

• Assess patient's cognitive ability before therapy and regularly thereafter.
• Monitor ALT levels weekly during first 18 weeks of therapy. If ALT is twice the upper limit of normal range after first 18 weeks, continue weekly monitoring. If no problems occur, decrease frequency of testing to q 3 months. Whenever dosage is increased, resume weekly monitoring for at least 6 weeks.
• For patients with ALT three to five times the upper limit of normal range, reduce dosage by 40 mg daily and monitor ALT weekly until normal. If ALT is more than five times upper limit of normal, stop therapy and monitor patient for signs and symptoms of hepatitis. May rechallenge when ALT returns to normal.

• Evaluate patient's and family's knowledge of drug therapy.

🔄 Nursing diagnoses

• Disturbed thought processes related to Alzheimer's disease
• Diarrhea related to drug-induced adverse GI reactions
• Deficient knowledge related to drug therapy

▶ Planning and implementation

• Give drug between meals. If GI upset becomes a problem, give drug with meals, although level may drop by 30% to 40%.
• If drug is stopped for 4 weeks or more, restart full dosage adjustment and monitoring schedule.
• Obtain order for antidiarrheal, if indicated.
Patient teaching
• Inform patient and family that drug doesn't alter underlying degenerative disease. Instead, it may alleviate symptoms of Alzheimer's disease.
• Explain to patient and family that the effect of therapy depends on taking the drug at regular intervals.
⚠ ALERT: Instruct caregivers when to give drug. Explain that dosage adjustment is integral to safe use. Abruptly stopping or reducing daily dose by 80 mg or more may trigger behavioral disturbances and cognitive decline.
• Advise patient and caregivers to report immediately any significant adverse effects or changes in status.

☑ Evaluation

• Patient exhibits improved cognitive ability.
• Patient or caregiver states that drug-induced diarrhea hasn't occurred.
• Patient and family state understanding of drug therapy.

tacrolimus
(tek-roh-LYE-mus)
Prograf

Pharmacologic class: bacteria-derived macrolide
Therapeutic class: immunosuppressant
Pregnancy risk category: C

Indications and dosages

▶ **Prophylaxis of organ rejection in allogenic liver transplantation.** *Adults:* 0.03 to 0.05 mg/kg I.V. daily as continuous infusion given at least 6 hours after transplantation. P.O. therapy should be substituted as soon as possible, with first dose given 8 to 12 hours after discontinuing I.V. infusion. Recommended initial P.O. dosage is 0.1 to 0.15 mg/kg daily in two divided doses q 12 hours. Adjust dosage according to response.
Children: Initially, 0.03 to 0.05 mg/kg I.V. daily, followed by 0.15 to 0.2 mg/kg P.O. daily on schedule similar to that for adults; adjust dosage, p.r.n.

▶ **Prophylaxis of organ rejection in allogenic kidney transplantation.** *Adults:* 0.03 to 0.05 mg/kg I.V. daily as continuous infusion given at least 6 hours after transplantation. P.O. therapy should be substituted as soon as possible. Recommended initial P.O. dosage is 0.2 mg/kg daily administered in two divided doses q 12 hours. Initial dose may be given within 24 hours of transplantation but delayed until creatinine equals or exceeds 4 mg/dl.

▼ I.V. administration

• Dilute drug with normal saline solution injection or D₅W injection to 0.004 to 0.02 mg/ml before use.
• Each required daily dose of diluted drug is infused continuously over 24 hours.
• Monitor patient continuously during first 30 minutes of infusion; then monitor frequently for anaphylaxis.
• Keep epinephrine 1:1,000 available to treat anaphylaxis.
• Store diluted solution for no more than 24 hours in glass or polyethylene containers. Don't store drug in polyvinyl chloride container.

Contraindications and precautions

• Contraindicated in patients hypersensitive to drug. I.V. form contraindicated in patients hypersensitive to castor oil derivatives.
※ Lifespan: In pregnant and breast-feeding women, drug isn't recommended.

Adverse reactions

CNS: *asthenia, headache, tremor, insomnia, paresthesia, delirium, **coma**, pain, fever, **neurotoxicity.***
CV: *hypertension, peripheral edema.*

GI: *ascites, diarrhea, nausea, constipation, anorexia, vomiting, abdominal pain.*
GU: *abnormal kidney function,* UTI, oliguria, *nephrotoxicity.*
Hematologic: *anemia,* leukocytosis, THROMBOCYTOPENIA.
Metabolic: *hyperkalemia,* hypokalemia, *hyperglycemia, hypomagnesemia.*
Musculoskeletal: *back pain.*
Respiratory: *pleural effusion, atelectasis, dyspnea.*
Skin: *photosensitivity reactions.*
Other: *anaphylaxis.*

Interactions

Drug-drug. *Bromocriptine, cimetidine, clarithromycin, clotrimazole, cyclosporine, danazol, diltiazem, erythromycin, ethinyl estradiol, fluconazole, itraconazole, ketoconazole, methylprednisolone, metoclopramide, nefazodone, nicardipine, nifedipine, omeprazole, protease inhibitors, verapamil:* May increase tacrolimus level. Monitor patient for adverse effects.
Carbamazepine, phenobarbital, phenytoin, rifabutin, rifampin: May decrease tacrolimus level. Monitor effectiveness of tacrolimus.
Cyclosporine: Increases risk of excess nephrotoxicity. Don't give together.
Immunosuppressants (except adrenocorticosteroids): May over-suppress immune system. Monitor patient closely, especially during times of stress.
Inducers of CYP enzyme system: May increase tacrolimus metabolism and decrease plasma level. Dosage adjustment may be needed.
Inhibitors of CYP enzyme system: May decrease tacrolimus metabolism and increase plasma level. Dosage adjustment may be needed.
Nephrotoxic drugs (such as aminoglycosides, amphotericin B, cisplatin, cyclosporine): May cause additive or synergistic effects. Monitor patient closely.
Viral vaccines: Tacrolimus may interfere with immune response to live virus vaccines.
Drug-herb. *St. John's wort:* May decrease tacrolimus level. Monitor effectiveness of tacrolimus.
Drug-food. *Any food:* Inhibits drug absorption. Tell patient to take drug on an empty stomach.
Grapefruit juice: Increases drug levels in liver transplant patients. Discourage use together.

Reactions may be *common,* uncommon, *life-threatening,* or COMMON AND LIFE-THREATENING.

Effects on lab test results

• May increase glucose, creatinine, and BUN levels. May decrease magnesium level. May increase or decrease potassium level.
• May increase WBC count and liver function test values. May decrease hemoglobin, hematocrit, and platelet count.

Pharmacokinetics

Absorption: Variable. Food reduces absorption and bioavailability of drug.
Distribution: Distribution between whole blood and plasma depends on several factors, such as hematocrit, temperature of separation of plasma, drug level, and protein level. Drug is 75% to 99% protein-bound.
Metabolism: Extensive.
Excretion: Primarily in bile; less than 1% excreted unchanged in urine. *Half-life:* 33 to 56 hours.

Route	Onset	Peak	Duration
P.O., I.V.	Unknown	1½-3½ hr	Unknown

Action

Chemical effect: Unknown; may inhibit T-lymphocyte activation, which results in immunosuppression.
Therapeutic effect: Prevents organ rejection.

Available forms

Capsules: 1 mg, 5 mg
Injection: 5 mg/ml

NURSING PROCESS

🔲 Assessment

• Obtain history of patient's organ transplant before therapy and reassess regularly.
• Monitor patient for signs of neurotoxicity and nephrotoxicity, especially in those receiving high dosage or those with renal dysfunction.
• Obtain potassium and glucose levels regularly. Monitor patient for hyperglycemia.
• Drug increases risk of infections, lymphomas, and other cancers.
• Be alert for adverse reactions and drug interactions.
• Evaluate patient's and family's knowledge of drug therapy.

🔲 Nursing diagnoses

• Risk for injury related to potential organ transplant rejection
• Ineffective protection related to drug-induced immunosuppression
• Deficient knowledge related to drug therapy

🔲 Planning and implementation

• Child with normal kidney and liver function may need higher dosage than adult.
• Patient with hepatic or renal dysfunction needs lowest possible dosage.
• Give adrenocorticosteroids with this drug.
• Give oral drug on empty stomach.
• Because of risk of anaphylaxis, use injection only in patient who can't take oral form.
• Don't use other immunosuppressants (except for adrenocorticosteroids) during therapy.
• Avoid potassium-sparing diuretics during therapy.
Patient teaching
• Instruct patient to take drug on empty stomach and not to take it with grapefruit juice.
• Explain need for repeated tests during therapy to monitor adverse reactions and drug effectiveness.
• Advise woman of childbearing age to notify prescriber if she becomes pregnant or plans to do so.
• Instruct patient to check with prescriber before taking other drugs.

🔲 Evaluation

• Patient doesn't exhibit signs and symptoms of organ rejection.
• Patient doesn't develop serious complications as result of drug-induced adverse reactions.
• Patient and family state understanding of drug therapy.

tacrolimus (topical)

(tack-row-LYE-mus)
Protopic

Pharmacologic class: macrolide
Therapeutic class: immunosuppressant
Pregnancy risk category: C

Indication and dosages

▶ **Moderate to severe atopic dermatitis in patients unresponsive to other therapies or** unable to use other therapies because of risks. *Adults:* Apply thin layer of 0.03% or 0.1% strength to affected areas twice daily and rub in completely. Continue for 1 week after affected area clears.

Children age 2 and older: Apply thin layer of 0.03% strength to affected areas twice daily and rub in completely. Continue for 1 week after affected area clears.

Contraindications and precautions

• Contraindicated in patients hypersensitive to drug.

• Don't use in patients with Netherton's syndrome or generalized erythroderma.

⚠ **Lifespan:** In pregnant women, use only if potential benefits outweigh risks to fetus. In breast-feeding women, weigh risks and benefits of drug therapy; drug appears in breast milk. In children ages 2 to 15, use only 0.03% ointment.

Adverse reactions

CNS: *headache, fever,* hyperesthesia, asthenia, insomnia, pain.
CV: face edema, peripheral edema.
EENT: *otitis media, pharyngitis,* rhinitis, sinusitis, conjunctivitis.
GI: diarrhea, vomiting, nausea, abdominal pain, gastroenteritis, dyspepsia.
GU: dysmenorrhea.
Hematologic: lymphadenopathy.
Musculoskeletal: back pain, myalgia.
Respiratory: *increased cough, asthma,* pneumonia, bronchitis.
Skin: *skin burning, pruritus, skin erythema, skin infection,* eczema herpeticum, pustular rash, *folliculitis,* urticaria, maculopapular rash, rash, fungal dermatitis, acne, sunburn, tingling, benign skin neoplasm, skin disorder, vesiculobullous rash, dry skin, herpes zoster, eczema, exfoliative dermatitis, contact dermatitis.
Other: *flulike symptoms, accidental injury, infection, lack of drug effect,* alcohol intolerance, periodontal abscess, cyst, *herpes simplex, allergic reaction.*

Interactions

Drug-drug. *Calcium channel blockers, cimetidine, CYP 3A4 inhibitors (erythromycin, itraconazole, ketoconazole, fluconazole):* May interfere with effects of tacrolimus. Use together cautiously.

Drug-lifestyle. *Sun exposure:* Risk of phototoxicity. Tell patient to avoid or minimize exposure to artificial or natural sunlight.

Effects on lab test results

None reported.

Pharmacokinetics

Absorption: Immediate, with no systemic accumulation.
Distribution: Unknown.
Metabolism: Unknown.
Excretion: Unknown. *Half-life:* Unknown.

Route	Onset	Peak	Duration
Topical	Unknown	Unknown	Unknown

Action

Chemical effect: May inhibit T-lymphocyte activation in the skin, which causes immunosuppression. Also inhibits the release of mediators from mast cells and basophils in skin.
Therapeutic effect: Improves skin condition.

Available forms

Ointment: 0.03%, 0.1%

NURSING PROCESS

🔬 Assessment

• Assess patient's underlying condition before therapy and reassess regularly.

• Evaluate patient with infected atopic dermatitis; clear infections at treatment site before using drug.

• Evaluate patient's and family's knowledge of drug therapy.

🔲 Nursing diagnoses

• Impaired skin integrity related to underlying skin condition

• Acute pain related to drug-induced adverse effects

• Deficient knowledge related to tacrolimus therapy

▶ Planning and implementation

• Drug is used only for short-term or intermittent long-term therapy.

⑧ ALERT: Don't use occlusive dressings over drug application. This may promote systemic absorption.

• Drug may increase the risk of varicella zoster, herpes simplex virus, and eczema herpeticum.
• Evaluate all cases of lymphadenopathy to determine etiology. If a clear etiology is unknown or acute mononucleosis is diagnosed, consider stopping drug.
• Monitor all cases of lymphadenopathy until resolution.
• Local adverse effects are most common during the first few days of therapy.

Patient teaching
• Tell patient to wash hands before and after applying drug and to avoid applying drug to wet skin. Skin should be completely dry before applying drug.
• Instruct patient not to use bandages or other occlusive dressings.
• Tell patient not to bathe, shower, or swim immediately after application because doing so could wash the ointment off.
• Advise patient to avoid or minimize exposure to natural or artificial sunlight.
• Tell patient that if he needs to be outdoors after applying drug, to wear loose-fitting clothing that covers the treated area. Check with prescriber regarding sunscreen use.
• Tell patient not to use drug for any disorder other than that for which it was prescribed.
• Instruct patient to report adverse reactions.
• Tell patient to store the ointment at room temperature.

☑ Evaluation
• Patient has improved skin condition.
• Patient states that pain management techniques are effective.
• Patient and family state understanding of drug therapy.

tadalafil
(tah-DAH-lah-phil)
Cialis

Pharmacologic class: selective inhibitor of cyclic guanosine monophosphate (cGMP)–specific phosphodiesterase type 5 (PDE5)
Therapeutic class: erectile dysfunction drug
Pregnancy risk category: B

Indications and dosages

▶ **Erectile dysfunction.** *Men:* 10 mg P.O. as a single dose, p.r.n., before sexual activity. Range is 5 to 20 mg based on effectiveness and tolerance. Maximum, one dose daily.

⊠ **Adjust-a-dose:** For patients with renal impairment, if creatinine clearance is 31 to 50 ml/minute, starting dosage is 5 mg once daily and maximum dosage is 10 mg taken once q 48 hours; if 30 ml/minute or less, maximum dosage is 5 mg once daily. For patients with mild to moderate hepatic impairment (Child-Pugh A or B), dosage shouldn't exceed 10 mg daily. For patients taking potent CYP 3A4 inhibitors (such as erythromycin, itraconazole, ketoconazole, ritonavir), don't exceed one 10-mg dose q 72 hours.

Contraindications and precautions

• Contraindicated in patients hypersensitive to drug or its components and in those taking nitrates or alpha-adrenergic blockers (other than tamsulosin 0.4 mg once daily). Drug isn't recommended for patients with severe hepatic impairment (Child-Pugh Class C), MI within 90 days, New York Heart Association Class II or greater heart failure within 6 months, CVA within 6 months, uncontrolled arrhythmias, blood pressure lower than 90/50 mm Hg or higher than 170/100 mm Hg, unstable angina, or angina that occurs during sexual intercourse. Drug also isn't recommended for patients whose cardiac status makes sexual activity inadvisable and for those with hereditary degenerative retinal disorders.
• Use cautiously in patients taking potent CYP 3A4 inhibitors and in patients with bleeding disorders, significant peptic ulceration, or renal or hepatic impairment. Use cautiously in patients with conditions that predispose them to priapism (such as sickle cell anemia, multiple myeloma, or leukemia), anatomical penis abnormalities, or left ventricular outflow obstruction.
⚕ **Lifespan:** Drug is for men only. In elderly men, consider a lower dose because they may be more sensitive to drug effects.

Adverse reactions

CNS: *headache.*
CV: flushing.
EENT: nasal congestion.
GI: *dyspepsia.*

Musculoskeletal: back pain, limb pain, myalgia.

Interactions

Drug-drug. *Alpha-blockers (except tamsulosin 0.4 mg daily), nitrates:* May enhance hypotensive effects. Avoid using together.
Potent CYP 3A4 inhibitors (such as erythromycin, itraconazole, ketoconazole, ritonavir): May increase tadalafil level. Patient shouldn't exceed 10 mg q 72 hours.
Rifampin and other CYP 3A4 inducers: May decrease tadalafil level. Monitor patient closely.
Drug-food. *Grapefruit:* May increase drug level. Discourage use together. Monitor patient closely.
Drug-lifestyle: *Alcohol use:* May increase risk of headache, dizziness, orthostatic hypotension, and increased heart rate. Discourage use together.

Effects on lab test results

None reported.

Pharmacokinetics

Absorption: Median effect occurs in 2 hours.
Distribution: Wide. 97% protein-bound.
Metabolism: Mainly through CYP 3A4 isoenzymes.
Excretion: In feces and urine. *Half-life:* 17½ hours.

Route	Onset	Peak	Duration
P.O.	Immediate	½-6 hr	Unknown

Action

Chemical effect: Prevents the breakdown of cGMP by phosphodiesterase, thus increasing cGMP levels.
Therapeutic effect: Prolongs smooth muscle relaxation and promotes blood flow into the corpus cavernosum.

Available forms

Tablets (film-coated): 5 mg, 10 mg, 20 mg

NURSING PROCESS

Assessment
⊛ ALERT: Sexual activity may increase cardiac risk. Evaluate patient's cardiac risk before starting drug.

• Before patient starts drug, assess for underlying causes of erectile dysfunction.
• Evaluate patient's and family's knowledge of drug therapy.

Nursing diagnoses
• Sexual dysfunction related to patient's underlying condition
• Risk for injury related to potential for prolonged erections or priapism
• Deficient knowledge related to drug therapy

Planning and implementation
• Drug may cause transient decreases in supine blood pressure.
• Drug increases risk of prolonged erections and priapism.
Patient teaching
• Warn patient that taking drug with nitrates could cause a serious drop in blood pressure, raising the risk of heart attack or stroke.
• Tell patient to seek immediate medical attention if he develops chest pain after taking the drug.
• Urge patient to seek emergency medical care if his erection lasts more than 4 hours.
• Tell patient to take drug about 60 minutes before anticipated sexual activity. Explain that drug has no effect without sexual stimulation.
• Warn patient not to change dosage unless directed by prescriber.
• Caution patient against drinking large amounts of alcohol while taking drug.

Evaluation
• Sexual activity improves with drug therapy.
• Patient doesn't experience injury from prolonged erection or priapism.
• Patient and family state understanding of drug therapy.

tamoxifen citrate

(teh-MOKS-uh-fen SIGH-trayt)
Apo-Tamox ♦ , Nolvadex, Nolvadex-D ♦ ◇ ,
Novo-Tamoxifen ♦ , Tamofen ♦ , Tamone ♦

Pharmacologic class: nonsteroidal antiestrogen
Therapeutic class: antineoplastic
Pregnancy risk category: D

Indications and dosages

▶ **Advanced postmenopausal breast cancer.** *Adults:* 20 to 40 mg P.O. b.i.d.
▶ **Adjunct treatment for breast cancer.** *Adults:* 10 mg P.O. b.i.d. to t.i.d. for no more than 5 years.
▶ **Reduction of breast cancer risk in high-risk women.** *Adults:* 20 mg P.O. daily for 5 years.
▶ **Ductal carcinoma in situ (DCIS).** *Adults:* 20 mg P.O. daily for 5 years.
▶ **Stimulation of ovulation‡.** *Adults:* 5 to 40 mg P.O. b.i.d. for 4 days.
▶ **McCune–Albright syndrome and precocious puberty‡.** *Children ages 2 to 10:* 20 mg P.O. daily. Treat for up to 12 months.
▶ **Mastalgia‡.** *Adults:* 10 mg P.O. daily for 10 months.

Contraindications and precautions

• Contraindicated in patients hypersensitive to drug, in women receiving coumarin-type anticoagulants, and in those with history of deep vein thrombosis or pulmonary emboli.
• Use cautiously in patients with leukopenia or thrombocytopenia.
Lifespan: In pregnant and breast-feeding women, drug isn't recommended. In children, safety of drug hasn't been established.

Adverse reactions

CNS: confusion, weakness, headache, sleepiness, ***CVA.***
CV: *hot flushes.*
EENT: corneal changes, cataracts, retinopathy.
GI: *nausea, vomiting, diarrhea.*
GU: *vaginal discharge* and bleeding, *irregular menses, amenorrhea,* ***endometrial cancer, uterine sarcoma.***
Hematologic: ***leukopenia, thrombocytopenia.***
Hepatic: fatty liver, cholestasis, ***hepatic necrosis.***
Metabolic: *hypercalcemia, weight changes, fluid retention.*
Musculoskeletal: brief exacerbation of pain from osseous metastases.
Respiratory: ***pulmonary embolism.***
Skin: *skin changes,* rash.
Other: temporary bone or tumor pain.

Interactions

Drug-drug. *Antacids:* May affect absorption of enteric-coated tablet. Don't use within 2 hours of tamoxifen dose.
Bromocriptine: May elevate tamoxifen level. Monitor patient for toxicity.
Coumadin-type anticoagulants: May cause significant increase in anticoagulant effect. Monitor patient, PT, and INR closely.

Effects on lab test results

• May increase BUN, creatinine, calcium, and liver enzyme levels.
• May decrease WBC and platelet counts.

Pharmacokinetics

Absorption: Appears to be well absorbed.
Distribution: Widely in total body water.
Metabolism: Extensive.
Excretion: Drug and metabolites excreted mainly in feces, mostly as metabolites. *Half-life:* Over 7 days.

Route	Onset	Peak	Duration
P.O.	4-10 wk	Unknown	Several wk

Action

Chemical effect: Exact antineoplastic action is unknown; acts as estrogen antagonist.
Therapeutic effect: Hinders function of breast cancer cells.

Available forms

Tablets: 10 mg, 20 mg
Tablets (enteric-coated)♦: 10 mg, 20 mg

NURSING PROCESS

Assessment

• Assess patient's breast cancer before therapy and regularly thereafter.
• Monitor CBC closely in patient with leukopenia or thrombocytopenia.
• Monitor lipid levels during long-term therapy in patients with hyperlipidemia.
• Monitor calcium level. Drug may compound hypercalcemia related to bone metastases during initiation of therapy.
• Be alert for adverse reactions.
• Monitor patient's hydration status if adverse GI reactions occur.
• Evaluate patient's and family's knowledge of drug therapy.

⊕ Nursing diagnoses
- Ineffective health maintenance related to presence of breast cancer
- Risk for deficient fluid volume related to drug-induced adverse GI reactions
- Deficient knowledge related to drug therapy

⟩ Planning and implementation
- Make sure patient swallows enteric-coated tablets whole.

⊗ **ALERT:** Serious, life-threatening, or fatal events are linked to drug in women at high risk for cancer and women with DCIS include endometrial cancer, uterine sarcoma, CVA, and pulmonary embolism. Prescribers should discuss potential benefits and risks of these serious events with women considering drug to reduce their risk of developing breast cancer. The benefits outweigh risks in women already diagnosed with breast cancer.

Patient teaching
- Instruct patient to report symptoms of pulmonary embolism (chest pain, difficulty breathing, rapid breathing, sweating or fainting).
- Tell patient to report symptoms of CVA (headache, vision changes, confusion, difficulty speaking or walking, and weakness of face, arm or leg, especially on one side of the body).
- Reassure patient that acute bone pain during drug therapy usually means that drug will produce good response. Tell her to take an analgesic for pain.
- Encourage patient who is taking or has taken drug to have regular gynecologic examinations because of increased risk of uterine cancer.
- If patient is taking drug to reduce risk of breast cancer, teach proper technique for breast self-examination.
- Tell patient that annual mammograms are important.
- Advise patient to use barrier form of contraception because short-term therapy induces ovulation in premenopausal women.
- Advise woman of childbearing age to avoid becoming pregnant during therapy and to consult with prescriber before becoming pregnant.

☑ Evaluation
- Patient responds well to drug.
- Patient maintains adequate hydration.
- Patient and family state understanding of drug therapy.

---

tamsulosin hydrochloride
(tam-soo-LOH-sin high-droh-KLOR-ighd)
Flomax

Pharmacologic class: alpha-1$_a$ antagonist
Therapeutic class: BPH drug
Pregnancy risk category: B

Indications and dosages
▶ **BPH.** *Men:* 0.4 mg P.O. once daily, given 30 minutes after same meal each day. If no response after 2 to 4 weeks, increase dosage to 0.8 mg P.O. once daily.

Contraindications and precautions
- Contraindicated in patients hypersensitive to drug or its components.
⚘ **Lifespan:** Drug is indicated for men only.

Adverse reactions
CNS: asthenia, *dizziness, headache,* insomnia, somnolence, syncope, vertigo.
CV: chest pain, orthostatic hypotension.
EENT: amblyopia, pharyngitis, *rhinitis,* sinusitis.
GI: diarrhea, nausea.
GU: abnormal ejaculation.
Musculoskeletal: back pain.
Respiratory: cough.
Other: decreased libido, *infection,* tooth disorder.

Interactions
Drug-drug. *Alpha-adrenergic blockers:* May interact with tamsulosin. Avoid using together.
Cimetidine: Decreases tamsulosin clearance. Use cautiously.
Warfarin: Study results are inconclusive. Use together cautiously.

Effects on lab test results
None reported.

Pharmacokinetics
Absorption: More than 90%. Food increases bioavailability by 30%.
Distribution: Distributed into extracellular fluids. Extensively bound to protein (94% to 99%).
Metabolism: Primarily metabolized by CYP enzymes in the liver.
Excretion: 76% of drug eliminated in urine; 21% in feces. *Half-life:* 9 to 13 hours.

Reactions may be *common,* uncommon, *life-threatening*, or COMMON AND LIFE-THREATENING.

Route	Onset	Peak	Duration
P.O.	Unknown	4-5 hr	9-15 hr

Action

Chemical effect: Selectively blocks alpha receptors in the prostate, leading to relaxation of smooth muscles in the bladder neck and prostate, which improves urine flow and reduces symptoms of BPH.
Therapeutic effect: Improves urine flow.

Available forms

Capsules: 0.4 mg

NURSING PROCESS

⚖ Assessment

• Assess patient for signs of prostatic hyperplasia, including frequency of urination, nocturnal urination, and urinary hesitancy.
• Monitor patient for decreases in blood pressure and notify prescriber.
• Evaluate patient's and family's knowledge of drug therapy.

✪ Nursing diagnoses

• Risk for injury related to decreased blood pressure and resulting syncope
• Impaired urinary elimination related to underlying prostatic hyperplasia
• Deficient knowledge related to drug therapy

▶ Planning and implementation

• Symptoms of BPH and cancer of the prostate are similar; cancer should be ruled out before therapy starts.
• If therapy is interrupted for several days or more, restart therapy at one capsule daily.
• Drug may cause a sudden drop in blood pressure, especially after the first dose or when changing doses.
⊛ **ALERT:** Don't confuse Flomax with Fosamax.
Patient teaching
• Instruct patient not to crush, chew, or open capsules.
• Tell patient to get up slowly from chair or bed when therapy starts and to avoid situations where injury could occur because of syncope. Advise him that drug may cause a sudden drop in blood pressure, especially after the first dose or when changing doses.
• Instruct patient not to drive or perform hazardous tasks for 12 hours after the initial dose or

changes in dose until response can be monitored.
• Tell patient to take drug about 30 minutes after same meal each day.

✓ Evaluation

• Patient doesn't experience sudden decreases in blood pressure.
• Patient experiences normal urinary elimination patterns.
• Patient and family state understanding of drug therapy.

tegaserod maleate
(teh-GAS-uh-rahd MALL-ee-ayt)
Zelnorm

Pharmacologic class: 5-HT$_4$ receptor partial agonist
Therapeutic class: irritable bowel drug
Pregnancy risk category: B

Indications and dosages

▶ **Short-term treatment for irritable bowel syndrome, when the primary bowel symptom is constipation.** *Women:* 6 mg P.O. b.i.d. before meals for 4 to 6 weeks. May add another 4- to 6-week course for patients who respond to therapy at 4 to 6 weeks.

Contraindications and precautions

• Contraindicated in patients hypersensitive to drug or its components and in those with severe renal impairment, moderate or severe hepatic impairment, a history of bowel obstruction, symptomatic gallbladder disease, suspected sphincter of Oddi dysfunction or abdominal adhesions, or frequent or current diarrhea.
⚠ **Lifespan:** In pregnant women, use drug only if clearly needed. Breast-feeding women should either stop the drug or stop breast-feeding, taking into account the importance of the drug to the mother. It isn't known whether drug appears in breast milk. In children, safety and efficacy of drug haven't been established.

Adverse reactions

CNS: *headache,* dizziness, migraine.
GI: *abdominal pain,* diarrhea, nausea, flatulence.

Musculoskeletal: back pain, arthropathy, leg pain.
Other: accidental injury.

Interactions

Drug-drug. *Digoxin:* Reduces peak level and exposure of digoxin by 15%. Use cautiously.
Drug-food. *Food:* Reduces bioavailability of drug. Advise patient to take drug on an empty stomach.

Effects on lab test results

None reported.

Pharmacokinetics

Absorption: Food reduces bioavailability by 40% to 65%.
Distribution: About 98% protein-bound.
Metabolism: By two pathways. The first is hydrolysis, followed by oxidation and conjugation. The second is direct glucuronidation.
Excretion: Two-thirds of dose unchanged in feces, with the remaining one-third in the urine, primarily as the metabolite. *Half-life:* Unknown.

Route	Onset	Peak	Duration
P.O.	Unknown	1 hr	Unknown

Action

Chemical effect: Binds with high affinity to 5-HT$_4$ receptors and acts as an agonist. Activating 5-HT$_4$ receptors in the GI tract stimulates the peristaltic reflex and intestinal secretion and inhibits visceral sensitivity.
Therapeutic effect: Relieves constipation.

Available forms

Tablets: 2 mg, 6 mg

NURSING PROCESS

Assessment
• Assess patient's condition before therapy and reassess regularly.
• Monitor patient for diarrhea and abdominal pain.
• Evaluate patient's and family's knowledge of drug therapy.

Nursing diagnoses
• Constipation related to irritable bowel syndrome

• Diarrhea related to adverse effect of tegaserod maleate therapy
• Deficient knowledge related to drug therapy

Planning and implementation
• Give drug on an empty stomach before a meal.
• If patient experiences new or sudden worsening of abdominal pain, stop drug.
• Some patients develop diarrhea during therapy. In most cases, diarrhea occurs within the first week of therapy and resolves with continued therapy.
Patient teaching
• Tell patient to take drug on an empty stomach, before a meal.
• Inform patient she may have diarrhea during therapy. Tell her to report severe diarrhea or diarrhea accompanied by severe cramping, abdominal pain, or dizziness.
• Tell patient not to take drug if she now has or often has diarrhea.
• Tell patient to report new or worsening abdominal pain.
• Tell patient not to use drug during pregnancy or breast-feeding.

Evaluation
• Patient expresses relief from constipation.
• Patient reports no diarrhea.
• Patient and family state understanding of drug therapy.

telmisartan
(tel-mih-SAR-tan)
Micardis

Pharmacologic class: angiotensin II receptor antagonist
Therapeutic class: antihypertensive
Pregnancy risk category: C (D in second and third trimesters)

Indications and dosages

▶ **Hypertension (used alone or with other antihypertensives).** *Adults:* 40 mg P.O. daily. Blood pressure response is dose-related between 20 and 80 mg daily.

Contraindications and precautions

• Contraindicated in patients hypersensitive to drug or its components.

• Use cautiously in patients with renal and hepatic insufficiency and in those with an activated renin-angiotensin system, such as volume- or salt-depleted patients (such as those being treated with high doses of diuretics).

⚖ **Lifespan:** In pregnant women, avoid use. If pregnancy is suspected, notify prescriber because drug should be stopped. Advise breast-feeding woman about the risk of adverse effects on her infant and the need to stop breast-feeding or drug therapy, taking into account importance of drug therapy. In children, safety and effectiveness haven't been established.

Adverse reactions

CNS: dizziness, pain, fatigue, headache.
CV: chest pain, hypertension, peripheral edema.
EENT: pharyngitis, sinusitis.
GI: abdominal pain, diarrhea, dyspepsia, nausea.
GU: UTI.
Musculoskeletal: back pain, myalgia.
Respiratory: cough, upper respiratory tract infection.
Other: flulike symptoms.

Interactions

Drug-drug. *Digoxin:* Increases digoxin level. Monitor digoxin level closely.
Warfarin: Slightly decreases warfarin level. Monitor INR.

Effects on lab test results

• May increase liver enzyme levels.

Pharmacokinetics

Absorption: Readily absorbed.
Distribution: Highly protein-bound; volume of distribution is about 500 L.
Metabolism: Metabolized by conjugation to an inactive metabolite.
Excretion: Mainly excreted unchanged in feces. *Half-life:* 24 hours.

Route	Onset	Peak	Duration
P.O.	Unknown	30 min-1 hr	24 hr

Action

Chemical effect: Blocks the vasoconstrictive and aldosterone-secreting effects of angiotensin II by selectively blocking the binding of angiotensin II to the AT_1 receptor in many tissues, such as vascular smooth muscle and the adrenal gland.
Therapeutic effect: Lowers blood pressure.

Available forms

Tablets: 40 mg, 80 mg

NURSING PROCESS

🔖 **Assessment**
• In patients whose renal function may depend on the activity of the renin-angiotensin-aldosterone system, such as those with severe heart failure, use of ACE inhibitors and angiotensin-receptor antagonists may be related to oliguria or progressive azotemia and (rarely) to acute renal failure or death.
• In patients with biliary obstruction, drug level may elevate because of inability to excrete drug.
• Drug isn't removed by hemodialysis. Patients undergoing dialysis may develop orthostatic hypotension. Closely monitor blood pressure.
• Evaluate patient's and family's knowledge of drug therapy.

🔖 **Nursing diagnoses**
• Risk for injury related to presence of hypertension
• Ineffective cerebral and cardiopulmonary tissue perfusion related to drug-induced hypotension
• Deficient knowledge related to drug therapy

▶ **Planning and implementation**
• Most of the antihypertensive effect is present within 2 weeks. Maximal blood pressure reduction is generally attained after 4 weeks. If blood pressure isn't controlled by drug alone, a diuretic may be added.
• If hypotension occurs, place patient in supine position and give normal saline solution I.V. if needed.
Patient teaching
• Inform woman of childbearing age of consequences of second- and third-trimester exposure to drug. Instruct patient to report suspected pregnancy to prescriber immediately.
• Tell patient that transient hypotension may occur. Instruct him to lie down if feeling dizzy and to climb stairs slowly and rise slowly to standing position.
• Instruct patient with heart failure to notify prescriber about decreased urine output.
• Teach patient other means to reduce blood pressure, such as diet control, exercise, smoking cessation, and stress reduction.

- Inform patient that drug shouldn't be removed from blister-sealed packet until immediately before use.

☑ Evaluation

- Patient doesn't experience injury from underlying disease.
- Patient doesn't experience hypotension and maintains adequate tissue perfusion.
- Patient and family state understanding of drug therapy.

temazepam
(teh-MAZ-ih-pam)
Euhypnos◇, Normison◇, Restoril, Temaze◇

Pharmacologic class: benzodiazepine
Therapeutic class: sedative-hypnotic
Pregnancy risk category: X
Controlled substance schedule: IV

Indications and dosages

▶ **Short-term treatment of insomnia.** *Adults age 65 and younger:* 7.5 to 30 mg P.O. 30 minutes before bedtime.
Adults older than age 65: 7.5 mg P.O. h.s.

Contraindications and precautions

- Contraindicated in patients hypersensitive to benzodiazepines.
- Use cautiously in patients with chronic pulmonary insufficiency, impaired liver or kidney function, severe or latent depression, suicidal tendencies, or history of drug abuse.
- ≛ Lifespan: In pregnant women, drug is contraindicated. In breast-feeding women, drug isn't recommended. In children, safety of drug hasn't been established.

Adverse reactions

CNS: *drowsiness, dizziness, lethargy,* disturbed coordination, daytime sedation, confusion, nightmares, vertigo, euphoria, weakness, headache, fatigue, nervousness, anxiety, depression.
EENT: blurred vision.
GI: diarrhea, nausea, dry mouth.
Other: physical or psychological dependence.

Interactions

Drug-drug. *CNS depressants, including opioid analgesics:* Increases CNS depression. Use together cautiously.
Drug-herb. *Calendula, catnip, hops, lady's slipper, lemon balm, passion flower, sassafras, skullcap, valerian, yerba maté:* May increase sedative effects. Monitor patient closely; discourage use together.
Kava: May cause excessive sedation. Discourage use together.
Drug-lifestyle. *Alcohol use:* May cause additive CNS effects. Strongly discourage use together.

Effects on lab test results

- May increase liver enzyme levels.

Pharmacokinetics

Absorption: Well absorbed.
Distribution: Distributed widely throughout body; 98% protein-bound.
Metabolism: Metabolized in liver to primarily inactive metabolites.
Excretion: Metabolites excreted in urine. *Half-life:* 10 to 17 hours.

Route	Onset	Peak	Duration
P.O.	Unknown	1-2 hr	Unknown

Action

Chemical effect: May act on limbic system, thalamus, and hypothalamus of CNS to produce hypnotic effects.
Therapeutic effect: Promotes sleep.

Available forms

Capsules: 7.5 mg, 15 mg, 20 mg◇, 30 mg

NURSING PROCESS

☡ Assessment

- Assess patient's sleeping disorder before therapy and regularly thereafter.
- Assess mental status before therapy. Geriatric patients are more sensitive to drug's adverse CNS effects.
- Be alert for adverse reactions and drug interactions.
- Evaluate patient's and family's knowledge of drug therapy.

🔲 Nursing diagnoses

- Disturbed sleep pattern related to presence of insomnia
- Risk for injury related to drug-induced adverse CNS reactions
- Deficient knowledge related to drug therapy

▶ Planning and implementation

- Prevent hoarding or intentional overdosing by patient who is depressed, suicidal, or drug-dependent or who has history of drug abuse.
- Make sure patient has swallowed capsule before leaving bedside.
- Supervise walking and raise bed rails, particularly for geriatric patients.

🛇 **ALERT:** Don't confuse Restoril with Vistaril.

Patient teaching

- Warn patient to avoid activities that require mental alertness or physical coordination.

☑ Evaluation

- Patient states that drug induces sleep.
- Patient doesn't experience injury from adverse CNS reactions.
- Patient and family state understanding of drug therapy.

---

tenecteplase
(te-NEK-te-plase)
TNKase

Pharmacologic class: recombinant tissue plasminogen activator
Therapeutic class: thrombolytic
Pregnancy risk category: C

Indications and dosages

▶ **Reduction of mortality from acute MI.**
Adults who weigh less than 60 kg (132 lb):
30 mg (6 ml) by I.V. bolus over 5 seconds.
Adults who weigh 60 to 69 kg (132 to 152 lb):
35 mg (7 ml) by I.V. bolus over 5 seconds.
Adults who weigh 70 to 79 kg (154 to 174 lb):
40 mg (8 ml) by I.V. bolus over 5 seconds.
Adults who weigh 80 to 89 kg (176 to 196 lb):
45 mg (9 ml) by I.V. bolus over 5 seconds.
Adults who weigh 90 kg (198 lb) or more:
50 mg (10 ml) by I.V. bolus over 5 seconds.
Maximum dose is 50 mg.

▼ I.V. administration

- Use syringe prefilled with sterile water for injection and inject entire contents into drug vial. Don't use bacteriostatic water for injection. Gently swirl solution once mixed. Don't shake. Make sure contents are completely dissolved. Draw up the appropriate dose needed from the reconstituted vial with the syringe and discard any unused portion.
- Give drug immediately once reconstituted, or refrigerate and use within 8 hours.
- Give drug in a designated line. Don't give drug in same I.V. line as dextrose. Flush dextrose-containing lines with normal saline solution before administration.
- Give heparin with tenecteplase, but not in the same I.V. line.

Contraindications and precautions

- Contraindicated in patients with active internal bleeding; history of CVA; intracranial or intraspinal surgery or trauma within the previous 2 months; intracranial neoplasm, aneurysm, or arteriovenous malformation; severe uncontrolled hypertension; or known bleeding diathesis.
- Use cautiously in patients who have had recent major surgery (such as coronary artery bypass graft), organ biopsy, or obstetrical delivery, or previous puncture of noncompressible vessels. Also use cautiously in patients with recent trauma, recent GI or GU bleeding, high risk of left ventricular thrombus, acute pericarditis, hypertension (systolic 180 mm Hg or above, diastolic 110 mm Hg or above), severe hepatic dysfunction, hemostatic defects, subacute bacterial endocarditis, septic thrombophlebitis, diabetic hemorrhagic retinopathy, or cerebrovascular disease.

⚖ **Lifespan:** In pregnant and breast-feeding women, use cautiously. In children, safety and effectiveness haven't been established. In patients age 75 and older, give cautiously; the drug benefit should be weighed against the risk of increased adverse effects.

Adverse reactions

CNS: *CVA, intracranial hemorrhage.*
CV: *major hematoma, minor hematoma.*
EENT: *pharyngeal bleeding,* epistaxis.
GI: *GI bleeding.*
GU: *hematuria.*
Hematologic: *bleeding at puncture sites.*

Interactions

Drug-drug. *Anticoagulants (heparin, vitamin K antagonists), drugs that alter platelet function (acetylsalicylic acid, dipyridamole, glycoprotein IIb/IIIa inhibitors):* Increases risk of bleeding when used before, during, or after therapy with tenecteplase. Use cautiously.

Effects on lab test results

• May increase PT, PTT, and INR.

Pharmacokinetics

Absorption: Administered I.V.
Distribution: Related to weight and is an approximation of plasma volume.
Metabolism: Primarily hepatic.
Excretion: Unknown. *Half-life:* 20 minutes to 2 hours.

Route	Onset	Peak	Duration
I.V.	Immediate	Immediate	20-24 min

Action

Chemical effect: Binds to fibrin and converts plasminogen to plasmin. Specificity to fibrin decreases systemic activation of plasminogen and the resulting breakdown of circulating fibrinogen.
Therapeutic effect: Dissolves blood clots.

Available forms

Injection: 50 mg

NURSING PROCESS

🏷 Assessment

• Assess underlying condition before therapy and reassess regularly thereafter.
• Monitor ECG for reperfusion arrhythmias.
• Evaluate pain before therapy and reassess regularly.
• Evaluate patient's and family's knowledge of drug therapy.

⊕ Nursing diagnoses

• Ineffective tissue perfusion, coronary, related to presence of blood clots
• Acute pain related to MI
• Deficient knowledge related to tenecteplase therapy

⊠ Planning and implementation

• Minimize arterial and venous punctures during therapy.

• Avoid noncompressible arterial punctures and internal jugular and subclavian venous punctures.
• Monitor patient for bleeding. If serious bleeding occurs, stop heparin and antiplatelet drugs immediately.
• Cholesterol embolism is rarely related to thrombolytic use, but may be lethal. Signs and symptoms may include livedo reticularis "purple toe" syndrome, acute renal failure, gangrenous digits, hypertension, pancreatitis, MI, cerebral infarction, spinal cord infarction, retinal artery occlusion, bowel infarction, and rhabdomyolysis.

Patient teaching
• Inform patient about proper dental care to avoid excessive gum bleeding.
• Advise patient to report any adverse effects or excess bleeding immediately.
• Explain use of drug to patient and family.

✓ Evaluation

• Patient regains tissue perfusion with dissolution of blood clots.
• Patient is relieved of pain.
• Patient and family state understanding of drug therapy.

teniposide (VM-26)
(teh-NIP-uh-sighd)
Vumon

Pharmacologic class: podophyllotoxin (specific to phase of cell cycle G_2 and late S phase)
Therapeutic class: antineoplastic
Pregnancy risk category: D

Indications and dosages

▶ **Refractory childhood acute lymphoblastic leukemia.** *Children:* Optimum dosage hasn't been established. One protocol reported by manufacturer is 165 mg/m^2 I.V. twice weekly for eight or nine doses. Usually used with other drugs.

▽ I.V. administration

• Follow institutional policy to reduce risks. Preparation and administration of parenteral form are linked to carcinogenic, mutagenic, and teratogenic risks for personnel.
• Dilute drug in D_5W or normal saline solution injection to level of 0.1, 0.2, 0.4, or 1 mg/ml.

Reactions may be *common,* uncommon, *life-threatening,* or COMMON AND LIFE-THREATENING.

Don't agitate vigorously; precipitation may form. Discard cloudy solutions.
• Don't mix with other drugs or solutions. Heparin is physically incompatible with drug.
• Don't give drug through membrane-type inline filter because diluent may dissolve filter.
• Infuse over 45 to 90 minutes to prevent hypotension. If hypotension occurs, stop infusion.
• Prepare and store in glass containers. Solutions containing 0.5 to 1 mg/ml teniposide are stable for 4 hours; those containing 0.1 to 0.2 mg/ml are stable for 6 hours at room temperature.

Contraindications and precautions

• Contraindicated in patients hypersensitive to drug or to polyoxyethylated castor oil (an injection vehicle).
☀ **Lifespan:** In pregnant and breast-feeding women, drug isn't recommended.

Adverse reactions

CV: hypotension from rapid infusion.
GI: *nausea, vomiting, mucositis, diarrhea.*
Hematologic: MYELOSUPPRESSION (dose-limiting), LEUKOPENIA, NEUTROPENIA, THROMBOCYTOPENIA, *anemia.*
Skin: alopecia.
Other: *hypersensitivity reactions* (chills, fever, urticaria, tachycardia, *bronchospasm,* dyspnea, hypotension, flushing), *phlebitis at injection site with extravasation.*

Interactions

Drug-drug. *Methotrexate:* May increase clearance and intracellular levels of methotrexate. Monitor patient closely.
Sodium salicylate, sulfamethizole, tolbutamide: May displace teniposide from protein-binding sites and increase toxicity. Monitor patient closely.

Effects on lab test results

• May increase uric acid level.
• May decrease hemoglobin, hematocrit, and RBC, WBC, platelet, and neutrophil counts.

Pharmacokinetics

Absorption: Administered I.V.
Distribution: Distributed mainly in liver, kidneys, small intestine, and adrenals. Drug crosses blood-brain barrier to limited extent; highly bound to plasma proteins.

Metabolism: Metabolized extensively in liver.
Excretion: About 40% eliminated through kidneys as unchanged drug or metabolites. *Half-life:* 5 hours.

Route	Onset	Peak	Duration
I.V.	Unknown	Unknown	Unknown

Action

Chemical effect: Acts in late S or early G2 phase of cell cycle, thus preventing cells from entering mitosis.
Therapeutic effect: Prevents reproduction of leukemic cells.

Available forms

Injection: 50 mg/5 ml

NURSING PROCESS

▨ Assessment

• Assess patient's condition before therapy and regularly thereafter.
• Obtain baseline blood counts and kidney and liver function tests, then monitor periodically.
• Monitor blood pressure before therapy and at 30-minute intervals during infusion.
• Be alert for adverse reactions and drug interactions.
• Evaluate patient's and family's knowledge of drug therapy.

▦ Nursing diagnoses

• Ineffective health maintenance related to presence of leukemia
• Ineffective protection related to drug-induced immunosuppression
• Deficient knowledge related to drug therapy

▷ Planning and implementation

• Some prescribers may decide to use drug despite patient's history of hypersensitivity because therapeutic benefits may outweigh risks. Give antihistamines and corticosteroids to these patients before infusion begins and monitor closely during drug administration.
⊛ **ALERT:** Have diphenhydramine, hydrocortisone, epinephrine, and appropriate emergency equipment available to establish airway in case of anaphylaxis.
• Ensure careful placement of I.V. catheter. Extravasation can cause local tissue necrosis or sloughing.

⊛ **ALERT:** Report systolic blood pressure below 90 mm Hg and stop infusion.

Patient teaching

• Tell patient to report discomfort at I.V. site immediately.

• Encourage adequate fluid intake to increase urine output and facilitate excretion of uric acid.

• Review infection-control and bleeding precautions to take during therapy.

• Reassure patient that hair should grow back after therapy stops.

• Instruct patient and parents to notify prescriber if adverse reactions occur.

☑ **Evaluation**

• Patient responds well to drug.

• Patient doesn't develop serious complications from immunosuppression.

• Patient and family state understanding of drug therapy.

---

tenofovir disoproxil fumarate
(teh-NAH-fuh-veer diso-PRAHK-sul FOO-mah-rate)
Viread

Pharmacologic class: nucleotide reverse transcriptase inhibitor
Therapeutic class: antiviral, antiretroviral
Pregnancy risk category: B

Indications and dosages

▶ **HIV-1 infection, with other antiretrovirals.**
Adults: 300 mg P.O. once daily with a meal. When given with didanosine, give 2 hours before or 1 hour after didanosine.

Contraindications and precautions

• Contraindicated in patients hypersensitive to any component of the drug. Don't use in patients with creatinine clearance less than 60 ml/minute.

• Use cautiously in patients with hepatic impairment or risk factors for liver disease.

⚖ Lifespan: In pregnant women, give drug only if benefits clearly outweigh the risks. Breast-feeding women shouldn't breast-feed. In children, safety and effectiveness haven't been established. In elderly patients, use cautiously because they are more likely to have renal impairment and to be receiving other drug therapy.

Adverse reactions

CNS: asthenia, headache.
GI: abdominal pain, anorexia, diarrhea, flatulence, *nausea,* vomiting.
GU: glycosuria.
Hematologic: *neutropenia.*
Metabolic: hyperglycemia.

Interactions

Drug-drug. *Acyclovir, cidofovir, ganciclovir, valacyclovir, valganciclovir (drugs that reduce renal function or compete for renal tubular secretion):* Increases level of tenofovir or other renally eliminated drugs. Monitor patient for adverse effects.
Atazanavir: Decreases atazanavir levels, causing resistance. Give both drugs with ritonavir.
Didanosine (buffered formulation): Increases didanosine bioavailability. Monitor patient for didanosine-related adverse effects, such as bone marrow suppression, GI distress, and peripheral neuropathy. Give tenofovir 2 hours before or 1 hour after didanosine.

Effects on lab test results

• May increase amylase, AST, ALT, creatinine kinase, serum and urine glucose, and triglyceride levels. May decrease HIV-1 RNA levels.

• May decrease neutrophil and CD4 cell counts.

Pharmacokinetics

Absorption: In fasting patients, tenofovir is poorly absorbed (bioavailability 25%) with peak level occurring in about 1 hour. A high-fat meal delays the peak by 1 hour but increases bioavailability to 40%.
Distribution: Tenofovir has low binding to plasma and proteins.
Metabolism: Neither tenofovir nor tenofovir disoproxil fumarate is metabolized by liver enzymes, including CYP enzymes.
Excretion: Renal, through glomerular filtration and active tubular secretion. *Half-life:* Unknown.

Route	Onset	Peak	Duration
P.O.	Unknown	1-2 hr	Unknown

Action

Chemical effect: Tenofovir disoproxil fumarate is hydrolyzed to produce tenofovir. Tenofovir undergoes sequential phosphorylations to yield tenofovir diphosphate. Tenofovir diphosphate is

---

a competitive antagonist of HIV reverse transcriptase.

Therapeutic effect: Inhibits HIV replication.

Available forms

Tablets: 300 mg as the fumarate salt (equivalent to 245 mg of tenofovir disoproxil)

NURSING PROCESS

Assessment

• Assess patient's viral infection before therapy and regularly thereafter.

• Evaluate patient for risk of severe adverse reactions. Antiretrovirals, alone or combined, have been linked to lactic acidosis and severe (including fatal) hepatomegaly with steatosis. These effects may occur without elevated transaminase levels. Risk is increased for women, obese patients, and those exposed to antiretrovirals long-term. Monitor all patients for hepatotoxicity, including lactic acidosis and hepatomegaly with steatosis.

• Evaluate patient's and family's knowledge of drug therapy.

Nursing diagnoses

• Noncompliance related to long-term therapy

• Risk for infection related to presence of HIV

• Deficient knowledge related to drug therapy

Planning and implementation

• Antiretrovirals have been linked to the accumulation and redistribution of body fat, resulting in central obesity, peripheral wasting, and development of a buffalo hump. The long-term effects of these changes are unknown. Monitor patients for changes in body fat.

• Tenofovir may be linked to bone abnormalities (osteomalacia and decreased bone mineral density) and renal toxicity (increased creatinine and phosphaturia levels). Monitor patient carefully during long-term therapy.

• Drug may lead to decreased HIV-1 RNA levels and CD4 cell counts.

• The effects of tenofovir on the progression of HIV infection are unknown.

• Due to a high rate of early virologic resistance, triple antiretroviral therapy with abacavir, lamivudine, and tenofovir shouldn't be used as new therapy regimen for untreated or pretreated patients. Monitor patients currently controlled with this combination and those who use

this combination in addition to other antiretrovirals, and consider modifying therapy.

Patient teaching

• Instruct patient to take tenofovir with a meal to enhance bioavailability.

• Tell patient to report adverse effects, including nausea, vomiting, diarrhea, flatulence, and headache.

Evaluation

• Patient complies with therapy regimen.

• Patient has reduced signs and symptoms of infection.

• Patient and family state understanding of drug therapy.

terazosin hydrochloride
(ter-uh-ZOH-sin high-droh-KLOR-ighd)
Hytrin

Pharmacologic class: selective alpha$_1$-adrenergic blocker
Therapeutic class: antihypertensive
Pregnancy risk category: C

Indications and dosages

▶ **Hypertension.** *Adults:* Initially, 1 mg P.O. h.s., increased gradually based on response. Usual dosage range is 1 to 5 mg daily. Maximum, 20 mg daily.

▶ **Symptomatic BPH.** *Adults:* Initially, 1 mg P.O. h.s. Dosage increased in stepwise manner to 2 mg, 5 mg, and 10 mg once daily to achieve optimal response. Most patients require 10 mg daily for optimal response.

Contraindications and precautions

• Contraindicated in patients hypersensitive to drug.

⚕ Lifespan: In pregnant and breast-feeding women, use cautiously. In children, safety of drug hasn't been established.

Adverse reactions

CNS: *asthenia, dizziness, headache,* nervousness, paresthesia, somnolence.
CV: palpitations, orthostatic hypotension, tachycardia, *peripheral edema,* atrial fibrillation.
EENT: nasal congestion, sinusitis, blurred vision.

GI: nausea.
GU: impotence, priapism.
Hematologic: *thrombocytopenia.*
Musculoskeletal: back pain, muscle pain.
Respiratory: dyspnea.
Other: decreased libido.

Interactions

Drug-drug. *Antihypertensives:* May cause excessive hypotension. Use together cautiously.
Clonidine: May decrease antihypertensive effect of clonidine. Monitor patient.
Drug-herb. *Butcher's broom:* Possible diminished effect. Discourage using together.

Effects on lab test results

• May decrease total protein and albumin levels.
• May decrease hematocrit, hemoglobin, and platelet and WBC counts.

Pharmacokinetics

Absorption: Rapid with about 90% of dose being bioavailable.
Distribution: About 90% to 94% plasma protein-bound.
Metabolism: In liver.
Excretion: About 40% in urine, 60% in feces, mostly as metabolites. Up to 30% may be unchanged. *Half-life:* About 12 hours.

Route	Onset	Peak	Duration
P.O.	≤ 15 min	2-3 hr	24 hr

Action

Chemical effect: Decreases blood pressure by vasodilation produced in response to blockade of alpha$_1$-adrenergic receptors. Improves urine flow by blocking alpha$_1$-adrenergic receptors in smooth muscle of bladder neck and prostate, thus relieving urethral pressure and reestablishing urine flow.
Therapeutic effect: Lowers blood pressure and relieves symptoms of BPH.

Available forms

Capsules: 1 mg, 2 mg, 5 mg, 10 mg

NURSING PROCESS

🔧 Assessment
• Assess patient's condition before therapy and regularly thereafter.
• Monitor blood pressure frequently.

• Be alert for adverse reactions and drug interactions.
• Evaluate patient's and family's knowledge of drug therapy.

🔲 Nursing diagnoses
• Risk for injury related to presence of hypertension
• Sexual dysfunction related to drug-induced impotence
• Deficient knowledge related to drug therapy

▶ Planning and implementation
⚠ **ALERT:** If drug is stopped for several days, dosage will need to be readjusted to initial regimen.
Patient teaching
• Tell patient not to stop drug but to call prescriber if adverse reactions occur.
• Tell patient to take the first dose at bedtime. If he must get up, he should do so slowly to prevent dizziness or blackouts.
• Warn patient to avoid activities that require mental alertness for 12 hours after first dose.
• Teach patient other means to reduce blood pressure, such as diet control, exercise, smoking cessation, and stress reduction.

☑ Evaluation
• Patient's blood pressure is normal.
• Patient develops and maintains positive attitude toward his sexuality despite impotence.
• Patient and family state understanding of drug therapy.

---

terbutaline sulfate
(ter-BYOO-tuh-leen SUL-fayt)
Brethine, Bricanyl

Pharmacologic class: beta$_2$-adrenergic agonist
Therapeutic class: bronchodilator
Pregnancy risk category: B

Indications and dosages

▶ **Bronchospasm in patients with reversible obstructive airway disease.** *Adults and children older than age 15:* 5 mg P.O. t.i.d. at 6-hour intervals while awake. Or, 0.25 mg S.C. may be repeated in 15 to 30 minutes; maximum 0.5 mg q 4 hours.
Children ages 12 to 15: 2.5 mg P.O. t.i.d.

Reactions may be *common,* uncommon, *life-threatening,* or **COMMON AND LIFE-THREATENING.**

▶ **Premature labor‡.** *Adults:* Initially, 2.5 to 10 mcg/minute I.V.; increase dose gradually as tolerated in 10- to 20-minute intervals until desired effects are achieved. Maximum dosages range from 17.5 to 30 mcg/minute, although dosages of up to 80 mcg/minute have been used cautiously. Continue infusion for at least 12 hours after uterine contractions stop. Maintenance therapy, 2.5 to 10 mg P.O. q 4 to 6 hours.

▼ I.V. administration

● Monitor uterine response, maternal blood pressure, and maternal and fetal heart rates. Also monitor patient for circulatory overload and pulmonary edema.
● Protect injection from light. If discolored, don't use.

Contraindications and precautions

● Contraindicated in patients hypersensitive to drug or sympathomimetic amines.
● Use cautiously in patient with CV disorders, hyperthyroidism, diabetes, or seizure disorders.
⚜ Lifespan: In pregnant and breast-feeding women, use cautiously. In children age 11 and younger, safety of drug hasn't been established.

Adverse reactions

CNS: *nervousness, tremor, headache, drowsiness, dizziness,* weakness.
CV: *palpitations,* tachycardia, ***arrhythmias,*** flushing.
GI: *vomiting, nausea,* heartburn.
Metabolic: hypokalemia.
Respiratory: ***paradoxical bronchospasm,*** dyspnea.
Skin: diaphoresis.

Interactions

Drug-drug. *Digoxin, cyclopropane, halogenated inhaled anesthetics, levodopa:* Increases risk of arrhythmias. Monitor patient closely.
CNS stimulants: Increases CNS stimulation. Avoid use together.
MAO inhibitors: May cause severe hypertension (hypertensive crisis). Don't use together.
Propranolol, other beta blockers: Blocks bronchodilating effects of terbutaline. Avoid use together.

Effects on lab test results

● May decrease potassium level.

Pharmacokinetics

Absorption: 33% to 50% of P.O. dose; unknown for S.C.
Distribution: Widely distributed throughout body.
Metabolism: Partially metabolized in liver to inactive compounds.
Excretion: Excreted primarily in urine. *Half-life:* Unknown.

Route	Onset	Peak	Duration
P.O.	30 min	2-3 hr	4-8 hr
S.C.	≤ 15 min	30-60 min	1½-4 hr

Action

Chemical effect: Relaxes bronchial smooth muscle by acting on beta$_2$-adrenergic receptors.
Therapeutic effect: Improves breathing ability.

Available forms

Injection: 1 mg/ml
Tablets: 2.5 mg, 5 mg

NURSING PROCESS

⚕ Assessment
● Assess patient's condition before therapy and regularly thereafter.
● Monitor patient closely for toxicity.
● Evaluate patient's and family's knowledge of drug therapy.

⊞ Nursing diagnoses
● Ineffective breathing pattern related to underlying respiratory condition
● Pain related to drug-induced headache
● Deficient knowledge related to drug therapy

▷ Planning and implementation
● For subcutaneous administration, inject in lateral deltoid area.
● If bronchospasm develops during therapy, notify prescriber immediately.
● Mild analgesic may be used to treat drug-induced headache.
● **⚠ ALERT:** Don't confuse terbutaline with tolbutamide or terbinafine.
Patient teaching
● Explain to patient and family why drug is needed.
● Instruct patient to report paradoxical bronchospasm, and tell him to stop drug if it happens.

- Warn patient that tolerance may develop with prolonged use.

☑ Evaluation
- Patient's breathing is improved.
- Patient's headache is relieved with mild analgesic.
- Patient and family state understanding of drug therapy.

terconazole
(ter-KON-uh-zohl)
Terazol 3, Terazol 7

Pharmacologic class: triazole derivative
Therapeutic class: antifungal
Pregnancy risk category: C

Indications and dosages
▶ **Vulvovaginal candidiasis.** *Women:* 1 applicator of cream or 1 suppository inserted into vagina h.s.; 0.4% cream used for 7 consecutive days; 0.8% cream or 80-mg suppository used for 3 consecutive days. Repeat course, if needed, after reconfirmation by smear or culture.

Contraindications and precautions
- Contraindicated in patients hypersensitive to drug or inactive ingredients in formulation.
- ⚠ Lifespan: In pregnant women, use cautiously. In breast-feeding women, drug isn't recommended. In girls, safety hasn't been established.

Adverse reactions
CNS: *headache,* fever.
GI: abdominal pain.
GU: dysmenorrhea, vulvovaginal pain or burning.
Skin: irritation, photosensitivity reactions, *pruritus.*
Other: chills, body aches.

Interactions
None significant.

Effects on lab test results
None reported.

Pharmacokinetics
Absorption: 5% to 16%.
Distribution: Mainly local.

Metabolism: Unknown.
Excretion: Unknown. *Half-life:* 4 to 11 hours.

Route	Onset	Peak	Duration
Intravaginal	Unknown	Unknown	Unknown

Action
Chemical effect: May increase fungal cell membrane permeability (*Candida* species only).
Therapeutic effect: Impairs function of *Candida* species.

Available forms
Vaginal cream: 0.4%, 0.8%
Vaginal suppositories: 80 mg

NURSING PROCESS

🗲 Assessment
- Assess patient's infection before therapy and regularly thereafter.
- Evaluate patient's and family's knowledge of drug therapy.

⊕ Nursing diagnoses
- Risk for infection related to presence of susceptible fungi
- Acute pain related to drug-induced burning
- Deficient knowledge related to drug therapy

▶ Planning and implementation
- Insert cream using supplied applicator.
- If vaginal suppository is used, have patient remain supine for about 30 minutes after insertion.
- Report fever, chills, other flulike symptoms, or sensitivity, and stop drug.
- ⓢ **ALERT:** Don't confuse terconazole with tioconazole.
Patient teaching
- Instruct patient how to insert cream or suppository.
- Advise patient to continue therapy during menstrual period. Tell her not to use tampons.
- Tell patient to use drug for the full amount of time it was prescribed. Explain how to prevent reinfection.

☑ Evaluation
- Patient is free from infection.
- Patient states that drug-induced burning is tolerable.

• Patient and family state understanding of drug therapy.

teriparatide (rDNA origin)
(tehr-ih-PAHR-uh-tyd)
Forteo

Pharmacologic class: recombinant human parathyroid hormone (PTH)
Therapeutic class: antiosteoporotic
Pregnancy risk category: C

Indications and dosages

▶ **Osteoporosis in postmenopausal women at high risk for fracture; to increase bone mass in men with primary or hypogonadal osteoporosis who are at high risk for fracture.**
Adults: 20 mcg S.C. in thigh or abdominal wall once daily.

Contraindications and precautions

• Contraindicated in patients hypersensitive to drug or its components. Don't give to patients who have had radiation to the skeleton, those with Paget's disease or unexplained alkaline phosphatase elevations, or those at increased risk for osteosarcoma, such as children. Don't give drug to patients with bone metastases, a history of skeletal malignancies, or metabolic bone diseases other than osteoporosis. Avoid use in patients with hypercalcemia. Don't continue therapy beyond 2 years.
• Use cautiously in patients with active or recent urolithiasis and in patients with hepatic, renal, or cardiac disease.
⚠ Lifespan: In pregnant and breast-feeding women, drug isn't recommended. In children, safety and effectiveness of drug haven't been established.

Adverse reactions

CNS: asthenia, depression, dizziness, headache, insomnia, syncope, vertigo, *pain.*
CV: angina pectoris, hypertension, orthostatic hypotension.
EENT: pharyngitis, rhinitis.
GI: constipation, diarrhea, dyspepsia, nausea, tooth disorder, vomiting.
Metabolic: hypercalcemia.

Musculoskeletal: *arthralgia,* leg cramps, neck pain.
Respiratory: dyspnea, cough, pneumonia.
Skin: rash, sweating.

Interactions

Drug-drug. *Calcium supplements:* May increase urinary calcium excretion. Dosage may need adjustment.
Digoxin: Hypercalcemia may predispose patient to digitalis toxicity. Use together cautiously.

Effects on lab test results

• May increase calcium and uric acid levels. May decrease phosphorus levels.
• May increase urinary calcium and phosphorus excretion.

Pharmacokinetics

Absorption: Rapid and extensive, with level peaking after about 30 minutes. Availability is about 95%.
Distribution: Unknown.
Metabolism: Unknown for drug, but PTH is metabolized in the liver.
Excretion: Unknown for drug, but PTH is excreted by the kidneys. Elimination is rapid.
Half-life: 1 hour.

Route	Onset	Peak	Duration
S.C.	Rapid	30 min	3 hr

Action

Chemical effect: Regulates calcium and phosphorus metabolism in bones and kidneys, increases calcium, and decreases phosphorus levels.
Therapeutic effect: Decreases risk of fractures in patients with osteoporosis.

Available forms

Injection: 750 mcg/3 ml in a prefilled pen

NURSING PROCESS

📝 **Assessment**
🔔 **ALERT:** Because of the risk of osteosarcoma, give drug only to patients for whom potential benefits outweigh risks.
• If patient could have urolithiasis or hypercalciuria, measure urinary calcium excretion before therapy.

- Evaluate patient's and family's knowledge of drug therapy.

🔛 Nursing diagnoses
- Risk for falls related to presence of osteoporosis
- Chronic pain related to adverse drug effects
- Deficient knowledge related to drug therapy

⟩ Planning and implementation
- Monitor patient for orthostatic hypotension, which may occur within 4 hours of dosing.
- Track calcium levels. If patient develops persistent hypercalcemia, stop drug and evaluate its possible cause.

Patient teaching
- Instruct patient on the proper use and disposal of the prefilled pen.
- Tell patient not to share pen with others.
- Advise patient to sit or lie down if drug causes a fast heart beat, light-headedness, or dizziness. Tell patient to report persistent or worsening symptoms.
- Instruct patient to report persistent symptoms of hypercalcemia (nausea, vomiting, constipation, lethargy, and muscle weakness).

✓ Evaluation
- Patient doesn't fall.
- Patient reports no pain or states that pain is controlled by therapy.
- Patient and family state understanding of drug therapy.

testolactone
(tes-tuh-LAK-tohn)
Teslac

Pharmacologic class: androgen
Therapeutic class: antineoplastic
Pregnancy risk category: C
Controlled substance schedule: III

Indications and dosages
▶ **Advanced postmenopausal breast cancer.**
Women: 250 mg P.O. q.i.d.

Contraindications and precautions
- Contraindicated in patients hypersensitive to drug and in men with breast cancer.

🔆 **Lifespan:** In pregnant women, use cautiously. In breast-feeding women, drug isn't recommended. In children, drug isn't indicated.

Adverse reactions
CNS: paresthesia, peripheral neuropathy.
CV: increased blood pressure, edema.
GI: nausea, vomiting, diarrhea, anorexia, glossitis.
Skin: erythema, nail changes, alopecia.

Interactions
Drug-drug. *Oral anticoagulants:* Increases pharmacologic effects. Monitor patient carefully.

Effects on lab test results
None reported.

Pharmacokinetics
Absorption: Good.
Distribution: Widely distributed in total body water.
Metabolism: Extensively metabolized in liver.
Excretion: Testolactone and its metabolites excreted primarily in urine. *Half-life:* Unknown.

Route	Onset	Peak	Duration
P.O.	6-12 wk	Unknown	Unknown

Action
Chemical effect: Unknown; may change tumor's hormonal environment and alter neoplastic process.
Therapeutic effect: Hinders breast cancer cell activity.

Available forms
Tablets: 50 mg

NURSING PROCESS

🗎 Assessment
- Assess patient's breast cancer before therapy and regularly thereafter.
- Monitor fluid and electrolyte levels, especially calcium level.
- Evaluate patient's and family's knowledge of drug therapy.

🔛 Nursing diagnoses
- Ineffective health maintenance related to presence of breast cancer

• Disturbed sensory perception (tactile) related to drug-induced paresthesia and peripheral neuropathy
• Deficient knowledge related to drug therapy

> **Planning and implementation**
• Encourage patient to drink fluids to aid calcium excretion, and encourage exercise to prevent hypercalcemia. Immobilized patients are prone to hypercalcemia.
• Higher-than-recommended doses don't promote remission.
• Continue therapy for at least 3 months unless there is active progression of the disease.
Patient teaching
• Inform patient that therapeutic response isn't immediate; it may take up to 3 months for benefit to be noted.
• Encourage patient to exercise and drink plenty of fluids to help prevent hypercalcemia.
• Tell patient to report adverse effects.

☑ Evaluation
• Patient responds well to drug.
• Patient lists ways to protect against risk of injury caused by diminished tactile sensation.
• Patient and family state understanding of drug therapy.

testosterone
(tes-TOS-teh-rohn)
Andronaq-50, Histerone-50, Histerone 100, Testamone 100, Testaqua, Testoject-50

testosterone cypionate
Andronate 100, Andronate 200, depAndro 100, depAndro 200, Depotest, Depo-Testosterone, Duratest-100, Duratest-200, T-Cypionate, Testred Cypionate 200, Virilon IM

testosterone enanthate
Andro L.A. 200, Andropository 200, Andryl 200, Delatest, Delatestryl, Durathate-200, Everone 200, Testrin-P.A.

testosterone propionate
Malogen in Oil ◆, Testex

Pharmacologic class: androgen

Therapeutic class: androgen replacement, antineoplastic
Pregnancy risk category: X
Controlled substance schedule: III

Indications and dosages

▶ **Hypogonadism.** *Men:* 10 to 25 mg testosterone I.M. two to three times weekly. Or, 50 to 400 mg testosterone cypionate or testosterone enanthate I.M. q 2 to 4 weeks. Or, 10 to 25 mg testosterone propionate I.M. two to three times weekly.
▶ **Delayed puberty.** *Boys:* 25 to 50 mg testosterone or testosterone propionate I.M. two or three times weekly for up to 6 months.
▶ **Metastatic breast cancer 1 to 5 years postmenopausal.** *Women:* 100 mg testosterone I.M. three times weekly. Or, 50 to 100 mg testosterone propionate I.M. three times weekly. Or, 200 to 400 mg testosterone cypionate or testosterone enanthate I.M. q 2 to 4 weeks.
▶ **Postpartum breast pain and engorgement.** *Adults:* 25 to 50 mg testosterone or testosterone propionate I.M. daily for 3 to 4 days.

Contraindications and precautions

• Contraindicated in men with breast or prostate cancer; patients with hypercalcemia; and those with cardiac, hepatic, or renal decompensation.
⚖ Lifespan: In pregnant and breast-feeding women, drug is contraindicated. In geriatric patients, use cautiously.

Adverse reactions

CNS: headache, anxiety, depression, paresthesia, sleep apnea syndrome.
CV: edema.
GI: nausea.
GU: hypoestrogenic effects in women (*acne; edema; oily skin; hirsutism; hoarseness; weight gain;* clitoral enlargement; decreased or increased libido; flushing; diaphoresis; vaginitis, including itching, drying, and burning; vaginal bleeding; menstrual irregularities), excessive hormonal effects in boys and men (prepubertal: premature epiphyseal closure, *acne,* priapism, *growth of body and facial hair,* phallic enlargement; postpubertal: testicular atrophy, oligospermia, decreased ejaculatory volume, impotence, gynecomastia, epididymitis), bladder irritability.
Hematologic: *polycythemia, suppression of clotting factors.*

Hepatic: reversible jaundice, *cholestatic hepatitis.*
Metabolic: hypercalcemia.
Skin: local edema, hypersensitivity skin signs and symptoms.
Other: androgenic effects in women, pain and induration at injection site.

Interactions

Drug-drug. *Hepatotoxic drugs:* Increases risk of hepatotoxicity. Monitor patient closely.
Insulin, oral antidiabetics: Alters dosage requirements. Monitor glucose level in diabetic patients.
Oral anticoagulants: Alters dosage requirements. Monitor PT and INR.

Effects on lab test results

• May increase sodium, potassium, phosphate, cholesterol, liver enzyme, calcium, and creatinine levels. May decrease thyroxine-binding globulin and total T_4 levels.
• May increase RBC count and resin uptake of T_3 and T_4 levels.

Pharmacokinetics

Absorption: Unknown.
Distribution: 98% to 99% protein-bound, primarily to testosterone–estradiol-binding globulin.
Metabolism: In liver.
Excretion: In urine. *Half-life:* 10 to 100 minutes.

Route	Onset	Peak	Duration
I.M.	Unknown	Unknown	Unknown

Action

Chemical effect: Stimulates target tissues to develop normally in androgen-deficient men. Drug may have some antiestrogen properties, making it useful to treat certain estrogen-dependent breast cancers. Its action in postpartum breast engorgement isn't known because drug doesn't suppress lactation.
Therapeutic effect: Increases testosterone level, inhibits some estrogen activity, and relieves postpartum breast pain and engorgement.

Available forms

testosterone
Injection (aqueous suspension): 25 mg/ml, 50 mg/ml, 100 mg/ml

testosterone cypionate
Injection (in oil): 100 mg/ml, 200 mg/ml
testosterone enanthate
Injection (in oil): 100 mg/ml, 200 mg/ml
testosterone propionate
Injection (in oil): 100 mg/ml

NURSING PROCESS

Assessment
• Assess patient's condition before therapy and regularly thereafter.
• Periodically monitor calcium level and liver function test results.
• Monitor hemoglobin and hematocrit for polycythemia.
• Monitor prepubertal boys by X-ray for rate of bone maturation.
• Be alert for adverse reactions and drug interactions.
• Evaluate patient's and family's knowledge of drug therapy.

Nursing diagnoses
• Ineffective health maintenance related to underlying condition
• Disturbed body image related to drug-induced adverse androgenic reactions
• Deficient knowledge related to drug therapy

Planning and implementation
• Give daily dose requirement in divided doses for best results.
• Store preparations at room temperature. If crystals appear, warm and shake bottle to disperse them.
• Inject deep into upper outer quadrant of gluteal muscle. Rotate sites to prevent muscle atrophy. Report soreness at site because of possibility of postinfection furunculosis.
• Unless contraindicated, use with diet high in calories and protein in small, frequent meals.
• Report signs of virilization in woman.
• Edema generally can be controlled with sodium restriction or diuretics.
ALERT: Therapeutic response in breast cancer usually appears within 3 months. If signs of disease progression appear, stop drug. In metastatic breast cancer, hypercalcemia usually signals progression of bone metastases. Report signs of hypercalcemia.

Reactions may be *common*, uncommon, *life-threatening*, or COMMON AND LIFE-THREATENING.

• Androgens may alter results of laboratory studies during therapy and for 2 to 3 weeks after therapy ends.

⊛ **ALERT:** Testosterone and methyltestosterone aren't interchangeable. Don't confuse testosterone with testolactone.

Patient teaching
• Tell patient to use effective nonhormonal form of contraception during therapy.
• Instruct man to report priapism, reduced ejaculatory volume, and gynecomastia. Drug may need to be stopped.
• Inform woman that virilization may occur. Tell her to report androgenic effects immediately. Stopping drug will prevent further androgenic changes but probably won't reverse those already present.
• Teach patient to recognize and report signs of hypoglycemia.
• Instruct patient to follow dietary measures to combat drug-induced adverse reactions.

☑ **Evaluation**
• Patient responds well to drug.
• Patient states acceptance of altered body image.
• Patient and family state understanding of drug therapy.

---

testosterone transdermal system
(tes-TOS-teh-rohn tranz-DER-mal SIHS-tum)
Androderm, Testoderm, Testoderm TTS

Pharmacologic class: androgen
Therapeutic class: androgen replacement
Pregnancy risk category: X
Controlled substance schedule: III

Indications and dosages

▶ **Primary or hypogonadotropic hypogonadism.** *Men:* One 6-mg Testoderm patch applied to scrotal area daily. If scrotal area is too small for 6-mg patch, start with 4-mg patch. Patch worn for 22 to 24 hours daily. Or, 5 mg Androderm daily either as two 2.5-mg systems or one 5-mg system applied h.s. to clean, dry skin on back, abdomen, upper arms, or thighs. Or, one 5-mg Testoderm TTS patch applied to arm, back, or upper buttock daily.

Contraindications and precautions

• Contraindicated in patients hypersensitive to drug and in patients with known or suspected breast or prostate cancer.
• Use cautiously in patients with renal, hepatic, or cardiac disease.
⚞ **Lifespan:** In women, drug is contraindicated. In children, drug isn't indicated. In geriatric men, use cautiously because they may be at greater risk for prostatic hyperplasia or prostate cancer.

Adverse reactions

CV: *CVA,* headache, depression.
GI: *GI bleeding.*
GU: prostatitis, prostate abnormalities, UTI.
Skin: acne, *pruritus,* irritation, *blister under system,* allergic contact dermatitis; burning, induration (at application site).
Other: gynecomastia, breast tenderness.

Interactions

Drug-drug. *Antidiabetics:* Alters antidiabetic dosage requirements. Monitor glucose level.
Oral anticoagulants: Alters anticoagulant dosage requirements. Monitor PT and INR.
Oxyphenbutazone: May elevate oxyphenbutazone levels. Monitor patient for adverse reactions.

Effects on lab test results

• May increase sodium, potassium, phosphate, cholesterol, liver enzyme, calcium, and creatinine levels.
• May increase RBC count.

Pharmacokinetics

Absorption: Absorbed from scrotal skin after application.
Distribution: Chiefly bound to sex–hormone-binding globulin.
Metabolism: Metabolized in liver.
Excretion: Excreted in urine. *Half-life:* 10 to 100 minutes.

Route	Onset	Peak	Duration
Transdermal	Unknown	2-4 hr	2 hr after removal

Action

Chemical effect: Stimulates target tissues to develop normally in androgen-deficient men.
Therapeutic effect: Increases testosterone in androgen-deficient men.

Available forms

Transdermal system: 2.5 mg/day, 4 mg/day, 5 mg/day, 6 mg/day

NURSING PROCESS

Assessment

• Assess patient's condition before therapy and regularly thereafter.
• Because long-term use of systemic androgens is linked to polycythemia, monitor hematocrit and hemoglobin values periodically in patient on long-term therapy.
• Periodically assess liver function tests, lipid profiles, and prostatic acid phosphatase and prostate-specific antigen levels.
• Be alert for adverse reactions and drug interactions.
• Evaluate patient's and family's knowledge of drug therapy.

Nursing diagnoses

• Sexual dysfunction related to androgen deficiency
• Risk for impaired skin integrity related to drug-induced irritation at application site
• Deficient knowledge related to drug therapy

Planning and implementation

• Apply Testoderm system on clean, dry scrotal skin. Dry shave scrotal hair (don't use chemical depilatories).
• Apply Androderm to clean, dry skin on back, abdomen, upper arms, or thighs.
• Apply Testoderm TTS to clean, dry skin on arm, back, or upper buttock.
③ ALERT: Don't confuse Testoderm with Estraderm.
Patient teaching
• Teach patient how to apply transdermal system.
• Tell patient that topical testosterone preparations can cause virilization in female partners. Advise these women to report acne or changes in body hair.
• Advise patient to report to prescriber persistent erections, nausea, vomiting, changes in skin color, or ankle edema.

Evaluation

• Patient states that he can resume normal sexual activity.
• Patient maintains normal skin integrity.

• Patient and family state understanding of drug therapy.

---

tetanus immune globulin, human
(TET-uh-nus ih-MYOON GLOH-byoo-lin)
BayTet

Pharmacologic class: immune serum
Therapeutic class: tetanus prophylaxis
Pregnancy risk category: C

Indications and dosages

▶ **Tetanus exposure.** *Adults and children age 7 and older:* 250 units I.M.
Children younger than age 7: 4 units/kg I.M.
▶ **Tetanus.** *Adults and children:* Single doses of 3,000 to 6,000 units I.M. Optimal dosage hasn't been established.

Contraindications and precautions

• In patients with thrombocytopenia or coagulation disorders, I.M. injection is contraindicated unless potential benefits outweigh risks.
※ **Lifespan:** In pregnant and breast-feeding women, use cautiously.

Adverse reactions

GU: slight fever, nephrotic syndrome.
Skin:
Other: hypersensitivity reactions; *anaphylaxis; angioedema;* pain, stiffness, erythema at injection site.

Interactions

Drug-drug. *Live-virus vaccines:* May interfere with response. Defer administration of live-virus vaccines for 3 months after administration of tetanus immune globulin.

Effects on lab test results

None reported.

Pharmacokinetics

Absorption: Slow.
Distribution: Unknown.
Metabolism: Unknown.
Excretion: Unknown. *Half-life:* About 28 days.

Route	Onset	Peak	Duration
I.M.	Unknown	2-3 days	4 wk

Reactions may be *common,* uncommon, *life-threatening*, or COMMON AND LIFE-THREATENING.

Action

Chemical effect: Provides passive immunity to tetanus.
Therapeutic effect: Prevents tetanus.

Available forms

Injection: 250 units per vial or syringe

NURSING PROCESS

⚖ Assessment

• Obtain history of injury, tetanus immunizations, last tetanus toxoid injection, allergies, and reaction to immunizations.
• Antibodies remain at effective level for about 4 weeks (several times the duration of antitoxin-induced antibodies), which protects patient for incubation period of most tetanus cases.
• Be alert for adverse reactions and drug interactions.
• Evaluate patient's and family's knowledge of drug therapy.

🔡 Nursing diagnoses

• Risk for injury related to potential for tetanus to occur
• Deficient knowledge related to drug therapy

▶ Planning and implementation

🔞 **ALERT:** Have epinephrine 1:1,000 available to treat hypersensitivity reactions.
• Use drug if wound is more than 24 hours old or if patient has had fewer than two tetanus toxoid injections.
• Thoroughly clean wound and remove all foreign matter.
• Inject drug into deltoid muscle for adult and child age 3 and older and into anterolateral aspect of thigh in neonate and child younger than age 3.
🔞 **ALERT:** Don't confuse drug with tetanus toxoid. Tetanus immune globulin isn't a substitute for tetanus toxoid, which should be given at same time to produce active immunization. Don't give at same site as toxoid.
Patient teaching
• Warn patient that pain and tenderness at injection site may occur. Suggest mild analgesic for pain relief.
• Tell patient to document date of tetanus immunization and encourage him to keep immunization current.

✅ Evaluation

• Patient doesn't develop tetanus.
• Patient and family state understanding of drug therapy.

tetracycline hydrochloride

(tet-ruh-SIGH-kleen high-droh-KLOR-ighd)
Achromycin†, Apo-Tetra ◆, Mysteclin ◇, Novo-Tetra ◆, Nu-Tetra ◆, Sumycin, Tetrex ◇, Topicycline

Pharmacologic class: tetracycline
Therapeutic class: antibiotic
Pregnancy risk category: NR

Indications and dosages

▶ **Infections caused by sensitive gram-negative and gram-positive organisms, including *Chlamydia*, *Mycoplasma*, *Rickettsia*, and organisms that cause trachoma.** *Adults:* 1 to 2 g P.O. divided into two to four doses.
Children older than age 8: 25 to 50 mg/kg P.O. daily divided into four doses.
▶ **Uncomplicated urethral, endocervical, or rectal infection caused by *Chlamydia trachomatis*.** *Adults:* 500 mg P.O. q.i.d. for at least 7 days.
▶ **Brucellosis.** *Adults:* 500 mg P.O. q 6 hours for 3 weeks combined with 1 g of streptomycin I.M. q 12 hours first week and daily the second week.
▶ **Gonorrhea in patients sensitive to penicillin.** *Adults:* Initially, 1.5 g P.O.; then 500 mg q 6 hours for 4 days.
▶ **Syphilis in nonpregnant patients sensitive to penicillin.** *Adults:* 500 mg P.O. q.i.d. for 15 days.
▶ **Acne.** *Adults and adolescents:* Initially, 125 to 250 mg P.O. q 6 hours; then 125 to 500 mg daily or q other day. Or, apply 3% ointment or 2.2% solution to affected areas daily or b.i.d.
▶ **Lyme disease‡.** *Adults:* 250 to 500 mg P.O. q.i.d. for 10 to 30 days.
▶ **Adjunct therapy for acute transmitted epididymitis (children older than age 8); pelvic inflammatory disease; and infection with *Helicobacter pylori*‡.** *Adults:* 500 mg P.O. q.i.d. for 10 to 14 days.

Contraindications and precautions

• Contraindicated in patients hypersensitive to tetracyclines.

• Use cautiously in patients with impaired kidney or liver function.

❧ **Lifespan:** In women in the last half of pregnancy and in children younger than age 8, use cautiously, if at all, because drug may cause permanent discoloration of teeth, enamel defects, and bone growth retardation. In breast-feeding women, drug isn't recommended.

Adverse reactions

CNS: dizziness, headache, *intracranial hypertension (pseudotumor cerebri).*
CV: *pericarditis.*
EENT: sore throat, glossitis, dysphagia.
GI: anorexia, *epigastric distress, nausea,* vomiting, *diarrhea,* esophagitis, oral candidiasis, stomatitis, enterocolitis, inflammatory lesions in anogenital region.
Hematologic: *neutropenia, thrombocytopenia,* eosinophilia.
Musculoskeletal: *retardation of bone growth if used in children younger than age 9.*
Skin: candidal superinfection, maculopapular and erythematous rashes, urticaria, photosensitivity reactions, increased pigmentation.
Other: *permanent discoloration of teeth, enamel defects,* **hypersensitivity reactions.**

Interactions

Drug-drug. *Antacids (including sodium bicarbonate); antidiarrheals containing bismuth subsalicylate, kaolin, or pectin; laxatives containing aluminum, calcium, or magnesium:* Decreases antibiotic absorption. Give tetracyclines 1 hour before or 2 hours after these drugs.
Ferrous sulfate, other iron products, zinc: Decreases antibiotic absorption. Give tetracyclines 2 hours before or 3 hours after iron.
Hormonal contraceptives: Decreases contraceptive effectiveness and increased risk of breakthrough bleeding. Recommend nonhormonal form of birth control.
Lithium carbonate: May alter lithium level. Monitor patient.
Methoxyflurane: May cause severe nephrotoxicity with tetracyclines. Monitor patient carefully.
Oral anticoagulants: Potentiates anticoagulant effects. Monitor PT and adjust anticoagulant dosage.

Penicillins: May interfere with bactericidal action of penicillins. Avoid using together.
Drug-food. *Milk, dairy products, other foods:* Decreases drug absorption. Give drug 1 hour before or 2 hours after these products.
Drug-lifestyle. *Sun exposure:* Photosensitivity reactions may occur. Urge patient to avoid prolonged or unprotected exposure to sunlight.

Effects on lab test results

• May increase BUN and liver enzyme levels.
• May increase eosinophil counts. May decrease platelet and neutrophil counts.
• May cause false-negative reading with glucose enzymatic tests (Diastix).

Pharmacokinetics

Absorption: 75% to 80%. Food or milk products significantly reduces.
Distribution: Distributed widely in body tissues and fluids. CSF penetration is poor. Drug is 20% to 67% protein-bound.
Metabolism: None.
Excretion: Excreted primarily unchanged in urine. *Half-life:* 6 to 11 hours.

Route	Onset	Peak	Duration
P.O.	Unknown	2-4 hr	Unknown

Action

Chemical effect: Unknown; may act by binding to 30S ribosomal subunit of microorganisms, thus inhibiting protein synthesis.
Therapeutic effect: Hinders bacterial activity.

Available forms

Capsules: 250 mg, 500 mg
Ointment†: 3%
Oral suspension: 125 mg/5 ml
Topical solution: 2.2 mg/ml

NURSING PROCESS

⚕ Assessment

• Assess patient's infection before therapy and regularly thereafter.
• Obtain specimen for culture and sensitivity tests before first dose. Therapy may begin pending results.
• If adverse GI reactions occur, monitor hydration.
• Be alert for adverse reactions and drug interactions.

Reactions may be *common,* uncommon, *life-threatening,* or COMMON AND LIFE-THREATENING.

- Evaluate patient's and family's knowledge of drug therapy.

🔁 Nursing diagnoses
- Risk for infection related to presence of susceptible bacteria
- Risk for deficient fluid volume related to drug-induced adverse GI reactions
- Deficient knowledge related to drug therapy

≫ Planning and implementation
⑤ ALERT: Check expiration date. Outdated or deteriorated tetracyclines have been linked to reversible nephrotoxicity (Fanconi's syndrome).
- Give drug on empty stomach.
- Don't expose drug to light or heat.

Patient teaching
- Tell patient to take drug with full glass of water on empty stomach, at least 1 hour before or 2 hours after meals. Also, tell him to take drug at least 1 hour before bedtime to prevent esophagitis. Explain that effectiveness of drug is reduced when taken with milk or other dairy products, food, antacids, or iron products.
- Tell patient to take drug exactly as prescribed, even after he feels better, and to take entire amount prescribed.
- Warn patient to avoid direct sunlight and ultraviolet light. Recommend sunscreen to help prevent photosensitivity reactions. Tell him that photosensitivity persists after drug is stopped.
- Advise patient that topical forms of the drug may stain skin and clothing.
- Tell patient using topical preparation to wash, rinse, and thoroughly dry the affected area before applying the drug. Also, advise him to avoid getting it in his eyes, nose, mouth, or other mucous membranes.

☑ Evaluation
- Patient is free from infection.
- Patient maintains adequate hydration.
- Patient and family state understanding of drug therapy.

theophylline
(thee-OF-ih-lin)
Immediate-release liquids
Accurbron*, Aquaphyllin, Asmalix*, Bronkodyl*, Elixomin*, Elixophyllin*, Lanophyllin*, Slo-Phyllin, Theolair

Immediate-release tablets and capsules
Bronkodyl, Elixophyllin, Nuelin ◊ , Slo-Phyllin

Timed-release capsules
Elixophyllin SR, Nuelin-SR ◊ , Slo-bid Gyrocaps, Slo-Phyllin, Theo-24, Theobid Duracaps, Theochron, Theospan-SR, Theovent Long-Acting

Timed-release tablets
Quibron-T/SR Dividose, Respbid, Sustaire, T-Phyl, Theochron, Theolair-SR, Theo-Sav, Theo-Time, Theo-X, Uniphyl

theophylline sodium glycinate

Pharmacologic class: xanthine derivative
Therapeutic class: bronchodilator
Pregnancy risk category: C

Indications and dosages

▶ **Oral theophylline for acute bronchospasm in patients not already receiving theophylline.** *Adults (nonsmokers):* Loading dose of 6 mg/kg P.O.; then 3 mg/kg q 6 hours for two doses. Maintenance dosage is 3 mg/kg q 8 hours.
Children ages 9 to 16 and young adult smokers: Loading dose of 6 mg/kg P.O.; then 3 mg/kg q 4 hours for three doses; then 3 mg/kg q 6 hours.
Children ages 6 months to 9 years: Loading dose of 6 mg/kg P.O.; then 4 mg/kg q 4 hours for three doses; then 4 mg/kg q 6 hours.
Older adults or those with cor pulmonale: Loading dose of 6 mg/kg P.O.; then 2 mg/kg q 6 hours for two doses; then 2 mg/kg q 8 hours.
⛔ Adjust-a-dose: For adults with heart failure or liver disease, give loading dose of 6 mg/kg P.O.; then 2 mg/kg q 8 hours for two doses; then 1 to 2 mg/kg q 12 hours.
▶ **Parenteral theophylline for patients not receiving theophylline.** *Adults (nonsmokers):* Loading dose of 4.7 mg/kg given slow I.V.; then maintenance infusion of 0.55 mg/kg/hour I.V. for 12 hours; then 0.39 mg/kg/hour.

Adults (otherwise healthy smokers): Loading dose of 4.7 mg/kg given slow I.V.; then maintenance infusion of 0.79 mg/kg/hour I.V. for 12 hours; then 0.63 mg/kg/hour.

Older adults or those with cor pulmonale: Loading dose of 4.7 mg/kg given slow I.V.; then maintenance infusion of 0.47 mg/kg/hour I.V. for 12 hours; then 0.24 mg/kg/hour.

Adults with heart failure or liver disease: Loading dose of 4.7 mg/kg given slow I.V.; then maintenance infusion of 0.39 mg/kg/hour I.V. for 12 hours; then 0.08 to 0.16 mg/kg/hour.

Children ages 9 to 16: Loading dose of 4.7 mg/kg given slow I.V.; then maintenance infusion of 0.79 mg/kg/hour I.V. for 12 hours; then 0.63 mg/kg/hour.

Children ages 6 months to 9 years: Loading dose of 4.7 mg/kg given slow I.V.; then maintenance infusion of 0.95 mg/kg/hour I.V. for 12 hours; then 0.79 mg/kg/hour.

▶ **Oral and parenteral theophylline for acute bronchospasm in patients receiving theophylline.** *Adults and children:* Each 0.5 mg/kg I.V. or P.O. (loading dose) increases plasma level by 1 mcg/ml. Ideally, dose is based on current theophylline level. In emergencies, some clinicians recommend 2.5 mg/kg P.O. dose of rapidly absorbed form if no obvious signs of theophylline toxicity are present.

▶ **Chronic bronchospasm.** *Adults and children:* 16 mg/kg or 400 mg P.O. daily (whichever is less) given in 3 or 4 divided doses at 6- to 8-hour intervals. Or, 12 mg/kg or 400 mg P.O. daily (whichever is less) using extended-release preparation given in 2 or 3 divided doses at 8- or 12-hour intervals. Dosage increased as tolerated at 2- to 3-day intervals to maximum dosage as follows:

Adults and children age 16 and older: 13 mg/kg or 900 mg P.O. daily (whichever is less) in divided doses.

Children ages 12 to 16: 18 mg/kg P.O. daily in divided doses.

Children ages 9 to 12: 20 mg/kg P.O. daily in divided doses.

Children ages 1 to 9: 24 mg/kg P.O. daily in divided doses.

Children younger than age 1‡: Loading dose is 1 mg/kg P.O. or I.V. for each 2 mcg/ml increase in theophylline level desired. Maintenance dosage for premature neonates up to 40 weeks postconception age is 1 mg/kg q 12 hours. Maintenance dosage for term neonates up to age 4

weeks is 1 to 2 mg/kg q 12 hours; 1 to 2 mg/kg q 8 hours in those age 4 to 8 weeks; and 1 to 3 mg/kg q 6 hours in those older than age 8 weeks.

▶ **Cystic fibrosis‡.** *Infants:* 10 to 20 mg/kg I.V. daily.

▶ **Promotion of diuresis; Cheyne-Stokes respirations; paroxysmal nocturnal dyspnea‡.** *Adults:* 200 to 400 mg I.V. bolus as a single dose.

▼ I.V. administration

• Use commercially available infusion solution, or mix drug in D₅W.
• Use infusion pump for continuous infusion.

Contraindications and precautions

• Contraindicated in patients with active peptic ulcer or seizure disorders and in those who are hypersensitive to xanthine compounds (caffeine, theobromine).
• Don't use extended-release forms for acute bronchospasm.
• Use cautiously in patients with COPD, cardiac failure, cor pulmonale, renal or hepatic disease, peptic ulceration, hyperthyroidism, diabetes mellitus, glaucoma, severe hypoxemia, hypertension, compromised cardiac or circulatory function, angina, acute MI, or sulfite sensitivity.
🔆 **Lifespan:** In pregnant women, use cautiously. In breast-fed infants, drug may cause irritability, insomnia, or fretting. In young children, infants, neonates, and geriatric patients, use cautiously.

Adverse reactions

CNS: *restlessness, dizziness,* headache, *insomnia,* irritability, *seizures,* muscle twitching.
CV: *palpitations, sinus tachycardia,* extrasystoles, flushing, *marked hypotension, arrhythmias.*
GI: *nausea, vomiting,* diarrhea, epigastric pain.
Respiratory: increased respiratory rate, *respiratory arrest.*

Interactions

Drug-drug. *Adenosine:* Decreases antiarrhythmic effectiveness. Higher doses of adenosine may be needed.
Barbiturates, carbamazepine, phenytoin, rifampin: Enhances metabolism and decreases theophylline blood level. Monitor patient for decreased effect.

Carteolol, pindolol, propranolol, timolol: May act antagonistically, reducing the effects of one or both drugs. The elimination of theophylline may also be reduced. Monitor theophylline level and patient closely.

Cimetidine, fluoroquinolone (such as ciprofloxacin), influenza virus vaccine, macrolide antibiotics (such as erythromycin), hormonal contraceptives: Decreases hepatic clearance of theophylline; elevates theophylline level. Monitor patient for toxicity.

Nadolol: Antagonizes drug; may cause bronchospasm in sensitive patients. Use together cautiously.

Drug-herb. *Cacao tree:* May inhibit drug metabolism. Discourage use together.

Cayenne: May increase drug absorption. Discourage use together.

St. John's wort: May decrease drug effectiveness. Discourage use together.

Drug-food. *Any food:* Accelerates absorption. Give drug on an empty stomach.

Caffeine: Decreases hepatic clearance of theophylline and elevates theophylline level. Monitor patient for toxicity.

Drug-lifestyle. *Smoking:* Increases drug elimination, increasing dosage requirements. Monitor drug response and level.

Effects on lab test results

• May increase free fatty acid level.

Pharmacokinetics

Absorption: Well absorbed. Food may further alter rate of absorption, especially of some extended-release preparations.

Distribution: Distributed throughout extracellular fluids; equilibrium between fluid and tissues occurs within 1 hour of I.V. loading dose.

Metabolism: In liver to inactive compounds.

Excretion: About 10% excreted unchanged in urine. *Half-life:* Adults, 7 to 9 hours; smokers, 4 to 5 hours; children, 3 to 5 hours; premature infants, 20 to 30 hours.

Route	Onset	Peak	Duration
P.O.			
regular	15-60 min	1-2 hr	Unknown
enteric-coated	15-60 min	1-2 hr	5 hr
extended-release	15-60 min	1-2 hr	4-7 hr
I.V.	15 min	15-30 min	Unknown

Action

Chemical effect: Inhibits phosphodiesterase, the enzyme that degrades cAMP, and relaxes smooth muscle of bronchial airways and pulmonary blood vessels.

Therapeutic effect: Improves breathing ability.

Available forms

theophylline
Capsules: 100 mg, 200 mg
Capsules (extended-release): 50 mg, 60 mg, 65 mg, 75 mg, 100 mg, 125 mg, 130 mg, 200 mg, 250 mg, 260 mg, 300 mg
D₅W injection: 200 mg in 50 ml or 100 ml; 400 mg in 100 ml, 250 ml, 500 ml, or 1,000 ml; 800 mg in 500 ml or 1,000 ml
Elixir: 27 mg/5 ml, 50 mg/5 ml*
Oral solution: 27 mg/5 ml, 50 mg/5 ml
Syrup: 27 mg/5 ml, 50 mg/5 ml
Tablets: 100 mg, 125 mg, 200 mg, 250 mg, 300 mg
Tablets (chewable): 100 mg
Tablets (extended-release): 100 mg, 200 mg, 250 mg, 300 mg, 400 mg, 500 mg, 600 mg
theophylline sodium glycinate
Elixir: 110 mg/5 ml (equivalent to 55 mg of anhydrous theophylline/5 ml)

NURSING PROCESS

🔁 Assessment

• Assess patient's condition before therapy and regularly thereafter.

• Monitor vital signs; measure fluid intake and output. Expect effects such as improvement in quality of pulse and respirations.

• Metabolism rate varies among individuals; dosage is determined by monitoring response, tolerance, pulmonary function, and drug level. Therapeutic level is 10 to 20 mcg/ml in adults and 5 to 15 mcg/ml in children.

• Be alert for adverse reactions and drug interactions.

⑤ ALERT: Monitor patient for signs and symptoms of toxicity including tachycardia, anorexia, nausea, vomiting, diarrhea, restlessness, irritability, and headache. The presence of any of these signs in patients taking theophylline warrants checking theophylline level and adjusting dose as indicated.

• If adverse GI reactions occur, monitor hydration.

• Evaluate patient's and family's knowledge of drug therapy.

Nursing diagnoses
• Impaired gas exchange related to presence of bronchospasm
• Risk for deficient fluid volume related to drug-induced adverse GI reactions
• Deficient knowledge related to drug therapy

Planning and implementation
• Give oral drug around-the-clock, using sustained-release product at bedtime.
ALERT: Don't confuse sustained-release forms with standard-release forms.
• Dosage may need to be increased in cigarette smokers and habitual marijuana smokers; smoking causes drug to be metabolized faster.
• Daily dose may need to be decreased in patients with heart failure or hepatic disease and in geriatric patients because metabolism and excretion may be decreased.
ALERT: Don't confuse Theolair with Thyrolar.
Patient teaching
• Instruct patient not to dissolve, crush, or chew sustained-release products. For child unable to swallow capsules, sprinkle contents of capsules over soft food and tell patient to swallow without chewing.
• Supply instructions for home care and dosage schedule.
• Tell patient to relieve GI symptoms by taking oral drug with full glass of water after meals, although food in stomach delays absorption.
• Instruct patient to take drug regularly, as directed.
• Inform geriatric patient that dizziness may occur at start of therapy.
• Have patient change position slowly and avoid hazardous activities.
• Tell patient to check with prescriber before taking other drugs, including OTC drugs. OTC drugs may contain ephedrine with theophylline salts; excessive CNS stimulation may result.
• If patient's dosage is stabilized while he is smoking and then he quits smoking, tell him to notify his prescriber; the dosage may need to be reduced.

Evaluation
• Patient demonstrates improved gas exchange, exhibited in arterial blood gas values and respiratory status.

• Patient maintains adequate hydration.
• Patient and family state understanding of drug therapy.

thiamine hydrochloride (vitamin B₁)

(THIGH-eh-min high-droh-KLOR-ighd)
Betamin◇, Beta-Sol◇, Biamine, Thiamilate†

Pharmacologic class: water-soluble vitamin
Therapeutic class: nutritional supplement
Pregnancy risk category: A

Indications and dosages

▶ **RDA.** *Men age 51 and older:* 1.2 mg P.O. daily.
Men ages 15 to 50: 1.5 mg P.O. daily.
Boys ages 11 to 14: 1.3 mg P.O. daily.
Women age 51 and older: 1 mg P.O. daily.
Women ages 11 to 50: 1.1 mg P.O. daily.
Pregnant women: 1.5 mg P.O. daily.
Breast-feeding women: 1.6 mg P.O. daily.
Children ages 7 to 10: 1 mg P.O. daily.
Children ages 4 to 6: 0.9 mg P.O. daily.
Children ages 1 to 3: 0.7 mg P.O. daily.
Infants age 6 months to 1 year: 0.4 mg P.O. daily.
Neonates and infants younger than age 6 months: 0.3 mg P.O. daily.
▶ **Beriberi.** *Adults:* Depending on severity, 10 to 20 mg I.M. t.i.d. for 2 weeks, followed by dietary correction and multivitamin supplement containing 5 to 10 mg of thiamine daily for 1 month.
Children: Depending on severity, 10 to 50 mg I.M. daily for several weeks with adequate diet.
▶ **Wet beriberi with myocardial failure.**
Adults and children: 10 to 30 mg I.V. for emergency therapy.
▶ **Wernicke's encephalopathy.** *Adults:* Initially, 100 mg I.V.; then 50 to 100 mg I.V. or I.M. daily until patient is consuming regular balanced diet.

I.V. administration

• Dilute drug before administration.
• Give large I.V. doses cautiously. Keep epinephrine available to treat anaphylaxis.
• Don't use with materials that yield alkaline solutions. Unstable in alkaline solutions.
• If patient has history of hypersensitivity reactions, apply skin test before starting therapy.

Contraindications and precautions

• Contraindicated in patients hypersensitive to thiamine products.
⚜ Lifespan: In pregnant women, use cautiously if dose exceeds RDA.

Adverse reactions

CNS: restlessness, weakness.
CV: *CV collapse,* cyanosis.
EENT: tightness of throat.
GI: nausea, *hemorrhage.*
Respiratory: *pulmonary edema.*
Skin: feeling of warmth, pruritus, urticaria, diaphoresis.
Other: tenderness and induration after I.M. administration, *hypersensitivity reactions (including anaphylactic shock).*

Interactions

None significant.

Effects on lab test results

None reported.

Pharmacokinetics

Absorption: Absorbed readily after small P.O. doses; after large P.O. dose, total amount absorbed is limited. In alcoholics and in patients with cirrhosis or malabsorption, GI absorption is decreased. When given with meals, drug's GI rate of absorption decreases, but total absorption remains same. After I.M. dose, rapid and complete.
Distribution: Wide. When intake exceeds minimal requirements, tissue stores become saturated.
Metabolism: In liver.
Excretion: In urine. *Half-life:* Unknown.

Route	Onset	Peak	Duration
P.O., I.V., I.M.	Unknown	Unknown	Unknown

Action

Chemical effect: Combines with adenosine triphosphate to form coenzyme needed for carbohydrate metabolism.
Therapeutic effect: Restores normal thiamine level.

Available forms

Elixir: 250 mcg/5 ml
Injection: 100 mg/ml, 200 mg/ml

Tablets: 5 mg†, 10 mg†, 25 mg†, 50 mg†, 100 mg†, 250 mg†, 500 mg†
Tablets (enteric-coated): 20 mg

NURSING PROCESS

🗟 Assessment
• Assess patient's condition before therapy and regularly thereafter.
• Be alert for adverse reactions.
• Evaluate patient's and family's knowledge of drug therapy.

🖅 Nursing diagnoses
• Imbalanced nutrition: less than body requirements related to presence of thiamine deficiency
• Diarrhea related to drug-induced adverse GI reactions
• Deficient knowledge related to drug therapy

▷ Planning and implementation
• Use parenteral route only when P.O. route isn't feasible.
• For treating alcoholic patient, give thiamine before dextrose infusions to prevent encephalopathy.
• Drug malabsorption is most likely in patients with alcoholism, cirrhosis, and GI disease.
• Significant deficiency can occur in about 3 weeks of thiamine-free diet. Thiamine deficiency usually requires simultaneous therapy for multiple deficiencies.
• If breast-fed infant develops beriberi, give drug to both mother and child.
⑤ ALERT: Don't confuse thiamine with Thorazine.
Patient teaching
• Stress proper nutritional habits to prevent recurrence of deficiency.

☑ Evaluation
• Patient regains normal thiamine level.
• Patient maintains normal bowel pattern.
• Patient and family state understanding of drug therapy.

thioguanine (6-thioguanine, 6-TG)
(thigh-oh-GWAH-neen)
Lanvis ♦ , Tabloid

Pharmacologic class: antimetabolite (specific to S phase of cell cycle)

Therapeutic class: antineoplastic
Pregnancy risk category: D

Indications and dosages

▶ **Acute nonlymphocytic leukemia, chronic myelogenous leukemia.** *Adults and children:* Initially, 2 mg/kg P.O. daily (usually calculated to nearest 20 mg). If needed, increase dosage gradually to 3 mg/kg daily, as tolerated.

Contraindications and precautions

• Contraindicated in patients whose disease has shown resistance to drug.
• Use cautiously in patients with renal or hepatic dysfunction.
⚠ **Lifespan:** In pregnant and breast-feeding women, drug isn't recommended.

Adverse reactions

GI: nausea, vomiting, stomatitis, diarrhea, anorexia.
Hematologic: *leukopenia, anemia, thrombocytopenia* (occurs slowly over 2 to 4 weeks).
Hepatic: *hepatotoxicity,* jaundice, hepatic fibrosis, *toxic hepatitis.*
Metabolic: hyperuricemia.

Interactions

Drug-drug. *Mercaptopurine:* Complete cross-resistance with Tabloid. Avoid use together.
Myelosuppressant drugs: Increases risk of toxicity, especially myelosuppression, hepatotoxicity, and bleeding. Use together cautiously.

Effects on lab test results

• May increase uric acid level and liver function test values.
• May decrease hemoglobin, hematocrit, and WBC, RBC, and platelet counts.

Pharmacokinetics

Absorption: Incomplete and variable; average bioavailability is 30%.
Distribution: Distributed well in bone marrow cells.
Metabolism: Extensively metabolized to less active form in liver and other tissues.
Excretion: Excreted in urine, mainly as metabolites. *Half-life:* Initial phase, 15 minutes; terminal phase, 11 hours.

Route	Onset	Peak	Duration
P.O.	Unknown	Unknown	Unknown

Action

Chemical effect: Inhibits purine synthesis.
Therapeutic effect: Inhibits selected leukemic cell reproduction.

Available forms

Tablets (scored): 40 mg

NURSING PROCESS

⚕ Assessment

• Assess patient's condition before therapy and regularly thereafter.
• Monitor CBC daily during induction and then weekly during maintenance therapy.
• Monitor uric acid level.
• Watch for jaundice.
• Be alert for adverse reactions and drug interactions.
• Evaluate patient's and family's knowledge of drug therapy.

⬱ Nursing diagnoses

• Ineffective health maintenance related to presence of leukemia
• Ineffective protection related to drug-induced immunosuppression
• Deficient knowledge related to drug therapy

▶ Planning and implementation

⚠ ALERT: Drug may be ordered as 6-thioguanine. The numeral 6 is part of drug name and doesn't signify dosage units.
• Report jaundice; it may be reversible if drug is stopped promptly. Also, drug must be stopped if hepatotoxicity or hepatic tenderness occurs.
• Encourage patient to drink fluids to prevent hyperuricemia.
Patient teaching
• Instruct patient to watch for signs of infection and bleeding, and teach him infection-control and bleeding precautions.
• Tell patient to increase fluid intake.
• Advise woman of childbearing age to avoid becoming pregnant during therapy, and to consult with prescriber before becoming pregnant.

☑ Evaluation

• Patient responds well to drug.
• Patient doesn't develop serious complications from drug-induced immunosuppression.
• Patient and family state understanding of drug therapy.

Reactions may be *common,* uncommon, *life-threatening,* or **COMMON AND LIFE-THREATENING.**

thioridazine hydrochloride

(thigh-oh-RIGH-duh-zeen high-droh-KLOR-ighd)
Aldazine ◊ , **Apo-Thioridazine** ✦ , **Mellaril***,
Mellaril Concentrate, Novo-Ridazine ✦ ,
PMS Thioridazine ✦

Pharmacologic class: phenothiazine (piperidine derivative)
Therapeutic class: antipsychotic
Pregnancy risk category: C

Indications and dosages

▶ **Schizophrenia in patients who have failed at least two trials with different antipsychotics.** *Adults:* Initially, 50 to 100 mg P.O. t.i.d., with gradual, incremental increases up to 800 mg daily in divided doses, if needed. Dosage varies.

▶ **Short-term treatment of moderate to marked depression with varying degrees of anxiety; dementia in geriatric patients; behavioral problems in children.** *Adults:* Initially, 25 mg P.O. t.i.d. Maximum, 200 mg daily. *Children ages 2 to 12:* 0.5 to 3 mg/kg P.O. daily in divided doses. Give 10 mg b.i.d. to t.i.d. to children with moderate disorders and 25 mg b.i.d. to t.i.d. to hospitalized, severely disturbed, or psychotic children.

Contraindications and precautions

• Contraindicated in patients hypersensitive to drug and in those with CNS depression, severe hypertensive or hypotensive cardiac disease, coma, reduced levels of CYP 2D6 isoenzyme, congenital long QT syndrome, or a history of cardiac arrhythmias.
• Don't give to patients taking fluvoxamine, propranolol, pindolol, fluoxetine, or drugs that inhibit the CYP 2D6 enzyme or that prolong the QT interval.
• Use cautiously in debilitated patients and in patients with hepatic disease, CV disease, respiratory disorder, hypocalcemia, seizure disorder, severe reactions to insulin or electroconvulsive therapy, and exposure to extreme heat or cold (including antipyretic therapy) or organophosphate insecticides.
⚠ **Lifespan:** In pregnant and breast-feeding women and in geriatric patients, use cautiously.

Adverse reactions

CNS: extrapyramidal reactions, *tardive dyskinesia, sedation,* EEG changes, dizziness, *neuroleptic malignant syndrome.*
CV: *orthostatic hypotension,* tachycardia, ECG changes.
EENT: *ocular changes, blurred vision,* retinitis pigmentosa.
GI: *dry mouth, constipation.*
GU: *urine retention,* dark urine, menstrual irregularities, inhibited ejaculation.
Hematologic: *transient leukopenia, agranulocytosis,* hyperprolactinemia.
Hepatic: cholestatic jaundice.
Metabolic: weight gain, increased appetite.
Skin: *mild photosensitivity reactions.*
Other: gynecomastia, allergic reaction.

Interactions

Drug-drug. *Antacids:* Inhibits absorption of oral phenothiazines. Separate doses by at least 2 hours.
Barbiturates, lithium: May decrease phenothiazine effect. Monitor patient.
Centrally acting antihypertensives: Decreases antihypertensive effect. Monitor blood pressure.
Fluvoxamine, propranolol, pindolol, fluoxetine, and any drug that inhibits the CYP 2D6 enzyme and drugs known to prolong the QT interval: Potential for serious, fatal cardiac arrhythmias. Don't use together.
Other CNS depressants: Increases CNS depression. Use together cautiously.
Drug-herb. *Dong quai, St. John's wort:* Increases photosensitivity reactions. Discourage use together.
Kava: Increases risk of dystonic reactions. Discourage use together.
Milk thistle: Decreases liver toxicity caused by phenothiazines. Monitor liver enzymes if used together.
Yohimbe: Increases risk for yohimbe toxicity when used together. Discourage use together.
Drug-lifestyle. *Alcohol use:* May increase CNS depression, particularly psychomotor skills. Strongly discourage use.
Sun exposure: Increases photosensitivity reactions. Advise patient to avoid prolonged or unprotected exposure to sunlight.

Effects on lab test results

• May increase liver enzyme and prolactin levels.
• May decrease granulocyte and WBC counts.

Pharmacokinetics

Absorption: Erratic and variable, although P.O. concentrates and syrups are more predictable than tablets.
Distribution: Distributed widely in body; 91% to 99% protein-bound.
Metabolism: Metabolized extensively by liver.
Excretion: Excreted mostly as metabolites in urine, some in feces. *Half-life:* 20 to 40 hours.

Route	Onset	Peak	Duration
P.O.	Varies	Unknown	Unknown

Action

Chemical effect: Unknown; probably blocks postsynaptic dopamine receptors in brain.
Therapeutic effect: Relieves signs of psychosis, depression, anxiety, stress, fears, and sleep disturbances.

Available forms

Oral concentrate: 30 mg/ml, 100 mg/ml* (3% to 4.2% alcohol)
Oral suspension: 25 mg/5 ml, 100 mg/5 ml
Tablets: 10 mg, 15 mg, 25 mg, 50 mg, 100 mg, 150 mg, 200 mg

NURSING PROCESS

Assessment

• Assess patient's condition before therapy and regularly thereafter.
• Monitor patient for tardive dyskinesia. It may occur after prolonged use, or may not appear until months or years later. It may disappear spontaneously or persist for life, despite stopping drug.
• Monitor therapy with weekly bilirubin tests during first month, periodic blood tests (CBC and liver function), and ophthalmologic tests (long-term therapy).
⊛ **ALERT:** Monitor patient for symptoms of neuroleptic malignant syndrome (extrapyramidal effects, hyperthermia, autonomic disturbance), which is rare but can be fatal. It isn't necessarily related to length of drug use or type of neuroleptic; however, more than 60% of patients are men.
• Before starting therapy, perform baseline ECG and measure potassium level. Don't give Mellaril to patients with a QTc interval longer than 450 msec. Stop drug in patients with a QTc longer than 500 msec.

• Evaluate patient's and family's knowledge of drug therapy.

🖭 Nursing diagnoses

• Disturbed thought processes related to underlying condition
• Risk for injury related to drug-induced adverse CNS reactions
• Deficient knowledge related to drug therapy

▶ Planning and implementation

⊛ **ALERT:** Different liquid formulations have different concentrations. Check dosage.
⊛ **ALERT:** Mellaril prolongs the QT interval in a dose-related manner.
• Prevent contact dermatitis by keeping drug away from skin and clothes. Wear gloves when preparing liquid forms.
• Dilute liquid concentrate with water or fruit juice just before giving.
• Shake suspension well before using.
• Don't withdraw drug abruptly unless patient experiences severe adverse reactions. Abrupt withdrawal of long-term therapy may cause gastritis, nausea, vomiting, dizziness, tremors, feeling of warmth or cold, diaphoresis, tachycardia, headache, or insomnia.
• Report jaundice, symptoms of blood dyscrasia (fever, sore throat, infection, cellulitis, weakness), or persistent extrapyramidal reactions (longer than a few hours), especially in pregnant women and in children, and withhold drug.
• Acute dystonic reactions may be treated with diphenhydramine.
⊛ **ALERT:** Don't confuse thioridazine with Thorazine; don't confuse Mellaril with Elavil.
Patient teaching
• Warn patient to avoid activities that require alertness until CNS effects of drug are known. Drowsiness and dizziness usually subside after a few weeks.
• Tell patient to watch for orthostatic hypotension, especially with parenteral administration. Advise patient to change position slowly.
• Tell patient to avoid alcohol while taking drug.
• Instruct patient to report urine retention or constipation.
• Inform patient that drug may discolor urine.
• Tell patient to watch for and notify prescriber of blurred vision.
• Advise patient to relieve dry mouth with sugarless gum or hard candy.

Reactions may be *common,* uncommon, *life-threatening,* or **COMMON AND LIFE-THREATENING.**

• Tell patient to use sun block and to wear protective clothing to avoid photosensitivity reactions.

☑ **Evaluation**

• Patient's behavior and communication exhibit improved thought processes.
• Patient doesn't experience injury from adverse CNS reactions.
• Patient and family state understanding of drug therapy.

thiotepa
(thigh-oh-TEE-puh)
Thioplex

Pharmacologic class: alkylating agent (not specific to phase of cell cycle)
Therapeutic class: antineoplastic
Pregnancy risk category: D

Indications and dosages

▶ **Breast and ovarian cancers, lymphoma, Hodgkin's disease.** *Adults and children older than age 12:* 0.3 to 0.4 mg/kg I.V. q 1 to 4 weeks or 0.2 mg/kg for 4 to 5 days at intervals of 2 to 4 weeks.
▶ **Bladder tumor.** *Adults and children older than age 12:* 60 mg in 30 to 60 ml of normal saline solution instilled in bladder for 2 hours once weekly for 4 weeks.
▶ **Neoplastic effusions.** *Adults and children older than age 12:* 0.6 to 0.8 mg/kg intracavitarily or intratumor q 1 to 4 weeks.
▶ **Malignant meningeal neoplasm‡.** *Adults:* 1 to 10 mg/m² intrathecally, once to twice weekly.

▼ I.V. administration

• Reconstitute drug with 1.5 ml of sterile water for injection. Don't reconstitute with other solutions.
• Further dilute solution with normal saline solution injection, D_5W, D_5NS solution for injection, Ringer's injection, or lactated Ringer's injection.
• Drug may be given by rapid I.V. administration in doses of 0.3 to 0.4 mg/kg at intervals of 1 to 4 weeks.

• If pain occurs at insertion site, dilute further or use local anesthetic. Make sure drug doesn't infiltrate.
• Refrigerate and protect dry powder from direct sunlight. Solutions are stable for up to 5 days if refrigerated. Solution should be clear to slightly opaque. Discard if solution appears very opaque or contains precipitate.

Contraindications and precautions

• Contraindicated in patients hypersensitive to drug and in those with severe bone marrow, hepatic, or renal dysfunction.
• Use cautiously in patients with mild bone marrow suppression or renal or hepatic dysfunction.
⚘ **Lifespan:** In pregnant and breast-feeding women, drug isn't recommended. In children age 12 and younger, safety of drug hasn't been established.

Adverse reactions

CNS: headache, dizziness, fatigue, weakness, fever.
EENT: blurred vision, *laryngeal edema,* conjunctivitis.
GI: *nausea, vomiting,* abdominal pain, anorexia, stomatitis.
GU: amenorrhea, decreased spermatogenesis, dysuria, urine retention, hemorrhagic cystitis.
Hematologic: *leukopenia* (begins within 5 to 10 days), *thrombocytopenia, neutropenia,* anemia.
Respiratory: *asthma.*
Skin: urticaria, rash, dermatitis, alopecia.
Other: hypersensitivity reactions, pain at injection site, *anaphylaxis.*

Interactions

Drug-drug. *Anticoagulants, aspirin:* Increases bleeding risk. Avoid using together.
Neuromuscular blockers: May prolong muscular paralysis. Monitor patient closely.
Other alkylating agents, irradiation therapy: May intensify toxicity rather than enhance therapeutic response. Avoid using together.
Succinylcholine: Increases apnea with use together. Monitor patient closely.

Effects on lab test results

• May increase uric acid level. May decrease pseudocholinesterase level.

Rapid onset   *Liquid form contains alcohol.   ◆Canada   ◇Australia   †OTC   ‡Off-label use

• May decrease hemoglobin, hematocrit, and lymphocyte, platelet, WBC, RBC, and neutrophil counts.

Pharmacokinetics

Absorption: Absorption from bladder after instillation ranges from 10% to 100% of instilled dose; also variable after intracavitary administration. Increased by certain pathologic conditions.
Distribution: Crosses blood-brain barrier.
Metabolism: Metabolized extensively in liver.
Excretion: Drug and its metabolites excreted in urine. *Half-life:* 2¼ hours.

Route	Onset	Peak	Duration
I.V., bladder instillation, intracavitary	Unknown	Unknown	Unknown

Action

Chemical effect: Cross-links strands of cellular DNA and interferes with RNA transcription, causing growth imbalance that leads to cell death.
Therapeutic effect: Kills certain cancer cells.

Available forms

Injection: 15-mg vials

NURSING PROCESS

🔲 Assessment
• Assess patient's condition before therapy and regularly thereafter.
• Adverse GU reactions are reversible in 6 to 8 months.
• Monitor CBC weekly for at least 3 weeks after last dose.
• Monitor uric acid level.
• Be alert for adverse reactions and drug interactions.
• Evaluate patient's and family's knowledge of drug therapy.

🔲 Nursing diagnoses
• Ineffective health maintenance related to presence of neoplastic disease
• Ineffective protection related to drug-induced immunosuppression
• Deficient knowledge related to drug therapy

🔲 Planning and implementation
• Follow facility policy to minimize risks. Preparation and administration of parenteral form are linked to mutagenic, teratogenic, and carcinogenic risks to personnel.
• Drug can be given by all parenteral routes, including direct injection into tumor.
• Dehydrate patient 8 to 10 hours before bladder instillation use. Instill drug into bladder by catheter; ask patient to retain solution for 2 hours. If discomfort is too great with 60 ml, reduce volume to 30 ml. Reposition patient q 15 minutes for maximum area contact.
• When intracavitary use is needed, for neoplastic effusions, mix drug with 2% procaine hydrochloride or epinephrine hydrochloride 1:1,000.
• Report WBC count below 3,000/mm³ or platelet count below 150,000/mm³ and stop drug.
• To prevent hyperuricemia with resulting uric acid nephropathy, allopurinol may be used with adequate hydration.
Patient teaching
• Tell patient to watch for signs of infection (fever, sore throat, fatigue) and bleeding (easy bruising, nosebleeds, bleeding gums, melena). Tell patient to take temperature daily and to report even mild infections.
• Instruct patient to avoid OTC products containing aspirin.
• Advise woman of childbearing age to avoid becoming pregnant during therapy and to consult with prescriber before becoming pregnant.

🔲 Evaluation
• Patient responds well to drug.
• Patient doesn't develop serious complications from drug-induced immunosuppression.
• Patient and family state understanding of drug therapy.

thiothixene
(thigh-oh-THIKS-een)
Navane

thiothixene hydrochloride
Navane*

Pharmacologic class: thioxanthene
Therapeutic class: antipsychotic
Pregnancy risk category: C

Indications and dosages

▶ **Mild to moderate psychosis.** *Adults:* Initially, 2 mg P.O. t.i.d. Increase gradually to 15 mg daily.

▶ **Severe psychosis.** *Adults:* Initially, 5 mg P.O. b.i.d. Increase gradually to 20 to 30 mg daily. Maximum recommended dosage is 60 mg daily. Or, 4 mg I.M. b.i.d. or q.i.d. Maximum dosage is 30 mg I.M. daily. Switch to P.O. form as soon as possible.

Contraindications and precautions

• Contraindicated in patients hypersensitive to drug and in those with circulatory collapse, coma, CNS depression, or blood dyscrasia.

• Use cautiously in patients with history of seizure disorder or during alcohol withdrawal. Also use cautiously in debilitated patients and in patients with CV disease (may cause sudden drop in blood pressure), glaucoma, prostatic hyperplasia, or exposure to extreme heat.

⚜ Lifespan: In pregnant and breast-feeding women and in geriatric patients, use cautiously. In children younger than age 12, drug isn't recommended.

Adverse reactions

CNS: *extrapyramidal reactions, tardive dyskinesia,* sedation, pseudoparkinsonism, EEG changes, dizziness, restlessness, agitation, insomnia, *neuroleptic malignant syndrome.*
CV: *orthostatic hypotension,* tachycardia, ECG changes.
EENT: ocular changes, *blurred vision,* nasal congestion.
GI: *dry mouth, constipation.*
GU: *urine retention,* menstrual irregularities, inhibited ejaculation.
Hematologic: *transient leukopenia,* leukocytosis, *agranulocytosis.*
Hepatic: jaundice.
Metabolic: weight gain.
Skin: *mild photosensitivity reactions.*
Other: pain and sterile abscesses at I.M. injection site, gynecomastia, allergic reaction.

Interactions

Drug-drug. *Other CNS depressants:* Increases CNS depression. Avoid using together.
Drug-herb. *Nutmeg:* Herb may cause a loss of symptom control or interfere with therapy for psychiatric illnesses. Discourage using together.

Drug-lifestyle. *Alcohol use:* Increases CNS depression. Discourage using together.
Sun exposure: Increases photosensitivity reactions. Advise patient to avoid prolonged or unprotected exposure to sunlight.

Effects on lab test results

• May increase liver enzyme levels.
• May decrease granulocyte count. May increase or decrease WBC count.

Pharmacokinetics

Absorption: Rapid.
Distribution: Distributed widely in body; 91% to 99% protein-bound.
Metabolism: Minimal.
Excretion: Most of drug excreted as parent drug in feces. *Half-life:* 20 to 40 hours

Route	Onset	Peak	Duration
P.O., I.M.	Several wk	Unknown	Unknown

Action

Chemical effect: Unknown; probably blocks postsynaptic dopamine receptors in brain.
Therapeutic effect: Relieves signs and symptoms of psychosis.

Available forms

thiothixene
Capsules: 1 mg, 2 mg, 5 mg, 10 mg, 20 mg
thiothixene hydrochloride
Injection: 2 mg/ml, 5 mg/ml
Oral concentrate: 5 mg/ml*

NURSING PROCESS

▣ Assessment

• Assess patient's psychosis before therapy and regularly thereafter.

• Watch for orthostatic hypotension, especially with parenteral route.

• Monitor patient for tardive dyskinesia. It may occur after prolonged use or may not appear until months or years later. It may disappear spontaneously or persist for life, despite stopping drug.

• Monitor therapy with weekly bilirubin tests during first month, periodic blood tests (CBC and liver function), and ophthalmologic tests (long-term therapy).

⑤ **ALERT:** Monitor patient for symptoms of neuroleptic malignant syndrome (extrapyramidal

effects, hyperthermia, autonomic disturbance), which is rare but can be fatal. It isn't necessarily related to length of drug use or type of neuroleptic; however, more than 60% of patients are men.
• Be alert for adverse reactions and drug interactions.
• Evaluate patient's and family's knowledge of drug therapy.

⊞ **Nursing diagnoses**
• Disturbed thought processes related to presence of psychosis
• Risk for injury related to drug-induced adverse CNS reactions
• Deficient knowledge related to drug therapy

▷ **Planning and implementation**
• Prevent contact dermatitis by keeping drug away from skin and clothes. Wear gloves when preparing liquid forms.
• Dilute liquid concentrate with water or fruit juice just before giving.
• Give I.M. only in upper outer quadrant of buttocks or midlateral thigh. Massage slowly afterward to prevent sterile abscess. Injection may sting.
• Keep patient in supine position for 1 hour after I.M. administration.
• Slight yellowing of injection or concentrate is common and doesn't affect potency. Discard markedly discolored solutions.
• Don't withdraw drug abruptly unless required by severe adverse reactions. Abrupt withdrawal of long-term therapy may cause gastritis, nausea, vomiting, dizziness, tremors, feeling of warmth or cold, diaphoresis, tachycardia, headache, or insomnia.
• Report jaundice, symptoms of blood dyscrasia (fever, sore throat, infection, cellulitis, weakness), or persistent extrapyramidal reactions (longer than a few hours), especially in pregnant woman or in child, and withhold dose.
• Acute dystonic reactions may be treated with diphenhydramine.
⊛ **ALERT:** Don't confuse Navane with Nubain or Norvasc.

Patient teaching
• Warn patient to avoid activities that require alertness until CNS effects of drug are known. Drowsiness and dizziness usually subside after a few weeks.

• Tell patient to avoid alcohol while taking drug.
• If urine retention or constipation occurs, instruct patient to notify prescriber.
• Tell patient to relieve dry mouth with sugarless gum or hard candy.
• Tell patient to use sun block and wear protective clothing to avoid photosensitivity reactions.
• Tell patient to watch for orthostatic hypotension, especially with parenteral administration. Advise patient to change position slowly.

☑ **Evaluation**
• Patient's behavior and communication exhibit improved thought processes.
• Patient doesn't experience injury from adverse CNS reactions.
• Patient and family state understanding of drug therapy.

thyroid
(THIGH-royd)
Armour Thyroid, Thyroid USP

Pharmacologic class: thyroid hormone
Therapeutic class: thyroid drug
Pregnancy risk category: A

Indications and dosages

▶ **Hypothyroidism.** *Adults:* Initially, 30 mg P.O. daily; increase by 15 mg q 14 to 30 days, depending on disease severity, until desired response is achieved. Usual maintenance dosage is 60 to 180 mg P.O. daily as a single dose.
▶ **Congenital hypothyroidism.** *Children older than age 12:* May approach adult dosage (60 to 180 mg daily), depending on response. *Children ages 6 to 12:* 60 to 90 mg P.O. daily. *Children ages 1 to 5:* 45 to 60 mg P.O. daily. *Children ages 6 to 12 months:* 30 to 45 mg P.O. daily. *Children up to age 6 months:* 15 to 30 mg P.O. daily.

Contraindications and precautions

• Contraindicated in patients hypersensitive to drug and those with acute MI uncomplicated by hypothyroidism, untreated thyrotoxicosis, or uncorrected adrenal insufficiency.
• Use cautiously in patients with renal insufficiency, an ischemic state, or angina pectoris,

hypertension, or other CV disorder. Also use cautiously in patients with myxedema, diabetes mellitus, or diabetes insipidus.

⚠ **Lifespan:** In breast-feeding women and in geriatric patients, use cautiously.

Adverse reactions

CNS: *nervousness, insomnia,* tremor, headache.
CV: *tachycardia,* **arrhythmias,** angina pectoris, increased blood pressure, **cardiac decompensation and collapse.**
GI: diarrhea, vomiting.
GU: menstrual irregularities.
Metabolic: weight loss, heat intolerance.
Musculoskeletal: accelerated rate of bone maturation in infants and children.
Skin: diaphoresis.
Other: allergic reactions.

Interactions

Drug-drug. *Cholestyramine:* Impairs thyroid absorption. Separate doses by 4 to 5 hours.
Insulin, oral antidiabetics: Alters glucose level. Monitor level and adjust dosage, p.r.n.
I.V. phenytoin: Free thyroid released. Monitor patient for tachycardia.
Oral anticoagulants: Alters PT. Monitor PT and INR; adjust dosage, p.r.n.
Sympathomimetics (such as epinephrine): Increases risk of coronary insufficiency. Monitor patient closely.

Effects on lab test results

None reported.

Pharmacokinetics

Absorption: Absorbed from GI tract.
Distribution: Highly protein-bound.
Metabolism: Not fully understood.
Excretion: Not fully understood. *Half-life:* T_4, 7 days; T_3, 2 days.

Route	Onset	Peak	Duration
P.O.	Unknown	Unknown	Unknown

Action

Chemical effect: Not clearly defined; stimulates metabolism of body tissues by accelerating cellular oxidation.
Therapeutic effect: Raises thyroid hormone level in body.

Available forms

Tablets: 15 mg, 30 mg, 60 mg, 90 mg, 120 mg, 180 mg, 240 mg, 300 mg
Tablets (enteric-coated): 60 mg, 120 mg

NURSING PROCESS

⚗ Assessment

• Assess patient's thyroid condition before therapy and regularly thereafter.
• Monitor pulse rate and blood pressure.
• In children, sleeping pulse rate and basal morning temperature guide therapy.
• In patient with coronary artery disease who must receive drug, watch for possible coronary insufficiency.
• Be alert for adverse reactions and drug interactions.
• Evaluate patient's and family's knowledge of drug therapy.

⊕ Nursing diagnoses

• Ineffective health maintenance related to presence of hypothyroidism
• Disturbed sleep pattern related to drug-induced insomnia
• Deficient knowledge related to drug therapy

▶ Planning and implementation

• Drug requirements are about 25% lower in patients older than age 60 than in young adults.
• Thyroid hormones alter thyroid function test results.
• Patient taking drug usually requires decreased anticoagulant dosage.
⚠ **ALERT:** Don't confuse Thyrolar with thyroid.
Patient teaching
• Tell patient to take drug at same time each day, preferably before breakfast, to maintain constant levels.
• Suggest that patient take drug in the morning to prevent insomnia.
• Advise patient who has achieved stable response not to change brands.
• Instruct patient (especially geriatric patient) to notify prescriber promptly if chest pain, palpitations, sweating, nervousness, or other signs of overdose occur or if dyspnea or tachycardia develop.
• Tell patient to report unusual bleeding and bruising.

☑ Evaluation

- Patient regains normal thyroid function.
- Patient expresses importance of taking thyroid in morning if insomnia occurs.
- Patient and family state understanding of drug therapy.

tiagabine hydrochloride
(tigh-AG-ah-been high-droh-KLOR-ighd)
Gabitril

Pharmacologic class: GABA uptake inhibitor
Therapeutic class: anticonvulsant
Pregnancy risk category: C

Indications and dosages

▶ **Adjunctive therapy in partial seizures.**
Adults: Initially, 4 mg P.O. once daily. Total daily dosage may be increased by 4 to 8 mg at weekly intervals until response is noted or up to 56 mg daily. Divide dose b.i.d. to q.i.d.
Children ages 12 to 18: Initially, 4 mg P.O. once daily. Total daily dosage may be increased by 4 mg at the beginning of week 2 and by 4 to 8 mg/week until response is noted or up to 32 mg daily. Divide dose b.i.d. to q.i.d.

Contraindications and precautions

- Contraindicated in patients hypersensitive to drug or its ingredients.
- ⚕ **Lifespan:** In pregnant women, use only if clearly needed. In breast-feeding women, use cautiously; drug may appear in breast milk. In children younger than age 12, safety hasn't been established.

Adverse reactions

CNS: generalized weakness, *dizziness, asthenia, somnolence, nervousness,* tremor, difficulty with concentration and attention, insomnia, ataxia, confusion, speech disorder, difficulty with memory, paresthesia, depression, emotional lability, abnormal gait, hostility, language problems, agitation, pain.
CV: vasodilation.
EENT: nystagmus, pharyngitis.
GI: abdominal pain, *nausea,* diarrhea, vomiting, increased appetite, mouth ulcerations.
Musculoskeletal: myasthenia.
Respiratory: increased cough.
Skin: rash, pruritus.

Interactions

Drug-drug. *Carbamazepine, phenobarbital, phenytoin:* Increases tiagabine clearance. Monitor patient for loss of therapeutic effect. May need to increase tiagabine dose.
CNS depressants: Enhances CNS effects. Use cautiously.
Drug-lifestyle. *Alcohol use:* Enhances CNS effects. Discourage using together.

Effects on lab test results

None reported.

Pharmacokinetics

Absorption: Rapid and more than 95%. Absolute bioavailability is 90%.
Distribution: About 96% bound to plasma protein.
Metabolism: Likely to be metabolized by CYP 3A isoenzymes.
Excretion: About 25% is excreted in urine (2% unchanged); 63% in feces. *Half-life:* 7 to 9 hours.

Route	Onset	Peak	Duration
P.O.	Rapid	45 min	7-9 hr

Action

Chemical effect: Unknown; may enhance the activity of GABA, the major inhibitory neurotransmitter in the CNS. It binds to recognition sites related to the GABA uptake carrier and may thus permit more GABA to be available for binding to receptors on postsynaptic cells.
Therapeutic effect: Prevents partial seizures.

Available forms

Tablets: 4 mg, 12 mg, 16 mg, 20 mg

NURSING PROCESS

☑ Assessment

- Assess patient's seizure disorder before therapy and regularly thereafter.
- Assess patient's compliance with therapy at each follow-up visit.
- ⑨ **ALERT:** Monitor patient carefully for status epilepticus because sudden death may occur in patients receiving anticonvulsant.
- Assess patient for adverse reactions and drug interactions.
- Evaluate patient's and family's knowledge of drug therapy.

Reactions may be *common,* uncommon, *life-threatening,* or COMMON AND LIFE-THREATENING.

🔡 Nursing diagnoses

- Risk for injury related to seizure disorder
- Impaired physical mobility related to drug-induced generalized weakness
- Deficient knowledge related to drug therapy

⟫ Planning and implementation

- In patients with impaired liver function, reduced initial and maintenance doses or longer dosing intervals may be needed.
- ⏀ **ALERT:** Never withdraw drug suddenly because seizure frequency may increase. Withdraw gradually unless safety concerns require a more rapid withdrawal.
- Patients who aren't receiving at least one enzyme-inducing antiepileptic when starting therapy may require lower doses or slower dosage adjustments.
- Report breakthrough seizure activity to prescriber.
- ⏀ **ALERT:** Don't confuse tiagabine with tizanidine; both have 4-mg starting doses.

Patient teaching

- Advise patient to take drug only as prescribed.
- Advise patient to take drug with food.
- Warn patient that drug may cause dizziness, somnolence, and other symptoms and signs of CNS depression. Advise patient to avoid driving and other potentially hazardous activities that require mental alertness until drug's CNS effects are known.
- Tell woman to notify prescriber if she becomes pregnant or plans to become pregnant during therapy.
- Tell woman to notify prescriber if planning to breast-feed because drug may appear in breast milk.

✅ Evaluation

- Patient is free from seizure activity.
- Patient receives therapeutic dose and doesn't experience muscle weakness.
- Patient and family state understanding of drug therapy.

ticarcillin disodium

(tigh-kar-SIL-in digh-SOH-dee-um)
Ticar, Ticillin ◇

Pharmacologic class: extended-spectrum penicillin, alpha-carboxypenicillin

Therapeutic class: antibiotic
Pregnancy risk category: B

Indications and dosages

▶ **Severe systemic infections caused by susceptible strains of gram-positive and especially gram-negative organisms (including** *Pseudomonas* **and** *Proteus***).** *Adults and children older than age 1 month:* 200 to 300 mg/kg I.V. daily in divided doses q 4 to 6 hours.
▶ **Uncomplicated UTI.** *Adults and children weighing 40 kg (88 lb) or more:* 1 g I.V. or I.M. q 6 hours.
Infants and children older than age 1 month and weighing less than 40 kg: 50 to 100 mg/kg I.V. or I.M. daily in divided doses q 6 to 8 hours.

▼ I.V. administration

- Reconstitute drug in vials using D₅W, normal saline solution injection, sterile water for injection, or other compatible solution.
- Reconstitute 3-g piggyback vials with a minimum of 30 ml compatible solution; if diluting with 50 ml diluent, dilute to a concentration of 60 mg/ml. If diluting with 100 ml diluent, dilute to a concentration of 30 mg/ml.
- Add 4 ml of diluent for each gram of drug to obtain 200 mg/ml concentration. May dilute further, if desired.
- ⏀ **ALERT:** Aminoglycoside antibiotics (such as gentamicin, amikacin, and tobramycin) are chemically incompatible. Don't mix in same I.V. container.
- For direct injection, give slowly to avoid vein irritation. For intermittent infusion, give over 30 minutes to 2 hours. Infusing with a concentration of 50 mg/ml may reduce vein irritation.
- Continuous infusion may cause vein irritation. Change site q 48 hours.

Contraindications and precautions

- Contraindicated in patients hypersensitive to penicillins.
- Use cautiously in patients with other drug allergies, especially to cephalosporins (possible cross-sensitivity); and those with impaired kidney function, hemorrhagic conditions, hypokalemia, or sodium restrictions (contains 5.2 to 6.5 mEq sodium/g).
- ♨ **Lifespan:** In pregnant and breast-feeding women, use cautiously.

Adverse reactions

CNS: *seizures,* neuromuscular excitability.
CV: vein irritation, phlebitis.
GI: nausea, diarrhea, vomiting.
Hematologic: *leukopenia, neutropenia,* eosinophilia, *thrombocytopenia,* hemolytic anemia.
Metabolic: hypokalemia.
Other: *hypersensitivity reactions* (rash, pruritus, urticaria, chills, fever, edema, *anaphylaxis*), overgrowth of nonsusceptible organisms, pain at injection site.

Interactions

Drug-drug. *Lithium:* Alters renal elimination of lithium. Monitor lithium level closely.
Hormonal contraceptives: Efficacy of hormonal contraceptives may be decreased. Recommend an additional form of contraception during penicillin therapy.
Probenecid: Increases level of ticarcillin and other penicillins. Probenecid may be used for this purpose.

Effects on lab test results

• May increase ALT, AST, alkaline phosphatase, LDH, and sodium levels. May decrease potassium level.
• May increase eosinophil count. May decrease hemoglobin, hematocrit, and platelet, WBC, neutrophil, and granulocyte counts.

Pharmacokinetics

Absorption: Unknown after I.M. administration.
Distribution: Distributed widely. Penetrates minimally into CSF with non-inflamed meninges; 45% to 65% protein-bound.
Metabolism: About 13% metabolized by hydrolysis to inactive compounds.
Excretion: Excreted mostly in urine; also in bile. *Half-life:* About 1 hour.

Route	Onset	Peak	Duration
I.V.	Immediate	Immediate	Unknown
I.M.	Unknown	30-75 min	Unknown

Action

Chemical effect: Inhibits cell wall synthesis during microorganism multiplication; bacteria resist penicillins by producing penicillinase en-zymes that convert penicillins to inactive penicilloic acid. Drug resists these enzymes.
Therapeutic effect: Kills bacteria.

Available forms

Injection: 1 g, 3 g, 6 g
I.V. infusion: 3 g

NURSING PROCESS

⚡ Assessment

• Assess patient's infection before therapy and regularly thereafter.
• Before giving drug, find out if patient is allergic to penicillin. Negative history of penicillin allergy is no guarantee against future allergic reaction.
• Obtain specimen for culture and sensitivity tests before giving first dose. Therapy may begin pending results.
• Monitor potassium level.
• Monitor CBC and platelet count.
• Monitor INR in patients receiving warfarin therapy because drug may prolong PT.
• Be alert for adverse reactions and drug interactions.
• If adverse GI reactions occur, monitor patient's hydration.
• Evaluate patient's and family's knowledge of drug therapy.

Nursing diagnoses

• Risk for infection related to presence of susceptible bacteria
• Risk for deficient fluid volume related to drug-induced adverse GI reactions
• Deficient knowledge related to drug therapy

▷ Planning and implementation

• Decrease dosage in patient with renal impairment.
• Reconstitute drug for I.M. use in vials with sterile water for injection, normal saline solution injection, or lidocaine 1% (without epinephrine). Use 2 ml of diluent per gram of drug.
• Inject I.M. dose deep into large muscle. Don't exceed 2 g per injection.
• Give drug at least 1 hour before bacteriostatic antibiotics.
• Drug is typically used with another antibiotic, such as gentamicin.

⊛ **ALERT:** Institute seizure precautions. Patient with high drug level may develop seizures.
Patient teaching
• Instruct patient to report adverse reactions.

☑ **Evaluation**
• Patient is free from infection.
• Patient maintains adequate hydration.
• Patient and family state understanding of drug therapy.

ticarcillin disodium and clavulanate potassium
(tigh-kar-SIL-in digh-SOH-dee-um and KLAV-yoo-lan-nayt poh-TAH-see-um)
Timentin

Pharmacologic class: extended-spectrum penicillin, beta-lactamase inhibitor
Therapeutic class: antibiotic
Pregnancy risk category: B

Indications and dosages
▶ **Systemic and urinary tract infections.**
Average-weight adult (60 kg [132 lb]): 3.1 g (3 g ticarcillin and 100 mg clavulanic acid) I.V. q 4 to 6 hours. Or, for UTI, 3.2 g (3 g ticarcillin and 200 mg clavulanic acid) I.V. q 8 hours.
▶ **Moderate gynecologic infections.** *Average-weight adult:* 200 mg/kg daily I.V. in divided doses q 6 hours.
▶ **Severe gynecologic infections.** *Average-weight adult:* 300 mg/kg daily I.V. in divided doses q 4 hours.
▶ **Systemic, urinary tract, and gynecologic infections.** *Adults weighing more than 60 kg:* 200 to 300 mg/kg I.V. daily (based on ticarcillin content) in divided doses q 4 to 6 hours.
Children age 3 months and older and weighing less than 60 kg: 200 mg/kg I.V. daily in divided doses q 6 hours for mild to moderate infections. 300 mg/kg daily in divided doses q 4 hours for severe infections.
Children age 3 months and older weighing 60 kg or more: 3.1 g (3 g ticarcillin and 100 mg clavulanic acid) I.V. q 6 hours for mild to moderate infections and q 4 hours for severe infections.
◪ **Adjust-a-dose:** For patients with renal impairment, if creatinine clearance is greater than

60 ml/minute, give 3.1 g q 4 hours; if 30 to 60 ml/minute, give 2 g q q 4 hours; if 10 to 30 ml/minute, give 2 g q 8 hours; if less than 10 ml/minute, give 2 g q 12 hours; and if less than 10 and the patient has hepatic dysfunction, give 2 g q 24 hours. If the patient is on peritoneal dialysis, give 3.1 g q 12 hours and if the patient is on hemodialysis, give 2 g q 12 hours and 3.1 g after hemodialysis.

▽ I.V. administration
• Reconstitute drug with 13 ml of sterile water for injection or normal saline solution injection.
• Further dilute to maximum of 10 to 100 mg/ml (based on ticarcillin component). In fluid-restricted patient, dilute to maximum of 48 mg/ml if using D_5W, 43 mg/ml if using normal saline solution injection, or 86 mg/ml if using sterile water for injection.
• Aminoglycoside antibiotics (such as gentamicin and tobramycin) are chemically incompatible. Don't mix in same I.V. container.
• Infuse over 30 minutes.

Contraindications and precautions
• Contraindicated in patients hypersensitive to penicillins.
• Use cautiously in patients with other drug allergies, especially to cephalosporins (possible cross-sensitivity), and those with impaired kidney function, hemorrhagic condition, hypokalemia, or sodium restrictions (contains 4.5 mEq sodium/g).
⚫ Lifespan: In pregnant and breast-feeding women, use cautiously.

Adverse reactions
CNS: *seizures,* neuromuscular excitability, headache, giddiness.
CV: vein irritation, phlebitis.
GI: nausea, diarrhea, stomatitis, vomiting, epigastric pain, flatulence, *pseudomembranous colitis,* taste and smell disturbances.
Hematologic: *leukopenia, neutropenia,* eosinophilia, *thrombocytopenia,* hemolytic anemia, anemia.
Metabolic: hypokalemia.
Other: *hypersensitivity reactions* (rash, pruritus, urticaria, chills, fever, edema, *anaphylaxis*), overgrowth of nonsusceptible organisms, pain at injection site.

Interactions

Drug-drug. *Hormonal contraceptives:* Efficacy of hormonal contraceptives may be decreased. Recommend an additional form of contraception during ticarcillin therapy.
Probenecid: Increases blood levels of ticarcillin. Probenecid may be used for this purpose.

Effects on lab test results

• May increase ALT, AST, alkaline phosphatase, LDH, and sodium levels. May decrease potassium level.
• May increase eosinophil count. May decrease hemoglobin, hematocrit, and platelet, WBC, neutrophil, and granulocyte counts.

Pharmacokinetics

Absorption: Administered I.V.
Distribution: Ticarcillin disodium distributed widely; penetrates minimally into CSF with noninflamed meninges. Clavulanic acid penetrates pleural fluid, lungs, and peritoneal fluid.
Metabolism: About 13% of ticarcillin dose metabolized by hydrolysis to inactive compounds; clavulanic acid is thought to undergo extensive metabolism but its fate is unknown.
Excretion: Ticarcillin excreted primarily in urine; also excreted in bile. Clavulanate's metabolites are excreted in urine. *Half-life:* About 1 hour.

Route	Onset	Peak	Duration
I.V.	Immediate	Immediate	Unknown

Action

Chemical effect: Inhibits cell wall synthesis during microorganism replication; clavulanic acid increases ticarcillin's effectiveness by inactivating beta lactamases, which destroy ticarcillin.
Therapeutic effect: Kills susceptible bacteria.

Available forms

Injection: 3 g ticarcillin and 100 mg clavulanic acid

NURSING PROCESS

⚕ Assessment
• Assess patient's infection before therapy and regularly thereafter.
• Before giving drug, find out if patient is allergic to penicillin. Negative history of penicillin

allergy is no guarantee against future allergic reaction.
• Obtain specimen for culture and sensitivity tests before giving first dose. Therapy may begin pending results.
• Monitor CBC and platelet count.
• Be alert for adverse reactions and drug interactions.
• If adverse GI reactions occur, monitor patient's hydration.
• Evaluate patient's and family's knowledge of drug therapy.

⚕ Nursing diagnoses
• Risk for infection related to presence of susceptible bacteria
• Risk for deficient fluid volume related to drug-induced adverse GI reactions
• Deficient knowledge related to drug therapy

⯈ Planning and implementation
• Decrease dosage in patient with renal impairment.
• Give drug at least 1 hour before bacteriostatic antibiotics.
Patient teaching
• Instruct patient to report adverse reactions immediately.

✓ Evaluation
• Patient is free from infection.
• Patient maintains adequate hydration.
• Patient and family state understanding of drug therapy.

ticlopidine hydrochloride
(tigh-KLOH-peh-deen high-droh-KLOR-ighd)
Ticlid

Pharmacologic class: platelet aggregation inhibitor
Therapeutic class: antithrombotic
Pregnancy risk category: B

Indications and dosages

▶ **To reduce risk of thrombotic CVA in patients with history of CVA or who have experienced CVA precursors.** *Adults:* 250 mg P.O. b.i.d. with meals.

Contraindications and precautions

• Contraindicated in patients hypersensitive to drug and those with hematopoietic disorders (such as neutropenia, thrombocytopenia, or disorders of hemostasis), active pathologic bleeding (such as peptic ulceration or active intracranial bleeding), or severe hepatic impairment.
• Drug is reserved for patients intolerant to aspirin.
⚠ Lifespan: In pregnant women, use cautiously. In breast-feeding women, drug isn't recommended. In children, safety of drug hasn't been established.

Adverse reactions

CNS: dizziness, *intracerebral bleeding.*
CV: vasculitis.
EENT: epistaxis, conjunctival hemorrhage.
GI: *diarrhea,* nausea, dyspepsia, vomiting, flatulence, anorexia, *abdominal pain, bleeding.*
GU: hematuria, nephrotic syndrome, dark-colored urine.
Hematologic: *neutropenia, agranulocytosis, pancytopenia, immune thrombocytopenia.*
Hepatic: *hepatitis,* cholestatic jaundice.
Metabolic: *hyponatremia.*
Musculoskeletal: arthropathy, myositis.
Respiratory: *allergic pneumonitis.*
Skin: *rash,* purpura, pruritus, urticaria, *thrombocytopenic purpura,* ecchymoses.
Other: *hypersensitivity reactions, postoperative bleeding,* systemic lupus erythematosus, *serum sickness.*

Interactions

Drug-drug. *Antacids:* Decreases ticlopidine level. Separate administration times by at least 2 hours.
Aspirin: Potentiates aspirin effects on platelets. Don't use together.
Cimetidine: Decreases clearance of ticlopidine and increases risk of toxicity. Avoid using together.
Digoxin: Slightly decreases digoxin level. Monitor level.
Theophylline: Decreases theophylline clearance and risk of toxicity. Monitor patient closely and adjust theophylline dosage.
Drug-herb. *Red clover:* May increase risk of bleeding. Caution against using together.

Effects on lab test results

• May increase ALT, AST, and alkaline phosphatase levels. May decrease sodium level.
• May decrease neutrophil, WBC, RBC, platelet, and granulocyte counts.

Pharmacokinetics

Absorption: Rapid and extensive; enhanced by food.
Distribution: 98% bound to proteins and lipoproteins.
Metabolism: Extensively metabolized by liver. More than 20 metabolites have been identified; unknown if parent drug or active metabolites are responsible for pharmacologic activity.
Excretion: 60% excreted in urine and 23% in feces. *Half-life:* 12½ hours after single dose; 4 to 5 days after multiple doses.

Route	Onset	Peak	Duration
P.O.	Unknown	2 hr	Unknown

Action

Chemical effect: Unknown; may block adenosine diphosphate–induced platelet-fibrinogen and platelet-platelet binding.
Therapeutic effect: Prevents blood clots from forming.

Available forms

Tablets: 250 mg

NURSING PROCESS

📋 Assessment
• Assess patient's condition before therapy and regularly thereafter.
• Obtain baseline liver function tests before therapy. Monitor test results closely, especially during first 4 months of therapy, and repeat when liver dysfunction is suspected.
• Determine baseline CBC and WBC differentials and then repeat at second week of therapy and q 2 weeks until end of third month. If patient shows signs of declining neutrophil count or if count falls 30% below baseline, test more frequently. After first 3 months, obtain CBC and WBC differential counts only in patient showing signs of infection.
• Be alert for adverse reactions and drug interactions.
• Evaluate patient's and family's knowledge of drug therapy.

🔲 Nursing diagnoses
• Impaired cerebral tissue perfusion related to CVA potential or history
• Ineffective protection related to drug-induced adverse hematologic reactions
• Deficient knowledge related to drug therapy

▶ Planning and implementation
• Thrombocytopenia may occur rarely. Report platelet count of 80,000/mm³ or less, and stop drug. Give 20 mg of methylprednisolone I.V. to normalize bleeding time within 2 hours. Platelet transfusions also may be used.
• When used preoperatively, drug may decrease risk of graft occlusion in patient receiving coronary artery bypass grafts and reduce severity of drop in platelet count in patient receiving extracorporeal hemoperfusion during open heart surgery.

Patient teaching
• Tell patient to take drug with meals; this substantially increases bioavailability and improves GI tolerance.
• Tell patient to avoid aspirin-containing products and to check with prescriber before taking OTC drugs.
• Explain that drug prolongs bleeding time but that patient should report unusual or prolonged bleeding. Advise him to tell dentist and other prescribers that he is taking this drug.
• Stress importance of regular blood tests.
• Because neutropenia can increase risk of infection, tell patient to promptly report such signs as fever, chills, and sore throat.
• If drug is substituted for a fibrinolytic or anticoagulant, tell patient to stop those drugs before starting this drug therapy.
• Advise patient to stop drug 10 to 14 days before elective surgery.
• Tell patient to report yellow skin or sclera, severe or persistent diarrhea, rashes, S.C. bleeding, light-colored stools, and dark urine.

✓ Evaluation
• Patient maintains adequate cerebral perfusion.
• Patient doesn't develop serious complications.
• Patient and family state understanding of drug therapy.

timolol maleate
(TIH-moh-lol MAL-ee-ayt)
Apo-Timol ◆ , Blocadren

Pharmacologic class: beta blocker
Therapeutic class: antihypertensive, adjunct in MI, antimigraine drug
Pregnancy risk category: C

Indications and dosages

▶ **Hypertension.** *Adults:* Initially, 10 mg P.O. b.i.d. Usual daily maintenance dosage is 20 to 40 mg. Maximum, 60 mg daily. Allow at least 7 days to elapse between increases in dosage.
▶ **MI (long-term prophylaxis in patients who have survived acute phase).** *Adults:* 10 mg P.O. b.i.d.
▶ **Prevention of migraine headache.** *Adults:* Usual dosage is 10 mg P.O. b.i.d. During maintenance therapy, 20-mg daily dose may be given. Maximum daily dose is 30 mg in divided doses (10 mg in morning and 20 mg in evening). If maximum dose for 6 to 8 weeks doesn't achieve an adequate response, use a different drug.
▶ **Angina‡.** *Adults:* 15 to 45 mg P.O. daily given in three or four divided doses.

Contraindications and precautions

• Contraindicated in patients hypersensitive to drug and in those with bronchial asthma, severe COPD, sinus bradycardia and heart block greater than first-degree, cardiogenic shock, or overt heart failure.
• Use cautiously in patients with compensated heart failure; hepatic, renal, or respiratory disease; diabetes; or hyperthyroidism.
⚖ Lifespan: In pregnant women, use cautiously. In breast-feeding women, drug isn't recommended. In children, safety of drug hasn't been established.

Adverse reactions

CNS: fatigue, lethargy, dizziness.
CV: *bradycardia,* hypotension, peripheral vascular disease, *arrhythmias, heart failure.*
GI: nausea, vomiting, diarrhea.
Respiratory: dyspnea, *bronchospasm, increased airway resistance.*
Skin: pruritus.

Interactions

Drug-drug. *Aminophylline, theophylline:* May act antagonistically reducing the effects of one or both drugs. Elimination of theophylline may also be reduced. Monitor theophylline level and patient closely.

Catecholamine-depleting drugs (such as reserpine): May have additive effects when given with beta blockers. Monitor patient for hypotension and bradycardia.

Cimetidine: May increase the drug effects of beta blocker. Consider another H_2 agonist or decrease the dose of beta blocker.

Digoxin, diltiazem, verapamil: Excessive bradycardia and increased depressant effect on myocardium. Use together cautiously.

Epinephrine: May cause an initial hypertensive episode followed by bradycardia. Stop beta blocker 3 days before anticipated epinephrine use. Monitor patient closely.

Insulin: May mask symptoms of hypoglycemia (such as tachycardia) as a result of beta blockade. Use cautiously in diabetic patients.

NSAIDs (ibuprofen, indomethacin): Decreases antihypertensive effect. Monitor blood pressure and adjust dosage.

Oral antidiabetics: May alter requirements for these drugs in previously stabilized diabetic patients. Monitor patient for hypoglycemia.

Prazosin: May increase the risk of orthostatic hypotension in the early phases of use together. Assist patient to stand slowly until effects are known.

Quinidine: May increase beta-adrenergic blockade. Monitor heart rate.

Verapamil: May increase the effects of both drugs. Monitor cardiac function closely and decrease dosages as necessary.

Effects on lab test results

• May increase BUN, potassium, uric acid, and glucose levels.

Pharmacokinetics

Absorption: About 90%.
Distribution: Distributed throughout body; depending on assay method, drug is 10% to 60% protein-bound.
Metabolism: About 80% metabolized in liver to inactive metabolites.
Excretion: Drug and its metabolites excreted primarily in urine. *Half-life:* About 4 hours.

Route	Onset	Peak	Duration
P.O.	15-30 min	1-2 hr	6-12 hr

Action

Chemical effect: Unknown. In MI, drug may decrease myocardial oxygen requirements. It also prevents arterial dilation through beta blockade for migraine headache prophylaxis.
Therapeutic effect: Lowers blood pressure and helps to prevent MI and migraine headaches.

Available forms

Tablets: 5 mg, 10 mg, 20 mg

NURSING PROCESS

⚕ Assessment

• Assess patient's condition before therapy and regularly thereafter.
• Monitor blood pressure frequently.
• Be alert for adverse reactions and drug interactions.
• Evaluate patient's and family's knowledge of drug therapy.

⊕ Nursing diagnoses

• Risk for injury related to history of hypertension or MI
• Acute pain related to migraine headache
• Deficient knowledge related to drug therapy

▷ Planning and implementation

• Check patient's apical pulse rate before giving drug. Report extreme pulse rate, and withhold drug.
• Don't stop drug abruptly; this can exacerbate angina and precipitate MI. Reduce dosage gradually over 1 to 2 weeks.
• **ALERT:** Don't confuse timolol with atenolol.
Patient teaching
• Explain importance of taking drug exactly as prescribed.
• Tell patient not to stop drug abruptly because serious complications can occur. Instead, tell him to report adverse reactions.
• Teach patient other means to reduce blood pressure such as diet control, weight reduction, exercise, smoking cessation, and stress reduction.

☑ Evaluation

• Patient doesn't experience injury from underlying disease.

- Patient doesn't develop migraine headaches.
- Patient and family state understanding of drug therapy.

tinzaparin sodium
(TIN-zuh-pear-in SOE-dee-um)
Innohep

Pharmacologic class: low–molecular-weight heparin
Therapeutic class: anticoagulant
Pregnancy risk category: B

Indications and dosages

▶ **Adjunct treatment (with warfarin sodium) of symptomatic deep vein thrombosis with or without pulmonary embolism.**
Adults: 175 anti-Xa IU per kg of body weight S.C. once daily for at least 6 days and until the patient is adequately anticoagulated with warfarin (INR at least 2) for 2 consecutive days. Begin warfarin when appropriate, usually within 1 to 3 days after tinzaparin starts. The volume to be given may be calculated as follows:

$$\frac{\text{Patient weight}}{\text{in kg}} \times 0.00875 \text{ ml/kg} = \frac{\text{volume to be}}{\text{given (in ml)}}$$

Contraindications and precautions

- Contraindicated in patients hypersensitive to drug or to heparin, sulfites, benzyl alcohol, or pork products. Also contraindicated in patients with active major bleeding and patients with current or previous heparin-induced thrombocytopenia.
- Use cautiously in patients with increased risk of hemorrhage, such as those with bacterial endocarditis, uncontrolled hypertension, diabetic retinopathy, or congenital or acquired bleeding disorders (such as hepatic failure, amyloidosis, GI ulceration, or hemorrhagic CVA). Also use cautiously in patients being treated with platelet inhibitors, in patients who have recently undergone brain, spinal, or ophthalmologic surgery, and in patients with renal insufficiency.
- ⚖ **Lifespan:** In pregnant women, use cautiously and only when clearly needed. In breast-feeding women, use cautiously; it isn't known whether drug appears in breast milk. In children, safety and effectiveness haven't been established. In geriatric patients, use cautiously

because they may have reduced elimination of drug.

Adverse reactions

CNS: headache, fever, dizziness, insomnia, confusion, *cerebral or intracranial bleeding,* pain.
CV: *arrhythmias,* chest pain, hypotension, hypertension, *MI, thromboembolism,* tachycardia, dependent edema, angina pectoris.
EENT: epistaxis, ocular hemorrhage.
GI: anorectal bleeding, constipation, flatulence, hematemesis, hemarthrosis, *GI hemorrhage,* melena, nausea, vomiting, dyspepsia, *retroperitoneal or intra-abdominal bleeding.*
GU: dysuria, hematuria, UTI, urine retention, *vaginal hemorrhage.*
Hematologic: *granulocytopenia, thrombocytopenia,* anemia, *agranulocytosis, pancytopenia, hemorrhage.*
Musculoskeletal: back pain.
Respiratory: pneumonia, respiratory disorder, *pulmonary embolism,* dyspnea.
Skin: bullous eruption, cellulitis, *injection site hematoma,* pruritus, purpura, rash, skin necrosis, wound hematoma.
Other: *hypersensitivity reactions, spinal or epidural hematoma,* infection, impaired healing, *allergic reaction,* congenital anomaly, *fetal death, fetal distress.*

Interactions

Drug-drug. *Oral anticoagulants, platelet inhibitors (such as dextran, dipyridamole, NSAIDs, salicylates, sulfinpyrazone), thrombolytics:* May increase the risk of bleeding. Use together cautiously and monitor patient.

Effects on lab test results

- May increase AST and ALT levels.
- May increase granular leukocyte count. May decrease hemoglobin, hematocrit, and granulocyte, platelet, RBC, and WBC counts.

Pharmacokinetics

Absorption: Plasma levels peak in 4 to 5 hours.
Distribution: The volume of distribution is similar in magnitude to that of blood volume, which suggests that distribution is limited to the central compartment.
Metabolism: Drug is partially metabolized by desulfation and depolymerization, similar to that seen by other low–molecular-weight heparins.

Reactions may be *common,* uncommon, *life-threatening,* or **COMMON AND LIFE-THREATENING.**

Excretion: The primary route of elimination is renal. *Half-life:* 3 to 4 hours.

Route	Onset	Peak	Duration
S.C.	2-3 hr	4-5 hr	Unknown

Action

Chemical effect: Inhibits reactions that lead to blood clotting, including the formation of fibrin clots. The drug also acts as a potent co-inhibitor of several activated coagulation factors, especially factors Xa and IIa (thrombin). It also induces release of tissue factor pathway inhibitor, which may contribute to the antithrombotic effect.
Therapeutic effect: Reduces the ability of the blood to clot.

Available forms

Injection: 20,000 anti-Xa IU per ml in 2-ml vials

NURSING PROCESS

Assessment

• Assess patient's condition before therapy and regularly thereafter.
• Monitor platelet count during therapy. If platelet count falls below 100,000/mm^3, stop drug.
• Monitor CBC and stool tests for occult blood periodically during therapy.
• Drug may affect PT and INR levels. Patients who also receive warfarin should have blood drawn for PT and INR tests just before the next scheduled dose of this drug.
• Drug contains sodium metabisulfite, which may cause allergic reactions in susceptible people.
• Assess weight before therapy to calculate accurate dose.
• Evaluate patient's and family's knowledge of drug therapy.

Nursing diagnoses

• Ineffective protection related to increased risk of bleeding
• Ineffective tissue perfusion, peripheral, related to deep vein thrombosis
• Deficient knowledge related to tinzaparin sodium therapy

Planning and implementation

• If patient develops serious bleeding or receives a large overdose, replace volume and hemostatic blood elements (such as RBCs, fresh frozen plasma, and platelets) p.r.n. If this is ineffective, consider giving protamine sulfate.
ALERT: Don't give I.M. or I.V., and don't mix with other injections or infusions.
ALERT: Drug can't be interchanged (unit for unit) with heparin or other low–molecular-weight heparins.
• During administration, have the patient lie or sit down. Give drug by deep S.C. injection into the abdominal wall. Insert the whole length of the needle into a skin fold held between thumb and forefinger. Hold skin fold throughout injection. To minimize bruising, don't rub the injection site after administration.
• Rotate injection sites between the right and left anterolateral and posterolateral abdominal wall.
• Use an appropriate calibrated syringe to ensure withdrawal of the correct volume of drug from vial.
ALERT: When neuraxial anesthesia (epidural or spinal anesthesia) or spinal puncture is used, the patient is at risk for spinal hematoma, which can result in long-term or permanent paralysis. Watch for evidence of neurologic impairment. Consider the risks and benefits of neuraxial intervention in patients being anticoagulated with low–molecular-weight heparins or heparinoids.
• Store drug at room temperature.
Patient teaching
• Inform patient that co-administration of warfarin will begin within 1 to 3 days of tinzaparin administration. Explain the importance of warfarin therapy.
• Stress the importance of laboratory monitoring to ensure effectiveness and safety of therapy.
• Instruct patient to take safety measures to prevent cuts and bruises (such as using a soft toothbrush and an electric razor).
• Review the warning signs of bleeding, and instruct the patient to report evidence of bleeding immediately.
• Warn patient about the risks of becoming pregnant while taking tinzaparin sodium. Cases of gasping syndrome have occurred in premature infants who received large amounts of benzyl alcohol.

☑ Evaluation

• Patient states appropriate bleeding precautions to take.

• Patient's peripheral neurovascular status returns to baseline.

• Patient and family state understanding of tinzaparin sodium therapy.

tirofiban hydrochloride
(ty-roh-FYE-ban high-droh-KLOR-ighd)
Aggrastat

Pharmacologic class: GP IIb/IIIa receptor antagonist
Therapeutic class: platelet aggregation inhibitor
Pregnancy risk category: B

Indications and dosages

▶ **Acute coronary syndrome, with heparin, aspirin, or both, including patients who are to be managed medically and those undergoing percutaneous transluminal coronary angioplasty (PTCA) or atherectomy.** *Adults:* I.V. loading dose of 0.4 mcg/kg/minute for 30 minutes; then continuous I.V. infusion of 0.1 mcg/kg/minute. Continue through angiography and for 12 to 24 hours after angioplasty or atherectomy.

⬛ **Adjust-a-dose:** For patients with renal impairment, if creatinine clearance is less than 30 ml/minute, give a loading dose of 0.2 mcg/kg/minute for 30 minutes; then continuous infusion of 0.05 mcg/kg/minute. Continue infusion through angiography and for 12 to 24 hours after angioplasty or atherectomy.

▼ I.V. administration

• Dilute 50-ml injection vials (250 mcg/ml) to same strength as 500-ml premixed vials (50 mcg/ml) as follows: Withdraw and discard 100 ml from a 500-ml bag of sterile saline solution or D₅W and replace this volume with 100 ml of tirofiban injection (from two 50-ml vials or four 25-ml vials) or withdraw 50 ml from a 250-ml bag of sterile saline solution or D₅W and replace this volume with 50 ml of tirofiban injection, to achieve 50 mcg/ml.

• Inspect solution for particulate matter before administration, and check for leaks by squeez-ing the inner bag firmly. If particles are visible or if leaks occur, discard solution.

⑤ **ALERT:** Don't mix in the same line as diazepam.

• Heparin and tirofiban can be given through same I.V. catheter.

• Store drug at room temperature, and protect from light. Discard unused solution 24 hours after the start of infusion.

Contraindications and precautions

• Contraindicated in patients hypersensitive to drug or its ingredients, in those with active internal bleeding or history of bleeding diathesis within the previous 30 days, and in those with history of intracranial hemorrhage, intracranial neoplasm, arteriovenous malformation, aneurysm, thrombocytopenia after prior exposure to tirofiban, CVA within 30 days, or hemorrhagic CVA. Also contraindicated in patients with history, symptoms, or findings suggestive of aortic dissection; severe hypertension (systolic blood pressure over 180 mm Hg or diastolic blood pressure over 110 mm Hg); acute pericarditis; patients who have had major surgical procedure or severe physical trauma within previous 30 days; or patients receiving another parenteral GP IIb/IIIa inhibitor.

• Use cautiously in patients with increased risk of bleeding, including those with hemorrhagic retinopathy or platelet count below 150,000/mm³.

⚜ **Lifespan:** In breast-feeding women, stop drug or breast-feeding because of potential adverse effects in infants. In children, safety and efficacy of drug haven't been established.

Adverse reactions

CNS: fever, dizziness, headache.
CV: *bradycardia, coronary artery dissection,* edema, vasovagal reaction.
GI: nausea, *occult bleeding.*
Hematologic: *minor bleeding, thrombocytopenia.*
Musculoskeletal: pelvic pain, leg pain.
Skin: sweating.
Other: *major bleeding at arterial access site.*

Interactions

Drug-drug. *Clopidogrel, dipyridamole, heparin, NSAIDs, oral anticoagulants such as warfarin, thrombolytics, ticlopidine:* Increases risk of bleeding. Monitor patient closely.

Levothyroxine, omeprazole: Increases renal clearance of tirofiban. Monitor patient.
Drug-herb. *Dong quai, feverfew, garlic, ginger:* May increase the risk of bleeding. Discourage use together.

Effects on lab test results

• May decrease hemoglobin, hematocrit, and platelet count.

Pharmacokinetics

Absorption: Administered I.V.
Distribution: 65% protein-bound. Volume ranges from 22 to 42 liters.
Metabolism: Limited. *Half-life:* 2 hours.
Excretion: Renal clearance accounts for 39 to 69% of elimination; feces accounts for 25%. *Half-life:* 2 hours.

Route	Onset	Peak	Duration
I.V.	Immediate	Immediate	4-8 hr after end of infusion

Action

Chemical effect: Reversibly binds to the glycoprotein IIb/IIIa (GP IIb/IIIa) receptor on human platelets and inhibits platelet aggregation.
Therapeutic effect: Prevents clot formation.

Available forms

Injection: 25- and 50-ml vials (250 mcg/ml), 250- and 500-ml premixed vials (50 mcg/ml)

NURSING PROCESS

Assessment

• Assess patient's condition before therapy and regularly thereafter.
• Monitor hemoglobin, hematocrit, and platelet count before starting therapy, 6 hours after loading dose, and at least daily during therapy.
• Monitor patient for bleeding.
• If thrombocytopenia occurs, notify prescriber
• Evaluate patient's and family's knowledge of drug therapy.

Nursing diagnoses

• Ineffective cardiopulmonary tissue perfusion related to presence of acute coronary syndrome
• Risk for injury related to increased bleeding tendencies
• Deficient knowledge related to drug therapy

Planning and implementation

• Minimize injection and avoid noncompressible I.V. sites.
• The most common adverse effect is bleeding at the arterial access site for cardiac catheterization.
ALERT: Don't confuse Aggrastat with Argatroban.

Patient teaching
• Explain that drug is a blood thinner used to prevent chest pain and heart attack.
• Explain that risk of serious bleeding is far outweighed by the benefits of drug.
• Instruct patient to report chest discomfort or other adverse events immediately.
• Inform patient that frequent blood sampling may be needed to evaluate therapy.

Evaluation

• Patient maintains adequate cardiopulmonary tissue perfusion.
• Patient doesn't experience life-threatening bleeding episode.
• Patient and family state understanding of drug therapy.

tobramycin sulfate
(toh-breh-MIGH-sin SUL-fayt)
Nebcin

Pharmacologic class: aminoglycoside
Therapeutic class: antibiotic
Pregnancy risk category: D

Indications and dosages

▶ **Serious infections caused by sensitive strains of** *Citrobacter, Enterobacter, Escherichia coli, Klebsiella, Proteus, Providencia, Pseudomonas, Serratia,* **and** *Staphylococcus aureus. Adults and children with normal renal function:* 3 mg/kg I.M. or I.V. daily divided q 8 hours. Up to 5 mg/kg daily divided q 6 to 8 hours for life-threatening infections.
Neonates younger than age 1 week or premature infants: Up to 4 mg/kg I.V. or I.M. daily in two equal doses q 12 hours.

I.V. administration

• Dilute in 50 to 100 ml of normal saline solution or D₅W for adults and in less volume for children.

• Infuse over 20 to 60 minutes. After I.V. infusion, flush line with normal saline solution or D₅W.

Contraindications and precautions

• Contraindicated in patients hypersensitive to aminoglycosides.
• Use cautiously in patients with impaired kidney function or neuromuscular disorders.
⚠ **Lifespan:** In pregnant and breast-feeding women, drug isn't recommended. In elderly patients, use cautiously.

Adverse reactions

CNS: headache, lethargy, confusion, disorientation.
EENT: *ototoxicity.*
GI: nausea, vomiting, diarrhea.
GU: *nephrotoxicity.*
Hematologic: anemia, eosinophilia, *leukopenia, thrombocytopenia, agranulocytosis.*
Other: hypersensitivity reactions *(anaphylaxis).*

Interactions

Drug-drug. *Acyclovir, amphotericin B, cephalothin, cisplatin, methoxyflurane, other aminoglycosides, vancomycin:* Increases nephrotoxicity. Use together cautiously.
Atracurium, doxacurium, mivacurium, pancuronium, rocuronium, tubocurarine, vecuronium: May increase the effects of nondepolarizing muscle relaxant including prolonged respiratory depression. Use together only when necessary. Dose of nondepolarizing muscle relaxant may need to be reduced.
Dimenhydrinate: May mask symptoms of ototoxicity. Use cautiously.
General anesthetics: May potentiate neuromuscular blockade. Monitor patient closely.
I.V. loop diuretics (such as furosemide): Increases ototoxicity. Use together cautiously.
Parenteral penicillins (such as ticarcillin): Tobramycin inactivation in vitro. Don't mix.

Effects on lab test results

• May increase BUN, creatinine, and nonprotein nitrogen and nitrogenous compound levels. May decrease calcium, magnesium, and potassium levels.
• May increase eosinophil count. May decrease hemoglobin, hematocrit, and WBC, platelet, and granulocyte counts.

Pharmacokinetics

Absorption: Unknown.
Distribution: Wide, although CSF penetration is low, even in patients with inflamed meninges. Protein-binding is minimal.
Metabolism: None.
Excretion: Excreted primarily in urine; small amount may be excreted in bile. *Half-life:* 2 to 3 hours.

Route	Onset	Peak	Duration
I.V.	Immediate	Immediate	8 hr
I.M.	Unknown	30-90 min	8 hr

Action

Chemical effect: Inhibits protein synthesis by binding directly to 30S ribosomal subunit.
Therapeutic effect: Kills susceptible bacteria.

Available forms

Injection: 40 mg/ml, 10 mg/ml (pediatric)
Powder for injection: 30 mg/ml after reconstitution
Premixed parenteral injection for I.V. infusion: 60 mg or 80 mg in normal saline solution

NURSING PROCESS

⬛ Assessment

• Assess patient's infection before therapy and regularly thereafter.
• Obtain specimen for culture and sensitivity tests before giving first dose. Therapy may begin pending results.
• Draw blood for peak tobramycin level 1 hour after I.M. injection and 30 minutes to 1 hour after infusion ends; draw blood for trough level just before next dose. Don't collect blood in heparinized tube because heparin is incompatible with drug.
• Weigh patient and review baseline kidney function studies before therapy.
• Evaluate patient's hearing before and during therapy. Report tinnitus, vertigo, or hearing loss.
⊗ **ALERT:** Peak levels higher than 12 mcg/ml and trough levels higher than 2 mcg/ml may be linked to increased risk of toxicity.
• Monitor kidney function (output, specific gravity, urinalysis, BUN and creatinine levels, and creatinine clearance).
• Be alert for adverse reactions and drug interactions.

• Evaluate patient's and family's knowledge of drug therapy.

⊞ **Nursing diagnoses**
• Risk for infection related to susceptible bacteria
• Risk for injury related to potential for drug-induced nephrotoxicity
• Deficient knowledge related to drug therapy

▶ **Planning and implementation**
• Notify prescriber of signs of decreasing kidney function.
• Keep patient well hydrated while taking drug to minimize chemical irritation of renal tubules.
• If no response occurs in 3 to 5 days, therapy may be stopped and new specimens obtained for culture and sensitivity testing.
⚕ **ALERT:** Don't confuse tobramycin with Trobicin.
Patient teaching
• Emphasize need to drink 2 L of fluid each day.
• Instruct patient to report adverse reactions.

☑ **Evaluation**
• Patient is free from infection.
• Patient maintains normal kidney function.
• Patient and family state understanding of drug therapy.

tocainide hydrochloride
(TOH-kay-nighd high-droh-KLOR-ighd)
Tonocard

Pharmacologic class: local anesthetic
Therapeutic class: ventricular antiarrhythmic
Pregnancy risk category: C

Indications and dosages

▶ **Suppression of symptomatic life-threatening ventricular arrhythmias, such as sustained ventricular tachycardia.** *Adults:* Initially, 400 mg P.O. q 8 hours. Usual dosage is between 1,200 and 1,800 mg daily in three divided doses.
▶ **Myotonic dystrophy‡.** *Adults:* 800 to 1,200 mg P.O. daily.

Contraindications and precautions

• Contraindicated in patients hypersensitive to lidocaine or other amide-type local anesthetics

and in those with second- or third-degree AV block in absence of artificial pacemaker.
• Use cautiously in patients with heart failure or diminished cardiac reserve and in those with hepatic or renal impairment. These patients often may be treated effectively with lower dose.
⚕ **Lifespan:** In breast-feeding women and in children, safety of drug hasn't been established. In geriatric patients, dizziness and falling are more likely to occur.

Adverse reactions

CNS: *light-headedness, tremor,* restlessness, paresthesia, *dizziness, vertigo,* drowsiness, fatigue, confusion, headache.
CV: hypotension, ***new or worsened arrhythmias, heart failure, bradycardia,*** palpitations.
EENT: blurred vision, tinnitus.
GI: *nausea,* vomiting, diarrhea, anorexia.
Hematologic: *blood dyscrasia.*
Hepatic: *hepatitis.*
Respiratory: ***respiratory arrest, pulmonary fibrosis,*** pneumonitis, ***pulmonary edema.***
Skin: rash, diaphoresis.

Interactions

Drug-drug. *Beta blockers:* Decreases myocardial contractility; increases CNS toxicity. Observe the patient closely.
Cimetidine: May decrease peak tocainide level. Monitor cardiac rhythm closely.
Disopyramide, lidocaine, mexiletine, phenytoin, procainamide, quinidine: May have additive effect and CNS toxicity. Monitor patient closely.
Rifampin: Increases clearance of tocainide. Monitor efficacy of tocainide.

Effects on lab test results

• May increase liver function test values. May decrease hemoglobin, hematocrit, and platelet and granulocyte counts.

Pharmacokinetics

Absorption: Rapid and complete.
Distribution: Not clearly defined, although drug appears to be widely distributed and apparently crosses blood-brain barrier. Only about 10% to 20% bound to plasma protein.
Metabolism: Metabolized, apparently in liver, to inactive metabolites.

Excretion: Excreted in urine. *Half-life:* About 11 to 23 hours.

Route	Onset	Peak	Duration
P.O.	Unknown	30 min-2 hr	8 hr

Action

Chemical effect: Class Ib antiarrhythmic that blocks fast sodium channel in cardiac tissues, especially Purkinje network, without involvement of autonomic nervous system.
Therapeutic effect: Restores normal sinus rhythm.

Available forms

Tablets: 400 mg, 600 mg

NURSING PROCESS

Assessment
• Assess patient's condition before therapy and regularly thereafter.
• Monitor therapeutic blood level. Therapeutic level ranges from 4 to 10 mcg/ml. Report any abnormalities.
⚠ ALERT: Monitor patient for tremors, which may indicate that maximum dosage has been reached.
• Monitor patient during transition from lidocaine to tocainide.
• Be alert for adverse reactions and drug interactions.
• Evaluate patient's and family's knowledge of drug therapy.

Nursing diagnoses
• Decreased cardiac output related to presence of cardiac arrhythmia
• Risk for injury related to drug-induced adverse reactions
• Deficient knowledge related to drug therapy

Planning and implementation
• Cardiologists commonly call drug "oral lidocaine." It may ease transition from I.V. lidocaine to oral antiarrhythmic therapy.
• Agranulocytosis and bone marrow suppression have been reported in patients taking usual doses of drug. Most cases have been reported within first 12 weeks of therapy. Look for unusual bruising or bleeding or signs of infection.
Patient teaching
• Instruct patient to take drug with food.

• Tell patient to report unusual bruising or bleeding or signs of infection.
• Tell patient to report sudden onset of pulmonary symptoms, such as coughing, wheezing, and exertional dyspnea. Drug has been linked to serious pulmonary toxicity.

Evaluation
• Patient exhibits normal cardiac output with abolishment of arrhythmia.
• Patient doesn't experience injury from adverse reactions.
• Patient and family state understanding of drug therapy.

tolcapone
(TOHL-cah-pohn)
Tasmar

Pharmacologic class: COMT inhibitor
Therapeutic class: antiparkinsonian
Pregnancy risk category: C

Indications and dosages

▶ **Adjunct to levodopa and carbidopa for signs and symptoms of idiopathic Parkinson's disease.** *Adults:* Initially, 100 mg P.O. t.i.d. (with levodopa-carbidopa). Recommended daily dosage is 100 mg P.O. t.i.d., although 200 mg P.O. t.i.d. may be given if the anticipated benefit is justified. If starting therapy with 200 mg t.i.d. and dyskinesia occurs, reduce dosage of levodopa. Maximum, 600 mg daily.

Contraindications and precautions

• Contraindicated in patients hypersensitive to drug or its components and in patients with liver disease, elevated ALT or AST values, or history of nontraumatic rhabdomyolysis, hyperpyrexia, or confusion possibly related to drug. Also contraindicated in patients withdrawn from drug because of evidence of drug-induced hepatocellular injury.
• Use cautiously in patients with severe renal impairment.
Lifespan: In pregnant women, use only if potential benefits outweigh risks. In breast-feeding women, use cautiously.

Reactions may be *common*, uncommon, *life-threatening*, or COMMON AND LIFE-THREATENING.

Adverse reactions

CNS: *dyskinesia, sleep disorder, dystonia, excessive dreaming, somnolence,* dizziness, *confusion, headache, hallucinations,* hyperkinesia, hypertonia, fatigue, falling, syncope, balance loss, depression, tremor, speech disorder, paresthesia, agitation, irritability, mental deficiency, hyperactivity, hypokinesia, fever.
CV: *orthostatic complaints,* chest pain, chest discomfort, palpitations, hypotension.
EENT: pharyngitis, tinnitus, sinus congestion.
GI: *nausea, anorexia, diarrhea,* flatulence, *vomiting,* constipation, abdominal pain, dyspepsia, dry mouth.
GU: UTI, urine discoloration, hematuria, micturition disorder, urinary incontinence, impotence.
Hematologic: *bleeding.*
Musculoskeletal: *muscle cramps,* stiffness, arthritis, neck pain.
Respiratory: bronchitis, dyspnea, upper respiratory tract infection.
Skin: increased sweating, rash.
Other: burning, influenza.

Interactions

Drug-drug. *CNS depressants:* Enhances sedative effects. Use cautiously.
Nonselective MAO inhibitors (phenelzine, tranylcypromine): Possible hypertensive crisis. Don't use together.

Effects on lab test results

• May increase liver function test values.

Pharmacokinetics

Absorption: Rapid. Absolute bioavailability is 65%.
Distribution: Not widely distributed into tissues; over 99.9% is bound to plasma proteins.
Metabolism: Almost complete, mainly by glucuronidation.
Excretion: 60% excreted in urine and 40% in feces. *Half-life:* 2 to 3 hours.

Route	Onset	Peak	Duration
P.O.	Unknown	2 hr	Unknown

Action

Chemical effect: Unknown; may reversibly inhibit human erythrocyte COMT when given with levodopa and carbidopa, resulting in a decrease in levodopa clearance and a twofold increase in levodopa bioavailability. Decreased clearance of levodopa prolongs half-life of levodopa from 2 to 3.5 hours.
Therapeutic effect: Improves physical mobility in patients with parkinsonism.

Available forms

Tablets: 100 mg, 200 mg

NURSING PROCESS

✒ Assessment

• Assess patient's history of Parkinson's disease, and reassess during therapy.
• Monitor liver enzyme levels before therapy, then q 2 weeks during first 3½ years of therapy, then q 8 weeks thereafter because of risk of liver toxicity. Stop drug if levels are elevated or if patient appears jaundiced. Assess patient's risk for physical injury because of drug's adverse CNS effects.
• Monitor patient for orthostatic hypotension and syncope.
• Evaluate patient's and family's knowledge of drug therapy.

⊕ Nursing diagnoses

• Impaired physical mobility related to underlying Parkinson's disease
• Disturbed thought processes related to drug-induced CNS adverse reactions
• Deficient knowledge related to drug therapy

❯ Planning and implementation

⚕ **ALERT:** Have patient provide written informed consent before drug is used. Give drug only to patients receiving levodopa and carbidopa who don't respond to or who aren't appropriate candidates for other adjunctive therapies because of risk of liver toxicity.
• Give first dose of day with first daily dose of levodopa and carbidopa.
• Patients with severe renal dysfunction may need a reduced dose.
• Withhold drug and notify prescriber if hepatic transaminases are elevated or if patient appears jaundiced.
• Because of risk of liver toxicity, stop drug if patient shows no benefit within 3 weeks.
• Because of highly protein-bound nature of drug, dialysis doesn't significantly remove drug.
• If severe diarrhea that is linked to drug therapy occurs, notify prescriber.

Patient teaching
- Advise patient to take drug exactly as prescribed.
- Teach patient signs of liver injury (jaundice, fatigue, loss of appetite, persistent nausea, pruritus, dark urine, or right upper quadrant tenderness) and instruct him to report them immediately.
- Warn patient about risk of orthostatic hypotension; tell him to use caution when rising from a seated or recumbent position.
- Instruct patient to avoid hazardous activities until CNS effects of drug are known.
- Tell patient that nausea may occur at the start of therapy.
- Inform patient about risk of increased dyskinesia or dystonia.
- Tell patient to report planned, suspected, or known pregnancy during therapy.
- Instruct patient to report to prescriber adverse effects, including diarrhea and hallucinations.
- Inform patient that drug may be taken without regard to meals.

☑ Evaluation
- Patient exhibits improved mobility with reduction of muscular rigidity and tremor.
- Patient remains mentally alert.
- Patient and family state understanding of drug therapy.

tolterodine tartrate
(tohl-TER-oh-deen TAR-trate)
Detrol, Detrol LA

Pharmacologic class: muscarinic receptor antagonist
Therapeutic class: anticholinergic
Pregnancy risk category: C

Indications and dosages

▶ **Overactive bladder in patients with symptoms of urinary frequency, urgency, or urge incontinence.** *Adults:* 2 mg P.O. b.i.d. Dosage may be lowered to 1 mg P.O. b.i.d. based on patient response and tolerance. Or, 4 mg of extended-release capsule P.O. daily; may be decreased to 2 mg P.O. daily.
◨ Adjust-a-dose: For patients with significantly reduced hepatic function and patients taking drug that inhibits CYP 3A4 isoenzyme system,

give 1 mg P.O. b.i.d. or 2 mg P.O. daily of extended-release capsules.

Contraindications and precautions

- Contraindicated in patients hypersensitive to drug or its components and in those with uncontrolled angle-closure glaucoma or urine or gastric retention.
- Use cautiously in patients with significant bladder outflow obstruction, GI obstructive disorders (such as pyloric stenosis), controlled angle-closure glaucoma, or hepatic or renal impairment.
⚠ Lifespan: Breast-feeding women should either stop drug or stop breast-feeding. In children, safety and efficacy of drug haven't been established.

Adverse reactions

CNS: fatigue, paresthesia, vertigo, dizziness, *headache,* nervousness, somnolence.
CV: hypertension, chest pain.
EENT: abnormal vision, xerophthalmia, pharyngitis, rhinitis, sinusitis.
GI: *dry mouth,* abdominal pain, constipation, diarrhea, dyspepsia, flatulence, nausea, vomiting.
GU: dysuria, micturition frequency, urine retention, UTI.
Metabolic: weight gain.
Musculoskeletal: arthralgia, back pain.
Respiratory: bronchitis, cough, upper respiratory tract infection.
Skin: pruritus, rash, erythema, dry skin.
Other: flulike syndrome, falls, fungal infection, infection.

Interactions

Drug-drug. *Antifungals (itraconazole, ketoconazole, miconazole), CYP 3A4 inhibitors (such as macrolide antibiotics clarithromycin and erythromycin), cyclosporin, vincristine:* May increase tolterodine concentration. Don't give tolterodine doses above 1 mg b.i.d. (2 mg daily of extended-release capsules) with these drugs.

Effects on lab test results

None reported.

Pharmacokinetics

Absorption: Well absorbed with about 77% bioavailability. Peak level occurs within 1 to

2 hours after administration. Food increases bioavailability by 53%.
Distribution: Volume of distribution is about 113 L, 96% protein-bound.
Metabolism: Primarily by oxidation by the CYP 2D6 pathway and forms an active 5-hydroxymethyl metabolite.
Excretion: Mostly recovered in urine; the rest in feces. Less than 1% of dose is recovered as unchanged drug, and 5% to 14% is recovered as the active metabolite. *Half-life:* 1¾ to 3½ hours.

Route	Onset	Peak	Duration
P.O.	Unknown	1-2 hr	Unknown

Action

Chemical effect: A competitive muscarinic receptor antagonist. Both urinary bladder contraction and salivation are mediated via cholinergic muscarinic receptors.
Therapeutic effect: Relieves symptoms of overactive bladder.

Available forms

Capsules (extended-release): 2 mg, 4 mg
Tablets: 1 mg, 2 mg

NURSING PROCESS

◢ Assessment
• Assess baseline bladder function and monitor therapeutic effects.
• Be alert for adverse reactions and drug interactions.
• Evaluate patient's and family's knowledge of drug therapy.

◕ Nursing diagnoses
• Impaired urinary elimination related to underlying medical condition
• Urine retention related to drug-induced adverse effects
• Deficient knowledge related to drug therapy

▶ Planning and implementation
• Food increases the absorption of tolterodine, but no dosage adjustment is needed.
• In the case of urine retention, notify prescriber and prepare for urinary catheterization.
• Dry mouth is the most frequently reported adverse reaction.

Patient teaching
• Tell patient that sugarless gum, hard candy, or saliva substitute may help relieve dry mouth.
• Advise patient to avoid driving or other potentially hazardous activities until visual effects of drug are known.
• Instruct patient to immediately report signs of infection, urine retention, or GI problems.

☑ Evaluation
• Patient experiences improved bladder function with drug therapy.
• Patient doesn't experience urine retention.
• Patient and family state understanding of drug therapy.

topiramate
(toh-PEER-uh-mayt)
Topamax

Pharmacologic class: sulfamate-substituted monosaccharide
Therapeutic class: antiepileptic
Pregnancy risk category: C

Indications and dosages

▶ **Partial onset seizures, primary generalized tonic-clonic seizures.** *Adults:* 200 to 400 mg P.O. daily in two divided doses. Initiate therapy at 25 to 50 mg daily followed by adjustment to an effective dose in increments of 25 to 50 mg weekly.
▶ **Adjunctive therapy for partial seizures, primary generalized tonic-clonic seizures, or Lennox-Gastaut syndrome.** *Children ages 2 to 16:* 5 to 9 mg/kg P.O. daily in two divided doses. Begin dosage adjustment at 1 to 3 mg/kg nightly for 1 week. Then increase at 1- to 2-week intervals by 1 to 3 mg/kg daily to achieve optimal response.

Contraindications and precautions

• Contraindicated in patients hypersensitive to drug or its components.
• Use cautiously in patients with hepatic and renal impairment. Also use cautiously with other drugs that predispose patients to heat-related disorders, including other carbonic anhydrase inhibitors and anticholinergics.
▲ **Lifespan:** In pregnant and breast-feeding women, use cautiously.

Adverse reactions

CNS: fever, *fatigue,* abnormal coordination, aggression, agitation, apathy, asthenia, *ataxia, confusion,* depression, depersonalization, *dizziness,* emotional lability, euphoria, *generalized tonic-clonic seizures,* hallucinations, hyperkinesia, hypertonia, hypesthesia, hypokinesia, insomnia, *nervousness, nystagmus, paresthesia,* personality disorder, *psychomotor slowing,* psychosis, *somnolence, speech disorders,* stupor, *suicide attempts, tremor,* vertigo, malaise, mood problems, difficulty with concentration, attention, language, or *memory.*
CV: chest pain, palpitations, edema, hot flushes.
EENT: *abnormal vision,* conjunctivitis, *diplopia,* eye pain, hearing problems, pharyngitis, sinusitis, tinnitus.
GI: taste perversion, abdominal pain, anorexia, constipation, diarrhea, dry mouth, dyspepsia, flatulence, gastroenteritis, gingivitis, *nausea,* vomiting.
GU: amenorrhea, dysuria, dysmenorrhea, hematuria, impotence, intermenstrual bleeding, menstrual disorder, menorrhagia, micturition frequency, renal calculi, urinary incontinence, UTI, vaginitis, leukorrhea.
Hematologic: anemia, epistaxis, *leukopenia.*
Metabolic: weight changes.
Musculoskeletal: arthralgia, back or leg pain, muscular weakness, myalgia, rigors.
Respiratory: bronchitis, cough, dyspnea, *upper respiratory tract infection.*
Skin: acne, alopecia, increased sweating, pruritus, rash.
Other: body odor, flulike syndrome, breast pain, decreased libido.

Interactions

Drug-drug. *Carbamazepine:* Decreases topiramate levels. Monitor patient.
Carbonic anhydrase inhibitors (acetazolamide, dichlorphenamide): Increases risk of renal calculus formation. Avoid use together.
CNS depressants: Possible topiramate-induced CNS depression, as well as other adverse cognitive and neuropsychiatric events. Use cautiously.
Hormonal contraceptives: Decreases efficacy. Report changes in bleeding patterns; urge patient to use other nonhormonal effective contraceptives.
Phenytoin: Decreases topiramate levels and increases phenytoin levels. Monitor levels.

Valproic acid: Decreases valproic acid and topiramate levels. Monitor patient.
Drug-lifestyle. *Alcohol use:* Possible topiramate-induced CNS depression, as well as other adverse cognitive and neuropsychiatric events. Discourage use together.

Effects on lab test results

• May increase liver enzyme levels. May decrease bicarbonate level.
• May decrease hemoglobin, hematocrit, and WBC count.

Pharmacokinetics

Absorption: Rapid.
Distribution: Up to 17% bound to plasma proteins.
Metabolism: Not extensive.
Excretion: Primarily eliminated unchanged in urine. *Half-life:* 21 hours.

Route	Onset	Peak	Duration
P.O.	Unknown	2 hr	Unknown

Action

Chemical effect: May block action potential, suggestive of a sodium channel blocking action. May also potentiate activity of GABA and antagonize ability of kainate to activate the amino acid (glutamate) receptor.
Therapeutic effect: Prevents partial-onset seizures.

Available forms

Capsules: 15 mg, 25 mg
Tablets: 25 mg, 100 mg, 200 mg

NURSING PROCESS

⚕ Assessment

• Assess patient's seizure disorder before therapy and regularly thereafter.
• Carefully monitor patient taking topiramate with other antiepileptic drugs; dosage adjustments may be needed to achieve optimal response.
• Oligohidrosis and hyperthermia have been infrequently reported, mainly in children. Monitor patient closely, especially in hot weather.
• Assess patient's compliance with therapy at each follow-up visit.
• Evaluate patient's and family's knowledge of drug therapy.

Reactions may be *common,* uncommon, *life-threatening,* or COMMON AND LIFE-THREATENING.

⊕ **Nursing diagnoses**
- Risk for injury related to seizure disorder
- Acute pain related to increased risk of renal calculi formation
- Deficient knowledge related to drug therapy

≫ **Planning and implementation**
- Renal insufficiency requires a reduced dose. For hemodialysis patients, supplemental doses may be needed to avoid rapid drops in drug levels during prolonged dialysis.
- **ALERT:** If an ocular adverse event, characterized by acute myopia and secondary angle-closure glaucoma, occurs, stop drug.
- **ALERT:** Don't confuse Topamax with Toprol XL.

Patient teaching
- Tell patient to maintain adequate fluid intake during therapy to minimize risk of forming renal calculi.
- Advise patient not to drive or operate hazardous machinery until CNS effects of drug are known.
- Tell patient that drug may decrease effectiveness of hormonal contraceptives and to use a barrier form of birth control.
- Tell patient to avoid crushing or breaking tablets because of bitter taste.
- Tell patient that drug can be taken without regard to food.
- Tell patient to notify prescriber immediately if he experiences changes in vision.

✓ **Evaluation**
- Patient is free from seizure activity.
- Patient maintains adequate hydration to prevent renal calculus formation.
- Patient and family state understanding of drug therapy.

topotecan hydrochloride
(toh-poh-TEE-ken high-droh-KLOR-ighd)
Hycamtin

Pharmacologic class: antitumor drug
Therapeutic class: antineoplastic
Pregnancy risk category: D

Indications and dosages

▶ **Metastatic carcinoma of ovary after failure of initial or subsequent chemotherapy;**

small-cell lung cancer after failure of first-line chemotherapy. *Adults:* 1.5 mg/m² by I.V. infusion over 30 minutes, daily for 5 consecutive days, starting on day 1 of a 21-day cycle, for minimum of four cycles in absence of tumor progression.

◩ **Adjust-a-dose:** For patients with renal impairment, if creatinine clearance is 20 to 39 ml/minute, decrease dosage to 0.75 mg/m². If severe neutropenia occurs, reduce dose by 0.25 mg/m² for subsequent courses. Or, in severe neutropenia, give granulocyte-colony stimulating factor (GSF) after subsequent course (before resorting to dose reduction) starting from day 6 of the course (24 hours after topotecan administration).

▼ **I.V. administration**

- Prepare drug under a vertical laminar flow hood while wearing gloves and protective clothing. If drug contacts skin, wash immediately and thoroughly with soap and water. If mucous membranes are affected, flush with water.
- Reconstitute drug in each 4-mg vial with 4 ml sterile water for injection.
- Dilute appropriate volume of reconstituted solution in normal saline solution or D₅W before use.
- Infuse over 30 minutes.
- Protect unopened vials of drug from light. Reconstituted vials stored at 68° to 77° F (20° to 25° C) and exposed to ambient lighting are stable for 24 hours.

Contraindications and precautions

- Contraindicated in patients hypersensitive to drug or its components and in patients with severe bone marrow depression.
- ⚖ **Lifespan:** In pregnant and breast-feeding women, drug is contraindicated.

Adverse reactions

CNS: *fever, fatigue, asthenia, headache,* paresthesia.
GI: *nausea, vomiting, diarrhea, constipation, abdominal pain, stomatitis, anorexia.*
Hematologic: NEUTROPENIA, LEUKOPENIA, THROMBOCYTOPENIA, *anemia.*
Respiratory: *dyspnea.*
Skin: *alopecia.*
Other: *sepsis.*

Interactions

Drug-drug. *Cisplatin:* Increases severity of myelosuppression. Use both drugs very cautiously.
Filgrastim (6-GSF): Prolongs duration of neutropenia. Don't give GSF until day 6 of regimen, 24 hours after completion of topotecan therapy.

Effects on lab test results

• May increase ALT, AST, and bilirubin levels.
• May decrease hemoglobin, hematocrit, and WBC, platelet, and neutrophil counts.

Pharmacokinetics

Absorption: Administered I.V.
Distribution: About 35% bound to plasma proteins.
Metabolism: Metabolized by liver.
Excretion: 30% excreted in urine. *Half-life:* 2 to 3 hours.

Route	Onset	Peak	Duration
I.V.	Unknown	Unknown	Unknown

Action

Chemical effect: Results from damage to DNA produced during DNA synthesis when replication enzymes interact with the complex formed.
Therapeutic effect: Kills certain cancer cells.

Available forms

Injection: 4-mg single-dose vial

NURSING PROCESS

⧉ Assessment
• Evaluate patient's and family's knowledge of drug therapy.
• Assess patient's underlying condition before and frequently during therapy.
• Monitor patient's CBC frequently during therapy.
• Be alert for adverse reactions and drug interactions.

⊞ Nursing diagnoses
• Ineffective health maintenance related to neoplastic disease
• Deficient knowledge related to drug therapy

▶ Planning and implementation
⊛ **ALERT:** Patient must have a baseline neutrophil count greater than 1,500/mm³ and platelet count greater than 100,000/mm³ before therapy can start.
• Frequent monitoring of peripheral blood cell count is critical. Don't give repeated doses until neutrophil count is greater than 1,000/mm³, platelet count is greater than 100,000/mm³, and hemoglobin is greater than 9 mg/dl.
Patient teaching
• Instruct patient to report promptly sore throat, fever, chills, or unusual bleeding or bruising.
• Advise woman of childbearing age to avoid pregnancy and breast-feeding during therapy.
• Tell patient and family about need for close monitoring of blood counts.

✓ Evaluation
• Patient shows positive response to drug.
• Patient and family state understanding of drug therapy.

torsemide
(TOR-seh-mighd)
Demadex

Pharmacologic class: loop diuretic
Therapeutic class: diuretic, antihypertensive
Pregnancy risk category: B

Indications and dosages

▶ **Diuresis in patients with heart failure.**
Adults: Initially, 10 to 20 mg P.O. or I.V. once daily. If response is inadequate, double dose until response is obtained. Maximum, 200 mg daily.
▶ **Diuresis in patients with chronic renal impairment.** *Adults:* Initially, 20 mg P.O. or I.V. once daily. If response is inadequate, double dose until response is obtained. Maximum, 200 mg daily.
▶ **Diuresis in patients with hepatic cirrhosis.** *Adults:* Initially, 5 to 10 mg P.O. or I.V. once daily with aldosterone antagonist or potassium-sparing diuretic. If response is inadequate, double dose until response is obtained. Maximum, 40 mg daily.
▶ **Hypertension.** *Adults:* Initially, 5 mg P.O. daily. Increase to 10 mg in 4 to 6 weeks if need-

ed and tolerated. If response is still inadequate, add another antihypertensive.

▼ I.V. administration

• Drug may be given by direct injection over at least 2 minutes. Rapid injection may cause ototoxicity. Don't give more than 200 mg at a time.
• Switch to oral form as soon as possible.

Contraindications and precautions

• Contraindicated in patients hypersensitive to drug or other sulfonylurea derivatives and in those with anuria.
• Use cautiously in patients with hepatic disease, cirrhosis, or ascites; sudden changes in fluid and electrolyte balance may precipitate hepatic coma.
• Lifespan: In pregnant and breast-feeding women, use cautiously. In children, safety of drug hasn't been established. In geriatric patients, use cautiously.

Adverse reactions

CNS: asthenia, dizziness, headache, nervousness, insomnia, syncope.
CV: ECG abnormalities, chest pain, edema, orthostatic hypertension.
EENT: rhinitis, sore throat.
GI: diarrhea, constipation, nausea, dyspepsia, HEMORRHAGE.
GU: *excessive urination,* impotence.
Metabolic: *dehydration,* electrolyte imbalances, including *hypokalemia, hypomagnesemia,* hypocalcemia, hyperuricemia, hyperglycemia; *hypochloremic alkalosis.*
Musculoskeletal: arthralgia, myalgia.
Respiratory: cough.
Other: *excessive thirst,* gout.

Interactions

Drug-drug. *Chlorothiazide, chlorthalidone, hydrochlorothiazide, indapamide, metolazone:* May cause excessive diuretic response resulting in serious electrolyte abnormalities or dehydration. Adjust doses carefully and monitor patient for this effect.
Cholestyramine: Decreases absorption of torsemide. Separate administration times by at least 3 hours.
Indomethacin: Decreases diuretic effectiveness in sodium-restricted patients. Avoid use together.

Lithium, ototoxic drugs (such as aminoglycosides, ethacrynic acid): Possible increased toxicity of these drugs. Avoid use together.
NSAIDs: May potentiate nephrotoxicity of NSAIDs. Use together cautiously.
Probenecid: Decreases diuretic effectiveness. Avoid use together.
Salicylates: Decreases excretion, possibly leading to salicylate toxicity. Avoid use together.
Spironolactone: Decreases renal clearance of spironolactone. Dosage adjustments isn't needed.
Drug-herb. *Licorice:* Potential for rapid potassium loss. Discourage use together.

Effects on lab test results

• May increase glucose, BUN, creatinine, cholesterol, and uric acid levels. May decrease calcium, potassium, and magnesium levels.

Pharmacokinetics

Absorption: Little first-pass metabolism.
Distribution: Extensively bound to plasma protein.
Metabolism: 80% hepatically metabolized.
Excretion: 22% to 34% excreted unchanged in urine. *Half-life:* 3½ hours.

Route	Onset	Peak	Duration
P.O.	1 hr	1-2 hr	6-8 hr
I.V.	≤ 10 min	≤ 1 hr	6-8 hr

Action

Chemical effect: Enhances excretion of sodium, chloride, and water by acting on ascending portion of loop of Henle.
Therapeutic effect: Promotes water and sodium excretion and lowers blood pressure.

Available forms

Injection: 10 mg/ml
Tablets: 5 mg, 10 mg, 20 mg, 100 mg

NURSING PROCESS

✍ Assessment

• Assess patient's condition before therapy and regularly thereafter.
• Monitor geriatric patients, who are especially susceptible to excessive diuresis, with potential for circulatory collapse and thromboembolic complications.

• During rapid diuresis and routinely with long-term use, monitor fluid intake and output, electrolyte levels, blood pressure, weight, and pulse rate. Drug may cause profound diuresis and water and electrolyte depletion.
• Watch for signs of hypokalemia, such as muscle weakness and cramps.
• Be alert for adverse reactions and drug interactions.
• Evaluate patient's and family's knowledge of drug therapy.

🔲 **Nursing diagnoses**
• Excess fluid volume related to presence of edema
• Risk for injury related to presence of hypertension
• Deficient knowledge related to drug therapy

▶ **Planning and implementation**
• Give oral drug in morning to prevent nocturia.
• Make sure patient is on a high-potassium diet; refer patient to a dietitian for guidance. Foods rich in potassium include citrus fruits, tomatoes, bananas, dates, and apricots.
⊛ **ALERT:** Don't confuse torsemide with furosemide.
Patient teaching
• Tell patient to take drug in morning to prevent sleep interruption.
• Advise patient to change position slowly to prevent dizziness and to limit alcohol intake and strenuous exercise in hot weather to prevent orthostatic hypotension.
• Advise patient to immediately report ringing in ears because it may indicate toxicity.
• Tell patient to check with prescriber or pharmacist before taking OTC drugs.

☑ **Evaluation**
• Patient shows no signs of edema.
• Patient's blood pressure is normal.
• Patient and family state understanding of drug therapy.

trace elements
(trays EL-uh-ments)

chromium (chromic chloride)
(KROH-mee-um)
Chroma-Pak, Chromic Chloride

copper (cupric sulfate)
(KAH-per)
Cupric Sulfate

iodine (sodium iodide)
(IGH-oh-dighn)
Iodopen

manganese (manganese chloride, manganese sulfate)
(MAN-geh-nees)

selenium (selenious acid)
(seh-LEHN-ee-um)
Sele-Pak, Selepen

zinc (zinc chloride, zinc sulfate)
(zink)
Zinca-Pak

Pharmacologic class: trace elements
Therapeutic class: nutritional agents
Pregnancy risk category: C

Indications and dosages

▶ **Prevention of individual trace element deficiencies in patients receiving long-term total parenteral nutrition (TPN).**
Adults: 10 to 15 mcg chromium I.V. daily. Or, 0.5 to 1.5 mg copper I.V. daily. Or, 1 to 2 mcg/kg iodine I.V. daily. Or, 0.15 to 0.8 mg manganese I.V. daily. Or, 20 to 40 mcg selenium I.V. daily. Or, 2.5 to 4 mg zinc I.V. daily.
Children: 0.14 to 0.20 mcg/kg chromium I.V. daily. Or, 20 mcg/kg copper I.V. daily. Or, 2 to 3 mcg/kg iodine I.V. daily. Or, 2 to 10 mcg/kg manganese I.V. daily. Or, 3 mcg/kg selenium I.V. daily.
Children age 5 and younger: 100 mcg/kg zinc I.V. daily.
Neonates: 300 mcg/kg zinc I.V. daily.

▽ I.V. administration

• Cautiously infuse diluted solution through patent I.V. line.

Contraindications and precautions

☀ **Lifespan:** In pregnant women, use cautiously.

Adverse reactions

GI: nausea, vomiting.

Interactions

None significant.

Effects on lab test results

None reported.

Pharmacokinetics

Absorption: Administered I.V.
Distribution: Unknown.
Metabolism: Unknown.
Excretion: Unknown. *Half-life:* Unknown.

Route	Onset	Peak	Duration
I.V.	Immediate	Immediate	Unknown

Action

Chemical effect: Participates in synthesis and stabilization of proteins and nucleic acids in subcellular and membrane transport systems.
Therapeutic effect: Restores normal body levels of trace elements.

Available forms

chromium
Injection: 4 mcg/ml, 20 mcg/ml
copper
Injection: 0.4 mg/ml, 2 mg/ml
iodine
Injection: 100 mcg/ml
manganese
Injection: 0.1 mg/ml
selenium
Injection: 40 mcg/ml
zinc
Injection: 1 mg/ml, 5 mg/ml

NURSING PROCESS

☕ Assessment

• Assess patient's trace element deficiency before therapy and regularly thereafter. Normal levels are 0.85 ng/ml chromium; 0.07 to 0.15 mg/ml copper; 4 to 20 mcg/dl manganese; 0.1 to 0.19 mcg/ml selenium; and 0.05 to 0.15 mg/dl zinc.

• Check levels of trace elements in patients who have received TPN for 2 months or longer. Call prescriber's attention to low levels of these elements because supplement may be needed.

• Evaluate patient's and family's knowledge of drug therapy.

ᗕ Nursing diagnoses

• Imbalanced nutrition: less than body requirements related to presence of deficiency of trace elements

• Deficient knowledge related to drug therapy

▷ Planning and implementation

⚠ **ALERT:** Don't give undiluted because of potential for phlebitis.

• Solutions of trace elements are compounded by pharmacy for addition to TPN solutions according to various formulas. One common trace element solution is Shils solution, which contains copper 1 mg/ml, iodide 0.06 mg/ml, manganese 0.4 mg/ml, and zinc 2 mg/ml.
Patient teaching
• Inform patient and family of need for trace elements.

☑ Evaluation

• Patient regains normal levels of trace elements.

• Patient and family state understanding of drug therapy.

---

tramadol hydrochloride
(TRAM-uh-dohl high-droh-KLOR-ighd)
Ultram

Pharmacologic class: synthetic analgesic
Therapeutic class: analgesic
Pregnancy risk category: C

Indications and dosages

▷ **Moderate to moderately severe pain.**
Adults: 50 to 100 mg P.O. q 4 to 6 hours, p.r.n. Maximum dosage is 400 mg daily.
◩ **Adjust-a-dose:** Maximum dosage in patients older than age 75 is 300 mg daily. For patients with cirrhosis, give 50 mg P.O. q 12 hours. For

patients with renal impairment, if creatinine clearance is less than 30 ml/minute, give dose q 12 hours. Maximum, 200 mg daily. Hemodialysis patients can receive their regular dose on same day of dialysis.

Contraindications and precautions

• Contraindicated in patients hypersensitive to drug and in those with acute intoxication from alcohol, hypnotics, centrally acting analgesics, opioids, or psychotropic drugs.

• Use cautiously in patients at risk for seizures or respiratory depression; patients with increased intracranial pressure or head injury, acute abdominal conditions, or renal or hepatic impairment; and patients physically dependent on opioids.

⚠ Lifespan: In pregnant women and in children, safety of drug hasn't been established. In breast-feeding women, drug isn't recommended.

Adverse reactions

CNS: *dizziness, vertigo, headache, somnolence, CNS stimulation, asthenia,* anxiety, confusion, coordination disturbance, malaise, euphoria, nervousness, sleep disorder, *seizures.*
CV: vasodilation.
EENT: visual disturbances.
GI: *nausea, constipation, vomiting,* dyspepsia, dry mouth, diarrhea, abdominal pain, anorexia, flatulence.
GU: urine retention, urinary frequency, menopausal symptoms.
Musculoskeletal: hypertonia.
Respiratory: *respiratory depression.*
Skin: *pruritus,* sweating, rash.

Interactions

Drug-drug. *Carbamazepine:* Increases tramadol metabolism. Patients receiving long-term carbamazepine therapy at dosage of up to 800 mg daily may require up to twice the recommended dose of tramadol.
CNS depressants: May have additive effects. Use together cautiously. Dosage of tramadol may need to be reduced.
MAO inhibitors, neuroleptics: Increases risk of seizures. Monitor patient closely.
Drug-herb. *5-hydroxytryptophan (5-HTP), SAMe, St. John's wort:* Increases serotonin levels. Discourage use together.

Effects on lab test results

• May increase liver enzyme levels.
• May decrease hemoglobin and hematocrit.

Pharmacokinetics

Absorption: Rapid and almost complete.
Distribution: About 20% bound to plasma proteins.
Metabolism: Extensively metabolized.
Excretion: 30% excreted in urine as unchanged drug and 60% as metabolites. *Half-life:* 6 to 7 hours.

Route	Onset	Peak	Duration
P.O.	Unknown	2 hr	Unknown

Action

Chemical effect: Unknown; centrally acting synthetic analgesic compound not chemically related to opioids that is thought to bind to opioid receptors and inhibit reuptake of norepinephrine and serotonin.
Therapeutic effect: Relieves pain.

Available forms

Tablets: 50 mg

NURSING PROCESS

✂ Assessment

• Assess patient's pain before therapy and regularly thereafter.
• Monitor CV and respiratory status.
③ **ALERT:** Closely monitor patient at risk for seizures. Drug has been reported to reduce seizure threshold.
• Monitor patient for drug dependence. Tramadol can produce dependence similar to that of codeine or dextropropoxyphene and thus has potential to be abused.
• Be alert for adverse reactions and drug interactions.
• Evaluate patient's and family's knowledge of drug therapy.

⊞ Nursing diagnoses

• Acute pain related to underlying condition
• Risk for constipation related to drug-induced adverse GI reactions
• Deficient knowledge related to drug therapy

Reactions may be *common,* uncommon, *life-threatening,* or COMMON AND LIFE-THREATENING.

⟩ Planning and implementation

• For better analgesic effect, give drug before onset of intense pain.

• If respiratory rate decreases or falls below 12 breaths/minute, withhold dose and notify prescriber.

• Because constipation is a common adverse effect, anticipate need for laxative therapy.

⊛ **ALERT:** Don't confuse tramadol with trazodone or trandolapril.

Patient teaching

• Instruct patient to take drug only as prescribed and not to increase dosage or dosage interval unless instructed by prescriber.

• Tell ambulatory patient to be careful when getting out of bed and walking. Warn outpatient to refrain from driving and performing other potentially hazardous activities that require mental alertness until drug's CNS effects are known.

• Instruct patient to check with prescriber before taking OTC drugs; drug interactions can occur.

☑ Evaluation

• Patient is free from pain.

• Patient regains normal bowel pattern.

• Patient and family state understanding of drug therapy.

---

trandolapril
(tran-DOH-luh-pril)
Mavik

Pharmacologic class: ACE inhibitor
Therapeutic class: antihypertensive
Pregnancy risk category: C (D in second and third trimesters)

Indications and dosages

▶ **Hypertension.** *Adults:* For patient not receiving a diuretic, initially 1 mg for a nonblack patient and 2 mg for a black patient P.O. once daily. If response isn't adequate, dosage may be increased at intervals of at least 1 week. Maintenance dosage is 2 to 4 mg daily for most patients. Some patients receiving 4-mg once-daily doses may need b.i.d. doses. For patient also receiving diuretic, initial dose is 0.5 mg P.O. once daily. Subsequent dosages adjusted based on blood pressure response.

▶ **Heart failure or left ventricular dysfunction after acute MI.** *Adults:* Initiate therapy 3 to 5 days after MI with 1 mg P.O. daily. Adjust as tolerated to target dosage of 4 mg daily.

Contraindications and precautions

• Contraindicated in patients hypersensitive to drug and in patients with a history of angioedema with previous therapy with ACE inhibitor.

• Use cautiously in patients with impaired renal function, heart failure, or renal artery stenosis.

⚖ **Lifespan:** In pregnant women, drug is contraindicated.

Adverse reactions

CNS: dizziness, headache, fatigue, drowsiness, insomnia, paresthesia, vertigo, anxiety.
CV: chest pain, first-degree AV block, *bradycardia*, edema, flushing, hypotension, palpitations.
EENT: epistaxis, throat irritation.
GI: diarrhea, dyspepsia, abdominal distention, abdominal pain or cramps, constipation, vomiting, *pancreatitis*.
GU: urinary frequency, impotence.
Hematologic: *neutropenia, leukopenia.*
Metabolic: *hyperkalemia*, hyponatremia.
Respiratory: dry, persistent, tickling, nonproductive cough; dyspnea; upper respiratory tract infection.
Skin: rash, pruritus, pemphigus.
Other: *anaphylaxis, angioedema,* decreased libido.

Interactions

Drug-drug. *Diuretics:* Increases risk of excessive hypotension. Monitor blood pressure closely.
Lithium: Increases lithium level and lithium toxicity. Avoid use together; monitor lithium level.
Potassium-sparing diuretics, potassium supplements: Increases risk of hyperkalemia. Monitor potassium level closely.
Drug-herb. *Licorice:* May increase sodium retention and blood pressure. Discourage use together.
Drug-food. *Salt substitutes containing potassium:* Increases risk of hyperkalemia. Monitor potassium level closely.

Effects on lab test results

• May increase BUN, creatinine, potassium, and liver enzyme levels. May decrease sodium level.
• May decrease neutrophil and WBC counts.

Pharmacokinetics

Absorption: Food slows absorption.
Distribution: 80% protein-bound.
Metabolism: Metabolized in liver.
Excretion: In urine and feces. *Half-life:* 5 to
10 hours. Longer in patients with renal impairment.

Route	Onset	Peak	Duration
P.O.			
drug	Unknown	1 hr	Unknown
metabolite	4-10 hr	1 hr	Unknown

Action

Chemical effect: Inhibits circulating and tissue
ACE activity, which reduces angiotensin II formation, decreases vasoconstriction and aldosterone secretion, and increases plasma renin.
Therapeutic effect: Lowers blood pressure.

Available forms

Tablets: 1 mg, 2 mg, 4 mg

NURSING PROCESS

Assessment

• Monitor patient's blood pressure and potassium level before and during drug therapy.
• Monitor patient for hypotension. If possible, stop diuretic therapy 2 to 3 days before starting drug.
• Monitor patient for jaundice and alert prescriber immediately if occurs.
• Monitor patient's compliance with therapy.
• Evaluate patient's and family's knowledge of drug therapy.

Nursing diagnoses

• Risk for injury related to hypertension
• Deficient knowledge related to drug therapy

Planning and implementation

• Take steps to prevent or minimize orthostatic hypotension.
• Maintain patient's nondrug therapies, such as sodium restriction, stress management, smoking cessation, and exercise program.
• **ALERT:** Angioedema that involves the tongue, glottis, or larynx may be fatal because of airway obstruction. Give appropriate therapy, including epinephrine 1:1,000 (0.3 to 0.5 ml) S.C.; have resuscitation equipment readily available for maintaining a patent airway.

Patient teaching

• Advise patient to report infection and other adverse reactions.
• Tell patient to avoid salt substitutes.
• Tell patient to use caution in hot weather and during exercise.
• Tell woman to report suspected pregnancy immediately.
• Advise patient about to undergo surgery or anesthesia to inform prescriber of use of drug.

Evaluation

• Patient's blood pressure is normal.
• Patient and family state understanding of drug therapy.

tranylcypromine sulfate
(tran-il-SIGH-proh-meen SUL-fayt)
Parnate

Pharmacologic class: MAO inhibitor
Therapeutic class: antidepressant
Pregnancy risk category: C

Indications and dosages

▶ **Depression.** *Adults:* 10 mg P.O. t.i.d. Increase by 10 mg daily at 1- to 3-week intervals to maximum of 60 mg daily, if needed, after 2 weeks of initial therapy.

Contraindications and precautions

• Contraindicated in patients receiving other MAO inhibitors or dibenzazepine derivatives; sympathomimetics (including amphetamines); some CNS depressants (including alcohol); some serotonin reuptake inhibitors; antihypertensive, diuretic, antihistaminic, sedative, or anesthetic drugs; bupropion hydrochloride, buspirone hydrochloride, dextromethorphan, meperidine; foods high in tyramine or tryptophan; or excessive quantities of caffeine. Also contraindicated in patients with confirmed or suspected cerebrovascular defect, CV disease, hypertension, or history of headache and in those undergoing elective surgery.
• Use cautiously with antiparkinsonians or spinal anesthetics; in patients with renal disease, diabetes, seizure disorder, Parkinson's disease, or hyperthyroidism; and in patients at risk for suicide.

⚘ **Lifespan:** In pregnant women, drug isn't recommended. In breast-feeding women and in children, safety of drug hasn't been established.

Adverse reactions

CNS: *dizziness, vertigo, headache,* anxiety, agitation, drowsiness, weakness, numbness, paresthesia, tremor, jitters, confusion.
CV: *orthostatic hypotension, tachycardia, paradoxical hypertension,* palpitations, *edema.*
EENT: blurred vision, tinnitus.
GI: dry mouth, *anorexia,* nausea, diarrhea, constipation, abdominal pain.
GU: impotence, urine retention, impaired ejaculation.
Hematologic: anemia, *leukopenia, agranulocytosis, thrombocytopenia.*
Hepatic: *hepatitis.*
Musculoskeletal: muscle spasm, myoclonic jerks.
Skin: rash.
Other: SIADH, chills.

Interactions

Drug-drug. *Amphetamines, antihistamines, meperidine, methylphenidate, sympathomimetics:* Enhances pressor effects of these drugs. Avoid use together.
Antiparkinsonians, barbiturates, dextromethorphan, methotrimeprazine, opioids, other sedatives, tricyclic antidepressants: Enhances adverse CNS effects. Use with caution and in reduced dosage.
Buspirone: May elevate blood pressure. Monitor patient's blood pressure closely.
Citalopram, fluoxetine, fluvoxamine, nefazodone, paroxetine, sertraline, venlafaxine: May cause serotonin syndrome involving CNS irritability, shivering, and altered consciousness. Don't give together. Wait at least 2 weeks after stopping an MAO inhibitor before giving an SSRI.
Dopamine, ephedrine, metaraminol, phenylephrine, pseudoephedrine: May cause severe headache, hypertension, fever and hypertensive crisis. Avoid use together.
Insulin, oral antidiabetics: Increases risk of hypoglycemia. Use cautiously and in reduced dosages; monitor patient's glucose level.
Levodopa: May cause a hypertensive reaction. Don't use together.
Drug-herb. *Cacao tree:* May have potential vasopressor effects. Discourage use together.

Ginseng: May cause headache, tremors, mania. Discourage use together.
Green tea: Contains caffeine. Discourage use together.
Scotch broom: Contains high levels of tyramine. Discourage use together.
St. John's wort: Has properties similar to those of SSRIs. Discourage use together.
Drug-food. *Caffeine:* May cause hypertensive crisis. Discourage use together.
Foods with high amine content and tyramine (such as aged, overripe and fermented foods and drinks, red wines, caviar, bologna, pepperoni, salami): May cause severe elevation of blood pressure, hypertensive crisis, or hemorrhagic CVA. Warn patient to avoid such foods for at least 1 month after stopping drug therapy.
Drug-lifestyle. *Alcohol use:* Enhances adverse CNS effects. Discourage use together.

Effects on lab test results

• May increase ALT and AST levels.
• May decrease hemoglobin, hematocrit, and WBC, granulocyte, and platelet counts.

Pharmacokinetics

Absorption: Rapid and complete.
Distribution: Unknown.
Metabolism: Metabolized in liver.
Excretion: Excreted primarily in urine; some excreted in feces. *Half-life:* 2½ hours.

Route	Onset	Peak	Duration
P.O.	Unknown	1-3½ hr	10 days after therapy stops

Action

Chemical effect: Unknown; probably promotes accumulation of neurotransmitters by inhibiting MAO.
Therapeutic effect: Relieves depression.

Available forms

Tablets: 10 mg

NURSING PROCESS

📋 **Assessment**
• Assess patient's condition before therapy and regularly thereafter.
• Assess patient for risk of self-harm.

- Obtain baseline blood pressure, heart rate, CBC, and liver function test results before beginning therapy; monitor throughout therapy.
- Be alert for adverse reactions and drug interactions.
- Evaluate patient's and family's knowledge of drug therapy.

Nursing diagnoses
- Disturbed thought processes related to presence of depression
- Risk for injury related to drug-induced adverse CNS reactions
- Deficient knowledge related to drug therapy

Planning and implementation
- Dosage usually is reduced to maintenance level as soon as possible.
- **ALERT:** Don't withdraw drug abruptly.
- In most patients, stop MAO inhibitors 14 days before elective surgery to avoid drug interactions that may occur during anesthetic procedure.
- If patient develops symptoms of overdose (palpitations, severe hypotension, or frequent headaches), withhold dose and notify prescriber.
- **ALERT:** Have phentolamine available to combat severe hypertension.
- Continue precautions for 10 days after stopping drug because it has long-lasting effects.

Patient teaching
- Warn patient to avoid foods high in tyramine or tryptophan and large amounts of caffeine. Tranylcypromine is the MAO inhibitor most often reported to cause hypertensive crisis with ingestion of foods high in tyramine, such as aged cheese, Chianti wine, beer, avocados, chicken livers, chocolate, bananas, soy sauce, meat tenderizers, salami, and bologna.
- Tell patient to avoid alcohol during drug therapy.
- Instruct patient to sit up for 1 minute before getting out of bed to avoid dizziness.
- Warn patient to avoid overexertion because MAO inhibitors may suppress angina.
- Advise patient to consult prescriber before taking other prescription or OTC drugs. If MAO inhibitors are taken with OTC cold, hay fever, or diet-aid drugs, severe adverse effects may occur.
- Instruct patient not to stop drug suddenly.

Evaluation
- Patient's behavior and communication exhibit improved thought processes.
- Patient doesn't experience injury from adverse CNS reactions.
- Patient and family state understanding of drug therapy.

trastuzumab
(trahs-TOO-zuh-mab)
Herceptin

Pharmacologic class: monoclonal antibody
Therapeutic class: antineoplastic
Pregnancy risk category: B

Indications and dosages
▶ **Monotherapy for patients with metastatic breast cancer whose tumors overexpress the human epidermal growth factor receptor 2 (HER2) protein and who have received one or more chemotherapy regimens for their metastatic disease; or with paclitaxel for metastatic breast cancer in patients whose tumors overexpress the HER2 protein and who haven't received chemotherapy for their metastatic disease.** *Adults:* Initial loading dose of 4 mg/kg I.V. over 90 minutes. If the initial loading dose is well tolerated, maintenance dosage is 2 mg/kg I.V. weekly as a 30-minute I.V. infusion.

I.V. administration
- Reconstitute drug in each vial with 20 ml of bacteriostatic water for injection, USP, 1.1% benzyl alcohol preserved, as supplied, to yield a multidose solution containing 21 mg/ml. Immediately after reconstitution, label vial for drug expiration 28 days from date of reconstitution.
- If patient is hypersensitive to benzyl alcohol, drug must be reconstituted with sterile water for injection. Drug reconstituted with sterile water for injection must be used immediately; unused portion must be discarded. Avoid other reconstitution diluents.
- Determine dose (mg) of drug needed, based on loading dose of 4 mg/kg or maintenance dose of 2 mg/kg. Calculate volume of 21 mg/ml solution and withdraw amount from vial; add it to an infusion bag containing 250 ml of normal saline solution. Don't use D_5W solution.

- Don't mix or dilute with other drugs.
- Don't give as an I.V. push or bolus.
- Vials of drug are stable at 36° to 46° F (2° to 8° C) before reconstitution. Discard reconstituted solution after 28 days. Store drug solution diluted in normal saline solution for injection at 36° to 46° F before use; it's stable for up to 24 hours.

Contraindications and precautions

- Use cautiously in patients with cardiac dysfunction and in patients hypersensitive to drug or its components.
- ☆ Lifespan: In pregnant women, use only if clearly needed. Breast-feeding women should stop breast-feeding during drug therapy and for 6 months after last dose. In children, safety and effectiveness haven't been established. In elderly patients, use cautiously.

Adverse reactions

CNS: *pain, fever, headache, asthenia, insomnia, dizziness,* paresthesia, depression, peripheral neuritis, neuropathy.
CV: tachycardia, **heart failure,** *peripheral edema,* edema, **left ventricular dysfunction.**
EENT: *rhinitis, pharyngitis,* sinusitis.
GI: *nausea, diarrhea, vomiting, anorexia, abdominal pain.*
GU: UTI.
Hematologic: anemia, **leukopenia.**
Musculoskeletal: bone pain, arthralgia, *back pain.*
Respiratory: *cough, dyspnea.*
Skin: *rash,* acne.
Other: *chills, infection, flulike syndrome,* allergic reaction, herpes simplex, **hypersensitivity reactions (including anaphylaxis).**

Interactions

Drug-drug. *Anthracyclines:* Increases potential for cardiotoxic effects. Monitor patient closely.
Paclitaxel: Decreases clearance of trastuzumab. Monitor patient closely when used together.

Effects on lab test results

- May decrease hemoglobin, hematocrit, and WBC count.

Pharmacokinetics

Absorption: Administered I.V.
Distribution: Volume is 44 ml/kg.
Metabolism: Unknown.

Excretion: Unknown. *Half-life:* 1 to 32 days.

Route	Onset	Peak	Duration
I.V.	Unknown	Unknown	Unknown

Action

Chemical effect: Recombinant DNA-derived monoclonal antibody that selectively binds to HER2. Shown to inhibit the proliferation of human tumor cells that overexpress HER2.
Therapeutic effect: Hinders function of specific breast cancer tumor cells that overexpress HER2.

Available forms

Injection: lyophilized sterile powder containing 440 mg per vial

NURSING PROCESS

⚗ Assessment
- Before beginning therapy, make sure patient has had a thorough baseline cardiac assessment, including history, physical examination, and evaluation, to see if he's at risk for developing cardiotoxicity.
- Use drug only in patients with metastatic breast cancer whose tumors have HER2 protein overexpression.
- Assess patient for chills and fever, especially during the first infusion.
- Monitor patient closely for signs and symptoms of cardiac dysfunction, especially if also receiving anthracyclines and cyclophosphamide.
- Monitor patient for dyspnea, increased cough, paroxysmal nocturnal dyspnea, peripheral edema, and S_3 gallop. Monitor patients also receiving chemotherapy closely for cardiac dysfunction or failure, anemia, leukopenia, diarrhea, and infection.
- Evaluate patient's and family's knowledge of drug therapy.

🔲 Nursing diagnoses
- Imbalanced nutrition: less than body requirements related to drug-induced GI adverse effects
- Decreased cardiac output related to drug-induced decreased left ventricular function
- Deficient knowledge related to drug therapy

▷ Planning and implementation
- Treat first infusion-related symptoms with acetaminophen, diphenhydramine, and meperidine (with or without reducing the rate of infusion).

• If patient experiences a significant decrease in cardiac function, notify prescriber.

Patient teaching

• Tell patient about possibility of first-dose, infusion-related adverse effects.

• Instruct patient to notify prescriber immediately if signs and symptoms of cardiac dysfunction develop, such as shortness of breath, increased cough, or peripheral edema.

• Instruct patient to report adverse effects to prescriber.

☑ Evaluation

• Patient doesn't experience adverse GI effects (nausea, vomiting, diarrhea).

• Patient doesn't exhibit dyspnea, increased cough, paroxysmal nocturnal dyspnea, peripheral edema, or S₃ gallop as result of drug-induced cardiac dysfunction.

• Patient and family state understanding of drug therapy.

---

travoprost
(TRA-voe-prost)
Travatan

Pharmacologic class: prostaglandin analogue
Therapeutic class: antiglaucoma drug, ocular antihypertensive
Pregnancy risk category: C

Indications and dosages

▶ **Reduction of elevated intraocular pressure (IOP) in patients with open-angle glaucoma or ocular hypertension who are intolerant of other IOP-lowering drugs, or in patients who have had insufficient responses to other IOP-lowering drugs.** *Adults:* 1 gtt in conjunctival sac of affected eye once daily in evening.

Contraindications and precautions

• Contraindicated in patients hypersensitive to drug, benzalkonium chloride, or other components.

• Use cautiously in patients with renal or hepatic impairment, active intraocular inflammation (iritis, uveitis), or risk factors for macular edema. Also use cautiously in aphakic patients and pseudophakic patients with a torn posterior lens capsule.

• Don't use in patients with angle-closure glaucoma or inflammatory or neovascular glaucoma.

☀ **Lifespan:** In pregnant women and in women attempting to become pregnant, drug isn't recommended. In breast-feeding women, use cautiously. In children, safety and effectiveness haven't been established.

Adverse reactions

CNS: anxiety, depression, headache, pain.
CV: angina pectoris, ***bradycardia,*** chest pain, hypertension, hypotension.
EENT: *ocular hyperemia, decreased visual acuity, eye discomfort, foreign body sensation, eye pain, eye pruritus,* conjunctival hyperemia, abnormal vision, blepharitis, blurred vision, cataracts, conjunctivitis, dry eyes, eye disorders, iris discoloration, keratitis, lid margin crusting, photophobia, subconjunctival hemorrhage, tearing, sinusitis.
GI: dyspepsia, GI disorder.
GU: prostate disorder, urinary incontinence, UTI.
Metabolic: hypercholesterolemia.
Musculoskeletal: arthritis, back pain.
Respiratory: bronchitis.
Other: accidental injury, cold syndrome, infection.

Interactions

Drug-herb. *Areca, jaborandi:* Possible additive effects. Avoid use together.

Effects on lab test results

• May increase cholesterol level.

Pharmacokinetics

Absorption: Absorbed through the cornea.
Distribution: Levels peak within 30 minutes.
Metabolism: Hydrolyzed by esterases in the cornea to its active free acid. The liver primarily metabolizes the active acid of drug reaching the systemic circulation.
Excretion: Within 1 hour. *Half-life:* 45 minutes.

Route	Onset	Peak	Duration
Ophthalmic	Unknown	30 min	Unknown

Action

Chemical effect: May increase uveoscleral outflow.
Therapeutic effect: Reduces IOP.

Reactions may be *common,* uncommon, *life-threatening,* or COMMON AND LIFE-THREATENING.

Available forms

Ophthalmic solution: 0.004%

NURSING PROCESS

Assessment
- Assess patient's condition before therapy and regularly thereafter.
- If a pregnant woman or a woman attempting to become pregnant accidentally comes in contact with drug, thoroughly cleanse the exposed area with soap and water immediately.
- Evaluate patient's and family's knowledge of drug therapy.

Nursing diagnoses
- Acute pain related to adverse EENT effects of drug
- Risk for activity intolerance related to decreased visual acuity
- Deficient knowledge related to travoprost therapy

Planning and implementation
- Have patient remove contact lenses before administration of drug. Lenses may be reinserted 15 minutes after administration.
- If multiple ophthalmic drugs are being used, separate administration times by least 5 minutes.
- Temporary or permanent increased pigmentation of the iris and eyelid may occur as well as increased pigmentation and growth of the eyelashes.

Patient teaching
- Teach patient to instill drops and advise him to wash hands before and after instilling solution. Warn him not to touch dropper or tip to eye or surrounding tissue.
- Tell patient receiving treatment to only one eye about the potential for increased brown pigmentation of the iris, eyelid skin darkening, and increased length, thickness, pigmentation, or number of lashes in the treated eye.
- Tell patient that, if eye trauma or infection occurs or if eye surgery is needed, he should seek medical advice before continuing to use the multidose container.
- Advise patient to immediately report conjunctivitis or lid reactions.
- Advise patient to apply light pressure on lacrimal sac for 1 minute after instillation to minimize systemic absorption of drug.

- Tell patient to remove contact lenses before administration of solution and that he can reinsert them 15 minutes after administration.
- Advise patient that, if more than one ophthalmic drug is being used, the drugs should be given at least 5 minutes apart.
- Stress importance of compliance with recommended therapy.
- Tell patient to discard container within 6 weeks of removing it from the sealed pouch.
- Tell pregnant woman or woman attempting to become pregnant that, if she accidentally comes in contact with drug, she should thoroughly cleanse the exposed area with soap and water immediately.

Evaluation
- Patient denies pain.
- Patient's activity level improves.
- Patient and family state understanding of travoprost therapy.

trazodone hydrochloride
(TRAYZ-oh-dohn high-droh-KLOR-ighd)
Desyrel, Desyrel Dividose

Pharmacologic class: triazolopyridine derivative
Therapeutic class: antidepressant
Pregnancy risk category: C

Indications and dosages

▶ **Depression.** *Adults:* Initially, 150 mg P.O. daily in divided doses. Increase by 50 mg daily q 3 to 4 days, p.r.n. Average daily dose ranges from 150 to 400 mg. Maximum, 600 mg daily for inpatients or 400 mg daily for outpatients.
▶ **Aggressive behavior‡.** *Adults:* 50 mg P.O. b.i.d.
▶ **Panic disorder‡.** *Adults:* 300 mg P.O. daily.

Contraindications and precautions

- Contraindicated in patients in initial recovery phase of MI and in patients hypersensitive to drug.
- Use cautiously in patients with cardiac disease and in those at risk for suicide.
- **Lifespan:** In pregnant and breast-feeding women and in children, safety of drug hasn't been established.

Adverse reactions

CNS: *drowsiness, dizziness,* nervousness, fatigue, confusion, tremor, weakness, hostility, syncope, anger, nightmares, vivid dreams, headache, insomnia.
CV: orthostatic hypotension, tachycardia, hypertension, shortness of breath.
EENT: blurred vision, tinnitus, nasal congestion.
GI: dry mouth, dysgeusia, constipation, nausea, vomiting, anorexia.
GU: urine retention; priapism, possibly leading to impotence; hematuria.
Hematologic: anemia.
Skin: rash, urticaria, diaphoresis.
Other: decreased libido.

Interactions

Drug-drug. *Antihypertensives:* Increases hypotensive effect of trazodone. Monitor blood pressure; antihypertensive dosage may have to be decreased.
Carbamazepine: May decrease plasma levels of trazodone. Monitor decreased therapeutic effect.
Clonidine, CNS depressants: Enhances CNS depression. Avoid use together.
Digoxin, phenytoin: May increase levels of these drugs. Monitor patient for toxicity.
MAO inhibitors: Unknown. Use together cautiously.
Phenothiazines: May increase trazodone level. Monitor toxic effects.
Venlafaxine, SSRIs: May cause serotonin syndrome. Don't use together.
Drug-herb. *St. John's wort:* Serotonin syndrome may occur. Discourage use together.
Drug-lifestyle. *Alcohol use:* Enhances CNS depression. Discourage use together.

Effects on lab test results

● May increase ALT and AST levels.
● May decrease hemoglobin and hematocrit.

Pharmacokinetics

Absorption: Well absorbed from GI tract. Food delays absorption but increases amount of drug absorbed by 20%.
Distribution: Distributed widely in body; isn't concentrated in any particular tissue.
Metabolism: Metabolized by liver.
Excretion: About 75% excreted in urine; remainder excreted in feces. *Half-life:* First phase, 3 to 6 hours; second phase, 5 to 9 hours.

Route	Onset	Peak	Duration
P.O.	Unknown	1-2 hr	Unknown

Action

Chemical effect: Unknown, although it inhibits serotonin uptake in brain; not a tricyclic derivative.
Therapeutic effect: Relieves depression.

Available forms

Tablets (film coated): 50 mg, 100 mg
Tablets (scored): 150 mg, 300 mg

NURSING PROCESS

▨ Assessment
● Assess patient's condition before therapy and regularly thereafter.
● Be alert for adverse reactions and drug interactions.
● Evaluate patient's and family's knowledge of drug therapy.

▣ Nursing diagnoses
● Disturbed thought processes related to presence of depression
● Risk for injury related to drug-induced adverse CNS reactions
● Deficient knowledge related to drug therapy

▷ Planning and implementation
● Give after meals or light snack for optimal absorption and to decrease risk of dizziness.
● Don't stop drug abruptly, but stop it at least 48 hours before surgery.
● If adverse reactions occur, notify prescriber.
● **ALERT:** Don't confuse trazodone with tramadol.
Patient teaching
● Instruct patient to take drug after meals or light snack.
● **ALERT:** Inform men that priapism may occur. Advise him to notify prescriber immediately; surgical intervention may be needed.
● Warn patient to avoid activities that require alertness and good psychomotor coordination until CNS effects of drug are known. Drowsiness and dizziness usually subside after first few weeks.
● Teach patient's family how to recognize signs of suicidal tendency or suicidal ideation.

Reactions may be *common,* uncommon, *life-threatening,* or COMMON AND LIFE-THREATENING.

☑ Evaluation
- Patient's behavior and communication exhibit improved thought processes.
- Patient doesn't experience adverse CNS reactions.
- Patient and family state understanding of drug therapy.

treprostinil sodium
(tre-PROSS-ti-nil soh-dee-UHM)
Remodulin

Pharmacologic class: vasodilator
Therapeutic class: antihypertensive
Pregnancy risk category: B

Indications and dosages

▶ **New York Heart Association Class II to IV pulmonary arterial hypertension (PAH) to reduce symptoms caused by exercise.**
Adults: Initially, 1.25 nanogram/kg/minute by continuous S.C. infusion. If the initial dose can't be tolerated, reduce infusion rate to 0.625 nanogram/kg/minute. Increase by no more than 1.25 nanogram/kg/minute increments each week for the first 4 weeks and then by no more than 2.5 nanogram/kg/minute each week for the duration of infusion. Maximum infusion rate is 40 nanogram/kg/minute. To determine infusion rate in ml/hour, use the following formula:

$$\frac{\text{infusion rate}}{\text{(ml/hour)}} = \frac{\text{(nanogram/} \times \text{weight} \times \text{body} \times 0.00006}{\text{kg/minute)} \qquad \text{(kg)} \qquad \text{drug strength (mg/ml)}}$$

▧ **Adjust-a-dose:** In patients with mild or moderate hepatic insufficiency, initial dose is 0.625 nanogram/kg of ideal body weight per minute; increase cautiously.

Contraindications and precautions

- Contraindicated in patients hypersensitive to drug or structurally related compounds.
- Use cautiously in patients with hepatic or renal impairment.
- ▲ **Lifespan:** In pregnant women, use only if clearly needed. In breast-feeding women, use cautiously; it isn't known whether drug appears in breast milk. In children, safety and effectiveness haven't been established; select dosage cautiously. In elderly patients, use cautiously.

Adverse reactions

CNS: dizziness, *headache*, fatigue.
CV: *vasodilation*, hypotension, edema, chest pain, *right ventricular heart failure.*
GI: *diarrhea, nausea.*
Respiratory: dyspnea.
Skin: *rash*, pruritus, pallor.
Other: *jaw pain, infusion site pain, infusion site reaction.*

Interactions

Drug-drug: *Anticoagulants:* May increase risk of bleeding. Monitor patient closely for bleeding.
Antihypertensives, diuretics, vasodilators: May exacerbate reduction in blood pressure. Monitor blood pressure.

Effects on lab test results

None reported.

Pharmacokinetics

Absorption: Rapid and complete. 100% bioavailable.
Distribution: 91% bound to plasma proteins.
Metabolism: By the liver. Five metabolites are known, but their activity isn't.
Excretion: In the urine, 4% as unchanged drug and 64% as metabolites. *Half-life:* 2 to 4 hours.

Route	Onset	Peak	Duration
S.C.	Unknown	Unknown	Unknown

Action

Chemical effect: Acts by direct vasodilation of pulmonary and systemic arterial vascular beds and inhibition of platelet aggregation.
Therapeutic effect: Reduces pulmonary artery pressure.

Available forms

Injection: 1 mg/ml, 2.5 mg/ml, 5 mg/ml, 10 mg/ml

NURSING PROCESS

☲ Assessment
- Assess patient's condition before therapy and regularly thereafter.
- Make sure adequate monitoring and emergency care are available when starting therapy.
- Assess patient's ability to accept, place, and care for S.C. catheter and use infusion pump.

• Be alert for adverse reactions and drug interactions.
• Evaluate patient's and family's knowledge of drug therapy.

Nursing diagnoses
• Activity intolerance related to presence of pulmonary hypertension
• Acute pain related to adverse drug effect of headache
• Deficient knowledge related to drug therapy

Planning and implementation
• Drug should be used only by prescribers experienced in the diagnosis and treatment of PAH.
• Give only by continuous S.C. infusion via a self-inserted S.C. catheter, using an infusion pump designed for S.C. drug delivery.
• The infusion pump should be small and light-weight; be adjustable to approximately 0.002 ml/hour; have occlusion or no-delivery, low-battery, programming-error, and motor-malfunction alarms; have delivery accuracy of ± 6% or better; and be positive pressure driven.
• The reservoir should be made of polyvinyl chloride, polypropylene, or glass.
• A single syringe can be given up to 72 hours at 99° F (37° C).
• Use a single vial no longer than 14 days after the initial introduction into the vial.
• Inspect for particulate matter and discoloration before giving.
• Unopened vials are stable until the date indicated when stored at 59° to 77° F (15° to 25° C).
• If patient doesn't improve or has worsening of symptoms, increase dose. If there are excessive effects or unacceptable infusion site symptoms, decrease dose.
• Avoid abrupt withdrawal or sudden large dose reductions, because PAH symptoms may worsen.
Patient teaching
• Tell patient drug is infused continuously through S.C. catheter, via an infusion pump.
• Inform patient that therapy will be needed for prolonged periods, possibly years.
• Tell patient that subsequent disease management may require I.V. therapy.
• Inform patient that many side effects may be related to the underlying disease (dyspnea, fatigue, chest pain, right ventricular failure, pallor).

• Tell patient that the most common local reactions are pain, erythema, induration, and rash at the infusion site.

Evaluation
• Patient states activity intolerance is improving.
• Patient doesn't have headache.
• Patient and family state understanding of drug therapy.

triamcinolone
(trigh-am-SIN-oh-lohn)
Aristocort, Atolone, Kenacort

triamcinolone acetonide
Kenaject-40, Kenalog-10, Kenalog-40, Tac-3, Tac-40, Triam-A, Triamonide 40, Tri-Kort, Trilog

triamcinolone diacetate
Amcort, Aristocort Forte, Aristocort Intralesional, Clinacort, Triam Forte, Trilone, Tristoject

triamcinolone hexacetonide
Aristospan Intra-Articular, Aristospan Intralesional

Pharmacologic class: glucocorticoid
Therapeutic class: anti-inflammatory, immunosuppressant
Pregnancy risk category: C

Indications and dosages

▶ **Severe inflammation or immunosuppression.** *Adults:* 4 to 48 mg triamcinolone P.O. daily, in one to four divided doses. Or, initially, 2.5 to 60 mg triamcinolone acetonide I.M. Additional doses of 20 to 100 mg may be given, p.r.n., at 6-week intervals. Or, 2.5 to 15 mg intra-articularly, or up to 1 mg intralesionally, p.r.n. Or, 40 mg triamcinolone diacetate I.M. weekly; or 5 to 48 mg by intralesional or sublesional injections (at 1- to 2-week intervals); or 2 to 40 mg by intra-articular, intrasynovial, or soft tissue injection (may repeat at 1- to 8-week intervals). Or, with triamcinolone hexacetonide, use up to 0.5 mg/in^2 of affected skin intralesionally, or 2 to 20 mg intra-articularly q 3 to 4 weeks, p.r.n.

Contraindications and precautions

• Contraindicated in patients hypersensitive to drug or its components and in those with systemic fungal infections.

• Use cautiously in patients with GI ulcer, renal disease, hypertension, osteoporosis, diabetes mellitus, hypothyroidism, cirrhosis, diverticulitis, nonspecific ulcerative colitis, recent intestinal anastomoses, thromboembolic disorders, seizures, myasthenia gravis, heart failure, tuberculosis, ocular herpes simplex, emotional instability, or psychotic tendencies.

⚘ Lifespan: In pregnant and breast-feeding women, use cautiously.

Adverse reactions

CNS: *euphoria, insomnia,* psychotic behavior, *pseudotumor cerebri,* vertigo, headache, paresthesia, *seizures.*

CV: *heart failure,* hypertension, edema, *arrhythmias,* thrombophlebitis, *thromboembolism.*

EENT: cataracts, glaucoma.

GI: *peptic ulceration,* GI irritation, increased appetite, *pancreatitis,* nausea, vomiting.

GU: menstrual irregularities.

Metabolic: hypokalemia, hyperglycemia, carbohydrate intolerance.

Musculoskeletal: muscular weakness, osteoporosis, growth suppression in children.

Skin: delayed wound healing, acne, various skin eruptions.

Other: *acute adrenal insufficiency* during times of increased stress such as infection, surgery, trauma, abrupt withdrawal; susceptibility to infections; hirsutism; cushingoid state (moonface, buffalo hump, central obesity).

Interactions

Drug-drug. *Aspirin, indomethacin, other NSAIDs:* Increases risk of GI distress and bleeding. Give together cautiously.

Barbiturates, phenytoin, rifampin: Decreases corticosteroid effect. Increase corticosteroid.

Drugs that deplete potassium (such as thiazide diuretics): Enhances potassium-wasting effects of triamcinolone. Monitor potassium level.

Oral anticoagulants: Alters dosage requirements. Monitor PT closely.

Skin-test antigens: Decreases response. Defer skin testing.

Toxoids, vaccines: Decreases antibody response and increases risk of neurologic complications. Avoid use together.

Effects on lab test results

• May increase glucose and cholesterol levels. May decrease potassium and calcium levels.

Pharmacokinetics

Absorption: Readily after P.O. administration. Variable after other routes of administration.

Distribution: To muscle, liver, skin, intestines, and kidneys. Extensively bound to plasma proteins. Only unbound portion is active.

Metabolism: In liver.

Excretion: In urine; insignificant quantities also excreted in feces. *Half-life:* 18 to 36 hours.

Route	Onset	Peak	Duration
P.O., I.M., intralesional, intra-articular, intrasynovial	Varies	Varies	Varies

Action

Chemical effect: Not clearly defined; decreases inflammation, mainly by stabilizing leukocyte lysosomal membranes; suppresses immune response; stimulates bone marrow; and influences protein, fat, and carbohydrate metabolism.

Therapeutic effect: Relieves inflammation and suppresses immune system function.

Available forms

triamcinolone
Syrup: 4 mg/5 ml
Tablets: 4 mg, 8 mg
triamcinolone acetonide
Injection (suspension): 3 mg/ml, 10 mg/ml, 40 mg/ml
triamcinolone diacetate
Injection (suspension): 25 mg/ml, 40 mg/ml
triamcinolone hexacetonide
Injection (suspension): 5 mg/ml, 20 mg/ml

NURSING PROCESS

⚕ **Assessment**

• Assess patient before and after therapy; monitor weight, blood pressure, and electrolyte level.

• Watch for adverse reactions, drug interactions, depression, or psychotic episodes, especially with high doses.

- Evaluate patient's and family's knowledge of drug therapy.

🔄 Nursing diagnoses
- Ineffective health maintenance related to underlying condition
- Risk for injury related to drug-induced adverse reactions
- Deficient knowledge related to drug therapy

➤ Planning and implementation
- Drug isn't used for alternate-day therapy.
- Always adjust to lowest effective dose.
- For better results and less toxicity, give once-daily dose in morning.
- Give oral dose with food when possible to reduce GI irritation.
- Give I.M. injection deep into gluteal muscle. Rotate injection sites to prevent muscle atrophy.
- Don't use 10 mg/ml strength for I.M. administration.
- Assist prescriber with intralesional, intraarticular, or intrasynovial administration.
- Don't use 40 mg/ml strength for I.D. or intralesional administration.
- ⑧ **ALERT:** Parenteral form isn't for I.V. use. Different salt formulations aren't interchangeable.
- Don't use diluents that contain preservatives; flocculation may occur.
- Unless contraindicated, give low-sodium diet high in potassium and protein. Give potassium supplements, p.r.n.
- Gradually reduce drug dosage after long-term therapy. After abrupt withdrawal, patient may experience rebound inflammation, fatigue, weakness, arthralgia, fever, dizziness, lethargy, depression, fainting, orthostatic hypotension, dyspnea, anorexia, or hypoglycemia. After prolonged use, sudden withdrawal may be fatal.
- ⑧ **ALERT:** Don't confuse triamcinolone with Triaminicin, Triaminic, or Triaminicol.

Patient teaching
- Tell patient not to stop drug abruptly or without prescriber's consent.
- Instruct patient to take oral drug with food.
- Teach patient signs of early adrenal insufficiency (fatigue, muscle weakness, joint pain, fever, anorexia, nausea, dyspnea, dizziness, and fainting).
- Instruct patient to wear or carry medical identification at all times.
- Warn patient receiving long-term therapy about cushingoid symptoms and tell him to report sudden weight gain and swelling to prescriber.
- Tell patient to report slow healing.
- Advise patient receiving long-term therapy to consider exercise or physical therapy. Also tell patient to ask prescriber about vitamin D or calcium supplements.

✓ Evaluation
- Patient responds well to drug.
- Patient doesn't experience injury from adverse reactions.
- Patient and family state understanding of drug therapy.

triamcinolone acetonide
(trigh-am-SIN-oh-lohn as-EE-tuh-nighd)
Azmacort

Pharmacologic class: glucocorticoid
Therapeutic class: anti-inflammatory, immunosuppressant
Pregnancy risk category: C

Indications and dosages
▶ **Corticosteroid-dependent asthma.** *Adults:* 2 inhalations t.i.d. to q.i.d. Maximum, 16 inhalations daily. In some patients, maintenance can be accomplished when total daily dose is given b.i.d.
Children ages 6 to 12: 1 or 2 inhalations t.i.d. to q.i.d. or 2 to 4 inhalations b.i.d. Maximum, 12 inhalations daily.

Contraindications and precautions
- Contraindicated in patients hypersensitive to drug or its components and in those with status asthmaticus.
- Use cautiously, if at all, in patients with tuberculosis of respiratory tract; untreated fungal, bacterial, or systemic viral infections; or ocular herpes simplex. Also use cautiously in patients receiving systemic corticosteroids.
- **Lifespan:** In pregnant women, use cautiously. In breast-feeding women, drug isn't recommended.

Adverse reactions
CV: *facial edema.*
EENT: dry or irritated nose or throat, hoarseness.

GI: *oral candidiasis,* dry or irritated tongue or mouth.
Respiratory: cough, wheezing.
Other: ***hypothalamic-pituitary-adrenal function suppression, adrenal insufficiency.***

Interactions

None significant.

Effects on lab test results

None reported.

Pharmacokinetics

Absorption: Slow.
Distribution: Without spacer, about 10% to 25% of dose goes to airways; remainder goes to mouth and throat and is swallowed. Spacer may help a greater percentage reach lungs.
Metabolism: Metabolized in liver. Some drug that reaches lungs may be metabolized locally.
Excretion: Excreted in urine and feces. *Half-life:* 18 to 36 hours.

Route	Onset	Peak	Duration
Inhalation	1-4 wk	Unknown	Unknown

Action

Chemical effect: May decrease inflammation by stabilizing leukocyte lysosomal membranes.
Therapeutic effect: Improves breathing ability.

Available forms

Inhalation aerosol: 100 mcg/metered spray

NURSING PROCESS

Assessment

- Assess patient's asthma before therapy and regularly thereafter.
- Be alert for adverse reactions.
- Evaluate patient's and family's knowledge of drug therapy.

Nursing diagnoses

- Ineffective breathing pattern related to presence of asthma
- Impaired tissue integrity related to drug's adverse effect on oral mucosa
- Deficient knowledge related to drug therapy

Planning and implementation

- Patient who has recently been transferred to oral inhaled steroids from systemic administration of steroids may need to be placed back on systemic steroids during periods of stress or severe asthma attacks.
- Taper oral therapy slowly.
- If patient is also to receive bronchodilator by inhalation, give bronchodilator first, wait several minutes, then give triamcinolone.
- If more than one inhalation is ordered for each dose, wait 1 minute between inhalations.
- Store drug between 36° and 86° F (2° and 30° C).

ALERT: Don't confuse triamcinolone with Triaminicin, Triaminic, or Triaminicol.

Patient teaching

- Inform patient that inhaled steroids don't provide relief for emergency asthma attacks.
- Instruct patient to use drug as prescribed, even when feeling well.
- Advise patient to ensure delivery of proper dose by gently warming canister to room temperature before using. Patients can carry canister in pocket to keep it warm.
- Instruct patient requiring bronchodilator to use it several minutes before triamcinolone. Tell him to allow 1 minute to elapse before repeat inhalations and to hold breath for a few seconds to enhance drug action.
- Teach patient to check mucous membranes frequently for signs of fungal infection.
- Tell patient to prevent oral fungal infections by gargling or rinsing mouth with water after each use of inhaler but not to swallow water.
- Tell patient to keep inhaler clean and unobstructed by washing it with warm water and drying it thoroughly after use.
- Instruct patient to contact prescriber if response to therapy decreases; prescriber may need to adjust dosage. Tell patient not to exceed recommended dosage on his own.
- Instruct patient to wear or carry medical identification at all times.

Evaluation

- Patient exhibits improved breathing ability.
- Patient maintains normal oral mucosa integrity.
- Patient and family state understanding of drug therapy.

triamterene

(trigh-AM-tuh-reen)
Dyrenium

Pharmacologic class: potassium-sparing diuretic
Therapeutic class: diuretic
Pregnancy risk category: B

Indications and dosages

▶ **Edema.** *Adults:* Initially, 100 mg P.O. b.i.d. after meals. Total daily dose shouldn't exceed 300 mg.

Contraindications and precautions

• Contraindicated in patients hypersensitive to drug and in those with anuria, severe or progressive renal disease or dysfunction, severe hepatic disease, or hyperkalemia.
• Use cautiously in patients with impaired liver function or diabetes mellitus, and in debilitated patients.
⚘ **Lifespan:** In pregnant women, use cautiously. In breast-feeding women, safety of drug hasn't been established. In geriatric patients, use cautiously.

Adverse reactions

CNS: dizziness, weakness, fatigue, headache.
CV: hypotension.
GI: dry mouth, nausea, vomiting, diarrhea.
GU: azotemia, interstitial nephritis, nephrolithiasis.
Hematologic: megaloblastic anemia related to low folic acid levels, *thrombocytopenia, agranulocytosis.*
Hepatic: jaundice.
Metabolic: HYPERKALEMIA, *acidosis,* hypokalemia, hyponatremia, hyperglycemia.
Musculoskeletal: muscle cramps.
Skin: photosensitivity reactions, rash.
Other: *anaphylaxis.*

Interactions

Drug-drug. *ACE inhibitors, potassium supplements:* Increases risk of hyperkalemia. Don't use together.
Amantadine: Increases risk of amantadine toxicity. Don't use together.

Lithium: Decreases lithium clearance, increasing risk of lithium toxicity. Monitor lithium level.
NSAIDs (indomethacin): May enhance risk of nephrotoxicity. Avoid use together.
Quinidine: May interfere with some laboratory tests that measure quinidine level. Inform laboratory that patient is taking triamterene.
Drug-food. *Potassium-containing salt substitutes, potassium-rich foods:* Increases risk of hyperkalemia. Discourage use together.
Drug-lifestyle. *Sun exposure:* Photosensitivity reactions may occur. Urge patient to avoid prolonged or unprotected exposure to sunlight.

Effects on lab test results

• May increase BUN, creatinine, glucose, and uric acid levels. May decrease sodium levels. May increase or decrease potassium level.
• May increase liver function test values. May decrease hemoglobin, hematocrit, and RBC, granulocyte, and platelet counts.

Pharmacokinetics

Absorption: Rapid; extent varies.
Distribution: About 67% protein-bound.
Metabolism: By hydroxylation and sulfation.
Excretion: In urine. *Half-life:* 100 to 150 minutes.

Route	Onset	Peak	Duration
P.O.	2-4 hr	6-8 hr	7-9 hr

Action

Chemical effect: Inhibits sodium reabsorption and potassium and hydrogen excretion by direct action on distal tubule.
Therapeutic effect: Promotes water and sodium excretion.

Available forms

Capsules: 50 mg, 100 mg

NURSING PROCESS

🔖 **Assessment**
• Assess patient's edema before therapy and regularly thereafter. Full effect of triamterene is delayed 2 to 3 days when used alone.
• Monitor blood pressure and BUN and electrolyte levels.
• Watch for blood dyscrasia.

• Be alert for adverse reactions and drug interactions.
• Evaluate patient's and family's knowledge of drug therapy.

🔄 Nursing diagnoses
• Excess fluid volume related to underlying condition
• Ineffective health maintenance related to drug-induced hyperkalemia
• Deficient knowledge related to drug therapy

▶ Planning and implementation
• Give drug after meals to minimize nausea.
• **⊛ ALERT:** Withdraw drug gradually to minimize excessive rebound potassium excretion.
• Drug is less potent than thiazides and loop diuretics and is useful as adjunct to other diuretic therapy. Triamterene is usually used with potassium-wasting diuretics.
• When used with other diuretics, lower initial dose of each drug and adjust to individual requirements.
⊛ ALERT: Don't confuse triamterene with trimipramine.

Patient teaching
• Tell patient to take drug after meals.
⊛ ALERT: Warn patient to avoid excessive ingestion of potassium-rich foods, potassium-containing salt substitutes, and potassium supplements to prevent serious hyperkalemia.
• Instruct patient to avoid direct sunlight, wear protective clothing, and use sunblock to prevent photosensitivity reactions.

☑ Evaluation
• Patient exhibits no signs of edema.
• Patient's potassium level is normal.
• Patient and family state understanding of drug therapy.

---

triazolam
(trigh-AH-zoh-lam)
Alti-Triazolam ♦ , Apo-Triazo ♦ , Halcion, Novo-Triolam ♦

Pharmacologic class: benzodiazepine
Therapeutic class: sedative-hypnotic
Pregnancy risk category: X
Controlled substance schedule: IV

Indications and dosages
▶ **Insomnia.** *Adults:* 0.125 to 0.5 mg P.O. h.s.
Adults older than age 65: 0.125 mg P.O. h.s.; increased, p.r.n., to 0.25 mg P.O. h.s.

Contraindications and precautions
• Contraindicated in patients hypersensitive to benzodiazepines.
• Use cautiously in patients with impaired liver or kidney function, chronic pulmonary insufficiency, sleep apnea, depression, suicidal tendencies, or history of drug abuse.
⚖ Lifespan: In pregnant women, drug is contraindicated. In breast-feeding women, drug isn't recommended. In children, safety of drug hasn't been established.

Adverse reactions
CNS: *drowsiness, dizziness, headache,* rebound insomnia, amnesia, light-headedness, lack of coordination, confusion, depression, nervousness, ataxia.
GI: nausea, vomiting.
Other: physical or psychological abuse.

Interactions
Drug-drug. *Cimetidine, erythromycin, hormonal contraceptives, isoniazid, ranitidine:* May cause prolonged triazolam blood levels. Monitor patient for increased sedation.
Diltiazem: May increase CNS depression and prolong effects of triazolam. Use lower dose of triazolam.
Fluconazole, itraconazole, ketoconazole, miconazole: May increase and prolong levels, CNS depression, and psychomotor impairment. Don't use together.
Other CNS depressants, including opioid analgesics, other psychotropic drugs, anticonvulsants, antihistamines: May cause excessive CNS depression. Use together cautiously.
Other potent CYP 3A inhibitors, such as nefazodone: Decreases clearance of triazolam. Don't use together.
Drug-herb. *Calendula, catnip, hops, lady's slipper, lemon balm, passion flower, sassafras, skullcap, valerian, yerba maté:* Potential for increased sedative effects. Monitor patient closely if used together.
Kava: May cause excessive sedation. Discourage use together.

Drug-food. *Grapefruit juice:* May delay drug onset and increase effects. Advise patient to avoid use together.
Drug-lifestyle. *Alcohol use:* May cause additive CNS effects. Strongly discourage use together.

Effects on lab test results

• May increase liver function test values.

Pharmacokinetics

Absorption: Good.
Distribution: Wide; 90% protein-bound.
Metabolism: In liver.
Excretion: In urine. *Half-life:* 1½ to 5½ hours.

Route	Onset	Peak	Duration
P.O.	Unknown	1-2 hr	Unknown

Action

Chemical effect: May act on limbic system, thalamus, and hypothalamus of CNS to produce hypnotic effects.
Therapeutic effect: Promotes sleep.

Available forms

Tablets: 0.125 mg, 0.25 mg

NURSING PROCESS

Assessment
• Assess patient's condition before therapy and regularly thereafter.
• Assess mental status before starting therapy. Geriatric patients are more sensitive to drug's CNS effects.
• Be alert for adverse reactions and drug interactions.
• Evaluate patient's and family's knowledge of drug therapy.

Nursing diagnoses
• Disturbed sleep pattern related to underlying disorder
• Risk for injury related to drug-induced adverse CNS reactions
• Deficient knowledge related to drug therapy

Planning and implementation
• Take precautions to prevent hoarding or intentional overdosing by patients who are depressed, suicidal, or drug-dependent, or who have a history of drug abuse.
• Store drug in cool, dry place away from light.

• Institute safety precautions once drug has been given.
⊗ ALERT: Don't confuse Halcion with Haldol or halcinonide.

Patient teaching
• Warn patient not to take more than prescribed amount because overdose can occur at total daily dosage of 2 mg (or four times the highest recommended amount).
• Warn patient about performing activities that require mental alertness or physical coordination. For inpatient, supervise walking and raise bed rails, particularly for geriatric patient.
• Inform patient that drug is very short-acting and therefore has less tendency to cause morning drowsiness.
• Tell patient that rebound insomnia may develop for 1 or 2 nights after stopping therapy.

Evaluation
• Patient states that drug produces sleep.
• Patient doesn't experience injury from adverse CNS reactions.
• Patient and family state understanding of drug therapy.

trifluoperazine hydrochloride
(trigh-floo-oh-PER-eh-zeen high-droh-KLOR-ighd)
Apo-Trifluoperazine ♦, Novo-Flurazine ♦, PMS Trifluoperazine ♦

Pharmacologic class: phenothiazine (piperazine derivative)
Therapeutic class: antipsychotic, antiemetic
Pregnancy risk category: C

Indications and dosages

▶ **Anxiety.** *Adults:* 1 to 2 mg P.O. b.i.d. Maximum, 6 mg daily. Don't use for longer than 12 weeks.
▶ **Schizophrenia and other psychotic disorders.** *Adult outpatients:* 1 to 2 mg P.O. b.i.d., increased p.r.n. Or, 1 to 2 mg deep I.M. q 4 to 6 hours, p.r.n.
Adult inpatients: 2 to 5 mg P.O. b.i.d.; may increase gradually to 40 mg daily.
Children ages 6 to 12 (hospitalized or under close supervision): 1 mg P.O. daily or b.i.d.; may increase gradually to 15 mg daily, if needed.

Contraindications and precautions

• Contraindicated in patients hypersensitive to phenothiazines or in patients experiencing coma, CNS depression, bone marrow suppression, or liver damage.

• Use cautiously in debilitated patients and in patients with CV disease (may cause drop in blood pressure), seizure disorder, glaucoma, or prostatic hyperplasia. Also use cautiously in patients exposed to extreme heat.

⚠ **Lifespan:** In pregnant and breast-feeding women and in children younger than age 6, safety of drug hasn't been established. In geriatric patients, use cautiously.

Adverse reactions

CNS: *extrapyramidal reactions, tardive dyskinesia,* pseudoparkinsonism, dizziness, drowsiness, insomnia, fatigue, headache, *neuroleptic malignant syndrome.*

CV: *orthostatic hypotension,* tachycardia, ECG changes.

EENT: ocular changes, *blurred vision.*

GI: *dry mouth, constipation,* nausea.

GU: *urine retention,* menstrual irregularities, inhibited lactation.

Hematologic: *transient leukopenia, agranulocytosis.*

Hepatic: cholestatic jaundice.

Metabolic: weight gain.

Skin: *photosensitivity reactions,* sterile abscesses, rash.

Other: allergic reaction, pain at I.M. injection site, gynecomastia.

Interactions

Drug-drug. *Antacids:* Inhibits absorption of oral phenothiazines. Separate doses by at least 2 hours.

Barbiturates, lithium: May decrease phenothiazine effect. Monitor patient.

Centrally acting antihypertensives: Decreases antihypertensive effect. Monitor blood pressure.

CNS depressants: Increases CNS depression. Use together cautiously.

Propranolol: Increases levels of both propranolol and trifluoperazine. Monitor patient closely.

Warfarin: Decreases effect of oral anticoagulants. Monitor PT and INR.

Drug-herb. *Dong quai, St. John's wort:* Increases photosensitivity reactions. Discourage use together.

Ginkgo: Potential decreased adverse effects of thioridazine. Monitor patient.

Kava: Increases risk of dystonic reactions. Discourage use together.

Milk thistle: Decreases liver toxicity caused by phenothiazines. Discourage use together; monitor liver enzymes if used together.

Yohimbe: Increases risk for yohimbe toxicity when used together. Discourage use together.

Drug-lifestyle. *Alcohol use:* May increase CNS depression, particularly psychomotor skills. Strongly discourage use together.

Effects on lab test results

• May increase liver enzyme levels.
• May decrease WBC and granulocyte counts.

Pharmacokinetics

Absorption: Variable with P.O. use; rapid after I.M. use.

Distribution: Wide; 91% to 99% protein-bound.

Metabolism: Extensively by liver.

Excretion: Primarily in urine; some in feces. *Half-life:* 20 to 40 hours.

Route	Onset	Peak	Duration
P.O., I.M.	Up to several wk	Unknown	Unknown

Action

Chemical effect: Unknown; probably blocks postsynaptic dopamine receptors in brain.

Therapeutic effect: Relieves anxiety and signs and symptoms of psychotic disorders.

Available forms

Injection: 2 mg/ml
Oral concentrate: 10 mg/ml
Tablets (regular and film-coated): 1 mg, 2 mg, 5 mg, 10 mg

NURSING PROCESS

🔖 **Assessment**

• Assess patient's condition before therapy and regularly thereafter.

• Watch for orthostatic hypotension, especially with parenteral use.

• Monitor patient for tardive dyskinesia, which may occur after prolonged use. It may not appear until months or years later and may disappear spontaneously or persist for life, despite stopping drug.

• Monitor therapy with weekly bilirubin tests during first month, periodic blood tests (CBC and liver function), and ophthalmologic tests (long-term use).

⊛ **ALERT:** Monitor patient for symptoms of neuroleptic malignant syndrome (extrapyramidal effects, hyperthermia, autonomic disturbance), which is rare but can be fatal. It isn't necessarily related to length of drug use or type of neuroleptic; however, more than 60% of patients are men.

• Evaluate patient's and family's knowledge of drug therapy.

⊞ Nursing diagnoses

• Anxiety related to underlying condition
• Disturbed thought processes related to underlying psychotic disorder
• Deficient knowledge related to drug therapy

▶ Planning and implementation

• Although there is little likelihood of contact dermatitis, those sensitive to phenothiazine drugs should avoid direct contact. Wear gloves when preparing liquid forms.

• Dilute liquid concentrate with 60 ml of tomato or fruit juice, carbonated beverage, coffee, tea, milk, water, or semisolid food.

• Give deep I.M. only in upper outer quadrant of buttocks. Massage slowly afterward to prevent sterile abscess. Injection may sting.

• Protect injection or concentrate from light. Slight yellowing of drug is common; it doesn't affect potency. Discard markedly discolored solutions.

• Keep patient supine for 1 hour after drug administration and advise him to change position slowly.

• Don't withdraw drug abruptly unless severe adverse reactions occur. Abrupt withdrawal of long-term therapy may cause gastritis, nausea, vomiting, dizziness, tremor, feeling of warmth or cold, diaphoresis, tachycardia, headache, insomnia, anorexia, muscle rigidity, altered mental status, or evidence of autonomic instability.

• Withhold dose and notify prescriber if patient develops jaundice, symptoms of blood dyscrasia (fever, sore throat, infection, cellulitis, weakness), or extrapyramidal reactions longer than a few hours, especially in pregnant women and in children.

• Acute dystonic reactions may be treated with diphenhydramine.

⊛ **ALERT:** Don't confuse trifluoperazine with triflupromazine.

Patient teaching

• Teach patient or caregiver how to prepare oral form of drug.

• Warn patient to avoid activities that require alertness or good psychomotor coordination until CNS effects of drug are known. Drowsiness and dizziness usually subside after a few weeks.

• Tell patient to avoid alcohol during drug therapy.

• Instruct patient to report urine retention or constipation.

• Tell patient to use sun block and wear protective clothing to avoid photosensitivity reactions.

• Tell patient to relieve dry mouth with sugarless gum or hard candy.

☑ Evaluation

• Patient's anxiety is reduced.
• Patient's behavior and communication exhibit improved thought processes.
• Patient and family state understanding of drug therapy.

---

trihexyphenidyl hydrochloride
(trigh-heks-eh-FEEN-ih-dil high-droh-KLOR-ighd)
Apo-Trihex ♦ , Trihexy-2, Trihexy-5

Pharmacologic class: anticholinergic
Therapeutic class: antiparkinsonian
Pregnancy risk category: C

Indications and dosages

▶ **All forms of parkinsonism and adjunct treatment to levodopa in management of parkinsonism.** *Adults:* 1 mg P.O. first day, then increased by 2 mg q 3 to 5 days until total of 6 to 10 mg is given daily. Usually given t.i.d. with meals. Sometimes given q.i.d. (last dose h.s.) Postencephalitic parkinsonism may require total daily dosage of 12 to 15 mg.

▶ **Drug-induced extrapyramidal reactions.** *Adults:* 5 to 15 mg P.O. daily. Initial dose of 1 mg may control some reactions.

Contraindications and precautions

• Contraindicated in patients hypersensitive to drug.

• Use cautiously in patients with glaucoma; cardiac, hepatic, or renal disorders; obstructive

---

disease of GI and GU tracts; or prostatic hyperplasia.

⚜ Lifespan: In pregnant women and in children, safety of drug hasn't been established. In breast-feeding women, drug isn't recommended. In geriatric patients, monitor for mental confusion or disorientation.

Adverse reactions

CNS: nervousness, dizziness, headache, hallucinations, drowsiness, weakness.
CV: tachycardia.
EENT: blurred vision, mydriasis, increased intraocular pressure.
GI: *dry mouth,* constipation, *nausea,* vomiting.
GU: urinary hesitancy, urine retention.

Interactions

Drug-drug. *Amantadine:* May have additive anticholinergic reactions, such as confusion and hallucinations. Reduce dosage of trihexyphenidyl before giving.
Levodopa: Increases drug effect. May require lower doses of both drugs.
Drug-lifestyle. *Alcohol use:* Increases sedative effects. Discourage use together.

Effects on lab test results

None reported.

Pharmacokinetics

Absorption: Readily absorbed.
Distribution: Unknown; crosses blood-brain barrier.
Metabolism: Unknown.
Excretion: In urine. *Half-life:* 5½ to 10¼ hours.

Route	Onset	Peak	Duration
P.O.	1 hr	2-3 hr	6-12 hr

Action

Chemical effect: Unknown; blocks central cholinergic receptors, helping to balance cholinergic activity in basal ganglia.
Therapeutic effect: Improves physical mobility in patients with parkinsonism.

Available forms

Tablets: 2 mg, 5 mg

NURSING PROCESS

📝 Assessment
• Assess patient's condition before therapy and regularly thereafter.
⑤ ALERT: Gonioscopic ocular evaluation and monitoring of intraocular pressure are needed, especially in patients older than age 40.
• Be alert for adverse reactions and drug interactions. Adverse reactions are dose-related and usually transient.
• Evaluate patient's and family's knowledge of drug therapy.

🔢 Nursing diagnoses
• Impaired physical mobility related to presence of parkinsonism
• Risk for injury related to drug-induced adverse CNS reactions
• Deficient knowledge related to drug therapy

▷ Planning and implementation
• Dosage may need to be increased gradually in patient who develops tolerance to drug.
• Give drug with meals.
Patient teaching
• Warn patient that drug may cause nausea if taken before meals.
• Tell patient to avoid activities that require alertness until CNS effects of drug are known.
• Advise patient to report urinary hesitancy or urine retention.
• Tell patient to relieve dry mouth with cool drinks, ice chips, sugarless gum, or hard candy.

☑ Evaluation
• Patient exhibits improved physical mobility.
• Patient doesn't experience injury from adverse reactions.
• Patient and family state understanding of drug therapy.

---

trimethobenzamide hydrochloride
(trigh-meth-oh-BEN-zuh-mighd high-droh-KLOR-ighd)
Tebamide, T-Gen, Tigan, Triban, Trimazide

Pharmacologic class: ethanolamine-related antihistamine
Therapeutic class: antiemetic
Pregnancy risk category: NR

Indications and dosages

▶ **Nausea, vomiting.** *Adults:* 250 mg P.O. t.i.d. or q.i.d.; or 200 mg I.M. or P.R. t.i.d. or q.i.d.

▶ **Prevention of postoperative nausea and vomiting.** *Adults:* 200 mg I.M. or P.R. as single dose before or during surgery; if needed, repeat 3 hours after termination of anesthesia. Limit use to prolonged vomiting from known cause. *Children weighing 13 to 40 kg (28 to 88 lb):* 100 to 200 mg P.O. or P.R. t.i.d. or q.i.d. *Children weighing less than 13 kg:* 100 mg P.R. t.i.d. or q.i.d. Don't use in premature or newborn infants.

Contraindications and precautions

• Contraindicated in patients hypersensitive to drug. Suppositories are contraindicated in patients hypersensitive to benzocaine hydrochloride or similar local anesthetics.

⚞ **Lifespan:** In pregnant and breast-feeding women, safety of drug hasn't been established. In children, use cautiously. In children with viral illness, drug isn't recommended because it may contribute to development of Reye's syndrome.

Adverse reactions

CNS: *drowsiness,* dizziness, headache, disorientation, depression, Parkinsonian-like symptoms, *coma, seizures.*
CV: hypotension.
EENT: blurred vision.
GI: diarrhea.
Hepatic: jaundice.
Musculoskeletal: muscle cramps.
Skin: hypersensitivity reaction (pain, stinging, burning, redness, swelling at I.M. injection site).

Interactions

Drug-drug. *CNS depressants:* May cause additive CNS depression. Avoid use together.
Drug-lifestyle. *Alcohol use:* May cause additive CNS depression. Discourage use together.

Effects on lab test results

None reported.

Pharmacokinetics

Absorption: About 60% after P.O. use; unknown after P.R. or I.M. use.
Distribution: Unknown.
Metabolism: About 50% to 70%, probably in liver.

Excretion: In urine and feces. *Half-life:* 7 to 9 hours.

Route	Onset	Peak	Duration
P.O.	10-20 min	Unknown	3-4 hr
I.M.	15-30 min	Unknown	2-3 hr
P.R.	Unknown	Unknown	Unknown

Action

Chemical effect: Unknown; may act on chemoreceptor trigger zone to inhibit nausea and vomiting.
Therapeutic effect: Prevents or relieves nausea and vomiting.

Available forms

Capsules: 100 mg, 250 mg
Injection: 100 mg/ml
Suppositories: 100 mg, 200 mg

NURSING PROCESS

✎ Assessment
• Assess patient's condition before therapy and regularly thereafter.
• Be alert for adverse reactions and drug interactions.
• Evaluate patient's and family's knowledge of drug therapy.

▣ Nursing diagnoses
• Risk for deficient fluid volume related to potential for or presence of nausea and vomiting
• Diarrhea related to drug-induced adverse GI reactions
• Deficient knowledge related to drug therapy

▶ Planning and implementation
• Inject I.M. dose deep into upper outer quadrant of gluteal region to reduce pain and local irritation.
• Refrigerate suppositories.
• If skin hypersensitivity reaction occurs, withhold drug.
⊛ ALERT: Don't confuse Tigan with Ticar.
Patient teaching
• Advise patient of possibility of drowsiness and dizziness, and caution against driving or performing other activities requiring alertness until CNS effects of drug are known.
• Warn patient that I.M. administration of drug may be painful.

• If patient will be using suppositories, instruct him to remove foil and, if needed, moisten suppository with water for 10 to 30 seconds before inserting. Tell him to store suppositories in refrigerator.

✓ Evaluation
• Patient maintains adequate hydration with cessation of nausea and vomiting.
• Patient maintains normal bowel pattern.
• Patient and family state understanding of drug therapy.

trimethoprim
(trigh-METH-uh-prim)
Alprim ◊, **Primsol, Proloprim, Trimpex, Triprim** ◊

Pharmacologic class: synthetic folate antagonist
Therapeutic class: antibiotic
Pregnancy risk category: C

Indications and dosages

▶ **Acute otitis media caused by susceptible strains of *S. pneumoniae* and *H. influenzae.*** *Children age 6 months and older:* 10 mg/kg Primsol daily in divided doses q 12 hours for 10 days.
▶ **Uncomplicated UTIs caused by *E. coli*, *P. mirabilis, Klebsiella pneumoniae, Enterobacter* species, coagulase-negative *Staphylococcus* species (including *S. saprophyticus*).** *Adults:* 100 mg (10 ml) q 12 hours, or 200 mg (20 ml) daily for 10 days.
▶ **Prophylaxis of chronic and recurrent urinary tract infections‡.** *Adults:* 100 mg P.O. h.s. for 6 weeks to 6 months.
▶ **Traveler's diarrhea‡.** *Adults:* 200 mg P.O. b.i.d. for 3 to 5 days.
▶ *Pneumocystis carinii* **pneumonia‡.** *Adults:* 5 mg/kg P.O. t.i.d. with dapsone 100 mg daily for 21 days.
⧉ Adjust-a-dose: For patients with renal impairment, if creatinine clearance is 15 to 30 ml/minute, give half of the recommended dose q 12 hours; if less than 15 ml/minute, don't use drug.

Contraindications and precautions

• Contraindicated in patients hypersensitive to drug and in those with documented megaloblastic anemia caused by folate deficiency.
• Use cautiously in patients with hepatic impairment.
⚘ Lifespan: In pregnant women, use cautiously. In breast-feeding women, drug isn't recommended. In children younger than age 12, safety of drug (other than Primsol) hasn't been established.

Adverse reactions

CNS: fever.
GI: epigastric distress, nausea, vomiting, diarrhea, glossitis.
Hematologic: *thrombocytopenia, leukopenia,* megaloblastic anemia, *methemoglobinemia.*
Skin: *rash, pruritus,* exfoliative dermatitis.

Interactions

Drug-drug. *Phenytoin:* May decrease phenytoin metabolism and increase its level. Monitor patient for toxicity.

Effects on lab test results

• May increase BUN, creatinine, bilirubin, and aminotransferase levels.
• May decrease hemoglobin, hematocrit, and platelet and WBC counts.

Pharmacokinetics

Absorption: Quick and complete.
Distribution: Wide; about 42% to 46% protein-bound.
Metabolism: Less than 20% in liver.
Excretion: Mostly in urine. *Half-life:* 8 to 11 hours.

Route	Onset	Peak	Duration
P.O.	Unknown	1-4 hr	Unknown

Action

Chemical effect: Interferes with action of dihydrofolate reductase, inhibiting bacterial synthesis of folic acid.
Therapeutic effect: Inhibits certain bacteria.

Available forms

Oral solution: 50 mg/5 ml
Tablets: 100 mg, 200 mg

NURSING PROCESS

☰ Assessment
• Assess patient's infection before therapy and regularly thereafter.
• Obtain urine specimen for culture and sensitivity tests before giving first dose. Therapy may begin pending results.
⚡ **ALERT:** Monitor CBC routinely. Signs and symptoms such as sore throat, fever, pallor, and purpura may be early indications of serious blood disorders. Prolonged use of trimethoprim at high doses may cause bone marrow suppression.
• Be alert for adverse reactions and drug interactions.
• If adverse GI reactions occur, monitor hydration.
• Evaluate patient's and family's knowledge of drug therapy.

▣ Nursing diagnoses
• Infection related to presence of susceptible bacteria
• Risk for deficient fluid volume related to drug-induced adverse GI reactions
• Deficient knowledge related to drug therapy

▶ Planning and implementation
• Because resistance to trimethoprim develops rapidly when given alone, it's usually given with other drugs.
⚡ **ALERT:** Trimethoprim is also used with sulfamethoxazole; don't confuse the two products.
Patient teaching
• Instruct patient to take drug as prescribed, even if he feels better.

☑ Evaluation
• Patient is free from infection.
• Patient maintains adequate hydration.
• Patient and family state understanding of drug therapy.

triptorelin pamoate
(trip-TOE-reh-lin PAM-o-eight)
Trelstar Depot, Trelstar LA

Pharmacologic class: synthetic luteinizing hormone-releasing hormone (LHRH) analogue
Therapeutic class: antineoplastic
Pregnancy risk category: X

Indications and dosages
▶ **Palliative treatment of advanced prostate cancer.** *Men:* 3.75 mg Trelstar Depot I.M. given monthly as a single injection, or 11.25 mg Trelstar LA I.M into either buttock q 12 weeks.

Contraindications and precautions
• Contraindicated in patients hypersensitive to drug, its components, other LHRH agonists, or LHRH.
• Use cautiously in patients with metastatic vertebral lesions or upper or lower urinary tract obstruction during the first few weeks of therapy.
• Use cautiously in patients with hepatic and renal impairment; they have a level of exposure to drug two to four times higher than normal.
⚘ **Lifespan:** Drug is used for men only. In boys, safety and efficacy haven't been studied.

Adverse reactions
CNS: pain, headache, dizziness, fatigue, insomnia, emotional lability.
CV: hypertension.
GI: diarrhea, vomiting.
GU: urine retention, UTI, impotence.
Hematologic: anemia.
Musculoskeletal: *skeletal pain,* leg pain.
Skin: pruritus.
Other: *hot flushes,* pain at injection site.

Interactions
Drug-drug. *Hyperprolactinemic drugs:* Decreases pituitary gonadotropin-releasing hormone (GnRH) receptors. Don't use together.

Effects on lab test results
• May increase glucose, BUN, AST, ALT, and alkaline phosphatase. May transiently increase testosterone level.
• May decrease hemoglobin and hematocrit.

Pharmacokinetics
Absorption: Maintains level over a period of a month.
Distribution: No evidence of protein-binding.
Metabolism: Unknown, but is unlikely to involve hepatic microsomal enzymes; no metabolites have been identified.
Excretion: By both liver and kidneys. *Half-life:* 2 to 3 hours.

Route	Onset	Peak	Duration
I.M.	Unknown	Unknown	1 mo

Reactions may be *common,* uncommon, *life-threatening,* or COMMON AND LIFE-THREATENING.

Action

Chemical effect: Is a potent inhibitor of gonadotropin secretion. In men, testosterone declines to a level typically seen in surgically castrated men. As a result, tissues and functions that depend on these hormones become inactive.
Therapeutic effect: Decreases effects of sex hormones on tumor growth in the prostate gland.

Available forms

Injection: 3.75 mg, 11.25 mg

NURSING PROCESS

⚕ Assessment

• Assess patient's condition before therapy and regularly thereafter.
• Monitor testosterone and prostate-specific antigen levels.
• Evaluate patient's and family's knowledge of drug therapy.

🔷 Nursing diagnoses

• Ineffective health maintenance related to underlying condition
• Acute pain related to adverse drug effects
• Deficient knowledge related to drug therapy

▶ Planning and implementation

• Give drug only under the supervision of a prescriber.
• **⚠ ALERT:** Only sterile water may be used as a diluent.
• Dilute vial with 2 ml of sterile water for injection. Shake well until suspension appears milky. Use 20 G needle.
• Change the injection site periodically.
• Monitor patients with metastatic vertebral lesions or upper or lower urinary tract obstruction during the first few weeks of therapy.
• Initially, drug causes a transient increase in testosterone levels. As a result, signs and symptoms of prostate cancer may worsen during the first few weeks of therapy.
• Patients may experience worsening of symptoms or onset of new symptoms, including bone pain, neuropathy, hematuria, or urethral or bladder outlet obstruction.
• **⚠ ALERT:** Spinal cord compression, which can lead to paralysis and possibly death, may occur. If spinal cord compression or renal impairment

develops, give standard treatment. In extreme cases, immediate orchiectomy is considered.
• If patient has a hypersensitivity reaction, stop drug immediately and give supportive and symptomatic care.
• Diagnostic tests of pituitary-gonadal function conducted during and after therapy may be misleading.
• Reconstitute powder with 2 ml sterile water, using a 20-gauge needle.

Patient teaching

• Inform the patient about adverse reactions.
• Tell patient that symptoms (including bone pain, neuropathy, hematuria, or urethral or bladder outlet obstruction) may worsen during the first few weeks of therapy.
• Inform patient that a blood test will be used to monitor response to therapy.

☑ Evaluation

• Patient responds well to drug.
• Patient denies pain.
• Patient and family state understanding of drug therapy.

---

tubocurarine chloride
(too-boh-kyoo-RAH-reen KLOR-ighd)
Tubarine ◆

Pharmacologic class: nondepolarizing neuromuscular blocker
Therapeutic class: skeletal muscle relaxant
Pregnancy risk category: C

Indications and dosages

▶ **Adjunct to general anesthesia.** Dosage depends on anesthetic used, individual needs, and response. *Adults:* 1 unit/kg or 0.165 mg/kg I.V. slowly over 60 to 90 seconds. Average dose is initially 6 to 9 mg I.V. or I.M., followed by 3 to 4.5 mg in 3 to 5 minutes, if needed. Additional doses of 3 mg may be given if needed during prolonged anesthesia.
Children: 0.6 mg/kg I.V. or I.M.
Neonates: 0.3 mg/kg I.V. or I.M.
▶ **To assist with mechanical ventilation.**
Adults and children: Initially, 0.0165 mg/kg I.V. (average 1 mg), then adjust subsequent doses to patient response.
▶ **To lessen muscle contractions in pharmacologically or electrically induced seizures.**

Adults and children: 1 unit/kg or 0.165 mg/kg
I.V. over 60 to 90 seconds. Initial dose is 3 mg
less than calculated dose.

► **Diagnosis of myasthenia gravis.** *Adults:*
0.004 to 0.033 mg/kg as single I.V. or I.M. dose.

▼ I.V. administration

- Don't mix drug with barbiturates, such as
methohexital and thiopental because precipitate
will form.
- Use only fresh solutions and discard if discolored.
- Give drug I.V. over 60 to 90 seconds.
- Don't use if more than a faint color develops.
- Don't store drug where it can be exposed to
excessive heat.

Contraindications and precautions

- Contraindicated in patients hypersensitive to
drug and in those for whom histamine release is
hazardous (such as asthmatic patients).
- Use cautiously in debilitated patients and in
those with hepatic or pulmonary impairment, hypothermia, respiratory depression, myasthenia
gravis, myasthenic syndrome of lung cancer or
bronchogenic carcinoma, dehydration, thyroid
disorders, collagen diseases, porphyria, electrolyte disturbances, fractures, or muscle spasms.
- ☆ **Lifespan:** In women undergoing cesarean
delivery and in breast-feeding women, use large
doses cautiously. In geriatric patients, use cautiously.

Adverse reactions

CV: hypotension, *arrhythmias, bradycardia,
cardiac arrest.*
GI: increased salivation.
Musculoskeletal: *profound and prolonged
muscle relaxation,* residual muscle weakness.
Respiratory: *respiratory depression or apnea,
bronchospasm.*
Other: *hypersensitivity reactions, anaphylaxis.*

Interactions

Drug-drug. *Amikacin, gentamicin, neomycin,
streptomycin, tobramycin:* May increase the
effects of nondepolarizing muscle relaxant, including prolonged respiratory depression. Use
together only when necessary. Dose of nondepolarizing muscle relaxant may need to be reduced.
*Amphotericin B, ethacrynic acid, furosemide,
methotrimeprazine, opioid analgesics, propranolol, thiazide diuretics:* Potentiates neuromus-

cular blockade, leading to increased skeletal
muscle relaxation and, possibly, respiratory
paralysis. Use cautiously during surgical and
postoperative periods.
Carbamazepine, phenytoin: May decrease the
effects of tubocurarine. May need to increase
the dose of the tubocurarine.
*Kanamycin, general anesthetics (such as enflu-
rane, halothane, isoflurane), polymyxin antibiotics (colistin, polymyxin B sulfate):* Potentiates
neuromuscular blockade, leading to increased
skeletal muscle relaxation and potentiation of
effect. Use cautiously during surgical and postoperative periods.
Quinidine: Prolongs neuromuscular blockade.
Use together cautiously. Monitor patient closely.

Effects on lab test results

None reported.

Pharmacokinetics

Absorption: Unknown.
Distribution: In extracellular fluid, rapidly
reaching its site of action; about 50% bound to
plasma proteins, mainly globulins.
Metabolism: Undergoes *N*-demethylation in
liver.
Excretion: About 33% to 75% excreted unchanged in urine in 24 hours; up to 11% excreted in bile. *Half-life:* Unknown.

Route	Onset	Peak	Duration
I.V., I.M.	≤ 1 min	2-5 min	20-40 min

Action

Chemical effect: Prevents acetylcholine from
binding to receptors on muscle end plate, thus
blocking depolarization.
Therapeutic effect: Relaxes skeletal muscles;
diagnostic aid for myasthenia gravis.

Available forms

Injection: 3 mg (20 units)/ml

NURSING PROCESS

☑ Assessment

- Assess patient's condition before therapy and
regularly thereafter.
- Monitor baseline electrolyte determinations
(imbalance can potentiate neuromuscular blocking effects).
- Check vital signs q 15 minutes.

• Measure fluid intake and output; renal dysfunction prolongs duration of action because much of drug is unchanged before excretion.
• Monitor respiratory rate closely until patient is fully recovered from neuromuscular blockade, as evidenced by tests of muscle strength (hand grip, head lift, and ability to cough).
• Be alert for adverse reactions and drug interactions.
• Evaluate patient's and family's knowledge of drug therapy.

Nursing diagnoses
• Ineffective health maintenance related to underlying condition
• Ineffective breathing pattern related to drug-induced respiratory depression
• Deficient knowledge related to drug therapy

Planning and implementation
• Allow succinylcholine effects to subside before giving tubocurarine.
• Give sedatives or general anesthetics before neuromuscular blockers. Neuromuscular blockers don't obtund consciousness or alter pain threshold.
• Only personnel skilled in airway management should give drug.
• Keep airway clear. Have emergency respiratory support equipment immediately available.
• If vital signs change, notify prescriber immediately.
ALERT: Nerve stimulator and train-of-four monitoring are recommended to confirm antagonism of neuromuscular blockade and recovery of muscle strength. Before attempting reversal with neostigmine, some evidence of spontaneous recovery should be evident.
ALERT: Careful drug calculation is essential. Don't confuse units with mg. Always verify dosage with another health care professional.
Patient teaching
• Explain all events and happenings to patient because he still can hear.
• Reassure patient that he is being monitored at all times.

Evaluation
• Patient responds well to drug.
• Patient maintains adequate breathing patterns with or without mechanical assistance.
• Patient and family state understanding of drug therapy.

U

unoprostone isopropyl
(yoo-noh-PROST-ohn igh-soh-PROH-pul)
Rescula

Pharmacologic class: docosanoid
Therapeutic class: antiglaucoma agent, ocular antihypertensive
Pregnancy risk category: C

Indications and dosages
▶ **Reduction of intraocular pressure (IOP) in patients with open-angle glaucoma or ocular hypertension who can't tolerate or who respond inadequately to other IOP-lowering drugs.** *Adults:* 1 gtt in the affected eye b.i.d.

Contraindications and precautions
• Contraindicated in patients hypersensitive to drug, benzalkonium chloride, or other ingredients in product.
• Use cautiously in patients with active intraocular inflammation (uveitis) or with angle-closure, inflammatory, or neovascular glaucoma. Also use cautiously in patients with renal or hepatic impairment.
Lifespan: In pregnant women, weigh risks and benefits before giving drug. In breast-feeding women, use cautiously. In children, safety hasn't been established.

Adverse reactions
CNS: dizziness, headache, insomnia, pain.
CV: hypertension.
EENT: abnormal vision, blepharitis, cataracts, conjunctivitis, corneal lesion, *dry eyes,* eye discharge, *eye burning or stinging,* eye discomfort, eye irritation, eye hemorrhage, decreased length of eyelashes, *increased length of eyelashes,* eyelid disorder, foreign body sensation, keratitis, lacrimal disorder, pharyngitis, photophobia, rhinitis, sinusitis, vitreous disorder, *eye itching, injection of eye.*
Metabolic: *diabetes mellitus.*
Musculoskeletal: back pain.

Respiratory: bronchitis, increased cough, pharyngitis, increased cough.
Other: accidental injury, allergic reaction, flu-like syndrome.

Interactions

None reported.

Effects on lab test results

None reported.

Pharmacokinetics

Absorption: Absorbed through the cornea and conjunctival epithelium. Systemic absorption is minimal.
Distribution: Unknown.
Metabolism: Hydrolyzed by esterases to form unoprostone free acid.
Excretion: Rapid. Metabolites are excreted mainly in urine. *Half-life:* 14 minutes.

Route	Onset	Peak	Duration
Ophthalmic	Unknown	Unknown	Unknown

Action

Chemical effect: Unknown. Thought to increase the outflow of aqueous humor.
Therapeutic effect: Reduces IOP.

Available forms

Ophthalmic solution: 0.15% (1.5 mg/ml)

NURSING PROCESS

⌦ Assessment
• Assess patient's condition before therapy and regularly thereafter.
• Assess solution carefully before instilling. Serious eye damage and blindness may result from using contaminated solutions.
• Evaluate patient's and family's knowledge of drug therapy.

⊕ Nursing diagnoses
• Noncompliance related to long-term therapy
• Risk for injury related to adverse EENT effects of drug
• Deficient knowledge related to drug therapy

▷ Planning and implementation
• Avoid touching the tip of the container to the eye because this may contaminate the applicator and cause infection.

• Have patient who wears contact lenses remove them before giving drug. Drug contains benzalkonium chloride, which may be absorbed by the lenses. He may reinsert them 15 minutes after drug use.
• When giving an additional ophthalmic drug, separate administration of the drugs by 5 minutes.
• Store drug at room temperature.
Patient teaching
• Instruct patient to avoid touching the tip of the container to the eye because this could contaminate the tip and cause an eye infection.
• Instruct patient who wears contact lenses to remove lenses before using drug and to wait at least 15 minutes before reinserting them.
• Tell patient that drug may permanently darken eye color. Change may be gradual, over months to years.
• Instruct patient to report adverse effects, especially conjunctivitis (pink eye) or eyelid reactions.
• If eye trauma or infection occur or if ocular surgery is planned, tell patient to notify prescriber before continuing to use a multidose container.
• Tell patient that drug may be used with other ocular drugs, but that doses should be separated by 5 minutes.
• Warn patient not to use if he's allergic to this drug, benzalkonium chloride, or any other ingredient in the product.
• Instruct woman to notify prescriber if she becomes pregnant or intends to breast-feed while taking drug.

☑ Evaluation
• Patient is compliant with drug therapy.
• Patient sustains no injury.
• Patient and family state understanding of drug therapy.

urokinase
(yoo-roh-KIGH-nays)
Abbokinase

Pharmacologic class: thrombolytic enzyme
Therapeutic class: thrombolytic enzyme
Pregnancy risk category: B

Indications and dosages

▶ **Lysis of acute massive pulmonary emboli and pulmonary emboli accompanied by unstable hemodynamics.** *Adults:* For I.V. infusion only by constant infusion pump; priming dose: 4,400 IU/kg over 10 minutes, followed with 4,400 IU/kg per hour for 12 hours. Flush through any drug remaining in the I.V. tubing with a volume of compatible I.V. solution approximately equal to that of the tubing at 15 ml/hr.
▶ **Coronary artery thrombosis‡.** *Adults:* 2 to 3 million units over 45 to 90 minutes, with half or all of the dose given as an initial rapid injection over 5 minutes and the remainder, if any, as a continuous infusion.
▶ **Venous catheter occlusion‡.** *Adults:* Instill 5,000 IU into occluded line.

▼ I.V. administration

• Add 5 ml of sterile water for injection to vial. Don't use bacteriostatic water for injection to reconstitute; it contains preservatives. Use immediately after reconstitution.
• Dilute further with normal saline solution or D_5W solution before infusion.
• Solution may be filtered through a 0.45 micron or smaller filter before administration.
• Give by infusion pump. Total volume of fluid given shouldn't exceed 200 ml.
• Store powder at 36° to 46° F (2° to 8° C).

Contraindications and precautions

• Contraindicated in patients with active internal bleeding; aneurysm; arteriovenous malformation; bleeding diathesis; visceral or intracranial cancer; ulcerative colitis; diverticulitis; severe hypertension; hemostatic defects, including those secondary to severe hepatic or renal insufficiency; uncontrolled hypocoagulation; subacute bacterial endocarditis or rheumatic valvular disease; history of CVA; recent trauma with possible internal injuries; or recent cerebral embolism, thrombosis, or hemorrhage.
• Also contraindicated within 10 days after intra-arterial diagnostic procedure or surgery (liver or kidney biopsy, lumbar puncture, thoracentesis, paracentesis, or extensive or multiple cutdowns); and within 2 months after intracranial or intraspinal surgery.
• I.M. injections and other invasive procedures are contraindicated during urokinase therapy.
≋ **Lifespan:** In pregnant women, drug should be used only when clearly needed. Drug is con-

traindicated during the first 10 days postpartum. In children, safety of drug hasn't been established.

Adverse reactions

CNS: fever, *CVA,* hemiplegia.
CV: *reperfusion arrhythmias,* tachycardia, transient hypotension or hypertension.
GI: nausea, vomiting.
Hematologic: *bleeding.*
Respiratory: *bronchospasm,* minor breathing difficulties.
Skin: phlebitis, rash.
Other: *anaphylaxis,* chills.

Interactions

Drug-drug. Anticoagulants: Increases risk of bleeding. Monitor patient closely.
Aspirin, dipyridamole, indomethacin, phenylbutazone, other drugs affecting platelet activity: Increases risk of bleeding. Monitor patient closely.

Effects on lab test results

• May increase PT, PTT, and INR. May decrease hemoglobin and hematocrit.

Pharmacokinetics

Absorption: Administered I.V.
Distribution: Rapidly cleared from circulation; most of drug accumulates in kidneys and liver.
Metabolism: Rapid, in liver.
Excretion: Small amount excreted in urine and bile. *Half-life:* 10 to 20 minutes.

Route	Onset	Peak	Duration
I.V.	Immediate	20 min-2 hr	4 hr

Action

Chemical effect: Activates plasminogen by directly cleaving peptide bonds at two sites.
Therapeutic effect: Dissolves blood clots in lungs, coronary arteries, and venous catheters.

Available forms

Injection: 250,000-IU vial

NURSING PROCESS

🗒 **Assessment**
• Assess patient's condition before therapy and regularly thereafter.

• Assess patient for any contraindications to the therapy.

• Monitor patient for excessive bleeding q 15 minutes for first hour; q 30 minutes for second through eighth hours; then once every shift. Pretreatment with drugs affecting platelets places patient at high risk for bleeding.

• Monitor pulse rates and color and sensation of limbs every hour.

• Keep laboratory flow sheet on patient's chart to monitor PTT, PT, INR, hemoglobin, and hematocrit.

• Be alert for adverse reactions and drug interactions.

• Evaluate patient's and family's knowledge of drug therapy.

⊞ Nursing diagnoses

• Ineffective tissue perfusion (cardiopulmonary, peripheral) related to presence of blood clot(s)

• Ineffective protection related to drug-induced bleeding

• Deficient knowledge related to drug therapy

▷ Planning and implementation

• Have typed and crossmatched RBCs, whole blood, and aminocaproic acid available to treat bleeding, and keep corticosteroids available to treat allergic reactions.

• Keep venipuncture sites to a minimum; use pressure dressing on puncture sites for at least 15 minutes.

• Keep limb being treated in alignment to prevent bleeding from infusion site.

• Avoid unnecessary handling of patient; pad side rails. Bruising is more likely during therapy.

• To prevent recurrent thrombosis, start heparin by continuous infusion when patient's thrombin time has decreased to less than twice the normal control value after urokinase has been stopped.

⊛ ALERT: Rare reports of orolingual edema, urticaria, cholesterol embolization, and infusion reactions causing hypoxia, cyanosis, acidosis, and back pain have occurred in patients receiving this drug.

Patient teaching

• Instruct patient to report symptoms of bleeding and other adverse reactions.

☑ Evaluation

• Patient regains normal tissue perfusion with dissolution of blood clots.

• Patient doesn't experience serious complications from drug-induced bleeding.

• Patient and family state understanding of drug therapy.

ursodiol
(ur-sih-DIGH-al)
Actigall

Pharmacologic class: bile acid
Therapeutic class: gallstone-solubilizing agent
Pregnancy risk category: B

Indications and dosages

▶ **Dissolution of gallstones smaller than 20 mm in diameter in patients who are poor candidates for surgery or who refuse surgery.**
Adults: 8 to 10 mg/kg P.O. daily in two or three divided doses.

▶ **Prevention of gallstone formation in obese patients experiencing rapid weight loss.**
Adults: 300 mg P.O. b.i.d.

Contraindications and precautions

• Contraindicated in patients hypersensitive to drug or other bile acids and in patients with chronic hepatic disease, unremitting acute cholecystitis, cholangitis, biliary obstruction, gallstone-induced pancreatitis, or biliary fistula.

⚖ Lifespan: In pregnant and breast-feeding women, use cautiously. In children, safety of drug hasn't been established.

Adverse reactions

CNS: *headache,* fatigue, anxiety, depression, *dizziness,* sleep disorders.
EENT: rhinitis.
GI: *nausea, vomiting, dyspepsia,* metallic taste, *abdominal pain,* biliary pain, cholecystitis, *diarrhea, constipation,* stomatitis, flatulence.
GU: UTI.
Musculoskeletal: arthralgia, myalgia, back pain.
Respiratory: cough.
Skin: pruritus, rash, dry skin, urticaria, hair thinning, diaphoresis.

Interactions

Drug-drug. *Antacids that contain aluminum, cholestyramine, colestipol:* Binds ursodiol and prevents its absorption. Avoid use together.

Clofibrate, estrogens, hormonal contraceptives: Increases hepatic cholesterol secretion; may counteract effects of ursodiol. Avoid use together.

Effects on lab test results

• May decrease liver enzyme levels in patients with liver disease.

Pharmacokinetics

Absorption: About 90%.
Distribution: Conjugated and then secreted into hepatic bile ducts. Drug in bile is concentrated in gallbladder and expelled into duodenum in gallbladder bile. A small amount appears in systemic circulation.
Metabolism: In liver. A small amount undergoes bacterial degradation with each cycle of enterohepatic circulation.
Excretion: Primarily in feces with very small amount in urine. *Half-life:* Unknown.

Route	Onset	Peak	Duration
P.O.	Unknown	1-3 hr	Unknown

Action

Chemical effect: Unknown; probably suppresses hepatic synthesis and secretion of cholesterol as well as intestinal cholesterol absorption. After long-term administration, ursodiol can solubilize cholesterol from gallstones.
Therapeutic effect: Dissolves cholesterol gallstones.

Available forms

Capsules: 300 mg

NURSING PROCESS

☑ Assessment

• Assess patient's condition before therapy and regularly thereafter.
• Usually, therapy is long-term and requires ultrasound images of gallbladder q 6 months. If partial stone dissolution doesn't occur within 12 months, it's unlikely that complete dissolution will. Safety of use for longer than 24 months hasn't been established.
• **⑤ ALERT:** Monitor liver function test results, including AST and ALT levels, at beginning of therapy, after 1 month, after 3 months, and then q 6 months during therapy. Abnormal test results may indicate worsening of disease. A he-

patotoxic metabolite of drug may form in some patients.
• Be alert for adverse reactions and drug interactions.
• If adverse GI reactions occur, monitor patient's hydration.
• Evaluate patient's and family's knowledge of drug therapy.

⊕ Nursing diagnoses

• Risk for injury related to presence of gallstones
• Risk for deficient fluid volume related to drug-induced adverse GI reactions
• Deficient knowledge related to drug therapy

▶ Planning and implementation

• Drug won't dissolve calcified cholesterol stones, radiolucent bile pigment stones, or radiopaque stones.

Patient teaching
• Tell patient about alternative therapies, including watchful waiting (with no intervention) and cholecystectomy because relapse rate after bile acid therapy may be as high as 50% after 5 years.

☑ Evaluation

• Patient is free from gallstones.
• Patient maintains adequate hydration.
• Patient and family state understanding of drug therapy.

valacyclovir hydrochloride
(val-ay-SIGH-kloh-veer high-droh-KLOR-ighd)
Valtrex

Pharmacologic class: synthetic purine nucleoside
Therapeutic class: antiviral
Pregnancy risk category: B

Indications and dosages

▶ **Herpes zoster (shingles) in immunocompetent patients.** *Adults:* 1 g P.O. q 8 hours for 7 days.

⧄ **Adjust-a-dose:** For patient with renal impairment, if creatinine clearance is 30 to 49 ml/ minute, give 1 g q 12 hours; if 10 to 29, give 1 g q 24 hours; if less than 10, give 500 mg q 24 hours.

▶ **Initial episodes of genital herpes in immunocompetent adults.** *Adults:* 1 g P.O. q 12 hours for 10 days.

⧄ **Adjust-a-dose:** For patients with renal impairment, if creatinine clearance is 10 to 29 ml/ minute, give 1 g q 24 hours; if less than 10, give 500 mg q 12 hours.

▶ **Recurrent genital herpes in immunocompetent patients.** *Adults:* 500 mg P.O. q 12 hours for 3 days.

⧄ **Adjust-a-dose:** For patients with renal impairment, if creatinine clearance is 29 ml/minute or less, give 500 mg q 24 hours.

▶ **Chronic suppression of recurrent genital herpes.** *Adults:* 1 g P.O. once daily.

⧄ **Adjust-a-dose:** For patients with renal impairment, if creatinine clearance is 29 ml/minute or less, give 500 mg q 24 hours.

▶ **Chronic suppression of genital herpes in patients with a history of 9 or fewer recurrences per year.** *Adults:* 500 mg P.O. daily.

⧄ **Adjust-a-dose:** For patients with renal impairment, if creatinine clearance is 29 ml/minute or less, give 500 mg q 48 hours.

▶ **Chronic suppression of recurrent genital herpes in HIV-infected individuals with CD4 count of 100/mm³ or more.** *Adults:* 500 mg P.O. twice daily. Safety and efficacy of therapy beyond 6 months hasn't been established.

⧄ **Adjust-a-dose:** For patients with renal impairment, if creatinine clearance is 29 ml/minute or less, give 500 mg q 24 hours.

▶ **Cold sores (herpes labialis).** *Adults:* 2 g P.O. for two doses, taken about 12 hours apart.

⧄ **Adjust-a-dose:** For patient with renal impairment, creatinine clearance is 30 to 49 ml/ minute, give 1 g q 12 hours; if 10 to 29 ml/ minute, give 500 mg q 12 hours; if less than 10 ml/minute, give 500 mg as a single dose.

Contraindications and precautions

● Contraindicated in patients hypersensitive to or intolerant of valacyclovir, acyclovir, or components of their formulations.

● Drug isn't recommended for immunocompromised patients. Thrombotic thrombocytopenic purpura and hemolytic uremic syndrome have been fatal in some patients with advanced HIV

disease and in bone marrow transplant and renal transplant recipients.

● Use cautiously in patients with renal impairment and in those receiving other nephrotoxic drugs.

⚘ Lifespan: In pregnant women, give drug only if potential benefits outweigh risk to the fetus. In breast-feeding women, use cautiously. In children, safety and effectiveness haven't been established.

Adverse reactions

CNS: *headache,* dizziness, depression.
GI: *nausea,* vomiting, diarrhea, abdominal pain.
GU: dysmenorrhea.
Musculoskeletal: arthralgia.

Interactions

Drug-drug. *Cimetidine, probenecid:* Reduces rate (but not extent) of conversion from valacyclovir to acyclovir and reduces renal clearance of acyclovir, thereby increasing acyclovir level. Monitor patient for possible toxicity.

Effects on lab test results

● May increase AST, ALT, alkaline phosphatase, and creatinine levels.
● May decrease hemoglobin and hematocrit and WBC and platelet counts.

Pharmacokinetics

Absorption: Rapid; absolute bioavailability of about 54.5%.
Distribution: Protein-binding ranges from 13.5% to 17.9%.
Metabolism: Rapid; nearly completely converted to acyclovir and L-valine by first-pass intestinal or hepatic metabolism.
Excretion: In urine and feces. *Half-life:* Averages 2½ to 3¼ hours.

Route	Onset	Peak	Duration
P.O.	30 min	Unknown	Unknown

Action

Chemical effect: Rapidly converted to acyclovir, which becomes incorporated into viral DNA and inhibits viral DNA polymerase, thereby inhibiting viral replication.
Therapeutic effect: Inhibits susceptible viral growth of herpes zoster.

Reactions may be *common,* uncommon, *life-threatening,* or COMMON AND LIFE-THREATENING.

Available forms

Caplets: 500 mg, 1,000 mg

NURSING PROCESS

✎ Assessment
- Assess patient's infection before therapy.
- Evaluate patient's and family's knowledge of drug therapy.

✺ Nursing diagnoses
- Risk for infection related to herpes zoster
- Deficient fluid volume related to adverse GI reactions
- Deficient knowledge related to drug therapy

▶ Planning and implementation
- Dosage adjustment may be needed in geriatric patient, depending on underlying renal status.
- Although overdose hasn't been reported, precipitation of acyclovir in renal tubules may occur when solubility (2.5 mg/ml) is exceeded in the intratubular fluid. In the event of acute renal failure and anuria, the patient may benefit from hemodialysis until kidney function is restored.
⊛ ALERT: Don't confuse valacyclovir with valganciclovir.
Patient teaching
- Inform patient that drug may be taken without regard to meals.
- Review signs and symptoms of herpes infection (rash, tingling, itching, and pain), and advise patient to notify prescriber immediately if they occur. Treatment should begin as soon as possible after symptoms appear, preferably within 48 hours.

☑ Evaluation
- Patient is free from infection.
- Patient maintains adequate hydration.
- Patient and family state understanding of drug therapy.

valdecoxib

(val-da-COX-ibb)
Bextra

Pharmacologic class: COX-2 inhibitor
Therapeutic class: nonsteroidal anti-inflammatory drug (NSAID)
Pregnancy risk category: C

Indications and dosages

▶ **Osteoarthritis, rheumatoid arthritis.**
Adults: 10 mg P.O. once daily.
▶ **Primary dysmenorrhea.** *Adults:* 20 mg P.O. b.i.d.

Contraindications and precautions

- Contraindicated in patients hypersensitive to drug or sulfonamides and in patients with aspirin sensitivity that results in aspirin-induced asthma. Don't give to patients who have experienced asthma, urticaria, or allergic-type reactions after taking aspirin or NSAIDs. Don't use in patients with advanced renal or hepatic disease.
- Use cautiously in patients with a history of GI bleeding or peptic ulcer disease; in debilitated patients; and in patients with conditions or on therapies that may increase the risk of GI bleeding, such as treatment with oral corticosteroids or anticoagulants, longer duration of NSAID therapy, smoking, alcoholism, or poor general health. Also use cautiously in dehydrated patients; those with fluid retention, mild to moderate hepatic impairment, renal impairment, heart failure, hypertension, or preexisting asthma; and those taking diuretics or ACE inhibitors.
- **Lifespan:** In early pregnancy, use only if benefits outweigh risks. In late pregnancy, don't use drug; it may cause premature closure of the ductus arteriosus. In breast-feeding woman, stop drug or tell her to stop breast-feeding, taking into account the importance of the drug to the mother; it isn't known whether drug appears in breast milk. In children, safety and effectiveness haven't been established. In geriatric patients, use cautiously.

Adverse reactions

CNS: dizziness, headache, *CVA.*
CV: hypertension, angina pectoris, *arrhythmias, heart failure, aneurysm,* peripheral edema.
EENT: sinusitis.
GI: abdominal fullness, abdominal pain, diarrhea, dyspepsia, flatulence, nausea.
Hematologic: *thrombocytopenia, leukopenia.*
Hepatic: *hepatitis.*
Musculoskeletal: back pain, myalgia.
Respiratory: upper respiratory tract infection, *bronchospasm.*
Skin: rash, *Stevens-Johnson syndrome.*

Other: flulike syndrome, accidental injury, *hypersensitivity reactions.*

Interactions

Drug-drug. *Aspirin:* Increases risk of GI ulceration. Use together cautiously.
ACE inhibitors: May diminish antihypertensive effect. Monitor blood pressure carefully.
Furosemide, thiazide diuretics: May reduce natriuretic effect. Monitor patient carefully.
Dextromethorphan: Increases level of dextromethorphan. Monitor patient carefully.
Fluconazole, ketoconazole: Enhances valdecoxib effects. Monitor patient closely.
Lithium: Delays lithium clearance. Monitor lithium level.
Warfarin: May increase anticoagulant activity. Monitor INR closely.

Effects on lab test results

• May increase ALT, AST, alkaline phosphatase, BUN, creatinine, cholesterol, glucose, potassium, lipid, uric acid, and LDH levels. May decrease calcium and potassium levels.
• May decrease hemoglobin, hematocrit, and platelet and WBC counts.

Pharmacokinetics

Absorption: Maximal concentrations achieved in 3 hours.
Distribution: 98% protein-bound.
Metabolism: Extensive.
Excretion: Eliminated predominantly via hepatic metabolism. Less than 5% of dose is excreted unchanged in urine and feces; 70% of dose is excreted via urine as metabolites. *Half-life:* 8 to 11 hours.

Route	Onset	Peak	Duration
P.O.	Unknown	3 hr	Unknown

Action

Chemical effect: May inhibit prostaglandin synthesis primarily through inhibition of cyclooxygenase-2 (COX-2). COX-1 doesn't appear to be inhibited at human therapeutic concentrations.
Therapeutic effect: Decreases pain, inflammation, and fever.

Available forms

Tablets: 10 mg, 20 mg

NURSING PROCESS

⚖ Assessment

• Assess patient's condition before therapy and regularly thereafter.
• Assess volume status before therapy. Rehydrate dehydrated patients before treatment starts.
• If used in advanced kidney disease, monitor kidney function.
• Monitor patient carefully for signs and symptoms of GI toxicity, such as bleeding or ulceration.
• Monitor patient for signs and symptoms of anemia.
• Monitor hemoglobin and hematocrit in patients on long-term therapy.
• Evaluate patient's and family's knowledge of drug therapy.

⊞ Nursing diagnoses

• Chronic pain related to underlying condition
• Impaired physical mobility related to underlying condition
• Deficient knowledge related to valdecoxib therapy

▷ Planning and implementation

• GI toxicity, as indicated by bleeding, ulceration, or perforation of the stomach, small intestine, or large intestine, can occur without warning. Risk increases with longer duration of treatment.
• When stopping therapy, taper drug slowly.
• Liver function test results may be elevated, and there may be progression to more serious hepatic abnormalities.
• If hepatic disease is suspected or if systemic symptoms such as eosinophilia or rash occur, stop drug.
⊛ **ALERT:** Stop drug at the first sign of a skin rash or a hypersensitivity reaction and immediately notify the prescriber.
• Symptoms of overdose may include lethargy, drowsiness, nausea, vomiting, and epigastric pain. These are usually reversible with supportive treatment. GI bleeding, hypertension, acute renal failure, respiratory depression, and coma may occur. Anaphylactoid reactions also may occur. Treatment is symptomatic and supportive. No antidote exists.
⊛ **ALERT:** Don't confuse Bextra with Arixtra.

Reactions may be *common*, uncommon, *life-threatening*, or **COMMON AND LIFE-THREATENING**.

Patient teaching
• Advise patient to notify prescriber if signs or symptoms of GI bleeding and ulceration, weight gain, edema, skin rash, or liver toxicity (nausea, fatigue, lethargy, jaundice, right upper quadrant tenderness, flulike symptoms) occur.
• Advise patient to seek emergency attention if he has trouble breathing, especially if he has a history of aspirin sensitivity.

☑ Evaluation
• Patient is free from pain.
• Patient states that physical mobility has improved.
• Patient and family state understanding of drug therapy.

valganciclovir
(val-gan-SYE-kloh-veer)
Valcyte

Pharmacologic class: synthetic nucleoside
Therapeutic class: antiviral drug
Pregnancy risk category: C

Indications and dosages

▶ **Active CMV retinitis in patients with AIDS.** *Adults:* Induction dose: 900 mg (two 450-mg tablets) P.O. b.i.d. with food for 21 days; maintenance dose: 900 mg (two 450-mg tablets) P.O. once daily with food.
▶ **Inactive CMV retinitis.** *Adults:* 900 mg (two 450-mg tablets) P.O. once daily with food.
▶ **Prevention of CMV in kidney, heart, and pancreas-kidney transplants.** *Adults:* 900 mg P.O. daily with food 10 days before through 100 days after transplant.
◩ **Adjust-a-dose:** Patients with renal impairment need adjusted dose.

Contraindications and precautions

• Contraindicated in patients hypersensitive to valganciclovir or ganciclovir.
• Don't use in patients receiving hemodialysis.
• Use cautiously in patients with preexisting cytopenias and in those who have received immunosuppressants or radiation.
⚞ **Lifespan:** In pregnant women, use only if potential benefits outweigh risks. In breast-feeding women, don't use drug; it's unknown whether drug appears in breast milk and serious adverse reactions may occur in infants. In children, safety and efficacy of drug haven't been established.

Adverse reactions

CNS: *pyrexia, headache, insomnia,* peripheral neuropathy, paresthesia, *seizures,* psychosis, hallucinations, confusion, agitation.
EENT: *retinal detachment.*
GI: *diarrhea, nausea, vomiting, abdominal pain.*
Hematologic: NEUTROPENIA, *anemia, thrombocytopenia, pancytopenia, bone marrow depression, aplastic anemia.*
Other: catheter-related infection, *sepsis,* local or systemic infections, *hypersensitivity reactions.*

Interactions

Drug-drug. *Didanosine:* Possible increased absorption of didanosine. Monitor patient closely for didanosine toxicity.
Immunosuppressants, zidovudine: Possible enhanced neutropenia, anemia, thrombocytopenia, and bone marrow depression when used together. Monitor CBC.
Mycophenolate mofetil: May increase levels of both drugs in renally impaired patients. Use together carefully.
Probenecid: Decreases renal clearance of ganciclovir. Monitor patient for ganciclovir toxicity.
Drug-food. *Any food:* Increases absorption of drug. Give drug with food.

Effects on lab test results

• May increase creatinine level.
• May decrease hemoglobin, hematocrit, and RBC, WBC, neutrophil, and platelet counts.

Pharmacokinetics

Absorption: Well absorbed from GI tract. Higher when taken with food.
Distribution: Minimal binding to proteins.
Metabolism: In intestinal wall and liver to ganciclovir.
Excretion: Eliminated renally. *Half-life:* 4 hours.

Route	Onset	Peak	Duration
P.O.	Unknown	1-3 hr	Unknown

Action

Chemical effect: Drug is a prodrug that is converted to ganciclovir, which inhibits replication of viral DNA synthesis of CMV.
Therapeutic effect: Inhibits CMV.

Available forms

Tablets: 450 mg

NURSING PROCESS

▨ Assessment
• Assess patient's condition before therapy and regularly thereafter.
• Obtain baseline laboratory studies before beginning therapy and reassess regularly.
• Evaluate patient's and family's knowledge of drug therapy.

▨ Nursing diagnoses
• Risk for imbalanced fluid volume related to adverse GI effects
• Ineffective protection related to adverse hematologic reactions
• Deficient knowledge related to valganciclovir therapy

▷ Planning and implementation
• Adhere to dosing guidelines for valganciclovir because ganciclovir and valganciclovir aren't interchangeable, and overdose may occur.
• Cytopenia may occur at any time during treatment and may increase with continued dosing. Cell counts usually recover 3 to 7 days after stopping drug. Monitor patient's CBC closely and frequently throughout therapy.
• No drug interaction studies have been conducted; however, because drug is converted to ganciclovir, it can be assumed that drug interactions would be similar.
• Drug may cause temporary or permanent inhibition of spermatogenesis.
⊛ ALERT: Severe leukopenia, neutropenia, anemia, pancytopenia, bone marrow depression, aplastic anemia and thrombocytopenia may occur. If patient's ANC is less than 500/mm^3, platelets are less than 25,000/mm^3, or hemoglobin is less than 8 g/dl, don't use drug.
• Overdose may cause severe, fatal bone marrow depression and renal toxicity; if overdose occurs, maintain adequate hydration and consider hematopoietic growth factors. Dialysis may be used to reduce level.

⊛ ALERT: Don't confuse valganciclovir with valacyclovir.
Patient teaching
• Instruct women of childbearing age to use contraception during treatment. Instruct men to use barrier contraception during and for 90 days after treatment.
• Inform patient about infection control and bleeding precautions.
• Tell patient to take drug with food.

☑ Evaluation
• Patient remains well hydrated throughout therapy.
• Patient has no serious adverse hematologic reactions.
• Patient and family state understanding of drug therapy.

---

valproate sodium
(val-PROH-ayt SOH-dee-um)
Depacon, Depakene, Epilim◇, Valpro◇

valproic acid
Depakene

divalproex sodium
Depakote, Depakote ER, Depakote Sprinkle, Epival ✦

Pharmacologic class: carboxylic acid derivative
Therapeutic class: anticonvulsant
Pregnancy risk category: D

Indications and dosages

▶ **Simple and complex absence seizures, mixed seizure types (including absence seizures).** *Adults and children:* Initially, 15 mg/kg P.O. or I.V. daily; then increase by 5 to 10 mg/kg daily at weekly intervals up to maximum of 60 mg/kg daily. Don't use Depakote ER in children younger than age 10.
▶ **Mania.** *Adults:* Initially, 750 mg divalproex sodium (delayed-release) P.O. daily in divided doses. Adjust dosage based on patient's response; maximum dosage is 60 mg/kg daily.
▶ **Prevention of migraine headache.** *Adults:* Initially, 250 mg divalproex sodium (delayed-release) P.O. b.i.d. Some patients may need up

---

to 1,000 mg daily. Or, 500 mg Depakote ER
P.O. daily for 1 week; then 1,000 mg P.O. daily.
► **Complex partial seizures.** *Adults and children age 10 and older:* 10 to 15 mg/kg P.O. or
I.V. daily; then increase by 5 to 10 mg/kg daily
at weekly intervals, up to 60 mg/kg daily.
 Adjust-a-dose: For elderly patients, use lower
initial dose and adjust more slowly.

▼ I.V. administration

• Dilute with at least 50 ml of a compatible
diluent (D_5W, saline solution, lactated Ringer's
injection).
• Give I.V. over 1 hour. Don't exceed 20 mg/
minute.
• Use of I.V. therapy for more than 14 days
hasn't been studied.

Contraindications and precautions

• Contraindicated in patients hypersensitive to
drug and in patients with hepatic dysfunction or
urea cycle disorder (UCD).
 Lifespan: In pregnant and breast-feeding
women, drug isn't recommended. In children
younger than age 10, safety of Depakote ER
hasn't been established. In elderly patients, start
at lower dose and adjust dosage more slowly.

Adverse reactions

CNS: *sedation,* emotional upset, depression,
psychosis, aggressiveness, hyperactivity, behavioral deterioration, muscle weakness, tremor,
ataxia, headache, dizziness, incoordination.
EENT: nystagmus, diplopia.
GI: *nausea, vomiting, indigestion,* diarrhea,
abdominal cramps, constipation, increased appetite and weight gain, anorexia, *pancreatitis.*
Hematologic: petechiae, bruising, eosinophilia,
hemorrhage, leukopenia, bone marrow suppression, thrombocytopenia.
Hepatic: *toxic hepatitis, hepatotoxicity.*
Skin: rash, alopecia, pruritus, photosensitivity
reactions, *erythema multiforme, Stevens-Johnson syndrome.*
Other: *flulike syndrome, infection.*

Interactions

Drug-drug. *Aspirin, chlorpromazine, cimetidine, felbamate:* May cause valproic acid toxicity. Use together cautiously and monitor levels.
Benzodiazepines, other CNS depressants: May
cause excessive CNS depression. Avoid use together.

Carbamazepine: May result in carbamazepine
CNS toxicity (acute psychotic reaction). Carefully monitor levels.
Cholestyramine: Decreases valproate level.
Monitor patient for decreased effect.
Erythromycin: Increases valproate level. Monitor patient for toxicity.
Lamotrigine: Inhibits lamotrigine metabolism.
Decrease lamotrigine dosage when valproic acid
therapy is initiated.
Phenobarbital: Increases phenobarbital level.
Monitor patient closely.
Phenytoin: Increases or decreases phenytoin
level and increases metabolism of valproic acid.
Monitor patient closely.
Rifampin: May decrease valproate level. Monitor level.
Warfarin: Valproic acid may displace warfarin
from binding sites. Monitor PT and INR.
Drug-herb. *Glutamine:* Increases risk of
seizures. Discourage use together.
White willow: Herb contains substances similar
to aspirin. Discourage use together.
Drug-lifestyle. *Alcohol use:* May cause excessive CNS depression. Discourage use together.

Effects on lab test results

• May increase ALT, AST, and bilirubin levels.
• May increase eosinophil count and bleeding
time. May decrease platelet and WBC counts.
• May produce false-positive test results for ketones in urine.

Pharmacokinetics

Absorption: Valproate sodium and divalproex
sodium quickly convert to valproic acid, which
is then quickly and almost completely absorbed.
Distribution: Rapid throughout body; 80% to
95% protein-bound.
Metabolism: In liver.
Excretion: Primarily in urine; some excreted in
feces and exhaled in air. *Half-life:* 6 to 16 hours
(may be considerably longer in patient with
liver function impairment, in geriatric patient,
and in child up to age 18 months; may be considerably shorter in patient receiving hepatic
enzyme-inducing anticonvulsants).

Route	Onset	Peak	Duration
P.O.	Unknown	1-4 hr	Unknown
I.V.	Unknown	Unknown	Unknown

Action

Chemical effect: Unknown; may increase brain levels of GABA, which transmits inhibitory nerve impulses in CNS.
Therapeutic effect: Prevents and treats certain types of seizure activity.

Available forms

valproate sodium
Injection: 100 mg/ml
Syrup: 250 mg/ml
valproic acid
Capsules: 250 mg
Syrup: 200 mg/5 ml ◆
Tablets (crushable): 100 mg ◆
Tablets (enteric-coated): 200 mg ◆, 500 mg ◆
divalproex sodium
Capsules (containing coated particles): 125 mg
Tablets (delayed-release): 125 mg, 250 mg, 500 mg
Tablets (extended-release): 500 mg

NURSING PROCESS

🖉 Assessment

• Assess patient's condition before therapy and regularly thereafter.
• Monitor drug level; therapeutic level is 50 to 100 mcg/ml.
• Before starting drug and periodically thereafter, monitor liver function studies, platelet counts, and PT.
• Be alert for adverse reactions and drug interactions.
• Evaluate patient's and family's knowledge of drug therapy.

🔡 Nursing diagnoses

• Risk for trauma related to seizure activity
• Disturbed thought processes related to drug-induced adverse CNS reactions
• Deficient knowledge related to drug therapy

❱ Planning and implementation

• To switch adults and children age 10 and older taking Depakote for seizures to Depakote ER, give dose of new drug that's 8% to 20% larger than previous drug dose.
• Don't give syrup to patient who needs sodium restriction. Check with prescriber.
• Give drug with food or milk to minimize adverse GI reactions.

• Sudden withdrawal may worsen seizures. If adverse reactions develop, call prescriber immediately.
• ⊛ **ALERT:** Serious or fatal hepatotoxicity may follow nonspecific symptoms, such as malaise, fever, and lethargy. If patient has suspected or apparently substantial hepatic dysfunction, notify prescriber immediately and stop drug.
• Patients at high risk for developing hepatotoxicity include those with congenital metabolic disorders, mental retardation, or organic brain disease; those taking other anticonvulsants; and children younger than age 2.
• Divalproex sodium carries a lower risk of adverse GI effects than other drug forms.
• If tremors occur, notify prescriber. Dosage may need to be reduced.
• ⊛ **ALERT:** Fatal hyperammonemic encephalopathy may occur in patients with a UCD, particularly one such as ornithine transcarbamylase deficiency. Evaluate patients with risk factors for UCD before starting therapy. In patients who develop symptoms of unexplained hyperammonemic encephalopathy during therapy, stop drug; give prompt, appropriate treatment; and evaluate for underlying UCD.
Patient teaching
• Tell patient that drug may be taken with food or milk to reduce adverse GI effects.
• Instruct patient not to chew capsules and not to crush or chew extended-release tablets.
• Tell patient and parents that syrup shouldn't be mixed with carbonated beverages.
• Tell patient and parents to keep drug out of children's reach.
• Warn patient and parents not to stop drug therapy abruptly.
• Advise patient to refrain from driving or performing other potentially hazardous activities that require mental alertness until drug's CNS effects are known.

☑ Evaluation

• Patient is free from seizure activity.
• Patient maintains normal thought processes.
• Patient and family state understanding of drug therapy.

---

valsartan

(val-SAR-tin)
Diovan

Pharmacologic class: angiotensin II receptor blocker
Therapeutic class: antihypertensive
Pregnancy risk category: C (D in second and third trimesters)

Indications and dosages

▶ **Hypertension, used alone or with other antihypertensives.** *Adults:* Initially, 80 mg P.O. once daily. Expect a reduction in blood pressure in 2 to 4 weeks. If additional antihypertensive effect is needed, increase dosage to 160 or 320 mg daily, or add a diuretic. (Addition of a diuretic has a greater effect than dose increases above 80 mg.) Usual dosage range is 80 to 320 mg daily.
▶ **Heart failure (New York Heart Association classes II to IV) in patients who are intolerant of ACE inhibitors.** *Adults:* Initially, 40 mg P.O. b.i.d. Increase as tolerated to 80 mg b.i.d. Maximum dosage is 160 mg b.i.d. Avoid using with ACE inhibitors or beta blockers.

Contraindications and precautions

• Contraindicated in patients hypersensitive to drug.
• Use cautiously in patients with severe renal or hepatic disease.
⚠ **Lifespan:** During second or third trimester of pregnancy or in breast-feeding women, don't give drug. In children, safety and effectiveness haven't been established.

Adverse reactions

CNS: fatigue, *dizziness,* headache, insomnia, vertigo.
CV: edema, hypotension, postural hypotension, syncope.
EENT: pharyngitis, rhinitis, sinusitis, blurred vision.
GI: abdominal pain, diarrhea, nausea, dyspepsia.
GU: renal impairment.
Hematologic: *neutropenia.*
Metabolic: *hyperkalemia.*
Musculoskeletal: arthralgia, back pain.
Respiratory: cough, upper respiratory tract infection.

Other: viral infection, *angioedema.*

Interactions

Drug-drug. *Other angiotensin II blockers, potassium sparing diuretics, potassium supplements:* Increases potassium level. Avoid use together.
Drug-food. *Salt substitutes containing potassium:* Increases potassium level. In heart failure patients, may also increase creatinine level. Discourage use together.

Effects on lab test results

• May increase potassium level.
• May decrease neutrophil count.

Pharmacokinetics

Absorption: Bioavailability about 25%; food decreases absorption.
Distribution: Not extensive; 95% bound to proteins.
Metabolism: In liver and kidneys.
Excretion: In urine and feces. *Half-life:* 6 hours.

Route	Onset	Peak	Duration
P.O.	Within 2 hr	2-4 hr	24 hr

Action

Chemical effect: Blocks binding of angiotensin II to receptor sites in vascular smooth muscle and adrenal gland.
Therapeutic effect: Inhibits pressor effects of renin-angiotensin system.

Available forms

Tablets: 80 mg, 160 mg, 320 mg

NURSING PROCESS

📝 **Assessment**
• Monitor patient for hypotension. Correct volume and sodium depletions before starting drug therapy.
• Evaluate patient's and family's knowledge of drug therapy.

🔲 **Nursing diagnoses**
• Risk for injury related to presence of hypertension
• Deficient knowledge related to drug therapy

▷ Planning and implementation
● Drug can be given without regard to meals.
Patient teaching
● Tell woman to notify prescriber if she becomes pregnant.
● Teach patient other means of reducing blood pressure, including proper diet, exercise, smoking cessation, and stress reduction.

☑ Evaluation
● Patient's blood pressure becomes normal.
● Patient and family state understanding of drug therapy.

---

vancomycin hydrochloride
(van-koh-MIGH-sin high-droh-KLOR-ighd)
Vancocin, Vancoled

Pharmacologic class: glycopeptide
Therapeutic class: antibiotic
Pregnancy risk category: C

Indications and dosages
▶ **Severe staphylococcal infections when other antibiotics are ineffective or contraindicated.** *Adults:* 500 mg I.V. q 6 hours, or 1 g q 12 hours.
Children: 40 mg/kg I.V. daily in divided doses q 6 hours.
Neonates: Initially, 15 mg/kg; then 10 mg/kg I.V. daily, divided q 12 hours for first week after birth; then q 8 hours up to age 1 month.
▶ **Endocarditis prophylaxis for dental procedures.** *Adults:* 1 g I.V. slowly over 1 hour, starting 1 hour before procedure.
Children: 20 mg/kg I.V. over 1 hour, starting 1 hour before procedure.
🔲 **Adjust-a-dose:** For patients with renal impairment, adjust I.V. dosage.
▶ **Antibiotic-related pseudomembranous and staphylococcal enterocolitis.** *Adults:* 125 to 500 mg P.O. q 6 hours for 7 to 10 days.
Children: 40 mg/kg P.O. daily in divided doses q 6 to 8 hours for 7 to 10 days. Maximum, 2 g daily.

▼ I.V. administration
● Dilute in 200 ml of saline solution injection or D_5W.
● Infuse over 60 minutes.

● Check site daily for phlebitis and irritation. Watch for irritation and infiltration; extravasation can cause tissue damage and necrosis. If red-neck or red-man syndrome occurs because drug is infused too rapidly, stop infusion and report to prescriber.
● Refrigerate I.V. solution after reconstitution and use within 96 hours.

Contraindications and precautions
● Contraindicated in patients hypersensitive to drug.
● Use cautiously in patients receiving other neurotoxic, nephrotoxic, or ototoxic drugs; patients older than age 60; and those with impaired liver or kidney function, hearing loss, or allergies to other antibiotics.
⚖ **Lifespan:** In pregnant women, use cautiously. In breast-feeding women, safety of drug hasn't been established.

Adverse reactions
CNS: fever, pain.
CV: hypotension.
EENT: tinnitus, ototoxicity.
GI: nausea.
GU: *nephrotoxicity, pseudomembranous colitis.*
Hematologic: eosinophilia, *leukopenia.*
Respiratory: wheezing, dyspnea.
Skin: "red-neck" or "red-man" syndrome (maculopapular rash on face, neck, trunk, and limbs with rapid I.V. infusion; pruritus and hypotension with histamine release).
Other: chills, *anaphylaxis,* superinfection, thrombophlebitis at injection site.

Interactions
Drug-drug. *Aminoglycosides, amphotericin B, cisplatin, pentamidine:* Increases risk of nephrotoxicity and ototoxicity. Monitor patient closely.

Effects on lab test results
● May increase BUN and creatinine levels.
● May increase eosinophil counts. May decrease neutrophil and WBC counts.

Pharmacokinetics
Absorption: Minimal systemic absorption with P.O. administration. (Drug may accumulate in patients with colitis or renal failure.)
Distribution: In body fluids; achieves therapeutic level in CSF if meninges inflamed.
Metabolism: Unknown.

Excretion: In urine with parenteral administration; in feces with P.O. administration. *Half-life:* 6 hours.

Route	Onset	Peak	Duration
P.O.	Unknown	Unknown	Unknown
I.V.	Immediate	Immediate	Unknown

Action

Chemical effect: Hinders bacterial cell wall synthesis, damaging bacterial plasma membrane and making cell more vulnerable to osmotic pressure.
Therapeutic effect: Kills susceptible bacteria.

Available forms

Capsules: 125 mg, 250 mg
Powder for injection: 500-mg, 1-g vials
Powder for oral solution: 1-g, 10-g bottles

NURSING PROCESS

🖎 Assessment
• Assess patient's infection before therapy and regularly thereafter.
• Obtain urine specimen for culture and sensitivity tests before giving first dose. Therapy may begin pending test results.
• Obtain hearing evaluation and kidney function studies before therapy and repeat during therapy.
• Check levels regularly, especially in geriatric patients, premature infants, and those with decreased renal function.
• Be alert for adverse reactions and drug interactions.
• Evaluate patient's and family's knowledge of drug therapy.

🔲 Nursing diagnoses
• Risk for infection related to presence of susceptible bacteria
• Risk for injury related to drug-induced adverse reactions
• Deficient knowledge related to drug therapy

▶ Planning and implementation
• In patient with renal dysfunction, adjust dosage.
• ⑤ **ALERT:** Oral administration is ineffective for systemic infections, and I.V. administration is ineffective for pseudomembranous (*Clostridium difficile*) diarrhea.
• Oral form is stable for 2 weeks when refrigerated.

• Don't give drug I.M.
• When using drug to treat staphylococcal endocarditis, give for at least 4 weeks.
Patient teaching
• Tell patient to take entire amount of drug exactly as directed, even after he feels better.
• Tell patient to stop drug immediately and report adverse reactions, especially fullness or ringing in ears.

☑ Evaluation
• Patient is free from infection.
• Patient doesn't experience injury from adverse reactions.
• Patient and family state understanding of drug therapy.

---

vardenafil hydrochloride
(var-DEN-ah-phill high-droh-KLOR-ighd)
Levitra

Pharmacologic class: selective inhibitor of cyclic guanosine monophosphate (cGMP)-specific phosphodiesterase type 5 (PDE5)
Therapeutic class: erectile dysfunction drug
Pregnancy risk category: B

Indications and dosages

▶ **Erectile dysfunction.** *Men:* 10 mg P.O. p.r.n., 1 hour before sexual activity. Dose range is 5 to 20 mg based on effectiveness and tolerance. Maximum is one dose daily.
Elderly men age 65 and older: Initial dose is 5 mg P.O. p.r.n., 1 hour before sexual activity. Maximum is one dose daily.
⊠ **Adjust-a-dose:** For patients with moderate hepatic impairment (Child-Pugh B), initial dose is 5 mg daily, p.r.n., Don't exceed 10 mg daily. For patients taking ritonavir, don't exceed 2.5 mg in a 72-hour period. For patients taking itraconazole 400 mg daily or ketoconazole 400 mg daily, don't exceed 2.5 mg daily. For patients taking erythromycin, itraconazole 200 mg daily or ketoconazole 200 mg daily, don't exceed 5 mg daily.

Contraindications and precautions

• Contraindicated in patients hypersensitive to drug or its components, and in those taking nitrates or alpha blockers.

Rapid onset   *Liquid form contains alcohol.*   ◆Canada   ◇ Australia   †OTC   ‡Off-label use

• Use cautiously in patients with unstable angina; hypotension (systolic lower than 90 mm Hg); uncontrolled hypertension (blood pressure higher than 170/110 mm Hg); CVA, life-threatening arrhythmia, or MI within 6 months; severe cardiac failure; severe hepatic impairment (Child-Pugh C); end stage renal disease requiring dialysis; hereditary degenerative retinal disorders; hepatic or renal dysfunction; anatomical deformation of the penis; or prolonged QT interval. Also use cautiously in patients taking Class IA or Class III antiarrhythmics and in those with conditions that predispose them to priapism (sickle cell anemia, multiple myeloma, or leukemia).

⚖ Lifespan: Drug is only indicated for adult men. Men age 65 and older have reduced drug clearance.

Adverse reactions

CNS: *headache,* dizziness.
CV: *flushing.*
EENT: rhinitis, sinusitis.
GI: dyspepsia, nausea.
Musculoskeletal: back pain.
Other: flulike syndrome.

Interactions

Drug-drug. *Alpha-adrenergic blockers:* Enhances hypotensive effects. Don't use together.
Erythromycin, itraconazole 200 mg daily, ketoconazole 200 mg daily: Increases vardenafil level. Don't exceed 5 mg daily.
Itraconazole 400 mg daily, ketoconazole 400 mg daily: Increases vardenafil level. Don't exceed 2.5 mg daily.
Nitrates: Enhances hypotensive effects. Don't use together.
Ritonavir: Increases vardenafil level. Don't exceed 2.5 mg in a 72-hour period.
Drug-food. *High-fat meals:* Reduces peak level of drug. Advise patient to take on empty stomach.

Effects on lab test results

• May increase CK level.

Pharmacokinetics

Absorption: Rapid. Absolute bioavailability is 15%.
Distribution: Both drug and its major active metabolite are 95% bound to proteins. Protein-binding is reversible and independent of drug level.
Metabolism: Primarily through CYP 3A4, along with CYP 3A5 and CYP 2c isoenzymes. N-desmethylation converts drug into the major metabolite, which accounts for 7% of drug.
Excretion: Predominately in feces. *Half-life:* 4 to 5 hours.

Route	Onset	Peak	Duration
P.O.	Immediate	30-120 min	Unknown

Action

Chemical effect: Selectively inhibits cGMP-specific phosphodiesterase type 5 and prevents the breakdown of cGMP by phosphodiesterase, leading to increased cGMP level and prolonged smooth muscle relaxation promoting the flow of blood into the corpus cavernosum.
Therapeutic effect: Stimulates penile erection.

NURSING PROCESS

🗟 Assessment
• Assess patient's erectile dysfunction before therapy and regularly thereafter.
• Be alert for adverse reactions and drug interactions.
• Evaluate patient's and family's knowledge of drug therapy.

🖏 Nursing diagnoses
• Sexual dysfunction related to process of erectile dysfunction
• Chronic low self-esteem related to erectile dysfunction
• Deficient knowledge related to drug therapy

▶ Planning and implementation
Ⓢ **ALERT:** Because of cardiac risk during sexual activity, drug increases risk for patients with underlying CV disease.
Patient teaching
• Tell patient that drug doesn't protect against sexually transmitted diseases and that he should use protective measures to prevent infection.
• Advise patient that drug is most rapidly absorbed if taken on an empty stomach.
• Tell patient to notify prescriber of visual changes.
• Instruct patient to seek medical attention if erection persists for more than 4 hours.

Reactions may be *common,* uncommon, *life-threatening,* or COMMON AND LIFE-THREATENING.

• Tell patient to take drug 60 minutes before anticipated sexual activity. The drug will have no effect in the absence of sexual stimulation.
• Tell patient not to take drug more than once per day.

☑ **Evaluation**
• Patient states improvement in sexual functioning.
• Patient demonstrates increased self-esteem.
• Patient and family state understanding of drug therapy.

vasopressin (ADH)
(VAY-soh-preh-sin)
Pitressin

Pharmacologic class: posterior pituitary hormone
Therapeutic class: ADH, peristaltic stimulant
Pregnancy risk category: C

Indications and dosages

▶ **Neurogenic diabetes insipidus.** *Adults:* 5 to 10 units I.M. or S.C. b.i.d. to q.i.d., p.r.n. Range 5 to 60 units daily. Or, intranasally (aqueous solution used as spray or applied to cotton balls) in individualized doses, based on response. *Children:* 2.5 to 10 units I.M. or S.C. b.i.d. to q.i.d., p.r.n. Or, intranasally (aqueous solution used as spray or applied to cotton balls) in individualized doses.
▶ **Postoperative abdominal distention.** *Adults:* Initially, 5 units (aqueous) I.M.; then q 3 to 4 hours, increasing dose to 10 units, if needed. Reduce dose proportionally for children.
▶ **To expel gas before abdominal X-ray.** *Adults:* 10 units S.C. 2 hours before X-ray; then again 30 minutes later.
▶ **Provocative testing for growth hormone and corticotropin release‡.** *Adults:* 10 units I.M. *Children:* 0.3 units/kg I.M.
▶ **G.I. hemorrhage‡.** *Adults:* 0.2 to 0.4 units/ minute I.V. Increase up to 0.9 units/minute p.r.n. Or, 0.1 to 0.5 units/minute intra-arterially.

▼ I.V. administration

• Drug is used I.V. for G.I. hemorrhage only.
• Dilute with normal saline solution or D₅W to concentration of 0.1 to 1 unit/ml.

Contraindications and precautions

• Contraindicated in patients with chronic nephritis accompanied by nitrogen retention.
• Use cautiously in preoperative and postoperative polyuric patients, and those with seizure disorders, migraine headache, asthma, CV disease, heart failure, renal disease, goiter with cardiac complications, arteriosclerosis, or fluid overload.
🛎 **Lifespan:** In pregnant and breast-feeding women, children, and geriatric patients, use cautiously.

Adverse reactions

CNS: tremor, vertigo, headache.
CV: angina in patients with vascular disease, vasoconstriction, *arrhythmias, cardiac arrest, myocardial ischemia,* circumoral pallor, decreased cardiac output.
GI: abdominal cramps, nausea, vomiting, flatulence.
Skin: cutaneous gangrene, diaphoresis.
Other: *water intoxication* (drowsiness, listlessness, headache, confusion, weight gain, *seizures, coma*), *hypersensitivity reactions* (urticaria, *angioedema, bronchoconstriction, anaphylaxis*).

Interactions

Drug-drug. *Carbamazepine, chlorpropamide, clofibrate, fludrocortisone, tricyclic antidepressants:* Increases antidiuretic response. Use together cautiously.
Demeclocycline, heparin, lithium, norepinephrine: Reduces antidiuretic activity. Use together cautiously.
Drug-lifestyle. *Alcohol use:* Reduces antidiuretic activity. Discourage use together.

Effects on lab test results

None reported.

Pharmacokinetics

Absorption: Unknown.
Distribution: Throughout extracellular fluid without evidence of protein-binding.
Metabolism: Most of drug is destroyed rapidly in liver and kidneys.
Excretion: In urine. *Half-life:* 10 to 20 minutes.

Route	Onset	Peak	Duration
S.C., I.M., intranasal	Unknown	Unknown	2-8 hr

Action

Chemical effect: Increases permeability of renal tubular epithelium to adenosine monophosphate and water; epithelium promotes reabsorption of water and produces concentrated urine (ADH effect).
Therapeutic effect: Promotes water reabsorption and stimulates GI motility.

Available forms

Injection: 0.5-, 1-, and 10-ml ampules (20 units/ml)

NURSING PROCESS

Assessment

• Assess patient's condition before therapy and regularly thereafter.
• Monitor specific gravity of urine and fluid intake and output to aid evaluation of drug effectiveness.
• To prevent possible seizures, coma, and death, observe patient closely for early signs of water intoxication.
• Monitor blood pressure of patient on vasopressin frequently. Watch for excessively elevated blood pressure or lack of response to drug, which may be indicated by hypotension. Also monitor daily weight.
• Be alert for adverse reactions and drug interactions.
• Evaluate patient's and family's knowledge of drug therapy.

Nursing diagnoses

• Risk for deficient fluid volume related to polyuria from diabetes insipidus
• Diarrhea related to drug-induced increased GI motility
• Deficient knowledge related to drug therapy

Planning and implementation

• Drug may be used for transient polyuria resulting from ADH deficiency related to neurosurgery or head injury.
• To reduce adverse reactions, use minimum effective dosage.
• Give drug with one to two glasses of water to reduce adverse reactions and to improve therapeutic response.
• A rectal tube facilitates gas expulsion after vasopressin injection.

⊛ **ALERT:** Never inject during first stage of labor; doing so may cause uterus to rupture.
• Aqueous solution can be used as a nasal spray or applied to cotton balls. Follow manufacturer's guidelines for intranasal use.
⊛ **ALERT:** Don't confuse vasopressin with desmopressin.
Patient teaching
• Instruct patient how to give drug. Tell patient taking drug S.C. to rotate injection sites to prevent tissue damage.
• Stress importance of monitoring fluid intake and output.
• Tell patient to notify prescriber immediately if adverse reactions occur.

Evaluation

• Patient maintains adequate hydration.
• Patient doesn't experience diarrhea.
• Patient and family state understanding of drug therapy.

vecuronium bromide
(veh-kyoo-ROH-nee-um BROH-mighd)
Norcuron

Pharmacologic class: nondepolarizing neuromuscular blocker
Therapeutic class: skeletal muscle relaxant
Pregnancy risk category: C

Indications and dosages

▶ **Adjunct to general anesthesia; to facilitate endotracheal intubation; to provide skeletal muscle relaxation during surgery or mechanical ventilation. Dosage depends on anesthetic used, individual needs, and response. Dosages are representative and must be adjusted.** *Adults and children age 10 and older:* Initially, 0.08 to 0.1 mg/kg I.V. bolus. During prolonged surgery give maintenance doses of 0.01 to 0.015 mg/kg within 25 to 40 minutes of initial dose. Maintenance doses may be given q 12 to 15 minutes in patients receiving balanced anesthesia. Or, drug may be given by continuous I.V. infusion of 1 mcg/kg/minute initially, then 0.8 to 1.2 mcg/kg/minute.
Children younger than age 10: May require slightly higher initial dose as well as supplementation slightly more often than adults.

▼ I.V. administration

• Give drug by rapid I.V. injection. Or, 10 to 20 mg may be added to 100 ml of compatible solution and given by I.V. infusion.
• Compatible solutions include D₅W, normal saline solution for injection, dextrose 5% in normal saline solution for injection, and lactated Ringer's injection.
• Don't mix drug with alkaline solutions.
• Store reconstituted solution in refrigerator. Discard after 24 hours.

Contraindications and precautions

• Contraindicated in patients hypersensitive to bromides.
• Use cautiously in patients with altered circulation caused by CV disease and edematous states, and in patients with hepatic disease, severe obesity, bronchogenic carcinoma, electrolyte disturbances, or neuromuscular disease.
⚹ Lifespan: In pregnant and breast-feeding women and geriatric patients, use cautiously.

Adverse reactions

Musculoskeletal: skeletal muscle weakness.
Respiratory: *prolonged, dose-related respiratory insufficiency or apnea.*

Interactions

Drug-drug. *Amikacin, gentamicin, neomycin, streptomycin, tobramycin:* May increase the effects of nondepolarizing muscle relaxant, including prolonged respiratory depression. Use together only when necessary. May need to reduce dose of nondepolarizing muscle relaxant.
Carbamazepine, phenytoin: May decrease the effects of vecuronium. May need to increase dose of the vecuronium.
Kanamycin; bacitracin; clindamycin; general anesthetics, such as enflurane, halothane, isoflurane; other skeletal muscle relaxants; polymyxin antibiotics such as colistin, polymyxin B sulfate; quinidine; tetracyclines: Potentiates neuromuscular blockade, leading to increased skeletal muscle relaxation and potentiation of effect. Use cautiously during surgical and postoperative periods.

Effects on lab test results

None reported.

Pharmacokinetics

Absorption: Administered I.V.

Distribution: In extracellular fluid; rapidly reaches its site of action (skeletal muscles); 60% to 90% protein-bound.
Metabolism: Hepatic; rapid and extensive.
Excretion: In feces and urine. *Half-life:* 20 minutes.

Route	Onset	Peak	Duration
I.V.	≤ 1 min	3-5 min	25-30 min

Action

Chemical effect: Prevents acetylcholine from binding to receptors on motor end plate, thus blocking depolarization.
Therapeutic effect: Relaxes skeletal muscle.

Available forms

Injection: 10 mg/vial, 20 mg/vial

NURSING PROCESS

⊡ Assessment
• Assess patient's condition before therapy and regularly thereafter.
• Monitor respiratory rate closely until patient is fully recovered from neuromuscular blockade as evidenced by tests of muscle strength (hand grip, head lift, and ability to cough).
• Be alert for adverse reactions and drug interactions.
• Evaluate patient's and family's knowledge of drug therapy.

⊡ Nursing diagnoses
• Ineffective health maintenance related to underlying condition
• Ineffective breathing pattern related to drug's effect on respiratory muscles
• Deficient knowledge related to drug therapy

▷ Planning and implementation
• Keep airway clear. Have emergency respiratory support equipment available immediately.
• Drug should be used only by personnel skilled in airway management.
• Previous administration of succinylcholine may enhance neuromuscular blocking effect and duration of action.
• Give sedatives or general anesthetics before neuromuscular blockers. Neuromuscular blockers don't obtund consciousness or alter pain threshold.
• Give analgesics for pain.

• Nerve stimulator and train-of-four monitoring are recommended to confirm antagonism of neuromuscular blockade and recovery of muscle strength. Before attempting pharmacologic reversal with neostigmine, some evidence of spontaneous recovery should be seen.

⊛ **ALERT:** Careful dosage calculation is essential. Always verify with another health care professional.

• Don't give by I.M. injection.

Patient teaching
• Explain all events and happenings to patient because he can still hear.
• Reassure patient that he is being monitored at all times.

☑ Evaluation
• Patient responds well to drug.
• Patient maintains effective breathing pattern with mechanical assistance.
• Patient and family state understanding of drug therapy.

venlafaxine hydrochloride
(ven-leh-FAKS-een high-droh-KLOR-ighd)
Effexor, Effexor XR

Pharmacologic class: neuronal serotonin, norepinephrine, and dopamine reuptake inhibitor
Therapeutic class: antidepressant
Pregnancy risk category: C

Indications and dosages

▶ **Depression.** *Adults:* Initially, 75 mg P.O. daily in two or three divided doses, or 75 mg (extended-release) P.O. once daily with food. With both forms, increase dosage as tolerated and needed in increments of 75 mg daily at intervals of no less than 4 days. For moderately depressed outpatients, usual maximum dosage is 225 mg daily; in certain severely depressed patients, dosage may be as high as 350 mg daily.

▶ **Generalized or social anxiety disorder.** *Adults:* 75 mg (extended-release) P.O. once daily. May increase p.r.n. in increments of 75 mg daily at intervals of no less than 4 days to maximum of 225 mg daily.

▶ **Prevention of major depressive disorder relapse‡.** *Adults:* 100 to 200 mg P.O. daily, or 75 to 225 mg (extended-release) P.O. daily.

⧄ **Adjust-a-dose:** For patients with hepatic impairment, reduce total daily dose by one-half. For patients with mild to moderate renal impairment (GFR of 10 to 70 ml/minute), reduce total daily dose by one-quarter to one-half. In patients undergoing hemodialysis, withhold dose until dialysis session is completed; reduce daily dose by one-half.

Contraindications and precautions

• Contraindicated in patients hypersensitive to drug and in those who took an MAO inhibitor within 14 days.
• Use cautiously in patients with renal impairment or diseases, in those with conditions that could affect hemodynamic responses or metabolism, and in those with a history of mania or seizures.

⚘ **Lifespan:** In pregnant and breast-feeding women, use cautiously. In children, safety of drug hasn't been established.

Adverse reactions

CNS: *asthenia, headache, somnolence, dizziness, nervousness, insomnia,* anxiety, tremor, abnormal dreams, paresthesia, agitation.
CV: hypertension.
EENT: blurred vision.
GI: *nausea, constipation,* vomiting, *dry mouth, anorexia,* diarrhea, dyspepsia, flatulence.
GU: *abnormal ejaculation,* impotence, urinary frequency, impaired urination.
Metabolic: weight loss.
Skin: *diaphoresis,* rash.
Other: yawning, chills, infection.

Interactions

Drug-drug. *Haloperidol:* Increases haloperidol level. Use together cautiously.
Phenelzine, selegiline, tranylcypromine: May cause serotonin syndrome, which includes CNS irritability, shivering, and altered consciousness. Don't give together. Wait at least 2 weeks after stopping an MAO inhibitor before giving any SSRI.
Trazodone: May cause serotonin syndrome. Avoid use together.
Drug-herb. *St. John's wort:* Increases sedative-hypnotic effects. Discourage use together.

Yohimbe: May cause additive stimulation. Discourage use together.

Effects on lab test results

None reported.

Pharmacokinetics

Absorption: About 92%.
Distribution: About 25% to 29% protein-bound in plasma.
Metabolism: Extensively metabolized in liver.
Excretion: Excreted in urine. *Half-life:* 5 hours.

Route	Onset	Peak	Duration
P.O.	Unknown	Unknown	Unknown

Action

Chemical effect: Blocks reuptake of norepinephrine and serotonin into neurons in CNS.
Therapeutic effect: Relieves depression.

Available forms

Capsules (extended-release): 37.5 mg, 75 mg, 150 mg
Tablets: 25 mg, 37.5 mg, 50 mg, 75 mg, 100 mg

NURSING PROCESS

Assessment

• Assess patient's depression before therapy and regularly thereafter.
• Carefully monitor blood pressure. Venlafaxine therapy is linked to sustained, dose-dependent increases in blood pressure. Greatest increases (averaging about 7 mm Hg above baseline) occur in patients taking 375 mg daily.
• Be alert for adverse reactions and drug interactions.
• Evaluate patient's and family's knowledge of drug therapy.

Nursing diagnoses

• Disturbed thought processes related to presence of depression
• Risk for injury related to drug-induced adverse CNS reactions
• Deficient knowledge related to drug therapy

Planning and implementation

• Give drug with food.
• ALERT: If given for 6 weeks or more, don't stop drug abruptly; taper dosage over a 2-week period.

Patient teaching

• Instruct patient to take drug with food.
• Warn patient to avoid hazardous activities until full effects of drug are known.
• Tell patient it may take several weeks before the full antidepressant effect is seen.
• Tell patient to avoid alcohol while taking drug and to notify prescriber before taking other medications, including OTC preparations, because of possible interactions.
• Instruct patient to notify prescriber if adverse reactions occur.

Evaluation

• Patient's behavior and communication exhibit improved thought processes.
• Patient doesn't experience injury from adverse CNS reactions.
• Patient and family state understanding of drug therapy.

verapamil hydrochloride
(veh-RAP-uh-mil high-droh-KLOR-ighd)
Anpec ◇, Anpec SR ◇, Apo-Verap ♦, Calan, Calan SR, Cordilox ◇, Cordilox SR ◇, Covera-HS, Isoptin ◇, Isoptin SR, Novo-Veramil ♦, Nu-Verap ♦, Veracaps SR ◇, Verahexal ◇, Verelan, Verelan PM

Pharmacologic class: calcium channel blocker
Therapeutic class: antianginal, antihypertensive, antiarrhythmic
Pregnancy risk category: C

Indications and dosages

▶ **Vasospastic angina; classic chronic, stable angina pectoris; unstable angina; chronic atrial fibrillation.** *Adults:* Starting dose is 80 mg P.O. q 6 to 8 hours. Increase at weekly intervals, p.r.n. Some patients may need up to 480 mg daily. Or, 180 mg Covera-HS P.O. h.s.; maximum, 480 mg P.O. daily h.s.
▶ **Supraventricular arrhythmias.** *Adults:* 0.075 to 0.15 mg/kg (5 to 10 mg) by I.V. push over 2 minutes with ECG and blood pressure monitoring. If no response occurs, give a second dose of 10 mg (0.15 mg/kg) 30 minutes after the initial dose.
Children ages 1 to 15: 0.1 to 0.3 mg/kg as I.V. bolus over 2 minutes. Repeat in 30 minutes if no response.

Children younger than age 1: 0.1 to 0.2 mg/kg as I.V. bolus over at least 2 minutes with continuous ECG monitoring. Repeat in 30 minutes if no response.

▶ **Prevention of recurrent PSVT.** *Adults:* 240 to 480 mg P.O. daily in three or four divided doses.

▶ **To control ventricular rate in digitalized patients with chronic atrial flutter or atrial fibrillation.** *Adults:* 240 to 320 mg P.O. in three or four divided doses.

▶ **Hypertension.** *Adults:* Start therapy with sustained-release capsules at 120 mg (240 mg for Verelan) P.O. daily in the morning. Adjust dosage based on effectiveness 24 hours after dosing. Increase in increments of 120 mg daily to a maximum of 480 mg daily. Or, Covera-HS 180 mg P.O. daily h.s. or Verelan PM 200 mg P.O. h.s.

▼ I.V. administration

● Give drug by direct injection into vein or into tubing of free-flowing, compatible I.V. solution.
● Compatible solutions include D₅W, half-normal and normal saline solutions, and Ringer's and lactated Ringer's solutions.
● Give I.V. doses slowly over at least 2 minutes (3 minutes for geriatric patients) to minimize risk of adverse reactions.
● Perform continuous ECG and blood pressure monitoring during administration.

Contraindications and precautions

● Contraindicated in patients hypersensitive to drug and those with severe left ventricular dysfunction; cardiogenic shock; second- or third-degree AV block or sick sinus syndrome, except in presence of functioning pacemaker; atrial flutter or fibrillation and accessory bypass tract syndrome; severe heart failure (unless secondary to verapamil therapy); or severe hypotension.
● I.V. verapamil is contraindicated in patients with ventricular tachycardia and in those receiving I.V. beta blockers.
● Use cautiously in patients with increased intracranial pressure or hepatic or renal disease.
⚰ Lifespan: In pregnant women and geriatric patients, use cautiously. In breast-feeding women, drug isn't recommended.

Adverse reactions

CNS: dizziness, headache, asthenia.

CV: transient hypotension, *heart failure, bradycardia, AV block, ventricular asystole, ventricular fibrillation,* peripheral edema.
GI: constipation, nausea.
Respiratory: *pulmonary edema.*
Skin: rash.

Interactions

Drug-drug. *Acebutolol, atenolol, betaxolol, carteolol, esmolol, metoprolol, nadolol, penbutolol, pindolol, propranolol, timolol:* May increase the effects of both drugs. Monitor cardiac function closely and decrease dosages, p.r.n.
Antihypertensives, quinidine: May cause hypotension. Monitor blood pressure.
Carbamazepine, digoxin: May increase levels of these drugs. Monitor patient for toxicity.
Cyclosporine: May increase cyclosporine level. Monitor cyclosporine level.
Disopyramide, flecainide, propranolol, other beta blockers: May cause heart failure. Use together cautiously.
Lithium: May decrease lithium level. Monitor patient closely.
Rifampin: May decrease oral bioavailability of verapamil. Monitor patient for lack of effect.
Drug-herb. *Black catechu:* May cause additive effects. Tell patient to use together cautiously.
Yerba maté: May decrease clearance of yerba maté methylxanthines and cause toxicity. Discourage concomitant use.
Drug-food. *Any food:* Increases drug absorption. Tell patient to take drug with food.
Drug-lifestyle. *Alcohol use:* May enhance effects of alcohol. Discourage use together.

Effects on lab test results

● May increase ALT, AST, alkaline phosphatase, and bilirubin levels.

Pharmacokinetics

Absorption: Rapid and complete from GI tract after P.O. administration; only about 20% to 35% reaches systemic circulation.
Distribution: About 90% of circulating drug is bound to proteins.
Metabolism: In liver.
Excretion: In urine as unchanged drug and active metabolites. *Half-life:* 6 to 12 hours.

Route	Onset	Peak	Duration
P.O.	1-2 hr	1-9 hr	8-24 hr
I.V.	Rapid	Immediate	1-6 hr

Reactions may be *common*, uncommon, *life-threatening*, or COMMON AND LIFE-THREATENING.

Action

Chemical effect: Not clearly defined; inhibits calcium ion influx across cardiac and smooth-muscle cells, thus decreasing myocardial contractility and oxygen demand. Drug also dilates coronary arteries and arterioles.
Therapeutic effect: Relieves angina, lowers blood pressure, and restores normal sinus rhythm.

Available forms

Capsules (extended-release): 120 mg, 180 mg, 240 mg
Capsules (sustained-release): 120 mg, 160 mg ◊, 180 mg, 200 mg, 240 mg, 360 mg
Injection: 2.5 mg/ml
Tablets: 40 mg, 80 mg, 120 mg, 160 mg ◊
Tablets (extended-release): 100 mg, 120 mg, 180 mg, 200 mg, 240mg, 300 mg
Tablets (sustained-release): 120 mg, 180 mg, 240 mg

NURSING PROCESS

⚖ Assessment

• Assess patient's condition before therapy and regularly thereafter.
• Monitor blood pressure at start of therapy and during dosage adjustments.
• Monitor liver function studies during prolonged treatment.
• Be alert for adverse reactions and drug interactions.
• Evaluate patient's and family's knowledge of drug therapy.

🔲 Nursing diagnoses

• Acute pain related to presence of angina
• Decreased cardiac output related to presence of arrhythmia
• Deficient knowledge related to drug therapy

▷ Planning and implementation

• Give lower doses to patient with severely compromised cardiac function or patient taking beta blockers.
• Give drug with food, but keep in mind that giving extended-release tablets with food may decrease rate and extent of absorption. It also produces smaller fluctuations of peak and trough levels.

• If drug is being used to terminate supraventricular tachycardia, prescriber may have patient perform vagal maneuvers after receiving drug.
• Assist patient with walking because dizziness may occur.
• If patient has signs of heart failure, such as swelling of hands and feet or shortness of breath, notify prescriber.
⚠ ALERT: Don't confuse Isoptin with Intropin; don't confuse Verelan with Vivarin, Voltaren, Ferralyn, or Virilon.
Patient teaching
• Instruct patient to take drug with food.
• If patient is kept on nitrate therapy during adjustment of oral verapamil dosage, urge continued compliance. S.L. nitroglycerin, especially, may be taken p.r.n. when angina is acute.
• Encourage patient to increase fluid and fiber intake to combat constipation. Give stool softener.
• Instruct patient to report adverse reactions, especially swelling of hands and feet and shortness of breath.

☑ Evaluation
• Patient has reduced severity or frequency of angina.
• Patient regains normal cardiac output with restoration of normal sinus rhythm.
• Patient and family state understanding of drug therapy.

vinblastine sulfate (VLB)

(vin-BLAH-steen SUL-fayt)
Velban, Velbe ♦ ◊

Pharmacologic class: vinca alkaloid (specific to M phase of cell cycle)
Therapeutic class: antineoplastic
Pregnancy risk category: D

Indications and dosages

▶ **Breast or testicular cancer, Hodgkin's and non-Hodgkin's lymphoma, choriocarcinoma, lymphosarcoma, mycosis fungoides, Kaposi's sarcoma, histiocytosis.** *Adults:* 0.1 mg/kg or 3.7 mg/m² I.V. weekly or q 2 weeks. May be increased to maximum of 0.5 mg/kg or 18.5 mg/m² weekly according to response. If WBC count is less than 4,000/mm³, don't repeat dose.

▶ **Letterer-Siwe disease (histiocytosis X).** *Children:* 6.5 mg/m². Dosage modifications should be made according to hematologic response.
▶ **Hodgkin's disease.** *Children:* 6 mg/ m² with other agents. Dosage modifications should be made according to hematologic response.
▶ **Testicular germ cell carcinoma.** *Children:* 3 mg/ m² with other agents. Dosage modifications should be made according to hematologic response.
🛇 **Adjust-a-dose:** If bilirubin level is greater than 3 mg/dl, decrease dosage by half.

▼ I.V. administration

• Follow facility policy to reduce risks. Preparation and administration of parenteral form are linked to carcinogenic, mutagenic, and teratogenic risks for personnel.
• Reconstitute drug in 10-mg vial with 10 ml of saline solution injection or sterile water. This yields 1 mg/ml.
• Inject drug directly into vein or running I.V. line over 1 minute. Drug also may be given in 50 ml of D₅W or normal saline solution infused over 15 minutes.
• If extravasation occurs, stop infusion immediately and notify prescriber. Manufacturer recommends that moderate heat be applied to area of leakage. Local injection of hyaluronidase may help disperse drug. Some clinicians prefer to apply ice packs on and off q 2 hours for 24 hours, with local injection of hydrocortisone or normal saline solution.
• Refrigerate reconstituted solution. Discard after 30 days.

Contraindications and precautions

• Contraindicated in patients with severe leukopenia or bacterial infection.
• Use cautiously in patients with hepatic dysfunction.
⚠ **Lifespan:** In pregnant and breast-feeding women, drug isn't recommended.

Adverse reactions

CNS: depression, *paresthesia, peripheral neuropathy and neuritis, numbness, loss of deep tendon reflexes, seizures, CVA,* headache.
CV: hypertension, *MI, phlebitis.*
EENT: pharyngitis.

GI: *nausea, vomiting,* ulcer, *bleeding, constipation, ileus, anorexia,* diarrhea, abdominal pain, *stomatitis.*
GU: oligospermia, aspermia, urine retention.
Hematologic: anemia, *leukopenia* (nadir on days 4 to 10; lasts another 7 to 14 days), *thrombocytopenia.*
Metabolic: hyperuricemia, *weight loss.*
Musculoskeletal: uric acid nephropathy, *muscle pain and weakness.*
Respiratory: *acute bronchospasm,* shortness of breath.
Skin: reversible alopecia, vesiculation, cellulitis, necrosis with extravasation.

Interactions

Drug-drug. *Erythromycin, other drugs that inhibit CYP pathway:* May increase toxicity of vinblastine. Monitor patient closely.
Mitomycin: Increases risk of bronchospasm and shortness of breath. Monitor patient closely.
Phenytoin: Decreases phenytoin level. Monitor patient closely.

Effects on lab test results

• May increase uric acid level.
• May decrease hemoglobin, hematocrit, and WBC and platelet counts.

Pharmacokinetics

Absorption: Administered I.V.
Distribution: Widely in body tissues; crosses blood-brain barrier but doesn't achieve therapeutic level in CSF.
Metabolism: Partially in liver to active metabolite.
Excretion: Primarily in bile as unchanged drug; smaller portion excreted in urine. *Half-life:* Alpha phase, 3¾ minutes; beta phase, 1½ hours; terminal phase, 25 hours.

Route	Onset	Peak	Duration
I.V.	Unknown	Unknown	Unknown

Action

Chemical effect: Arrests mitosis in metaphase, blocking cell division.
Therapeutic effect: Inhibits replication of certain cancer cells.

Available forms

Injection: 10-mg vials (lyophilized powder), 1 mg/ml in 10-ml vials

---

⚕ Assessment
• Assess patient's condition before therapy and regularly thereafter.
③ ALERT: After giving drug, monitor patient for development of life-threatening acute bronchospasm. Reaction is most likely if patient also receives mitomycin.
• Be alert for adverse reactions and drug interactions.
• Assess for numbness and tingling in hands and feet. Assess gait for early evidence of footdrop. Drug is less neurotoxic than vincristine.
• Evaluate patient's and family's knowledge of drug therapy.

⊞ Nursing diagnoses
• Ineffective health maintenance related to presence of neoplastic disease
• Ineffective protection related to drug-induced adverse hematologic reactions
• Deficient knowledge related to drug therapy

⊠ Planning and implementation
• Give antiemetic before giving drug.
• Don't give drug into limb with compromised circulation.
③ ALERT: Drug is fatal if given intrathecally; it's for I.V. use only.
• If acute bronchospasm occurs after administration, notify prescriber immediately.
• Make sure patient maintains adequate fluid intake to facilitate excretion of uric acid.
• If stomatitis occurs, stop drug and notify prescriber.
• Don't repeat dose more frequently than q 7 days to prevent severe leukopenia.
③ ALERT: Don't confuse vinblastine with vincristine or vindesine.
Patient teaching
• Teach patient about infection-control and bleeding precautions.
• Warn patient that alopecia may occur, but that it's usually reversible.
• Tell patient to report adverse reactions promptly.
• Encourage adequate fluid intake to increase urine output and facilitate excretion of uric acid.

☑ Evaluation
• Patient responds well to drug.

• Patient doesn't develop serious complications from adverse hematologic reactions.
• Patient and family state understanding of drug therapy.

vincristine sulfate
(vin-KRIH-steen SUL-fayt)
Oncovin, Vincasar PFS

Pharmacologic class: vinca alkaloid (specific to M phase of cell cycle)
Therapeutic class: antineoplastic
Pregnancy risk category: D

Indications and dosages
▶ **Breast cancer‡, acute lymphoblastic and other leukemias, Hodgkin's disease, non-Hodgkin's lymphoma, neuroblastoma, rhabdomyosarcoma, Wilms' tumor.** *Adults:* 1.4 mg/m² I.V. weekly. Maximum, 2 mg weekly.
Children weighing more than 10 kg (22 lb): 1.5 to 2 mg/m² I.V. weekly. Maximum single dose is 2 mg.
Children weighing 10 kg or less: 0.05 mg/kg I.V. once weekly.

▼ I.V. administration
• Follow facility policy to reduce risks. Preparation and administration of parenteral form are linked to carcinogenic, mutagenic, and teratogenic risks for personnel.
• Inject drug directly into vein or running I.V. line slowly over 1 minute. Drug also may be given in 50 ml of D₅W or normal saline solution infused over 15 minutes.
• If drug extravasates, stop infusion immediately and notify prescriber. Apply heat on and off q 2 hours for 24 hours. Give 150 units of hyaluronidase to area of infiltrate.
• All vials (1-, 2-, and 5-mg) contain 1 mg/ml solution and should be refrigerated.

Contraindications and precautions
• Contraindicated in patients hypersensitive to drug and in those with demyelinating form of Charcot-Marie-Tooth syndrome. Don't give drug to patients who are receiving radiation therapy through ports that include the liver.
• Use cautiously in patients with hepatic dysfunction, neuromuscular disease, or infection.

⚸ **Lifespan:** In pregnant and breast-feeding women, drug isn't recommended.

Adverse reactions

CNS: fever, *peripheral neuropathy,* sensory loss, *loss of deep tendon reflexes, paresthesia, wristdrop and footdrop,* headache, ataxia, cranial nerve palsies, *jaw pain,* hoarseness, vocal cord paralysis, *seizures, coma, permanent neurotoxicity.*
CV: hypotension, hypertension, *phlebitis.*
EENT: visual disturbances, diplopia, optic and extraocular neuropathy, ptosis.
GI: diarrhea, *constipation, cramps,* ileus that mimics surgical abdomen, *nausea, vomiting,* anorexia, dysphagia, *intestinal necrosis, stomatitis.*
GU: urine retention, dysuria, acute uric acid neuropathy, polyuria.
Hematologic: anemia, *leukopenia, thrombocytopenia.*
Metabolic: hyponatremia, hyperuricemia, weight loss.
Musculoskeletal: *muscle weakness and cramps.*
Respiratory: *acute bronchospasm.*
Skin: rash, *reversible alopecia,* cellulitis at injection site, severe local reaction with extravasation.
Other: SIADH.

Interactions

Drug-drug. *Asparaginase:* Decreases hepatic clearance of vincristine. Monitor patient closely for toxicity.
Calcium channel blockers: Enhances vincristine accumulation. Monitor patient for toxicity.
Digoxin: Decreases digoxin effects. Monitor digoxin level.
Mitomycin: Possible increased frequency of bronchospasm and acute pulmonary reactions. Monitor patient closely.
Phenytoin: May reduce phenytoin level. Monitor patient closely.

Effects on lab test results

● May increase uric acid level. May decrease sodium level.
● May decrease hemoglobin, hematocrit, and WBC and platelet counts.

Pharmacokinetics

Absorption: Administered I.V.

Distribution: Wide. Bound to erythrocytes and platelets; crosses blood-brain barrier but doesn't achieve therapeutic level in CSF.
Metabolism: Extensively in liver.
Excretion: Primarily in bile; smaller portion excreted in urine. *Half-life:* First phase, 4 minutes; second phase, 2¼ hours; terminal phase, 85 hours.

Route	Onset	Peak	Duration
I.V.	Unknown	Unknown	Unknown

Action

Chemical effect: Arrests mitosis in metaphase, blocking cell division.
Therapeutic effect: Inhibits replication of certain cancer cells.

Available forms

Injection: 1 mg/ml in 1-, 2-, and 5-ml multiple-dose vials; 1 mg/ml in 1- and 2-ml preservative-free vials

NURSING PROCESS

✍ Assessment

● Assess patient's condition before therapy and regularly thereafter.
🛈 **ALERT:** After giving drug, monitor patient for development of life-threatening acute bronchospasm. Reaction is most likely to occur if patient also receives mitomycin.
● Monitor patient for hyperuricemia, especially if he has leukemia or lymphoma.
● Be alert for adverse reactions and drug interactions.
● Check for depression of Achilles tendon reflex, numbness, tingling, footdrop or wristdrop, difficulty in walking, ataxia, and slapping gait. Also check ability to walk on heels.
● Monitor bowel function. Constipation may be early sign of neurotoxicity.
● Evaluate patient's and family's knowledge of drug therapy.

🔲 Nursing diagnoses

● Ineffective health maintenance related to presence of neoplastic disease
● Ineffective protection related to drug-induced adverse hematologic reactions
● Deficient knowledge related to drug therapy

Reactions may be *common,* uncommon, *life-threatening,* or **COMMON AND LIFE-THREATENING.**

⟩ Planning and implementation
- Give antiemetic before drug.
- Don't give drug to one patient as single dose. The 5-mg vials are for multiple-dose use.
- ⚇ **ALERT:** Drug is fatal if given intrathecally; it's for I.V. use only.
- Because of risk of neurotoxicity, don't give drug more than once a week. Children are more resistant to neurotoxicity than adults. Neurotoxicity is dose-related and usually reversible.
- If acute bronchospasm occurs after administration, notify prescriber immediately.
- Maintain good hydration and give allopurinol to prevent uric acid nephropathy.
- If SIADH develops, fluid restriction may be needed.
- Give stool softener, laxative, or water before dosing to help prevent constipation.
- ⚇ **ALERT:** Don't confuse vincristine with vinblastine or vindesine.

Patient teaching
- Instruct patient on infection control and bleeding precautions.
- Warn patient that alopecia may occur, but that it's usually reversible.
- Tell patient to report adverse reactions promptly.
- Encourage fluid intake to facilitate excretion of uric acid.
- Advise woman of childbearing age to avoid becoming pregnant during therapy. Also recommend that she consult with prescriber before becoming pregnant.

☑ Evaluation
- Patient responds well to drug.
- Patient doesn't develop serious complications from adverse hematologic reactions.
- Patient and family state understanding of drug therapy.

vinorelbine tartrate
(vin-oh-REL-been TAR-trayt)
Navelbine

Pharmacologic class: semisynthetic vinca alkaloid
Therapeutic class: antineoplastic
Pregnancy risk category: D

Indications and dosages

▶ **Alone or as adjunct therapy with cisplatin for first-line treatment of ambulatory patients with nonresectable advanced non–small-cell lung cancer; alone or with cisplatin in stage IV of non–small-cell lung cancer; with cisplatin in stage III of non–small-cell lung cancer.** *Adults:* 30 mg/m^2 I.V. weekly. In combination treatment, same dosage used along with 120 mg/m^2 of cisplatin, given on days 1 and 29, and then q 6 weeks.
▶ **Breast cancer‡.** *Adults:* 20 to 30 mg/m^2 I.V. over 20 to 60 minutes weekly. Or, 30 mg/m^2 over 3 to 5 minutes. If used in combination therapy, give 25 or 30 mg/m^2 I.V. in periodic doses. If used with mitoxantrone and ifosfamide, give 12 mg/m^2 I.V. in periodic doses.

▼ I.V. administration
- Drug must be diluted.
- Give drug I.V. over 6 to 10 minutes into side port of free-flowing I.V. line that is closest to I.V. bag. Afterward, flush with 75 to 125 ml of D$_5$W or normal saline solution.

Contraindications and precautions
- Contraindicated in patients with pretreatment granulocyte counts below 1,000 cells/mm^3.
- Use cautiously in patients whose bone marrow may have been compromised by previous exposure to radiation therapy or chemotherapy or whose bone marrow is still recovering from previous chemotherapy. Also use cautiously in patients with hepatic impairment.
- ☀ Lifespan: In pregnant and breast-feeding women, drug isn't recommended. In children, safety of drug hasn't been established.

Adverse reactions
CNS: *peripheral neuropathy, asthenia, fatigue.*
GI: *nausea, vomiting, anorexia, diarrhea, constipation, stomatitis.*
Hematologic: **bone marrow suppression** *(agranulocytosis,* LEUKOPENIA, *thrombocytopenia, anemia).*
Hepatic: *bilirubinemia.*
Musculoskeletal: jaw pain, chest pain, myalgia, arthralgia, loss of deep tendon reflexes.
Respiratory: *dyspnea.*
Skin: *alopecia, rash.*
Other: SIADH, *injection site pain or reaction.*

Interactions

Drug-drug. *Cisplatin:* Increases risk of bone marrow suppression when given with cisplatin. Monitor patient's hematologic status closely. *Mitomycin:* May cause pulmonary reactions. Monitor patient's respiratory status closely.

Effects on lab test results

• May increase bilirubin level.

• May decrease liver function test values, hemoglobin, hematocrit, and granulocyte, WBC, and platelet counts.

Pharmacokinetics

Absorption: Administered I.V.
Distribution: Widely in body tissues and bound to lymphocytes and platelets.
Metabolism: Extensively in liver.
Excretion: Primarily in bile; smaller portion excreted in urine. *Half-life:* 27¾ to 43½ hours.

Route	Onset	Peak	Duration
I.V.	Unknown	Unknown	Unknown

Action

Chemical effect: Arrests mitosis in metaphase, blocking cell division.
Therapeutic effect: Inhibits replication of selected cancer cells.

Available forms

Injection: 10 mg/ml, 50 mg/5 ml

NURSING PROCESS

Assessment

• Assess patient's condition before therapy and regularly thereafter.

• Monitor patient closely for hypersensitivity reactions.

• To judge effects of therapy, monitor patient's peripheral blood count and bone marrow.

• Be alert for adverse reactions and drug interactions.

• Assess patient for numbness and tingling in hands and feet. Assess gait for early evidence of footdrop.

• **ALERT:** Monitor patient's deep tendon reflexes; loss may indicate cumulative toxicity.

• Evaluate patient's and family's knowledge of drug therapy.

Nursing diagnoses

• Ineffective health maintenance related to presence of neoplastic disease

• Ineffective protection related to drug-induced adverse hematologic reactions

• Deficient knowledge related to drug therapy

Planning and implementation

• Give antiemetic before giving drug.

• Check patient's granulocyte count before administration; it should be 1,000/mm³ or more. If it's less, withhold drug and notify prescriber.

• Take care to avoid extravasation during administration because drug can cause considerable irritation, localized tissue necrosis, and thrombophlebitis. If extravasation occurs, stop drug immediately and inject remaining portion of dose into a different vein.

• **ALERT:** Drug is fatal if given intrathecally; it's for I.V. use only.

• Dosage adjustments are made according to hematologic toxicity or hepatic insufficiency, whichever results in lower dosage. If patient's granulocyte count falls between 1,000 and 1,500 cells/mm³, reduce dosage by half. If three consecutive doses are skipped because of agranulocytosis, stop drug.

• Drug may be a contact irritant, and solution must be handled and given with care. Gloves are recommended. Avoid inhaling vapors and allowing drug to contact skin or mucous membranes, especially those of eyes. In case of contact, wash with copious amounts of water for at least 15 minutes.

Patient teaching

• Instruct patient on infection control and bleeding precautions.

• Warn patient that alopecia may occur, but that it's usually reversible.

• Instruct patient not to take other drugs, including OTC preparations, unless approved by prescriber.

• Instruct patient to tell prescriber about signs and symptoms of infection (fever, chills, malaise) because drug may have immunosuppressant activity.

Evaluation

• Patient responds well to drug.

• Patient doesn't develop serious complications from adverse hematologic reactions.

• Patient and family state understanding of drug therapy.

Reactions may be *common,* uncommon, *life-threatening,* or COMMON AND LIFE-THREATENING.

vitamin A (retinol)
(VIGH-tuh-min ay)
Aquasol A, Palmitate-A 5000

Pharmacologic class: fat-soluble vitamin
Therapeutic class: vitamin
Pregnancy risk category: A (C at higher-than-recommended doses)

Indications and dosages

▶ **RDA.** RDAs have been converted to retinol equivalents (RE). One RE has activity of 1 mcg of all-trans retinol, 6 mcg of beta carotene, or 12 mcg of carotenoid provitamins.
Men older than age 11: 1,000 mcg RE or 5,000 IU
Pregnant women and women older than age 11: 800 mcg RE or 4,000 IU
Breast-feeding women (first 6 months): 1,300 mcg RE or 6,500 IU
Breast-feeding women (second 6 months): 1,200 mcg RE or 6,000 IU
Children ages 7 to 10: 700 mcg RE or 3,500 IU
Children ages 4 to 6: 500 mcg RE or 2,500 IU
Children ages 1 to 3: 400 mcg RE or 2,000 IU
Neonates and infants younger than age 1: 375 mcg RE or 1,875 IU
▶ **Severe vitamin A deficiency.** *Adults and children older than age 8:* 100,000 IU I.M. or P.O. daily for 3 days, followed by 50,000 IU I.M. or P.O. daily for 2 weeks; then 10,000 to 20,000 IU P.O. daily for 2 months. Follow with adequate dietary nutrition and RE vitamin A supplements.
Children ages 1 to 8: 17,500 to 35,000 IU I.M. daily for 10 days.
Infants younger than age 1: 7,500 to 15,000 IU I.M. daily for 10 days.
▶ **Maintenance dosage to prevent recurrence of vitamin A deficiency.** *Children ages 1 to 8:* 5,000 to 10,000 IU P.O. daily for 2 months; then adequate dietary nutrition and RE vitamin A supplements.

Contraindications and precautions

• Contraindicated for oral administration in patients with malabsorption syndrome; if malabsorption is from inadequate bile secretion, oral route may be used with administration of bile salts (dehydrocholic acid). Also contraindicated

in patients hypersensitive to other ingredients in product and in those with hypervitaminosis A.
• I.V. administration contraindicated except for special water-miscible forms intended for infusion with large parenteral volumes. I.V. push of vitamin A of any type is also contraindicated (anaphylaxis or anaphylactoid reactions and death have resulted).
⚱ **Lifespan:** In pregnant and breast-feeding women, use cautiously, avoiding doses exceeding RE.

Adverse reactions

CNS: irritability, headache, *increased intracranial pressure,* fatigue, lethargy, malaise.
EENT: papilledema, exophthalmos.
GI: anorexia, epigastric pain, vomiting, polydipsia.
GU: hypomenorrhea, polyuria.
Hepatic: jaundice, hepatomegaly, *cirrhosis.*
Metabolic: slow growth, decalcification of bone, hypercalcemia, periostitis, premature closure of epiphyses, migratory arthralgia, cortical thickening over radius and tibia.
Skin: alopecia; dry, cracked, scaly skin; pruritus; lip fissures; erythema; inflamed tongue, lips, and gums; massive desquamation; increased pigmentation; night sweats.
Other: splenomegaly, *anaphylactic shock.*

Interactions

Drug-drug. *Cholestyramine resin, mineral oil:* Reduces GI absorption of fat-soluble vitamins. If needed, give mineral oil h.s.
Hormonal contraceptives: May increase vitamin A level. Monitor patient.
Isotretinoin, multivitamins containing vitamin A: Increases risk of toxicity. Avoid use together.
Neomycin (oral): Decreases vitamin A absorption. Avoid use together.
Warfarin: Increases risk of bleeding. Monitor PT and INR closely; monitor patient for bleeding.

Effects on lab test results

• May increase liver enzyme and calcium levels.

Pharmacokinetics

Absorption: Absorbed readily and completely if fat absorption is normal; larger doses or regular dose in patients with fat malabsorption, low protein intake, or hepatic or pancreatic disease

---

may be absorbed incompletely. Because vitamin A is fat-soluble, absorption requires bile salts, pancreatic lipase, and dietary fat.

Distribution: Stored (primarily as palmitate) in liver. Normal adult liver stores are sufficient to provide vitamin A requirements for 2 years. Lesser amounts of retinyl palmitate are stored in kidneys, lungs, adrenal glands, retinas, and intraperitoneal fat. Vitamin A circulates bound to specific alpha-1 protein, retinol-binding protein.

Metabolism: In liver.

Excretion: Retinol (fat-soluble) combines with glucuronic acid and is metabolized to retinal and retinoic acid. Retinoic acid undergoes biliary excretion in feces. Retinal, retinoic acid, and other water-soluble metabolites are excreted in urine and feces. *Half-life:* Unknown.

Route	Onset	Peak	Duration
P.O., I.M.	Unknown	3-5 hr	Unknown

Action

Chemical effect: Stimulates retinal function, bone growth, reproduction, and integrity of epithelial and mucosal tissues.

Therapeutic effect: Raises vitamin A level in body.

Available forms

Capsules: 10,000 IU, 15,000 IU, 25,000 IU, 50,000 IU

Drops: 30 ml with dropper (50,000 IU/0.1 ml)

Injection: 2-ml vials (50,000 IU/ml with 0.5% chlorobutanol, polysorbate 80, butylated hydroxyanisole, and butylated hydroxytoluene)

Tablets: 5,000 IU, 10,000 IU

NURSING PROCESS

▓ Assessment

• Assess patient's vitamin A intake from fortified foods, dietary supplements, self-administered drugs, and prescription drug sources before therapy and reassess regularly thereafter.

• If dose is high, watch for adverse reactions. Acute toxicity may result from a single dose of 25,000 IU/kg; 350,000 IU in infants and over 2 million IU in adults may also be acutely toxic. Doses that don't exceed RE are usually nontoxic.

• Chronic toxicity in infants (age 3 to 6 months) may result from doses of 18,500 IU daily for 1 to 3 months. In adults, chronic toxicity has re-

sulted from doses of 50,000 IU daily for more than 18 months; 500,000 IU daily for 2 months, and 1 million IU daily for 3 days.

• Be alert for drug interactions.

• Evaluate patient's and family's knowledge of drug therapy.

▣ Nursing diagnoses

• Imbalanced nutrition: less than body requirements related to inadequate intake

• Ineffective health maintenance related to vitamin A toxicity caused by excessive intake

• Deficient knowledge related to drug therapy

▶ Planning and implementation

• Adequate vitamin A absorption requires suitable protein, vitamin E, zinc intake, and bile secretion; give supplemental salts, if necessary. Zinc supplements may be necessary in patient receiving long-term total parenteral nutrition.

• Liquid preparations may be mixed with cereal or fruit juice to be given NG.

• I.M. absorption is fastest and most complete with aqueous preparations, intermediate with emulsions, and slowest with oil suspensions.

ⓢ **ALERT:** Give parenteral form by I.M. route or continuous I.V infusion in total parenteral nutrition. Never give as I.V. bolus.

• Protect drug from light.

Patient teaching

• Warn patient against taking megadoses of vitamins without specific indications. Also stress that he not share prescribed vitamins with others.

• Explain importance of avoiding prolonged use of mineral oil while taking this drug because mineral oil reduces vitamin A absorption.

• Review the signs and symptoms of vitamin A toxicity, and tell patient to report them immediately.

• Advise patient to consume adequate protein, vitamin E, and zinc, which, along with bile, are necessary for vitamin A absorption.

• Instruct patient to store vitamin A in tight, light-resistant container.

☑ Evaluation

• Patient regains normal vitamin A level.

• Patient doesn't exhibit signs and symptoms of vitamin A toxicity.

• Patient and family state understanding of drug therapy.

Reactions may be *common*, uncommon, *life-threatening*, or COMMON AND LIFE-THREATENING.

vitamin C (ascorbic acid)

(VIGH-tuh-min see)
Ascorbicap†, Cebid Timecelles†, Cecon†, Cenolate†, Cetane†, Cevalin†, Cevi-Bid, Ce-Vi-Sol*, Dull-C†, Flavorcee†, N'ice Vitamin C Drops†, Penta-vite ◇, Redoxon ♦, Vita-C†

Pharmacologic class: water-soluble vitamin
Therapeutic class: vitamin
Pregnancy risk category: A (C at higher-than-recommended doses)

Indications and dosages

▶ **RDA.** *Men:* 90 mg.
Women: 75 mg.
Pregnant women ages 14 to 18: 80 mg.
Pregnant women ages 19 to 50: 85 mg.
Breast-feeding women ages 14 to 18: 115 mg.
Breast-feeding women ages 19 to 50: 120 mg.
Boys ages 9 to 13: 45 mg.
Boys ages 14 to 18: 75 mg.
Girls ages 9 to 13: 45 mg.
Girls ages 14 to 18: 65 mg.
Children ages 4 to 8: 25 mg.
Children ages 1 to 3: 15 mg.
Infants ages 6 months to 1 year: 50 mg.
Neonates and infants younger than age 6 months: 40 mg.
▶ **Frank and subclinical scurvy.** *Adults:* Depending on severity, 300 mg to 1 g P.O., S.C., I.M., or I.V. daily; then at least 50 mg daily for maintenance.
Children: Depending on severity, 100 to 300 mg P.O., S.C., I.M., or I.V. daily, then at least 30 mg daily for maintenance.
Premature infants: 75 to 100 mg P.O., I.M., I.V., or S.C. daily.
▶ **Extensive burns, delayed fracture or wound healing, postoperative wound healing, severe febrile or chronic disease states.**
Adults: 300 to 500 mg P.O., S.C., I.M., or I.V. daily for 7 to 10 days. For extensive burns, 1 to 2 g daily.
Children: 100 to 200 mg P.O., S.C., I.M., or I.V. daily.
▶ **Prevention of vitamin C deficiency in patients with poor nutritional habits or increased requirements.** *Adults:* 70 to 150 mg P.O., S.C., I.M., or I.V. daily.

Pregnant or breast-feeding women: 70 to 150 mg P.O., S.C., I.M., or I.V. daily.
Children: at least 40 mg P.O., S.C., I.M., or I.V. daily.
Infants: at least 35 mg P.O., S.C., I.M., or I.V. daily.
▶ **Potentiation of methenamine in urine acidification.** *Adults:* 4 to 12 g P.O. daily in divided doses.

▼ I.V. administration

- Avoid rapid I.V. administration. It may cause faintness or dizziness.
- Give I.V. infusion cautiously in patients with renal insufficiency.
- Protect solution from light and refrigerate ampules.

Contraindications and precautions

🜊 **Lifespan:** In pregnant women, give if clearly needed. In breast-feeding women, use cautiously.

Adverse reactions

CNS: faintness, dizziness with rapid I.V. administration.
GI: diarrhea.
GU: acid urine, oxaluria, renal calculi.
Other: discomfort at injection site.

Interactions

Drug-drug. *Aspirin (high doses):* Increases risk of ascorbic acid deficiency. Monitor patient closely.
Hormonal contraceptives, estrogen: Increases level of estrogen. Monitor patient.
Oral iron supplements: Increases iron absorption. A beneficial drug interaction. Encourage use together.
Warfarin: Decreases anticoagulant effect. Monitor patient closely.
Drug-herb. *Bearberry:* Inactivates bearberry in urine. Discourage use together.

Effects on lab test results

None reported.

Pharmacokinetics

Absorption: After P.O. use, absorbed readily; may be reduced with very large doses or in patients with diarrhea or GI diseases. Unknown for I.M and S.C. use.

Distribution: Widely in body with high levels in liver, leukocytes, platelets, glandular tissues, and lens of eyes. Protein-binding is low.
Metabolism: In liver.
Excretion: In urine. Renal excretion is directly proportional to blood levels. *Half-life:* Unknown.

Route	Onset	Peak	Duration
P.O., I.V., I.M., S.C.	Unknown	Unknown	Unknown

Action

Chemical effect: Stimulates collagen formation and tissue repair; involved in oxidation-reduction reactions throughout body.
Therapeutic effect: Raises vitamin C level in body.

Available forms

Capsules (timed-release): 500 mg†
Crystals: 100 g (4 g/tsp)†, 500 g (4 g/tsp)†
Injection: 100 mg/ml; 250 mg/ml; 500 mg/ml
Lozenges: 60 mg†
Oral liquid: 50 ml (35 mg/0.6 ml)*†
Oral solution: 60 mg/ml†, 100 mg/ml†
Powder: 100 g (4 g/tsp)†, 500 g (4 g/tsp)†
Syrup: 20 mg/ml in 120 ml†, 480 ml†; 500 mg/5 ml in 5 ml†, 120 ml†, 480 ml†
Tablets: 25 mg†, 50 mg†, 100 mg†, 250 mg†, 500 mg†, 1,000 mg†
Tablets (chewable): 50 mg, 100 mg†, 250 mg†, 500 mg†, 1,000 mg†
Tablets (effervescent): 1,000 mg sugar-free†
Tablets (timed-release): 500 mg†, 1,000 mg†, 1,500 mg

NURSING PROCESS

⚞ Assessment

• Assess patient's condition before therapy and regularly thereafter.
• When giving for urine acidification, check urine pH to ensure efficacy.
• Be alert for adverse reactions and drug interactions.
• If adverse GI reactions occur, monitor patient's hydration.
• Evaluate patient's and family's knowledge of drug therapy.

⊕ Nursing diagnoses

• Imbalanced nutrition: less than body requirements related to inadequate intake

• Risk for deficient fluid volume related to drug-induced adverse GI reactions
• Deficient knowledge related to drug therapy

⧁ Planning and implementation

• Give P.O. solution directly into mouth or mix with food.
• Dissolve effervescent tablets in glass of water immediately before giving.
• Utilization of vitamin may be better with I.M. route, the preferred parenteral route.
Patient teaching
• Stress proper nutritional habits to prevent recurrence of deficiency.
• Advise patient with vitamin C deficiency to decrease or stop smoking.

☑ Evaluation

• Patient regains normal vitamin C level.
• Patient maintains adequate hydration.
• Patient and family state understanding of drug therapy.

vitamin D

cholecalciferol (vitamin D₃)
(koh-lih-kal-SIF-eh-rol)
Delta-D, Vitamin D₃

ergocalciferol (vitamin D₂)
(er-goh-kal-SIF-er-ohl)
Calciferol, Drisdol, Radiostol Forte ◆

Pharmacologic class: fat-soluble vitamin
Therapeutic class: vitamin
Pregnancy risk category: C

Indications and dosages

▶ **RDA for cholecalciferol.** *Adults age 50 and younger and children:* 200 IU.
Adults ages 51 to 70: 400 IU.
Adults older than age 70: 600 IU.
Pregnant or breast-feeding women: 400 IU.
▶ **Rickets and other vitamin D deficiency diseases.** *Adults:* Initially, 12,000 IU P.O. or I.M. daily, usually increased according to response up to 500,000 IU daily. After correction of deficiency, maintenance includes adequate diet and RDA supplements.

▶ **Hypoparathyroidism.** *Adults and children:* 50,000 to 200,000 IU P.O. or I.M. daily with calcium supplement.

▶ **Familial hypophosphatemia.** *Adults:* 10,000 to 80,000 IU P.O. or I.M. daily with phosphorus supplement.

Contraindications and precautions

• Contraindicated in patients with hypercalcemia, hypervitaminosis A, or renal osteodystrophy with hyperphosphatemia.

• Use cautiously in cardiac patients, especially those receiving digoxin, and in patients with increased sensitivity to these drugs.

• Give ergocalciferol cautiously, if at all, to patients with impaired kidney function, heart disease, renal calculi, or arteriosclerosis.

⚠ Lifespan: In pregnant and breast-feeding women, give cautiously.

Adverse reactions

Adverse reactions listed are usually seen only in vitamin D toxicity.

CNS: headache, weakness, somnolence, overt psychosis, irritability.

CV: *calcifications of soft tissues including heart, arrhythmias;* hypertension.

EENT: rhinorrhea, conjunctivitis (calcific), photophobia.

GI: anorexia, nausea, vomiting, constipation, dry mouth, metallic taste, polydipsia.

GU: polyuria, albuminuria, hypercalciuria, nocturia, impaired kidney function, reversible azotemia.

Metabolic: hypercalcemia, hyperthermia, weight loss.

Musculoskeletal: bone and muscle pain, bone demineralization.

Skin: pruritus.

Other: decreased libido.

Interactions

Drug-drug. *Cholestyramine resin, mineral oil:* Inhibits GI absorption of oral vitamin D. Space doses. Use together cautiously.

Corticosteroids: Antagonizes effect of vitamin D. Monitor vitamin D level closely.

Digoxin: Increases risk of arrhythmias. Monitor calcium level.

Phenobarbital, phenytoin: Increases vitamin D metabolism, which decreases half-life as well as drug's effectiveness. Monitor patient closely.

Thiazide diuretics: May cause hypercalcemia in patients with hypoparathyroidism. Monitor patient closely.

Verapamil: Atrial fibrillation has occurred because of increased calcium. Monitor patient closely.

Effects on lab test results

• May increase BUN, creatinine, AST, ALT, urine urea, albumin, calcium, and cholesterol levels.

Pharmacokinetics

Absorption: From small intestine with P.O. administration; unknown for I.M. administration.
Distribution: Throughout body; bound to proteins stored in liver.
Metabolism: In liver and kidneys.
Excretion: Primarily in bile; small amount excreted in urine. *Half-life:* 24 hours.

Route	Onset	Peak	Duration
P.O., I.M.	2-24 hr	3-12 hr	Varies

Action

Chemical effect: Promotes absorption and utilization of calcium and phosphate, helping to regulate calcium homeostasis.
Therapeutic effect: Helps to maintain normal calcium and phosphate levels in body.

Available forms

Capsules: 1.25 mg (50,000 IU)
Injection: 12.5 mg (500,000 IU)/ml
Oral liquid: 8,000 IU/ml in 60-ml dropper bottle
Tablets: 400 IU, 1,000 IU

NURSING PROCESS

🔖 Assessment

• Assess patient's condition before therapy and regularly thereafter.

⚠ **ALERT:** Monitor patient's eating and bowel habits; dry mouth, nausea, vomiting, metallic taste, and constipation may be early evidence of toxicity.

• Monitor serum and urine calcium, potassium, and urea levels when high therapeutic dosages are used.

• Be alert for adverse reactions and drug interactions.

• Evaluate patient's and family's knowledge of drug therapy.

⊞ Nursing diagnoses
• Imbalanced nutrition: less than body requirements related to inadequate intake
• Ineffective health maintenance related to vitamin D toxicity
• Deficient knowledge related to drug therapy

▷ Planning and implementation
• Use I.M. injection of vitamin D dispersed in oil for patient unable to absorb P.O. form.
• Dosages of 60,000 IU daily can cause hypercalcemia.
• Malabsorption from inadequate bile or hepatic dysfunction may require addition of exogenous bile salts with oral form.
• Patient with hyperphosphatemia requires dietary phosphate restrictions and binding agents to avoid metastatic calcifications and renal calculus formation.
Patient teaching
• Warn patient of dangers of increasing dosage without consulting prescriber. Vitamin D is fat-soluble.
• Tell patient taking vitamin D to restrict his intake of magnesium-containing antacids.

☑ Evaluation
• Patient regains normal vitamin D level.
• Patient doesn't develop vitamin D toxicity.
• Patient and family state understanding of drug therapy.

---

vitamin E (tocopherol)
(VIGH-tuh-min ee)
Amino-Opti-E†, Aquasol E Drops†, Aquavit-E, d'ALPHA E 400 Softgels, d'ALPHA E 1000 Softgels, Dry E 400, E-Complex-600†, E-200 I.U. Softgels†, E-400 I.U. Softgels†, E-Vitamin Succinate†, Mixed E 400 Softgels, Mixed E 1000 Softgels, Vitamin E with Mixed Tocopherols, Vita-Plus E Softgels†

Pharmacologic class: fat-soluble vitamin
Therapeutic class: vitamin
Pregnancy risk category: A

Indications and dosages
▶ **RDA.** RDAs for vitamin E have been converted to α-tocopherol equivalents (α-TE). One α-TE equals 1 mg of D-α tocopherol or 1.49 IU
Infants age 6 months and younger: 4 α-TE
Infants ages 7 to 12 months: 5 α-TE
Children ages 1 to 3: 6 α-TE
Children ages 4 to 8: 7 α-TE
Children ages 9 to 13: 11 α-TE
Children ages 14 to 18: 15 α-TE
Adults, pregnant women: 15 α-TE
Breast-feeding women: 19 α-TE
▶ **Vitamin E deficiency in adults and in children with malabsorption syndrome.** *Adults:* Depending on severity, 60 to 75 IU P.O. daily. *Children:* 1 IU/kg P.O. daily.

Contraindications and precautions
No known contraindications.

Adverse reactions
None reported with recommended dosages.

Interactions
Drug-drug. *Cholestyramine resin, mineral oil:* Inhibits GI absorption of oral vitamin E. Space doses. Use together cautiously.
Iron: May catalyze oxidation and increase daily requirements. Give separately.
Oral anticoagulants: Hypoprothrombinemic effects may be increased, possibly causing bleeding. Monitor patient closely.
Vitamin K: Antagonizes effects of vitamin K possible with large doses of vitamin E. Avoid use together.

Effects on lab test results
None reported.

Pharmacokinetics
Absorption: GI absorption depends on presence of bile. Only 20% to 60% of vitamin obtained from dietary sources is absorbed. As dosage increases, fraction of vitamin E absorbed decreases.
Distribution: To all tissues and stored in adipose tissues.
Metabolism: In liver.
Excretion: Primarily in bile; small amount excreted in urine. *Half-life:* Unknown.

Route	Onset	Peak	Duration
P.O.	Unknown	Unknown	Unknown

Action

Chemical effect: Unknown; thought to act as an antioxidant and protect RBC membranes against hemolysis.
Therapeutic effect: Raises vitamin E level in body.

Available forms

Capsules: 100 IU, 200 IU†, 400 IU†, 600 IU†, 1,000 IU†
Drops: 15 IU/ 0.3 ml
Liquid: 15 IU/30 ml
Oral Solution: 50 IU/ml
Tablets (chewable): 100 IU, 200 IU†, 400 IU†, 500 IU, 600 IU, 800 IU, 1000 IU

NURSING PROCESS

Assessment
• Assess patient's condition before therapy and regularly thereafter.
• Monitor patient with liver or gallbladder disease for response to therapy. Adequate bile is essential for vitamin E absorption.
• Be alert for drug interactions.
• Evaluate patient's and family's knowledge of drug therapy.

Nursing diagnoses
• Imbalanced nutrition: less than body requirements related to inadequate intake
• Deficient knowledge related to drug therapy

Planning and implementation
• Requirements increase with rise in dietary polyunsaturated acids.
• Make sure patient swallows tablets or capsules whole.
• Store drug in tightly closed, light-resistant container.
• If patient has malabsorption caused by lack of bile, give vitamin E with bile salts.
• Hypervitaminosis E symptoms include fatigue, weakness, nausea, headache, blurred vision, flatulence, diarrhea.
Patient teaching
• Tell patient not to crush tablets or open capsules. An oral solution and chewable tablets are commercially available.

• Discourage patient from taking megadoses, which can cause thrombophlebitis. Vitamin E is fat-soluble.

Evaluation
• Patient regains normal vitamin E level.
• Patient and family state understanding of drug therapy.

voriconazole
(vhor-i-KHAN-a-zawl)
Vfend

Pharmacologic class: synthetic triazole
Therapeutic class: antifungal
Pregnancy risk category: D

Indications and dosages

▶ **Invasive aspergillosis; serious infections caused by *Fusarium* species and *Scedosporium apiospermum* in patients intolerant of or refractory to other therapy.** *Adults:* Initially, 6 mg/kg I.V. q 12 hours for two doses, then 4 mg/kg I.V. q 12 hours for maintenance. Switch to P.O. form as tolerated, using the following maintenance dosages:
Adults weighing 40 kg (88 lb) or more: Maintenance dosage, 200 mg P.O. q 12 hours. May increase to 300 mg P.O. q 12 hours, if necessary.
Adults weighing less than 40 kg: Maintenance dosage, 100 mg P.O. q 12 hours. May increase to 150 mg P.O. q 12 hours, if necessary.
Adjust-a-dose: In patients with mild to moderate hepatic cirrhosis, decrease the maintenance dosage by one-half.

I.V. administration
• Reconstitute powder with 19 ml of sterile water for injection to obtain a volume of 20 ml of clear concentrate containing 10 mg/ml of drug. If a vacuum doesn't pull the diluent into the vial, discard the vial. Shake vial until all the powder is dissolved.
• Further dilute the 10-mg/ml solution to a concentration of 5 mg/ml or less. Follow the manufacturer's instructions for diluting.
• Don't dilute with 4.2% sodium bicarbonate infusion.
• Infuse over 1 to 2 hours, at a concentration of 5 mg/ml or less and a maximum of 3 mg/kg hourly.

• Monitor creatinine level in patient with moderate to severe renal dysfunction (creatinine clearance less than 50 ml/minute). If creatinine level increases, consider changing to P.O. form.
• Don't infuse with blood products or any electrolyte supplementation.
• Store unreconstituted vials at controlled room temperature (59° to 86° F [15° to 30° C]). Use reconstituted solution immediately.

Contraindications and precautions

• Contraindicated in patients hypersensitive to drug or its components and in those with rare hereditary problems of galactose intolerance, Lapp lactase deficiency, or glucose-galactose malabsorption. Also contraindicated in patients taking rifampin, carbamazepine, long-acting barbiturates, sirolimus, rifabutin, ergot alkaloids, pimozide, or quinidine.
• Use cautiously in patients hypersensitive to other azoles. Use I.V. form cautiously in patients with creatinine clearance less than 50 ml/minute.
⚠ Lifespan: In pregnant women, avoid using. Drug can cause harm to fetus. In breast-feeding women, don't use drug unless benefits clearly outweigh risks. In children younger than age 12, safety and effectiveness haven't been established.

Adverse reactions

CNS: fever, headache, hallucinations, dizziness.
CV: tachycardia, hypertension, hypotension, peripheral edema, vasodilation.
EENT: *abnormal vision,* photophobia, chromatopsia, dry mouth.
GI: abdominal pain, nausea, vomiting, diarrhea.
GU: *acute renal failure.*
Hepatic: cholestatic jaundice.
Metabolic: hypokalemia, hypomagnesemia.
Skin: rash, pruritus.
Other: chills.

Interactions

Drug-drug. *Benzodiazepines, calcium channel blockers, lovastatin, omeprazole, sulfonylureas, vinca alkaloids:* Increases levels of these drugs. Adjust dosages of these drugs and monitor patient for adverse effects.
Carbamazepine, long-acting barbiturates, rifampin, rifabutin: Decreases voriconazole level. Avoid use together.

Coumarin anticoagulants, warfarin: Significantly increases PT. Monitor PT or other appropriate anticoagulant test results.
Cyclosporine, tacrolimus: Increases levels of these drugs. Reduce dosages of these drugs and monitor levels. Adjust doses and monitor levels of these drugs when voriconazole is stopped.
Ergot alkaloids (such as ergotamine), sirolimus: Increases concentrations of these drugs. Avoid use together.
HIV protease inhibitors (amprenavir, nelfinavir, saquinavir), nonnucleoside reverse transcriptase inhibitors (delavirdine, efavirenz): May increase levels of both drugs. Monitor patient for adverse effects.
Phenytoin: Decreases voriconazole level and increases phenytoin level. Increase voriconazole maintenance dose and monitor phenytoin level.
Pimozide, quinidine: Increases levels of these drugs, possibly leading to QT prolongation and torsades de pointes. Avoid use together.

Effects on lab test results

• May increase AST, ALT, bilirubin, alkaline phosphatase, and creatinine levels. May decrease potassium and magnesium levels.
• May decrease hemoglobin, hematocrit, and platelet, WBC, and RBC counts.

Pharmacokinetics

Absorption: Oral bioavailability is about 96%.
Distribution: Extensive. Protein-binding is 58%.
Metabolism: By the CYP 2C19, 2C9, and 3A4.
Excretion: Via hepatic metabolism, with less than 2% excreted unchanged in the urine. *Half-life:* Depends on dose.

Route	Onset	Peak	Duration
P.O., I.V.	Immediate	1-2 hr	12 hr

Action

Chemical effect: Inhibits an essential step in fungal ergosterol biosynthesis.
Therapeutic effect: Kills susceptible fungi.

Available forms

Injection: 200 mg
Tablets: 50 mg, 200 mg

Reactions may be *common,* uncommon, *life-threatening*, or COMMON AND LIFE-THREATENING.

NURSING PROCESS

🔍 Assessment
- Assess patient's condition before therapy and regularly thereafter.
- Monitor liver function test results throughout therapy. Monitor patient who develops abnormal liver function test results for more severe hepatic injury.
- Monitor renal function during treatment.
- If treatment lasts more than 28 days, monitor visual acuity, visual fields, and color perception.
- Evaluate patient's and family's knowledge of drug therapy.

🔲 Nursing diagnoses
- Risk for infection related to presence of fungus
- Risk for injury related to adverse CNS effects of drug
- Deficient knowledge related to drug therapy

▷ Planning and implementation
- Use oral form in patients with moderate to severe renal impairment unless the benefit outweighs the risk of I.V. use.
- Infusion reactions, including flushing, fever, sweating, tachycardia, chest tightness, dyspnea, faintness, nausea, pruritus, and rash, may occur as soon as infusion starts. If reaction occurs, notify prescriber. Infusion may need to be stopped.
- If patient develops signs and symptoms of liver disease that may be caused by therapy, stop drug.

Patient teaching
- Tell patient to take oral drug at least 1 hour before or 1 hour after a meal.
- Advise patient to avoid driving or operating machinery while taking drug, especially at night, because vision changes, including blurring and photophobia, may occur.
- Tell patient to avoid strong, direct sunlight during therapy.
- Tell woman of childbearing potential to use effective contraception during treatment.

✅ Evaluation
- Infection is successfully treated.
- Patient doesn't sustain any injury.
- Patient and family state understanding of drug therapy.

warfarin sodium
(WAR-feh-rin SOH-dee-um)
Coumadin, Warfilone ◆

Pharmacologic class: coumarin derivative
Therapeutic class: anticoagulant
Pregnancy risk category: X

Indications and dosages

▶ **Pulmonary embolism related to deep vein thrombosis, MI, rheumatic heart disease with heart valve damage, prosthetic heart valves, chronic atrial fibrillation.** *Adults:* Initially, 2 to 5 mg P.O. or I.V daily for 2 to 4 days. PT and INR determinations then can be used to establish optimal dose. Usual maintenance dosage is 2 to 10 mg daily.

▼ I.V. administration

- Reconstitute by adding 2.7 ml of sterile water for injection to vial of 5 mg of warfarin. Resulting solution contains 2 mg/ml.
- Inject dose slowly over 1 to 2 minutes.

Contraindications and precautions

- Contraindicated in patients with bleeding or hemorrhagic tendencies, GI ulcerations, severe hepatic or renal disease, severe uncontrolled hypertension, subacute bacterial endocarditis, polycythemia vera, or vitamin K deficiency. Also contraindicated in patients who have had recent eye, brain, or spinal cord surgery.
- Use cautiously in patients with diverticulitis, colitis, mild-or-moderate hypertension, mild-or-moderate hepatic or renal disease, drainage tubes in any orifice, or regional or lumbar block anesthesia. Also use cautiously if patient has any condition that increases the risk of hemorrhage.
- ⚖ Lifespan: In pregnant women, drug is contraindicated. In breast-feeding women, use cautiously. Infants, especially neonates, may be more susceptible to anticoagulants because of vitamin K deficiency. Geriatric patients have an increased risk of bleeding and usually receive lower dosages.

Rapid onset   *Liquid form contains alcohol.   ◆Canada   ◇ Australia   †OTC   ‡Off-label use

Adverse reactions

CNS: headache, *fever.*
GI: anorexia, nausea, vomiting, cramps, *diarrhea,* mouth ulcerations, sore mouth, melena.
GU: hematuria, excessive menstrual bleeding.
Hematologic: *hemorrhage* with excessive dosage.
Hepatic: *hepatitis,* jaundice.
Skin: dermatitis, urticaria, necrosis, gangrene, alopecia, *rash.*

Interactions

Drug-drug. *Acetaminophen:* May increase bleeding with more than 2 weeks of acetaminophen therapy at dosages of more than 2 g/day. Monitor patient carefully.
Allopurinol, amiodarone, anabolic steroids, cephalosporins, chloramphenicol, cimetidine, clofibrate, danazol, diazoxide, diflunisal, disulfiram, erythromycin, ethacrynic acid, fluoroquinolones, glucagon, heparin, influenza virus vaccine, isoniazid, lovastatin, meclofenamate, methimazole, methylthiouracil, metronidazole, miconazole, nalidixic acid, neomycin (oral), pentoxifylline, propafenone, propoxyphene, quinidine, sulfonamides, tamoxifen, tetracyclines, thiazides, thrombolytics, thyroid drugs, tricyclic antidepressants, vitamin E: Increases PT. Monitor patient for bleeding. Reduce anticoagulant dosage.
Anticonvulsants: Increases levels of phenytoin and phenobarbital. Monitor patient for toxicity.
Barbiturates, carbamazepine, corticosteroids, corticotropin, mercaptopurine, methaqualone, nafcillin, hormonal contraceptives containing estrogen, rifampin, spironolactone, sucralfate, trazodone: Decreases PT with reduced anticoagulant effect. Monitor patient carefully.
Chloral hydrate, glutethimide, propylthiouracil, sulfinpyrazone: May increase or decrease PT. Avoid use, if possible. Monitor patient carefully.
Cholestyramine: Decreases response when given too close together. Give 6 hours after oral anticoagulants.
NSAIDs, salicylates: Increases PT and ulcerogenic effects. Don't use together.
Sulfonylureas (oral antidiabetics): Increases hypoglycemic response. Monitor glucose level.
Drug-herb. *Angelica:* Significantly prolongs PT when used together. Discourage use together.
Motherwort, red clover, arnica, ginkgo biloba, ginseng, pau d'arco: May increase risk of bleeding. Discourage use together.

Drug-food. *Foods or enteral products containing vitamin K:* May impair anticoagulation. Tell patient to maintain consistent daily intake of leafy green vegetables.
Drug-lifestyle. *Alcohol use:* Enhances anticoagulant effects. Discourage alcohol intake; however, one or two drinks daily are unlikely to affect warfarin response.

Effects on lab test results

• May increase ALT and AST levels.
• May increase INR, PT, and PTT.

Pharmacokinetics

Absorption: Rapid and complete.
Distribution: Highly bound to proteins, especially albumin.
Metabolism: In liver.
Excretion: Metabolites reabsorbed from bile and excreted in urine. *Half-life:* 1 to 3 days.

Route	Onset	Peak	Duration
P.O.	½-3 days	Unknown	2-5 days
I.V.	Unknown	Unknown	2-5 days

Action

Chemical effect: Inhibits vitamin K-dependent activation of clotting factors II, VII, IX, and X, formed in liver.
Therapeutic effect: Reduces ability of blood to clot.

Available forms

Powder for injection: 5 mg
Tablets: 1 mg, 2 mg, 2.5 mg, 3 mg, 4 mg, 5 mg, 6 mg, 7.5 mg, 10 mg

NURSING PROCESS

⚕ Assessment

• Assess patient's condition before therapy and regularly thereafter.
• Draw blood to establish baseline coagulation parameters before therapy.
⑤ ALERT: INR determinations are essential for proper control. Clinicians typically try to maintain INR at two to three times normal; risk of bleeding is high when INR exceeds six times normal.
• Be alert for adverse reactions and drug interactions. Elderly patients and patients with renal or hepatic failure are especially sensitive to warfarin effect.

• Regularly inspect patient for bleeding gums, bruises on arms or legs, petechiae, nosebleeds, melena, tarry stools, hematuria, and hematemesis.
• Observe breast-feeding infants of mothers taking drug for unexpected bleeding.
• Evaluate patient's and family's knowledge of drug therapy.

🔯 **Nursing diagnoses**
• Risk for injury related to potential for blood clot formation from underlying condition
• Ineffective protection related to increased risk of bleeding
• Deficient knowledge related to drug therapy

▶ **Planning and implementation**
• Give drug at same time daily.
• I.V. form may be obtained from manufacturer for rare patient who can't have oral therapy. Follow guidelines carefully for preparation and administration.
• Because onset of action is delayed, heparin sodium is commonly given during first few days of treatment. When heparin is given simultaneously, blood for PT shouldn't be drawn within 5 hours of intermittent I.V. heparin administration. However, blood for PT may be drawn at any time during continuous heparin infusion.
⑤ **ALERT:** Withhold drug and call prescriber immediately if fever and rash occur; they may signal severe adverse reactions.
• The drug's anticoagulant effect can be neutralized by vitamin K injections.
• Drug is best oral anticoagulant for patient taking antacids or phenytoin.
Patient teaching
• Stress importance of compliance with prescribed dosage and follow-up appointments. Patient should wear or carry medical identification that indicates his increased risk of bleeding.
• Instruct patient and family to watch for signs of bleeding and to notify prescriber immediately if they occur.
• Warn patient to avoid OTC products containing aspirin, other salicylates, or drugs that may interact with warfarin.
• Tell patient to notify prescriber if menses are heavier than usual; dosage adjustment may be necessary.
• Tell patient to use electric razor when shaving to avoid scratching skin and to use soft toothbrush.

• Instruct patient to read food labels. Food and enteral feedings that contain vitamin K may impair anticoagulation.
• Tell patient to eat a daily, consistent amount of leafy green vegetables that contain vitamin K. Eating varying amounts may alter anticoagulant effects.

☑ **Evaluation**
• Patient doesn't develop blood clots.
• Patient states appropriate bleeding precautions to take.
• Patient and family state understanding of drug therapy.

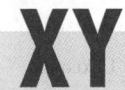

xylometazoline hydrochloride
(zigh-loh-met-uh-ZOH-leen high-droh-KLOR-ighd)
Otrivin

Pharmacologic class: sympathomimetic
Therapeutic class: decongestant, vasoconstrictor
Pregnancy risk category: NR

Indications and dosages

▶ **Nasal congestion.** *Adults and children age 12 and older:* 2 to 3 gtt or sprays of 0.1% solution in each nostril q 8 to 10 hours.
Children ages 6 months to 12 years: 2 to 3 gtt of 0.05% solution in each nostril q 8 to 10 hours.
Children younger than age 6 months: 1 gtt of 0.05% solution in each nostril q 6 hours, p.r.n. Drug shouldn't be used for more than 3 to 5 days.

Contraindications and precautions

• Contraindicated in patients hypersensitive to drug and in those with angle-closure glaucoma.
• Use cautiously in patients with hyperthyroidism, cardiac disease, hypertension, diabetes mellitus, or advanced arteriosclerosis.
⚜ **Lifespan:** In pregnant and breast-feeding women, safety of drug hasn't been established. In children younger than age 2, give drug under prescriber's direction and supervision.

Adverse reactions

EENT: transient burning, stinging; dryness or ulceration of nasal mucosa; sneezing; rebound nasal congestion or irritation (with excessive or long-term use).

Interactions

None significant.

Effects on lab test results

None reported.

Pharmacokinetics

Absorption: Intranasal. Enough may be absorbed to produce systemic effects.
Distribution: Unknown.
Metabolism: Unknown.
Excretion: Unknown. *Half-life:* Unknown.

Route	Onset	Peak	Duration
Intranasal	5-10 min	Unknown	5-6 hr

Action

Chemical effect: Unknown; may cause local vasoconstriction of dilated arterioles, reducing blood flow and nasal congestion.
Therapeutic effect: Relieves nasal congestion.

Available forms

Nasal solution: 0.05%, 0.1%.

NURSING PROCESS

⚗ Assessment
• Assess patient's condition before therapy and regularly thereafter.
• Be alert for adverse reactions.
• Evaluate patient's and family's knowledge of drug therapy.

⊕ Nursing diagnoses
• Ineffective health maintenance related to presence of nasal congestion
• Impaired tissue integrity related to drug's adverse effect on nasal mucosa
• Deficient knowledge related to drug therapy

▶ Planning and implementation
• When giving more than one spray, allow 3 to 5 minutes to elapse between sprays. Have patient clear his nose before each spray.

Patient teaching
• Teach patient how to use drug. Have him hold his head upright to minimize swallowing of the drug; tell him to sniff spray briskly. Instruct him to wait 3 to 5 minutes between sprays and to clear his nose before each spray.
• Tell patient not to share drug to prevent spread of infection.
• Tell patient not to exceed recommended dosage, to use only as needed, and to use for only 3 to 5 days.

☑ Evaluation
• Patient's nasal congestion is eliminated.
• Patient maintains normal intranasal mucosa.
• Patient and family state understanding of drug therapy.

Z

zafirlukast
(zay-FEER-loo-kast)
Accolate

Pharmacologic class: synthetic, selective peptide leukotriene receptor antagonist
Therapeutic class: antiasthmatic, bronchodilator
Pregnancy risk category: B

Indications and dosages

▶ **Prophylaxis and long-term treatment of chronic asthma.** *Adults and children age 12 and older:* 20 mg P.O. b.i.d. taken 1 hour before or 2 hours after meals.
Children ages 5 to 11: 10 mg P.O. b.i.d. taken 1 hour before or 2 hours after meals.
▶ **Prophylaxis for seasonal allergic rhinitis.** *Adults:* 20 to 40 mg P.O. as a single dose before exposure to allergen.

Contraindications and precautions

• Contraindicated in patients hypersensitive to drug.
• Use cautiously in patients with hepatic impairment.
⚖ **Lifespan:** In pregnant women, drug should be used only if clearly needed. In breast-feeding

women, drug shouldn't be given. In children younger than age 5, safety and effectiveness haven't been established. In geriatric patients, use cautiously.

Adverse reactions

CNS: *headache,* asthenia, dizziness, pain, fever.
GI: nausea, diarrhea, abdominal pain, vomiting, dyspepsia.
Musculoskeletal: myalgia, back pain.
Other: infection, accidental injury.

Interactions

Drug-drug. *Aspirin:* Increases zafirlukast level. Monitor patient.
Erythromycin, theophylline: Decreases zafirlukast level. Monitor patient.
Warfarin: Increases PT. Monitor PT and INR levels, and adjust dosage of anticoagulant.
Drug-food. *Any food:* Reduces rate and extent of drug absorption. Give drug 1 hour before or 2 hours after meals.

Effects on lab test results

• May increase liver enzyme levels.

Pharmacokinetics

Absorption: Rapid.
Distribution: Unknown.
Metabolism: Extensive.
Excretion: Mainly in feces; 10% in urine. *Half-life:* 10 hours.

Route	Onset	Peak	Duration
P.O.	Unknown	3 hr	Unknown

Action

Chemical effect: Selectively competes for leukotriene receptor sites. Blocks inflammatory action and inhibits bronchoconstriction.
Therapeutic effect: Improves breathing.

Available forms

Tablets: 10 mg, 20 mg

NURSING PROCESS

Assessment

• Evaluate patient's and family's understanding of drug therapy.

Nursing diagnoses

• Impaired gas exchange related to broncho-spasm
• Deficient knowledge related to drug therapy

Planning and implementation

ALERT: Don't use drug for reversing broncho-spasm in acute asthma attack.
ALERT: Reduction in oral steroid dose has been followed in rare cases by eosinophilia, vasculitic rash, worsening pulmonary symptoms, cardiac complications, or neuropathy, sometimes presenting as Churg-Strauss syndrome.
Patient teaching
• Tell patient to keep taking drug even if symptoms disappear.
• Advise patient to continue taking other anti-asthmatics.
• Instruct patient to take drug 1 hour before or 2 hours after meals.

Evaluation

• Patient demonstrates improved gas exchange.
• Patient and family state understanding of drug therapy.

zalcitabine (ddC, dideoxycytidine)
(zal-SIGH-tuh-been)
Hivid

Pharmacologic class: nucleoside analogue
Therapeutic class: antiviral
Pregnancy risk category: C

Indications and dosages

▶ **Advanced HIV infection (CD4+ T-cell count below 300 cells/mm³) in patients with significant deterioration.** *Adults and children age 13 and older weighing at least 30 kg (66 lb):* 0.75 mg P.O. q 8 hours given with other antiretrovirals.

Contraindications and precautions

• Contraindicated in patients hypersensitive to drug or its components.
• Use cautiously in patients with peripheral neuropathy, baseline cardiomyopathy, or history of heart failure. Use cautiously in patients with creatinine clearance less than 55 ml/minute because they may be at increased risk for toxicity. Use cautiously in patients with hepatic failure;

drug regimen (zalcitabine and zidovudine) may worsen hepatic dysfunction in patients with hepatic impairment. Use cautiously in patients with history of pancreatitis; rarely, pancreatitis is fatal in patients receiving zalcitabine.

⚠ Lifespan: In pregnant women and in children younger than age 13, safety of drug hasn't been established.

Adverse reactions

CNS: *peripheral neuropathy, headache, fatigue,* dizziness, confusion, *seizures,* impaired concentration, amnesia, insomnia, depression, tremor, hypertonia, asthenia, agitation, abnormal thinking, anxiety, *fever.*
CV: *cardiomyopathy, heart failure,* chest pain.
EENT: pharyngitis, ocular pain, abnormal vision, ototoxicity, nasal discharge.
GI: nausea, vomiting, diarrhea, abdominal pain, anorexia, constipation, stomatitis, esophageal ulcer, glossitis, *pancreatitis.*
Hematologic: anemia, *neutropenia, leukopenia, thrombocytopenia.*
Respiratory: cough.
Musculoskeletal: myalgia, arthralgia.
Skin: pruritus; night sweats; *erythematous, maculopapular, or follicular rash;* urticaria.

Interactions

Drug-drug. *Aminoglycosides, amphotericin B, foscarnet, other drugs that may impair kidney function:* Increases risk of nephrotoxicity. Avoid use together.
Antacids containing aluminum or magnesium: Decreases absorption of zalcitabine. Separate administration times.
Chloramphenicol, cisplatin, dapsone, disulfiram, ethionamide, glutethimide, gold salts, hydralazine, iodoquinol, isoniazid, metronidazole, nitrofurantoin, phenytoin, ribavirin, vincristine, and other drugs that can cause peripheral neuropathy: Increases risk of peripheral neuropathy. Avoid use together.
Cimetidine, probenecid: Increases zalcitabine level. Monitor patient carefully.
Pentamidine: Increases risk of pancreatitis. Avoid use together.
Drug-food. *Any food:* Decreases rate of drug absorption. Give drug on empty stomach.

Effects on lab test results

● May increase alkaline phosphatase, ALT, and AST levels. May alter glucose level.

● May decrease hemoglobin, hematocrit, and neutrophil, WBC, and platelet counts.

Pharmacokinetics

Absorption: Mean absolute bioavailability is above 80%. Administering drug with food decreases rate and extent of absorption.
Distribution: Enters CNS.
Metabolism: Doesn't appear to undergo significant hepatic metabolism; phosphorylation to active form occurs within cells.
Excretion: Primarily in urine. *Half-life:* 2 hours.

Route	Onset	Peak	Duration
P.O.	Unknown	1-2 hr	Unknown

Action

Chemical effect: Inhibits replication of HIV by blocking viral DNA synthesis.
Therapeutic effect: Reduces symptoms linked to advanced HIV infection.

Available forms

Tablets: 0.375 mg, 0.75 mg

NURSING PROCESS

🖎 Assessment
● Assess patient's condition before therapy and regularly thereafter.
● Assess patient for signs of peripheral neuropathy, characterized by numbness and burning in limbs.
● Be alert for adverse reactions and drug interactions.
● Evaluate patient's and family's knowledge of drug therapy.

🖏 Nursing diagnoses
● Risk for infection related to presence of HIV
● Disturbed sensory perceptions (tactile) related to drug-induced peripheral neuropathy
● Deficient knowledge related to drug therapy

▶ Planning and implementation
● Adjust dosage in patient with moderate to severe renal failure.
● Don't give drug with food because it decreases rate and extent of absorption.
● If signs and symptoms of peripheral neuropathy occur, notify prescriber. If symptoms are bilateral and persist beyond 72 hours, stop drug.

If symptoms persist or worsen beyond 1 week, stop drug permanently. If peripheral neuropathy resolves to minor symptoms, drug may be reintroduced at 0.375 mg P.O. q 8 hours. If drug isn't withdrawn, peripheral neuropathy may progress to sharp, shooting pain or severe continuous burning pain requiring opioid analgesics and may not be reversible.

• If this drug is stopped because of toxicity, resume recommended dose for zidovudine (100 mg q 4 hours).

⊛ **ALERT:** Don't confuse drug with other antivirals that use initials for identification.

Patient teaching

• Inform patient that drug doesn't cure HIV infection and that opportunistic infections may occur despite continued use. Review safe sex practices with patient.

• Inform patient that peripheral neuropathy is the major toxicity linked to this drug and that pancreatitis is the major life-threatening toxicity. Review signs and symptoms of these adverse reactions, and instruct patient to call prescriber promptly if they appear.

• Instruct woman of childbearing age to use effective contraceptive during drug therapy.

☑ **Evaluation**

• Patient responds well to drug.
• Patient doesn't develop peripheral neuropathy.
• Patient and family state understanding of drug therapy.

zaleplon
(ZAL-eh-plon)
Sonata

Pharmacologic class: pyrazolopyrimidine
Therapeutic class: hypnotic
Pregnancy risk category: C
Controlled substance schedule: IV

Indications and dosages

▶ **Short-term treatment of insomnia.** *Adults:* 10 mg P.O. h.s.; may increase dose to 20 mg if needed. Low-weight adults may respond to 5-mg dose.

Elderly and debilitated patients: Initially, 5 mg P.O. h.s.; doses over 10 mg aren't recommended.

⊠ **Adjust-a-dose:** For patients with mild to moderate hepatic impairment and those taking cimetidine, give 5 mg P.O. daily.

Contraindications and precautions

• Don't use in patients with severe hepatic impairment.
• Use cautiously in debilitated patients, in those with compromised respiratory function, and in those with signs and symptoms of depression.
⚖ Lifespan: In elderly patients, use cautiously.

Adverse reactions

CNS: *headache,* amnesia, dizziness, somnolence, depression, hypertonia, nervousness, depersonalization, hallucinations, vertigo, difficulty concentrating, anxiety, paresthesia, hypesthesia, tremor, asthenia, migraine, malaise, fever.
CV: chest pain, peripheral edema.
EENT: abnormal vision, conjunctivitis, eye pain, ear pain, hyperacusis, epistaxis, parosmia.
GI: constipation, dry mouth, anorexia, dyspepsia, nausea, abdominal pain, colitis.
GU: dysmenorrhea.
Musculoskeletal: arthritis, myalgia, back pain.
Respiratory: bronchitis.
Skin: pruritus, rash, photosensitivity reactions.

Interactions

Drug-drug. *Carbamazepine, phenobarbital, phenytoin, rifampin, other drugs that induce CYP 3A4:* May reduce efficacy of zaleplon. Consider a different hypnotic.
Cimetidine: Potential pharmacokinetic interaction. For patient taking cimetidine, use an initial zaleplon dose of 5 mg.
CNS depressants (imipramine, thioridazine): May produce additive CNS effects. Use cautiously together.
Drug-food. *High-fat foods, heavy meals:* Prolongs absorption, delaying peak zaleplon levels by about 2 hours; sleep onset may be delayed. Separate administration from meals.
Drug-lifestyle. *Alcohol use:* May increase CNS effects. Discourage use together.

Effects on lab test results

None reported.

Pharmacokinetics

Absorption: Rapid and almost complete. Levels peak within 1 hour. Dosing after a high-fat or heavy meal delays peak levels by about 2 hours.

Distribution: Substantially into extravascular tissues. Protein-binding is about 60%.

Metabolism: Extensive, primarily by aldehyde oxidase and, to a lesser extent, CYP 3A4 to inactive metabolites. Less than 1% of dose is excreted unchanged in urine.

Excretion: Rapid. *Half-life:* 1 hour.

Route	Onset	Peak	Duration
P.O.	1 hr	1 hr	3-4 hr

Action

Chemical effect: Has a chemical structure unrelated to benzodiazepines but interacts with the GABA and benzodiazepine receptor complex in the CNS. Modulation of this complex is hypothesized to be responsible for sedative, anxiolytic, muscle relaxant, and anticonvulsant effects of benzodiazepines.

Therapeutic effect: Promotes sleep.

Available forms

Capsules: 5 mg, 10 mg

NURSING PROCESS

Assessment
- Carefully evaluate patient because sleep disturbances may be a symptom of an underlying physical or psychiatric disorder.
- Closely monitor elderly or debilitated patients and patients with compromised respiratory function because of illness.
- Monitor patient for drug abuse and dependence.
- Evaluate patient's and family's knowledge of drug therapy.

Nursing diagnoses
- Disturbed sleep pattern related to presence of insomnia
- Risk for injury related to drug-induced adverse CNS reactions
- Deficient knowledge related to drug therapy

Planning and implementation
- Don't give drug with or following a high-fat or heavy meal.
- Because drug works rapidly, give only immediately before bedtime or after patient has been unable to sleep.

- Adverse reactions are usually dose-related. Give lowest effective dose.
- Limit hypnotic use to 7 to 10 days. If hypnotics will be taken for more than 3 weeks, prescriber should reevaluate patient.
- The potential for drug abuse and dependence exists. Drug shouldn't be given as more than a 1-month supply.

Patient teaching
- Advise patient that zaleplon works rapidly and should be taken immediately before bedtime or after trying to sleep but being unable to.
- Advise patient to take drug only if he can sleep undisturbed for at least 4 hours.
- Warn patient that drowsiness, dizziness, lightheadedness, and difficulty with coordination occur most often within 1 hour after taking drug.
- Advise patient to avoid performing activities that require mental alertness until CNS effects of drug are known.
- Advise patient to avoid alcohol while taking drug and to notify prescriber before taking any prescription or OTC drugs.
- Tell patient not to take drug after a high-fat or heavy meal.
- Advise patient to report any continued sleep problems despite use of drug.
- Inform patient that dependence can occur, and that drug is recommended for short-term use only.
- Warn patient not to abruptly stop drug because withdrawal symptoms, including unpleasant feelings, stomach and muscle cramps, vomiting, sweating, shakiness, and seizures, may occur.
- Tell patient that insomnia may recur for a few nights after stopping drug, but should resolve on its own.
- Advise patient that zaleplon may cause changes in behavior and thinking, including outgoing or aggressive behavior, loss of personal identity, confusion, strange behavior, agitation, hallucinations, worsening of depression, or suicidal thoughts. Tell patient to notify prescriber immediately if any of these symptoms occur.

Evaluation
- Patient states that drug effectively promotes sleep.
- Patient doesn't experience injury as a result of drug-induced adverse CNS reactions.
- Patient and family state understanding of drug therapy.

Reactions may be *common*, uncommon, *life-threatening*, or **COMMON AND LIFE-THREATENING**.

zanamivir

(zah-NAM-ah-veer)
Relenza

Pharmacologic class: neuraminidase inhibitor
Therapeutic class: antiviral
Pregnancy risk category: C

Indications and dosages

▶ **Uncomplicated acute illness caused by influenza A and B virus in patients who have been symptomatic for no more than 2 days.**
Adults and children age 7 and older: 2 oral inhalations (one 5-mg blister per inhalation for a total dose of 10 mg) b.i.d. using the Diskhaler inhalation device for 5 days. Give two doses on the first day of treatment with at least 2 hours between doses. Subsequent doses should be about 12 hours apart (in the morning and evening) at about the same time each day.

Contraindications and precautions

• Contraindicated in patients hypersensitive to drug or its components.
• Use cautiously in patients with severe or decompensated COPD, asthma, or other underlying respiratory disease.
⚖ Lifespan: In breast-feeding women, use cautiously. In children younger than age 7, safety and effectiveness haven't been established.

Adverse reactions

CNS: headache, dizziness.
EENT: nasal signs and symptoms; sinusitis; ear, nose, and throat infections.
GI: diarrhea, nausea, vomiting.
Respiratory: bronchitis, cough.

Interactions

None reported.

Effects on lab test results

None reported.

Pharmacokinetics

Absorption: About 4% to 17%, with peak levels occurring 1 to 2 hours following a 10-mg dose.
Distribution: Less than 10% protein binding.
Metabolism: Not metabolized.

Excretion: Excreted unchanged in the urine within 24 hours. Unabsorbed drug is excreted in feces. *Half-life:* 2½ to 5¼ hours.

Route	Onset	Peak	Duration
Inhalation	Unknown	1-2 hr	Unknown

Action

Chemical effect: Probably inhibits the enzyme neuraminidase on the surface of the influenza virus, possibly altering virus particle aggregation and release. When neuraminidase is inhibited, the virus can't escape from its host cell to attack others, thereby inhibiting the process of viral proliferation.
Therapeutic effect: Lessens the symptoms of influenza.

Available forms

Powder for inhalation: 5 mg per blister

NURSING PROCESS

✎ Assessment
• Obtain accurate patient medical history before starting therapy.
• Lymphopenia, neutropenia, and a rise in liver enzyme and CK levels may occur during treatment. Monitor patient appropriately.
• Monitor patient for bronchospasm and decline in lung function. If they occur, stop the drug.
• Evaluate patient's and family's knowledge of drug therapy.

⊞ Nursing diagnoses
• Risk for infection related to influenza virus
• Imbalanced nutrition: less than body requirements related to drug's adverse GI effects
• Deficient knowledge related to drug therapy

▷ Planning and implementation
• Have patient exhale fully before inserting the mouthpiece. Then, keeping the Diskhaler level, have patient close his lips around the mouthpiece, and have him breathe in steadily and deeply. Instruct patient to hold his breath for a few seconds after inhaling to help keep the drug in his lungs.
• Have a fast-acting bronchodilator available in case of wheezing for patients with underlying respiratory disease. Have patient scheduled to use an inhaled bronchodilator for asthma use his bronchodilator before starting therapy.

• Safety and effectiveness of drug haven't been established for influenza prophylaxis. Use of drug shouldn't affect the evaluation of patient for annual influenza vaccination.

• No data are available to support safety and effectiveness of zanamivir in patients who begin treatment after 48 hours of symptoms.

Patient teaching

• Teach patient how to properly administer drug using the Diskhaler inhalation device and tell him to carefully read the instructions.

• Advise patient to keep the Diskhaler level when loading and inhaling zanamivir. Tell patient to always check inside the mouthpiece of the Diskhaler before each use to make sure it's free of foreign objects.

• Instruct patient with respiratory disease who has an impending scheduled dose of inhaled bronchodilator to take it before taking zanamivir. Tell patient with asthma to have a fast-acting bronchodilator available in case of wheezing while taking zanamivir.

• Tell patient to finish the entire 5-day course of treatment even if he feels better and symptoms improve before the fifth day.

• Inform patient that use of zanamivir hasn't been shown to reduce the risk of transmission of influenza virus to others.

☑ Evaluation

• Patient recovers from influenza.

• Patient doesn't experience adverse GI effects.

• Patient and family state understanding of drug therapy.

---

zidovudine (azidothymidine, AZT)
(zigh-DOH-vyoo-deen)
Apo-Zidovudine ♦ , Novo-AZT ♦ , Retrovir

Pharmacologic class: thymidine analogue
Therapeutic class: antiviral
Pregnancy risk category: C

Indications and dosages

▶ **HIV infection.** *Adults:* 600 mg P.O. daily in divided doses given with other antiretrovirals. Or, for patients who can't take the oral form, 1 mg/kg I.V. over 1 hour, q 4 hours around-the-clock until oral therapy can be used.
Children age 6 weeks to 12 years: 160 mg/m²
P.O. q 8 hours (480 mg/m² daily up to a maxi-

mum of 200 mg q 8 hours) given with other antiretrovirals.

⌧ **Adjust-a-dose:** Patients with end stage renal disease (creatinine clearance less than 15 ml/minute) maintained on dialysis should receive 1 mg/kg I.V. q 6 to 8 hours.

▶ **Prevention of maternal-fetal HIV transmission.** *Pregnant women past 14 weeks' gestation:* 100 mg P.O. five times daily until the start of labor. Then, 2 mg/kg I.V. over 1 hour followed by a continuous I.V. infusion of 1 mg/kg/hour until the umbilical cord is clamped.
Neonates: 2 mg/kg P.O. q 6 hours starting within 12 hours after birth and continuing until age 6 weeks. Or, give 1.5 mg/kg via I.V. infusion over 30 minutes q 6 hours.

⌧ **Adjust-a-dose:** For patients on hemodialysis or peritoneal dialysis, give 100 mg P.O. q 6 to 8 hours.

For patients with mild to moderate hepatic dysfunction or liver cirrhosis, reduce daily dose.

▶ **Post-exposure prophylaxis after occupational exposure to HIV‡.** *Adults:* 600 mg P.O. daily in two or three divided doses for 4 weeks given with other antiretrovirals.

▼ I.V. administration

• Dilute drug before use. Remove calculated dose from vial; add to D₅W to yield no more than 4 mg/ml.

• Infuse drug over 1 hour at constant rate; give q 4 hours around the clock. Avoid rapid infusion or bolus injection.

• After drug is diluted, solution is physically and chemically stable for 24 hours at room temperature and for 48 hours if refrigerated at 36° to 46° F (2° to 8° C). Store undiluted vials at 59° to 77° F (15° to 25° C) and protect them from light.

• Adding mixture to biological or colloidal fluids (such as blood products and protein solutions) isn't recommended.

Contraindications and precautions

• Contraindicated in patients hypersensitive to drug.

• Use cautiously and with close monitoring in patients with advanced symptomatic HIV infection and in those with severe bone marrow depression. Also use cautiously in patients with hepatomegaly, hepatitis, or other known risk factors for hepatic disease.

⚞ **Lifespan:** In breast-feeding women, drug shouldn't be used. In geriatric patients, use cautiously.

Adverse reactions

CNS: *asthenia, headache, **seizures,** paresthesia, malaise,* insomnia, *dizziness,* somnolence, *fever.*
GI: *nausea, anorexia, abdominal pain, vomiting,* constipation, *diarrhea,* dyspepsia, taste perversion.
Hematologic: *severe bone marrow suppression (resulting in anemia), agranulocytosis, thrombocytopenia.*
Metabolic: *lactic acidosis.*
Musculoskeletal: myalgia.
Skin: *rash,* diaphoresis.

Interactions

Drug-drug. *Atovaquone, fluconazole, methadone, probenecid, valproic acid:* May increase levels of zidovudine. Dosage adjustment may be needed.
Doxorubicin, ribavirin, stavudine: In vitro, these drugs, when used with zidovudine, have been shown to be antagonists. Avoid use together.
Ganciclovir, interferon alfa, and other bone marrow–suppressive or cytotoxic drugs: May increase hematologic toxicity of zidovudine. Use cautiously as with other reverse transcriptase inhibitors.
Nelfinavir, rifampin, ritonavir: Decreased bioavailability of zidovudine may occur. Dosage adjustment isn't needed.
Phenytoin: Altered phenytoin level and 30% decrease in zidovudine clearance. Monitor patient closely.

Effects on lab test results

• May increase ALT, AST, alkaline phosphatase, and LDH levels.
• May decrease hemoglobin, hematocrit, and granulocyte and platelet counts.

Pharmacokinetics

Absorption: Rapid.
Distribution: Preliminary data reveal good CSF penetration; about 36% protein-bound.
Metabolism: Rapid, to inactive compound.
Excretion: In urine. *Half-life:* 1 hour.

Route	Onset	Peak	Duration
P.O.	Unknown	30-90 min	Unknown
I.V.	Immediate	30-90 min	Unknown

Actions

Chemical effect: Prevents replication of HIV by inhibiting the enzyme reverse transcriptase.
Therapeutic effect: Reduces symptoms of HIV infection.

Available forms

Capsules: 100 mg
Injection: 10 mg/ml
Syrup: 50 mg/5 ml
Tablets: 300 mg

NURSING PROCESS

⚕ Assessment
• Assess patient's condition before therapy and regularly thereafter.
• Monitor blood studies q 2 weeks to detect anemia or agranulocytosis.
• Be alert for adverse reactions and drug interactions.
• Evaluate patient's and family's knowledge of drug therapy.

⊞ Nursing diagnoses
• Infection related to presence of HIV
• Ineffective protection related to drug-induced adverse hematologic reactions
• Deficient knowledge related to drug therapy

▶ Planning and implementation
• Drug temporarily decreases morbidity and mortality in certain patients with AIDS or AIDS-related complex.
• Optimum duration of treatment and optimum dosage for effectiveness with minimum toxicity aren't yet known.
⚠ ALERT: Notify prescriber of abnormal hematologic study results. Significant anemia (hemoglobin of less than 7.5 g/dl or reduction of more than 25% of baseline) or significant neutropenia (granulocyte count of less than 750/mm^3 or reduction of more than 50% from baseline) may require a dose interruption until evidence of marrow recovery is observed.
Patient teaching
• Advise patient that blood transfusions may be needed during treatment. Drug often causes low RBC count.
• Stress importance of compliance with every-4-hour dosage schedule. Suggest ways to avoid missing doses, perhaps by using an alarm clock.

• Warn patient not to take other drugs for AIDS (especially street drugs) unless approved by prescriber. Some supposed AIDS cures may interfere with drug's effectiveness.

• Advise pregnant HIV-infected women that drug therapy only reduces risk of HIV transmission to neonates. Long-term risks to infants are unknown.

• Advise health care worker considering zidovudine prophylaxis after occupational exposure (such as after needle-stick injury) that drug's safety and effectiveness haven't been proven.

☑ **Evaluation**

• Patient exhibits reduced severity and frequency of symptoms linked to HIV infection.

• Patient doesn't develop complications from therapy.

• Patient and family state understanding of drug therapy.

ziprasidone
(zi-PRAY-si-done)
Geodon

Pharmacologic class: atypical antipsychotic
Therapeutic class: psychotropic
Pregnancy risk category: C

Indications and dosage

▶ **Symptomatic schizophrenia.** *Adults:* Initially, 20 mg P.O. b.i.d. with food. Dosages are highly individualized. Dosage adjustments should occur no sooner than q 2 days, but to allow for lowest possible doses, the interval should be several weeks. Effective dosage range is usually 20 to 80 mg b.i.d. Maximum recommended dosage is 100 mg b.i.d.

▶ **Rapid control of acute agitation in schizophrenic patients.** *Adults:* 10 to 20 mg I.M. as a single dose. Doses of 10 mg may be given q 2 hours; doses of 20 mg may be given q 4 hours. Maximum cumulative dose is 40 mg daily.

Contraindications and precautions

• Contraindicated in patients hypersensitive to drug. Also contraindicated in patients taking drugs that prolong QT interval and in those who have a QTc interval longer than 500 msec. Contraindicated in patients with a history of QT-interval prolongation, congenital QT-interval

syndrome, recent MI, and uncompensated heart failure.

• Use cautiously in patients with acute diarrhea and in patients with a history of bradycardia, hypokalemia, seizures, aspiration pneumonia, or hypomagnesemia.

• Give I.M. ziprasidone with caution to patients with impaired renal function.

☼ **Lifespan:** Breast-feeding women shouldn't take ziprasidone. In elderly patients, safety and effectiveness of I.M. use haven't been established

Adverse reactions

P.O. use
CNS: dystonia.
CV: tachycardia.
EENT: abnormal vision.
Musculoskeletal: myalgia.
Respiratory: cough.
Skin: rash.
I.M. use
CNS: speech disorders.
CV: vasodilation.
GU: priapism.
Musculoskeletal: back pain.
Skin: sweating.
Other: flulike syndrome, tooth disorder.
Both routes
CNS: *somnolence,* akathisia, dizziness, extrapyramidal symptoms, hypertonia, asthenia; *headache, dizziness,* anxiety, insomnia, agitation, cogwheel rigidity, paresthesia, personality disorder, psychosis, *suicide attempt.*
CV: orthostatic hypotension; hypertension, *bradycardia.*
EENT: rhinitis.
GI: *nausea,* constipation, dyspepsia, diarrhea, dry mouth, anorexia; abdominal pain, rectal hemorrhage, vomiting, dyspepsia.
GU: dysmenorrhea.
Skin: injection site pain, furunculosis.

Interactions

Drug-drug. *Antihypertensives:* May enhance hypotensive effects. Monitor blood pressure.
Carbamazepine: May decrease levels of ziprasidone. Higher doses of ziprasidone may be needed to achieve desired effect.
Drugs that increase dopamine level, such as levodopa and dopamine agonists: May have antagonistic effect on ziprasidone. Use together cautiously.

Reactions may be *common,* uncommon, *life-threatening,* or COMMON AND LIFE-THREATENING.

Drugs that lower potassium and magnesium levels, such as diuretics: May increase risk of arrhythmias. If giving together, monitor potassium and magnesium levels.

Drugs that prolong QT interval, including arsenic trioxide, chlorpromazine, dofetilide, dolasetron mesylate, droperidol, gatifloxacin, halofantrine, levomethadyl acetate, mefloquine, mesoridazine, moxifloxacin, pentamidine, pimozide, probucol, quinidine, sotalol, sparfloxacin, tacrolimus, thioridazine, or other class Ia and III antiarrhythmics: May increase risk of arrhythmias when used together. Don't give together.

Itraconazole, ketoconazole: May increase ziprasidone level. Lower doses of ziprasidone may be needed to achieve desired effect.

Effects on lab test results

None reported.

Pharmacokinetics

Absorption: Doubled when taken with food, which is recommended. Peak concentrations reached in about 6 to 8 hours.
Distribution: Highly protein-bound.
Metabolism: Hepatic metabolism; no active metabolites. Less than one-third of the drug is metabolized through the CYP system. CYP 3A4 (major) and CYP 1A2 (minor) are the pathways involving the CYP system.
Excretion: Unknown. *Half-life:* 2½ to 7 hours.

Route	Onset	Peak	Duration
P.O.	1-3 days	6-8 hr	12 hr
I.M.	Unknown	1 hour	Unknown

Action

Chemical effect: Unknown; may work through dopamine and serotonin antagonism. These neurotransmitters are generally targeted for treatment of positive and negative symptoms of schizophrenia. Blocking these neurotransmitters allows symptomatic improvement with minimal adverse effects in the extrapyramidal system.
Therapeutic effect: Relieves psychotic signs and symptoms of schizophrenia.

Available forms

Capsules: 20 mg, 40 mg, 60 mg, 80 mg
Injection: 20 mg/ml single-dose vials (after reconstitution)

NURSING PROCESS

✍ Assessment

• Assess patient's condition before therapy and regularly thereafter.
• Evaluate and monitor patient who experiences dizziness, palpitations, or syncope.
• Drug may prolong QT interval. Other antipsychotics should be considered in patient with a history of QT interval prolongation, acute MI, congenital QT interval syndrome, and other conditions that place the patient at risk for life-threatening arrhythmias. Don't give other drugs that prolong the QT interval with ziprasidone.
• Patient taking antipsychotics is at risk for developing neuroleptic malignant syndrome or tardive dyskinesia.
• Electrolyte disturbances, such as hypokalemia or hypomagnesemia, increase the risk of arrhythmias. Before starting therapy, monitor potassium and magnesium levels and correct imbalances.
• Evaluate patient's and family's knowledge of drug therapy.

🔟 Nursing diagnoses

• Disturbed thought processes related to underlying condition
• Risk for fall related to adverse CNS effects of drug
• Deficient knowledge related to ziprasidone therapy

▶ Planning and implementation

• Don't adjust dosage sooner than q 2 days. Longer intervals may be necessary because symptom response may not be seen for up to 4 to 6 weeks.
• Monitor patient for prolonged QT interval during therapy. Further monitor patient with symptoms of arrhythmias. If QTc interval is greater than 500 msec, stop drug.
• Immediately treat patient with symptoms of neuroleptic malignant syndrome, which can be life-threatening.
• Monitor patient for tardive dyskinesia.
• If long-term therapy of ziprasidone is indicated, switch to P.O. as soon as possible. Effect of I.M. administration for more than 3 consecutive days isn't known.
• Don't give ziprasidone I.M. to schizophrenic patient already taking ziprasidone P.O.

• Give oral drug with food, which increases the effect.
• For I.M. use, add 1.2 ml of sterile water for injection to vial and shake vigorously until entire drug is dissolved.
• Don't mix I.M. injection with any other product besides sterile water for injection.
• Inspect for particulate matter and discoloration before administration, whenever solution and container permit.
• Store dry form at room temperature. Store reconstituted form for up to 24 hours at room temperature or up to 7 days refrigerated (36° to 46° F [2° to 8° C]). Protect from light.

Patient teaching
• Tell patient to take drug with food.
• Tell patient to immediately report to prescriber symptoms of dizziness, fainting, irregular heart beat, or relevant cardiac problems.
• Advise patient to report to prescriber any recent episodes of diarrhea.
• Advise patient to report to prescriber abnormal movements.
• Tell patient to report to prescriber sudden fever, muscle rigidity, or change in mental status.

☑ **Evaluation**
• Patient demonstrates reduced psychotic symptoms with drug therapy.
• Patient doesn't fall.
• Patient and family state understanding of drug therapy.

zoledronic acid
(zoe-LEH-druh-nick ASS-id)
Zometa

Pharmacologic class: bisphosphonate
Therapeutic class: antihypercalcemic
Pregnancy risk category: D

Indications and dosages

▶ **Hypercalcemia related to malignancy.**
Adults: 4 mg by I.V. infusion over at least 15 minutes. If albumin-corrected calcium level doesn't return to normal, consider retreatment with 4 mg. Allow at least 7 days to pass before retreatment to allow a full response to the initial dose.

▶ **Multiple myeloma and bone metastases of solid tumors given with standard antineoplastic therapy. Prostate cancer should have progressed after treatment with at least one hormonal therapy.** *Adults:* 4 mg infused over 15 minutes q 3 or 4 weeks. Duration of treatment in studies was 15 months for prostate cancer, 12 months for breast cancer and multiple myeloma, and 9 months for other solid tumors.

▼ I.V. administration
• Reconstitute by adding 5 ml of sterile water to each vial. Powder must be completely dissolved.
• Withdraw 4 mg of drug and mix in 100 ml of normal saline solution or D_5W.
• The drug must be given as an I.V. infusion over at least 15 minutes. Give drug as a single I.V. solution in a line separate from all other drugs.
• If not used immediately after reconstitution, solution must be refrigerated and given within 24 hours.
• Inspect solution for particulate matter and discoloration before giving it.
• Don't mix drug with solutions that contain calcium (such as lactated Ringer's solution).

Contraindications and precautions
• Contraindicated in patients with significant hypersensitivity to drug, other bisphosphonates, or ingredients in formulation.
• Not recommended in patients with hypercalcemia of malignancy with creatinine greater than 4.5 mg/dl. Not recommended in patients with bone metastases with creatinine greater than 3.0 mg/dl.
• Use cautiously in patients with aspirin-sensitive asthma because other bisphosphonates have been linked to bronchoconstriction in these patients.
  ⚕ Lifespan: In pregnant women, avoid use. Caution women of childbearing age to avoid becoming pregnant. In breast-feeding women, give cautiously; it isn't known whether drug appears in breast milk. In children, safety and effectiveness haven't been established. In geriatric patients, give cautiously.

Adverse reactions
Hypercalcemia
CNS: headache, somnolence, anxiety, confusion, agitation, insomnia, fever.

CV: *hypotension.*
GI: *nausea, constipation, diarrhea, abdominal pain, vomiting,* anorexia, dysphagia.
GU: *UTI, candidiasis.*
Hematologic: anemia, *granulocytopenia, thrombocytopenia, pancytopenia.*
Metabolic: dehydration.
Musculoskeletal: *skeletal pain,* arthralgia.
Respiratory: *dyspnea, cough,* pleural effusion.
Other: PROGRESSION OF CANCER, infection.

Bone metastases
CNS: headache, anxiety, insomnia, depression, paresthesia, hypesthesia, fatigue, weakness, dizziness, fever.
CV: *hypotension, leg edema.*
GI: *nausea, constipation, diarrhea, abdominal pain, vomiting, anorexia, increased appetite.*
GU: *UTI.*
Hematologic: anemia, *neutropenia.*
Metabolic: *dehydration, weight loss.*
Musculoskeletal: *skeletal pain, arthralgia, myalgia, back pain.*
Respiratory: *dyspnea, cough.*
Skin: alopecia, dermatitis.
Other: PROGRESSION OF CANCER, rigors, infection.

Interactions

Drug-drug. *Aminoglycosides, loop diuretics:* May have additive effects to lower calcium level. Give together cautiously, and monitor calcium level.
Thalidomide: In multiple myeloma patients, the risk of renal dysfunction may increase. Use together cautiously.

Effects on lab test results

● May increase creatinine level. May decrease calcium, phosphorus, magnesium, and potassium levels.
● May decrease hemoglobin, hematocrit, and RBC, WBC, and platelet counts.

Pharmacokinetics

Absorption: Administered I.V.
Distribution: Protein binding of about 22%. Post-infusion decline of level is consistent with a triphasic process: Low level observed up to 28 days after a dose.
Metabolism: Doesn't inhibit CYP enzymes or undergo biotransformation in vivo.

Excretion: Primarily via the kidneys. *Half-life:* Alpha is 0.23 hours; beta is 1.75 hours for early distribution. *Terminal half-life:* 167 hours.

Route	Onset	Peak	Duration
I.V.	Unknown	Unknown	7-28 days

Action

Chemical effect: Inhibits bone resorption, probably by inhibiting osteoclast activity and osteoclastic resorption of mineralized bone and cartilage, decreasing calcium release induced by the stimulatory factors produced by tumors.
Therapeutic effect: Lowers calcium level in malignant disease.

Available forms

Injection: 4 mg zoledronic acid, 220 mg mannitol, and 24 mg sodium citrate

NURSING PROCESS

Assessment
● Assess patient's condition before therapy and regularly thereafter.
● Assess kidney function before and during therapy because drug is excreted mainly via the kidneys. The risk of adverse reactions may be greater in patients with impaired renal function. If patient has renal impairment, give drug only if benefits outweigh risks and at an adjusted dosage.
● Measure creatinine level before each dose.
● Make sure patient is adequately hydrated before giving drug; urine output should be about 2 liters daily.
● Evaluate patient's and family's knowledge of drug therapy.

Nursing diagnoses
● Ineffective protection related to adverse hematologic effects
● Ineffective health maintenance related to underlying condition
● Deficient knowledge related to drug therapy

Planning and implementation
⊕ ALERT: A significant decline in renal function could progress to renal failure; single doses shouldn't exceed 4 mg and infusion should last at least 15 minutes.

⊛ ALERT: After giving drug, carefully monitor renal function and calcium, phosphate, magnesium, and creatinine levels.

• Other bisphosphonates have been linked to bronchoconstriction in patients with asthma and aspirin sensitivity.

• Give patient an oral calcium supplement of 500 mg and a multiple vitamin containing 400 IU of vitamin D daily.

Patient teaching

• Review the use and administration of drug with patient and family.

• Instruct patient to report adverse effects promptly.

• Explain the importance of periodic laboratory tests to monitor therapy and renal function.

• Advise patient to notify prescriber if she is pregnant.

✓ Evaluation

• Patient has no adverse hematologic reactions.

• Patient shows improvement in condition.

• Patient and family state understanding of drug therapy.

zolmitriptan
(zohl-muh-TRIP-tan)
Zomig, Zomig-ZMT

Pharmacologic class: selective 5-hydroxytryptamine receptor agonist
Therapeutic class: antimigraine drug
Pregnancy risk category: C

Indications and dosages

▶ **Acute migraine headache.** *Adults:* Initially, 2.5 mg or less P.O. increased to 5 mg per dose, p.r.n. If headache returns after initial dose, second dose may be given after 2 hours. Maximum dose is 10 mg in 24-hour period. Or, give 2.5 mg P.O. of orally disintegrating tablets; don't break tablets in half. If headache returns after initial dose, a second dose may be given after 2 hours. Maximum dose is 10 mg in 24-hour period.

⊠ Adjust-a-dose: For patients with liver disease, use doses under 2.5 mg. Don't use orally disintegrating tablets.

Contraindications and precautions

• Contraindicated in patients hypersensitive to drug or its components; in those with uncontrolled hypertension, ischemic heart disease (angina pectoris, history of MI or documented silent ischemia); and in those with symptoms or findings consistent with ischemic heart disease, coronary artery vasospasm, including Prinzmetal's variant angina, or other significant heart disease.

• Avoid use within 24 hours of other 5-HT$_1$ agonists or drugs containing ergot, or within 2 weeks of stopping MAO inhibitor therapy. Also avoid use in patients with hemiplegic or basilar migraine.

• Use cautiously in patients with liver disease and in patients who may be at risk for coronary artery disease (CAD), such as postmenopausal women, men older than age 40, or patients with hypertension, hypercholesterolemia, obesity, diabetes, smoking, or family history of CAD.

⚖ Lifespan: In pregnant and breast-feeding women, use cautiously.

Adverse reactions

CNS: somnolence, vertigo, *dizziness,* hypesthesia, paresthesia, asthenia, pain.
CV: palpitations, *coronary artery vasospasm, transient myocardial ischemia, MI, ventricular tachycardia, ventricular fibrillation;* pain, tightness, pressure, or heaviness in chest.
EENT: *pain, tightness, or pressure in the neck, throat, or jaw.*
GI: dry mouth, dyspepsia, dysphagia, nausea.
Musculoskeletal: myalgia, myasthenia.
Skin: sweating.
Other: warm or cold sensations.

Interactions

Drug-drug. *Cimetidine:* Doubles half-life of zolmitriptan. Monitor patient closely.
Ergot-containing drugs, serotonin$_{1B/1D}$ agonists: May cause additive effects. Avoid use within 24 hours of almotriptan.
Hormonal contraceptives: May increase levels of zolmitriptan. Monitor patient closely.
MAO inhibitors: Increased levels of zolmitriptan. Avoid use of drug within 2 weeks of stopping MAO inhibitor therapy.
SSRIs: May cause additive serotonin effects, resulting in weakness, hyperreflexia, or incoordination. If given together, monitor patient closely.

Effects on lab test results

• May increase glucose level.

Pharmacokinetics

Absorption: Well absorbed following P.O. administration, with an absolute bioavailability of 40%.
Distribution: 25% bound to protein.
Metabolism: Converted to active N-desmethyl metabolite.
Excretion: About 65% of dose is recovered in urine (8% unchanged) and 30% in feces. *Half-life:* 3 hours.

Route	Onset	Peak	Duration
P.O.	Unknown	2 hr	3 hr
P.O. orally disintegrating	Unknown	2 hr	Unknown

Action

Chemical effect: Selective serotonin receptor agonist causes constriction of cranial blood vessels and inhibits proinflammatory neuropeptide release.
Therapeutic effect: Relieves migraine headache pain.

Available forms

Tablets: 2.5 mg, 5 mg
Tablets (orally disintegrating): 2.5 mg, 5 mg

NURSING PROCESS

🔍 Assessment

• Assess patient's history of migraine headaches and drug's effectiveness.
• Assess patient for history of coronary artery disease, hypertension, arrhythmias, or presence of risk factors for coronary artery disease.
• Monitor liver function test results before starting drug therapy, and report abnormalities.
• Use drug only when a clear diagnosis of migraine has been established.
• Evaluate patient's and family's knowledge of drug therapy.

🔷 Nursing diagnoses

• Acute pain related to presence of migraine headache
• Impaired cardiopulmonary tissue perfusion related to drug-induced adverse cardiac events
• Deficient knowledge related to drug therapy

▶ Planning and implementation

• Use a lower dose in patients with moderate-to-severe hepatic impairment; don't give them orally disintegrating tablets because those tablets can't be broken in half.
• Don't give drug to prevent migraine headaches or to treat hemiplegic migraines, basilar migraines, or cluster headaches.
⑤ ALERT: Don't give drug within 24 hours of ergot-containing drugs or within 2 weeks of MAO inhibitor.
Patient teaching
• Tell patient that drug is intended to relieve the symptoms of migraines, not to prevent them.
• Advise patient to take drug as prescribed. Caution against taking a second dose unless instructed by prescriber. Tell patient that if a second dose is indicated and permitted, he should take it at least 2 hours after initial dose.
• Advise patient to immediately report pain or tightness in chest or throat, heart throbbing, rash, skin lumps, or swelling of face, lips, or eyelids.
• Tell woman not to take drug if she plans or suspects pregnancy.
• Instruct patient to release the orally disintegrating tablets from the blister pack just before administration. Open the pack and dissolve on tongue.
• Advise patient not to break the orally disintegrating tablets in half.

✓ Evaluation

• Patient has relief from migraine headache.
• Patient doesn't experience pain or tightness in the chest or throat, arrhythmias, increases in blood pressure, or MI.
• Patient and family state understanding of drug therapy.

zolpidem tartrate

(ZOHL-peh-dim TAR-trayt)
Ambien

Pharmacologic class: imidazopyridine
Therapeutic class: hypnotic
Pregnancy risk category: B
Controlled substance schedule: IV

Indications and dosages

▶ **Short-term management of insomnia.**
Adults: 10 mg P.O. h.s.
☒ **Adjust-a-dose:** For elderly and debilitated patients and patients with hepatic insufficiency, give 5 mg P.O. h.s. Maximum, 10 mg daily.

Contraindications and precautions

• Use cautiously in patients with conditions that could affect metabolism or hemodynamic responses and in those with compromised respiratory status, because hypnotics may depress respiratory drive. Also use cautiously in patients with depression or history of alcohol or drug abuse.
⚕ **Lifespan:** In pregnant women, use cautiously. In breast-feeding women, drug isn't recommended. In children, safety of drug hasn't been established.

Adverse reactions

CNS: daytime drowsiness, light-headedness, abnormal dreams, amnesia, dizziness, *headache,* hangover effect, sleep disorder, lethargy, depression.
CV: palpitations.
EENT: sinusitis, pharyngitis.
GI: nausea, vomiting, diarrhea, dyspepsia, constipation, abdominal pain, dry mouth.
Musculoskeletal: back or chest pain, myalgia, arthralgia.
Skin: rash.
Other: flulike syndrome, hypersensitivity reactions.

Interactions

Drug-drug. *CNS depressants:* Enhances CNS depression. Use together cautiously.
Drug-food. *Any food:* Decreases rate and extent of absorption. Take drug on an empty stomach.
Drug-lifestyle. *Alcohol use:* May cause excessive CNS depression. Discourage use together.

Effects on lab test results

None reported.

Pharmacokinetics

Absorption: Rapid. Food delays drug absorption.
Distribution: Protein-binding is about 92.5%.
Metabolism: In liver.
Excretion: Primarily in urine. *Half-life:* 2½ hours.

Route	Onset	Peak	Duration
P.O.	Rapid	30 min-2 hr	Unknown

Action

Chemical effect: Interacts with one of three identified GABA and benzodiazepine receptor complexes but isn't a benzodiazepine. It exhibits hypnotic activity but no muscle relaxant or anticonvulsant properties.
Therapeutic effect: Promotes sleep.

Available forms

Tablets: 5 mg, 10 mg

NURSING PROCESS

🔍 **Assessment**
• Assess patient's condition before therapy and regularly thereafter.
• Be alert for adverse reactions and drug interactions.
• Evaluate patient's and family's knowledge of drug therapy.

🔢 **Nursing diagnoses**
• Disturbed sleep pattern related to presence of insomnia
• Risk for injury related to drug-induced adverse CNS reactions
• Deficient knowledge related to drug therapy

▶ **Planning and implementation**
• Drug has a rapid onset of action; give when patient is ready to sleep.
• Use hypnotics only for short-term management of insomnia, usually 7 to 10 days. Persistent insomnia may indicate primary psychiatric or medical disorder.
• Because most adverse reactions are dose-related, use smallest effective dose in all patients, especially those who are elderly or debilitated.
• Give drug at least 1 hour before meals or 2 hours after meals.
• **⚠ ALERT:** Don't confuse Ambien with Amen.
Patient teaching
• Tell patient to take drug immediately before going to bed.
• For faster onset, instruct patient not to take drug with or immediately after meals. Food decreases drug's absorption.
• Warn patient about performing activities that require mental alertness or physical coordina-

tion. For inpatient, supervise walking and raise bed rails, particularly for geriatric patient.

☑ **Evaluation**
• Patient states that drug effectively promotes sleep.
• Patient doesn't experience injury from adverse CNS reactions.
• Patient and family state understanding of drug therapy.

zonisamide
(zon-ISS-a-mide)
Zonegran

Pharmacologic class: sulfonamide
Therapeutic class: anticonvulsant
Pregnancy risk category: C

Indications and dosages

▶ **Adjunct therapy for partial seizures in adults with epilepsy.** *Adults:* Initially, 100 mg P.O. as a single daily dose for 2 weeks. After 2 weeks, the dose may be increased to 200 mg daily for at least 2 weeks. It can be increased to 300 mg and 400 mg P.O. daily, with the dose stable for at least 2 weeks to achieve steady state at each level. Doses larger than 100 mg can be divided. Can be taken with or without food.

Contraindications and precautions

• Contraindicated in patients hypersensitive to drug or other sulfonamides.
• Rarely, patients receiving sulfonamides have died because of severe reactions such as Stevens-Johnson syndrome, fulminant hepatic necrosis, aplastic anemia, otherwise unexplained rashes, and agranulocytosis. If signs of hypersensitivity or other serious reactions occur, stop drug immediately.
• Use cautiously in patients with renal or hepatic dysfunction. If GFR is less than 50 ml/minute, don't use drug. If patient develops acute renal failure or a significant sustained increase in creatinine or BUN levels, stop drug.
• Use caution when drug is prescribed with other drugs that predispose patients to heat-related disorders (such as carbonic anhydrase inhibitors and anticholinergics).
⚠ **Lifespan:** In pregnant women, avoid use; use only if potential benefits outweigh risks to

fetus. Advise breast-feeding women to stop breast-feeding or avoid giving drug, taking into consideration the importance of the drug to the mother. In children, safety and effectiveness haven't been established.

Adverse reactions

CNS: *headache, dizziness,* ataxia, nystagmus, paresthesia, confusion, difficulties in concentration and memory, mental slowing, agitation, irritability, depression, insomnia, anxiety, nervousness, schizophrenic or schizophreniform behavior, *somnolence,* fatigue, speech abnormalities, difficulties in verbal expression.
EENT: diplopia, rhinitis.
GI: *anorexia,* nausea, diarrhea, dyspepsia, constipation, dry mouth, taste perversion, abdominal pain.
Metabolic: weight loss.
Skin: ecchymoses, *rash.*
Other: flulike symptoms.

Interactions

Drug-drug. *Drugs that induce or inhibit CYP 3A4:* Alters zonisamide level. Zonisamide clearance is increased by phenytoin, carbamazepine, phenobarbital, and valproate. Monitor patient closely.

Effects on lab test results

• May increase BUN and creatinine levels.

Pharmacokinetics

Absorption: Level peaks in 2 to 6 hours; food delays but doesn't affect bioavailability.
Distribution: Extensively binds to erythrocytes. Drug is about 40% bound to proteins. Protein-binding is unaffected in the presence of therapeutic levels of phenytoin, phenobarbital, or carbamazepine.
Metabolism: By CYP 3A4. Drug clearance increases in patients who are also taking enzyme-inducing drugs.
Excretion: Primarily in urine as parent drug and as glucuronide of a metabolite. *Half-life:* About 63 hours.

Route	Onset	Peak	Duration
P.O.	Unknown	Unknown	Unknown

Action

Chemical effect: May produce antiseizure effects through action at the sodium and calcium channels, thereby stabilizing neuronal membranes and suppressing neuronal hypersynchronization. May also suppress GABA synaptic activity without help or may facilitate dopaminergic and serotonergic neurotransmission. **Therapeutic effect:** Prevents and stops seizure activity.

Available forms

Capsules: 100 mg

NURSING PROCESS

⚗ Assessment

• Assess patient's condition before therapy and regularly thereafter.
• Monitor patient for symptoms of hypersensitivity.
• Monitor body temperature, especially in summer, because decreased sweating may occur (especially in children age 17 and younger), resulting in heatstroke and dehydration.
• Monitor renal function periodically.
• Evaluate patient's and family's knowledge of drug therapy.

⊕ Nursing diagnoses

• Risk for trauma related to seizures
• Risk for injury related to drug-induced adverse CNS effects
• Deficient knowledge related to drug therapy

▷ Planning and implementation

• Drug may be taken with or without food. Don't break capsule.
• Use cautiously in patient with hepatic and renal disease; may need slower adjustment and more frequent monitoring. If GFR is less than 50 ml/minute, don't use drug.
• Abrupt zonisamide withdrawal may cause increased frequency of seizures or status epilepticus; reduce dose or stop drug gradually.
• Increase fluid intake and urine output to help prevent renal calculi, especially in patient with predisposing factors.
• Children appear to be at an increased risk for drug-associated oligohidrosis and hyperthermia. Closely monitor patients, especially children, for evidence of decreased sweating and increased body temperature, especially in warm or hot weather.

Patient teaching

• Tell patient medication can be taken with or without food. Warn against biting or breaking the capsule.
• Instruct patient to contact prescriber immediately if a skin rash develops or seizures worsen.
• Tell patient to contact prescriber immediately if he develops sudden back pain, abdominal pain, pain when urinating, bloody or dark urine, fever, sore throat, mouth sores, easy bruising, decreased sweating, increased body temperature, depression, or speech or language problems.
• Tell patient to drink 6 to 8 glasses of water a day.
• Tell patient to avoid hazardous activities until full effects of drug are known. It may cause drowsiness.
• Instruct patient not to stop taking drug without prescriber's approval.
• Tell patient to notify prescriber about planned, suspected, or known pregnancy. Also tell her to notify prescriber if she's breast-feeding.
• Advise woman of childbearing age to use contraception while taking drug.

✓ Evaluation

• Patient is free from seizure activity.
• Patient doesn't experience adverse CNS effects.
• Patient and family state understanding of drug therapy.

Reactions may be *common,* uncommon, *life-threatening,* or COMMON AND LIFE-THREATENING.

Herbal
Medicines

aloe

(AH-loh)

Reported uses

Used externally as a topical gel for minor burns, sunburn, cuts, frostbite, skin irritation, and other wounds and abrasions.

Used to treat amenorrhea, asthma, colds, seizures, bleeding, and ulcers.

Preparations also are used to treat acne, AIDS, arthritis, asthma, blindness, bursitis, cancer, colitis, depression, diabetes, glaucoma, hemorrhoids, multiple sclerosis, peptic ulcers, and varicose veins.

Dosages

▶ **Pruritus, skin irritation, burns, and other wounds (external forms).** Apply liberally, p.r.n. Although internal use isn't recommended, some sources suggest 100 to 200 mg aloe or 50 to 100 mg aloe extract P.O., taken in the evening. Information about dosages for aloe juice is inadequate.

Cautions

● External preparations contraindicated in patients hypersensitive to herb and in those with history of allergic reactions to plants in the Liliaceae family (such as garlic, onions, and tulips).

● Oral use is contraindicated in patients with cardiac or kidney disease (because of risk of hypokalemia and disturbance of cardiac rhythm); in those with intestinal obstruction; in those with Crohn's disease, ulcerative colitis, appendicitis, or abdominal pain of unknown origin; in women who are pregnant or breast-feeding; and in children.

⚘ **Lifespan:** None reported.

Adverse reactions

CV: *arrhythmias.*
GI: painful intestinal spasms, damage to intestinal mucosa, harmless brown discoloration of intestinal mucous membranes, *severe hemorrhagic diarrhea.*
GU: *kidney damage,* red discoloration of urine, *reflex stimulation of uterine musculature causing miscarriage or premature birth.*

Metabolic: fluid and electrolyte loss, hypokalemia.
Musculoskeletal: muscle weakness, accelerated bone deterioration.
Skin: contact dermatitis, delayed healing of deep wounds.

Interactions

Herb-drug. *Antiarrhythmics, cardiac glycosides such as digoxin:* Oral form may lead to toxic reaction. Monitor patient closely.
Corticosteroids, diuretics: Increases potassium loss. Monitor patient for signs of hypokalemia.
Disulfiram: Tincture contains alcohol and could precipitate a disulfiram reaction. Discourage use together.
Herb-herb. *Licorice:* Increases risk of potassium deficiency. Discourage use together.

Action

When taken internally, aloe produces a metabolite that irritates the large intestine and stimulates colonic activity. It also causes active secretion of fluids and electrolytes and inhibits reabsorption of fluids from the colon, resulting in a feeling of distention and increased peristalsis. The cathartic effect occurs 8 to 12 hours after ingestion.

When used externally, besides acting as a moisturizer on burns and other wounds, herb reduces inflammation. Its antipruritic effect may result from blockage of the conversion of histidine to histamine. Wound healing may result from increased blood flow to the wound area.

Common forms

In capsules or as cream, hair conditioner, jelly, juice, liniment, lotion, ointment, shampoo, skin cream, soap, sunscreen, and in facial tissues.
Also as an ingredient in Benzoin Compound Tincture.
Capsules: 75 mg, 100 mg, 200 mg aloe vera extract or aloe vera powder.
Gel: 98%, 99.5%, 99.6% aloe vera gel.
Juice: 99.6%, 99.7% aloe vera juice.
Tincture*: 1:10, 50% alcohol.

Nursing considerations

● Oral use can cause severe abdominal discomfort and serious hypokalemia and electrolyte imbalance.

---

*Liquid may contain alcohol.

• Studies on the use of injections for cancer have shown a link to death.
• Use of injectable preparations of herb or its chemical constituents isn't recommended.

Patient teaching

• Warn patient against ingesting aloe vera gel or aloe vera juice.
• Advise patient to consult prescriber before using an herbal preparation because another treatment may be available.
• Instruct patient to tell the pharmacist of any herbal or dietary supplement he's taking when filling a new prescription.
• Tell patient that if he uses herb and delays seeking medical diagnosis and treatment, his condition could worsen.
• Warn patient not to take herb without medical advice if he's also taking digoxin, another drug to control his heart rate, a diuretic, or a corticosteroid.
• Herb may cause feelings of dehydration, weakness, and confusion, especially if used for a prolonged period. Instruct patient to seek medical help immediately if any of these signs or symptoms appear.
• Tell patient that FDA doesn't recognize laxatives containing aloe to be safe or effective.

angelica
(an-JEL-ih-kah)

Reported uses

To treat gynecologic disorders, postmenopausal symptoms, menstrual discomfort, and anemia. Also used to treat mild peptic discomfort, such as GI spasms, flatulence, bloating, colic and loss of appetite; to strengthen the heart; to improve circulation in the limbs; and to relieve osteoporosis, hay fever, cough, asthma, bronchitis, acne, and eczema.

Dosages

No consensus exists.

Cautions

• Urge caution in diabetic patients because various species of this plant contain polysaccharides that may disrupt glucose-level control.

⚠ Lifespan: In pregnant and breast-feeding women, herb is contraindicated because of potential stimulant effects on the uterus.

Adverse reactions

CV: hypotension.
Skin: photodermatitis, phototoxicity.

Interactions

Herb-drug. *Antacids, H_2-receptor antagonists, proton pump inhibitors, sucralfate:* Herb may increase acid production in the stomach and may interfere with absorption of these drugs. Discourage use together.
Anticoagulants: Potentiates effects with excessive doses of herb. Monitor patient for bleeding.
Herb-lifestyle. *Sun exposure:* Photosensitivity reaction may occur. Advise patient to avoid unprotected or prolonged exposure to sunlight.

Action

Root extracts may have antitumor properties by inhibiting cancer cells; also may have anti-inflammatory and analgesic actions.
Isolated substances extracted from the root inhibit platelet aggregation, exert antimicrobial action, and decrease myocardial injury and the risk of PVCs and arrhythmias induced by myocardial reperfusion.

Improved pulmonary function and decreased mean arterial pulmonary pressures may occur when compounds are used with nifedipine in patient with COPD and pulmonary hypertension.

Common forms

Fluid extract, tincture, essential oil, and cut, dried, and powdered root.

Nursing considerations

• Monitor patients using herb for signs of bleeding—especially those also taking anticoagulants.
• Find out why patient is using the herb.
• Monitor patient for persistent diarrhea, which may be a sign of something more serious.
• Monitor patient for dermatologic reaction.
• Photodermatosis is possible after contact with the plant juice or plant extract.

Bold italic type indicates that reaction may be life-threatening.

Patient teaching

- Instruct patient to tell the pharmacist of any herbal or dietary supplement he's taking when filling a new prescription.
- Warn patient not to treat symptoms with herb before seeking appropriate medical evaluation because doing so may delay diagnosis of a potentially serious medical condition.
- Advise patient not to take herb if pregnant or if taking an acid blocker or blood-thinning drug.
- Advise patient to report skin rash.

bilberry
(BIL-beh-ree)
bilberries, bog bilberries, European blueberries, huckleberries, whortleberries

Reported uses

Used to treat visual and circulatory problems, glaucoma, cataracts, diabetic retinopathy, macular degeneration, varicose veins, and hemorrhoids. Also used to improve night vision.

Dosages

Suggested dosages vary considerably. Most herbalists recommend using standardized products consisting of 25% anthocyanoside content.
▶ **Improve night vision.** 60 to 120 mg of bilberry extract P.O. daily.
▶ **Visual and circulatory problems.** 240 to 480 mg P.O. daily in two or three divided doses.

Cautions

- Urge caution in patients taking anticoagulants. Herb may be unsuitable for those with a bleeding disorder.
- ⚖ Lifespan: In pregnant and breast-feeding women, herb is contraindicated.

Adverse reactions

Other: *toxic reaction.*

Interactions

Herb-drug. *Anticoagulants, antiplatelets:* Inhibits platelet aggregation, possibly increasing the risk of bleeding. Monitor patient.
Disulfiram: May cause disulfiram reaction if herb preparation contains alcohol. Advise patient to avoid use together.

Action

May reduce vascular permeability and tissue edema. Also may aid blood flow. Exerts potent antioxidant effects and a protective effect on LDLs.
 Chemical components of herb may exert changes in the retina (allowing better adaptation to darkness and light), decrease excessive platelet aggregation, and exert preventive and curative antiulcer actions.

Common forms

Capsules: 60 mg, 80 mg, 120 mg, 450 mg. Also available in liquid, tincture, fluid extract, and dried root, leaves, and berries.

Nursing considerations

⊛ **ALERT:** Long-term consumption of large doses of bilberry leaves can be poisonous. Doses of 1.5 g/kg or more in a day may be fatal.
- Herb may reduce glucose level in diabetics. Dosage may need to be adjusted in those taking antidiabetic drugs.
- For treatment of vascular and ocular conditions, consistent dosing is required.

Patient teaching

- Instruct patient to tell the pharmacist of any herbal or dietary supplement he's taking when filling a new prescription.
- Warn patient not to treat symptoms with herb before seeking appropriate medical evaluation because doing so may delay diagnosis of a potentially serious medical condition.
- Herb may be taken without regard to meals or food.
- Advise any patient using the dried fruit to take each dose with a full glass of water.

capsicum
(KAP-sih-kem)

Reported uses

Used to treat bowel disorders, chronic laryngitis, and peripheral vascular disease. Various preparations are applied topically as counterirritants and external analgesics. The FDA has approved topical capsaicin for temporary relief of pain from rheumatoid arthritis, osteoarthritis, postherpetic neuralgia (shingles), and diabetic

---

*Liquid may contain alcohol.

neuropathy. It's being tested for treatment of psoriasis, intractable pruritus, vitiligo, phantom limb pain, mastectomy pain, Guillain-Barré syndrome, neurogenic bladder, vulvar vestibulitis, apocrine chromhidrosis, and reflex sympathetic dystrophy. It's also used in personal defense sprays and to treat refractory pruritus and pruritus caused by renal failure.

Dosages

Topical preparations range from 0.025% to 0.25%. Most effective when applied t.i.d. or q.i.d.; duration of action is about 4 to 6 hours. Less frequent applications typically produce incomplete analgesia.

Cautions

• Contraindicated in patients hypersensitive to herb or chili pepper products. Patients with irritable bowel syndrome should avoid use because herb has irritant and peristaltic effects.
• Patients with asthma who use herb may experience more bronchospasms.
⚠ Lifespan: In pregnant women, herb is contraindicated because of possible uterine stimulant effects.

Adverse reactions

EENT: blepharospasm, extreme burning pain, lacrimation, conjunctival edema, hyperemia, burning pain in nose, sneezing, serous discharge.
GI: oral burning, diarrhea, gingival irritation, bleeding gums.
Respiratory: *bronchospasm,* cough, retrosternal discomfort.
Skin: transient skin irritation, itching, stinging, erythema without vesicular eruption, contact dermatitis.

Interactions

Herb-drug. *ACE inhibitors:* Increases risk of cough when applied topically. Monitor patient closely.
Anticoagulants: May alter anticoagulant effects. Monitor PT and INR closely; tell patient to avoid use together.
Antiplatelets, heparin and low–molecular-weight heparin, warfarin: Increases risk of bleeding. Advise patient to avoid use together. If they must be used together, monitor patient for bleeding.

Aspirin, salicylic acid compounds: Reduces bioavailability of these drugs. Discourage use together.
MAO inhibitors: Herb increases catecholamine secretion and increases risk of hypertensive crisis. Discourage use together.
Theophylline: Increases absorption when given with herb. Discourage use together.
Herb-herb. *Feverfew, garlic, ginger, ginkgo, ginseng:* Increases anticoagulant effects of capsicum, and increases risk of bleeding. Discourage use together; if these herbs must be used together, monitor patient closely for bleeding.

Action

Topical herb produces an extremely intense irritation at the contact point. Initial dose causes profound pain; however, repeated applications cause desensitization, with analgesic and anti-inflammatory effects.

Juices from the fruits may have antibacterial properties in vitro.

Common forms

Cream: 0.025%, 0.075%, 0.25%.
Gel: 0.025%.
Lotion: 0.025%, 0.075%.
Roll-on: 0.075%.
Self-defense spray: 5%, 10%.
Also available as the vegetable, pepper.

Nursing considerations

• Find out why patient is using the herb.
• Topical product shouldn't be used on broken or irritated skin or covered with a tight bandage.
• Washing the area thoroughly with soap and water treats adverse skin reaction to topically applied herb. Soaking the area in vegetable oil after washing provides a slower onset but longer duration of relief than cold water. Vinegar water irrigation is moderately successful. Rubbing alcohol also may help.
• EMLA, an emulsion of lidocaine and prilocaine, provides pain relief in about 1 hour to skin that has been severely irritated by herb.
• Herb shouldn't be taken orally for more than 2 days and shouldn't be used again for 2 weeks.
• After topical application, relief may occur in 3 days but may take as long as 14 to 28 days, depending on the condition requiring analgesia.

Bold italic type indicates that reaction may be life-threatening.

Patient teaching

- Tell patient to avoid contact with eyes, mucous membranes, and broken skin.
- If patient is using herb topically, instruct him to wash his hands before and immediately after applying it. Advise contact lens wearers to wash hands and to use gloves or an applicator if handling lenses after applying capsicum.
- If incidental contact occurs, instruct patient to flush exposed area with cool running water for as long as necessary.
- Warn patient taking MAO inhibitor not to use this herb.

cat's claw
(KATS klaw)

Reported uses

Used to treat GI problems, including Crohn's disease, colitis, inflammatory bowel disease, diverticulitis, gastritis, dysentery, ulcerations and hemorrhoids, and to enhance immunity. Used to treat systemic inflammatory diseases (such as arthritis and rheumatism). Used by cancer patients for its antimutagenic effects. Used with zidovudine to stimulate the immune system by patients with HIV infection. Used as a contraceptive.

Dosages

No consensus exists. Herbal literature suggests 500 to 1,000 mg P.O. t.i.d. Other sources suggest different dosages depending on condition and form of herbal product.
Capsules: 2 capsules (175 mg/capsule) P.O. daily or 3 capsules P.O. t.i.d.; dosage varies by manufacturer.
Decoction: 2 to 3 cups/day made from 10 to 30 g inner stalk bark or root in 1 quart (1 L) of water for 30 to 60 minutes.
Extract (alcohol-free): 7 to 10 gtt t.i.d. up to 15 gtt five times a day.
Liquid or alcohol extract*: 10 to 15 gtt b.i.d. to t.i.d., to 1 to 3 ml t.i.d.
Powdered extract: 1 to 3 capsules (500 mg/capsule) P.O. b.i.d. to q.i.d.

Cautions

- Patients who have had transplant surgery, and patients who have autoimmune disease, multiple sclerosis, or tuberculosis should avoid use. Patients with coagulation disorders and those receiving anticoagulants should also avoid use.
- Patients with a history of peptic ulcer disease or gallstones should use caution when taking this herb because it stimulates stomach acid secretion.

⚱ **Lifespan:** In pregnant and breast-feeding women, herb is contraindicated.

Adverse reactions

CV: hypotension.

Interactions

Herb-drug. *Antihypertensives:* May potentiate hypotensive effects. Discourage use together. *Immunosuppressants:* May counteract the therapeutic effects because herb has immunostimulant properties. Discourage use together.
Herb-food. *Food:* Enhances absorption of herb. Patient can take herb with food.

Action

Some chemical components stimulate immune system function and exert antitumor activity. Other components may inhibit platelet aggregation and the sympathetic nervous system, reduce the heart rate, decrease peripheral vascular resistance, and lower blood pressure. They also may exhibit antiviral activity and antioxidant properties in vitro. One component has weak diuretic properties.

Common forms

In tablets and capsules; as teas and tinctures; as cut, dried, and powdered bark, roots, and leaves.
Tablets, capsules: 25 mg, 150 mg, 175 mg, 300 mg, 350 mg (standard extract), 400 mg, 500 mg, 800 mg, 1 g, 5 g (raw herb).

Nursing considerations

- Find out why patient is using the herb.
- Some liquid extracts contain alcohol and may be unsuitable for children or patients with liver disease.
- This herb and its contents vary from manufacturer to manufacturer; the alkaloid concentration varies from season to season.

Patient teaching

- Instruct patient to tell the pharmacist of any herbal or dietary supplement he's taking when filling a new prescription.

*Liquid may contain alcohol.

• Inform patient that herb shouldn't be used for more than 8 weeks without a 2- to 3-week rest period from the herb.
• Instruct patient to promptly report adverse reactions and new signs or symptoms.
• Recommend another method of contraception if herb is being used for this purpose.
• Tell patient to rise slowly from a sitting or lying position to avoid dizziness from possible hypotension.
• Advise patient to watch for signs of bleeding, especially if anticoagulants are also being taken.

chamomile
(KAH-meh-mighl)

Reported uses

Used to treat stomach disorders, such as GI spasms and other GI inflammatory conditions. Used to treat insomnia. Used to treat menstrual disorders, migraine, epidermolysis bullosa, eczema, eye irritation, throat discomfort, and hemorrhoids. Used as a topical bacteriostat and mouthwash. Teas are mainly used for sedation or relaxation.

Dosages

Usually taken as a tea, prepared by adding 1 tbs (3 g) of the flower head to hot water and steeping for 10 to 15 minutes; it is then taken up to q.i.d.

Cautions

• Herb is believed to be an abortifacient, and some of its components may have teratogenic effects.
• Urge caution in patients hypersensitive to components of volatile oils and in those at risk for contact dermatitis.
• Safety in patients with liver or kidney disorders hasn't been established, so these patients should avoid use.
⚗ Lifespan: In pregnant and breast-feeding women, discourage use. In teething babies or in children younger than age 2, herb shouldn't be used.

Adverse reactions

EENT: conjunctivitis, eyelid angioedema.
GI: nausea, vomiting.

Skin: eczema, contact dermatitis.
Other: *anaphylaxis.*

Interactions

Herb-drug. *Anticoagulants:* May potentiate effects. Discourage use together.
Other drugs: Potential for decreased absorption of drugs because of antispasmodic activity of herb in the GI tract. Discourage use together.

Action

Exhibits anti-inflammatory, antiallergenic, antidiuretic, sedative, antibacterial, and antifungal properties. May lower urea level. Some compounds may stimulate liver regeneration after oral use; others have in vitro antitumor activity. One component may have antiulcer effects.

Common forms

As capsules, liquid, and tea, and as an ingredient in many cosmetic products.
Capsules: 354 mg, 360 mg

Nursing considerations

• Find out why patient is using the herb.
⊛ ALERT: People sensitive to ragweed and chrysanthemums or other Compositae family members (arnica, yarrow, feverfew, tansy, artemisia) may be more susceptible to contact allergies and anaphylaxis. Those with hay fever or bronchial asthma caused by pollens are more susceptible to anaphylactic reaction.
• Signs and symptoms of anaphylaxis include shortness of breath, swelling of the tongue, rash, tachycardia, and hypotension.

Patient teaching

• Advise patient to consult prescriber before using an herbal preparation because a treatment with proven effectiveness may be available.
• Instruct patient to tell the pharmacist of any herbal or dietary supplement he's taking when filling a new prescription.
• If patient is pregnant or is planning pregnancy, advise her not to use herb.
• If patient is taking an anticoagulant, advise him not to use herb because of possibly enhanced anticoagulant effects.
• Advise patient that herb may enhance an allergic reaction or make existing symptoms worse in susceptible individuals.
• Instruct parent not to give herb to child before checking with a knowledgeable practitioner.

Bold italic type indicates that reaction may be life-threatening.

echinacea

(eh-kih-NAY-zyah)

Reported uses

Used as a wound-healing agent for abscesses, burns, eczema, varicose ulcers of the leg and other skin wounds, and as a nonspecific immunostimulant for the supportive treatment of upper respiratory tract infections, the common cold, and urinary tract infections.

Dosages

Capsules containing powdered herb: Equivalent to 900 mg to 1 g P.O. t.i.d.; doses can vary.
Expressed juice: 6 to 9 ml P.O. daily.
Tea: ½ tsp (500 mg) of coarsely powdered herb simmered in 1 cup (240 ml) of boiling water for 10 minutes. Advise patient to avoid this method of administration because some active compounds are water-insoluble.
Tincture: 0.75 to 1.5 ml (15 to 30 gtt) P.O. two to five times daily. May be used as 60 gtt P.O. t.i.d.

Cautions

• Contraindicated in patients with severe illnesses, such as HIV infection, collagen disease, leukosis, multiple sclerosis, tuberculosis, or autoimmune diseases.
⚘ **Lifespan:** In pregnant and breast-feeding women, discourage use because effects are unknown.

Adverse reactions

CNS: fever.
GI: nausea, vomiting, unpleasant taste, minor GI symptoms.
GU: diuresis.
Other: tachyphylaxis, allergic reaction in patients allergic to plants belonging to the daisy family.

Interactions

Herb-drug. *Disulfiram, metronidazole:* Herbal products that contain alcohol may cause a disulfiram reaction. Discourage use together.
Immunosuppressants such as cyclosporine: Decreases effectiveness of these drugs. Discourage use together.

Herb-lifestyle. *Alcohol use:* Echinacea preparations containing alcohol may enhance CNS depression. Discourage use together.

Action

Extract stimulates the immune system and reduces growth of bacteria responsible for vaginal infections. Components may exert local anesthetic effects and anti-inflammatory activities. Essential oil components produce a tingling sensation on the tongue. Some compounds also exhibit direct antitumor activity and insecticidal activity. Conjugates in the plant activate adrenal cortex activity. The fresh-pressed juice of the aerial portion and the extract of the roots may inhibit influenza, herpes infections, and vesicular stomatitis virus.

Common forms

Capsules and tablets; also as hydroalcoholic extracts, fresh-pressed juice, glycerite, lozenges, and tinctures.
Capsules: 125 mg, 355 mg (85 mg herbal extract powder), 500 mg.
Tablets: 335 mg.

Nursing considerations

• Daily dose depends on the preparation and potency.
• Echinacea shouldn't be taken for more than 8 weeks.
• Echinacea is considered supportive treatment for infection; it shouldn't be used in place of antibiotic therapy.
• Echinacea is usually taken at the first sign of illness and continued for up to 14 days. Regular prophylactic use isn't recommended.
• Herbalists recommend using liquid preparations because it's believed that echinacea functions in the mouth and should have direct contact with the lymph tissues at the back of the throat.
• Some tinctures contain 15% to 90% alcohol, which may be unsuitable for children and adolescents, alcoholics, and patients with hepatic disease.

Patient teaching

• Instruct patient to tell the pharmacist of any herbal or dietary supplement he's taking when filling a new prescription.
• Advise patient not to delay seeking appropriate medical evaluation for a prolonged illness.

*Liquid may contain alcohol.

⚛ **ALERT:** Advise patient taking herb for prolonged time that overstimulation of the immune system and possible immune suppression may occur.
• Advise woman to avoid use of herb during pregnancy and when breast-feeding.

eucalyptus
(yoo-kah-LIP-tes)

Reported uses

Used internally and externally as an expectorant. Used to treat infections and fevers. Also used topically to treat sore muscles and rheumatism.

Dosages

Essential oil: Oil is used in massage blends for sore muscles and in foot baths or saunas, steam inhalations, chest rubs, room sprays, bath blends, and air diffusions. For external use only.
Leaf: Average daily dose is 4 to 16 g P.O. divided every 3 to 4 hours.
Oil: For internal use, average dose is 0.3 to 0.6 g P.O. daily. For external use, oil with 5% to 20% concentration or a semisolid preparation with 5% to 10% concentration.
Tea: Prepared using one of two methods. For the infusion method, 6 oz (180 ml) of dried herb is steeped in boiling water for 2 to 3 minutes, and then strained. For the decoction method, 6 to 8 oz (180 to 240 ml) of dried herb is placed in boiling water, boiled for 3 to 5 minutes and then strained.
Tincture: 3 to 4 g P.O. daily.

Cautions

• Patients who have had an allergic reaction to eucalyptus or its vapors should avoid use.
• Patients who have liver disease, or have intestinal tract inflammation should avoid use.
• Essential oil preparations shouldn't be applied to an infant's or child's face because of risk of severe bronchial spasm.
⚘ Lifespan: Pregnant and breast-feeding women should avoid use.

Adverse reactions

CNS: delirium, dizziness, *seizures.*
EENT: miosis.

GI: epigastric burning, nausea, vomiting.
Musculoskeletal: muscular weakness.
Respiratory: *asthma-like attacks.*

Interactions

Herb-drug. *Antidiabetics:* Enhances effects. Discourage use together, except under direct medical supervision.
Other drugs: Eucalyptus oil induces detoxication enzyme systems in the liver; therefore, the oil may affect any drug metabolized in liver. Monitor patient for effect and toxic reaction.
Herb-herb. *Other herbs that cause hypoglycemia (basil, Glucomannan, Queen Anne's lace):* Decreases glucose level. Monitor patient for effect and advise caution.

Action

Produces a stimulant effect on nasal cold receptors. Acts as a counterirritant and causes an increase in cutaneous blood flow. Also exhibits antimicrobial, antifungal, and anti-inflammatory effects.

Common forms

As an oil and a lotion.

Nursing considerations

• In susceptible patients, particularly infants and children, application of eucalyptus to the face or the inhalation of vapors can cause asthma-like attacks.
• Monitor glucose level in diabetic patient taking eucalyptus.
⚛ **ALERT:** The oil shouldn't be taken internally unless it has been diluted. As little as a few drops of oil for children and 4 to 5 ml of oil for adults can cause poisoning. Signs include hypotension, circulatory dysfunction, and cardiac and respiratory failure.
• If poisoning or overdose occurs, don't induce vomiting because of risk of aspiration. Administer activated charcoal and treat symptomatically.

Patient teaching

• Instruct patient to tell the pharmacist of any herbal or dietary supplement he's taking when filling a new prescription.
• Advise patient to stop taking eucalyptus immediately and to notify prescriber if he has hives, skin rash, or trouble breathing.
• Inform patient of potential adverse effects.

Bold italic type indicates that reaction may be life-threatening.

• Instruct caregiver not to apply to the face of a child or infant, especially around the nose.

fennel
(FEN-el)

Reported uses

Used to increase milk secretion, promote menses, facilitate birth, and increase libido. Used as an expectorant to manage cough and bronchitis. Also used to treat mild spastic disorders of the GI tract, feelings of fullness, and flatulence. Fennel syrup has been used to treat upper respiratory tract infections in children.

Dosages

▶ **GI complaints.** Herbalists recommend 0.1 to 0.6 ml P.O. of the oil daily, or 5 to 7 g of the fruit daily.

Cautions

• Urge caution in patients allergic to other members of the Umbelliferae family, such as celery, carrots, or mugwort.
• Discourage use in those with a history of seizures.
☙ Lifespan: In pregnant women, discourage use.

Adverse reactions

CNS: *seizures,* hallucinations.
GI: nausea, vomiting.
Respiratory: *pulmonary edema.*
Skin: photodermatitis, contact dermatitis.
Other: allergic reaction.

Interactions

Herb-drug. *Drugs that lower the seizure threshold, anticonvulsants:* Increases risk of seizure. Monitor patient very closely.
Herb-lifestyle. *Sun exposure:* Increases risk of photosensitivity reactions. Advise patient to wear protective clothing and sunscreen and to limit exposure to direct sunlight.

Action

May exhibit stimulant and antiflatulent properties. Fennel oil with methylparaben inhibits the growth of *Salmonella enteritidis* and, to a lesser extent, *Listeria monocytogenes.*

Common forms

Volatile oil in water: 2% (sweet fennel), 4% (bitter fennel).

Nursing considerations

• Find out why patient is using the herb.
• Verify that the patient doesn't have an allergic response to celery, fennel, or similar spices and herbs.

Patient teaching

• Inform patient that herb can't be recommended for any use because of insufficient evidence.
• Instruct patient to tell the pharmacist of any herbal or dietary supplement he's taking when filling a new prescription.
⚠ **ALERT:** Don't mistake poison hemlock for fennel. Hemlock can cause vomiting, paralysis, and death. Know the source of preparation before taking fennel.
• Tell patient to stop taking this herb and contact prescriber immediately if he experiences hives, rash, or difficulty breathing.
• Advise patient to avoid sun exposure if photodermatitis occurs.

feverfew
(FEE-ver-fyoo)

Reported uses

Used as an antipyretic and to treat psoriasis, toothache, insect bites, rheumatism, asthma, stomachache, menstrual problems, and threatened miscarriage. Also used for migraine prophylaxis.

Dosages

Infusion: Prepared by steeping 2 tsp in a cup of water for 15 minutes. For stronger infusion, double the amount and allow it to steep for 25 minutes. Infusion dose in folk medicine is 1 cup (240 ml) t.i.d.; stronger infusions are used for washes.
Powder: Daily dose recommended by herbalists is 50 mg to 1.2 g.
▶ **Migraine treatment.** Average dose of 543 mcg P.O. parthenolide (a component of feverfew) daily.
▶ **Migraine prophylaxis.** 25 mg of freeze-dried leaf extract P.O. daily, or 50 mg of leaf

P.O. daily with food, or 50 to 200 mg of aerial parts of plant P.O. daily.

Cautions

• Patients allergic to members of the daisy, or Asteraceae, family—including yarrow, southernwood, wormwood, chamomile, marigold, goldenrod, coltsfoot, and dandelion—and patients who have had previous reactions to herb shouldn't take it internally.

• Those taking anticoagulants such as warfarin and heparin should use cautiously.

⚶ **Lifespan:** Pregnant women should avoid use because of herb's potential abortifacient properties; breast-feeding women also should avoid use. Children shouldn't use herb.

Adverse reactions

CNS: dizziness.
CV: tachycardia.
GI: GI upset, mouth ulcerations.
Skin: contact dermatitis.

Interactions

Herb-drug. *Anticoagulants, antiplatelet drugs including aspirin and thrombolytics:* Herb inhibits prostaglandin synthesis and platelet aggregation. Monitor patient for increased bleeding.

Action

Main active ingredients may inhibit serotonin release by platelets. Extracts of herb contain chemicals that inhibit activation of leukocytes and the synthesis of leukotrienes and prostaglandins.

Common forms

As capsules, dried leaves, liquid, powder, seeds, and tablets.
Capsules: 250 mg (leaf extract), 380 mg (pure leaf).

Nursing considerations

• Find out why patient is using the herb.
• Rash or contact dermatitis may indicate sensitivity to herb. Tell patient to discontinue use immediately.
• Potency is often based on the parthenolide content in the preparation, which varies.

Patient teaching

• Assure patient that several other strategies for migraine treatment and prophylaxis exist and that these should be attempted before taking products with unknown benefits and risks.

• Instruct patient not to withdraw herb abruptly, but to taper its use gradually because of risk of post-feverfew syndrome. Symptoms include tension headaches, insomnia, joint stiffness and pain, and lethargy.

• Tell patient to report promptly unusual signs and symptoms, such as mouth sores or skin ulcerations.

• Instruct patient to tell the pharmacist of any herbal or dietary supplement he's taking when filling a new prescription.

• Educate patient about risk of increased bleeding when combining herb with an anticoagulant, such as warfarin or heparin, or an antiplatelet, such as aspirin or an NSAID.

• Warn patient that a rash or abnormal skin condition may indicate an allergy to herb. Instruct patient to stop taking the herb if a rash appears.

flax
(flaks)

Reported uses

Used to treat constipation, functional disorders of the colon resulting from laxative abuse, irritable bowel syndrome, and diverticulitis. Also used as a supplement to decrease the risk of hypercholesterolemia and atherosclerosis. Externally, herb may be made into a poultice and used to treat areas of local inflammation.

Dosages

▶ **For all systemic uses.** 1 to 2 tbs (15 to 30 ml) of oil or mature seeds daily in two or three divided doses. Average dose is 1 oz (30 ml) of oil or 1 oz mature seeds daily.
▶ **For topical use.** 30 to 50 g of flax meal applied as a hot, moist poultice or compress, as needed.

Cautions

• Patients with an ileus or esophageal stricture and those experiencing an acute inflammatory illness of the GI tract should avoid use.

Bold italic type indicates that reaction may be life-threatening.

≛ Lifespan: Pregnant and breast-feeding women and those planning to become pregnant should avoid use.

Adverse reactions

GI: diarrhea, flatulence, nausea.

Interactions

Herb-drug. *Laxatives, stool softeners:* Possible increase in laxative actions of herb. Discourage use together.
Oral medications: Because of its fibrous content and binding potential, drug absorption may be altered or prevented. Advise patient to avoid using herb within 2 hours of a drug.

Action

Decreases total cholesterol and low-density lipoprotein levels. May decrease thrombin-mediated platelet aggregation. Herb contains lignins, which may have weak estrogenic, anti-estrogenic, and steroid-like activity. Diets high in flax may lower the risk of breast and other hormone-dependent cancers. Linolenic acid supplement, derived from flax, arginine, and yeast RNA, may improve weight gain in some patients with HIV.

Common forms

As a powder, capsules, softgel capsules, and an oil.
Softgel capsules: 1,000 mg.

Nursing considerations

• Find out why patient is using the herb.
⊛ **ALERT:** Immature seedpods are especially poisonous. Overdose symptoms include, but aren't limited to, shortness of breath, tachypnea, cyanosis, weakness, and unstable gait, progressing to paralysis and seizures.

Patient teaching

• Encourage patient to drink plenty of fluids to minimize flatulence.
• Instruct patient to refrigerate flaxseed oil to prevent breakdown of essential fatty acids.
• Remind patient that other cholesterol-lowering therapies exist that have been proven to improve survival and lower the risk of cardiac disease; herb has no such support.
• Warn patient not to treat chronic constipation, other GI disturbances, or ophthalmic injury with

herb before seeking appropriate medical evaluation, because doing so may delay diagnosis of a potentially serious medical condition.
• Instruct patient never to ingest immature seeds and to keep herb away from children and pets.
• Tell patient to report decreased effects of other drugs being taken if patient continues to use the herb.

garlic
(GAR-lik)

Reported uses

Used most commonly to decrease total cholesterol level, decrease triglyceride level, and increase high-density lipoprotein cholesterol level. Also used to help prevent atherosclerosis because of its effect on blood pressure and platelet aggregation. Used to decrease the risk of cancer, especially cancer of the GI tract. Used to decrease the risk of CVA and MI and to treat cough, colds, fevers, and sore throats.

Used to treat asthma, diabetes, inflammation, heavy metal poisoning, constipation, and athlete's foot. Also used as an antimicrobial and to reduce symptoms in patients with AIDS.

Dosages

▶ **Lower cholesterol level.** 600 to 900 mg of dried power, 2 to 5 mg of allicin, or 2 to 5 g of fresh clove. Average dose is 4 g of fresh garlic or 8 mg of essential oil daily.

Cautions

• Contraindicated in patients sensitive to garlic or other members of the Lilaceae family and in those with GI disorders, such as peptic ulcer or reflux disease.
≛ Lifespan: In pregnant women, herb is contraindicated because of its oxytocic effects.

Adverse reactions

CNS: dizziness.
GI: halitosis; irritation of mouth, esophagus, and stomach; nausea; vomiting.
Hematologic: decreased hemoglobin production and lysis of RBCs (with long-term use or excessive dosages).

Skin: contact dermatitis, diaphoresis.
Other: allergic reaction, *anaphylaxis,* garlic odor.

Interactions

Herb-drug. *Anticoagulants, NSAIDs, prostacy-clin:* May increase bleeding time. Discourage use together.
Antidiabetics: Glucose level may be decreased further. Advise caution if using together, and tell patient to monitor glucose level closely.
Drugs metabolized by the enzyme CYP 2E1, a member of the CYP system (such as aceta-minophen): Decreases metabolism of these drugs. Monitor patient for clinical effects and toxic reaction.
Herb-herb. *Herbs with anticoagulant effects:* Increases bleeding time. Discourage use together.
Herbs with antihyperglycemic effects: Glucose level may be further decreased. Tell patient to use caution and to monitor glucose level closely.

Action

May exhibit antithrombotic, lipid-lowering, cholesterol-lowering, antitumor, and antimicrobial effects. May have hypoglycemic activity and hypotensive properties, as well as antibacterial, antifungal, larvicidal, insecticidal, amebicidal, and antiviral activities. A component in garlic oil may inhibit adenosine diphosphate-induced platelet aggregation. Also may decrease a type of carcinogen and nitrite accumulation.

Common forms

In tablets; also as fresh bulb, antiseptic oil, fresh extract, powdered, freeze-dried garlic powder, and garlic oil (essential oil).
Dried powder: 400 to 1,200 mg.
Fresh bulb: 2 to 5 g.
Tablets (allicin total potential): 2 to 5 mg.
Tablets (garlic extract): 100 mg, 320 mg, 400 mg, 600 mg.

Nursing considerations

• Herb isn't recommended for patients with diabetes, insomnia, pemphigus, organ transplants, or rheumatoid arthritis, or in postsurgical patients.
• Herb may lower glucose level. If patient is taking an antihyperglycemic, watch for signs

and symptoms of hypoglycemia and monitor his glucose level.

Patient teaching

• Advise patient that cholesterol-lowering drugs are commonly used for hypercholesterolemia because of their proven survival data and ability to lower cholesterol levels more effectively than herb.
• Instruct patient to watch for signs of bleeding (bleeding gums, easy bruising, tarry stools, petechiae) if herb supplements are taken with antiplatelet drugs.
• Instruct patient to tell the pharmacist of any herbal or dietary supplement he's taking when filling a new prescription.
• Advise patient not to delay seeking appropriate medical evaluation because doing so may delay diagnosis of a potentially serious medical condition.
• Discourage heavy use of herb before surgery.
• If patient is using herb to lower his cholesterol level, advise him to notify his prescriber and to have his cholesterol level monitored.
• If patient is using herb as a topical antiseptic, tell him to avoid prolonged exposure to the skin because burns can occur.

ginger
(JIN-jer)

Reported uses

Used as an antiemetic, GI protectant, anti-inflammatory agent useful for arthritis treatment, CV stimulant, antitumor agent, antioxidant, and as therapy for microbial and parasitic infestations. Also used to treat seasickness, morning or motion sickness, and postoperative nausea and vomiting, and to provide relief from pain and swelling caused by rheumatoid arthritis, osteoarthritis, or muscular discomfort.

Dosages

Infusion: Prepared by steeping 0.5 to 1 g of herb in boiling water and then straining after 5 minutes. (1 tsp is equal to 3 g of drug.) Dosage forms and strengths vary with the condition.

Bold italic type indicates that reaction may be life-threatening.

► **As an antiemetic.** 500 to 1,000 mg powdered ginger P.O., or 1,000 mg fresh ginger root P.O.

► **Arthritis.** 1 to 2 g daily.

► **Nausea caused by chemotherapy.** 1 g P.O. before chemotherapy.

► **Migraine headache or arthritis.** Up to 2 g P.O. daily.

► **Motion sickness.** 1 g P.O. 30 minutes before travel, then 0.5 to 1 g q 4 hours. Also could begin 1 to 2 days before trip.

Cautions

• Patients with gallstones or with an allergy to herb should avoid use.

• Patients with bleeding disorders should avoid using large amounts of herb.

• Patients taking a CNS depressant or an antiarrhythmic should use cautiously.

⚠ **Lifespan:** Pregnant women should avoid using large amounts of herb.

Adverse reactions

CNS: CNS depression.
CV: *arrhythmias,* increased bleeding time.
GI: heartburn.

Interactions

Herb-drug. *Anticoagulants and other drugs that can increase bleeding time:* May further increase bleeding time. Discourage use together.

Herb-herb. *Herbs that may increase bleeding time:* May further increase bleeding time. Discourage use together.

Action

Inhibits platelet aggregation induced by adenosine diphosphate and epinephrine. May exhibit anti-inflammatory and positive inotropic effects. Specific components of herb produce varying CV effects.

Common forms

As root, extract, liquid, powder, capsules, tablets, and teas.
Extract: 250 mg.
Liquid, powder, capsules: 100 mg, 465 mg.
Root: 530 mg.
Tablets (chewable): 67.5 mg.

Nursing considerations

• Find out why patient is using the herb.

• Herb may interfere with the intended therapeutic effect of conventional drugs.

• If overdose occurs, monitor patient for arrhythmias and CNS depression.

Patient teaching

• Advise patient to consult prescriber before using an herbal preparation because a treatment with proven efficacy may be available.

• Instruct patient to tell the pharmacist of any herbal or dietary supplement he's taking when filling a new prescription.

• Advise pregnant woman to consult with a knowledgeable practitioner before using herb medicinally.

• Educate patient to look for signs and symptoms of bleeding, such as nosebleeds or excessive bruising.

ginkgo
(GIN-koh)

Reported uses

Primarily used to manage cerebral insufficiency, dementia, and circulatory disorders such as intermittent claudication. Also used to treat headaches, asthma, colitis, impotence, depression, altitude sickness, tinnitus, cochlear deafness, vertigo, premenstrual syndrome, macular degeneration, diabetic retinopathy, and allergies. Used as an adjunctive treatment for pancreatic cancer and schizophrenia. Also used in addition to physical therapy for Fontaine stage IIb peripheral arterial disease to decrease pain during ambulation with a minimum of 6 weeks of treatment.

Dosages

► **Dementia syndromes.** 120 to 240 mg P.O. daily in two or three divided doses.

► **Peripheral arterial disease, vertigo, and tinnitus.** 120 to 160 mg P.O. daily in two or three divided doses.

Cautions

• Patients with a history of an allergic reaction to gingko or any of its components and patients

*Liquid may contain alcohol.

with increased risk of intracranial hemorrhage (hypertension, diabetes) should avoid use.
• Patients receiving an antiplatelet or an anticoagulant should avoid use because of the increased risk of bleeding.
• Herb should be avoided before surgery.
⚱ **Lifespan:** Herb should be avoided before childbirth.

Adverse reactions

CNS: headache, *seizures, subarachnoid hemorrhage.*
GI: diarrhea, flatulence, nausea, vomiting.
Skin: contact hypersensitivity reaction, dermatitis.

Interactions

Herb-drug. *Anticoagulants, antiplatelets, high-dose vitamin E:* May increase the risk of bleeding. Discourage use together.
MAO inhibitors: Theoretically, herb can potentiate the activity of these drugs. Advise patient to stop taking herb.
SSRIs: Herb extracts may reverse the sexual dysfunction caused by these drugs. Urge patient to consult prescriber before using together.
Warfarin: Possibly increases INR when taken together. Monitor INR.
Herb-herb. *Garlic and other herbs that increase bleeding time:* Potentiates anticoagulant effects. Advise patient to use together cautiously.

Action

Produces arterial and venous vasoactive changes that increase tissue perfusion and cerebral blood flow. Also produces arterial vasodilation, inhibits arterial spasms, decreases capillary permeability, reduces capillary fragility, decreases blood viscosity, and reduces erythrocyte aggregation. Ginkgo biloba extract acts as an antioxidant, and ginkgolide B (a component of gingko) may be a potent inhibitor of platelet activating factor.

Common forms

As ginkgo biloba extract in capsules, tablets, and sublingual sprays (standardized to contain 24% flavone glycosides and 6% terpenes) and as concentrated alcoholic extract of fresh leaf.
Capsules: 30 mg, 40 mg, 60 mg, 120 mg, 260 mg, 420 mg.

Capsules (ginkgo biloba extract [24% standardized extract] bound to phosphatidylcholine): 80 mg.
S.L. sprays: 15 mg/spray, 40 mg/spray.
Tablets: 30 mg, 40 mg, 60 mg, 120 mg, 260 mg, 420 mg.

Nursing considerations

• Herb extracts are considered standardized if they contain 24% ginkgo flavonoid glycosides and 6% terpene lactones.
• Treatment period ranges from 6 to 8 weeks, but therapy beyond 3 months isn't recommended.
⑤ **ALERT:** Seizures may occur in children after ingestion of more than 50 seeds.
• Monitor patient for possible adverse reactions, such as GI problems, headaches, dizziness, allergic reaction, and serious bleeding.

Patient teaching

• Inform patient that the therapeutic and toxic components of gingko can vary significantly from product to product. Advise him to obtain gingko from a reliable source.
• Advise patient to discontinue use at least 2 weeks before surgery.
• Advise patient to report unusual bleeding or bruising.
• Instruct patient to keep seeds out of reach of children because of potential risk of seizures with ingestion.
• Advise patient to avoid contact with the fruit pulp or seed coats because of the risk of contact dermatitis. More potent preparations may cause irritation or blistering of skin or mucous membranes if applied externally.

ginseng
(JIN-sehng)

Reported uses

Used to minimize or reduce the activity of the thymus gland. Also used as a sedative, demulcent (soothes irritated or inflamed internal tissues or organs), aphrodisiac, antidepressant, sleep aid, and diuretic. May be used to improve stamina, concentration, healing, stress-resistance, vigilance, and work efficiency and to

---

Bold italic type indicates that reaction may be life-threatening.

improve well-being in geriatric patients with debilitated or degenerative conditions.

Also used to decrease fasting blood glucose and hemoglobin A1c in diabetic and nondiabetic patients, and to treat hyperlipidemia, hepatic dysfunction, and impaired cognitive function.

Dosages

Dosages vary with the disease state; usually, 0.5 to 2 g dry ginseng root daily or 200 to 600 mg ginseng extract daily, in one or two equal doses.

▶ **Improved well-being in debilitated geriatric patients.** 0.4 to 0.8 g root P.O. daily on a continual basis.

Cautions

• Urge caution in patients with CV disease, hypertension, hypotension, or diabetes, and in those receiving steroid therapy.

✢ **Lifespan:** In pregnant or breast-feeding women, discourage use; effects are unknown.

Adverse reactions

CNS: headache, insomnia, nervousness.
CV: chest pain, palpitations, hypertension.
EENT: epistaxis.
GI: diarrhea, nausea, vomiting.
GU: impotence, vaginal bleeding.
Skin: pruritus, skin eruptions (with ginseng abuse).
Other: breast pain.

Interactions

Herb-drug. *Anticoagulants, antiplatelet drugs:* May decrease the effects of these drugs. Monitor PT and INR.
Antidiabetics, insulin: Increases hypoglycemic effects. Monitor glucose level.
Drugs metabolized by CYP 3A4: Herb may inhibit this enzyme system. Monitor patient for clinical effects and toxicity.
Phenelzine, other MAO inhibitors: May cause headache, irritability, visual hallucinations, and other interactions. Discourage use together.
Warfarin: Herb may decrease drug effect. Discourage using herb.

Action

Ginseng compounds may exert opposing effects. For example, one compound has CNS-depressant, anticonvulsant, analgesic, and anti-

psychotic effects and stress-ulcer–preventing action. Another compound has CNS-stimulating, antifatigue, hypertensive, and stress-ulcer–aggravating effects. Some components enhance cardiac performance, whereas others depress cardiac function.

Oral herb may reduce cholesterol and triglycerides, decrease platelet adhesiveness, impair coagulation, and increase fibrinolysis. It may also reduce stress by acting on the adrenal gland.

Extracts of herb may exhibit antioxidant activity.

Common forms

As capsules, teas, extract, root powder, whole root (by the pound), and oil.
Capsules: 100 mg, 250 mg, 500 mg.
Extract*: 2 oz root extract (in alcohol base).
Root powder: 1 oz, 4 oz.
Tea bags: 1,500 mg ginseng root.

Nursing considerations

• Some debate exists concerning a possible ginseng abuse syndrome. It reportedly occurs when large doses of the herb are taken with other psychomotor stimulants, such as tea and coffee; symptoms include diarrhea, hypertension, restlessness, insomnia, skin eruptions, depression, appetite suppression, euphoria, and edema. However, some reputable herbal sources discredit such reports.

• Considering the high level of bioactivity for herb components, herb may not be safe for patients with a serious or chronic medical condition.

• Monitor diabetic patient for signs and symptoms of hypoglycemia.

Patient teaching

• Tell patient with medical conditions to check with prescriber before taking herb.

• Advise diabetic patient to check glucose level closely until effects are known.

• Instruct patient to watch for unusual symptoms (nervousness, insomnia, palpitations, diarrhea) because of risk of herb toxicity.

• Inform patient that the therapeutic and toxic components of herb can vary significantly from product to product. Advise him to obtain herb from a reliable source.

---

*Liquid may contain alcohol.

goldenseal
(GOHL-den-seel)

Reported uses

Used to treat GI disorders, gastritis, peptic ulceration, anorexia, postpartum hemorrhage, dysmenorrhea, eczema, pruritus, tuberculosis, cancer, mouth ulcerations, otorrhea, tinnitus, and conjunctivitis; also used as a wound antiseptic, diuretic, laxative, and anti-inflammatory agent.

Used to shorten the duration of acute *Vibrio* cholera diarrhea and diarrhea caused by some species of *Giardia, Salmonella, Shigella,* and some *Enterobacteriaceae.* May be used to improve biliary secretion and function in patients with hepatic cirrhosis.

Dosages

Alcohol and water extract: 250 mg P.O. t.i.d.
Dried rhizome: 0.5 to 1 g P.O. t.i.d.

Cautions

• Patients with hypertension, heart failure, or arrhythmias, or severe renal or hepatic disease should avoid use.
⚠ Lifespan: Pregnant and breast-feeding women should avoid use. In infants, herb shouldn't be used.

Adverse reactions

CNS: sedation, reduced mental alertness, hallucinations, delirium, paresthesia, paralysis.
CV: hypotension, hypertension, *asystole, heart block.*
GI: nausea, vomiting, diarrhea, GI cramping, mouth ulcerations.
Hematologic: megaloblastic anemia from decreased vitamin B absorption, *leukopenia.*
Respiratory: *respiratory depression.*
Skin: contact dermatitis.

Interactions

Herb-drug. *Anticoagulants:* May reduce anticoagulant effect. Discourage use together.
Antidiabetics, insulin: Increases hypoglycemic effects. Discourage use together; advise patient to monitor glucose levels closely.

Antihypertensives: May reduce or enhance hypotensive effect. Discourage use together.
Beta blockers, calcium channel blockers, digoxin: May interfere or enhance cardiac effects. Discourage use together.
CNS depressants such as benzodiazepines: May enhance sedative effects. Discourage use together.
Cephalosporins, disulfiram, metronidazole: May cause disulfiram-like reaction when taken with liquid herbal preparations. Discourage use together.
Herb-lifestyle. *Alcohol use:* May enhance sedative effects. Discourage use together.

Action

May have astringent, anti-inflammatory, oxytocic, antihemorrhagic, and laxative properties. Inhibits muscular contractions.

Decreases the anticoagulant effect of heparin and acts as a cardiac stimulant (at lower dosages), increases coronary perfusion, and inhibits cardiac activity (at higher dosages). May exhibit antipyretic activity (greater than aspirin) and antimuscarinic, antihistaminic, antitumor, antimicrobial, antiparasitic, and hypotensive effects.

Causes vasoconstriction and produces significant changes in blood pressure.

Common forms

In capsules and tablets; also as alcohol and water extracts, dried ground root powder, tinctures, and teas.
Capsules, tablets: 250 mg, 350 mg, 400 mg, 404 mg, 470 mg, 500 mg, 535 mg, 540 mg.

Nursing considerations

• German Commission E hasn't endorsed the use of herb for any condition because of its potential toxicity and lack of well-documented effectiveness.
• Berberine, a chemical constitute of herb, increases bilirubin levels in infants and thus shouldn't be given to them.
• Monitor patient for signs and symptoms of vitamin B deficiency such as megaloblastic anemia, paresthesia, seizures, cheilosis, glossitis, and seborrheic dermatitis.
• Monitor patient for adverse CV, respiratory, and neurologic effects. If patient has a toxic reaction, induce vomiting and perform gastric

---

Bold italic type indicates that reaction may be life-threatening.

lavage. After lavage, administer activated charcoal and treat symptomatically.

Patient teaching

• Instruct patient to tell the pharmacist of any herbal or dietary supplement he's taking when filling a new prescription.

• Advise patient not to use herb because of its toxicity and lack of documented effectiveness, especially if the patient has CV disease.

⊛ **ALERT:** High doses may lead to vomiting, bradycardia, hypertension, respiratory depression, exaggerated reflexes, seizures, and death.

grapeseed, pinebark
(GRAYP-seed, PIGHN-bahrk)

Reported uses

Used as an antioxidant to treat circulatory disorders (hypoxia from atherosclerosis, inflammation, and cardiac or cerebral infarction). Also used to treat pain, limb heaviness, and swelling in patients with peripheral circulatory disorders and to treat inflammatory conditions, varicose veins, and cancer.

Dosages

Tablets, capsules: 25 to 300 mg P.O. daily for up to 3 weeks; maintenance dosage of 40 to 80 mg P.O. once daily.

Cautions

• Patients with liver dysfunction should use cautiously.

≋ Lifespan: No considerations reported.

Adverse reactions

Hepatic: *hepatotoxicity.*

Interactions

None reported.

Action

Demonstrates antilipoperoxidant activity and xanthine oxidase inhibition. Inhibits enzymes responsible for skin turnover. Extract exhibits therapeutic effects in Ehrlich ascites carcinoma and inhibits growth of *Streptococcus mutans.*

Common forms

Tablets, capsules: 25 mg to 300 mg.

Nursing considerations

• Grapeseed may interfere with the intended therapeutic effect of conventional drugs.

• Grapeseed extract may have antiplatelet effects. If a patient is having elective surgery, it may be prudent to stop the supplement 2 to 3 days before surgery. Monitor PT and INR.

Patient teaching

• Warn patient not to treat symptoms of venous insufficiency or circulatory disorders before seeking appropriate medical evaluation because doing so may delay diagnosis of a potentially serious medical condition.

• Instruct patient to tell the pharmacist of any herbal or dietary supplement he's taking when filling a new prescription.

kava
(KAH-veh)

Reported uses

Used to treat nervous anxiety, stress, and restlessness. Used orally as a sedative, to promote wound healing, and to treat headaches, seizure disorders, the common cold, respiratory tract infection, tuberculosis, and rheumatism. Also used to treat urogenital infections, including chronic cystitis, venereal disease, uterine inflammation, menstrual problems, and vaginal prolapse. Some herbal practitioners consider herb an aphrodisiac. Kava juice is used to treat skin diseases, including leprosy. Also used as a poultice for intestinal problems, otitis, and abscesses.

Dosages

▶ **Anxiety.** 50 to 70 mg purified kava lactones P.O. t.i.d., equivalent to 100 to 250 mg of dried kava root extract per dose. (By comparison, the traditional bowl of raw kava beverage contains about 250 mg of kava lactones.)

▶ **Restlessness.** 180 to 210 mg of kava lactones taken as a tea 1 hour before bedtime. The typical dose in this form is 1 cup t.i.d. Prepare by simmering 2 to 4 g of the root in 5 oz boiling water for 5 to 10 minutes and then straining.

Cautions

• Patients hypersensitive to herb or any of its components should avoid this herb. Depressed patients should avoid the herb because of possible sedative activity; those with endogenous depression should avoid it because of increased risk of suicide.

• Patients with renal disease, thrombocytopenia, or neutropenia should use cautiously.

≋ **Lifespan:** Pregnant women should avoid the herb because of possible loss of uterine tone; breast-feeding women also should avoid it. Children shouldn't use this herb.

Adverse reactions

CNS: mild euphoric changes characterized by feelings of happiness, fluent and lively speech, and increased sensitivity to sounds; morning fatigue.
EENT: visual accommodation disorders, pupil dilation, disorders of oculomotor equilibrium.
GI: mild GI disturbances, mouth numbness.
GU: hematuria.
Hematologic: increased RBC count, decreased platelets and lymphocytes.
Metabolic: reduced levels of albumin, total protein, bilirubin, and urea; increased HDL cholesterol.
Respiratory: *pulmonary hypertension.*
Skin: scaly rash.

Interactions

Herb-drug. *Antiplatelet drugs, type B MAO inhibitors:* Possible additive effects. Monitor patient closely.
Barbiturates, benzodiazepines: Kava lactones potentiate the effects of CNS depressants, leading to toxicity. Discourage use together.
Levodopa: Possible reduced effectiveness of levodopa therapy in patients with Parkinson's disease, apparently because of dopamine antagonism. Advise patient to use cautiously.
Herb-herb. *Calamus, calendula, California poppy, capsicum, catnip, celery, couch grass, elecampane, German chamomile, goldenseal, gotu kola, hops, Jamaican dogwood, lemon balm, sage, sassafras, shepherd's purse, Siberian ginseng, skullcap, stinging nettle, St. John's wort, valerian, wild lettuce, yerba maté:* Addi-

tive sedative effects may occur. Monitor patient closely.
Herb-lifestyle. *Alcohol use:* Increases risk of CNS depression and liver damage. Discourage use together.

Action

Components of the root may cause local anesthetic activity that is similar to cocaine but lasts longer than benzocaine. Some components show fungistatic properties against several fungi.

Induces muscular relaxation and inhibits the limbic system, an effect linked to suppression of emotional excitability and mood enhancement. Produces mild euphoria with no effect on thoughts and memory during the intoxication. Other effects include analgesia, sedation, hyporeflexia, impaired gait, and pupil dilation.

Common forms

A drink from pulverized roots, tablets, capsules, or extract.

Nursing considerations

• Heavy herb users are more likely to complain of poor health. About 20% are underweight with reduced levels of albumin, total protein, bilirubin, urea, platelets, and lymphocytes; increased HDL cholesterol and RBCs; hematuria; puffy faces; scaly rashes; and some evidence of pulmonary hypertension. These symptoms resolve several weeks after the herb is stopped. Toxic doses can cause progressive ataxia, muscle weakness, and ascending paralysis, all of which resolve when herb is stopped. Extreme use (more than 300 g/week) may increase gamma-glutamyl transferase levels.

• Patient shouldn't use herb with conventional sedative-hypnotics, anxiolytics, MAO inhibitors, other psychopharmacologic drugs, levodopa, or antiplatelet drugs without first consulting prescriber.

• Adverse effects of herb may occur at start of therapy but are usually transient.

Patient teaching

Ⓧ **ALERT:** Tell patient to report jaundice, dark urine, easy bruising, and abdominal pain. Herb has been linked to liver damage including cirrhosis, hepatitis, and liver failure.

Bold italic type indicates that reaction may be life-threatening.

• Advise patient that usual doses can affect motor function; caution against performing hazardous activities.
• Warn patient to avoid taking herb with alcohol because of increased risk of CNS depression and liver damage.
• Instruct patient to tell the pharmacist of any herbal or dietary supplement he's taking when filling a new prescription.

milk thistle
(MILK THIH-sel)

Reported uses

Used to treat dyspepsia, liver damage from chemicals, *Amanita* mushroom poisoning, supportive therapy for inflammatory liver disease and cirrhosis, loss of appetite, and gallbladder and spleen disorders. It's also used as a liver protectant.

Dosages

Dried fruit or seed: 12 to 15 g P.O. daily.
Oral: Doses of milk thistle extract vary from 200 to 400 mg of silibinin (70% silymarin extract) P.O. daily.
Tea: 3 to 5 g freshly crushed fruit or seed steeped in 5 oz (148 ml) of boiling water for 10 to 15 minutes. One cup of tea t.i.d. to q.i.d., 30 minutes before meals.

Cautions

• Herb shouldn't be used by patients hypersensitive to it or to plants in the Asteraceae family. Use in decompensated cirrhosis isn't recommended.
⚝ **Lifespan:** Pregnant or breast-feeding women shouldn't use herb.

Adverse reactions

GI: nausea, vomiting, diarrhea.

Interactions

Herb-drug. *Aspirin:* Herb may improve aspirin metabolism in patients with liver cirrhosis. Advise patient to consult prescriber before use.

Cisplatin: Herb may prevent kidney damage by cisplatin. Advise patient to consult prescriber before use.
Disulfiram: Products that contain alcohol may cause a disulfiram-like reaction. Discourage use together.
Hepatotoxic drugs: May prevent liver damage from butyrophenones, phenothiazines, phenytoin, acetaminophen, and halothane. Advise patient to consult prescriber before use.
Tacrine: Silymarin reduces adverse cholinergic effects when given together. Advise patient to consult prescriber before use.

Action

Exerts hepatoprotective and antihepatotoxic actions over liver toxins by altering the outer liver membrane cell structure so that toxins cannot enter the cell. Also leads to activation of the regenerative capacity of the liver through cell development.

Common forms

As capsules, tablets, and extract.
Capsules: 50 mg, 100 mg, 175 mg, 200 mg, 505 mg.
Tablets: 85 mg (standardized to contain 80% silymarin with the flavonoid silibinin).

Nursing considerations

• Warn patient not to take herb for liver inflammation or cirrhosis before seeking appropriate medical evaluation because doing so may delay diagnosis of a potentially serious medical condition.
• Mild allergic reaction may occur, especially in people allergic to members of the Asteraceae family, including ragweed, chrysanthemums, marigolds, and daisies.
• Don't confuse milk thistle seeds or fruit with other parts of the plant or with blessed thistle (*Cnictus benedictus*).
• Silymarin has poor water solubility; therefore, effectiveness when prepared as a tea is questionable.

Patient teaching

• Instruct patient to tell the pharmacist of any herbal or dietary supplement he's taking when filling a new prescription.
• Although no chemical interactions have been reported in clinical studies, advise patient that

herb may interfere with therapeutic effect of conventional drugs.

• Warn patient not to take this herb while pregnant or breast-feeding.

• Tell patient to stay alert for possible allergic reaction, especially if allergic to ragweed, chrysanthemums, marigolds, or daisies.

nettle
(NEH-tel)

Reported uses

Used to treat allergic rhinitis, osteoarthritis, rheumatoid arthritis, kidney stones, asthma, and BPH. Also used as a diuretic, an expectorant, a general health tonic, a blood builder and purifier, a pain reliever and anti-inflammatory, and a lung tonic for ex-smokers. Also used for eczema, hives, bursitis, tendinitis, laryngitis, sciatica, and premenstrual syndrome. Herb is being investigated for treatment of hay fever and irrigation of the urinary tract.

Dosages

▶ **Allergic rhinitis.** 600 mg freeze-dried leaf P.O. at onset of symptoms.
▶ **BPH.** 4 g root extract P.O. daily, or 600 to 1,200 mg P.O. encapsulated extract daily.
Fresh juice: 5 to 10 ml P.O. t.i.d.
Infusion: 1.5 g powdered nettle in cold water; heated to boiling for 1 minute, then steeped covered for 10 minutes and strained (1 tsp is equal to 1.3 g herb).
Liquid extract (1:1 in 25% alcohol)*: 2 to 6 ml P.O. t.i.d.
▶ **Osteoarthritis.** 1 leaf applied to affected area daily.
▶ **Rheumatoid arthritis.** 8 to 12 g leaf extract P.O. daily.
Tea: 1 tbs fresh young plant steeped in 1 cup (240 ml) boiled water for 15 minutes. Three or more cups taken daily.
Tincture (1:5 in 45% alcohol)*: 2 to 6 ml P.O. t.i.d.

Cautions

⚘ **Lifespan:** In pregnant or breast-feeding women herb is contraindicated because of its di-uretic and uterine stimulation properties. In children, herb is also contraindicated.

Adverse reactions

CV: edema.
GI: gastric irritation, gingivostomatitis.
GU: decreased urine formation; oliguria; increased diuresis in patients with arthritic conditions and those with myocardial or chronic venous insufficiency.
Skin: topical irritation, burning sensation.

Interactions

Herb-drug. *Disulfiram:* Possible adverse reaction if taken with liquid extract or tincture. Discourage use together.
Herb-lifestyle. *Alcohol use:* Possible additive effect from liquid extract and tincture. Discourage alcohol use.

Action

Acts primarily as a diuretic by increasing urine volume and decreasing systolic blood pressure. May stimulate uterine contractions. Extract reduces urine flow, nocturia, and residual urine.

Common forms

As capsules, dried leaf, root extract, and tincture.
Capsules: 150 mg, 300 mg.

Nursing considerations

• Herb is reported to be an abortifacient and may affect the menstrual cycle.
• Internal adverse effects are rare and allergic in nature.

Patient teaching

• Advise patient to consult prescriber before using an herbal preparation because a treatment with proven effectiveness may be available.
• Instruct patient to tell the pharmacist of any herbal or dietary supplement he's taking when filling a new prescription.
• Recommend caution if patient takes an antihypertensive or antidiabetic.
• Warn patient that external adverse effects result from skin contact and include burning and stinging that may persist for 12 hours or more.

Bold italic type indicates that reaction may be life-threatening.

- Advise patient to eat foods high in potassium, such as bananas and fresh vegetables, to replenish electrolytes lost through diuresis.
- Caution patient against using herb for BPH or to relieve fluid accumulation caused by heart failure without medical approval and supervision.
- Tell patient to wash thoroughly with soap and water, use antihistamines and steroid creams, and wear heavy gloves if plant will be handled. If rubbed against the skin, herb can cause intense burning for 12 hours or more.

passion flower
(PAH-shen FLOW-er)

Reported uses

Used as a sedative, a hypnotic, an analgesic, and an antispasmodic for treating muscle spasms caused by indigestion, menstrual cramping, pain, or migraines. Also used for neuralgia, generalized seizures, hysteria, nervous agitation, and insomnia. Crushed leaves and flowers are used topically for cuts and bruises.

Dosages

Dried herb: 250 mg to 1 g P.O., two to three 100-mg capsules P.O. b.i.d., or one 400-mg capsule P.O. daily.
Extract in vegetable glycerin base (alcohol-free): 10 to 15 gtt P.O., b.i.d. or t.i.d.
▶ **Cuts and bruises.** Crushed leaves and flowers are applied topically, p.r.n.
▶ **Hemorrhoids.** Prepare by soaking 20 g dried herb in 200 ml of simmering water, straining, then cooling before use. Apply topically, as indicated.
Infusion: 150 ml of hot water poured over 1 tsp of herb. Strain after standing for 10 minutes. Take b.i.d. or t.i.d., with a final dose about 30 minutes before h.s.
Liquid extract (1:1 in 25% alcohol)*: 0.5 to 1 ml P.O. t.i.d.
Solid extract: Taken in doses of 150 to 300 mg P.O. daily
Tincture (1:8 in 45% alcohol)*: 0.5 to 2 ml (½ to 1 tsp) P.O. t.i.d.
▶ **Parkinson's disease.** 10 to 30 gtt P.O. (0.7% flavonoids) t.i.d.

Dried herb: 0.25 to 1 g P.O. t.i.d.
Liquid extract: 0.5 to 1 ml P.O. t.i.d.
Tea: 4 to 8 g (3 to 6 tsp) daily in divided doses.
Tincture: 0.5 to 2 ml P.O. t.i.d.

Cautions

- Excessive doses may cause sedation and may potentiate MAO inhibitor therapy.
- Those with liver disease or a history of alcoholism should avoid products that contain alcohol.
⚹ Lifespan: Pregnant and breast-feeding women shouldn't take this herb.

Adverse reactions

CNS: drowsiness, headache, flushing, agitation, confusion, psychosis.
CV: *shock*, tachycardia, hypotension, *ventricular arrhythmias*.
GI: nausea, vomiting.
Respiratory: *asthma*.
Other: allergic reaction.

Interactions

Herb-drug. *Disulfiram, metronidazole:* Herbal products that contain alcohol may cause a disulfiram-like reaction. Discourage use together.
Hexobarbital: Increases sleeping time and other barbiturate effects may be potentiated. Monitor patient's level of consciousness carefully.
MAO inhibitors: Actions can be potentiated by herb. Discourage use together.

Action

Obtained from leaves, fruits, and flowers of *Passiflora incarnata.* Contains indole alkaloids, including harman and harmine, flavonoids, and maltol. Indole alkaloids are the basis of many biologically active substances, such as serotonin and tryptophan. Exact effect of these alkaloids is unknown; however, they can cause CNS stimulation via MAO inhibition, thereby decreasing intracellular metabolism of norepinephrine, serotonin, and other biogenic amines. Flavonoids can reduce capillary permeability and fragility. Maltol can cause sedative effects and potentiate hexobarbital and anticonvulsive activity.

*Liquid may contain alcohol.

Common forms

As liquid extract, crude extract, tincture, dried herb, and in several homeopathic remedies.
Liquid extract*: 1:1 in 25% alcohol.
Tincture*: 1:8 in 45% alcohol, or containing 0.7% flavonoids.

Nursing considerations

• Monitor patient for possible adverse CNS effects.

❧ **ALERT:** A disulfiram-like reaction may produce nausea, vomiting, flushing, headache, hypotension, tachycardia, and possibly ventricular arrhythmias and shock, leading to death.

• Patients with liver disease or alcoholism shouldn't use herbal products that contain alcohol.

Patient teaching

• Warn patient not to take herb for chronic pain or insomnia before seeking medical attention because doing so may delay diagnosis of a potentially serious medical condition.

• Instruct patient to tell the pharmacist of any herbal or dietary supplement he's taking when filling a new prescription.

• Tell patient to avoid activities that require alertness and coordination until CNS effects are known.

primrose, evening
(PRIHM-rohz, EEV-ning)

Reported uses

Infusion used for sedative and astringent properties. Used to treat asthmatic coughs, GI disorders, whooping cough, psoriasis, multiple sclerosis, asthma, Raynaud's disease, and Sjögren's syndrome. Poultices made with evening primrose oil may be used to speed wound healing.

Used to treat pruritic symptoms of atopic dermatitis and eczema, breast pain and tenderness from premenstrual syndrome, benign breast disease, and diabetic neuropathy.

Used in rheumatoid arthritis to improve patients' symptoms and reduce the need for pain medication; also used to lower serum cholesterol, improve hypertension, and decrease platelet aggregation.

Also may be used to calm hyperactive children and to reduce mammary tumors from baseline size.

Dosages

The following dosages are based on a standardized gamma linoleic acid content of 8%.
▶ **Eczema.** *Adults:* 6 to 8 g P.O. daily in divided doses.
Children: 2 to 4 g P.O. daily in divided doses.
▶ **Breast pain.** 3 to 4 g P.O. daily.
No consensus exists for all other disorders.

Cautions

• Urge caution or discourage use in schizophrenic patients and in those taking antiseizure drugs.
❧ **Lifespan:** In pregnant women, discourage use; effects are unknown.

Adverse reactions

CNS: headache, *temporal lobe epilepsy.*
CV: *thrombosis.*
GI: nausea.
Skin: rash.
Other: inflammation, *immunosuppression.*

Interactions

Herb-drug. *Phenothiazines:* May increase risk of seizures. Discourage use together.

Action

Aids prostaglandin synthesis.

Common forms

Capsules: 50 mg, 500 mg, 1,300 mg.
Gelcaps: 500 mg, 1,300 mg.

Nursing considerations

• Find out why patient is using the herb.
• Monitor patient for adverse effects, especially with long-term use.

Patient teaching

• Instruct patient with seizure disorders to reconsider need to use herb.
• Tell parents to use herb for a hyperactive child only under medical supervision.

Bold italic type indicates that reaction may be life-threatening.

Saint John's wort
(SAYNT JAHNS WART)

Reported uses

Used to treat depression, bronchial inflammation, burns, cancer, enuresis, gastritis, hemorrhoids, hypothyroidism, insect bites and stings, insomnia, kidney disorders, and scabies, and has been used as a wound-healing agent. Herb can be used to treat HIV infection; also can be used topically for phototherapy of skin diseases, including psoriasis, cutaneous T-cell lymphoma, warts, and Kaposi's sarcoma.

Dosages

▶ **Depression.** 300 mg standardized extract preparations (standardized to 0.3% hypericin) P.O. t.i.d. for 4 to 6 weeks; or 2 to 4 g tea that has been steeped in 1 to 2 cups (240 to 480 ml) of water for about 10 minutes and taken P.O. daily for 4 to 6 weeks.
▶ **Burns and skin lesions.** Cream applied topically; strength isn't standardized.

Cautions

• Transplant patients maintained on cyclosporine therapy should avoid this herb because of the risk of organ rejection.
⚕ Lifespan: Pregnant women and both men and women planning pregnancy shouldn't take herb because of mutagenic risk to sperm cells and oocytes and adverse effects on reproductive cells.

Adverse reactions

CNS: fatigue, neuropathy, restlessness, headache.
GI: digestive complaints, fullness sensation, constipation, diarrhea, nausea, abdominal pain, dry mouth.
Skin: photosensitivity reactions, pruritus.
Other: delayed hypersensitivity.

Interactions

Herb-drug. *Amitriptyline, chemotherapy drugs, cyclosporine, digoxin, drugs metabolized by the CYP enzyme system, hormonal contraceptives, protease inhibitors, theophylline, and warfarin:* Decreases effectiveness of these drugs. May require drug dosage adjustment. Monitor patient closely; discourage use together.

Barbiturates: Decreases sedative effects. Monitor patient closely.
Indinavir: Substantially reduces drug level, causing loss of therapeutic effects. Discourage use together.
MAO inhibitors, including phenelzine and tranylcypromine: May increase effects and cause toxicity and hypertensive crisis. Discourage use together.
Opioids: Increases sedative effects. Discourage use together.
Reserpine: Antagonizes effects of reserpine. Discourage use together.
SSRIs, such as citalopram, fluoxetine, paroxetine, sertraline: Increases risk of serotonin syndrome. Discourage use together.
Herb-herb. *Herbs with sedative effects, such as calamus, calendula, California poppy, capsicum, catnip, celery, couch grass, elecampane, German chamomile, goldenseal, gotu kola, Jamaican dogwood, kava, lemon balm, sage, sassafras, shepherd's purse, Siberian ginseng, skullcap, stinging nettle, valerian, wild carrot, and wild lettuce:* May enhance effects of herbs. Monitor patient closely; discourage use together.
Herb-food. *Tyramine-containing foods such as beer, cheese, dried meats, fava beans, liver, wine, and yeast:* May cause hypertensive crisis when used together. Advise patient to separate administration times.
Herb-lifestyle. *Alcohol use:* May increase sedative effects. Discourage use together.
Sun exposure: Increases risk of photosensitivity reaction. Advise patient to avoid unprotected or prolonged exposure to sunlight.

Action

Inhibits stress-induced increase in corticotropin-releasing hormone, corticotropin, and cortisol. Also has antiviral activity, including action against retroviruses.

Common forms

As capsules, sublingual capsules, and liquid tinctures.
Capsules: 100 mg, 300 mg, 500 mg (standardized to 0.3% hypericin); 250 mg (standardized to 0.14% hypericin).

*Liquid may contain alcohol.

Nursing considerations

• Monitor patient for response to herbal therapy, as evidenced by improved mood and lessened depression.

• By using standardized extracts, patient can better control the dosage. Clinical studies have used formulations of standardized 0.3% hypericin as well as hyperforin-stabilized version of the extract.

• Herb interacts with many other products; they must be considered before patient takes it with other prescription or OTC products.

• Signs and symptoms of serotonin syndrome include dizziness, nausea, vomiting, headache, epigastric pain, anxiety, confusion, restlessness, and irritability.

• Because herb decreases the effect of certain prescription drugs, watch for signs of drug toxicity if patient stops herb. Drug dosage may need reduction.

Patient teaching

• Instruct patient to tell the pharmacist of any herbal or dietary supplement he's taking when filling a new prescription.

• Instruct patient to consult a health care provider for a thorough medical evaluation before using herb.

• If patient takes herb for mild-to-moderate depression, explain that the effects may not be felt for 4 to 6 weeks. Tell him that a new therapy may be needed if no improvement occurs after this time.

• ⊕ ALERT: If patient wants to switch from an SSRI to herb, tell him he may need to wait a few weeks for the SSRI to leave his system before it's safe to start taking the herb. The exact time required depends on which SSRI he's taking.

• Inform patient that herb interacts with many other prescription and OTC products.

saw palmetto
(SAW pal-MEH-toh)

Reported uses

Used as a mild diuretic; also used to treat such GU problems as BPH and to increase sperm production, breast size, and sexual vigor.

Dosages

▶ **BPH.** 320 mg P.O. daily in two divided doses for 3 months. Other recommendations include 1 to 2 g fresh saw palmetto berries or 0.5 to 1 g dried berry in decoction P.O. t.i.d.

Cautions

• Those with breast cancer or hormone-dependent illnesses other than BPH should avoid this herb.

⚞ Lifespan: Pregnant and breast-feeding women and women of childbearing age shouldn't use this herb.

Adverse reactions

CNS: headache.
CV: hypertension.
GI: abdominal pain, constipation, diarrhea, nausea.
GU: dysuria, impotence, urine retention.
Musculoskeletal: back pain.
Other: decreased libido.

Interactions

Herb-drug. *Adrenergics, hormones, hormone-like drugs:* May cause estrogen, androgen, and alpha-blocking effects. Drug dosages may need adjustment if patient takes this herb. Monitor patient closely.

Action

Has an anti-inflammatory effect and inhibits prolactin and growth-factor–induced prostatic cell proliferation. May inhibit hormonally induced prostate enlargement.

Common forms

As tablets, capsules, teas, berries (fresh or dried), and liquid extract.

Nursing considerations

• Find out why patient is using the herb.

• Herb should be used cautiously for conditions other than BPH because data about its effectiveness in other conditions is lacking.

• Obtain a baseline prostate-specific antigen (PSA) test before patient starts taking herb because it may cause a false-negative PSA result.

• Herb may not alter prostate size.

Bold italic type indicates that reaction may be life-threatening.

Patient teaching

- Instruct patient to tell the pharmacist of any herbal or dietary supplement he's taking when filling a new prescription.
- Warn patient not to take herb for bladder or prostate problems before seeking medical attention because doing so could delay diagnosis of a potentially serious medical condition.
- Tell patient to take herb with food to minimize GI effects.

valerian

(veh-LEHR-ee-ehn)

Reported uses

Used to treat menstrual cramps, restlessness and sleep disorders from nervous conditions, and other symptoms of psychological stress, such as anxiety, nervous headaches, and gastric spasms. Used topically as a bath additive for restlessness and sleep disorders.

Dosages

Bath additive: 100 g of root mixed with 2 L of hot water and added to one full bath.
Standardized tinctures: 2% essential oil.
Tea: 1 cup (240 ml) P.O. b.i.d. to t.i.d., and h.s.
Tincture (1:5 in 45% to 50% alcohol)*: 15 to 20 gtt in water several times daily.
▶ **Hastening sleep and improving sleep quality.** 400 to 800 mg root P.O. up to 2 hours before bedtime. Some patients need 2 to 4 weeks of use for significant improvement. Maximum, 15 g daily.
▶ **Restlessness.** 220 mg of extract P.O. t.i.d.

Cautions

- Patients with hepatic impairment shouldn't use this herb because of the risk of hepatotoxicity.
- Patients with acute or major skin injuries, fever, infectious diseases, cardiac insufficiency, or hypertonia shouldn't bathe with valerian products.
- ※ **Lifespan:** Pregnant and breast-feeding women should avoid this herb; effects are unknown.

Adverse reactions

CNS: excitability, headache, insomnia.
CV: cardiac disturbance.
EENT: blurred vision.
GI: nausea.
Other: hypersensitivity reaction.

Interactions

Herb-drug. *Barbiturates, benzodiazepines:* May have additive effects. Monitor patient closely.
CNS depressants: May have additive effects. Discourage use together.
Disulfiram: Disulfiram reaction may occur if herbal extract or tincture contains alcohol. Discourage use together.
Herb-herb. *Herbs with sedative effects, such as catnip, hops, kava, passion flower, skullcap:* May increase sedative effects. Monitor patient closely.
Herb-lifestyle. *Alcohol use:* May increase sedative effects. Advise patient to avoid use together.

Action

May exhibit a sedative effect and weak anticonvulsant and antidepressant properties. Also has antispasmodic effects on GI smooth muscle, produces coronary dilation, and has antiarrhythmic activity.

Common forms

As standardized capsules, tablets, and tinctures; also as tinctures and teas containing crude dried herb and in combination with other dietary supplements.
Standardized capsules, tablets (0.8% valerenic acid): 250 mg, 400 mg, 450 mg, 493 mg, 530 mg, 550 mg.
Standardized tincture: 2% essential oil.

Nursing considerations

- Herb seems to have a more pronounced effect on those with disturbed sleep or sleep disorders.
- Evidence of herb toxicity includes difficulty walking, hypothermia, and increased muscle relaxation.
- Withdrawal symptoms, such as increased agitation and decreased sleep, can occur if herb is stopped abruptly after prolonged use.

---

*Liquid may contain alcohol.

Patient teaching

• Warn patient not to take herb for insomnia before seeking medical attention because doing so may delay diagnosis of a potentially serious medical condition.

• Instruct patient to tell the pharmacist of any herbal or dietary supplement he's taking when filling a new prescription.

• If patient takes herb, explain that herb may take 2 to 4 weeks to take effect.

• Inform patient that many extract products contain 40% to 60% alcohol and may not be appropriate for all patients.

• Inform patient that most adverse effects occur only after long-term use.

Bold italic type indicates that reaction may be life-threatening.

Glossary

Agranulocytosis: an abnormal blood condition, characterized by a severe reduction in the number of granulocytes, basophils, eosinophils, and neutrophils, resulting in high fever, exhaustion, and bleeding ulcers of the throat, mucous membranes and GI tract. It's an acute disease and may be an adverse reaction to drug or radiation therapy.

Allergic reaction: a local or general reaction after exposure to an allergen to which the patient has already been exposed and sensitized. Reaction may range from localized dermatitis to anaphylaxis.

Alopecia: absence or loss of hair.

Angioedema: a potentially life-threatening condition characterized by sudden swelling of tissue involving the face, neck, lips, tongue, throat, hands, feet, genitals, or intestine.

Aplastic anemia: a deficiency of all of the formed elements of the blood related to bone marrow failure. It may be caused by neoplastic bone marrow disease or by destruction of the bone marrow by exposure to toxic chemicals, radiation, or certain medications. Also known as pancytopenia.

Arthralgia: any pain that affects a joint.

Azotemia: a toxic condition caused by renal insufficiency and subsequent retention of urea in the blood. Also called uremia.

Cushing's syndrome: a metabolic disorder caused by an increased production of adrenocorticotropic hormone from a tumor of the adrenal cortex or of the anterior lobe of the pituitary gland, or by excessive intake of glucocorticoids. It is characterized by central obesity, "moon face," glucose intolerance, growth suppression in children, and weakening of the muscles.

Disseminated intravascular coagulation (DIC): a life-threatening coagulopathy resulting from overstimulation of the body's clotting and anticlotting processes in response to disease, septicemia, neoplasms, obstetric emergencies,
severe trauma, prolonged surgery, and hemorrhage.

Eosinophilia: an increase in the number of eosinophils in the blood accompanying many inflammatory conditions. Substantial increases are considered a reflection of an allergic response.

Erythema: redness of the skin caused by dilation and congestion of the superficial capillaries, often a sign of inflammation or infection.

Gray baby syndrome: a possibly fatal condition that can occur in newborns (especially premature babies) who are given chloramphenicol for a bacterial infection, like meningitis. Symptoms usually appear 2 to 9 days after therapy has been initiated. They include vomiting, loose green stools, refusal to suck, hypotension, cyanosis, low body temperature, and CV collapse. The baby becomes limp and has a gray coloring.

Hemolytic anemia: a disorder characterized by the premature destruction of RBCs. Anemia may be minimal or absent, reflecting the ability of the bone marrow to increase production of RBCs.

Hepatitis: inflammation of the liver usually from a viral infection but sometimes from toxic agents.

Hirsutism: excessive growth of dark, coarse body hair, distributed in a male characteristic pattern.

Hypercalcemia: greater-than-normal amounts of calcium in the blood. Signs and symptoms include confusion, anorexia, abdominal pain, muscle pain, and weakness.

Hyperglycemia: greater-than-normal amounts of glucose in the blood. Classic signs and symptoms include excessive hunger, thirst, and frequent urination. Others include fatigue, weight loss, blurred vision, and poor wound healing.

Hyperkalemia: greater-than-normal amounts of potassium in the blood. Signs and symptoms include nausea, fatigue, weakness, and palpitations or irregular pulse.

Hypermagnesemia: greater-than-normal amounts of magnesium in the blood. Toxic levels in the blood may cause cardiac arrhythmias and may depress deep tendon reflexes and respiration.

Hypernatremia: greater-than-normal amounts of sodium in the blood. Signs and symptoms include confusion, seizures, coma, dysrhythmic muscle twitching, lethargy, tachycardia, and irritability.

Hyperplasia: an increase in the number of cells.

Hypersensitivity reaction: an abnormal and undesireable reaction in response to a foreign agent. Classified by the mechanism involved and the time it takes to occur, these reactions are assigned a rating of 1 through 4 (Types I, II, III, IV).

Hypocalcemia: less-than-normal amounts of calcium in the blood. Signs and symptoms of severe hypocalcemia include cardiac arrhythmias and muscle cramping and twitching as well as numbness and tingling of the hands, feet, lips, and tongue.

Hypoglycemia: less-than-normal amounts of glucose in the blood. Signs and symptoms include weakness, drowsiness, confusion, hunger, and dizziness. Patients may be pale, irritable, shaky, sweaty, and have a cold, clammy feeling and complain of headache and a rapid heart beat. Left untreated, delirium, coma, and death may occur.

Hypokalemia: less-than-normal amounts of potassium in the blood. Signs and symptoms include palpitations, muscle weakness or cramping, paresthesias, GI complaints such as constipation, nausea or vomiting, and abdominal cramping. Patient may also experience frequent urination, delirium, and depression.

Hypomagnesemia: less-than-normal amounts of magnesium in the blood. Signs and symp-

toms include nausea, vomiting, muscle weakness, tremors, tetany, and lethargy.

Hyponatremia: less-than-normal amounts of sodium in the blood. Signs and symptoms may range from mild anorexia, headache, or muscle cramps to obtundation, coma, or seizures.

Leukocytosis: an abnormal increase in the number of circulating WBCs. Kinds of leukocytosis include basophilia, eosinophilia, and neutrophilia.

Leukopenia: an abnormal decrease in the number of WBCs to fewer than 5,000 cells/mm^3.

Myalgia: diffuse muscle pain, usually associated with malaise.

Nephrotic syndrome: an abnormal kidney condition characterized by marked proteinuria, hypoalbuminemia, and edema.

Neuroleptic malignant syndrome: the rarest and most serious of the neuroleptic-induced movement disorders. It is a neurologic emergency in most cases. Signs and symptoms include fever, rigidity, and tremor. Mental status changes such as drowsiness and confusion can progress to stupor and coma. Other symptoms may include seizures and cardiac arrhythmias.

Neutropenia: an abnormal decrease in the number of circulating neutrophils in the blood.

Pancytopenia: a deficiency of all of the formed elements of the blood related to bone marrow failure. It may be caused by neoplastic bone marrow disease or by destruction of the bone marrow after exposure to toxic chemicals, radiation, or certain medications. Also known as aplastic anemia.

Pharmacodynamics: the study of drug action in the body at the tissue site including uptake, movement, binding, and interactions.

Pharmacokinetics: the study of the action of drugs within the body, including the routes and mechanisms of absorption and excretion, the rate at which a drug's action begins and the duration of the effect, the biotransformation of the substance in the body, and the effects and routes of excretions of the metabolites of the drug.

Pseudomembranous colitis: a complication of antibiotic therapy that causes severe local tissue inflammation of the colon. Signs and symptoms include watery diarrhea, abdominal pain or cramping, and low-grade fever.

Pseudotumor cerebri: benign intracranial hypertension, most common in women between the ages of 20 and 50, caused by increased pressure within the brain. Symptoms include headache, dizziness, nausea, vomiting, and ringing or rushing sound in the ears.

Pruritus: itching.

Psoriasis: a common skin disorder characterized by the eruption of red, silvery-scaled maculopapules, predominantly on the elbows, knees, scalp, and trunk.

Reye's syndrome: an encephalopathy that affects children of all ages. While the cause and cure are unknown, research has established a link between the use of aspirin and other salicylate-containing medications, as well as other causes. The syndrome may follow an upper respiratory infection or chicken pox. Its onset is rapid, usually starting with irritable, combative behavior and vomiting, and progressing to semiconsciousness, seizures, coma, and possibly death.

Serotonin syndrome: a typically mild, yet potentially serious drug-related condition most often reported in patients taking two or more medications that increase CNS serotonin levels. The most common drug combinations associated with serotonin syndrome involve the MAO inhibitors, SSRIs, and the tricyclic antidepressants. Signs and symptoms include confusion, agitation, restlessness, rapid heart rate, muscle rigidity or twitching, tremors, and nausea.

Serum sickness: an immune complex disease appearing 1 or 2 weeks after infection of a foreign serum or serum protein, with local and systemic reactions, such as urticaria, fever, general lymphadenopathy, edema, arthritis, and occasionally albuminuria or severe nephritis.

Syncope: a brief loss of consciousness caused by oxygen deficiency to the brain, often preceded by a feeling of dizziness. Having the patient lie down or place his head between his knees may prevent it.

Thrombocytopenia: an abnormal decrease in the number of platelets in the blood, predisposing the patient to bleeding disorders.

Thrombocytopenic purpura: a bleeding disorder characterized by a marked decrease in the number of platelets, causing multiple bruises, petechiae, and hemorrhage into the tissues.

Tinnitus: sound in one or both ears, such as buzzing, ringing, or whistling, occurring without external stimuli. It may be due to an ear infection, the use of certain drugs, a blocked auditory tube or canal, or head trauma.

Urticaria: an itchy skin condition characterized by pale wheals with well-defined red edges. This may be the result of an allergic response to insect bites, food, or drugs.

Pregnancy risk categories

The Food and Drug Administration has assigned a pregnancy risk category to each systemically absorbed drug based on available clinical and preclinical information. The five categories (A, B, C, D, and X) reflect a drug's potential to cause birth defects. Although drugs are best avoided during pregnancy, this rating system permits rapid assessment of the risk-benefit ratio if giving a drug to a pregnant woman becomes necessary. Drugs in category A are generally considered safe to use in pregnancy; drugs in category X are generally contraindicated.

- A: Adequate studies in pregnant women haven't shown a risk to fetus.
- B: Animal studies haven't shown a risk to fetus, but controlled studies haven't been conducted in pregnant women; or animal studies have shown an adverse effect on fetus, but adequate studies in pregnant women haven't shown a risk to fetus.
- C: Animal studies have shown an adverse effect on fetus, but adequate studies haven't been conducted in humans. The benefits from use in pregnant women may be acceptable despite potential risks.

- D: The drug may cause risk to human fetus, but the potential benefits of use in pregnant women may be acceptable despite the risks (such as in a life-threatening situation or a serious disease for which safer drugs can't be used or are ineffective).
- X: Studies in animals or humans show fetal abnormalities, or adverse-reaction reports indicate evidence of fetal risk. The risks involved clearly outweigh potential benefits.
- NR: Not rated.

Controlled substance schedules

Drugs regulated under the jurisdiction of the Controlled Substances Act of 1970 are divided into the following groups or schedules:

- Schedule I (C-I): High abuse potential and no accepted medical use. Examples include heroin, cocaine, and LSD.
- Schedule II (C-II): High abuse potential with severe dependence liability. Examples include opioids, amphetamines, and some barbiturates.
- Schedule III (C-III): Less abuse potential than schedule II drugs and moderate dependence liability. Examples include nonbarbiturate sedatives, non-amphetamine stimulants, anabolic steroids, dronabinol, and limited amounts of certain opioids.
- Schedule IV (C-IV): Less abuse potential than schedule III drugs and limited dependence liability. Examples include some sedatives, anxiolytics, and non-opioid analgesics.

- Schedule V (C-V): Limited abuse potential. This category includes mainly small amounts of opioids, such as codeine, used as antitussives or antidiarrheals. Under federal law, limited quantities of certain C-V drugs may be purchased without a prescription directly from a pharmacist if allowed under specific state laws. The purchaser must be at least age 18 and must furnish suitable identification. All such transactions must be recorded by the dispensing pharmacist.

Dialyzable drugs

The amount of a drug removed by dialysis differs among patients and depends on several factors, including the patient's condition, the drug's properties, length of dialysis and dialysate used, rate of blood flow or dwell time, and purpose of dialysis. This table indicates the effect of hemodialysis on selected drugs.

Drug	Level reduced by hemodialysis?	Drug	Level reduced by hemodialysis?
acetaminophen	Yes (may not influence toxicity)	cefoxitin	Yes
		cefpodoxime	Yes
acetazolamide	No	ceftazidime	Yes
acyclovir	Yes	ceftibuten	Yes
allopurinol	Yes	ceftizoxime	Yes
alprazolam	No	ceftriaxone	No
amikacin	Yes	cefuroxime	Yes
amiodarone	No	cephalexin	Yes
amitriptyline	No	cephradine	Yes
amlodipine	No	chloral hydrate	Yes
amoxicillin	Yes	chlorambucil	No
amoxicillin and clavulanate potassium	Yes	chloramphenicol	Yes (very small amount)
		chlordiazepoxide	No
amphotericin B	No	chloroquine	No
ampicillin	Yes	chlorpheniramine	No
ampicillin and sulbactam sodium	Yes	chlorpromazine	No
aspirin	Yes	chlorthalidone	No
atenolol	Yes	cimetidine	Yes
azathioprine	Yes	ciprofloxacin	Yes (only by 20%)
aztreonam	Yes	cisplatin	No
captopril	Yes	clindamycin	No
carbamazepine	No	clofibrate	No
carbenicillin	Yes	clonazepam	No
carmustine	No	clonidine	No
cefaclor	Yes	clorazepate	No
cefadroxil	Yes	codeine	No
cefazolin	Yes	colchicine	No
cefepime	Yes	cortisone	No
cefoperazone	Yes	co-trimoxazole	Yes
cefotaxime	Yes	cyclophosphamide	Yes
cefotetan	Yes (only by 20%)		

(continued)

Drug	Level reduced by hemodialysis?	Drug	Level reduced by hemodialysis?
diazepam	No	glutethimide	Yes
diazoxide	No	glyburide	No
diclofenac	No	guanfacine	No
dicloxacillin	No	haloperidol	No
didanosine	Yes	heparin	No
digoxin	No	hydralazine	No
diltiazem	No	hydrochlorothiazide	No
diphenhydramine	No	hydroxyzine	No
dipyridamole	No	ibuprofen	No
disopyramide	Yes	imipenem and cilastatin	Yes
doxazosin	No	imipramine	No
doxepin	No	indapamide	No
doxorubicin	No	indomethacin	No
doxycycline	No	insulin	No
enalapril	Yes	irbesartan	No
erythromycin	Yes (only by 20%)	iron dextran	No
ethacrynic acid	No	isoniazid	Yes
ethambutol	Yes (only by 20%)	isosorbide	No
ethosuximide	Yes	isradipine	No
famciclovir	Yes	kanamycin	Yes
famotidine	No	ketoconazole	No
fenoprofen	No	ketoprofen	Yes
flecainide	No	labetalol	No
fluconazole	Yes	levofloxacin	No
flucytosine	Yes	lidocaine	No
fluorouracil	Yes	lisinopril	Yes
fluoxetine	No	lithium	Yes
flurazepam	No	lomefloxacin	No
foscarnet	Yes	lomustine	No
fosinopril	No	loracarbef	Yes
furosemide	No	loratadine	No
gabapentin	Yes	lorazepam	No
ganciclovir	Yes	mechlorethamine	No
gemfibrozil	No	mefenamic acid	No
gentamicin	Yes	meperidine	No
glipizide	No	mercaptopurine	Yes

Drug	Level reduced by hemodialysis?	Drug	Level reduced by hemodialysis?
meropenem	Yes	pentamidine	No
methadone	No	pentazocine	Yes
methotrexate	Yes	perindopril	Yes
methyldopa	Yes	phenobarbital	Yes
methylprednisolone	No	phenylbutazone	No
metoclopramide	No	phenytoin	No
metolazone	No	piperacillin	Yes
metoprolol	No	piperacillin and tazobactam	Yes
metronidazole	Yes	piroxicam	No
mexiletine	Yes	prazosin	No
miconazole	No	prednisone	No
midazolam	No	primidone	Yes
minocycline	No	procainamide	Yes
minoxidil	Yes	promethazine	No
misoprostol	No	propoxyphene	No
morphine	No	propranolol	No
nabumetone	No	protriptyline	No
nadolol	Yes	pyridoxine	Yes
nafcillin	No	quinapril	No
naproxen	No	quinidine	Yes
nelfinavir	Yes	quinine	Yes
nifedipine	No	ranitidine	Yes
nimodipine	No	rifampin	No
nitrofurantoin	Yes	rofecoxib	No
nitroglycerin	No	sertraline	No
nitroprusside	Yes	sotalol	Yes
nizatidine	No	stavudine	Yes
norfloxacin	No	streptomycin	Yes
nortriptyline	No	sucralfate	No
ofloxacin	Yes	sulbactam	Yes
olanzapine	No	sulindac	No
omeprazole	No	temazepam	No
oxacillin	No	theophylline	Yes
oxazepam	No	ticarcillin	Yes
paroxetine	No	ticarcillin and clavulanate	Yes
penicillin G	Yes		

(continued)

Drug	Level reduced by hemodialysis?
timolol	No
tobramycin	Yes
tocainide	Yes
tolbutamide	No
topiramate	Yes
trazodone	No
triazolam	No
trimethoprim	Yes
valacyclovir	Yes
valproic acid	No
valsartan	No
vancomycin	No
verapamil	No
warfarin	No

Table of equivalents

Metric measures

Metric weight equivalents

1 kilogram (kg)	=	1,000 grams (g)
1 gram	=	1,000 milligrams (mg)
1 milligram	=	1,000 micrograms (mcg)
0.6 g	=	600 mg
0.3 g	=	300 mg
0.1 g	=	100 mg
0.06 g	=	60 mg
0.03 g	=	30 mg
0.015 g	=	15 mg
0.001 g	=	1 mg

Metric volume equivalents

1 liter (L)	=	1,000 milliliters (ml)
1 milliliter	=	1,000 microliters (mcl)

Metric weight conversions

Household		Metric
1 ounce	=	30 grams
1 pound	=	453.6 grams
2.2 pounds	=	1 kilogram

Metric volume conversions

Household		Metric
1 teaspoon (tsp)	=	5 ml
1 tablespoon (tbs)	=	15 ml
2 tablespoons	=	30 ml
8 ounces	=	240 ml
1 pint (pt)	=	473 ml
1 quart (qt)	=	946 ml
1 gallon (gal)	=	3,785 ml

Temperature conversions

Fahrenheit degrees	Centigrade degrees	Fahrenheit degrees	Centigrade degrees	Fahrenheit degrees	Centigrade degrees
106.0	41.1	100.6	38.1	95.2	35.1
105.8	41.0	100.4	38.0	95.0	35.0
105.6	40.9	100.2	37.9	94.8	34.9
105.4	40.8	100.0	37.8	94.6	34.8
105.2	40.7	99.8	37.7	94.4	34.7
105.0	40.6	99.6	37.6	94.2	34.6
104.8	40.4	99.4	37.4	94.0	34.4
104.6	40.3	99.2	37.3	93.8	34.3
104.4	40.2	99.0	37.2	93.6	34.2
104.2	40.1	98.8	37.1	93.4	34.1
104.0	40.0	98.6	37.0	93.2	34.0
103.8	39.9	98.4	36.9	93.0	33.9
103.6	39.8	98.2	36.8	92.8	33.8
103.4	39.7	98.0	36.7	92.6	33.7
103.2	39.6	97.8	36.5	92.4	33.6
103.0	39.4	97.6	36.4	92.2	33.4
102.8	39.3	97.4	36.3	92.0	33.3
102.6	39.2	97.2	36.2	91.8	33.2
102.4	39.1	97.0	36.1	91.6	33.1
102.2	39.0	96.8	36.0	91.4	33.0
102.0	38.9	96.6	35.9	91.2	32.9
101.8	38.8	96.4	35.8	91.0	32.8
101.6	38.7	96.2	35.7	90.8	32.7
101.4	38.6	96.0	35.6	90.6	32.6
101.2	38.4	95.8	35.4	90.4	32.4
101.0	38.3	95.6	35.3	90.2	32.3
100.8	38.2	95.4	35.2	90.0	32.2

*1 ml = 1 cubic centimeter (cc); however, ml is the preferred measurement term.

Look-alike and sound-alike drug names

Watch out for the following drug names that resemble other drug names either in the way they're spelled or the way they sound. Don't confuse antivirals that use abbreviations for identification. Also, don't mix up different iron salts because their elemental content may vary.

abciximab and infliximab

acetazolamide and acetohexamide

acetylcholine and acetylcysteine

acetylcysteine and acetylcholine

Aciphex and Aricept

Aggrastat and argatroban

albuterol and atenolol or Albutein

Aldactone and Aldactazide

Aldomet and Aldoril or Anzemet

alitretinoin and tretinoin

alprazolam and alprostadil

amantadine and rimantadine

Ambien and Amen

Amicar and Amikin

Amikin and Amicar

amiloride and amiodarone

aminophylline and amitriptyline or ampicillin

Aminosyn and Amikacin

amiodarone and amiloride

amitriptyline and nortriptyline or aminophylline

amlodipine and amiloride

Anafranil and enalapril, nafarelin, or alfentanil

anakinra and amikacin

Antabuse and Anturane

Anturane and Accutane or Artane

Anzemet and Aldomet

Apresoline and Apresazide

Aquasol A and AquaMEPHYTON

Aricept and Ascriptin

Artane and Anturane or Altace

Asacol and Os-Cal

atenolol and timolol or albuterol

Atrovent and Alupent

Avinza and Invanz

azathioprine and azidothymidine, Azulfidine, or azatadine

bacitracin and Bactroban

baclofen and Bactroban

BCG intravesical and BCG vaccine

Benadryl and Bentyl or Benylin

Benemid and Beminal

Bentyl and Aventyl or Benadryl

benztropine and bromocriptine or brimonidine

Betagan and BetaGen or Betapen

Bumex and Buprenex

bupropion and buspirone

calcifediol and calcitriol

Carbatrol and carvedilol

carboplatin and cisplatin

Cardene and Cardura or codeine

Cardizem SR and Cardene SR

Cardura and Coumadin, K-Dur, Cardene, or Cordarone

Catapres and Cetapred or Combipres

Celebrex and Cerebyx or Celexa

Celexa and Celebrex or Cerebyx

Cerebyx and Cerezyme, Celexa, or Celebrex

Chloromycetin and chlorambucil

chlorpromazine and chlorpropamide

Ciloxan and Cytoxan or cinoxacin

cimetidine and simethicone

Citrucel and Citracal

clomiphene and clomipramine or clonidine

clonidine and quinidine or clomiphene

clorazepate and clofibrate

clotrimazole and co-trimoxazole

clozapine and Cloxapen, clofazimine, or Klonopin

codeine and Cardene, Lodine, or Cordran

corticotropin and cosyntropin

Cozaar and Zocor

cyclosporine and cycloserine

cyproheptadine and cyclobenzaprine

dacarbazine and Dicarbosil or procarbazine

Dantrium and Daraprim

Demerol and Demulen, Dymelor, or Temaril

desipramine and disopyramide or imipramine

desmopressin and vasopressin

desonide and Desogen or Desoxyn

Desoxyn and digoxin or digitoxin

dexamethasone and desoximetasone

Dexedrine and dextran or Excedrin

Diamox and Diabinese

diazepam and diazoxide

diazoxide and Dyazide

diclofenac and Diflucan or Duphalac

dicyclomine and dyclonine or doxycycline

digoxin and doxepin, Desoxyn, or digitoxin

Dilantin and Dilaudid

dimenhydrinate and diphenhydramine

Diprivan and Ditropan

dipyridamole and disopyramide

disopyramide and desipramine or dipyridamole

Ditropan and Diazepam

dobutamine and dopamine

doxapram and doxorubicin, doxepin, or doxazosin

doxepin and doxazosin, digoxin, doxapram, or Doxidan

doxycycline, and doxylamine or dicyclomine

d-penicillamine and penicillin

dronabinol and droperidol

droperidol and dronabinol

DynaCirc and Dynacin

Elavil and Equanil or Mellaril

Eldepryl and enalapril

enalapril and Anafranil or Eldepryl

Endep and Depen

ephedrine and epinephrine

epinephrine and ephedrine or norepinephrine

Epogen and Neupogen

Estratab and Estratest

Ethmozine and Erythrocin

ethosuximide and methsuximide

etidronate and etretinate, etidocaine, or etomidate

Eurax and Serax or Urex

Femara and FemHRT

fentanyl and alfentanil

Flexeril and Floxin or Flaxedil

Flomax and Fosamax or Volmax

floxuridine and fludarabine or flucytosine

flunisolide and fluocinonide

fluorouracil and fludarabine, flucytosine, or floxuridine

fluoxetine and fluvoxamine or fluvastatin

fluticasone and fluconazole

fluvastatin and fluoxetine

folic acid and folinic acid

fosinopril and lisinopril

furosemide and torsemide

glimepiride and glyburide or glipizide

guanabenz and guanadrel or guanfacine

guaifenesin and guanfacine

Haldol and Halcion or Halog

hydralazine and hydroxyzine

hydrocortisone and hydroxychloroquine

hydromorphone and morphine

hydroxyzine and hydroxyurea or hydralazine

HyperHep and Hyperstat or Hyper-Tet

Hyperstat and Nitrostat

idarubicin and daunorubicin or doxorubicin

ifosfamide and cyclophosphamide

imipramine and desipramine

Imodium and Ionamin

Imuran and Inderal

Inderal and Inderide, Isordil, Adderall, or Imuran

Isoptin and Intropin

Isordil and Isuprel or Inderal

K-Phos-Neutral and Neutra-Phos-K

Lamictal and Lamisil

lamotrigine and lamivudine

Lanoxin and Levoxyl or levothyroxine

Lantus and Lente

Leukeran and leucovorin

Levatol or Lipitor

levothyroxine and liothyronine or liotrix

Lithobid and Levbid

Lithonate and Lithostat

Lithotabs and Lithobid or Lithostat

Lodine and codeine, iodine, or Iopidine

Lorabid and Lortab

lorazepam and alprazolam

Lotensin and Loniten or lovastatin

Luvox and Lasix

magnesium sulfate and manganese sulfate

Maxidex and Maxzide

Mellaril and Elavil

melphalan and Mephyton

Mestinon and Mesantoin or Metatensin

metaproterenol and metoprolol or metipranolol

methicillin and mezlocillin

methimazole and mebendazole or methazolamide

methocarbamol and mephobarbital

methylprednisolone and medroxyprogesterone

methyltestosterone and medroxyprogesterone

metoprolol and metaproterenol or metolazone

Mevacor and Mivacron

Micronor and Micro-K or Micronase

Minocin and niacin or Mithracin

mitomycin and mithramycin

Monopril and Monurol

Nalfon and Naldecon

naloxone and naltrexone

Navane and Nubain or Norvasc

nelfinavir and nevirapine

Nicoderm and Nitro-Dur

Nicorette and Nordette

nifedipine and nimodipine or nicardipine

Nitro-Bid and Nicobid

nitroglycerine and nitroprusside

norepinephrine and epinephrine

Noroxin and Neurontin

nortriptyline and amitriptyline

Nubain and Navane

nystatin and Nitrostat

Ocuflox and Ocufen

olsalazine and olanzapine

opium tincture and camphorated opium tincture

oxaprozin and oxazepam

oxymorphone and oxymetholone

pancuronium and pipecuronium

Parlodel and pindolol

paroxetine and paclitaxel

Paxil and Doxil, paclitaxel, or Taxol

pemoline and Pelamine

penicillin G benzathine and Polycillin, penicillamine, or other types of penicillin

penicillin G potassium and Polycillin, penicillamine, or other types of penicillin

penicillin G procaine and Polycillin, penicillamine, or other types of penicillin

penicillin G sodium and Polycillin, penicillamine, or other types of penicillin

penicillin V potassium and Polycillin, penicillamine, or other types of penicillin

pentobarbital and phenobarbital

pentostatin and pentosan

Persantine and Periactin

phentermine and phentolamine

phenytoin and mephenytoin

pindolol and Parlodel, Panadol, or Plendil

Pitocin and Pitressin

Plendil and pindolol

pralidoxime and pramoxine or pyridoxine

Pravachol and Prevacid or propranolol

prednisolone and prednisone

Premarin and Primaxin

Prilosec and Prozac, Prinivil, or Plendil

primidone and prednisone

Prinivil and Proventil or Prilosec

ProAmatine and protamine

probenecid and Procanbid

procainamide and probenecid

promethazine and promazine

propranolol and Pravachol

ProSom and Proscar or Prozac

protamine and Protopam or Protropin

Prozac and Proscar, Prilosec, or ProSom

pyridoxine and pralidoxime or Pyridium

Questran and Quarzan

quinidine and quinine or clonidine

ranitidine and ritodrine or rimantadine

Reminyl and Robinul

Restoril and Vistaril

riboflavin and ribavirin

rifabutin and rifampin or rifapentine

Rifater and Rifadin or Rifamate

risperidone and reserpine or Risperdal

Ritalin and Rifadin

ritodrine and ranitidine

ritonavir and Retrovir

Sandimmune and Sandoglobulin or Sandostatin

saquinavir and saquinavir mesylate (the dosages are
different)

Sarafem and Serophene

selegiline and Stelazine or Sertraline

Serentil and Serevent or Aventyl

Serzone and Seroquel

simethicone and cimetidine

Sinequan and saquinavir

Solu-Cortef and Solu-Medrol

somatropin and somatrem or sumatriptan

sotalol and Stadol

streptozocin and streptomycin

sufentanil and alfentanil or fentanyl

sulfadiazine and sulfasalazine

sulfamethoxazole and sulfamethizole

sulfamethoxazole alone and combination products

sulfasalazine and sulfisoxazole, salsalate, or sulfadiazine

sulfisoxazole and sulfasalazine

sulfisoxazole alone and combination products

sulfonamide drugs

sumatriptan and somatropin

Survanta and Sufenta

Tegretol and Toradol

Tenex and Xanax, Entex, or Ten-K

terbinafine and terbutaline

terbutaline and tolbutamide or terbinafine

terconazole and tioconazole

Testoderm and Estraderm

testosterone and testolactone

thiamine and Thorazine

thioridazine and Thorazine

Tigan and Ticar

timolol and atenolol

Timoptic and Viroptic

tobramycin and Trobicin

Tobrex and Tobradex

tolnaftate and Tornalate

Toradol and Tegretol

Trandate and Trental

Trental and Trendar or Trandate

triamcinolone and Triaminicin or Triaminicol

triamterene and trimipramine

trifluoperazine and triflupromazine

trimipramine and triamterene or trimeprazine

Ultracet and Ultracef

Urispas and Urised

valacyclovir and valganciclovir

Vancenase and Vanceril

Vanceril and Vansil

Verelan and Vivarin, Ferralyn, or Virilon

Versed and VePesid

vidarabine and cytarabine

vinblastine and vincristine, vindesine, or vinorelbine

Visine and Visken

Volmax and Flomax

Voltaren and Ventolin or Verelan

Wellbutrin and Wellcovorin or Wellferon

Xanax and Zantac, Tenex, or Zyrtec

Xenical and Xeloda

Zarontin and Zaroxolyn

Zaroxolyn and Zarontin

Zebeta and DiaBeta

Zestril and Zostrix

Zocor and Zoloft

Zofran and Zosyn, Zantac, or Zoloft

Zyprexa and Zyrtec

Zyrtec and Zyprexa

Drugs that shouldn't be crushed

Many drug forms, such as slow-release, enteric-coated, encapsulated beads, wax-matrix, sublingual, and buccal forms, are made to release their active ingredients over a certain period of time or at preset points after administration. The disruptions caused by crushing these drug forms can dramatically affect the absorption rate and increase the risk of adverse reactions.

Other reasons not to crush these drug forms include such considerations as taste, tissue irritation, and unusual formulation—for example, a capsule within a capsule, a liquid within a capsule, or a multiple-compressed tablet. Avoid crushing the following drugs, listed by brand name, for the reasons noted beside them.

Accutane (irritant)

Aciphex (delayed-release)

Adalat CC (sustained-release)

Advicor (extended-release)

Aggrenox (extended-release)

Allegra D (extended-release)

Altocor (extended-release)

Amnesteem (irritant)

Arthrotec (delayed-release)

Asacol (delayed-release)

Augmentin XR (extended-release)

Avinza (extended-release)

Azulfidine EN-tabs (enteric-coated)

Bellergal-S (slow-release)

Biaxin XL (extended-release)

Bisacodyl (enteric-coated)

Bontril Slow-Release (slow-release)

Breonesin (liquid-filled)

Brexin L.A. (slow-release)

Bromfed (slow-release)

Bromfed-PD (slow-release)

Calan SR (sustained-release)

Carbatrol (extended release)

Cardizem CD, LA, SR (slow-release)

Cartia XT (extended-release)

Ceclor CD (slow-release)

Ceftin (strong, persistent taste)

Charcoal Plus DS (enteric-coated)

Chloral Hydrate (liquid within a capsule, taste)

Chlor-Trimeton Allergy 8-hour and 12-hour (slow-release)

Choledyl SA (slow-release)

Cipro XR (extended-release)

Claritin-D 12-hour (slow-release)

Claritin-D 24-hour (slow-release)

Colace (liquid within a capsule)

Colazal (granules within capsules must reach colon intact)

Colestid (protective coating)

Compazine Spansules (slow-release)

Concerta (extended release)

Congess SR (sustained-release)

Contac 12 Hour, Maximum Strength 12 Hour (slow-release)

Cotazym-S (enteric-coated)

Covera-HS (extended release)

Creon (enteric-coated)

Cytovene (irritant)

Dallergy, Dallergy-Jr (slow-release)

Deconamine SR (slow-release)

Depakene (slow-release, mucous membrane irritant)

Depakote (enteric-coated)

Depakote ER (extended-release)

Desyrel (taste)

Dexedrine Spansule (slow-release)

Diamox Sequels (slow-release)

Dilacor XR (extended-release)

Dilatrate-SR (slow-release)

Diltia XT (extended-release)

Dimetapp Extentabs (slow-release)

Ditropan XL (slow-release)

Dolobid (irritant)

Drisdol (liquid-filled)

Dristan (protective coating)

Drixoral (slow-release)

Dulcolax (enteric-coated)

DynaCirc CR (slow-release)

Easprin (enteric-coated)

Ecotrin (enteric-coated)

Ecotrin Maximum Strength (enteric-coated)

E.E.S. 400 Filmtab (enteric-coated)

Effexor XR (extended-release)

Emend (hard gelatin capsule)

E-Mycin (enteric-coated)

Entex LA (slow-release)

Entex PSE (slow-release)

Eryc (enteric-coated)

Ery-Tab (enteric-coated)

Erythrocin Stearate (enteric-coated)

Erythromycin Base (enteric-coated)

Eskalith CR (slow-release)

Extendryl JR, SR (slow-release)

Feldene (mucous membrane irritant)

Feosol (enteric-coated)

Feratab (enteric-coated)

Fergon (slow-release)

Fero-Folic 500 (slow-release)

Fero-Grad-500 (slow-release)

Ferro-Sequel (slow-release)

Feverall Children's Capsules, Sprinkle (taste)

Flomax (slow-release)

Fumatinic (slow-release)

Geocillin (taste)

Glucophage XR (extended-release)

Glucotrol XL (slow-release)

Guaifed (slow-release)

Guaifed-PD (slow-release)

Guaifenex LA (slow-release)

Guaifenex PSE (slow-release)

Humibid DM, LA, Pediatric (slow-release)

Hydergine LC (liquid within a capsule)

Hytakerol (liquid-filled)

Iberet (slow-release)

ICAPS Plus (slow-release)

ICAPS Time Release (slow-release)

Imdur (slow-release)

Inderal LA (slow-release)

Indocin SR (slow-release)

InnoPran XL (extended-release)

Ionamin (slow-release)

Isoptin SR (sustained-release)

Isordil Sublingual (sublingual)

Isordil Tembids (slow-release)

Isosorbide Dinitrate Sublingual (sublingual)

Kaon-Cl (slow-release)

K-Dur (slow-release)

Klor-Con (slow-release)

Klotrix (slow-release)

K-Tab (slow-release)

Levbid (slow-release)

Levsinex Timecaps (slow-release)

Lithobid (slow-release)

Macrobid (slow-release)

Mestinon Timespans (slow-release)

Metadate CD, ER (extended-release)

Methylin ER (extended release)

Micro-K Extencaps (slow-release)

Motrin (taste)

MS Contin (slow-release)

Mucinex (extended-release)

Naprelan (slow-release)

Nexium (sustained-release)

Niaspan (extended-release)

Nitroglyn (slow-release)

Nitrong (slow-release)

Nitrostat (sublingual)

Norflex (slow-release)

Norpace CR (slow-release)

Oramorph SR (slow-release)

Oruvail (extended-release)

OxyContin (slow-release)

Pancrease (enteric-coated)

Pancrease MT (enteric-coated)

Paxil CR (controlled-release)

PCE (slow-release)

Pentasa (controlled release)

Phazyme (slow-release)

Phazyme 95 (slow-release)

Phenytex (extended-release)

Plendil (slow-release)

Prelu-2 (slow-release)

Prevacid, Prevacid SoluTab (delayed-release)

Prilosec (slow-release)

Prilosec OTC (delayed-release)

Pro-Banthine (taste)

Procanbid (slow-release)

Procardia (delayed absorption)

Procardia XL (slow-release)

Protonix (delayed-release)

Proventil Repetabs (slow-release)

Prozac Weekly (slow-release)

Quibron-T/SR (slow-release)

Quinidex Extentabs (slow-release)

Respaire SR (slow-release)

Respbid (slow-release)

Risperdal M-Tab (delayed-release)

Ritalin-LA, -SR (slow-release)

Rondec-TR (slow-release)

Sinemet CR (slow-release)

Slo-bid Gyrocaps (slow-release)

Slo-Niacin (slow-release)

Slo-Phyllin GG, Gyrocaps (slow-release)

Slow FE (slow-release)

Slow-K (slow-release)

Slow-Mag (slow-release)

Sorbitrate (sublingual)

Sotret (irritant)

Sudafed 12 Hour (slow-release)

Sustaire (slow-release)

Tegretol-XR (extended-release)

Ten-K (slow-release)

Tenuate Dospan (slow-release)

Tessalon Perles (slow-release)

Theobid Duracaps (slow-release)

Theochron (slow-release)

Theoclear LA (slow-release)

Theolair-SR (slow-release)

Theo-Sav (slow-release)

Theospan-SR (slow-release)

Theo-24 (slow-release)

Theovent (slow-release)

Theo-X (slow-release)

Thorazine Spansules (slow-release)

Tiazac (sustained-release)

Topamax (taste)

Toprol XL (extended-release)

T-Phyl (slow-release)

Trental (slow-release)

Trinalin Repetabs (slow-release)

Tylenol Extended Relief (slow-release)

Uniphyl (slow-release)

Vantin (taste)

Verelan, Verelan PM (slow-release)

Volmax (slow-release)

Voltaren (enteric-coated)

Voltaren-XR (extended-release)

Wellbutrin SR (sustained-release)

Xanax XR (extended-release)

Zerit XR (extended-release)

Zomig-ZMT (delayed-release)

ZORprin (slow-release)

Zyban (slow-release)

Zyrtec-D 12 hour (extended-release)

Normal laboratory test values

Normal values may differ from laboratory to laboratory. Standard International units are abbreviated SI.

Hematology

Activated partial thromboplastin time
21-35 sec (SI, 21-35 sec)

Bleeding time
Duke: 1-3 min (SI, 1-3 m)
Ivy: 3-6 min (SI, 3-6 m)
Template: 3-6 min (SI, 3-6 m)

Fibrinogen, plasma
200-400 mg/dl (SI, 2-4 g/L)

Hematocrit
Men: 42%-52% (SI, 0.42-0.52)
Women: 36%-48% (SI, 0.36-0.48)

Hemoglobin, total
Men: 14-17.4 g/dl (SI, 140-174 g/L)
Women: 12-16 g/dl (SI, 120-160 g/L)

Platelet aggregation
3-5 min (SI, 3-5 min)

Platelet count
140,000-400,000/mm³ (SI, 140-400 × 10⁹/L)

Prothrombin time
10-14 sec (SI, 10-14 sec); INR for patients on warfarin therapy, 2-3 (SI, 2-3) (those with prosthetic heart valve, 2.5-3.5 [SI, 2.5-3.5])

Red blood cell count
Men: 4.5-5.5 million/mm³ (SI, 4.5-5.5 × 10¹²/L) venous blood
Women: 4-5 million/ mm³ (SI, 4-5 × 10¹²/L) venous blood

Red blood cell indices
Mean corpuscular volume: 82-98 femtoliter
Mean corpuscular hemoglobin: 26-34 picograms/cell
Mean corpuscular hemoglobin concentration: 31-37 g/dl

Reticulocyte count
0.5%-1.5% (SI, 0.005-0.025) of total RBC count

White blood cell count
4,500-10,500 cells/mm³

White blood cell differential, blood
Neutrophils: 54%-75% (SI, 0.54-0.75)
Lymphocytes: 25%-40% (SI, 0.25-0.4)
Monocytes: 2%-8% (SI, 0.02-0.08)
Eosinophils: up to 4% (SI, up to 0.04)
Basophils: up to 1% (SI, up to 0.01)

Blood chemistry

Alanine aminotransferase
Adults: 10-35 units/L (SI, 0.17-0.6 mu kat/L)
Neonates: 13-45 units/L (SI, 0.22-0.77 mu kat/L)

Amylase, serum
Adults ≥ age 18: 25-85 units/L (SI, 0.39-1.45 mu kat/L)

Arterial blood gases
pH: 7.35-7.45 (SI, 7.35-7.45)
Paco₂: 35-45 mm Hg (SI, 4.7-5.3 kPa)
Pao₂: 80-100 mm Hg (SI, 10.6-13.3 kPa)
HCO₃⁻: 22-26 mEq/L (SI, 22-25 mmol/L)
Sao₂: 94%-100% (SI, 0.94-1.00)

Aspartate aminotransferase
Men: 14-20 units/L (SI, 0.23-0.33 mu kat/L)
Women: 7-34 units/L (SI, 0.12-0.58 mkat/L)

Bilirubin, serum
Adults, total: 0.2-1 mg/dl (SI, 3.5-17 micromol/L)
Neonates, total: 1-10 mg/dl (SI, 17-170 micromol/L)
Neonates, unconjugated indirect: 0-10 mg/dl (SI, 0-170 micromol/L)

Blood urea nitrogen
8-20 mg/dl (SI, 2.9-7.5 mmol/L)

Calcium, serum
  Adults: 8.2-10.2 mg/dl (SI, 2.05-
  2.54 mmol/L)
  Children: 8.6-11.2 mg/dl (SI, 2.15-
  2.79 mmol/L)

Carbon dioxide, total, blood
  22-26 mEq/L (SI, 22-26 mmol/L)

Cholesterol, total, serum
  Men: < 205 mg/dl (SI, < 5.30 mmol/L)
  (desirable)
  Women: < 190 mg/dl (SI, < 4.90 mmol/L)
  (desirable)

Creatine kinase, isoenzymes
  CK-BB: none
  CK-MB: 0-7%
  CK-MM: 96-100%

Creatinine, serum
  Adults: 0.6-1.3 mg/dl (SI, 53-115 micro-
  mol/L)

Glucose, plasma, fasting
  70-110 mg/dl (SI, 3.9-6.1 mmol/L)

Glucose, plasma, 2-hour postprandial
  < 145 mg/dl (SI, < 8 mmol/L)

Lactate dehydrogenase
  Total: 71-207 units/L in adults (SI, 1.2-
  3.52 mu kat/L)
  LD1: 14%-26% (SI, 0.14-0.26)
  LD2: 29%-39% (SI, 0.29-0.39)
  LD3: 20%-26% (SI, 0.20-0.26)
  LD4: 8%-16% (SI, 0.08-0.16)
  LD5: 6%-16% (SI, 0.06-0.16)

Lipase
  < 160 units/L (SI, < 2.72 mu kat/L)

Magnesium, serum
  1.8-2.6 mg/dl (SI, 0.74-1.07 mmol/L)

Phosphates, serum
  2.7-4.5 mg/dl (SI, 0.87-1.45 mmol/L)

Potassium, serum
  3.8-5 mEq/L (SI, 3.5-5 mmol/L)

Protein, serum
  Total: 6.3-8.3 g/dl (SI, 64-83 g/L)
  Albumin fraction: 3.5-5 g/dl (SI, 35-50 g/L)

Sodium, serum
  135-145 mEq/L (SI, 135-145 mmol/L)

Triglycerides, serum
  Men > age 20: 40-180 mg/dl (SI, 0.11-2.01
  mmol/L)
  Women > age 20: 10-190 mg/dl (SI, 0.11-
  2.21 mmol/L)

Uric acid, serum
  Men: 3.4-7 mg/dl (SI, 202-416 micromol/L)
  Women: 2.3-6 mg/dl (SI, 143-357 micro-
  mol/L)

Selected opioid analgesic combination products

Many common analgesics are combinations of two or more generic drugs. This table reviews common opioid analgesics.

Trade names and controlled substance schedule (CSS)	Generic drugs	Indications and adult dosages
Aceta with Codeine, Tylenol with Codeine #3 *CSS III*	• acetaminophen 300 mg • codeine phosphate 30 mg	For fever, mild to moderate pain. Give 1 or 2 tablets q 4 hours. Maximum, 12 tablets in 24 hours.
Alor 5/500, Damason-P, Lortab ASA *CSS III*	• aspirin 500 mg • hydrocodone bitartrate 5 mg	For moderate to moderately severe pain. Give 1 or 2 tablets q 4 hours. Maximum, 8 tablets in 24 hours.
Anexsia 7.5/650, Lorcet Plus *CSS III*	• acetaminophen 650 mg • hydrocodone bitartrate 7.5 mg	For arthralgia, bone pain, dental pain, headache, migraine, moderate pain. Give 1 or 2 tablets q 4 hours. Maximum, 6 tablets in 24 hours.
Capital with Codeine Suspension, Tylenol with Codeine Elixir *CSS V*	• acetaminophen 120 mg • codeine phosphate 12 mg/5 ml	For mild to moderate pain. Give 15 ml q 4 hours.
Darvocet-N 50 *CSS IV*	• acetaminophen 325 mg • propoxyphene napsylate 50 mg	For mild to moderate pain. Give 1 or 2 tablets q 4 hours. Maximum, 12 tablets in 24 hours.
Darvocet-N 100, Propacet 100 *CSS IV*	• acetaminophen 650 mg • propoxyphene napsylate 100 mg	For mild to moderate pain. Give 1 tablet q 4 hours. Maximum, 6 tablets in 24 hours.
Empirin with Codeine No. 3 *CSS III*	• aspirin 325 mg • codeine phosphate 30 mg	For fever, mild to moderate pain. Give 1 or 2 tablets q 4 hours. Maximum, 12 tablets in 24 hours.
Empirin with Codeine No. 4 *CSS III*	• aspirin 325 mg • codeine phosphate 60 mg	For fever, mild to moderate pain. Give 1 tablet q 4 hours. Maximum, 6 tablets in 24 hours.
Fioricet with Codeine *CSS III*	• acetaminophen 325 mg • butalbital 50 mg • caffeine 40 mg • codeine phosphate 30 mg	For headache, mild to moderate pain. Give 1 or 2 capsules q 4 hours. Maximum, 6 capsules in 24 hours.
Fiorinal with Codeine No. 3 *CSS III*	• aspirin 325 mg • butalbital 50 mg • caffeine 40 mg • codeine phosphate 30 mg	For headache, mild to moderate pain. Give 1 or 2 tablets or capsules q 4 hours. Maximum, 6 tablets or capsules in 24 hours.
Lorcet 10/650 *CSS III*	• acetaminophen 650 mg • hydrocodone bitartrate 10 mg	For moderate to moderately severe pain. Give 1 tablet q 4 hours. Maximum, 6 tablets in 24 hours.
Lortab 2.5/500 *CSS III*	• acetaminophen 500 mg • hydrocodone bitartrate 2.5 mg	For moderate to moderately severe pain. Give 1 or 2 tablets q 4 hours. Maximum, 8 tablets in 24 hours.

Trade names and controlled substance schedule (CSS)	Generic drugs	Indications and adult dosages
Lortab 5/500, Vicodin *CSS III*	• acetaminophen 500 mg • hydrocodone bitartrate 5 mg	For moderate to moderately severe pain. Give 1 or 2 tablets q 4 hours. Maximum, 8 tablets in 24 hours.
Lortab 7.5/500 *CSS III*	• acetaminophen 500 mg • hydrocodone bitartrate 7.5 mg	For moderate to moderately severe pain. Give 1 tablet q 4 hours. Maximum, 8 tablets in 24 hours.
Lortab 10/500 *CSS III*	• acetaminophen 500 mg • hydrocodone bitartrate 10 mg	For moderate to moderately severe pain. Give 1 tablet q 4-6 hours. Maximum, 6 tablets in 24 hours.
Percocet 2.5/325 *CSS II*	• acetaminophen 325 mg • oxycodone hydrochloride 2.5 mg	For moderate to moderately severe pain. Give 1 or 2 tablets q 4-6 hours. Maximum, 12 tablets in 24 hours.
Percocet 5/325, Roxicet *CSS II*	• acetaminophen 325 mg • oxycodone hydrochloride 5 mg	For moderate to moderately severe pain. Give 1 or 2 tablets q 4 hours. Maximum, 12 tablets in 24 hours.
Percocet 7.5/500 *CSS II*	• acetaminophen 500 mg • oxycodone hydrochloride 7.5 mg	For moderate to moderately severe pain. Give 1 or 2 tablets q 4-6 hours. Maximum, 8 tablets in 24 hours.
Percocet 10/650 *CSS II*	• acetaminophen 650 mg • oxycodone hydrochloride 10 mg	For moderate to moderately severe pain. Give 1 or 2 tablets q 4-6 hours. Maximum, 6 tablets in 24 hours.
Percodan-Demi *CSS II*	• aspirin 325 mg • oxycodone hydrochloride 2.25 mg • oxycodone terephthalate 0.19 mg	For moderate to moderately severe pain. Give 1 or 2 tablets q 6 hours. Maximum, 8 tablets in 24 hours.
Percodan, Roxiprin *CSS II*	• aspirin 325 mg • oxycodone hydrochloride 4.5 mg • oxycodone terephthalate 0.38 mg	For moderate to moderately severe pain. Give 1 tablet q 6 hours. Maximum, 4 tablets in 24 hours.
Roxicet 5/500, Roxilox *CSS II*	• acetaminophen 500 mg • oxycodone hydrochloride 5 mg	For moderate to moderately severe pain. Give 1 or 2 tablets q 4-6 hours. Maximum, 8 tablets in 24 hours.
Roxicet Oral Solution *CSS II*	• acetaminophen 325 mg • oxycodone hydrochloride 5 mg/ 5 ml	For moderate to moderately severe pain. Give 5–10 ml q 4-6 hours. Maximum, 60 ml in 24 hours.
Talacen *CSS IV*	• acetaminophen 650 mg • pentazocine hydrochloride 25 mg	For mild to moderate pain. Give 1 tablet q 4 hours. Maximum, 6 tablets in 24 hours.
Talwin Compound *CSS IV*	• aspirin 325 mg • pentazocine hydrochloride 12.5 mg	For moderate pain. Give 2 tablets q 6 hours. Maximum, 8 tablets in 24 hours.
Tylenol with Codeine No. 2 *CSS III*	• acetaminophen 300 mg • codeine phosphate 15 mg	For fever, mild to moderate pain. Give 1 or 2 tablets q 4 hours. Maximum, 12 tablets in 24 hours.

(continued)

Trade names and controlled substance schedule (CSS)	Generic drugs	Indications and adult dosages
Tylenol with Codeine No. 4 *CSS III*	• acetaminophen 300 mg • codeine phosphate 60 mg	For fever, mild to moderate pain. Give 1 tablet q 4 hours. Maximum, 6 tablets in 24 hours.
Tylox *CSS II*	• acetaminophen 500 mg • oxycodone hydrochloride 5 mg	For moderate to moderately severe pain. Give 1 or 2 tablets q 4 hours. Maximum, 12 tablets in 24 hours.
Vicodin ES *CSS III*	• acetaminophen 750 mg • hydrocodone bitartrate 7.5 mg	For moderate to moderately severe pain. Give 1 tablet q 4-6 hours. Maximum, 5 tablets in 24 hours.
Wygesic *CSS IV*	• acetaminophen 650 mg • propoxyphene napsylate 65 mg	For mild to moderate pain. Give 1 tablet q 4 hours. Maximum, 6 tablets in 24 hours.
Zydone *CSS III*	• acetaminophen 400 mg • hydrocodone bitartrate 10 mg	For moderate to moderately severe pain. Give 1 tablet q 4-6 hours. Maximum, 6 tablets in 24 hours.

English-to-Spanish drug phrase translator

Medication history

Do you take any medications?	**¿Toma Ud. medicamentos?**
– Prescription?	– ¿De receta?
– Over-the-counter?	– ¿Sin necesidad de receta?
– Other?	– ¿Otro?

Which prescription medications do you take routinely?
- How often do you take them?
  - Once daily?
  - Twice daily?
  - Three times daily?
  - Four times daily?
  - More often?

¿Qué medicamentos de receta toma Ud. por rutina?
- ¿Con qué frecuencia los toma?
  - ¿Una vez al día?
  - ¿Dos veces al día?
  - ¿Tres veces al día?
  - ¿Cuátro veces al día?
  - ¿Con más frecuencia?

Which over-the-counter medications do you take routinely?
- How often do you take them?
- Once daily?
- Twice daily?
- Three times daily?
- Four times daily?
- More often?

¿Qué medicamentos que no necesitan receta toma Ud. por rutina?
- ¿Con que frecuencia los toma?
- ¿Una vez al día?
- ¿Dos veces al día?
- ¿Tres veces al día?
- ¿Cuatro veces al día?
- ¿Con más frecuencia?

Which medications do you take periodically?

¿Qué medicamentos toma Ud. periódicamente?

Why do you take these medications?

¿Por qué toma Ud. estos medicamentos?

What is the dosage for each medication?

¿Cuál es la dosis para cada uno de los medicamentos?

How does each medication make you feel?

¿Cómo le hace sentirse cada medicamento?

Are you allergic to any medications?

¿Está Ud. alérgico(a) a algúnos medicamentos?

- Which medications?
- What happens when you have an allergic reaction?

- ¿A qué medicamentos?
- ¿Qué pasa cuando Ud. tiene una reacción alérgica?

Medication teaching

Purpose of the medication

This medication will:
- elevate your blood pressure.
- improve circulation to your _____.
- lower your blood pressure.
- lower your blood sugar.

Este medicamento hará que:
- su presión sanguínea suba.
- la circulación por _____ mejore.
- su presión sanguínea baje.
- el nivel de azucar en la sangre baje.

– make your heart rhythm more even.
– raise your blood sugar.
– reduce or prevent the formation of blood clots.
– remove fluid from your body.
– remove fluid from your feet, ankles, or legs.
– remove fluid from your lungs so that they work better.
– remove fluid from your pancreas so that it works better.

– el ritmo del corazón sea más uniforme.
– su nivel de azucar en la sangre suba.
– se reduzca o evite la formación de coágulos de sangre.
– se le quite fluido en el cuerpo.
– se le quite fluido de los pies, tobillos o piernas.
– se le quite fluido de los pulmones para que funcionen mejor.
– se le quite fluido de la páncreas para que funcione mejor.

This medication will help your body to:
– kill the bacteria in your _____.
– slow down your heart rate.
– soften your bowel movements.
– speed up your heart rate.
– use insulin more efficiently.

Este medicamento le ayudará a su cuerpo a:
– destruir la bacteria de la _____.
– reducir el latir del corazón.
– ablandar sus evacuaciones.
– acelerar el latir del corazón.
– usar la insulina más eficazmente.

This medication will help you to:
– breathe better.
– fight infections.
– relax.
– sleep.
– think more clearly.

Este medicamento le ayudará a Ud. a:
– respirar con mayor facilidad.
– luchar contra infecciones.
– relajarse.
– dormir.
– pensar con mayor claridad.

This medication will relieve or reduce:
– the acid production in your stomach.
– anxiety.
– bladder spasms.
– burning in your stomach or chest.
– burning when you urinate.
– diarrhea.
– muscle cramps.
– nausea.
– pain in your _____.

Este medicamento le aliviará o disminuirá:
– la producción de acido en el estómago.
– la angustia.
– espasmos en la vejiga.
– sensación ardiente en el estómago o tórax.
– sensación ardiente al orinar.
– diarrea.
– espasmos en los músculos.
– nausea.
– dolor en la (el) _____.

This medication will help your body to produce more or less:
– antibodies.
– clotting factors.
– insulin.
– platelets.
– red blood cells.
– white blood cells.

Este medicamento le ayudará a su cuerpo a producir más o menos:
– anticuerpos.
– factores o agentes coagulantes.
– insulina.
– plaquetas.
– células rojas de sangre.
– células blancas de sangre.

This medication or treatment will destroy:
– antibodies.
– bacteria.
– cancer cells.
– clotting factors.
– platelets.
– red blood cells.
– white blood cells.

Este medicamento o tratamiento destruirá:
– anticuerpos.
– bacteria.
– células cancerosas.
– factores o agentes coagulantes.
– plaquetas.
– células rojas de sangre.
– células blancas de sangre.

Medication administration

I would like to give you:
– an injection.
– an I.V. medication.
– a liquid medication.
– a medicated cream or powder.
– a medication through your epidural catheter.
– a medication through your rectum.
– a medication through your _____ tube.
– a medication under your tongue.
– your pill(s).
– a suppository.

Quisiera darle a Ud. un(a):
– inyección.
– medicamento por vía intravenosa.
– medicamento en forma líquida.
– medicamento en pomada o polvo.
– medicamento por el catéter epidural.
– medicamento por el recto.
– medicamento por su _____ tubo.
– medicamento debajo de la lengua.
– su(s) píldora(s).
– supositorio.

This is how you take this medication.

Así se toma este medicamento.

If you can't swallow this pill, I can crush it and mix it in some food or liquid such as:

– applesauce.
– pudding.
– yogurt.

Si Ud. no se puede tragar esta píldora, puedo aplastarla y mezclarla en un alimento/líquido, tal como:
– puré de manzana.
– pudín.
– yogur.

If you can't swallow this pill, I can get it in another form.

Si Ud. no puede tragarse esta píldora, puede obtenerla en otra forma.

If you can't swallow a pill, you can crush it and mix it in soft food.

Si Ud. no se puede tragar la píldora, la puede moler y mezclarla en un alimento blando.

I need to mix this medication in juice or water.

Tengo que mezclar este medicamento en jugo (zumo) o agua.

I need to give you this injection in your:
– abdomen.
– buttocks.
– hip.
– outer arm.
– thigh.

Tengo que ponerle esta inyección:
– en el abdomen.
– en las nalgas.
– en la cadera.
– en el brazo.
– en el muslo.

I need to give you this medication I.V.

Tengo que darle este medicamento por via intravenosa (I.V.).

Place it under your tongue.

Póngaselo debajo de la lengua.

You should feel some burning when it is under your tongue.

Ud. debiera sentir un ardor cuando se lo pone debajo de la lengua.

This indicates that it is working.

Esto indica que está tomando efecto.

Some medications are coated with a special substance to protect your stomach from getting upset.

Algunos medicamentos están cubiertos con una sustancia especial para protegerle contra un trastorno estomacal.

Do not chew:
– enteric-coated pills.
– long-acting pills.
– capsules.
– sublingual medication.

No masque Ud.:
– píldoras con recubrimientoentérico.
– píldoras de efecto prolongado.
– cápsulas.
– medicamentos sublinguales.

Ask your doctor or pharmacist whether you can:
– mix your medication with food or fluids.
– take your medication with or without food.

Pregúntele Ud. a su doctor o farmacéutico si debiera:
– mezclar su medicamento con un alimento o con líquidos.
– tomar su medicamento con o sin alimento.

You need to take your medication:
– after meals.
– before meals.
– on an empty stomach.
– with meals or food.

Ud. tiene que tomarse el medicamento:
– después de las comidas.
– antes de las comidas.
– con el estómago vacío.
– con las comidas o con un alimento.

Skipping doses

If you skip or miss a dose:
– Take it as soon as you remember it.
– Wait until the next dose.
– Call the doctor if you are not sure.
– Do not take an extra dose.

Si Ud. omite o se salta una dosis:
– Tómesela encuanto se acuerde.
– Espérese hasta la siguiente dosis.
– Llame al doctor si Ud. no está seguro(a).
– No se tome una dosis extra.

Adverse effects

Some common adverse effects of _____ are:
– constipation
– diarrhea
– difficulty sleeping
– dry mouth
– fatigue
– headache
– itching
– light-headedness
– nausea
– poor appetite
– rash
– upset stomach
– weight loss or gain
– frequent urination.

Unos efectos adversos comunes a _____ son:
– estreñimiento
– diarrea
– dificultad en dormir
– boca seca
– fatiga
– dolor de cabeza
– comezón (picazón)
– mareo
– nausea
– poco apetito
– erupción
– trastorno estomacal
– perdida o aumento de peso
– orinar con frecuencia.

These adverse effects:
– will go away after your body gets used to the medication.
– may persist as long as you take the medication.

Estos efectos adversos:
– desaparecerán una vez que su cuerpo se acostumbre al medicamento.
– puede continuar mientras Ud. tome el medicamento.

If they bother you, speak to your doctor about changing your medication.

Si le molestan a Ud., hable con su doctor acerca de que le cambie el medicamento.

If you have an adverse reaction to your medication, call your doctor right away.

Si Ud. tiene una reacción adversa a su medicamento, llame a su doctor inmediatamente.

Other concerns

Tell your doctor if you are pregnant or breast-feeding.

While you are taking this medication, ask your doctor if:
- you can safely take other over-the-counter medications.
- you can drink alcoholic beverages.
- your medications interact with each other.

Dígale a su doctor si Ud. está ebarazada o si cría a los pechos.

Mientras Ud. tome este medicamento, pregúntele a su doctor si:
- puede tomar otros medicamentos que no necesitan receta.
- puede tomar bebidas alcohólicas.
- sus medicamentos interaccionan uno con el otro.

Storing medication

You should keep your medication:
- in a cool, dry place.
- in the refrigerator.
- at room temperature.
- out of direct sunlight.
- away from heat.
- away from children.

Ud. debiera guardar sus medicamentos:
- en un lugar fresco, seco.
- en el refrigerador.
- al tiempo.
- fuera de la luz de sol.
- lejos de la calefacción.
- lejos del alcance de los niños.

Do not keep your medication:
- in a warm place or near heat.

- in the sun.
- in your pocket.
- in the bathroom medicine cabinet.

No guarde Ud. su medicamento:
- en un lugar caliente ni cerca de la calefacción.
- en el sol.
- en su bolsillo.
- en el botiquín del baño.

Teaching a patient to give a subcutaneous injection

To give yourself an injection, follow these steps:
- Draw up the medication.
- Replace the cap carefully.
- Decide where you are going to give the injection.
- Clean the skin area with alcohol.
- Gently pinch up a little skin over the area.

- Using a dartlike motion, stab the needle into your skin.
- Gently pull back on the plunger to see if there is any blood in the syringe.
- Steadily push the medication into your skin.

- Pull the needle out.
- Apply gentle pressure with the alcohol wipe.

- Dispose of the needle in a proper receptacle.

Así es como uno se pone una inyección a sí mismo(a):
- Saque el medicamento.
- Coloque de nuevo la tapa con cuidado.
- Decida Ud. donde va a ponerse la inyección.
- Limpie el área de la piel con alcohol.
- Suavemente pellizque un poco de piel sobre el área.

- Con un movimiento rápido, penetre la aguja en su piel.
- Con cuidado retire el émbolo para ver si hay sangre en la jeringa.
- Constantemente empuje el medicamento dentro de su piel.
- Saque la aguja.
- Ejerza presión suavemente con un limpión de alcohol.
- Deshagase de la aguja en un recipiente apropiado.

Insulin preparation and administration

The doctor has ordered insulin for you.

To draw up insulin, follow these steps:

- Wipe the rubber top of the insulin bottle with alcohol.
- Remove the needle cap.
- Pull out the plunger until the end of the plunger in the barrel aligns with the number of units of insulin that you need.

- Push the needle through the rubber top of the insulin bottle.
- Inject the air into the bottle.
- Without removing the needle from the bottle, turn it upside down.
- Withdraw the plunger until the end of the plunger aligns with the number of units you need.
- Gently pull the needle out of the bottle.

To mix insulin, follow these steps:

- Wipe the rubber tops of the insulin bottles with alcohol.
- Gently roll the cloudy insulin between your palms.
- Remove the needle cap.
- Pull out the plunger until the end of the plunger in the barrel aligns with the number of units of NPH or Lente insulin that you need.
- Push the needle through the rubber top of the cloudy insulin bottle.
- Inject the air into the bottle.
- Remove the needle.
- Pull out the plunger until the end of the plunger in the barrel aligns with the number of units of clear regular insulin that you need.

- Push the needle through the rubber top of the clear insulin bottle.
- Inject the air into the bottle.
- Without removing the needle, turn the bottle upside down.
- Withdraw the plunger until it aligns with the number of units of clear regular insulin that you need.
- Gently pull the needle out of the bottle.
- Push the needle into the cloudy (NPH or Lente) insulin without injecting it into the bottle.

El doctor ha recetado insulina para Ud.

Para extraer la insulina siga las siguientes pasos:

- Limpie la tapa de hule (goma) de la botella de la insulina con alcohol.
- Quítele el capuchón a la aguja.
- Saque el émbolo hasta el otro extremo del émbolo en la cuba esté al nivel de la dosis de insulina (número de unidades) que Ud. necesita.
- Empuje la aguja por la tapa de hule (goma) de la botella de insulina.
- Inyecte el aire dentro de la botella.
- Sin sacar la aguja de la botella, póngala al revés.
- Retire el émbolo hasta que llegue la insulina al número de unidades que Ud. necesita.

- Retire Ud. la aguja de la botella suavemente.

Para mezclar la insulina siga los siguientes pasos:

- Limpie la tapa de hule (goma) de las botellas de insulina con alcohol.
- Suavemente mueva la insulina turbia entre las palmas de la mano.
- Retire el capuchón de la aguja.
- Saque el émbolo hasta que el otro extremo del émbolo en el barril esté al nivel con la dosis de insulina turbia (NPH o insulina Lente) (número de unidades) que Ud. necesita.
- Empuje la aguja por la tapa de goma (hule) de la botella de insulina turbia.
- Inyecte el aire dentro de la botella.
- Saque la aguja.
- Retire el émbolo hasta que el otro extremo del émbolo en el barril esté al nivel con la dosis de insulina clara (regular) (número de unidades) que Ud. necesita.
- Empuje Ud. la aguja por la tapa de goma de la botella de insulna clara.
- Inyecte el aire dentro de la botella.
- Sin sacar la aguja, vuelva la botella al revés.
- Retire el émbolo hasta que llegue a la dosis de insulina (regular) clara (número de unidades) que Ud. necesita.
- Suavemente saque Ud. la aguja de la botella.
- Empuje la aguja en la insulina turbia (NPH o insulina Lente) sin inyectarla dentro de la botella.

– Withdraw the plunger until you reach your total dosage of insulin in units (regular combined with NPH or Lente).

– We will practice again.

– Retire el émbolo hasta que llegue a su dosis total de insulina en unidades (regular y NPH o Lente conbinadas).

– Practicaremos juntos(as) otra vez.

Home care phrases

Wash your hands before touching medications.	Lávese Ud. las manos antes de tocar los medicamentos.
Check the medication bottle for name, dose, and frequency (how often it's supposed to be taken).	En el envase del medicamento verifique Ud. el nombre, la dosis y la frecuencia (con que frequencia se debe tomar).
Check the expiration date on all medications.	Verifique Ud. la fecha en la que el medicamento expira.
Store medications according to pharmacy instructions.	Guarde Ud. los medicamentos según las instrucciones de la farmacia.
Under adequate lighting, read medication labels carefully before taking doses.	Bajo luz adequada, lea Ud. la etiqueta del medicamento con mucho cuidado antes de tomar las dosis.
Don't crush medication without first asking the doctor or pharmacist.	No machaque Ud. el medicamento sin antes preguntárselo al doctor o al farmaceútico.
Contact your doctor if a new or unexpected symptom or another problem appears.	Póngase Ud. en contacto con su doctor si un síntoma nuevo o inesperado u otros problemas aparecen.
Do not stop taking medication unless instructed by your doctor.	No deje Ud. de tomar el medicamento sólo que se lo ordene su doctor.
Discard outdated medications.	Deshágase Ud. de medicamentos caducos.
Never take someone else's medications.	Nunca tome Ud. los medicamentos de otra persona.
Keep a record of your current medications.	Apunte Ud. (tome nota de) sus medicamentos actuales.

General drug therapy phrases

Drug classes

Analgesic	Analgésico
Anesthetic	Anestético
Antacid	Antiácido
Antianginal	Agente antianginal
Anxiolytic	Agente ansiolítico
Antiarrhythmic	Agente antiarrítmico
Antibiotic	Antibiótico
Anticancer agent	Agente anticarcinógeno
Anticoagulant	Anticoagulante
Anticonvulsant	Anticonvulsivante

Antidepressant	Antidepresivo
Antidiarrheal	Antidiarreico
Antifungal	Agente antifúngico
Antigout agent	Agente antigota
Antihistamine	Antihistamínico
Antihyperlipemic	Agente hiperlipémico
Antihypertensive	Agente antihipertenso
Anti-inflammatory	Agente antiinflamatorio
Antimalarial	Agente antimalárico
Antiparkinsonian	Agente antiparkinsoniano
Antipsychotic	Agente antipsicótico
Antipyretic	Antipirético
Antiseptic	Antiséptico
Antispasmodic	Antiespasmódico
Antithyroid agent	Agente antitiroideo
Antituberculosis agent	Agente antituberculoso
Antitussive	Agente antitusígeno
Antiviral	Agente antiviral
Appetite stimulant	Estimulante para el apetito
Appetite suppressant	Supresor de apetito
Bronchodilator	Broncodilatador
Decongestant	Descongestivo
Digestant	Digestivo (agente que estimula la digestión)
Diuretic	Diurético
Emetic	Emético
Fertility agent	Agente para la fertilidad
Hypnotic	Hipnótico
Insulin	Insulina
Laxative	Laxante
Muscle relaxant	Relajante de músculos
Oral contraceptive	Anticonceptivo oral
Oral hypoglycemic agent	Agente hipoglucémico oral
Sedative	Sedante
Steroid	Esteroide
Thyroid hormone	Hormona de la glándula tiroides
Vaccine	Vacuna
Vasodilator	Vasodilatador
Vitamin	Vitamina

Routes

Intradermal	Intradérmica
Intramuscular	Intramuscular
Intravenous	Intravenosa
Oral	Oral
Rectal	Rectal
Subcutaneous	Subcutánea
Topical	Tópica
Vaginal	Vaginal

Preparations

Capsule	Cápsula
Cream	Pomada
Drops	Gotas
Elixir	Elixir
Injection	Inyección
Inhaler	Inhalador
Lotion	Loción
Lozenge	Pastilla
Powder	Polvo
Spray	Atomizador
Suppository	Supositorio
Suspension	Suspensión
Syrup	Jarabe
Tablet	Tableta

Frequency

Once daily	Una vez al día
Twice daily	Dos veces al día
Three times daily	Tres veces al día
Four times daily	Cuatro veces al día
In the morning	Por la mañana
With meals	Con las comidas
Before meals	Antes de las comidas
After meals	Después de las comidas
Before bedtime	Antes de acostarse
When you have _____	Cuando Ud. tome _____
Only when you need it	Sólo cuando lo necesite
Every four hours	Cada cuatro horas
Every six hours	Cada seis horas
Every eight hours	Cada ocho horas

Acknowledgments

We would like to thank the following companies for granting us permission to include their drugs in the full-color photoguide.

Abbott Laboratories
Depakote®
Hytrin®

AstraZeneca LP
Arimidex®
Crestor®
Prilosec®
Tenormin®
Toprol-XL®

Aventis Pharmaceuticals
DiaBeta®
Lasix®

Bayer Corporation
Cipro®
Levitra®

Biovail Pharmaceuticals, Inc.
Cardizem®
Cardizem CD®
Cardizem LA®
Vasotec®

Bristol-Myers Squibb Company
Capoten®
Coumadin®
Monopril®
Pravachol®
Serzone®

Elan Pharmaceuticals, Inc.
Frova®

Forest Pharmaceuticals, Inc.
Celexa®

GlaxoSmithKline
Copyright GlaxoSmithKline.
Used with permission.
Amoxil®
Augmentin®
Avandia®
Ceftin®
Compazine®
Coreg®
Lanoxin®
Paxil®
Relafen®
Wellbutrin SR®

Janssen Pharmaceutica, Inc.
Risperdal®
Risperdal® M-Tab™

King Pharmaceuticals, Inc.
Levoxyl®

Eli Lilly and Company
Prozac®

Mallinckrodt, Inc.
Pamelor®

Merck & Co., Inc.
Used with permission of
Merck & Co., Inc.
Cozaar®
Fosamax®
Mevacor®
Pepcid®
Prinivil®
Singulair®
Vioxx®
Zocor®

Merck Santé
An associate of Merck KGaA,
Darmstadt, Germany
Glucophage®
Glucophage XR®

Novartis Pharmaceuticals, Inc.
Ritalin®

Ortho-McNeil Pharmaceutical
Levaquin®

Pfizer, Inc.
Registered Trademarks of
Pfizer, Inc. All Rights Reserved. Courtesy of Pfizer Inc.
Accupril®
Celebrex®
Diflucan®
Dilantin® Kapseals®
Glucotrol®
Glucotrol XL®
Lipitor®
Neurontin®
Norvasc®
Procardia XL®
Viagra®
Zantac®
Zithromax®
Zoloft®

Pharmacia Corporation, a Pfizer, Inc. corporation
Registered Trademarks of
Pharmacia Corporation, a
Pfizer Inc. corporation. All
rights reserved. Courtesy of
Pfizer Inc.
Bextra®
Micronase®
Provera®
Xanax®

Procter & Gamble Pharmaceuticals, Inc.
Actonel®

Purdue Pharma L.P.
OxyContin®

Acknowledgments 1401

Roche Laboratories, Inc.
Valium®

Sanofi-Synthelabo, Inc.
Ambien®

Schering Corporation and Key Pharmaceuticals, Inc.
Clarinex®
K-Dur®

Tap Pharmaceuticals, Inc.
Prevacid®

Warner Chilcott Laboratories, Inc.
Duricef®
Eryc®
Estrace®
Ovcon® 35

Wyeth Pharmaceuticals
The appearance of these tablets and capsules is a trademark of Wyeth Pharmaceuticals, Philadelphia, Pa.
Effexor XR®
Phenergan®
Premarin®

Index

A

abacavir sulfate, 58, **89-90**
Abbocillin VK ◇, 991
Abbokinase, 1284
Abbreviating drug names, 33
abciximab, **90-92**
Abdominal distention, postoperative
  neostigmine for, 906
  vasopressin for, 1299
Abdominal radiation therapy adverse effects
  granisetron for, 658
  ondansetron for, 943
Abdominal radiography, vasopressin to express gas before, 1299
Abdominal surgery patients
  dalteparin for, 400
  enoxaparin for, 507
Abdominal trauma during pregnancy, Rh₀(D) immune globulin, human, for, 1102
Abelcet, 153
Abenol, 95
Abilify, 175
Abortion
  carboprost tromethamine for, 286
  ertapenem for, 525
  oxytocin, synthetic injection, for, 960
  Rh₀(D) immune globulin, human, for Rh exposure from, 1102
Abreva, 462
Abscess, metronidazole for, 850
acarbose, 72, **92-93**
Accolate, 1322
AccuNeb, 110
Accupril, 1085
Accurbron, 1221
Accutane, 730
Accutane Roche ♦, 730
acebutolol, 44, 52, 60, **93-95**
Aceon, 1003
Aceta Elixir, 95
acetaminophen, **95-97**
Acetaminophen toxicity, acetylcysteine for, 99
Acetaminophen Uniserts, 95
Aceta Tablets, 95
Aceta with Codeine, 1388t

Acetazolam, 97
acetazolamide, **97-99**
acetazolamide sodium, 48, **97-99**
acetylcysteine, **99-101**
acetylsalicylic acid, **181-183**
Achromycin, 1219
Aciclovir ◇, 102
Acid indigestion
  aluminum hydroxide for, 130
  calcium carbonate for, 269
  magaldrate for, 791
  magnesium citrate for, 794
  magnesium oxide for, 795
  ranitidine for, 1097
  sodium bicarbonate for, 1158
Acihexal ◇, 102
Aciphex, 1091
Aclin ◇, 1188
Acne
  clindamycin for, 356
  doxycycline for, 485
  finasteride for, 582
  hormonal contraceptives for, 550
  isotretinoin for, 730
  spironolactone for, 1173
  tetracycline for, 1219
Acromegaly
  bromocriptine for, 246
  octreotide for, 932
ACT-3 ◇, 680
Actamin, 95
ACTH, **377-378**
Acthar, 377
Actidose, 101
Actidose-Aqua, 101
Actigall, 1286
Actimmune, 717
Actimol, 95
Actinic keratoses
  diclofenac for, 436
  fluorouracil for, 593
Actiq, 575
activated charcoal, **101-102**
Activated partial thromboplastin time, 1386t
Actonel, 1115
Actos, 1024
Actraphane HM ◇, 709
Actraphane HM Penfill ◇, 709
Actraphane MC ◇, 709
Actrapid HM ◇, 709
Actrapid HM Penfill ◇, 709

Actrapid MC ◇, 709
Actrapid MC Penfill ◇, 709
Actron caplets, 737
Acute coronary syndrome
  clopidogrel for, 367
  eptifibatide for, 522
  tirofiban for, 1244
Acute dystonic reaction, benztropine for, 221
Acute intermittent porphyria, chlorpromazine for, 336
Acute lymphoblastic leukemia
  cyclophosphamide for, 386
  doxorubicin for, 480
  mercaptopurine for, 816
  methotrexate for, 833
  pegaspargase for, 974
  sargramostim for, 1138
  teniposide for, 1206
  vincristine for, 1307
Acute lymphocytic leukemia
  asparaginase for, 179
  cytarabine for, 393
  daunorubicin for, 410
  ifosfamide for, 685
Acute mountain sickness, acetazolamide for, 97
Acute myeloid leukemia
  cyclophosphamide for, 386
  doxorubicin for, 480
  gemtuzumab ozogamicin for, 642
  idarubicin for, 684
  mercaptopurine for, 816
  sargramostim for, 1138
Acute promyelocytic leukemia, arsenic trioxide for, 177
acyclovir sodium, 58, **102-104**
Adalat, 914
Adalat CC, 914
Adalat P.A., 914
Adalat XL, 914
adalimumab, **104-105**
adefovir dipivoxil, **106-107**
Adenocard, 107
adenosine, **107-108**
ADH, **1299-1300**
Adipex-P, 1010
Adoxa, 485
Adrenalin, 513
Adrenalin Chloride, 513
adrenaline, **513-516**

t refers to a table; **boldface** refers to the drug's monograph; ***boldface italic*** refers to a full-color photograph.

t refers to a table; **boldface** refers to the drug's monograph; ***boldface italic*** refers to a full-color photograph.

---

t refers to a table; **boldface** refers to the drug's monograph; ***boldface italic*** refers to a full-color photograph.

---

t refers to a table; **boldface** refers to the drug's monograph; ***boldface italic*** refers to a full-color photograph.

t refers to a table; **boldface** refers to the drug's monograph; ***boldface italic*** refers to a full-color photograph.

---

t refers to a table; **boldface** refers to the drug's monograph; ***boldface italic*** refers to a full-color photograph.

---

t refers to a table; **boldface** refers to the drug's monograph; ***boldface italic*** refers to a full-color photograph.

---

t refers to a table; **boldface** refers to the drug's monograph; ***boldface italic*** refers to a full-color photograph.

---

t refers to a table; **boldface** refers to the drug's monograph; ***boldface italic*** refers to a full-color photograph.

---

t refers to a table; **boldface** refers to the drug's monograph; ***boldface italic*** refers to a full-color photograph.

---

t refers to a table; **boldface** refers to the drug's monograph; ***boldface italic*** refers to a full-color photograph.

THE SKY'S THE LIMIT

Nursing Students

- ■ Career Planning
- ■ Educational Programs
- ■ Involvement in Activities
- ■ Benefits and Money-Saving Programs
- ■ Leadership Opportunities
- ■ Networking

Nursing students in associate degree, diploma, baccalaureate,* generic masters, generic doctoral, or pre-nursing programs are invited to join the National Student Nurses' Association (NSNA), a pre-professional organization for nursing students. Over 35,000 nursing students are already taking advantage of the many programs, benefits, and leadership opportunities that NSNA has to offer: discounts on products and services, representation in the annual House of Delegates, opportunities to run for state and national office, a chance to win contests and prizes, and an opportunity to influence nursing practice in the future. "The Sky's the Limit." Join NSNA today!

*RNs in degree completion programs are also eligible for membership.

For more information contact:
NATIONAL STUDENT NURSES'
ASSOCIATION, INC (NSNA).
45 Main Street, Suite 606
Brooklyn, NY 11201
Tel: (718) 210-0705 • Fax: (718) 210-0710
e-mail: nsna@nsna.org • Website: www.nsna.org
Earn academic credit; visit *nsnaleadershipu.org*

VISIT THE NSNA WEBSITE
http://www.nsna.org

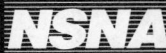

National Student Nurses' Association, Inc.

Visit eDrugInfo.com

This Web site gives you:
- updates on recently approved drugs, new indications, and new warnings
- patient-teaching aids on new drugs, administration techniques, and supportive measures
- news summaries on recent drug developments
- information on herbal medicines
- links to pharmaceutical companies and government agencies
- a drug information bookstore.

About PharmDisk 6.0

PharmDisk 6.0 mini-CD contains:
- a Pharmacology Self-Test—a self-paced test complete with rationales for correct and incorrect answers
- a Match Game—an engaging game that helps you learn to identify drug classes
- a direct link to **eDrugInfo.com** for drug updates and important drug news.

Windows minimum system requirements
- Windows 98
- Pentium 166
- 64 MB RAM
- 30 MB free hard-disk space
- SVGA monitor with High Color (16-bit) and Small Fonts
- CD-ROM drive and mouse

CAUTION: Do not attempt to use this mini-CD in a floppy disk drive, Zip drive, certain slot drives, or a car stereo. Do not insert the mini-CD into a CD-ROM drive that requires the mini-CD to be in a vertical position. Placing the CD into such a drive may result in jamming.

Before installing this program, make sure your monitor is set to the minimum display requirements. If it isn't, consult your user's manual for instructions about changing the display settings.

To install on Windows 98 or higher:
- Place the mini-CD on the inner ring of the CD-ROM drive tray. Close the tray.
- In a few moments, the CD should automatically start. Once it starts, click the "Install" button to install on your computer.
- Click "Start" and select "Run" if the CD doesn't start automatically.
- Type **d:\setup** (where **d** is the letter of your CD-ROM drive), and click *OK*. Follow on-screen instructions for installing the CD.

Special note: Before using *PharmDisk 6.0*, read the file *Readme.txt* for important information about operating the program.

For technical support, call toll free 1-800-638-3030, Monday through Friday, 8:30 am to 5 pm Eastern Time.